Robbins
BASIC PATHOLOGY

Robbins
BASIC
PATHOLOGY

TENTH EDITION

Vinay Kumar, MBBS, MD, FRCPath

Alice Hogge and Arthur A. Baer Distinguished Service Professor of Pathology
Biological Sciences Division and The Pritzker Medical School
University of Chicago
Chicago, Illinois

Abul K. Abbas, MBBS

Distinguished Professor and Chair
Department of Pathology
University of California, San Francisco
San Francisco, California

Jon C. Aster, MD, PhD

Professor of Pathology
Brigham and Women's Hospital and Harvard Medical School
Boston, Massachusetts

ARTIST James A. Perkins, MS, MFA

ELSEVIER

ELSEVIER

1600 John F. Kennedy Blvd.
Philadelphia, Pennsylvania 19103-2899

ROBBINS BASIC PATHOLOGY, TENTH EDITION

ISBN: 978-0-323-35317-5
International Edition: 978-0-323-48054-3

Notices

Knowledge and best practice in this field are constantly changing. As new research and experience broaden our understanding, changes in research methods, professional practices, or medical treatment may become necessary.

Practitioners and researchers must always rely on their own experience and knowledge in evaluating and using any information, methods, compounds, or experiments described herein. In using such information or methods they should be mindful of their own safety and the safety of others, including parties for whom they have a professional responsibility.

With respect to any drug or pharmaceutical products identified, readers are advised to check the most current information provided (i) on procedures featured or (ii) by the manufacturer of each product to be administered, to verify the recommended dose or formula, the method and duration of administration, and contraindications. It is the responsibility of practitioners, relying on their own experience and knowledge of their patients, to make diagnoses, to determine dosages and the best treatment for each individual patient, and to take all appropriate safety precautions.

To the fullest extent of the law, neither the Publisher nor the authors, contributors, or editors assume any liability for any injury and/or damage to persons or property as a matter of products liability, negligence or otherwise, or from any use or operation of any methods, products, instructions, or ideas contained in the material herein.

Library of Congress Cataloging-in-Publication Data

Names: Kumar, Vinay, 1944- editor. | Abbas, Abul K., editor. | Aster, Jon C.,
   editor. | Perkins, James A., illustrator.
Title: Robbins basic pathology / [edited by] Vinay Kumar, Abul K. Abbas,
   Jon C. Aster ; artist, James A. Perkins.
Other titles: Basic pathology
Description: Tenth edition. | Philadelphia, Pennsylvania : Elsevier, [2018]
   | Includes bibliographical references and index.
Identifiers: LCCN 2017002902 | ISBN 9780323353175 (hardcover : alk. paper)
Subjects: | MESH: Pathologic Processes
Classification: LCC RB111 | NLM QZ 140 | DDC 616.07–dc23 LC record available at
   https://lccn.loc.gov/2017002902

Executive Content Strategist: James Merritt
Director, Content Development: Rebecca Gruliow
Publishing Services Manager: Julie Eddy
Book Production Specialist: Clay S. Broeker
Design Direction: Brian Salisbury

Printed in Canada

Last digit is the print number: 9   8   7   6   5   4   3   2   1

  Working together to grow libraries in developing countries

www.elsevier.com • www.bookaid.org

DEDICATION

Dedicated to

Our Grandchildren

Kiera, Nikhil, and Kavi

And Our Children

Jonathan and Rehana Abbas

Michael and Meghan Aster

Contributors

Anthony Chang, MD
Professor
Department of Pathology
The University of Chicago
Chicago, Illinois

Lora Hedrick Ellenson, MD
Professor and Chief of Gynecologic Pathology
Department of Pathology and Laboratory Medicine
Weill Cornell Medicine–New York Presbyterian
   Hospital
New York, New York

Jonathan I. Epstein, MD
Professor
Departments of Pathology, Urology, and Oncology
The Johns Hopkins Medical Institutions
Baltimore, Maryland

Karen M. Frank, MD, PhD, D(ABMM)
Chief of Microbiology Service
Department of Laboratory Medicine
Clinical Center
National Institutes of Health
Bethesda, Maryland

Matthew P. Frosch, MD, PhD
Lawrence J. Henderson Associate Professor
Department of Pathology
Massachusetts General Hospital and Harvard Medical
   School
Boston, Massachusetts

Andrew Horvai, MD, PhD
Clinical Professor
Department of Pathology
University of California, San Francisco
San Francisco, California

Aliya N. Husain, MBBS
Professor
Department of Pathology
The University of Chicago
Chicago, Illinois

Zoltan G. Laszik, MD, PhD
Professor of Pathology
University of California, San Francisco
San Francisco, California

Alexander J. Lazar, MD, PhD
Professor
Departments of Pathology, Genomic Medicine, and
   Translational Molecular Pathology
The University of Texas MD Anderson Cancer Center
Houston, Texas

Susan C. Lester, MD, PhD
Assistant Professor and Chief of Breast Pathology
   Services
Department of Pathology
Harvard Medical School
Brigham and Women's Hospital
Boston, Massachusetts

Mark W. Lingen, DDS, PhD, FRCPath
Professor
Department of Pathology
The University of Chicago
Chicago, Illinois

Tamara L. Lotan, MD
Associate Professor of Pathology
The Johns Hopkins Hospital
Baltimore, Maryland

Anirban Maitra, MBBS
Professor
Pathology and Translational Molecular Pathology
University of Texas MD Anderson Cancer Center
Houston, Texas

Alexander J. McAdam, MD, PhD
Associate Professor of Pathology
Department of Pathology
Harvard Medical School
Medical Director
Clinical Microbiology Laboratory
Boston Children's Hospital
Boston, Massachusetts

Richard N. Mitchell, MD, PhD
Lawrence J. Henderson Professor of Pathology
Member of the Harvard/MIT Health Sciences and
   Technology Faculty
Department of Pathology
Brigham and Women's Hospital
Harvard Medical School
Boston, Massachusetts

Peter Pytel, MD
Professor
Department of Pathology
University of Chicago
Chicago, Illinois

Neil D. Theise, MD
Professor
Department of Pathology
Icahn School of Medicine at Mount Sinai
New York, New York

Jerrold R. Turner, MD, PhD
Departments of Pathology and Medicine (GI)
Brigham and Women's Hospital
Harvard Medical School
Boston, Massachusetts

Clinical Consultants

Harold J. Burstein, MD
Dana-Farber Cancer Institute and Harvard Medical
School
Boston, Massachusetts
Diseases of the Breast

Vanja Douglas, MD
University of California, San Francisco
San Francisco, California
Diseases of the Central Nervous System

Hilary J. Goldberg, MD
Brigham and Women's Hospital, Harvard Medical
School
Boston, Massachusetts
Diseases of the Lung

Ira Hanan, MD
University of Chicago
Chicago, Illinois
Diseases of the Gastrointestinal Tract

Cadence Kim, MD
Urologic Associates
Philadelphia, Pennsylvania
Diseases of the Male Genital System

Anne LaCase, MD
Dana Farber Cancer Institute and Harvard Medical
School
Boston, Massachusetts
Diseases of Hematopoietic and Lymphoid Systems

Joyce Liu, MD, MPH
Dana-Farber Cancer Institute and Harvard Medical
School
Boston, Massachusetts
Diseases of the Female Genital Tract

Graham McMahon, MD, MMSC
Brigham and Women's Hospital and Harvard Medical
School
Boston, Massachusetts
Diseases of the Endocrine System

Meyeon Park, MD
University of California, San Francisco
San Francisco, California
Disease of the Kidney

Anna E. Rutherford, MD, MPH
Brigham and Women's Hospital and Harvard Medical
School
Boston, Massachusetts
Diseases of the Liver

Matthew J. Sorrentino, MD
University of Chicago
Chicago, Illinois
Diseases of the Blood Vessels and Diseases of the
Heart

Preface

The tenth edition is an important milestone in the life of a text-book. This occasion is a propitious time to look back on the origins of *Basic Pathology*, which are summed up best by quoting Stanley Robbins from the preface of the first edition (1971):

"Of books as well as men, it may be observed that fat ones contain thin ones struggling to get out. In a sense, this book bears such a relationship to its more substantial progenitor, *Robbins Pathology*. It arose from an appreciation of the modern medical student's dilemma. As the curriculum has become restructured to place greater emphasis on clinical experience, time for reading is correspondingly curtailed....In writing this book, rare and esoteric lesions are omitted without apology, and infrequent or trivial ones described only briefly. We felt it important, however, to consider rather fully the major disease entities."

While the goals of "baby Robbins" remain true to the vision of Stanley Robbins, this edition has been revised on the basis of a few additional principles.

- First, it is obvious that an understanding of disease mechanisms is based more than ever on a strong foundation of basic science. In keeping with this, we have always woven the relevant basic cell and molecular biology into the sections on pathophysiology in various chapters. *In this edition we go one step further and introduce a new chapter titled "The Cell as a Unit of Health and Disease" at the very beginning of the book.* In this chapter we have attempted to encapsulate aspects of cell and molecular biology that we believe are helpful in preparing readers for discussions of specific diseases. It is, in essence, a refresher course in cell biology.

- Second, as teachers, we are acutely aware that medical students feel overwhelmed by the rapid growth of information about the molecular basis of disease. We have therefore excluded those new "breakthroughs" in the laboratory that have not yet reached the bedside. Thus, for example, the drugs developed for targeting cancer mutations that are still in clinical trials have not been discussed except in those rare instances in which the evidence of efficacy is close to hand. Similarly, in genetically heterogeneous disorders, we have focused on the most common mutations without providing a catalog of all the genes and polymorphisms involved. Thus, we have tried to balance discussions of advancement in sciences with the needs of students in the early stages of their careers. This effort required us to read each chapter as if it was written de novo and in many cases to remove parts of the text that had been present in the previous edition. It is our hope that these changes will unburden the students and that the tenth edition will be seen as an up to date yet simple to comprehend book.

- Third, because illustrations facilitate the understanding of difficult concepts such as control of the cell cycle and the actions of cancer genes, the art has been significantly revised and enhanced by adding depth so that the four-color figures are seen in three dimensions.

- Finally, we have added a board of clinical consultants to help us in keeping the clinical content accurate and up to date.

As an additional "tool" to help students focus on the fundamentals, we have continued the use of Summary boxes designed to provide key "take home" messages. These have been retained at the risk of adding a few additional pages to the book because students have uniformly told us that they find them useful.

Although we have entered the genomic era, the time-honored tools of gross and microscopic analysis remain useful, and morphologic changes are highlighted for ready reference. The strong emphasis on clinicopathologic correlations is maintained, and, wherever understood, the impact of molecular pathology on the practice of medicine is emphasized. We are pleased that all of this was accomplished without a significant "bulge" in the waistline of the text.

We continue to firmly believe that clarity of writing and proper use of language enhance comprehension and facilitate the learning process. Those familiar with the previous editions will notice significant reorganization of the text in many chapters to improve the flow of information and make it more logical. We are now in the digital age, so the text will be available online. In addition, over 100 updated and revised cases developed by one of us (VK) will also be available, linked to the electronic version of the text. We hope that these interactive cases will enhance and reinforce learning of pathology through application to clinical cases.

It is a privilege for us to edit this book, and we realize the considerable trust placed in us by students and teachers of pathology. We remain acutely conscious of this responsibility and hope that this edition will be worthy of and possibly enhance the tradition of its forebears.

Acknowledgments

Any large endeavor of this type cannot be completed without the help of many individuals. We thank the contributors of various chapters. Many are veterans of the older sibling of this text, the so-called "Big Robbins," and they are listed in the table of contents. To each of them, a special thanks. In addition, we are also very grateful to our clinical consultants for their input. They are listed separately after the contributor names. We are fortunate to continue our collaboration with Jim Perkins, whose illustrations bring abstract ideas to life and clarify difficult concepts, and we welcome members of our clinical advisory board who read various chapters for accuracy and appropriateness of the clinical content; they are listed on a separate page. Our assistants, Trinh Nu and Thelma Wright from Chicago, Ana Narvaez from San Francisco, and Muriel Goutas from Boston, deserve thanks for coordinating the tasks.

Many colleagues have enhanced the text by providing helpful critiques in their areas of interest. These include Dr. Rick Aster, who provided "late-breaking news" in the area of climate change science. Many others offered critiques of various chapters; they include Drs. Jerry Turner, Jeremy Segal, Nicole Cipriani, and Alex Gallan at the University of Chicago. Alex Gallan single handedly reviewed and updated over 100 clinical cases available online. Others have provided us with photographic gems from their personal collections; they are individually acknowledged in the credits for their contribution(s). For any unintended omissions, we offer our apologies.

Many at Elsevier deserve recognition for their roles in the production of this book. This text was fortunate to be in the hands of Rebecca Gruliow (Director, Content Development), who has been our partner for several editions. Others deserving of our thanks are Bill Schmitt, Executive Content Strategist, who has been our friend and cheerleader for the past many editions. Upon his well-earned retirement, he handed over the charge to Jim Merritt, who had previously worked on the immunology texts authored by one of us (AKA). Jim is a consummate professional and took over the "book" effortlessly. We are especially grateful to the entire production team, in particular Clay Broeker, Book Production Specialist, for tolerating our sometimes next to "impossible" demands and for putting up with our idiosyncrasies during the periods of extreme exhaustion that afflict all authors who undertake what seems like an endless task. We are thankful to the entire Elsevier team for sharing our passion for excellence, including Karen Giacomucci, Brian Salisbury, Tim Santner, Kristine McKercher, and Melissa Darling. We also thank numerous students and teachers scattered across the globe for raising questions about the clarity of content and serving as the ultimate "copyeditors." Their efforts reassured us that the book is read seriously by them.

Ventures such as this exact a heavy toll from the families of the authors. We thank them for their tolerance of our absences, both physical and emotional. We are blessed and strengthened by their unconditional support and love and by their sharing with us the belief that our efforts are worthwhile and useful. We are especially grateful to our wives Raminder Kumar, Ann Abbas, and Erin Malone, who continue to provide steadfast support.

And finally, we the editors salute each other; our partnership thrives because of a shared vision of excellence in teaching despite differences in opinions and individual styles.

VK
AKA
JCA

Online Resources for Instructors and Students

Resources for Instructors

The following resources for instructors are available for use when teaching via Evolve. Contact your local sales representative for more information, or go directly to the Evolve website to request access: https://evolve.elsevier.com. Note: *It may take 1-3 days for account access setup and verification upon initial account setup.*

Image Collection

To assist in the classroom, we have made the images available for instructors for teaching purposes. The images are provided in JPEG, PowerPoint, and PDF versions with labels on/off and may be downloaded for use in lecture presentations.

Test Bank

Instructors can access a complete test bank of over 250 multiple-choice questions for use in teaching.

Resources for Students

The following resources are available at StudentConsult.com to students with purchase of *Robbins Basic Pathology* (10th edition).

Textbook Online

The complete textbook is available online at StudentConsult.com. The online version is fully searchable and provides all figures from the print book, with enhanced functionality for many, including clickable enlargements and slideshow views of multiple-part images.

Targeted Therapy Boxes

Students have access online at StudentConsult.com to 14 targeted therapy boxes on clinical therapy topics, including statins, targeted therapy for breast cancer, vitamin D, aspirin and NSAIDs, treatment of Marfan syndrome, and more. These exemplify how the understanding of molecular pathogenesis has led to the development of therapy.

Videos

Students can access 30 videos online at StudentConsult.com. The videos cover acute appendicitis, adenomyosis, arteriosclerosis, Barrett's esophagus, basal cell carcinoma, breast cancer, chronic obstructive pyelonephritis, CML, cystic fibrosis with bronchiectatsis, diabetic glomerulosclerosis, ectopic pregnancy, eczematous dermatitis, familial adenomatous polyposis syndrome, giardiasis, hemochromatosis, Hirschsprung's disease, ischemic cardiomyopathy, massive hepatocellular necrosis, mature cystic teratoma, metastatic squamous cell carcinoma, mucinous colorectal adenocarcinoma, multiple sclerosis, necrotizing vasculitis, osteoarthritis, pancreatic cancer, renal cell carcinoma, sarcoidosis, seminoma, tuberculosis, and ulcerative colitis.

Clinical Cases

Students can study over 100 clinical cases available online on Studentconsult.com. The clinical cases are designed to enhance clinical pathologic correlations and pathophysiology.

Self-Assessment Questions

Students can test and score themselves with interactive multiple-choice questions linked to chapters online at StudentConsult.com.

Contents

CHAPTER 1   The Cell as a Unit of Health and Disease   1
Richard N. Mitchell

CHAPTER 2   Cell Injury, Cell Death, and Adaptations   31

CHAPTER 3   Inflammation and Repair   57

CHAPTER 4   Hemodynamic Disorders, Thromboembolism, and Shock   97

CHAPTER 5   Diseases of the Immune System   121

CHAPTER 6   Neoplasia   189

CHAPTER 7   Genetic and Pediatric Diseases   243
Anirban Maitra

CHAPTER 8   Environmental and Nutritional Diseases   299

CHAPTER 9   General Pathology of Infectious Diseases   341
Alexander J. McAdam, Karen M. Frank

CHAPTER 10   Blood Vessels   361
Richard N. Mitchell

CHAPTER 11   Heart   399
Richard N. Mitchell

CHAPTER 12   Hematopoietic and Lymphoid Systems   441

CHAPTER 13   Lung   495
Aliya N. Husain

CHAPTER 14   Kidney and Its Collecting System   549
Anthony Chang, Zoltan G. Laszik

CHAPTER 15   Oral Cavities and Gastrointestinal Tract   583
Jerrold R. Turner, Mark W. Lingen

Chapters without author names were written by the editors.

CHAPTER 16   Liver and Gallbladder   637
              Neil D. Theise

CHAPTER 17   Pancreas   679
              Anirban Maitra

CHAPTER 18   Male Genital System and Lower Urinary Tract   691
              Jonathan I. Epstein, Tamara L. Lotan

CHAPTER 19   Female Genital System and Breast   713
              Lora Hedrick Ellenson, Susan C. Lester

CHAPTER 20   Endocrine System   749
              Anirban Maitra

CHAPTER 21   Bones, Joints, and Soft Tissue Tumors   797
              Andrew Horvai

CHAPTER 22   Peripheral Nerves and Muscles   835
              Peter Pytel

CHAPTER 23   Central Nervous System   849
              Matthew P. Frosch

CHAPTER 24   Skin   889
              Alexander J. Lazar

              Index   909

The Cell as a Unit of Health and Disease

CHAPTER OUTLINE

The Genome 1
Noncoding DNA 1
Histone Organization 3
Micro-RNA and Long Noncoding RNA 4
Cellular Housekeeping 6
Plasma Membrane: Protection and Nutrient Acquisition 8
Cytoskeleton 11
Cell-Cell Interactions 12
Biosynthetic Machinery: Endoplasmic Reticulum and Golgi Apparatus 12

Waste Disposal: Lysosomes and Proteasomes 13
Cellular Metabolism and Mitochondrial Function 13
Cellular Activation 16
Cell Signaling 16
Signal Transduction Pathways 16
Modular Signaling Proteins, Hubs, and Nodes 18
Transcription Factors 19
Growth Factors and Receptors 19

Extracellular Matrix 21
Components of the Extracellular Matrix 22
Maintaining Cell Populations 24
Proliferation and the Cell Cycle 24
Stem Cells 25
Concluding Remarks 28

Pathology literally translates to the study of *suffering* (Greek *pathos* = suffering, *logos* = study); as applied to modern medicine, it is the study of *disease*. Virchow was certainly correct in asserting that disease originates at the cellular level, but we now realize that cellular disturbances arise from alterations in molecules (genes, proteins, and others) that influence the survival and behavior of cells. Thus, the foundation of modern pathology is understanding the *cellular* and molecular abnormalities that give rise to diseases. It is helpful to consider these abnormalities in the context of *normal* cellular structure and function, which is the theme of this introductory chapter.

It is unrealistic (and even undesirable) to condense the vast and fascinating field of cell biology into a single chapter. Consequently, rather than attempting a comprehensive review, the goal here is to survey basic principles and highlight recent advances that are relevant to the mechanisms of disease that are emphasized throughout the rest of the book.

THE GENOME

The sequencing of the human genome at the beginning of the 21st century represented a landmark achievement of biomedical science. Since then, the rapidly dropping cost of sequencing and the computational capacity to analyze vast amounts of data promise to revolutionize our understanding of health and disease. At the same time, the emerging information has also revealed a breathtaking level of complexity far beyond the linear sequencing of the genome. The potential for these new powerful tools to expand our understanding of pathogenesis and drive therapeutic innovation excites and inspires scientists and the lay public alike.

Noncoding DNA

The human genome contains about 3.2 billion DNA base pairs. Yet, within the genome there are only roughly 20,000 protein-encoding genes, comprising just 1.5% of the genome. The proteins encoded by these genes are the fundamental constituents of cells, functioning as enzymes, structural elements, and signaling molecules. Although 20,000 underestimates the actual number of proteins encoded (many genes produce multiple RNA transcripts that encode distinct protein isoforms), it is nevertheless startling that worms composed of fewer than 1000 cells — and with genomes 30-fold smaller — are also assembled from roughly 20,000 protein-encoding genes. Perhaps even more unsettling is that many of these proteins are recognizable homologs of molecules expressed in humans. What then separates humans from worms?

The answer is not completely known, but evidence supports the assertion that the difference lies in the 98.5% of the human genome that does not encode proteins. The function of such long stretches of DNA (which has been called the "dark matter" of the genome) was mysterious for many years. However, it is now clear that more than 85% of the human genome is ultimately transcribed, with almost 80% being devoted to the regulation of gene expression. It follows that whereas proteins provide the building blocks

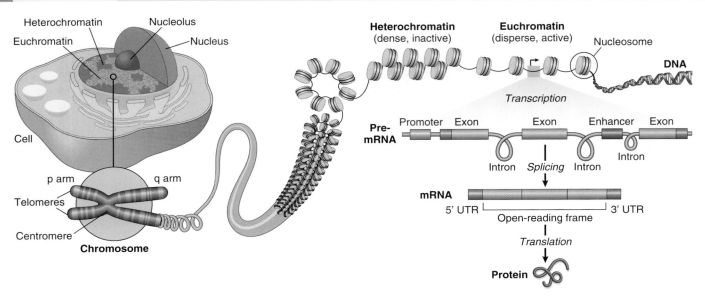

Fig. 1.1 The organization of nuclear DNA. At the light microscopic level, the nuclear genetic material is organized into dispersed, transcriptionally active *euchromatin* or densely packed, transcriptionally inactive *heterochromatin*; chromatin can also be mechanically connected with the nuclear membrane, and nuclear membrane perturbation can thus influence transcription. Chromosomes (as shown) can only be visualized by light microscopy during cell division. During mitosis, they are organized into paired chromatids connected at *centromeres*; the centromeres act as the locus for the formation of a *kinetochore* protein complex that regulates chromosome segregation at metaphase. The *telomeres* are repetitive nucleotide sequences that cap the termini of chromatids and permit repeated chromosomal replication without loss of DNA at the chromosome ends. The chromatids are organized into short "P" ("petite") and long "Q" ("next letter in the alphabet") arms. The characteristic banding pattern of chromatids has been attributed to relative GC content (less GC content in bands relative to interbands), with genes tending to localize to interband regions. Individual chromatin fibers are composed of a string of nucleosomes—DNA wound around octameric histone cores—with the nucleosomes connected via DNA linkers. Promoters are noncoding regions of DNA that initiate gene transcription; they are on the same strand and upstream of their associated gene. Enhancers are regulatory elements that can modulate gene expression across distances of 100 kB or more by looping back onto promoters and recruiting additional factors that are needed to drive the expression of pre-mRNA species. The intronic sequences are subsequently spliced out of the pre-mRNA to produce the definitive message that includes exons that are translated into protein and 3'- and 5'-untranslated regions (UTR) that may have regulatory functions. In addition to the enhancer, promoter, and UTR sequences, noncoding elements are found throughout the genome; these include short repeats, regulatory factor binding regions, noncoding regulatory RNAs, and transposons.

and machinery required for assembling cells, tissues, and organisms, it is the noncoding regions of the genome that provide the critical "architectural planning."

The major classes of functional non–*protein-coding DNA sequences* found in the human genome include (Fig. 1.1):

- *Promoter* and *enhancer* regions that bind protein transcription factors
- Binding sites for proteins that organize and maintain higher order *chromatin structures*
- *Noncoding regulatory RNAs.* Of the 80% of the genome dedicated to regulatory functions, the vast majority is transcribed into RNAs—micro-RNAs and long noncoding RNAs (described later)—that are never translated into protein, but can regulate gene expression
- *Mobile genetic elements* (e.g., *transposons*). Remarkably, more than one-third of the human genome is composed of such "jumping genes." These segments can cruise around the genome, and are implicated in gene regulation and chromatin organization.
- Special structural regions of DNA, including *telomeres* (chromosome ends) and *centromeres* (chromosome "tethers")

Importantly, **many genetic variations (*polymorphisms*) associated with diseases are located in non–protein-coding regions of the genome**. Thus, variation in gene

regulation may prove to be more important in disease causation than structural changes in specific proteins. Another surprise that emerged from genome sequencing is that any two humans are typically >99.5% DNA-identical (and are 99% sequence-identical with chimpanzees)! Thus, individual variation, including differential susceptibility to diseases and environmental exposures, is encoded in <0.5% of our DNA (importantly, this still represents about 15 million base pairs).

The two most common forms of DNA variation in the human genome are *single-nucleotide polymorphisms (SNPs)* and *copy number variations (CNVs)*.

- SNPs are variants at single nucleotide positions and are almost always *biallelic* (only two choices exist at a given site within the population, such as A or T). More than 6 million human SNPs have been identified, with many showing wide variation in frequency in different populations. The following features are worthy of note:
  - SNPs occur across the genome—within exons, introns, intergenic regions, and coding regions.
  - Roughly 1% of SNPs occur in coding regions, which is about what would be expected by chance, because coding regions comprise about 1.5% of the genome.
  - SNPs located in noncoding regions can occur in regulatory elements in the genome, thereby altering gene

expression; in such instances the SNP may have a direct influence on disease susceptibility.

- SNPs can also be "neutral" variants with no effect on gene function or carrier phenotype.
- Even "neutral" SNPs may be useful markers if they happen to be coinherited with a disease-associated gene as a result of physical proximity. In other words, the SNP and the causative genetic factor are in *linkage disequilibrium*.
- The effect of most SNPs on disease susceptibility is weak, and it remains to be seen if the identification of such variants, alone or in combination, can be used to develop effective strategies for disease prediction or prevention.
- CNVs are a form of genetic variation consisting of different numbers of large contiguous stretches of DNA; these can range from 1000 base pairs to millions of base pairs. In some instances these loci are, like SNPs, biallelic and simply duplicated or deleted in a subset of the population. In other instances there are complex rearrangements of genomic material, with multiple alleles in the human population. CNVs are responsible for several million base pairs of sequence difference between any

two individuals. Approximately 50% of CNVs involve gene-coding sequences; thus, CNVs may underlie a large portion of human phenotypic diversity.

It is important to note that *alterations in DNA sequence cannot by themselves explain the diversity of phenotypes in human populations*; moreover, classical genetic inheritance cannot explain differing phenotypes in monozygotic twins. The answers to these conundrums probably lie in *epigenetics*—heritable changes in gene expression that are not caused by alterations in DNA sequence (see later).

Histone Organization

Even though virtually all cells in the body have the same genetic composition, differentiated cells have distinct structures and functions arising through lineage-specific programs of gene expression. Such cell type–specific differences in DNA transcription and translation are regulated by *epigenetic* modifications that consist of several changes that profoundly influence gene expression, including:

- *Chromatin organization* (Fig. 1.2). Genomic DNA is packed into nucleosomes, which are composed of 147

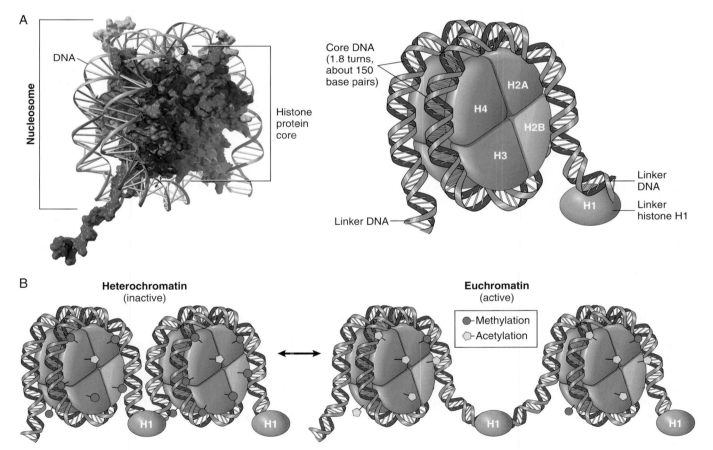

Fig. 1.2 Chromatin organization. (A) Nucleosomes are comprised of octamers of histone proteins (two each of histone subunits H2A, H2B, H3, and H4) encircled by 1.8 loops of 147 base pairs of DNA; histone H1 sits on the 20 to 80 nucleotide linker DNA between nucleosomes and helps stabilize the overall chromatin architecture. The histone subunits are positively charged, thus allowing the compaction of the negatively charged DNA. (B) The relative state of DNA unwinding (and thus access for transcription factors) is regulated by histone modification, for example, by acetylation, methylation, and/or phosphorylation (so-called "marks"); marks are dynamically written and erased. Certain marks such as histone acetylation "open up" the chromatin structure, whereas others, such as methylation of particular histone residues, tend to condense the DNA and lead to gene silencing. DNA itself can also be also be methylated, a modification that is associated with transcriptional inactivation.

base pair DNA segments wrapped around a central core of proteins called *histones*. Nucleosomes resemble beads joined by short DNA linkers; the entire structure is generically called *chromatin*. Importantly, the winding and compaction of chromatin in any given cell varies in different genomic regions. Thus, nuclear chromatin exists in two basic forms (visualizable by standard histology): (1) histochemically dense and transcriptionally inactive *heterochromatin* and (2) histochemically dispersed and transcriptionally active *euchromatin*. Because only euchromatin permits gene expression and thereby dictates cellular identity and activity, there are a host of mechanisms that tightly regulate the state of chromatin (described below).

- *DNA methylation.* High levels of DNA methylation in gene regulatory elements typically result in chromatin condensation and transcriptional silencing. Like histone modifications (see later), DNA methylation is tightly regulated by methyltransferases, demethylating enzymes, and methylated-DNA-binding proteins.

- *Histone modifying factors.* Nucleosomes are highly dynamic structures regulated by an array of nuclear proteins and post-translational modifications:
  - *Chromatin remodeling complexes* can reposition nucleosomes on DNA, exposing (or obscuring) gene regulatory elements such as promoters.
  - *"Chromatin writer" complexes* carry out more than 70 different covalent histone modifications generically denoted as *marks*. These include methylation, acetylation, and phosphorylation of specific histone amino acid residues: *Histone methylation* of lysines and arginines is accomplished by specific writer enzymes; methylation of histone lysine residues can lead to transcriptional activation or repression, depending on which histone residue is "marked." *Histone acetylation* of lysine residues (occurring through histone acetyl transferases) tends to open up chromatin and increase transcription; histone deacetylases (HDAC) reverse this process, leading to chromatin condensation. *Histone phosphorylation* of serine residues can variably open or condense chromatin, to increase or decrease transcription, respectively.
  - Histone marks are reversible through the activity of *"chromatin erasers."* Other proteins function as *"chromatin readers,"* binding histones that bear particular marks and thereby regulating gene expression.

The mechanisms involved in the cell-specific epigenetic regulation of genomic organization and gene expression are undeniably complex. Despite the intricacies, learning to manipulate these processes will likely bear significant therapeutic benefits because many diseases are associated with inherited or acquired epigenetic alterations, and dysregulation of the "epigenome" has a central role in the genesis of benign and malignant neoplasms (Chapter 6). Moreover—unlike genetic changes—epigenetic alterations (e.g., histone acetylation and DNA methylation) are readily reversible and are therefore amenable to intervention; indeed, HDAC inhibitors and DNA methylation inhibitors are already being used in the treatment of various forms of cancer.

Micro-RNA and Long Noncoding RNA

Another mechanism of gene regulation depends on the functions of noncoding RNAs. As the name implies, these are encoded by genes that are transcribed but not translated. Although many distinct families of noncoding RNAs exist, only two examples are discussed here: small RNA molecules called *microRNAs* and *long noncoding RNAs* >200 nucleotides in length.

- *Micro-RNAs (miRNAs)* are relatively short RNAs (22 nucleotides on average) that function primarily to modulate the translation of target mRNAs into their corresponding proteins. **Posttranscriptional silencing of gene expression by miRNA is a fundamental and evolutionarily conserved mechanism of gene regulation present in all eukaryotes (plants and animals).** Even bacteria have a primitive version of the same general machinery that they use to protect themselves against foreign DNA (e.g., from phages and viruses).

- The human genome contains almost 6000 miRNA genes, only 3.5-fold less than the number of protein-coding genes. Moreover, individual miRNAs appear to regulate multiple protein-coding genes, allowing each miRNA to coregulate entire programs of gene expression. Transcription of miRNA genes produces a primary transcript (pri-miRNA) that is processed into progressively smaller segments, including trimming by the enzyme *Dicer*. This generates mature single-stranded miRNAs of 21 to 30 nucleotides that associate with a multiprotein aggregate called RNA-induced silencing complex (RISC; Fig. 1.3). Subsequent base pairing between the miRNA strand and its target mRNA directs the RISC to either induce mRNA cleavage or to repress its translation. In this way, the target mRNA is *posttranscriptionally silenced*.

Taking advantage of the same pathway, *small interfering RNAs (siRNAs)* are short RNA sequences that can be introduced into cells. These serve as substrates for Dicer and interact with the RISC complex in a manner analogous to endogenous miRNAs. Synthetic siRNAs that can target specific mRNA species are therefore powerful laboratory tools to study gene function (so-called knockdown technology); they also are promising as therapeutic agents to silence pathogenic genes, e.g., oncogenes involved in neoplastic transformation.

- *Long noncoding RNA (lncRNA).* The human genome also contains a very large number of lncRNAs—at least 30,000, with the total number potentially exceeding coding mRNAs by 10- to 20-fold. lncRNAs modulate gene expression in many ways (Fig. 1.4); for example, they can bind to regions of chromatin, restricting RNA polymerase access to coding genes within the region. The best-known example of a repressive function involves XIST, which is transcribed from the X chromosome and plays an essential role in physiologic X chromosome inactivation. XIST itself escapes X inactivation, but forms a repressive "cloak" on the X chromosome from which it is transcribed, resulting in gene silencing. Conversely, it has been appreciated that many enhancers are sites of lncRNA synthesis, with the lncRNAs expanding transcription from gene promoters through

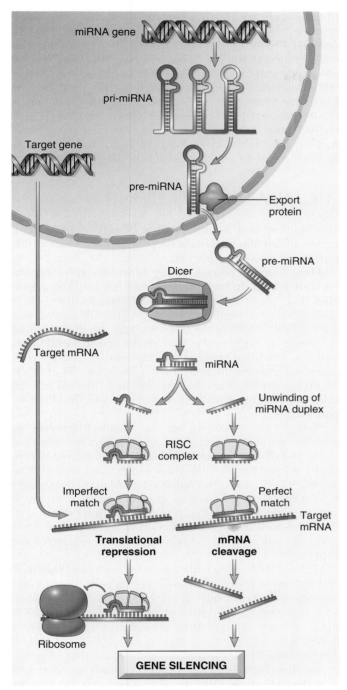

Fig. 1.3 Generation of microRNAs (miRNA) and their mode of action in regulating gene function. miRNA genes are transcribed to produce a primary miRNA (pri-miRNA), which is processed within the nucleus to form *pre-miRNA* composed of a single RNA strand with secondary hairpin loop structures that form stretches of double-stranded RNA. After this pre-miRNA is exported out of the nucleus via specific transporter proteins, the cytoplasmic enzyme *Dicer* trims the pre-miRNA to generate mature double-stranded miRNAs of 21 to 30 nucleotides. The miRNA subsequently unwinds, and the resulting single strands are incorporated into the multiprotein *RISC*. Base pairing between the single-stranded miRNA and its target mRNA directs RISC to either cleave the mRNA target or to repress its translation. In either case, the target mRNA gene is silenced posttranscriptionally.

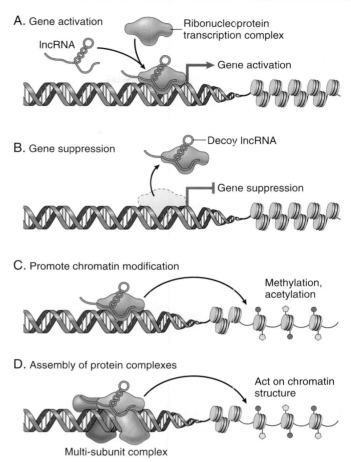

Fig. 1.4 Roles of long noncoding RNAs (lncRNAs). (A) Long noncoding RNAs (lncRNAs) can facilitate transcription factor binding and thus promote gene activation. (B) Conversely, lncRNAs can preemptively bind transcription factors and thus prevent gene transcription. (C) Histone and DNA modification by acetylases or methylases (or deacetylases and demethylases) may be directed by the binding of lncRNAs. (D) In other instances lncRNAs may act as scaffolding to stabilize secondary or tertiary structures and/or multisubunit complexes that influence general chromatin architecture or gene activity. *(Adapted from Wang KC, Chang HY: Molecular mechanisms of long noncoding RNAs, Mol Cell 43:904, 2011.)*

a variety of mechanisms (Fig. 1.4). Ongoing studies are exploring the role of lncRNAs in diseases like atherosclerosis and cancer.

Gene Editing

Exciting new developments that permit exquisitely specific genome editing stand to usher in an era of molecular revolution. These advances come from a wholly unexpected source: the discovery of clustered regularly interspaced short palindromic repeats (CRISPRs) and Cas (or CRISPR-associated genes). These are linked genetic elements that endow prokaryotes with a form of acquired immunity to phages and plasmids. Bacteria use this system to sample the DNA of infecting agents, incorporating it into the host genome as CRISPRs. CRISPRs are transcribed and processed into an RNA sequence that binds and directs the nuclease Cas9 to a sequences (e.g., a phage), leading to its cleavage and the destruction of the phage. Gene editing repurposes this process by using artificial guide RNAs (gRNAs) that bind Cas9 and are complementary to a DNA sequence of interest. Once directed to the target sequence by the gRNA, Cas9 induces double-strand DNA breaks.

Repair of the resulting highly specific cleavage sites can lead to somewhat random disruptive mutations in the targeted sequences (through nonhomologous end joining [NHEJ]), or the precise introduction of new sequences of interest (by homologous recombination). Both the gRNAs and the Cas9 enzyme can be delivered to cells with a single easy-to-build plasmid (Fig. 1.5). However, the real beauty of the system (and the excitement about its genetic engineering potential) comes from its impressive flexibility and specificity, which is substantially better than other previous editing systems. Applications include inserting specific mutations into the genomes of cells to model cancers and other diseases, and rapidly generating transgenic animals from edited embryonic stem cells. On the flip side, it now is feasible to selectively "correct" mutations that cause heritable disease, or—perhaps more worrisome—to just eliminate less "desirable" traits. Predictably, the technology has inspired a vigorous debate regarding its application.

CELLULAR HOUSEKEEPING

The viability and normal activity of cells depend on a variety of fundamental housekeeping functions that all differentiated cells must perform.

Many normal housekeeping functions are compartmentalized within membrane-bound intracellular organelles (Fig. 1.6). By isolating certain cellular functions within distinct compartments, potentially injurious degradative enzymes or reactive metabolites can be concentrated or stored at high concentrations in specific organelles without risking damage to other cellular constituents. Moreover, compartmentalization allows for the creation of unique intracellular environments (e.g., low pH or high calcium) that are optimal for certain enzymes or metabolic pathways.

New proteins destined for the plasma membrane or secretion are synthesized in the *rough endoplasmic reticulum (RER)* and physically assembled in the *Golgi apparatus*; proteins intended for the cytosol are synthesized on free ribosomes. *Smooth endoplasmic reticulum (SER)* may be abundant in certain cell types such as gonads and liver where it serves as the site of steroid hormone and lipoprotein synthesis, as well as the modification of hydrophobic compounds such as drugs into water-soluble molecules for export.

Cells catabolize the wide variety of molecules that they endocytose, as well as their own repertoire of proteins and organelles—all of which are constantly being degraded and renewed. Breakdown of these constituents takes place at three different sites, ultimately serving different functions.

- *Proteasomes* are "disposal" complexes that degrade denatured or otherwise "tagged" cytosolic proteins and release short peptides. In some cases the peptides so generated are presented in the context of class I major histocompatibility molecules to help drive the adaptive immune response (Chapter 5). In other cases, proteasomal degradation of regulatory proteins or transcription factors can trigger or shut down cellular signaling pathways.
- *Lysosomes* are intracellular organelles that contain enzymes that digest a wide range of macromolecules, including proteins, polysaccharides, lipids, and nucleic acids. They are the organelle in which phagocytosed microbes and damaged or unwanted cellular organelles are degraded and eliminated.
- *Peroxisomes* are specialized cell organelles that contain catalase, peroxidase and other oxidative enzymes. They

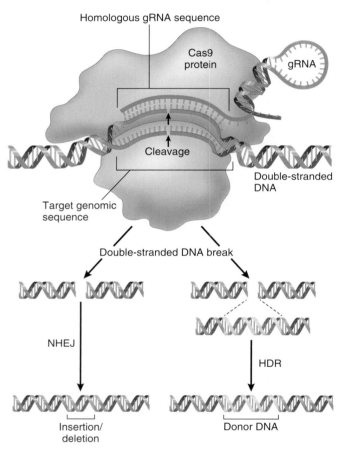

Fig. 1.5 Gene editing with clustered regularly interspersed short palindromic repeats (CRISPRs)/Cas9. In bacteria, DNA sequences consisting of CRISPRs are transcribed into guide RNAs (gRNAs) with a constant region and a variable sequence of about 20 bases. The constant regions of gRNAs bind to Cas9, permitting the variable regions to form heteroduplexes with homologous host cell DNA sequences. The Cas9 nuclease then cleaves the bound DNA, producing a double-stranded DNA break. To perform gene editing, gRNAs are designed with variable regions that are homologous to a target DNA sequence of interest. Coexpression of the gRNA and Cas9 in cells leads to efficient cleavage of the target sequence. In the absence of homologous DNA, the broken DNA is repaired by nonhomologous end joining (NHEJ), an error-prone method that often introduces disruptive insertions or deletions (indels). By contrast, in the presence of a homologous "donor" DNA spanning the region targeted by CRISPR/Cas9, cells instead may use homologous DNA recombination (HDR) to repair the DNA break. HDR is less efficient than NHEJ, but has the capacity to introduce precise changes in DNA sequence. Potential applications of CRISPR/Cas9 coupled with HDR include the repair of inherited genetic defects and the creation of pathogenic mutations.

Relative volumes of intracellular organelles (hepatocyte)

Compartment	% total volume	number/cell	role in the cell
Cytosol	54%	1	metabolism, transport, protein translation
Mitochondria	22%	1700	energy generation, apoptosis
Rough ER	9%	1*	synthesis of membrane and secreted proteins
Smooth ER, Golgi	6%	1*	protein modification, sorting, catabolism
Nucleus	6%	1	cell regulation, proliferation, DNA transcription
Endosomes	1%	200	intracellular transport and export, ingestion of extracellular substances
Lysosomes	1%	300	cellular catabolism
Peroxisomes	1%	400	very long-chain fatty acid metabolism

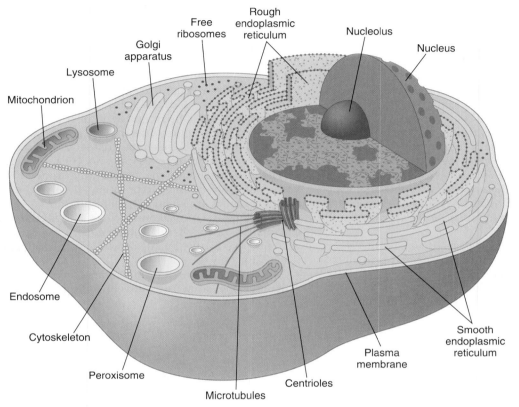

Fig. 1.6 Basic subcellular constituents of cells. The table presents the number of various organelles within a typical hepatocyte, as well as their volume within the cell. The figure shows geographic relationships but is not intended to be accurate to scale. *Rough and smooth ER form a single compartment; the Golgi apparatus is organized as a set of discrete stacked cisternae interconnected by transport vesicles. *(Adapted from Weibel ER, Stäubli W, Gnägi HR, et al: Correlated morphometric and biochemical studies on the liver cell. I. Morphometric model, stereologic methods, and normal morphometric data for rat liver, J Cell Biol 42:68, 1969.)*

play a specialized role in the breakdown of very long chain fatty acids, generating hydrogen peroxide in the process.

The contents and position of cellular organelles also are subject to regulation. *Endosomal vesicles* shuttle internalized material to the appropriate intracellular sites or direct newly synthesized materials to the cell surface or targeted organelle. Movement of both organelles and proteins within the cell and of the cell in its environment is orchestrated by the cytoskeleton. These structural proteins also regulate cellular shape and intracellular organization, requisites for maintaining *cell polarity*. This is particularly critical in epithelia, in which the top of the cell *(apical)* and the bottom and side of the cell *(basolateral)* are often exposed to different environments and have distinct functions.

Most of the adenosine triphosphate (ATP) that powers cells is made through oxidative phosphorylation in the mitochondria. However, mitochondria also serve as an important source of metabolic intermediates that are needed for anabolic metabolism. They also are sites of synthesis of certain macromolecules (e.g., heme), and contain important sensors of cell damage that can initiate and regulate the process of apoptotic cell death.

Cell growth and maintenance require a constant supply of both energy and the building blocks that are needed for synthesis of macromolecules. In growing and dividing cells, all of these organelles have to be replicated *(organellar biogenesis)* and correctly apportioned in daughter cells following mitosis. Moreover, because the macromolecules and organelles have finite life spans (mitochondria, e.g., last only about 10 days), mechanisms also must exist that allow for the recognition and degradation of "worn out" cellular components. The final catabolism occurs in lysosomes.

With this as a primer, we now move on to discuss cellular components and their function in greater detail.

Plasma Membrane: Protection and Nutrient Acquisition

Plasma membranes (and all other organellar membranes) are more than just static lipid sheaths. Rather, they are fluid bilayers of amphipathic phospholipids with hydrophilic head groups that face the aqueous environment and hydrophobic lipid tails that interact with each other to form a barrier to passive diffusion of large or charged molecules (Fig. 1.7A). The bilayer is composed of a heterogeneous collection of different phospholipids, which are distributed asymmetrically—for example, certain membrane lipids preferentially associate with extracellular or cytosolic faces. Asymmetric partitioning of phospholipids is important in several cellular processes:

- *Phosphatidylinositol* on the inner membrane leaflet can be phosphorylated, serving as an electrostatic scaffold for intracellular proteins; alternatively, polyphosphoinositides can be hydrolyzed by phospholipase C to generate intracellular second signals such as diacylglycerol and inositol trisphosphate.
- *Phosphatidylserine* is normally restricted to the inner face where it confers a negative charge and is involved in electrostatic interactions with proteins; however, when it flips to the extracellular face, which happens in

cells undergoing apoptosis (programmed cell death), it becomes an "eat me" signal for phagocytes. In the special case of platelets, it serves as a cofactor in the clotting of blood.
- *Glycolipids* and *sphingomyelin* are preferentially expressed on the extracellular face; glycolipids (and particularly gangliosides, with complex sugar linkages and terminal sialic acids that confer negative charges) are important in cell–cell and cell–matrix interactions, including inflammatory cell recruitment and sperm–egg interactions.

Certain membrane components associate laterally with each other in the bilayer, leading to distinct domains called *lipid rafts*. Because inserted membrane proteins have different intrinsic solubilities in various lipid domains, they tend to accumulate in certain regions of the membrane (e.g., rafts) and to become depleted from others. Such nonrandom distributions of lipids and membrane proteins impact cell–cell and cell–matrix interactions, as well as intracellular signaling and the generation of specialized membrane regions involved in secretory or endocytic pathways.

The plasma membrane is liberally studded with a variety of proteins and glycoproteins involved in (1) ion and metabolite transport, (2) fluid-phase and receptor-mediated uptake of macromolecules, and (3) cell–ligand, cell–matrix, and cell–cell interactions. Proteins interact with the lipid bilayer by one of four general arrangements (Fig. 1.7B):
- Most proteins are transmembrane (*integral*) proteins, having one or more relatively hydrophobic α-helical

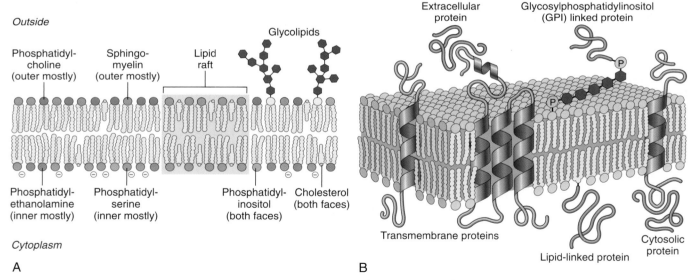

Fig. 1.7 Plasma membrane organization and asymmetry. (A) The plasma membrane is a bilayer of phospholipids, cholesterol, and associated proteins. The phospholipid distribution within the membrane is asymmetric; *phosphatidylcholine* and *sphingomyelin* are overrepresented in the outer leaflet, and *phosphatidylserine* (negative charge) and *phosphatidylethanolamine* are predominantly found on the inner leaflet; glycolipids occur only on the outer face where they contribute to the extracellular glycocalyx. Non-random partitioning of certain membrane components such as cholesterol creates membrane domains known as lipid rafts. (B) Membrane-associated proteins may traverse the membrane (singly or multiply) via α-helical hydrophobic amino acid sequences; depending on the sequence and hydrophobicity of these domain, such proteins may be enriched or excluded from lipid rafts and other membrane domain. Proteins on the cytosolic face may associate with membranes through posttranslational modifications, for example, farnesylation or addition of palmitic acid. Proteins on the extracytoplasmic face may associate with the membrane via glycosyl phosphatidyl inositol linkages. Besides protein–protein interactions within the membrane, membrane proteins can also associate with extracellular and/or intracytoplasmic proteins to generate large, relatively stable complexes (e.g., the *focal adhesion complex*). Transmembrane proteins can translate mechanical forces (e.g., from the cytoskeleton or ECM) as well as chemical signals across the membrane. It is worth remembering that a similar organization of lipids and associated proteins also occurs within the various organellar membranes.

segments that traverse the lipid bilayer. Integral membrane proteins typically contain positively charged amino acids in their cytoplasmic domains that anchor the proteins to the negatively charged head groups of membrane phospholipids.

- Proteins may be synthesized in the cytosol and post-translationally attached to prenyl groups (e.g., farnesyl, related to cholesterol) or fatty acids (e.g., palmitic or myristic acid) that insert into the cytosolic side of the plasma membrane.
- Attachment to membranes can occur through glyco-sylphosphatidylinositol (GPI) anchors on the extracellular face of the membrane.
- Extracellular proteins can noncovalently associate with transmembrane proteins, which serve to anchor them to the cell.

Many plasma membrane proteins function together as larger complexes; these may assemble under the control of chaperone molecules in the RER or by lateral diffusion in the plasma membrane. The latter mechanism is characteristic of many protein receptors (e.g., cytokine receptors) that dimerize or trimerize in the presence of ligand to form functional signaling units. Although lipid bilayers are fluid in the two-dimensional plane of the membrane, membrane components can nevertheless be constrained to discrete domains. This can occur by localization to lipid rafts (discussed earlier), or through intercellular protein–protein interactions (e.g., at *tight junctions*) that establish discrete boundaries; indeed, this strategy is used to maintain *cell polarity* (e.g., top/apical versus bottom/basolateral) in epithelial layers. Alternatively, unique domains can be formed through the interaction of membrane proteins with cytoskeletal molecules or an extracellular matrix (ECM).

The extracellular face of the plasma membrane is diffusely studded with carbohydrates, not only as complex oligosaccharides on glycoproteins and glycolipids, but also as polysaccharide chains attached to integral membrane proteoglycans. This *glycocalyx* functions as a chemical and mechanical barrier, and is also involved in *cell–cell* and *cell–matrix interactions*.

Passive Membrane Diffusion

Small, nonpolar molecules such as O_2 and CO_2 readily dissolve in lipid bilayers and therefore rapidly diffuse across them, as do hydrophobic molecules (e.g., steroid-based molecules such as estradiol or vitamin D). Similarly, small polar molecules (<75 daltons in mass, such as water, ethanol, and urea) readily cross membranes. In contrast, the lipid bilayer is an effective barrier to the passage of larger polar molecules, even those only slightly greater than 75 daltons, such as glucose. Lipid bilayers also are impermeant to ions, no matter how small, because of their charge and high degree of hydration. We will next discuss specialized mechanisms that regulate traffic across plasma membranes.

Carriers and Channels

For each of the larger polar molecules that must cross membranes to support normal cellular functions (e.g., for nutrient uptake and waste disposal), unique plasma membrane protein complexes are typically required. For low-molecular-weight species (ions and small molecules up to approximately 1000 daltons), *channel proteins* and *carrier proteins* may be used (although this discussion focuses on plasma membranes, it should be noted that similar pores and channels are needed for transport across organellar membranes). Each transported molecule (e.g., ion, sugar, nucleotide) requires a transporter that is typically highly specific (e.g., glucose but not galactose):

- *Channel proteins* create hydrophilic pores that, when open, permit rapid movement of solutes (usually restricted by size and charge; Fig. 1.8).
- *Carrier proteins* bind their specific solute and undergo a series of conformational changes to transfer the ligand across the membrane; their transport is relatively slow.

In many cases, a concentration and/or electrical gradient between the inside and outside of the cell drives solute movement via *passive transport* (virtually all plasma membranes have an electrical potential difference across them, with the inside negative relative to the outside). In other cases, *active transport* of certain solutes *against* a concentration gradient is accomplished by carrier molecules (not channels) using energy released by ATP hydrolysis or a coupled ion gradient. Transporter ATPases include the notorious *multidrug resistance (MDR) protein*, which pumps polar compounds (e.g., chemotherapeutic drugs) out of cells and may render cancer cells resistant to treatment.

Because membranes are freely permeable to water, it moves into and out of cells by osmosis, depending on relative solute concentrations. Thus, extracellular salt in excess of that in the cytosol *(hypertonicity)* causes a net movement of water out of cells, whereas *hypotonicity* causes a net movement of water into cells. The cytosol is rich in charged metabolites and protein species, which attract a large number of counterions that tend to increase the intracellular osmolarity. As a consequence, to prevent overhydration cells must constantly pump out small inorganic ions (e.g., Na^+)—typically through the activity of membrane ion-exchanging ATPases. Loss of the ability to generate energy (e.g., in a cell injured by toxins or ischemia) therefore results in osmotic swelling and eventual rupture of cells. Similar transport mechanisms also regulate intracellular and intraorganellar pH; most cytosolic enzymes prefer to work at pH 7.4, whereas lysosomal enzymes function best at pH 5 or less.

Receptor-Mediated and Fluid-Phase Uptake

Uptake of fluids or macromolecules by the cell, called *endocytosis,* occurs by two fundamental mechanisms (Fig. 1.8). Certain small molecules—including some vitamins—are taken up by invaginations of the plasma membrane called *caveolae.* For larger molecules, uptake occurs after binding to specific cell-surface receptors; internalization occurs through a membrane invagination process driven by an intracellular matrix of *clathrin* proteins. Clathrin is a hexamer of proteins that spontaneously assembles into a basketlike lattice to drive the invagination process. We shall come back to these later.

The process by which large molecules are exported from cells is called *exocytosis.* In this process, proteins synthesized and packaged within the RER and Golgi apparatus

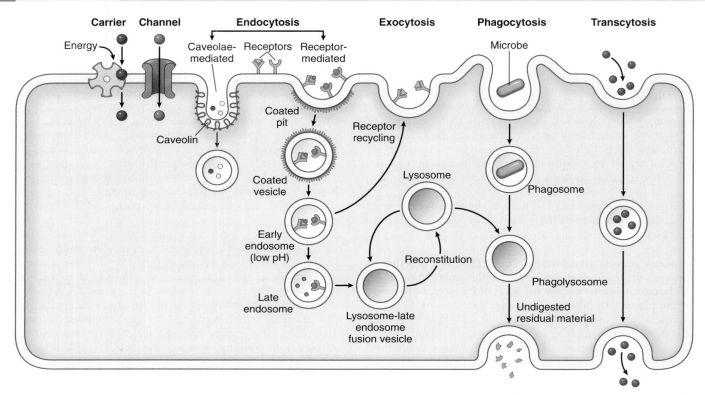

Fig. 1.8 Movement of small molecules and larger structures across membranes. The lipid bilayer is relatively impermeable to all but the smallest and/or most hydrophobic molecules. Thus, the import or export of charged species requires specific transmembrane transporter proteins; the internalization or externalization of large proteins, complex particles, or even cells requires encircling them with segments of the membrane. Small charged solutes can move across the membrane using either channels or carriers; in general, each molecule requires a unique transporter. *Channels* are used when concentration gradients can drive the solute movement. *Carriers* are required when solute is moved *against* a concentration gradient. Receptor-mediated and fluid-phase uptake of material involves membrane-bound vacuoles. *Caveolae* endocytose extracellular fluid, membrane proteins, and some receptor-bound molecules (e.g., folate) in a process driven by caveolin proteins concentrated within lipid rafts. *Pinocytosis* of extracellular fluid and most surface receptor–ligand pairs involves *clathrin-coated pits and vesicles*. After internalization, the clathrin dissociates and can be reused, whereas the resulting vesicle progressively matures and acidifies. In the early and/or late endosome, ligand can be released from its receptor (e.g., iron released from transferrin bound to the transferrin receptor) with receptor recycling to the cell surface for another round. Alternatively, receptor and ligand within endosomes can be targeted to fuse with lysosomes (e.g., epidermal growth factor bound to its receptor); after complete degradation, the late endosome–lysosome fusion vesicle can reconstitute lysosomes. *Phagocytosis* involves the non–clathrin-mediated membrane invagination of large particles—typically by specialized phagocytes (e.g., macrophages or neutrophils). The resulting phagosomes eventually fuse with lysosomes to facilitate the degradation of the internalized material. *Transcytosis* involves the transcellular endocytotic transport of solute and/or bound ligand from one face of a cell to another. *Exocytosis* is the process by which membrane-bound vesicles fuse with the plasma membrane and discharge their contents to the extracellular space.

are concentrated in secretory vesicles, which then fuse with the plasma membrane and expel their contents.

Transcytosis is the movement of endocytosed vesicles between the apical and basolateral compartments of cells; this is a mechanism for transferring large amounts of intact proteins across epithelial barriers (e.g., ingested antibodies in maternal milk across intestinal epithelia) or for the rapid movement of large volumes of solute. In fact, increased transcytosis probably plays a role in the increased vascular permeability seen in tumors.

We now return to the two forms of endocytosis mentioned earlier.

- *Caveolae-mediated endocytosis.* Caveolae ("little caves") are *noncoated* plasma membrane invaginations associated with GPI-linked molecules, cyclic adenosine monophosphate (cAMP)-binding proteins, SRC-family kinases, and the folate receptor. Caveolin is the major structural protein of caveolae. Internalization of caveolae with any bound molecules and associated extracellular fluid is denoted *potocytosis*—literally "cellular

sipping." Although caveolae likely participate in the transmembrane delivery of some molecules (e.g., folate), they also appear to contribute to the regulation of transmembrane signaling and/or cellular adhesion via the internalization of receptors and integrins. Mutations in caveolin are associated with muscular dystrophy and electrical abnormalities in the heart.

- *Pinocytosis and receptor-mediated endocytosis* (Fig. 1.8). *Pinocytosis* ("cellular drinking") is a fluid-phase process. The plasma membrane invaginates and is pinched off to form a cytoplasmic vesicle; after delivering their cargo, endocytosed vesicles recycle back to the plasma membrane *(exocytosis)* for another round of ingestion. Endocytosis and exocytosis are tightly balanced and highly active, as a cell typically pinocytoses 10% to 20% of its own cell volume each hour, or about 1% to 2% of its plasma membrane each minute. Pinocytosis and receptor-mediated endocytosis begin with the formation of a *clathrin-coated pit* containing the ligand to be internalized (by itself or bound to the receptor), which rapidly invaginates and pinches off to form a *clathrin-coated vesicle*. Thus, trapped within the vesicle is a gulp of the extracellular milieu, as well as receptor-bound macromolecules as described below. The vesicles then rapidly uncoat and fuse with an acidic intracellular structure called the *early endosome*, which progressively matures to late endosomes and ultimately fuses with lysosomes.

Receptor-mediated endocytosis is the major uptake mechanism for certain macromolecules, as exemplified by transferrin and low-density lipoprotein (LDL). These macromolecules bind to receptors that localize to clathrin-coated pits. After binding to their specific receptors, LDL and transferrin are endocytosed in vesicles that mature into early and late endosomes. In the acidic environment of the endosome, LDL and transferrin release their bound ligands (cholesterol and iron, respectively), which then exit into the cytosol, and the LDL receptor and transferrin receptor subsequently recycle to the plasma membrane. Defects in receptor-mediated transport of LDL are responsible for familial hypercholesterolemia, as described in Chapter 7.

Cytoskeleton

The ability of cells to adopt a particular shape, maintain polarity, organize the intracellular organelles, and move about depends on the intracellular scaffolding of proteins called the *cytoskeleton* (Fig. 1.9). In eukaryotic cells, there are three major classes of cytoskeletal proteins:

- *Actin microfilaments* are fibrils 5- to 9-nm in diameter formed from the **g**lobular protein actin (G-actin), the most abundant cytosolic protein in cells. G-actin monomers noncovalently polymerize into long **f**ilaments (**F**-actin) that intertwine to form double-stranded helices. In muscle cells, the filamentous protein *myosin* binds to actin and moves along it, driven by ATP hydrolysis (the basis of muscle contraction). In non-muscle cells, F-actin assembles via an assortment of actin-binding proteins into well-organized bundles and networks that control cell shape and movement.

- *Intermediate filaments* are fibrils 10-nm in diameter that comprise a large and heterogeneous family. Members include *lamins A, B,* and *C*, which contribute to the structure of nuclear lamina. Individual types of intermediate filaments have characteristic tissue-specific patterns of expression that are useful for identifying the cellular origin of poorly differentiated tumors.
  - *Vimentin:* Mesenchymal cells (fibroblasts, endothelium) anchoring intracellular organelles
  - *Desmin:* Muscle cells, forming the scaffold on which actin and myosin contract
  - *Neurofilaments:* Axons of neurons, imparting strength and rigidity
  - *Glial fibrillary acidic protein:* Glial cells that support neurons
  - *Cytokeratins:* Epithelial cells express more than 30 distinct varieties with distinct patterns of expression in different lineages (e.g., lung versus gastrointestinal epithelia). These can serve as histochemical markers for various epithelia

  Intermediate filaments are found predominantly in a ropelike polymerized form and primarily serve to impart tensile strength and allow cells to bear mechanical stress. The nuclear membrane lamins are important not only for maintaining nuclear morphology but also for regulating nuclear gene transcription. The critical roles of lamins is emphasized by rare but fascinating disorders caused by lamin mutations, which range from certain forms of muscular dystrophy to progeria, a disease of premature aging. Intermediate filaments also form the major structural proteins of epidermis and hair.

- *Microtubules* are 25-nm-thick fibrils composed of noncovalently polymerized dimers of α- and β-tubulin arrayed in constantly elongating or shrinking hollow tubes with a defined polarity; the ends are designated "+" or "−." The "−" end is typically embedded in a *microtubule organizing center (MTOC* or *centrosome)* near the nucleus where it is associated with paired *centrioles*, while the "+" end elongates or recedes in response to various stimuli by the addition or subtraction of tubulin dimers. Microtubules are involved in several important cellular functions:
  - Support cables for "molecular motor" proteins that allow the movement of vesicles and organelles around cells. *Kinesins* are the motors for anterograde (− to +) transport, whereas *dyneins* move cargo in a retrograde direction (+ to −).
  - The mechanical support for sister chromatid separation during mitosis
  - The core of *primary* cilia, single nonmotile projections on nucleated cells that help regulate proliferation and differentiation
  - The core of motile cilia (e.g., in bronchial epithelium) or flagella (in sperm)

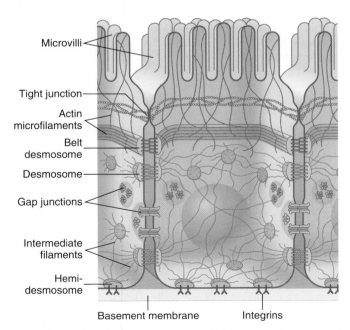

Microvilli
Tight junction
Actin microfilaments
Belt desmosome
Desmosome
Gap junctions
Intermediate filaments
Hemidesmosome
Basement membrane   **Integrins**

Fig. 1.9 Cytoskeletal elements and cell–cell interactions. Interepithelial adhesion involves several different surface protein interactions, including *tight junctions* and *desmosomes*; adhesion to the ECM involves cellular integrins (and associated proteins) within *hemidesmosomes*. See text for details.

Cell-Cell Interactions

Cells interact and communicate with one another by forming junctions that provide mechanical links and enable surface receptors to recognize ligands on other cells. *Cell junctions* are organized into three basic types (Fig. 1.9):

- *Occluding junctions (tight junctions)* seal adjacent cells together to create a continuous barrier that restricts the paracellular (between cells) movement of ions and other molecules. Viewed *en face*, occluding junctions form a tight meshlike network of macromolecular contacts between neighboring cells. The complexes that mediate these cell–cell interactions are composed of multiple proteins, including *occludin* and *claudin*. In addition to being a high-resistance barrier to solute movement, occluding junctions also maintain cellular polarity by forming the boundary between apical and basolateral domains of cells. Significantly, these junctions (as well as the desmosomes described later) are dynamic structures that can dissociate and reform as required to facilitate epithelial proliferation or inflammatory cell migration.

- *Anchoring junctions (desmosomes)* mechanically attach cells—and their intracellular cytoskeletons—to other cells or to the ECM. When the adhesion focus is between cells, and is small and rivetlike, it is designated a *spot desmosome*. When such a focus attaches the cell to the ECM, it is called a *hemidesmosome*. Similar adhesion domains can also occur as broad bands between cells, where they are denoted as *belt desmosomes*. Cell–cell desmosomal junctions are formed by the homotypic association of transmembrane glycoproteins called *cadherins*.

  - In spot desmosomes, the cadherins are linked to intracellular intermediate filaments and allow extracellular forces to be mechanically communicated (and dissipated) over multiple cells.
  - In belt desmosomes, the transmembrane adhesion molecules are associated with intracellular actin microfilaments, by which they can influence cell shape and/or motility.
  - In hemidesmosomes, the transmembrane connector proteins are called *integrins*; like cadherins, these attach to intracellular intermediate filaments, and thus they functionally link the cytoskeleton to the ECM. *Focal adhesion complexes* are large macromolecular complexes that localize at hemidesmosomes, and include proteins that can generate intracellular signals when cells are subjected to increased shear stress, for example, endothelium in the bloodstream, or cardiac myocytes in a failing heart.

- *Communicating junctions (gap junctions)* mediate the passage of chemical or electrical signals from one cell to another. The junction consists of a dense planar array of 1.5- to 2-nm pores (called *connexons*) formed by hexamers of transmembrane protein *connexins*. These pores permit the passage of ions, nucleotides, sugars, amino acids, vitamins, and other small molecules; the permeability of the junction is rapidly reduced by lowered intracellular pH or increased intracellular calcium. Gap junctions play a critical role in cell–cell communication; in cardiac myocytes, for example, cell-to-cell calcium fluxes through gap junctions allowing the myocardium to behave as a functional syncytium capable of coordinated waves of contraction—the beating of the heart.

Biosynthetic Machinery: Endoplasmic Reticulum and Golgi Apparatus

The structural proteins and enzymes of the cell are constantly renewed by a balance between ongoing synthesis and intracellular degradation. The endoplasmic reticulum (ER) is the site of synthesis of all transmembrane proteins and lipids needed for the assembly of plasma membrane and cellular organelles, including the ER itself. It is also the initial site of synthesis of all molecules destined for export out of the cell. The ER is organized into a mesh-like interconnected maze of branching tubes and flattened lamellae forming a continuous sheet around a single lumen that is topologically contiguous with the extracellular environment. The ER is composed of distinct domains that are distinguished by the presence or absence of ribosomes (Fig. 1.6).

Rough ER (RER): Membrane-bound ribosomes on the cytosolic face of the RER translate mRNA into proteins that are extruded into the ER lumen or become integrated into the ER membrane. This process is directed by specific *signal sequences* on the N-termini of nascent proteins. Proteins insert into the ER fold and must fold properly in order to assume a functional conformation and assemble into higher order complexes. Proper folding of the extracellular domains of many proteins involves the formation of disulfide bonds. A number of inherited disorders, including many cases of familial hypercholesterolemia (Chapter 6), are cause by mutations that disrupt disulfide bond formation. In addition, N-linked oligosaccharides (sugar moieties attached to asparagine residues) are added in the ER. *Chaperone molecules* retain proteins in the ER until these modifications are complete and the proper conformation is achieved. If a protein fails to fold and assemble into complexes appropriately, it is retained and degraded within the ER. Moreover, excess accumulation of misfolded proteins—exceeding the capacity of the ER to edit and degrade them—leads to the *ER stress response* (also called the *unfolded protein response* or the *UPR*), which triggers cell death through *apoptosis* (Chapter 2).

As an example of the importance of the ER editing function, the disease *cystic fibrosis* most commonly results from misfolding of the CFTR membrane transporter protein. In cystic fibrosis, the most common mutation in the *CFTR* gene results in the loss of a single amino acid residue (phenylalanine 508), leading in turn to misfolding, ER retention, and degradation of the CFTR protein. The loss of CFTR function leads to abnormal epithelial chloride transport, hyperviscous bronchial secretions and recurrent airway infections (Chapter 7).

Golgi apparatus: From the RER, proteins and lipids destined for other organelles or for extracellular export are shuttled into the Golgi apparatus. This organelle consists of stacked cisternae that progressively modify proteins in an orderly fashion from *cis* (near the ER) to *trans* (near the plasma membrane); macromolecules are shuttled between the various cisternae within membrane-bound vesicles. As molecules move from *cis* to *trans*, the N-linked oligosaccharides originally added to proteins in the ER are pruned and further modified in a stepwise fashion; O-linked oligosaccharides (sugar moieties linked to serine or threonine) are also appended. Some of this glycosylation is important in directing molecules to lysosomes (via the mannose-6-phosphate receptor); other glycosylation adducts may be important for cell–cell or cell–matrix interactions, or for clearing senescent cells (e.g., platelets and red cells). In addition to the stepwise glycosylation of lipids and proteins, the *cis Golgi network* is where proteins are recycled back to the ER, and the *trans Golgi network* is where proteins and lipids are dispatched to other organelles (including the plasma membrane), or to secretory vesicles destined for extracellular release. The Golgi complex is especially prominent in cells specialized for secretion, including goblet cells of the intestine, bronchial epithelium (secreting large amounts of polysaccharide-rich mucus), and plasma cells (secreting large quantities of antibodies).

Smooth ER (SER): The SER in most cells is relatively sparse, forming the transition zone from RER to transport vesicles moving to the Golgi. However, in cells that synthesize steroid hormones (e.g., in the gonads or adrenals), or that catabolize lipid-soluble molecules (e.g., in the liver), the SER may be particularly conspicuous. Indeed, repeated exposure to compounds that are metabolized by the SER (e.g., phenobarbital, which is catabolized by the cytochrome P-450 system) leads to a reactive hyperplasia of the SER. The SER also is responsible for sequestering intracellular calcium; subsequent release from the SER into the cytosol can mediate a number of responses to extracellular signals. In addition, in muscle cells, a specialized SER called the *sarcoplasmic reticulum* is responsible for the cyclical release and sequestration of calcium ions that regulate muscle contraction and relaxation, respectively.

Waste Disposal: Lysosomes and Proteasomes

As already mentioned briefly, **cellular waste disposal depends on the activities of lysosomes and proteasomes** (Fig. 1.10).

- *Lysosomes* are membrane-bound organelles containing roughly 40 different acid hydrolases (i.e., enzymes that function best in acidic pH ≤5), including proteases, nucleases, lipases, glycosidases, phosphatases, and sulfatases. Lysosomal enzymes are initially synthesized in the ER lumen and then tagged with a mannose-6-phosphate (M6P) residue within the Golgi apparatus. Such M6P-modified proteins are subsequently delivered to lysosomes through trans-Golgi vesicles that express M6P receptors. The other macromolecules destined for catabolism in the lysosomes arrive by one of three other pathways (Fig. 1.10):
  - Material internalized by fluid-phase pinocytosis or receptor-mediated endocytosis passes from plasma membrane to early endosome to late endosome, and ultimately into the lysosome, becoming progressively more acidic in the process. The early endosome is the first acidic compartment encountered, whereas

proteolytic enzymes only begin significant digestion in the late endosome; late endosomes mature into lysosomes.
  - Senescent organelles and large protein complexes can be shuttled into lysosomes by a process called *autophagy*. Through poorly understood mechanisms, obsolete organelles are corralled by a double membrane derived from the ER; the membrane progressively expands to encircle a collection of structures and forms an *autophagosome*, which then fuses with lysosomes where the contents are catabolized. In addition to facilitating the turnover of aged and defunct cellular constituents, autophagy also is used to preserve cell viability during nutrient depletion. The significance of autophagy in cell biology was recognized by the award of the 2016 Nobel Prize to Yoshinori Ohsumi for his discoveries relating to the mechanism of autophagy. This topic is discussed in more detail in Chapter 2.
  - *Phagocytosis* of microorganisms or large fragments of matrix or debris occur primarily in professional phagocytes (macrophages and neutrophils). The material is engulfed to form a *phagosome* that subsequently fuses with a lysosome.
- *Proteasomes* play an important role in degrading cytosolic proteins (Fig. 1.10); these include denatured or misfolded proteins (akin to what occurs within the ER), as well as other proteins whose levels and half-life need to be tightly regulated (e.g., transcription factors). Many (but not all) proteins destined for proteasome destruction are targeted after covalent addition of a protein called *ubiquitin*. Polyubiquitinated molecules are progressively unfolded and funneled into the polymeric proteasome complex, a cylinder containing multiple different protease activities, each with its active site pointed at the hollow core. Proteasomes digest proteins into small (6–12 amino acids) fragments that can subsequently be further degraded to their constituent amino acids and recycled, or presented to immune cells in the context of major histocompatibility complex class I molecules, an important component of host immune surveillance.

CELLULAR METABOLISM AND MITOCHONDRIAL FUNCTION

Mitochondria evolved from ancestral prokaryotes that were engulfed by primitive eukaryotes about 1.5 billion years ago. Their origin explains why mitochondria contain their own DNA genome (circularized, about 1% of the total cellular DNA), which encodes roughly 1% of the total cellular proteins and approximately 20% of the proteins involved in *oxidative phosphorylation*. Although their genomes are small, mitochondria can nevertheless perform all the steps of DNA replication, transcription, and translation. Interestingly, the mitochondrial machinery is similar to present-day bacteria; for example, mitochondria initiate protein synthesis with N-formylmethionine and are sensitive to anti-bacterial antibiotics.

Mitochondria are dynamic, constantly undergoing fission and fusion with other mitochondria; in this way,

A LYSOSOMAL DEGRADATION

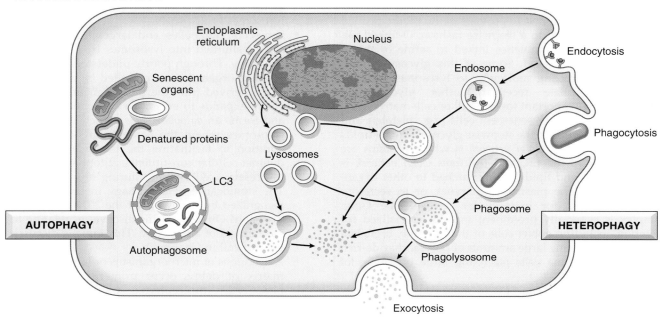

B PROTEASOMAL DEGRADATION

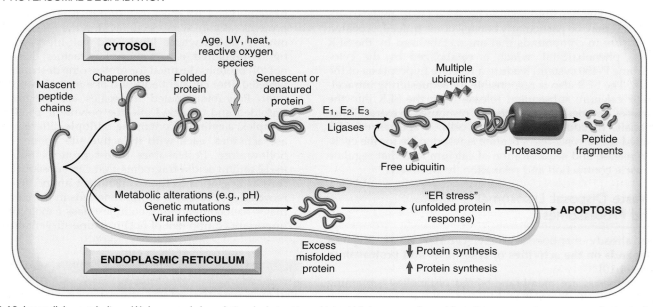

Fig. 1.10 Intracellular catabolism. (A) Lysosomal degradation. In *heterophagy (right side)*, lysosomes fuse with endosomes or phagosomes to facilitate the degradation of their internalized contents (see Fig. 1.8). The end products may be released into the cytosol for nutrition or discharged into the extracellular space *(exocytosis)*. In *autophagy (left side)*, senescent organelles or denatured proteins are targeted for lysosome-driven degradation by encircling them with a double membrane derived from the ER and marked by LC3 proteins (microtubule-associated protein 1A/1B-light chain 3). Cell stressors such as nutrient depletion or certain intracellular infections can also activate the autophagocytic pathway. (B) Proteasome degradation. Cytosolic proteins destined for turnover (e.g., transcription factors or regulatory proteins), senescent proteins, or proteins that have become denatured because of extrinsic mechanical or chemical stresses can be tagged by multiple ubiquitin molecules (through the activity of E_1, E_2, and E_3 ubiquitin ligases). This marks the proteins for degradation by proteasomes, cytosolic multisubunit complexes that degrade proteins to small peptide fragments. High levels of misfolded proteins within the ER trigger a protective unfolded protein response engendering a broad reduction in protein synthesis, but specific increases in chaperone proteins that can facilitate protein refolding. If this is inadequate to cope with the levels of misfolded proteins, apoptosis is induced.

mitochondria can undergo regular renewal to stave off degenerative changes that might occur because of genetic disorders or oxygen free radical damage. Mitochondria turn over rapidly, with estimated half-lives ranging from 1 to 10 days, depending on the tissue, nutritional status, metabolic demands, and intercurrent injury. Because the ovum contributes the vast majority of cytoplasmic organelles to the fertilized zygote, mitochondrial DNA is virtually entirely *maternally inherited*. However, because the protein constituents of mitochondria derive from both nuclear and mitochondrial genetic transcription, mitochondrial disorders may be X-linked, autosomal, or maternally inherited.

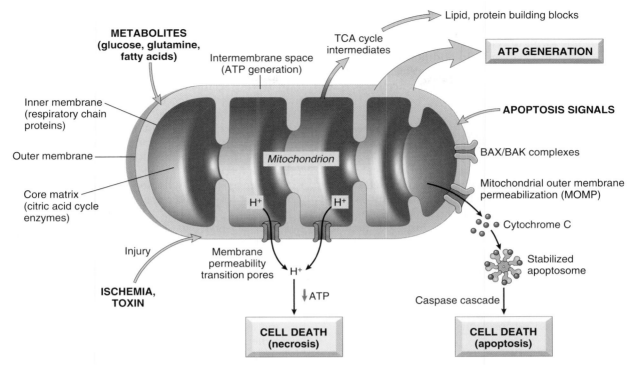

Fig. 1.11 Roles of the mitochondria. Besides the efficient generation of ATP from carbohydrate and fatty acid substrates, mitochondria play an important role in intermediary metabolism, serving as the source of molecules used to synthesize lipids and proteins, and they also are centrally involved in cell life-and-death decisions.

Mitochondria provide the enzymatic machinery for oxidative phosphorylation (and thus the relatively efficient generation of energy from glucose and fatty acid substrates). They also have central roles in anabolic metabolism and the regulation programmed cell death, so-called "apoptosis" (Fig. 1.11).

Energy Generation. Each mitochondrion has two separate and specialized membranes. The inner membrane contains the enzymes of the respiratory chain folded into cristae. This encloses a core matrix space that harbors the bulk of certain metabolic enzymes, such as the enzymes of the citric acid cycle. Outside the inner membrane is the intermembrane space, site of ATP synthesis, which is, in turn, enclosed by the outer membrane; the latter is studded with porin proteins that form aqueous channels permeable to small (<5000 daltons) molecules. Larger molecules (and even some smaller polar species) require specific transporters.

The major source of the energy needed to run all basic cellular functions derives from oxidative metabolism. Mitochondria oxidize substrates to CO_2, and in the process transfer high-energy electrons from the original molecule (e.g., gluocse) to molecular oxygen to water. The oxidation of various metabolites drives hydrogen ion (proton) pumps that transfer H^+ ions from the core matrix into the intermembrane space. As these H^+ ions flow back down their electrochemical gradient, the energy released is used to synthesize *ATP*.

It should be noted that the electron transport chain need not necessarily be coupled to ATP generation. Thus, an inner membrane protein enriched in brown fat called thermogenin (or UCP-1 = uncoupling protein 1) is a proton transporter that can dissipate the proton gradient (uncouple it from oxidative phosphorylation) in the form of heat (nonshivering thermogenesis). As a natural (albeit usually low-level) byproduct of substrate oxidation and electron transport, mitochondria also are an important source of reactive oxygen species (e.g., oxygen free radicals, hydrogen peroxide); importantly, hypoxia, toxic injury, or even mitochondrial aging can lead to significantly increased levels of intracellular oxidative stress.

Intermediate Metabolism. Pure oxidative phosphorylation produces abundant ATP, but also "burns" glucose to CO_2 and H_2O, leaving no carbon moieties for use as building blocks for lipids or proteins. For this reason, rapidly growing cells (both benign and malignant) increase glucose and glutamine uptake and decrease their production of ATP per glucose molecule—forming lactic acid in the presence of adequate oxygen—a phenomenon called the Warburg effect (or aerobic glycolysis). Both glucose and glutamine provide carbon moieties that prime the mitochondrial tricarboxylic acid (TCA) cycle, but instead of being used to make ATP, intermediates are "spun off" to make lipids, nucleic acids, and proteins. Thus, depending on the growth state of the cell, mitochondrial metabolism can be modulated to support either cellular maintenance or cellular growth. Ultimately, growth factors, nutrient supplies, and oxygen availability, as well as cellular signaling pathways and sensors that respond to these exogenous factors, govern these metabolic decisions.

Cell Death. Mitochondria are like the proverbial Dr. Jekyll and Mr. Hyde. On the one hand, they are factories of energy production in the form of ATP that allow the cells to survive; on the other hand, they participate in driving cell death when the cells are exposed to noxious stimuli that the cells cannot adapt to. The role of mitochondria in the two principle forms of cell death, necrosis and apoptosis, are discussed in Chapter 2. In addition to providing ATP and metabolites that enable the bulk of cellular activity, mitochondria also regulate the balance of cell survival and death.

CELLULAR ACTIVATION

Cell communication is critical in multicellular organisms. At the most basic level, extracellular signals determine whether a cell lives or dies, whether it remains quiescent, or whether it is stimulated to perform a specific function. Intercellular signaling is important in the developing embryo, in maintaining tissue organization, and in ensuring that tissues respond in an adaptive and effective fashion to various threats, such as local tissue trauma or a systemic infection. Loss of cellular communication and the "social controls" that maintain normal relationships of cells can variously lead to unregulated growth (cancer) or an ineffective response to an extrinsic stress (as in shock).

Cell Signaling

An individual cell is constantly exposed to a remarkable cacophony of signals, which must be "interpeted" and integrated into responses that benefit the organism as a whole. Some signals may induce a given cell type to differentiate, others may stimulate proliferation, and yet others may direct the cell to perform a specialized function. Multiple signals received in combination may trigger yet another totally unique response. Many cells require certain inputs just to continue living; in the absence of appropriate exogenous signals, they die by apoptosis.

The sources of the signals that most cells respond to can be classified into several groups:
- *Pathogens and damage to neighboring cells.* Many cells have an innate capacity to sense and respond to damaged cells (*danger signals*), as well as foreign invaders such as microbes. The receptors that generate these danger signals are discussed in Chapters 3 and 5.
- *Cell-cell contacts,* mediated through adhesion molecules and/or gap junctions. As mentioned previously, *gap junction signaling* is accomplished between adjacent cells via hydrophilic connexons that permit the movement of small ions (e.g., calcium), various metabolites, and potential second messenger molecules such as cAMP.
- *Cell-ECM contacts,* mediated through integrins, which are discussed in Chapter 3 in the context of leukocyte attachment to other cells during inflammation.
- *Secreted molecules.* The most important secreted molecules include *growth factors,* discussed later; *cytokines,* a term reserved for mediators of inflammation and immune responses (also discussed in Chapters 3 and 5); and *hormones,* which are secreted by endocrine organs and act on different cell types (Chapter 20).

Signaling pathways also can be classified into different types based on the spatial relationships between the sending and receiving cells:

- *Paracrine signaling.* Cells in just the immediate vicinity are affected. Paracrine signaling may involve transmembrane "sending" molecules that activate receptors on adjacent cells or secreted factors that diffuse for only short distances. In some instances, the latter is achieved by having secreted factors bind tightly to ECM.
- *Autocrine signaling* occurs when molecules secreted by a cell affect that same cell. This can serve as a means to entrain groups of cells undergoing synchronous differentiation during development, or it can be used to amplify (positive feedback) or dampen (negative feedback) a response.
- *Synaptic signaling.* Activated neurons secrete *neurotransmitters* at specialized cell junctions *(synapses)* onto target cells.
- *Endocrine signaling.* A hormone is released into the bloodstream and acts on target cells at a distance.

Regardless of the nature of an extracellular stimulus (paracrine, synaptic, or endocrine), the signal it conveys is transmitted to the cell via a specific *receptor* protein. Signaling molecules *(ligands)* bind their respective receptors and initiate a cascade of intracellular events culminating in the desired cellular response. Ligands usually have high affinities for receptors and at physiologic concentrations bind receptors with exquisite specificity. Receptors may be present on the cell surface or located within the cell (Fig. 1.12):
- *Intracellular receptors* include transcription factors that are activated by lipid-soluble ligands that easily transit plasma membranes. Examples include vitamin D and steroid hormones, which activate nuclear hormone receptors. In other settings, a small and/or nonpolar signaling ligand can diffuse into adjacent cells. Such is the case for nitric oxide (NO), through which endothelial cells regulate intravascular pressure. NO is generated by an activated endothelial cell and then diffuses into adjacent vascular smooth muscle cells; there it activates guanylyl cyclase to generate cyclic GMP, an intracellular second signal that causes smooth muscle relaxation.
- *Cell-surface receptors* are generally transmembrane proteins with extracellular domains that bind activating ligands. Depending on the receptor, ligand binding may (1) open ion channels (typically at the synapse between electrically excitable cells), (2) activate an associated GTP-binding regulatory protein (*G protein*), (3) activate an endogenous or associated enzyme, often a tyrosine kinase, or (4) trigger a proteolytic event or a change in protein binding or stability that activates a latent transcription factor. Activities (2) and (3) are associated with growth factor signaling pathways that drive cell proliferation, whereas activity (4) is a common feature of multiple pathways (e.g., Notch, Wnt, and Hedgehog) that regulate normal development. Understandably, signals transduced by cell surface receptors are often deranged in developmental disorders and in cancers.

Signal Transduction Pathways

Binding of a ligand to a cell surface receptor mediates signaling by inducing clustering of the receptor *(receptor*

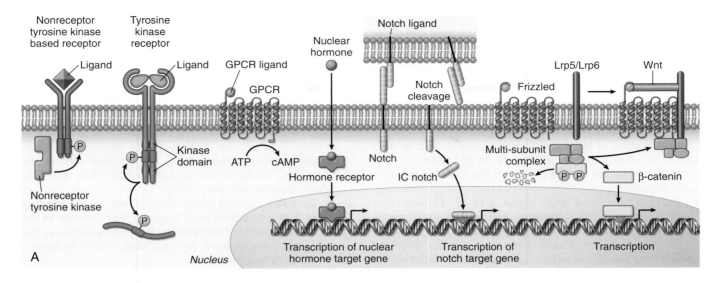

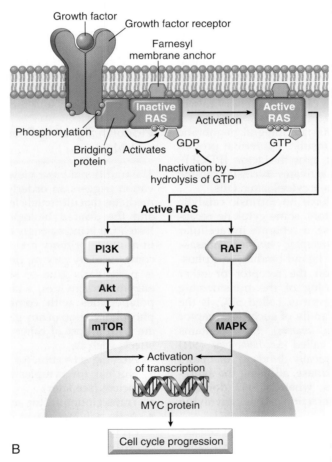

Fig. 1.12 Receptor-mediated signaling. (A) Categories of signaling receptors, including receptors that use a nonreceptor tyrosine kinase; a receptor tyrosine kinase; a nuclear receptor that binds its ligand and can then influence transcription; a seven-transmembrane receptor linked to heterotrimeric G proteins; Notch, which recognizes a ligand on a distinct cell and is cleaved yielding an intracellular fragment that can enter the nucleus and influence transcription of specific target genes; and the Wnt/Frizzled pathway where activation releases intracellular β-catenin from a protein complex that normally drives its constitutive degradation. The released β-catenin can then migrate to the nucleus and act as a transcription factor. Lrp5/Lrp6, low-density lipoprotein (LDL) receptor-related proteins 5 and 6, are highly homologous and act as coreceptors in Wnt/Frizzled signaling. (B) Signaling from a tyrosine kinase-based receptor. Binding of the growth factor (ligand) causes receptor dimerization and autophosphorylation of tyrosine residues. Attachment of adapter (or bridging) proteins couples the receptor to inactive, GDP-bound RAS, allowing the GDP to be displaced in favor of GTP and yielding activated RAS. Activated RAS interacts with and activates RAF (also known as *MAP kinase kinase kinase*). This kinase then phosphorylates mitogen-activated protein kinase (MAPK), and activated MAP kinase phosphorylates other cytoplasmic proteins and nuclear transcription factors, generating cellular responses. Activated RAS can also interact with other components, such as phosphatidyl 3-kinase (PI3 kinase), which activates other signaling systems. The cascade is turned off when the activated RAS eventually hydrolyzes GTP to GDP converting RAS to its inactive form. Mutations in RAS that lead to delayed GTP hydrolysis can thus lead to augmented proliferative signaling. *GDP*, Guanosine diphosphate; *GTP*, guanosine triphosphate; *mTOR*, mammalian target of rapamycin.

crosslinking) or other conformational changes (Fig. 1.12). The common theme is that all of these perturbations cause a change in the physical state of the intracellular domain of the receptor, which then triggers additional biochemical events that lead to signal transduction.

Cellular receptors are grouped into several types based on the signaling mechanisms they use and the intracellular biochemical pathways they activate (Fig. 1.12). Receptor signaling most commonly leads to the formation or modification of biochemical intermediates and/or activation of enzymes, and ultimately to the generation of active transcription factors that enter the nucleus and alter gene expression:

- *Receptors associated with kinase activity.* Downstream phosphorylation is a common pathway of signal transduction. Changes in receptor geometry can stimulate intrinsic receptor *protein kinase* activity or promote the enzymatic activity of recruited intracellular kinases. These kinases add charged phosphate residues to target molecules. *Tyrosine kinases* phosphorylate specific tyrosine residues, whereas *serine/threonine kinases* add phosphates to distinct serine or threonine residues, and *lipid kinases* phosphorylate lipid substrates. For every phosphorylation event, there is also a potential counter-regulatory *phosphatase*, an enzyme that can remove the phosphate residue and thus modulate signaling; usually, phosphatases play an inhibitory role in signal transduction.
- *Receptor tyrosine kinases (RTKs)* are integral membrane proteins (e.g., receptors for insulin, epidermal growth factor, and platelet-derived growth factor [PDGF]); ligand-induced crosslinking activates intrinsic tyrosine kinase domains located in their cytoplasmic tails.
- Several kinds of receptors have no intrinsic catalytic activity (e.g., immune receptors, some cytokine receptors, and integrins). For these, a separate intracellular protein—known as a *nonreceptor tyrosine kinase*—interacts with receptors after ligand binding and phosphorylates specific motifs on the receptor or other proteins. The cellular homolog of the transforming protein of the Rous sarcoma virus, called SRC, is the prototype for an important family of such nonreceptor tyrosine kinases *(Src-family kinases)*. SRC contains unique functional regions called *Src-homology (SH)* domains; SH2 domains typically bind to receptors phosphorylated by another kinase, allowing the aggregation of multiple enzymes, whereas SH3 domains mediate protein–protein interactions, often involving proline-rich domains.
- *G-protein coupled receptors* are polypeptides that characteristically traverse the plasma membrane seven times (hence their designation as seven-transmembrane or serpentine receptors); more than 1500 such receptors have been identified. After ligand binding, the receptor associates with an intracellular guanosine triphosphate (GTP)-binding protein (G protein). At baseline, these G proteins contain guanosine diphosphate (GDP); interaction with a receptor-ligand complex results in G protein activation through the exchange of GDP for GTP. Downstream signaling typically involves the generation of cAMP, and inositol-1,4,5,-triphosphate (IP_3), the latter releasing calcium from the ER.

- *Nuclear receptors.* Lipid-soluble ligands can diffuse into cells where they interact with intracellular proteins to form a receptor-ligand complex that directly binds to nuclear DNA; the results can be either activation or repression of gene transcription.
- *Other classes of receptors.* Other receptors—originally recognized as important for embryonic development and cell fate determination—have since been shown to participate in the functions of mature cells, particularly within the immune system. These pathways rely on protein:protein interactions, rather than enzymatic activities, to transduce signals, which may serve to allow for very precise control.
  - Receptor proteins of the *Notch* family: ligand binding to Notch receptors leads to proteolytic cleavage of the receptor and subsequent nuclear translocation of the cytoplasmic domain (intracellular Notch) to form a transcription complex.
  - *Wnt* protein ligands act through a pathway involving transmembrane *Frizzled* family receptors, which regulate the intracellular levels of β-catenin. In the absence of Wnt, β-catenin is targeted for ubiquitin-directed proteasome degradation. Wnt binding to Frizzled (and other coreceptors) recruits other proteins that disrupt the degradation-targeting complex. This stabilizes β-catenin, allowing it to translocate to the nucleus and form a transcription complex.

Modular Signaling Proteins, Hubs, and Nodes

The traditional *linear* view of signaling—that receptor activation triggers an orderly sequence of biochemical intermediates that ultimately leads to changes in gene expression and the desired biological response—is oversimplified. Instead, it is increasingly clear that any initial signal results in multiple primary and secondary effects, each of which contributes in varying degrees to the final outcome. This is particularly true of signaling pathways that rely on enzymatic activities, which typically modulate a web of polypeptides with complex interactions. For example, phosphorylation of any given protein can allow it to associate with a host of other molecules, resulting in multiple effects such as:

- Enzyme activation (or inactivation)
- Nuclear (or cytoplasmic) localization of transcription factors (see later)
- Transcription factor activation (or inactivation)
- Actin polymerization (or depolymerization)
- Protein degradation (or stabilization)
- Activation of feedback inhibitory (or stimulatory) loops

Adaptor proteins play a key role in organizing intracellular signaling pathways. These proteins function as molecular connectors that physically link different enzymes and promote the assembly of complexes; adaptors can be integral membrane proteins or cytosolic proteins. A typical adaptor may contain a few specific domains (e.g., SH2 or SH3) that mediate protein–protein interactions. By influencing the proteins that are recruited to signaling complexes, adaptors can determine downstream signaling events.

By analogy with computer networks, the protein–protein complexes can be considered *nodes* and the biochemical events feeding into or emanating from these nodes can be thought of as *hubs*. Signal transduction can therefore be visualized as a kind of networking phenomenon; understanding this higher-order complexity is the province of *systems biology*, involving a "marriage" of biology and computation.

Transcription Factors

Most signal transduction pathways ultimately influence cellular function by modulating gene transcription through the activation and nuclear localization of transcription factors. Conformational changes of transcription factors (e.g., following phosphorylation) can allow their translocation into the nucleus or can expose specific DNA or protein-binding motifs. Transcription factors may drive the expression of a relatively limited set of genes or may have much more widespread effects on gene expression. Among the transcription factors that regulate the expression of genes that are needed for growth are MYC and JUN, whereas a transcription factor that triggers the expression of genes that lead to growth arrest is p53. Transcription factors have a modular design, often containing domains that bind DNA and others that interact with other proteins, such as components of the RNA polymerase complex required for transcription.

- DNA-binding domains permit specific binding to short DNA sequences. Whereas some transcription factor binding sites are found in promoters, close to the site where transcription starts, it is now appreciated that most transcription factors bind widely throughout genomes, including to long-range regulatory elements such as enhancers. Enhancers function by looping back to gene promoters, and therefore are spatially located close to the genes that they regulate, even though it terms of genomic sequence they may appear to be far away. These insights highlight the importance of chromatin organization in regulating gene expression, both normal and pathologic.
- For a transcription factor to induce transcription, it must also possess protein:protein interaction domains that directly or indirectly recruit histone-modifying enzymes, chromatin-remodeling complexes, and (most importantly) RNA polymerase—the large multiprotein enzymatic complex that is responsible for RNA synthesis.

GROWTH FACTORS AND RECEPTORS

A major role of growth factors is to stimulate the activity of proteins that are required for cell survival, growth and division. Growth factor activity is mediated through binding to specific receptors, ultimately influencing the expression of genes that can:

- Promote entry of cells into the cell cycle
- Relieve blocks on cell-cycle progression (thus promoting replication)
- Prevent apoptosis
- Enhance biosynthesis of cellular components (nucleic acids, proteins, lipids, carbohydrates) required for a mother cell to give rise to two daughter cells

Although some growth factors are proteins that "just" stimulate cell proliferation and/or survival, it is important to remember that they also can drive a host of other activities, including migration, differentiation, and synthetic capacity. Some of the important growth factors relevant to tissue regeneration and repair are listed in Table 1.1 and described further in Chapter 3.

Growth factors can be involved in the proliferation of cells at steady state as well as after injury, when irreversibly damaged cells must be replaced. Uncontrolled

Table 1.1 Growth Factors Involved in Regeneration and Repair

Growth Factor	Sources	Functions
Epidermal growth factor (EGF)	Activated macrophages, salivary glands, keratinocytes, and many other cells	Mitogenic for keratinocytes and fibroblasts; stimulates keratinocyte migration; stimulates formation of granulation tissue
Transforming growth factor-α (TGF-α)	Activated macrophages, keratinocytes, many other cell types	Stimulates proliferation of hepatocytes and many other epithelial cells
Hepatocyte growth factor (HGF) (scatter factor)	Fibroblasts, stromal cells in the liver, endothelial cells	Enhances proliferation of hepatocytes and other epithelial cells; increases cell motility
Vascular endothelial growth factor (VEGF)	Mesenchymal cells	Stimulates proliferation of endothelial cells; increases vascular permeability
Platelet-derived growth factor (PDGF)	Platelets, macrophages, endothelial cells, smooth muscle cells, keratinocytes	Chemotactic for neutrophils, macrophages, fibroblasts, and smooth muscle cells; activates and stimulates proliferation of fibroblasts, endothelial, and other cells; stimulates ECM protein synthesis
Fibroblast growth factors (FGFs), including acidic (FGF-1) and basic (FGF-2)	Macrophages, mast cells, endothelial cells, many other cell types	Chemotactic and mitogenic for fibroblasts; stimulates angiogenesis and ECM protein synthesis
Transforming growth factor-β (TGF-β)	Platelets, T lymphocytes, macrophages, endothelial cells, keratinocytes, smooth muscle cells, fibroblasts	Chemotactic for leukocytes and fibroblasts; stimulates ECM protein synthesis; suppresses acute inflammation
Keratinocyte growth factor (KGF) (i.e., FGF-7)	Fibroblasts	Stimulates keratinocyte migration, proliferation, and differentiation

ECM, Extracellular membrane.

proliferation can result when the growth factor activity is dysregulated, or when growth factor signaling pathways are altered to become constitutively active. Thus, many growth factor pathway genes are *proto-oncogenes*, and gain-of-function mutations in these genes can convert them into oncogenes capable of driving unfettered cell proliferation and tumor formation. The following discussion summarizes selected growth factors that are involved in the important proliferative processes of tissue repair and regeneration; by virtue of their proliferative effects they can also drive tumorigenesis. Although the growth factors described here all involve receptors with intrinsic kinase activity, other growth factors may signal through each of the various pathways shown in Fig. 1.12.

- *Epidermal growth factor and transforming growth factor-α.* Both of these factors belong to the EGF family and bind to the same receptors, explaining their shared biologic activities. EGF and TGF-α are produced by macrophages and a variety of epithelial cells, and are mitogenic for hepatocytes, fibroblasts, and a host of epithelial cells. The "EGF receptor family" includes four membrane receptors with intrinsic tyrosine kinase activity; the best-characterized is EGFR1, also known as ERB-B1, or simply EGFR. EGFR1 mutations and/or amplification frequently occur in a number of cancers including those of the lung, head and neck, breast, and brain. The ERBB2 receptor (also known as HER2) is overexpressed in a subset of breast cancers. To treat malignancies, many of these receptors have been successfully targeted by antibodies and small molecule antagonists.

- *Hepatocyte growth factor.* Hepatocyte growth factor (HGF; also known as scatter factor) has mitogenic effects on hepatocytes and most epithelial cells. HGF acts as a morphogen during embryonic development (i.e., it influences the pattern of tissue differentiation), promotes cell migration (hence its designation as scatter factor), and enhances hepatocyte survival. HGF is produced by fibroblasts and most mesenchymal cells, as well as endothelium and nonhepatocyte liver cells. It is synthesized as an inactive precursor (pro-HGF) that is proteolytically activated by serine proteases released at sites of injury. The receptor for HGF is MET, which has intrinsic tyrosine kinase activity. It is frequently overexpressed or mutated in tumors, particularly renal and thyroid papillary carcinomas. Consequently, MET inhibitors are being evaluated as cancer therapies.

- *Platelet-derived growth factor.* PDGF is a family of several closely related proteins, each consisting of two chains (designated by pairs of letters). Three isoforms of PDGF (AA, AB, and BB) are constitutively active, while PDGF-CC and PDGF-DD must be activated by proteolytic cleavage. PDGF is stored in platelet granules and is released on platelet activation. Although originally isolated from platelets (hence the name), it also is produced by many other cells, including activated macrophages, endothelium, smooth muscle cells, and a variety of tumors. All PDGF isoforms exert their effects by binding to two cell surface receptors (PDGFR α and β), both having intrinsic tyrosine kinase activity. PDGF induces fibroblast, endothelial, and smooth muscle cell proliferation and matrix synthesis, and is chemotactic for these cells (and inflammatory cells), thus promoting

recruitment of the cells into areas of inflammation and tissue injury.

- *Vascular endothelial growth factor.* Vascular endothelial growth factors (VEGFs)—VEGF-A, -B, -C, and -D, and PIGF (placental growth factor)—are a family of homodimeric proteins. VEGF-A is generally referred to simply as VEGF; it is the major factor responsible for *angiogenesis*, inducing blood vessel development, after injury and in tumors. In comparison, VEGF-B and PIGF are involved in embryonic vessel development, and VEGF-C and -D stimulate both angiogenesis and lymphatic development *(lymphangiogenesis)*. VEGFs also are involved in the maintenance of endothelial cells lining mature vessels. Its expression is highest in epithelial cells adjacent to fenestrated endothelium (e.g., podocytes in the kidney, pigment epithelium in the retina, and choroid plexus in the brain). VEGF induces angiogenesis by promoting endothelial cell migration and proliferation (capillary sprouting), and the formation of the vascular lumina. VEGFs also induce vascular dilation and increase vascular permeability. As might be anticipated, hypoxia is the most important inducer of VEGF production through pathways that involve activation of the transcription factor hypoxia-inducible factor (HIF-1). Other VEGF inducers—produced at sites of inflammation or wound healing—include PDGF and TGF-α.

  VEGFs bind to a family of receptor tyrosine kinases (VEGFR-1, -2, and -3). VEGFR-2 is highly expressed in endothelium and is the most important for angiogenesis. Antibodies against VEGF are approved for the treatment of several tumors such as renal and colon cancers because cancers require angiogenesis for their spread and growth. Anti-VEGF antibodies also are used in the treatment of a number of ophthalmic diseases, including: "wet" age-related macular degeneration (AMD a disorder of inappropriate angiogenesis and vascular permeability that causes adult-onset blindness); the retinopathy of prematurity; and the leaky vessels that lead to diabetic macular edema. Finally, increased levels of soluble versions of VEGFR-1 (s-FLT-1) in pregnant women may contribute to preeclampsia (hypertension and proteinuria) by "sopping up" the free VEGF required for maintaining normal endothelium.

- *Fibroblast growth factor.* Fibroblast growth factor (FGF) is a family of growth factors with more than 20 members. Acidic FGF (aFGF, or FGF-1) and basic FGF (bFGF, or FGF-2) are the best characterized; FGF-7 is also referred to as keratinocyte growth factor (KGF). Released FGFs associate with heparan sulfate in the ECM, which serves as a reservoir for inactive factors that can be subsequently released by proteolysis (e.g., at sites of wound healing). FGFs transduce signals through four tyrosine kinase receptors (FGFR 1–4). FGFs contribute to wound healing responses, hematopoiesis, and development; bFGF has all the activities necessary for angiogenesis as well.

- *Transforming growth factor-β.* TGF-β has three isoforms (TGF-β1, TGF-β2, and TGF-β3) that belong to a family with about 30 members, including bone morphogenetic proteins (BMPs), activins, inhibins, and Müllerian inhibiting substance. TGF-β1 has the most widespread distribution, and it is more commonly referred to simply as

TGF-β. It is a homodimeric protein produced by multiple cell types, including platelets, endothelium, and mononuclear inflammatory cells. TGF-β is secreted as a precursor that requires proteolysis to yield the biologically active protein. There are two TGF-β receptors, both with serine/threonine kinase activity that induces the phosphorylation of several downstream cytoplasmic transcription factors called *Smads*. Phosphorylated Smads form heterodimers with Smad4, allowing nuclear translocation and association with other DNA-binding proteins to activate or inhibit gene transcription. TGF-β produces multiple and often opposing effects depending on the tissue type and concurrent signals. Agents with such multiplicity of effects are called *pleiotropic*, and TGF-β is "pleiotropic with a vengeance." Primarily, TGF-β drives scar formation by stimulating matrix synthesis through decreased matrix metalloproteinase (MMP) activity and increased activity of tissue inhibitors of proteinases (TIMPs). TGF-β also applies brakes to the inflammation that accompanies wound healing by inhibiting lymphocyte proliferation and the activity of other leukocytes.

EXTRACELLULAR MATRIX

The ECM is a network of interstitial proteins that constitutes a significant proportion of any tissue. **Cell interactions with ECM are critical for development and healing, as well as for maintaining normal tissue architecture** (Fig. 1.13). Much more than a simple "space filler" around cells, ECM serves several key functions:

- *Mechanical support* for cell anchorage and cell migration, and maintenance of cell polarity.
- *Control of cell proliferation,* by binding and displaying growth factors and by signaling through cellular receptors of the integrin family. The ECM provides a depot

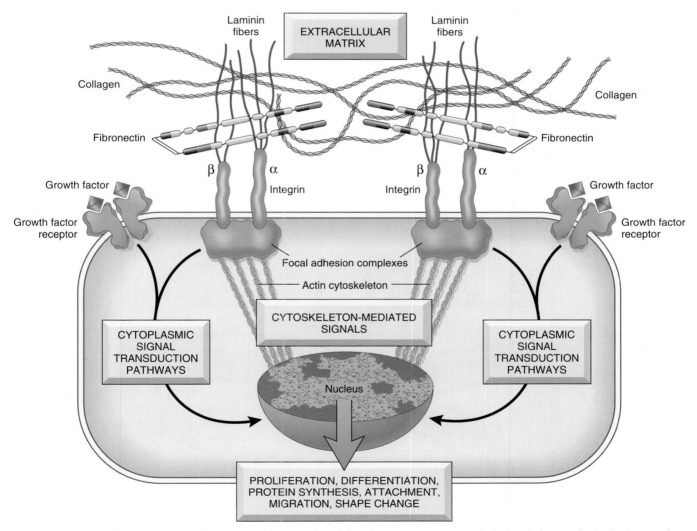

Fig. 1.13 Interactions of ECM and growth factor–mediated cell signaling. Cell surface integrins interact with the cytoskeleton at focal adhesion complexes (protein aggregates that include vinculin, α-actinin, and talin; see Fig. 1.16C). This can initiate the production of intracellular messengers or can directly transduce signals to the nucleus. Cell surface receptors for growth factors can activate signal transduction pathways that overlap with those mediated through integrins. Signals from ECM components and growth factors can be integrated by the cells to produce a given response, including changes in proliferation, locomotion, and/or differentiation.

for a variety of latent growth factors that can be activated within a focus of injury or inflammation.

- *Scaffolding for tissue renewal.* Because maintenance of normal tissue structure requires a basement membrane or stromal scaffold, the integrity of the basement membrane or the stroma of parenchymal cells is critical for the organized regeneration of tissues. Thus, ECM disruption results in defective tissue regeneration and repair, for example, cirrhosis of the liver resulting from the collapse of the hepatic stroma in various forms of hepatitis.
- *Establishment of tissue microenvironments.* The basement membrane acts as a boundary between the epithelium and underlying connective tissue; it does not just provide support to the epithelium but is also functional, for example, in the kidney, forming part of the filtration apparatus.

The ECM is constantly being remodeled; its synthesis and degradation accompany morphogenesis, tissue regeneration and repair, chronic fibrosis, and tumor invasion and metastasis. ECM occurs in two basic forms: interstitial matrix and basement membrane (Fig. 1.14

- *Interstitial matrix* is present in the spaces between cells in connective tissue, and between the parenchymal epithelium and the underlying supportive vascular and smooth muscle structures. The interstitial matrix is synthesized by mesenchymal cells (e.g., fibroblasts), forming an amorphous three-dimensional gel. Its major constituents are fibrillar and nonfibrillar collagens, as well as fibronectin, elastin, proteoglycans, hyaluronate, and other constituents (see later).
- *Basement membrane.* The seemingly random array of interstitial matrix in connective tissues becomes highly

organized around epithelial cells, endothelial cells, and smooth muscle cells, forming the specialized *basement membrane.* This is synthesized conjointly by the overlying epithelium and the underlying mesenchymal cells, forming a flat lamellar "chicken wire" mesh (although labeled as a *membrane*, it is quite porous). The major constituents are amorphous nonfibrillar type IV collagen and laminin.)

Components of the Extracellular Matrix

The components of the ECM fall into three groups of proteins (Fig. 1.15):

- *Fibrous structural proteins* such as collagens and elastins that confer tensile strength and recoil
- *Water-hydrated gels* such as proteoglycans and hyaluronan that permit compressive resistance and lubrication
- *Adhesive glycoproteins* that connect ECM elements to one another and to cells

Collagens. Collagens are composed of three separate polypeptide chains braided into a ropelike triple helix. About 30 collagen types have been identified, some of which are unique to specific cells and tissues.

- Some collagen types (e.g., types I, II, III, and V collagens) form linear fibrils stabilized by interchain hydrogen bonding; such *fibrillar collagens* form a major proportion of the connective tissue in structures such as bone, tendon, cartilage, blood vessels, and skin, as well as in healing wounds and scars. The tensile strength of the fibrillar collagens derives from lateral crosslinking of the triple helices by covalent bonds, an unusual

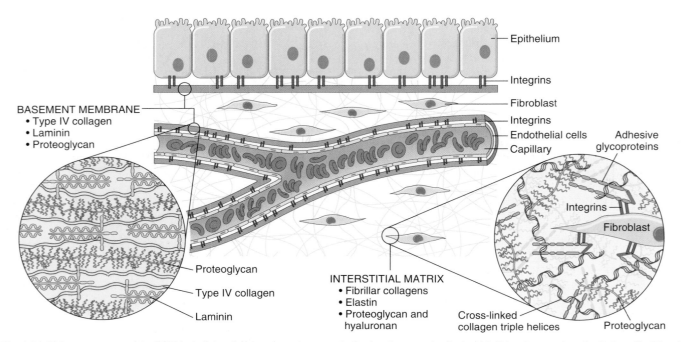

Fig. 1.14 Main components of the ECM, including collagens, proteoglycans, and adhesive glycoproteins. Both epithelial and mesenchymal cells (e.g., fibroblasts) interact with ECM via integrins. Basement membranes and the interstitial ECM have different architecture and general composition, although certain components are present in both. For the sake of clarity, many ECM components (e.g., elastin, fibrillin, hyaluronan, and syndecan) are not included.

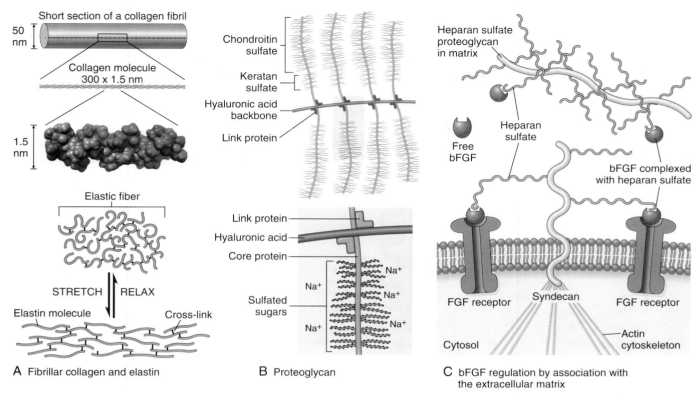

Fig. 1.15 ECM components. (A) Fibrillar collagen, and elastic tissue structures. Because of rodlike fibril stacking and extensive lateral crosslinking, collagen fibers have marked tensile strength but little elasticity. Elastin also is crosslinked but differs in having large hydrophobic segments that form a dense globular configuration at rest. As stretch is exerted, the hydrophobic domains are pulled open, but the crosslinks keep the molecules intact; release of the tension allows the hydrophobic domains of the proteins to refold. (B) Proteoglycan structure. The highly negatively charged sulfated sugars on the proteoglycan "bristles" attract sodium and water to generate a viscous compressible matrix. (C) Regulation of basic FGF (bFGF, FGF-2) activity by ECM and cellular proteoglycans. Heparan sulfate binds bFGF secreted in the ECM. Syndecan is a cell surface proteoglycan with a transmembrane core protein and extracellular glycosaminoglycan side chains that bind bFGF, and a cytoplasmic tail that interacts with the intracellular actin cytoskeleton. Syndecan side chains bind bFGF released from damaged ECM, thus facilitating bFGF interaction with cell surface receptors.

post-translational modification that requires hydroxylation of lysine residues in collagen by the enzyme lysyl oxidase. Because lysyl oxidase is a vitamin C–dependent enzyme, children with ascorbate deficiency have skeletal deformities, and people of any age with vitamin C deficiency heal poorly and bleed easily because of "weak" collagen. Genetic defects in collagens cause diseases such as *osteogenesis imperfecta* and certain forms of *Ehlers-Danlos syndrome* (Chapter 7).

• *Nonfibrillar* collagens variously contribute to the structures of planar basement membranes (type IV collagen); help regulate collagen fibril diameters or collagen-collagen interactions via so-called "**f**ibril-**a**ssociated **c**ollagen with **i**nterrupted **t**riple helices" (FACITs, such as type IX collagen in cartilage); and provide anchoring fibrils within basement membrane beneath stratified squamous epithelium (type VII collagen).

Elastin. The ability of tissues to recoil and recover their shape after physical deformation is conferred by elastin (Fig. 1.15). Elasticity is especially important in cardiac valves and large blood vessels, which must accommodate recurrent pulsatile flow, as well as in the uterus, skin, and ligaments. Morphologically, elastic fibers consist of a central core of elastin with an associated meshlike network composed of fibrillin. The latter relationship partially

explains why fibrillin defects lead to skeletal abnormalities and weakened aortic walls, as in individuals with Marfan syndrome. Fibrillin also controls the availability of TGF-β (Chapter 7).

Proteoglycans and hyaluronan (Fig. 1.15). Proteoglycans form highly hydrated gels that confer resistance to compressive forces; in joint cartilage, proteoglycans also provide a layer of lubrication between adjacent bony surfaces. Proteoglycans consist of long polysaccharides called glycosaminoglycans (examples are keratan sulfate and chondroitin sulfate) attached to a core protein; these are then linked to a long hyaluronic acid polymer called hyaluronan in a manner reminiscent of the bristles on a test-tube brush. The highly negatively charged, densely packed sulfated sugars attract cations (mostly sodium) and abundant water molecules, producing a viscous, gelatin-like matrix. Besides providing compressibility to tissues, proteoglycans also serve as reservoirs for secreted growth factors (e.g., FGF and HGF). Some proteoglycans are integral cell membrane proteins that have roles in cell proliferation, migration, and adhesion, for example, by binding and concentrating growth factors and chemokines (Fig. 1.15).

Adhesive glycoproteins and adhesion receptors. These are structurally diverse molecules variously involved in cell-cell, cell-ECM, and ECM-ECM interactions (Fig. 1.16). Prototypical adhesive glycoproteins include fibronectin (a

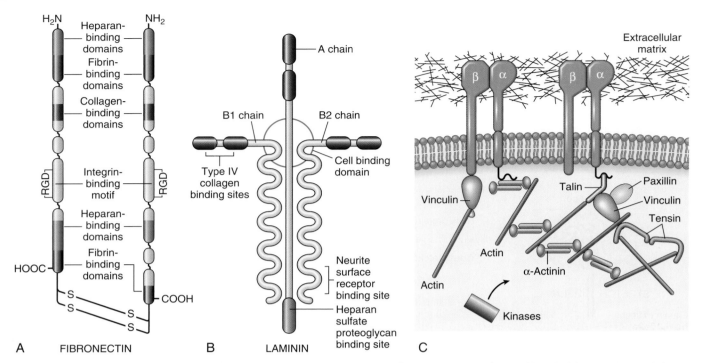

Fig. 1.16 Cell and ECM interactions: adhesive glycoproteins and integrin signaling. (A) *Fibronectin* consists of a disulfide-linked dimer, with several distinct domains that allow binding to ECM and integrins, the latter through arginine-glycine-aspartic acid (RGD) motifs. (B) The cross-shaped *laminin* molecule is one of the major components of basement membranes; its multidomain structure allows interactions between type IV collagen, other ECM components, and cell-surface receptors. (C) Integrins and integrin-mediated signaling events at focal adhesion complexes. Each α–β heterodimeric integrin receptor is a transmembrane dimer that links ECM and the intracellular cytoskeleton. It is also associated with a complex of linking molecules (e.g., vinculin and talin) that can recruit and activate kinases that ultimately trigger downstream signaling cascades.

major component of the interstitial ECM) and laminin (a major constituent of basement membrane). Integrins are representative of the adhesion receptors, also known as cell adhesion molecules (CAMs); the CAMs also include immunoglobulins family members, cadherins, and selectins.

- *Fibronectin* is a large (450 kD) disulfide-linked heterodimer that exists in tissue and plasma forms; it is synthesized by a variety of cells, including fibroblasts, monocytes, and endothelium. Fibronectin has specific domains that bind to distinct ECM components (e.g., collagen, fibrin, heparin, and proteoglycans), as well as integrins (Fig. 1.16). In healing wounds, tissue and plasma fibronectin provide a scaffold for subsequent ECM deposition, angiogenesis, and reepithelialization.
- *Laminin* is the most abundant glycoprotein in the basement membrane. It is an 820-kD cross-shaped heterotrimer that connects cells to underlying ECM components such as type IV collagen and heparan sulfate (Fig. 1.16). Besides mediating the attachment to the basement membrane, laminin can also modulate cell proliferation, differentiation, and motility.
- *Integrins* are a large family of transmembrane heterodimeric glycoproteins composed of α- and β-subunits that allow cells to attach to ECM constituents such as laminin and fibronectin, thus functionally and structurally linking the intracellular cytoskeleton with the outside world. Integrins also mediate cell-cell adhesive interactions. For instance, integrins on the surface of leukocytes are essential in mediating firm adhesion to and transmigration across the endothelium at sites of inflammation

(Chapter 3), and they play a critical role in platelet aggregation (Chapter 4). Integrins attach to ECM components via a tripeptide arginine-glycine-aspartic acid motif (abbreviated RGD). In addition to providing focal attachment to underlying substrates, binding through the integrin receptors can also trigger signaling cascades that influence cell locomotion, proliferation, shape, and differentiation (Fig. 1.16).

MAINTAINING CELL POPULATIONS

Proliferation and the Cell Cycle

Cell proliferation is fundamental to development, maintenance of steady-state tissue homeostasis, and replacement of dead or damaged cells. The key elements of cellular proliferation are accurate DNA replication accompanied by the coordinated synthesis of all other cellular constituents, followed by equal apportionment of DNA and other cellular constituents (e.g., organelles) to daughter cells through mitosis and cytokinesis.

The sequence of events that results in cell division is called the *cell cycle*. The cell cycle consists of G_1 (presynthetic growth), S (DNA synthesis), G_2 (premitotic growth), and M (mitotic) phases; quiescent cells that are not actively cycling are in the G_0 state. (Fig. 1.17). Cells can enter G_1 either from the G_0 quiescent cell pool or after completing a round of mitosis. Each stage requires completion of the previous step, as well as activation of

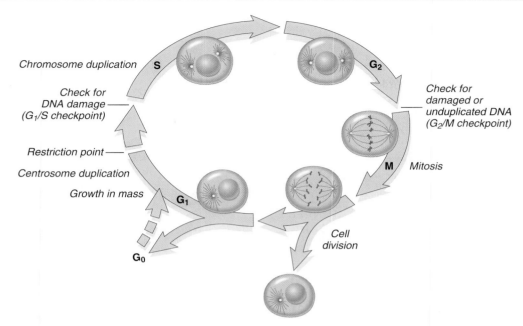

Fig. 1.17 Cell-cycle landmarks. The figure shows the cell-cycle phases (G_0, G_1, G_2, S, and M), the location of the G_1 restriction point, and the G_1/S and G_2/M cell-cycle checkpoints. G1 restriction point refers to the phase in G1 at which the cell gets committed to the cell cycle without further need of the growth factor that initiated cell division. Cells from labile tissues such as the epidermis and the gastrointestinal tract may cycle continuously; stable cells such as hepatocytes are quiescent but can enter the cell cycle; permanent cells such as neurons and cardiac myocytes have lost the capacity to proliferate. *(Modified from Pollard TD, Earnshaw WC: Cell biology, Philadelphia, 2002, Saunders.)*

necessary factors (see later); nonfidelity of DNA replication or cofactor deficiency results in arrest at the various transition points.

The cell cycle is regulated by numerous activators and inhibitors. Cell-cycle progression is driven by proteins called *cyclins*—named for the cyclic nature of their production and degradation—and cyclin-associated enzymes called *cyclin-dependent kinases* (CDKs) (Fig. 1.18). CDKs acquire the ability to phosphorylate protein substrates (i.e., kinase activity) by forming complexes with the relevant cyclins. Transiently increased synthesis of a particular cyclin leads to increased kinase activity of the appropriate CDK binding partner; as the CDK completes its round of phosphorylation, the associated cyclin is degraded and the CDK activity abates. Thus, as cyclin levels rise and fall, the activity of associated CDKs likewise waxes and wanes.

More than 15 cyclins have been identified; cyclins D, E, A, and B appear sequentially during the cell cycle and bind to one or more CDKs. The cell cycle thus resembles a relay race in which each leg is regulated by a distinct set of cyclins: as one collection of cyclins leaves the track, the next set takes over.

Embedded in the cell cycle are surveillance mechanisms primed to sense DNA or chromosomal damage. These quality-control *checkpoints* ensure that cells with genetic imperfections do not complete replication. Thus, the G_1-S checkpoint monitors the integrity of DNA before irreversibly committing cellular resources to DNA replication. Later in the cell cycle, the G_2-M check point ensures that there has been accurate DNA replication before the cell actually divides. When cells do detect DNA irregularities, checkpoint activation delays cell-cycle progression and triggers DNA repair mechanisms. If the genetic derangement is too severe to be repaired, the cells either undergo

apoptosis or enter a nonreplicative state called *senescence*—primarily through p53-dependent mechanisms (see later).

Enforcing the cell-cycle checkpoints is the job of *CDK inhibitors (CDKIs)*; they accomplish this by modulating CDK-cyclin complex activity. There are several different CDKIs:

- One family of CDKIs—composed of three proteins called *p21* (CDKN1A), *p27* (CDKN1B), and *p57* (CDKN1C)—broadly inhibits multiple CDKs
- Another family of CDKIs has selective effects on cyclin CDK4 and cyclin CDK6; these proteins are called *p15* (CDKN2B), *p16* (CDKN2A), *p18* (CDKN2C), and *p19* (CDKN2D)
- Defective CDKI checkpoint proteins allow cells with damaged DNA to divide, resulting in mutated daughter cells at risk for malignant transformation

An equally important aspect of cell growth and division is the biosynthesis of other cellular components needed to make two daughter cells, such as membranes and organelles. Thus when growth factor receptor signaling stimulates cell-cycle progression, it also activates events that promote changes in cellular metabolism that support growth. Chief among these is the Warburg effect, mentioned earlier, marked by increased cellular uptake of glucose and glutamine, increased glycolysis, and (counterintuitively) decreased oxidative phosphorylation. These changes are major elements of cancer-cell growth and are discussed in greater detail in Chapter 6.

Stem Cells

Not all stem cells are created equal. During development, *totipotent stem cells* can give rise to *all* types of

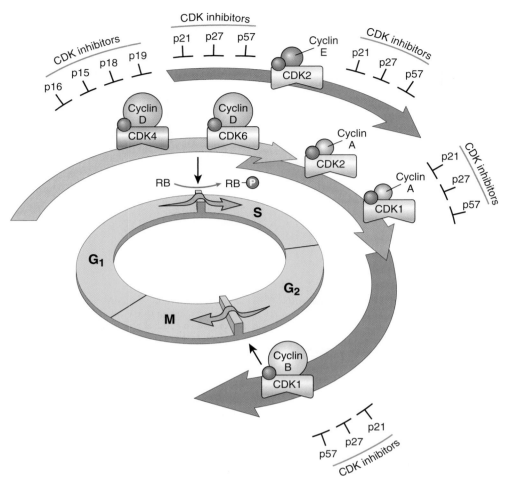

Fig. 1.18 Role of cyclins, CDKs, and CDK inhibitors in regulating the cell cycle. *Shaded arrows* represent the phases of the cell cycle during which specific cyclin-CDK complexes are active. As illustrated, cyclin D-CDK4, cyclin D-CDK6, and cyclin E-CDK2 regulate the G_1-to-S transition by phosphorylating the Rb protein (pRb). Cyclin A-CDK2 and cyclin A-CDK1 are active in the S phase. Cyclin B-CDK1 is essential for the G_2-to-M transition. Two families of CDK inhibitors can block activity of CDKs and progression through the cell cycle. The so-called "INK4 inhibitors," composed of p16, p15, p18, and p19, act on cyclin D-CDK4 and cyclin D-CDK6. The other family of three inhibitors, p21, p27, and p57, can inhibit all CDKs.

differentiated tissues; in the mature organism, *adult stem cells* in various tissues only have the capacity to replace damaged cells and maintain cell populations within the tissues where they reside. There also are populations of stem cells between these extremes with varying capacities to differentiate into multiple cell lineages. Thus, depending on the source and stage of development, there may be limits on the cell types that a stem cell population can generate.

In normal tissues (without neoplasia, degeneration, or healing), there is a homeostatic equilibrium between the replication, self-renewal, and differentiation of stem cells and the death of the mature, fully differentiated cells (Fig. 1.19). The dynamic relationship between stem cells and terminally differentiated parenchyma is nicely exemplified by the continuously dividing epithelium of the skin. Thus, stem cells at the basal layer of the epithelium progressively differentiate as they migrate to the upper layers of the epithelium before dying and being shed.

Under conditions of homeostasis, stem cells are characterized by two important properties:
• *Self-renewal*, which permits stem cells to maintain their numbers. Self-renewal may follow asymmetric or symmetric division.
• *Asymmetric division* refers to cell replication in which one daughter cell enters a differentiation pathway and gives rise to mature cells, whereas the other remains undifferentiated and retains its self-renewal capacity. By contrast, in symmetric division, both daughter cells retain self renewal capacity. Such divisions are seen early in embryogenesis (when stem cell populations are expanding) and under conditions of stress, such as in the bone marrow following chemotherapy.

Although there is a tendency in the scientific literature to partition stem cells into several different subsets, fundamentally there are only two varieties:
• *Embryonic stem cells (ES cells)* are the most undifferentiated. They are present in the inner cell mass of the

blastocyst, have virtually limitless cell renewal capacity, and can give rise to every cell in the body; they are thus said to be *totipotent* (Fig. 1.20). ES cells can be maintained for extended periods without differentiating; thereafter, appropriate culture conditions allow them to form specialized cells of all three germ cell layers,

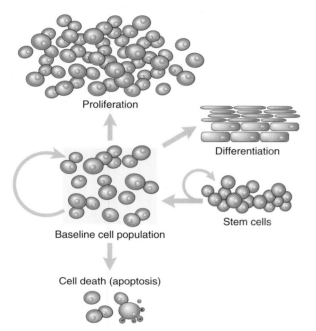

Fig. 1.19 Mechanisms regulating cell populations. Cell numbers can be altered by increased or decreased rates of stem cell input, cell death resulting from apoptosis, or changes in the rates of proliferation or differentiation. *(Modified from McCarthy NJ, et al: Apoptosis in the development of the immune system: growth factors, clonal selection and bcl-2, Cancer Metastasis Rev 11:157, 1992.)*

including neurons, cardiac muscle, liver cells, and pancreatic islet cells.

- *Tissue stem cells* (also called *adult stem cells*) are found in intimate association with the differentiated cells of a given tissue. They are normally protected within specialized tissue microenvironments called *stem cell niches*. Such niches have been demonstrated in many organs, most notably the bone marrow, where hematopoietic stem cells congregate in a perivascular niche. Other niches for stem cells include the bulge region of hair follicles; the limbus of the cornea; the crypts of the gut; the canals of Hering in the liver; and the subventricular zone in the brain. Soluble factors and other cells within the niches keep the stem cells quiescent until there is a need for expansion and differentiation of the precursor pool (Fig. 1.21).

Adult stem cells have a limited repertoire of differentiated cells that they can generate. Thus, although adult stem cells can maintain tissues with high (e.g., skin and gastrointestinal tract) or low (e.g., endothelium) cell turnover, the adult stem cells in any given tissue can usually only produce cells that are normal constituents of that tissue.

Hematopoietic stem cells are the most extensively studied; they continuously replenish all the cellular elements of the blood as they are consumed. They can be isolated directly from bone marrow, as well as from the peripheral blood after administration of certain colony stimulating factors (CSF) that induce their release from bone marrow niches. Although rare, hematopoietic stem cells can be purified to virtual homogeneity based on cell surface markers. Clinically, these stem cells can be used to repopulate marrows depleted after chemotherapy (e.g., for leukemia), or to provide normal precursors to correct various blood cell defects (e.g., sickle cell disease; see Chapter 12).

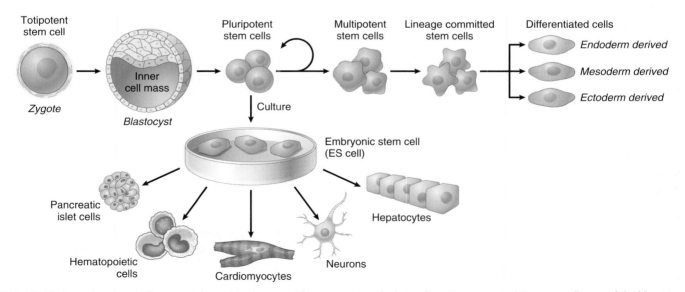

Fig. 1.20 Embryonal stem cells. The zygote, formed by the union of sperm and egg, divides to form blastocysts, and the inner cell mass of the blastocyst generates the embryo. The pluripotent cells of the inner cell mass, known as embryonic stem (ES) cells, can be induced to differentiate into cells of multiple lineages. In the embryo, pluripotent stem cells can asymmetrically divide to yield a residual stable pool of ES cells in addition to generating populations that have progressively more restricted developmental capacity, eventually generating stem cells that are committed to just specific lineages. ES cells can be cultured in vitro and induced to give rise to cells of all three germ layers.

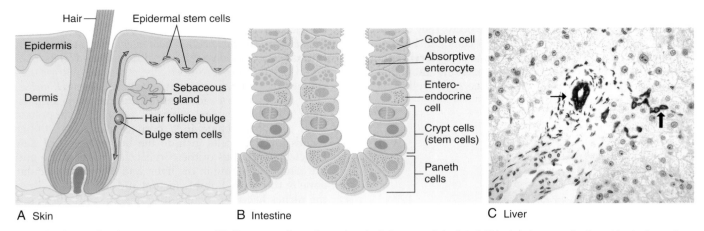

A Skin   B Intestine   C Liver

Fig. 1.21 Stem cell niches in various tissues. (A) Skin stem cells are located in the bulge area of the hair follicle, in sebaceous glands, and in the lower layer of the epidermis. (B) Small intestine stem cells are located near the base of the crypt, above Paneth cells. (C) Liver stem cells *(oval cells)* are located in the canals of Hering *(thick arrow)*, structures that connect bile ductules *(thin arrow)* to parenchymal hepatocytes. Bile duct cells and canals of Hering are stained here with an immunohistochemical stain for cytokeratin 7. *(C, Courtesy Tania Roskams, MD, University of Leuven, Belgium.)*

Besides hematopoietic stem cells, the bone marrow (and notably, other tissues such as fat) also contains a population of *mesenchymal stem cells*. These are multipotent cells that can differentiate into a variety of stromal cells including chondrocytes (cartilage), osteocytes (bone), adipocytes (fat), and myocytes (muscle). Because these cells can be expanded to large numbers, they represent a potential means of manufacturing the stromal scaffolding needed for tissue regeneration.

Regenerative Medicine

The ability to identify, isolate, expand, and transplant stem cells has given birth to the new field of regenerative medicine. Theoretically, the differentiated progeny of ES or adult stem cells can be used to repopulate damaged tissues or to construct entire organs for replacement. In particular, there is considerable excitement about the therapeutic opportunities for restoring damaged tissues that have low intrinsic regenerative capacity, such as myocardium after a myocardial infarct or neurons after a stroke. Unfortunately, despite an improving ability to purify and expand stem cell populations, much of the initial enthusiasm has been tempered by difficulties encountered in introducing and functionally integrating the replacement cells into sites of damage.

More recently it has been possible to generate pluripotential cells, resembling ES cells, that are derived from the patient into whom they will be implanted. To accomplish this, a handful of genes have been identified whose products can—remarkably—reprogram somatic cells to achieve the "stem-ness" of ES cells. When such genes are introduced into fully differentiated cells (e.g., fibroblasts), *induced pluripotent stem cells (iPS cells)* are generated (Fig. 1.22), albeit at low frequency. Because these cells are derived from the patient, their differentiated progeny (e.g., insulin-secreting β-cells in a patient with diabetes) can be engrafted without eliciting an immunologically mediated rejection reaction that would occur if the differentiated cells were derived from ES cells obtained from another donor.

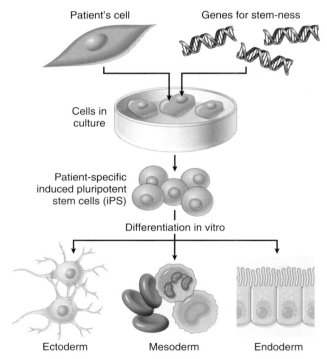

Fig. 1.22 The production of induced pluripotent stem cells (iPS cells). Genes that confer stem cell properties are introduced into a patient's differentiated cells, giving rise to stem cells that can be induced to differentiate into various lineages. *(Modified from Hochedlinger K, Jaenisch R: Nuclear transplantation, embryonic stem cells, and the potential for cell therapy,* N Engl J Med *349:275–286, 2003.)*

Concluding Remarks

This survey of selected topics in cell biology serves as a basis for our later discussions of pathology, and we will refer back to it throughout the book. Students should, however, remember that this summary is intentionally brief, and more information about some of the fascinating topics reviewed here can be readily found in textbooks devoted to cell and molecular biology.

SUGGESTED READINGS

Genetics and Epigenetics

Batista PJ, Chang HY: Long noncoding RNAs: cellular address codes in development and disease, *Cell* 152:1298, 2013. *[Good review regarding lncRNA biology.]*

Cech TR, Steitz JA: The noncoding RNA revolution trashing old rules to forge new ones, *Cell* 157:77, 2014. *[An excellent review of the roles played by noncoding RNAs.]*

Hübner MR, Eckersley-Maslin MA, Spector DL: Chromatin organization and transcriptional regulation, *Curr Opin Genet Dev* 23:89, 2013. *[A nice discussion of genome organization and chromatin structure–function relationships that regulate cell type–specific nuclear transcription.]*

Jarovcevski M, Akbarian S: Epigenetic mechanisms in neurologic disease, *Nat Med* 18:1194, 2012. *[A well-written overview of genomic organization and transcriptional regulation, with a specific focus on neurologic disease.]*

Meller VH, Joshi SS, Deshpande N: Modulation of chromatin by noncoding RNA, *Annu Rev Genet* 49:673, 2015. *[An excellent overview of the roles played by noncoding RNAs in nuclear organization.]*

Minarovits J, Banati F, Szenthe K, et al: Epigenetic regulation, *Adv Exp Med Biol* 879:1, 2016. *[A brief primer on the pathways that regulate chromatin structure and accessibility.]*

Rowley MJ, Corces VG: The three-dimensional genome: principles and roles of long-distance interactions, *Curr Opin Cell Biol* 40:8, 2016. *[An interesting discussion regarding the mechanisms by which three-dimensional conformations can influence nuclear transcription.]*

Teperino R, Lempradl A, Pospisilik JA: Bridging epigenomics and complex disease: the basics, *Cell Mol Life Sci* 70:1609, 2013. *[An introductory review of the epigenetic basis for human disease.]*

Cellular Housekeeping

Andersson ER: The role of endocytosis in activating and regulating signal transduction, *Cell Mol Life Sci* 69:1755, 2011. *[Overview of endocytosis with specific emphasis on its role in modulating intracellular signaling.]*

Choi AM, Ryter SW, Levine B: Autophagy in human health and disease, *N Engl J Med* 368:651, 2013. *[A superb review concerning the physiologic and pathophysiologic aspects of autophagy.]*

English AR, Zurek N, Voeltz GK: Peripheral ER structure and function, *Curr Opin Cell Biol* 21:596, 2009. *[An overview of the structural and functional organization of the endoplasmic reticulum and its relationship to other cellular organelles.]*

Guillot C, Lecuit T: Mechanics of epithelial tissue homeostasis and morphogenesis, *Science* 340:1185, 2013. *[A topical discussion about cellular interactions and the mechanical basis of tissue maintenance.]*

Hetz C, Chevet E, Oakes SA: Proteostasis control by the unfolded protein response, *Nat Cell Biol* 17:829, 2015. *[Mechanisms underlying endoplasmic reticulum editing and cellular homeostasis.]*

Kaur J, Debnath J: Autophagy at the crossroads of catabolism and anabolism, *Nat Rev Mol Cell Biol* 16:461, 2015. *[An excellent review of the mechanisms and consequences of cellular autophagy.]*

Simons K, Sampaio JL: Membrane organization and lipid rafts, *Cold Spring Harb Perspect Biol* 3:1, 2013. *[A nice review of the general principles of membrane architecture and emphasizing domain organization.]*

Wong E, Cuervo AM: Integration of clearance mechanisms: the proteasome and autophagy, *Cold Spring Harb Perspect Biol* 2:1, 2010. *[An overview of intracellular degradation pathways, specifically focusing on the elimination of aberrant or abnormal constituents.]*

Cellular Metabolism and Mitochondrial Function

Andersen JL, Kornbluth S: The tangled circuitry of metabolism and apoptosis, *Mol Cell* 49:399, 2013. *[A solid review of the interplay between cell metabolism, cell proliferation, and cell death.]*

Dang CV: Links between metabolism and cancer, *Genes Dev* 26:877, 2012. *[An excellent review on metabolic functions of mitochondria.]*

Friedman JR, Nunnari J: Mitochondrial form and function, *Nature* 505:335, 2014. *[A good overview of mitochondrial replication, and response to cellular injury.]*

Tait SW, Green DR: Mitochondria and cell death: outer membrane permeabilization and beyond, *Nat Rev Mol Cell Biol* 11:621, 2010. *[A review of the role of mitochondria in cell death pathways.]*

Cellular Activation

Duronio RJ, Xiong Y: Signaling pathways that control cell proliferation, *Cold Spring Harb Perspect Biol* 5:1, 2013. *[An excellent overall review of cell signaling and proliferation.]*

Morrison DK: MAP kinase pathways, *Cold Spring Harb Perspect Biol* 4:1, 2012. *[A review of mitogen-activated kinase signaling pathways.]*

Perona R: Cell signalling: growth factors and tyrosine kinase receptors, *Clin Transl Oncol* 8:77, 2011. *[An overview of signaling pathways with an emphasis on how these become dysregulated in malignancy.]*

Maintaining Cell Populations

Alvarado AS, Yamanaka S: Rethinking differentiation: stem cells, regeneration, and plasticity, *Cell* 157:110, 2014.

Fuchs E, Chen T: A matter of life and death: self-renewal in stem cells, *EMBO Rep* 14:39, 2013. *[A scholarly review on the conceptual framework and experimental underpinnings of our understanding regarding stem cell renewal, using cutaneous stem cells as a paradigm.]*

Li M, Liu GH, Izpisua-Belmonte JC: Navigating the epigenetic landscape of pluripotent stem cells, *Nat Rev Mol Cell Biol* 13:524, 2012. *[A good discussion of the epigenetic regulation of stem cell proliferation and subsequent differentiation.]*

Martello G, Smith A: The nature of embryonic stem cells, *Annu Rev Cell Dev Biol* 30:647, 2014. *[A good, comprehensive overview of cell plasticity and stemness.]*

Cell Injury, Cell Death, and Adaptations

2

CHAPTER OUTLINE

Introduction to Pathology 31
Overview of Cellular Responses
  to Stress and Noxious
  Stimuli 31
Causes of Cell Injury 32
Sequence of Events in Cell Injury
  and Cell Death 33
Reversible Cell Injury 33
Cell Death 34
Necrosis 35
Apoptosis 37

Other Pathways of Cell Death 40
Autophagy 40
Mechanisms of Cell Injury and Cell
  Death 41
Hypoxia and Ischemia 42
Ischemia-Reperfusion Injury 43
Oxidative Stress 43
Cell Injury Caused by Toxins 45
Endoplasmic Reticulum Stress 45
DNA Damage 47
Inflammation 47

Common Events in Cell Injury From Diverse
  Causes 47
Cellular Adaptations to Stress 48
Hypertrophy 48
Hyperplasia 49
Atrophy 50
Metaplasia 50
Intracellular Accumulations 51
Pathologic Calcification 53
Cellular Aging 54

INTRODUCTION TO PATHOLOGY

The field of pathology is devoted to understanding the causes of disease and the changes in cells, tissues, and organs that are associated with disease and give rise to the presenting signs and symptoms in patients. There are two important terms that students will encounter throughout their study of pathology and medicine:

- *Etiology* refers to the underlying causes and modifying factors that are responsible for the initiation and progression of disease. It is now clear that many common diseases, such as hypertension, diabetes, and cancer, are caused by a combination of inherited genetic susceptibility and various environmental triggers. Elucidating the genetic and environmental factors underlying diseases is a major theme of modern medicine.
- *Pathogenesis* refers to the mechanisms of development and progression of disease, which account for the cellular and molecular changes that give rise to the specific functional and structural abnormalities that characterize any particular disease. Thus, etiology refers to why a disease arises and pathogenesis describes how a disease develops (Fig. 2.1).

Defining the etiology and pathogenesis of disease not only is essential for understanding disease but also is the basis for developing rational treatments and effective preventive measures. Thus, pathology provides the scientific foundation for the practice of medicine.

To render diagnoses and guide therapy in clinical practice, pathologists identify changes in the gross or microscopic appearance (morphology) of cells and tissues, and biochemical alterations in body fluids (such as blood and urine). Pathologists also use a variety of morphologic, molecular, and other techniques to define the biochemical, structural, and functional changes that occur in cells, tissues, and organs in response to injury. We begin, in this chapter, with a discussion of cellular abnormalities induced by a variety of internal (e.g., genetic) and external (e.g., environmental) abnormalities and stresses.

OVERVIEW OF CELLULAR RESPONSES TO STRESS AND NOXIOUS STIMULI

Cells actively interact with their environment, constantly adjusting their structure and function to accommodate changing demands and extracellular stresses. The intracellular milieu of cells is normally tightly regulated such that it remains fairly constant, a state referred to as homeostasis. As cells encounter physiologic stresses (such as increased workload in the heart) or potentially injurious conditions (such as nutrient deprivation), they can undergo *adaptation*, achieving a new steady state and preserving viability and function. If the adaptive capability is exceeded or if the external stress is inherently harmful or excessive, *cell injury* develops (Fig. 2.2). Within certain limits, injury is *reversible*, and cells return to their stable baseline; however, if the stress is severe, persistent, or rapid in onset, it results in *irreversible injury* and death of the affected cells. *Cell death* is one of the most crucial events in the evolution

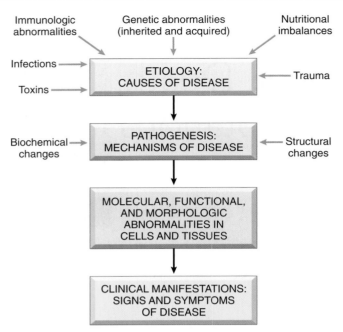

Fig. 2.1 Steps in the evolution of disease. Only selected major causes (etiologies) are shown.

of disease in any tissue or organ. It results from diverse causes, including ischemia (lack of blood flow), infections, toxins, and immune reactions. Cell death also is a normal and essential process in embryogenesis, the development of organs, and the maintenance of tissue homeostasis.

Because damage to cells is the basis of all disease, in this chapter we discuss first the causes, mechanisms, and consequences of the various forms of acute cell injury, including reversible injury and cell death. We then consider cellular adaptations to stress and conclude with two other processes that affect cells and tissues: the deposition of abnormal substances and cell aging.

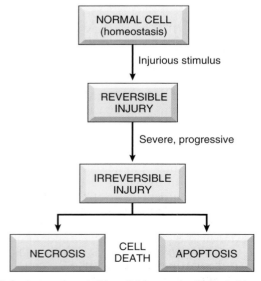

Fig. 2.2 Sequence of reversible cell injury and cell death. Necrosis and apoptosis are the two major pathways of cell death and are discussed in detail later.

CAUSES OF CELL INJURY

The causes of cell injury span a range from gross physical trauma, such as after a motor vehicle accident, to a single gene defect that results in a nonfunctional enzyme in a specific metabolic disease. Most injurious stimuli can be grouped into the following categories.

Hypoxia and ischemia. Hypoxia, which refers to oxygen deficiency, and ischemia, which means reduced blood supply, are among the most common causes of cell injury. Both deprive tissues of oxygen, and ischemia, in addition, results in a deficiency of essential nutrients and a build up of toxic metabolites. The most common cause of hypoxia is ischemia resulting from an arterial obstruction, but oxygen deficiency also can result from inadequate oxygenation of the blood, as in a variety of diseases affecting the lung, or from reduction in the oxygen-carrying capacity of the blood, as with anemia of any cause, and carbon monoxide (CO) poisoning.

Toxins. Potentially toxic agents are encountered daily in the environment; these include air pollutants, insecticides, CO, asbestos, cigarette smoke, ethanol, and drugs. Many drugs in therapeutic doses can cause cell or tissue injury in a susceptible patient or in many individuals if used excessively or inappropriately (Chapter 7). Even innocuous substances, such as glucose, salt, water and oxygen, can be toxic.

Infectious agents. All types of disease-causing pathogens, including viruses, bacteria, fungi, and protozoans, injure cells. The mechanisms of cell injury caused by these diverse agents are discussed in Chapter 9.

Immunologic reactions. Although the immune system defends the body against pathogenic microbes, immune reactions also can result in cell and tissue injury. Examples are autoimmune reactions against one's own tissues, allergic reactions against environmental substances, and excessive or chronic immune responses to microbes (Chapter 5). In all of these situations, immune responses elicit inflammatory reactions, which are often the cause of damage to cells and tissues.

Genetic abnormalities. Genetic aberrations can result in pathologic changes as conspicuous as the congenital malformations associated with Down syndrome or as subtle as the single amino acid substitution in hemoglobin giving rise to sickle cell anemia (Chapter 7). Genetic defects may cause cell injury as a consequence of deficiency of functional proteins, such as enzymes in inborn errors of metabolism, or accumulation of damaged DNA or misfolded proteins, both of which trigger cell death when they are beyond repair.

Nutritional imbalances. Protein–calorie insufficiency among impoverished populations remains a major cause of cell injury, and specific vitamin deficiencies are not uncommon even in developed countries with high standards of living (Chapter 8). Ironically, excessive dietary intake may result in obesity and also is an important underlying factor in many diseases, such as type 2 diabetes mellitus and atherosclerosis.

Physical agents. Trauma, extremes of temperature, radiation, electric shock, and sudden changes in atmospheric pressure all have wide-ranging effects on cells (Chapter 8).

Aging. Cellular senescence results in a diminished ability of cells to respond to stress and, eventually, the death of cells and of the organism. The mechanisms underlying cellular aging are discussed at the end of this chapter.

With this introduction, we proceed to a discussion of the progression and morphologic manifestations of cell injury, and then to the biochemical mechanisms in injury caused by different noxious stimuli.

SEQUENCE OF EVENTS IN CELL INJURY AND CELL DEATH

Although various injurious stimuli damage cells through diverse biochemical mechanisms, all tend to induce a stereotypic sequence of morphologic and structural alterations in most types of cells.

Reversible Cell Injury

Reversible injury is the stage of cell injury at which the deranged function and morphology of the injured cells can return to normal if the damaging stimulus is removed (Fig. 2.3). In reversible injury, cells and intracellular organelles typically become swollen because they take in water as a result of the failure of energy-dependent ion pumps in the plasma membrane, leading to an inability to maintain ionic and fluid homeostasis. In some forms of injury, degenerated organelles and lipids may accumulate inside the injured cells.

> ## MORPHOLOGY
>
> The two main morphologic correlates of reversible cell injury are cellular swelling and fatty change.
> - **Cellular swelling** (Fig. 2.4B) is commonly seen in cell injury associated with increased permeability of the plasma membrane. It may be difficult to appreciate with the light microscope, but it is often apparent at the level of the whole organ. When it affects many cells in an organ, it causes pallor (as a result of compression of capillaries), increased turgor, and an increase in organ weight. Microscopic examination may show small, clear vacuoles within the cytoplasm; these represent distended and pinched-off segments of the endoplasmic reticulum (ER). This pattern of nonlethal injury is sometimes called hydropic change or vacuolar degeneration.
> - **Fatty change** is manifested by the appearance of triglyceride containing lipid vacuoles in the cytoplasm. It is principally encountered in organs that are involved in lipid metabolism, such as the liver, and hence it is discussed in Chapter 16.
>
> The cytoplasm of injured cells also may become redder (eosinophilic), a change that becomes much more pronounced with progression to necrosis (described later). Other intracellular changes associated with cell injury (Fig. 2.3) include (1) plasma membrane alterations such as blebbing, blunting, or distortion of microvilli, and loosening of intercellular attachments; (2) mitochondrial changes such as swelling and the appearance of phospholipid-rich amorphous densities; (3) dilation of the ER

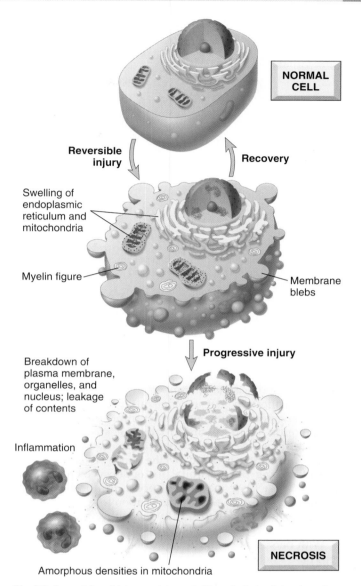

Fig. 2.3 Reversible cell injury and necrosis. The principal cellular alterations that characterize reversible cell injury and necrosis are illustrated. By convention, reversible injury is considered to culminate in necrosis if the injurious stimulus is not removed.

> with detachment of ribosomes and dissociation of polysomes; and (4) nuclear alterations, such as clumping of chromatin. The cytoplasm may contain so-called "myelin figures," which are collections of phospholipids resembling myelin sheaths that are derived from damaged cellular membranes.

In some situations, potentially injurious insults induce specific alterations in cellular organelles, such as the ER. The smooth ER is involved in the metabolism of various chemicals, and cells exposed to these chemicals show hypertrophy of the ER as an adaptive response that may have important functional consequences. For instance, many drugs, including barbiturates, which were commonly used as sedatives in the past and are still used as a treatment for some forms of epilepsy, are metabolized in the liver by the cytochrome P-450 mixed-function oxidase system found in the smooth ER. Protracted use of

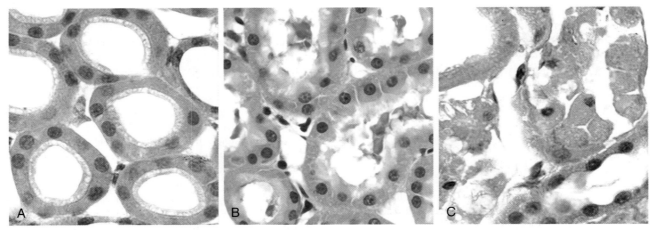

Fig. 2.4 Morphologic changes in reversible and irreversible cell injury (necrosis). (A) Normal kidney tubules with viable epithelial cells. (B) Early (reversible) ischemic injury showing surface blebs, increased eosinophilia of cytoplasm, and swelling of occasional cells. (C) Necrotic (irreversible) injury of epithelial cells, with loss of nuclei and fragmentation of cells and leakage of contents. *(Courtesy of Drs. Neal Pinckard and M.A. Venkatachalam, University of Texas Health Sciences Center, San Antonio, Texas.)*

barbiturates leads to a state of tolerance, marked by the need to use increasing doses of the drug to achieve the same effect. This adaptation stems from hypertrophy (an increase in volume) of the smooth ER of hepatocytes and a consequent increase in P-450 enzymatic activity. P-450–mediated modification of compounds sometimes leads to their detoxification, but in other instances converts them into a dangerous toxin; one such example involves carbon tetrachloride (CCl_4), discussed later. Cells adapted to one drug demonstrate an increased capacity to metabolize other compounds handled by the same system. Thus, if patients taking phenobarbital for epilepsy increase their alcohol intake, they may experience a drop in blood concentration of the anti-seizure medication to subtherapeutic levels because of smooth ER hypertrophy in response to the alcohol.

With persistent or excessive noxious exposures, injured cells pass a nebulous "point of no return" and undergo cell death. The clinical relevance of defining this transition point is obvious—if the biochemical and molecular changes that predict cell death can be identified, it may be possible to devise strategies for preventing the transition from reversible to irreversible cell injury. Although there are no definitive morphologic or biochemical correlates of irreversibility, it is consistently characterized by three phenomena: the *inability to restore mitochondrial function* (oxidative phosphorylation and adenosine triphosphate [ATP] generation) even after resolution of the original injury; the *loss of structure and functions of the plasma membrane and intracellular membranes*; and the *loss of DNA and chromatin structural integrity*. As discussed in more detail later, injury to lysosomal membranes results in the enzymatic dissolution of the injured cell, which is the culmination of necrosis.

Cell Death

When cells are injured they die by different mechanisms, depending on the nature and severity of the insult.
- Severe disturbances, such as loss of oxygen and nutrient supply and the actions of toxins, cause a rapid and

uncontrollable form of death that has been called "accidental" cell death. The morphological manifestation of accidental cell death is **necrosis** (Greek, *necros* = death) (Table 2.1). Necrosis is the major pathway of cell death in many commonly encountered injuries, such as those resulting from ischemia, exposure to toxins, various infections, and trauma. Necrosis is traditionally considered the inevitable end result of severe damage that is beyond salvage and is not thought to be regulated by specific signals or biochemical mechanisms; in other words, necrosis happens accidentally because the injury is too severe to be repaired and many cellular constituents simply fail or fall apart.
- In contrast, when the injury is less severe, or cells need to be eliminated during normal processes, they activate a precise set of molecular pathways that culminate in death. Because this kind of cell death can be manipulated

Table 2.1 Features of Necrosis and Apoptosis

Feature	Necrosis	Apoptosis
Cell size	Enlarged (swelling)	Reduced (shrinkage)
Nucleus	Pyknosis → karyorrhexis → karyolysis	Fragmentation into nucleosome-sized fragments
Plasma membrane	Disrupted	Intact; altered structure, especially orientation of lipids
Cellular contents	Enzymatic digestion; may leak out of cell	Intact; may be released in apoptotic bodies
Adjacent inflammation	Frequent	No
Physiologic or pathologic role	Invariably pathologic (culmination of irreversible cell injury)	Often physiologic means of eliminating unwanted cells; may be pathologic after some forms of cell injury, especially DNA and protein damage

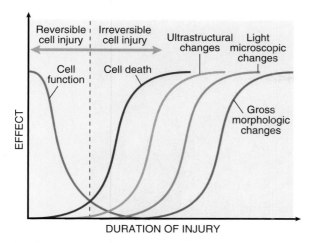

Reversible | Irreversible
cell injury | cell injury

Cell death

Ultrastructural changes

Light microscopic changes

Cell function

EFFECT

Gross morphologic changes

DURATION OF INJURY

Fig. 2.5 The relationship among cellular function, cell death, and the morphologic changes of cell injury. Note that cells may rapidly become nonfunctional after the onset of injury, although they are still viable, with potentially reversible damage; with a longer duration of injury, irreversible injury and cell death may result. Note also that cell death typically precedes ultrastructural, light microscopic, and grossly visible morphologic changes.

by therapeutic agents or genetic mutations, it is said to be "regulated" cell death. The morphologic appearance of most types of regulated cell death is **apoptosis** (see Table 2.1). In some instances, regulated cell death shows features of both necrosis and apoptosis, and has been called *necroptosis*. The discovery of these previously unrecognized forms of cell death that were regulated by identifiable genes and signaling pathways showed that cell death can be a controlled process. The idea of regulated cell death also raises the possibility that specific molecular pathways can be targeted therapeutically to prevent the loss of cells in pathologic conditions. Apoptosis is a process that eliminates cells with a variety of intrinsic abnormalities and promotes clearance of the fragments of the dead cells without eliciting an inflammatory reaction. This "clean" form of cell suicide occurs in pathologic situations when a cell's DNA or proteins are damaged beyond repair or the cell is deprived of necessary survival signals. **But unlike necrosis, which is always an indication of a pathologic process, apoptosis also occurs in healthy tissues.** It serves to eliminate unwanted cells during normal development and to maintain constant cell numbers, so it is not necessarily associated with pathologic cell injury. These types of physiologic cell death are also called *programmed cell death*.

It is important to point out that **cellular function may be lost long before cell death occurs, and that the morphologic changes of cell injury (or death) lag far behind loss of function and viability** (Fig. 2.5). For example, myocardial cells become noncontractile after 1 to 2 minutes of ischemia, but may not die until 20 to 30 minutes of ischemia have elapsed. Morphologic features indicative of the death of ischemic myocytes appear by electron microscopy within 2 to 3 hours after the death of the cells, but are not evident by light microscopy until 6 to 12 hours later.

Necrosis

Necrosis is a form of cell death in which cellular membranes fall apart, and cellular enzymes leak out and ultimately digest the cell (Fig. 2.3). Necrosis elicits a local host reaction, called *inflammation*, that is induced by substances released from dead cells and which serves to eliminate the debris and start the subsequent repair process (Chapter 3). The enzymes responsible for digestion of the cell are derived from lysosomes and may come from the dying cells themselves or from leukocytes recruited as part of the inflammatory reaction. Necrosis often is the culmination of reversible cell injury that cannot be corrected.

The biochemical mechanisms of necrosis vary with different injurious stimuli. These mechanisms include: failure of energy generation in the form of ATP because of reduced oxygen supply or mitochondrial damage; damage to cellular membranes, including the plasma membrane and lysosomal membranes, which results in leakage of cellular contents including enzymes; irreversible damage to cellular lipids, proteins, and nucleic acids, which may be caused by reactive oxygen species (ROS); and others. These biochemical mechanisms are discussed later when we consider the individual causes of cell necrosis.

MORPHOLOGY

Necrosis is characterized by changes in the cytoplasm and nuclei of the injured cells (Figs. 2.3 and 2.4C).

- **Cytoplasmic changes.** Necrotic cells show increased eosinophilia (i.e., they are stained red by the dye eosin—the E in the hematoxylin and eosin [H&E] stain), attributable partly to increased binding of eosin to denatured cytoplasmic proteins and partly to loss of basophilic ribonucleic acid (RNA) in the cytoplasm (basophilia stems from binding of the blue dye hematoxylin—the H in "H&E"). Compared with viable cells, the cell may have a glassy, homogeneous appearance, mostly because of the loss of lighter staining glycogen particles. Myelin figures are more prominent in necrotic cells than in cells with reversible injury. When enzymes have digested cytoplasmic organelles, the cytoplasm becomes vacuolated and appears "moth-eaten." By electron microscopy, necrotic cells are characterized by discontinuities in plasma and organelle membranes, marked dilation of mitochondria associated with the appearance of large amorphous intramitrochondrial densities, disruption of lysosomes, and intracytoplasmic myelin figures.
- **Nuclear changes.** Nuclear changes assume one of three patterns, all resulting from a breakdown of DNA and chromatin. **Pyknosis** is characterized by nuclear shrinkage and increased basophilia; the DNA condenses into a dark shrunken mass. The pyknotic nucleus can undergo fragmentation; this change is called **karyorrhexis**. Ultimately, the nucleus may undergo **karyolysis**, in which the basophilia fades because of digestion of DNA by deoxyribonuclease (DNase) activity. In 1 to 2 days, the nucleus in a dead cell may completely disappear.
- **Fates of necrotic cells.** Necrotic cells may persist for some time or may be digested by enzymes and disappear. Dead cells may be replaced by myelin figures, which are either phagocytosed by other cells or further degraded into fatty acids. These fatty acids bind calcium salts, which may result in the dead cells ultimately becoming calcified.

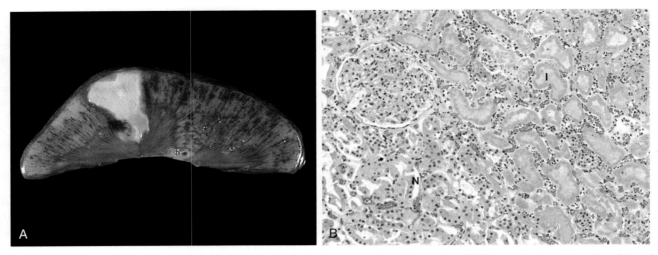

Fig. 2.6 Coagulative necrosis. (A) A wedge-shaped kidney infarct *(yellow)* with preservation of the outlines. (B) Microscopic view of the edge of the infarct, with normal kidney *(N)* and necrotic cells in the infarct *(I)*. The necrotic cells show preserved outlines with loss of nuclei, and an inflammatory infiltrate is present (difficult to discern at this magnification).

Morphologic Patterns of Tissue Necrosis

In severe pathologic conditions, large areas of a tissue or even entire orgrans may undergo necrosis. This may happen in association with marked ischemia, infections, and certain inflammatory reactions. There are several morphologically distinct patterns of tissue necrosis that may provide etiologic clues. Although the terms that describe these patterns do not reflect underlying mechanisms, such terms are commonly used and their implications are understood by pathologists and clinicians.

MORPHOLOGY

Most of the types of necrosis described here have distinctive gross appearances; the exception is fibrinoid necrosis, which is detected only by histologic examination.

- **Coagulative necrosis** is a form of necrosis in which the underlying tissue architecture is preserved for at least several days after death of cells in the tissue (Fig. 2.6). The affected tissues take on a firm texture. Presumably the injury denatures not only structural proteins but also enzymes, thereby blocking the proteolysis of the dead cells; as a result, eosinophilic, anucleate cells may persist for days or weeks. Leukocytes are recruited to the site of necrosis, and the dead cells are ultimately digested by the action of lysosomal enzymes of the leukocytes. The cellular debris is then removed by phagocytosis mediated primarily by infiltrating neutrophils and macrophages. Coagulative necrosis is characteristic of infarcts (areas of necrosis caused by ischemia) in all solid organs except the brain.
- **Liquefactive necrosis** is seen in focal bacterial and, occasionally, fungal infections because microbes stimulate rapid accumulation of inflammatory cells, and the enzymes of leukocytes digest ("liquefy") the tissue. For obscure reasons, hypoxic death of cells within the central nervous system often evokes liquefactive necrosis (Fig. 2.7). Whatever the pathogenesis, the dead cells are completely digested, transforming the tissue into a viscous liquid that is eventually removed by phagocytes. If the process is initiated by acute inflammation, as in a bacterial

infection, the material is frequently creamy yellow and is called **pus** (Chapter 3).

- Although **gangrenous necrosis** is not a distinctive pattern of cell death, the term is still commonly used in clinical practice. It usually refers to the condition of a limb (generally the lower leg) that has lost its blood supply and has undergone coagulative necrosis involving multiple tissue layers. When bacterial infection is superimposed, the morphologic appearance changes to liquefactive necrosis because of the destructive contents of the bacteria and the attracted leukocytes (resulting in so-called "wet gangrene").
- **Caseous necrosis** is most often encountered in foci of tuberculous infection. Caseous means "cheeselike," referring to the friable yellow-white appearance of the area of necrosis on gross examination (Fig. 2.8). On microscopic examination, the necrotic focus appears as a collection of fragmented or lysed cells with an amorphous granular pink appearance in H&E-stained tissue sections. Unlike coagulative necrosis, the tissue

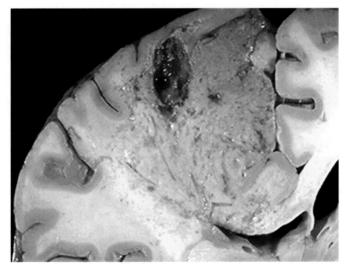

Fig. 2.7 Liquefactive necrosis. An infarct in the brain shows dissolution of the tissue.

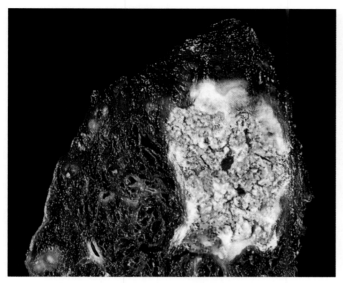

Fig. 2.8 Caseous necrosis. Tuberculosis of the lung, with a large area of caseous necrosis containing yellow-white (cheesy) debris.

architecture is completely obliterated and cellular outlines cannot be discerned. Caseous necrosis is often surrounded by a collection of macrophages and other inflammatory cells; this appearance is characteristic of a nodular inflammatory lesion called a granuloma (Chapter 3).

• **Fat necrosis** refers to focal areas of fat destruction, typically resulting from the release of activated pancreatic lipases into the substance of the pancreas and the peritoneal cavity. This occurs in the calamitous abdominal emergency known as acute pancreatitis (Chapter 17). In this disorder, pancreatic enzymes that have leaked out of acinar cells and ducts liquefy the membranes of fat cells in the peritoneum, and lipases split the triglyceride esters contained within fat cells. The released fatty acids combine with calcium to produce grossly visible chalky white areas (fat saponification), which enable the surgeon and the pathologist to identify the lesions (Fig. 2.9). On histologic examination, the foci of necrosis contain shadowy outlines of necrotic fat cells surrounded by basophilic calcium deposits and an inflammatory reaction.

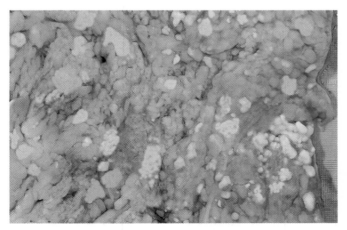

Fig. 2.9 Fat necrosis in acute pancreatitis. The areas of white chalky deposits represent foci of fat necrosis with calcium soap formation (saponification) at sites of lipid breakdown in the mesentery.

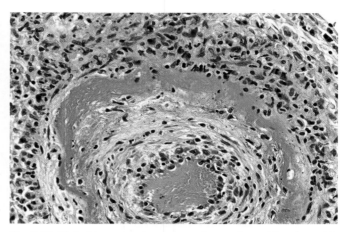

Fig. 2.10 Fibrinoid necrosis in an artery in a patient with polyarteritis nodosa. The wall of the artery shows a circumferential bright pink area of necrosis with protein deposition and inflammation.

• **Fibrinoid necrosis** is a special form of necrosis. It usually occurs in immune reactions in which complexes of antigens and antibodies are deposited in the walls of blood vessels, but it also may occur in severe hypertension. Deposited immune complexes and plasma proteins that leak into the wall of damaged vessels produce a bright pink, amorphous appearance on H&E preparations called fibrinoid (fibrinlike) by pathologists (Fig. 2.10). The immunologically mediated diseases (e.g., polyarteritis nodosa) in which this type of necrosis is seen are described in Chapter 5.

Leakage of intracellular proteins through the damaged cell membrane and ultimately into the circulation provides a means of detecting tissue-specific necrosis using blood or serum samples. Cardiac muscle, for example, contains a unique isoform of the enzyme creatine kinase and of the contractile protein troponin, whereas hepatic bile duct epithelium contains the enzyme alkaline phosphatase, and hepatocytes contain transaminases. Irreversible injury and cell death in these tissues elevate the serum levels of these proteins, which makes them clinically useful markers of tissue damage.

Apoptosis

Apoptosis is a pathway of cell death in which cells activate enzymes that degrade the cells' own nuclear DNA and nuclear and cytoplasmic proteins (Fig. 2.11). Fragments of the apoptotic cells then break off, giving the appearance that is responsible for the name (*apoptosis*, "falling off"). The plasma membrane of the apoptotic cell remains intact, but the membrane is altered in such a way that the fragments, called apoptotic bodies, become highly "edible," leading to their rapid consumption by phagocytes. The dead cell and its fragments are cleared with little leakage of cellular contents, so apoptotic cell death does not elicit an inflammatory reaction. Thus, apoptosis differs in many respects from necrosis (Table 2.1).

Causes of Apoptosis

Apoptosis occurs in many normal situations and serves to eliminate potentially harmful cells and cells that have

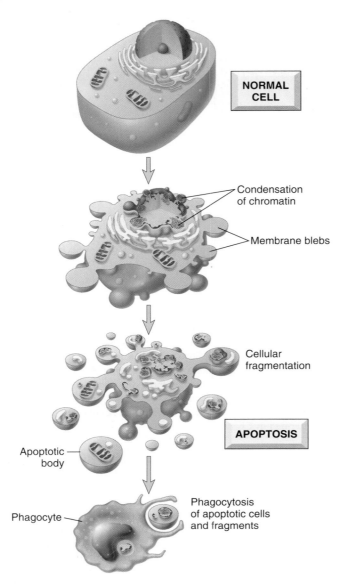

NORMAL CELL

Condensation of chromatin

Membrane blebs

Cellular fragmentation

APOPTOSIS

Apoptotic body

Phagocyte

Phagocytosis of apoptotic cells and fragments

Fig. 2.11 Apoptosis. The cellular alterations in apoptosis are illustrated. Contrast these with the changes that characterize necrotic cell death, shown in Fig. 2.3.

Table 2.2 Physiologic and Pathologic Conditions Associated With Apoptosis

Condition	Mechanism of Apoptosis
Physiologic	
During embryogenesis	Loss of growth factor signaling (presumed mechanism)
Turnover of proliferative tissues (e.g., intestinal epithelium, lymphocytes in bone marrow, and thymus)	Loss of growth factor signaling (presumed mechanism)
Involution of hormone-dependent tissues (e.g., endometrium)	Decreased hormone levels lead to reduced survival signals
Decline of leukocyte numbers at the end of immune and inflammatory responses	Loss of survival signals as stimulus for leukocyte activation is eliminated
Elimination of potentially harmful self-reactive lymphocytes	Strong recognition of self antigens induces apoptosis by both the mitochondrial and death receptor pathways
Pathologic	
DNA damage	Activation of proapoptotic proteins by BH3-only sensors
Accumulation of misfolded proteins	Activation of proapoptotic proteins by BH3-only sensors, possibly direct activation of caspases
Infections, especially certain viral infections	Activation of the mitochondrial pathway by viral proteins Killing of infected cells by cytotoxic T lymphocytes, which activate caspases

- *Apoptosis in pathologic conditions.* Apoptosis eliminates cells that are damaged beyond repair. This is seen when there is severe DNA damage, for example, after exposure to radiation and cytotoxic drugs. The accumulation of misfolded proteins also triggers apoptotic death; the underlying mechanisms of this cause of cell death and its significance in disease are discussed later, in the context of ER stress. Certain infectious agents, particularly some viruses, induce apoptotic death of infected cells.

Mechanisms of Apoptosis

Apoptosis is regulated by biochemical pathways that control the balance of death- and survival-inducing signals and ultimately the activation of enzymes called *caspases*. Caspases were so named because they are cysteine proteases that cleave proteins after aspartic acid residues. Two distinct pathways converge on caspase activation: the mitochondrial pathway and the death receptor pathway (Fig. 2.12). Although these pathways can intersect, they are generally induced under different conditions, involve different molecules, and serve distinct roles in physiology and disease. The end result of apoptotic cell death is the clearance of apoptotic bodies by phagocytes.

- **The mitochondrial (intrinsic) pathway seems to be responsible for apoptosis in most physiologic and pathologic situations.** Mitochondria contain several proteins that are capable of inducing apoptosis, including cytochrome c. When mitochondrial membranes

outlived their usefulness (Table 2.2). It also occurs as a pathologic event when cells are damaged, especially when the damage affects the cell's DNA or proteins; thus, the irreparably damaged cell is eliminated.

- *Physiologic apoptosis.* During normal development of an organism, some cells die and are replaced by new ones. In mature organisms, highly proliferative and hormone-responsive tissues undergo cycles of proliferation and cell loss that are often determined by the levels of growth factors. In these situations, the cell death is always by apoptosis, ensuring that unwanted cells are eliminated without eliciting potentially harmful inflammation. In the immune system, apoptosis eliminates excess leukocytes left at the end of immune responses as well as lymphocytes that recognize self-antigens and could cause autoimmune diseases if they were not purged.

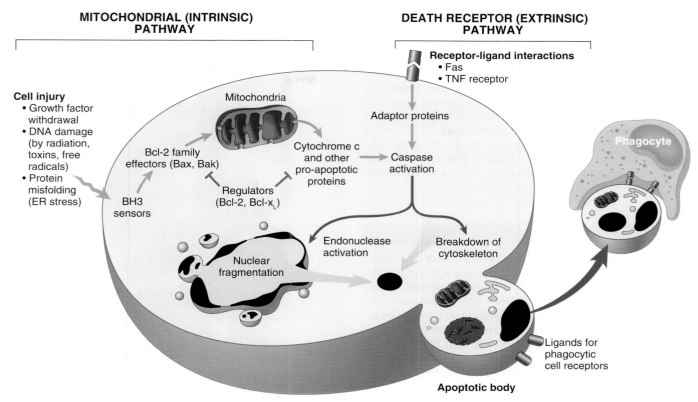

MITOCHONDRIAL (INTRINSIC) PATHWAY

DEATH RECEPTOR (EXTRINSIC) PATHWAY

Receptor-ligand interactions
• Fas
• TNF receptor

Cell injury
• Growth factor withdrawal
• DNA damage (by radiation, toxins, free radicals)
• Protein misfolding (ER stress)

Mitochondria

Adaptor proteins

BH3 sensors

Bcl-2 family effectors (Bax, Bak)

Cytochrome c and other pro-apoptotic proteins

Caspase activation

Regulators (Bcl-2, Bcl-x$_L$)

Nuclear fragmentation

Endonuclease activation

Breakdown of cytoskeleton

Phagocyte

Ligands for phagocytic cell receptors

Apoptotic body

Fig. 2.12 Mechanisms of apoptosis. The two pathways of apoptosis differ in their induction and regulation, and both culminate in the activation of caspases. In the mitochondrial pathway, BH3-only proteins, which are related to members of the Bcl-2 family, sense a lack of survival signals or DNA or protein damage. These BH3-only proteins activate effector molecules that increase mitochondrial permeability. In concert with a deficiency of Bcl-2 and other proteins that maintain mitochondrial permeability, the mitochondria become leaky and various substances, such as cytochrome c, enter the cytosol and activate caspases. Activated caspases induce the changes that culminate in cell death and fragmentation. In the death receptor pathway, signals from plasma membrane receptors lead to the assembly of adaptor proteins into a "death-inducing signaling complex," which activates caspases, and the end result is the same.

become permeable, cytochrome c leaks out into the cytoplasm, triggering caspase activation and apoptotic death. A family of more than 20 proteins, the prototype of which is Bcl-2, controls the permeability of mitochondria. In healthy cells, Bcl-2 and the related protein Bcl-xL, which are produced in response to growth factors and other stimuli, maintain the integrity of mitochondrial membranes, in large part by holding two proapoptotic members of the family, Bax and Bak, in check. When cells are deprived of growth factors and survival signals, or are exposed to agents that damage DNA, or accumulate unacceptable amounts of misfolded proteins, a number of sensors are activated. These sensors are called BH3 proteins because they contan the third domain seen in Bcl-family proteins. They in turn shift this delicate, life-sustaining balance in favor of pro-apoptotic Bak and Bax. As a result, Bak and Bax dimerize, insert into the mitochondrial membrane, and form channels through which cytochrome c and other mitochondrial proteins escape into the cytosol. After cytochrome c enters the cytosol, it, together with certain cofactors, activates caspase-9. The net result is the activation of a caspase cascade, ultimately leading to nuclear fragmentation and formation of apoptotic bodies.

• **The death receptor (extrinsic) pathway of apoptosis.** Many cells express surface molecules, called death receptors, that trigger apoptosis. Most of these are members of the tumor necrosis factor (TNF) receptor family, which contain in their cytoplasmic regions a conserved "death domain," so named because it mediates interaction with other proteins involved in cell death. The prototypic death receptors are the type I TNF receptor and Fas (CD95). Fas ligand (FasL) is a membrane protein expressed mainly on activated T lymphocytes. When these T cells recognize Fas-expressing targets, Fas molecules are crosslinked by FasL and bind adaptor proteins via the death domain. These then recruit and activate caspase-8, which, in turn, activates downstream caspases. The death receptor pathway is involved in the elimination of self-reactive lymphocytes and in the killing of target cells by some cytotoxic T lymphocytes (CTLs) that express FasL.

In either pathway, after caspase-9 or caspase-8 is activated, it cleaves and thereby activates additional caspases that cleave numerous targets and ultimately activate enzymes that degrade the cells' proteins and nucleus. The end result is the characteristic cellular fragmentation of apoptosis.

• **Clearance of apoptotic cells.** Apoptotic cells and their fragments entice phagocytes by producing a number of "eat-me" signals. For instance, in normal cells, phosphatidylserine is present on the inner leaflet of the plasma membrane, but in apoptotic cells this phospholipid "flips" to the outer leaflet, where it is recognized by tissue macrophages, leading to phagocytosis of the apoptotic cells. Cells that are dying by apoptosis also secrete soluble factors that recruit phagocytes. The plasma membrane alterations and secreted proteins facilitate prompt clearance of the dead cells before the cells undergo membrane damage and release their contents (which can induce inflammation). Numerous macrophage receptors have been shown to be involved in the binding and engulfment of apoptotic cells. The phagocytosis of apoptotic cells is so efficient that dead cells disappear without leaving a trace, and inflammation is virtually absent.

MORPHOLOGY

In H&E-stained tissue sections, the nuclei of apoptotic cells show various stages of chromatin condensation and aggregation and, ultimately, karyorrhexis (Fig. 2.13); at the molecular level, this is reflected in the fragmentation of DNA into nucleosome-sized pieces. The cells rapidly shrink, form cytoplasmic buds, and fragment into apoptotic bodies that are composed of membrane-bound pieces of cytosol and organelles (Fig. 2.11). Because these fragments are quickly extruded and phagocytosed without eliciting an inflammatory response, even substantial apoptosis may be histologically undetectable.

Other Pathways of Cell Death

In addition to necrosis and apoptosis, two other patterns of cell death have been described that have unusual features. Although the importance of these pathways in disease remains to be established, they are the subjects of considerable current research, and it is useful to be aware of the basic concepts.

- *Necroptosis.* This form of cell death is initiated by engagement of TNF receptors as well as other, poorly defined triggers. Unlike the extrinsic pathway of apoptosis, which also is downstream of TNF receptors, in necroptosis, kinases called receptor-interacting protein (RIP) kinases are activated, initiating a series of events that result in the dissolution of the cell, much like necrosis. The name necroptosis implies that there are features of both necrosis and apoptosis. Some infections are believed to kill cells by this pathway, and it has been hypothesized to play a role in ischemic injury and other pathologic situations, especially those associated with inflammatory reactions in which the cytokine TNF is produced. However, when and why it occurs and how significant it is in human diseases is not well understood.
- *Pyroptosis.* This form of cell death is associated with activation of a cytosolic danger-sensing protein complex called the inflammasome (Chapter 5). The net result of inflammasome activation is the activation of caspases, some of which induce the production of cytokines that induce inflammation, often manifested by fever, and others trigger apoptosis. Thus, apoptosis and inflammation coexist. The name pyroptosis stems from the association of apoptosis with fever (Greek, *pyro* = fire). It is thought to be one mechanism by which some infectious microbes cause the death of infected cells. Its role in other pathologic situations is unknown.

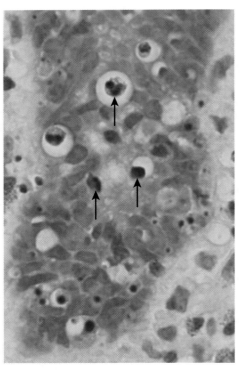

Fig. 2.13 Morphologic appearance of apoptotic cells. Apoptotic cells (some indicated by *arrows*) in colonic epithelium are shown. (Some preparative regimens for colonoscopy may induce apoptosis in epithelial cells, which explains the presence of dead cells in this biopsy.) Note the fragmented nuclei with condensed chromatin and the shrunken cell bodies, some with pieces falling off. *(Courtesy of Dr. Sanjay Kakar, Department of Pathology, University of California San Francisco, San Francisco, California.)*

Autophagy

Autophagy ("self-eating") refers to lysosomal digestion of the cell's own components. It is a survival mechanism in times of nutrient deprivation, so that the starved cell can live by eating its own contents and recycling these contents to provide nutrients and energy. In this process, intracellular organelles and portions of cytosol are first sequestered within an ER-derived autophagic vacuole, whose formation is initiated by cytosolic proteins that sense nutrient deprivation (Fig. 2.14). The vacuole fuses with lysosomes to form an autophagolysosome, in which lysosomal enzymes digest the cellular components. In some circumstances, autophagy may be associated with atrophy of tissues (discussed later) and may represent an adaptation that helps cells survive lean times. If, however, the starved cell can no longer cope by devouring its contents, autophagy may eventually lead to apoptotic cell death.

Extensive autophagy is seen in ischemic injury and some types of myopathies. Polymorphisms in a gene involved in autophagy have been associated with inflammatory bowel disease, but the mechanistic link between autophagy and intestinal inflammation is not known. The role of autophagy in cancer is discussed in Chapter 6. Thus, a once little-appreciated survival pathway in cells may prove to have wide-ranging roles in human disease.

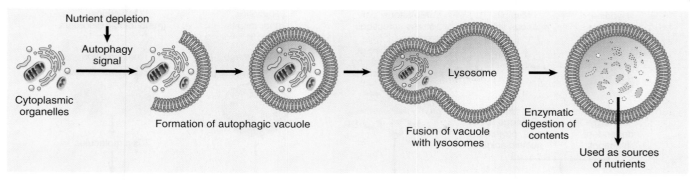

Fig. 2.14 Autophagy. Cellular stresses, such as nutrient deprivation, activate autophagy genes, which initiate the formation of membrane-bound vesicles in which cellular organelles are sequestered. These vesicles fuse with lysosomes, in which the organelles are digested, and the products are used to provide nutrients for the cell. The same process can trigger apoptosis by mechanisms that are not well defined.

SUMMARY

PATTERNS OF CELL INJURY AND CELL DEATH

- Reversible cell injury: cell swelling, fatty change, plasma membrane blebbing and loss of microvilli, mitochondrial swelling, dilation of the ER, eosinophilia (resulting from decreased cytoplasmic RNA)
- Necrosis: Accidental cell death manifested by increased cytoplasmic eosinophilia; nuclear shrinkage, fragmentation, and dissolution; breakdown of plasma membrane and organellar membranes; abundant myelin figures; leakage and enzymatic digestion of cellular contents
- Morphologic types of tissue necrosis: under different conditions, necrosis in tissues may assume specific patterns: coagulative, liquefactive, gangrenous, caseous, fat, and fibrinoid.
- Apoptosis: regulated mechanism of cell death that serves to eliminate unwanted and irreparably damaged cells, with the least possible host reaction, characterized by enzymatic degradation of proteins and DNA, initiated by caspases; and by rapid recognition and removal of dead cells by phagocytes
- Apoptosis is initiated by two major pathways:
  - Mitochondrial (intrinsic) pathway is triggered by loss of survival signals, DNA damage, and accumulation of misfolded proteins (ER stress); associated with leakage of proapoptotic proteins from mitochondrial membrane into the cytoplasm, where they trigger caspase activation; inhibited by anti-apoptotic members of the Bcl family, which are induced by survival signals including growth factors.
  - Death receptor (extrinsic) pathway is responsible for elimination of self-reactive lymphocytes and damage by CTLs; is initiated by engagement of death receptors (members of the TNF receptor family) by ligands on adjacent cells.
- Two other unusual pathways of cell death are necroptosis (which, as the name implies, includes features of both necrosis and apoptosis and is regulated by particular signaling pathways) and pyroptosis, which can lead to the release of proinflammatory cytokines and may initiate apoptosis.
- Autophagy is an adaptation to nutrient deprivation in which cells digest their own organelles and recycle them to provide energy and substrates. If the stress is too severe for the process to cope with it, it results in cell death by apoptosis.

MECHANISMS OF CELL INJURY AND CELL DEATH

Before discussing individual mechanisms of cell injury and death, some general principles should be emphasized.

- **The cellular response to injurious stimuli depends on the type of injury, its duration, and its severity.** Thus, low doses of toxins or a brief period of ischemia may lead to reversible cell injury, whereas larger toxin doses or longer ischemic times may result in irreversible injury and cell death.
- **The consequences of an injurious stimulus also depend on the type, status, adaptability, and genetic makeup of the injured cell.** The same injury has vastly different outcomes depending on the cell type. For instance, striated skeletal muscle in the leg tolerates complete ischemia for 2 to 3 hours without irreversible injury, whereas cardiac muscle dies after only 20 to 30 minutes of ischemia. The nutritional (or hormonal) status also can be important; understandably, a glycogen-replete hepatocyte will survive ischemia better than one that has just burned its last glucose molecule. Genetically determined diversity in metabolic pathways can contribute to differences in responses to injurious stimuli. For instance, when exposed to the same dose of a toxin, individuals who inherit variants in genes encoding cytochrome P-450 may catabolize the toxin at different rates, leading to different outcomes. Much effort is now directed toward understanding the role of genetic polymorphisms in responses to drugs and toxins, a field of study called pharmacogenomics. In fact, genetic variations influence susceptibility to many complex diseases as well as responsiveness to various therapeutic agents. Using the genetic makeup of the individual patient to guide therapy is one example of "precision medicine."
- **Cell injury usually results from functional and biochemical abnormalities in one or more of a limited number of essential cellular components** (Fig. 2.15). As we discuss in more detail later, different external insults and endogenous perturbations typically affect different cellular organelles and biochemical pathways. For instance, deprivation of oxygen and nutrients (as

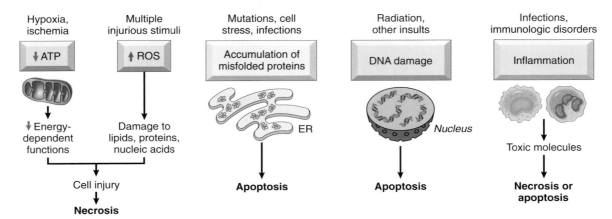

Fig. 2.15 The principal biochemical mechanisms and sites of damage in cell injury. Note that causes and mechanisms of cell death by necrosis and apoptosis are shown as being independent but there may be overlap; for instance, both may contribute to cell death caused by ischemia, oxidative stress, or radiation. *ATP*, Adenosine triphosphate; *ROS*, reactive oxygen species.

in hypoxia and ischemia) primarily impairs energy-dependent cellular functions, culminating in necrosis, whereas damage to proteins and DNA triggers apoptosis. However, it should be emphasized that the very same injurious agent may trigger multiple and overlapping biochemical pathways. Not surprisingly, therefore, it has proved difficult to prevent cell injury by targeting an individual pathway.

As we discussed in the beginning of this chapter and have alluded to throughout, there are numerous and diverse causes of cell injury and cell death. Similarly, there are many biochemical pathways that can initiate the sequence of events that lead to cell injury and culminate in cell death. Some of these pathways are recognized to play important roles in human diseases. In the following section, we organize our discussion of the mechanisms of cell injury along its major causes and pathways, and discuss the principal biochemical alterations in each. For the sake of clarity and simplicity, we emphasize the unique mechanisms in each pathway, but it is important to point out that any initiating trigger may activate one or more of these mechanisms, and several mechanisms may be active simultaneously.

Hypoxia and Ischemia

Deficiency of oxygen leads to failure of many energy-dependent metabolic pathways, and ultimately to death of cells by necrosis. Most cellular ATP is produced from adenosine diphosphate (ADP) by oxidative phosphorylation during reduction of oxygen in the electron transport system of mitochondria. High-energy phosphate in the form of ATP is required for membrane transport, protein synthesis, lipogenesis, and the deacylation-reacylation reactions necessary for phospholipid turnover. It is estimated that in total, the cells of a healthy human burn 50 to 75 kg of ATP every day! Not surprisingly, therefore, cells deprived of oxygen are at risk of suffering catastrophic failure of many essential functions. Oxygen deprivation is one of the most frequent causes of cell injury and necrosis in clinical medicine.

Cells subjected to the stress of hypoxia that do not immediately die activate compensatory mechanisms that are induced by transcription factors of the hypoxia-inducible factor 1 (HIF-1) family. HIF-1 simulates the synthesis of several proteins that help the cell to survive in the face of low oxygen. Some of these proteins, such as vascular endothelial growth factor (VEGF), stimulate the growth of new vessels and thus attempt to increase blood flow and the supply of oxygen. Other proteins induced by HIF-1 cause adaptive changes in cellular metabolism by stimulating the uptake of glucose and glycolysis and dampening mitochondrial oxidative phosphorylation. Anaerobic glycolysis can generate ATP in the absence of oxygen using glucose derived either from the circulation or from the hydrolysis of intracellular glycogen. Understandably, normal tissues with a greater glycolytic capacity because of the presence of glycogen (e.g., the liver and striated muscle) are more likely to survive hypoxia and decreased oxidative phosphorylation than tissues with limited glucose stores (e.g., the brain). Although it seems counterintuitive, rapidly proliferating normal cells and cancer cells rely on aerobic glycolysis to produce much of their energy, a phenomenon referred to as the Warburg effect. The reason for this is that although glycolysis yields less ATP per molecule of glucose burned than oxidative phosphorylation, metabolites generated by glycolysis and the TCA cycle serve as precursors for the synthesis of cellular constituents (e.g., proteins, lipids, and nucleic acids) that are needed for cell growth and division. Alterations in cellular metabolism are frequently seen in cancer cells, so they are discussed in more detail in Chapter 6.

Persistent or severe hypoxia and ischemia ultimately lead to failure of ATP generation and depletion of ATP in cells. Loss of this critical energy store has deleterious effects on many cellular systems (Fig. 2.16).

- *Reduced activity of plasma membrane ATP-dependent sodium pumps*, resulting in intracellular accumulation of sodium and efflux of potassium. The net gain of solute is accompanied by isoosmotic gain of water, causing *cell swelling* and dilation of the ER.
- The compensatory *increase in anaerobic glycolysis* leads to lactic acid accumulation, decreased intracellular pH, and decreased activity of many cellular enzymes.
- Prolonged or worsening depletion of ATP causes *structural disruption of the protein synthetic apparatus,*

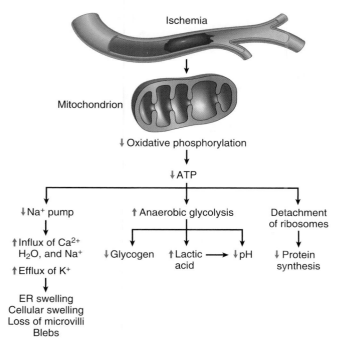

Ischemia

Mitochondrion

↓ Oxidative phosphorylation

↓ ATP

↓ Na⁺ pump

↑ Influx of Ca²⁺
H₂O, and Na⁺

↑ Efflux of K⁺

ER swelling
Cellular swelling
Loss of microvilli
Blebs

↑ Anaerobic glycolysis

↓ Glycogen   ↑ Lactic ⟶ ↓ pH
acid

Detachment
of ribosomes

↓ Protein
synthesis

Fig. 2.16 The functional and morphologic consequences of hypoxia and ischemia. *ER*, Endoplasmic reticulum.

manifested as detachment of ribosomes from the rough ER (RER) and dissociation of polysomes into monosomes, with a consequent reduction in protein synthesis.

- It also has been suggested that hypoxia *per se* increases the accumulation of ROS. Whether this is true is a matter of debate; however, there is ample evidence that hypoxia predisposes cells to ROS-mediated damage if blood flow (and oxygen delivery) is reestablished, a phenomenon called reperfusion injury (described later).
- Ultimately, there is irreversible *damage to mitochondrial and lysosomal membranes*, and the cell undergoes necrosis. Membrane damage is a late event in cell injury caused by diverse mechanisms, and is discussed later. Although necrosis is the principal form of cell death caused by hypoxia, apoptosis by the mitochondrial pathway is also thought to contribute.

The functional consequences of hypoxia and ischemia depend on the severity and duration of the deficit. For instance, the heart muscle ceases to contract within 60 seconds of coronary occlusion. If hypoxia continues, worsening ATP depletion causes further deterioration, undergoing the sequence of changes illustrated in Fig. 2.3 and described earlier.

Ischemia-Reperfusion Injury

Under certain circumstances, the restoration of blood flow to ischemic but viable tissues results, paradoxically, in increased cell injury. This is the reverse of the expected outcome of the restoration of blood flow, which normally results in the recovery of reversibly injured cells. This so-called "ischemia-reperfusion injury" is a clinically important process that may contribute significantly to

tissue damage, especially after myocardial and cerebral ischemia.

Several mechanisms may account for the exacerbation of cell injury resulting from reperfusion of ischemic tissues:
- New damage may be initiated during reoxygenation by increased generation of ROS (described in more detail below). Some of the ROS may be generated by injured cells with damaged mitochondria that cannot carry out the complete reduction of oxygen, and at the same time cellular anti-oxidant defense mechanisms may be compromised by ischemia, exacerbating the situation. ROS generated by infiltrating leukocytes also may contribute to the damage of vulnerable injured cells.
- The inflammation that is induced by ischemic injury may increase with reperfusion because it enhances the influx of leukocytes and plasma proteins. The products of activated leukocytes may cause additional tissue injury (Chapter 3). Activation of the complement system also may contribute to ischemia-reperfusion injury. Complement proteins may bind to the injured tissues, or to antibodies that are deposited in the tissues, and subsequent complement activation generates byproducts that exacerbate the cell injury and inflammation.

Oxidative Stress

Oxidative stress refers to cellular abnormalities that are induced by ROS, which belong to a group of molecules known as free radicals. Free radical-mediated cell injury is seen in many circumstances, including chemical and radiation injury, hypoxia, cellular aging, tissue injury caused by inflammatory cells, and ischemia-reperfusion injury. In all these cases, cell death may be by necrosis, apoptosis, or the mixed pattern of necroptosis.

Free radicals are chemical species with a single unpaired electron in an outer orbit. Such chemical states are extremely unstable, and free radicals readily react with inorganic and organic molecules; when generated in cells, they avidly attack nucleic acids as well as a variety of cellular proteins and lipids. In addition, free radicals initiate reactions in which molecules that react with the free radicals are themselves converted into other types of free radicals, thereby propagating the chain of damage.

Generation and Removal of Reactive Oxygen Species

The accumulation of ROS is determined by their rates of production and removal (Fig. 2.17). ROS are produced by two major pathways.
- **ROS are produced normally in small amounts in all cells during the reduction-oxidation (redox) reactions** that occur during mitochondrial respiration and energy generation. In this process, molecular oxygen is reduced in mitochondria to generate water by the sequential addition of four electrons. This reaction is imperfect, however, and small amounts of highly reactive but short-lived toxic intermediates are generated when oxygen is only partially reduced. These intermediates include superoxide ($O_2^{\cdot-}$), which is converted to hydrogen peroxide (H_2O_2) spontaneously and by the action of the enzyme superoxide dismutase (SOD). H_2O_2 is more stable than $O_2^{\cdot-}$ and can cross biologic membranes. In the presence of metals, such as Fe^{2+}, H_2O_2 is converted to the

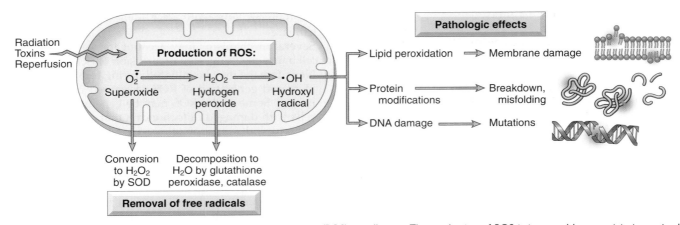

Fig. 2.17 The generation, removal, and role of reactive oxygen species (ROS) in cell injury. The production of ROS is increased by many injurious stimuli. These free radicals are removed by spontaneous decay and by specialized enzymatic systems. Excessive production or inadequate removal leads to accumulation of free radicals in cells, which may damage lipids (by peroxidation), proteins, and DNA, resulting in cell injury. *SOD,* Superoxide dismutase.

highly reactive hydroxyl radical $\cdot OH$ by the Fenton reaction. The properties and pathologic effects of the major ROS are summarized in Table 2.3.

- **ROS are produced in phagocytic leukocytes, mainly neutrophils and macrophages,** as a weapon for destroying ingested microbes and other substances during inflammation and host defense (Chapter 3). The ROS are generated in the phagosomes and phagolysosomes of leukocytes by a process that is similar to mitochondrial respiration and is called the *respiratory burst* (or oxidative burst). In this process, a phagosome membrane enzyme catalyzes the generation of superoxide, which is converted to H_2O_2. H_2O_2 is in turn converted to a highly reactive compound, hypochlorite (the major component of household bleach), by the enzyme myeloperoxidase, which is present in leukocytes. The role of ROS in inflammation is described in Chapter 3.
- Nitric oxide (NO) is another reactive free radical produced in macrophages and other leukocytes. It can react with O_2^- to form a highly reactive compound, peroxynitrite, which also participates in cell injury.

The generation of free radicals is increased under several circumstances:
- The absorption of radiant energy (e.g., ultraviolet (UV) light, x-rays). Ionizing radiation can hydrolyze water into hydroxyl ($\cdot OH$) and hydrogen ($H\cdot$) free radicals.

- The enzymatic metabolism of exogenous chemicals (e.g., carbon tetrachloride—see later)
- Inflammation, in which free radicals are produced by leukocytes (Chapter 3)
- Reperfusion of ischemic tissues, as already described.

Cells have developed mechanisms to remove free radicals and thereby minimize their injurious effects. Free radicals are inherently unstable and decay spontaneously. There also are nonenzymatic and enzymatic systems, sometimes called free radical scavengers, serving to inactivate free radicals (Fig. 2.17).
- The rate of decay of superoxide is significantly increased by the action of superoxide dismutase (SOD).
- Glutathione (GSH) peroxidases are a family of enzymes whose major function is to protect cells from oxidative damage. The most abundant member of this family, GSH peroxidase 1, is found in the cytoplasm of all cells. It catalyzes the breakdown of H_2O_2 by the reaction $2GSH + H_2O_2 \rightarrow GS\text{-}SG + 2H_2O$. The intracellular ratio of oxidized GSH to reduced GSH is a reflection of this enzyme's activity and thus of the cell's ability to catabolize free radicals.
- Catalase, present in peroxisomes, catalyzes the decomposition of hydrogen peroxide ($2H_2O_2 \rightarrow O_2 + 2H_2O$). It is one of the most active enzymes known, capable of degrading millions of molecules of H_2O_2 per second.

Table 2.3 Principal Free Radicals Involved in Cell Injury

Free Radical	Mechanisms of Production	Mechanisms of Removal	Pathologic Effects
Superoxide (O_2^-)	Incomplete reduction of O_2 during mitochondrial oxidative phosphorylation; by phagocyte oxidase in leukocytes	Conversion to H_2O_2 and O_2 by superoxide dismutase	Direct damaging effects on lipids (peroxidation), proteins, and DNA
Hydrogen peroxide (H_2O_2)	Mostly from superoxide by action of superoxide dismutase	Conversion to H_2O and O_2 by catalase, glutathione peroxidase	Can be converted to $\cdot OH$ and OCl^-, which destroy microbes and cells
Hydroxyl radical ($\cdot OH$)	Produced from H_2O, H_2O_2, and O_2^- by various chemical reactions	Conversion to H_2O by glutathione peroxidase	Direct damaging effects on lipids, proteins, and DNA
Peroxynitrite ($ONOO\cdot$)	Interaction of O_2^- and NO mediated by NO synthase	Conversion to nitrite by enzymes in mitochondria and cytosol	Direct damaging effects on lipids, proteins, and DNA

- Endogenous or exogenous anti-oxidants (e.g., vitamins E, A, and C and β-carotene) may either block the formation of free radicals or scavenge them after they have formed.

Cell Injury Caused by Reactive Oxygen Species

ROS causes cell injury by damaging multiple components of cells (Fig. 2.17):

- *Lipid peroxidation of membranes.* Double bonds in membrane polyunsaturated lipids are vulnerable to attack by oxygen-derived free radicals. The lipid–radical interactions yield peroxides, which are themselves unstable and reactive, and an autocatalytic chain reaction ensues. Damage to plasma membranes as well as mitochondrial and lysosomal membranes can have devastating consequences, as discussed earlier in the context of ischemia and hypoxia.
- *Crosslinking and other changes in proteins.* Free radicals promote sulfhydryl-mediated protein crosslinking, resulting in enhanced degradation or loss of enzymatic activity. Free radical reactions also may directly cause polypeptide fragmentation. Damaged proteins may fail to fold properly, triggering the unfolded protein response, described later.
- *DNA damage.* Free radical reactions with thymine residues in nuclear and mitochondrial DNA produce single-strand breaks. Such DNA damage has been implicated in apoptotic cell death, aging, and malignant transformation of cells.
- In addition to the role of ROS in cell injury and the killing of microbes, low concentrations of ROS are involved in numerous signaling pathways in cells and thus in many physiologic reactions. Therefore, these molecules are produced normally but, to avoid their harmful effects, their intracellular concentrations are tightly regulated in healthy cells.

Cell Injury Caused by Toxins

Toxins, including environmental chemicals and substances produced by infectious pathogens, induce cell injury that culminates primarily in necrotic cell death. Different types of toxins induce cell injury by two general mechanism:

- *Direct-acting toxins.* Some toxins act directly by combining with a critical molecular component or cellular organelle. For example, in mercuric chloride poisoning (as may occur from ingestion of contaminated seafood) (Chapter 8), mercury binds to the sulfhydryl groups of various cell membrane proteins, causing inhibition of ATP-dependent transport and increased membrane permeability. Many anti-neoplastic chemotherapeutic agents also induce cell damage by direct cytotoxic effects. Also included in this class are toxins made by microorganisms (described in Chapter 9). These often cause damage by targeting host cell molecules that are needed for essential functions, such as protein synthesis and ion transport.
- *Latent toxins.* Many toxic chemicals are not intrinsically active but must first be converted to reactive metabolites, which then act on target cells. Understandably, such toxins typically affect the cells in which they are activated. This is usually accomplished by cytochrome

P-450 in the smooth ER of the liver and other organs. Although the metabolites might cause membrane damage and cell injury by direct covalent binding to protein and lipids, the most important mechanism of cell injury involves the formation of free radicals. *Carbon tetrachloride* (CCl_4)—once widely used in the dry cleaning industry but now banned—and the analgesic *acetaminophen* belong in this category. The effect of CCl_4 is still instructive as an example of chemical injury. CCl_4 is converted to a toxic free radical, principally in the liver, and this free radical is the cause of cell injury, mainly by membrane phospholipid peroxidation. In less than 30 minutes after exposure to CCl_4, there is sufficient damage to the ER membranes of hepatocytes to cause a decline in the synthesis of enzymes and plasma proteins; within 2 hours, swelling of the smooth ER and dissociation of ribosomes from the RER have occurred. There also is decreased synthesis of apoproteins that form complexes with triglycerides and thereby facilitate triglyceride secretion; this defect results in the accumulation of lipids in hepatocytes and other cells and the "fatty liver" of CCl_4 poisoning. Mitochondrial injury follows, and subsequently diminished ATP stores result in defective ion transport and progressive cell swelling; the plasma membranes are further damaged by fatty aldehydes produced by lipid peroxidation in the ER. The end result can be cell death.

Endoplasmic Reticulum Stress

The accumulation of misfolded proteins in a cell can stress compensatory pathways in the ER and lead to cell death by apoptosis. During normal protein synthesis, chaperones in the ER control the proper folding of newly synthesized proteins, and misfolded polypeptides are ubiquitinated and targeted for proteolysis. If unfolded or misfolded proteins accumulate in the ER, they first induce a protective cellular response that is called the *unfolded protein response* (Fig. 2.18). This adaptive response activates signaling pathways that increase the production of chaperones and decrease protein translation, thus reducing the levels of misfolded proteins in the cell. When a large amount of misfolded protein accumulates and cannot be handled by the adaptive response, the signals that are generated result in activation of proapoptotic sensors of the BH3-only family as well as direct activation of caspases, leading to apoptosis by the mitochondrial (intrinsic) pathway.

Intracellular accumulation of misfolded proteins may be caused by abnormalities that increase the production of misfolded proteins or reduce the ability to eliminate them. This may result from gene mutations that lead to the production of proteins that cannot fold properly; aging, which is associated with a decreased capacity to correct misfolding; infections, especially viral infections, when large amounts of microbial proteins are synthesized within cells, more than the cell can handle; increased demand for secretory proteins such as insulin in insulin-resistant states; and changes in intracellular pH and redox state. Protein misfolding is thought to be the fundamental cellular abnormality in several neurodegenerative diseases (Chapter 23). Deprivation of glucose and oxygen, as in ischemia and hypoxia, also may increase the burden of misfolded proteins.

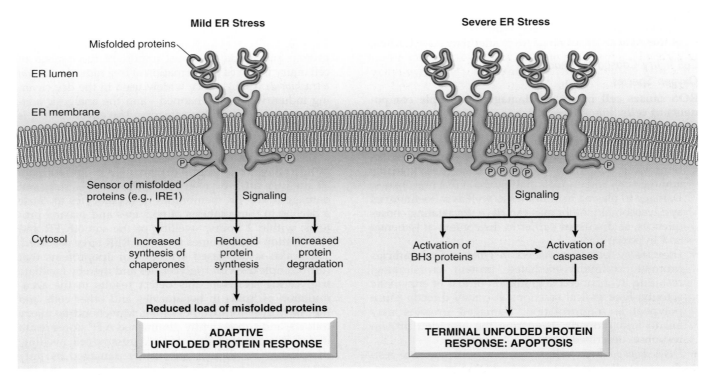

Fig. 2.18 The unfolded protein response and endoplasmic reticulum (ER) stress. The presence of misfolded proteins in the ER is detected by sensors in the ER membrane, such as the kinase IRE-1, which form oligomers that are activated by phosphorylation. This triggers an adaptive unfolded protein response, which can protect the cell from the harmful consequences of the misfolded proteins. When the amount of misfolded proteins is too great to be corrected, excessive activation of ER sensors activates the mitochondrial pathway of apoptosis and the irreparably damaged cell dies; this is also called the terminal unfolded protein response.

Protein misfolding within cells may cause disease by creating a deficiency of an essential protein or by inducing apoptosis (Table 2.4).
- Misfolded proteins often lose their activity and are rapidly degraded, both of which can contribute to a loss of function. If this function is essential, cellular injury ensues. One important disease in which this occurs is cystic fibrosis, which is caused by inherited mutations in a membrane transport protein that prevent its normal folding.

- Cell death as a result of protein misfolding is recognized as a feature of a number of diseases, including the neurodegenerative disorders Alzheimer disease, Huntington disease, and Parkinson disease, and may underlie type 2 diabetes as well (Table 2.4).

As discussed later in the chapter, improperly folded proteins can also accumulate in extracellular tissues, as in amyloidosis.

Table 2.4 Diseases Caused by Misfolded Proteins[a]

Disease	Affected Protein	Pathogenesis
Diseases Caused by Mutant Proteins That Are Degraded, Leading to Their Deficiency		
Cystic fibrosis	CFTR	Loss of CFTR leads to defects in chloride transport and death of affected cells
Familial hypercholesterolemia	LDL receptor	Loss of LDL receptor leads to hypercholesterolemia
Tay-Sachs disease	Hexosaminidase β subunit	Lack of the lysosomal enzyme leads to storage of GM2 gangliosides in neurons
Diseases Caused by Misfolded Proteins That Result in ER Stress-Induced Cell Loss		
Retinitis pigmentosa	Rhodopsin	Abnormal folding of rhodopsin causes photoreceptor loss and cell death, resulting in blindness
Creutzfeldt-Jacob disease	Prions	Abnormal folding of PrPsc causes neuronal cell death
Alzheimer disease	Aβ peptide	Abnormal folding of Aβ peptide causes aggregation within neurons and apoptosis
Diseases Caused by Misfolded Proteins That Result From Both ER Stress-Induced Cell Loss and Functional Deficiency of the Protein		
Alpha-1-anti-trypsin deficiency	α-1 anti-trypsin	Storage of nonfunctional protein in hepatocytes causes apoptosis; absence of enzymatic activity in lungs causes destruction of elastic tissue giving rise to emphysema

[a]Selected illustrative examples of diseases are shown in which protein misfolding is thought to be the major mechanism of functional derangement or cell or tissue injury.
CFTR, Cystic fibrosis transmembrane conductance regulator; *LDL*, low-density lipoprotein.

DNA Damage

Exposure of cells to radiation or chemotherapeutic agents, intracellular generation of ROS, and acquisition of mutations may all induce DNA damage, which if severe may trigger apoptotic death. Damage to DNA is sensed by intracellular sentinel proteins, which transmit signals that lead to the accumulation of p53 protein. p53 first arrests the cell cycle (at the G1 phase) to allow the DNA to be repaired before it is replicated (Chapter 6). However, if the damage is too great to be repaired successfully, p53 triggers apoptosis, mainly by stimulating BH3-only sensor proteins that ultimately activate Bax and Bak, proapoptotic members of the Bcl-2 family. When p53 is mutated or absent (as it is in certain cancers), cells with damaged DNA that would otherwise undergo apoptosis survive. In such cells, the DNA damage may result in mutations or DNA rearrangements (e.g., translocations) that lead to neoplastic transformation (Chapter 6).

Inflammation

A common cause of injury to cells and tissues is the inflammatory reaction that is elicited by pathogens, necrotic cells, and dysregulated immune responses, as in autoimmune diseases and allergies. In all these situations, **inflammatory cells, including neutrophils, macrophages, lymphocytes, and other leukocytes, secrete products that evolved to destroy microbes but also may damage host tissues.** These injurious immune reactions are classified under hypersensitivity. Their mechanisms and significance are discussed in Chapter 5.

Common Events in Cell Injury From Diverse Causes

In the previous discussion, we addressed the mechanisms of cell injury according to the initiating cause, and highlighted the principal pathways of injury that are triggered in different pathophysiologic situations. Some abnormalities characterize cell injury regardless of the cause, and are thus seen in a variety of pathologic situations. Two of these changes are described next.

Mitochondrial Dysfunction

Mitochondria may be viewed as "mini-factories" that produce life-sustaining energy in the form of ATP. Not surprisingly, therefore, they also are critical players in cell injury and death. Mitochondria are sensitive to many types of injurious stimuli, including hypoxia, chemical toxins, and radiation (Fig. 2.19). Mitochondrial changes occur in necrosis and apoptosis. They may result in several biochemical abnormalities:

- Failure of oxidative phosphorylation leads to progressive depletion of ATP, culminating in necrosis of the cell, as described earlier.
- Abnormal oxidative phosphorylation also leads to the formation of ROS, which have many deleterious effects, as already described.
- Damage to mitochondria is often associated with the formation of a high-conductance channel in the mitochondrial membrane, called the mitochondrial

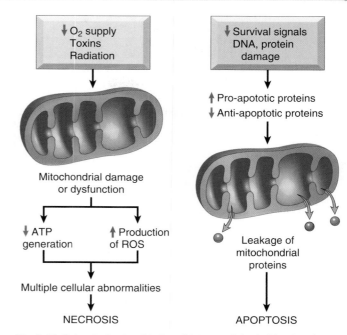

Fig. 2.19 Role of mitochondria in cell injury and death. Mitochondria are affected by a variety of injurious stimuli and their abnormalities lead to necrosis or apoptosis. This pathway of apoptosis is described in more detail later. *ATP*, Adenosine triphosphate; *ROS*, reactive oxygen species.

permeability transition pore. The opening of this channel leads to the loss of mitochondrial membrane potential and pH changes, further compromising oxidative phosphorylation.

- Mitochondria also contain proteins such as cytochrome c that, when released into the cytoplasm, tell the cell there is internal injury and activate a pathway of apoptosis, as discussed earlier.

Defects in Membrane Permeability

Increased membrane permeability leading ultimately to overt membrane damage is a feature of most forms of cell injury that culminate in necrosis. The most important sites of membrane damage during cell injury are the mitochondrial membrane, the plasma membrane, and membranes of lysosomes. As noted earlier, increased permeability of the plasma membrane and lysosomal membranes is not a feature of apoptosis.

- *Mitochondrial membrane damage.* As discussed earlier, damage to mitochondrial membranes results in decreased production of ATP, with many deleterious effects culminating in necrosis.
- *Plasma membrane damage.* Plasma membrane damage leads to loss of osmotic balance and influx of fluids and ions, as well as loss of cellular contents. The cells may also leak metabolites that are vital for the reconstitution of ATP, thus further depleting energy stores.
- *Injury to lysosomal membranes* results in leakage of their enzymes into the cytoplasm and activation of the acid hydrolases in the acidic intracellular pH of the injured (e.g., ischemic) cell. Activation of these enzymes leads to enzymatic digestion of cell components, and the cells die by necrosis.

SUMMARY

MECHANISMS OF CELL INJURY

- Different initiating events cause cell injury and death by diverse mechanisms.
- Hypoxia and ischemia lead to ATP depletion and failure of many energy-dependent functions, resulting first in reversible injury and, if not corrected, in necrosis.
- In ischemia-reperfusion injury, restoration of blood flow to an ischemic tissue exacerbates damage by increasing production of ROS and by inflammation.
- Oxidative stress refers to accumulation of ROS, which can damage cellular lipids, proteins, and DNA, and is associated with numerous initiating causes.
- Protein misfolding depletes essential proteins and, if the misfolded proteins accumulate within cells, results in apoptosis.
- DNA damage (e.g., by radiation) also can induce apoptosis if it is not repaired.
- Inflammation is associated with cell injury because of the damaging actions of the products of inflammatory leukocytes.

We have now concluded the discussion of cell injury and cell death. As we have seen, these processes are the root cause of many common diseases. We end this chapter with brief considerations of three other processes: cellular adaptations to stresses; intracellular accumulations of various substances and extracellular deposition of calcium, both of which are often associated with cell injury; and aging.

CELLULAR ADAPTATIONS TO STRESS

Adaptations are reversible changes in the number, size, phenotype, metabolic activity, or functions of cells in response to changes in their environment. *Physiologic adaptations* usually represent responses of cells to normal stimulation by hormones or endogenous chemical mediators (e.g., the hormone-induced enlargement of the breast and uterus during pregnancy), or to the demands of mechanical stress (in the case of bones and muscles). *Pathologic adaptations* are responses to stress that allow cells to modulate their structure and function and thus escape injury, but at the expense of normal function, such as squamous metaplasia of bronchial epithelium in smokers. Physiologic and pathologic adaptations can take several distinct forms, as described in the following text.

Hypertrophy

Hypertrophy is an increase in the size of cells resulting in an increase in the size of the organ. In contrast, hyperplasia (discussed next) is an increase in cell number. Stated another way, in pure hypertrophy there are no new cells, just bigger cells containing increased amounts of structural proteins and organelles. Hyperplasia is an adaptive response in cells capable of replication, whereas hypertrophy occurs when cells have a limited capacity to divide. Hypertrophy and hyperplasia also can occur together, and obviously both result in an enlarged organ.

Hypertrophy can be physiologic or pathologic and is caused either by increased functional demand or by growth factor or hormonal stimulation.

- The massive physiologic enlargement of the uterus during pregnancy occurs as a consequence of estrogen-stimulated smooth muscle hypertrophy and smooth muscle hyperplasia (Fig. 2.20). In contrast, in response to increased workload the striated muscle cells in both the skeletal muscle and the heart undergo only hypertrophy because adult muscle cells have a limited capacity to divide. Therefore, the chiseled physique of the avid weightlifter stems solely from the hypertrophy of individual skeletal muscles.
- An example of pathologic hypertrophy is the cardiac enlargement that occurs with hypertension or aortic valve disease (Fig. 2.21). The differences between normal, adapted, and irreversibly injured cells are illustrated by the responses of the heart to different types of

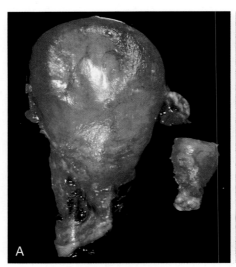
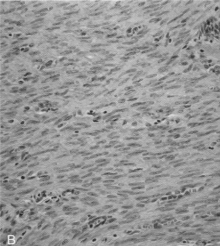
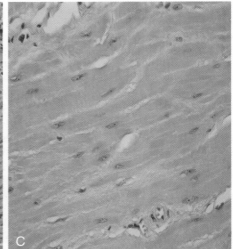

Fig. 2.20 Physiologic hypertrophy of the uterus during pregnancy. (A) Gross appearance of a normal uterus *(right)* and a gravid uterus *(left)* that was removed for postpartum bleeding. (B) Small spindle-shaped uterine smooth muscle cells from a normal uterus. (C) Large, plump hypertrophied smooth muscle cells from a gravid uterus; compare with B. (*B* and *C*, Same magnification.)

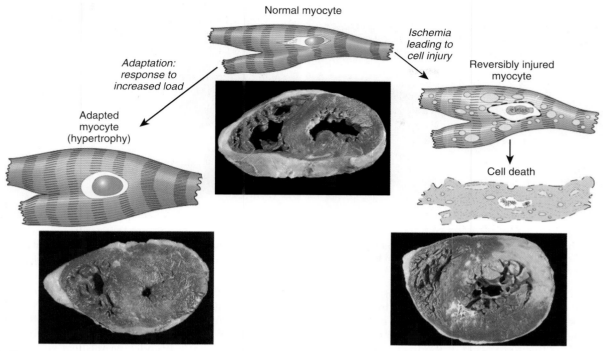

Fig. 2.21 The relationship among normal, adapted, reversibly injured, and dead myocardial cells. The cellular adaptation depicted here is hypertrophy, the cause of reversible injury is ischemia, and the irreversible injury is ischemic coagulative necrosis. In the example of myocardial hypertrophy *(lower left)*, the left ventricular wall is thicker than 2 cm (normal, 1–1.5 cm). Reversibly injured myocardium shows functional effects without any gross or light microscopic changes, or reversible changes such as cellular swelling and fatty change *(shown here)*. In the specimen showing necrosis *(lower right)* the transmural light area in the posterolateral left ventricle represents an acute myocardial infarction. All three transverse sections of myocardium were stained with triphenyltetrazolium chloride, an enzyme substrate that colors viable myocardium magenta. Failure to stain is due to enzyme loss after cell death.

stress. Myocardium subjected to a persistently increased workload, as in hypertension or with a narrowed (stenotic) valve, adapts by undergoing hypertrophy to generate the required higher contractile force. If, on the other hand, the myocardium is subjected to reduced blood flow (ischemia) due to an occluded coronary artery, the muscle cells may undergo injury.

The mechanisms driving cardiac hypertrophy involve at least two types of signals: mechanical triggers, such as stretch, and soluble mediators that stimulate cell growth, such as growth factors and adrenergic hormones. These stimuli turn on signal transduction pathways that lead to the induction of a number of genes, which in turn stimulate synthesis of many cellular proteins, including growth factors and structural proteins. The result is the synthesis of more proteins and myofilaments per cell, which increases the force generated with each contraction, enabling the cell to meet increased work demands. There may also be a switch of contractile proteins from adult to fetal or neonatal forms. For example, during muscle hypertrophy, the α-myosin heavy chain is replaced by the fetal β form of the myosin heavy chain, which produces slower, more energetically economical contraction.

An adaptation to stress such as hypertrophy can progress to functionally significant cell injury if the stress is not relieved. Whatever the cause of hypertrophy, a limit is reached beyond which the enlargement of muscle mass can no longer compensate for the increased burden. When this happens in the heart, several degenerative changes occur in the myocardial fibers, of which the most important are fragmentation and loss of myofibrillar contractile elements. Why hypertrophy progresses to these regressive changes is incompletely understood. There may be finite limits on the abilities of the vasculature to adequately supply the enlarged fibers, the mitochondria to supply ATP, or the biosynthetic machinery to provide sufficient contractile proteins or other cytoskeletal elements. The net result of these degenerative changes is ventricular dilation and ultimately cardiac failure.

Hyperplasia

Hyperplasia is an increase in the number of cells in an organ that stems from increased proliferation, either of differentiated cells or, in some instances, less differentiated progenitor cells. As discussed earlier, hyperplasia takes place if the tissue contains cell populations capable of replication; it may occur concurrently with hypertrophy and often in response to the same stimuli.

Hyperplasia can be physiologic or pathologic; in both situations, cellular proliferation is stimulated by growth factors that are produced by a variety of cell types.

- The two types of physiologic hyperplasia are (1) hormonal hyperplasia, exemplified by the proliferation of the glandular epithelium of the female breast at puberty and during pregnancy, and (2) compensatory hyperplasia, in which residual tissue grows after removal or loss of part of an organ. For example, when part of a liver is resected, mitotic activity in the remaining cells begins as

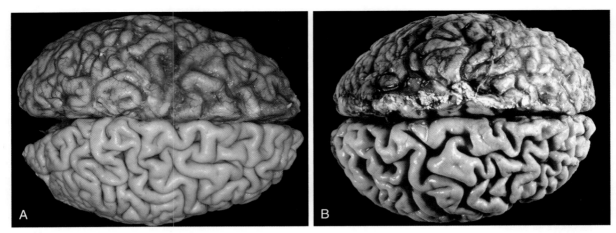

Fig. 2.22 Atrophy as seen in the brain. (A) Normal brain of a young adult. (B) Atrophy of the brain in an 82-year-old man with atherosclerotic disease. Atrophy of the brain is caused by aging and reduced blood supply. Note that loss of brain substance narrows the gyri and widens the sulci. The meninges have been stripped from the bottom half of each specimen to show the surface of the brain.

early as 12 hours later, eventually restoring the liver to its normal size. The stimuli for hyperplasia in this setting are polypeptide growth factors produced by uninjured hepatocytes as well as nonparenchymal cells in the liver (Chapter 3). After restoration of the liver mass, various growth inhibitors turn off cell proliferation.

- Most forms of pathologic hyperplasia are caused by excessive hormonal or growth factor stimulation. For example, after a normal menstrual period there is a burst of uterine epithelial proliferation that is normally tightly regulated by the stimulatory effects of pituitary hormones and ovarian estrogen and the inhibitory effects of progesterone. A disturbance in this balance leading to increased estrogenic stimulation causes endometrial hyperplasia, which is a common cause of abnormal menstrual bleeding. Benign prostatic hyperplasia is another common example of pathologic hyperplasia induced in responses to hormonal stimulation by androgens. Stimulation by growth factors also is involved in the hyperplasia that is associated with certain viral infections; for example, papillomaviruses cause skin warts and mucosal lesions that are composed of masses of hyperplastic epithelium. Here the growth factors may be encoded by viral genes or by the genes of the infected host cells.

An important point is that in all of these situations, **the hyperplastic process remains controlled; if the signals that initiate it abate, the hyperplasia disappears**. It is this responsiveness to normal regulatory control mechanisms that distinguishes pathologic hyperplasias from cancer, in which the growth control mechanisms become permanently dysregulated or ineffective (Chapter 6). Nevertheless, in many cases, pathologic hyperplasia constitutes a fertile soil in which cancers may eventually arise. For example, patients with hyperplasia of the endometrium are at increased risk of developing endometrial cancer (Chapter 19).

Atrophy

Atrophy is shrinkage in the size of cells by the loss of cell substance. When a sufficient number of cells are

involved, the entire tissue or organ is reduced in size, or atrophic (Fig. 2.22). Although atrophic cells may have diminished function, they are not dead.

Causes of atrophy include a decreased workload (e.g., immobilization of a limb to permit healing of a fracture), loss of innervation, diminished blood supply, inadequate nutrition, loss of endocrine stimulation, and aging (senile atrophy). Although some of these stimuli are physiologic (e.g., the loss of hormone stimulation in menopause) and others are pathologic (e.g., denervation), the fundamental cellular changes are similar. They represent a retreat by the cell to a smaller size at which survival is still possible; a new equilibrium is achieved between cell size and diminished blood supply, nutrition, or trophic stimulation.

Cellular atrophy results from a combination of decreased protein synthesis and increased protein degradation.

- Protein synthesis decreases because of reduced metabolic activity.
- The degradation of cellular proteins occurs mainly by the ubiquitin-proteasome pathway. Nutrient deficiency and disuse may activate ubiquitin ligases, which attach multiple copies of the small peptide ubiquitin to cellular proteins and target them for degradation in proteasomes. This pathway is also thought to be responsible for the accelerated proteolysis seen in a variety of catabolic conditions, including the cachexia associated with cancer.
- In many situations, atrophy also is associated with autophagy, with resulting increases in the number of autophagic vacuoles. As discussed previously, autophagy is the process in which the starved cell eats its own organelles in an attempt to survive.

Metaplasia

Metaplasia is a change in which one adult cell type (epithelial or mesenchymal) is replaced by another adult cell type. In this type of cellular adaptation, a cell type sensitive to a particular stress is replaced by another cell type better able to withstand the adverse environment. Metaplasia is thought to arise by the reprogramming of stem cells

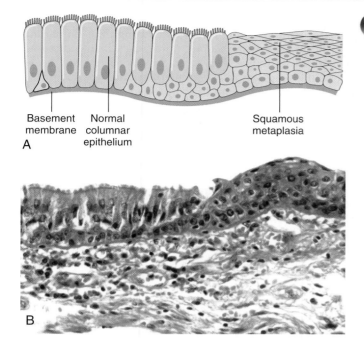

Fig. 2.23 Metaplasia of normal columnar *(left)* to squamous epithelium *(right)* in a bronchus, shown schematically (A) and histologically (B).

to differentiate along a new pathway rather than a phenotypic change (transdifferentiation) of already differentiated cells.

Epithelial metaplasia is exemplified by the change that occurs in the respiratory epithelium of habitual cigarette smokers, in whom the normal ciliated columnar epithelial cells of the trachea and bronchi often are replaced by stratified squamous epithelial cells (Fig. 2.23). The rugged stratified squamous epithelium may be able to survive the noxious chemicals in cigarette smoke that the more fragile specialized epithelium would not tolerate. Although the metaplastic squamous epithelium has survival advantages, important protective mechanisms are lost, such as mucus secretion and ciliary clearance of particulate matter. Epithelial metaplasia is therefore a double-edged sword. Because vitamin A is essential for normal epithelial differentiation, its deficiency also may induce squamous metaplasia in the respiratory epithelium.

Metaplasia need not always occur in the direction of columnar to squamous epithelium; in chronic gastric reflux, the normal stratified squamous epithelium of the lower esophagus may undergo metaplastic transformation to gastric or intestinal-type columnar epithelium. Metaplasia also may occur in mesenchymal cells, but in these situations it is generally a reaction to some pathologic alteration and not an adaptive response to stress. For example, bone is occasionally formed in soft tissues, particularly in foci of injury.

The influences that induce metaplastic change in an epithelium, if persistent, may predispose to malignant transformation. In fact, squamous metaplasia of the respiratory epithelium often coexists with lung cancers composed of malignant squamous cells. It is thought that cigarette smoking initially causes squamous metaplasia, and cancers arise later in some of these altered foci.

SUMMARY

CELLULAR ADAPTATIONS TO STRESS

- Hypertrophy: increased cell and organ size, often in response to increased workload; induced by growth factors produced in response to mechanical stress or other stimuli; occurs in tissues incapable of cell division
- Hyperplasia: increased cell numbers in response to hormones and other growth factors; occurs in tissues whose cells are able to divide or contain abundant tissue stem cells
- Atrophy: decreased cell and organ size, as a result of decreased nutrient supply or disuse; associated with decreased synthesis of cellular building blocks and increased breakdown of cellular organelles and autophagy
- Metaplasia: change in phenotype of differentiated cells, often in response to chronic irritation, that makes cells better able to withstand the stress; usually induced by altered differentiation pathway of tissue stem cells; may result in reduced functions or increased propensity for malignant transformation

INTRACELLULAR ACCUMULATIONS

Under some circumstances, cells may accumulate abnormal amounts of various substances, which may be harmless or may cause varying degrees of injury. The substance may be located in the cytoplasm, within organelles (typically lysosomes), or in the nucleus, and it may be synthesized by the affected cells or it may be produced elsewhere.

The main pathways of abnormal intracellular accumulations are inadequate removal and degradation or excessive production of an endogenous substance, or deposition of an abnormal exogenous material (Fig. 2.24). Selected examples of each are described as follows.

Fatty Change. Fatty change, also called steatosis, refers to any accumulation of triglycerides within parenchymal cells. It is most often seen in the liver, since this is the major organ involved in fat metabolism, but also may occur in heart, skeletal muscle, kidney, and other organs. Steatosis may be caused by toxins, protein malnutrition, diabetes mellitus, obesity, or anoxia. Alcohol abuse and diabetes associated with obesity are the most common causes of fatty change in the liver (fatty liver) in industrialized nations. This process is discussed in more detail in Chapter 16.

Cholesterol and Cholesteryl Esters. Cellular cholesterol metabolism is tightly regulated to ensure normal generation of cell membranes (in which cholesterol is a key component) without significant intracellular accumulation. However, phagocytic cells may become overloaded with lipid (triglycerides, cholesterol, and cholesteryl esters) in several different pathologic processes, mostly characterized by increased intake or decreased catabolism of lipids. Of these, atherosclerosis is the most important. The role of lipid and cholesterol deposition in the pathogenesis of atherosclerosis is discussed in Chapter 10.

Proteins. Morphologically visible protein accumulations are less common than lipid accumulations; they may occur when excesses are presented to the cells or if the cells

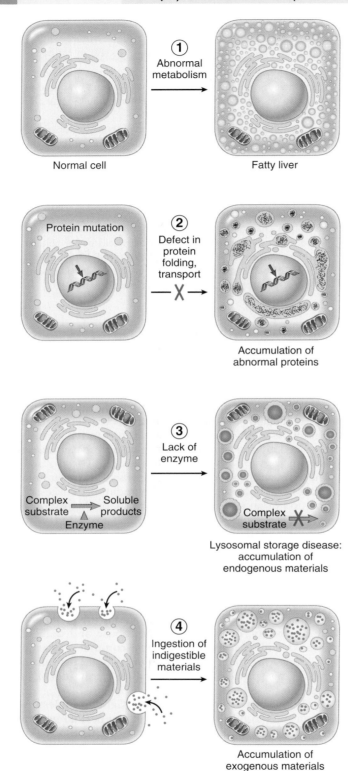

Fig. 2.24 Mechanisms of intracellular accumulation: *(1)* Abnormal metabolism, as in fatty change in the liver. *(2)* Mutations causing alterations in protein folding and transport, so that defective molecules accumulate intracellularly. *(3)* A deficiency of critical enzymes responsible for breaking down certain compounds, causing substrates to accumulate in lysosomes, as in lysosomal storage diseases. *(4)* An inability to degrade phagocytosed particles, as in carbon pigment accumulation.

synthesize excessive amounts. In the kidney, for example, trace amounts of albumin filtered through the glomerulus are normally reabsorbed by pinocytosis in the proximal convoluted tubules. However, in disorders with heavy protein leakage across the glomerular filter (e.g., nephrotic syndrome), much more of the protein is reabsorbed, and vesicles containing this protein accumulate, giving the histologic appearance of pink, hyaline cytoplasmic droplets. The process is reversible: if the proteinuria abates, the protein droplets are metabolized and disappear. Another example is the marked accumulation of newly synthesized immunoglobulins that may occur in the RER of some plasma cells, forming rounded, eosinophilic Russell bodies. Other examples of protein aggregation are discussed elsewhere in this book (e.g., "alcoholic hyaline" in the liver in Chapter 16; neurofibrillary tangles in neurons in Chapter 23).

Glycogen. Excessive intracellular deposits of glycogen are associated with abnormalities in the metabolism of either glucose or glycogen. In poorly controlled diabetes mellitus, the prime example of abnormal glucose metabolism, glycogen accumulates in renal tubular epithelium, cardiac myocytes, and β cells of the islets of Langerhans. Glycogen also accumulates within cells in a group of related genetic disorders collectively referred to as glycogen storage diseases, or glycogenoses (Chapter 7).

Pigments. Pigments are colored substances that are either exogenous, coming from outside the body, such as carbon, or are endogenous, synthesized within the body itself, such as lipofuscin, melanin, and certain derivatives of hemoglobin.

The most common exogenous pigment is *carbon*, a ubiquitous air pollutant of urban life. When inhaled, it is phagocytosed by alveolar macrophages and transported through lymphatic channels to the regional tracheobronchial lymph nodes. Aggregates of the pigment blacken the draining lymph nodes and pulmonary parenchyma (*anthracosis*) (Chapter 13).

- *Lipofuscin*, or "wear-and-tear pigment," is an insoluble brownish-yellow granular intracellular material that accumulates in a variety of tissues (particularly the heart, liver, and brain) with aging or atrophy. Lipofuscin represents complexes of lipid and protein that are produced by the free radical–catalyzed peroxidation of polyunsaturated lipids of subcellular membranes. It is not injurious to the cell but is a marker of past free radical injury. The brown pigment (Fig. 2.25), when present in large amounts, imparts an appearance to the tissue that is called brown atrophy.
- *Melanin* is an endogenous, brown-black pigment that is synthesized by melanocytes located in the epidermis and acts as a screen against harmful UV radiation. Although melanocytes are the only source of melanin, adjacent basal keratinocytes in the skin can accumulate the pigment (e.g., in freckles), as can dermal macrophages.
- *Hemosiderin* is a hemoglobin-derived granular pigment that is golden yellow to brown and accumulates in tissues when there is a local or systemic excess of iron. Iron is normally stored within cells in association with the protein apoferritin, forming ferritin micelles. Hemosiderin pigment represents large aggregates of these

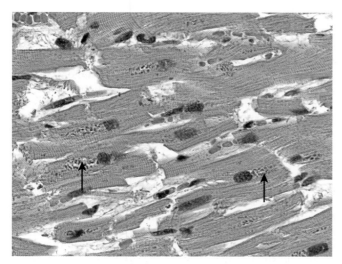

Fig. 2.25 Lipofuscin granules in cardiac myocytes (deposits indicated by *arrows*).

ferritin micelles, readily visualized by light and electron microscopy; the iron can be unambiguously identified by the Prussian blue histochemical reaction (Fig. 2.26). Although hemosiderin accumulation is usually pathologic, small amounts of this pigment are normal in the mononuclear phagocytes of the bone marrow, spleen, and liver, where aging red cells are normally degraded. Excessive deposition of hemosiderin, called hemosiderosis, and more extensive accumulations of iron seen in hereditary hemochromatosis are described in Chapter 16.

PATHOLOGIC CALCIFICATION

Pathologic calcification, a common process in a wide variety of disease states, is the result of an abnormal deposition of calcium salts, together with smaller amounts of iron, magnesium, and other minerals. It can occur in two ways.

* *Dystrophic calcification*. In this form, calcium metabolism is normal but it *deposits in injured or dead tissue*, such as

areas of necrosis of any type. It is virtually ubiquitous in the arterial lesions of advanced atherosclerosis (Chapter 10). Although dystrophic calcification may be an incidental finding indicating insignificant past cell injury, it also may be a cause of organ dysfunction. For example, calcification can develop in aging or damaged heart valves, resulting in severely compromised valve motion. Dystrophic calcification of the aortic valves is an important cause of aortic stenosis in elderly persons (Chapter 11).

Dystrophic calcification is initiated by the extracellular deposition of crystalline calcium phosphate in membrane-bound vesicles, which may be derived from injured cells, or the intracellular deposition of calcium in the mitochondria of dying cells. It is thought that the extracellular calcium is concentrated in vesicles by its affinity for membrane phospholipids, whereas phosphates accumulate as a result of the action of membrane-bound phosphatases. The crystals are then propagated, forming larger deposits.

* *Metastatic calcification*. This form is *associated with hypercalcemia* and can occur in normal tissues. The major causes of hypercalcemia are (1) *increased secretion of parathyroid hormone*, due to either primary parathyroid tumors or production of parathyroid hormone–related protein by other malignant tumors; (2) *destruction of bone* due to the effects of accelerated turnover (e.g., Paget disease), immobilization, or tumors (increased bone catabolism associated with multiple myeloma, leukemia, or diffuse skeletal metastases); (3) *vitamin D–related disorders* including vitamin D intoxication and *sarcoidosis* (in which macrophages activate a vitamin D precursor); and (4) renal failure, in which phosphate retention leads to secondary hyperparathyroidism.

MORPHOLOGY

Regardless of the site, calcium salts are seen on gross examination as fine white granules or clumps, often felt as gritty deposits. Dystrophic calcification is common in areas of caseous necrosis in tuberculosis. Sometimes a tuberculous lymph node is essentially converted to radiopaque stone. On histologic examination,

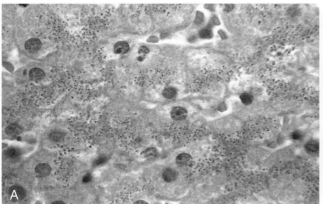
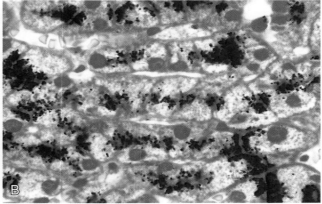

Fig. 2.26 Hemosiderin granules in liver cells. (A) Hematoxylin-eosin–stained section showing golden-brown, finely granular pigment. (B) Iron deposits shown by a special staining process called the Prussian blue reaction.

calcification appears as intracellular and/or extracellular basophilic deposits. With time, heterotopic bone may form in foci of calcification.

Metastatic calcification can occur widely throughout the body but principally affects the interstitial tissues of the vasculature, kidneys, lungs, and gastric mucosa. The calcium deposits morphologically resemble those described in dystrophic calcification. Although they generally do not cause clinical dysfunction, extensive calcifications in the lungs may be evident on radiographs and may produce respiratory deficits, and massive deposits in the kidney (nephrocalcinosis) can lead to renal damage.

SUMMARY

ABNORMAL INTRACELLULAR DEPOSITIONS AND CALCIFICATIONS

- Abnormal deposits of materials in cells and tissues are the result of excessive intake or defective transport or catabolism.
  - Depositions of lipids
    - Fatty change: accumulation of free triglycerides in cells, resulting from excessive intake or defective transport (often because of defects in synthesis of transport proteins); manifestation of reversible cell injury
    - Cholesterol deposition: result of defective catabolism and excessive intake; seen in macrophages and smooth muscle cells of vessel walls in atherosclerosis
  - Deposition of proteins: reabsorbed proteins in kidney tubules; immunoglobulins in plasma cells
  - Deposition of glycogen: in macrophages of patients with defects in lysosomal enzymes that break down glycogen (glycogen storage diseases)
  - Deposition of pigments: typically indigestible pigments, such as carbon, lipofuscin (breakdown product of lipid peroxidation), or iron (usually resulting from overload, as in hemosiderosis)
- Pathologic calcifications
  - Dystrophic calcification: deposition of calcium at sites of cell injury and necrosis
  - Metastatic calcification: deposition of calcium in normal tissues, caused by hypercalcemia (usually a consequence of parathyroid hormone excess)

CELLULAR AGING

Individuals age because their cells age. Although public attention on the aging process has traditionally focused on its cosmetic manifestations, aging has important health consequences, because age is one of the strongest independent risk factors for many chronic diseases, such as cancer, Alzheimer disease, and ischemic heart disease. Perhaps one of the most striking discoveries about cellular aging is that it is not simply a consequence of cells' "running out of steam," but in fact is regulated by a limited number of genes and signaling pathways that are evolutionarily conserved from yeast to mammals.

Cellular aging is the result of a progressive decline in the life span and functional activity of cells. Several abnormalities contribute to the aging of cells (Fig. 2.27):

- *Accumulation of mutations in DNA.* A variety of metabolic insults over time may result in damage to nuclear and mitochondrial DNA. ROS induced by toxins and radiation exposure contribute to DNA damage associated with aging. Although most DNA damage is repaired by DNA repair enzymes, some persists and accumulates as cells age, especially if repair mechanisms become inefficient over time. Accumulation of mutations in nuclear and mitochondrial DNA ultimately compromise the functional activities and survival of cells.
- *Decreased cellular replication.* Normal cells (other than stem cells) have a limited capacity for replication, and after a fixed number of divisions, they become arrested in a terminally nondividing state, known as replicative senescence. Aging is associated with progressive replicative senescence of cells. Cells from children have the capacity to undergo more rounds of replication than do cells from older people. In contrast, cells from patients with Werner syndrome, a rare disease characterized by premature aging, have a markedly reduced in vitro life span.

Replicative senescence occurs in aging cells because of progressive shortening of telomeres, which ultimately results in cell cycle arrest. *Telomeres* are short repeated sequences of DNA present at the ends of chromosomes that are important for ensuring the complete replication of chromosome ends and for protecting the ends from fusion and degradation. Telomeric DNA also binds proteins that shield it, preventing activation of a DNA damage response. When somatic cells replicate, a small section of the telomere is not duplicated, and telomeres become progressively shortened. As they shorten, the ends of chromosomes cannot be protected and are sensed in cells as broken DNA, which signals cell cycle arrest. Telomere length is maintained by nucleotide addition mediated by an enzyme called *telomerase*. Telomerase is a specialized RNA-protein complex that uses its own RNA as a template for adding nucleotides to the ends of chromosomes. Telomerase is expressed in germ cells and is present at low levels in stem cells, but absent in most somatic cells (Fig. 2.28). Therefore, as mature somatic cells age, their telomeres become shorter and they exit the cell cycle, resulting in an inability to generate new cells to replace damaged ones. Conversely, in immortalized cancer cells, telomerase is usually reactivated and telomere length is stabilized, allowing the cells to proliferate indefinitely. This is discussed more fully in Chapter 6. Telomere shortening also may decrease the regenerative capacity of stem cells, further contributing to cellular aging. Despite such alluring observations, however, the relationship of telomerase activity and telomere length to aging has yet to be fully established. Abnormalities in telomere maintenance have been implicated in many diseases, such as aplastic anemia and other cytopenias (thought to be caused by a failure of hematopoietic stem cells), premature greying of hair, skin pigment and nail abnormalities, pulmonary and liver fibrosis, and others.

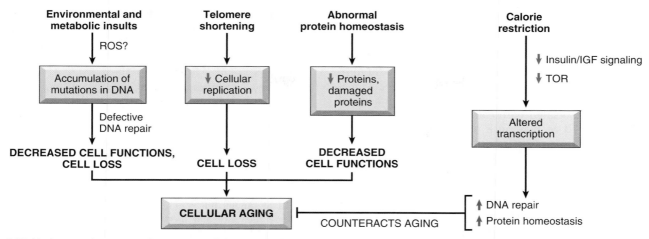

Fig. 2.27 Mechanisms that cause and counteract cellular aging. DNA damage, replicative senescence, and decreased and misfolded proteins are among the best-described mechanisms of cellular aging. Some environmental influences, such as calorie restriction, counteract aging by activating various signaling pathways and transcription factors. *IGF,* Insulin-like growth factor; *ROS,* reactive oxygen species; *TOR,* target of rapamycin.

These disorders are sometimes considered the prototypic "telomeropathies."

- *Defective protein homeostasis.* With the passage of time, cells are unable to maintain normal protein homeostasis, because of increased turnover and decreased synthesis caused by reduced translation of proteins and defective activity of chaperones (which promote normal protein folding) and proteasomes (which destroy misfolded

proteins). The resultant decrease in intracellular proteins can have many deleterious effects on cell survival, replication, and functions. The concomitant accumulation of misfolded proteins exacerbates the loss of functional proteins and can trigger apoptosis.

- There has been great interest in defining biochemical signaling pathways that counteract the aging process, not only because of their obvious therapeutic potential

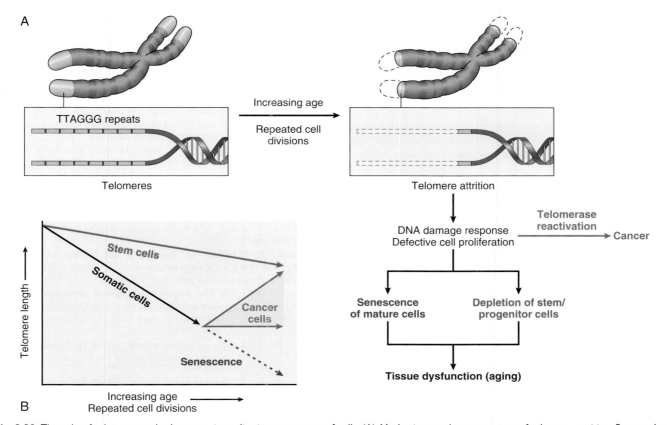

Fig. 2.28 The role of telomeres and telomerase in replicative senescence of cells. (A) Mechanisms and consequences of telomere attrition. Repeated cell division associated with aging leads to progressive shortening of telomeres, which triggers senescence and loss of stem cell pools. (B) Telomere attrition is characteristic of somatic cells. Stem cells maintain their telomeres and are, therefore, capable of more cycles of replication. Cancer cells frequently activate telomerase and are thus able to maintain telomeres.

(the search for the "elixir of youth") but also because elucidating these pathways might tell us about the mechanisms that cause aging. Calorie restriction has been found to slow down aging and prolong life in every species tested from flies to mice. It is now thought that calorie restriction alters signaling pathways that influence aging (Fig. 2.27). Among the biochemical alterations associated with calorie restriction that have been described as playing a role in counteracting the aging process is reduced activation of insulin-like growth factor receptor signaling, which involves a downstream network of kinases and transcription factors. Reduced IGF-1 signaling leads to lower rates of cell growth and metabolism and possibly reduced errors in DNA replication, better DNA repair and improve protein homeostasis. Calorie restriction also serves to improve immunity. All of these inhibit aging.

- *Persistent inflammation.* As individuals age, the accumulation of damaged cells, lipids, and other endogenous substances may activate the inflammasome pathway (Chapter 5), resulting in persistent low-level inflammation. Inflammation in turn induces chronic diseases, such as atherosclerosis and type 2 diabetes. Cytokines produced during inflammatory reactions may themselves induce cellular alterations that exacerbate aging, and chronic metabolic disorders may accelerate the aging process.

Clinical observations and epidemiologic studies have shown that physical activity and, as mentioned previously, calorie restriction slow the aging process, whereas stresses, perhaps acting via increased production of glucocorticoids, accelerate aging. Alas, the precise mechanisms underlying these effects remain to be defined, and for now we all remain vulnerable to the ravages of age.

SUMMARY

CELLULAR AGING

- Results from a combination of multiple, progressive cellular alterations, including:
- Accumulation of DNA damage and mutations
- Replicative senescence: reduced capacity of cells to divide secondary to progressive shortening of chromosomal ends (telomeres)
- Defective protein homeostasis: loss of normal proteins and accumulation of misfolded proteins
- Aging is exacerbated by chronic diseases, especially those associated with prolonged inflammation, and by stress, and is slowed down by calorie restriction and exercise.

It should be apparent that the various forms of cellular derangements and adaptations described in this chapter cover a wide spectrum, ranging from reversible and irreversible forms of acute cell injury, to adaptations in cell size, growth, and function, to largely unavoidable consequences of aging. Reference is made to these many different alterations throughout this book, because all instances of organ injury and ultimately all cases of clinical disease arise from derangements in cell structure and function.

SUGGESTED READINGS

Calado RT, Young NS: Telomere diseases, *N Engl J Med* 361:2353, 2009. *[An excellent review of the basic biology of telomeres, and how their abnormalities may contribute to cancer, aging, and other diseases.]*

Chipuk JE, Moldoveanu T, Llambl F, et al: The BCL-2 family reunion, *Mol Cell* 37:299, 2010. *[A review of the biochemistry and biology of the BCL-2 family of apoptosis-regulating proteins.]*

Choi AMK, Ryter S, Levine B: Autophagy in human health and disease, *N Engl J Med* 368:7, 2013. *[An excellent discussion of the mechanisms and significance of autophagy.]*

Conrad M, Angeli JPF, Vandenabeele P, et al: Regulated necrosis: disease relevance and therapeutic opportunities, *Nat Rev Drug Discov*, 15:348, 2016. *[A review of newly discovered pathways of cell death and possible therapeutic interventions.]*

Dong Z, Saikumar P, Weinberg JM, et al: Calcium in cell injury and death, *Ann Rev Pathol* 1:405, 2006. *[A review of the links between calcium and cell injury.]*

Frey N, Olson EN: Cardiac hypertrophy: the good, the bad, and the ugly, *Annu Rev Physiol* 65:45, 2003. *[Excellent discussion of the mechanisms of muscle hypertrophy, using the heart as the paradigm.]*

Hotchkiss RS, Strasser A, McDunn JE, et al: Cell death, *N Engl J Med* 361:1570, 2009. *[Excellent review of the major pathways of cell death (necrosis, apoptosis, and autophagy-associated death), and their clinical implications and therapeutic targeting.]*

Kenyon CJ: The genetics of ageing, *Nature* 464:504, 2010. *[An excellent review of the genes that influence aging, based on human genetic syndromes and studies with mutant model organisms.]*

Lambeth JD, Neish AS: Nox enzymes and new thinking on reactive oxygen: a double-edged sword revisited, *Ann Rev Pathol Mech Dis* 9:47, 2014. *[A discussion of reactive oxygen species and their roles in physiology and cell injury.]*

Lopez-Otin C, Blasco MA, Partridge L, et al: The hallmarks of aging, *Cell* 153:1194, 2013. *[A landmark review that suggests nine hallmarks of aging and directions for future research.]*

Marquez FC, Volovik Y, Cohen E: The roles of cellular and organismal aging in the development of late-onset maladies, *Ann Rev Pathol Mech Dis* 10:1, 2015. *[A review of the many ways by which cellular aging contributes to the development of chronic diseases.]*

McKinnell IW, Rudnicki MA: Molecular mechanisms of muscle atrophy, *Cell* 119:907, 2004. *[Discussion of the mechanisms of cellular atrophy.]*

Nathan C, Cunningham-Bussel A: Beyond oxidative stress: an immunologist's guide to reactive oxygen species, *Nat Rev Immunol* 13:349, 2013. *[An excellent modern review of the production, catabolism, targets, and actions of reactive oxygen species, and their roles in inflammation.]*

Newgard CB, Sharpless NE: Coming of age: molecular drivers of aging and therapeutic opportunities, *J Clin Invest* 3:946, 2013. *[A summary of key molecular pathways in aging.]*

Oakes SA, Papa FR: The role of endoplasmic reticulum stress in human pathology, *Ann Rev Pathol Mech Dis* 10:173, 2015. *[An up-to-date review of the unfolded protein response and the pathogenic importance of cell injury caused by misfolded proteins.]*

Tosh D, Slack JM: How cells change their phenotype, *Nat Rev Mol Cell Biol* 3:187, 2002. *[Review of metaplasia and the roles of stem cells and genetic reprogramming.]*

Vanden Berghe T, Linkermann A, Jouan-Lanhouet S, et al: Regulated necrosis: the expanding network of non-apoptotic cell death pathways, *Nat Rev Mol Cell Biol* 15:135, 2014. *[A current review of various forms of programmed non-apoptotic pathways of cell death.]*

Inflammation and Repair

CHAPTER OUTLINE

Overview of Inflammation: Definitions
  and General Features 57
Causes of Inflammation 59
Recognition of Microbes and Damaged
  Cells 59
Acute Inflammation 60
*Reactions of Blood Vessels in Acute
  Inflammation 60*
*Leukocyte Recruitment to Sites of
  Inflammation 62*
*Phagocytosis and Clearance of the Offending
  Agent 66*
Leukocyte-Mediated Tissue Injury 69
*Other Functional Responses of Activated
  Leukocytes 70*

*Termination of the Acute Inflammatory
  Response 70*
Mediators of Inflammation 70
Vasoactive Amines: Histamine and Serotonin 71
Arachidonic Acid Metabolites 71
Cytokines and Chemokines 73
Complement System 75
Other Mediators of Inflammation 77
Morphologic Patterns of Acute
  Inflammation 78
Serous Inflammation 78
Fibrinous Inflammation 78
Purulent (Suppurative) Inflammation, Abscess 78
Ulcers 79
Outcomes of Acute Inflammation 79

Chronic Inflammation 81
Causes of Chronic Inflammation 81
Morphologic Features 81
*Cells and Mediators of Chronic
  Inflammation 82*
Systemic Effects of Inflammation 86
Tissue Repair 87
Overview of Tissue Repair 87
Cell and Tissue Regeneration 88
Repair by Scarring 89
Factors That Impair Tissue Repair 93
*Clinical Examples of Abnormal Wound Healing
  and Scarring 93*

OVERVIEW OF INFLAMMATION: DEFINITIONS AND GENERAL FEATURES

Inflammation is a response of vascularized tissues to infections and tissue damage that brings cells and molecules of host defense from the circulation to the sites where they are needed, to eliminate the offending agents. Although in common medical and lay parlance, inflammation suggests a harmful reaction, it is actually a protective response that is essential for survival. It serves to rid the host of both the initial cause of cell injury (e.g., microbes, toxins) and the consequences of such injury (e.g., necrotic cells and tissues). The mediators of defense include phagocytic leukocytes, antibodies, and complement proteins (Fig. 3.1). Most of these normally circulate in the blood, where they are sequestered so they cannot damage normal tissues but can be rapidly recruited to any site in the body. Some of the cells involved in inflammatory responses also reside in tissues, where they function as sentinels on the lookout for threats. The process of inflammation delivers leukocytes and proteins to foreign invaders, such as microbes, and to damaged or necrotic tissues, and it activates the recruited cells and molecules, which then function to eliminate the harmful or unwanted substances. Without inflammation, infections would go unchecked, wounds would never

heal, and injured tissues might remain permanent festering sores.

The typical inflammatory reaction develops through a series of sequential steps:
- The offending agent, which is located in extravascular tissues, is recognized by host cells and molecules.
- Leukocytes and plasma proteins are recruited from the circulation to the site where the offending agent is located.
- The leukocytes and proteins are activated and work together to destroy and eliminate the offending substance.
- The reaction is controlled and terminated.
- The damaged tissue is repaired.

Inflammation may be of two types, acute and chronic (Table 3.1). The initial, rapid response to infections and tissue damage is called *acute inflammation*. It typically develops within minutes or hours and is of short duration, lasting for several hours or a few days. Its main characteristics are the exudation of fluid and plasma proteins (edema) and the emigration of leukocytes, predominantly neutrophils (also called polymorphonuclear leukocytes). When acute inflammation achieves its desired goal of eliminating the offenders, the reaction subsides and residual injury is repaired. But if the initial response fails to clear the stimulus, the reaction progresses to a protracted type

STIMULUS

PRODUCTION OF MEDIATORS

INFLUX OF LEUKOCYTES, PLASMA PROTEINS

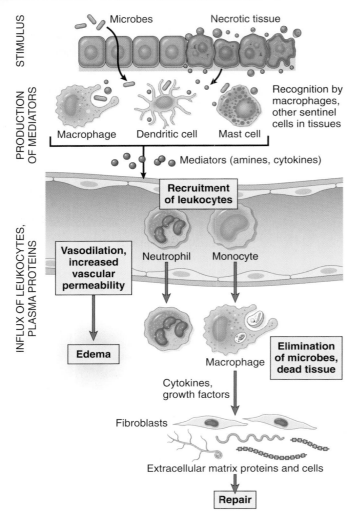

Microbes   Necrotic tissue

Recognition by macrophages, other sentinel cells in tissues

Macrophage   Dendritic cell   Mast cell

Mediators (amines, cytokines)

Recruitment of leukocytes

Vasodilation, increased vascular permeability

Neutrophil   Monocyte

Edema

Macrophage

Elimination of microbes, dead tissue

Cytokines, growth factors

Fibroblasts

Extracellular matrix proteins and cells

Repair

Fig. 3.1 Sequence of events in an inflammatory reaction. Macrophages and other cells in tissues recognize microbes and damaged cells and liberate mediators, which trigger the vascular and cellular reactions of inflammation. Recruitment of plasma proteins from the blood is not shown.

Table 3.1 Features of Acute and Chronic Inflammation

Feature	Acute	Chronic
Onset	Fast: minutes or hours	Slow: days
Cellular infiltrate	Mainly neutrophils	Monocytes/macrophages and lymphocytes
Tissue injury, fibrosis	Usually mild and self-limited	May be severe and progressive
Local and systemic signs	Prominent	Less

injured, the presence of the infection or damage is sensed by resident cells, including macrophages, dendritic cells, mast cells, and other cell types. These cells secrete molecules (cytokines and other mediators) that induce and regulate the subsequent inflammatory response. Inflammatory mediators are also produced from plasma proteins that react to the microbes or to products of necrotic cells. Some of these mediators promote the efflux of plasma and the recruitment of circulating leukocytes to the site where the offending agent is located. Mediators also activate the recruited leukocytes, enhancing their ability to destroy and remove the offending agent. Understanding the role of chemical mediators is important because most anti-inflammatory drugs target specific mediators. We shall discuss the mediators of inflammation in detail later, after we review the main steps in inflammatory reactions.

The external manifestations of inflammation, often called its cardinal signs, are heat (calor in Latin), redness (rubor), swelling (tumor), pain (dolor), and loss of function (functio laesa). The first four of these were described more than 2000 years ago by a Roman encyclopedist named Celsus, who wrote the then-famous text De Medicina, and the fifth was added in the late 19th century by Rudolf Virchow, known as the "father of modern pathology." These manifestations occur as consequences of the vascular changes and leukocyte recruitment and activation, as will be evident from the discussion that follows.

Although normally protective, **in some situations, the inflammatory reaction becomes the cause of disease, and the damage it produces is its dominant feature.** For example, inflammatory reactions to infections are often accompanied by local tissue damage and its associated signs and symptoms (e.g., pain and functional impairment). Typically, however, these harmful consequences are self-limited and resolve as the inflammation abates, leaving little or no permanent damage. In contrast, there are many diseases in which the inflammatory reaction is misdirected (e.g., against self tissues in autoimmune diseases), occurs against normally harmless environmental substances that evoke an immune response (e.g., in allergies), or is excessively prolonged (e.g., in infections by microbes that resist eradication).

Inflammatory reactions underlie common chronic diseases, such as rheumatoid arthritis, atherosclerosis, and lung fibrosis, as well as life-threatening hypersensitivity reactions to insect bites, drugs, and toxins (Table 3.2). For this reason our pharmacies abound with anti-inflammatory drugs, which ideally would control the harmful sequelae of inflammation yet not interfere with its beneficial effects. In fact, inflammation may contribute to a variety of diseases that are thought to be primarily metabolic, degenerative, or genetic disorders, such as type 2 diabetes, Alzheimer disease, and cancer. Hence, anti-inflammatory drugs may well have a broader role than currently indicated. In recognition of the wide-ranging harmful consequences of inflammation, the lay press has rather melodramatically referred to it as "the silent killer."

Not only excessive inflammation but also defective inflammation is responsible for serious illness. Too little inflammation, which is typically manifested by increased susceptibility to infections, is most often caused by a reduced number of leukocytes resulting from replacement of the bone marrow by cancers and suppression of the

of inflammation that is called *chronic inflammation*. As discussed later in this chapter, chronic inflammation may follow acute inflammation or arise de novo. It is of longer duration and is associated with more tissue destruction, the presence of lymphocytes and macrophages, the proliferation of blood vessels, and fibrosis.

Inflammation is induced by chemical mediators that are produced by host cells in response to injurious stimuli. When a microbe enters a tissue or the tissue is

Table 3.2 Disorders Caused by Inflammatory Reactions

Disorders	Cells and Molecules Involved in Injury
Acute	
Acute respiratory distress syndrome	Neutrophils
Asthma	Eosinophils; IgE antibodies
Glomerulonephritis	Antibodies and complement; neutrophils, monocytes
Septic shock	Cytokines
Chronic	
Arthritis	Lymphocytes, macrophages; antibodies?
Asthma	Eosinophils; IgE antibodies
Atherosclerosis	Macrophages; lymphocytes
Pulmonary fibrosis	Macrophages; fibroblasts

Listed are selected examples of diseases in which the inflammatory response plays a significant role in tissue injury. Some, such as asthma, can present with acute inflammation or a chronic illness with repeated bouts of acute exacerbation. These diseases and their pathogenesis are discussed in relevant chapters.

marrow by therapies for cancer and graft rejection. Recall that leukocytes, the cells of the inflammatory response, arise from progenitors in the bone marrow, hence any compromise of marrow function will diminish the generation of mature leukocytes. Inherited genetic abnormalities of leukocyte function are rare disorders but they provide valuable information about the mechanisms of leukocyte responses. These conditions are described in Chapter 5, in the context of immunodeficiency diseases.

Inflammation is terminated when the offending agent is eliminated. The reaction resolves because mediators are broken down and dissipated, and leukocytes have short life spans in tissues. In addition, anti-inflammatory mechanisms are activated, serving to control the response and prevent it from causing excessive damage to the host. After inflammation has achieved its goal of eliminating the offending agents, it sets into motion the process of *tissue repair*. Repair consists of a series of events that heal damaged tissue. In this process, the injured tissue is replaced through *regeneration* of surviving cells and filling of residual defects with connective tissue *(scarring)*.

This chapter describes the etiology of and stimuli for inflammation, and then the sequence of events, mediators, and morphologic patterns of acute inflammation. This is followed by a discussion of chronic inflammation, and then the process of tissue repair.

CAUSES OF INFLAMMATION

Inflammatory reactions may be triggered by a variety of stimuli:

- **Infections** (bacterial, viral, fungal, parasitic) and microbial toxins are among the most common and medically important causes of inflammation. Different infectious pathogens elicit distinct inflammatory responses, from mild acute inflammation that causes little or no lasting damage and successfully eradicates the infection, to severe systemic reactions that can be fatal, to prolonged chronic reactions that cause extensive tissue injury. The

morphologic pattern of the response can be useful in identifying its etiology, as discussed later in this chapter.

- **Tissue necrosis** elicits inflammation regardless of the cause of cell death, which may include *ischemia* (reduced blood flow, the cause of myocardial infarction), *trauma*, and *physical and chemical injury* (e.g., thermal injury, as in burns or frostbite; irradiation; exposure to some environmental chemicals). Several molecules released from necrotic cells are known to trigger inflammation; some of these are described later.
- **Foreign bodies** (splinters, dirt, sutures) may elicit inflammation by themselves or because they cause traumatic tissue injury or carry microbes. Even some endogenous substances stimulate potentially harmful inflammation if large amounts are deposited in tissues; such substances include urate crystals (in the disease gout), and cholesterol crystals (in atherosclerosis).
- **Immune reactions** (also called *hypersensitivity*) are reactions in which the normally protective immune system damages the individual's own tissues. The injurious immune responses may be directed against self antigens, causing *autoimmune diseases*, or may be inappropriate reactions against environmental substances, as in *allergies*, or against microbes. Inflammation is a major cause of tissue injury in these diseases (Chapter 5). Because the stimuli for the inflammatory responses in autoimmune and allergic diseases (self and environmental antigens) cannot be eliminated, these reactions tend to be persistent and difficult to cure, are often associated with chronic inflammation, and are important causes of morbidity and mortality.

RECOGNITION OF MICROBES AND DAMAGED CELLS

The first step in inflammatory responses is the recognition of microbes and necrotic cells by cellular receptors and circulating proteins. The cells and receptors that recognize invaders evolved as adaptations of multicellular organisms to the presence of microbes in the environment, and the responses they trigger are critical for survival.

- *Cellular receptors for microbes.* Phagocytes, dendritic cells (cells in epithelia and all tissues whose function is to capture microbes), and many other cells express receptors that detect the presence of infectious pathogens. The best defined of these receptors belong to the family of *Toll-like receptors (TLRs)*, which are named for the founding member, *Toll*, a gene that was discovered in Drosophila (Chapter 5). TLRs are located in plasma membranes and endosomes, so they are able to detect extracellular and ingested microbes. Other microbial sensors are present in the cytoplasm of cells. TLRs recognize motifs common to many microbes, often called pathogen-associated molecular patterns (PAMPs). Recognition of microbes by these receptors stimulates the production and expression of a number of secreted and membrane proteins. These proteins include cytokines that induce inflammation, anti-viral cytokines (interferons), and cytokines and membrane proteins that promote lymphocyte activation and even more potent immune responses. We will return to TLRs in more detail in Chapter 5, when we discuss innate immunity, the early defense against infections.

- *Sensors of cell damage.* All cells have cytosolic receptors that recognize molecules that are liberated or altered as a consequence of cell damage, and are hence appropriately called damage-associated molecular patterns (DAMPs). These molecules include uric acid (a product of DNA breakdown), ATP (released from damaged mitochondria), reduced intracellular K^+ concentrations (reflecting loss of ions because of plasma membrane injury), DNA (when it is released into the cytoplasm and not sequestered in nuclei, as it should be normally), and many others. The receptors activate a multiprotein cytosolic complex called the *inflammasome*, which induces the production of the cytokine interleukin-1 (IL-1). IL-1 recruits leukocytes and thus induces inflammation (discussed later). Gain-of-function mutations in the cytosolic receptors are the cause of rare diseases known as *autoinflammatory syndromes* that are characterized by spontaneous inflammation; IL-1 antagonists are effective treatments for these disorders. The inflammasome also has been implicated in inflammatory reactions to urate crystals (the cause of gout), cholesterol crystals (in atherosclerosis), lipids (in metabolic syndrome and obesity-associated diabetes), and amyloid deposits in the brain (in Alzheimer disease). These disorders are discussed in relevant chapters.
- *Circulating proteins.* Several plasma proteins recognize microbes and function to destroy blood-borne microbes and to stimulate inflammation at tissue sites of infection. The *complement system* reacts against microbes and produces mediators of inflammation (discussed later). A circulating protein called *mannose-binding lectin* recognizes microbial sugars and promotes ingestion of microbes and activation of the complement system. Other proteins called *collectins* also bind to microbes and promote their phagocytosis.

SUMMARY

GENERAL FEATURES AND CAUSES OF INFLAMMATION

- Inflammation is a beneficial host response to foreign invaders and necrotic tissue, but also may cause tissue damage.
- The main components of inflammation are a vascular reaction and a cellular response; both are activated by mediators that are derived from plasma proteins and various cells.
- The steps of the inflammatory response can be remembered as the five Rs: (1) recognition of the injurious agent, (2) recruitment of leukocytes, (3) removal of the agent, (4) regulation (control) of the response, and (5) resolution (repair).
- The causes of inflammation include infections, tissue necrosis, foreign bodies, trauma, and immune responses.
- Epithelial cells, tissue macrophages and dendritic cells, leukocytes, and other cell types express receptors that sense the presence of microbes and necrotic cells. Circulating proteins recognize microbes that have entered the blood.
- The outcome of acute inflammation is either elimination of the noxious stimulus followed by decline of the reaction and repair of the damaged tissue, or persistent injury resulting in chronic inflammation.

ACUTE INFLAMMATION

Acute inflammation has three major components: (1) dilation of small vessels, leading to an increase in blood flow, (2) increased permeability of the microvasculature, enabling plasma proteins and leukocytes to leave the circulation, and (3) emigration of the leukocytes from the microcirculation, their accumulation in the focus of injury, and their activation to eliminate the offending agent (Fig. 3.1). When an injurious agent, such as an infectious microbe or dead cells, is encountered, phagocytes that reside in all tissues try to eliminate these agents. At the same time, phagocytes and other sentinel cells in the tissues recognize the presence of the foreign or abnormal substance and react by liberating soluble molecules that mediate inflammation. Some of these mediators act on small blood vessels in the vicinity and promote the efflux of plasma and the recruitment of circulating leukocytes to the site where the offending agent is located.

Reactions of Blood Vessels in Acute Inflammation

The vascular reactions of acute inflammation consist of changes in the flow of blood and the permeability of vessels, both designed to maximize the movement of plasma proteins and leukocytes out of the circulation and into the site of infection or injury. The escape of fluid, proteins, and blood cells from the vascular system into interstitial tissues or body cavities is known as *exudation* (Fig. 3.2). An *exudate* is an extravascular fluid that has a high protein concentration and contains cellular debris. Its presence implies that there is an increase in the permeability of small blood vessels, typically during an inflammatory reaction. In contrast, a *transudate* is a fluid with low protein content, little or no cellular material, and low specific gravity. It is essentially an ultrafiltrate of blood plasma that is produced as a result of osmotic or hydrostatic imbalance across vessels with normal vascular permeability (Chapter 4). *Edema* denotes an excess of fluid in the interstitial tissue or serous cavities; it can be either an exudate or a transudate. *Pus*, a *purulent* exudate, is an inflammatory exudate rich in leukocytes (mostly neutrophils), the debris of dead cells, and, in many cases, microbes.

Changes in Vascular Flow and Caliber

Changes in vascular flow and caliber begin early after injury and consist of the following:

- Vasodilation is induced by the action of several mediators, notably histamine, on vascular smooth muscle. It is one of the earliest manifestations of acute inflammation, and may be preceded by transient vasoconstriction. Vasodilation first involves the arterioles and then leads to the opening of new capillary beds in the area. The result is *increased blood flow*, which is the cause of heat and redness (*erythema*) at the site of inflammation.
- Vasodilation is quickly followed by increased permeability of the microvasculature, with the outpouring of protein-rich fluid (an exudate) into the extravascular tissues.
- The loss of fluid and increased vessel diameter lead to slower blood flow, concentration of red cells in small

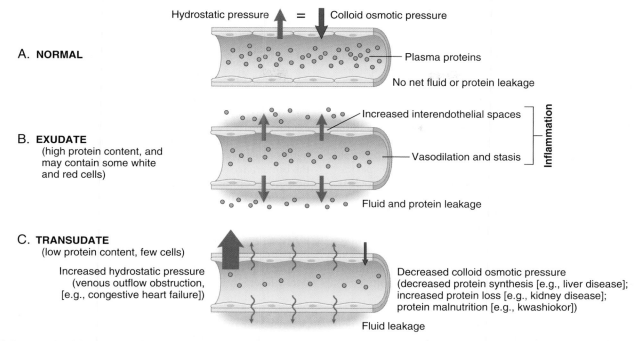

Hydrostatic pressure ⬆ = ⬇ Colloid osmotic pressure

A. **NORMAL**

Plasma proteins

No net fluid or protein leakage

B. **EXUDATE**
(high protein content, and
may contain some white
and red cells)

Increased interendothelial spaces

Vasodilation and stasis

Inflammation

Fluid and protein leakage

C. **TRANSUDATE**
(low protein content, few cells)

Increased hydrostatic pressure
(venous outflow obstruction,
[e.g., congestive heart failure])

Decreased colloid osmotic pressure
(decreased protein synthesis [e.g., liver disease];
increased protein loss [e.g., kidney disease];
protein malnutrition [e.g., kwashiokor])

Fluid leakage

Fig. 3.2 Formation of exudates and transudates. (A) Normal hydrostatic pressure *(blue arrow)* is about 32 mm Hg at the arterial end of a capillary bed and 12 mm Hg at the venous end; the mean colloid osmotic pressure of tissues is approximately 25 mm Hg *(green arrow)*, which is equal to the mean capillary pressure. Therefore, the net flow of fluid across the vascular bed is almost nil. (B) An exudate is formed in inflammation because vascular permeability increases as a result of retraction of endothelial cells, creating spaces through which fluid and proteins can pass. (C) A transudate is formed when fluid leaks out because of increased hydrostatic pressure or decreased osmotic pressure.

vessels, and increased viscosity of the blood. These changes result in stasis of blood flow, engorgement of small vessels jammed with slowly moving red cells, seen histologically as *vascular congestion* and externally as localized redness (*erythema*) of the involved tissue.

- As stasis develops, blood leukocytes, principally neutrophils, accumulate along the vascular endothelium. At the same time endothelial cells are activated by mediators produced at sites of infection and tissue damage, and express increased levels of adhesion molecules. Leukocytes then adhere to the endothelium, and soon afterward they migrate through the vascular wall into the interstitial tissue, in a sequence that is described later.

Increased Vascular Permeability (Vascular Leakage)

Several mechanisms are responsible for increased vascular permeability in acute inflammation (Fig. 3.3), which include:

- *Retraction of endothelial cells* resulting in opening of interendothelial spaces is the most common mechanism of vascular leakage. It is elicited by histamine, bradykinin, leukotrienes, and other chemical mediators. It occurs rapidly after exposure to the mediator (within 15 to 30 minutes) and is usually short-lived; hence, it is referred to as the immediate transient response, to distinguish it from the delayed prolonged response that follows endothelial injury, described next. The main sites for this rapid increase in vascular permeability are postcapillary venules.

- *Endothelial injury,* resulting in endothelial cell necrosis and detachment. Direct damage to the endothelium is encountered in severe injuries, for example, in burns, or is induced by the actions of microbes and microbial

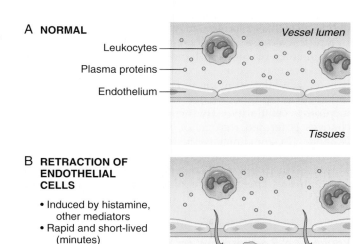

A **NORMAL**

Leukocytes

Plasma proteins

Endothelium

Vessel lumen

Tissues

B **RETRACTION OF ENDOTHELIAL CELLS**

- Induced by histamine, other mediators
- Rapid and short-lived (minutes)

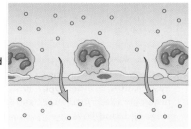

C **ENDOTHELIAL INJURY**

- Caused by burns, some microbial toxins
- Rapid; may be long-lived (hours to days)

Fig. 3.3 Principal mechanisms of increased vascular permeability in inflammation and their features and underlying causes.

toxins that target endothelial cells. Neutrophils that adhere to the endothelium during inflammation may also injure the endothelial cells and thus amplify the reaction. In most instances leakage starts immediately after injury and is sustained for several hours until the damaged vessels are thrombosed or repaired.

- Increased transport of fluids and proteins, called *transcytosis*, through the endothelial cell. This process, documented in experimental models, may involve intracellular channels that open in response to certain factors, such as vascular endothelial growth factor (VEGF), that promote vascular leakage. Its contribution to the vascular permeability seen in acute inflammation in humans is unclear.

Although these mechanisms of increased vascular permeability are described separately, all probably contribute in varying degrees in responses to most stimuli. For example, at different stages of a thermal burn, leakage results from endothelial retraction caused by inflammatory mediators and direct and leukocyte-dependent endothelial injury.

Responses of Lymphatic Vessels and Lymph Nodes

In addition to blood vessels, lymphatic vessels also participate in acute inflammation. The system of lymphatics and lymph nodes filters and polices the extravascular fluids. Lymphatics drain the small amount of extravascular fluid that seeps out of capillaries under normal circumstances. In inflammation, lymph flow is increased to help drain edema fluid that accumulates because of increased vascular permeability. In addition to fluid, leukocytes and cell debris, as well as microbes, may find their way into lymph. Lymphatic vessels, like blood vessels, proliferate during inflammatory reactions to handle the increased load. The lymphatics may become secondarily inflamed (*lymphangitis*), as may the draining lymph nodes (*lymphadenitis*). Inflamed lymph nodes are often enlarged because of increased cellularity. This constellation of pathologic changes is termed *reactive*, or *inflammatory*, *lymphadenitis* (Chapter 12). For clinicians the presence of red streaks near a skin wound is a telltale sign of an infection in the wound. This streaking follows the course of the lymphatic channels and indicates the presence of lymphangitis; it may be accompanied by painful enlargement of the draining lymph nodes, indicating lymphadenitis.

Leukocyte Recruitment to Sites of Inflammation

Leukocytes that are recruited to sites of inflammation perform the key function of eliminating the offending

- Increased vascular permeability allows plasma proteins and leukocytes, the mediators of host defense, to enter sites of infection or tissue damage. Fluid leak from blood vessels (exudation) results in edema.
- Lymphatic vessels and lymph nodes also are involved in inflammation, and often show redness and swelling.

agents. The most important leukocytes in typical inflammatory reactions are the ones capable of phagocytosis, namely, neutrophils and macrophages. Neutrophils are produced in the bone marrow and rapidly recruited to sites of inflammation. Macrophages are slower responders. The principal functions of these cell types differ in subtle but important ways—neutrophils use cytoskeletal rearrangements and enzyme assembly to mount rapid, transient responses, whereas macrophages, being long-lived, make slower but more prolonged responses that often rely on new gene transcription (Table 3.3). Macrophages are discussed in more detail later, in the context of chronic inflammation. These leukocytes ingest and destroy bacteria and other microbes, as well as necrotic tissue and foreign substances. Macrophages also produce growth factors that aid in repair. A price that is paid for the defensive potency of leukocytes is that, when strongly activated, they may induce tissue damage and prolong inflammation, because the leukocyte products that destroy microbes and help "clean up" necrotic tissues can also produce "collateral damage" of normal host tissues. When there is systemic activation of inflammation, as may occur when there is invasion of the bloodstream by bacteria, the resulting systemic inflammatory response may even be lethal.

The journey of leukocytes from the vessel lumen to the tissue is a multistep process that is mediated and controlled by adhesion molecules and cytokines. Leukocytes normally flow rapidly in the blood, and in inflammation, they have to be stopped and then brought to the offending agent or the site of tissue damage, outside the vessels. This process can be divided into phases, consisting first of adhesion of leukocytes to endothelium at the site of inflammation, then transmigration of the leukocytes through the vessel wall, and movement of the cells toward the offending agent. Different molecules play important roles in each of these steps (Fig. 3.4).

Leukocyte Adhesion to Endothelium

When blood flows from capillaries into postcapillary venules, circulating cells are swept by laminar flow against the vessel wall. Red cells, being smaller, tend to move faster than the larger white cells. As a result, red cells are confined to the central axial column, and leukocytes are pushed out toward the wall of the vessel, but the flow prevents the cells from attaching to the endothelium. As the blood flow slows early in inflammation (stasis), hemodynamic conditions change (wall shear stress decreases), and more white cells assume a peripheral position along the endothelial surface. This process of leukocyte redistribution is called *margination*. By moving close to the vessel wall, leukocytes are able to detect and react to changes in the endothelium. If the endothelial cells are activated by cytokines and other mediators produced locally, they express adhesion molecules to which the

> ## SUMMARY
>
> ### VASCULAR REACTIONS IN ACUTE INFLAMMATION
>
> - Vasodilation is induced by inflammatory mediators such as histamine (described later), and is the cause of erythema and stasis of blood flow.
> - Increased vascular permeability is induced by histamine, kinins, and other mediators that produce gaps between endothelial cells, by direct or leukocyte-induced endothelial injury, and by increased passage of fluids through the endothelium.

Table 3.3 Properties of Neutrophils and Macrophages

	Neutrophils	Macrophages
Origin	HSCs in bone marrow	• HSCs in bone marrow (in inflammatory reactions) • Many tissue-resident macrophages: stem cells in yolk sac or fetal liver (early in development)
Life span in tissues	1–2 days	Inflammatory macrophages: days or weeks Tissue-resident macrophages: years
Responses to activating stimuli	Rapid, short-lived, mostly degranulation and enzymatic activity	More prolonged, slower, often dependent on new gene transcription
• Reactive oxygen species	Rapidly induced by assembly of phagocyte oxidase (respiratory burst)	Less prominent
• Nitric oxide	Low levels or none	Induced following transcriptional activation of iNOS
• Degranulation	Major response; induced by cytoskeletal rearrangement	Not prominent
• Cytokine production	Low levels or none	Major functional activity, requires transcriptional activation of cytokine genes
• NET formation	Rapidly induced, by extrusion of nuclear contents	No
• Secretion of lysosomal enzymes	Prominent	Less

HSC, Hematopoietic stem cells; *iNOS,* inducible nitric oxide synthase; *NET,* neutrophil extracellular traps.
This table lists the major differences between neutrophils and macrophages. The reactions summarized above are described in the text. Note that the two cell types share many features, such as phagocytosis, ability to migrate through blood vessels into tissues, and chemotaxis.

leukocytes attach loosely. These cells bind and detach and thus begin to tumble on the endothelial surface, a process called rolling. The cells finally come to rest at some point where they *adhere* firmly (resembling pebbles over which a stream runs without disturbing them).

The attachment of leukocytes to endothelial cells is mediated by complementary adhesion molecules on the two cell types whose expression is enhanced by cytokines. Cytokines are secreted by cells in tissues in response to microbes and other injurious agents, thus ensuring that leukocytes are recruited to the tissues where these stimuli are present. The two major families of molecules involved in leukocyte adhesion and migration are the selectins and integrins (Table 3.4). These molecules are expressed on leukocytes and endothelial cells, as are their ligands.

• *Selectins* **mediate the initial weak interactions between leukocytes and endothelium.** Selectins are receptors expressed on leukocytes and endothelium that contain an extracellular domain that binds sugars (hence the lectin part of the name). The three members of this family are E-selectin (also called CD62E), expressed on endothelial cells; P-selectin (CD62P), present on platelets and endothelium; and L-selectin (CD62L), found on the surface of most leukocytes. The ligands for selectins are sialic acid-containing oligosaccharides bound to glycoprotein backbones. The endothelial selectins are typically expressed at low levels or not at all on unactivated endothelium, and are upregulated after stimulation by cytokines and other mediators. Therefore, binding of leukocytes is largely restricted to the endothelium at sites of infection or tissue injury (where the mediators are produced). For example, in unactivated endothelial cells, P-selectin is found primarily in intracellular Weibel-Palade bodies; however, within minutes of exposure to mediators such as histamine or thrombin, P-selectin is distributed to the cell surface. Similarly, E-selectin and the ligand for L-selectin are expressed on endothelium only after stimulation by IL-1 and tumor

necrosis factor (TNF), cytokines that are produced by tissue macrophages, dendritic cells, mast cells, and endothelial cells themselves following encounters with microbes and dead tissues. (These and other cytokines are described in more detail later.) Leukocytes express L-selectin at the tips of their microvilli and also express ligands for E- and P-selectins, all of which bind to the complementary molecules on the endothelial cells. These are low-affinity interactions with a fast off rate, and they are easily disrupted by the flowing blood. As a result, the bound leukocytes bind, detach, and bind again, and thus begin to roll along the endothelial surface. These weak selectin-mediated rolling interactions slow down the leukocytes and give them the opportunity to recognize additional adhesion molecules on the endothelium.

• **Firm adhesion of leukocytes to endothelium is mediated by a family of leukocyte surface proteins called** *integrins.* Integrins are transmembrane two-chain glycoproteins that mediate the adhesion of leukocytes to endothelium and of various cells to the extracellular matrix. They are normally expressed on leukocyte plasma membranes in a low-affinity form and do not adhere to their specific ligands until the leukocytes are activated by chemokines. Chemokines are chemoattractant cytokines that are secreted by many cells at sites of inflammation, bind to endothelial cell proteoglycans, and are displayed at high concentrations on the endothelial surface. When the rolling leukocytes encounter the displayed chemokines, the cells are activated, and their integrins undergo conformational changes and cluster together, thus converting to a high-affinity form. At the same time, other cytokines, notably TNF and IL-1, activate endothelial cells to increase their expression of ligands for integrins. These ligands include intercellular adhesion molecule-1 (ICAM-1), which binds to the integrins leukocyte function–associated antigen-1 (LFA-1) (also called CD11aCD18) and macrophage-1

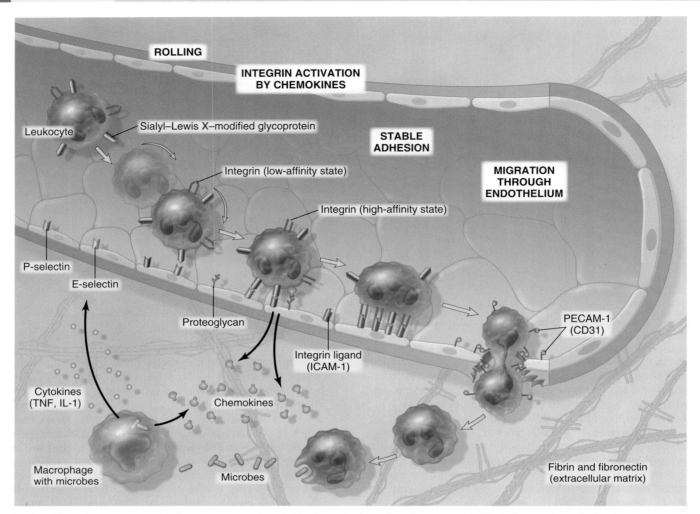

Fig. 3.4 The multistep process of leukocyte migration through blood vessels, shown here for neutrophils. The leukocytes first roll, then become activated and adhere to endothelium, then transmigrate across the endothelium, pierce the basement membrane, and move toward chemoattractants emanating from the source of injury. Different molecules play predominant roles at each step of this process: selectins in rolling; chemokines (usually displayed bound to proteoglycans) in activating the neutrophils to increase avidity of integrins; integrins in firm adhesion; and CD31 (PECAM-1) in transmigration. *ICAM-1,* Intercellular adhesion molecule-1; *PECAM-1 (CD31),* platelet endothelial cell adhesion molecule-1; *TNF,* tumor necrosis factor.

Table 3.4 Endothelial and Leukocyte Adhesion Molecules

Family	Molecule	Distribution	Ligand
Selectin	L-selectin (CD62L)	Neutrophils, monocytes T cells (naïve and central memory) B cells (naïve)	Sialyl-Lewis X/PNAd on GlyCAM-1, CD34, MAdCAM-1, others; expressed on endothelium (HEV)
	E-selectin (CD62E)	Endothelium activated by cytokines (TNF, IL-1)	Sialyl-Lewis X (e.g., CLA) on glycoproteins; expressed on neutrophils, monocytes, T cells (effector, memory)
	P-selectin (CD62P)	Endothelium activated by cytokines (TNF, IL-1), histamine, or thrombin; platelets	Sialyl-Lewis X on PSGL-1 and other glycoproteins; expressed on neutrophils, monocytes, T cells (effector, memory)
Integrin	LFA-1 (CD11aCD18)	Neutrophils, monocytes, T cells (naïve, effector, memory)	ICAM-1 (CD54), ICAM-2 (CD102); expressed on endothelium (upregulated on activated endothelium)
	MAC-1 (CD11bCD18)	Monocytes, DCs	ICAM-1 (CD54), ICAM-2 (CD102); expressed on endothelium (upregulated on activated endothelium)
	VLA-4 (CD49aCD29)	Monocytes T cells (naïve, effector, memory)	VCAM-1 (CD106); expressed on endothelium (upregulated on activated endothelium)
	α4β7 (CD49DCD29)	Monocytes T cells (gut homing naïve effector, memory)	VCAM-1 (CD106), MAdCAM-1; expressed on endothelium in gut and gut-associated lymphoid tissues
Ig	CD31	Endothelial cells, leukocytes	CD31 (homotypic interaction)

CLA, Cutaneous lymphocyte antigen-1; *GlyCAM-1,* glycan-bearing cell adhesion molecule-1; *HEV,* high endothelial venule; *ICAM,* intercellular adhesion molecule; *Ig,* immunoglobulin; *IL-1,* interleukin-1; *MAdCAM-1,* mucosal adhesion cell adhesion molecule-1; *PSGL-1,* P-selectin glycoprotein ligand-1; *TNF,* tumor necrosis factor; *VCAM,* vascular cell adhesion molecule.

antigen (Mac-1) (CD11bCD18), and vascular cell adhesion molecule-1 (VCAM-1), which binds to the integrin very late antigen-4 (VLA-4) (Table 3.4). The combination of cytokine-induced expression of integrin ligands on the endothelium and increased affinity of integrins on the leukocytes results in firm integrin-mediated binding of the leukocytes to the endothelium at the site of inflammation. The leukocytes stop rolling, and engagement of integrins by their ligands delivers signals leading to cytoskeletal changes that arrest the leukocytes and firmly attach them to the endothelium.

The most telling proof of the importance of leukocyte adhesion molecules is the existence of genetic deficiencies in these molecules that result in recurrent bacterial infections as a consequence of impaired leukocyte adhesion and defective inflammation. These leukocyte adhesion deficiencies are described in Chapter 5.

Leukocyte Migration Through Endothelium

After being arrested on the endothelial surface, leukocytes migrate through the vessel wall primarily by squeezing between cells at intercellular junctions. This extravasation of leukocytes, called *transmigration*, occurs mainly in postcapillary venules, the site at which there is maximal retraction of endothelial cells. Further movement of leukocytes is driven by chemokines produced in extravascular tissues, which stimulate leukocytes to travel along a chemical gradient (described shortly). In addition, platelet endothelial cell adhesion molecule-1 (PECAM-1) (also called CD31), an adhesion molecule of the immunoglobulin (Ig) superfamily expressed on leukocytes and endothelial cells, mediates the binding events needed for leukocytes to traverse the endothelium. After traversing the endothelium, leukocytes pierce the basement membrane, probably by secreting collagenases, and they enter the extravascular tissue. Typically, the vessel wall is not injured during leukocyte transmigration.

Chemotaxis of Leukocytes

After exiting the circulation, leukocytes move in the tissues toward the site of injury by a process called *chemotaxis*, which is defined as locomotion along a chemical gradient. Both exogenous and endogenous substances can act as chemoattractants, including the following:

- Bacterial products, particularly peptides with N-formylmethionine termini
- Cytokines, especially those of the chemokine family
- Components of the complement system, particularly C5a
- Products of the lipoxygenase pathway of arachidonic acid (AA) metabolism, particularly leukotriene B4 (LTB$_4$)

These chemoattractants are produced by microbes and by host cells in response to infections and tissue damage and during immunologic reactions. All act by binding to seven-transmembrane G protein-coupled receptors on the surface of leukocytes. Signals initiated from these receptors activate second messengers that induce polymerization of actin, resulting in increased amounts at the leading edge of the cell and localization of myosin filaments at the back. The leukocyte moves by extending filopodia that pull the back of the cell in the direction of extension, much like the front wheels

pull an automobile with front-wheel drive. The net result is that leukocytes migrate toward the inflammatory stimulus in the direction of the locally produced chemoattractants.

The nature of the leukocyte infiltrate varies with the age of the inflammatory response and the type of stimulus. In most forms of acute inflammation, neutrophils predominate in the inflammatory infiltrate during the first 6 to 24 hours and are gradually replaced by monocyte-derived macrophages over 24 to 48 hours (Fig. 3.5). There are several reasons for the early preponderance of neutrophils: they are more numerous in the blood than other leukocytes, they respond more rapidly to chemokines, and they may attach more firmly to the adhesion molecules that are rapidly induced on endothelial cells, such as P- and E-selectins. After entering tissues, neutrophils are short-lived; they undergo apoptosis and disappear within 24 to 48 hours. Macrophages not only survive longer but also may proliferate in the tissues, and thus they become the dominant population in prolonged inflammatory reactions. There are, however, exceptions to this stereotypic pattern of cellular infiltration. In certain infections—for example, those produced by *Pseudomonas* bacteria—the cellular infiltrate is dominated by neutrophils for several days; in viral infections, lymphocytes may be the first cells to arrive; some hypersensitivity reactions are dominated by activated lymphocytes, macrophages, and plasma cells (reflecting the immune response); and in allergic reactions, eosinophils may be a prominent cell type.

The molecular understanding of leukocyte recruitment and migration has provided a large number of potential therapeutic targets for controlling harmful inflammation. **Agents that block TNF, one of the major cytokines in leukocyte recruitment, are among the most successful therapeutics ever developed for chronic inflammatory diseases,** and antagonists of leukocyte integrins are approved for inflammatory diseases and are being tested in clinical trials. Predictably, these antagonists not only have the desired effect of controlling the inflammation but can also compromise the ability of treated patients to defend themselves against microbes, which, of course, is the physiologic function of the inflammatory response.

SUMMARY

LEUKOCYTE RECRUITMENT TO SITES OF INFLAMMATION

- Leukocytes are recruited from the blood into the extravascular tissue where infectious pathogens or damaged tissues may be located, migrate to the site of infection or tissue injury, and are activated to perform their functions.
- Leukocyte recruitment is a multistep process consisting of loose attachment to and rolling on endothelium (mediated by selectins); firm attachment to endothelium (mediated by integrins); and migration through interendothelial gaps.
- Various cytokines promote the expression of selectins and integrin ligands on endothelium (TNF, IL-1), increase the avidity of integrins for their ligands (chemokines), and promote directional migration of leukocytes (also chemokines). Tissue macrophages and other cells responding to the pathogens or damaged tissues produce many of these cytokines.
- Neutrophils predominate in the early inflammatory infiltrate and are later replaced by monocytes and macrophages.

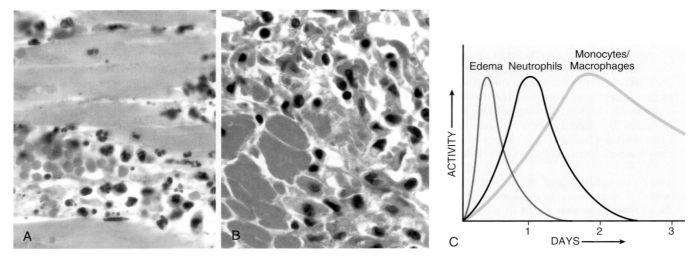

Fig. 3.5 Nature of leukocyte infiltrates in inflammatory reactions. The photomicrographs show an inflammatory reaction in the myocardium after ischemic necrosis (infarction). (A) Early (neutrophilic) infiltrates and congested blood vessels. (B) Later (mononuclear) cellular infiltrates. (C) The approximate kinetics of edema and cellular infiltration. For simplicity, edema is shown as an acute transient response, although secondary waves of delayed edema and neutrophil infiltration also can occur.

Phagocytosis and Clearance of the Offending Agent

Recognition of microbes or dead cells induces several responses in leukocytes that are collectively called *leukocyte activation* (Fig. 3.6). After leukocytes (particularly neutrophils and monocytes) have been recruited to a site

of infection or tissue injury they must be activated to perform their functions. This makes perfect sense because, while we want our defenders to patrol our body constantly, it would be wasteful to keep them at a high level of alert and expending energy before they are required. The functional responses that are most important for destruction of microbes and other offenders are phagocytosis and

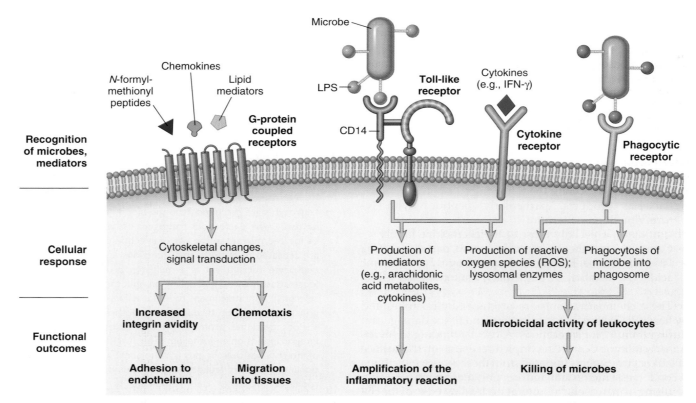

Fig. 3.6 Leukocyte activation. Various types of leukocyte cell surface receptors recognize different agonists. Once stimulated, the receptors initiate responses that mediate leukocyte functions. Only some receptors are depicted (see text for details). LPS first binds to a circulating LPS-binding protein (not shown). *IFN-γ,* Interferon-γ; *LPS,* lipopolysaccharide.

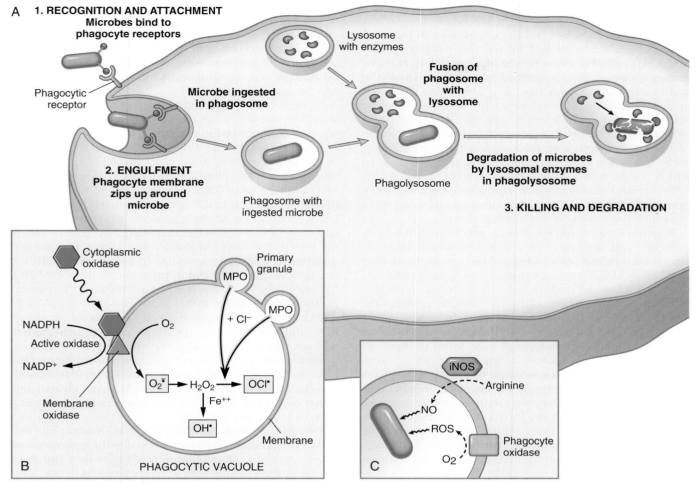

Fig. 3.7 Phagocytosis and intracellular destruction of microbes. (A) Phagocytosis of a particle (e.g., a bacterium) involves binding to receptors on the leukocyte membrane, engulfment, and fusion of the phagocytic vacuoles with lysosomes. This is followed by destruction of ingested particles within the phagolysosomes by lysosomal enzymes and by reactive oxygen and nitrogen species. (B) In activated phagocytes, cytoplasmic components of the phagocyte oxidase enzyme assemble in the membrane of the phagosome to form the active enzyme, which catalyzes the conversion of oxygen into superoxide (O_2^-) and H_2O_2. Myeloperoxidase, present in the granules of neutrophils, converts H_2O_2 to hypochlorite. (C) Microbicidal reactive oxygen species (ROS) and nitric oxide (NO) kill ingested microbes. During phagocytosis, granule contents may be released into extracellular tissues (not shown). *iNOS*, Inducible NO synthase; *MPO*, myeloperoxidase; *ROS*, reactive oxygen species.

intracellular killing. Several other responses aid in the defensive functions of inflammation and may contribute to its injurious consequences.

Phagocytosis

Phagocytosis involves three sequential steps: (1) recognition and attachment of the particle to be ingested by the leukocyte; (2) engulfment, with subsequent formation of a phagocytic vacuole; and (3) killing or degradation of the ingested material (Fig. 3.7). These steps are triggered by activation of phagocytes by microbes, necrotic debris, and various mediators.

Recognition by Phagocytic Receptors. Mannose receptors, scavenger receptors, and receptors for various opsonins bind and ingest microbes. The macrophage mannose receptor is a lectin that binds terminal mannose and fucose residues of glycoproteins and glycolipids. These sugars are typically part of molecules found on microbial cell walls, whereas mammalian glycoproteins and glycolipids contain terminal sialic acid or N-acetylgalactosamine. Therefore, the

mannose receptor recognizes microbes and not host cells. Scavenger receptors bind and ingest low-density lipoprotein (LDL) particles as well as a variety of microbes. The efficiency of phagocytosis is greatly enhanced when microbes are opsonized (coated) by specific proteins (opsonins) for which the phagocytes express high-affinity receptors. The major opsonins are immunoglobulin (Ig)G antibodies, the C3b breakdown product of complement activation, and certain plasma lectins, notably mannose-binding lectin, all of which are recognized by specific receptors on leukocytes.

Engulfment. After a particle is bound to phagocyte receptors, extensions of the cytoplasm (pseudopods) flow around it, and the plasma membrane pinches off to form a cytosolic vesicle (phagosome) that encloses the particle. The phagosome then fuses with lysosomes, resulting in the discharge of lysosomal contents into the phagolysosome (Fig. 3.7). During this process the phagocyte also may release some granule contents into the extracellular space, thereby damaging innocent bystander normal cells.

Intracellular Destruction of Microbes and Debris

The killing of microbes and the destruction of ingested materials are accomplished by reactive oxygen species (ROS, also called reactive oxygen intermediates), reactive nitrogen species, mainly derived from nitric oxide (NO), and lysosomal enzymes (Fig. 3.7). This is the final step in the elimination of infectious agents and necrotic cells. The killing and degradation of microbes and elimination of dead-cell debris within neutrophils and macrophages occur most efficiently after their activation. All these killing mechanisms are normally sequestered in lysosomes, to which phagocytosed materials are brought. Thus, potentially harmful substances are segregated from the cell's cytoplasm and nucleus to avoid damage to the phagocyte while it is performing its normal function.

Reactive Oxygen Species. ROS are produced by the rapid assembly and activation of a multicomponent enzyme, phagocyte oxidase (also called NADPH oxidase), which oxidizes NADPH (reduced nicotinamide-adenine dinucleotide phosphate) and, in the process, reduces oxygen to the superoxide anion ($O_2^{\cdot-}$) (Fig. 3.7B). In neutrophils, this oxidative reaction is tightly linked to phagocytosis, and is called the *respiratory burst*. Phagocyte oxidase is an enzyme complex consisting of at least seven proteins. In resting neutrophils, different components of the enzyme are located in the plasma membrane and the cytoplasm. In response to activating stimuli, the cytosolic protein components translocate to the phagosomal membrane, where they assemble and form the functional enzyme complex. Thus, the ROS are produced within the phagolysosome, where they can act on ingested particles without damaging the host cell. $O_2^{\cdot-}$ so produced is then converted into hydrogen peroxide (H_2O_2), mostly by spontaneous dismutation, a process of simultaneous oxidation and reduction. H_2O_2 is not able to kill microbes efficiently by itself. However, the azurophilic granules of neutrophils contain the enzyme *myeloperoxidase* (MPO), which, in the presence of a halide such as Cl^-, converts H_2O_2 to hypochlorite (OCl_2^-, the active ingredient in household bleach). The latter is a potent anti-microbial agent that destroys microbes by *halogenation* (in which the halide is bound covalently to cellular constituents) or by *oxidation* of proteins and lipids (lipid peroxidation). The H_2O_2-MPO-halide system is the most efficient bactericidal system of neutrophils. Nevertheless, inherited deficiency of MPO only causes a modest increase in susceptibility to infection, emphasizing the redundancy of microbicidal mechanisms in leukocytes. H_2O_2 also is converted to hydroxyl radical ($OH\bullet$), another powerful destructive agent. As discussed in Chapter 2, these oxygen-derived free radicals bind to and modify cellular lipids, proteins, and nucleic acids, and thus destroy cells such as microbes.

Oxygen-derived radicals may be released extracellularly from leukocytes after exposure to microbes, chemokines, and antigen–antibody complexes, or following a phagocytic challenge. These ROS are implicated in tissue damage accompanying inflammation.

Serum, tissue fluids, and host cells possess *anti-oxidant mechanisms* that protect against these potentially harmful oxygen-derived radicals. These anti-oxidants are discussed in Chapter 2; they include (1) the enzyme *superoxide dismutase*, which is found in or can be activated in a variety of cell types; (2) *catalase*, which detoxifies H_2O_2; and (3) *glutathione peroxidase,* another powerful H_2O_2 detoxifier. The role of oxygen-derived free radicals in any given inflammatory reaction depends on the balance between production and inactivation of these metabolites by cells and tissues.

Genetic defects in the generation of ROS are the cause of an immunodeficiency disease called *chronic granulomatous disease*, described in Chapter 5.

Nitric Oxide. NO, a soluble gas produced from arginine by the action of nitric oxide synthase (NOS), also participates in microbial killing. There are three different types of NOS: endothelial (eNOS), neuronal (nNOS), and inducible (iNOS). eNOS and nNOS are constitutively expressed at low levels, and the NO they generate acts to maintain vascular tone and as a neurotransmitter, respectively. iNOS, the type that is involved in microbial killing, is expressed when macrophages are activated by cytokines (e.g., IFN-γ) or microbial products, and induces the production of NO. In macrophages, NO reacts with superoxide ($O_2^{\cdot-}$) to generate the highly reactive free radical peroxynitrite ($ONOO^\bullet$) (Fig. 3.7C). These nitrogen-derived free radicals, similar to ROS, attack and damage the lipids, proteins, and nucleic acids of microbes and host cells.

In addition to its role as a microbicidal substance, NO produced by endothelial cells relaxes vascular smooth muscle and promotes vasodilation. It is not clear if this action of NO plays an important role in the vascular reactions of acute inflammation.

Granule Enzymes and Other Proteins. **Neutrophils and monocytes contain granules packed with enzymes and anti-microbial proteins that degrade microbes and dead tissues and may contribute to tissue damage.** These granules are actively secretory and thus distinct from classical lysosomes. Neutrophils have two main types of granules. The smaller *specific* (or secondary) granules contain lysozyme, collagenase, gelatinase, lactoferrin, plasminogen activator, histaminase, and alkaline phosphatase. The larger *azurophil* (or primary) granules contain MPO, bactericidal factors (such as defensins), acid hydrolases, and a variety of neutral proteases (elastase, cathepsin G, nonspecific collagenases, proteinase 3). Phagocytic vesicles containing engulfed material may fuse with these granules (and with lysosomes, as described earlier), and the ingested materials are destroyed. In addition, both types of granules also undergo exocytosis (degranulation), leading to the extracellular release of granule contents.

Different granule enzymes serve different functions. *Acid proteases* degrade bacteria and debris within phagolysosomes, which are acidified by membrane-bound proton pumps. *Neutral proteases* are capable of degrading various extracellular components, such as collagen, basement membrane, fibrin, elastin, and cartilage, resulting in the tissue destruction that accompanies inflammatory processes. Neutrophil elastase combats infections by degrading virulence factors of bacteria. Macrophages also contain acid hydrolases, collagenase, elastase, phospholipase, and plasminogen activator.

Because of the destructive effects of granule enzymes, the initial leukocytic infiltration, if unchecked, can potentiate further inflammation by damaging tissues. These harmful proteases, however, are normally controlled by a system of *anti-proteases* in the serum and tissue fluids. Foremost among these is α_1-anti-trypsin, which is the major inhibitor of neutrophil elastase. A deficiency of these inhibitors may lead to sustained action of leukocyte proteases, as is the case in patients with α_1-anti-trypsin deficiency (Chapter 13).

Neutrophil Extracellular Traps

Neutrophil extracellular traps (NETs) are extracellular fibrillar networks that concentrate anti-microbial substances at sites of infection and prevent the spread of the microbes by trapping them in the fibrils. They are produced by neutrophils in response to infectious pathogens (mainly bacteria and fungi) and inflammatory mediators (e.g., chemokines, cytokines, and complement proteins). The extracellular traps consist of a viscous meshwork of nuclear chromatin that binds and concentrates granule proteins such as anti-microbial peptides and enzymes (Fig. 3.8). NETs provide an additional mechanism of killing microbes that does not involve phagocytosis. In the process of NET formation, the nuclei of the neutrophils are lost, leading to the death of the cells, sometimes called NETosis, representing a distinctive form of cell death affecting neutrophils. NETs also have been detected in the blood during sepsis. The nuclear chromatin in the NETs, which includes histones and associated DNA, may be a source of nuclear antigens in systemic autoimmune diseases, particularly lupus, in which individuals react against their own DNA and nucleoproteins (Chapter 5).

Leukocyte-Mediated Tissue Injury

Leukocytes are important mediators of injury to normal cells and tissues under several circumstances:

- As part of a normal defense reaction against infectious microbes, when tissues at or near the site of infection suffer collateral damage. In some infections that are difficult to eradicate, such as tuberculosis and certain viral diseases such as hepatitis, the prolonged host response contributes more to the pathology than does the microbe itself.
- When the inflammatory response is inappropriately directed against host tissues, as in certain autoimmune diseases.
- When the host "hyper-reacts" against usually harmless environmental substances, as in allergic diseases, including asthma, and some drug reactions.

Leukocytes damage tissues by releasing injurious molecules. The potentially toxic contents of granules are released by leukocytes into the extracellular milieu by several mechanisms. Controlled secretion of granule contents following degranulation is a normal response of activated leukocytes. If phagocytes encounter materials that cannot be easily ingested, such as immune complexes deposited on immovable flat surfaces (e.g., glomerular basement membrane), the inability of the leukocytes to surround and ingest these substances ("frustrated phagocytosis") triggers strong activation and also the release of large amounts of granule enzymes into the extracellular environment. Some phagocytosed substances, such as urate and

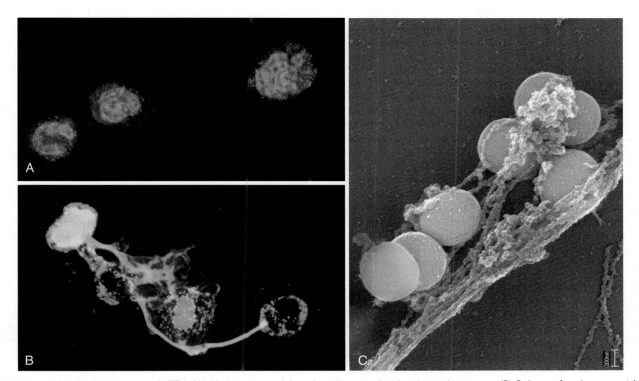

Fig. 3.8 Neutrophil extracellular traps (NETs). (A) Healthy neutrophils with nuclei stained red and cytoplasm green. (B) Release of nuclear material from neutrophils (note that two have lost their nuclei), forming extracellular traps. (C) An electron micrograph of bacteria (staphylococci) trapped in NETs. *(From Brinkmann V, Zychlinsky A: Beneficial suicide: why neutrophils die to make NETs, Nat Rev Microbiol 5:577, 2007, with permission.)*

silica crystals, may damage the membrane of the phagolysosome and also lead to the release of damaging contents.

Other Functional Responses of Activated Leukocytes

In addition to eliminating microbes and dead cells, activated leukocytes play several other roles in host defense. Importantly, these cells, especially macrophages, produce cytokines that can either amplify or limit inflammatory reactions, growth factors that stimulate the proliferation of endothelial cells and fibroblasts and the synthesis of collagen, and enzymes that remodel connective tissues. Because of these activities, macrophages also have central roles in orchestrating chronic inflammation and tissue repair, after the inflammation has subsided. These functions of macrophages are discussed later in the chapter.

In this discussion of acute inflammation, we emphasize the importance of neutrophils and macrophages. However, it has become clear that some T lymphocytes, which are cells of adaptive immunity, also contribute to acute inflammation. The most important of these cells are those that produce the cytokine IL-17 (so-called "T_H17 cells"), which are discussed in more detail in Chapter 5. IL-17 induces the secretion of chemokines that recruit other leukocytes. In the absence of effective T_H17 responses, individuals are susceptible to fungal and bacterial infections, and the skin abscesses that develop are "cold abscesses," lacking the classic features of acute inflammation, such as warmth and redness.

Termination of the Acute Inflammatory Response

Such a powerful system of host defense, with its inherent capacity to cause tissue injury, needs tight controls to minimize damage. In part, inflammation declines after the offending agents are removed simply because the mediators of inflammation are produced in rapid bursts, only as long as the stimulus persists, have short half-lives, and are degraded after their release. Neutrophils also have short half-lives in tissues and die by apoptosis within hours to a day or two after leaving the blood. In addition, as inflammation develops, the process itself triggers a variety of stop signals that actively terminate the reaction. These active termination mechanisms include a switch in the type of arachidonic acid metabolite produced, from proinflammatory leukotrienes to anti-inflammatory lipoxins (described later), and the liberation of anti-inflammatory cytokines, including transforming growth factor-β (TGF-β) and IL-10, from macrophages and other cells. Other control mechanisms that have been demonstrated experimentally include neural impulses (cholinergic discharge), which inhibit the production of TNF in macrophages.

SUMMARY

LEUKOCYTE ACTIVATION AND REMOVAL OF OFFENDING AGENTS

- Leukocytes can eliminate microbes and dead cells by phagocytosis, followed by their destruction in phagolysosomes.
- Destruction is caused by free radicals (ROS, NO) generated in activated leukocytes and by granule enzymes.
- Neutrophils can extrude their nuclear contents to form extracellular nets that trap and destroy microbes.
- Granule enzymes may be released into the extracellular environment.
- The mechanisms that function to eliminate microbes and dead cells (the physiologic role of inflammation) also are capable of damaging normal tissues (the pathologic consequences of inflammation).
- Anti-inflammatory mediators terminate the acute inflammatory reaction when it is no longer needed.

MEDIATORS OF INFLAMMATION

The mediators of inflammation are the substances that initiate and regulate inflammatory reactions. Although the harried student may find the list of mediators daunting (as do professors!), it is worthy of note that this knowledge has been used to design a large armamentarium of anti-inflammatory agents that are used every day by many people and which include familiar drugs such as aspirin and acetaminophen. The most important mediators of acute inflammation are vasoactive amines, lipid products (prostaglandins and leukotrienes), cytokines (including chemokines), and products of complement activation (Table 3.5). We begin by summarizing the general properties of the

Table 3.5 Principal Mediators of Inflammation

Mediator	Source	Action
Histamine	Mast cells, basophils, platelets	Vasodilation, increased vascular permeability, endothelial activation
Prostaglandins	Mast cells, leukocytes	Vasodilation, pain, fever
Leukotrienes	Mast cells, leukocytes	Increased vascular permeability, chemotaxis, leukocyte adhesion, and activation
Cytokines (TNF, IL-1, IL-6)	Macrophages, endothelial cells, mast cells	Local: endothelial activation (expression of adhesion molecules). Systemic: fever, metabolic abnormalities, hypotension (shock)
Chemokines	Leukocytes, activated macrophages	Chemotaxis, leukocyte activation
Platelet-activating factor	Leukocytes, mast cells	Vasodilation, increased vascular permeability, leukocyte adhesion, chemotaxis, degranulation, oxidative burst
Complement	Plasma (produced in liver)	Leukocyte chemotaxis and activation, direct target killing (membrane attack complex), vasodilation (mast cell stimulation)
Kinins	Plasma (produced in liver)	Increased vascular permeability, smooth muscle contraction, vasodilation, pain

mediators of inflammation and then discuss some of the more important molecules.

- **Mediators may be produced locally by cells at the site of inflammation, or may be derived from circulating inactive precursors that are activated at the site of inflammation.** *Cell-derived mediators* are rapidly released from intracellular granules (e.g., amines) or are synthesized de novo (e.g., prostaglandins, leukotrienes, cytokines) in response to a stimulus. **The major cell types that produce mediators of acute inflammation are tissue macrophages, dendritic cells, and mast cells,** but platelets, neutrophils, endothelial cells, and most epithelia also can be induced to elaborate some of the mediators. Therefore, cell-derived mediators are most important for reactions against offending agents in tissues. *Plasma-derived mediators* (e.g., complement proteins) are present in the circulation as inactive precursors that must be activated, usually by a series of proteolytic cleavages, to acquire their biologic properties. They are produced mainly in the liver, are effective against circulating microbes, and also can be recruited into tissues.
- **Active mediators are produced only in response to various molecules that stimulate inflammation, including microbial products and substances released from necrotic cells.** Many of these stimuli trigger well-defined receptors and signaling pathways, as described earlier. The usual requirement for microbes or dead tissues as the initiating stimulus ensures that inflammation is normally triggered only when and where it is needed.
- **Most of the mediators are short-lived.** They quickly decay, or are inactivated by enzymes, or they are otherwise scavenged or inhibited. There is thus a system of checks and balances that regulates mediator actions. These built-in control mechanisms are discussed with each class of mediator.
- **One mediator can stimulate the release of other mediators.** For instance, products of complement activation stimulate the release of histamine, and the cytokine TNF acts on endothelial cells to stimulate the production of another cytokine, IL-1, and many chemokines. The secondary mediators may have the same actions as the initial mediators but also may have different and even opposing activities, thus providing mechanisms for amplifying—or, in certain instances, counteracting—the initial action of a mediator.

Vasoactive Amines: Histamine and Serotonin

The two major vasoactive amines, so named because they have important actions on blood vessels, are *histamine* **and** *serotonin.* They are stored as preformed molecules in cells and are therefore among the first mediators to be released during inflammation. The richest sources of histamine are mast cells, which are normally present in the connective tissue adjacent to blood vessels. Histamine also is found in blood basophils and platelets. It is stored in mast cell granules and is released by degranulation in response to a variety of stimuli, including (1) physical injury, such as trauma, cold, or heat, by unknown mechanisms; (2) binding of antibodies to mast cells, which

underlies immediate hypersensitivity (allergic) reactions (Chapter 5); and (3) products of complement called *anaphylatoxins* (C3a and C5a), described later. Antibodies and complement products bind to specific receptors on mast cells and trigger signaling pathways that induce rapid degranulation. Neuropeptides (e.g., substance P) and cytokines (IL-1, IL-8) also may trigger release of histamine.

Histamine causes dilation of arterioles and increases the permeability of venules. Histamine is considered the principal mediator of the immediate transient phase of increased vascular permeability, producing interendothelial gaps in postcapillary venules, as discussed earlier. Its vasoactive effects are mediated mainly via binding to receptors, called H_1 receptors, on microvascular endothelial cells. The antihistamine drugs that are commonly used to treat some inflammatory reactions, such as allergies, are H_1 receptor antagonists that bind to and block the receptor. Histamine also causes contraction of some smooth muscles, but leukotrienes, described later, are much more potent and relevant for causing spasms of bronchial muscles, for example, in asthma.

Serotonin (5-hydroxytryptamine) is a preformed vasoactive mediator present in platelets and certain neuroendocrine cells, such as in the gastrointestinal tract, and in mast cells in rodents but not humans. Its primary function is as a neurotransmitter in the gastrointestinal tract. It also is a vasoconstrictor, but the importance of this action in inflammation is unclear.

Arachidonic Acid Metabolites

The lipid mediators *prostaglandins* **and** *leukotrienes* **are produced from arachidonic acid present in membrane phospholipids, and they stimulate vascular and cellular reactions in acute inflammation.** Arachidonic acid is a 20-carbon polyunsaturated fatty acid that is derived from dietary sources or by conversion from the essential fatty acid linoleic acid. Most cellular arachidonic acid is esterified and incorporated into membrane phospholipids. Mechanical, chemical, and physical stimuli or other mediators (e.g., C5a) trigger the release of arachidonic acid from membranes by activating cellular phospholipases, mainly phospholipase A_2. Once freed from the membrane, arachidonic acid is rapidly converted to bioactive mediators. These mediators, also called *eicosanoids* (because they are derived from 20-carbon fatty acids; Greek *eicosa* = 20), are synthesized by two major classes of enzymes: cyclooxygenases (which generate prostaglandins) and lipoxygenases (which produce leukotrienes and lipoxins) (Fig. 3.9). Eicosanoids bind to G protein-coupled receptors on many cell types and can mediate virtually every step of inflammation (Table 3.6).

Prostaglandins

Prostaglandins (PGs) are produced by mast cells, macrophages, endothelial cells, and many other cell types, and are involved in the vascular and systemic reactions of inflammation. They are generated by the actions of two *cyclooxygenases* called COX-1 and COX-2. COX-1 is produced in response to inflammatory stimuli and also is constitutively expressed in most tissues, where it may serve a homeostatic function (e.g., fluid and electrolyte balance in

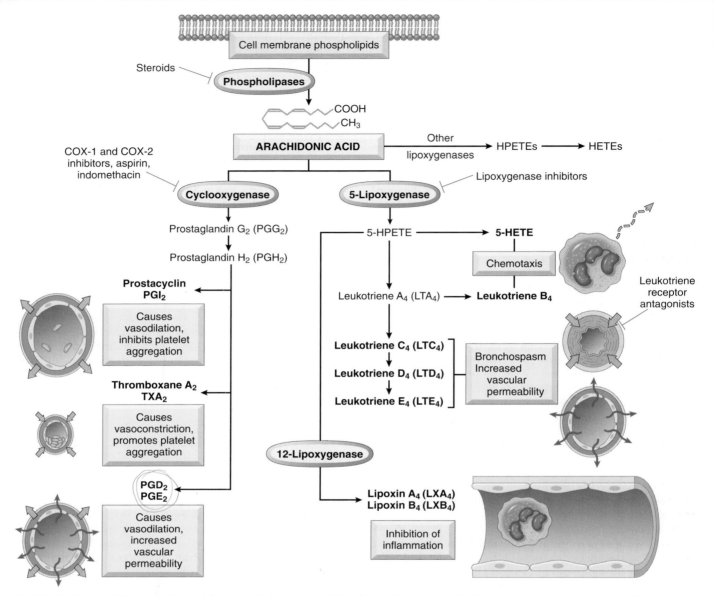

Fig. 3.9 Production of AA metabolites and their roles in inflammation. Clinically useful antagonists of different enzymes and receptors are indicated in *red*. While leukotriene receptor antagonists inhibit all actions of leukotrienes, they are used in the clinic to treat asthma, as shown. *COX-1, COX-2,* Cyclooxygenase 1 and 2; *HETE,* hydroxyeicosatetraenoic acid; *HPETE,* hydroperoxyeicosatetraenoic acid.

the kidneys, cytoprotection in the gastrointestinal tract). In contrast, COX-2 is induced by inflammatory stimuli and thus generates the PGs that are involved in inflammatory reactions, but it is low or absent in most normal tissues.

Table 3.6 Principal Actions of Arachidonic Acid Metabolites in Inflammation

Action	Eicosanoid
Vasodilation	Prostaglandins PGI$_2$ (prostacyclin), PGE$_1$, PGE$_2$, PGD$_2$
Vasoconstriction	Thromboxane A$_2$, leukotrienes C$_4$, D$_4$, E$_4$
Increased vascular permeability	Leukotrienes C$_4$, D$_4$, E$_4$
Chemotaxis, leukocyte adhesion	Leukotriene B$_4$
Smooth muscle contraction	Prostaglandins PGC4, PGD4, PGE4

Prostaglandins are named based on structural features coded by a letter (e.g., PGD, PGE, PGF, PGG, and PGH) and a subscript numeral (e.g., 1, 2), which indicates the number of double bonds in the compound. The most important prostaglandins in inflammation are PGE$_2$, PGD$_2$, PGF$_{2a}$, PGI$_2$ (prostacyclin), and TXA$_2$ (thromboxane A$_2$), each of which is derived by the action of a specific enzyme on an intermediate in the pathway. Some of these enzymes have restricted tissue distribution and functions.

- PGD$_2$ is the major prostaglandin made by mast cells; along with PGE$_2$ (which is more widely distributed), it causes vasodilation and increases the permeability of postcapillary venules, thus potentiating exudation and resultant edema. PGD$_2$ also is a chemoattractant for neutrophils.
- Platelets contain the enzyme thromboxane synthase, which is responsible for synthesizing TXA2, the major

platelet eicosanoid. TXA_2 is a potent platelet-aggregating agent and vasoconstrictor, and thus promotes thrombosis.

- In contrast, vascular endothelium contains prostacyclin synthase, which is responsible for the formation of prostacyclin (PGI_2) and its stable end product PGF_{1a}. Prostacyclin is a vasodilator and a potent inhibitor of platelet aggregation, and thus serves to prevent thrombus formation on normal endothelial cells. A thromboxane–prostacyclin imbalance has been implicated in coronary and cerebral artery thrombosis (Chapter 4).
- In addition to their local effects, prostaglandins are involved in the pathogenesis of *pain* and *fever*, two common systemic manifestations of inflammation. PGE_2 makes the skin hypersensitive to painful stimuli, and causes fever during infections (described later).

Leukotrienes

Leukotrienes are produced in leukocytes and mast cells by the action of lipoxygenase and are involved in vascular and smooth muscle reactions and leukocyte recruitment. The synthesis of leukotrienes involves multiple steps, the first of which generates leukotriene A_4 (LTA_4), which in turn gives rise to LTB_4 or LTC_4. LTB_4 is produced by neutrophils and some macrophages, and is a potent chemotactic agent and activator of neutrophils, causing aggregation and adhesion of the cells to venular endothelium, generation of ROS, and release of lysosomal enzymes. The cysteinyl-containing leukotriene LTC_4 and its metabolites, LTD_4 and LTE_4, are produced mainly in mast cells and cause intense vasoconstriction, bronchospasm (important in asthma), and increased permeability of venules.

Lipoxins

Lipoxins also are generated from arachidonic acid by the lipoxygenase pathway, but unlike prostaglandins and leukotrienes, the lipoxins suppress inflammation by inhibiting the recruitment of leukocytes. They inhibit neutrophil chemotaxis and adhesion to endothelium. They also are unusual in that two cell populations are required for the transcellular biosynthesis of these mediators. Leukocytes, particularly neutrophils, produce intermediates in lipoxin synthesis, and these are converted to lipoxins by platelets interacting with the leukocytes.

Pharmacologic Inhibitors of Prostaglandins and Leukotrienes

The importance of eicosanoids in inflammation has driven attempts to develop drugs that inhibit their production or actions and thus suppress inflammation. These anti-inflammatory drugs include the following:

- **Cyclooxygenase inhibitors** include aspirin and other nonsteroidal anti-inflammatory drugs (NSAIDs), such as ibuprofen. They inhibit both COX-1 and COX-2 and thus block all prostaglandin synthesis (hence their efficacy in treating pain and fever); aspirin does this by irreversibly inactivating cyclooxygenases. Selective COX-2 inhibitors are a newer class of these drugs that are 200- to 300-fold more potent in blocking COX-2 than COX-1. There has been great interest in COX-2 as a therapeutic target because of the possibility that COX-1 is responsible for the production of prostaglandins that are involved in both inflammation and physiologic

functions such as protecting gastric epithelial cells from acid-induced injury, whereas COX-2 generates prostaglandins that are involved only in inflammation. If this idea is correct, the selective COX-2 inhibitors should be anti-inflammatory without having the toxicities of the nonselective inhibitors, such as gastric ulceration. However, these distinctions are not absolute, as COX-2 also seems to play some role in normal homeostasis. Furthermore, selective COX-2 inhibitors may increase the risk of cardiovascular and cerebrovascular events, possibly because they impair endothelial cell production of prostacyclin (PGI_2), which prevents thrombosis, while leaving intact the COX-1-mediated production by platelets of TXA_2, which induces platelet aggregation. Thus, selective COX-2 inhibition may tilt the balance toward vascular thrombosis, especially in combination with other factors that increase the risk of thrombosis. Nevertheless, these drugs are used in individuals who do not have risk factors for cardiovascular disease and when the drugs' benefits outweigh their risks.
- **Lipoxygenase inhibitors.** 5-lipoxygenase is not affected by NSAIDs, and many new inhibitors of this enzyme pathway have been developed. Pharmacologic agents that inhibit leukotriene production (e.g., zileuton) are useful in the treatment of asthma.
- **Corticosteroids** are broad-spectrum anti-inflammatory agents that reduce the transcription of genes encoding COX-2, phospholipase A_2, proinflammatory cytokines (e.g., IL-1 and TNF), and iNOS.
- **Leukotriene receptor antagonists** block leukotriene receptors and prevent the actions of the leukotrienes. These drugs (e.g., Montelukast) are useful in the treatment of asthma.

Cytokines and Chemokines

Cytokines are proteins secreted by many cell types (principally activated lymphocytes, macrophages, and dendritic cells, but also endothelial, epithelial, and connective tissue cells) that mediate and regulate immune and inflammatory reactions. By convention, growth factors that act on epithelial and mesenchymal cells are not grouped under cytokines. The general properties and functions of cytokines are discussed in Chapter 5. Here the cytokines involved in acute inflammation are reviewed (Table 3.7).

Tumor Necrosis Factor and Interleukin-1

TNF and IL-1 serve critical roles in leukocyte recruitment by promoting adhesion of leukocytes to endothelium and their migration through vessels. Activated macrophages and dendritic cells mainly produce these cytokines; TNF also is produced by T lymphocytes and mast cells, and some epithelial cells produce IL-1 as well. Microbial products, foreign bodies, necrotic cells, and a variety of other inflammatory stimuli can stimulate the secretion of TNF and IL-1. The production of TNF is induced by signals through TLRs and other microbial sensors, and the synthesis of IL-1 is stimulated by the same signals, but the generation of the biologically active form of this cytokine is dependent on the inflammasome, described earlier.

Table 3.7 Cytokines in Inflammation

Cytokine	Principal Sources	Principal Actions in Inflammation
In Acute Inflammation		
TNF	Macrophages, mast cells, T lymphocytes	Stimulates expression of endothelial adhesion molecules and secretion of other cytokines; systemic effects
IL-1	Macrophages, endothelial cells, some epithelial cells	Similar to TNF; greater role in fever
IL-6	Macrophages, other cells	Systemic effects (acute phase response)
Chemokines	Macrophages, endothelial cells, T lymphocytes, mast cells, other cell types	Recruitment of leukocytes to sites of inflammation; migration of cells in normal tissues
IL-17	T lymphocytes	Recruitment of neutrophils and monocytes
In Chronic Inflammation		
IL-12	Dendritic cells, macrophages	Increased production of IFN-γ
IFN-γ	T lymphocytes, NK cells	Activation of macrophages (increased ability to kill microbes and tumor cells)
IL-17	T lymphocytes	Recruitment of neutrophils and monocytes

The most important cytokines involved in inflammatory reactions are listed. Many other cytokines may play lesser roles in inflammation. There is also considerable overlap between the cytokines involved in acute and chronic inflammation. Specifically, all the cytokines listed under acute inflammation may also contribute to chronic inflammatory reactions.
IFN-γ, Interferon-γ; *IL-1*, interleukin-1; *NK*, natural killer; *TNF*, tumor necrosis factor.

The actions of TNF and IL-1 contribute to the local and systemic reactions of inflammation (Fig. 3.10). The most important roles of these cytokines in inflammation are the following:

- **Endothelial activation.** Both TNF and IL-1 act on endothelium to induce a spectrum of changes referred to as *endothelial activation*. These changes include increased expression of endothelial adhesion molecules, mostly E- and P-selectins and ligands for leukocyte integrins; increased production of various mediators, including other cytokines and chemokines, and eicosanoids; and increased procoagulant activity of the endothelium.
- **Activation of leukocytes and other cells.** TNF augments responses of neutrophils to other stimuli such as bacterial endotoxin and stimulates the microbicidal activity of macrophages. IL-1 activates fibroblasts to synthesize collagen and stimulates proliferation of synovial cells and other mesenchymal cells. IL-1 and IL-6 also stimulate the generation of a subset of CD4+ helper T cells called T_H17 cells, described later and in Chapter 5.
- **Systemic acute-phase response.** IL-1 and TNF (as well as IL-6) induce the systemic acute-phase responses associated with infection or injury, including fever (described later in the chapter). They also are implicated in the pathogenesis of the systemic inflammatory response

syndrome (SIRS), resulting from disseminated bacterial infection (sepsis) and other serious conditions, described later.
- TNF regulates energy balance by promoting lipid and protein catabolism and by suppressing appetite. Therefore, sustained production of TNF contributes to *cachexia*, a pathologic state characterized by weight loss, muscle atrophy, and anorexia that accompanies some chronic infections and cancers.

As mentioned earlier, **TNF antagonists have been remarkably effective in the treatment of chronic inflammatory diseases,** particularly rheumatoid arthritis, psoriasis, and some types of inflammatory bowel disease. One complication of this therapy is increased susceptibility to mycobacterial infection, resulting from reduced ability of macrophages to kill intracellular microbes. Although many of the actions of TNF and IL-1 are overlapping, IL-1 antagonists are not as effective, for reasons that remain obscure. Also, blocking either cytokine has no effect on the outcome of sepsis, perhaps because other cytokines contribute to this serious systemic inflammatory reaction.

Chemokines

Chemokines are a family of small (8–10 kD) proteins that act primarily as chemoattractants for specific types of leukocytes. About 40 different chemokines and 20 different receptors for chemokines have been identified. They are classified into four major groups, according to the arrangement of cysteine (C) residues in the proteins:

- *C-X-C chemokines* have one amino acid residue separating the first two of the four conserved cysteines. These chemokines act primarily on neutrophils. IL-8 (now called CXCL8) is typical of this group. It is secreted by activated macrophages, endothelial cells, and other cell types, and causes activation and chemotaxis of neutrophils, with limited activity on monocytes and eosinophils. Its most important inducers are microbial products and cytokines, mainly IL-1 and TNF.
- *C-C chemokines* have the first two conserved cysteine residues adjacent. The C-C chemokines, which include monocyte chemoattractant protein (MCP-1, CCL2), eotaxin (CCL11), and macrophage inflammatory protein-1α (MIP-1α, CCL3), mainly serve as chemoattractants for monocytes, eosinophils, basophils, and lymphocytes. Although most of the chemokines in this class have overlapping actions, eotaxin selectively recruits eosinophils.
- *C chemokines* lack the first and third of the four conserved cysteines. The C chemokines (e.g., lymphotactin, XCL1) are relatively specific for lymphocytes.
- *CX_3C chemokines* contain three amino acids between the first two cysteines. The only known member of this class is called *fractalkine* (CX_3CL1). This chemokine exists in two forms: a cell surface-bound protein induced on endothelial cells by inflammatory cytokines that promotes strong adhesion of monocytes and T cells, and a soluble form, derived by proteolysis of the membrane-bound protein, that has potent chemoattractant activity for the same cells.

Chemokines mediate their activities by binding to seven-transmembrane G protein–coupled receptors. These

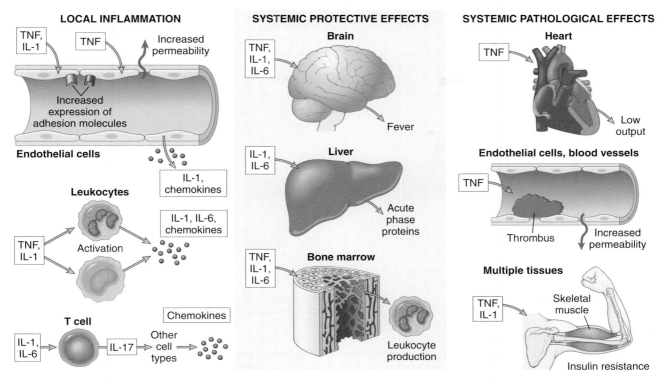

Fig. 3.10 Major roles of cytokines in acute inflammation. *PDGF,* Platelet-derived growth factor; *PGE,* prostaglandin E; *PGI,* prostaglandin I.

receptors usually exhibit overlapping ligand specificities, and leukocytes generally express multiple receptors. As discussed in Chapter 5, certain chemokine receptors (CXCR4, CCR5) act as coreceptors for a viral envelope glycoprotein of human immunodeficiency virus (HIV), the cause of AIDS, and are thus involved in binding and entry of the virus into cells.

Chemokines bind to proteoglycans and are displayed at high concentrations on the surface of endothelial cells and in the extracellular matrix. They have two main functions:

- **Acute inflammation.** Most chemokines stimulate leukocyte attachment to endothelium by acting on leukocytes to increase the affinity of integrins, and also serve as chemoattractants, thereby guiding leukocytes to sites of infection or tissue damage. Because they mediate aspects of the inflammatory reaction, they are sometimes called *inflammatory chemokines.* Their production is induced by microbes and other stimuli.
- **Maintenance of tissue architecture.** Some chemokines are produced constitutively by stromal cells in tissues and are sometimes called *homeostatic chemokines.* These organize various cell types in different anatomic regions of the tissues, such as T and B lymphocytes in discrete areas of the spleen and lymph nodes (Chapter 5).

Although the role of chemokines in inflammation is well established, it has proved difficult to develop chemokine antagonists that suppress inflammation, perhaps because of the functional redundancy of these proteins.

Other Cytokines in Acute Inflammation

The list of cytokines implicated in inflammation is huge and constantly growing. In addition to the ones described

earlier, two that have received considerable interest are IL-6, made by macrophages and other cells, which is involved in local and systemic reactions, and IL-17, produced mainly by T lymphocytes, which promotes neutrophil recruitment. IL-6 receptor antagonists are used in the treatment of rheumatoid arthritis, and IL-17 antagonists are very effective in psoriasis and other inflammatory diseases. Type I interferons, whose normal function is to inhibit viral replication, contribute to some of the systemic manifestations of inflammation. Cytokines also play key roles in chronic inflammation; these are described later in the chapter.

Complement System

The complement system is a collection of soluble proteins and their membrane receptors that function mainly in host defense against microbes and in pathologic inflammatory reactions. There are more than 20 complement proteins, some of which are numbered C1 through C9. They function in both innate and adaptive immunity for defense against microbial pathogens. In the process of complement activation, several cleavage products of complement proteins are elaborated that cause increased vascular permeability, chemotaxis, and opsonization. The activation and functions of complement are outlined in Fig. 3.11.

Complement proteins are present in inactive forms in the plasma, and many of them are activated to become proteolytic enzymes that degrade other complement proteins, thus forming an enzymatic cascade capable of tremendous amplification. The critical step in complement activation is the proteolysis of the third (and most

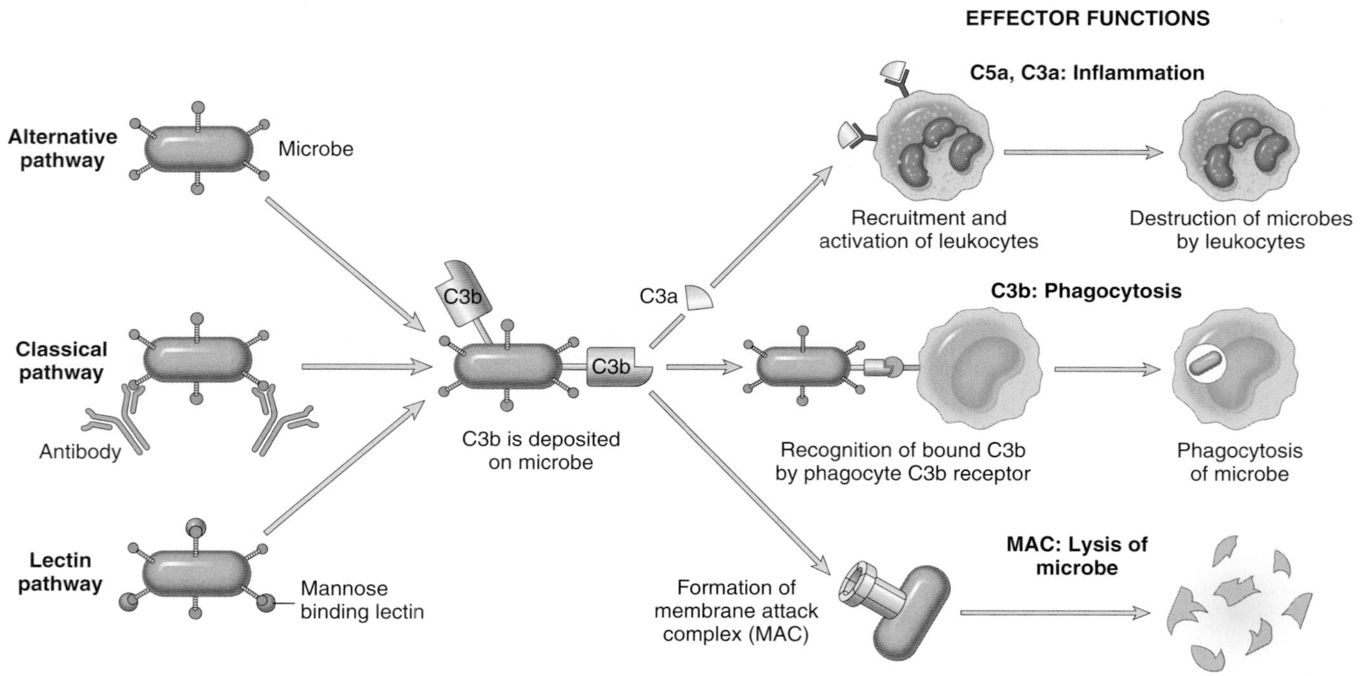

Fig. 3.11 The activation and functions of the complement system. Activation of complement by different pathways leads to cleavage of C3. The functions of the complement system are mediated by breakdown products of C3 and other complement proteins, and by the membrane attack complex (MAC).

abundant) component, C3. **Cleavage of C3 can occur by one of three pathways**:

- The *classical pathway*, which is triggered by fixation of C1 to antibody (IgM or IgG) that has combined with antigen
- The *alternative pathway*, which can be triggered by microbial surface molecules (e.g., endotoxin, or LPS), complex polysaccharides, and other substances, in the absence of antibody
- The *lectin pathway*, in which plasma mannose-binding lectin binds to carbohydrates on microbes and directly activates C1

All three pathways of complement activation lead to the formation of an enzyme called the *C3 convertase*, which splits C3 into two functionally distinct fragments, C3a and C3b. C3a is released, and C3b becomes covalently attached to the cell or molecule where the complement is being activated. More C3b then binds to the previously generated fragments to form *C5 convertase*, which cleaves C5 to release C5a and leave C5b attached to the cell surface. C5b binds the late components (C6–C9), culminating in the formation of the membrane attack complex (MAC, composed of multiple C9 molecules). The enzymatic activity of complement proteins provides such tremendous amplification that millions of molecules of C3b can deposit on the surface of a microbe within 2 or 3 minutes!

The complement system has three main functions (Fig. 3.11):

- **Inflammation.** *C5a,* and, to a lesser extent, *C4a* and *C3a,* are cleavage products of the corresponding complement components that stimulate histamine release from mast cells and thereby increase vascular permeability and cause vasodilation. They are called *anaphylatoxins*

because they have effects similar to those of mast cell mediators that are involved in the reaction called *anaphylaxis* (Chapter 5). C5a also is a chemotactic agent for neutrophils, monocytes, eosinophils, and basophils. In addition, C5a activates the lipoxygenase pathway of arachidonic acid metabolism in neutrophils and monocytes, causing release of more inflammatory mediators.

- **Opsonization and phagocytosis.** *C3b* and its cleavage product *iC3b* (inactive C3b), when fixed to a microbial cell wall, act as opsonins and promote phagocytosis by neutrophils and macrophages, which bear cell surface receptors for these complement fragments.
- **Cell lysis.** The deposition of the MAC on cells drills holes in the cell membrane, making the cells permeable to water and ions and resulting in their osmotic death (lysis). This function of complement is important mainly for the killing of microbes with thin cell walls, such as *Neisseria* bacteria. Hence, deficiency of the terminal components of complement predisposes to infections by the *Neisseria* species meningococci and gonococci. In patients with complement deficiencies, these microbes can cause serious disseminated infections.

The activation of complement is tightly controlled by cell-associated and circulating regulatory proteins. Different regulatory proteins inhibit the production of active complement fragments or remove fragments that deposit on cells. These regulators are expressed on normal host cells and thus prevent healthy tissues from being injured at sites of complement activation. Regulatory proteins can be overwhelmed when large amounts of complement are deposited on host cells and in tissues, as happens in autoimmune diseases, in which individuals produce complement-fixing antibodies against their own cell and tissue antigens (Chapter 5). The most important of these regulatory proteins are the following:

- **C1 inhibitor** blocks the activation of C1, the first protein of the classical complement pathway. Inherited deficiency of this inhibitor is the cause of *hereditary angioedema*.
- **Decay accelerating factor (DAF)** and **CD59** are two proteins that are linked to plasma membranes by a glycophosphatidyl (GPI) anchor. DAF prevents formation of C3 convertases and CD59 inhibits formation of the MAC. An acquired deficiency of the enzyme that creates GPI anchors leads to deficiency of these regulators and excessive complement activation and lysis of red cells (which are sensitive to complement-mediated cell lysis). This gives rise to a disease called *paroxysmal nocturnal hemoglobinuria (PNH)* (Chapter 12).
- Other complement regulatory proteins proteolytically cleave active complement components. For instance, Factor H is a plasma protein that serves as a cofactor for the proteolysis of the C3 convertase; its deficiency results in excessive complement activation. Mutations in Factor H are associated with a kidney disease called the hemolytic uremic syndrome (Chapter 14), as well as increased permeability of retinal vessels in *wet* macular degeneration of the eye.

The complement system contributes to disease in several ways. The activation of complement by antibodies or antigen–antibody complexes deposited on host cells and tissues is an important mechanism of cell and tissue injury (Chapter 5). Inherited deficiencies of complement proteins cause increased susceptibility to infections, and, as mentioned earlier, deficiencies of regulatory proteins cause a variety of disorders.

Other Mediators of Inflammation

Platelet-Activating Factor

PAF is a phospholipid-derived mediator that was discovered as a factor that caused platelet aggregation, but it is now known to have multiple inflammatory effects. A variety of cell types, including platelets themselves, basophils, mast cells, neutrophils, macrophages, and endothelial cells, can elaborate PAF. In addition to platelet aggregation, PAF causes vasoconstriction and bronchoconstriction, and at low concentrations it induces vasodilation and increased vascular permeability. Despite these documented actions, trials of PAF antagonists in various inflammatory conditions have been disappointing.

Products of Coagulation

Studies performed more than 50 years ago suggested that inhibiting coagulation reduced the inflammatory reaction to some microbes, leading to the idea that coagulation and inflammation are linked processes. This concept was supported by the discovery of protease-activated receptors (PARs), which are activated by thrombin (the protease that cleaves fibrinogen to produce a fibrin clot). PARs are expressed on leukocytes, suggesting a role in inflammation, but their clearest role is in platelets, in which thrombin activation of a PAR known as the thrombin receptor is a potent trigger of platelet aggregation during the process of clot formation (Chapter 4). In fact, it is difficult to dissociate clotting and inflammation, because virtually all forms of tissue injury that lead to clotting also induce inflammation, and inflammation causes changes in endothelial cells that increase the likelihood of abnormal clotting (thrombosis, described in Chapter 4). Whether the products of coagulation, per se, have a significant role in stimulating inflammation is still not established.

Kinins

Kinins are vasoactive peptides derived from plasma proteins, called kininogens, by the action of specific proteases called kallikreins. The enzyme kallikrein cleaves a plasma glycoprotein precursor, high-molecular-weight kininogen, to produce *bradykinin*. **Bradykinin increases vascular permeability and causes contraction of smooth muscle, dilation of blood vessels, and pain when injected into the skin.** These effects are similar to those of histamine. The action of bradykinin is short-lived, because it is quickly inactivated by an enzyme called kininase. Bradykinin has been implicated as a mediator in some forms of allergic reaction, such as anaphylaxis.

Neuropeptides

Neuropeptides are secreted by sensory nerves and various leukocytes, and may play a role in the initiation and regulation of inflammatory responses. These small peptides, including substance P and neurokinin A, are produced in the central and peripheral nervous systems. Nerve fibers containing substance P are prominent in the lung and gastrointestinal tract. Substance P has many biologic functions, including the transmission of pain signals, regulation of blood pressure, stimulation of hormone secretion by endocrine cells, and in increasing vascular permeability.

When Lewis discovered the role of histamine in inflammation, one mediator was thought to be enough. Now, we are wallowing in them! Yet, from this large compendium, it is likely that a few mediators are most important for the reactions of acute inflammation in vivo, and these are summarized in Table 3.8. This list is compiled in part from the

Table 3.8 Role of Mediators in Different Reactions of Inflammation

Reaction of Inflammation	Principal Mediators
Vasodilation	Histamine Prostaglandins
Increased vascular permeability	Histamine C3a and C5a (by liberating vasoactive amines from mast cells, other cells) Leukotrienes C_4, D_4, E_4
Chemotaxis, leukocyte recruitment and activation	TNF, IL-1 Chemokines C3a, C5a Leukotriene B_4
Fever	IL-1, TNF Prostaglandins
Pain	Prostaglandins Bradykinin
Tissue damage	Lysosomal enzymes of leukocytes Reactive oxygen species

observed anti-inflammatory effects of antagonists to these molecules, thus highlighting the importance of basic biology to the practice of medicine. The redundancy of the mediators and their actions ensures that this protective response remains robust and is not readily subverted.

SUMMARY

ACTIONS OF THE PRINCIPAL MEDIATORS OF INFLAMMATION

- Vasoactive amines, mainly histamine: vasodilation and increased vascular permeability
- Arachidonic acid metabolites (prostaglandins and leukotrienes): several forms exist and are involved in vascular reactions, leukocyte chemotaxis, and other reactions of inflammation; antagonized by lipoxins
- Cytokines: proteins produced by many cell types; usually act at short range; mediate multiple effects, mainly in leukocyte recruitment and migration; principal ones in acute inflammation are TNF, IL-1, and chemokines
- Complement proteins: Activation of the complement system by microbes or antibodies leads to the generation of multiple breakdown products, which are responsible for leukocyte chemotaxis, opsonization and phagocytosis of microbes and other particles, and cell killing
- Kinins: produced by proteolytic cleavage of precursors; mediate vascular reaction, pain

MORPHOLOGIC PATTERNS OF ACUTE INFLAMMATION

The morphologic hallmarks of acute inflammatory reactions are dilation of small blood vessels and accumulation of leukocytes and fluid in the extravascular tissue. The vascular and cellular reactions account for the signs and symptoms of the inflammatory response. Increased blood flow to the injured area and increased vascular permeability lead to the accumulation of extravascular fluid rich in plasma proteins (*edema*) and account for the redness (*rubor*), warmth (*calor*), and swelling (*tumor*) that accompany acute inflammation. Leukocytes that are recruited and activated by the offending agent and by endogenous mediators may release toxic metabolites and proteases extracellularly, causing tissue damage and loss of function (*functio laesa*). During the damage, and in part as a result of the liberation of prostaglandins, neuropeptides, and cytokines, one of the local symptoms is pain (*dolor*).

Although these general features are characteristic of most acute inflammatory reactions, special morphologic patterns are often superimposed on them, depending on the severity of the reaction, its specific cause, and the particular tissue and site involved. The importance of recognizing distinct gross and microscopic patterns of inflammation is that they often provide valuable clues about the underlying cause.

Serous Inflammation

Serous inflammation is marked by the exudation of cell-poor fluid into spaces created by injury to surface epithelia

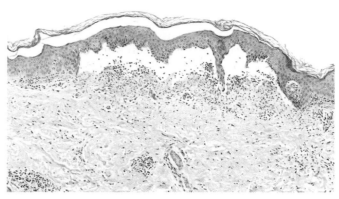

Fig. 3.12 Serous inflammation. Low-power view of a cross section of a skin blister showing the epidermis separated from the dermis by a focal collection of serous effusion.

or into body cavities lined by the peritoneum, pleura, or pericardium. Typically, the fluid in serous inflammation is not infected by destructive organisms and does not contain large numbers of leukocytes (which tend to produce purulent inflammation, described later). In body cavities the fluid may be derived from the plasma (as a result of increased vascular permeability) or from the secretions of mesothelial cells (as a result of local irritation); accumulation of fluid in these cavities is called an *effusion*. (Effusions consisting of transudates also occur in noninflammatory conditions, such as reduced blood outflow in heart failure, or reduced plasma protein levels in some kidney and liver diseases.) The skin blister resulting from a burn or viral infection represents accumulation of serous fluid within or immediately beneath the damaged epidermis of the skin (Fig. 3.12).

Fibrinous Inflammation

A fibrinous exudate develops when the vascular leaks are large or there is a local procoagulant stimulus. With a large increase in vascular permeability, higher-molecular-weight proteins such as fibrinogen pass out of the blood, and fibrin is formed and deposited in the extracellular space. A fibrinous exudate is characteristic of inflammation in the lining of body cavities, such as the meninges, pericardium (Fig. 3.13A), and pleura. Histologically, fibrin appears as an eosinophilic meshwork of threads or sometimes as an amorphous coagulum (Fig. 3.13B). Fibrinous exudates may be dissolved by fibrinolysis and cleared by macrophages. If the fibrin is not removed, with time, it may stimulate the ingrowth of fibroblasts and blood vessels and thus lead to scarring. Conversion of the fibrinous exudate to scar tissue (*organization*) within the pericardial sac leads to opaque fibrous thickening of the pericardium and epicardium in the area of exudation and, if the fibrosis is extensive, obliteration of the pericardial space.

Purulent (Suppurative) Inflammation, Abscess

Purulent inflammation is characterized by the production of pus, an exudate consisting of neutrophils, the liquefied debris of necrotic cells, and edema fluid. The most frequent cause of purulent (also called *suppurative*)

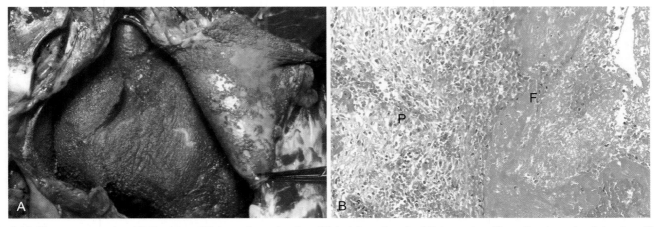

Fig. 3.13 Fibrinous pericarditis. (A) Deposits of fibrin on the pericardium. (B) A pink meshwork of fibrin exudate *(F)* overlies the pericardial surface *(P)*.

inflammation is infection with bacteria that cause liquefactive tissue necrosis, such as staphylococci; these pathogens are referred to as *pyogenic* (pus-producing) bacteria. A common example of an acute suppurative inflammation is acute appendicitis. ***Abscesses* are localized collections of pus** caused by suppuration buried in a tissue, an organ, or a confined space. They are produced by seeding of pyogenic bacteria into a tissue (Fig. 3.14). Abscesses have a central region that appears as a mass of necrotic leukocytes and tissue cells. There is usually a zone of preserved neutrophils around this necrotic focus, and outside this region there may be vascular dilation and parenchymal and fibroblastic proliferation, indicating chronic inflammation and repair. In time the abscess may become walled off and ultimately replaced by connective tissue. When persistent or at critical locations (such as the brain), abscesses may have to be drained surgically.

Ulcers

An ulcer is a local defect, or excavation, of the surface of an organ or tissue that is produced by the sloughing (shedding) of inflamed necrotic tissue (Fig. 3.15). Ulceration can occur only when tissue necrosis and resultant inflammation exist on or near a surface. It is most commonly encountered in (1) the mucosa of the mouth, stomach, intestines, or genitourinary tract, and (2) the skin and subcutaneous tissue of the lower extremities in older persons who have circulatory disturbances that predispose to extensive ischemic necrosis. Acute and chronic inflammation often coexist in ulcers, such as peptic ulcers of the stomach or duodenum and diabetic ulcers of the legs. During the acute stage there is intense polymorphonuclear infiltration and vascular dilation in the margins of the defect. With chronicity, the margins and base of the ulcer develop fibroblast proliferation, scarring, and the accumulation of lymphocytes, macrophages, and plasma cells.

OUTCOMES OF ACUTE INFLAMMATION

Although, as might be expected, many variables may modify the basic process of inflammation, including the

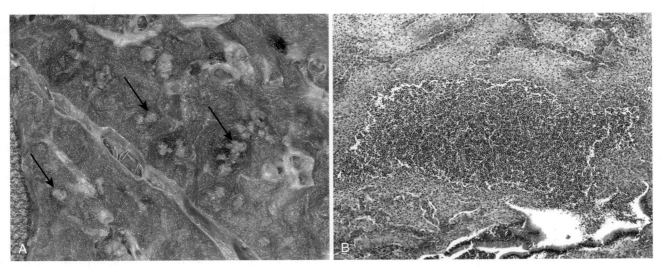

Fig. 3.14 Purulent inflammation. (A) Multiple bacterial abscesses *(arrows)* in the lung in a case of bronchopneumonia. (B) The abscess contains neutrophils and cellular debris, and is surrounded by congested blood vessels.

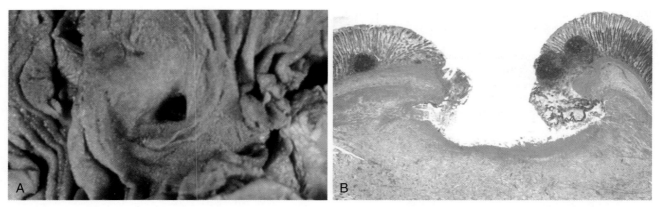

Fig. 3.15 The morphology of an ulcer. (A) A chronic duodenal ulcer. (B) Low-power cross-section view of a duodenal ulcer crater with an acute inflammatory exudate in the base.

nature and intensity of the injury, the site and tissue affected, and the responsiveness of the host, **acute inflammatory reactions typically have one of three outcomes** (Fig. 3.16):

- **Complete resolution.** In a perfect world, all inflammatory reactions, after they have succeeded in eliminating the offending agent, should end with restoration of the site of acute inflammation to normal. This is called *resolution* and is the usual outcome when the injury is limited or short-lived or when there has been little tissue destruction and the damaged parenchymal cells can regenerate. Resolution involves removal of cellular debris and microbes by macrophages, and resorption of edema fluid by lymphatics.

- **Healing by connective tissue replacement (scarring, or fibrosis).** This occurs after substantial tissue destruction, when the inflammatory injury involves tissues that are incapable of regeneration, or when there is abundant fibrin exudation in tissue or in serous cavities (pleura, peritoneum) that cannot be adequately cleared. In all

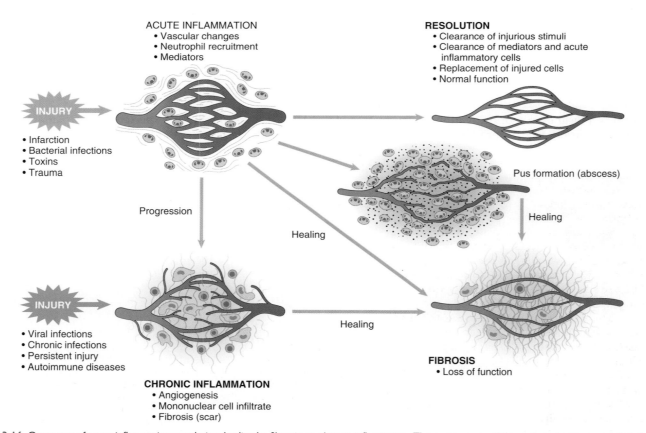

Fig. 3.16 Outcomes of acute inflammation: resolution, healing by fibrosis, or chronic inflammation. The components of the various reactions and their functional outcomes are listed.

these situations, connective tissue grows into the area of damage or exudate, converting it into a mass of fibrous tissue.

- Progression of the response to **chronic inflammation.** Acute to chronic transition occurs when the acute inflammatory response cannot be resolved, as a result of either the persistence of the injurious agent or some interference with the normal process of healing.

CHRONIC INFLAMMATION

Chronic inflammation is a response of prolonged duration (weeks or months) in which inflammation, tissue injury, and attempts at repair coexist, in varying combinations. It may follow acute inflammation, as described earlier, or may begin insidiously, as a smoldering, sometimes progressive, process without any signs of a preceding acute reaction.

Causes of Chronic Inflammation

Chronic inflammation arises in the following settings:

- **Persistent infections** by microorganisms that are difficult to eradicate, such as mycobacteria and certain viruses, fungi, and parasites. These organisms often evoke an immune reaction called *delayed-type hypersensitivity* (Chapter 5). The inflammatory response sometimes takes a specific pattern called *granulomatous inflammation* (discussed later). In other cases, unresolved acute inflammation evolves into chronic inflammation, such as when an acute bacterial infection of the lung progresses to a chronic lung abscess.
- **Hypersensitivity diseases.** Chronic inflammation plays an important role in a group of diseases that are caused by excessive and inappropriate activation of the immune system (Chapter 5). In *autoimmune diseases*, self (auto) antigens evoke a self-perpetuating immune reaction that results in chronic inflammation and tissue damage; examples of such diseases are rheumatoid arthritis and multiple sclerosis. In *allergic diseases*, chronic inflammation is the result of excessive immune responses against common environmental substances, as in bronchial asthma. Because these autoimmune and allergic reactions are triggered against antigens that are normally harmless, the reactions serve no useful purpose and only cause disease. Such diseases may show morphologic patterns of mixed acute and chronic inflammation because they are characterized by repeated bouts of inflammation. Fibrosis may dominate the late stages.
- **Prolonged exposure to potentially toxic agents, either exogenous or endogenous.** An example of an exogenous agent is particulate silica, a nondegradable inanimate material that, when inhaled for prolonged periods, results in an inflammatory lung disease called *silicosis* (Chapter 13). *Atherosclerosis* (Chapter 10) is a chronic inflammatory process affecting the arterial wall that is thought to be induced, at least in part, by excessive production and tissue deposition of endogenous cholesterol and other lipids.
- Some forms of chronic inflammation may be important in the pathogenesis of diseases that are not conventionally thought of as inflammatory disorders. These include neurodegenerative diseases such as Alzheimer disease, metabolic syndrome and the associated type 2 diabetes, and certain cancers in which inflammatory reactions promote tumor development. The role of inflammation in these conditions is discussed in the relevant chapters.

Morphologic Features

In contrast to acute inflammation, which is manifested by vascular changes, edema, and predominantly neutrophilic infiltration, chronic inflammation is characterized by the following:

- **Infiltration with mononuclear cells,** which include macrophages, lymphocytes, and plasma cells (Fig. 3.17)
- **Tissue destruction,** induced by the persistent offending agent or by the inflammatory cells
- **Attempts at healing** by connective tissue replacement of damaged tissue, accomplished by *angiogenesis* (proliferation of small blood vessels) and, in particular, *fibrosis*

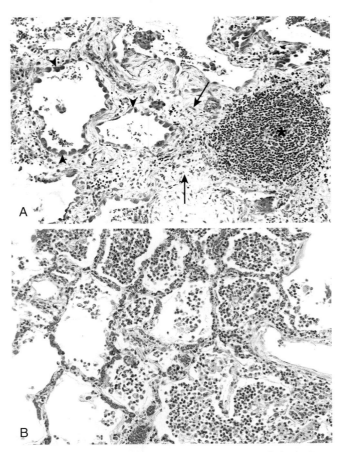

Fig. 3.17 (A) Chronic inflammation in the lung, showing all three characteristic histologic features: (1) collection of chronic inflammatory cells (*), (2) destruction of parenchyma (normal alveoli are replaced by spaces lined by cuboidal epithelium, *arrowheads*), and (3) replacement by connective tissue (fibrosis, *arrows*). (B) In contrast, in acute inflammation of the lung (acute bronchopneumonia), neutrophils fill the alveolar spaces and blood vessels are congested.

Because angiogenesis and fibrosis are also components of wound healing and repair, they are discussed later, in the context of tissue repair.

Cells and Mediators of Chronic Inflammation

The combination of leukocyte infiltration, tissue damage, and fibrosis that characterize chronic inflammation is the result of the local activation of several cell types and the production of mediators.

Role of Macrophages

The dominant cells in most chronic inflammatory reactions are macrophages, which contribute to the reaction by secreting cytokines and growth factors that act on various cells, by destroying foreign invaders and tissues, and by activating other cells, notably T lymphocytes. Macrophages are professional phagocytes that act as filters for particulate matter, microbes, and senescent cells. They also function as effector cells that eliminate microbes in cellular and humoral immune responses (Chapter 5). But they serve many other roles in inflammation and repair. Here we review the basic biology of macrophages, including their development and functional responses.

Macrophages are tissue cells derived from hematopoietic stem cells in the bone marrow and from progenitors in the embryonic yolk sac and fetal liver during early development (Fig. 3.18). Circulating cells of this lineage are known as *monocytes*. Macrophages are normally diffusely scattered in most connective tissues. In addition, they are found in specific locations in organs such as the liver (where they are called Kupffer cells), spleen and lymph nodes (sinus histiocytes), central nervous system (microglial cells), and lungs (alveolar macrophages). Together these cells comprise the *mononuclear phagocyte system*, also known by the older (and inaccurate) name of reticuloendothelial system.

In inflammatory reactions, progenitors in the bone marrow give rise to monocytes, which enter the blood, migrate into various tissues, and differentiate into macrophages. Entry of blood monocytes into tissues is governed by the same factors that are involved in neutrophil emigration, such as adhesion molecules and chemokines. The half-life of blood monocytes is about 1 day, whereas the life span of tissue macrophages is several months or years. Thus, macrophages often become the dominant cell population in inflammatory reactions within 48 hours of onset. The macrophages that reside in tissues in the steady state (in the absence of tissue injury or inflammation), such as microglia, Kupffer cells, and alveolar macrophages, arise from the yolk sac or fetal liver very early in embryogenesis, populate the tissues, stay for long periods, and are replenished mainly by the proliferation of resident cells.

There are two major pathways of macrophage activation, called *classical* **and** *alternative* (Fig. 3.19). Which of these two pathways is taken by a given macrophage depends on the nature of the activating signals.

- **Classical macrophage activation** may be induced by microbial products such as endotoxin, which engage TLRs and other sensors, and by T cell–derived signals,

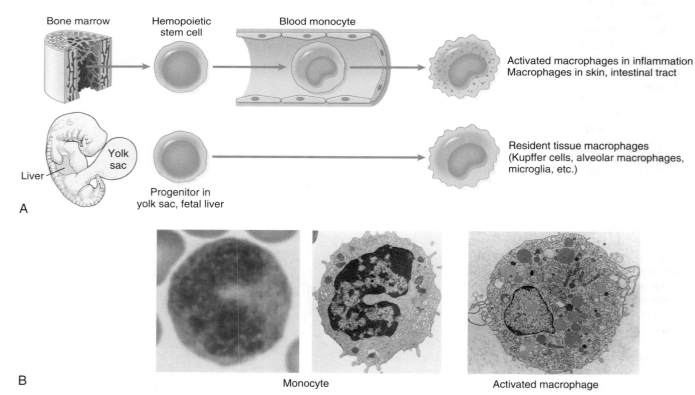

Fig. 3.18 Maturation of mononuclear phagocytes. (A) During inflammatory reactions, the majority of tissue macrophages are derived from hematopoietic precursors. Some long-lived resident tissue macrophages are derived from embryonic precursors that populate the tissues early in development. (B) The morphology of a monocyte and activated macrophage.

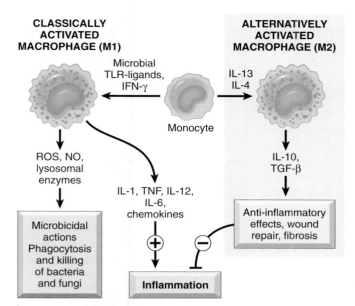

Fig. 3.19 Classical and alternative macrophage activation. Different stimuli activate monocytes/macrophages to develop into functionally distinct populations. Classically activated macrophages are induced by microbial products and cytokines, particularly IFN-γ. They phagocytose and destroy microbes and dead tissues and can potentiate inflammatory reactions. Alternatively activated macrophages are induced by other cytokines and are important in tissue repair and the resolution of inflammation.

importantly the cytokine IFN-γ, in immune responses. Classically activated (also called M1) macrophages produce NO and ROS and upregulate lysosomal enzymes, all of which enhance their ability to kill ingested organisms, and secrete cytokines that stimulate inflammation. These macrophages are important in host defense against microbes and in many inflammatory reactions.

- **Alternative macrophage activation** is induced by cytokines other than IFN-γ, such as IL-4 and IL-13, produced by T lymphocytes and other cells. These macrophages are not actively microbicidal; instead, the principal function of alternatively activated (M2) macrophages is in tissue repair. They secrete growth factors that promote angiogenesis, activate fibroblasts, and stimulate collagen synthesis.

It seems plausible that in response to most injurious stimuli, the first activation pathway is the classical one, designed to destroy the offending agents, and this is followed by alternative activation, which initiates tissue repair. However, such a precise sequence is not well documented in most inflammatory reactions. In addition, although the concept of M1 and M2 macrophages provides a useful framework for understanding macrophage heterogeneity, numerous other subpopulations have been described and the M1 and M2 subsets are not fixed.

The products of activated macrophages eliminate injurious agents such as microbes and initiate the process of repair, but are also responsible for much of the tissue injury in chronic inflammation. Several functions of macrophages are central to the development and persistence of chronic inflammation and the accompanying tissue injury.

- **Macrophages secrete mediators of inflammation,** such as cytokines (TNF, IL-1, chemokines, and others) and eicosanoids. Thus, macrophages are central to the initiation and propagation of inflammatory reactions.
- Macrophages **display antigens to T lymphocytes and respond to signals from T cells,** thus setting up a feedback loop that is essential for defense against many microbes by cell-mediated immune responses. These interactions are described further in the discussion of the role of lymphocytes in chronic inflammation, later in this chapter, and in more detail in Chapter 5 where cell-mediated immunity is considered.

Their impressive arsenal of mediators makes macrophages powerful allies in the body's defense against unwanted invaders, but the same weaponry can also induce considerable tissue destruction when macrophages are inappropriately or excessively activated. It is because of these activities of macrophages that tissue destruction is one of the hallmarks of chronic inflammation.

In some instances if the irritant is eliminated, macrophages eventually disappear (either dying off or making their way via lymphatics into lymph nodes). In others, macrophage accumulation persists, as a result of continuous recruitment from the circulation and local proliferation at the site of inflammation.

Role of Lymphocytes

Microbes and other environmental antigens activate T and B lymphocytes, which amplify and propagate chronic inflammation. Although the major function of these lymphocytes is as the mediators of adaptive immunity, which provides defense against infectious pathogens (Chapter 5), these cells are often present in chronic inflammation and, when they are activated, the inflammation tends to be persistent and severe. Some of the strongest chronic inflammatory reactions, such as granulomatous inflammation, described later, are dependent on lymphocyte responses. Lymphocytes may be the dominant population in the chronic inflammation seen in autoimmune and other hypersensitivity diseases.

By virtue of their ability to secrete cytokines, CD4+ T lymphocytes promote inflammation and influence the nature of the inflammatory reaction. These T cells greatly amplify the early inflammatory reaction that is induced by recognition of microbes and dead cells as part of the innate immune response. There are three subsets of CD4+ T cells that secrete different cytokines and elicit different types of inflammation.

- T$_H$1 cells produce the cytokine IFN-γ, which activates macrophages by the classical pathway.
- T$_H$2 cells secrete IL-4, IL-5, and IL-13, which recruit and activate eosinophils and are responsible for the alternative pathway of macrophage activation.
- T$_H$17 cells secrete IL-17 and other cytokines, which induce the secretion of chemokines responsible for recruiting neutrophils into the reaction.

Both T$_H$1 and T$_H$17 cells are involved in defense against many types of bacteria and viruses and in autoimmune diseases. T$_H$2 cells are important in defense against helminthic parasites and in allergic inflammation. These T cell

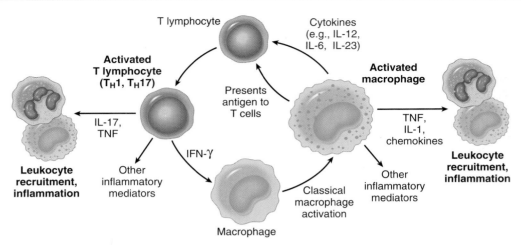

Fig. 3.20 Macrophage–lymphocyte interactions in chronic inflammation. Activated T cells produce cytokines that recruit macrophages (TNF, IL-17, chemokines) and others that activate macrophages (IFN-γ). Activated macrophages in turn stimulate T cells by presenting antigens and via cytokines such as IL-12.

subsets and their functions are described in more detail in Chapter 5.

Lymphocytes and macrophages interact in a bidirectional way, and these interactions play an important role in propagating chronic inflammation (Fig. 3.20). Macrophages display antigens to T cells, express membrane molecules (called costimulators) that activate T cells, and produce cytokines (IL-12 and others) that also stimulate T cell responses (Chapter 5). Activated T lymphocytes, in turn, produce cytokines, described earlier, which recruit and activate macrophages, promoting more antigen presentation and cytokine secretion. The result is a cycle of cellular reactions that fuel and sustain chronic inflammation.

Activated B lymphocytes and antibody-producing plasma cells are often present at sites of chronic inflammation. The antibodies may be specific for persistent foreign or self antigens in the inflammatory site or against altered tissue components. However, the specificity and even the importance of antibodies in most chronic inflammatory disorders are unclear.

In some chronic inflammatory reactions, the accumulated lymphocytes, antigen-presenting cells, and plasma cells cluster together to form lymphoid structures resembling the follicles found in lymph nodes. These are called *tertiary lymphoid organs*; this type of lymphoid organogenesis is often seen in the synovium of patients with long-standing rheumatoid arthritis, in the thyroid in Hashimoto thyroiditis, and in the gastric mucosa in the setting of *Helicobacter pylori* infection. It has been postulated that the local formation of lymphoid organs may perpetuate the immune reaction, but the significance of these structures is not established.

Other Cells in Chronic Inflammation

Other cell types may be prominent in chronic inflammation induced by particular stimuli.

- **Eosinophils** are abundant in immune reactions mediated by IgE and in parasitic infections (Fig. 3.21). Their recruitment is driven by adhesion molecules similar to those used by neutrophils, and by specific chemokines (e.g., eotaxin) derived from leukocytes and epithelial cells. Eosinophils have granules that contain *major basic protein*, a highly cationic protein that is toxic to parasites but also injures host epithelial cells. This is why eosinophils are of benefit in controlling parasitic infections, yet also contribute to tissue damage in immune reactions such as allergies (Chapter 5).
- **Mast cells** are widely distributed in connective tissues and participate in both acute and chronic inflammatory reactions. Mast cells arise from precursors in the bone marrow. They have many similarities with circulating basophils, but they do not arise from basophils, are tissue-resident, and therefore play more significant roles in inflammatory reactions in tissues than basophils do. Mast cells (and basophils) express on their surface the receptor FcεRI, which binds the Fc portion of IgE antibody. In immediate hypersensitivity reactions, IgE bound to the mast cells' Fc receptors specifically recognizes antigen, and in response the cells degranulate and release mediators, such as histamine and prostaglandins (Chapter 5). This type of response occurs during allergic reactions to foods, insect venom, or drugs, sometimes with catastrophic results (e.g., anaphylactic shock). Mast cells also are present in chronic inflammatory reactions, and because they secrete a

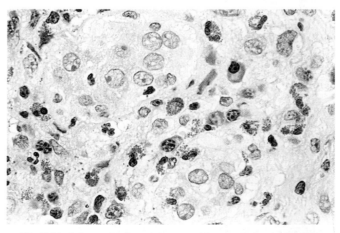

Fig. 3.21 A focus of inflammation containing numerous eosinophils.

plethora of cytokines, they can promote inflammatory reactions.

- Although **neutrophils** are characteristic of acute inflammation, many forms of chronic inflammation, lasting for months, continue to show large numbers of neutrophils, induced either by persistent microbes or by cytokines and other mediators produced by activated macrophages and T lymphocytes. In chronic bacterial infection of bone (osteomyelitis), a neutrophilic exudate can persist for many months. Neutrophils also are important in the chronic damage induced in lungs by smoking and other irritant stimuli (Chapter 13). This pattern of inflammation has been called *acute on chronic.*

Granulomatous Inflammation

Granulomatous inflammation is a form of chronic inflammation characterized by collections of activated macrophages, often with T lymphocytes, and sometimes associated with central necrosis. The activated macrophages may develop abundant cytoplasm and begin to resemble epithelial cells, and are called *epithelioid cells.* Some activated macrophages may fuse, forming multinucleate *giant cells.* Granuloma formation is a cellular attempt to contain an offending agent that is difficult to eradicate. In this attempt there is often strong activation of T lymphocytes leading to macrophage activation, which can cause injury to normal tissues.

There are two types of granulomas, which differ in their pathogenesis.

- **Immune granulomas** are caused by a variety of agents that are capable of inducing a persistent T cell–mediated immune response. This type of immune response produces granulomas usually when the inciting agent cannot be readily eliminated, such as a persistent microbe or a self antigen. In such responses, macrophages activate T cells to produce cytokines, such as IL-2, which activates other T cells, perpetuating the response, and IFN-γ, which activates the macrophages.
- **Foreign body granulomas** are seen in response to relatively inert foreign bodies, in the absence of T cell–mediated immune responses. Typically, foreign body granulomas form around materials such as talc (associated with intravenous drug abuse), sutures, or other fibers that are large enough to preclude phagocytosis by a macrophage but are not immunogenic. Epithelioid cells and giant cells are apposed to the surface of the foreign body. The foreign material can usually be identified in the center of the granuloma, particularly if viewed with polarized light, in which it may appear refractile.

MORPHOLOGY

In the usual H&E stained tissue samples (Fig. 3.22), the activated macrophages in granulomas have pink granular cytoplasm with indistinct cell boundaries and are called **epithelioid cells.** A collar of lymphocytes surrounds the aggregates of epithelioid macrophages. Older granulomas may have a rim of fibroblasts and connective tissue. Frequently, but not invariably, multinucleated **giant cells** 40 to 50 μm in diameter are found in

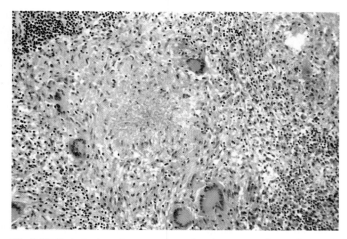

Fig. 3.22 Typical tuberculous granuloma showing an area of central necrosis surrounded by multiple multinucleate giant cells, epithelioid cells, and lymphocytes.

granulomas; these are called Langhans giant cells. They consist of a large mass of cytoplasm and many nuclei. Granulomas associated with certain infectious organisms (classically *Mycobacterium tuberculosis*) often contain a central zone of necrosis. Grossly, this has a granular, cheesy appearance and is therefore called **caseous necrosis.** Microscopically, this necrotic material appears as amorphous, structureless, eosinophilic, granular debris, with loss of cellular details. The granulomas in Crohn disease, sarcoidosis, and foreign body reactions tend to not have necrotic centers and are said to be *noncaseating.* Healing of granulomas is accompanied by fibrosis that may be extensive.

Granulomas are encountered in certain specific pathologic states; recognition of the granulomatous pattern is important because of the limited number of conditions (some life threatening) that cause it (Table 3.9). In the setting of persistent T cell responses to certain microbes (e.g., *M. tuberculosis, Treponema pallidum,* or fungi), T cell–derived cytokines are responsible for chronic macrophage activation and granuloma formation. Granulomas may also develop in some immune-mediated inflammatory diseases, notably Crohn disease, which is one type of inflammatory bowel disease and an important cause of granulomatous inflammation in the United States, and in a disease of unknown etiology called *sarcoidosis.* **Tuberculosis is the prototype of a granulomatous disease caused by infection and should always be excluded as the cause when granulomas are identified.** In this disease the granuloma is referred to as a *tubercle.* The morphologic patterns in the various granulomatous diseases may be sufficiently different to allow a reasonably accurate diagnosis (Table 3.9), but it is always necessary to identify the specific etiologic agent by special stains for organisms (e.g., acid-fast stains for tubercle bacilli), by culture methods (e.g., in tuberculosis and fungal diseases), by molecular techniques (e.g., the polymerase chain reaction in tuberculosis), and by serologic studies (e.g., in syphilis).

Table 3.9 Examples of Diseases With Granulomatous Inflammation

Disease	Cause	Tissue Reaction
Tuberculosis	Mycobacterium tuberculosis	Caseating granuloma (tubercle): focus of activated macrophages (epithelioid cells), rimmed by fibroblasts, lymphocytes, histiocytes, occasional Langhans giant cells; central necrosis with amorphous granular debris; acid-fast bacilli
Leprosy	Mycobacterium leprae	Acid-fast bacilli in macrophages; noncaseating granulomas
Syphilis	Treponema pallidum	Gumma: microscopic to grossly visible lesion, enclosing wall of macrophages; plasma cell infiltrate; central cells are necrotic without loss of cellular outline; organisms difficult to identify in tissue
Cat-scratch disease	Gram-negative bacillus	Rounded or stellate granuloma containing central granular debris and recognizable neutrophils; giant cells uncommon
Sarcoidosis	Unknown etiology	Noncaseating granulomas with abundant activated macrophages
Crohn disease (inflammatory bowel disease)	Immune reaction against undefined gut microbes and, possibly, self antigens	Occasional noncaseating granulomas in the wall of the intestine, with dense chronic inflammatory infiltrate

SUMMARY

CHRONIC INFLAMMATION

- Chronic inflammation is a prolonged host response to persistent stimuli that may follow unresolved acute inflammation or be chronic from the outset.
- It is caused by microbes that resist elimination, immune responses against self and environmental antigens, and some toxic substances (e.g., silica); underlies many medically important diseases.
- It is characterized by coexisting inflammation, tissue injury, attempted repair by scarring, and immune response.
- The cellular infiltrate consists of macrophages, lymphocytes, plasma cells, and other leukocytes.
- It is mediated by cytokines produced by macrophages and lymphocytes (notably T lymphocytes); bidirectional interactions between these cells tend to amplify and prolong the inflammatory reaction.
- Granulomatous inflammation is a morphologically specific pattern of chronic inflammation induced by T cell and macrophage activation in response to an agent that is resistant to eradication.

SYSTEMIC EFFECTS OF INFLAMMATION

Inflammation, even if it is localized, is associated with cytokine-induced systemic reactions that are collectively called the acute-phase response. Anyone who has suffered through a severe bout of a bacterial or viral illness (e.g., pneumonia or influenza) has experienced the systemic manifestations of acute inflammation. These changes are reactions to cytokines whose production is stimulated by bacterial products such as LPS, viral double stranded RNA and by other inflammatory stimuli. The cytokines TNF, IL-1, and IL-6 are important mediators of the acute-phase reaction; other cytokines, notably type I interferons, also contribute to the reaction.

The acute-phase response consists of several clinical and pathologic changes:

- **Fever,** characterized by an elevation of body temperature, usually by 1° to 4°C, is one of the most prominent manifestations of the acute-phase response, especially when inflammation is associated with infection. Substances that induce fever are called *pyrogens.* The increase in body temperature is caused by prostaglandins that are produced in the vascular and perivascular cells of the hypothalamus. Bacterial products, such as LPS (called *exogenous pyrogens*), stimulate leukocytes to release cytokines such as IL-1 and TNF (called *endogenous pyrogens*) that increase the enzymes (cyclooxygenases) that convert arachadonic acid into prostaglandins. In the hypothalamus, the prostaglandins, especially PGE_2, stimulate the production of neurotransmitters that reset the temperature set point at a higher level. NSAIDs, including aspirin, reduce fever by inhibiting prostaglandin synthesis. How, and even if, fever contributes to the protective host response remains unclear.
- **Acute-phase proteins** are plasma proteins, mostly synthesized in the liver, whose plasma concentrations may increase several hundred-fold as part of the response to inflammatory stimuli. Three of the best-known of these proteins are C-reactive protein (CRP), fibrinogen, and serum amyloid A (SAA) protein. Synthesis of these molecules in hepatocytes is stimulated by cytokines. Many acute-phase proteins, such as CRP and SAA, bind to microbial cell walls, and they may act as opsonins and fix complement. Fibrinogen binds to red cells and causes them to form stacks (rouleaux) that sediment more rapidly at unit gravity than do individual red cells. This is the basis for measuring the *erythrocyte sedimentation rate* as a simple test for an inflammatory response caused by any stimulus. Acute-phase proteins have beneficial effects during acute inflammation, but prolonged production of these proteins (especially SAA) in states of chronic inflammation can, in some cases, cause *secondary amyloidosis* (Chapter 5). Elevated serum levels of CRP serve as a marker for increased risk of myocardial infarction in patients with coronary artery disease. It is postulated that inflammation involving atherosclerotic plaques in the coronary arteries predisposes to

thrombosis and subsequent infarction. Another peptide whose production is increased in the acute-phase response is the iron-regulating peptide *hepcidin*. Chronically elevated plasma concentrations of hepcidin reduce the availability of iron and are responsible for the *anemia* associated with chronic inflammation (Chapter 12).

- **Leukocytosis** is a common feature of inflammatory reactions, especially those induced by bacterial infections. The leukocyte count usually climbs to 15,000 or 20,000 cells/mL, but sometimes it may reach extraordinarily high levels of 40,000 to 100,000 cells/mL. These extreme elevations are referred to as *leukemoid reactions*, because they are similar to (and must be distinguished from) the white cell counts observed in leukemia. The leukocytosis occurs initially because of accelerated release of cells from the bone marrow postmitotic reserve pool (caused by cytokines, including TNF and IL-1) and is therefore associated with a rise in the number of more immature neutrophils in the blood, referred to as a *shift to the left*. Prolonged infection also induces proliferation of precursors in the bone marrow, caused by increased production of colony-stimulating factors (CSFs). Thus, if inflammation is sustained the bone marrow output of leukocytes increases, an effect that usually more than conpensates for the loss of these cells in the inflammatory reaction. (See also the discussion of leukocytosis in Chapter 12.) Most bacterial infections induce an increase in the blood neutrophil count, called *neutrophilia*. Viral infections, such as infectious mononucleosis, mumps, and German measles, cause an absolute increase in the number of lymphocytes (*lymphocytosis*). In some allergies and parasitic infestations, there is an increase in the number of blood eosinophils, creating an *eosinophilia*. Certain infections (typhoid fever and infections caused by some viruses, rickettsiae, and certain protozoa) are associated with a decreased number of circulating white cells (*leukopenia*).
- Other manifestations of the acute-phase response include increased heart rate and blood pressure; decreased sweating, mainly because of redirection of blood flow from cutaneous to deep vascular beds, to minimize heat loss through the skin; rigors (shivering), chills (search for warmth), anorexia, somnolence, and malaise, probably because of the actions of cytokines on brain cells.

In severe bacterial infections (**sepsis**), the large amounts of bacteria and their products in the blood stimulate the production of enormous quantities of several cytokines, notably TNF and IL-1. High blood levels of cytokines cause widespread clinical and pathologic abnormalities such as disseminated intravascular coagulation, hypotensive shock, and metabolic disturbances including insulin resistance and hyperglycemia. This clinical triad is known as *septic shock*; it is discussed in more detail in Chapter 4. A syndrome similar to septic shock may occur as a complication of noninfectious disorders, such as severe burns, trauma, pancreatitis, and other serious conditions. Collectively these reactions are called *systemic inflammatory response syndrome (SIRS)*.

We next consider the process of repair, which is a healing response to tissue destruction resulting from inflammation or other causes.

SUMMARY

SYSTEMIC EFFECTS OF INFLAMMATION

- Fever: Cytokines (TNF, IL-1) stimulate production of PGs in hypothalamus
- Production of acute-phase proteins: C-reactive protein, others; synthesis stimulated by cytokines (IL-6, others) acting on liver cells
- Leukocytosis: Cytokines (CSFs) stimulate production of leukocytes from precursors in the bone marrow
- In some severe infections, septic shock: Fall in blood pressure, disseminated intravascular coagulation, metabolic abnormalities; induced by high levels of TNF and other cytokines

TISSUE REPAIR

Overview of Tissue Repair

Critical to the survival of an organism is the ability to repair the damage caused by toxic insults and inflammation. In fact, the inflammatory response to microbes and injured tissues not only serves to eliminate these dangers but also sets into motion the process of repair.

Repair of damaged tissues occurs by two types of reactions: regeneration by proliferation of residual (uninjured) cells and maturation of tissue stem cells, and the deposition of connective tissue to form a scar (Fig. 3.23).

- **Regeneration.** Some tissues are able to replace the damaged components and essentially return to a normal

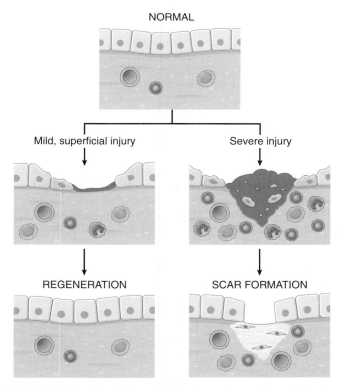

Fig. 3.23 Mechanisms of tissue repair: regeneration and scar formation. Following mild injury, which damages the epithelium but not the underlying tissue, resolution occurs by regeneration, but after more severe injury with damage to the connective tissue, repair is by scar formation.

state; this process is called *regeneration*. Regeneration occurs by proliferation of cells that survive the injury and retain the capacity to proliferate, for example, in the rapidly dividing epithelia of the skin and intestines, and in some parenchymal organs, notably the liver. In other cases, tissue stem cells may contribute to the restoration of damaged tissues. However, whereas lower animals such as salamanders and fish can regenerate entire limbs or appendages, mammals have a limited capacity to regenerate damaged tissues and organs, and only some components of most tissues are able to fully restore themselves.

- **Connective tissue deposition (scar formation).** If the injured tissues are incapable of complete restitution, or if the supporting structures of the tissue are severely damaged, repair occurs by the laying down of connective (fibrous) tissue, a process that may result in formation of a *scar*. Although the fibrous scar is not normal, it provides enough structural stability that the injured tissue is usually able to function. The term *fibrosis* is most often used to describe the extensive deposition of collagen that occurs in the lungs, liver, kidney, and other organs as a consequence of chronic inflammation, or in the myocardium after extensive ischemic necrosis (infarction). If fibrosis develops in a tissue space occupied by an inflammatory exudate, it is called *organization* (as in organizing pneumonia affecting the lung).

After many common types of injury, both regeneration and scar formation contribute in varying degrees to the ultimate repair. Both processes involve the proliferation of various cells, and close interactions between cells and the extracellular matrix (ECM). We first discuss the general mechanisms of cellular proliferation and regeneration, and then the salient features of regeneration and healing by scar formation, and conclude with a description of cutaneous wound healing and fibrosis (scarring) in parenchymal organs as illustrations of the repair process.

Cell and Tissue Regeneration

The regeneration of injured cells and tissues involves cell proliferation, which is driven by growth factors and is critically dependent on the integrity of the extracellular matrix, and by the development of mature cells from stem cells. Before describing examples of repair by regeneration, we discuss the control of cell proliferation in this process. The general principles of cell proliferation were summarized in Chapter 1.

Cell Proliferation: Signals and Control Mechanisms

Several cell types proliferate during tissue repair. These include the remnants of the injured tissue (which attempt to restore normal structure), vascular endothelial cells (to create new vessels that provide the nutrients needed for the repair process), and fibroblasts (the source of the fibrous tissue that forms the scar to fill defects that cannot be corrected by regeneration).

The ability of tissues to repair themselves is determined, in part, by their intrinsic proliferative capacity. In some tissues (sometimes called *labile* tissues), cells are constantly being lost and must be continually replaced by new cells

that are derived from tissue stem cells and rapidly proliferating immature progenitors. These types of tissues include hematopoietic cells in the bone marrow and many surface epithelia, such as the basal layers of the squamous epithelia of the skin, oral cavity, vagina, and cervix; the cuboidal epithelia of the ducts draining exocrine organs (e.g., salivary glands, pancreas, biliary tract); the columnar epithelium of the gastrointestinal tract, uterus, and fallopian tubes; and the transitional epithelium of the urinary tract. These tissues can readily regenerate after injury as long as the pool of stem cells is preserved.

Other tissues (called *stable* tissues) are made up of cells that are normally in the G_0 stage of the cell cycle and hence not proliferating, but they are capable of dividing in response to injury or loss of tissue mass. These tissues include the parenchyma of most solid organs, such as liver, kidney, and pancreas. Endothelial cells, fibroblasts, and smooth muscle cells are also normally quiescent but can proliferate in response to growth factors, a reaction that is particularly important in wound healing.

Some tissues (called *permanent* tissues) consist of terminally differentiated nonproliferative cells, such as the majority of neurons and cardiac muscle cells. Injury to these tissues is irreversible and results in a scar, because the cells cannot regenerate. Skeletal muscle cells are usually considered nondividing, but satellite cells attached to the endomysial sheath provide some regenerative capacity for muscle.

Cell proliferation is driven by signals provided by growth factors and from the extracellular matrix. Many different growth factors have been described, some of which act on multiple cell types, while others are cell-type specific (Chapter 1). Growth factors are typically produced by cells near the site of damage. The most important sources of these growth factors are macrophages that are activated by the tissue injury, but epithelial and stromal cells also produce some of these factors. Several growth factors bind to ECM proteins and are displayed at the site of tissue injury at high concentrations. All growth factors activate signaling pathways that ultimately induce changes in gene expression that drive cells through the cell cycle and support the biosynthesis of molecules and organelles that are needed for cell division (Chapter 1). In addition to responding to growth factors, cells use integrins to bind to ECM proteins, and signals from the integrins can also stimulate cell proliferation.

In the process of regeneration, proliferation of residual cells is supplemented by development of mature cells from stem cells. In Chapter 1 we introduced the major types of stem cells. In adults, the most important stem cells for regeneration after injury are tissue stem cells. These stem cells live in specialized niches, and it is believed that injury triggers signals in these niches that activate quiescent stem cells to proliferate and differentiate into mature cells that repopulate the injured tissue.

Mechanisms of Tissue Regeneration

The importance of regeneration in the replacement of injured tissues varies in different types of tissues and with the severity of injury.

- In epithelia of the intestinal tract and skin, injured cells are rapidly replaced by proliferation of residual cells and differentiation of cells derived from tissue stem cells, providing the underlying basement membrane is intact. The residual epithelial cells produce the growth factors involved in these processes. The newly generated cells migrate to fill the defect created by the injury, and tissue integrity is restored (Fig. 3.23).

- Tissue regeneration can occur in parenchymal organs whose cells are capable of proliferation, but with the exception of the liver, this is usually a limited process. Pancreas, adrenal, thyroid, and lung have some regenerative capacity. The surgical removal of a kidney elicits in the remaining kidney a compensatory response that consists of both hypertrophy and hyperplasia of proximal duct cells. The mechanisms underlying this response are not understood, but they likely involve local production of growth factors and interactions of cells with the ECM. The extraordinary capacity of the liver to regenerate has made it a valuable model for studying this process, as described below.

Restoration of normal tissue architecture can occur only if the residual tissue is structurally intact, for example after partial surgical resection of the liver. By contrast, if the entire tissue is damaged by infection or inflammation, regeneration is incomplete and is accompanied by scarring. For example, extensive destruction of the liver with collapse of the reticulin framework, as occurs in a liver abscess, leads to scar formation even though the remaining liver cells have the capacity to regenerate.

Liver Regeneration

The human liver has a remarkable capacity to regenerate, as demonstrated by its growth after partial hepatectomy, which may be performed for tumor resection or for living-donor hepatic transplantation. The mythologic image of liver regeneration is the regrowth of the liver of Prometheus, which was eaten every day by an eagle sent by Zeus as punishment for stealing the secret of fire, and regrew every night. The reality, although less dramatic, is still quite impressive.

Regeneration of the liver occurs by two major mechanisms: proliferation of remaining hepatocytes and repopulation from progenitor cells. Which mechanism plays the dominant role depends on the nature of the injury.

- **Proliferation of hepatocytes following partial hepatectomy.** In humans, resection of up to 90% of the liver can be corrected by proliferation of the residual hepatocytes. This process is driven by cytokines such as IL-6 produced by Kupffer cells, and by growth factors such as hepatocyte growth factor (HGF) produced by many cell types.
- **Liver regeneration from progenitor cells.** In situations in which the proliferative capacity of hepatocytes is impaired, such as after chronic liver injury or inflammation, progenitor cells in the liver contribute to repopulation. In rodents, these progenitor cells have been called *oval cells* because of the shape of their nuclei. Some of these progenitor cells reside in specialized niches called *canals of Hering*, where bile canaliculi connect with larger bile ducts. The signals that drive proliferation of progenitor cells and their differentiation into mature hepatocytes are topics of active investigation.

SUMMARY

REPAIR BY REGENERATION

- Different tissues consist of continuously dividing cells (epithelia, hematopoietic tissues), normally quiescent cells that are capable of proliferation (most parenchymal organs), and nondividing cells (neurons, skeletal and cardiac muscle). The regenerative capacity of a tissue depends on the proliferative potential of its constituent cells.
- Cell proliferation is controlled by the cell cycle, and is stimulated by growth factors and interactions of cells with the extracellular matrix.
- Regeneration of the liver is a classic example of repair by regeneration. It is triggered by cytokines and growth factors produced in response to loss of liver mass and inflammation. In different situations, regeneration may occur by proliferation of surviving hepatocytes or repopulation from progenitor cells.

Repair by Scarring

If repair cannot be accomplished by regeneration alone, it occurs by replacement of the injured cells with connective tissue, leading to the formation of a scar, or by a combination of regeneration of some residual cells and scar formation. As discussed earlier, scarring may happen if the tissue injury is severe or chronic and results in damage to parenchymal cells and epithelia as well as to the connective tissue framework, or if nondividing cells are injured. In contrast to regeneration, which involves the restitution of tissue components, scar formation is a response that "patches" rather than restores the tissue. The term *scar* is most often used in connection to *wound healing* in the skin, but also may be used to describe the replacement of parenchymal cells in any tissue by collagen, as in the heart after myocardial infarction.

Steps in Scar Formation

Repair by connective tissue deposition consists of a series of sequential steps that follow tissue injury (Fig. 3.24).

- Within minutes after injury, a hemostatic plug comprised of platelets (Chapter 4) is formed, which stops bleeding and provides a scaffold for infiltrating inflammatory cells.
- **Inflammation.** This step is comprised of the typical acute and chronic inflammatory responses. Breakdown products of complement activation, chemokines released from activated platelets, and other mediators produced at the site of injury function as chemotactic agents to recruit neutrophils and then monocytes during the next 6 to 48 hours. As described earlier, these inflammatory cells eliminate the offending agents, such as microbes that may have entered through the wound, and clear the debris. **Macrophages are the central cellular players in the repair process**—M1 macrophages clear microbes and necrotic tissue and promote inflammation in a positive feedback loop, and M2 macrophages produce growth factors that stimulate the proliferation of many cell types in the next stage of repair. As the injurious agents and necrotic cells are cleared, the

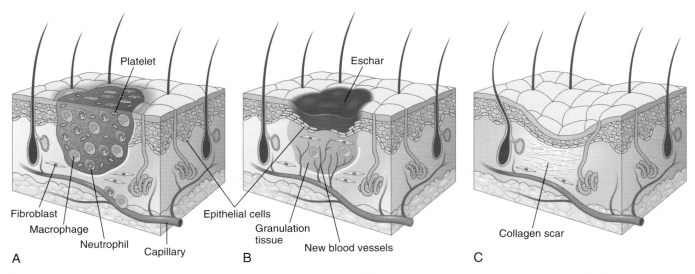

Fig. 3.24 Steps in repair by scar formation: healing of a large wound in the skin. This is an example of healing by second intention. (A) Hemostatic plug and inflammation. (B) Proliferation of epithelial cells; formation of granulation tissue by vessel growth and proliferating fibroblasts. (C) Remodeling to produce the fibrous scar.

inflammation resolves; how this inflammatory flame is extinguished in most situations of injury is still not well defined.

- **Cell proliferation.** In the next stage, which takes up to 10 days, several cell types, including epithelial cells, endothelial and other vascular cells, and fibroblasts, proliferate and migrate to close the now-clean wound. Each cell type serves unique functions.
  - *Epithelial cells* respond to locally produced growth factors and migrate over the wound to cover it.
  - *Endothelial and other vascular cells* proliferate to form new blood vessels, a process known as **angiogenesis**. Because of the importance of this process in physiologic host responses and in many pathologic conditions, it is described in more detail later.
  - *Fibroblasts* proliferate and migrate into the site of injury and lay down collagen fibers that form the scar.
  - The combination of proliferating fibroblasts, loose connective tissue, new blood vessels and scattered chronic inflammatory cells, forms a type of tissue that is unique to healing wounds and is called *granulation tissue*. This term derives from its pink, soft, granular gross appearance, such as that seen beneath the scab of a skin wound.
- **Remodeling.** The connective tissue that has been deposited by fibroblasts is reorganized to produce the stable fibrous *scar*. This process begins 2 to 3 weeks after injury and may continue for months or years.

Healing of skin wounds can be classified into *healing by first intention (primary union)*, referring to epithelial regeneration with minimal scarring, as in well-apposed surgical incisions, and *healing by second intention (secondary union)*, referring to larger wounds that heal by a combination of regeneration and scarring. Because the fundamental processes involved in both types of wound healing represent a continuum from regeneration to scarring, we do not make this distinction in our discussion of the key events in tissue repair.

Angiogenesis

Angiogenesis is the process of new blood vessel development from existing vessels. It is critical in healing at sites of injury, in the development of collateral circulations at sites of ischemia, and in allowing tumors to increase in size beyond the constraints of their original blood supply. Much work has been done to understand the mechanisms of angiogenesis, and therapies have been developed either to augment the process (e.g., to improve blood flow to a heart ravaged by coronary atherosclerosis) or to inhibit it (to frustrate tumor growth or block pathologic vessel growth, as in wet macular degeneration of the eye).

Angiogenesis involves sprouting of new vessels from existing ones, and consists of the following steps (Fig. 3.25):

- Vasodilation in response to NO and increased permeability induced by VEGF
- Separation of pericytes from the abluminal surface and breakdown of the basement membrane to allow formation of a vessel sprout
- Migration of endothelial cells toward the area of tissue injury
- Proliferation of endothelial cells just behind the leading front ("tip") of migrating cells
- Remodeling into capillary tubes
- Recruitment of periendothelial cells (pericytes for small capillaries and smooth muscle cells for larger vessels) to form the mature vessel
- Suppression of endothelial proliferation and migration and deposition of the basement membrane

It has been suggested that endothelial progenitor cells are present in the bone marrow and can be recruited to promote new vessel formation. However, these cells likely play a minor, if any, role in the angiogenesis associated with the healing of most wounds.

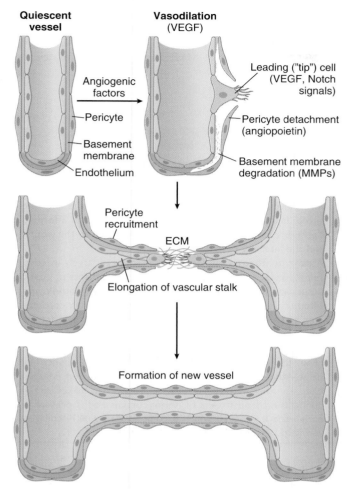

Quiescent vessel

Vasodilation (VEGF)

Angiogenic factors

Leading ("tip") cell (VEGF, Notch signals)

Pericyte

Pericyte detachment (angiopoietin)

Basement membrane

Endothelium

Basement membrane degradation (MMPs)

Pericyte recruitment

ECM

Elongation of vascular stalk

Formation of new vessel

Fig. 3.25 Angiogenesis. In tissue repair, angiogenesis occurs mainly by the sprouting of new vessels. The steps in the process, and the major signals involved, are illustrated. The newly formed vessel joins up with other vessels (not shown) to form the new vascular bed.

The process of angiogenesis involves several signaling pathways, cell–cell interactions, ECM proteins, and tissue enzymes.

- **Growth factors.** *VEGFs*, mainly VEGF-A (Chapter 1), stimulates both migration and proliferation of endothelial cells, thus initiating the process of capillary sprouting in angiogenesis. It promotes vasodilation by stimulating the production of NO and contributes to the formation of the vascular lumen. *Fibroblast growth factors (FGFs)*, mainly FGF-2, stimulate the proliferation of endothelial cells. They also promote the migration of macrophages and fibroblasts to the damaged area, and stimulate epithelial cell migration to cover epidermal wounds. Newly formed vessels need to be stabilized by the recruitment of pericytes and smooth muscle cells and by the deposition of connective tissue. Multiple growth factors, including PDGF and TGF-β, likely participate in the stabilization process: PDGF recruits smooth muscle cells and TGF-β suppresses endothelial proliferation and migration, and enhances the production of ECM proteins.

- **Notch signaling.** Through "cross talk" with VEGF, the Notch signaling pathway regulates the sprouting and branching of new vessels and thus ensures that the new vessels that are formed have the proper spacing to effectively supply the healing tissue with blood.
- **ECM proteins** participate in the process of vessel sprouting in angiogenesis, largely through interactions with integrin receptors of endothelial cells and by providing the scaffold for vessel growth.
- **Enzymes** in the ECM, notably the matrix metalloproteinases (MMPs), degrade the ECM to permit remodeling and extension of the vascular tube.

Newly formed vessels are leaky because of incomplete interendothelial junctions and because VEGF, the growth factor that drives angiogenesis, increases vascular permeability. This leakiness accounts in part for the edema that may persist in healing wounds long after the acute inflammatory response has resolved.

Activation of Fibroblasts and Deposition of Connective Tissue

The laying down of connective tissue occurs in two steps: (1) migration and proliferation of fibroblasts into the site of injury and (2) deposition of ECM proteins produced by these cells. These processes are orchestrated by locally produced cytokines and growth factors, including PDGF, FGF-2, and TGF-β. The major sources of these factors are inflammatory cells, particularly alternatively activated (M2) macrophages that infiltrate sites of injury.

In response to cytokines and growth factors, fibroblasts enter the wound from the edges and migrate toward the center. Some of these cells may differentiate into cells called *myofibroblasts*, which contain smooth muscle actin and have increased contractile activity, and serve to close the wound by pulling its margins toward the center. Activated fibroblasts and myofibroblasts also increase their synthetic activity and produce connective tissue proteins, mainly collagen, which is the major component of the fully developed scar.

TGF-β is the most important cytokine for the synthesis and deposition of connective tissue proteins. It is produced by most of the cells in granulation tissue, including alternatively activated macrophages. The levels of TGF-β in tissues are primarily regulated not by the transcription of the gene but by the post-transcriptional activation of latent TGF-β, the rate of secretion of the active molecule, and factors in the ECM, notably integrins, that enhance or diminish TGF-β activity. In addition, microfibrils made up of fibrillin also regulate the bioavailability of TGF-β (Chapter 6). TGF-β stimulates fibroblast migration and proliferation, increases the synthesis of collagen and fibronectin, and decreases the degradation of ECM by inhibiting metalloproteinases. TGF-β is involved not only in scar formation after injury but also in the development of fibrosis in lung, liver, and kidneys that follows chronic inflammation. TGF-β also has anti-inflammatory effects that serve to limit and terminate inflammatory responses. It does this by inhibiting lymphocyte proliferation and the activity of other leukocytes.

As healing progresses, the number of proliferating fibroblasts and new vessels decreases, but the fibroblasts progressively assume a more synthetic phenotype, and hence there is increased deposition of ECM. Collagen synthesis, in particular, is necessary for the healing wound to become strong and mechanically stable. Collagen synthesis by fibroblasts begins early in wound healing (days 3–5) and continues for several weeks, depending on the size of the wound. Net collagen accumulation depends not only on increased synthesis but also on diminished collagen degradation (discussed later). As the scar matures, there is progressive vascular regression, which eventually transforms the highly vascularized granulation tissue into a pale, largely avascular scar.

Remodeling of Connective Tissue

After the scar is formed, it is remodeled to increase its strength and contract it. Wound strength increases because of cross-linking of collagen and increased size of collagen fibers. In addition, there is a shift of the type of collagen deposited, from type III collagen early in repair to more resilient type I collagen. In well-sutured skin wounds, strength may recover to 70% to 80% of normal skin by 3 months. Wound contraction is initially caused by myofibroblasts and later by cross-linking of collagen fibers.

With time, the connective tissue is degraded and the scar shrinks. The degradation of collagens and other ECM components is accomplished by a family of *matrix metalloproteinases* (MMPs), so called because they are dependent on metal ions (e.g., zinc) for their enzymatic activity. MMPs are produced by a variety of cell types (fibroblasts, macrophages, neutrophils, synovial cells, and some epithelial cells), and their synthesis and secretion are regulated by growth factors, cytokines, and other agents. They include interstitial collagenases, which cleave fibrillar collagen (MMP-1, -2, and -3); gelatinases (MMP-2 and 9), which degrade amorphous collagen and fibronectin; and stromelysins (MMP-3, -10, and -11), which degrade a variety of ECM constituents, including proteoglycans, laminin, fibronectin, and amorphous collagen. Neutrophil elastase, cathepsin G, plasmin, and other serine proteinases can also degrade ECM but are less important in wound remodeling than the MMPs. In addition, activated collagenases can be rapidly inhibited by specific tissue inhibitors of metalloproteinases (TIMPs), produced by most mesenchymal cells. Thus, a balance of MMPs and TIMPs regulates the size and nature of the scar.

MOROPHOLOGY

- **Granulation tissue** is characterized by proliferation of fibroblasts and new thin-walled, delicate capillaries in a loose extracellular matrix, often with admixed inflammatory cells, mainly macrophages (Fig. 3.26A). This tissue progressively invades the site of injury; the amount of granulation tissue that is formed depends on the size of the tissue deficit created by the wound and the intensity of inflammation.
- A **scar** or **fibrosis** in tissues is composed of largely inactive, spindle-shaped fibroblasts, dense collagen, fragments of elastic tissue, and other ECM components (Fig. 3.26B). Pathologists often use special stains to identify different protein constituents of scars and fibrotic tissues. The trichrome stain detects collagen fibers, and the elastin stain identifies delicate fibers of elastin, which is the major component of pliable elastic tissue. (The trichrome actually contains three stains—hence its name—that stain red cells orange, muscle red, and collagen blue.) Another extracellular matrix protein that makes up the connective tissue stroma of normal organs and is present in early scars is reticulin, which is composed of type III collagen, and it too can be identified with a special stain.

SUMMARY

REPAIR BY SCAR FORMATION

- Repair occurs by deposition of connective tissue and scar formation if the injured tissue is not capable of regeneration or if the structural framework is damaged and cannot support regeneration.

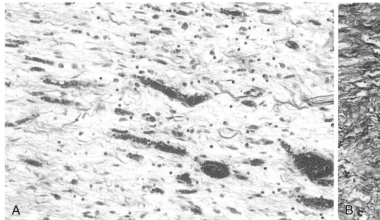 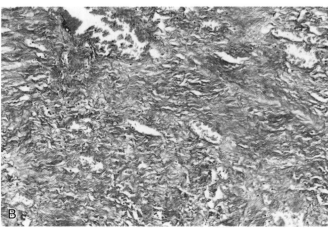

Fig. 3.26 (A) Granulation tissue showing numerous blood vessels, edema, and a loose extracellular matrix containing occasional inflammatory cells. Collagen is stained blue by the trichrome stain; minimal mature collagen can be seen at this point. (B) Trichrome stain of mature scar, showing dense collagen (stained blue) and scattered vascular channels.

- The main steps in repair by scarring are clot formation, inflammation, angiogenesis and formation of granulation tissue, migration and proliferation of fibroblasts, collagen synthesis, and connective tissue remodeling.
- Macrophages are critical for orchestrating the repair process, by eliminating offending agents and producing cytokines and growth factors that stimulate the proliferation of the cell types involved in repair.
- TGF-β is a potent fibrogenic agent; ECM deposition depends on the balance among fibrogenic agents, matrix metalloproteinases (MMPs) that digest ECM, and the tissue inhibitors of MMPs (TIMPs).

Factors That Impair Tissue Repair

Tissue repair may be impaired by a variety of factors that reduce the quality or adequacy of the reparative process. Factors that interfere with healing may be extrinsic (e.g., infection) or intrinsic to the injured tissue, and systemic or local:

- **Infection** is one of the most important causes of delayed healing; it prolongs inflammation and potentially increases the local tissue injury.
- **Diabetes** is a metabolic disease that compromises tissue repair for many reasons (Chapter 24), and is an important systemic cause of abnormal wound healing.
- **Nutritional status** has profound effects on repair; protein malnutrition and vitamin C deficiency, for example, inhibit collagen synthesis and retard healing.
- **Glucocorticoids (steroids)** have well-documented anti-inflammatory effects, and their administration may result in weak scars because they inhibit TGF-β production and diminish fibrosis. In some instances, however, the anti-inflammatory effects of glucocorticoids are desirable. For example, in corneal infections, glucocorticoids may be prescribed (along with antibiotics) to reduce the likelihood of opacity due to collagen deposition.
- **Mechanical factors** such as increased local pressure or torsion may cause wounds to pull apart (dehisce).
- **Poor perfusion,** resulting either from arteriosclerosis and diabetes or from obstructed venous drainage (e.g., in varicose veins), also impairs healing.
- **Foreign bodies** such as fragments of steel, glass, or even bone impede healing.
- **The type and extent of tissue injury** affects the subsequent repair. Complete restoration can occur only in tissues composed of cells capable of proliferating; even then, extensive injury will probably result in incomplete tissue regeneration and at least partial loss of function. Injury to tissues composed of nondividing cells must inevitably result in scarring; such is the case with healing of a myocardial infarct.
- **The location of the injury** and the character of the tissue in which the injury occurs also are important. For example, in inflammation arising in tissue spaces (e.g., pleural, peritoneal, synovial cavities), small exudates may be resorbed and digested by the proteolytic enzymes of leukocytes, resulting in resolution of the inflammation and restoration of normal tissue architecture. However, when the exudate is too large to be fully resorbed it undergoes organization, a process during which granulation tissue grows into the exudate, and a fibrous scar ultimately forms.

Clinical Examples of Abnormal Wound Healing and Scarring

Complications in tissue repair can arise from abnormalities in any of the basic components of the process, including deficient scar formation, excessive formation of the repair components, and formation of contractures.

Defects in Healing: Chronic Wounds

These are seen in numerous clinical situations, as a result of local and systemic factors. The following are some common examples.

- *Venous leg ulcers* (Fig. 3.27A) develop most often in elderly people as a result of chronic venous hypertension, which may be caused by severe varicose veins or congestive heart failure. Deposits of iron pigment (hemosiderin) are common, resulting from red cell breakdown, and there may be accompanying chronic inflammation. These ulcers fail to heal because of poor delivery of oxygen to the site of the ulcer.
- *Arterial ulcers* (Fig. 3.27B) develop in individuals with atherosclerosis of peripheral arteries, especially associated with diabetes. The ischemia results in atrophy and then necrosis of the skin and underlying tissues. These lesions can be quite painful.
- *Pressure sores* (Fig. 3.27C) are areas of skin ulceration and necrosis of underlying tissues caused by prolonged compression of tissues against a bone, for example, in bedridden, immobile elderly individuals with numerous morbidities. The lesions are caused by mechanical pressure and local ischemia.
- *Diabetic ulcers* (Fig. 3.27D) affect the lower extremities, particularly the feet. Tissue necrosis and failure to heal are the result of small vessel disease causing ischemia, neuropathy, systemic metabolic abnormalities, and secondary infections. Histologically, these lesions are characterized by epithelial ulceration (Fig. 3.27E) and extensive granulation tissue in the underlying dermis (Fig. 3.27F).

In some cases failure of healing may lead to dehiscence (wound rupture). Although not common, this occurs most frequently after abdominal surgery and is a result of increased abdominal pressure, such as may occur with vomiting, coughing, or ileus.

Excessive Scarring

Excessive formation of the components of the repair process can give rise to hypertrophic scars and keloids. The accumulation of excessive amounts of collagen may result in a raised scar known as a *hypertrophic scar*. These often grow rapidly and contain abundant myofibroblasts, but they tend to regress over several months (Fig. 3.28A). Hypertrophic scars generally develop after thermal or traumatic injury that involves the deep layers of the dermis. If the scar tissue grows beyond the boundaries of the

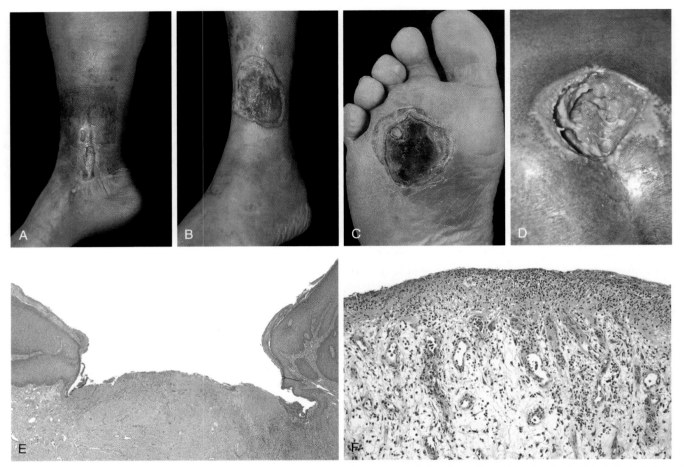

Fig. 3.27 Chronic wounds illustrating defects in wound healing. (A–D) External appearance of skin ulcers. *(From Eming SA, Margin P, Tomic-Canic M: Wound repair and regeneration: mechanisms, signaling, and translation,* Sci Transl Med 6:265, 2014.) (A) Venous leg ulcer; (B) arterial ulcer, with more extensive tissue necrosis; (C) diabetic ulcer; and (D) pressure sore. (E–F) Histologic appearance of a diabetic ulcer. (E) ulcer crater; (F) chronic inflammation and granulation tissue.

original wound and does not regress, it is called a *keloid* (Fig. 3.28B). Certain individuals seem to be predisposed to keloid formation, particularly those of African descent.

Exuberant granulation is another deviation in wound healing characterized by the formation of excessive amounts of granulation tissue, which protrudes above the level of the surrounding skin and blocks reepithelialization (this process has been called, with more literary fervor, *proud flesh*). Excessive granulation must be removed by cautery or surgical excision to permit restoration of epithelial continuity. Rarely, incisional scars or traumatic injuries may be followed by exuberant proliferation of fibroblasts and other connective tissue elements that may, in fact, recur after excision. Called *desmoids*, or *aggressive fibromatoses*, these neoplasms lie at the gray zone of benign and malignant low-grade tumors.

Wound contraction is an important part of the normal healing process. An exaggeration of this process gives rise to *contracture* and results in deformities of the wound and the surrounding tissues. Contractures are particularly prone to develop on the palms, the soles, and the anterior aspect of the thorax. Contractures are commonly seen after serious burns and can compromise the movement of joints.

Fibrosis in Parenchymal Organs

The term fibrosis is used to denote the excessive deposition of collagen and other ECM components in a tissue. The terms *scar* and *fibrosis* may be used interchangeably, but *fibrosis* most often refers to the abnormal deposition of collagen that occurs in internal organs in chronic diseases. The basic mechanisms of fibrosis are the same as those of scar formation in the skin during tissue repair. Fibrosis is a pathologic process induced by persistent injurious stimuli such as chronic infections and immunologic reactions, and is typically associated with loss of tissue (Fig. 3.29). It may be responsible for substantial organ dysfunction and even organ failure.

As discussed earlier, the major cytokine involved in fibrosis is TGF-β. The mechanisms that lead to increased TGF-β activity in fibrosis are not precisely known, but cell death by necrosis or apoptosis and the production of ROS seem to be important triggers, regardless of the tissue. The cells that produce collagen in response to TGF-β stimulation may vary depending on the tissue. In most organs, such as in the lung and kidney, myofibroblasts are the main source of collagen, but stellate cells are the major collagen producers in liver cirrhosis.

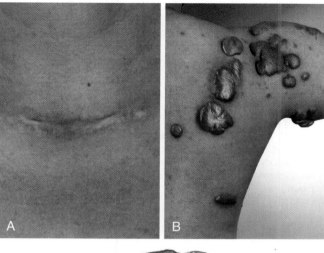

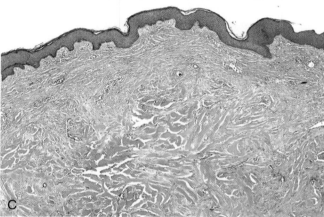

Fig. 3.28 Clinical examples of excessive scarring and collagen deposition. (A) Hypertrophic scar. (B) Keloid. (C) Microscopic appearance of a keloid. Note the thick connective tissue deposition in the dermis. *(A–B from Eming SA, Margin P, Tomic-Canic M: Wound repair and regeneration: mechanisms, signaling, and translation, Sci Transl Med 6:265, 2014, p. 2.)*

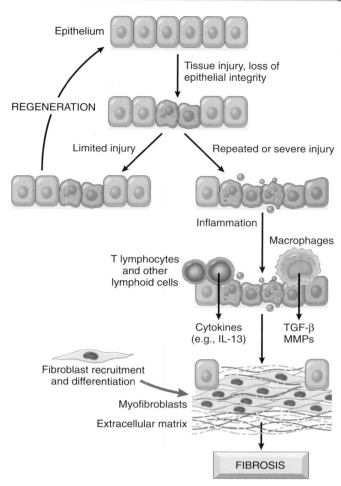

Fig. 3.29 Mechanisms of fibrosis. Persistent tissue injury leads to chronic inflammation and loss of tissue architecture. Cytokines produced by macrophages and other leukocytes stimulate the migration and proliferation of fibroblasts and myofibroblasts and the deposition of collagen and other extracellular matrix proteins. The net result is replacement of normal tissue by fibrosis.

Fibrotic disorders include diverse chronic and debilitating diseases such as liver cirrhosis, systemic sclerosis (scleroderma), fibrosing diseases of the lung (idiopathic pulmonary fibrosis, pneumoconioses, and drug- or radiation-induced pulmonary fibrosis), end-stage kidney disease, and constrictive pericarditis. These conditions are discussed in the relevant chapters later in the book. Because fibrosis is the major cause of morbidity and death in these conditions, there is great interest in the development of anti-fibrotic drugs.

- Wound healing can be altered by many conditions, particularly infection and diabetes; the type, volume, and location of the injury are important factors that influence the healing process.
- Excessive production of ECM can cause keloids in the skin.
- Persistent stimulation of collagen synthesis in chronic inflammatory diseases leads to tissue fibrosis, often with extensive loss of the tissue and functional impairment.

SUMMARY

CUTANEOUS WOUND HEALING AND PATHOLOGIC ASPECTS OF REPAIR

- The main phases of cutaneous wound healing are inflammation, formation of granulation tissue, and ECM remodeling.
- Cutaneous wounds can heal by primary union (first intention) or secondary union (secondary intention); secondary healing involves more extensive scarring and wound contraction.

SUGGESTED READINGS

Alitalo K: The lymphatic vasculature in disease, *Nat Med* 17:1371–1380, 2011. [*An excellent review of the cell biology of lymphatic vessels, their functions in immune and inflammatory reactions, and their roles in inflammatory, neoplastic, and other diseases.*]

Dennis EA, Norris PC: Eicosanoid storm in infection and inflammation, *Nat Rev Immunol* 15:511, 2015. [*A review of the pro- and antiinflammatory activities of eicosanoids.*]

Duffield JS, Lupher M, Thannickal VJ, et al: Host responses in tissue repair and fibrosis, *Ann Rev Pathol Mech Dis* 8:241, 2013. [*An overview of the cellular mechanisms of fibrosis, with an emphasis on the role of the immune system in fibrotic reactions to chronic infections.]*

Eming SA, Martin P, Tomic-Canic M: Wound repair and regeneration: mechanisms, signaling, and translation, *Sci Transl Med* 6:265r6, 2014. *[A modern review of host responses that contribute to tissue repair.]*

Flannagan RS, Jaumouillé V, Grinstein S: The cell biology of phagocytosis, *Ann Rev Pathol Mech Dis* 7:61–98, 2012. *[A modern discussion of the receptors involved in phagocytosis, the molecular control of the process, and the biology and functions of phagosomes.]*

Friedman SL, Sheppard D, Duffield JS, et al: Therapy for fibrotic diseases: nearing the starting line, *Sci Transl Med* 5:167sr1, 2013. *[An excellent review of the current concepts of the pathogenesis of fibrosis, emphasizing the roles of different cell populations and the extracellular matrix, and the potential for translating basic knowledge to the development of new therapies.]*

Gabay C, Lamacchia C, Palmer G: IL-1 pathways in inflammation and human diseases, *Nat Rev Rheumatol* 6:232, 2010. *[An excellent review of the biology of IL-1 and the therapeutic targeting of this cytokine in inflammatory diseases.]*

Hubmacher D, Apte SS: The biology of the extracellular matrix: novel insights, *Curr Opin Rheumatol* 25:65–70, 2013. *[A brief review of the structural and biochemical properties of the ECM.]*

Kalliolias GD, Ivashkiv LB: TNF biology, pathogenic mechanisms and emerging therapeutic strategies, *Nat Rev Rheumatol* 12:49, 2016. *[An excellent review of TNF and its signaling pathways, and the development and clinical efficacy of TNF inhibitors.]*

Khanapure SP, Garvey DS, Janero DR, et al: Eicosanoids in inflammation: biosynthesis, pharmacology, and therapeutic frontiers, *Curr Top Med Chem* 7:311, 2007. *[A summary of the properties of this important class of inflammatory mediators.]*

Kolaczkowska E, Kubes P: Neutrophil recruitment and function in health and inflammation, *Nat Rev Immunol* 13:159–175, 2013. *[An excellent review of neutrophil generation, recruitment, functions and fates, and their roles in different types of inflammatory reactions.]*

Kopp JL, Grompe M, Sander M: Stem cell versus plasticity in liver and pancreas regeneration, *Nat Cell Biol* 18:238, 2016. *[An excellent review of the relative contributions of parenchymal cells and stem cells to organ regeneration.]*

Mayadas TN, Cullere X, Lowell CA: The multifaceted functions of neutrophils, *Ann Rev Pathol Mech Dis* 9:181, 2014. *[An excellent review of neutrophil biology.]*

McAnully RJ: Fibroblasts and myofibroblasts: their source, function, and role in disease, *Int J Biochem Cell Biol* 39:666, 2007. *[A discussion of the two major types of stroma cells and their roles in tissue repair and fibrosis.]*

Nathan C, Ding A: Nonresolving inflammation, *Cell* 140:871, 2010. *[A discussion of the abnormalities that lead to chronic inflammation.]*

Okin D, Medzhitov R: Evolution of inflammatory diseases, *Curr Biol* 22:R733–R740, 2012. *[An interesting conceptual discussion of the balance between the high potential cost and benefit of the inflammatory response and how this balance may be disturbed by environmental changes, accounting for the association between inflammation and many of the diseases of the modern world.]*

Page-McCaw A, Ewald AJ, Werb Z: Matrix metalloproteinases and the regulation of tissue remodelling, *Nat Rev Mol Cell Biol* 8:221, 2007. *[A review of the function of matrix modifying enzymes in tissue repair.]*

Ricklin D, Lambris JD: Complement in immune and inflammatory disorders, *J Immunol* 190:3831–3838, 3839–3847, 2013. *[Two companion articles on the biochemistry and biology of the complement system, and the development of therapeutic agents to alter complement activity in disease.]*

Rock KL, Latz E, Ontiveros F, et al: The sterile inflammatory response, *Annu Rev Immunol* 28:321–342, 2010. *[An excellent discussion of how the immune system recognizes necrotic cells and other noninfectious harmful agents.]*

Romito A, Cobellis G: Pluripotent stem cells: current understanding and future directions, *Stem Cells Int* 2016. [Epub 2015] *[A cogent summary of endogenous and induced pluripotent stem cells.]*

Schmidt S, Moser M, Sperandio M: The molecular basis of leukocyte recruitment and its deficiencies, *Mol Immunol* 55:49–58, 2013. *[A review of the mechanisms of leukocyte recruitment and leukocyte adhesion deficiencies.]*

Sica A, Mantovani A: Macrophage plasticity and polarization: in vivo veritas, *J Clin Invest* 122:787–795, 2012. *[An excellent review of macrophage subpopulations, their generation, and their roles in inflammation, infections, cancer, and metabolic disorders.]*

Stappenbeck TS, Miyoshi H: The role of stromal stem cells in tissue regeneration and wound repair, *Science* 324:1666, 2009. *[An excellent review of the role of tissue stem cells in repair.]*

Stearns-Kurosawa DJ, Osuchowski MF, Valentine C, et al: The pathogenesis of sepsis, *Ann Rev Pathol Mech Dis* 6:19, 2011. *[A discussion of the current concepts of pathogenic mechanisms in sepsis and septic shock.]*

Welti J, Loges S, Dimmeler S, et al: Recent molecular discoveries in angiogenesis and antiangiogenic therapies in cancer, *J Clin Invest* 123:3190, 2013. *[A review of new advances in elucidating the stimuli and control of angiogenesis, and the development of therapies targeting the process.]*

Zlotnik A, Yoshie O: The chemokine superfamily revisited, *Immunity* 36:705–716, 2012. *[An excellent update on the classification, functions, and clinical relevance of chemokines and their receptors.]*

Hemodynamic Disorders, Thromboembolism, and Shock

4

Hyperemia and Congestion 97
Edema 98
Increased Hydrostatic Pressure 99
Reduced Plasma Osmotic Pressure 99
Lymphatic Obstruction 99
Sodium and Water Retention 100
Hemorrhage 100
Hemostasis and Thrombosis 101

Normal Hemostasis 101
Thrombosis 106
Disseminated Intravascular Coagulation
(DIC) 111
Embolism 112
Pulmonary Thromboembolism 112
Systemic Thromboembolism 112
Fat Embolism 112

Amniotic Fluid Embolism 113
Air Embolism 113
Infarction 114
Factors That Influence Infarct Development 115
Shock 115
Pathogenesis of Septic Shock 116
Stages of Shock 118

The health of cells and tissues depends on the circulation of blood, which delivers oxygen and nutrients and removes wastes generated by cellular metabolism. Under normal conditions, as blood passes through capillary beds, proteins in the plasma are retained within the vasculature and there is little net movement of water and electrolytes into the tissues. This balance is often disturbed by pathologic conditions that alter endothelial function, increase vascular hydrostatic pressure, or decrease plasma protein content, all of which promote edema—the accumulation of fluid in tissues resulting from a net movement of water into extravascular spaces. Depending on its severity and location, edema may have minimal or profound effects. In the lower extremities, it may only make one's shoes feel snugger after a long sedentary day; in the lungs, however, edema fluid can fill alveoli, causing life-threatening hypoxia.

The structural integrity of blood vessels is frequently compromised by trauma. *Hemostasis* is the process of blood clotting that prevents excessive bleeding after blood-vessel damage. Inadequate hemostasis may result in hemorrhage, which can compromise regional tissue perfusion and, if massive and rapid, may lead to hypotension, shock, and death. Conversely, inappropriate clotting (thrombosis) or migration of clots (embolism) can obstruct blood vessels, potentially causing ischemic cell death (infarction). Indeed, thromboembolism lies at the heart of three major causes of morbidity and death in developed countries: myocardial infarction, pulmonary embolism (PE), and cerebrovascular accident (stroke).

With this as a preface, we begin our discussion of hemodynamic disorders with conditions that increase tissue blood volumes.

HYPEREMIA AND CONGESTION

Hyperemia and congestion both refer to an increase in blood volume within a tissue, but have different underlying mechanisms. *Hyperemia* is an active process resulting from arteriolar dilation and increased blood inflow, as occurs at sites of inflammation or in exercising skeletal muscle. Hyperemic tissues are redder than normal because of engorgement with oxygenated blood. *Congestion* is a passive process resulting from impaired outflow of venous blood from a tissue. It can occur systemically, as in cardiac failure, or locally as a consequence of an isolated venous obstruction. Congested tissues have an abnormal blue-red color (*cyanosis*) that stems from the accumulation of deoxygenated hemoglobin in the affected area. In long-standing chronic congestion, inadequate tissue perfusion and persistent hypoxia may lead to parenchymal cell death and secondary tissue fibrosis, and the elevated intravascular pressures may cause edema or sometimes rupture capillaries, producing focal hemorrhages.

MORPHOLOGY

Cut surfaces of hyperemic or congested tissues feel wet and typically ooze blood. On microscopic examination, **acute pulmonary congestion** is marked by blood-engorged alveolar capillaries and variable degrees of alveolar septal edema and intraalveolar hemorrhage. In **chronic pulmonary congestion,** the septa become thickened and fibrotic, and the alveolar spaces contain numerous macrophages laden with hemosiderin ("heart failure cells") derived from phagocytosed red cells. In **acute**

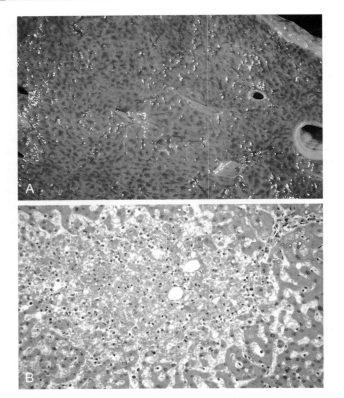

Fig. 4.1 Liver with chronic passive congestion and hemorrhagic necrosis. (A) In this autopsy specimen, central areas are red and slightly depressed compared with the surrounding tan viable parenchyma, creating "nutmeg liver" (so called because it resembles the cut surface of a nutmeg). (B) Microscopic preparation shows centrilobular hepatic necrosis with hemorrhage and scattered inflammatory cells. *(Courtesy of Dr. James Crawford.)*

hepatic congestion, the central vein and sinusoids are distended with blood, and there may even be necrosis of centrally located hepatocytes. The periportal hepatocytes, better oxygenated because of their proximity to hepatic arterioles, experience less severe hypoxia and may develop only reversible fatty change. In **chronic passive congestion of the liver,** the central regions of the hepatic lobules, viewed on gross examination, are red-brown and slightly depressed (owing to cell loss) and are accentuated against the surrounding zones of uncongested tan, sometimes fatty, liver **(nutmeg liver)** (Fig. 4.1A). Microscopic findings include centrilobular hepatocyte necrosis, hemorrhage, and hemosiderin-laden macrophages (Fig. 4.1B).

EDEMA

Approximately 60% of lean body weight is water, two-thirds of which is intracellular. Most of the remaining water is found in extracellular compartments in the form of interstitial fluid; only 5% of the body's water is in blood plasma. As noted earlier, edema is an accumulation of interstitial fluid within tissues. Extravascular fluid can also collect in body cavities and such accumulations are often referred to collectively as effusions. Examples include effusions in the pleural cavity (*hydrothorax*), the pericardial cavity (*hydropericardium*), or the peritoneal cavity (hydroperitoneum, or *ascites*). Anasarca is severe, generalized

edema marked by profound swelling of subcutaneous tissues and accumulation of fluid in body cavities.

Table 4.1 lists the major causes of edema. The mechanisms of inflammatory edema are largely related to increased vascular permeability and are discussed in Chapter 3; the noninflammatory causes are described in the following discussion.

Fluid movement between the vascular and interstitial spaces is governed mainly by two opposing forces—the vascular hydrostatic pressure and the colloid osmotic pressure produced by plasma proteins. Normally, the outflow of fluid produced by hydrostatic pressure at the arteriolar end of the microcirculation is nearly balanced by inflow at the venular end owing to slightly elevated osmotic pressure; hence there is only a small net outflow of fluid into the interstitial space, which is drained by lymphatic vessels. Either increased hydrostatic pressure or diminished colloid osmotic pressure causes increased movement of water into the interstitium (Fig. 4.2). This in turn increases the tissue's hydrostatic pressure, and eventually a new equilibrium is achieved. Excess edema fluid is removed by lymphatic drainage and is returned to the bloodstream by way of the thoracic duct (Fig. 4.2).

The edema fluid that accumulates in the setting of increased hydrostatic pressure or reduced intravascular

Table 4.1 Causes of Edema

Increased Hydrostatic Pressure
Impaired Venous Return
Congestive heart failure
Constrictive pericarditis
Ascites (liver cirrhosis)
Venous obstruction or compression
Thrombosis
External pressure (e.g., mass)
Lower extremity inactivity with prolonged dependency
Arteriolar Dilation
Heat
Neurohumoral dysregulation
Reduced Plasma Osmotic Pressure (Hypoproteinemia)
Protein-losing glomerulopathies (nephrotic syndrome)
Liver cirrhosis (ascites)
Malnutrition
Protein-losing gastroenteropathy
Lymphatic Obstruction
Inflammatory
Neoplastic
Postsurgical
Postirradiation
Sodium Retention
Excessive salt intake with renal insufficiency
Increased tubular reabsorption of sodium
Renal hypoperfusion
Increased renin-angiotensin-**aldosterone** secretion
Inflammation
Acute inflammation
Chronic inflammation
Angiogenesis

Data from Leaf A, Cotran RS: *Renal pathophysiology*, ed 3, New York, 1985, Oxford University Press, p 146.

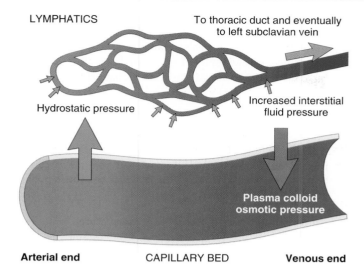

LYMPHATICS

To thoracic duct and eventually
to left subclavian vein

Hydrostatic pressure

Increased interstitial
fluid pressure

Plasma colloid
osmotic pressure

Arterial end   CAPILLARY BED   Venous end

Fig. 4.2 Factors influencing fluid movement across capillary walls. Capillary hydrostatic and osmotic forces are normally balanced so there is little net movement of fluid into the interstitium. However, increased hydrostatic pressure or diminished plasma osmotic pressure leads to extravascular fluid accumulation (edema). Tissue lymphatics drain much of the excess fluid back to the circulation by way of the thoracic duct; however, if the capacity for lymphatic drainage is exceeded, tissue edema results.

colloid typically is a protein-poor transudate; by contrast, because of increased vascular permeability, inflammatory edema fluid is a protein-rich exudate with a high specific gravity. The usual cutoffs for specific gravity (<1.012 for transudates and >1.020 for exudates) illustrate the point but are not clinically useful. We will now discuss the various causes of edema.

Increased Hydrostatic Pressure

Increases in hydrostatic pressure are mainly caused by disorders that impair venous return. Local increases in intravascular pressure caused, for example, by deep venous thrombosis in the lower extremity can cause edema restricted to the distal portion of the affected leg. Generalized increases in venous pressure, with resultant systemic edema, occur most commonly in congestive heart failure (Chapter 11). Fig. 4.3 illustrates the interlocking mechanisms that underlie generalized edema resulting from cardiac, renal, and hepatic failure. Several factors increase venous hydrostatic pressure in patients with congestive heart failure (Fig. 4.3). The reduced cardiac output leads to systemic venous congestion and resultant increase in capillary hydrostatic pressure. At the same time reduction in cardiac output results in hypoperfusion of the kidneys, triggering the renin-angiotensin-aldosterone axis and inducing sodium and water retention (secondary hyperaldosteronism). In patients with normal heart function, this adaptation increases cardiac filling and cardiac output, thereby improving renal perfusion. However, the failing heart often cannot increase its cardiac output in response to the compensatory increases in blood volume. Instead, a vicious cycle of fluid retention, increased venous hydrostatic pressures, and worsening edema ensues. Unless cardiac output is restored or renal water retention is reduced (e.g., by salt restriction or treatment with diuretics or aldosterone

antagonists), this downward spiral continues. Because secondary hyperaldosteronism is a common feature of generalized edema, salt restriction, diuretics, and aldosterone antagonists also are of value in the management of generalized edema resulting from non-cardiac causes.

Reduced Plasma Osmotic Pressure

Reduction of plasma albumin concentrations leads to decreased colloid osmotic pressure of the blood and loss of fluid from the circulation. Under normal circumstances, albumin accounts for almost half of the total plasma protein. Therefore, conditions in which albumin is either lost from the circulation or synthesized in inadequate amounts are common causes of reduced plasma osmotic pressure. *Nephrotic syndrome* is the most important cause of albumin loss from the blood. In diseases that are characterized by nephrotic syndrome (Chapter 14), the glomerular capillaries become leaky, leading to the loss of albumin (and other plasma proteins) in the urine and the development of generalized edema. Reduced albumin synthesis occurs in the setting of severe liver disease (e.g., cirrhosis) (Chapter 16) and protein malnutrition (Chapter 8). Regardless of cause, low albumin levels lead in a stepwise fashion to edema, reduced intravascular volume, renal hypoperfusion, and secondary hyperaldosteronism. Unfortunately, increased salt and water retention by the kidney not only fails to correct the plasma volume deficit but also exacerbates the edema, because the primary defect—low serum protein—persists.

Lymphatic Obstruction

Edema may result from lymphatic obstruction that compromises resorption of fluid from interstitial spaces. Impaired lymphatic drainage and consequent lymphedema usually results from a localized obstruction caused by an inflammatory or neoplastic condition. For example, the parasitic infection filariasis can cause massive edema of the lower extremity and external genitalia (so-called

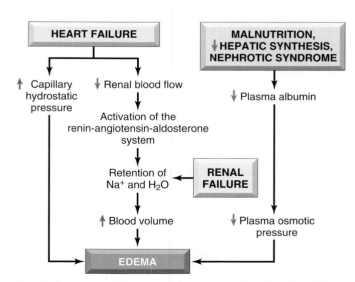

Fig. 4.3 Pathways leading to systemic edema resulting from heart failure, renal failure, or reduced plasma osmotic pressure.

"elephantiasis") by producing inguinal lymphatic and lymph node fibrosis. Infiltration and obstruction of superficial lymphatics by breast cancer may cause edema of the overlying skin; the characteristic finely pitted appearance of the skin of the affected breast is called *peau d'orange* (orange peel). Lymphedema also may occur as a complication of therapy. One relatively common setting for this clinical entity is in women with breast cancer who undergo axillary lymph node resection and/or irradiation, both of which can disrupt and obstruct lymphatic drainage, resulting in severe lymphedema of the arm.

Sodium and Water Retention

Excessive retention of salt (and its obligate associated water) can lead to edema by increasing hydrostatic pressure (because of expansion of the intravascular volume) and reducing plasma osmotic pressure. Excessive salt and water retention are seen in a wide variety of diseases that compromise renal function, including poststreptococcal glomerulonephritis and acute renal failure (Chapter 14).

MORPHOLOGY

Edema is easily recognized on gross inspection; microscopic examination shows clearing and separation of the extracellular matrix (ECM) elements. Although any tissue can be involved, edema most commonly is encountered in subcutaneous tissues, lungs, and brain.

Subcutaneous edema can be diffuse but usually accumulates preferentially in parts of the body positioned the greatest distance below the heart, where hydrostatic pressures are highest. Thus, edema typically is most pronounced in the legs with standing and the sacrum with recumbency, a relationship termed **dependent edema.** Finger pressure over edematous subcutaneous tissue displaces the interstitial fluid, leaving a finger-shaped depression; this appearance is called **pitting edema.** Edema resulting from **renal dysfunction** or **nephrotic syndrome** often manifests first in loose connective tissues (e.g., the eyelids, causing periorbital edema). With **pulmonary edema,** the lungs often are two to three times their normal weight, and sectioning shows frothy, sometimes blood-tinged fluid consisting of a mixture of air, edema fluid, and extravasated red cells. **Brain edema** (Chapter 23) can be localized (e.g., because of abscess or tumor) or generalized, depending on the nature and extent of the pathologic process or injury. With generalized edema, the sulci are narrowed as the gyri swell and become flattened against the skull.

Clinical Features

The effects of edema vary, ranging from merely annoying to rapidly fatal. Subcutaneous edema is important to recognize primarily because it signals potential underlying cardiac or renal disease; however, when significant, it also can impair wound healing and the clearance of infections. Pulmonary edema is a common clinical problem. It is seen most frequently in the setting of left ventricular failure, but also may occur in renal failure, acute respiratory distress syndrome (Chapter 11), and inflammatory and infectious disorders of the lung. It can cause death by interfering with

normal ventilatory function; besides impeding oxygen diffusion, alveolar edema fluid also creates a favorable environment for infections. Brain edema is life threatening; if the swelling is severe, the brain can herniate (extrude) through the foramen magnum. With increased intracranial

SUMMARY

EDEMA

- Edema results from the movement of fluid from the vasculature into the interstitial spaces; the fluid may be protein poor (transudate) or protein rich (exudate).
- Edema may be caused by:
  - Increased hydrostatic pressure (e.g., heart failure)
  - Increased vascular permeability (e.g., inflammation)
  - Decreased colloid osmotic pressure resulting from reduced plasma albumin
    - Decreased synthesis (e.g., liver disease, protein malnutrition)
    - Increased loss (e.g., nephrotic syndrome)
  - Lymphatic obstruction (e.g., inflammation or neoplasia)
  - Sodium retention (e.g., renal failure)

pressure, the brain stem vascular supply can be compressed, leading to death due to injury to the medullary centers controlling respiration and other vital functions (Chapter 23).

HEMORRHAGE

Hemorrhage, defined as the extravasation of blood from vessels, is most often the result of damage to blood vessels or defective clot formation. As described earlier, capillary bleeding can occur in chronically congested tissues. Trauma, atherosclerosis, or inflammatory or neoplastic erosion of a vessel wall also may lead to hemorrhage, which may be extensive if the affected vessel is a large vein or artery.

The risk of hemorrhage (often after a seemingly insignificant injury) is increased in a wide variety of clinical disorders collectively called hemorrhagic diatheses. These have diverse causes, including inherited or acquired defects in vessel walls, platelets, or coagulation factors, all of which must function properly to ensure homeostasis. These are discussed in the next section. Here we focus on clinical features of hemorrhages, regardless of the cause.

Hemorrhage may be manifested by different appearances and clinical consequences.

- Hemorrhage may be external or accumulate within a tissue as a *hematoma*, which ranges in significance from trivial (e.g., a bruise) to fatal (e.g., a massive retroperitoneal hematoma resulting from rupture of a dissecting aortic aneurysm) (Chapter 10). Large bleeds into body cavities are described variously according to location— *hemothorax, hemopericardium, hemoperitoneum,* or *hemarthrosis* (in joints). Extensive hemorrhages can occasionally result in jaundice from the massive breakdown of red cells and hemoglobin.

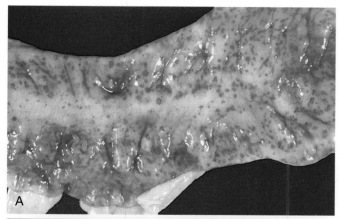

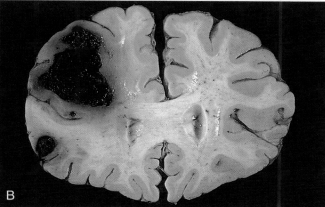

Fig. 4.4 (A) Punctate petechial hemorrhages of the colonic mucosa, a consequence of thrombocytopenia. (B) Fatal intracerebral hemorrhage.

- *Petechiae* are minute (1 to 2 mm in diameter) hemorrhages into skin, mucous membranes, or serosal surfaces (Fig. 4.4A); causes include low platelet counts (thrombocytopenia), defective platelet function, and loss of vascular wall support, as in vitamin C deficiency (Chapter 8).
- *Purpura* are slightly larger (3 to 5 mm) hemorrhages. Purpura can result from the same disorders that cause petechiae, as well as trauma, vascular inflammation (vasculitis), and increased vascular fragility.
- *Ecchymoses* are larger (1 to 2 cm) subcutaneous hematomas (colloquially called bruises). Extravasated red cells are phagocytosed and degraded by macrophages; the characteristic color changes of a bruise result from the enzymatic conversion of hemoglobin (red-blue color) to bilirubin (blue-green color) and eventually hemosiderin (golden-brown).

The clinical significance of any particular hemorrhage depends on the volume of blood that is lost and the rate of bleeding. Rapid loss of up to 20% of the blood volume, or slow losses of even larger amounts, may have little impact in healthy adults; greater losses, however, can cause hemorrhagic (hypovolemic) shock (discussed later). The site of hemorrhage also is important; bleeding that would be trivial in the subcutaneous tissues can cause death if located in the brain (Fig. 4.4B). Finally, chronic or recurrent external blood loss (e.g., due to peptic ulcer or menstrual bleeding)

frequently culminates in iron deficiency anemia as a consequence of a loss of iron in hemoglobin. By contrast, iron is efficiently recycled from phagocytosed red cells, so internal bleeding (e.g., a hematoma) does not lead to iron deficiency.

HEMOSTASIS AND THROMBOSIS

Normal hemostasis comprises a series of regulated processes that culminate in the formation of a blood clot that limits bleeding from an injured vessel. The pathologic counterpart of hemostasis is thrombosis, the formation of blood clot (thrombus) within non-traumatized, intact vessels. This discussion begins with normal hemostasis and its regulation, to be followed by causes and consequences of thrombosis.

Normal Hemostasis

Hemostasis is a precisely orchestrated process involving platelets, clotting factors, and endothelium that occurs at the site of vascular injury and culminates in the formation of a blood clot, which serves to prevent or limit the extent of bleeding. The general sequence of events leading to hemostasis at a site of vascular injury is shown in Fig. 4.5.
- *Arteriolar vasoconstriction* occurs immediately and markedly reduces blood flow to the injured area (Fig. 4.5A). It is mediated by reflex neurogenic mechanisms and augmented by the local secretion of factors such as *endothelin*, a potent endothelium-derived vasoconstrictor. This effect is transient, however, and bleeding would resume if not for activation of platelets and coagulation factors.
- *Primary hemostasis: the formation of the platelet plug.* Disruption of the endothelium exposes subendothelial von Willebrand factor (vWF) and collagen, which promote platelet adherence and activation. Activation of platelets results in a dramatic shape change (from small rounded discs to flat plates with spiky protrusions that markedly increased surface area), as well as the release of secretory granules. Within minutes the secreted products recruit additional platelets, which undergo *aggregation* to form a *primary hemostatic plug* (Fig. 4.5B).
- *Secondary hemostasis: deposition of fibrin.* Vascular injury exposes *tissue factor* at the site of injury. Tissue factor is a membrane-bound procoagulant glycoprotein that is normally expressed by subendothelial cells in the vessel wall, such as smooth muscle cells and fibroblasts. Tissue factor binds and activates factor VII (see later), setting in motion a cascade of reactions that culminates in *thrombin* generation. Thrombin cleaves circulating fibrinogen into insoluble *fibrin*, creating a fibrin meshwork, and also is a potent activator of platelets, leading to additional platelet aggregation at the site of injury. This sequence, referred to as *secondary hemostasis*, consolidates the initial platelet plug (Fig. 4.5C).
- *Clot stabilization and resorption.* Polymerized fibrin and platelet aggregates undergo contraction to form a solid, *permanent plug* that prevents further hemorrhage. At this stage, counterregulatory mechanisms (e.g., *tissue plasminogen activator, t-PA made by endothelial cells*) are set into motion that limit clotting to the site of injury (Fig. 4.5D) and eventually lead to clot resorption and tissue repair.

A. VASOCONSTRICTION

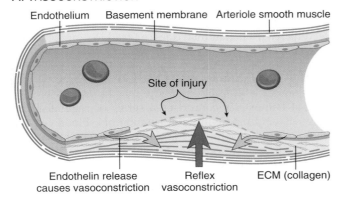

Endothelium   Basement membrane   Arteriole smooth muscle

Site of injury

Endothelin release causes vasoconstriction

Reflex vasoconstriction

ECM (collagen)

B. PLATELET ACTIVATION AND AGGREGATION

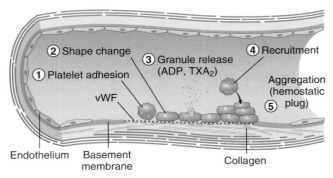

② Shape change

③ Granule release (ADP, TXA$_2$)

④ Recruitment

① Platelet adhesion

vWF

Aggregation (hemostatic ⑤ plug)

Endothelium   Basement membrane

Collagen

C. ACTIVATION OF CLOTTING FACTORS AND FORMATION OF FIBRIN

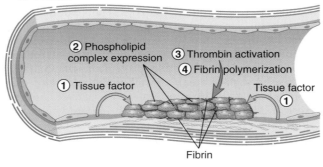

② Phospholipid complex expression

③ Thrombin activation

④ Fibrin polymerization

① Tissue factor

Tissue factor ①

Fibrin

D. CLOT RESORPTION

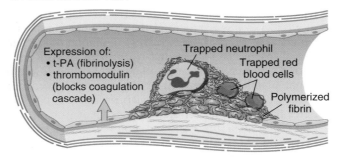

Expression of:
• t-PA (fibrinolysis)
• thrombomodulin (blocks coagulation cascade)

Trapped neutrophil

Trapped red blood cells

Polymerized fibrin

Fig. 4.5 Normal hemostasis. (A) After vascular injury, local neurohumoral factors induce a transient vasoconstriction. (B) Platelets bind via glycoprotein Ib (GpIb) receptors to von Willebrand factor (VWF) on exposed ECM and are activated, undergoing a shape change and granule release. Released ADP and thromboxane A$_2$ (TXA$_2$) induce additional platelet aggregation through platelet GpIIb-IIIa receptor binding to fibrinogen, and form the *primary* hemostatic plug. (C) Local activation of the coagulation cascade (involving tissue factor and platelet phospholipids) results in fibrin polymerization, "cementing" the platelets into a definitive *secondary* hemostatic plug. (D) Counterregulatory mechanisms, mediated by tissue plasminogen activator (t-PA, a fibrinolytic product) and thrombomodulin, confine the hemostatic process to the site of injury.

It should be emphasized that endothelial cells are central regulators of hemostasis; the balance between the anti-thrombic and prothrombotic activities of endothelium determines whether thrombus formation, propagation, or dissolution occurs. Normal endothelial cells express a variety of *anticoagulant* factors that inhibit platelet aggregation and coagulation and promote fibrinolysis; after injury or activation, however, this balance shifts, and endothelial cells acquire numerous *procoagulant* activities (activation of platelets and clotting factor, described above, see also Fig. 4.11). Besides trauma, endothelium can be activated by microbial pathogens, hemodynamic forces, and a number of pro-inflammatory mediators. We will return to the pro-coagulant and anti-coagulant roles of endothelium after a detailed discussion of the role of platelets and coagulation factors in hemostasis since endothelium modulates the functions of platelets and can trigger coagulation.

The following sections describe roles of platelets, coagulation factors and endothelium in hemostasis in greater detail, following the scheme illustrated in Fig. 4.5.

Platelets

Platelets play a critical role in hemostasis by forming the primary plug that initially seals vascular defects and by providing a surface that binds and concentrates activated coagulation factors. Platelets are disc-shaped anucleate cell fragments that are shed from megakaryocytes in the bone marrow into the bloodstream. Their function depends on several glycoprotein receptors, a contractile cytoskeleton, and two types of cytoplasmic granules. *α-Granules* have the adhesion molecule P-selectin on their membranes (Chapter 3) and contain proteins involved in coagulation, such as fibrinogen, coagulation factor V, and vWF, as well as protein factors that may be involved in wound healing, such as fibronectin, platelet factor 4 (a heparin-binding chemokine), platelet-derived growth factor (PDGF), and transforming growth factor-β. *Dense* (or δ) *granules* contain adenosine diphosphate (ADP) and adenosine triphosphate, ionized calcium, serotonin, and epinephrine.

After a traumatic vascular injury, platelets encounter constituents of the subendothelial connective tissue, such as vWF and collagen. On contact with these proteins, platelets undergo a sequence of reactions that culminate in the formation of a platelet plug (Fig. 4.5B).

• *Platelet adhesion* is mediated largely via interactions with vWF, which acts as a bridge between the platelet surface receptor glycoprotein Ib (GpIb) and exposed collagen

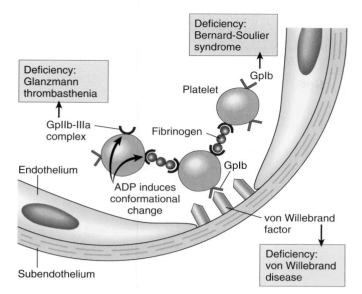

Fig. 4.6 Platelet adhesion and aggregation. VWF functions as an adhesion bridge between subendothelial collagen and the glycoprotein Ib (GpIb) platelet receptor. Platelet aggregation is accomplished by fibrinogen binding to platelet GpIIb-IIIa receptors on different platelets. Congenital deficiencies in the various receptors or bridging molecules lead to the diseases indicated in the colored boxes. *ADP,* Adenosine diphosphate.

(Fig. 4.6). Notably, genetic deficiencies of vWF (von Willebrand disease, Chapter 14) or GpIb (Bernard-Soulier syndrome) result in bleeding disorders, attesting to the importance of these factors.

- *Platelets rapidly change shape* following adhesion, being converted from smooth discs to spiky "sea urchins" with greatly increased surface area. This change is accompanied by alterations in *glycoprotein IIb/IIIa* that increase its affinity for fibrinogen (see later), and by the translocation of *negatively charged phospholipids* (particularly phosphatidylserine) to the platelet surface. These phospholipids bind calcium and serve as nucleation sites for the assembly of coagulation factor complexes.

- *Secretion (release reaction) of granule contents* occurs along with changes in shape; these two events are often referred to together as *platelet activation.* Platelet activation is triggered by a number of factors, including he coagulation factor thrombin and ADP. Thrombin activates platelets through a special type of G-protein–coupled receptor referred to as a *protease-activated receptor* (PAR), which is switched on by a proteolytic cleavage carried out by thrombin. ADP is a component of dense-body granules; thus, platelet activation and ADP release begets additional rounds of platelet activation, a phenomenon referred to as *recruitment.* Activated platelets also produce the prostaglandin *thromboxane A2* (TXA2), a potent inducer of platelet aggregation. *Aspirin* inhibits platelet aggregation and produces a mild bleeding defect by inhibiting cyclooxygenase, a platelet enzyme that is required for TXA2 synthesis. Although the phenomenon is less well characterized, it is also suspected that growth factors released from platelets contribute to the repair of the vessel wall following injury.

- *Platelet aggregation* follows their activation. The conformational change in glycoprotein IIb/IIIa that occurs with platelet activation allows binding of fibrinogen, a large bivalent plasma polypeptide that forms bridges between adjacent platelets, leading to their aggregation. Predictably, inherited deficiency of GpIIb-IIIa results in a bleeding disorder called *Glanzmann thrombasthenia.* The initial wave of aggregation is reversible, but concurrent activation of thrombin stabilizes the platelet plug by causing further platelet activation and aggregation, and by promoting irreversible *platelet contraction.* Platelet contraction is dependent on the cytoskeleton and consolidates the aggregated platelets. In parallel, thrombin also converts fibrinogen into insoluble *fibrin,* cementing the platelets in place and creating the definitive *secondary hemostatic plug.* Entrapped red cells and leukocytes are also found in hemostatic plugs, in part due to adherence of leukocytes to P-selectin expressed on activated platelets.

SUMMARY

PLATELET ADHESION, ACTIVATION, AND AGGREGATION

- Endothelial injury exposes the underlying basement membrane ECM; platelets adhere to the ECM primarily through the binding of platelet GpIb receptors to VWF.
- Adhesion leads to platelet activation, an event associated with secretion of platelet granule contents, including calcium (a cofactor for several coagulation proteins) and ADP (a mediator of further platelet activation); dramatic changes in shape and membrane composition; and activation of GpIIb/IIIa receptors.
- The GpIIb/IIIa receptors on activated platelets form bridging crosslinks with fibrinogen, leading to platelet aggregation.
- Concomitant activation of thrombin promotes fibrin deposition, cementing the platelet plug in place.

Coagulation Cascade

The coagulation cascade is a series of amplifying enzymatic reactions that lead to the deposition of an insoluble fibrin clot. As discussed later, the dependency of clot formation on various factors differs in the laboratory test tube and in blood vessels in vivo (Fig. 4.7). However, clotting in vitro and in vivo both follow the same general principles, as follows.

The cascade of reactions in the pathway can be likened to a "dance," in which coagulation factors are passed from one partner to the next (Fig. 4.8). Each reaction step involves an enzyme (an activated coagulation factor), a substrate (an inactive proenzyme form of a coagulation factor), and a cofactor (a reaction accelerator). These components are assembled on a negatively charged phospholipid surface, which is provided by activated platelets. Assembly of reaction complexes also depends on calcium, which binds to γ-carboxylated glutamic acid residues that are present in factors II, VII, IX, and X. The enzymatic reactions that produce γ-carboxylated glutamic acid use vitamin K as a cofactor and are antagonized by drugs such as Coumadin, a widely used anti-coagulant.

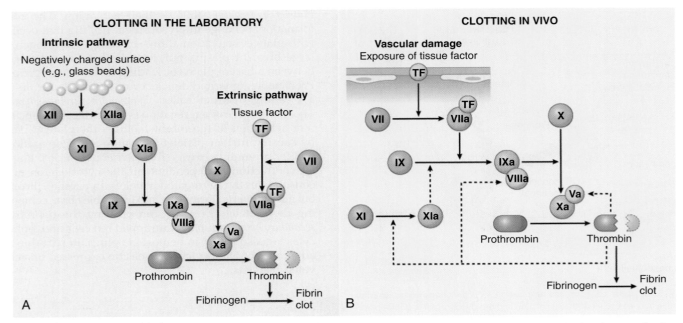

Fig. 4.7 The coagulation cascade in the laboratory and in vivo. (A) Clotting is initiated in the laboratory by adding phospholipids, calcium, and either a negative-charged substance such as glass beads (intrinsic pathway) or a source of tissue factor (extrinsic pathway). (B) In vivo, tissue factor is the major initiator of coagulation, which is amplified by feedback loops involving thrombin *(dotted lines)*. The red polypeptides are inactive factors, the *dark green* polypeptides are active factors, whereas the *light green* polypeptides correspond to cofactors.

Based on assays performed in clinical laboratories, the coagulation cascade has traditionally been divided into the *extrinsic* and *intrinsic* pathways (Fig. 4.7A).

- The *prothrombin time* (PT) assay assesses the function of the proteins in the extrinsic pathway (factors VII, X, V, II (prothrombin), and fibrinogen). In brief, tissue factor, phospholipids, and calcium are added to plasma and the time for a fibrin clot to form is recorded.

- The *partial thromboplastin time* (PTT) assay screens the function of the proteins in the intrinsic pathway (factors XII, XI, IX, VIII, X, V, II, and fibrinogen). In this assay, clotting of plasma is initiated by the addition of negative-charged particles (e.g., ground glass) that activate factor XII (Hageman factor) together with phospholipids and calcium, and the time to fibrin clot formation is recorded.

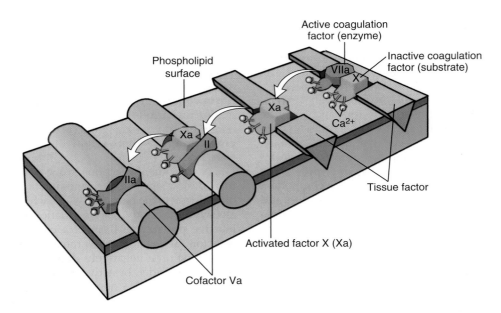

Fig. 4.8 Sequential conversion of factor X to factor Xa by way of the extrinsic pathway, followed by conversion of factor II (prothrombin) to factor IIa (thrombin). The initial reaction complex consists of a protease (factor VIIa), a substrate (factor X), and a reaction accelerator (tissue factor) assembled on a platelet phospholipid surface. Calcium ions hold the assembled components together and are essential for the reaction. Activated factor Xa then becomes the protease component of the next complex in the cascade, converting prothrombin to thrombin (factor IIa) in the presence of a different reaction accelerator, factor Va.

Although the PT and PTT assays are of great utility in evaluating coagulation factor function in patients, they do not recapitulate the events that lead to coagulation in vivo. This point is most clearly made by considering the clinical effects of deficiencies of various coagulation factors. Deficiencies of factors V, VII, VIII, IX, and X are associated with moderate to severe bleeding disorders, and prothrombin deficiency is likely incompatible with life. In contrast, factor XI deficiency is only associated with mild bleeding, and individuals with factor XII deficiency do not bleed and in fact may be susceptible to thrombosis. The paradoxical effect of factor XII deficiency may be explained by involvement of factor XII in the fibrinolysis pathway (discussed later); although there is also some evidence from experimental models suggesting that factor XII may promote thrombosis under certain circumstances, the relevance of these observations to human thrombotic disease remains to be determined.

Based on the effects of various factor deficiencies in humans, it is believed that, in vivo, factor VIIa/tissue factor complex is the most important activator of factor IX and that factor IXa/factor VIIIa complex is the most important activator of factor X (Fig. 4.7B). The mild bleeding tendency seen in patients with factor XI deficiency is likely explained by the ability of thrombin to activate factor XI (as well as factors V and VIII), a feedback mechanism that amplifies the coagulation cascade.

Among the coagulation factors, thrombin is the most important, because its various enzymatic activities control diverse aspects of hemostasis and link clotting to inflammation and repair. Among thrombin's most important activities are the following:

- *Conversion of fibrinogen into crosslinked fibrin.* Thrombin directly converts soluble fibrinogen into fibrin monomers that polymerize into an insoluble fibril, and also amplifies the coagulation process, not only by activating factor XI, but also by activating two critical cofactors: factors V and VIII. It also stabilizes the secondary hemostatic plug by activating factor XIII, which covalently crosslinks fibrin.
- *Platelet activation.* Thrombin is a potent inducer of platelet activation and aggregation through its ability to activate PARs, thereby linking platelet function to coagulation.
- *Proinflammatory effects.* PARs also are expressed on inflammatory cells, endothelium, and other cell types (Fig. 4.9), and activation of these receptors by thrombin is believed to mediate proinflammatory effects that contribute to tissue repair and angiogenesis.
- *Anti-coagulant effects.* Remarkably, through mechanisms described later, on encountering normal endothelium, thrombin changes from a procoagulant to an anticoagulant; this reversal in function prevents clots from extending beyond the site of the vascular injury.

Factors That Limit Coagulation. Once initiated, coagulation must be restricted to the site of vascular injury to prevent deleterious consequences. One limiting factor is simple dilution; blood flowing past the site of injury washes out activated coagulation factors, which are rapidly removed by the liver. A second is the requirement for negatively charged phospholipids, which, as mentioned, are mainly provided by platelets that have been

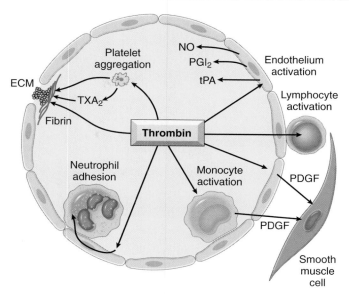

Fig. 4.9 Role of thrombin in hemostasis and cellular activation. Thrombin generates fibrin by cleaving fibrinogen, activates factor XIII (which is responsible for crosslinking fibrin into an insoluble clot), and also activates several other coagulation factors, thereby amplifying the coagulation cascade (Fig. 4.7). Through protease-activated receptors (PARs), thrombin activates (*1*) platelet aggregation and TxA$_2$ secretion; (*2*) endothelium, which responds by generating leukocyte adhesion molecules and a variety of fibrinolytic (t-PA), vasoactive (NO, PGI$_2$), or cytokine (PDGF) mediators; and (*3*) leukocytes, increasing their adhesion to activated endothelium. *ECM,* Extracellular matrix; *NO,* nitric oxide; *PDGF,* platelet-derived growth factor; *PGI$_2$,* prostaglandin I$_2$ (prostacyclin); *TXA2,* thromboxane A2; *t-PA,* tissue-type plasminogen activator. See Fig. 4.11 for anticoagulant activities mediated by thrombin via thrombomodulin. *(Courtesy of Shaun Coughlin, MD, PhD, Cardiovascular Research Institute, University of California at San Francisco, San Francisco, California.)*

activated by contact with subendothelial matrix at sites of vascular injury. However, the most important counterregulatory mechanisms involve factors that are expressed by intact endothelium adjacent to the site of injury (described later).

Activation of the coagulation cascade also sets into motion a *fibrinolytic cascade* that limits the size of the clot and contributes to its later dissolution (Fig. 4.10). Fibrinolysis is largely accomplished through the enzymatic activity of *plasmin,* which breaks down fibrin and interferes with its polymerization. An elevated level of breakdown products of fibrinogen (often called fibrin split products), most notably fibrin-derived *D-dimers,* are a useful clinical markers of several thrombotic states (described later). Plasmin is generated by enzymatic catabolism of the inactive circulating precursor *plasminogen,* either by a factor XII–dependent pathway (possibly explaining the association of factor XII deficiency and thrombosis) or by plasminogen activators. The most important plasminogen activator is t-PA; it is synthesized principally by endothelium and is most active when bound to fibrin. This characteristic makes t-PA a useful therapeutic agent, since its fibrinolytic activity is largely confined to sites of recent thrombosis. Once activated, plasmin is in turn tightly controlled by counterregulatory factors such as α$_2$-plasmin inhibitor, a plasma protein that binds and rapidly inhibits free plasmin.

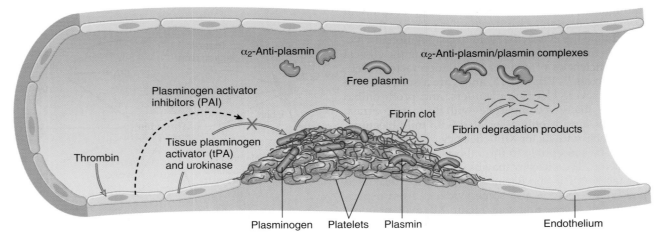

Fig. 4.10 The fibrinolytic system, illustrating various plasminogen activators and inhibitors (see text).

SUMMARY

COAGULATION FACTORS

- Coagulation occurs via the sequential enzymatic conversion of a cascade of circulating and locally synthesized proteins.
- Tissue factor elaborated at sites of injury is the most important initiator of the coagulation cascade in vivo.
- At the final stage of coagulation, thrombin converts fibrinogen into insoluble fibrin that contributes to formation of the definitive hemostatic plug.
- Coagulation normally is restricted to sites of vascular injury by:
  - limiting enzymatic activation to phospholipid surfaces provided by activated platelets or endothelium,
  - circulating inhibitors of coagulation factors, such as antithrombin III, whose activity is augmented by heparin-like molecules expressed on endothelial cells
  - expression of thrombomodulin on normal endothelial cells, which bind thrombin and convert it into an anti-coagulant,
  - activation of fibrinolytic pathways (e.g., by association of tissue plasminogen activator with fibrin).

Endothelium

The balance between the anticoagulant and procoagulant activities of endothelium often determines whether clot formation, propagation, or dissolution occurs (Fig. 4.11). Normal endothelial cells express a multitude of factors that inhibit the procoagulant activities of platelets and coagulation factors and that augment fibrinolysis. These factors act in concert to prevent thrombosis and to limit clotting to sites of vascular damage. However, if injured or exposed to proinflammatory factors, endothelial cells lose many of their antithrombotic properties. Here, we complete the discussion of hemostasis by focusing on the antithrombotic activities of normal endothelium; we return to the "dark side" of endothelial cells later when discussing thrombosis.

The antithrombotic properties of endothelium can be divided into activities directed at platelets, coagulation factors, and fibrinolysis.

- *Platelet inhibitory effects.* An obvious effect of intact endothelium is to serve as a barrier that shields platelets from subendothelial vWF and collagen. However, normal endothelium also releases a number of factors that inhibit platelet activation and aggregation. Among the most important are *prostacyclin (PGI₂), nitric oxide (NO),* and *adenosine diphosphatase;* the latter degrades ADP, already discussed as a potent activator of platelet aggregation. Finally, endothelial cells bind and alter the activity of thrombin, which is one of the most potent activators of platelets.
- *Anticoagulant effects.* Normal endothelium shields coagulation factors from tissue factor in vessel walls and expresses multiple factors that actively oppose coagulation, most notably thrombomodulin, endothelial protein C receptor, heparin-like molecules, and tissue factor pathway inhibitor. *Thrombomodulin* and *endothelial protein C receptor* bind thrombin and protein C, respectively, in a complex on the endothelial cell surface. When bound in this complex, thrombin loses its ability to activate coagulation factors and platelets, and instead cleaves and activates *protein C,* a vitamin K–dependent protease that requires a cofactor, protein S. Activated protein C/protein S complex is a potent inhibitor of coagulation factors Va and VIIIa. *Heparin-like molecules* on the surface of endothelium bind and activate antithrombin III, which then inhibits thrombin and factors IXa, Xa, XIa, and XIIa. The clinical utility of heparin and related drugs is based on their ability to stimulate antithrombin III activity. *Tissue factor pathway inhibitor* (TFPI), like protein C, requires protein S as a cofactor and, as the name implies, binds and inhibits tissue factor/factor VIIa complexes.
- *Fibrinolytic effects.* Normal endothelial cells synthesize t-PA, already discussed, as a key component of the fibrinolytic pathway.

Thrombosis

The primary abnormalities that lead to intravascular thrombosis are (1) endothelial injury, (2) stasis or turbulent blood flow, and (3) hypercoagulability of the blood (the so-called "Virchow triad") (Fig. 4.12). Thrombosis is

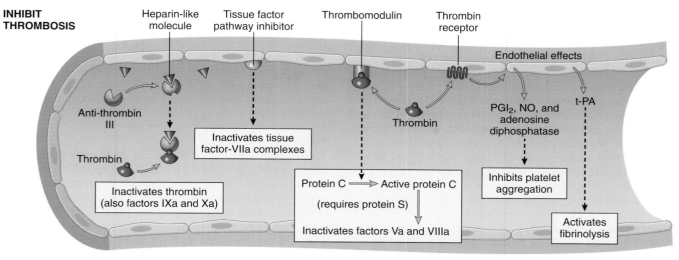

INHIBIT THROMBOSIS

FAVOR THROMBOSIS

Fig. 4.11 Anti-coagulant properties of normal endothelium (top) and procoagulant properties of injured or activated endothelium (bottom). *NO*, Nitric oxide; *PGI₂*, prostaglandin I2 (prostacyclin); *t-PA*, tissue plasminogen activator; *VWF*, von Willebrand factor. Thrombin receptors are also called protease-activated receptors (PARs).

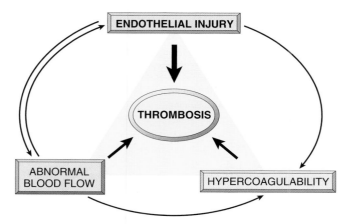

Fig. 4.12 Virchow's triad in thrombosis. Endothelial integrity is the most important factor. Abnormalities of procoagulants or anti-coagulants can tip the balance in favor of thrombosis. Abnormal blood flow (stasis or turbulence) can lead to hypercoagulability directly and also indirectly through endothelial dysfunction.

one of the scourges of modern man, because it underlies the most serious and common forms of cardiovascular disease. Here, the focus is on its causes and consequences; its role in cardiovascular disorders is discussed in detail in Chapters 10 and 11.

Endothelial Injury

Endothelial injury leading to platelet activation almost inevitably underlies thrombus formation in the heart and the arterial circulation, where the high rates of blood flow impede clot formation. Notably, cardiac and arterial clots are typically rich in platelets, and it is believed that platelet adherence and activation is a necessary prerequisite for thrombus formation under high shear stress, such as exists in arteries. This insight provides part of the reasoning behind the use of aspirin and other platelet inhibitors in coronary artery disease and acute myocardial infarction.

Obviously, severe endothelial injury may trigger thrombosis by exposing VWF and tissue factor. However, inflammation and other noxious stimuli also promote thrombosis by shifting the pattern of gene expression in endothelium to one that is "prothrombotic." This change is sometimes referred to as *endothelial activation* or *dysfunction* and can be produced by diverse exposures, including physical injury, infectious agents, abnormal blood flow, inflammatory mediators, metabolic abnormalities, such as hypercholesterolemia or homocystinemia, and toxins absorbed from cigarette smoke. Endothelial activation is believed to have an important role in triggering arterial thrombotic events.

The role of endothelial cell activation and dysfunction in arterial thrombosis is also discussed in Chapters 10 and 11. Here it suffices to mention several of the major prothrombotic alterations:

- *Procoagulant changes.* Endothelial cells activated by cytokines downregulate the expression of *thrombomodulin*, already described as a key modulator of thrombin activity. This may result in sustained activation of thrombin, which can in turn stimulate platelets and augment inflammation through PARs expressed on platelets and inflammatory cells. In addition, inflamed endothelium also downregulates the expression of other anticoagulants, such as protein C and tissue factor protein inhibitor, changes that further promote a procoagulant state.
- *Anti-fibrinolytic effects.* Activated endothelial cells secrete Plasminogen activator inhibitors (PAI), which limit fibrinolysis and downregulate the expression of t-PA, alterations that also favor the development of thrombi.

Abnormal Blood Flow

Turbulence (chaotic blood flow) contributes to arterial and cardiac thrombosis by causing endothelial injury or dysfunction, as well as by forming countercurrents and local pockets of stasis. Stasis is a major factor in the development of venous thrombi. Under conditions of normal laminar blood flow, platelets (and other blood cells) are found mainly in the center of the vessel lumen, separated from the endothelium by a slower-moving layer of plasma. By contrast, stasis and turbulence have the following deleterious effects:

- Both promote endothelial cell activation and enhanced procoagulant activity, in part through flow-induced changes in endothelial gene expression.
- Stasis allows platelets and leukocytes to come into contact with the endothelium when the flow is sluggish.
- Stasis also slows the washout of activated clotting factors and impedes the inflow of clotting factor inhibitors.

Turbulent and static blood flow contributes to thrombosis in a number of clinical settings. Ulcerated atherosclerotic plaques not only expose subendothelial ECM but also cause turbulence. Abnormal aortic and arterial dilations called aneurysms create local stasis and consequently are fertile sites for thrombosis (Chapter 9). Acute myocardial infarction results in focally noncontractile myocardium. Ventricular remodeling after more remote infarction can lead to aneurysm formation. In both cases, cardiac mural thrombi are more easily formed because of the local blood stasis (Chapter 11). Mitral valve stenosis (e.g., after rheumatic heart disease) results in left atrial

dilation. In conjunction with atrial fibrillation, a dilated atrium also produces stasis and is a prime location for the development of thrombi. Hyperviscosity syndromes (such as polycythemia vera, Chapter 12) increase resistance to flow and cause small vessel stasis; the deformed red cells in sickle cell anemia (Chapter 12) cause vascular occlusions, and the resultant stasis also predisposes to thrombosis.

Hypercoagulability

Hypercoagulability refers to an abnormally high tendency of the blood to clot, and is typically caused by alterations in coagulation factors. It contributes infrequently to arterial or intracardiac thrombosis but is an important underlying risk factor for venous thrombosis. The alterations of the coagulation pathways that predispose affected persons to thrombosis can be divided into primary (genetic) and secondary (acquired) disorders (Table 4.2).

Primary (inherited) hypercoagulability is most often caused by mutations in the factor V and prothrombin genes:

- Approximately 2% to 15% of whites carry a specific factor V mutation (called the Leiden mutation, after the Dutch city where it was first described). Among those with recurrent deep venous thrombosis (DVT), the frequency of this mutation approaches 60%. The mutation alters an amino acid residue in factor V and renders it

Table 4.2 Hypercoagulable States

Primary (Genetic)
Common (>1% of the Population)
Factor V mutation (G1691A mutation; factor V Leiden)
Prothrombin mutation (G20210A variant)
Increased levels of factor VIII, IX, or XI or fibrinogen
Rare
Anti-thrombin III deficiency
Protein C deficiency
Protein S deficiency
Very Rare
Fibrinolysis defects
Homozygous homocystinuria (deficiency of cystathione β-synthetase)
Secondary (Acquired)
High Risk for Thrombosis
Prolonged bed rest or immobilization
Myocardial infarction
Atrial fibrillation
Tissue injury (surgery, fracture, burn)
Cancer
Prosthetic cardiac valves
Disseminated intravascular coagulation
Heparin-induced thrombocytopenia
Anti-phospholipid antibody syndrome
Lower Risk for Thrombosis
Cardiomyopathy
Nephrotic syndrome
Hyperestrogenic states (pregnancy and postpartum)
Oral contraceptive use
Sickle cell anemia
Smoking

resistant to proteolysis by protein C. Thus, an important anti-thrombotic counterregulatory mechanism is lost. Heterozygotes carry a fivefold increased risk for venous thrombosis, with homozygotes having a 50-fold increased risk.

- A single-nucleotide substitution (G to A) in the 3′-untranslated region of the prothrombin gene is a fairly common allele (found in 1%–2% of the general population). This variant results in increased prothrombin transcription and is associated with a nearly threefold increased risk for venous thromboses.
- Elevated levels of *homocysteine* contribute to arterial and venous thrombosis, as well as to the development of atherosclerosis (Chapter 10). The prothrombotic effects of homocysteine may be due to thioester linkages formed between homocysteine metabolites and a variety of proteins, including fibrinogen. Marked elevations of homocysteine may be caused by an inherited deficiency of cystathione β-synthetase.
- Less common primary hypercoagulable states include inherited deficiencies of anti-coagulants such as anti-thrombin III, protein C, or protein S; affected patients typically present with venous thrombosis and recurrent thromboembolism in adolescence or in early adult life.

Although the risk of thrombosis is only mildly increased in heterozygous carriers of factor V Leiden and the prothrombin gene variant, these genetic factors carry added significance for two reasons. First, both abnormal alleles are sufficiently frequent that homozygous and compound heterozygous persons are not uncommon, and these individuals are at much higher risk for thrombosis. More importantly, heterozygous individuals are at higher risk for venous thrombosis in the setting of other acquired risk factors, such as pregnancy, prolonged bed rest, and lengthy airplane flights. Consequently, inherited causes of hypercoagulability should be considered in young patients (<50 years of age), even when other acquired risk factors are present.

Secondary (acquired) hypercoagulability is seen in many settings (Table 4.2). In some situations (e.g., cardiac failure or trauma), stasis or vascular injury may be the most important factor. The hypercoagulability associated with oral contraceptive use and the hyperestrogenic state of pregnancy may be related to increased hepatic synthesis of coagulation factors and reduced synthesis of anti-thrombin III. In disseminated cancers, release of procoagulant tumor products (e.g., mucin from adenocarcinoma) predisposes to thrombosis. The hypercoagulability seen with advancing age has been attributed to increased platelet aggregation and reduced release of PGI2 from endothelium. Smoking and obesity promote hypercoagulability by unknown mechanisms.

Among the acquired thrombophilic states, two are particularly important clinical problems and deserve special mention:

- *Heparin-induced thrombocytopenia* (HIT) *syndrome.* This syndrome occurs in up to 5% of patients treated with unfractionated heparin (for therapeutic anti-coagulation). It is marked by the development of autoantibodies that bind complexes of heparin and platelet membrane protein (platelet factor-4) (Chapter 12). Although the mechanism is unclear, it appears that these antibodies may also bind similar complexes present on platelet and endothelial surfaces, resulting in platelet activation, aggregation, and consumption (hence thrombocytopenia), as well as causing endothelial cell injury. The overall result is a prothrombotic state, even in the face of heparin administration and low platelet counts. Newer low-molecular-weight fractionated heparin preparations induce autoantibodies less frequently but can still cause *thrombosis if antibodies have already formed.*

- *Anti-phospholipid antibody syndrome.* This syndrome (previously called the lupus anti-coagulant syndrome) has protean clinical manifestations, including recurrent thromboses, repeated miscarriages, cardiac valve vegetations, and thrombocytopenia. Depending on the vascular bed involved, the clinical presentations can include pulmonary embolism (following lower extremity venous thrombosis), pulmonary hypertension (from recurrent subclinical pulmonary emboli), stroke, bowel infarction, or renovascular hypertension. Fetal loss does not appear to be explained by thrombosis, but rather seems to stem from antibody-mediated interference with the growth and differentiation of trophoblasts, leading to a failure of placentation. Anti-phospholipid antibody syndrome is also a cause of renal microangiopathy, resulting in renal failure associated with multiple capillary and arterial thromboses (Chapter 14).

The name anti-phospholipid antibody syndrome came from the detection in patients of circulating antibodies that bind to phospholipids. But this name is misleading, as it is believed that the most important pathologic effects are mediated through binding of the antibodies to epitopes on proteins that are somehow induced or "unveiled" by phospholipids. Suspected antibody targets include β_2-glycoprotein I, a plasma protein that associates with the surfaces of endothelial cells and trophoblasts, and prothrombin. In vivo, it is suspected that these antibodies bind to these and perhaps other proteins, thereby inducing a hypercoagulable state through uncertain mechanisms. However, in vitro, the antibodies interfere with phospholipids and thus inhibit coagulation (hence the name lupus anticoagulant, also a misnomer). The antibodies also frequently provide a false-positive serologic test for syphilis because the antigen in the standard assay for syphilis is embedded in cardiolipin.

Anti-phospholipid antibody syndrome has primary and secondary forms. Individuals with a well-defined autoimmune disease, such as systemic lupus erythematosus (Chapter 5), are designated as having *secondary antiphospholipid syndrome* (hence the earlier term *lupus anticoagulant syndrome*). In *primary anti-phospholipid syndrome*, patients exhibit only the manifestations of a hypercoagulable state and lack evidence of other autoimmune disorders; occasionally, it appears following exposure to certain drugs or infections. Therapy involves anti-coagulation and immunosuppression. Although anti-phospholipid antibodies are clearly associated with thrombotic diatheses, they have also been identified in 5% to 15% of apparently normal individuals, implying that they are necessary but not sufficient to cause the full-blown syndrome.

MORPHOLOGY

Thrombi can develop anywhere in the cardiovascular system. Arterial or cardiac thrombi typically arise at sites of endothelial injury or turbulence; venous thrombi characteristically occur at sites of stasis. Thrombi are focally attached to the underlying vascular surface and tend to propagate toward the heart; thus, arterial thrombi grow in a retrograde direction from the point of attachment, whereas venous thrombi extend in the direction of blood flow. The propagating portion of a thrombus tends to be poorly attached and therefore prone to fragmentation and migration through the blood as an **embolus.**

Thrombi can have grossly (and microscopically) apparent laminations called **lines of Zahn;** these represent pale platelet and fibrin layers alternating with darker red cell–rich layers. Such lines are significant in that they are only found in thrombi that form in flowing blood; their presence can therefore usually distinguish antemortem thrombosis from the bland nonlaminated clots that form in the postmortem state. Although thrombi formed in the "low-flow" venous system superficially resemble postmortem clots, careful evaluation generally shows ill-defined laminations.

Thrombi occurring in heart chambers or in the aortic lumen are designated as **mural thrombi.** Abnormal myocardial contraction (arrhythmias, dilated cardiomyopathy, or myocardial infarction) or endomyocardial injury (myocarditis, catheter trauma) promote cardiac mural thrombi (Fig. 4.13A), whereas ulcerated atherosclerotic plaques and aneurysmal dilation promote aortic thrombosis (Fig. 4.13B).

Arterial thrombi are frequently occlusive. They are typically rich in platelets, as the processes underlying their development (e.g., endothelial injury) lead to platelet activation. Although usually superimposed on a ruptured atherosclerotic plaque, other vascular injuries (vasculitis, trauma) can also be underlying causes. **Venous thrombi (phlebothrombosis)** are almost invariably occlusive; they frequently propagate some distance toward the heart, forming a long cast within the vessel lumen that is prone to give rise to emboli. Because these thrombi form in the sluggish venous circulation, they tend to contain more enmeshed red cells, leading to the moniker **red, or stasis, thrombi.** The veins of the lower extremities are most commonly affected (90% of venous thromboses); however, venous thrombi also can occur in the upper extremities, periprostatic plexus, or ovarian and periuterine veins, and under special circumstances they may be found in the dural sinuses, portal vein, or hepatic vein.

At autopsy, **postmortem clots** can sometimes be mistaken for venous thrombi. However, the former are gelatinous and because of red cell settling they have a dark red dependent portion and a yellow "chicken fat" upper portion; they also are usually not attached to the underlying vessel wall. By contrast, red thrombi typically are firm, focally attached to vessel walls, and they contain gray strands of deposited fibrin.

Thrombi on heart valves are called **vegetations.** Bacterial or fungal bloodborne infections can cause valve damage, leading to the development of large thrombotic masses **(infective endocarditis)** (Chapter 11). Sterile vegetations also can develop on noninfected valves in hypercoagulable states—the lesions of so-called **"nonbacterial thrombotic endocarditis"** (Chapter 11). Less commonly, sterile, **verrucous endocarditis (Libman-Sacks endocarditis)** can occur in the setting of systemic lupus erythematosus (Chapter 5).

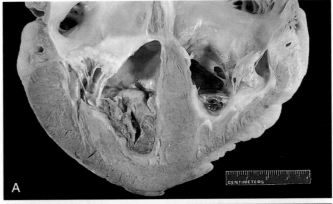

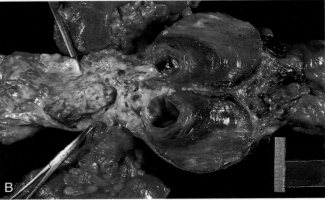

Fig. 4.13 Mural thrombi. (A) Thrombus in the left and right ventricular apices, overlying white fibrous scar. (B) Laminated thrombus in a dilated abdominal aortic aneurysm. Numerous friable mural thrombi are also superimposed on advanced atherosclerotic lesions of the more proximal aorta *(left side of photograph).*

Fate of the Thrombus

If a patient survives an initial thrombotic event, during the ensuing days to weeks the thrombus evolves through some combination of the following four processes:

- *Propagation.* The thrombus enlarges through the accretion of additional platelets and fibrin, increasing the odds of vascular occlusion or embolization.
- *Embolization.* Part or all of the thrombus is dislodged and transported elsewhere in the vasculature.
- *Dissolution.* If a thrombus is newly formed, activation of fibrinolytic factors may lead to its rapid shrinkage and complete dissolution. With older thrombi, extensive fibrin polymerization renders the thrombus substantially more resistant to plasmin-induced proteolysis, and lysis is ineffectual. This acquisition of resistance to lysis has clinical significance, as therapeutic administration of fibrinolytic agents (e.g., t-PA in the setting of acute coronary thrombosis) generally is not effective unless administered within a few hours of thrombus formation.
- *Organization and recanalization.* Older thrombi become organized by the ingrowth of endothelial cells, smooth muscle cells, and fibroblasts (Fig. 4.14). In time, capillary channels are formed that—to a limited extent—create conduits along the length of the thrombus, thereby reestablishing the continuity of the original lumen. Further recanalization can sometimes convert a thrombus into a

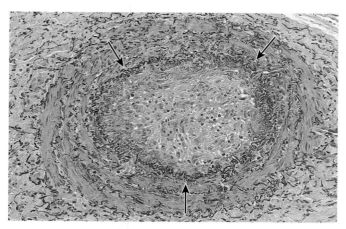

Fig. 4.14 An organized thrombus. Low-power view of a thrombosed artery stained for elastic tissue. The original lumen is delineated by the internal elastic lamina (arrows) and is completely filled with organized thrombus.

vascularized mass of connective tissue that is eventually incorporated into the wall of the remodeled vessel. Occasionally, instead of organizing, the center of a thrombus undergoes enzymatic digestion, presumably because of the release of lysosomal enzymes from entrapped leukocytes. If bacterial seeding occurs, the contents of degraded thrombi serve as an ideal culture medium, and the resulting infection may weaken the vessel wall, leading to the formation of a *mycotic aneurysm* (Chapter 10).

Clinical Features

Thrombi are significant because they cause obstruction of arteries and veins and may give rise to emboli. The effect that is of the greatest clinical importance depends on the site of thrombosis. Thus, although venous thrombi can cause congestion and edema in vascular beds distal to an obstruction, they are most worrisome because of their potential to embolize to the lungs and cause death. Conversely, whereas arterial thrombi can embolize and cause tissue infarction, their tendency to obstruct vessels (e.g., in coronary and cerebral vessels) is considerably more important.

Venous Thrombosis (Phlebothrombosis)

Most venous thrombi occur in the superficial or the deep veins of the leg. Superficial venous thrombi usually arise in the saphenous system, particularly in the setting of varicosities; these rarely embolize but they can be painful and can cause local congestion and swelling from impaired venous outflow, predisposing the overlying skin to the development of infections and varicose ulcers. Deep venous thromboses (DVTs) in the larger leg veins at or above the knee joint (e.g., popliteal, femoral, and iliac veins) are more serious because they are prone to embolize. Although such DVTs may cause local pain and edema, collateral channels often circumvent the venous obstruction. Consequently, DVTs are entirely asymptomatic in approximately 50% of patients and are recognized only after they have embolized to the lungs.

Lower-extremity DVTs are associated with stasis and hypercoagulable states, as described earlier (Table 4.2). Thus, common predisposing factors include congestive

heart failure, bed rest, and immobilization; the latter two factors reduce the milking action of leg muscles and thus slow venous return. Trauma, surgery, and burns not only immobilize a patient but also are associated with vascular injury, procoagulant release, increased hepatic synthesis of coagulation factors, and reduced t-PA production. Many factors contribute to the thrombotic diathesis of pregnancy; in addition to the potential for amniotic fluid infusion into the circulation at the time of delivery, pressure produced by the enlarging fetus and uterus can produce stasis in the veins of the legs, and late pregnancy and the postpartum period are associated with hypercoagulability. Tumor-associated procoagulant release is largely responsible for the increased risk of thromboembolic phenomena seen in disseminated cancers. These are sometimes referred to as *migratory thrombophlebitis*, because of the tendency to involve several different venous beds transiently, or as Trousseau syndrome, for the physician who both described the disorder and suffered from it. Regardless of the specific clinical setting, the risk of DVT is increased in persons older than 50 years.

Arterial and Cardiac Thrombosis

Atherosclerosis is a major cause of arterial thromboses because it is associated with the loss of endothelial integrity and with abnormal blood flow (Fig. 4.13B). Myocardial infarction can predispose to cardiac mural thrombi by causing dyskinetic myocardial contraction and endocardial injury (Fig. 4.13A), and rheumatic heart disease may engender atrial mural thrombi by causing atrial dilation and fibrillation. Both cardiac and aortic mural thrombi are prone to embolization. Although any tissue can be affected, the brain, kidneys, and spleen are particularly likely targets because of their rich blood supply.

● SUMMARY

THROMBOSIS

- Thrombus development is usually related to one or more components of Virchow's triad:
  - endothelial injury (e.g., by toxins, hypertension, inflammation, or metabolic products)
  - abnormal blood flow, stasis, or turbulence (e.g., resulting from aneurysms, atherosclerotic plaque)
  - hypercoagulability: either primary (e.g., factor V Leiden, increased prothrombin synthesis, anti-thrombin III deficiency) or secondary (e.g., bed rest, tissue damage, malignancy)
- Thrombi may propagate, resolve, become organized, or embolize.
- Thrombosis causes tissue injury by local vascular occlusion or by distal embolization.

Disseminated Intravascular Coagulation (DIC)

DIC is widespread thrombosis within the microcirculation that may be of sudden or insidious onset. It may be seen in disorders ranging from obstetric complications to advanced malignancy. To complicate matters, the widespread microvascular thrombosis consumes platelets and coagulation proteins (hence the synonym consumptive coagulopathy), and at the same time, fibrinolytic mechanisms are activated.

The net result is that excessive clotting and bleeding may co-exist in the same patient. It is discussed in greater detail along with other bleeding diatheses in Chapter 12.

EMBOLISM

An embolus is a detached intravascular solid, liquid, or gaseous mass that is carried by the blood from its point of origin to a distant site, where it often causes tissue dysfunction or infarction. The vast majority of emboli derive from a dislodged thrombus—hence the term thromboembolism. Less commonly, emboli are composed of fat droplets, bubbles of air or nitrogen, atherosclerotic debris (cholesterol emboli), tumor fragments, bits of bone marrow, or amniotic fluid. Inevitably, emboli lodge in vessels too small to permit further passage, resulting in partial or complete vascular occlusion; depending on the site of origin, emboli can arrest anywhere in the vascular tree. The primary consequence of systemic embolization is ischemic necrosis (infarction) of downstream tissues, whereas embolization in the pulmonary circulation leads to hypoxia, hypotension, and right-sided heart failure.

Pulmonary Thromboembolism

Pulmonary emboli originate from deep venous thromboses and are responsible for the most common form of thromboembolic disease. The incidence of pulmonary embolism (PE) is 2 to 4 per 1000 hospitalized patients. Although the rate of fatal PE has declined considerably since the early 1990s, PE still causes about 100,000 deaths per year in the United States. In more than 95% of cases, venous emboli originate from thrombi within deep leg veins proximal to the popliteal fossa; embolization from lower leg thrombi is uncommon.

Fragmented thrombi from DVTs are carried through progressively larger channels and usually pass through the right side of the heart before arresting in the pulmonary vasculature. Depending on size, a PE can occlude the main pulmonary artery, lodge at the bifurcation of the right and left pulmonary arteries (saddle embolus), or pass into the smaller, branching arterioles (Fig. 4.15). Frequently, multiple emboli occur, either sequentially or as a shower of smaller emboli from a single large thrombus; a patient who has had one pulmonary embolus is at increased risk for having more. Rarely, an embolus passes through an atrial or ventricular defect and enters the systemic circulation (paradoxical embolism). A more complete discussion of PE is found in Chapter 13; the major clinical and pathologic features are the following:

- Most pulmonary emboli (60%–80%) are small and clinically silent. With time, they undergo organization and become incorporated into the vascular wall; in some cases, organization of thromboemboli leaves behind bridging fibrous webs.
- At the other end of the spectrum, a large embolus that blocks a major pulmonary artery can cause sudden death.
- Embolic obstruction of medium-sized arteries and subsequent rupture of downstream capillaries rendered anoxic can cause pulmonary hemorrhage. Such emboli do not usually cause pulmonary infarction because the

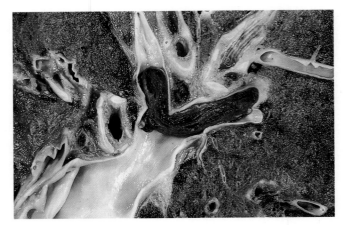

Fig. 4.15 Embolus derived from a lower-extremity deep venous thrombus lodged in a pulmonary artery branch.

area also receives blood through an intact bronchial circulation (dual circulation). However, a similar embolus in the setting of left-sided cardiac failure (and diminished bronchial artery perfusion) can lead to a pulmonary infarct.
- Embolism to small end-arteriolar pulmonary branches usually causes infarction.
- Multiple emboli occurring through time can cause pulmonary hypertension and right ventricular failure (cor pulmonale).

Systemic Thromboembolism

Most systemic emboli (80%) arise from intracardiac mural thrombi; two-thirds of these are associated with left ventricular infarcts and another 25% with dilated left atria (e.g., secondary to mitral valve disease). The remainder originate from aortic aneurysms, thrombi overlying ulcerated atherosclerotic plaques, fragmented valvular vegetations (Chapter 11), or the venous system (paradoxical emboli); 10% to 15% of systemic emboli are of unknown origin.

By contrast with venous emboli, which lodge primarily in the lung, arterial emboli can travel virtually anywhere; their final resting place understandably depends on their point of origin and the relative flow rates of blood to the downstream tissues. Common arteriolar embolization sites include the lower extremities (75%) and central nervous system (10%); intestines, kidneys, and spleen are less common targets. The consequences of embolization depend on the caliber of the occluded vessel, the collateral supply, and the affected tissue's vulnerability to anoxia; arterial emboli often lodge in end arteries and cause infarction.

Fat Embolism

Soft tissue crush injury or rupture of marrow vascular sinusoids (eg, due to a long bone fracture) release microscopic fat globules into the circulation. Fat and marrow emboli are common incidental findings after vigorous cardiopulmonary resuscitation but probably are of little clinical significance. Similarly, although fat and marrow embolism occurs in some 90% of individuals with severe skeletal injuries (Fig. 4.16A), less than 10% show any clinical findings. However, a minority of patients develop a

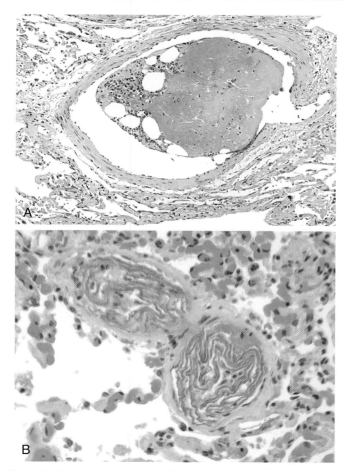

Fig. 4.16 Unusual types of emboli. (A) Bone marrow embolus. The embolus is composed of hematopoietic marrow and marrow fat cells *(clear spaces)* attached to a thrombus. (B) Amniotic fluid emboli. Two small pulmonary arterioles are packed with laminated swirls of fetal squamous cells. The surrounding lung is edematous and congested. *(Courtesy of Dr. Beth Schwartz, Baltimore, MD.)*

demonstration of fat microglobules (i.e., in the absence of accompanying marrow elements) requires specialized techniques (frozen sections and fat stains).

Amniotic Fluid Embolism

Amniotic fluid embolism is an uncommon, grave complication of labor and the immediate postpartum period occurring in 1 in 40,000 deliveries. The mortality rate approaches 80%, making it the most common cause of maternal death in the developed world and the fifth most common cause of maternal death in the United States, accounting for 10% of maternal deaths in this country; 85% of survivors suffer some form of permanent neurologic deficit. Onset is characterized by sudden severe dyspnea, cyanosis, and hypotensive shock, followed by seizures and coma. If the patient survives the initial crisis, pulmonary edema typically develops, along with (in about half the patients) disseminated intravascular coagulation secondary to release of thrombogenic substances from amniotic fluid. Indeed it is thought that morbidity and mortality in such cases results not from mechanical obstruction of pulmonary vessels but from biochemical activation of the coagulation system and the innate immune system caused by substances in the amniotic fluid.

The underlying cause is the entry of amniotic fluid (and its contents) into the maternal circulation via tears in the placental membranes and/or uterine vein rupture. Histologic analysis shows squamous cells shed from fetal skin, lanugo hair, fat from vernix caseosa, and mucin derived from the fetal respiratory or gastrointestinal tracts in the maternal pulmonary microcirculation (Fig. 4.16B). Other findings include marked pulmonary edema, diffuse alveolar damage (Chapter 13), and systemic fibrin thrombi generated by disseminated intravascular coagulation.

Air Embolism

Gas bubbles within the circulation can coalesce and obstruct vascular flow and cause distal ischemic injury. Thus, a small volume of air trapped in a coronary artery during bypass surgery or introduced into the cerebral arterial circulation by neurosurgery performed in an upright "sitting position" can occlude flow, with dire consequences. Small venous gas emboli generally have no deleterious effects, but sufficient air can enter the pulmonary circulation inadvertently during obstetric or laproscopic procedures or as a consequence of a chest wall injury to cause hypoxia, and very large venous emboli may arrest in the heart and cause death.

A particular form of gas embolism called decompression sickness is caused by sudden changes in atmospheric pressure. Scuba divers, underwater construction workers, and persons in unpressurized aircraft who undergo rapid ascent are at risk. When air is breathed at high pressure (e.g., during a deep sea dive), increased amounts of gas (particularly nitrogen) become dissolved in the blood and tissues. If the diver then ascends (depressurizes) too rapidly, the nitrogen expands in the tissues and bubbles out of solution in the blood to form gas emboli, which cause tissue ischemia. Rapid formation of gas bubbles within skeletal muscles and supporting tissues in and about joints is responsible for

symptomatic fat embolism syndrome characterized by pulmonary insufficiency, neurologic symptoms, anemia, thrombocytopenia, and a diffuse petechial rash that is fatal in 10% of cases. Clinical signs and symptoms appear 1 to 3 days after injury as the sudden onset of tachypnea, dyspnea, tachycardia, irritability, and restlessness, which can progress rapidly to delirium or coma. Thrombocytopenia is attributed to platelet adhesion to fat globules and subsequent aggregation or splenic sequestration; anemia can result from similar red cell aggregation and/or hemolysis. A diffuse petechial rash (seen in 20%–50% of cases) is related to rapid onset of thrombocytopenia and can be a useful diagnostic feature.

The pathogenesis of fat emboli syndrome involves both mechanical obstruction and biochemical injury. Fat microemboli occlude pulmonary and cerebral microvasculature, both directly and by triggering platelet aggregation. This deleterious effect is exacerbated by fatty acid release from lipid globules, which causes local toxic endothelial injury. Platelet activation and granulocyte recruitment (with free radical, protease, and eicosanoid release) (Chapter 3) complete the vascular assault. Because lipids are dissolved by the solvents used during tissue processing, microscopic

the painful condition called the bends (so named in the 1880s because the afflicted person arches the back in a manner reminiscent of a then-popular women's fashion pose called the Grecian bend). Gas bubbles in the pulmonary vasculature cause edema, hemorrhages, and focal atelectasis or emphysema, leading to respiratory distress, the so-called "chokes". Bubbles in the central nervous system can cause mental impairment and even sudden onset of coma. A more chronic form of decompression sickness is called caisson disease (named for pressurized underwater vessels used during bridge construction), in which recurrent or persistent gas emboli in the bones lead to multifocal ischemic necrosis; the heads of the femurs, tibiae, and humeri are most commonly affected.

Placing affected persons in a high-pressure chamber, to force the gas back into solution, treats acute decompression sickness. Subsequent slow decompression permits gradual gas resorption and exhalation so that obstructive bubbles do not re-form.

SUMMARY

EMBOLISM

- An embolus is a solid, liquid, or gaseous mass carried by the blood to a site distant from its origin; most are dislodged thrombi.
- Pulmonary emboli derive primarily from lower-extremity deep vein thrombi. Their effects depend mainly on the size of the embolus and the location in which it lodges. Consequences may include right-sided heart failure, pulmonary hemorrhage, pulmonary infarction, or sudden death.
- Systemic emboli derive primarily from cardiac mural or valvular thrombi, aortic aneurysms, or atherosclerotic plaques; whether an embolus causes tissue infarction depends on the site of embolization and the presence or absence of collateral circulation.
- Fat embolism can occur after crushing injuries to the bones; symptoms include pulmonary insufficiency and neurological damage. Amniotic fluid embolism may follow childbirth and can give rise to fatal pulmonary and cerebral manifestations. Air embolism can occur upon rapid decompression, most commonly in divers; it results from sudden bubbling of nitrogen dissolved in blood at higher pressures.

INFARCTION

An infarct is an area of ischemic necrosis caused by occlusion of the vascular supply to the affected tissue. Infarction primarily affecting the heart and the brain is a common and extremely important cause of clinical illness. Roughly 40% of all deaths in the United States are a consequence of cardiovascular disease, with most of these deaths stemming from myocardial or cerebral infarction. Pulmonary infarction is a common clinical complication, bowel infarction often is fatal, and ischemic necrosis of distal extremities (gangrene) causes substantial morbidity in the diabetic population.

Arterial thrombosis or arterial embolism underlies the vast majority of infarctions. Less common causes of arterial obstruction include vasospasm, expansion of an atheroma secondary to intraplaque hemorrhage, and extrinsic compression of a vessel, such as by tumor, a dissecting aortic aneurysm, or edema within a confined space (e.g., in anterior tibial compartment syndrome). Other uncommon causes of tissue infarction include vessel twisting (e.g., in testicular torsion or bowel volvulus), traumatic vascular rupture, and entrapment in a hernia sac. Although venous thrombosis can cause infarction, the more common outcome is simply congestion; typically, bypass channels rapidly open to provide sufficient outflow to restore the arterial inflow. Infarcts caused by venous thrombosis thus usually occur only in organs with a single efferent vein (e.g., testis or ovary).

MORPHOLOGY

Infarcts are classified based on their color (reflecting the amount of hemorrhage) and the presence or absence of microbial infection. Thus, infarcts may be either **red (hemorrhagic)** or **white (anemic)** and may be either **septic** or **bland.**

Red infarcts (Fig. 4.17A) occur (*1*) as a result of venous occlusions (such as in ovarian torsion); (*2*) in loose tissues (e.g., lung) where blood can collect in infarcted zones; (*3*) in tissues with dual circulations such as lung and small intestine, where partial, albeit

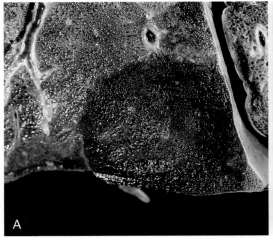
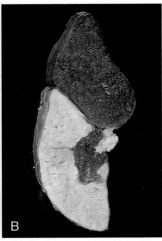

Fig. 4.17 Red and white infarcts. (A) Hemorrhagic, roughly wedge-shaped pulmonary infarct *(red infarct)*. (B) Sharply demarcated pale infarct in the spleen *(white infarct)*.

inadequate perfusion by collateral arterial supplies is typical; (4) in previously congested tissues (as a consequence of sluggish venous outflow); and (5) when flow is reestablished after infarction has occurred (e.g., after angioplasty of an arterial obstruction).

White infarcts occur with arterial occlusions in solid organs with end-arterial circulations (e.g., heart, spleen, and kidney), and where tissue density limits the seepage of blood from adjoining patent vascular beds (Fig. 4.17B). Infarcts tend to be wedge-shaped, with the occluded vessel at the apex and the organ periphery forming the base (Fig. 4.17); when the base is a serosal surface, there is often an overlying fibrinous exudate. Lateral margins may be irregular, reflecting flow from adjacent vessels. The margins of acute infarcts typically are indistinct and slightly hemorrhagic; with time, the edges become better defined by a narrow rim of hyperemia attributable to inflammation.

Infarcts resulting from arterial occlusions in organs without a dual circulation typically become progressively paler and more sharply defined with time (Fig. 4.17B). By comparison, hemorrhagic infarcts are the rule in the lung and other spongy organs (Fig. 4.17A). Extravasated red cells in hemorrhagic infarcts are phagocytosed by macrophages, and the heme iron is converted to intracellular hemosiderin. Small amounts do not impart any appreciable color to the tissue, but extensive hemorrhages leave a firm, brown residue.

In most tissues, the main histologic finding associated with infarcts is **ischemic coagulative necrosis** (Chapter 2). An inflammatory response begins to develop along the margins of infarcts within a few hours and usually is well defined within 1 to 2 days. Eventually, inflammation is followed by repair, beginning in the preserved margins (Chapter 3). In some tissues, parenchymal regeneration can occur at the periphery of the infarct, where the underlying stromal architecture has been spared. Most infarcts, however, are ultimately replaced by scar (Fig. 4.18). The brain is an exception to these generalizations; ischemic tissue injury in the central nervous system results in **liquefactive necrosis** (Chapter 2).

Septic infarctis occur when infected cardiac valve vegetations embolize, or when microbes seed necrotic **tissue**. In these cases the infarct is converted into an abscess, with a correspondingly greater inflammatory response and healing by organization and fibrosis (Chapter 3).

Factors That Influence Infarct Development

The effects of vascular occlusion range from inconsequential to tissue necrosis leading to organ dysfunction and sometimes death. The range of outcomes is influenced by the following three variables:

- *Anatomy of the vascular supply.* The presence or absence of an alternative blood supply is the most important factor in determining whether occlusion of an individual vessel causes damage. The dual supply of the lung by the pulmonary and bronchial arteries means that obstruction of the pulmonary arterioles does not cause lung infarction unless the bronchial circulation also is compromised. Similarly, the liver, which receives blood from the hepatic artery and the portal vein, and the hand and forearm, with its parallel radial and ulnar arterial supply, are resistant to infarction. By contrast, the kidney and the spleen both have end-arterial circulations, and arterial obstruction generally leads to infarction in these tissues.

- *Rate of occlusion.* Slowly developing occlusions are less likely to cause infarction because they allow time for the development of collateral blood supplies. For example, small interarteriolar anastomoses, which normally carry minimal blood flow, interconnect the three major coronary arteries. If one coronary artery is slowly occluded (e.g., by encroaching atherosclerotic plaque), flow in this collateral circulation may increase sufficiently to prevent infarction—even if the original artery becomes completely occluded.

- *Tissue vulnerability to hypoxia.* Neurons undergo irreversible damage when deprived of their blood supply for only 3 to 4 minutes. Myocardial cells, although hardier than neurons, still die after only 20 to 30 minutes of ischemia. By contrast, fibroblasts within myocardium remain viable after many hours of ischemia.

● SUMMARY

INFARCTION

- Infarcts are areas of ischemic necrosis most commonly caused by arterial occlusion (typically resulting from thrombosis or embolization); venous outflow obstruction is a less frequent cause.
- Infarcts caused by venous occlusion or occurring in spongy tissues typically are hemorrhagic (red); those caused by arterial occlusion in compact tissues typically are pale (white).
- Whether or not vascular occlusion causes tissue infarction is influenced by collateral blood supplies, the rate at which an obstruction develops, intrinsic tissue susceptibility to ischemic injury, and blood oxygenation.

SHOCK

Shock is a state in which diminished cardiac output or reduced effective circulating blood volume impairs tissue perfusion and leads to cellular hypoxia. At the outset, the cellular injury is reversible; however, prolonged shock eventually leads to irreversible tissue injury and is often fatal.

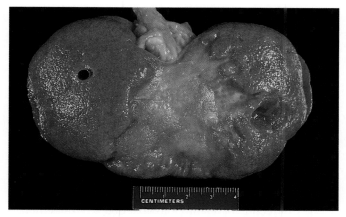

Fig. 4.18 Remote kidney infarct, now replaced by a large fibrotic scar.

Table 4.3 Three Major Types of Shock

Type of Shock	Clinical Examples	Principal Pathogenic Mechanisms
Cardiogenic	Myocardial infarction Ventricular rupture Arrhythmia Cardiac tamponade Pulmonary embolism	Failure of myocardial pump resulting from intrinsic myocardial damage, extrinsic pressure, or obstruction to outflow
Hypovolemic	Hemorrhage Fluid loss (e.g., vomiting, diarrhea, burns, trauma)	Inadequate blood or plasma volume
Septic	Overwhelming microbial infections Gram-negative sepsis Gram-positive septicemia Fungal sepsis Superantigens (e.g., toxic shock syndrome)	Peripheral vasodilation and pooling of blood; endothelial activation/injury; leukocyte-induced damage; disseminated intravascular coagulation; activation of cytokine cascades

Shock may complicate severe hemorrhage, extensive trauma or burns, myocardial infarction, pulmonary embolism, and microbial sepsis. Its causes fall into three general categories (Table 4.3):

- *Cardiogenic shock* results from low cardiac output as a result of myocardial pump failure. It may be caused by myocardial damage (infarction), ventricular arrhythmias, extrinsic compression (cardiac tamponade) (Chapter 12), or outflow obstruction (e.g., pulmonary embolism).
- *Hypovolemic shock* results from low cardiac output due to loss of blood or plasma volume (e.g., resulting from hemorrhage or fluid loss from severe burns).
- *Septic shock is triggered by microbial infections and is associated with severe systemic inflammatory response syndrome (SIRS).* In addition to microbes, SIRS may be triggered by a variety of insults, including burns, trauma, and/or pancreatitis. The common pathogenic mechanism is a massive outpouring of inflammatory mediators from innate and adaptive immune cells that produce arterial vasodilation, vascular leakage, and venous blood pooling. These cardiovascular abnormalities result in tissue hypoperfusion, cellular hypoxia, and metabolic derangements that lead to organ dysfunction and, if severe and persistent, organ failure and death. The pathogenesis of shock is discussed in detail below.

Less commonly, shock can result from a loss of vascular tone associated with anesthesia or secondary to a spinal cord injury *(neurogenic shock)*. Anaphylactic shock results from systemic vasodilation and increased vascular permeability that is triggered by an immunoglobulin E–mediated hypersensitivity reaction (Chapter 5).

Pathogenesis of Septic Shock

Septic shock is responsible for 2% of all hospital admissions in the United States. Of these, 50% require treatment in intensive care units. The number of cases in the United States exceeds 750,000/year and the incidence is rising, which is ironically due to improvements in life support for critically ill patients, as well as the growing ranks of immunocompromised hosts (because of chemotherapy, immunosuppression, advanced age, or human immunodeficiency virus infection) and the increasing prevalence of multidrug-resistant organisms in the hospital setting. Despite improvements in care, the mortality remains at a staggering 20% to 30%.

Septic shock is most frequently triggered by gram-positive bacterial infections, followed by gram-negative bacteria and fungi. Hence, an older synonym, "endotoxic shock," is no longer appropriate.

The ability of diverse microorganisms to cause septic shock is consistent with the idea that a variety of microbial constituents can trigger the process. As mentioned in Chapter 3, macrophages, neutrophils, dendritic cells, endothelial cells, and soluble components of the innate immune system (e.g., complement) recognize and are activated by several substances derived from microorganisms. After activation, these cells and factors initiate a number of inflammatory responses that interact in a complex, incompletely understood fashion to produce septic shock and multiorgan dysfunction (Fig. 4.19).

Factors believed to play major roles in the pathophysiology of septic shock include the following:

- *Inflammatory and counterinflammatory responses.* In sepsis, various microbial cell wall constituents engage receptors on cells of the innate immune system, triggering proinflammatory responses. Likely initiators of inflammation in sepsis are signaling pathways that lie downstream of Toll-like receptors (TLRs) (Chapter 5), which recognize a host of microbe-derived substances containing so-called "pathogen-associated molecular patterns" (PAMPs), as well as G-protein–coupled receptors that detect bacterial peptides, and C-type lectin receptors such as Dectins. On activation, innate immune cells produce numerous *cytokines*, including TNF, IL-1, IFN-γ, IL-12, and IL-18, as well as other inflammatory mediators such as high-mobility group box 1 protein (HMGB1). Markers of acute inflammation such as C-reactive protein and procalcitonin are also elevated. The latter is a clinically useful indicator of septic shock. Reactive oxygen species and lipid mediators such as prostaglandins and platelet-activating factor (PAF) are also elaborated. These effector molecules induce endothelial cells (and other cell types) to upregulate adhesion molecule expression and further stimulate cytokine and chemokine production. The *complement cascade* is also activated by microbial components, both directly and through the proteolytic activity of plasmin (Chapter 3), resulting in the production of anaphylotoxins (C3a, C5a), chemotactic fragments (C5a), and opsonins (C3b), all of which

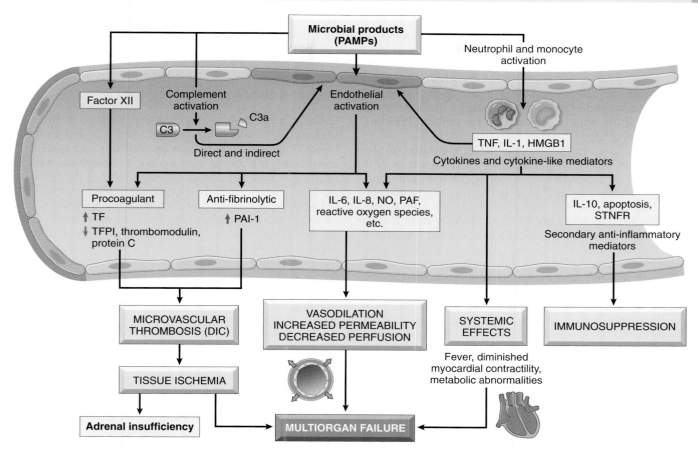

Fig. 4.19 Major pathogenic pathways in septic shock. Microbial products activate endothelial cells and cellular and humoral elements of the innate immune system, initiating a cascade of events that lead to end-stage multiorgan failure. Additional details are provided in the text. *DIC*, Disseminated intravascular coagulation; *HMGB1*, high-mobility group box 1 protein; *NO*, nitric oxide; *PAF*, platelet-activating factor; *PAI-1*, plasminogen activator inhibitor-1; *PAMP*, pathogen-associated molecular pattern; *STNFR*, soluble tumor necrosis factor receptor; *TF*, tissue factor; *TFPI*, tissue factor pathway inhibitor.

contribute to the proinflammatory state. In addition, microbial components can activate coagulation directly through factor XII and indirectly through altered endothelial function (discussed later). The accompanying widespread activation of thrombin may further augment inflammation by triggering protease activated receptors on inflammatory cells.

The hyperinflammatory state, initiated by sepsis, triggers counterregulatory immunosuppressive mechanisms, which may involve both innate and adaptive immune cells. As a result, septic patients may oscillate between hyperinflammatory and immunosuppressed states during their clinical course. Proposed mechanisms for the immune suppression include a shift from proinflammatory (T_H1) to anti-inflammatory (T_H2) cytokines (Chapter 5), production of anti-inflammatory mediators (e.g., soluble TNF receptor, IL-1 receptor antagonist, and IL-10), lymphocyte apoptosis, the immunosuppressive effects of apoptotic cells, and the induction of cellular anergy. In some patients the counterregulatory mechanisms overshoot the inflammatory responses and the resultant immune suppression renders such patients susceptible to superinfections.

• *Endothelial activation and injury.* The proinflammatory state and endothelial cell activation associated with sepsis lead to widespread vascular leakage and tissue edema, which have deleterious effects on both nutrient delivery and waste removal. One effect of inflammatory cytokines is to loosen endothelial cell tight junctions, making vessels leaky and resulting in the accumulation of protein-rich edema fluid throughout the body. This alteration impedes tissue perfusion and may be exacerbated by attempts to support the patient with intravenous fluids. Activated endothelium also upregulates production of nitric oxide (NO) and other vasoactive inflammatory mediators (e.g., C3a, C5a, and PAF), which may contribute to vascular smooth muscle relaxation and systemic hypotension.

• *Induction of a procoagulant state.* The derangement in coagulation is sufficient to produce the formidable complication of *disseminated intravascular coagulation* in up to half of septic patients. Sepsis alters the expression of many factors so as to favor coagulation. Proinflammatory cytokines increase tissue factor production by monocytes and possibly endothelial cells as well, and decrease the production of endothelial anti-coagulant factors, such as tissue factor pathway inhibitor, thrombomodulin, and protein C (see Fig. 4.11). They also dampen fibrinolysis by increasing plasminogen activator inhibitor-1 expression (see Fig. 4.10). The vascular leak and tissue edema decrease blood flow at the level of small vessels, producing stasis and diminishing the washout of activated coagulation factors. Acting in concert, these effects lead to systemic activation of thrombin and the deposition of fibrin-rich thrombi in small vessels, often throughout the body, further compromising tissue perfusion. In full-blown disseminated intravascular coagulation, the consumption of coagulation factors and platelets is so great that deficiencies of these factors appear, leading to concomitant bleeding and hemorrhage (Chapter 12).

- *Metabolic abnormalities.* Septic patients exhibit insulin resistance and hyperglycemia. Cytokines such as TNF and IL-1, stress-induced hormones (such as glucagon, growth hormone, and glucocorticoids), and catecholamines all drive gluconeogenesis. At the same time, the proinflammatory cytokines suppress insulin release while simultaneously promoting insulin resistance in the liver and other tissues, likely by impairing the surface expression of GLUT-4, a glucose transporter. Hyperglycemia decreases neutrophil function—thereby suppressing bactericidal activity—and causes increased adhesion molecule expression on endothelial cells. Although sepsis is initially associated with an acute surge in glucocorticoid production, this phase may be followed by adrenal insufficiency and a functional deficit of glucocorticoids. This may stem from depression of the synthetic capacity of intact adrenal glands or frank adrenal necrosis resulting from disseminated intravascular dissemination *(Waterhouse-Friderichsen syndrome)* (Chapter 20). Finally, cellular hypoxia and diminished oxidative phosphorylation lead to increased lactate production and lactic acidosis.
- *Organ dysfunction.* Systemic hypotension, interstitial edema, and small vessel thrombosis all decrease the delivery of oxygen and nutrients to the tissues that, because of cellular hypoxia, fail to properly use those nutrients that are delivered. Mitochondrial damage resulting from oxidative stress impairs oxygen use. High levels of cytokines and secondary mediators diminish myocardial contractility and cardiac output, and increased vascular permeability and endothelial injury can lead to the *acute respiratory distress syndrome* (Chapter 13). Ultimately, these factors may conspire to cause the failure of multiple organs, particularly the kidneys, liver, lungs, and heart, culminating in death.

The severity and outcome of septic shock are likely dependent on the extent and virulence of the infection; the immune status of the host; the presence of other comorbid conditions; and the pattern and level of mediator production. The multiplicity of factors and the complexity of the interactions that underlie sepsis explain why most attempts to intervene therapeutically with antagonists of specific mediators have not been effective and may even have had deleterious effects in some cases. The standard of care remains antibiotics to treat the underlying infection and intravenous fluids, pressors, and supplemental oxygen to maintain blood pressure and limit tissue hypoxia. Suffice it to say that even in the best of clinical centers, septic shock remains an obstinate clinical challenge.

An additional group of secreted bacterial proteins called *superantigens* also cause a syndrome similar to septic shock (e.g., *toxic shock syndrome*). Superantigens are polyclonal T-lymphocyte activators that induce the release of high levels of cytokines that result in a variety of clinical manifestations, ranging from a diffuse rash to vasodilation, hypotension, shock, and death.

Stages of Shock

Shock is a progressive disorder that leads to death if the underlying problems are not corrected. The exact mechanisms of sepsis-related death are still unclear; aside from increased lymphocyte and enterocyte apoptosis, cellular necrosis is minimal. Death typically follows the failure of multiple organs, which usually offer no morphological clues to explain their dysfunction. For hypovolemic and cardiogenic shock, however, the pathways leading to a patient's demise are reasonably well understood. Unless the insult is massive and rapidly lethal (e.g., exsanguination from a ruptured aortic aneurysm), shock tends to evolve through three general (albeit somewhat artificial) stages. These stages have been documented most clearly in hypovolemic shock but are common to other forms as well:

- An initial nonprogressive stage during which reflex compensatory mechanisms are activated and vital organ perfusion is maintained,
- A progressive stage characterized by tissue hypoperfusion and onset of worsening circulatory and metabolic derangement, including acidosis,
- An irreversible stage in which cellular and tissue injury is so severe that even if the hemodynamic defects are corrected, survival is not possible.

In the early nonprogressive phase of shock, various neurohumoral mechanisms help maintain cardiac output and blood pressure. These mechanisms include baroreceptor reflexes, release of catecholamines and anti-diuretic hormone, activation of the renin-angiotensin-alderosterone axis, and generalized sympathetic stimulation. The net effect is tachycardia, peripheral vasoconstriction, and renal fluid conservation; cutaneous vasoconstriction causes the characteristic "shocky" skin coolness and pallor (notably, septic shock can initially cause cutaneous vasodilation, so the patient may present with warm, flushed skin). Coronary and cerebral vessels are less sensitive to sympathetic signals and maintain relatively normal caliber, blood flow, and oxygen delivery. Thus, blood is shunted away from the skin to the vital organs such as the heart and the brain.

If the underlying causes are not corrected, shock passes imperceptibly to the progressive phase, which as noted is characterized by widespread tissue hypoxia. In the setting of persistent oxygen deficit, intracellular aerobic respiration is replaced by anaerobic glycolysis with excessive production of lactic acid. The resultant metabolic lactic acidosis lowers the tissue pH, which blunts the vasomotor response; arterioles dilate, and blood begins to pool in the microcirculation. Peripheral pooling not only worsens the cardiac output but also puts endothelial cells at risk for the development of anoxic injury with subsequent DIC. With widespread tissue hypoxia, vital organs are affected and begin to fail.

In the absence of appropriate intervention, or in severe cases, the process eventually enters an irreversible stage. Widespread cell injury is reflected in lysosomal enzyme leakage, further aggravating the shock state. Myocardial contractile function worsens, in part because of increased NO synthesis. The ischemic bowel may allow intestinal flora to enter the circulation, and thus bacteremic shock may be superimposed. Commonly, further progression to renal failure occurs as a consequence of ischemic injury of the kidney (Chapter 14), and despite the best therapeutic interventions, the downward spiral frequently culminates in death.

MORPHOLOGY

The cellular and tissue effects of shock are essentially those of hypoxic injury (Chapter 2) and are caused by a combination of **hypoperfusion** and **microvascular thrombosis**. Although any organ can be affected, the brain, heart, kidneys, adrenals, and gastrointestinal tract are most commonly involved. **Fibrin thrombi** can form in any tissue but typically are most readily visualized in kidney glomeruli. **Adrenal cortical cell lipid depletion** is akin to that seen in all forms of stress and reflects increased use of stored lipids for steroid synthesis. Whereas the lungs are resistant to hypoxic injury in hypovolemic shock occurring after hemorrhage, sepsis or trauma can precipitate diffuse alveolar damage (Chapter 13), leading to so-called **"shock lung."** Except for neuronal and cardiomyocyte loss, affected tissues can recover completely if the patient survives.

Clinical Features

The clinical manifestations of shock depend on the precipitating insult. In hypovolemic and cardiogenic shock, patients exhibit hypotension, a weak rapid pulse, tachypnea, and cool, clammy, cyanotic skin. As already noted, *in septic shock, the skin may be warm and flushed owing to peripheral vasodilation.* The primary threat to life is the underlying initiating event (e.g., myocardial infarction, severe hemorrhage, bacterial infection). However, the cardiac, cerebral, and pulmonary changes rapidly aggravate the situation. If patients survive the initial period, worsening renal function can provoke a phase dominated by progressive oliguria, acidosis, and electrolyte imbalances.

Prognosis varies with the origin of shock and its duration. Thus, more than 90% of young, otherwise healthy patients with hypovolemic shock survive with appropriate management; by comparison, septic or cardiogenic shock is associated with substantially worse outcomes, even with state-of-the-art care.

SUMMARY
SHOCK

- Shock is defined as a state of systemic tissue hypoperfusion resulting from reduced cardiac output and/or reduced effective circulating blood volume.

- The major types of shock are cardiogenic (e.g., myocardial infarction), hypovolemic (e.g., blood loss), and septic (e.g., infections).
- Shock of any form can lead to hypoxic tissue injury if not corrected.
- Septic shock is caused by the host response to bacterial or fungal infections; it is characterized by endothelial cell activation, vasodilation, edema, disseminated intravascular coagulation, and metabolic derangements.

SUGGESTED READINGS

Akhtar S: Fat embolism, *Anesthesiol Clin* 27:533, 2009. *[Recent overview of the pathogenesis and clinical issues in fat embolism syndrome.]*

Alberelli MA, De Candia E: Functional role of protease activated receptors in vascular biology, *Vascul Pharmacol* 62:72–81, 2014. *[An exhaustive review of the role played by PARs in hemostasis.]*

Angus DC, van der Poll T: Severe sepsis and septic shock, *N Engl J Med* 840:2013. *[An excellent review of clinical features, pathogenesis, and outcome of septic shock.]*

Benson MD: Current concepts of immunology and diagnosis in amniotic fluid embolism, *Clin Dev Immunol* doi:10.1155/2012/946576: 2012. *[Discussion of the pathophysiology of amniotic fluid embolism.]*

Cawcutt KA, Peters SG: Severe sepsis and septic shock: clinical overview and update on management, *Mayo Clin Proc* 89:1572, 2014. *[A brief clinical review of sepsis.]*

Chapman JC, Hajjar KA: Fibrinolysis and the control of blood coagulation, *Blood Rev* 29:17, 2015. *[An updated discussion of fibrinolysis and its role in the regulation of coagulation.]*

Chaturvedi S, McCrae KR: Recent advances in the antiphospholipid antibody syndrome, *Curr Opin Hematol* 21:371, 2014. *[A discussion of the pathophysiology of this important and complex entity.]*

Coleman DM, Obi A, Henke PK: Update in venous thromboembolism: pathophysiology, diagnosis, and treatment for surgical patients, *Curr Probl Surg* 52:233, 2015. *[An exhaustive review of this common clinical condition.]*

Ellery PE, Adams MJ: Tissue factor pathway inhibitor: then and now, *Semin Thromb Hemost* 40:881, 2014. *[Advances in understanding the role of tissue factor in coagulation.]*

Esmon CT, Esmon NL: The link between vascular features and thrombosis, *Annu Rev Physiol* 2011. *[An excellent review of the interactions of endothelium, blood flow, and hemostasis/thrombosis.]*

Greinacher A: Heparin induced thrombocytopenia, *N Engl J Med* 373:3, 2015. *[A nice review on this common and enigmatic condition.]*

Osinbowale O, Ali L, Chi YW: Venous thromboembolism: a clinical review, *Postgrad Med* 122:54, 2010. *[Good review at a medical student/house officer level.]*

Rao LVM, Esom CT, Pendurthi UR: Endothelial cell protein C receptor: a multiliganded and multifunctional receptor, *Blood* 124:1553, 2014. *[A discussion of this novel receptor in limiting coagulation.]*

Renne T, Schmaier AH, Nickel KF, et al: In vivo roles of factor XII, *Blood* 120:4296–4303, 2012. *[A review summarizing new insights into the still-uncertain in vivo functions of factor XII in thrombosis and vascular biology.]*

Versteeg HH, Heemskerk JWM, Levi M, et al: New fundamentals in hemostasis, *Physiol Rev* 93:327, 2013. *[An update in several issues in hemostasis.]*

Diseases of the Immune System

5

CHAPTER OUTLINE

The Normal Immune Response 121
Innate Immunity 122
Adaptive Immunity 124
Cells and Tissues of the Immune System 124
Lymphocytes 124
Antigen-Presenting Cells 128
Lymphoid Tissues 129
Overview of Lymphocyte Activation and Adaptive Immune Responses 130
Capture and Display of Antigens 130
Cell-Mediated Immunity: Activation of T Lymphocytes and Elimination of Intracellular Microbes 132
Humoral Immunity: Activation of B Lymphocytes and Elimination of Extracellular Microbes 132
Decline of Immune Responses and Immunologic Memory 134
Hypersensitivity: Immunologically Mediated Tissue Injury 134
Causes of Hypersensitivity Reactions 135
Classification of Hypersensitivity Reactions 135

Immediate (Type I) Hypersensitivity 136
Antibody-Mediated Diseases (Type II Hypersensitivity) 139
Immune Complex–Mediated Diseases (Type III Hypersensitivity) 140
T Cell–Mediated Diseases (Type IV Hypersensitivity) 142
Autoimmune Diseases 145
Immunologic Tolerance 145
Mechanisms of Autoimmunity: General Principles 147
Systemic Lupus Erythematosus 150
Rheumatoid Arthritis 158
Sjögren Syndrome 158
Systemic Sclerosis (Scleroderma) 159
Inflammatory Myopathies 162
Mixed Connective Tissue Disease 162
Polyarteritis Nodosa and Other Vasculitides 162
IgG4-Related Disease 162
Rejection of Transplants 162
Recognition and Rejection of Allografts 162

Transplantation of Hematopoietic Stem Cells 166
Immunodeficiency Syndromes 168
Primary (Inherited) Immunodeficiencies 168
Defects in Innate Immunity 172
Secondary (Acquired) Immunodeficiencies 173
Acquired Immunodeficiency Syndrome 173
Epidemiology 173
Properties of HIV 174
Pathogenesis of HIV Infection and AIDS 175
Natural History and Course of HIV Infection 178
Clinical Features of AIDS 180
Amyloidosis 182
Pathogenesis of Amyloid Deposition 183
Classification of Amyloidosis and Mechanisms of Amyloid Formation 183

Immunity refers to protection against infections. The immune system is the collection of cells and molecules that are responsible for defending the body against the countless pathogens that individuals encounter. Defects in the immune system render individuals easy prey to infections and are the cause of *immunodeficiency diseases*. But the immune system is itself capable of causing tissue injury and disease, which are often referred to as *hypersensitivity disorders*.

This chapter is devoted to diseases caused by too little immunity or too much immunologic reactivity. We also consider amyloidosis, a disease in which an abnormal protein, usually derived from fragments of antibodies or produced during chronic inflammatory disorders, is deposited in tissues. First, we review some important features of normal immune responses, to provide a foundation for understanding the abnormalities that give rise to immunologic diseases.

THE NORMAL IMMUNE RESPONSE

Defense against pathogens consists of two types of reactions (Fig. 5.1). *Innate immunity* (also called *natural*, or *native*, immunity) **is mediated by cells and proteins that are always present** (hence the term *innate*), **poised to react against infectious pathogens**. These mechanisms are called into action immediately in response to infection, and thus provide the first line of defense. Some of these mechanisms also are involved in clearing damaged cells and tissues. A major reaction of innate immunity is *inflammation* (Chapter 3).

Many pathogens have evolved to resist innate immunity, and protection against these infections requires the more specialized and powerful mechanisms of *adaptive immunity* (also called *acquired*, or *specific*, immunity). **Adaptive immunity is normally silent and responds** (or *adapts*)

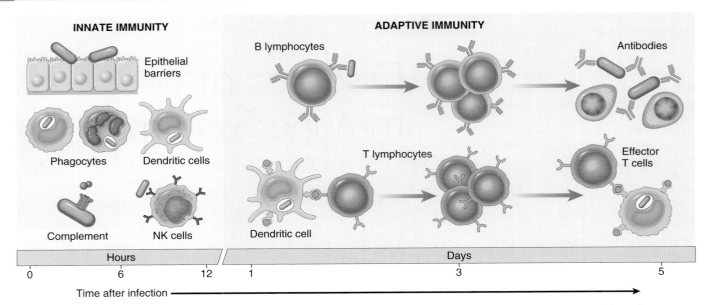

INNATE IMMUNITY

Epithelial barriers

Phagocytes   Dendritic cells

Complement   NK cells

ADAPTIVE IMMUNITY

B lymphocytes   Antibodies

T lymphocytes   Effector T cells

Dendritic cell

Hours   Days

0   6   12   1   3   5

Time after infection

Fig. 5.1 The principal components and kinetics of response of the innate and adaptive immune systems. *NK cells*, Natural killer cells.

to the presence of infectious agents by generating potent mechanisms for neutralizing and eliminating the pathogens. By convention, the terms *immune system* and *immune response* generally refer to adaptive immunity.

Innate Immunity

The major components of innate immunity are epithelial barriers that block the entry of microbes, phagocytic cells (mainly neutrophils and macrophages), dendritic cells (DCs), natural killer (NK) cells and other innate lymphoid cells, and several plasma proteins, including the proteins of the complement system. The various cells are discussed later in this chapter; the complement system was discussed in Chapter 3.

Phagocytes, dendritic cells and many other cells, such as epithelial cells, express receptors that sense the presence of infectious agents and substances released from dead cells. The microbial structures recognized by these receptors are called *pathogen-associated molecular patterns*; they are shared among microbes of the same type, and they are essential for the survival and infectivity of the microbes (so the microbes cannot evade innate immune recognition by mutating these molecules). The substances released from injured and necrotic cells are called *damage-associated molecular patterns*. The cellular receptors that recognize these molecules are often called *pattern recognition receptors*. It is estimated that innate immunity uses about 100 different receptors to recognize 1000 molecular patterns.

Receptors of Innate Immunity

Pattern recognition receptors are located in all the cellular compartments where pathogens may be present: plasma membrane receptors detect extracellular pathogens, endosomal receptors detect ingested microbes, and cytosolic receptors detect microbes in the cytoplasm (Fig. 5.2). Several classes of these receptors have been identified.

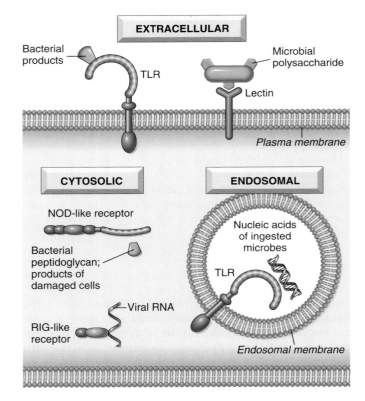

Fig. 5.2 Cellular receptors for microbes and products of cell injury. Phagocytes, dendritic cells, and many types of epithelial cells express different classes of receptors that sense the presence of microbes and dead cells. Toll-like receptors (TLRs) located in different cellular compartments, as well as other cytoplasmic and plasma membrane receptors, recognize products of different classes of microbes. The major classes of innate immune receptors are TLRs, NOD-like receptors in the cytosol (NLRs), C-type lectin receptors, RIG-like receptors for viral RNA, named after the founding member RIG-I, and cytosolic DNA sensors.

Toll-Like Receptors

The best known of the pattern recognition receptors are the *Toll-like receptors (TLRs)*. There are 10 TLRs in mammals that recognize a wide range of microbial molecules. The plasma membrane TLRs recognize bacterial products such as lipopolysaccharide (LPS), and endosomal TLRs recognize viral and bacterial RNA and DNA (see Fig. 5.2). Recognition of microbes by these receptors activates transcription factors that stimulate the production of several secreted and membrane proteins, including mediators of inflammation, anti-viral cytokines (interferons), and proteins that promote lymphocyte activation and the even more potent adaptive immune responses.

NOD-Like Receptors and the Inflammasome

NOD-like receptors (NLRs) are cytosolic receptors named after the founding members NOD-1 and NOD-2. They recognize a wide variety of substances, including products of necrotic cells (e.g., uric acid and released ATP), ion disturbances (e.g., loss of K⁺), and some microbial products. How this family of sensors detects so many diverse signs of danger or damage is not known. Several of the NLRs signal via a cytosolic multiprotein complex called the *inflammasome,* which activates an enzyme (caspase-1) that cleaves a precursor form of the cytokine interleukin-1 (IL-1) to generate the biologically active form (Fig. 5.3). As discussed in Chapter 3, IL-1 is a mediator of inflammation that recruits leukocytes and induces fever. Gain-of-function mutations in one of the NLRs result in periodic fever syndromes, called *autoinflammatory syndromes,* which respond very well to treatment with IL-1 antagonists. The NLR-inflammasome pathway also may play a role in a number of chronic disorders marked by inflammation. For example, recognition of urate crystals by a class of NLRs underlies the inflammation associated with gout. These receptors may detect and respond to lipids and cholesterol crystals that are deposited in abnormally large amounts in tissues; the resulting inflammation may contribute to obesity-associated type 2 diabetes and atherosclerosis, respectively.

Other Receptors for Microbial Products

C-type lectin receptors (CLRs) expressed on the plasma membrane of macrophages and DCs detect fungal glycans and elicit inflammatory reactions to fungi. Several cytosolic receptors detect the nucleic acids of viruses that replicate in the cytoplasm of infected cells, and stimulate the production of anti-viral cytokines. G protein–coupled receptors on neutrophils, macrophages, and most other types of leukocytes recognize short bacterial peptides containing N-formylmethionyl residues. Because all bacterial proteins and few mammalian proteins (only those synthesized within mitochondria) are initiated by N-formylmethionine, this receptor enables neutrophils to detect bacterial proteins and stimulates chemotactic responses. Mannose receptors recognize microbial sugars (which often contain terminal mannose residues, unlike mammalian glycoproteins) and induce phagocytosis of the microbes. In addition, two families of cytosolic receptors, one named after the founding member RIG-I and the other called cytosolic DNA sensors, recognize microbial RNA and DNA, respectively.

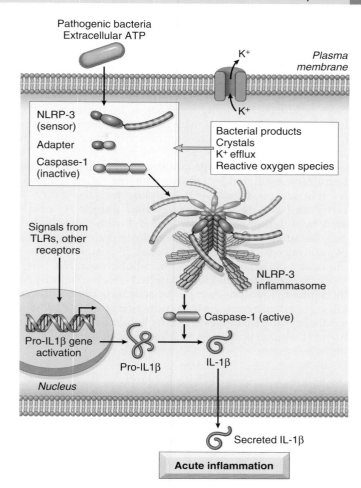

Fig. 5.3 The inflammasome. The inflammasome is a protein complex that recognizes products of dead cells and some microbes and induces the secretion of biologically active interleukin-1. It is a complex of multiple copies of a sensor protein (a leucine-rich protein called *NLRP3*), an adapter, and the enzyme caspase-1, which is converted from an inactive to an active form. The structure of the inflammasome as shown is simplified from known crystal structures. The formation of the inflammasome complex proceeds by a prion-like mechanism of propagation, in which one protein altered by activation induces conformational changes in other proteins of the same type. The net result is the activation and assembly of a large number of identical polypeptides, forming filament-like bundles of adapters and enzymes.

Reactions of Innate Immunity

The innate immune system provides host defense by the following two main reactions:

- *Inflammation.* Cytokines and products of complement activation, as well as other mediators, are produced during innate immune reactions and trigger the vascular and cellular components of inflammation. The recruited leukocytes destroy pathogens and ingest and eliminate damaged cells. This reaction was described in Chapter 3.
- *Anti-viral defense.* Type I interferons produced in response to viruses act on infected and uninfected cells and activate enzymes that degrade viral nucleic acids and inhibit viral replication.

In addition to these defensive functions, the innate immune system generates signals that stimulate the subsequent, more powerful adaptive immune response. Some of these signals are described later.

Adaptive Immunity

The adaptive immune system consists of lymphocytes and their products, including antibodies. In contrast to the limited repertoire of the innate immune system, the adaptive immune system can recognize a vast array of foreign substances.

There are two types of adaptive immunity: humoral immunity, mediated by soluble proteins called antibodies that are produced by B lymphocytes (also called **B cells**), **and cell-mediated (or cellular) immunity, mediated by T lymphocytes** (also called **T cells**). Antibodies provide protection against extracellular pathogens in the blood, mucosal surfaces, and tissues. T lymphocytes are important in defense against intracellular microbes. They work by either directly killing infected cells (accomplished by cytotoxic T lymphocytes) or by activating phagocytes to kill ingested microbes, via the production of soluble protein mediators called *cytokines* (made by helper T cells). We next turn to the main properties and functions of the cells of the immune system.

CELLS AND TISSUES OF THE IMMUNE SYSTEM

The cells of the immune system consist of lymphocytes, most of which have specific receptors for antigens and mount adaptive immune responses; specialized APCs, which capture and display microbial and other antigens to the lymphocytes; and various effector cells, whose function is to eliminate microbes and other antigens. Some of the remarkable features of the immune system are the expression of highly diverse and specific antigen receptors on B and T cells, the specialization of the cells that that enable them to perform many different functions, and the precise control mechanisms that permit useful responses when needed and prevent potentially harmful ones.

Lymphocytes

Lymphocytes are present in the circulation and in various lymphoid organs. Although all lymphocytes are morphologically similar, they actually consist of several functionally and phenotypically distinct populations (Fig. 5.4). Lymphocytes develop from precursors in the generative (primary) lymphoid organs; *T lymphocytes* mature in the thymus, whereas *B lymphocytes* mature in the bone marrow. Each T or B lymphocyte and its progeny, which constitute a *clone*, express a single antigen receptor, and the total population of lymphocytes (numbering about 10^{12} in humans) can recognize tens or hundreds of millions of antigens. The enormous diversity of antigen receptors is encoded by variant DNA sequences that are created during lymphocyte maturation by the joining and diversification of different gene segments to form functional antigen receptor genes, a process that occurs only in B cells and T cells. Hence the presence of rearranged antigen receptor genes is a reliable marker of these cells. As already mentioned, the antigen

receptors that are expressed in B cells are called *antibodies,* while their T-cell counterparts are called *T-cell receptors.*

Mature T and B lymphocytes recirculate through peripheral (secondary) lymphoid organs—the lymph nodes, spleen and mucosal tissues—and reside in these organs and in most tissues. Foreign antigens are concentrated in these organs, where they bind to and activate the clones of lymphocytes that express receptors for those antigens, a process known as clonal *selection*. All mature lymphocytes go through distinct phases during their lives— *naïve lymphocytes* express antigen receptors but have not responded to antigens and do not serve any functions; *effector lymphocytes* are induced by lymphocyte activation and perform the functions that eliminate microbes; and *memory lymphocytes,* induced during activation, survive in a functionally silent state even after the antigen is eliminated and respond rapidly upon subsequent encounters with the antigen.

T Lymphocytes

Thymus-derived T lymphocytes develop into the effector cells of cellular immunity and "help" B cells to produce antibodies against protein antigens. T cells constitute 60% to 70% of the lymphocytes in peripheral blood and are the major lymphocyte population in splenic periarteriolar sheaths and lymph node interfollicular zones. T cells cannot recognize free or circulating antigens; instead, the vast majority (>95%) of T cells sense only peptide fragments of proteins displayed by molecules of the major histocompatibility complex (MHC), discussed in more detail later. Because T cell antigen receptors have evolved to see MHC-bound peptides on cell surfaces, T cells only recognize antigens presented by other cells. The outcome of this interaction varies dramatically depending on the type of T cell that is involved and the identity of the other interacting cell, ranging from the killing of virus-infected cells to the activation of phagocytes or B lymphocytes that have ingested protein antigens.

Peptide antigens presented by MHC molecules are recognized by the *T-cell receptor (TCR)*, a heterodimer that in most T cells is composed of disulfide-linked α and β protein chains (Fig. 5.5). Each chain has a variable region that participates in binding a particular peptide antigen and a constant region that interacts with associated signaling molecules. TCRs are noncovalently linked to a cluster of five invariant polypeptide chains, the γ, δ, and ε proteins of the CD3 molecular complex and two ζ chains (see Fig. 5.5). The CD3 proteins and ζ chains do not bind antigens; instead, they are attached to the TCR and initiate intracellular biochemical signals after TCR recognition of antigen.

T cells also express a number of other molecules that serve important functions in immune responses. CD4 and CD8 are expressed on distinct T-cell subsets and act as coreceptors during T-cell activation. During antigen recognition, CD4 molecules on T cells bind to invariant portions of class II MHC molecules (described later) on selected antigen-presenting cells (APCs); in an analogous fashion, CD8 binds to class I MHC molecules. CD4 is expressed on 50% to 60% of T cells, whereas CD8 is expressed on about 40% of T cells. The CD4- and CD8-expressing T cells— called *CD4+* and *CD8+* cells, respectively—perform different but overlapping functions. CD4+ T cells are called *helper T cells* because they secrete soluble molecules

ANTIGEN RECOGNITION

FUNCTION

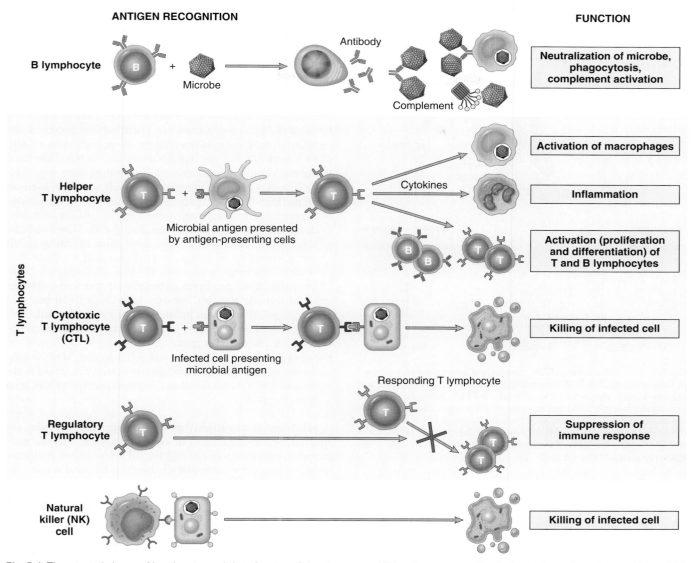

Fig. 5.4 The principal classes of lymphocytes and their functions. B lymphocytes and T lymphocytes are cells of adaptive immunity, and natural killer (NK) cells are cells of innate immunity. Several more classes of lymphocytes have been identified, including NK-T cells and so-called "innate lymphoid cells" *(ILCs);* the functions of these cells are not established.

(cytokines) that help B cells to produce antibodies and also help macrophages to destroy phagocytosed microbes. The central role of CD4+ helper cells in immunity is highlighted by the severe compromise that results from destruction of these cells by human immunodeficiency virus (HIV) infection (described later). CD8+ T cells also can secrete cytokines, but their most important role is to directly kill virus-infected cells and tumor cells; hence, they are called *cytotoxic T lymphocytes (CTLs).* Other important invariant proteins on T cells include CD28, which functions as the receptor for molecules called *costimulators* that are induced on APCs by microbes, and various adhesion molecules that strengthen the bond between the T cells and APCs and control the migration of the T cells to different tissues.

T cells that function to suppress immune responses are called *regulatory T lymphocytes.* This cell type is described later, in the context of tolerance of self antigens.

While most T cells express TCRs composed of α and β chains, a minority of peripheral blood T cells and many T cells associated with mucosal surfaces (e.g., lung, gastrointestinal tract) express TCRs that are composed of γ and δ chains, which are similar but not identical to α and β chains. Such *γδ T cells,* which do not express CD4 or CD8, recognize nonprotein molecules (e.g., bacterial lipoglycans), but their functional roles are not well understood. Another small population of T cells expresses markers of both T cells and NK cells. These so-called *NKT cells* recognize microbial glycolipids and may play a role in defense against some infections. The antigen receptors of γδ T cells and NKT cells recognize antigens independently of MHC molecules, and are much less diverse than the receptors of the more abundant CD4+ and CD8+ T cells. We will not discuss these rare lymphocyte populations further.

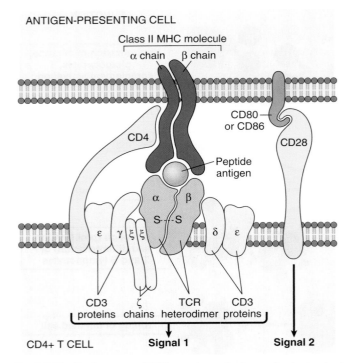

ANTIGEN-PRESENTING CELL

Fig. 5.5 The T-cell receptor (TCR) complex and other molecules involved in T-cell activation. The TCR heterodimer, consisting of an α chain and a β chain, recognizes antigen (in the form of peptide-MHC complexes expressed on antigen-presenting cells), and the linked CD3 complex and ζ chains initiate activating signals. CD4 and CD28 are also involved in T-cell activation. (Note that some T cells express CD8 and not CD4; these molecules serve analogous roles.) The sizes of the molecules are not drawn to scale. *MHC*, Major histocompatibility complex.

Major Histocompatibility Complex Molecules: The Peptide Display System of Adaptive Immunity

MHC molecules are fundamental to T-cell recognition of antigens, and genetic variations in MHC molecules are associated with many immunologic diseases; hence, it is important to review the structure and function of these molecules. The MHC was discovered on the basis of studies of graft rejection and acceptance (tissue, or *"histo,"* compatibility). It is now known that **the normal function of MHC molecules is to display peptides for recognition by CD4+ and CD8+ T lymphocytes.** In each person, T cells recognize only peptides displayed by that person's MHC molecules, which, of course, are the only MHC molecules that the T cells normally encounter. This phenomenon is called *MHC restriction.*

The human MHC, known as the human leukocyte antigen (HLA) complex, consists of a cluster of genes on chromosome 6 (Fig. 5.6). On the basis of their chemical structure, tissue distribution, and function, MHC gene products fall into two main categories:

- *Class I MHC* molecules are expressed on all nucleated cells and are encoded by three closely linked loci, designated HLA-A, HLA-B, and HLA-C (see Fig. 5.6). Each of these molecules consists of a polymorphic α chain noncovalently associated with an invariant β_2-microglobulin polypeptide (encoded by a separate gene on chromosome 15). The extracellular portion of the α

chain contains a cleft where the polymorphic residues are located and where foreign peptides bind to MHC molecules for presentation to T cells, and a conserved region that binds CD8, ensuring that only CD8+ T cells can respond to peptides displayed by class I molecules. In general, class I MHC molecules bind and display peptides derived from protein antigens present in the cytosol of the cell (e.g., viral and tumor antigens).

- *Class II MHC* molecules are encoded by genes in the HLA-D region, which contains three subregions: DP, DQ, and DR. Class II molecules are heterodimers of noncovalently linked α and β subunits (see Fig. 5.6). Unlike class I MHC molecules, which are expressed on all nucleated cells, expression of class II MHC molecules is restricted to a few cell types, mainly APCs (notably, dendritic cells), macrophages, and B cells. The extracellular portion of class II MHC molecules contains a cleft for the binding of antigenic peptides and a region that binds CD4. In general, class II MHC molecules bind to peptides derived from extracellular proteins synthesized outside the cell, for example, from microbes that are ingested and then broken down inside the cell. This property allows CD4+ T cells to recognize the presence of extracellular pathogens.

- Several other proteins are encoded in the MHC locus, including complement components (C2, C3, and Factor B) and the cytokines tumor necrosis factor (TNF) and lymphotoxin.

HLA genes are highly polymorphic; that is, there are alternative forms (alleles) of each gene at each locus (estimated to number over 10,000 for all HLA genes and over 3500 for HLA-B alleles alone). Each individual expresses only one set of HLA genes. It is believed that the polymorphism of MHC genes evolved to enable display of and response to any conceivable microbial peptide encountered in the environment. As a result of the polymorphism, a virtually infinite number of combinations of HLA molecules exists in the population. The HLA genes are closely linked on chromosome 6, so they are passed from parent to offspring *en bloc* and behave like a single locus with respect to their inheritance patterns. Each set of maternal and paternal HLA genes is referred to as an *HLA haplotype*. Because of this mode of inheritance, the probability that siblings will share the same two HLA haplotypes is 25%. By contrast, in most populations the probability that an unrelated donor will share the same two HLA haplotypes is very low. The implications of HLA polymorphism for transplantation are obvious; because each person has HLA alleles that differ to some extent from those of every other unrelated individual, grafts from unrelated donors will elicit immune responses in the recipient and be rejected. Only identical twins can accept grafts from one another, without fear of rejection. Even grafts from a donor to a sibling with the same HLA haplotype may be rejected because of differences in so-called "minor histocompatibility loci", other sets of polymorphic genes that are likely to differ by chance. (The only exception to this rule, of course, are identical twins) In fact, HLA molecules were discovered in the course of early attempts at tissue transplantation, because HLA molecules of the graft evoke immune responses that eventually lead to graft destruction

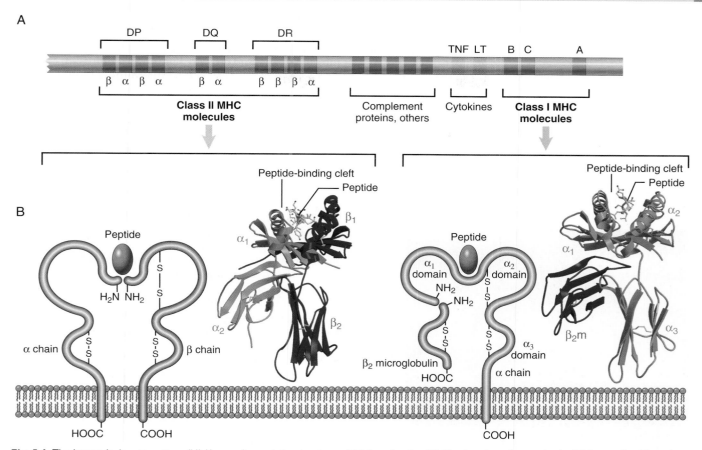

Fig. 5.6 The human leukocyte antigen (HLA) complex and the structure of HLA molecules. (A) The location of genes in the HLA complex. The relative locations, sizes, and distances between genes are not to scale. Genes that encode several proteins involved in antigen processing (the TAP transporter, components of the proteasome, and HLA-DM) are located in the class II region *(not shown)*. (B) Schematic diagrams and crystal structures of class I and class II HLA molecules. *(Crystal structures are courtesy of Dr. P. Bjorkman, California Institute of Technology, Pasadena, California.)*

(discussed later). This ability of MHC molecules to trigger immune responses is the reason these molecules are often called *antigens*.

The inheritance of particular MHC alleles influences both protective and harmful immune responses. The ability of any given MHC allele to bind the peptide antigens generated from a particular pathogen will determine whether a specific person's T cells can recognize and mount a protective response to that pathogen. Conversely, if the antigen is ragweed pollen and the response is an allergic reaction, inheritance of some HLA genes may make individuals susceptible to hay fever, the colloquial name for ragweed allergy.

Finally, many autoimmune diseases are associated with particular HLA alleles. We return to a discussion of these associations when we consider autoimmunity.

B Lymphocytes

B (bone marrow–derived) lymphocytes are the cells that produce antibodies, the mediators of humoral immunity. B cells make up 10% to 20% of the circulating peripheral lymphocyte population. They also are present in bone marrow and in the follicles of peripheral (secondary) lymphoid organs.

B cells recognize antigen by means of membrane-bound antibody of the immunoglobulin M (IgM) class, expressed on the surface together with signaling molecules to form the B-cell receptor (BCR) complex (Fig. 5.7). Whereas T cells recognize only MHC-associated peptides, B cells recognize and respond to many more chemical structures, including soluble or cell-associated proteins, lipids, polysaccharides, nucleic acids, and small chemicals, without a requirement for the MHC. As with TCRs, each antibody has a unique amino acid sequence. This sequence diversity is a consequence of the rearrangement and assembly of a multitude of immunoglobulin (Ig) gene segments, a process that creates functional Ig genes. B cells express several invariant molecules that are responsible for signal transduction and B-cell activation (see Fig. 5.7). Some are signaling molecules attached to the BCR; another example is CD21 (also known as the *type 2 complement receptor*, or CR2), which recognizes a complement breakdown product that frequently is deposited on microbes and promotes B-cell responses to microbial antigens. Interestingly, the ubiquitous Epstein-Barr virus has cleverly evolved to use CD21 as a receptor for binding to B cells and infecting them.

After stimulation, B cells differentiate into *plasma cells*, which secrete large amounts of antibodies. There are five classes, or isotypes, of immunoglobulins: IgG, IgM, and IgA constitute more than 95% of circulating antibodies. IgA is the major isotype in mucosal secretions; IgE is present in

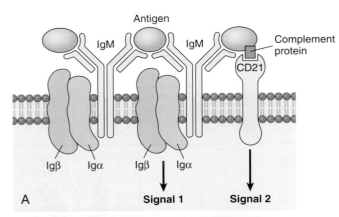

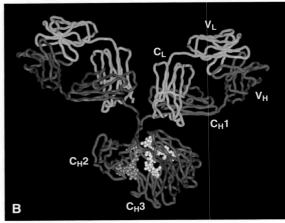

Fig. 5.7 Structure of antibodies and the B-cell antigen receptor. (A) The B-cell antigen receptor complex is composed of membrane immunoglobulin M (IgM; or IgD, *not shown*), which recognizes antigens, and the associated signaling proteins Igα and Igβ. CD21 is a receptor for a complement component that also promotes B-cell activation. (B) Crystal structure of a secreted IgG molecule, showing the arrangement of the variable (V) and constant (C) regions of the heavy (H) and light (L) chains. *(Courtesy of Dr. Alex McPherson, University of California, Irvine, California.)*

the circulation at very low concentrations and also is found attached to the surfaces of tissue mast cells; and IgD is expressed on the surfaces of B cells but is secreted at very low levels. These isotypes differ in their ability to activate complement and recruit inflammatory cells, and thus have different roles in host defense and disease states.

Natural Killer Cells and Innate Lymphoid Cells

NK cells are lymphocytes that arise from the same common lymphoid progenitor that gives rise to T lymphocytes and B lymphocytes. However, **NK cells are innate immune cells, as they are functional without prior activation and do not express highly variable and clonally distributed receptors for antigens**. Instead, NK cells have two types of receptors—inhibitory and activating. *Inhibitory receptors* recognize self class I MHC molecules, which are expressed on all healthy cells, whereas *activating receptors* recognize molecules that are expressed or upregulated on stressed or infected cells. Normally, the effects of inhibitory receptors dominate over those of activating receptors, preventing spontaneous activation of the NK cells. Infections (especially viral infections) and stress are associated with

reduced expression of class I MHC molecules and increased expression of proteins that engage activating receptors. The net result is that the NK cells are activated and the infected or stressed cells are killed and eliminated. NK cells also secrete cytokines such as interferon-γ (IFN-γ), which activates macrophages to destroy ingested microbes, and thus NK cells provide early defense against intracellular microbial infections.

Innate lymphoid cells (ILCs) are populations of lymphocytes that lack TCRs but produce cytokines similar to those that are made by T cells. They are classified into three groups, which produce IFN-γ, IL-5, or IL-17, cytokines that are characteristic of T_H1, T_H2, and T_H17 subsets of T cells, respectively (described later). NK cells are related to group 1 ILCs based on their production of IFN-γ, a cytokine also made by T_H1 cells. Because ILCs mostly reside in tissues, they are thought to provide early defense against infections in the tissues, before T cells are activated and can migrate into tissues. ILCs also may be early participants in inflammatory diseases.

Antigen-Presenting Cells

The immune system contains several cell types that are specialized to capture antigens and display these to lymphocytes. Foremost among these APCs are dendritic cells, the major cells for displaying protein antigens to naïve T cells. Several other cell types present antigens to lymphocytes at various stages of immune responses.

Dendritic Cells

Dendritic cells (DCs) are the most important antigen-presenting cells for initiating T-cell responses against protein antigens. These cells have numerous fine cytoplasmic processes that resemble dendrites, from which they derive their name. Several features of DCs account for their key role in antigen capture and presentation.

- These cells are located at the right place to capture antigens—under epithelia, the common site of entry of microbes and foreign antigens, and in the interstitia of all tissues, where antigens may be produced. DCs within the epidermis are called *Langerhans cells*.
- DCs express many receptors for capturing and responding to microbes (and other antigens), including TLRs and C-type lectin receptors.
- In response to microbes, DCs are recruited to the T-cell zones of lymphoid organs, where they are ideally positioned to present antigens to T cells.
- DCs express high levels of MHC and other molecules needed for antigen presentation and activation of T cells.

One subset of DCs is called *plasmacytoid DCs* because of their resemblance to plasma cells. These cells are present in the blood and lymphoid organs, and are major sources of the anti-viral cytokine type I interferon, produced in response to many viruses.

A second type of cell with dendritic morphology is present in the germinal centers of lymphoid follicles in the spleen and lymph nodes and is called the *follicular dendritic cell (FDC)*. These cells bear Fc receptors for IgG and receptors for C3b and can trap antigen bound to antibodies or

Table 5.1 Distribution of Lymphocytes in Tissues*

Tissue	Number of Lymphocytes × 10⁹
Lymph nodes	190
Spleen	70
Bone marrow	50
Blood	10
Skin	20
Intestines	50
Liver	10
Lungs	30

*Approximate numbers of lymphocytes in different tissues in a healthy adult.

complement proteins. These cells display antigens to B lymphocytes in lymphoid follicles and promote antibody responses, but are not involved in capturing antigens for display to T cells.

Other Antigen-Presenting Cells

Macrophages (Chapter 3) ingest microbes and other particulate antigens and display peptides for recognition by T lymphocytes. These T cells in turn activate the macrophages to kill the microbes, the central reaction of cell-mediated immunity. B cells present peptides to helper T cells and receive signals that stimulate antibody responses to protein antigens, critical steps in humoral immune responses.

Lymphoid Tissues

The tissues of the immune system consist of the *generative* (also called *primary,* or *central*) *lymphoid organs,* in which T lymphocytes and B lymphocytes mature and become competent to respond to antigens, and the *peripheral* (or *secondary*) *lymphoid organs,* in which adaptive immune responses to microbes are initiated. The principal generative lymphoid organs are the thymus, where T cells develop, and the bone marrow, the site of production of all blood cells and where B lymphocytes mature. The major peripheral organs are briefly described in the following sections.

Peripheral Lymphoid Organs

The peripheral lymphoid organs are organized to concentrate antigens, APCs, and lymphocytes in a way that optimizes interactions among these cells and the development of adaptive immune responses. Most of the body's lymphocytes are located in these organs (Table 5.1).

- *Lymph nodes* are encapsulated, highly organized collections of lymphoid cells and innate immune cells that are located along lymphatic channels throughout the body (Fig. 5.8A). As lymph passes through lymph nodes, resident APCs are able to sample antigens that are carried to the node in lymph derived from the interstitial fluids of tissues. In addition, DCs transport antigens from nearby epithelial surfaces and tissues by migrating through lymphatic vessels to the lymph nodes. Thus, antigens (e.g., of microbes that enter through epithelia or colonize tissues) become concentrated in draining lymph nodes.
- The *spleen* has an important role in immune responses to bloodborne antigens. Blood entering the spleen flows through a network of sinusoids, which enables the

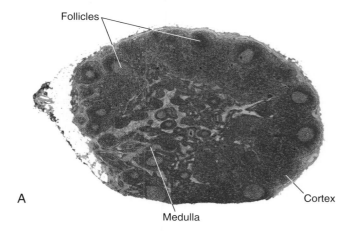

A

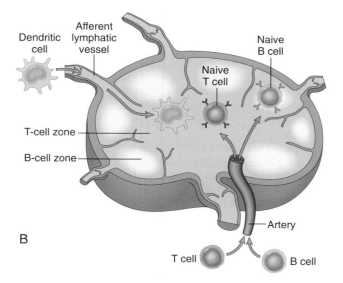

B

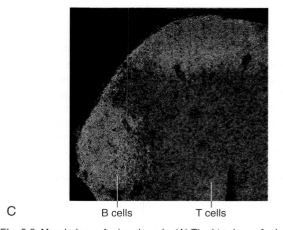

C

Fig. 5.8 Morphology of a lymph node. (A) The histology of a lymph node, with an outer cortex containing follicles and an inner medulla. (B) The segregation of B cells and T cells in different regions of the lymph node, illustrated schematically. (C) The location of B cells (*stained green,* using the immunofluorescence technique) and T cells *(stained red)* in a lymph node. *(Courtesy of Drs. Kathryn Pape and Jennifer Walter, University of Minnesota School of Medicine, Minneapolis, Minnesota.)*

trapping of bloodborne antigens by resident DCs and macrophages.

- The *cutaneous and mucosal lymphoid systems* are located under the epithelia of the skin and the gastrointestinal and respiratory tracts, respectively. They respond to antigens that enter through breaches in the epithelium. Pharyngeal tonsils and Peyer's patches of the intestine are two anatomically defined mucosal lymphoid tissues. The large number of lymphocytes in mucosal organs (second only to lymph nodes) reflects the huge surface area of these organs.

Within the peripheral lymphoid organs, T lymphocytes and B lymphocytes are segregated into different regions (Fig. 5.8B, C). In lymph nodes, the B cells are concentrated in discrete structures, called *follicles,* located around the periphery, or cortex, of each node. If the B cells in a follicle have recently responded to an antigen, the follicle develops a central pale-staining region called a *germinal center.* The T lymphocytes are concentrated in the parafollicular cortex. The follicles contain the FDCs that are involved in the activation of B cells, and the paracortex contains the DCs that present antigens to T lymphocytes. In the spleen, T lymphocytes are concentrated in periarteriolar lymphoid sheaths surrounding small arterioles, and B cells reside in the follicles.

Lymphocytes constantly travel between tissues and home to particular sites. Naive lymphocytes circulate through peripheral lymphoid organs where antigens are concentrated and immune responses are initiated, and effector lymphocytes migrate to sites of infection. The process of *lymphocyte recirculation* is most important for T cells, because naïve T cells have to "patrol" widely distributed peripheral lymphoid organs to find antigens, and effector T cells have to home to sites of infection to eliminate microbes. In contrast, plasma cells do not need to migrate to sites of infection because they secrete antibodies that are transported via the blood and lymph to distant tissues.

Cytokines: Messenger Molecules of the Immune System

Cytokines are secreted proteins that mediate immune and inflammatory reactions. Molecularly defined cytokines are called *interleukins,* a name implying a role in communication between leukocytes. Most cytokines have a wide spectrum of effects, and some are produced by several different cell types. The majority of these cytokines act on the cells that produce them or on neighboring cells, but some (like IL-1) have systemic effects.

Different cytokines contribute to specific types of immune responses.

- In innate immune responses, cytokines are produced rapidly after microbes and other stimuli are encountered, and function to induce inflammation and inhibit virus replication. These cytokines include TNF, IL-1, IL-12, type I IFNs, IFN-γ, and chemokines (Chapter 3). Their major sources are macrophages, DCs, ILCs, and NK cells, but endothelial and epithelial cells also can produce them.
- In adaptive immune responses, cytokines are produced principally by CD4+ T lymphocytes activated by antigen and other signals, and function to promote lymphocyte proliferation and differentiation and to activate effector cells. The main ones in this group are IL-2, IL-4, IL-5, IL-17, and IFN-γ; their roles in immune responses are described later. Some cytokines serve mainly to limit and terminate immune responses; these include TGF-β and IL-10.
- Some cytokines stimulate hematopoiesis and are called *colony-stimulating factors* because they stimulate formation of blood cell colonies from bone marrow progenitors (Chapter 12). Their functions are to increase leukocyte numbers during immune and inflammatory responses, and to replace leukocytes that are consumed during such responses. They are produced by marrow stromal cells, T lymphocytes, macrophages, and other cells. Examples include GM-CSF and IL-7.

The knowledge gained about cytokines has numerous practical therapeutic applications. Inhibiting cytokine production or actions can control the harmful effects of inflammation and tissue-damaging immune reactions. Patients with rheumatoid arthritis often show dramatic responses to TNF antagonists, an elegant example of rationally designed and molecularly targeted therapy. Many other cytokine antagonists are now approved for the treatment of various inflammatory disorders. Conversely, administration of cytokines is used to boost reactions that are normally dependent on these proteins, such as hematopoiesis and defense against some viruses.

OVERVIEW OF LYMPHOCYTE ACTIVATION AND ADAPTIVE IMMUNE RESPONSES

Adaptive immune responses develop in steps, consisting of: antigen recognition; activation, proliferation and differentiation of specific lymphocytes into effector and memory cells; elimination of the antigen; and decline of the response, with memory cells being the long-lived survivors. The major events in each step are summarized next; these general principles apply to protective responses against microbes as well as pathologic responses that injure the host.

Capture and Display of Antigens

Microbes and other foreign antigens can enter the body virtually anywhere, and it is obviously impossible for lymphocytes of every specificity to patrol every possible portal of antigen entry. To overcome this problem, microbes and their protein antigens in epithelia and other tissues are captured by resident dendritic cells, which then carry their antigenic cargo to draining lymph nodes through which T cells constantly recirculate (Fig. 5.9). Here the antigens are processed and displayed complexed with MHC molecules on the cell surface, where the antigens are recognized by T cells. Similarly, soluble antigens are captured and concentrated in follicles in lymph nodes and the spleen, where they may be recognized by B cells via their antigen receptors.

At the same time as microbial antigens are recognized by T lymphocytes and B lymphocytes, the microbe

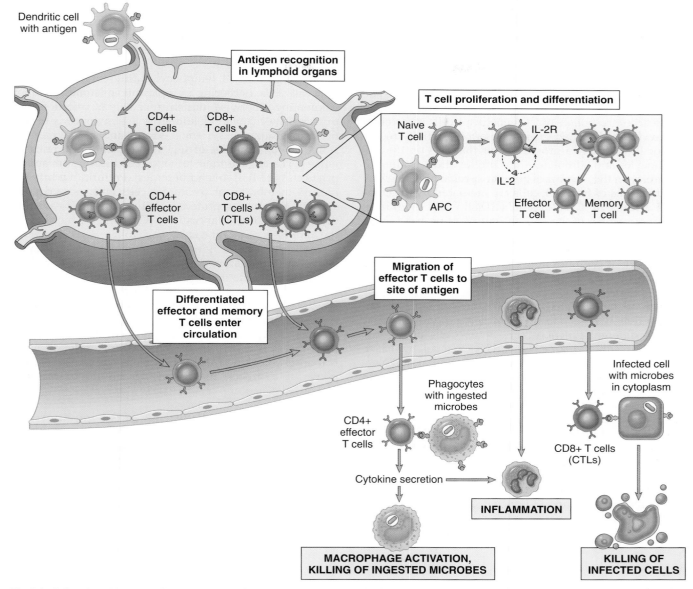

Fig. 5.9 Cell-mediated immunity. Dendritic cells (DCs) capture microbial antigens from epithelia and tissues and transport the antigens to lymph nodes. During this process, the DCs mature, and express high levels of MHC molecules and costimulators. Naïve T cells recognize MHC-associated peptide antigens displayed on DCs. The T cells are activated to proliferate and to differentiate into effector and memory cells, which migrate to sites of infection and serve various functions in cell-mediated immunity. CD4+ effector T cells of the T$_H$1 subset recognize the antigens of microbes ingested by phagocytes, and activate the phagocytes to kill the microbes; other subsets of effector cells enhance leukocyte recruitment and stimulate different types of immune responses. CD8+ cytotoxic T lymphocytes (CTLs) kill infected cells harboring microbes in the cytoplasm. Some activated T cells remain in the lymphoid organs and help B cells to produce antibodies, and some T cells differentiate into long-lived memory cells (not shown). APC, Antigen-presenting cell.

activates innate immune cells expressing pattern recognition receptors. In the case of immunization with a protein antigen, as in a vaccine, a microbial mimic called an *adjuvant* that stimulates innate immune responses is given with the antigen. During the innate response, the microbe or adjuvant activates APCs to express molecules called *costimulators* and to secrete cytokines that stimulate the proliferation and differentiation of T lymphocytes. The principal costimulators for T cells are the B7 proteins (CD80 and CD86), which are expressed on APCs and are recognized by the CD28 receptor on naïve T cells. Antigen ("signal 1") and costimulatory molecules produced during innate immune responses to microbes ("signal 2") function cooperatively to activate antigen-specific lymphocytes. The requirement for microbe-triggered signal 2 ensures that the adaptive immune response is induced by microbes and not by harmless substances. In immune responses to tumors and transplants, "signal 2" may be provided by substances released from necrotic cells (the damage-associated molecular patterns mentioned earlier).

The reactions and functions of T lymphocytes and B lymphocytes differ in important ways and are best considered separately.

Cell-Mediated Immunity: Activation of T Lymphocytes and Elimination of Intracellular Microbes

Naïve T lymphocytes are activated by antigen and costimulators in peripheral lymphoid organs, and proliferate and differentiate into effector cells that migrate to any site where the antigen (microbe) is present (see Fig. 5.9). One of the earliest responses of CD4+ helper T cells is secretion of the cytokine IL-2 and expression of high-affinity receptors for IL-2. IL-2 is a growth factor that acts on these T lymphocytes and stimulates their proliferation, leading to an increase in the number of antigen-specific lymphocytes. **The functions of helper T cells are mediated by the combined actions of CD40-ligand (CD40L) and cytokines.** CD40 is a member of the TNF-receptor family, and CD40L is a membrane protein homologous to TNF. When CD4+ helper T cells recognize antigens being displayed by macrophages or B lymphocytes, the T cells express CD40L, which engages CD40 on the macrophages or B cells and activates these cells.

Some of the activated CD4+ T cells differentiate into effector cells that secrete different sets of cytokines and perform different functions (Fig. 5.10). Cells of the T_H1 subset secrete the cytokine IFN-γ, which is a potent macrophage activator. The combination of CD40- and IFN-γ–mediated activation results in "classical" macrophage activation (Chapter 3), leading to the induction of microbicidal substances in macrophages and the destruction of ingested microbes. T_H2 cells produce IL-4, which stimulates B cells to differentiate into IgE-secreting plasma cells; IL-5, which activates eosinophils; and IL-13, which activates mucosal epithelial cells to secrete mucus, and induces the "alternative" pathway of macrophage activation, which is associated with tissue repair and fibrosis (Chapter 3). Eosinophils bind to and kill IgE-coated pathogens such as

helminthic parasites. T_H17 cells, so called because the signature cytokine of these cells is IL-17, recruit neutrophils and monocytes, which destroy some extracellular bacteria and fungi and are involved in certain inflammatory diseases.

Activated CD8+ T lymphocytes differentiate into CTLs that kill cells harboring cytoplasmic microbes, thereby eliminating otherwise hidden reservoirs of infection. The principal mechanism of killing by CTLs depends on the perforin–granzyme system. Perforin and granzymes are stored in the granules of CTLs and are rapidly released when CTLs engage their targets (cells bearing the appropriate class I MHC–bound peptides). Perforin binds to the plasma membrane of the target cells and promotes the entry of granzymes, proteases that specifically cleave and thereby activate cellular caspases (Chapter 2), which induce the apoptosis of target cells.

The responses of T cells are regulated by a balance between costimulatory and inhibitory receptors. The major costimulatory receptor is CD28, mentioned earlier as the molecule that recognizes B7 ligands on APCs and provides second signals that work together with antigen recognition. Other proteins of the CD28 family include two "coinhibitory" receptors, CTLA-4 and PD-1, which block signals from the TCR and from CD28 and thus terminate T cell responses. Blocking these coinhibitors has proved to be a powerful approach for enhancing anti-tumor immune responses (Chapter 6).

Humoral Immunity: Activation of B Lymphocytes and Elimination of Extracellular Microbes

Upon activation, B lymphocytes proliferate and then differentiate into plasma cells that secrete different classes of antibodies with distinct functions (Fig. 5.11). There are two major pathways of B-cell activation.

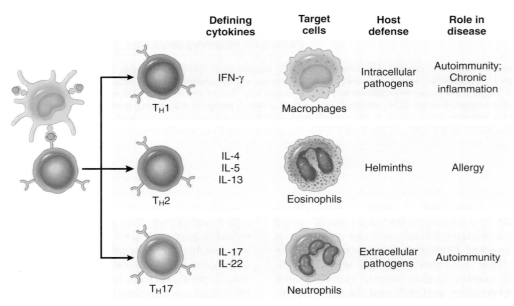

	Defining cytokines	Target cells	Host defense	Role in disease
T_H1	IFN-γ	Macrophages	Intracellular pathogens	Autoimmunity; Chronic inflammation
T_H2	IL-4 IL-5 IL-13	Eosinophils	Helminths	Allergy
T_H17	IL-17 IL-22	Neutrophils	Extracellular pathogens	Autoimmunity

Fig. 5.10 Subsets of helper T (T_H) cells. In response to stimuli (mainly cytokines) present at the time of antigen recognition, naive CD4+ T cells may differentiate into populations of effector cells that produce distinct sets of cytokines that act on different cells (indicated as target cells) and mediate different functions. The roles of these subsets in host defense and immunologic diseases are summarized. These populations may be capable of converting from one to another. Some activated T cells produce multiple cytokines and do not fall into a distinct subset.

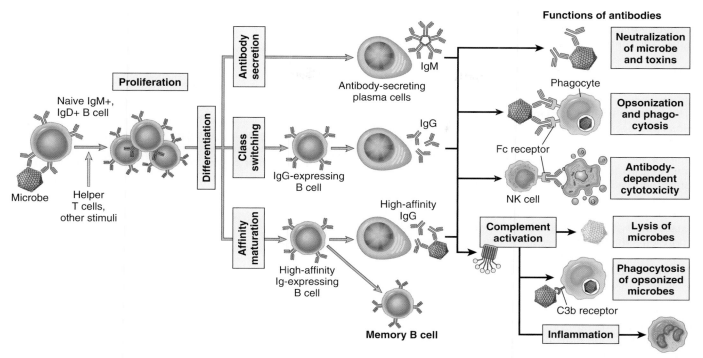

Fig. 5.11 Humoral immunity. Naive B lymphocytes recognize antigens, and under the influence of Th cells and other stimuli *(not shown)*, the B cells are activated to proliferate and to differentiate into antibody-secreting plasma cells. Some of the activated B cells undergo heavy-chain class switching and affinity maturation, and some become long-lived memory cells. Antibodies of different heavy-chain classes (isotypes) perform different effector functions, *shown on the right.* Note that the antibodies shown are IgG; these and IgM activate complement; and the specialized functions of IgA (mucosal immunity) and IgE (mast cell and eosinophil activation) are *not shown.*

- *T cell–independent.* Many polysaccharide and lipid antigens have multiple identical antigenic determinants (epitopes) that are able to simultaneously engage and cross-link several antibody molecules on each B cell and initiate the process of B-cell activation.
- *T cell–dependent.* Typical globular protein antigens are not able to bind to multiple antigen receptors, and the full response of B cells to protein antigens requires help from CD4+ T cells. B cells also act as APCs — they ingest protein antigens, degrade them, and display peptides bound to class II MHC molecules for recognition by helper T cells. The helper T cells express CD40L and secrete cytokines, which work together to activate the B cells.

Some of the progeny of the expanded B-cell clones differentiate into antibody-secreting plasma cells. Each plasma cell secretes antibodies with the same specificity as the cell surface antibodies (B-cell antigen receptors) that first recognized the antigen. Polysaccharides and lipids stimulate secretion mainly of IgM antibody. Protein antigens, by virtue of CD40L- and cytokine-mediated helper T-cell actions, induce the production of antibodies of different classes (IgG, IgA, IgE). **Production of functionally different antibodies, all with the same specificity, relies on heavy-chain class (isotype) switching, which increases the range of functions that antibodies serve.** Some of the isotype-specific functions of antibodies include opsonization and transplacental transfer of IgG, IgA secretion into mucosal lumens, and binding of IgE to mast cells. Helper T cells also stimulate the production of antibodies with

higher affinity for the antigen. This process, called *affinity maturation,* improves the quality of the humoral immune response. Some activated B cells migrate into follicles and form germinal centers, which are the major sites of isotype switching and affinity maturation. The helper T cells that stimulate these processes in B lymphocytes also migrate to and reside in the germinal centers and are called *follicular helper T (Tfh) cells.*

The humoral immune response combats microbes in numerous ways (see Fig. 5.11).

- Antibodies bind to microbes and prevent them from infecting cells, thereby neutralizing the microbes.
- IgG antibodies coat (opsonize) microbes and target them for phagocytosis, since phagocytes (neutrophils and macrophages) express receptors for the Fc tails of IgG molecules.
- IgG and IgM activate the complement system by the classical pathway, and complement products promote phagocytosis and destruction of microbes.
- IgA is secreted in mucosal tissues and neutralizes microbes in the lumens of the respiratory and gastrointestinal tracts (and other mucosal tissues).
- IgG is actively transported across the placenta and protects the newborn until the immune system becomes mature. This is a form of *passive immunity.*
- IgE coats helminthic parasites and functions with mast cells and eosinophils to kill them.

Circulating IgG antibodies have half-lives of about 3 weeks, which is much longer than the half-lives of most blood proteins, as a consequence of special mechanisms for recycling IgG and reducing its catabolism. Some antibody-secreting plasma cells migrate to the bone marrow and live for years, continuing to produce low levels of antibodies.

Decline of Immune Responses and Immunologic Memory

The majority of effector lymphocytes induced by an infectious pathogen die by apoptosis after the pathogen is eliminated, thus returning the immune system to its basal resting state. The initial activation of lymphocytes generates long-lived *memory cells,* which may survive for years after the infection. Memory cells are an expanded pool of antigen-specific lymphocytes (more numerous than the naïve cells specific for any antigen that are present before encounter with that antigen), and they respond faster and more effectively when reexposed to the antigen than do naïve cells. This is why the generation of memory cells is an important goal of vaccination.

SUMMARY

THE NORMAL IMMUNE RESPONSE: OVERVIEW OF CELLS, TISSUES, RECEPTORS, AND MEDIATORS

- The innate immune system uses several families of receptors, such as the Toll-like receptors, to recognize molecules present in various types of microbes and produced by damaged cells.
- Lymphocytes are the mediators of adaptive immunity and the only cells that produce specific and diverse receptors for antigens.
- T (thymus-derived) lymphocytes express antigen receptors called *T-cell receptors (TCRs)* that recognize peptide fragments of protein antigens that are displayed by MHC molecules on the surface of antigen-presenting cells.
- B (bone marrow–derived) lymphocytes express membrane-bound antibodies that recognize a wide variety of antigens. B cells are activated to become plasma cells, which secrete antibodies.
- Natural killer (NK) cells kill cells that are infected by some microbes, or are stressed and damaged beyond repair. NK cells express inhibitory receptors that recognize MHC molecules that are normally expressed on healthy cells, and are thus prevented from killing normal cells.
- Antigen-presenting cells (APCs) capture microbes and other antigens, transport them to lymphoid organs, and display them for recognition by lymphocytes. The most efficient APCs are DCs, which live in epithelia and most tissues.
- The cells of the immune system are organized in tissues, some of which are the sites of production of mature lymphocytes (the generative lymphoid organs, the bone marrow, and thymus), and others are the sites of immune responses (the peripheral lymphoid organs, including lymph nodes, spleen, and mucosal lymphoid tissues).
- The early reaction to microbes is mediated by the innate immune system, which is ready to respond to microbes. Components of the innate immune system include epithelial barriers, phagocytes, NK cells, and plasma proteins, for example, of the complement system. Innate immune reactions are often manifested as inflammation. Innate immunity, unlike adaptive immunity, does not have fine antigen specificity or memory.

- The defense reactions of adaptive immunity develop slowly, but are more potent and specialized.
- Microbes and other foreign antigens are captured by DCs and transported to lymph nodes, where the antigens are recognized by naïve lymphocytes. The lymphocytes are activated to proliferate and differentiate into effector and memory cells.
- Cell-mediated immunity is the reaction of T lymphocytes, designed to combat cell-associated microbes (e.g., phagocytosed microbes and microbes in the cytoplasm of infected cells). Humoral immunity is mediated by antibodies and is effective against extracellular microbes (in the circulation and mucosal lumens).
- CD4+ helper T cells help B cells to make antibodies, activate macrophages to destroy ingested microbes, stimulate recruitment of leukocytes, and regulate all immune responses to protein antigens. The functions of CD4+ T cells are mediated by secreted proteins called *cytokines.*
- CD8+ cytotoxic T lymphocytes kill cells that express antigens in the cytoplasm that are seen as foreign (e.g., virus-infected and tumor cells) and can also produce cytokines.
- Antibodies secreted by plasma cells neutralize microbes and block their infectivity, and promote the phagocytosis and destruction of pathogens. Antibodies also confer passive immunity to neonates.

The brief outline of basic immunology presented here provides a foundation for considering the diseases of the immune system. We first discuss the immune reactions that cause injury, called *hypersensitivity reactions,* and then disorders caused by the failure of tolerance to self antigens, called *autoimmune disorders,* and the rejection of transplants. This is followed by diseases caused by a defective immune system, called *immunodeficiency diseases.* We close with a consideration of amyloidosis, a disorder that is often associated with immune and inflammatory diseases.

HYPERSENSITIVITY: IMMUNOLOGICALLY MEDIATED TISSUE INJURY

Immune responses that normally are protective also are capable of causing tissue injury. Injurious immune reactions are grouped under *hypersensitivity,* and the resulting diseases are called *hypersensitivity diseases.* This term originated from the idea that persons who mount immune responses against an antigen are sensitized to that antigen, so pathologic or excessive reactions represent manifestations of a hypersensitive state. Normally, an exquisite system of checks and balances optimizes the eradication of infecting organisms without serious injury to host tissues. However, immune responses may be inadequately controlled or directed against normally harmless antigens or inappropriately targeted to host tissues, and in such situations, the normally beneficial response is the cause of disease. In this section, we describe the causes and general mechanisms of hypersensitivity diseases and then discuss specific situations in which the immune response is responsible for the disease.

Causes of Hypersensitivity Reactions

Pathologic immune responses may be directed against different types of antigens and may result from various underlying abnormalities.

- *Autoimmunity: reactions against self antigens.* Normally, the immune system does not react against one's own antigens. This phenomenon is called *self tolerance,* implying that the body "tolerates" its own antigens. On occasion, self-tolerance fails, resulting in reactions against one's own cells and tissues. Collectively, such reactions constitute *autoimmunity,* and diseases caused by autoimmunity are referred to as *autoimmune diseases.* We will return to the mechanisms of self-tolerance and autoimmunity later in this chapter.
- *Reactions against microbes.* There are many types of reactions against microbial antigens that may cause disease. In some cases, the reaction appears to be excessive or the microbial antigen is unusually persistent. If antibodies are produced against such antigens, the antibodies may bind to the microbial antigens to produce immune complexes, which deposit in tissues and trigger inflammation; this is the underlying mechanism of poststreptococcal glomerulonephritis (Chapter 14). T-cell responses against persistent microbes may give rise to severe inflammation, sometimes with the formation of granulomas (Chapter 3); this is the cause of tissue injury in tuberculosis and other infections. Rarely, antibodies or T cells reactive with a microbe cross-react with a host tissue; such cross-reactivity is believed to be the basis for rheumatic heart disease (Chapter 11). In some instances, the disease-causing immune response may be entirely normal, but in the process of eradicating the infection, host tissues are injured. In viral hepatitis, the virus that infects liver cells is not cytopathic, but it is recognized as foreign by the immune system. Cytotoxic

T cells try to eliminate infected cells, and this normal immune response damages liver cells.
- *Reactions against environmental antigens.* Almost 20% of the population is allergic to common environmental substances (e.g., pollens, animal danders, and dust mites), as well as some metal ions and therapeutic drugs. Such individuals are genetically predisposed to make unusual immune responses to noninfectious, typically harmless antigens to which all persons are exposed but against which only some react.

In all of these conditions, tissue injury is mediated by the same mechanisms that normally function to eliminate infectious pathogens—namely, antibodies, effector T lymphocytes, and various other effector cells. The fundamental problem in these diseases is that the immune response is triggered and maintained inappropriately. Because the stimuli for these abnormal immune responses are difficult or impossible to eliminate (e.g., self antigens, persistent microbes, or environmental antigens), and the immune system has many intrinsic positive feedback loops (which normally promote protective immunity), once a hypersensitivity reaction starts, it is difficult to control or terminate it. Therefore, these diseases tend to be chronic and debilitating, and are therapeutic challenges. Since inflammation is a major component of the pathology of these disorders, they are sometimes grouped under the term *immune-mediated inflammatory diseases.*

Classification of Hypersensitivity Reactions

Hypersensitivity reactions can be subdivided into four types based on the principal immune mechanism responsible for injury; three are variations on antibody-mediated injury, and the fourth is T-cell mediated (Table 5.2). The rationale for this classification is that the mechanism of

Table 5.2 Mechanisms of Hypersensitivity Reactions

Type	Immune Mechanisms	Histopathologic Lesions	Prototypical Disorders
Immediate (type I) hypersensitivity	Production of IgE antibody → immediate release of vasoactive amines and other mediators from mast cells; later recruitment of inflammatory cells	Vascular dilation, edema, smooth muscle contraction, mucus production, tissue injury, inflammation	Anaphylaxis; allergies; bronchial asthma (atopic forms)
Antibody-mediated (type II) hypersensitivity	Production of IgG, IgM → binds to antigen on target cell or tissue → phagocytosis or lysis of target cell by activated complement or Fc receptors; recruitment of leukocytes	Phagocytosis and lysis of cells; inflammation; in some diseases, functional derangements without cell or tissue injury	Autoimmune hemolytic anemia; Goodpasture syndrome
Immune complex–mediated (type III) hypersensitivity	Deposition of antigen-antibody complexes → complement activation → recruitment of leukocytes by complement products and Fc receptors → release of enzymes and other toxic molecules	Inflammation, necrotizing vasculitis (fibrinoid necrosis)	Systemic lupus erythematosus; some forms of glomerulonephritis; serum sickness; Arthus reaction
Cell-mediated (type IV) hypersensitivity	Activated T lymphocytes → (1) release of cytokines, inflammation and macrophage activation; (2) T cell–mediated cytotoxicity	Perivascular cellular infiltrates; edema; granuloma formation; cell destruction	Contact dermatitis; multiple sclerosis; type I diabetes; tuberculosis

Ig, Immunoglobulin.

immune injury is often a good predictor of the clinical manifestations and may help to guide the therapy. However, this classification of immune-mediated diseases is not perfect, because several immune reactions may coexist in any one disease.

The main types of hypersensitivity reactions are as follows:

- In *immediate (type I) hypersensitivity*, often called *allergy*, the injury is caused by T_H2 cells, IgE antibodies, and mast cells and other leukocytes. Mast cells release mediators that act on blood vessels and smooth muscle as well as cytokines that recruit and activate inflammatory cells.
- *Antibody-mediated disorders (type II hypersensitivity)* are caused by secreted IgG and IgM antibodies that bind to fixed tissue or cell surface antigens. Antibodies injure cells by promoting their phagocytosis or lysis and injure tissues by inducing inflammation. Antibodies also may interfere with cellular functions and cause disease without cell or tissue injury.
- In *immune complex–mediated disorders (type III hypersensitivity)*, IgG and IgM antibodies bind antigens, usually in the circulation, and form antigen-antibody complexes that deposit in vascular beds and induce inflammation. The leukocytes that are recruited (neutrophils and monocytes) produce tissue damage by release of lysosomal enzymes and generation of toxic free radicals.
- *T cell–mediated (type IV) hypersensitivity disorders* are caused mainly by immune responses in which T lymphocytes of the T_H1 and T_H17 subsets produce cytokines that induce inflammation and activate neutrophils and macrophages, which are responsible for tissue injury. CD8+ CTLs also may contribute to injury by directly killing host cells.

Immediate (Type I) Hypersensitivity

Immediate hypersensitivity is a tissue reaction that occurs rapidly (typically within minutes) after the interaction of antigen with IgE antibody bound to the surface of mast cells. The reaction is initiated by entry of an antigen, which is called an *allergen* because it triggers allergy. Many allergens are environmental substances that certain individuals are predisposed to developing allergic reactions against. T_H2 cells and IgE are responsible for the clinical and pathologic manifestations of the reaction. Immediate hypersensitivity may occur as a local reaction that is merely annoying (e.g., seasonal rhinitis, hay fever), severely debilitating (asthma), or even fatal (anaphylaxis).

Sequence of Events in Immediate Hypersensitivity Reactions

Most hypersensitivity reactions follow a stereotypic sequence of cellular responses (Fig. 5.12):

- *Activation of T_H2 cells and production of IgE antibody.* Allergens may be introduced by inhalation, ingestion, or injection. Variables that probably contribute to the strong T_H2 responses to allergens include the route of entry, dose, and chronicity of antigen exposure, and the genetic makeup of the host. It is not clear if allergenic substances also have unique structural or chemical properties that endow them with the ability to elicit T_H2

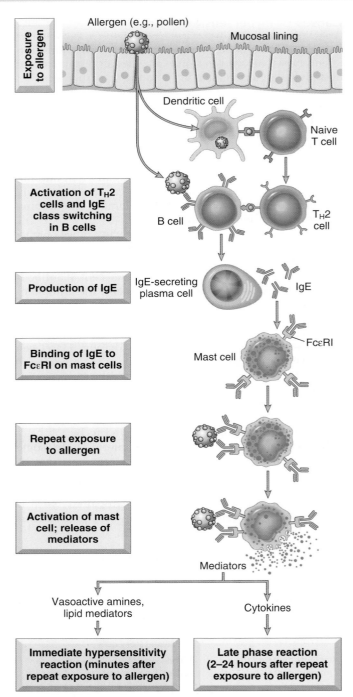

Fig. 5.12 Sequence of events in immediate (type I) hypersensitivity. Immediate hypersensitivity reactions are initiated by the introduction of an allergen, which stimulates T_H2 responses and IgE production in genetically susceptible individuals. IgE binds to Fc receptors (FcεRI) on mast cells, and subsequent exposure to the allergen activates the mast cells to secrete the mediators that are responsible for the pathologic manifestations of immediate hypersensitivity. See text for abbreviations.

responses. Immediate hypersensitivity is the prototypical T_H2-mediated reaction. The T_H2 cells that are induced secrete several cytokines, including IL-4, IL-5, and IL-13, which are responsible for essentially all the reactions of immediate hypersensitivity. IL-4 stimulates B cells specific for the allergen to undergo heavy-chain class switching to IgE and to secrete this immunoglobulin isotype. IL-5 activates eosinophils that are recruited to the reaction, and IL-13 acts on epithelial cells and stimulates mucus secretion. T_H2 cells often are recruited to the site of allergic reactions in response to chemokines that are produced locally; one of these chemokines, eotaxin, also recruits eosinophils to the same site.

- *Sensitization of mast cells by IgE antibody.* Mast cells are derived from precursors in the bone marrow and widely distributed in tissues, often residing near blood vessels and nerves and in subepithelial locations. Mast cells express a high-affinity receptor for the Fc portion of the ε heavy chain of IgE, called *FcεRI*. Even though the serum concentration of IgE is very low (in the range of 1 to 100 μg/mL), the affinity of the mast cell FcεRI receptor is so high that the receptors are always occupied by IgE. These antibody-bearing mast cells are sensitized to react if the specific antigen (the allergen) binds to the antibody molecules. Basophils are circulating cells that resemble mast cells. They also express FcεRI, but their role in most immediate hypersensitivity reactions is not established (since these reactions occur in tissues and most basophils are in the circulation). The third cell type that expresses FcεRI is eosinophils, which often are present in these reactions.
- *Activation of mast cells and release of mediators.* When a person who was sensitized by exposure to an allergen is reexposed to the allergen, the allergen binds to antigen-specific IgE molecules on mast cells, usually at or near the site of allergen entry. Cross-linking of these IgE molecules triggers a series of biochemical signals that culminate in the secretion of various mediators from the mast cells.

Three groups of mediators are important in different immediate hypersensitivity reactions:
- *Vasoactive amines* released from granule stores. The granules of mast cells contain histamine, which is released within seconds or minutes of activation. Histamine causes vasodilation, increased vascular permeability, smooth muscle contraction, and increased secretion of mucus. Other rapidly released mediators include chemotactic factors for neutrophils and eosinophils as well as neutral proteases (e.g., tryptase), which may damage tissues and also generate kinins and cleave complement components to produce additional chemotactic and inflammatory factors (e.g., C5a) (Chapter 3). The granules also contain acidic proteoglycans (heparin, chondroitin sulfate), the main function of which seems to be as a storage matrix for the amines.
- Newly synthesized *lipid mediators.* Mast cells synthesize and secrete prostaglandins and leukotrienes by the same pathways as do other leukocytes (Chapter 3). These lipid mediators have several actions that are important in immediate hypersensitivity reactions. Prostaglandin D2 (PGD_2) is the most abundant mediator generated by the cyclooxygenase pathway in mast cells. It causes intense bronchospasm as well as increased mucus secretion. The leukotrienes LTC_4 and LTD_4 are the most potent vasoactive and spasmogenic agents known; on a molar basis, they are several thousand times more active than histamine in increasing vascular permeability and in causing bronchial smooth muscle contraction. LTB_4 is highly chemotactic for neutrophils, eosinophils, and monocytes.
- *Cytokines.* Activation of mast cells results in the synthesis and secretion of several cytokines that are important for the late-phase reaction. These include TNF and chemokines, which recruit and activate leukocytes (Chapter 3), and IL-4 and IL-5, which amplify the T_H2-initiated immune reaction.

The reactions of immediate hypersensitivity clearly did not evolve to cause human discomfort and disease. The T_H2 response plays an important protective role in combating parasitic infections. IgE antibodies target helminths for destruction by eosinophils and mast cells. Mast cells also are involved in defense against bacterial infections. And snake aficionados will be relieved to hear that their mast cells may protect them from some snake venoms by releasing granule proteases that degrade the toxins. Why these beneficial responses are inappropriately activated by harmless environmental antigens, giving rise to allergies, remains a puzzle.

Development of Allergies

Susceptibility to immediate hypersensitivity reactions is genetically determined. An increased propensity to develop immediate hypersensitivity reactions is called *atopy.* Atopic individuals tend to have higher serum IgE levels and more IL-4–producing T_H2 cells than does the general population. A positive family history of allergy is found in 50% of atopic individuals. The basis of familial predisposition is not clear, but genes that are implicated in susceptibility to asthma and other atopic disorders include those encoding HLA molecules (which may confer immune responsiveness to particular allergens), cytokines (which may control T_H2 responses), a component of the FcεRI, and ADAM33, a metalloproteinase that may be involved in tissue remodeling in the airways.

Environmental factors are also important in the development of allergic diseases. Exposure to environmental pollutants, all too common in industrialized societies, is an important predisposing factor for allergy. It is notable that dogs and cats living in the same environment as humans develop allergies, whereas chimps living in the wild do not despite their much closer genetic similarity to humans. This simple observation suggests that environmental factors may be more important in the development of allergic disease than genetics. Viral infections of the airways are important triggers for bronchial asthma, an allergic disease affecting the lungs (Chapter 13). Bacterial skin infections are strongly associated with atopic dermatitis.

It is estimated that 20% to 30% of immediate hypersensitivity reactions are triggered by nonantigenic stimuli such as temperature extremes and exercise, and do not involve T_H2 cells or IgE. It is believed that in these cases mast cells are abnormally sensitive to activation by various nonimmune stimuli.

The incidence of many allergic diseases is increasing in developed countries and seems to be related to a decrease in infections during early life. These observations have

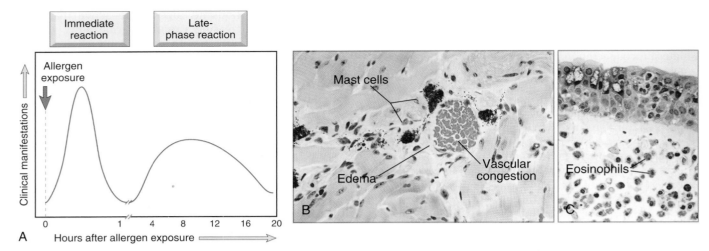

Fig. 5.13 Phases of immediate hypersensitivity reactions. (A) Kinetics of the immediate and late-phase reactions. The immediate vascular and smooth muscle reaction to allergen develops within minutes after challenge (allergen exposure in a previously sensitized individual), and the late-phase reaction develops 2 to 24 hours later. The immediate reaction (B) is characterized by vasodilation, congestion, and edema, and the late-phase reaction (C) is characterized by an inflammatory infiltrate rich in eosinophils, neutrophils, and T cells. *(Courtesy of Dr. Daniel Friend, Department of Pathology, Brigham and Women's Hospital, Boston, Massachusetts.)*

led to an idea, sometimes called the *hygiene hypothesis,* that early childhood and even prenatal exposure to microbial antigens educates the immune system in such a way that subsequent pathologic responses against common environmental allergens are prevented. Thus, too much hygiene in childhood may increase allergies later in life. The idea that early childhood exposure to antigens may reduce later allergies against those antigens has received support from clinical trials demonstrating that exposing infants to peanuts reduces the incidence of peanut allergy later in life.

Clinical and Pathologic Manifestations

Often, the IgE-triggered reaction has two well-defined phases (Fig. 5.13): (1) *the immediate response,* which is stimulated by mast cell granule contents and lipid mediators and is characterized by vasodilation, vascular leakage, and smooth muscle spasm, usually evident within 5 to 30 minutes after exposure to an allergen and subsiding by 60 minutes; and (2) *a second, late-phase reaction* stimulated mainly by cytokines, which usually sets in 2 to 8 hours later, may last for several days, and is characterized by inflammation as well as tissue destruction, such as mucosal epithelial cell damage. The dominant inflammatory cells in the late-phase reaction are neutrophils, eosinophils, and lymphocytes, especially T_H2 cells. Neutrophils are recruited by various chemokines; their roles in inflammation were described in Chapter 3. Eosinophils are recruited by eotaxin and other chemokines released from epithelium and are important effectors of tissue injury in the late-phase response. Eosinophils produce major basic protein and eosinophil cationic protein, which are toxic to epithelial cells, and LTC_4 and platelet-activating factor, which promote inflammation. The T_H2 cells produce cytokines that have multiple actions, as described earlier. These recruited leukocytes can amplify and sustain the inflammatory response, even in the absence of continuous allergen exposure. In addition, inflammatory leukocytes are responsible for much of the epithelial cell injury in

immediate hypersensitivity. Because inflammation is a major component of many allergic diseases, notably asthma and atopic dermatitis, therapy includes anti-inflammatory drugs such as corticosteroids.

An immediate hypersensitivity reaction may occur as a systemic disorder or as a local reaction (Table 5.3). The route of antigen exposure often determines the nature of the reaction. Systemic exposure to protein antigens (e.g., in bee venom) or drugs (e.g., penicillin) may result in systemic *anaphylaxis.* Within minutes of the exposure in a sensitized host, itching, urticaria (hives), and skin erythema appear, followed in short order by profound respiratory difficulty caused by pulmonary bronchoconstriction and accentuated by hypersecretion of mucus. Laryngeal edema may exacerbate matters by causing upper airway obstruction. In addition, the musculature of the entire gastrointestinal tract may be affected, with resultant vomiting, abdominal cramps, and diarrhea. Without immediate intervention, there may be systemic vasodilation with a fall

Table 5.3 Examples of Disorders Caused by Immediate Hypersensitivity

Clinical Syndrome	Clinical and Pathologic Manifestations
Anaphylaxis (may be caused by drugs, bee sting, food)	Fall in blood pressure (shock) caused by vascular dilation; airway obstruction due to laryngeal edema
Bronchial asthma	Airway obstruction caused by bronchial smooth muscle hyperactivity; inflammation and tissue injury caused by late-phase reaction
Allergic rhinitis, sinusitis (hay fever)	Increased mucus secretion; inflammation of upper airways and sinuses
Food allergies	Increased peristalsis due to contraction of intestinal muscles, resulting in vomiting and diarrhea

in blood pressure (anaphylactic shock), and the patient may progress to circulatory collapse and death within minutes.

Local reactions generally occur when the antigen is confined to a particular site, such as the skin (following contact), the gastrointestinal tract (following ingestion), or the lung (following inhalation). *Atopic dermatitis, food allergies, hay fever,* and certain forms of *asthma* are examples of localized allergic reactions. However, ingestion or inhalation of allergens also can trigger systemic reactions.

SUMMARY

IMMEDIATE (TYPE I) HYPERSENSITIVITY

- Immediate (type I) sensitivity is also called an *allergic reaction,* or *allergy.*
- Type I hypersensitivity is induced by environmental antigens (allergens) that stimulate strong T_H2 responses and IgE production in genetically susceptible individuals.
- IgE coats mast cells by binding to the FcεRI receptor; reexposure to the allergen leads to cross-linking of the IgE and FcεRI, activation of mast cells, and release of mediators.
- Principal mediators are histamine, proteases, and other granule contents; prostaglandins and leukotrienes; and cytokines.
- Mediators are responsible for the immediate vascular and smooth muscle reactions and the late-phase reaction (inflammation).
- The clinical manifestations may be local or systemic, and range from mildly annoying rhinitis to fatal anaphylaxis.

Antibody-Mediated Diseases (Type II Hypersensitivity)

Antibody-mediated (type II) hypersensitivity disorders are caused by antibodies directed against target antigens on the surface of cells or other tissue components. The antigens may be normal molecules intrinsic to cell membranes or in the extracellular matrix, or they may be adsorbed exogenous antigens (e.g., a drug metabolite). These reactions are the cause of several important diseases (Table 5.4).

Mechanisms of Antibody-Mediated Diseases

Antibodies cause disease by targeting cells for phagocytosis, activating the complement system, or interfering with normal cellular functions (Fig. 5.14). The antibodies that are responsible typically are high-affinity antibodies capable of activating complement and binding to the Fc receptors of phagocytes.

- *Opsonization and phagocytosis.* When circulating cells, such as red blood cells or platelets, are coated (opsonized) with autoantibodies, with or without complement proteins, the cells become targets for phagocytosis by neutrophils and macrophages (Fig. 5.14A). These phagocytes express receptors for the Fc tails of IgG antibodies and for breakdown products of the C3 complement protein, and use these receptors to bind and ingest opsonized particles. Opsonized cells are usually eliminated in the spleen, and this is why splenectomy is of clinical benefit in some antibody-mediated diseases.

Antibody-mediated cell destruction and phagocytosis occur in the following clinical situations: (1) transfusion reactions, in which cells from an incompatible

Table 5.4 Examples of Antibody-Mediated Diseases (Type II Hypersensitivity)

Disease	Target Antigen	Mechanisms of Disease	Clinicopathologic Manifestations
Autoimmune hemolytic anemia	Red blood cell membrane proteins	Opsonization and phagocytosis of red blood cells	Hemolysis, anemia
Autoimmune thrombocytopenic purpura	Platelet membrane proteins (GpIIb:IIIa integrin)	Opsonization and phagocytosis of platelets	Bleeding
Pemphigus vulgaris	Proteins in intercellular junctions of epidermal cells (desmogleins)	Antibody-mediated activation of proteases, disruption of intercellular adhesions	Skin vesicles (bullae)
Vasculitis caused by ANCA	Neutrophil granule proteins, presumably released from activated neutrophils	Neutrophil degranulation and inflammation	Vasculitis
Goodpasture syndrome	Protein in basement membranes of kidney glomeruli and lung alveoli	Complement- and Fc receptor–mediated inflammation	Nephritis, lung hemorrhage
Acute rheumatic fever	Streptococcal cell wall antigen; antibody cross-reacts with myocardial antigen	Inflammation, macrophage activation	Myocarditis, arthritis
Myasthenia gravis	Acetylcholine receptor	Antibody inhibits acetylcholine binding, down-modulates receptors	Muscle weakness, paralysis
Graves disease (hyperthyroidism)	TSH receptor	Antibody-mediated stimulation of TSH receptors	Hyperthyroidism
Pernicious anemia	Intrinsic factor of gastric parietal cells	Neutralization of intrinsic factor, decreased absorption of vitamin B_{12}	Abnormal erythropoiesis, anemia

ANCA, Anti-neutrophil cytoplasmic antibodies; *TSH,* thyroid-stimulating hormone.

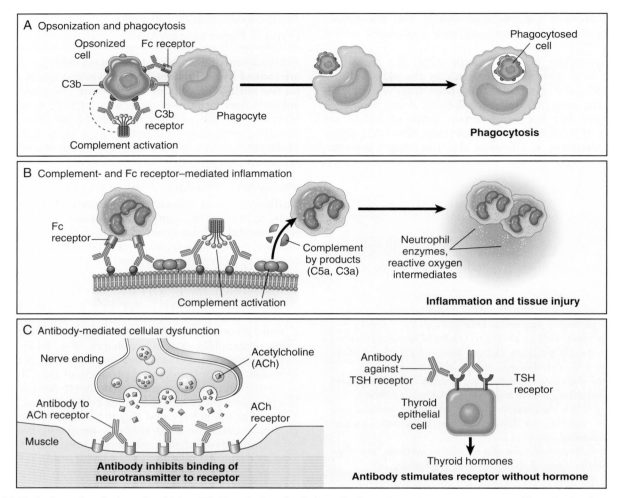

Fig. 5.14 Mechanisms of antibody-mediated injury. (A) Opsonization of cells by antibodies and complement components and ingestion by phagocytes. (B) Inflammation induced by antibody binding to Fc receptors of leukocytes and by complement breakdown products. (C) Anti-receptor antibodies disturb the normal function of receptors. In these examples, antibodies to the acetylcholine (ACh) receptor impair neuromuscular transmission in myasthenia gravis, and antibodies against the thyroid-stimulating hormone (TSH) receptor activate thyroid cells in Graves disease.

donor react with preformed antibody in the host (Chapter 12); (2) hemolytic disease of the newborn (erythroblastosis fetalis), in which IgG anti–red blood cell antibodies from the mother cross the placenta and cause destruction of fetal red blood cells (Chapter 7); (3) autoimmune hemolytic anemia, agranulocytosis, and thrombocytopenia, in which individuals produce antibodies to their own blood cells (Chapter 12); and (4) certain drug reactions, in which a drug attaches to plasma membrane proteins of red blood cells and antibodies are produced against the drug-protein complex.

• *Inflammation*. Antibodies bound to cellular or tissue antigens activate the complement system by the classical pathway (Fig. 5.14B). Products of complement activation serve several functions (see Fig. 3.11, Chapter 3), one of which is to recruit neutrophils and monocytes, triggering inflammation in tissues. Leukocytes also may be activated by engagement of Fc receptors, which recognize the bound antibodies. Antibody-mediated inflammation is responsible for tissue injury in some forms of glomerulonephritis, vascular rejection in organ grafts, and other disorders.

• *Antibody-mediated cellular dysfunction*. In some cases, antibodies directed against a host protein impair or dysregulate important functions without directly causing cell injury or inflammation (Fig. 5.14C). In myasthenia gravis, antibodies against acetylcholine receptors in the motor end plates of skeletal muscles inhibit neuromuscular transmission, with resultant muscle weakness. Antibodies also can stimulate cellular responses excessively. In Graves disease, antibodies against the thyroid-stimulating hormone receptor stimulate thyroid epithelial cells to secrete thyroid hormones, resulting in hyperthyroidism. Antibodies against hormones and other essential proteins can neutralize and block the actions of these molecules, causing functional derangements.

Immune Complex–Mediated Diseases (Type III Hypersensitivity)

Antigen–antibody (immune) complexes that are formed in the circulation may deposit in blood vessels, leading to complement activation and acute inflammation. Less

Table 5.5 Examples of Immune Complex–Mediated Diseases

Disease	Antigen Involved	Clinicopathologic Manifestations
Systemic lupus erythematosus	Nuclear antigens (circulating or "planted" in kidney)	Nephritis, skin lesions, arthritis, others
Poststreptococcal glomerulonephritis	Streptococcal cell wall antigen(s); may be "planted" in glomerular basement membrane	Nephritis
Polyarteritis nodosa	Hepatitis B virus antigens in some cases	Systemic vasculitis
Reactive arthritis	Bacterial antigens (e.g., *Yersinia*)	Acute arthritis
Serum sickness	Various proteins (e.g., foreign serum protein) (horse anti-thymocyte globulin)	Arthritis, vasculitis, nephritis
Arthus reaction (experimental)	Various foreign proteins	Cutaneous vasculitis

frequently, the complexes may be formed at sites where antigen has been "planted" previously (called *in situ immune complexes*). The antigens that form immune complexes may be exogenous, such as a foreign protein that is injected or produced by an infectious microbe, or endogenous, if the individual produces antibody against self antigens (autoimmunity). Examples of immune complex disorders and the antigens involved are listed in Table 5.5. Immune complex–mediated diseases tend be systemic, but often preferentially involve the kidney (glomerulonephritis), joints (arthritis), and small blood vessels (vasculitis), all of which are common sites of immune complex deposition.

Systemic Immune Complex Disease

Acute serum sickness is the prototype of a systemic immune complex disease; it was once a frequent sequela to the administration of large amounts of foreign serum (e.g., serum from immunized horses used for protection against diphtheria). In modern times, the disease is infrequent and usually seen in individuals who receive antibodies from other individuals or species, e.g. horse or rabbit antithymocyte globulin administered to deplete T cells in recipients of organ grafts. Nevertheless, it is an informative model that has taught us a great deal about immune complex disorders.

The pathogenesis of systemic immune complex disease can be divided into three phases (Fig. 5.15).

Formation of Immune Complexes. The introduction of a protein antigen triggers an immune response that results in the formation of antibodies, typically about 1 week after the injection of the protein. These antibodies are secreted into the blood, where they react with the antigen still present in the circulation and form antigen-antibody complexes.

Deposition of Immune Complexes. In the next phase, the circulating antigen-antibody complexes are deposited in various tissues. The factors that determine whether immune complex formation will lead to tissue deposition and disease are not fully understood, but the major influences seem to be the characteristics of the complexes and local vascular alterations. In general, complexes of medium size that are formed when antigen is in slight excess are the most pathogenic. Organs where blood is filtered at high

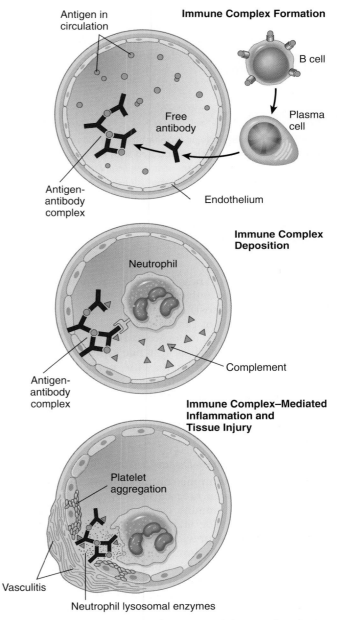

Fig. 5.15 Immune complex disease. The sequential phases in the induction of systemic immune complex–mediated diseases (type III hypersensitivity).

pressure to form other fluids, like urine and synovial fluid, are sites where immune complexes become concentrated and deposit; hence, immune complex disease often affects glomeruli and joints.

Inflammation and Tissue Injury. Once deposited in tissues, immune complexes initiate an acute inflammatory reaction via complement activation and engagement of leukocyte Fc receptors. Typically, the antibodies are IgG or IgM. Deposition of complement proteins can be detected at the site of injury. Consumption of complement during the active phase of the disease decreases serum levels of C3, which can be used as a marker for disease activity. During this phase (approximately 10 days after antigen administration), clinical features such as fever, urticaria, joint pain (arthralgia), lymph node enlargement, and proteinuria appear. Wherever complexes deposit, the tissue damage is similar. The resultant inflammatory lesion is termed *vasculitis* if it occurs in blood vessels, *glomerulonephritis* if it occurs in renal glomeruli, *arthritis* if it occurs in the joints, and so on.

MORPHOLOGY

The principal morphologic manifestation of immune complex injury is **acute vasculitis,** associated with fibrinoid necrosis of the vessel wall and intense neutrophilic infiltration (Fig. 3.12, Chapter 3). When deposited in the kidney, the complexes can be seen on immunofluorescence microscopy as granular deposits of immunoglobulin and complement and on electron microscopy as electron-dense deposits along the glomerular basement membrane (see Fig. 5.24).

In acute serum sickness induced by administration of a single large dose of antigen, the lesions tend to resolve as a result of phagocytosis and degradation of the immune complexes. A form of *chronic serum sickness* results from repeated or prolonged exposure to an antigen. This occurs in several diseases, such as systemic lupus erythematosus (SLE), which is associated with persistent antibody responses to autoantigens. In many diseases, the morphologic changes and other findings suggest immune complex deposition, but the inciting antigens are unknown. Included in this category are membranous glomerulonephritis and several vasculitides.

Local Immune Complex Disease (Arthus Reaction)

A model of local immune complex diseases is the *Arthus reaction,* in which an area of tissue necrosis appears as a result of acute immune complex vasculitis. The reaction is produced experimentally by injecting an antigen into the skin of a previously immunized animal with preformed antibody. Immune complexes form as the antigen diffuses into the vascular wall at the site of injection, triggering the same inflammatory reaction and histologic appearance as in systemic immune complex disease. Arthus lesions evolve over a few hours and reach a peak 4 to 10 hours after injection, when the injection site develops edema and hemorrhage, occasionally followed by ulceration.

SUMMARY

PATHOGENESIS OF DISEASES CAUSED BY ANTIBODIES AND IMMUNE COMPLEXES

- Antibodies can coat (opsonize) cells, with or without complement proteins, and target these cells for phagocytosis by phagocytes (macrophages), which express receptors for the Fc tails of IgG and for complement proteins. The result is depletion of the opsonized cells.
- Antibodies and immune complexes may deposit in tissues or blood vessels, and elicit an acute inflammatory reaction by activating complement, with release of breakdown products, or by engaging Fc receptors of leukocytes. The inflammatory reaction causes tissue injury.
- Antibodies can bind to cell surface receptors or other essential molecules and cause functional derangements (either inhibition or unregulated activation) without cell injury.

T Cell–Mediated Diseases (Type IV Hypersensitivity)

Several autoimmune disorders, as well as pathologic reactions to environmental chemicals and persistent microbes, are now known to be caused by T cells (Table 5.6). Two types of T cell reactions are capable of causing tissue injury and disease: (1) cytokine-mediated inflammation, in which the cytokines are produced mainly by CD4+ T cells, and (2) direct cell cytotoxicity, mediated by CD8+ T cells (Fig. 5.16). This group of diseases is of great clinical interest because T cells are increasingly recognized as the basis of chronic inflammatory diseases, and many of the new rationally designed therapies for these diseases have been developed to target the abnormal T cell reactions.

CD4+ T Cell–Mediated Inflammation

In CD4+ T cell–mediated hypersensitivity reactions, cytokines produced by the T cells induce inflammation that may be chronic and destructive. The prototype of T cell–mediated inflammation is *delayed-type hypersensitivity (DTH),* a tissue reaction to antigens given to immune individuals. In this reaction, an antigen administered into the skin of a previously immunized individual results in a detectable cutaneous reaction within 24 to 48 hours (hence the term *delayed,* in contrast to *immediate* hypersensitivity).

As described earlier, naïve T cells are activated in secondary lymphoid organs by recognition of peptide antigens displayed by dendritic cells. The T cells differentiate into effector cells under the influence of various cytokines (see Figs. 5.9 and 5.10). Classical T cell–mediated hypersensitivity is a reaction of T_H1 effector cells, but T_H17 cells also may contribute to the reaction, especially when neutrophils are prominent in the inflammatory infiltrate. T_H1 cells secrete cytokines, mainly IFN-γ, which are responsible for many of the manifestations of delayed-type hypersensitivity. IFN-γ-activated (classically activated) macrophages produce substances that destroy microbes and damage tissues, and mediators that promote inflammation (Chapter 3).

Table 5.6 T Cell–Mediated Diseases

Disease	Specificity of Pathogenic T Cells	Principal Mechanisms of Tissue Injury	Clinicopathologic Manifestations
Rheumatoid arthritis	Collagen? Citrullinated self proteins?	Inflammation mediated by T_H17 (and T_H1?) cytokines; role of antibodies and immune complexes?	Chronic arthritis with inflammation, destruction of articular cartilage
Multiple sclerosis	Protein antigens in myelin (e.g., myelin basic protein)	Inflammation mediated by T_H1 and T_H17 cytokines, myelin destruction by activated macrophages	Demyelination in CNS with perivascular inflammation; paralysis
Type I diabetes mellitus	Antigens of pancreatic islet β cells (insulin, glutamic acid decarboxylase, others)	T cell–mediated inflammation, destruction of islet cells by CTLs	Insulitis (chronic inflammation in islets), destruction of β cells; diabetes
Inflammatory bowel disease	Enteric bacteria; self antigens?	Inflammation mediated by T_H1 and T_H17 cytokines	Chronic intestinal inflammation, obstruction
Psoriasis	Unknown	Inflammation mediated mainly by T_H17 cytokines	Destructive plaques in the skin
Contact sensitivity	Various environmental chemicals (e.g., urushiol from poison ivy or poison oak, therapeutic drugs)	Inflammation mediated by T_H1 (and T_H17?) cytokines	Epidermal necrosis, dermal inflammation, causing skin rash and blisters

Examples of human T cell–mediated diseases are listed. In many cases, the specificity of the T cells and the mechanisms of tissue injury are inferred based on the similarity with experimental animal models of the diseases.

Activated T_H17 cells secrete cytokines that recruit neutrophils and monocytes.

Clinical Examples of CD4+ T Cell–Mediated Inflammatory Reactions

The classic example of DTH is the *tuberculin reaction* (known in clinical medicine as the *PPD skin test*), which is produced by the intracutaneous injection of purified protein derivative (PPD, also called *tuberculin*), a protein-containing antigen of the *Mycobacterium tuberculosis* bacillus. In a previously exposed individual, reddening and induration of the site appear in 8 to 12 hours, reach a peak in 24 to 72 hours, and thereafter slowly subside. Morphologically, delayed-type hypersensitivity is characterized by the

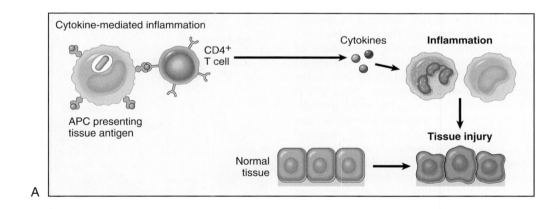

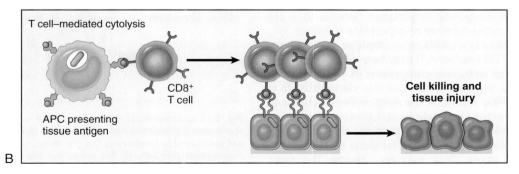

Fig. 5.16 Mechanisms of T-cell–mediated (type IV) hypersensitivity reactions. (A) CD4+ T_H1 cells (and sometimes CD8+ T cells, *not shown*) respond to tissue antigens by secreting cytokines that stimulate inflammation and activate phagocytes, leading to tissue injury. CD4+ T_H17 cells contribute to inflammation by recruiting neutrophils (and, to a lesser extent, monocytes). (B) In some diseases, CD8+ cytotoxic T lymphocytes (CTLs) directly kill tissue cells expressing intracellular antigens (shown as orange bars inside cells). *APC,* Antigen-presenting cell.

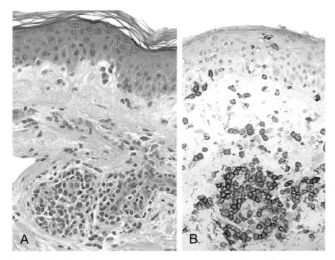

Fig. 5.17 Delayed hypersensitivity reaction in the skin. (A) Perivascular accumulation ("cuffing") of mononuclear inflammatory cells (lymphocytes and macrophages), with associated dermal edema and fibrin deposition. (B) Immunoperoxidase staining reveals a predominantly perivascular cellular infiltrate that marks positively with anti-CD4 antibodies. *(Courtesy of Dr. Louis Picker, Department of Pathology, Oregon Health Sciences University, Portland, Oregon.)*

accumulation of mononuclear cells, mainly CD4+ T cells and macrophages, around venules, producing perivascular "cuffing" (Fig. 5.17).

Prolonged DTH reactions against persistent microbes or other stimuli may result in a special pattern of reaction called *granulomatous inflammation*. The initial perivascular CD4+ T cell infiltrate is progressively replaced by macrophages over a period of 2 to 3 weeks. These accumulated macrophages typically exhibit morphologic evidence of activation; that is, they become large, flat, and eosinophilic, and are called *epithelioid cells*. The epithelioid cells occasionally fuse under the influence of cytokines (e.g., IFN-γ) to form multinucleate *giant cells*. An aggregate of epithelioid cells, typically surrounded by a collar of lymphocytes, is called a *granuloma* (Fig. 5.18A). The process is essentially a chronic form of T$_H$1-mediated inflammation and macrophage activation (see Fig. 5.18B). Older granulomas develop an enclosing rim of fibroblasts and connective tissue. In certain situations, such as infection by helminths known as schistosomes, T$_H$2 cells also are involved, and as a result eosinophils are prominent in the lesions. Recognition of granulomas is of diagnostic importance because they are seen only in a limited number of conditions (Chapter 3).

Contact dermatitis is a common example of tissue injury resulting from DTH reactions. It may be evoked by contact with urushiol, the antigenic component of poison ivy or poison oak, and presents as a vesicular dermatitis. It is thought that in these reactions, the environmental chemical binds to and structurally modifies self proteins, and peptides derived from these modified proteins are recognized by T cells and elicit the reaction. The same mechanism is responsible for many *drug reactions*, among the most common hypersensitivity reactions of humans. The responsible drug (often a reactive chemical) alters self proteins, including MHC molecules, and these neoantigens are recognized as foreign by T cells, leading to cytokine produc-

tion and inflammation. Drug reactions often manifest as skin rashes.

CD4+ T cell–mediated inflammation is the basis of tissue injury in many organ-specific and systemic autoimmune diseases, such as rheumatoid arthritis and multiple sclerosis, as well as diseases probably caused by uncontrolled reactions to bacterial commensals, such as inflammatory bowel disease (see Table 5.6).

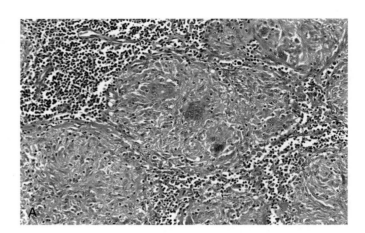

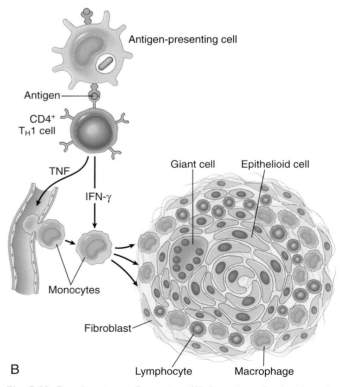

Fig. 5.18 Granulomatous inflammation. (A) A section of a lymph node shows several granulomas, each made up of an aggregate of epithelioid cells and surrounded by lymphocytes. The granuloma in the center shows several multinucleate giant cells. (B) The events that give rise to the formation of granulomas in type IV hypersensitivity reactions, illustrating the role of T$_H$1 cytokines. In some granulomatous disorders (e.g., schistosomiasis), T$_H$2 cells also contribute to the lesions. The role of T$_H$17 cells in granuloma formation is not proven. *(A, Courtesy of Dr. Trace Worrell, Department of Pathology, University of Texas Southwestern Medical School, Dallas, Texas.)*

CD8+ T Cell–Mediated Cytotoxicity

In this type of T cell–mediated reaction, CD8+ CTLs kill antigen-expressing target cells. Tissue destruction by CTLs may be an important component of some T cell–mediated diseases, such as type 1 diabetes. CTLs directed against cell surface histocompatibility antigens play an important role in graft rejection, which is discussed later. They also play a role in reactions against viruses. In a virus-infected cell, viral peptides are displayed by class I MHC molecules and the complex is recognized by the TCR of CD8+ T lymphocytes. The killing of infected cells leads to elimination of the infection, but in some cases, it is responsible for cell damage that accompanies the infection (e.g., in viral hepatitis). CD8+ T cells also produce cytokines, notably IFN-γ, and are involved in inflammatory reactions resembling DTH, especially following virus infections and exposure to some contact sensitizing agents.

SUMMARY

MECHANISMS OF T CELL–MEDIATED HYPERSENSITIVITY REACTIONS

- *Cytokine-mediated inflammation:* CD4+ T cells are activated by exposure to a protein antigen and differentiate into T_H1 and T_H17 effector cells. Subsequent exposure to the antigen results in the secretion of cytokines. IFN-γ activates macrophages to produce substances that cause tissue damage and promote fibrosis, and IL-17 and other cytokines recruit leukocytes, thus promoting inflammation.
- The classical T cell–mediated inflammatory reaction is **delayed-type hypersensitivity.** Chronic T_H1 reactions associated with macrophage activation often lead to granuloma formation.
- *T cell–mediated cytotoxicity:* CD8+ cytotoxic T lymphocytes (CTLs) specific for an antigen recognize cells expressing the target antigen and kill these cells. CD8+ T cells also secrete IFN-γ.

Now that we have described how the immune system can cause tissue damage, we turn to diseases in which normal control mechanisms fail. The prototypes of such diseases are autoimmune disorders, which are the result of failure of tolerance to self antigens.

AUTOIMMUNE DISEASES

Autoimmunity refers to immune reactions against self ("auto") antigens. Autoimmune diseases are estimated to affect at least 1% to 2% of the U.S. population. The evidence that these diseases are indeed the result of autoimmune reactions is more persuasive for some than for others. For instance, in many of these disorders, high-affinity autoantibodies have been identified, and in some cases these antibodies are known to cause pathologic abnormalities. There is also growing evidence for the activation of pathogenic self-reactive T cells in some of these diseases. In addition, experimental models have proved very informative, providing circumstantial evidence supporting an autoimmune etiology. Nevertheless, it is fair to say that for many

Table 5.7 Autoimmune Diseases

Organ-Specific	Systemic
Diseases Mediated by Antibodies	
Autoimmune hemolytic anemia	Systemic lupus erythematosus
Autoimmune thrombocytopenia	
Autoimmune atrophic gastritis of pernicious anemia	
Myasthenia gravis	
Graves disease	
Goodpasture syndrome	
Diseases Mediated by T Cells*	
Type I diabetes mellitus	Rheumatoid arthritis
Multiple sclerosis	Systemic sclerosis (scleroderma)† Sjögren syndrome†
Diseases Postulated to Be Autoimmune	
Inflammatory bowel diseases (Crohn disease, ulcerative colitis)‡	
Primary biliary cirrhosis†	Polyarteritis nodosa†
Autoimmune (chronic active) hepatitis	Inflammatory myopathies†

*A role for T cells has been demonstrated in these disorders, but antibodies may also be involved in tissue injury.
†An autoimmune basis of these disorders is suspected, but the supporting evidence is not strong.
‡These disorders may result from excessive immune responses to commensal enteric microbes, autoimmunity, or a combination of the two.

disorders traditionally classified as autoimmune, this etiology is suspected but not proved.

Autoimmune diseases may be *organ-specific,* in which the immune responses are directed against one particular organ or cell type and result in localized tissue damage, or *systemic,* characterized by lesions in many organs (Table 5.7). In systemic diseases that are caused by immune complexes and autoantibodies, the lesions principally affect the connective tissues and blood vessels of involved organs. Therefore, these diseases are often referred to as *collagen vascular diseases* or *connective tissue diseases,* even though the immunologic reactions are not specifically directed against constituents of connective tissue or blood vessels.

Normal persons are unresponsive (tolerant) to their own (self) antigens, and autoimmunity results from a failure of self-tolerance. Therefore, understanding the pathogenesis of autoimmunity requires familiarity with the mechanisms of normal immunologic tolerance.

Immunologic Tolerance

Immunologic tolerance is a state of unresponsiveness to an antigen that is induced by exposure of specific lymphocytes to that antigen. *Self-tolerance* refers to lack of immune responsiveness to one's own tissue antigens. Billions of different antigen receptors are randomly generated in developing T lymphocytes and B lymphocytes, and it is not surprising that during this process, receptors are produced that can recognize self antigens. Since these antigens cannot all be concealed from the immune system, there must be a means of eliminating or controlling self-recognizing lymphocytes. Several mechanisms work in

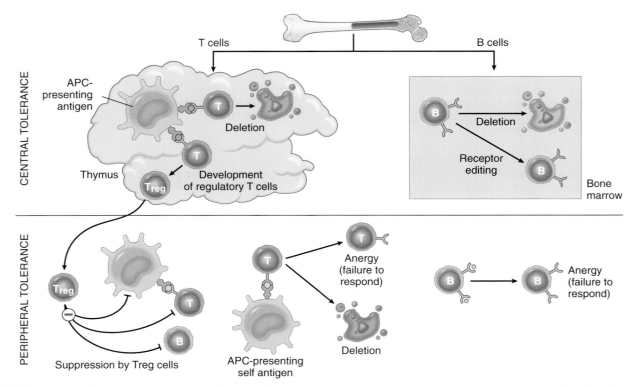

Fig. 5.19 Mechanisms of immunologic tolerance to self antigens. The principal mechanisms of central and peripheral self-tolerance in T cells and B cells are illustrated. *APC,* Antigen-presenting cell; *Treg cells,* regulatory T cells.

concert to select against self-reactivity and to thus prevent immune reactions against the body's own antigens. Two broad mechanisms are recognized: *central tolerance* and *peripheral tolerance* (Fig. 5.19).

Central Tolerance

The principal mechanism of central tolerance is the antigen-induced deletion (death) of self-reactive T lymphocytes and B lymphocytes during their maturation in central (generative) lymphoid organs (i.e., in the thymus for T cells and in the bone marrow for B cells). In the thymus, many autologous (self) protein antigens are processed and presented by thymic APCs. Any immature T cell that encounters such a self antigen undergoes apoptosis (a process called *deletion,* or *negative selection*), and the T cells that complete their maturation are thereby depleted of self-reactive cells. An exciting advance has been the identification of a protein called AIRE (autoimmune regulator), which stimulates expression of some peripheral tissue-restricted self antigens in the thymus and is thus critical for deletion of immature T cells specific for these antigens. Mutations in the *AIRE* gene are the cause of an autoimmune polyendocrinopathy (Chapter 20). Not all immature T cells that see self antigens in the thymus are deleted. Some CD4+ T cells survive and develop into regulatory T cells (described later).

Immature B cells that recognize self antigens with high affinity in the bone marrow also may die by apoptosis. Other self-reactive B cells are not deleted but instead undergo a second round of rearrangement of antigen receptor genes and then express new receptors that are no longer self-reactive (a process called *receptor editing*).

Central tolerance, however, is imperfect. Not all self antigens are present in the thymus or bone marrow, and hence lymphocytes bearing receptors for such autoantigens escape into the periphery. Self-reactive lymphocytes that escape negative selection can inflict tissue injury unless they are eliminated or muzzled in the peripheral tissues.

Peripheral Tolerance

Several mechanisms silence potentially autoreactive T cells and B cells in peripheral tissues; these are best defined for T cells. These mechanisms include the following:

- *Anergy.* This term refers to functional inactivation (rather than death) of lymphocytes that is induced by encounter with antigens under certain conditions. As described previously, activation of T cells requires two signals: recognition of peptide antigen in association with MHC molecules on APCs, and a set of second costimulatory signals (e.g., through B7 molecules) provided by the APCs. If the costimulatory signals are not delivered, or if an inhibitory receptor on the T cell (rather than the costimulatory receptor) is engaged when the cell encounters self antigen, the T cell becomes anergic and cannot respond to the antigen. Because costimulatory molecules are expressed at low levels or not at all on APCs presenting self antigens, the encounter between autoreactive T cells and self antigens in tissues may result in anergy.

  It is believed that if mature B cells encounter self antigen in peripheral tissues, especially in the absence of specific helper T cells, these B cells become unable to respond to the antigen. B lymphocytes also express inhibitory receptors that may play a role in limiting their activation and preventing responses to self antigens.

- *Suppression by regulatory T cells.* A population of T cells called *regulatory T cells* functions to prevent immune reactions against self antigens. Regulatory T cells develop mainly in the thymus, but they also may be induced in peripheral lymphoid tissues. The best-defined regulatory T cells are CD4+ cells that express high levels of CD25, the α chain of the IL-2 receptor, and a transcription factor of the forkhead family, called FOXP3. Both IL-2 and FOXP3 are required for the development and maintenance of functional CD4+ regulatory T cells. Mutations in the *FOXP3* gene result in severe autoimmunity in humans and mice; in humans, these mutations are the cause of a systemic autoimmune disease called *IPEX* (an acronym for immune dysregulation, polyendocrinopathy, enteropathy, X-linked).

  The mechanisms by which regulatory T cells suppress immune responses are not fully defined, but their inhibitory activity may be mediated in part by the secretion of immunosuppressive cytokines such as IL-10 and TGF-β, which inhibit lymphocyte activation and effector functions. Regulatory T cells also express CTLA-4, which may bind to B7 molecules on APCs and reduce their ability to activate T cells via CD28.

- *Deletion by apoptosis.* T cells that recognize self antigens may receive signals that promote their death by apoptosis. Two mechanisms of deletion of mature T cells have been proposed, based mainly on studies in mice. It is postulated that if T cells recognize self antigens, they upregulate a pro-apoptotic member of the Bcl-2 family called Bim, which triggers apoptosis by the mitochondrial pathway (Chapter 2). Another mechanism of apoptosis involves the death receptor Fas (a member of the TNF receptor family), which can be engaged by its ligand coexpressed on the same or neighboring cells. The importance of this pathway of self-tolerance is illustrated by the discovery that *FAS* mutations are responsible for an autoimmune disease called the *autoimmune lymphoproliferative syndrome* (ALPS), characterized by lymphadenopathy and production of autoantibodies.

- Some self antigens are hidden (sequestered) from the immune system, because the tissues in which these antigens are located do not communicate with the blood and lymph. As a result, unless released into the circulation, these antigens fail to elicit immune responses and are essentially ignored by the immune system. This is believed to be the case for antigens that are only found in the testis, eye, and brain, all of which are called *immune-privileged sites* because antigens located in these sites tend to be shielded from the immune system. If the antigens are released from these tissues, for example, as a consequence of trauma or infection, the result may be an immune response that leads to prolonged tissue inflammation and injury. This is the postulated mechanism for post-traumatic orchitis and uveitis.

Mechanisms of Autoimmunity: General Principles

Now that we have summarized the principal mechanisms of self-tolerance, we can ask how these mechanisms might break down to give rise to pathologic autoimmunity.

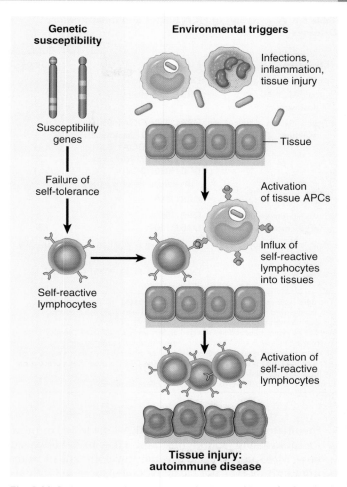

Fig. 5.20 Pathogenesis of autoimmunity. Autoimmunity results from multiple factors, including susceptibility genes that may interfere with self-tolerance and environmental triggers (such as infections, tissue injury, and inflammation) that promote lymphocyte entry into tissues, activation of self-reactive lymphocytes, and tissue damage.

Unfortunately, there are no simple answers to this question, and the underlying causes of most human autoimmune diseases remain to be determined. The best guess is that **breakdown of self-tolerance and development of autoimmunity result from the combined effects of susceptibility genes, which influence lymphocyte tolerance, and environmental factors, such as infections or tissue injury, that alter the display of and responses to self antigens** (Fig. 5.20).

Genetic Factors in Autoimmunity

Most autoimmune diseases are complex multigenic disorders. There is abundant evidence that inherited genes play a role in the development of autoimmune diseases.

- Autoimmune diseases have a tendency to run in families, and there is a greater incidence of the same disease in monozygotic than in dizygotic twins.
- Several autoimmune diseases are linked to the HLA locus, especially class II alleles (HLA-DR, HLA-DQ). The frequency of a disease in individuals with a particular HLA allele compared with those who do not inherit that allele, is called the *odds ratio* or *relative risk* (Table 5.8). The relative risk ranges from 3 or 4 for

Table 5.8 Association of HLA Alleles and Inflammatory Diseases

Disease	HLA Allele	Odds Ratio[†]
Rheumatoid arthritis (anti-CCP Ab positive)[‡]	DRB1, 1 SE allele[¶]	4
	DRB1, 2 SE alleles	12
Type 1 diabetes mellitus	DRB1*0301-DQA1*0501-DQB1*0201 haplotype	4
	DRB1*0401-DQA1*0301-DQB1*0302 haplotype	8
	DRB1*0301/0401 haplotype heterozygotes	35
Multiple sclerosis	DRB1*1501	3
Systemic lupus erythematosus	DRB1*0301	2
	DRB1*1501	1.3
Ankylosing spondylitis	B*27 (mainly B*2705 and B*2702)	100–200
Celiac disease	DQA1*0501-DQB1*0201 haplotype	7

[†]The odds ratio reflects approximate values of increased risk for the disease associated with the inheritance of particular HLA alleles. The data are from European-derived populations.
[‡]Anti-CCP Ab refers to antibodies directed against cyclic citrullinated peptides. Data are from patients who test positive for these antibodies in the serum.
[¶]SE refers to shared epitope, so called because the susceptibility alleles map to one region of the DRB1 protein (positions 70–74). The DRB1 protein is the product of the β chain of the HLA DR molecule.
Courtesy of Dr. Michelle Fernando, Imperial College London.

rheumatoid arthritis (RA) and HLA-DR4 to 100 or more for ankylosing spondylitis and HLA-B27. However, how *MHC* genes influence the development of autoimmunity is still not clear. Notably, most individuals with a susceptibility-related *MHC* allele never develop disease, and, conversely, individuals without the relevant *MHC* gene may get it. Expression of a particular *MHC* gene is therefore but one variable that contributes to autoimmunity.

• Genome-wide association (GWAS) studies and linkage studies in families are revealing many genetic polymorphisms that are associated with different autoimmune diseases (Table 5.9). Some of these genetic variants are disease-specific, but many of the associations are seen in multiple disorders, suggesting that they affect general mechanisms of immune regulation and self-tolerance. However, the mechanism by which most of these genetic variants contribute to particular autoimmune diseases is not established.

Role of Infections, Tissue Injury, and Other Environmental Factors

A variety of microbes, including bacteria, mycoplasmas, and viruses, have been implicated as triggers for autoimmunity. Microbes may induce autoimmune reactions by several mechanisms (Fig. 5.21):
• Microbial infections with resultant tissue necrosis and inflammation can stimulate expression of costimulatory molecules on APCs in the tissue, thus favoring a breakdown of T cell tolerance and subsequent T cell activation.
• Viruses and other microbes may share cross-reacting epitopes with self antigens, and as a result responses induced by the microbe may extend to self tissues, a phenomenon called *molecular mimicry*. The best example of a pathogenic immunologic cross-reaction is rheumatic heart disease, in which an antibody response against streptococci cross-targets cardiac antigens. It is not known if mimicry has a role in more common autoimmune diseases.

Recently, there has been great interest in the idea that the development of autoimmunity is influenced by the normal gut and skin *microbiome* (the diverse collection of commensal microbes that live with us in a symbiotic relationship). It is possible that different commensal microbes

Table 5.9 Selected Non–HLA Gene Variants Associated With Autoimmune Diseases

Putative Gene Involved	Diseases	Postulated Function of Encoded Protein and Role of Mutation/Polymorphism in Disease
Genes Involved in Immune Regulation		
PTPN22	RA, T1D, IBD	Protein tyrosine phosphatase; may affect signaling in lymphocytes and may alter negative selection or activation of self-reactive T cells
IL23R	IBD, PS, AS	Receptor for the T$_H$17-inducing cytokine IL-23; may alter differentiation of CD4+ T cells into pathogenic T$_H$17 effector cells
CTLA4	T1D, RA	Inhibits T-cell responses by terminating activation and promoting activity of regulatory T cells; may interfere with self-tolerance
IL2RA	MS, T1D	α chain of the receptor for IL-2, which is a growth and survival factor for activated and regulatory T cells; may affect development of effector cells and/or regulation of immune responses
Genes Involved in Immune Responses to Microbes		
NOD2	IBD	Cytoplasmic sensor of bacteria expressed in Paneth and other intestinal epithelial cells; may control resistance to gut commensal bacteria
ATG16	IBD	Involved in autophagy; possible role in defense against microbes and maintenance of epithelial barrier function
IRF5, IFIH1	SLE	Role in type I interferon production; type I IFN is involved in the pathogenesis of SLE (see text)

AS, Ankylosing spondylitis; IBD, inflammatory bowel disease; IFN, interferon; MS, multiple sclerosis; PS, psoriasis; RA, rheumatoid arthritis; SLE, systemic lupus erythematosus; T1D, type 1 diabetes.
The probable linkage of these genes with various autoimmune diseases has been defined by genome-wide association studies (GWAS) and other methods for studying disease-associated polymorphisms.
Adapted from Zenewicz LA, Abraham C, Flavell RA, et al: Unraveling the genetics of autoimmunity, Cell 140:791, 2010.

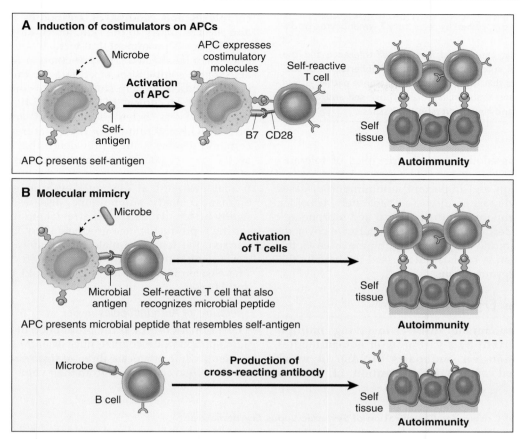

Fig. 5.21 Postulated role of infections in autoimmunity. Infections may promote activation of self-reactive lymphocytes by inducing the expression of costimulators (A), or microbial antigens may mimic self antigens and activate self-reactive lymphocytes as a cross-reaction (B).

affect the relative proportions of effector and regulatory T cells, and shape the host response toward or away from aberrant activation. However, it is still not clear which microbes contribute to specific diseases in humans, or if the microbiome can be manipulated to prevent or treat these disorders.

Adding to the complexity of the link between microbes and autoimmunity are recent observations suggesting that infections paradoxically protect individuals from some autoimmune diseases, notably type 1 diabetes, multiple sclerosis, and Crohn disease. The possible mechanisms underlying this effect are not understood.

In addition to infections, the display of tissue antigens also may be altered by a variety of environmental insults. As discussed later, *ultraviolet (UV) radiation* causes cell death and may lead to the exposure of nuclear antigens, which elicit pathologic immune responses in lupus; this mechanism is the proposed explanation for the association of lupus flares with exposure to sunlight. *Smoking* is a risk factor for RA, perhaps because it leads to chemical modification of self antigens. Local tissue injury for any reason may lead to the release of self antigens and autoimmune responses.

Finally, there is a strong *gender bias* of autoimmunity, with many of these diseases being more common in women than in men. The underlying mechanisms are not well understood, but may involve the effects of hormones and other factors.

An autoimmune response may itself promote further autoimmune attack. Tissue injury caused by an autoimmune response or any other cause may lead to exposure of self antigen epitopes that were previously concealed but are now presented to T cells in an immunogenic form. The activation of such autoreactive T cells is called *epitope spreading,* because the immune response spreads to epitopes that were not recognized initially. This is one of the mechanisms that may contribute to the chronicity of autoimmune diseases.

● SUMMARY

IMMUNOLOGIC TOLERANCE AND AUTOIMMUNITY

- Tolerance (unresponsiveness) to self antigens is a fundamental property of the immune system, and breakdown of tolerance is the basis of autoimmune diseases.
  - *Central tolerance:* immature T and B lymphocytes that recognize self antigens in the central (generative) lymphoid organs are killed by apoptosis; in the B-cell lineage, some of the self-reactive lymphocytes switch to new antigen receptors that are not self-reactive.
  - *Peripheral tolerance:* mature lymphocytes that recognize self antigens in peripheral tissues become functionally inactive

(anergic), are suppressed by regulatory T lymphocytes, or die by apoptosis.

- The factors that lead to a failure of self-tolerance and the development of autoimmunity include (1) inheritance of susceptibility genes that disrupt different tolerance pathways, and (2) infections and tissue injury that expose self antigens and activate APCs and lymphocytes in the tissues.

Having discussed the general principles of tolerance and autoimmunity, we proceed to a discussion of some of the most common and important autoimmune diseases. Although each disease is discussed separately, considerable overlap is apparent in their clinical and morphologic features and underlying pathogenesis. Here we cover the systemic autoimmune diseases; autoimmune diseases that affect single organ systems are discussed in chapters that deal with the relevant organs.

Systemic Lupus Erythematosus

SLE is an autoimmune disease involving multiple organs, characterized by a vast array of autoantibodies, particularly antinuclear antibodies (ANAs), in which injury is caused mainly by deposition of immune complexes and binding of antibodies to various cells and tissues. Injury to the skin, joints, kidney, and serosal membranes is prominent, but virtually every organ in the body may be affected. The presentation of SLE is so variable that a complex set of criteria for this disorder have been proposed, to help clinicians and for the design and assessment of clinical trials (Table 5.10). However, the disease is very heterogeneous, and any patient may present with any number of these features. SLE is a fairly common disease, with a prevalence that may be as high as 400 per 100,000 in certain populations. Although SLE often presents when a person is in the twenties or thirties, it may manifest at any age, even in early childhood. Similar to many autoimmune diseases, SLE predominantly affects women, with a female-to-male ratio of 9:1 for the reproductive age group of 17 to 55 years. By comparison, the female-to-male ratio is only 2:1 for disease developing during childhood or after 65 years of age. The prevalence of the disease is 2- to 3-fold higher in blacks and Hispanics than in whites.

Spectrum of Autoantibodies in SLE

The hallmark of SLE is the production of autoantibodies. Some antibodies recognize nuclear and cytoplasmic components, while others are directed against cell surface antigens of blood cells. Apart from their value in the diagnosis

Table 5.10 Revised Criteria for Classification of Systemic Lupus Erythematosus*

Criterion	Definition
Clinical Criteria	
Acute cutaneous lupus	Malar rash (fixed erythema, flat or raised, over the malar eminences), photosensitivity
Chronic cutaneous lupus	Discoid rash: erythematous raised patches with adherent keratotic scaling and follicular plugging
Nonscarring alopecia	Diffuse thinning or hair fragility in the absence of other causes
Oral or nasal ulcers	Oral or nasopharyngeal ulceration, usually painless
Joint disease	Nonerosive synovitis involving two or more peripheral joints, characterized by tenderness, swelling, or effusion
Serositis	Pleuritis (pleuritic pain or rub or evidence of pleural effusion), pericarditis
Renal disorder	Persistent proteinuria >0.5 g/24 hours, or red cell casts
Neurologic disorder	Seizures, psychosis, myelitis, or neuropathy, in the absence of offending drugs or other known causes
Hemolytic anemia	Hemolytic anemia
Leukopenia or lymphopenia	Leukopenia—<4.0 × 10^9 cells/L (4000 cells/mm^3) total on two or more occasions, *or* Lymphopenia—<1.5 × 10^9 cells/L (1500 cells/mm^3) on two or more occasions
Thrombocytopenia	Thrombocytopenia—<100 × 10^9 cells/L (100 × 10^3 cells/mm^3) in the absence of offending drugs and other conditions
Immunologic Criteria	
Antinuclear antibody (ANA)	Abnormal titer of antinuclear antibody by immunofluorescence
Anti-dsDNA antibody	Abnormal titer
Anti-Sm antibody	Presence of antibody to Sm nuclear antigen
Antiphospholipid antibody	Positive finding of antiphospholipid antibodies based on (1) an abnormal serum level of IgG or IgM anti-cardiolipin antibodies, (2) a positive test for lupus anticoagulant using a standard test, or (3) a false-positive serologic test for syphilis known to be positive for at least 6 months and confirmed by negative *Treponema pallidum* immobilization or fluorescent treponemal antibody absorption test
Low complement	Low C3, C4 or CH50
Direct Coombs test	Assay for anti-red cell antibody, in the absence of clinically evident hemolytic anemia

*This classification was initially proposed in 1997 by the American College of Rheumatology for the purpose of identifying patients in clinical studies. It has been updated in 2012 by the Systemic Lupus International Collaborating Clinics. A patient is classified as having SLE if four of the clinical and immunologic criteria are present at any time (not necessarily concurrently), including at least one clinical and one immunologic criterion. Some details have been omitted from the table.
Modified from Petri M, Orbai AM, Alarcón GS, et al: Derivation and validation of the Systemic Lupus International Collaborating Clinics classification criteria for systemic lupus erythematosus. *Arthritis Rheum* 64:2677, 2012.

Table 5.11 Autoantibodies in Systemic Autoimmune Diseases

Disease	Specificity of Autoantibody	% Positive	Disease Associations
Systemic lupus erythematosus (SLE)	Double-stranded DNA	40–60	Nephritis; specific for SLE
	U1-RNP	30–40	
	Smith (Sm) antigen (core protein of small RNP particles)	20–30	Specific for SLE
	Ro (SS-A) nucleoprotein	30–50	Congenital heart block; neonatal lupus
	Phospholipid-protein complexes (anti-PL)	30–40	Anti-phospholipid syndrome (in ~10% of SLE patients)
	Multiple nuclear antigens ("generic ANAs")	95–100	Found in other autoimmune diseases, not specific
Systemic sclerosis	DNA topoisomerase I	30–70	Diffuse skin disease, lung disease; specific for systemic sclerosis
	Centromeric proteins (CENPs) A, B, C	20–40	Limited skin disease, ischemic digital loss, pulmonary hypertension
	RNA polymerase III	15–20	Acute onset, scleroderma renal crisis, cancer
Sjögren syndrome	Ro/SS-A	75	More sensitive
	La/SS-B	50	More specific
Autoimmune myositis	Histidyl aminoacyl-tRNA synthetase, Jo1	25	Interstitial lung disease, Raynaud phenomenon
	Mi-2 nuclear antigen	5–10	Dermatomyositis, skin rash
	MDA5 (cytoplasmic receptor for viral RNA)	20–35 (Japanese)	Vascular skin lesions, interstitial lung disease
	TIF1γ nuclear protein	15–20	Dermatomyositis, cancer
Rheumatoid arthritis	CCP (cyclic citrullinated peptides); various citrullinated proteins	60–80	Specific for rheumatoid arthritis
	Rheumatoid factor	60–70	Not specific

"Generic" anti-nuclear antibodies (ANAs), which may react against many nuclear antigens, are positive in a large fraction of patients with SLE but also are positive in other autoimmune diseases. % *positive* refers to the approximate % of patients who test positive for each antibody.
Table compiled with the assistance of Dr. Antony Rosen, Johns Hopkins University, and Dr. Andrew Gross, University of California San Francisco.

and management of patients with SLE, these autoantibodies are of major pathogenic significance, as, for example, in the immune complex–mediated glomerulonephritis so typical of this disease. Autoantibodies also are found in other autoimmune diseases, many of which tend to be associated with specific types of autoantibodies (Table 5.11).

Anti-Nuclear Antibodies

ANAs can be grouped into four categories: (1) antibodies to DNA, (2) antibodies to histones, (3) antibodies to nonhistone proteins bound to RNA, and (4) antibodies to nucleolar antigens. The most widely used method for detecting ANAs is indirect immunofluorescence, which can identify antibodies that bind to a variety of nuclear antigens, including DNA, RNA, and proteins (collectively called *generic ANAs*). The pattern of nuclear fluorescence suggests the type of antibody present in the patient's serum. Several basic patterns are recognized (Fig. 5.22):

- A *homogeneous* or *diffuse* staining pattern usually reflects the presence of antibodies to chromatin, histones, and, occasionally, double-stranded DNA.
- A *rim* or *peripheral* staining pattern is most often indicative of antibodies to double-stranded DNA and sometimes to nuclear envelope proteins.
- A *centromeric* pattern is indicative of antibodies specific for centromeres. This pattern is often observed in patients with systemic sclerosis.
- A *speckled pattern* refers to the presence of uniform or variable-sized speckles. This is one of the most commonly observed patterns of fluorescence and therefore the least specific. It reflects the presence of antibodies to non-DNA nuclear constituents such as Sm antigen, ribonucleoprotein, and SS-A and SS-B reactive antigens.

- A *nucleolar* pattern refers to the presence of a few discrete spots of fluorescence within the nucleus and represents antibodies to RNA. This pattern is reported most often in patients with systemic sclerosis.

The fluorescence patterns are not absolutely specific for the type of antibody, and because many autoantibodies may be present, combinations of patterns are frequent. Attempts are ongoing to replace microscopic assays with quantitative assays for antibodies against specific nuclear and other antigens. Indeed, antibodies to double-stranded DNA and the so-called "Smith (Sm) antigen" can be detected by more quantitative assays and are virtually diagnostic of SLE. Nevertheless, the staining pattern has diagnostic value, and the test remains in use.

Other Autoantibodies

In addition to ANAs, lupus patients have a host of other autoantibodies. Some are directed against blood cells, such as red cells, platelets, and lymphocytes. *Anti-phospholipid antibodies* are present in 30% to 40% of lupus patients. They are actually directed against epitopes of various plasma proteins that are revealed when the proteins are in complex with phospholipids. Antibodies against the phospholipid–β_2-glycoprotein complex also bind to cardiolipin antigen, used in syphilis serology, and therefore lupus patients may have a false-positive test result for syphilis. Because these antibodies bind to phospholipids, they may prolong the partial thromboplastin time, an in vitro clotting test that requires phospholipids. Therefore, these antibodies are sometimes referred to as *lupus anti-coagulant*. Despite the observed clotting delays in vitro, patients with anti-phospholipid antibodies have complications related to excessive clotting (a hypercoagulable state), such as thrombosis (Chapter 4).

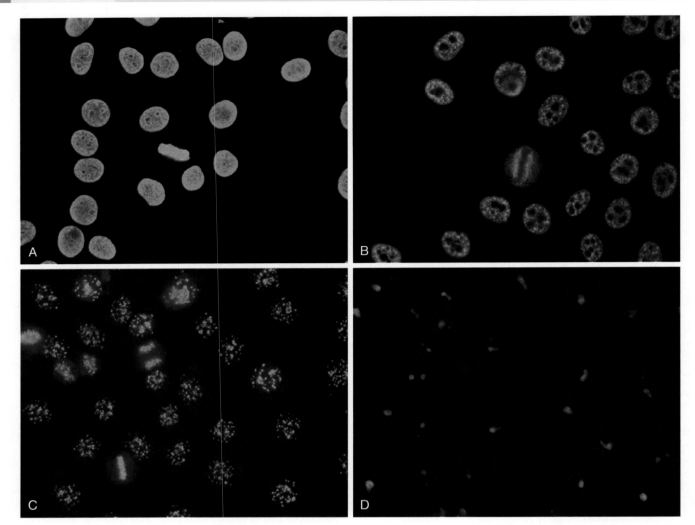

Fig. 5.22 Staining patterns of anti-nuclear antibodies. (A) Homogeneous or diffuse staining of nuclei is typical of antibodies reactive with dsDNA, nucleosomes, and histones, and is common in SLE. (B) A speckled pattern is seen with antibodies against various nuclear antigens, including Sm and RNPs. (C) The pattern of staining of anti-centromere antibodies is seen in some cases of systemic sclerosis, Sjögren syndrome, and other diseases. (D) A nucleolar pattern is typical of antibodies against nucleolar proteins. *(From Wiik AS, Høier-Madsen M, Forslid J, et al: Antinuclear antibodies: a contemporary nomenclature using HEp-2 cells. J Autoimm 35:276, 2010.)*

Pathogenesis

The fundamental defect in SLE is a failure of the mechanisms that maintain self-tolerance. Although what causes this failure of self-tolerance remains unknown, as is true of most autoimmune diseases, both genetic and environmental factors play a role.

Genetic Factors

Many lines of evidence support a genetic predisposition to SLE.

- *Familial association.* Family members have an increased risk for the development of SLE, and up to 20% of unaffected first-degree relatives have autoantibodies. There is a higher rate of concordance in monozygotic twins (25%) than in dizygotic twins (1%–3%).
- *HLA association.* The odds ratio (relative risk) for persons with HLA-DR2 or HLA-DR3 is 2 to 3, and if both haplotypes are present, the risk is about 5.

- *Other genes.* Genetic deficiencies of classical pathway complement proteins, especially C1q, C2, or C4, are seen in about 10% of patients with SLE. The complement deficiencies may result in defective clearance of immune complexes and apoptotic cells, and failure of B-cell tolerance. A polymorphism in the inhibitory Fc receptor, FcγRIIb, has been described in some patients; this may contribute to inadequate control of B-cell activation. Additional genes have been implicated by genome-wide association studies, but their contribution to the development of the disease remains unclear.

Environmental Factors

There are many indications that environmental factors also are involved in the pathogenesis of SLE.

- Exposure to UV light exacerbates the disease in many individuals. UV irradiation may induce apoptosis and also may alter DNA and make it immunogenic, perhaps by enhancing its recognition by TLRs. In addition, UV light may modulate the immune response, for example, by stimulating keratinocytes to produce IL-1, a cytokine that promotes inflammation.

- The gender bias of SLE is partly attributable to actions of sex hormones and partly related to genes on the X chromosome, independent of hormone effects.
- Drugs such as hydralazine, procainamide, and D-penicillamine can induce an SLE-like disorder.

Immunologic Factors

Recent studies in animal models and patients have revealed several immunologic aberrations that collectively may result in the persistent and uncontrolled activation of self-reactive lymphocytes.

- Failure of self-tolerance in B cells results from defective elimination of self-reactive B cells in the bone marrow or defects in peripheral tolerance mechanisms.
- CD4+ helper T cells specific for nucleosomal antigens also escape tolerance and contribute to the production of high-affinity pathogenic autoantibodies. The autoantibodies in SLE show characteristics of T cell–dependent antibodies produced in germinal centers, and increased numbers of follicular helper T cells have been detected in the blood of SLE patients.
- Type I interferons. Blood cells show a striking molecular signature that indicates exposure to interferon-α (IFN-α), a type I interferon that is produced mainly by plasmacytoid DCs. Some studies have shown that such cells from SLE patients produce abnormally large amounts of IFN-α.
- TLR signals. Studies in animal models have shown that TLRs that recognize DNA and RNA, notably the DNA-recognizing TLR9 and the RNA-recognizing TLR7, produce signals that activate B cells specific for self nuclear antigens.
- Other cytokines that may play a role in unregulated B-cell activation include the TNF family member BAFF, which promotes survival of B cells. In some patients and animal models, increased production of BAFF has been reported, and this has led to modest success of an antibody that blocks BAFF as a therapy for SLE.

A Model for the Pathogenesis of SLE

It is clear from this discussion that the immunologic abnormalities in SLE—both documented and postulated—are varied and complex. Nevertheless, an attempt can be made to synthesize results from human studies and animal models into a hypothetical model of the pathogenesis of SLE (Fig. 5.23). UV irradiation and other environmental insults lead to the apoptosis of cells. Inadequate clearance of the nuclei of these cells results in a large burden of nuclear antigens. Underlying abnormalities in B lymphocytes and T lymphocytes are responsible for defective tolerance, because of which self-reactive lymphocytes survive and remain functional. These lymphocytes are stimulated by nuclear self antigens, and antibodies are produced against the antigens. Complexes of the antigens and antibodies bind to Fc receptors on B cells and dendritic cells, and may be internalized. The nucleic acid components engage TLRs and stimulate B cells to produce more autoantibodies. TLR stimuli also activate dendritic cells to

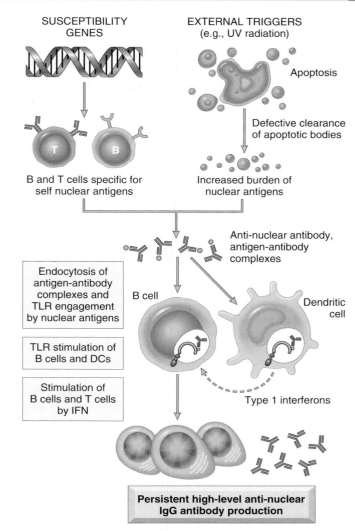

Fig. 5.23 Model for the pathogenesis of systemic lupus erythematosus. In this hypothetical model, susceptibility genes interfere with the maintenance of self-tolerance, and external triggers lead to persistence of nuclear antigens. The result is an antibody response against self nuclear antigens, which is amplified by the action of nucleic acids on dendritic cells (DCs) and B cells, and the production of type I interferons. *TLRs,* Toll-like receptors.

produce interferons and other cytokines, which further enhance the immune response and cause more apoptosis. The net result is a cycle of antigen release and immune activation resulting in the production of high-affinity autoantibodies.

Mechanisms of Tissue Injury

Different autoantibodies are the cause of most of the lesions of SLE.

- **Most of the systemic lesions are caused by immune complexes (type III hypersensitivity).** DNA-anti-DNA complexes can be detected in the glomeruli and small blood vessels. Low levels of serum complement (secondary to consumption of complement proteins) and granular deposits of complement and immunoglobulins in the glomeruli further support the immune complex nature of the disease. T cell infiltrates are also frequently seen in the kidneys, but the role of these cells in tissue damage is not established.

- **Autoantibodies of different specificities contribute to the pathology and clinical manifestations of SLE (type II hypersensitivity).** Autoantibodies specific for red blood cells, white blood cells, and platelets opsonize these cells and promote their phagocytosis, resulting in cytopenias. There is no evidence that ANAs, which are involved in immune complex formation, can penetrate intact cells. If cell nuclei are exposed, however, the ANAs can bind to them. In tissues, nuclei of damaged cells react with ANAs, lose their chromatin pattern, and become homogeneous, producing so-called "LE bodies" or hematoxylin bodies. Related to this phenomenon are *LE cells,* which are readily seen when blood is agitated in vitro. An LE cell is a phagocyte (neutrophil or macrophage) that has engulfed the denatured nucleus of an injured cell. The demonstration of LE cells in vitro was used in the past as a test for SLE. With new techniques for detection of ANAs, however, this test is now only of historic interest. Sometimes, LE cells are found in pericardial or pleural effusions in patients.
- *Anti-phospholipid antibody syndrome.* Patients with anti-phospholipid antibodies may develop venous and arterial thromboses, which may be associated with recurrent spontaneous miscarriages and focal cerebral or ocular ischemia. This constellation of clinical features, in association with lupus, is referred to as the *secondary anti-phospholipid antibody syndrome.* The mechanisms of thrombosis are not defined, and antibodies against clotting factors, platelets, and endothelial cells have all been proposed as being responsible for thrombosis (Chapter 4). Some patients develop these autoantibodies and the clinical syndrome without associated SLE. They are said to have the *primary anti-phospholipid antibody syndrome* (Chapter 4).
- The *neuropsychiatric manifestations* of SLE have been attributed to antibodies that cross the blood-brain barrier and react with neurons or receptors for various neurotransmitters. However, this is not established in all cases, and mechanisms involving other immune factors, such as cytokines, also may underlie the cognitive dysfunction and other CNS abnormalities that are associated with SLE.

MORPHOLOGY

The morphologic changes in SLE are extremely variable. The frequency of individual organ involvement is shown in Table 5.12. The most characteristic lesions result from immune complex deposition in blood vessels, kidneys, connective tissue, and skin.

Blood Vessels. An acute necrotizing vasculitis involving capillaries, small arteries, and arterioles may be present in any tissue. The arteritis leads to fibrinoid necrosis of the vessel walls. In chronic stages, vessels undergo fibrous thickening with luminal narrowing.

Kidney. Up to 50% of SLE patients have clinically significant renal involvement, and the kidney virtually always shows evidence of abnormality if examined by electron microscopy and immunofluorescence. Renal involvement takes a number of forms, all

Table 5.12 Clinical and Pathologic Manifestations of Systemic Lupus Erythematosus

Clinical Manifestation	Prevalence in Patients (%)*
Hematologic	100
Arthritis, arthralgia, or myalgia	80–90
Skin	85
Fever	55–85
Fatigue	80–100
Weight loss	60
Renal	50–70
Neuropsychiatric	25–35
Pleuritis	45
Pericarditis	25
Gastrointestinal	20
Raynaud phenomenon	15–40
Ocular	5–15
Peripheral neuropathy	15

*Percentages are approximate and may vary with age, ethnicity, and other factors. Table compiled with the assistance of Dr. Meenakshi Jolly, Rush Medical Center, Chicago.

of which are associated with the deposition of immune complexes within the glomeruli. According to the currently accepted classification, six patterns of glomerular disease are recognized. It should be noted that there is overlap within these classes and that lesions may evolve from one class to another over time. Thus, the exact percentage of patients with each of the six classes of lesions is difficult to determine. Suffice it to say that class I is the least common and class IV is the most common pattern.

- **Minimal mesangial lupus nephritis** (class I) is very uncommon, and is characterized by immune complex deposition in the mesangium, identified by immunofluorescence and by electron microscopy, but without structural changes by light microscopy.
- **Mesangial proliferative lupus nephritis** (class II) is characterized by mesangial cell proliferation, often accompanied by accumulation of mesangial matrix, and granular mesangial deposits of immunoglobulin and complement without involvement of glomerular capillaries.
- **Focal lupus nephritis** (class III) is defined by involvement of fewer than 50% of all glomeruli. The lesions may be segmental (affecting only a portion of the glomerulus) or global (involving the entire glomerulus). Affected glomeruli may exhibit swelling and proliferation of endothelial and mesangial cells associated with leukocyte accumulation, capillary necrosis, and hyaline thrombi. Often, there also is extracapillary proliferation associated with focal necrosis and crescent formation (Fig. 5.24A). The clinical presentation ranges from mild hematuria and proteinuria to acute renal insufficiency. Red blood cell casts in the urine are common when the disease is active. Some patients progress to diffuse glomerulonephritis. The active (or proliferative) inflammatory lesions can heal completely or lead to chronic global or segmental glomerular scarring.
- **Diffuse lupus nephritis** (class IV) is the most common and severe form of lupus nephritis. The lesions are identical to those in class III, but differ in extent; in diffuse lupus

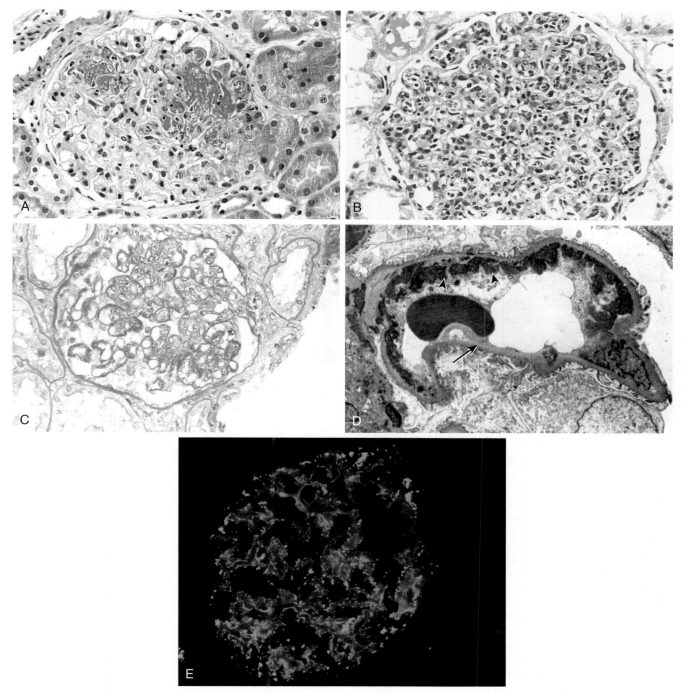

Fig. 5.24 Lupus nephritis. (A) Focal proliferative glomerulonephritis, with two focal necrotizing lesions at the 11 o'clock and 2 o'clock positions (H&E stain). Extracapillary proliferation is not prominent in this case. (B) Diffuse proliferative glomerulonephritis. Note the marked increase in cellularity throughout the glomerulus (H&E stain). (C) Lupus nephritis showing a glomerulus with several "wire-loop" lesions representing extensive subendothelial deposits of immune complexes (periodic acid-Schiff stain). (D) Electron micrograph of a renal glomerular capillary loop from a patient with SLE nephritis. Subendothelial dense deposits *(arrowheads)* on basement membrane *(arrow)* correspond to "wire loops" seen by light microscopy. (E) Deposition of IgG antibody in a granular pattern, detected by immunofluorescence. *(A to C, Courtesy of Dr. Helmut Rennke, Department of Pathology, Brigham and Women's Hospital, Boston, Massachusetts. D, Courtesy of Dr. Edwin Eigenbrodt, Department of Pathology, University of Texas, Southwestern Medical School, Dallas, Texas. E, Courtesy of Dr. Jean Olson, Department of Pathology, University of California, San Francisco, California.)*

nephritis, half or more of the glomeruli are affected. Involved glomeruli show proliferation of endothelial, mesangial, and epithelial cells (see Fig. 5.24B), with the latter producing cellular crescents that fill Bowman's space. Subendothelial immune complex deposits may create a circumferential thickening of the capillary wall, forming "wire-loop" structures on light microscopy (see Fig. 5.24C). Immune complexes can be readily detected by electron microscopy (see Fig. 5.24D) and immunofluorescence (see Fig. 5.24E). Lesions may progress to scarring of glomeruli. Patients with diffuse glomerulonephritis are usually symptomatic, showing hematuria as well as proteinuria. Hypertension and mild to severe renal insufficiency also are common.

- **Membranous lupus nephritis** (class V) is characterized by diffuse thickening of the capillary walls due to deposition of subepithelial immune complexes, similar to idiopathic membranous nephropathy, described in Chapter 14. The immune complexes are usually accompanied by increased production of basement membrane-like material, resulting in "holes" and "spikes" on silver stain. This lesion is usually accompanied by severe proteinuria or nephrotic syndrome, and may occur concurrently with focal or diffuse lupus nephritis.
- **Advanced sclerosing lupus nephritis** (class VI) is characterized by sclerosis of more than 90% of the glomeruli, and represents end-stage renal disease.

Changes in the **interstitium and tubules** are frequently present. Rarely, tubulointerstitial lesions may be the dominant abnormality. Discrete immune complexes similar to those in glomeruli are present in the tubular or peritubular capillary basement membranes in many lupus nephritis patients. Sometimes, there are well-organized B-cell follicles in the interstitium, associated with plasma cells that may be sources of autoantibodies.

Skin. Characteristic erythema affects the face along the bridge of the nose and cheeks (the **butterfly rash**) in approximately 50% of patients, but a similar rash also may be seen on the extremities and trunk. Urticaria, bullae, maculopapular lesions, and ulcerations also occur. Exposure to sunlight incites or accentuates the erythema. Histologically the involved areas show vacuolar degeneration of the basal layer of the epidermis (Fig. 5.25A). In the dermis, there is variable edema and perivascular inflammation. Vasculitis with fibrinoid necrosis may be prominent. Immunofluorescence microscopy shows deposits of immunoglobulin and complement along the dermoepidermal junction (Fig. 5.25B); these also may be present in uninvolved skin. This finding is not diagnostic of SLE and is sometimes seen in scleroderma and dermatomyositis.

Joints. Joint involvement is typically a nonerosive synovitis with little deformity, which contrasts with rheumatoid arthritis.

Central Nervous System. Although it was suggested in the past that the neuropsychiatric manifestations of SLE may be due to acute vasculitis, in histologic studies of the nervous system in such patients, significant vasculitis is rarely present. Instead, noninflammatory occlusion of small vessels by intimal proliferation is sometimes noted, which may be due to endothelial damage caused by autoantibodies or immune complexes.

Pericarditis and Other Serosal Cavity Involvement. Inflammation of the serosal lining membranes may be acute, subacute, or chronic. During the acute phase, the mesothelial surfaces are sometimes covered with fibrinous exudate. Later they become thickened, opaque, and coated with shaggy fibrous

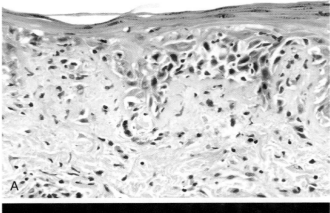

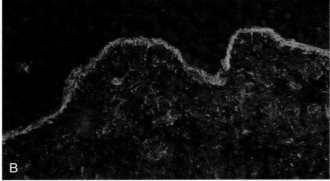

Fig. 5.25 Systemic lupus erythematosus involving the skin. (A) An H&E-stained section shows liquefactive degeneration of the basal layer of the epidermis and edema at the dermoepidermal junction. (B) An immunofluorescence micrograph stained for IgG reveals deposits of Ig along the dermoepidermal junction. (A, *Courtesy of Dr. Jag Bhawan, Boston University School of Medicine, Boston, Massachusetts. B, Courtesy of Dr. Richard Sontheimer, Department of Dermatology, University of Texas Southwestern Medical School, Dallas, Texas.*)

tissue that may lead to partial or total obliteration of the serosal cavity. Pleural and pericardial effusions may be present.

Cardiovascular system involvement may manifest as damage to any layer of the heart. Symptomatic or asymptomatic pericardial involvement is present in up to 50% of patients. Myocarditis is less common and may cause resting tachycardia and electrocardiographic abnormalities. **Valvular** (so-called "Libman-Sacks") **endocarditis** was more common prior to the widespread use of steroids. This sterile endocarditis takes the form of single or multiple 1- to 3-mm verrucous deposits, which may form on either surface of any heart valve, distinctively on either surface of the leaflets (Fig. 5.26). By comparison, the vegetations in infective endocarditis are larger, while those in rheumatic heart disease (Chapter 11) are smaller and confined to the lines of closure of the valve leaflets.

An increasing number of patients are affected by **coronary artery disease** manifesting as angina or myocardial infarction. This complication may be seen in young patients with long-standing disease, and is especially prevalent in those who have been treated with corticosteroids. The pathogenesis of accelerated coronary atherosclerosis is unclear but is probably multifactorial. Risk factors for atherosclerosis, including hypertension, obesity, and hyperlipidemia, are more commonly present in SLE patients than in the population at large. In addition, immune

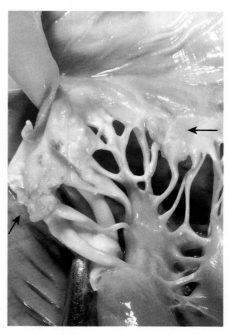

Fig. 5.26 Libman-Sacks endocarditis of the mitral valve in lupus erythematosus. The vegetations attached to the margin of the thickened valve leaflet are indicated by *arrows*. *(Courtesy of Dr. Fred Schoen, Department of Pathology, Brigham and Women's Hospital, Boston, Massachusetts.)*

complexes and anti-phospholipid antibodies may cause endothelial damage and promote atherosclerosis.

Spleen. Splenomegaly, capsular thickening, and follicular hyperplasia are common features. Central penicilliary arteries may show concentric intimal and smooth muscle cell hyperplasia, producing so-called **onion-skin lesions.**

Lungs. In addition to pleuritis and accompanying pleural effusions, some cases are complicated by chronic interstitial fibrosis and secondary pulmonary hypertension.

Other Organs and Tissues. LE, or hematoxylin, bodies in the bone marrow or other organs are strongly indicative of SLE. Lymph nodes may be enlarged due to hyperplasia of B cell follicles or even demonstrate necrotizing lymphadenitis due to vasculitis.

Clinical Features

SLE is a highly variable multisystem disease, and its diagnosis relies on a constellation of clinical, serologic, and morphologic findings (see Table 5.10). It may be acute or insidious in its onset. Often, the patient is a young woman with some or all of the following features: a butterfly rash on the face; fever; pain without deformity in one or more joints; pleuritic chest pain; and photosensitivity. In many patients, however, the presentation is subtle and puzzling, taking forms such as fever of unknown origin, abnormal urinary findings, or joint disease masquerading as rheumatoid arthritis or rheumatic fever. Generic ANAs, detected by immunofluorescence assays, are found in virtually 100% of patients, but these are not specific for SLE. Renal involvement may produce a variety of findings, including hematuria, red blood cell casts, proteinuria, and nephrotic syndrome (Chapter 14). Anemia or thrombocytopenia are

presenting manifestations in some patients and may be dominant clinical problems. In others, neuropsychiatric manifestations including psychosis or convulsions, or coronary artery disease may be prominent. Infections also are common, presumably because of the immune dysfunction that underlies SLE as well as treatment with immunosuppressive drugs.

The course of SLE is variable and unpredictable. Rare acute cases result in death within weeks to months. More often, with appropriate therapy, SLE follows a relapsing and remitting course over a period of years or decades. During acute flares, increased formation of immune complexes results in complement activation, often leading to hypocomplementemia. Disease flares are usually treated with corticosteroids or other immunosuppressive drugs. Even without therapy, in some patients the disease runs an indolent course for years with relatively mild manifestations, such as skin changes and mild hematuria. The overall 5-year and 10-year survivals are approximately 90% and 80%, respectively. The most common causes of death are renal failure and intercurrent infections. Coronary artery disease also is becoming an important cause of death. Patients treated with steroids and immunosuppressive drugs incur the usual risks associated with such therapy.

As mentioned earlier, involvement of skin along with multisystem disease is fairly common in SLE. The following sections describe two syndromes in which the cutaneous involvement is the exclusive or most prominent feature.

Chronic Discoid Lupus Erythematosus

Chronic discoid lupus erythematosus is a disease in which the skin manifestations may mimic SLE, but systemic manifestations are rare. It is characterized by the presence of skin plaques, most often on the face and scalp, showing varying degrees of edema, erythema, scaliness, follicular plugging, and skin atrophy surrounded by an elevated erythematous border. It progresses to SLE in 5% to 10% of patients, usually after many years. Conversely, some patients with SLE may have prominent discoid lesions in the skin. Approximately 35% of patients have a positive test for generic ANAs, but antibodies to double-stranded DNA are rarely present. Immunofluorescence studies of skin biopsy specimens show deposition of immunoglobulin and C3 at the dermoepidermal junction similar to that in SLE.

The term *subacute cutaneous lupus erythematosus* refers to a group intermediate between SLE and lupus erythematosus localized only to skin. The skin rash in this disease tends to be widespread and superficial. Most patients have mild systemic symptoms similar to those in SLE. There is a strong association with antibodies to the SS-A antigen and with the HLA-DR3 genotype.

Drug-Induced Lupus Erythematosus

An SLE-like syndrome may develop in patients receiving a variety of drugs, including hydralazine, procainamide, isoniazid, and D-penicillamine. Surprisingly, anti-TNF therapy, which is effective in rheumatoid arthritis and other autoimmune diseases, also can cause drug-induced lupus. Many of these drugs are associated with the development of ANAs, especially antibodies specific for histones. The disease remits after withdrawal of the offending drug.

SUMMARY

SYSTEMIC LUPUS ERYTHEMATOSUS

- SLE is a systemic autoimmune disease caused by autoantibodies produced against numerous self antigens and the formation of immune complexes.
- The major autoantibodies, and the ones responsible for the formation of circulating immune complexes, are directed against nuclear antigens. Other autoantibodies react with red blood cells, platelets, and various phospholipid-proteins complexes.
- Disease manifestations include nephritis, skin lesions, and arthritis (caused by the deposition of immune complexes), hematologic abnormalities (caused by antibodies against red cells, white cells and platelets) and neurologic abnormalities (caused by obscure mechanisms).
- The underlying cause of the breakdown in self-tolerance in SLE is unknown; non-exclusive possiblities include excessive generation or persistence of nuclear antigens, in individuals with inherited susceptibility genes, and environmental triggers (e.g., UV irradiation, which results in cellular apoptosis and release of nuclear antigens).

Rheumatoid Arthritis

Rheumatoid arthritis is an autoimmune disease that affects primarily the joints but also may involve extraarticular tissues such as the skin, blood vessels, lungs, and heart. Because the principal manifestations of the disease are in the joints, it is discussed in Chapter 21.

Sjögren Syndrome

Sjögren syndrome is a chronic disease characterized by dry eyes (*keratoconjunctivitis sicca*) **and dry mouth** (*xerostomia*) **resulting from immunologically mediated destruction of the lacrimal and salivary glands.** It occurs as an isolated disorder (primary form), also known as the *sicca syndrome,* or more often in association with another autoimmune disease (secondary form). Rheumatoid arthritis is the most common associated disorder, while other patients have SLE, polymyositis, scleroderma, vasculitis, mixed connective tissue disease, or autoimmune thyroid disease.

The lacrimal and salivary glands characteristically show dense lymphocytic infiltration consisting mainly of activated CD4+ helper T cells and some B cells, including plasma cells. Serologic studies frequently reveal autoantibodies. Antibodies against two ribonucleoprotein antigens, SS-A (Ro) and SS-B (La) (see Table 5.11), can be detected in as many as 90% of patients by sensitive techniques. High titers of antibodies to SS-A are associated with early disease onset, longer disease duration, and extraglandular manifestations, such as cutaneous vasculitis and nephritis. These autoantibodies also are present in a smaller percentage of patients with SLE and hence are not diagnostic of Sjögren syndrome. In addition, about 75% of patients have rheumatoid factor (an antibody reactive with self IgG), and 50% to 80% of patients have ANAs.

Pathogenesis

The pathogenesis of Sjögren syndrome remains obscure, but the pathology and serology, as well as an association, albeit weak, with HLA alleles, all point to activation of autoreactive T cells and B cells. The initiating trigger may be a viral infection of the salivary glands, which causes local cell death and release of tissue self antigens. In genetically susceptible individuals, CD4+ T cells and B cells specific for these self antigens may escape tolerance and participate in immune reactions that lead to tissue damage and, eventually, fibrosis. However, the role of particular cytokines or T cell subsets, and the nature of the autoantigens recognized by these lymphocytes, remain mysterious.

MORPHOLOGY

Lacrimal and salivary glands are the major targets of the disease, but other exocrine glands, including those lining the respiratory and gastrointestinal tracts and the vagina, also may be involved. The earliest histologic finding in both the major and the minor salivary glands is periductal and perivascular lymphocytic infiltration. Eventually the lymphocytic infiltrate becomes extensive (Fig. 5.27), and in the larger salivary glands, lymphoid follicles with germinal centers may be seen. The epithelial cells lining the ducts may become hyperplastic and obstruct the ducts. Later there is atrophy of the acini, fibrosis, and hyalinization; still later in the course, the atrophic parenchyma may be replaced with fat. In some cases, the lymphoid infiltrate may be so intense as to give the appearance of a lymphoma. Indeed, these patients are at high risk for development of B-cell lymphomas of the salivary gland and other extranodal sites (Chapter 12). The histologic findings are not specific or diagnostic and may be mimicked by chronic sialdenitis caused by ductal obstruction due to calculi.

The lack of tears leads to drying of the corneal epithelium, which becomes inflamed, eroded, and ulcerated; the oral mucosa may atrophy, with inflammatory fissuring and ulceration; and dryness and crusting of the nose may lead to ulcerations and even perforation of the nasal septum.

Clinical Features

Sjögren syndrome occurs most commonly in women between 50 and 60 years of age. As might be expected, symptoms result from inflammatory destruction of the exocrine glands. Keratoconjunctivitis produces blurred vision, burning, and itching, and thick secretions that accumulate in the conjunctival sac. Xerostomia results in difficulty in swallowing solid foods, a decrease in taste, cracks and fissures in the mouth, and dryness of the buccal mucosa. Parotid gland enlargement is present in half the patients; dryness of the nasal mucosa, epistaxis, recurrent bronchitis, and pneumonitis are other symptoms. Manifestations of extraglandular disease are seen in one third of patients and include synovitis, pulmonary fibrosis, and peripheral neuropathy. In contrast to SLE, glomerular lesions are rare in Sjögren syndrome. Defects of tubular function, however, including renal tubular acidosis, uricosuria, and phosphaturia, often are seen and are associated with tubulointerstitial nephritis (Chapter 14). About 60% of patients have another accompanying autoimmune disorder, such as rheumatoid arthritis.

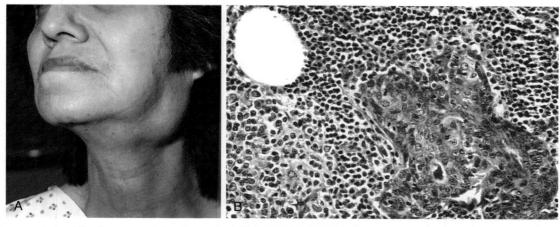

Fig. 5.27 Sjögren syndrome. (A) Enlargement of the salivary gland. (B) Intense lymphocytic and plasma cell infiltration with ductal epithelial hyperplasia in a salivary gland. *(A, Courtesy of Dr. Richard Sontheimer, Department of Dermatology, University of Texas Southwestern Medical School, Dallas, Texas. B, Courtesy of Dr. Dennis Burns, Department of Pathology, University of Texas Southwestern Medical School, Dallas, Texas.)*

SUMMARY

SJÖGREN SYNDROME

- Sjögren syndrome is an inflammatory disease that primarily affects the salivary and lacrimal glands, causing dryness of the mouth and eyes.
- The disease is believed to be caused by an autoimmune T-cell reaction against an unknown self antigen expressed in these glands, or immune reactions against the antigens of a virus that infects the tissues.

Systemic Sclerosis (Scleroderma)

Systemic sclerosis is an immunologic disorder characterized by excessive fibrosis in multiple tissues, obliterative vascular disease, and evidence of autoimmunity, mainly the production of multiple autoantibodies. Although the term *scleroderma* is ingrained in clinical medicine, the name *systemic sclerosis* is preferred because excessive fibrosis is seen in multiple organs. Cutaneous involvement is the usual presenting manifestation and eventually appears in approximately 95% of cases, but it is the visceral involvement—of the gastrointestinal tract, lungs, kidneys, heart, and skeletal muscles—that is responsible for most of the morbidity and mortality. Disease limited to the skin is also called *localized scleroderma.*

Systemic sclerosis is classified into two groups on the basis of its course:

- *Diffuse systemic sclerosis,* characterized by initial widespread skin involvement, with rapid progression and early visceral involvement
- *Limited systemic sclerosis,* with relatively mild skin involvement, often confined to the fingers and face. Involvement of the viscera occurs late, so the disease generally follows a fairly benign course. This presentation also is called *CREST syndrome* because of its frequent features of calcinosis, Raynaud phenomenon, esophageal dysmotility, sclerodactyly, and telangiectasia.

Pathogenesis

The cause of systemic sclerosis is not known, but **the disease likely results from three interrelated processes—autoimmune responses, vascular damage, and collagen deposition** (Fig. 5.28).

- *Autoimmunity.* It is proposed that CD4+ T cells responding to an as yet unidentified antigen accumulate in the skin and release cytokines that activate inflammatory cells and fibroblasts. Although inflammatory infiltrates in the affected skin typically are sparse, they include activated CD4+ T_H2 cells. Several cytokines, including IL-13 produced by T_H2 cells and TGF-β produced by macrophages and other cell types, stimulate synthesis of collagen and extracellular matrix proteins (e.g., fibronectin) in fibroblasts. Other cytokines recruit leukocytes and propagate the chronic inflammation.

  The presence of various autoantibodies, notably ANAs, provides diagnostic and prognostic information. It has been postulated that these antibodies stimulate fibrosis, but the evidence in support of this idea is not convincing.

- *Vascular damage.* Microvascular disease is consistently present early in the course of systemic sclerosis. Telltale signs of endothelial activation and injury and increased platelet activation have been noted. However, the cause of the vascular injury is not known; it could be the initiating event or the result of chronic inflammation, with mediators released by inflammatory cells inflicting damage on microvascular endothelium. Repeated cycles of endothelial injury followed by platelet aggregation lead to release of platelet and endothelial factors (e.g., PDGF, TGF-β) that trigger endothelial proliferation and intimal and perivascular fibrosis. Eventually, widespread narrowing of the microvasculature leads to ischemic injury and scarring. The pulmonary vasculature is frequently involved, and the resulting pulmonary hypertension is a serious complication of the disease.

- *Fibrosis.* The progressive fibrosis characteristic of the disease may be the culmination of multiple abnormalities, including the accumulation of alternatively

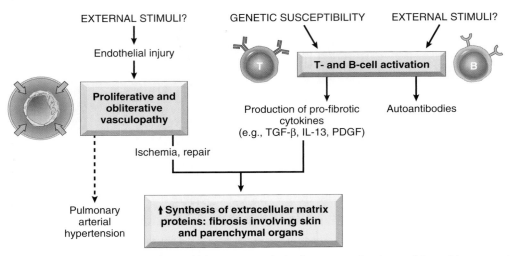

Fig. 5.28 A model for the pathogenesis of systemic sclerosis. Unknown external stimuli cause vascular abnormalities and immune activation in genetically susceptible individuals, and both contribute to the excessive fibrosis.

activated macrophages, actions of fibrogenic cytokines produced by infiltrating leukocytes, hyperresponsiveness of fibroblasts to these cytokines, and scarring following ischemic damage caused by the vascular lesions. Studies with cultured fibroblasts from patients have suggested an intrinsic abnormality that causes the cells to produce excessive amounts of collagen.

MORPHOLOGY

In systemic sclerosis, the most prominent changes occur in the skin, alimentary tract, musculoskeletal system, and kidney, but lesions also are often present in the blood vessels, heart, lungs, and peripheral nerves.

Skin. Most patients have diffuse fibrosis of the skin and associated atrophy, which usually begins in the fingers and distal regions of the upper extremities and extends proximally to involve the upper arms, shoulders, neck, and face. Edema and perivascular infiltrates containing CD4+ T cells are seen, together with swelling and degeneration of collagen fibers, which become eosinophilic. Capillaries and small arteries (150–500 µm in diameter) may show thickening of the basal lamina, endothelial damage, and partial occlusion. With disease progression, there is increasing fibrosis of the dermis, which becomes tightly bound to the subcutaneous structures. Fibrosis often is accompanied by thinning of the epidermis, loss of rete pegs, atrophy of the dermal appendages, and hyaline thickening of the walls of dermal arterioles and capillaries (Fig. 5.29B). Subcutaneous calcifications may develop, especially in patients with CREST syndrome. In advanced stages the fingers take on a tapered, clawlike appearance and have limited joint mobility, and the face becomes a drawn mask. Loss of blood supply may lead to cutaneous ulcerations and atrophic changes (Fig. 5.29C) or even autoamputation of the terminal phalanges.

Alimentary Tract. The alimentary tract is affected in approximately 90% of patients. Progressive atrophy and fibrous replacement of the muscularis may develop at any level of the gut but are most severe in the esophagus. The lower two thirds of the esophagus often develops a rubber-hose–like inflexibility.

The associated dysfunction of the lower esophageal sphincter gives rise to gastroesophageal reflux and its complications, including Barrett metaplasia (Chapter 15) and strictures. The mucosa is thinned and may ulcerate, and there is excessive collagenization of the lamina propria and submucosa. Loss of villi and microvilli in the small bowel is the anatomic basis for a malabsorption syndrome that sometimes is encountered.

Musculoskeletal System. Inflammation of the synovium, associated with synoviocyte hypertrophy, is common in the early stages; fibrosis later ensues. These changes are reminiscent of rheumatoid arthritis, but joint destruction is not common in systemic sclerosis. In a small subset of patients (approximately 10%), inflammatory myositis indistinguishable from polymyositis may develop.

Kidneys. Renal abnormalities occur in two-thirds of patients. The most prominent are the vascular lesions. Interlobular arteries show intimal thickening as a result of deposition of mucinous material containing glycoproteins and acid mucopolysaccharides and concentric proliferation of intimal cells. These changes resemble those seen in malignant hypertension, but in systemic sclerosis the alterations are restricted to vessels 150 to 500 µm in diameter and are not always associated with hypertension. Hypertension, however, does occur in 30% of patients, and in 20% it takes an ominously rapid, downhill course (malignant hypertension). In hypertensive patients, vascular alterations are more pronounced and are often associated with fibrinoid necrosis of arterioles that can lead to thrombosis and infarction. Such patients often die of renal failure, which accounts for about 50% of deaths. There are no specific glomerular changes.

Lungs. The lungs are affected in more than 50% of cases. This involvement may manifest as pulmonary hypertension and interstitial fibrosis. Pulmonary vasospasm secondary to endothelial dysfunction is considered important in the pathogenesis of pulmonary hypertension. Pulmonary fibrosis, when present, is indistinguishable from that seen in idiopathic pulmonary fibrosis (Chapter 13).

Heart. Pericarditis with effusion, myocardial fibrosis, and thickening of intramyocardial arterioles occur in one third of patients. Because of the changes in the lung, right ventricular hypertrophy and failure (cor pulmonale) are frequent.

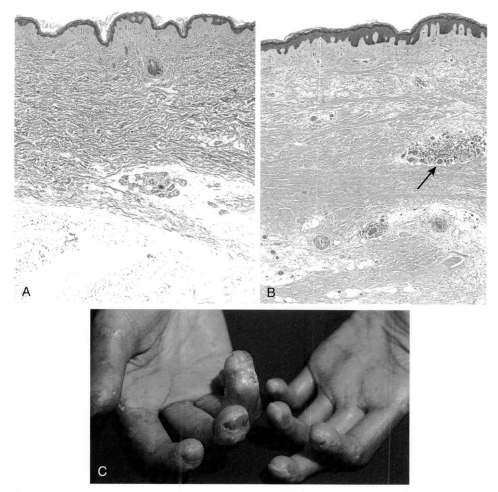

Fig. 5.29 Systemic sclerosis. (A) Normal skin. (B) Skin biopsy from a patient with systemic sclerosis. Note the extensive deposition of dense collagen in the dermis, the virtual absence of appendages (e.g., hair follicles), and foci of inflammation *(arrow)*. (C) The extensive subcutaneous fibrosis has virtually immobilized the fingers, creating a clawlike flexion deformity. Loss of blood supply has led to cutaneous ulcerations. *(C, Courtesy of Dr. Richard Sontheimer, Department of Dermatology, University of Texas Southwestern Medical School, Dallas, Texas.)*

Clinical Features

Systemic sclerosis has a female-to-male ratio of 3:1 and a peak incidence in the 50- to 60-year age group. Although systemic sclerosis shares features with SLE, rheumatoid arthritis (Chapter 21), and polymyositis (Chapter 22), it is distinguished by the striking cutaneous changes, notably skin thickening. Raynaud phenomenon, caused by episodic vasoconstriction of the arteries and arterioles of the extremities, is seen in virtually all patients and precedes other symptoms in 70% of cases. Progressive collagen deposition in the skin leads to increasing stiffness, especially of the hands, with eventually complete immobilization of the joints. Nailfold capillary loops are distorted early in the disease, and later disappear. Dysphagia attributable to esophageal fibrosis and its resultant hypomotility are present in more than 50% of patients. Eventually, destruction of the esophageal wall leads to atony and dilation, especially at its lower end. Abdominal pain, intestinal obstruction, or malabsorption syndrome reflect involvement of the small intestine. Respiratory difficulties caused by the pulmonary fibrosis may result in right-sided cardiac dysfunction, and myocardial fibrosis may cause either arrhythmias or cardiac failure. Mild proteinuria occurs in as many as 30% of patients, but rarely is severe enough to cause nephrotic syndrome. The most ominous manifestation is malignant hypertension, with the subsequent development of fatal renal failure (Chapter 14), but in its absence progression of the disease may be slow. In most patients the disease pursues a steady downhill course over the span of many years, although life span is improving with better treatment of the complications. The disease tends to be more severe in blacks, especially black women. As treatment of the renal complications has improved, pulmonary and cardiac complications have become the major cause of death.

Virtually all patients have ANAs that react with a variety of nuclear antigens (see Table 5.11). Two ANAs are strongly associated with systemic sclerosis. One directed against DNA topoisomerase I (anti-Scl 70) is highly specific and is associated with a greater likelihood of pulmonary fibrosis and peripheral vascular disease. The other, an anti-centromere antibody, is associated with a higher likelihood of CREST syndrome. Patients with this syndrome have relatively limited skin disease, often confined to fingers, forearms and face, and subcutaneous calcifications. Involvement of the viscera, including esophageal lesions, pulmonary hypertension, and biliary cirrhosis, may not occur at all or occur late. In general, these patients live longer than those with systemic sclerosis with diffuse visceral involvement from the outset.

SUMMARY

SYSTEMIC SCLEROSIS

- Systemic sclerosis (commonly called *scleroderma*) is characterized by progressive fibrosis involving the skin, gastrointestinal tract, and other tissues.
- Fibrosis may be the result of activation of fibroblasts by cytokines produced by T cells, but what triggers T cell responses is unknown.
- Endothelial injury and microvascular disease are commonly present in the lesions of systemic sclerosis, perhaps causing chronic ischemia, but the pathogenesis of vascular injury is not known.

Inflammatory Myopathies

Inflammatory myopathies comprise an uncommon, heterogeneous group of disorders characterized by injury and inflammation of mainly the skeletal muscles that are probably immunologically mediated. Based on clinical, morphologic, and immunologic features, three disorders—polymyositis, dermatomyositis, and inclusion body myositis—have been described. Each may occur alone or with other immune-mediated diseases, particularly systemic sclerosis. These diseases are described in Chapter 22.

Mixed Connective Tissue Disease

Mixed connective tissue disease is a disorder with clinical features that overlap those of SLE, systemic sclerosis, and polymyositis. The disease is characterized serologically by high titers of antibodies to U1 ribonucleoprotein. Typically, it presents with synovitis of the fingers, Raynaud phenomenon, and mild myositis. Renal involvement is modest, and there is a favorable response to corticosteroids, at least in the short term. Because these clinical features are shared with other diseases, mixed connective tissue disease may not be a distinct entity, and in fact it may evolve over time into classic SLE or systemic sclerosis. However, progression to other autoimmune disorders is not universal, and there may be a form of mixed connective tissue disease that is distinct from other autoimmune diseases. Serious complications of mixed connective tissue disease include pulmonary hypertension, interstitial lung disease, and renal disease.

Polyarteritis Nodosa and Other Vasculitides

Polyarteritis nodosa belongs to a group of disorders characterized by necrotizing inflammation of the walls of blood vessels that show strong evidence of an immunologic basis. Any type of vessel may be involved—arteries, arterioles, veins, or capillaries. These vasculitides are discussed in Chapter 10.

IgG4-Related Disease

IgG4-related disease (IgG4-RD) is a newly recognized constellation of fibro-inflammatory disorders characterized by tissue infiltrates rich in IgG4 antibody-producing plasma cells and lymphocytes, particularly T cells, associated with fibrosis and obliterative phlebitis (Fig. 5.30). The disorder is often, but not always, associated with elevated serum IgG4 concentrations. Increased numbers of IgG4-producing plasma cells in tissue are a sine qua non of this disorder. IgG4-related disease has now been described in virtually every organ system, including the biliary tree, salivary glands, periorbital tissues, kidneys, lungs, lymph nodes, meninges, aorta, breast, prostate, thyroid, pericardium, and skin. Many conditions long viewed as disorders of single organs are now part of the IgG4-RD spectrum. These include *Mikulicz syndrome* (enlargement and fibrosis of salivary and lacrimal glands), *Riedel thyroiditis, idiopathic retroperitoneal fibrosis, autoimmune pancreatitis,* and *inflammatory pseudotumors* of the orbit, lungs, and kidneys, to name a few. The disease most often affects middle-aged and older men.

The pathogenesis of this condition is not understood, and although IgG4 production in lesions is a hallmark of the disease, it is not known if this antibody type contributes to the pathology. The key role of B cells is supported by clinical trials in which depletion of B cells by anti–B-cell reagents such as rituximab provided clinical benefit.

REJECTION OF TRANSPLANTS

A major barrier to transplantation is the process of *rejection*, in which the recipient's immune system recognizes the graft as foreign and attacks it. The key to successful transplantation has been the development of therapies that prevent or minimize rejection. Transplant rejection is discussed here because it involves several of the immunologic reactions that underlie immune-mediated inflammatory diseases.

Recognition and Rejection of Allografts

Rejection is a process in which T lymphocytes and antibodies produced against graft antigens react against and destroy the grafts. We next discuss how this occurs.

Recognition of Graft Alloantigens

The major antigenic differences between a donor and recipient that result in rejection of transplants are differences in HLA alleles. Grafts exchanged between individuals of the same species are called *allografts*. Because HLA genes are highly polymorphic, there are always some differences between individuals (except, of course, identical twins). Following transplantation, the recipient's T cells recognize donor antigens from the graft (the allogeneic antigens, or alloantigens) by two pathways. The graft

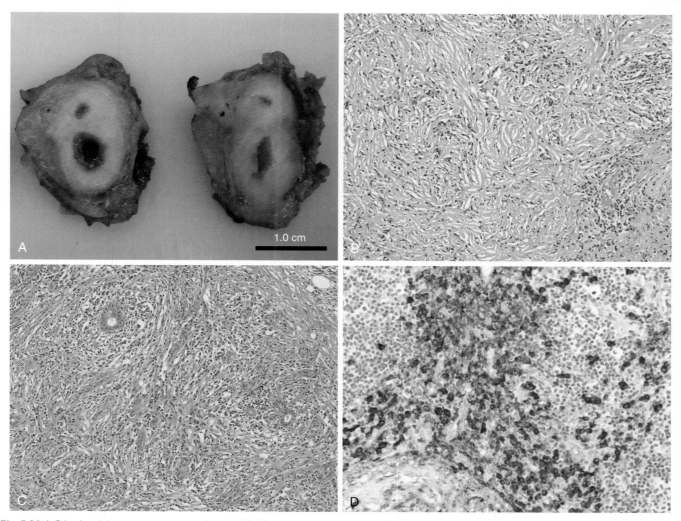

Fig. 5.30 IgG4-related disease: representative lesions. (A) Bile duct showing sclerosing cholangitis. (B) Sclerotic area of the bile duct with storiform fibrosis. (C) Submandibular gland with infiltrates of lymphocytes and plasma cells and whorls of fibrosis. (D) Section of an involved lacrimal gland stained with an antibody against IgG4, showing large numbers of IgG4-producing plasma cells. *(From Kamisawa T, Zen Y, Pillai S, et al: IgG4-related disease. Lancet 385:1460, 2015.)*

antigens are either presented directly to recipient T cells by graft APCs, or the graft antigens are picked up by host APCs, processed (like any other foreign antigen), and presented to host T cells. These are called the direct and indirect pathways of recognition of alloantigens. Both lead to the activation of CD8+ T cells, which develop into CTLs, and CD4+ T cells, which become cytokine-producing effector cells, mainly T_H1 cells. We do not know the relative importance of these pathways in the rejection of allografts. The direct pathway may be most important for CTL-mediated acute rejection, and the indirect pathway may play a greater role in chronic rejection, described later.

The frequency of T cells that can recognize the foreign antigens in a graft is much higher than the frequency of T cells specific for any microbe. For this reason, immune responses to allografts are stronger than responses to pathogens. Predictably, these strong reactions can destroy grafts rapidly, and their control requires powerful immunosuppressive agents.

Mechanisms of Graft Rejection

Graft rejection is classified into hyperacute, acute, and chronic, on the basis of clinical and pathologic features. This classification was devised by nephrologists and pathologists based on rejection of kidney allografts, and has stood the test of time remarkably well. Each type of rejection is mediated by a particular kind of immune response. In the following discussion, the description of the morphology of rejection is limited to kidney allografts, but similar changes are seen in other organ transplants.

- **Hyperacute rejection is mediated by preformed antibodies specific for antigens on graft endothelial cells.** The preformed antibodies may be natural IgM antibodies specific for blood group antigens, or may be antibodies specific for allogeneic MHC molecules that were induced by prior exposure through blood transfusions, pregnancy, or organ transplantation. Immediately after the graft is implanted and blood flow is restored, the antibodies bind to antigens on the graft

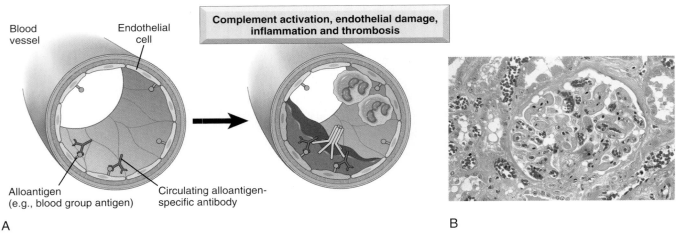

Fig. 5.31 Hyperacute rejection. (A) Deposition of antibody on endothelium and activation of complement causes thrombosis. (B) Hyperacute rejection of a kidney allograft showing platelet fibrin thrombi and severe ischemic injury in a glomerulus.

endothelium and activate the complement and clotting systems, leading to endothelial injury, thrombus formation, and ischemic necrosis of the graft (Fig. 5.31A). Hyperacute rejection is not a common problem, because every donor and recipient are matched for blood type and potential recipients are tested for antibodies against the cells of the prospective donor, a test called a *cross-match.*

MORPHOLOGY

In hyperacute rejection, the affected kidney rapidly becomes cyanotic, mottled, and anuric. Virtually all arterioles and arteries exhibit acute fibrinoid necrosis of their walls and narrowing or complete occlusion of their lumens by thrombi (Fig. 5.31B). Neutrophils rapidly accumulate within arterioles, glomeruli, and peritubular capillaries. As these changes intensify and become diffuse, the glomerular capillaries also undergo thrombotic occlusion, and eventually the kidney cortex undergoes outright necrosis (infarction). Affected kidneys are nonfunctional and have to be removed.

- **Acute rejection is mediated by T cells and antibodies that are activated by alloantigens in the graft.** It occurs within days or weeks after transplantation, and is the principal cause of early graft failure. It also may appear suddenly months or even years later, after immunosuppression is tapered or terminated. Based on the role of T cells or antibodies, acute rejection is divided into two types, although in most rejecting grafts, both patterns are present.

  In *acute cellular rejection,* CD8+ CTLs may directly destroy graft cells, or CD4+ cells secrete cytokines and induce inflammation, which damages the graft (Fig. 5.32A). T cells also may react against graft vessels, leading to vascular damage. Current immunosuppressive therapy is designed mainly to prevent and reduce acute rejection by blocking the activation of alloreactive T cells.

MORPHOLOGY

Acute cellular (T cell–mediated) rejection may produce two different patterns of injury.
- In the *tubulointerstitial pattern* (sometimes called type I), there is extensive interstitial inflammation and tubular inflammation (tubulitis) associated with focal tubular injury (Fig. 5.32B). As might be expected, the inflammatory infiltrates contain activated CD4+ and CD8+ T lymphocytes.
- The *vascular pattern* shows inflammation of vessels (type II) (Fig. 5.32C) and sometimes necrosis of vessel walls (type III). The affected vessels have swollen endothelial cells, and at places lymphocytes are seen between the endothelium and the vessel wall, a finding termed *endotheliitis* or *intimal arteritis.* The recognition of cellular rejection is important because, in the absence of accompanying humoral rejection, most patients respond well to immunosuppressive therapy.

  In acute *antibody-mediated (vascular* or *humoral) rejection,* antibodies bind to vascular endothelium and activate complement via the classical pathway (Fig. 5.33A). The resultant inflammation and endothelial damage cause graft failure.

MORPHOLOGY

Acute antibody-mediated rejection is manifested mainly by damage to glomeruli and small blood vessels. Typically, there is inflammation of glomeruli and peritubular capillaries (Fig. 5.33B) associated with deposition of complement products, which is due to activation of the complement system by the antibody-dependent classical pathway (Fig. 5.33C). Small vessels also may show focal thrombosis.

- **Chronic rejection is an indolent form of graft damage that occurs over months or years, leading to progressive loss of graft function.** Chronic rejection manifests

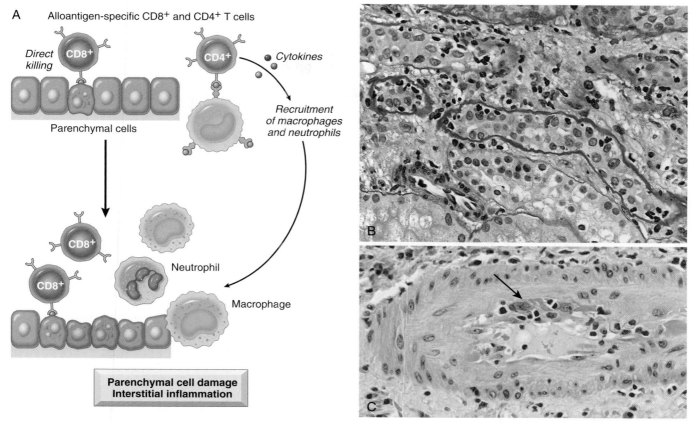

Fig. 5.32 Acute cellular rejection. (A) Destruction of graft cells by T cells. Acute T cell–mediated rejection involves direct killing of graft cells by CD8+ CTLs and inflammation caused by cytokines produced by CD4 T cells. (B) Acute cellular rejection of a kidney graft, manifested by inflammatory cells in the interstitium and between epithelial cells of the tubules (tubulitis). Collapsed tubules are outlined by wavy basement membranes. (C) Rejection vasculitis in a kidney graft. An arteriole is shown with inflammatory cells attacking and undermining the endothelium (endotheliitis) *(arrow)*. *(Courtesy of Drs. Zoltan Laszik and Kuang-Yu Jen, Department of Pathology, University of California, San Francisco, California.)*

as interstitial *fibrosis* and gradual narrowing of graft blood vessels *(graft arteriosclerosis).* In both lesions, the culprits are believed to be T cells that react against graft alloantigens and secrete cytokines, which stimulate the proliferation and activities of fibroblasts and vascular smooth muscle cells in the graft (Fig. 5.34A). Alloantibodies also contribute to chronic rejection. Although treatments to prevent or curtail acute rejection have steadily improved, leading to longer than 1-year survival of transplants, chronic rejection is refractory to most therapies and is becoming the principal cause of graft failure.

MORPHOLOGY

Chronic rejection is dominated by vascular changes, often with intimal thickening and vascular occlusion (Fig. 5.34B). Chronically rejecting kidney grafts show glomerulopathy, with duplication of the basement membrane, likely secondary to chronic endothelial injury (Fig. 5.34C) and peritubular capillaritis with multilayering of peritubular capillary basement membranes. Interstitial fibrosis and tubular atrophy with loss of renal parenchyma may occur secondary to the vascular lesions (Fig. 5.34D). Interstitial mononuclear cell infiltrates are typically sparse.

Methods of Increasing Graft Survival

Because HLA molecules are the major targets in transplant rejection, better matching of the donor and the recipient improves graft survival. HLA matching is more beneficial for living related kidney transplants than for other kinds of transplants, and survival improves with increasing number of loci matched. However, as drugs for immunosuppression have improved, HLA matching is no longer done for heart, lung, liver, and islet transplantation; in such instances, the recipient often needs a transplant urgently and other considerations, such as anatomic compatibility, are of greater importance.

Immunosuppression of the recipient is a necessity in all organ transplantation, except in the case of identical twins. At present, drugs such as cyclosporine, the related FK506, mofetil mycophenolate (MMF), rapamycin, azathioprine, corticosteroids, anti-thymocyte globulin, and monoclonal antibodies (e.g., monoclonal anti-CD3) are used. Cyclosporine and FK506 suppress T cell–mediated immunity by inhibiting transcription of cytokine genes, in particular, the gene for IL-2. Although immunosuppression has made transplantation of many organs feasible, it has its own problems. Suppression of the immune system results in increased susceptibility to opportunistic fungal, viral, and other infections. Reactivation of latent viruses,

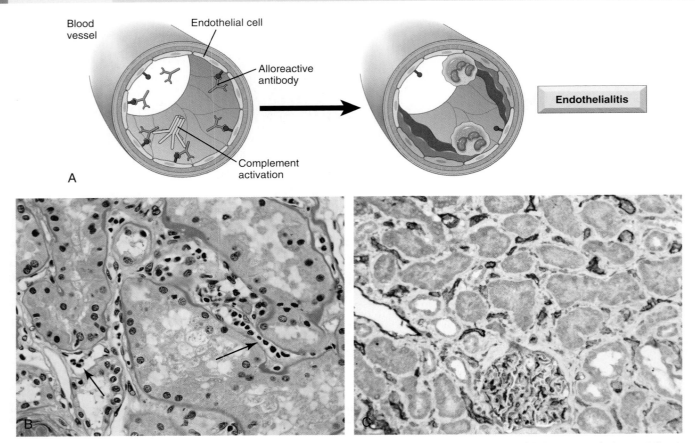

Fig. 5.33 Acute antibody-mediated (humoral) rejection. (A) Graft damage caused by antibody deposition in vessels. (B) Light micrograph showing inflammation (capillaritis) in peritubular capillaries *(arrows)* in a kidney graft. (C) Immunoperoxidase stain shows C4d deposition in peritubular capillaries and a glomerulus. *(Courtesy of Dr. Zoltan Laszik, Department of Pathology, University of California, San Francisco, California.)*

such as cytomegalovirus (CMV) and polyoma virus, are frequent complications. Immunosuppressed patients also are at increased risk for developing virus-induced tumors, such as Epstein-Barr virus (EBV)–induced lymphomas and human papillomavirus (HPV)–induced squamous cell carcinomas. To circumvent the untoward effects of immunosuppression, much effort is being devoted to induce donor-specific tolerance in host T cells. One strategy is to prevent host T cells from receiving costimulatory signals from donor DCs during the initial phase of sensitization. This can be accomplished by administration of agents that block the interaction of the B7 molecules on the DCs of the graft and the CD28 receptor on host T cells, which, by interrupting the second signal for T cell activation, induces either T cell apoptosis or anergy. Other approaches include injecting into recipients regulatory T cells enriched for cells specific for donor alloantigens; these trials are in their infancy.

Transplantation of Hematopoietic Stem Cells

Use of hematopoietic stem cell (HSC) transplants for hematologic malignancies, bone marrow failure syndromes (such as aplastic anemia), and disorders caused by inherited HSC defects (such as sickle cell anemia, thalassemia, and immunodeficiency states) is increasing in number each year. Transplantation of genetically "reengineered" hema-

topoietic stem cells obtained from affected patients may be useful in treating inherited forms of immunodeficiency. Historically, HSCs were obtained from the bone marrow, but now they usually are harvested from peripheral blood after they are mobilized from the bone marrow by administration of hematopoietic growth factors, or from the umbilical cord blood of newborn infants, a rich source of HSCs. In most of the conditions in which HSC transplantation is indicated, the recipient is irradiated or treated with chemotherapy to destroy the immune system (and sometimes, cancer cells) and to "open up" niches in the microenvironment of the marrow that nurture HSCs, thus allowing the transplanted HSCs to engraft. Two major problems complicate this form of transplantation and distinguish it from solid organ transplants: graft-versus-host disease and immune deficiency.

Graft-Versus-Host Disease

GVHD occurs when immunologically competent cells or their precursors are transplanted into immunologically crippled recipients, and the transferred cells recognize alloantigens in the host and attack host tissues. It is seen most commonly in the setting of HSC transplantation but, rarely, may occur following transplantation of solid organs rich in lymphoid cells (e.g., the liver). On receiving allogeneic HSCs, an immunologically compromised host cannot reject the graft, but T cells present in the

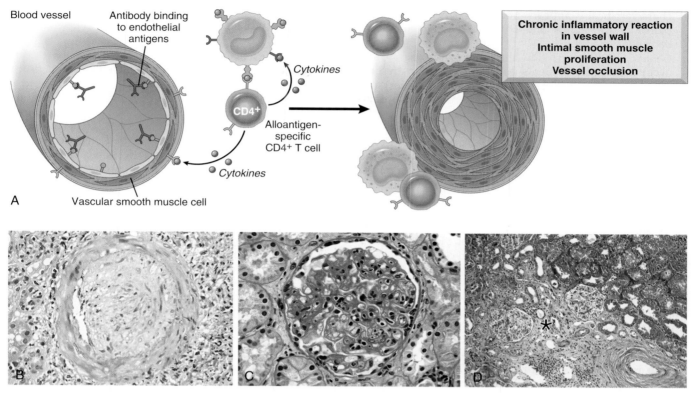

Fig. 5.34 Chronic rejection. (A) Graft arteriosclerosis caused by T-cell cytokines and antibody deposition. (B) Graft arteriosclerosis in a cardiac transplant. (C) Transplant glomerulopathy, the characteristic manifestation of chronic antibody-mediated rejection in the kidney. The glomerulus shows inflammatory cells within the capillary loops (glomerulitis), accumulation of mesangial matrix, and duplication of the capillary basement membrane. (D) Interstitial fibrosis and tubular atrophy, resulting from arteriosclerosis of arteries and arterioles in a chronically rejecting kidney allograft. In this trichrome stain, the blue area *(asterisk)* shows fibrosis, contrasted with the normal kidney *(top right)*. An artery showing prominent arteriosclerosis is shown *(bottom right)*. (**B,** *Courtesy of Dr. Richard Mitchell, Department of Pathology, Brigham and Women's Hospital, Boston, Massachusetts. C and D, Courtesy of Dr. Zoltan Laszik, Department of Pathology, University of California, San Francisco, California.)*

donor graft perceive the host's tissue as foreign and react against it. This results in the activation of donor CD4+ and CD8+ T cells, ultimately causing inflammation and killing recipient cells. To try to minimize GVHD, HSC transplants are done between donor and recipient that are carefully HLA-matched using precise DNA sequencing–based methods.

There are two forms of GVHD.
- *Acute GVHD* (occurring days to weeks after transplantation) causes epithelial cell necrosis in three principal target organs: liver, skin, and gut. Destruction of small bile ducts gives rise to jaundice, and mucosal ulceration of the gut results in bloody diarrhea. Cutaneous involvement (Fig. 5.35) manifests as a rash, which

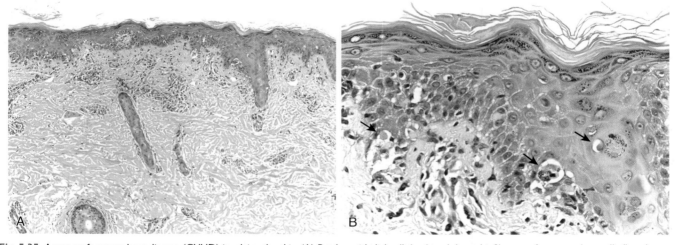

Fig. 5.35 Acute graft-versus-host disease (GVHD) involving the skin. (A) Patchy epithelial cell death and dermal infiltrates of mononuclear cells (lymphocytes and macrophages). (B) Focally dead epithelial cells *(arrows).*

characteristically appears first on the neck, ears, and palms of the hands and soles of the feet and then becomes generalized.

- *Chronic GVHD* may follow the acute syndrome or may occur insidiously. Patients develop skin lesions resembling those of systemic sclerosis (discussed earlier) and manifestations mimicking other autoimmune disorders.

Because GVHD is mediated by T lymphocytes contained in the transplanted donor cells, depletion of donor T cells before transplantation virtually eliminates the disease. This approach, however, has proven to be a mixed blessing: GVHD is ameliorated, but the recurrence of tumor in leukemic patients as well as the incidence of graft failures and EBV-related B-cell lymphoma increase. It seems that the multifaceted T cells not only mediate GVHD but also are required for engraftment of the transplanted HSCs, suppression of EBV-infected B-cell clones, and control of leukemia cells.

Immune Deficiencies

These are often of prolonged duration in recipients of HSC transplants. Among the many reasons for this impairment is the slow reconstitution of the adaptive immune system (derived from donor HSC), after the recipient's immune system is destroyed or suppressed to allow the graft to take. During the many months that may be needed for immune reconstitution, recipients are susceptible to a variety of infections, mostly with viruses, such as CMV and EBV.

SUMMARY

RECOGNITION AND REJECTION OF TRANSPLANTS

- Rejection of solid organ transplants is initiated mainly by host T cells that recognize the foreign HLA antigens of the graft, either directly (on APCs in the graft) or indirectly (after uptake and presentation by host APCs).
- Types and mechanisms of rejection of solid organ grafts are as follows:
  - *Hyperacute rejection:* Preformed anti-donor antibodies bind to graft endothelium immediately after transplantation, leading to thrombosis, ischemic damage, and rapid graft failure.
  - *Acute cellular rejection:* T cells destroy graft parenchyma (and vessels) by cytotoxicity and inflammatory reactions.
  - *Acute antibody-mediated (humoral) rejection:* Antibodies damage graft vasculature.
  - *Chronic rejection:* Dominated by arteriosclerosis, this type is caused by T cell activation and antibodies. The T cells may secrete cytokines that induce proliferation of vascular smooth muscle cells, and the antibodies cause endothelial injury. The vascular lesions and T cell reactions cause parenchymal fibrosis.
- Treatment of graft rejection relies on immunosuppressive drugs, which inhibit immune responses against the graft.
- Transplantation of hematopoietic stem cells (HSCs) requires careful matching of donor and recipient and is often complicated by graft-vs-host disease (GVHD) and immune deficiency.

IMMUNODEFICIENCY SYNDROMES

Immune deficiencies can be divided into *primary* (or *congenital*) *immunodeficiency disorders,* which are genetically determined, and *secondary* (or *acquired*) *immunodeficiencies,* which may arise as complications of cancers, infections, malnutrition, or side effects of immunosuppression, irradiation, or chemotherapy for cancer and other diseases. **Immunodeficiencies are manifested clinically by increased infections, which may be newly acquired or reactivation of latent infections.** The primary immunodeficiency syndromes are accidents of nature that provide valuable insights into some of the molecules critical in the development of the immune system. Paradoxically, several immunodeficiencies also are associated with autoimmune disorders, perhaps because the deficiency results in loss of regulatory mechanisms or persistence of infections that promote autoimmunity. Here we briefly discuss the more important and best-defined primary immunodeficiencies, to be followed by a more detailed description of acquired immunodeficiency syndrome (AIDS), the most devastating example of secondary immunodeficiency.

Primary (Inherited) Immunodeficiencies

Primary immunodeficiency diseases are inherited genetic disorders that impair mechanisms of innate immunity (phagocytes, NK cells, or complement) or the humoral and/or cellular arms of adaptive immunity (mediated by B lymphocytes and T lymphocytes, respectively). These immunodeficiencies are usually detected in infancy, between 6 months and 2 years of age, the telltale signs being susceptibility to recurrent infections. With advances in genetic analyses, the mutations responsible for many of these diseases are now known (Fig. 5.36). Here we present selected examples of immunodeficiencies, beginning with the more common defects in the maturation and activation of B lymphocytes and T lymphocytes, followed by disorders of innate immunity.

Severe Combined Immunodeficiency

Severe combined immunodeficiency (SCID) spans a constellation of genetically distinct syndromes, all having in common impaired development of mature T lymphocytes and/or B lymphocytes and defects in both humoral and cell-mediated immunity. Affected infants present with thrush (oral candidiasis), severe diaper rash, and failure to thrive. Some infants develop a generalized rash shortly after birth because maternal T cells are transferred across the placenta and attack the fetus, causing GVHD. Children with SCID are extremely susceptible to recurrent, severe infections by a wide range of pathogens, including *Candida albicans, Pneumocystis jiroveci, Pseudomonas,* cytomegalovirus, varicella, and a whole host of bacteria. Without HSC transplantation, death occurs within the first year of life. The overall prevalence of the disease is approximately 1 in 65,000 to 1 in 100,000, but it is 20 to 30 times more frequent in some Native American populations.

Despite the common clinical manifestations, of different forms of SCID the underlying defects are quite varied.

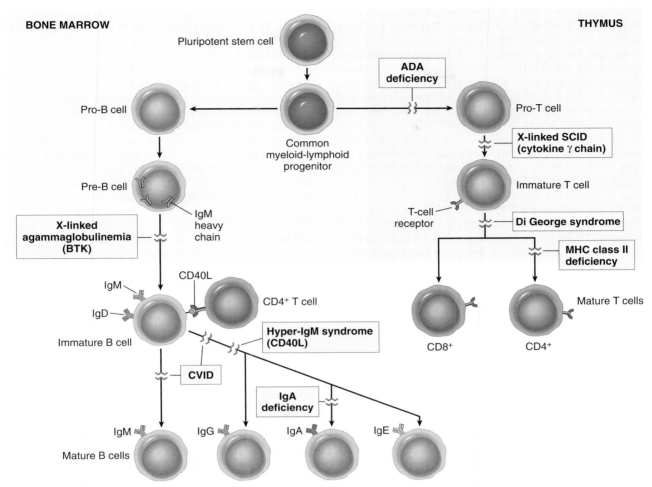

Fig. 5.36 Primary immune deficiency diseases. Shown are the principal pathways of lymphocyte development and the blocks in these pathways in selected primary immune deficiency diseases. The affected genes are indicated in parentheses for some of the disorders. *ADA,* Adenosine deaminase; *CD40L,* CD40 ligand (also known as *CD154*); *CVID,* common variable immunodeficiency; *SCID,* severe combined immunodeficiency.

Often, the defect resides in the T-cell compartment, with a secondary impairment of humoral immunity. Two major forms are described next.

- *X-linked SCID.* **Approximately half of the cases of SCID are X-linked; these are caused by mutations in the gene encoding the common γ (γc) chain shared by the receptors for the cytokines IL-2, IL-4, IL-7, IL-9, and IL-15.** Of these cytokines, defective IL-7 signaling is the most important underlying basis of SCID because this cytokine is responsible for stimulating the survival and expansion of immature B and T cell precursors in the generative lymphoid organs.
- *Autosomal recessive SCID.* **Another 40% to 50% of SCID cases follow autosomal recessive pattern of inheritance, with approximately half of these caused by mutations in adenosine deaminase (ADA), an enzyme involved in purine metabolism.** ADA deficiency results in accumulation of adenosine and deoxyadenosine triphosphate metabolites, which inhibit DNA synthesis and are toxic to lymphocytes. Other autosomal recessive forms of SCID result variously from defects in another purine metabolic pathway, primary failure of class II MHC expression, or mutations in genes encoding the

recombinase responsible for the rearrangement of lymphocyte antigen-receptor genes.

MORPHOLOGY

The histologic findings in SCID depend on the underlying defect. In the two most common forms (γc mutation and ADA deficiency), the thymus is small and devoid of lymphoid cells. In X-linked SCID, the thymus contains lobules of undifferentiated epithelial cells resembling fetal thymus, whereas in SCID caused by ADA deficiency, remnants of Hassall's corpuscles can be found. In both diseases, other lymphoid tissues are hypoplastic as well, with marked depletion of T cell areas and in some cases both T cell and B cell zones.

Currently, HSC transplantation is the mainstay of treatment. X-linked SCID is the first disease in which gene therapy has been successful. For gene therapy, a normal γc gene is expressed using a viral vector in HSCs taken from patients, and the cells are then transplanted back into the patients. The clinical experience is small, but some patients have shown reconstitution of their immune systems for several years after therapy. Unfortunately, however, about

20% of patients receiving a first-generation viral vector developed T cell acute lymphoblastic leukemia (T-ALL), highlighting the dangers of this particular approach to gene therapy. The uncontrolled T-cell proliferation is likely the result of the virus integrating into the genome close to an oncogene, leading to the activation of the oncogene, and possibly also because of the growth advantage conferred by the introduced normal γc gene. Current trials are using new vectors with safety features built in. Patients with ADA deficiency also have been treated with HSC transplantation and, more recently, with administration of the enzyme or gene therapy involving the introduction of a normal ADA gene into T-cell precursors.

X-Linked Agammaglobulinemia

X-linked agammaglobulinemia (XLA), or Bruton disease, is characterized by the failure of pre–B cells to differentiate into mature B cells and, as the name implies, a resultant absence of antibodies (gamma globulin) in the blood. It is one of the more common forms of primary immunodeficiency, occurring at a frequency of about 1 in 100,000 male infants. During normal B-cell maturation, immunoglobulin (Ig) heavy chain genes are rearranged first, followed by light chain genes. At each stage, signals are received from the expressed components of the antigen receptor that drive maturation to the next stage; these signals act as quality controls, to ensure that the correct receptor proteins are being produced. In XLA, B-cell maturation stops after the initial heavy chain gene rearrangement because of mutations in a tyrosine kinase that is associated with the pre–B-cell receptor and is involved in pre-B-cell signal transduction. This kinase is called *Bruton tyrosine kinase (BTK)*. When BTK is nonfunctional, the pre–B-cell receptor cannot signal the cells to proceed along the maturation pathway. As a result, Ig light chains are not produced, and the complete Ig molecule containing heavy and light chains cannot be assembled and transported to the cell membrane, although free heavy chains can be found in the cytoplasm. Because the *BTK* gene is on the X chromosome, the disorder is only seen in males. Sporadic cases with the same features have been described in females, possibly due to mutations in other genes that function in the same pathway.

Classically, the disease is characterized by a profound reduction in the number of B cells in the blood and secondary lymphoid organs and an absence of germinal centers and plasma cells in these organs. T-cell numbers and responses may be normal.

The disease usually does not become apparent until about 6 months of age, as maternal antibodies that were transported via the placenta are depleted. In most cases, recurrent bacterial infections of the respiratory tract, such as acute and chronic pharyngitis, sinusitis, otitis media, bronchitis, and pneumonia, call attention to the underlying immune defect. Almost always, the causative organisms are *Haemophilus influenzae, Streptococcus pneumoniae,* or *Staphylococcus aureus,* organisms that are normally opsonized by antibodies and cleared by phagocytosis. Because antibodies are important for neutralizing certain infectious viruses, individuals with this disease also are susceptible to some viral infections, especially those caused by enteroviruses. These viruses infect the gastrointestinal tract, and from

there they can disseminate to the nervous system via the blood. Thus, immunization with live poliovirus carries the risk for paralytic poliomyelitis, and infections with echovirus can cause fatal encephalitis. For similar reasons, *Giardia lamblia,* an intestinal protozoan that is normally resisted by secreted IgA, causes persistent infections in individuals with this disorder. Many intracellular viral, fungal, and protozoal infections are handled quite well by the intact T cell–mediated immunity. For unclear reasons, autoimmune diseases (such as rheumatoid arthritis and dermatomyositis) occur in as many as 35% of patients with this disease.

The treatment of X-linked agammaglobulinemia is replacement therapy with intravenous immunoglobulin (IVIG) from pooled human serum.

DiGeorge Syndrome (Thymic Hypoplasia)

DiGeorge syndrome is caused by a congenital defect in thymic development resulting in deficient T-cell maturation. T cells are absent in the lymph nodes, spleen, and peripheral blood, and infants with this defect are extremely vulnerable to viral, fungal, and protozoal infections. Patients also are susceptible to infection with intracellular bacteria, because of defective T cell–mediated immunity. B cells and serum immunoglobulins are generally unaffected.

The disorder is a consequence of a developmental malformation affecting the third and fourth pharyngeal pouches, structures that give rise to the thymus, parathyroid glands, and portions of the face and aortic arch. Thus, in addition to the thymic and T-cell defects, there may be parathyroid gland hypoplasia, resulting in hypocalcemic tetany, as well as additional midline developmental abnormalities. In 90% of cases of DiGeorge syndrome, there is a deletion affecting chromosomal region 22q11, discussed in Chapter 7. Transplantation of thymic tissue has successfully treated some affected infants. In patients with partial defects, immunity may improve spontaneously with age.

Hyper-IgM Syndrome

This disease is characterized by the production of normal (or even supranormal) levels of IgM antibodies and decreased levels of the IgG, IgA, and IgE isotypes; the underlying defect is an inability of T cells to activate B cells. As discussed earlier, many of the functions of CD4+ helper T cells require the engagement of CD40 on B cells, macrophages, and dendritic cells by CD40L (also called *CD154*) expressed on antigen-activated T cells. This interaction triggers Ig class switching and affinity maturation in the B cells, and stimulates the microbicidal functions of macrophages. Approximately 70% of individuals with hyper-IgM syndrome have the X-linked form of the disease, caused by mutations in the gene encoding CD40L located on Xq26. In the remaining patients, the disease is inherited in an autosomal recessive pattern caused by loss-of-function mutations involving either CD40 or an enzyme called *activation-induced cytidine deaminase (AID)*, a DNA-editing enzyme that is required for Ig class switching and affinity maturation.

Patients present with recurrent pyogenic infections because of low levels of opsonizing IgG antibodies. Those with CD40L mutations also are susceptible to pneumonia caused by the intracellular organism *Pneumocystis jiroveci*, because CD40L-mediated macrophage activation, a key reaction of cell-mediated immunity, is compromised. Occasionally, the IgM antibodies react with blood cells, giving rise to autoimmune hemolytic anemia, thrombocytopenia, and neutropenia. In older patients, there may be a proliferation of IgM-producing plasma cells that infiltrate the mucosa of the gastrointestinal tract.

Common Variable Immunodeficiency

This relatively frequent but poorly defined entity encompasses **a heterogeneous group of disorders in which the common feature is hypogammaglobulinemia, generally affecting all the antibody classes but sometimes only IgG.** The diagnosis of common variable immunodeficiency is based on exclusion of other well-defined causes of decreased antibody production. The estimated prevalence of the disease is about 1 in 50,000.

Although most patients have normal numbers of mature B cells, plasma cells are absent, suggesting a block in B-cell differentiation. In keeping with this idea, B cell areas of the lymphoid tissues (i.e., lymphoid follicles in nodes, spleen, and gut) tend to be hyperplastic. The enlargement of B cell areas may reflect incomplete activation, such that B cells can proliferate in response to antigen but do not differentiate into antibody-producing plasma cells. The defective antibody production has been variably attributed to intrinsic B-cell defects, deficient T-cell help, or excessive T-cell suppressive activity. Paradoxically, these patients are prone to develop a variety of autoimmune disorders (hemolytic anemia, pernicious anemia) as well as lymphoid tumors. Common variable immunodeficiency may be genetic or acquired. Different genetic causes have been discovered, including mutations in a receptor for BAFF, a cytokine that promotes the survival and differentiation of B cells, and in a molecule called ICOS (inducible costimulator), a homologue of CD28 that contributes to the function of T follicular helper cells. However, in the majority of cases, the genetic basis is unknown.

Patients typically present with recurrent sinopulmonary bacterial infections. About 20% of patients have recurrent herpesvirus infections, and serious enterovirus infections causing meningoencephalitis also may occur. Individuals with this disorder also are prone to the development of persistent diarrhea caused by *G. lamblia*. In contrast to X-linked agammaglobulinemia, common variable immunodeficiency affects both sexes equally, and the onset of symptoms is later, in childhood or adolescence. As in X-linked agammaglobulinemia, these patients have a high frequency of autoimmune diseases (approximately 20%), including rheumatoid arthritis. The risk for lymphoid malignancy also is increased, and an increase in gastric cancer has been reported.

Isolated IgA Deficiency

This is the most common primary immune deficiency disease, affecting about 1 in 700 whites. As noted previously, IgA is the major immunoglobulin in mucosal secretions and is thus involved in defending the airways and the gastrointestinal tract. Weakened mucosal defenses due to IgA deficiency predispose patients to recurrent sinopulmonary infections and diarrhea. There also is a significant

(but unexplained) association with autoimmune diseases. The pathogenesis of IgA deficiency seems to involve a block in the terminal differentiation of IgA-secreting B cells to plasma cells; IgM and IgG subclasses of antibodies are present in normal or even supranormal levels. The molecular basis for this defect is not understood.

Other Defects in Lymphocyte Activation

Many rare cases of lymphocyte activation defects have been described that affect antigen receptor signaling and various biochemical pathways. Defects in T_H1 responses are associated with atypical mycobacterial infections, and defective T_H17 responses are the cause of chronic mucocutaneous candidiasis as well as bacterial infections of the skin (a disorder called *Job syndrome*).

Immunodeficiencies Associated With Systemic Diseases

In some inherited systemic disorders, immune deficiency is a prominent clinical problem. Two representative examples of such diseases are described next.

*   *Wiskott-Aldrich syndrome* is an X-linked disease characterized by thrombocytopenia, eczema, and a marked vulnerability to recurrent infection that results in early death. The thymus is normal, at least early in the disease course, but there is progressive loss of T lymphocytes from the blood and the T cell zones (paracortical areas) of lymph nodes, with variable defects in cellular immunity. Patients do not make antibodies to polysaccharide antigens, and the response to protein antigens is poor. IgM levels in the serum are low, but levels of IgG are usually normal and, paradoxically, IgA and IgE are often elevated. The syndrome is caused by mutations in an X-linked gene encoding Wiskott-Aldrich syndrome protein (WASP). WASP belongs to a family of signaling proteins that link membrane receptors, such as antigen receptors, to cytoskeletal elements. The WASP protein is involved in cytoskeleton-dependent responses, including cell migration and signal transduction, but how this contributes to the functions of lymphocytes and platelets is unclear. The only treatment is HSC transplantation.

*   *Ataxia telangiectasia* is an autosomal-recessive disorder characterized by abnormal gait (ataxia), vascular malformations (telangiectases), neurologic deficits, increased incidence of tumors, and immunodeficiency. The immunologic defects are of variable severity and may affect both B cells and T cells. The most prominent humoral immune abnormalities are defective production of isotype-switched antibodies, mainly IgA and IgG2. The T-cell defects are usually less pronounced, and may be associated with thymic hypoplasia. Patients experience upper and lower respiratory tract bacterial infections, multiple autoimmune phenomena, and increasingly frequent cancers, particularly lymphoid tumors, with advancing age. The gene responsible for this disorder encodes a protein called ATM (ataxia telangiectasia mutated), a sensor of DNA damage that activates cell cycle checkpoints and apoptosis in cells with damaged DNA. Lack of ATM also leads to abnormalities in antigen gene recombination (and therefore defects in the generation of antigen receptors) and abnormal antibody isotype switching.

Defects in Innate Immunity

Inherited defects in the early innate immune response typically affect leukocyte functions or the complement system and lead to increased vulnerability to infections (Table 5.13). Some defects whose molecular bases are defined are summarized next.

Defects in Leukocyte Function

- *Leukocyte adhesion deficiencies (LADs)* stem from inherited defects in adhesion molecules that impair leukocyte recruitment to sites of infection, resulting in recurrent bacterial infections. LAD1 is caused by defects in the β_2 chain that is shared by the integrins LFA-1 and Mac-1, while LAD2 is caused by a defect in a fucosyl transferase that is required to synthesize functional sialyl-Lewis X, the ligand for E- and P-selectins.
- *Chronic granulomatous disease* results from inherited defects in the genes encoding components of phagocyte oxidase, the phagolysosomal enzyme that generates ROS such as superoxide ($O_2^{\cdot-}$), resulting in defective bacterial killing and susceptibility to recurrent bacterial infection. The name of this disease comes from the macrophage-rich chronic inflammatory reaction that appears at sites of infection if the initial neutrophil defense is inadequate. These collections of activated macrophages form granulomas in an effort to wall off the microbes.
- *Chédiak-Higashi syndrome* is characterized by defective fusion of phagosomes and lysosomes, resulting in defective phagocyte function and susceptibility to infections. The main leukocyte abnormalities are neutropenia, defective degranulation, and delayed microbial killing. The affected leukocytes contain giant granules, which are readily seen in peripheral blood smears and are thought to result from aberrant phagolysosome fusion. In addition, there are abnormalities in melanocytes (leading to albinism), cells of the nervous system (associated with nerve defects), and platelets (causing bleeding disorders). The gene associated with this disorder encodes a large cytosolic protein called LYST, which is believed to regulate lysosomal trafficking.
- *TLR defects* are rare but informative. Mutations in *TLR3*, a receptor for viral RNA, result in recurrent herpes simplex encephalitis, and mutations in *MYD88*, an adaptor protein needed for signaling downstream of multiple TLRs, are associated with destructive bacterial pneumonias.

Table 5.13 Common Inherited Immune Deficiencies of Phagocytic Leukocytes and the Complement System

Disease	Defect
Defects in Leukocyte Function	
Leukocyte adhesion deficiency 1	Defective leukocyte adhesion because of mutations in the β chain of CD11/CD18 integrins
Leukocyte adhesion deficiency 2	Defective leukocyte adhesion because of mutations in fucosyl transferase required for synthesis of sialylated oligosaccharide (receptor for selectins)
Chédiak-Higashi syndrome	Decreased leukocyte functions because of mutations affecting protein involved in lysosomal membrane traffic
Chronic granulomatous disease	Decreased oxidative burst
X-linked	Phagocyte oxidase (membrane component)
Autosomal recessive	Phagocyte oxidase (cytoplasmic components)
Myeloperoxidase deficiency	Decreased microbial killing because of defective MPO-H_2O_2 system
Defects in the Complement System	
C2, C4 deficiency	Defective classical pathway activation; results in reduced resistance to infection and reduced clearance of immune complexes
C3 deficiency	Defects in all complement functions
Deficiency of complement regulatory proteins	Excessive complement activation; clinical syndromes include angioedema, paroxysmal hemoglobinuria, and others

Modified in part from Gallin JI: Disorders of phagocytic cells. In Gallin JI, et al, editors: *Inflammation: basic principles and clinical correlates*, ed 2, New York, 1992, Raven Press, pp 860–861.

Deficiencies Affecting the Complement System

- Deficiency of several *complement components* have been described, with C2 deficiency being the most common. Deficiencies of *C2* or *C4*, early components of the classical pathway, are associated with increased bacterial or viral infections; however, many patients are asymptomatic, presumably because the alternative complement pathway is able to control most infections. Surprisingly, in some patients with C2, C4, or C1q deficiency, the dominant manifestation is an SLE-like autoimmune disease, possibly because these factors are involved in clearance of immune complexes. Deficiency of C3 is rare. It is associated with severe pyogenic infections as well as immune complex–mediated glomerulonephritis. Deficiency of the late components C5 to C9 results in increased susceptibility to recurrent neisserial (gonococcal and meningococcal) infections, as *Neisseria* bacteria have thin cell walls and are especially susceptible to the lytic actions of complement.
- Defects in *complement regulatory proteins* result in excessive inflammation or cell injury. A deficiency of *C1 inhibitor (C1 INH)* gives rise to an autosomal dominant disorder called *hereditary angioedema*, C1 INH is an inhibitor of many proteases, including kallikrein and coagulation factor XII, both of which are involved in the production of vasoactive peptides such as bradykinin. Therefore, defective C1 INH activity leads to over-production of bradykinin, which is a potent vasodilator. Affected patients have episodes of edema affecting skin and mucosal surfaces such as the larynx and the gastrointestinal tract. Acquired deficiencies of other complement regulatory proteins are the cause of *paroxysmal nocturnal hemoglobinuria* (Chapter 12), while some cases of *hemolytic uremic syndrome* (Chapter 14) stem from inherited defects in complement regulatory proteins.

SUMMARY

PRIMARY (INHERITED) IMMUNE DEFICIENCY DISEASES

- These diseases are caused by inherited mutations in genes involved in lymphocyte maturation or function, or in innate immunity.
- Some of the more common disorders affecting lymphocytes and the adaptive immune response are:
  - *X-SCID:* Failure of T cell and B cell maturation; mutation in the common γ chain of a cytokine receptor, leading to failure of IL-7 signaling and defective lymphopoiesis
  - *Autosomal recessive SCID:* Failure of T cell development; secondary defect in antibody responses; approximately 50% of cases caused by mutation in the gene encoding ADA, leading to accumulation of toxic metabolites during lymphocyte maturation and proliferation
  - *X-linked agammaglobulinemia (XLA):* Failure of B-cell maturation, absence of antibodies; caused by mutations in the *BTK* gene, which encodes B-cell tyrosine kinase, required for maturation signals from the pre–B-cell and B-cell receptors
  - *Di George syndrome:* Failure of development of thymus, with T cell deficiency
  - *X-linked hyper-IgM syndrome:* Failure to produce isotype-switched high-affinity antibodies (IgG, IgA, IgE); mutations in genes encoding CD40L or activation-induced cytosine deaminase
  - *Common variable immunodeficiency:* Defects in antibody production; cause unknown in most cases.
  - *Selective IgA deficiency:* Failure of IgA production; cause unknown
- Deficiencies in innate immunity include defects of leukocyte function, complement, and innate immune receptors.
- These diseases present clinically with increased susceptibility to infections in early life.

Secondary (Acquired) Immunodeficiencies

Secondary (acquired) immune deficiencies may be encountered in individuals with cancer, diabetes and other metabolic diseases, malnutrition, chronic infection, and in patients receiving chemotherapy or radiation therapy for cancer, or immunosuppressive drugs to prevent graft rejection or to treat autoimmune diseases (Table 5.14). As a group, the secondary immune deficiencies are more common than the disorders of primary genetic origin. Discussed next is perhaps the most important secondary immune deficiency disease, AIDS, which has become one of the great scourges of humankind.

ACQUIRED IMMUNODEFICIENCY SYNDROME

AIDS is a disease caused by the retrovirus human immunodeficiency virus (HIV) and is characterized by profound immunosuppression that leads to opportunistic

Table 5.14 Causes of Secondary (Acquired) Immunodeficiencies

Cause	Mechanism
Human immunodeficiency virus infection	Depletion of CD4+ helper T cells
Irradiation and chemotherapy treatments for cancer	Decreased bone marrow precursors for all leukocytes
Involvement of bone marrow by cancers (metastases, leukemias)	Reduced leukocyte development due to displacement of progenitors
Protein-calorie malnutrition	Metabolic derangements inhibit lymphocyte maturation and function
Removal of spleen	Decreased phagocytosis of microbes

infections, secondary neoplasms, and neurologic manifestations. Although AIDS was first recognized as a distinct entity as recently as the 1980s, it has become one of the most devastating afflictions in history. Of the estimated 36 million HIV-infected individuals worldwide, about 70% are in Africa and 20% in Asia. More than 25 million deaths are attributable to HIV/AIDS, with 1 to 2 million deaths annually. Effective anti-retroviral drugs have been developed, but the infection continues to spread in parts of the world where these therapies are not widely available, and in some African countries, more than 30% of the population is HIV infected. Despite the remarkable progress in drug therapy of AIDS, cure is still a distant goal. The advent of these drugs also raises its own tragic concern; because more individuals are living with HIV, the risk of spreading the infection will increase if vigilance is relaxed.

The enormous medical and social burden of AIDS has led to an explosion of research aimed at understanding this modern plague and its remarkable ability to cripple host defenses. The literature on HIV and AIDS is vast. Here we summarize the currently available data on the epidemiology, pathogenesis, and clinical features of HIV infection.

Epidemiology

Epidemiologic studies in the United States have identified five groups of adults at high risk for developing AIDS.
- Homosexual or bisexual men constitute the largest group, accounting for about 50% of the reported cases. This includes about 5% who also are intravenous drug abusers.
- Heterosexual contacts of members of other high-risk groups constituted about 20% of infections from 2001 to 2004. In Africa and Asia, this is by far the largest group of patients with new infections, most of which occur in women who are infected by male partners.
- Intravenous drug abusers with no previous history of homosexuality represented about 20% of infected individuals and 9% of new cases in 2009.
- Surviving hemophiliacs, especially those who received large amounts of factor VIII or factor IX concentrates before 1985, make up about 0.5% of all cases.
- Other recipients of HIV-infected whole blood or components (e.g., platelets, plasma) account for about 1% of patients.

- HIV infection of the newborn. Close to 2% of all AIDS cases occur in this pediatric population. The vast majority acquires the infection by transmission of the virus from mother to child (discussed later).
- In approximately 5% of cases, the risk factors cannot be determined.

It should be apparent from the preceding discussion that **transmission of HIV occurs under conditions that facilitate exchange of blood or body fluids containing the virus or virus-infected cells.** The three major routes of transmission are sexual contact, parenteral inoculation, and passage of the virus from infected mothers to their newborns.

- *Sexual transmission* is the dominant mode of infection worldwide, accounting for more than 75% of all cases of HIV transmission. Because most infected individuals in the United States are men who have sex with men, sexual transmission has mainly occurred among homosexual men. The virus is carried in the semen, and it enters the recipient's body through abrasions in rectal or oral mucosa or by direct contact with mucosal lining cells. Viral spread occurs in two ways: (1) direct inoculation into the blood vessels breached by trauma and (2) infection of DCs or CD4+ cells within the mucosa. Sexual transmission of HIV is enhanced by coexisting sexually transmitted diseases, especially those associated with genital ulceration.
- *Parenteral transmission* of HIV has occurred in intravenous drug abusers, hemophiliacs who received contaminated factor VIII and factor IX concentrates, and other recipients of contaminated blood products. In the United States at present, parenteral transmission is common only among intravenous drug users. Transmission occurs by sharing of needles, syringes, and other paraphernalia contaminated with HIV-containing blood. Transmission of HIV by transfusion of blood or blood products, such as lyophilized factor VIII and factor IX concentrates, has been virtually eliminated by public health measures, including screening of donated blood and plasma for antibody to HIV, stringent purity criteria for factor VIII and factor IX preparations, and screening of donors on the basis of history. An extremely small risk for acquiring AIDS through transfusion of seronegative blood persists, because a recently infected individual may be antibody-negative. Currently, this risk is estimated to be 1 in more than 2 million units of blood transfused.
- As alluded to earlier, *mother-to-infant transmission* is the major cause of pediatric AIDS. Infected mothers can transmit the infection to their offspring by three routes: (1) in utero by transplacental spread; (2) during delivery through an infected birth canal; and (3) after birth by ingestion of breast milk. Of these, transmission during birth (intrapartum) and in the immediate period thereafter (peripartum) is considered to be the most common mode in the United States. The reported transmission rates vary from 7% to 49% in different parts of the world. Higher risk of transmission is associated with high maternal viral load and low CD4+ T cell counts as well as chorioamnionitis. Fortunately, anti-retroviral therapy given to infected pregnant women in the United

States has virtually eliminated mother-to-child transmission, but it remains a major source of infection in areas where these treatments are not available.

Much concern has arisen in the lay public and among healthcare workers about the spread of HIV infection outside the high-risk groups. Extensive studies indicate that HIV infection cannot be transmitted by casual personal contact in the household, workplace, or school. Spread by insect bites is virtually impossible. Regarding transmission of HIV infection to healthcare workers, an extremely small but definite risk is present. Seroconversion has been documented after accidental needle-stick injury or exposure of nonintact skin to infected blood in laboratory accidents. After needle-stick accidents, the risk for seroconversion is believed to be about 0.3%, and anti-retroviral therapy given within 24 to 48 hours of a needle stick can greatly reduce the risk of infection. By comparison, approximately 30% of those accidentally exposed to hepatitis B–infected blood become seropositive.

Properties of HIV

HIV is a nontransforming human retrovirus belonging to the lentivirus family. Included in this group are feline immunodeficiency virus, simian immunodeficiency virus, visna virus of sheep, bovine immunodeficiency virus, and the equine infectious anemia virus.

Two genetically different but related forms of HIV, called HIV-1 and HIV-2, have been isolated from patients. HIV-1 is the most common type associated with AIDS in the United States, Europe, and Central Africa, whereas HIV-2 causes a similar disease principally in West Africa and India. The ensuing discussion relates primarily to HIV-1, but is generally applicable to HIV-2 as well.

Structure of HIV

Similar to most retroviruses, the HIV-1 virion is spherical and contains an electron-dense, cone-shaped core surrounded by a lipid envelope derived from the host cell membrane (Fig. 5.37). The virus core contains (1) the major capsid protein p24; (2) nucleocapsid protein p7/p9; (3) two copies of viral genomic RNA; and (4) the three viral enzymes (protease, reverse transcriptase, and integrase). p24 is the most abundant viral antigen and is the antigen detected by an assay widely used to diagnose HIV infection. The viral core is surrounded by a matrix protein called *p17,* which lies underneath the virion envelope. Studding the viral envelope are two viral glycoproteins, gp120 and gp41, which are critical for HIV infection of cells.

The HIV-1 RNA genome contains the *gag, pol,* and *env* genes, which are typical of retroviruses. The products of the *gag* and *pol* genes are large precursor proteins that are cleaved by the viral protease to yield the mature proteins. In addition to these three standard retroviral genes, HIV contains several accessory genes, including *tat, rev, vif, nef, vpr,* and *vpu,* which regulate the synthesis and assembly of infectious viral particles and the pathogenicity of the virus.

Molecular analysis of different HIV-1 isolates has revealed considerable variability in certain parts of the viral genome, mostly within sequences that encode particular regions of the envelope glycoproteins. Because the

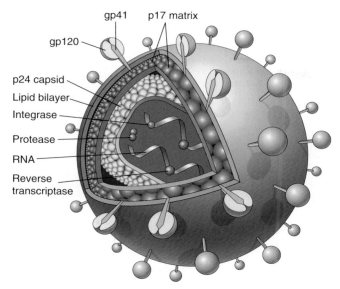

gp41   p17 matrix
gp120
p24 capsid
Lipid bilayer
Integrase
Protease
RNA
Reverse transcriptase

Fig. 5.37 The structure of the human immunodeficiency virus (HIV)-1 virion. The viral particle is covered by a lipid bilayer derived from the host cell and studded with viral glycoproteins gp41 and gp120.

antibody response against HIV-1 is targeted against its envelope, such variability poses problems for the development of a single-antigen vaccine. Based on genetic variation, HIV-1 can be divided into three subgroups, designated M (major), O (outlier), and N (neither M nor O). Group M viruses are the most common form worldwide, and they are further divided into several subtypes, or clades, designated A through K. Various subtypes differ in their geographic distribution; for example, subtype B is the most common form in western Europe and the United States, whereas subtype E is the most common clade in Thailand. Currently, clade C is the fastest spreading clade worldwide, being present in India, Ethiopia, and Southern Africa.

Pathogenesis of HIV Infection and AIDS

While HIV can infect many tissues, the two major targets of HIV infection are the immune system and the central nervous system. The effects of HIV infection on each of these two systems are discussed separately.

Profound immune deficiency, primarily affecting cell-mediated immunity, is the hallmark of AIDS. This results chiefly from infection and subsequent loss of CD4+ T cells as well as impaired function of surviving helper T cells and other immune cells. We first describe the mechanisms involved in viral entry into T cells and macrophages and the replicative cycle of the virus within cells. This is followed by a more detailed review of the interaction between HIV and its cellular targets.

Life Cycle of HIV

The life cycle of HIV consists of infection of cells, integration of the provirus into the host cell genome, activation of viral replication, and production and release of infectious virus (Fig. 5.38). The molecules and mechanisms of each of these steps are understood in considerable detail.

Infection of Cells by HIV

HIV infects cells by using the CD4 molecule as a receptor and various chemokine receptors as coreceptors (see Fig. 5.38). Binding of HIV gp120 to CD4 is essential for infection and accounts for the tropism of the virus for CD4+ T cells and for CD4+ monocytes/macrophages and DCs. However, binding to CD4 is not sufficient for infection, as HIV gp120 also must bind to other cell surface molecules (coreceptors) for entry into the cell. Chemokine receptors, particularly CCR5 and CXCR4, serve this role. HIV isolates can be distinguished by their use of these coreceptors: R5 strains use CCR5, X4 strains use CXCR4, and some strains (R5X4) are dual-tropic. R5 strains preferentially infect cells of the monocyte/macrophage lineage and are thus referred to as *M-tropic*, whereas X4 strains are *T-tropic*, preferentially infecting T cells, but these distinctions are not absolute.

Polymorphisms in the gene encoding CCR5 are associated with altered susceptibility to HIV infection. About 1% of white Americans inherit two mutated copies of the *CCR5* gene and are resistant to R5 HIV isolates. About 20% of individuals are heterozygous for this protective *CCR5* allele; these individuals are not protected from AIDS, but the onset of their disease after infection is delayed. Only rare homozygotes for the mutation have been found in African and East Asian populations.

Molecular details of the deadly handshake between HIV glycoproteins and their cell surface receptors have been elucidated. The HIV envelope contains two noncovalently associated glycoproteins, surface gp120 and the transmembrane protein gp41. The initial step in infection is the binding of the gp120 envelope glycoprotein to CD4 molecules, which leads to a conformational change that creates a new recognition site on gp120 for the coreceptors CCR5 or CXCR4. Binding to the coreceptors induces conformational changes in gp41 that exposes a hydrophobic region called the fusion peptide at the tip of gp41. This peptide inserts into the cell membrane of the target cells (e.g., T cells or macrophages), leading to fusion of the virus with the host cell. After fusion, the virus core containing the HIV genome enters the cytoplasm of the cell.

Viral Replication

Once internalized, the RNA genome of the virus undergoes reverse transcription, leading to the synthesis of double-stranded complementary DNA (cDNA; proviral DNA) (see Fig. 5.38). In quiescent T cells, HIV cDNA may remain in the cytoplasm in a linear episomal form. In dividing T cells, the cDNA circularizes, enters the nucleus, and is then integrated into the host genome. After integration, the provirus may be silent for months or years, a form of *latent infection*. Alternatively, proviral DNA may be transcribed, leading to the expression of viral proteins that are required for the formation of complete viral particles. HIV infects memory cells and activated T cells but is inefficient at productively infecting naïve (resting) T cells.

Completion of the viral life cycle in latently infected cells occurs only after cell activation, and in the case of most CD4+ T cells, virus activation results in death of the infected cells. Activation of T cells by antigens or cytokines upregulates several transcription factors, including NF-κB, which moves from the cytosol into the nucleus. In

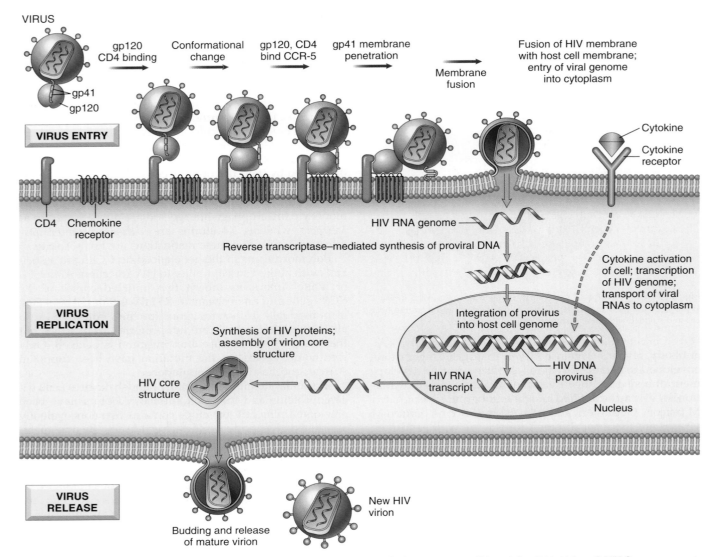

Fig. 5.38 The life cycle of HIV showing the steps from viral entry to production of infectious virions. *(Adapted from Wain-Hobson S: HIV. One on one meets two. Nature 384:117, 1996.)*

the nucleus, NF-κB binds to regulatory sequences within several genes, including genes for cytokines and other immune mediators, promoting their transcription. The long-terminal-repeat sequences that flank the HIV genome also contain NF-κB–binding sites, so binding of the transcription factor activates viral gene expression. Imagine now a latently infected CD4+ cell that encounters an environmental antigen. Induction of NF-κB in such a cell (a physiologic response) activates the transcription of HIV proviral DNA (a pathologic outcome) and leads ultimately to the production of virions and to cell death. Furthermore, TNF and other cytokines produced by activated macrophages also stimulate NF-κB activity and thus lead to production of HIV RNA. Thus, it seems that HIV thrives when the host T cells and macrophages are physiologically activated, a situation that can be described as "subversion from within." Such activation in vivo may result from antigenic stimulation by HIV itself or by other infecting microorganisms. HIV-positive individuals are at increased risk

for recurrent infections, which leads to increased lymphocyte activation and production of proinflammatory cytokines. These, in turn, stimulate more HIV production, loss of additional CD4+ T cells, and more infections. Thus, it is easy to see how HIV infection sets up a vicious cycle that culminates in inexorable destruction of the immune system.

Mechanism of T-Cell Depletion in HIV Infection

Loss of CD4+ T cells is mainly caused by the direct cytopathic effects of the replicating virus. In infected individuals, approximately 100 billion new viral particles are produced and 1 to 2 billion CD4+ T cells die each day. Death of these cells is a major cause of the relentless, and eventually profound, T cell immunodeficiency. Up to a point, the immune system can replace the dying T cells, but as the disease progresses, renewal of CD4+ T cells cannot keep up with their loss. Possible mechanisms by which the virus directly kills infected cells include increased plasma membrane permeability associated with budding of virus particles and defects in protein synthesis stemming from interference by viral proteins involved in viral replication.

In addition to direct killing of cells by the virus, other mechanisms may contribute to the loss or functional impairment of T cells. These include:

- Chronic activation of uninfected cells, responding to HIV itself or to infections that are common in individuals with AIDS, leading to apoptosis of these cells.
- HIV infection of cells in lymphoid organs (spleen, lymph nodes, tonsils) causing progressive destruction of the architecture and cellular composition of lymphoid tissues.
- Fusion of infected and uninfected cells, leading to formation of syncytia (giant cells). In tissue culture the gp120 expressed on productively infected cells binds to CD4 molecules on uninfected T cells, followed by cell fusion. Fused cells usually die within a few hours.
- Qualitative defects in T cell function. Even in asymptomatic HIV-infected individuals, defects have been reported, including a reduction in antigen-induced T cell proliferation, a decrease in T_H1-type responses relative to the T_H2 type, defects in intracellular signaling, and many more. The loss of T_H1 responses results in a profound deficiency in cell-mediated immunity. There also is a selective loss of the memory subset of CD4+ helper T cells early in the course of disease, which explains poor recall responses to previously encountered antigens.

Low-level chronic or latent infection of T cells is an important feature of HIV infection. Integrated provirus, without viral gene expression (latent infection), can persist in cells for months or years. Even with potent antiviral therapy, which practically sterilizes the peripheral blood, latent virus lurks within CD4+ cells (both T cells and macrophages) in lymph nodes. According to some estimates, 0.05% of CD4+ T cells in the lymph nodes are latently infected. Because most of these CD4+ T cells are memory cells, they are long-lived, with a life span of months to years, and thus provide a persistent reservoir of virus.

HIV Infection of Non–T Immune Cells

In addition to infection and loss of CD4+ T cells, infection of macrophages and DCs also is important in the pathogenesis of HIV infection.

Macrophages. Similar to T cells, most macrophages infected by HIV are found in tissues, and in certain tissues, such as the lungs and brain, as many as 10% to 50% of macrophages are infected. Although cell division is required for nuclear entry and replication of most retroviruses, HIV-1 can infect and multiply in terminally differentiated nondividing macrophages, which may contain large numbers of virus particles. Even though macrophages allow viral replication, they are quite resistant to the cytopathic effects of HIV, in contrast to CD4+ T cells. Thus, macrophages may be reservoirs of infection, and in late stages of HIV infection, when CD4+ T-cell numbers decline greatly, macrophages may be an important site of continued viral replication.

Dendritic Cells. Mucosal DCs may be infected by the virus and transport it to regional lymph nodes, where the virus is transmitted to CD4+ T cells. Follicular DCs in the germinal centers of lymph nodes also are potential reservoirs of HIV. Although some follicular DCs may be susceptible to HIV infection, most virus particles are found on the surface of their dendritic processes.

B Cell Function in HIV Infection. Although B cells cannot be infected by HIV, they may show profound abnormalities. Paradoxically, there is spontaneous B-cell activation and hypergammaglobulinemia in association with an inability to mount antibody responses to newly encountered antigens. The defective antibody responses may be due to lack of T-cell help as well as acquired defects in B cells.

Pathogenesis of Central Nervous System Involvement

Like the lymphoid system, the nervous system is a target of HIV infection. Macrophages and microglia, cells in the CNS that belong to the macrophage lineage, are the predominant cell types in the brain that are infected with HIV. It is believed that HIV is carried into the brain by infected monocytes. In keeping with this, the HIV isolates from the brain are almost exclusively M-tropic. The mechanism of HIV-induced damage of the brain, however, remains obscure. Because neurons are not infected and the extent of neuropathologic changes is often less than might be expected from the severity of neurologic symptoms, most clinicians believe that the neurologic deficit is caused indirectly by viral products and by soluble factors produced by infected microglia, such as the cytokines IL-1, TNF, and IL-6.

● SUMMARY

HUMAN IMMUNODEFICIENCY VIRUS LIFE CYCLE AND THE PATHOGENESIS OF AIDS

- *Virus entry into cells:* Requires CD4 and coreceptors, which are receptors for chemokines; involves binding of viral gp120 and fusion with the cell mediated by viral gp41 protein; main cellular targets: CD4+ helper T cells, macrophages, DCs
- *Viral replication:* Integration of provirus genome into host cell DNA; triggering of viral gene expression by stimuli that activate infected cells (e.g., infectious microbes, cytokines produced during normal immune responses)
- *Progression of infection:* Acute infection of mucosal T cells and DCs; viremia with dissemination of virus; latent infection of cells in lymphoid tissue; continuing viral replication and progressive loss of CD4+ T cells
- *Mechanisms of immune deficiency:*
  - Loss of CD4+ T cells: T cell death during viral replication and budding (similar to other cytopathic infections); apoptosis occurring as a result of chronic stimulation; decreased thymic output; functional defects
  - Defective macrophage and DC functions
  - Destruction of architecture of lymphoid tissues (late)

Natural History and Course of HIV Infection

HIV disease begins with acute infection, which is only partly controlled by the host immune response, and advances to chronic progressive infection of peripheral lymphoid tissues (Figs. 5.39 and 5.40).

- *Acute phase.* **Virus typically enters through mucosal surfaces, and acute (early) infection is characterized by infection of memory CD4+ T cells (which express CCR5) in mucosal lymphoid tissues, and the death of many of these infected cells.** Because the mucosal tissues are the largest reservoir of T cells in the body, and a major site of residence of memory T cells, this local loss results in considerable depletion of lymphocytes. At this stage, few infected cells are detectable in the blood and other tissues.

  Mucosal infection is followed by dissemination of the virus and the development of host immune responses. DCs in epithelia at sites of virus entry capture the virus and then migrate into the lymph nodes. Once in lymphoid tissues, DCs pass HIV on to CD4+ T cells through direct cell–cell contact. Within days after the first exposure to HIV, viral replication can be detected in lymph nodes. This replication leads to viremia, during which high numbers of HIV particles are present in the patient's blood. The virus disseminates throughout the body and infects helper T cells, macrophages, and DCs in peripheral lymphoid tissues.

  Within 3 to 6 weeks after initial infection, 40% to 90% of infected individuals develop an *acute HIV syndrome*, which is triggered by the initial spread of the virus and the host response. This phase is associated with a self-limited acute illness with nonspecific symptoms, including sore throat, myalgias, fever, weight loss, and fatigue, resembling a flulike syndrome. Rash, lymphadenopathy, diarrhea, and vomiting also may occur. This typically resolves spontaneously in 2 to 4 weeks.

  As the infection spreads, the individual mounts antiviral humoral and cell-mediated immune responses. These responses are evidenced by seroconversion (usually within 3 to 7 weeks of presumed exposure) and by the appearance of virus-specific CD8+ cytotoxic T cells. HIV-specific CD8+ T cells are detected in the blood at about the time viral titers begin to fall and are most likely responsible for the initial containment of HIV infection. These immune responses partially control the infection and viral production, and such control is reflected by a drop in viremia to low but detectable levels by about 12 weeks after the primary exposure.

- *Chronic phase.* **In the next, chronic phase of the disease, lymph nodes and the spleen are sites of continuous HIV replication and cell destruction.** During this period of the disease, few or no clinical manifestations of the HIV infection are present. Therefore, this phase of HIV disease is called the *clinical latency period*. Although few peripheral blood T cells harbor the virus, destruction of CD4+ T cells within lymphoid tissues (up to 10% of which may be infected) continues during this phase, and the number of circulating blood CD4+ T cells steadily declines. Eventually, over a period of years, the continuous cycle of virus infection, T-cell death, and new infection leads to a steady decline in the number of

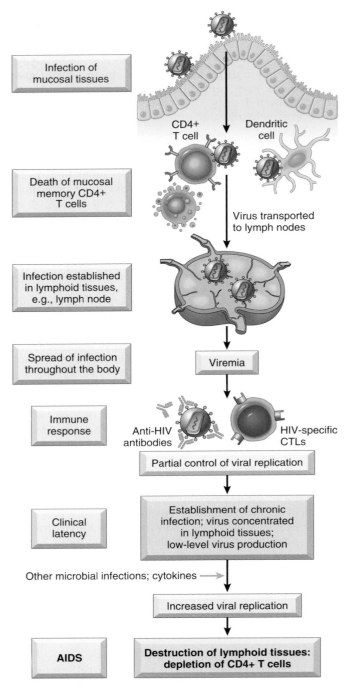

Fig. 5.39 Pathogenesis of HIV-1 infection. The initial infection starts in mucosal tissues, involving mainly memory CD4+ T cells and dendritic cells, and spreads to lymph nodes. Viral replication leads to viremia and widespread seeding of lymphoid tissue. The viremia is controlled by the host immune response, and the patient then enters a phase of clinical latency. During this phase, viral replication in both T cells and macrophages continues unabated, but there is some immune containment of virus *(not shown)*. A gradual erosion of CD4+ cells continues, and, ultimately, CD4+ T-cell numbers decline and the patient develops clinical symptoms of full-blown AIDS. *CTL,* Cytotoxic T lymphocyte.

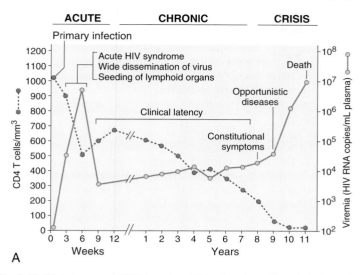

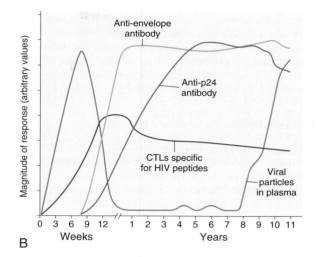

Fig. 5.40 Clinical course of HIV infection. (A) During the early period after primary infection, there is dissemination of virus, development of an immune response to HIV, and often an acute viral syndrome. During the period of clinical latency, viral replication continues and the CD4+ T-cell count gradually decreases, until it reaches a critical level below which there is a substantial risk for AIDS-associated diseases. (B) Immune response to HIV infection. A cytotoxic T-lymphocyte (CTL) response to HIV is detectable by 2 to 3 weeks after the initial infection, and it peaks by 9 to 12 weeks. Marked expansion of virus-specific CD8+ T-cell clones occurs during this time, and up to 10% of a patient's CTLs may be HIV specific at 12 weeks. The humoral immune response to HIV peaks at about 12 weeks. (*A,* Redrawn from Fauci AS, Lane HC: Human immunodeficiency virus disease: AIDS and related conditions. In Fauci AS, et al, editors: Harrison's principles of internal medicine, ed 14, New York, 1997, McGraw-Hill, p 1791.)

CD4+ T cells in the lymphoid tissues and the circulation.

- *AIDS.* **The final phase is progression to AIDS, characterized by a breakdown of host defense, a dramatic increase in plasma virus, and severe, life-threatening clinical disease.** Typically the patient presents with long-lasting fever (>1 month), fatigue, weight loss, and diarrhea. After a variable period, serious opportunistic infections, secondary neoplasms, or clinical neurologic disease (grouped under the rubric *AIDS indicator diseases* or *AIDS-defining illnesses,* discussed later) emerge, and the patient is said to have developed AIDS.

The extent of viremia, measured as HIV-1 RNA levels in the blood, is a useful marker of HIV disease progression and is of value in the management of HIV-infected individuals. The viral load at the end of the acute phase reflects the equilibrium reached between the virus and the host response, and in a given patient it may remain fairly stable for several years. This level of steady-state viremia, called the *viral set point,* is a predictor of the rate of decline of CD4+ T cells and, therefore, progression of HIV disease.

Because the loss of immune containment is associated with declining CD4+ T cell counts, the Centers for Disease Control and Prevention (CDC) classification of HIV infection stratifies patients into three groups based on CD4+ cell counts: greater than or equal to 500 cells/μL, 200 to 499 cells/μL, and fewer than 200 cells/μL (Table 5.15).

In the absence of treatment, most patients with HIV infection progress to AIDS after a chronic phase lasting from 7 to 10 years, but there are exceptions. In *rapid progressors,* the middle, chronic phase is telescoped to 2 to 3 years after primary infection. About 5% to 15% of infected individuals are *long-term nonprogressors,* defined as untreated HIV-1–infected individuals who remain asymptomatic for

10 years or more, with stable CD4+ T cell counts and low levels of plasma viremia (usually <500 viral RNA copies/mL). Remarkably, about 1% of infected individuals have undetectable plasma virus (<50 to 75 RNA copies/mL); these have been called *elite controllers.* Individuals with such an uncommon clinical course have attracted great attention in the hope that studying them may shed light on host and viral factors that influence disease progression. Studies thus far indicate that this group is heterogeneous with respect to the variables that influence the course of the disease. In most cases, the viral isolates do not show qualitative abnormalities, suggesting that the uneventful course cannot be attributed to a "wimpy" virus. In all cases, there is evidence of a vigorous anti-HIV immune

Table 5.15 CDC Classification Categories of HIV Infection

| | CD4+ T-Cell Categories | | |
| | **1** | **2** | **3** |
Clinical Categories	**≥500 Cells/μL**	**200–499 Cells/μL**	**<200 Cells/μL**
A. Asymptomatic: acute (primary) HIV, or persistent generalized lymphadenopathy	A1	A2	A3
B. Symptomatic: no A or C conditions	B1	B2	B3
C. AIDS indicator conditions: including constitutional disease, neurologic disease, or neoplasm			

Data from Centers for Disease Control and Prevention: 1993 revised classification system and expanded surveillance definition for AIDS among adolescents and adults. *MMWR* 41(RR-17):1, 1992.

response, but the immune correlates of protection are still unknown. Some of these individuals have high levels of HIV-specific CD4+ and CD8+ T-cell responses, and these levels are maintained over the course of infection. The inheritance of particular *HLA* alleles seems to correlate with resistance to disease progression, perhaps reflecting the ability to mount anti-viral T cell responses.

Clinical Features of AIDS

In the following section, we summarize the clinical manifestations of the terminal phase of the disease, full-blown AIDS.

In the United States, the typical adult patient with AIDS presents with fever, weight loss, diarrhea, generalized lymphadenopathy, multiple opportunistic infections, neurologic disease, and, in many cases, secondary neoplasms.

Opportunistic Infections

Opportunistic infections account for the majority of deaths in untreated patients with AIDS. Many of these infections represent reactivation of latent infections, which are normally kept in check by a robust immune system but are not completely eradicated because the infectious agents have evolved to coexist with their hosts. The actual frequency of infections varies in different regions of the world, and has been markedly reduced by the advent of highly active anti-retroviral therapy (called HAART or ART), which relies on a combination of three or four drugs that block different steps of the HIV life cycle.

- Approximately 15% to 30% of untreated HIV-infected individuals develop *pneumonia* caused by the fungus *Pneumocystis jiroveci* at some time during the course of the disease. Before the advent of HAART, this infection was the presenting feature in about 20% of cases, but the incidence is much less in patients who respond to HAART.
- *Candidiasis* is the most common fungal infection in patients with AIDS, and infection of the oral cavity, vagina, and esophagus are its most common clinical manifestations. In HIV-infected individuals, oral candidiasis is a sign of immunologic decompensation, and often heralds the transition to AIDS. Invasive candidiasis is infrequent in patients with AIDS, and it usually occurs when there is drug-induced neutropenia or use of indwelling catheters.
- *Cytomegalovirus* (CMV) may cause disseminated disease, but more commonly affects the eye and gastrointestinal tract. Chorioretinitis used to be seen in approximately 25% of patients, but has decreased dramatically after the initiation of HAART. CMV retinitis occurs almost exclusively in patients with CD4+ T cell counts less than 50 per microliter. Gastrointestinal CMV infection, seen in 5% to 10% of cases, manifests as esophagitis and colitis, the latter associated with multiple mucosal ulcerations.
- Disseminated bacterial infection with *nontuberculous*, or *atypical, mycobacteria* (mainly *Mycobacterium avium-intracellulare*) also occurs late, in the setting of severe immunosuppression. Coincident with the AIDS epidemic, the incidence of tuberculosis has risen dramatically. Worldwide, almost one third of all deaths in AIDS patients are attributable to *tuberculosis,* but this compli-

cation remains uncommon in the United States. Both reactivation of latent pulmonary disease and new primary infection contribute to this toll. As with tuberculosis in other settings, the infection may be confined to lungs or may involve multiple organs. Most worrisome are reports indicating that a growing number of isolates are resistant to multiple anti-mycobacterial drugs.

- *Cryptococcosis* occurs in about 10% of AIDS patients. As in other settings with immunosuppression, meningitis is the major clinical manifestation of cryptococcosis. *Toxoplasma gondii,* another frequent invader of the CNS in AIDS, causes encephalitis and is responsible for 50% of all mass lesions in the CNS.
- *JC virus,* a human papovavirus, is another important cause of CNS infections in HIV-infected patients. It causes progressive multifocal leukoencephalopathy (Chapter 23). *Herpes simplex virus infection* is manifested by mucocutaneous ulcerations involving the mouth, esophagus, external genitalia, and perianal region. Persistent diarrhea, which is common in untreated patients with advanced AIDS, is often caused by infections with protozoans or enteric bacteria.

Tumors

Patients with AIDS have a high incidence of certain tumors, notably Kaposi sarcoma, B cell lymphoma, cervical cancer in women, and anal cancer in men. These tumors are often considered *AIDS-defining malignancies.* It is estimated that 25% to 40% of untreated HIV-infected individuals will eventually develop a malignancy. Many of these tumors are caused by *oncogenic DNA viruses,* including Kaposi sarcoma herpesvirus (Kaposi sarcoma), EBV (B cell lymphoma), and human papillomavirus (cervical and anal carcinoma). These viruses establish latent infections that are kept in check in healthy individuals by a competent immune system. The increased risk for malignancy in AIDS patients exists mainly because of failure to contain the infection following reactivation of the viruses and decreased cellular immunity against virally infected cells undergoing malignant transformation. The incidence of many of these tumors, especially Kaposi sarcoma, is decreasing as treatment has improved and patients have less immune compromise. Nevertheless, HIV-infected individuals remain more susceptible to tumors that occur in the general population, such as lung and skin cancers and certain forms of lymphoma.

Kaposi Sarcoma. Kaposi sarcoma (KS), a vascular tumor that is otherwise rare in the United States, is considered an AIDS-defining malignancy. The morphology of KS and its occurrence in patients not infected with HIV are discussed in Chapter 10. At the onset of the AIDS epidemic, up to 30% of infected homosexual or bisexual men had KS, but with use of HAART there has been a dramatic decline in its incidence in recent years. In contrast, in areas of sub-Saharan Africa where HIV infection is both frequent and largely untreated, Kaposi sarcoma is one of the most common tumors.

The lesions of KS are characterized by a proliferation of spindle-shaped cells that express markers of both endothelial cells (vascular or lymphatic) and smooth muscle cells.

In addition, KS lesions contain chronic inflammatory cell infiltrates. Many of the features of KS suggest that it is not a malignant tumor (despite its ominous name).

There is compelling evidence that KS is caused by the *KS herpesvirus (KSHV)*, also called *human herpesvirus 8 (HHV8)*. Exactly how KSHV infection leads to KS is still unclear. Like other herpesviruses, KSHV establishes latent infection, during which several proteins are produced with potential roles in stimulating spindle cell proliferation and preventing apoptosis. These include a viral homologue of the cell cycle regulator cyclin D (an oncogene) and several inhibitors of p53 (a key tumor suppressor gene), both of which have been implicated in tumor development (Chapter 6). The spindle cells produce proinflammatory and angiogenic factors, which recruit the inflammatory and neovascular components of the lesion, and the latter components supply signals that aid in spindle cell survival and growth. However, KSHV infection, while necessary for KS development, is not sufficient, and additional cofactors are needed. In the AIDS-related form, that cofactor is clearly HIV. HIV-mediated immune suppression may aid in widespread dissemination of KSHV in the host.

Clinically, AIDS-associated KS is quite different from the sporadic form (Chapter 10). In HIV-infected individuals, the tumor is usually widespread, affecting the skin, mucous membranes, gastrointestinal tract, lymph nodes, and lungs. These tumors also tend to be more aggressive than sporadic KS.

Lymphomas. Lymphoma occurs at a markedly increased rate in individuals with AIDS, making it another AIDS-defining tumor. Roughly 5% of AIDS patients present with lymphoma, and approximately another 5% develop lymphoma during their subsequent course. Even in the era of anti-retroviral therapy, lymphoma continues to occur in HIV-infected individuals at an incidence that is at least 10-fold greater than the population average. Based on molecular characterization of HIV-associated lymphomas and the epidemiologic considerations above, at least two mechanisms appear to underlie the increased risk for B-cell tumors in HIV-infected individuals.

- *Tumors Induced by Oncogenic Viruses.* T-cell immunity is required to restrain the proliferation of B cells latently infected with oncogenic viruses such as EBV and KSHV. With the appearance of severe T-cell depletion in the course of HIV infection, this control is lost, and the infected B cells undergo unchecked proliferation that predispose to mutations and the development of B-cell tumors. As a result, AIDS patients are at high risk for developing aggressive B-cell lymphomas composed of tumor cells infected by oncogenic viruses, particularly EBV. The tumors often occur in extranodal sites, such as the CNS, gut, orbit, and lungs, and elsewhere. AIDS patients also are prone to rare lymphomas that present as malignant effusions (so-called "primary effusion lymphoma"), which are remarkable in that the tumor cells are usually coinfected by both EBV and KSHV, a highly unusual example of cooperativity between two oncogenic viruses.
- *Germinal Center B-Cell Hyperplasia.* The majority of the lymphomas that arise in patients with preserved CD4 T-cell counts are not associated with EBV or KSHV. The

increased risk for lymphoma in these patients may be related to the profound germinal center B cell hyperplasia that occurs in HIV infection. The high level of proliferation and somatic mutations that occur in germinal center B cells set the stage for chromosomal translocations and mutations involving tumor-causing genes. In fact, the aggressive B-cell tumors that arise outside the setting of severe T cell depletion in HIV-infected individuals, such as Burkitt lymphoma and diffuse large B cell lymphoma, often are associated with mutations in oncogenes such as MYC and BCL6 that bear the molecular hallmarks of "mistakes" during the attempted diversification of immunoglobulin genes in germinal center B cells.

Several other EBV-related proliferations also merit mention. *Hodgkin lymphoma*, an unusual B-cell tumor associated with a pronounced tissue inflammatory response (Chapter 12), also occurs at increased frequency in HIV-infected individuals. In virtually all instances of HIV-associated Hodgkin lymphoma, the characteristic tumor cells (Reed-Sternberg cells) are infected with EBV. Many (but not all) HIV patients with Hodgkin lymphoma have low CD4 counts at the time of disease presentation. EBV infection also is responsible for oral hairy leukoplakia (white projections on the tongue), which results from EBV-driven squamous cell proliferation of the oral mucosa (Chapter 15).

Other Tumors. In addition to KS and lymphomas, patients with AIDS also have an increased occurrence of *carcinoma of the uterine cervix* and of *anal cancer*. Both of these tumors are highly associated with *human papilloma virus* infection, which is poorly controlled in the setting of immunosuppression.

Central Nervous System Disease

Involvement of the CNS is a common and important manifestation of AIDS. Ninety percent of patients demonstrate some form of neurologic involvement at autopsy, and 40% to 60% have clinically apparent neurologic dysfunction. Importantly, in some patients, neurologic manifestations may be the sole or earliest presenting feature of HIV infection. Lesions include a self-limited presumed viral meningoencephalitis or aseptic meningitis, vacuolar myelopathy, peripheral neuropathies, and, most commonly, a progressive encephalopathy called *HIV-associated neurocognitive disorder* (Chapter 23).

Effect of Anti-Retroviral Drug Therapy on the Course of HIV Infection

The advent of new drugs that target the viral reverse transcriptase, protease, and integrase enzymes has changed the clinical face of AIDS. When a combination of at least three effective drugs is used in a motivated, compliant patient, HIV replication is reduced to below the threshold of detection (<50 RNA copies/mL) and remains there as long as the patient adheres to therapy. Once the virus is suppressed, the progressive loss of CD4+ T cells is halted, and the peripheral CD4+ T-cell count slowly increases, often returning to a normal level. With the use of these drugs, the annual death rate from AIDS in the United States has decreased from a peak of 16 to 18 per 100,000 individuals in 1995–1996 to less than 4 per 100,000. Many AIDS-associated disorders, such as opportunistic infections with *P. jiroveci* and Kaposi sarcoma, now are uncommon. Effective anti-retroviral therapy also has reduced the transmission of the virus, especially from infected mothers to newborns.

Despite these dramatic improvements, several new complications associated with HIV infection and its treatment have emerged. Some patients with advanced disease who are given anti-retroviral therapy develop a paradoxical clinical deterioration during the period of recovery of the immune system despite increasing CD4+ T-cell counts and decreasing viral load. This disorder, called the *immune reconstitution inflammatory syndrome,* is not understood but is postulated to be a poorly regulated host response to the high antigenic burden of persistent microbes. Perhaps a more important complication of long-term anti-retroviral therapy pertains to adverse side effects of the drugs. These include lipoatrophy (loss of facial fat), lipoaccumulation (excess fat deposition centrally), elevated lipids, insulin resistance, peripheral neuropathy, and premature cardiovascular, kidney, and liver disease. Finally, non-AIDS morbidity is far more common than classic AIDS-related morbidity in long-term HAART-treated patients. Major causes of morbidity are cancer and accelerated cardiovascular disease. The mechanism for these non-AIDS–related complications is not known, but persistent inflammation and T-cell dysfunction may have a role.

MORPHOLOGY

Changes in the tissues (with the exception of the brain) are neither specific nor diagnostic. Common pathologic features of AIDS include opportunistic infections, Kaposi sarcoma, and B-cell lymphomas. Most of these lesions are discussed elsewhere, because they also occur in individuals who do not have HIV infection. Lesions in the central nervous system are described in Chapter 23.

Biopsy specimens from enlarged lymph nodes in the early stages of HIV infection reveal a marked hyperplasia of B-cell follicles, which often take on unusual, serpiginous shapes. The mantle zones that surround the follicles are attenuated, and the germinal centers impinge on interfollicular T cell areas. This hyperplasia of B cells is the morphologic reflection of the polyclonal B cell activation and hypergammaglobulinemia seen in HIV-infected individuals.

With disease progression, the frenzy of B cell proliferation subsides and gives way to a pattern of severe lymphoid involution. The lymph nodes are depleted of lymphocytes, and the organized network of follicular dendritic cells is disrupted. The germinal centers may even become hyalinized. During this advanced stage, viral burden in the nodes is reduced, in part because of the disruption of the follicular dendritic cells. These "burnt-out" lymph nodes are atrophic and small and may harbor numerous opportunistic pathogens, often within macrophages. Because of profound immunosuppression, the inflammatory response to infections both in the lymph nodes and at extranodal sites may be sparse or atypical. For example, mycobacteria often fail to

evoke granuloma formation because CD4+ cells are deficient, and the presence of these and other infectious agents may not be apparent without special stains. As might be expected, lymphoid involution is not confined to the nodes; in later stages of AIDS, the spleen and thymus also are converted to "wastelands" that are virtually devoid of lymphocytes.

Despite impressive advances in our understanding and treatment of HIV infection, the long-term prognosis of patients with AIDS remains a concern. Although with effective drug therapy the mortality rate has declined in the United States, the treated patients still carry viral DNA in their lymphoid tissues. Truly curative therapy remains elusive. Similarly, although considerable effort has been mounted to develop a protective vaccine, many hurdles remain before this becomes a reality. Molecular analyses have revealed an alarming degree of variation in viral isolates from patients; this renders the task of producing a vaccine extremely difficult. Recent efforts have focused on producing broadly neutralizing antibodies against relatively invariant portions of HIV proteins. At present, therefore, prevention, public health measures, and anti-retroviral drugs remain the mainstays in the fight against AIDS.

SUMMARY

CLINICAL COURSE AND COMPLICATIONS OF HIV INFECTION

- *Progression of disease.* HIV infection progresses through phases.
  - *Acute HIV infection.* Manifestations of acute viral illness
  - *Chronic (latent) phase.* Dissemination of virus, host immune response, progressive destruction of immune cells.
  - *AIDS.* Severe immune deficiency.
- *Clinical features.* Full-blown AIDS manifests with several complications, mostly resulting from immune deficiency.
  - Opportunistic infections
  - Tumors, especially tumors caused by oncogenic viruses
  - Neurologic complications of unknown pathogenesis
- Antiretroviral therapy has greatly decreased the incidence of opportunistic infections and tumors but also has numerous complications.

AMYLOIDOSIS

Amyloidosis is a condition associated with a number of disorders in which extracellular deposits of fibrillar proteins are responsible for tissue damage and functional compromise. These abnormal fibrils are produced by the aggregation of improperly folded proteins (which are soluble in their normal folded configuration). The fibrillar deposits bind a wide variety of proteoglycans and glycosaminoglycans, which contain charged sugar groups that give the deposits staining characteristics thought to resemble those of starch (amylose). Therefore, the deposits were called *amyloid,* a name that is firmly entrenched despite the realization that the deposits are unrelated to starch.

Pathogenesis of Amyloid Deposition

Amyloid deposits can occur in a variety of conditions, in each of which the protein composition is different. Although amyloid always has the same morphologic appearance, it is biochemically heterogeneous. In fact, at least 30 different proteins can aggregate to form fibrils with the appearance of amyloid. Regardless of their derivation, all amyloid deposits are composed of nonbranching fibrils, each formed of intertwined polypeptides in a β pleated sheet conformation (Fig. 5.41). Approximately 95% of the amyloid material consists of fibril proteins, the remaining 5% being various glycoproteins.

The three most common forms of amyloid are the following:

- *AL (amyloid light chain) amyloid* is made up of complete immunoglobulin light chains, the amino-terminal fragments of light chains, or both.
- *AA (amyloid-associated) amyloid* is composed of an 8500-dalton protein derived by proteolysis from a larger precursor in the blood called SAA (serum amyloid-associated) protein, which is synthesized in the liver.
- *β-amyloid protein (Aβ)* is a 4000-dalton peptide that is derived by proteolysis from a much larger transmembrane glycoprotein, called *amyloid precursor protein.*

Many other proteins also can deposit as amyloid in a variety of clinical settings. Some of the most clinically important examples are mentioned in the following section.

Classification of Amyloidosis and Mechanisms of Amyloid Formation

Amyloidosis results from abnormal folding of proteins, which assume a β pleated sheet conformation, aggregate, and deposit as fibrils in extracellular tissues. Normally, intracellular misfolded proteins are degraded in proteasomes and extracellular protein aggregates are taken up and degraded by macrophages. In amyloidosis, these quality control mechanisms fail and fibrillar proteins accumulate outside of cells. The proteins that form amyloid fall into two general categories (Fig. 5.42): (1) normal proteins that have an inherent tendency to associate and form fibrils, particularly when produced in increased amounts; and (2) mutant proteins that are prone to misfolding and aggregation. The mechanisms of deposition of different types of amyloid are discussed next along with classification.

Because a given form of amyloid (e.g., AA) may be associated with diverse clinical settings, we will follow a classification that takes into account clinical and biochemical features (Table 5.16). Amyloid may be systemic (generalized), involving several organ systems, or it may be localized to a single organ, such as the heart. On clinical grounds, the systemic pattern is subclassified into primary amyloidosis when it is associated with a clonal plasma cell proliferation, or secondary amyloidosis when it occurs as a complication of an underlying chronic inflammatory or tissue-destructive process. Hereditary or familial amyloidosis constitutes a separate, heterogeneous group with several distinctive patterns of organ involvement.

Primary Amyloidosis: Plasma Cell Proliferations Associated With Amyloidosis. Amyloid in this category is of the *AL type* and is usually systemic in distribution. This is the most common form of amyloidosis, with approximately 2000 to 3000 new cases each year in the United States. It is caused by a **clonal proliferation of plasma cells** that synthesize abnormal Ig molecules. The AL type of systemic amyloidosis occurs in 5% to 15% of individuals with multiple myeloma, a plasma-cell tumor characterized by excessive production of free immunoglobulin light chains (Chapter 12). The free, unpaired κ or λ light chains (referred to as *Bence Jones protein*) are prone to aggregating and depositing in tissues as amyloid. Since the majority of myeloma patients do not develop amyloidosis, however, it is clear that not all free light chains are equally likely to produce amyloid. For unknown reasons, λ light chains are approximately six times more likely to deposit as amyloid than κ light chains.

Most persons with AL amyloid do not have multiple myeloma or any other overt B cell neoplasm; such cases have been traditionally classified as primary amyloidosis, because their clinical features derive solely from the effects of amyloid deposition rather than formation of tumor masses. In virtually all such cases, however, monoclonal immunoglobulins or free light chains, or both, can be found in the blood or urine. Most of these patients also have a

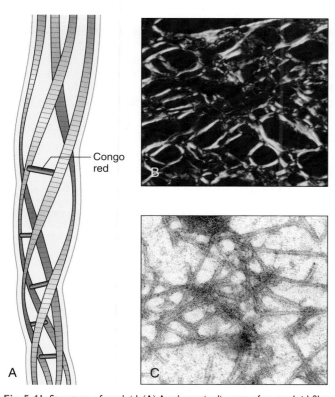

Congo red

Fig. 5.41 Structure of amyloid. (A) A schematic diagram of an amyloid fiber showing four fibrils (there can be as many as six in each fiber) wound around one another with regularly spaced binding of the Congo red dye. (B) Congo red staining shows apple-green birefringence under polarized light, a diagnostic feature of amyloid. (C) Electron micrograph of 7.5- to 10-nm amyloid fibrils. *(From Merlini G, Bellotti V: Molecular mechanisms of amyloidosis. N Engl J Med 349:583–596, 2003.)*

PRODUCTION OF ABNORMAL
AMOUNTS OF PROTEIN

PRODUCTION OF NORMAL
AMOUNTS OF MUTANT
PROTEIN (e.g., transthyretin)

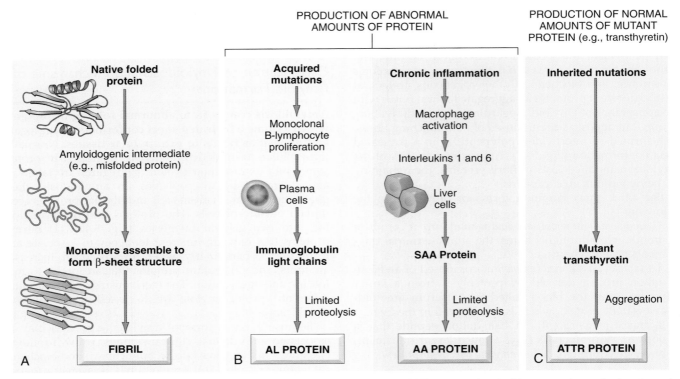

Fig. 5.42 Pathogenesis of amyloidosis. (A) General mechanism of formation of amyloid fibrils. (B) Formation of amyloid from excessive production of proteins prone to misfolding. (C) Formation of amyloid from mutant protein.

modest increase in the number of plasma cells in the bone marrow, which presumably secrete the precursors of AL protein.

Reactive Systemic Amyloidosis. The amyloid deposits in this pattern are systemic in distribution and are composed of *AA protein.* This category was previously referred to as secondary amyloidosis because it is **secondary to an associated inflammatory condition.** At one time, tuberculosis, bronchiectasis, and chronic osteomyelitis were the most important underlying conditions, but currently, these conditions frequently resolve with antibiotic treatment and less often lead to amyloidosis. More commonly now, reactive systemic amyloidosis complicates rheumatoid arthritis, other connective tissue disorders such as ankylosing spondylitis, and inflammatory bowel disease, particularly

Table 5.16 Classification of Amyloidosis

Clinicopathologic Category	Associated Diseases	Major Fibril Protein	Chemically Related Precursor Protein
Systemic (Generalized) Amyloidosis			
Plasma cell proliferations with amyloidosis (primary amyloidosis)	Multiple myeloma and other monoclonal plasma cell proliferations	AL	Immunoglobulin light chains, chiefly λ type
Reactive systemic amyloidosis (secondary amyloidosis)	Chronic inflammatory conditions	AA	SAA
Hemodialysis-associated amyloidosis	Chronic renal failure	$A\beta_2m$	β_2-microglobulin
Hereditary Amyloidosis			
Familial Mediterranean fever		AA	SAA
Familial amyloidotic neuropathies (several types)		ATTR	Transthyretin
Systemic senile amyloidosis		ATTR	Transthyretin
Localized Amyloidosis			
Senile cerebral	Alzheimer disease	Aβ	APP
Endocrine	Type 2 diabetes		
Medullary carcinoma of thyroid		A Cal	Calcitonin
Islets of Langerhans		AIAPP	Islet amyloid peptide
Isolated atrial amyloidosis		AANF	Atrial natriuretic factor

Crohn disease and ulcerative colitis. Among these, the most frequent associated condition is rheumatoid arthritis. Amyloidosis is reported to occur in approximately 3% of patients with rheumatoid arthritis and is clinically significant in one half of those affected. Heroin abusers who inject the drug subcutaneously also have a high occurrence rate of generalized AA amyloidosis. The chronic skin infections, which cause the "skin-popping" associated with injection of narcotics, seem to be responsible for the amyloidosis. Reactive systemic amyloidosis also may occur in association with certain cancers, the most common being renal cell carcinoma and Hodgkin lymphoma.

In AA amyloidosis, SAA synthesis by liver cells is stimulated by cytokines such as IL-6 and IL-1 that are produced during inflammation; thus, long-standing inflammation leads to a sustained elevation of SAA levels. While SAA levels are increased in all cases of inflammation, only a small subset get amyloidosis. It seems that in some patients SAA breakdown produces intermediates that are prone to forming fibrils.

Heredofamilial Amyloidosis.

A variety of familial forms of amyloidosis have been described. Most are rare and occur in limited geographic areas. The most common and best studied is an autosomal recessive condition called *familial Mediterranean fever,* which is encountered largely in individuals of Armenian, Sephardic Jewish, and Arabic origins. This is an "autoinflammatory" syndrome associated with excessive production of the cytokine IL-1 in response to inflammatory stimuli. It is characterized by attacks of fever accompanied by inflammation of serosal surfaces that manifests as peritonitis, pleuritis, and synovitis. The gene for familial Mediterranean fever encodes a protein called pyrin that is important in dampening the response of innate immune cells, particularly neutrophils, to inflammatory mediators. The amyloid seen in this disorder is of the AA type, suggesting that it is related to the recurrent bouts of inflammation.

In contrast to familial Mediterranean fever, a group of autosomal dominant familial disorders is characterized by deposition of amyloid made up of fibrils derived from mutant transthyretin (TTR). TTR is a transporter of the hormone thyroxine. Remarkably, specific TTR mutant polypeptides tend to form amyloid in different organs; thus, in some families, deposits are seen mainly in peripheral nerves (familial amyloidotic polyneuropathies), whereas in others cardiac deposits predominate. The mutated form of the *TTR* gene that leads to cardiac amyloidosis is carried by approximately 4% of the black population in the United States, and cardiomyopathy has been identified in both homozygous and heterozygous patients. The precise prevalence of patients with this mutation who develop clinically manifest cardiac disease is not known.

Hemodialysis-Associated Amyloidosis.

Patients on long-term hemodialysis for renal failure can develop amyloid deposits derived from β_2-microglobulin. This protein is present in high concentrations in the serum of individuals with renal disease, and in the past it was retained in the circulation because it could not be filtered through dialysis membranes. With new dialysis filters, the incidence of this complication has decreased substantially. The classical features of this form of amyloidosis are the triad of scapulohumeral periarthritis, carpal tunnel syndrome, and flexor tenosynovitis of the hand.

Localized Amyloidosis.

Sometimes, amyloid deposits are limited to a single organ or tissue without involvement of any other site in the body. The deposits may produce grossly detectable nodular masses or be evident only on microscopic examination. Nodular deposits of amyloid are most often encountered in the lung, larynx, skin, urinary bladder, tongue, and the region about the eye. Frequently, there are infiltrates of lymphocytes and plasma cells associated with these amyloid masses. At least in some cases, the amyloid consists of AL protein and may therefore represent a localized form of plasma cell–derived amyloid.

Endocrine Amyloid.

Microscopic deposits of localized amyloid may be found in certain endocrine tumors, such as medullary carcinoma of the thyroid gland, islet tumors of the pancreas, pheochromocytomas, and undifferentiated carcinomas of the stomach, and in the islets of Langerhans in individuals with type 2 diabetes mellitus. In these settings, the amyloidogenic proteins seem to be derived either from polypeptide hormones (e.g., medullary carcinoma) or from unique proteins (e.g., islet amyloid polypeptide).

Amyloid of Aging.

Several well-documented forms of amyloid deposition occur with aging. Senile systemic amyloidosis refers to the systemic deposition of amyloid in elderly patients (usually in their seventies and eighties). Because of the dominant involvement and related dysfunction of the heart, this form was previously called *senile cardiac amyloidosis.* Those who are symptomatic present with a restrictive cardiomyopathy and arrhythmias (Chapter 11). The amyloid in this form, in contrast to familial forms, is derived from normal TTR.

MORPHOLOGY

There are no consistent or distinctive patterns of organ or tissue distribution of amyloid deposits in any of the categories cited, but a few generalizations can be made. In AA amyloidosis secondary to chronic inflammatory disorders, kidneys, liver, spleen, lymph nodes, adrenal glands, thyroid glands, and many other tissues are typically affected. Although AL amyloidosis associated with plasma cell proliferations cannot reliably be distinguished from the AA form by its organ distribution, it more often involves the heart, gastrointestinal tract, respiratory tract, peripheral nerves, skin, and tongue. The localization of amyloid deposits in the hereditary syndromes is varied. In familial Mediterranean fever, the amyloidosis is of the AA type and accordingly may be widespread, involving the kidneys, blood vessels, spleen, respiratory tract, and (rarely) liver.

Amyloid may be appreciated macroscopically when it accumulates in large amounts. The organ is frequently enlarged, and the tissue appears gray and has a waxy, firm consistency. Histologically, the amyloid deposition is always extracellular and begins between cells, often closely adjacent to basement membranes

(Fig. 5.43A). As the amyloid accumulates, it encroaches on the cells, in time surrounding and destroying them. In the form associated with plasma cell proliferation, perivascular and vascular deposits are common.

The diagnosis of amyloidosis is based on histopathology. With the light microscope and hematoxylin and eosin stains, amyloid appears as an amorphous, eosinophilic, hyaline, extracellular substance. To differentiate amyloid from other hyaline materials (e.g., collagen, fibrin), a variety of histochemical stains are used. The most widely used is the Congo red stain, which under ordinary light gives a pink or red color to tissue deposits, but far more striking and specific is the green birefringence of the stained amyloid when observed by polarizing microscopy (Fig. 5.43B). This staining reaction is shared by all forms of amyloid and is imparted by the crossed β-pleated sheet configuration of amyloid fibrils. Confirmation can be obtained by electron microscopy, which reveals amorphous nonoriented thin fibrils. Subtyping of amyloid is most reliably done by mass spectroscopy, as immunohistochemical stains are not entirely sensitive or specific.

The pattern of organ involvement in different forms of amyloidosis is variable.

Kidney. Amyloidosis of the kidney is the most common and potentially the most serious form of organ involvement. Grossly, the kidneys may be of normal size and color, or in advanced cases they may be shrunken because of ischemia caused by vascular narrowing induced by the deposition of amyloid within arterial and arteriolar walls. Histologically, the amyloid is deposited primarily in the glomeruli, but the interstitial peritubular tissue, arteries, and arterioles are also affected. The glomerular deposits first appear as subtle thickenings of the mesangial matrix, accompanied usually by uneven widening of the basement membranes of the glomerular capillaries. In time, deposits in the mesangium and along the basement membranes cause capillary narrowing and distortion of the glomerular vascular tuft. With progression of the glomerular amyloidosis, the capillary lumens are obliterated and the obsolescent glomerulus is replaced by confluent masses or interlacing broad ribbons of amyloid.

Spleen. Amyloidosis of the spleen may be inapparent grossly or may cause moderate to marked splenomegaly (up to 800 g). For mysterious reasons, two distinct patterns of deposition are seen. In one, the deposits are largely limited to the splenic follicles, producing tapioca-like granules on gross inspection, designated *sago spleen.* In the other pattern, the amyloid involves the walls of the splenic sinuses and connective tissue framework in the red pulp. Fusion of the early deposits gives rise to large, maplike areas of amyloidosis, creating what has been designated *lardaceous spleen.*

Liver. The deposits may be inapparent grossly or may cause moderate to marked hepatomegaly. Amyloid appears first in the space of Disse and then progressively encroaches on adjacent hepatic parenchymal cells and sinusoids. In time, deformity, pressure atrophy, and disappearance of hepatocytes occur, causing total replacement of large areas of liver parenchyma. Vascular involvement and deposits in Kupffer cells are frequent. Liver function is usually preserved despite sometimes quite extensive involvement.

Heart. Amyloidosis of the heart (Chapter 11) may occur in any form of systemic amyloidosis. It also is the major organ involved in senile systemic amyloidosis. The heart may be enlarged and firm, but more often it shows no appreciable change on gross inspection. Histologically the deposits begin as focal subendocardial accumulations and within the myocardium between the muscle fibers. Expansion of these myocardial deposits eventually causes pressure atrophy of myocardial fibers. When the amyloid deposits are subendocardial, the conduction system may be damaged, accounting for the electrocardiographic abnormalities noted in some patients.

Other Organs. Nodular depositions in the **tongue** may cause macroglossia, giving rise to the designation tumor-forming amyloid of the tongue. The **respiratory tract** may be involved focally or diffusely from the larynx down to the smallest bronchioles. A distinct form of amyloid is found in the **brains** of patients with Alzheimer disease. It may be present in so-called "plaques" as well as blood vessels (Chapter 23). Amyloidosis of peripheral and autonomic **nerves** is a feature of several familial amyloidotic neuropathies.

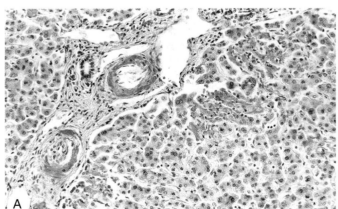
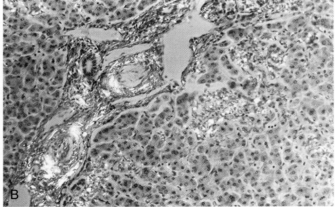

Fig. 5.43 Amyloidosis. (A) A section of liver stained with Congo red reveals pink-red deposits of amyloid in the walls of blood vessels and along sinusoids. (B) Note the yellow-green birefringence of the deposits when observed by a polarizing microscope. (*B, Courtesy of Dr. Trace Worrell and Sandy Hinton, Department of Pathology, University of Texas Southwestern Medical School, Dallas, Texas.*)

Clinical Features

Amyloidosis may be found as an unsuspected anatomic change, having produced no clinical manifestations, or it may cause serious clinical problems and even death. The symptoms depend on the magnitude of the deposits and on the sites or organs affected. Clinical manifestations at first are often entirely nonspecific, such as weakness, weight loss, lightheadedness, or syncope. Somewhat more specific findings appear later and most often relate to renal, cardiac, and gastrointestinal involvement.

Renal involvement gives rise to proteinuria that may be severe enough to cause the nephrotic syndrome (Chapter 14). Progressive obliteration of glomeruli in advanced cases ultimately leads to renal failure and uremia. Renal failure is a common cause of death. Cardiac amyloidosis may present insidiously as congestive heart failure. The most serious aspects of cardiac amyloidosis are conduction disturbances and arrhythmias, which may prove fatal. Occasionally, cardiac amyloidosis produces a restrictive pattern of cardiomyopathy and masquerades as chronic constrictive pericarditis (Chapter 11). Gastrointestinal amyloidosis may be asymptomatic, or it may present in a variety of ways. Amyloidosis of the tongue may cause sufficient enlargement and inelasticity to hamper speech and swallowing. Depositions in the stomach and intestine may lead to malabsorption, diarrhea, and disturbances in digestion. Vascular amyloidosis causes vascular fragility that may lead to bleeding, sometimes massive, that can occur spontaneously or following seemingly trivial trauma. Additionally, in some cases AL amyloid binds and inactivates factor X, a critical coagulation factor, leading to a life-threatening bleeding disorder.

The diagnosis of amyloidosis depends on the histologic demonstration of amyloid deposits in tissues. The most common sites biopsied are the kidney, when renal manifestations are present, or rectal or gingival tissues in patients suspected of having systemic amyloidosis. Examination of abdominal fat aspirates stained with Congo red can also be used for the diagnosis of systemic amyloidosis. The test is quite specific, but its sensitivity is low. In suspected cases of AL amyloidosis, serum and urine protein electrophoresis and immunoelectrophoresis should be performed. Bone marrow aspirates in such cases often show a monoclonal population of plasma cells, even in the absence of overt multiple myeloma. Scintigraphy with radiolabeled serum amyloid P (SAP) component is a rapid and specific test, since SAP binds to the amyloid deposits and reveals their presence. It also gives a measure of the extent of amyloidosis and can be used to follow patients undergoing treatment. Mass spectroscopy is a useful tool for identification of the protein component of amyloid. It can be performed on paraffin embedded tissues.

The prognosis for individuals with generalized amyloidosis is poor. Those with AL amyloidosis (not including multiple myeloma) have a median survival of 2 years after diagnosis. Individuals with myeloma-associated amyloidosis have an even poorer prognosis. The outlook for individuals with reactive systemic amyloidosis is somewhat better and depends to some extent on the control of the underlying condition. Resorption of amyloid after treatment of the associated condition has been reported, but this is a rare occurrence. New therapeutic strategies aimed at correcting protein misfolding and inhibiting fibrillogenesis are being developed.

SUMMARY

AMYLOIDOSIS

- Amyloidosis is a disorder characterized by the extracellular deposits of proteins that are prone to aggregate and form insoluble fibrils.
- The deposition of these proteins may result from: excessive production of proteins that are prone to aggregation; mutations that produce proteins that cannot fold properly and tend to aggregate; defective or incomplete proteolytic degradation of extracellular proteins.
- Amyloidosis may be localized or systemic. It is seen in association with a variety of primary disorders, including monoclonal B-cell proliferations (in which the amyloid deposits consist of immunoglobulin light chains); chronic inflammatory diseases such as rheumatoid arthritis (deposits of amyloid A protein, derived from an acute-phase protein produced in inflammation); Alzheimer disease (amyloid β protein); familial conditions in which the amyloid deposits consist of mutated proteins (e.g., transthyretin in familial amyloid polyneuropathies); and hemodialysis (deposits of β_2-microglobulin, whose clearance is defective).
- Amyloid deposits cause tissue injury and impair normal function by causing pressure on cells and tissues. They do not evoke an inflammatory response.

SUGGESTED READINGS

Bonnelykke K, Sparks R, Waage J, et al: Genetics of allergy and allergic sensitization: common variants, rare mutations, *Curr Opin Immunol* 36:115, 2015. [*An update on the genes associated with allergic diseases.*]

Broderick L, De Nardo D, Franklin BS, et al: The inflammasomes and autoinflammatory syndromes, *Annu Rev Pathol* 10:395, 2015. [*A discussion of the inflammasome and its role in inflammatory diseases.*]

Chaudhry A, Rudensky AY: Control of inflammation by integration of environmental cues by regulatory T cells, *J Clin Invest* 123:939–944, 2013. [*A thoughtful discussion of how regulatory T cells control inflammatory responses and maintain homeostasis in the immune system.*]

Cheng MH, Anderson MS: Monogenic autoimmunity, *Annu Rev Immunol* 30:393–427, 2012. [*An excellent review of autoimmune syndromes caused by single-gene mutations, and what they teach us about pathways of immunologic tolerance.*]

Conley ME, Casanova JL: Discovery of single-gene inborn errors of immunity by next generation sequencing, *Curr Opin Immunol* 30:17, 2014. [*A review of modern approaches for identifying the genetic basis of immunodeficiency diseases.*]

Craft JE: Follicular helper T cells in immunity and systemic autoimmunity, *Nat Rev Rheumatol* 8:337–347, 2012. [*A discussion of the properties and generation of follicular helper T cells and their roles in antibody production and autoimmunity.*]

Douek DC, Roederer M, Koup RA: Emerging concepts in the immunopathogenesis of AIDS, *Annu Rev Med* 60:471, 2009. [*A balanced discussion of the pathogenesis of AIDS, and the still unresolved issues.*]

Galli SJ: The development of allergic inflammation, *Nature* 454:445, 2008. [*An excellent review of the mechanisms of inflammation in allergic diseases.*]

Galli SJ: The mast cell-IgE paradox: from homeostasis to anaphylaxis, *Am J Pathol* 186:212, 2016. [*A fascinating discussion of the evolution of mast cell responses and their roles in host defense and disease.*]

Goodnow CC: Multistep pathogenesis of autoimmune disease, *Cell* 130:25, 2007. [*An excellent discussion of the checkpoints that prevent autoimmunity and why these might fail.*]

Holgate ST: Innate and adaptive immune responses in asthma, *Nat Med* 18:673–683, 2012. [*A comprehensive discussion of the roles of T_H2 cells, cytokines, and other cells of the immune system in the development and resolution of asthma.*]

Jancar S, Sanchez Crespo M: Immune complex–mediated tissue injury: a multistep paradigm, *Trends Immunol* 26:48, 2005. [*A summary of the mechanisms of immune complex–mediated tissue injury.*]

Jennette JC, Falk RJ, Hu P, et al: Pathogenesis of antineutrophil cytoplasmic autoantibody-associated small-vessel vasculitis, *Annu Rev Pathol* 8:139–160, 2013. [*A comprehensive review of the clinical and pathologic features and pathogenesis of small-vessel vasculitis.*]

Pandey S, Kawai T, Akira S: Microbial sensing by Toll-like receptors and intracellular nucleic acid sensors, *Cold Spring Harb Perspect Biol* 7:a016246, 2014. [*An excellent review of the receptors used by the innate immune system to sense microbes.*]

Klein L, Kyewski B, Allen PM, et al: Positive and negative selection of the T cell repertoire: what thymocytes see (and don't see), *Nat Rev Immunol* 14:377, 2014. [*A discussion of the mechanisms of T cell maturation and central tolerance induced in the thymus.*]

Lamkanfi M, Dixit VM: Mechanisms and functions of inflammasomes, *Cell* 157:1013, 2014. [*An excellent update on the inflammasome and its role in inflammation and host defense.*]

Liu Z, Davidson A: Taming lupus—a new understanding of pathogenesis is leading to clinical advances, *Nat Med* 18:871–882, 2012. [*An excellent review of recent advances in understanding the genetics of lupus and the roles of innate and adaptive immune responses in the disease, and how these advances are shaping the development of novel therapies.*]

Mahajan VS, Mattoo H, Deshpande V, et al: IgG4-related disease, *Annu Rev Pathol* 9:315, 2014. [*A comprehensive discussion of the features and likely pathogenesis of this recently recognized entity.*]

Mathis D, Benoist C: Microbiota and autoimmune disease: the hosted self, *Cell Host Microbe* 10:297–301, 2011. [*A review of the evidence that the microbiome influences immune activation and autoimmunity, and the relevance of these findings to human autoimmune diseases.*]

Mavragani CP, Moustsopoulos HM: Sjögren's syndrome, *Annu Rev Pathol* 9:273, 2014. [*A review of the pathogenesis and clinical features of Sjögren's syndrome.*]

Mitchell RN: Graft vascular disease: immune response meets the vessel wall, *Annu Rev Pathol* 4:19, 2009. [*A review of the mechanisms that lead to vascular disease in chronic graft rejection.*]

Moir S, Chun TW, Fauci AS: Pathogenic mechanisms of HIV disease, *Annu Rev Pathol* 6:223, 2011. [*A discussion of current concepts of the mechanisms by which HIV causes immunodeficiency.*]

Nankivell BJ, Alexander SI: Rejection of the kidney allograft, *N Engl J Med* 363:1451, 2010. [*A good review of the mechanisms of recognition and rejection of allografts and the development of new strategies for treating rejection.*]

O'Shea JJ, Paul WE: Mechanisms underlying lineage commitment and plasticity of helper CD4+ T cells, *Science* 327:1098, 2010. [*An excellent review of the development and functions of helper T cell subsets, and the uncertainties in the field.*]

Ohkura N, Kitagawa Y, Sakaguchi S: Development and maintenance of regulatory T cells, *Immunity* 38:414–423, 2013. [*An excellent review of the molecular mechanisms underlying the generation, maintenance, and stability of regulatory T cells.*]

Pattanaik D, Brown M, Postlethwaite BC, et al: Pathogenesis of systemic sclerosis, *Front Immunol* 6:272, 2015. [*A discussion of current concepts of the pathogenesis of systemic sclerosis.*]

Parvaneh N, Casanova JL, Notarangelo LD, et al: Primary immunodeficiencies: a rapidly evolving story, *J Allergy Clin Immunol* 131:314–323, 2013. [*An excellent review of newly described primary immunodeficiency syndromes.*]

Schwartz RH: Historical overview of immunological tolerance, *Cold Spring Harb Perspect Biol* 4:a006908, 2012. [*A thoughtful summary of the mechanisms of tolerance, the experimental studies behind the elucidation of these mechanisms, and how they may be disrupted to give rise to autoimmunity.*]

Tsokos GC: Systemic lupus erythematosus, *N Engl J Med* 365:2110, 2011. [*An excellent review of the clinical features and pathogenesis of lupus.*]

Westermark GT, Fandrich M, Westermark P: AA amyloidosis: pathogenesis and targeted therapies, *Annu Rev Pathol* 10:321, 2015. [*An excellent review of the pathogenesis and clinical features of a major form of amyloidosis.*]

Victora GD, Nussenzweig MC: Germinal centers, *Annu Rev Immunol* 30:429–457, 2012. [*An excellent review of the properties and formation of germinal centers and their roles in antibody responses and autoimmune diseases.*]

Voight BF, Cotsapas C: Human genetics offers an emerging picture of common pathways and mechanisms in autoimmunity, *Curr Opin Immunol* 24:552–557, 2012. [*A discussion of the genetic associations with autoimmune diseases and the implications for understanding pathways of autoimmunity.*]

Weaver CT, Elson CO, Fouser LA, et al: The T_H17 pathway and inflammatory diseases of the intestines, lungs, and skin, *Annu Rev Pathol* 8:477, 2013. [*An excellent review of the development and lineage relationships of T_H17 cells and their roles in autoimmune and other inflammatory diseases.*]

Zenewicz L, Abraham C, Flavell RA, et al: Unraveling the genetics of autoimmunity, *Cell* 140:791, 2010. [*An update on susceptibility genes for autoimmune diseases, how these are identified, and their significance.*]

Neoplasia 6

Nomenclature 190
Benign Tumors 190
Malignant Tumors 190
**Characteristics of Benign and Malignant
   Neoplasms 192**
Differentiation and Anaplasia 192
Local Invasion 194
Metastasis 195
Epidemiology 196
Cancer Incidence 197
Environmental Factors 197
Age and Cancer 199
Acquired Predisposing Conditions 199
*Interactions Between Environmental and Genetic
   Factors 200*

Cancer Genes 200
Genetic Lesions in Cancer 201
Driver and Passenger Mutations 201
Epigenetic Modifications and Cancer 203
Carcinogenesis: A Multistep Process 204
Hallmarks of Cancer 204
Self-Sufficiency in Growth Signals 205
*Insensitivity to Growth Inhibitory Signals: Tumor
   Suppressor Genes 208*
Altered Cellular Metabolism 214
Evasion of Cell Death 217
Limitless Replicative Potential (Immortality) 218
Sustained Angiogenesis 219
Invasion and Metastasis 220
Evasion of Immune Surveillance 223

*Tumor-Promoting Inflammation as an Enabler of
   Malignancy 228*
**Etiology of Cancer: Carcinogenic
   Agents 228**
Chemical Carcinogens 228
Radiation Carcinogenesis 231
Viral and Microbial Oncogenesis 231
Clinical Aspects of Neoplasia 235
Effects of Tumor on Host 235
Grading and Staging of Cancer 236
Laboratory Diagnosis of Cancer 237

Cancer is the second leading cause of death in the United States; only cardiovascular diseases exact a higher toll. Even more agonizing than the associated mortality is the emotional and physical suffering inflicted by neoplasms. Patients and the public often ask, "When will there be a cure for cancer?" The answer to this simple question is difficult, because cancer is not one disease but rather many disorders that share a profound growth dysregulation. Some cancers, such as Hodgkin lymphoma, are highly curable, whereas others, such as cancer of the pancreas, are virtually always fatal. The only hope for controlling cancer lies in learning more about its pathogenesis, and great strides have been made in understanding the molecular basis of cancer. This chapter deals with the basic biology of neoplasia—the nature of benign and malignant neoplasms and the molecular basis of neoplastic transformation. The host response to tumors and the clinical features of neoplasia also are discussed.

Before we discuss the features of cancer cells and the mechanisms of carcinogenesis, it is useful to summarize the fundamental and shared characteristics of cancers:

- **Cancer is a genetic disorder caused by DNA mutations.** Most pathogenic mutations are either induced by exposure to mutagens or occur spontaneously as part of aging. In addition, cancers frequently show epigenetic changes, such as focal increases in DNA methylation and alterations in histone modifications, which may themselves stem from acquired mutations in genes that regulate such modifications. These genetic and epigenetic changes alter the expression or function of key genes that regulate fundamental cellular processes, such as growth, survival, and senescence.

- **Genetic alterations in cancer cells are heritable, being passed to daughter cells upon cell division. As a result, cells harboring these alterations are subject to Darwinian selection (survival of the fittest, arguably the most important scientific concept in biology).** Cells bearing mutations that provide a growth or survival advantage outcompete their neighbors and thus come to dominate the population. At the time of tumor initiation, these selective advantages are conferred on a single cell, and as a result all tumors are *clonal* (i.e., the progeny of one cell). However, even beyond the point of initiation, Darwinian selection continues to shape the evolution of cancers by favoring the emergence of genetically distinct subclones with more aggressive characteristics, an important concept referred to as *progression* and discussed in more detail later in this chapter.

- **Mutations and epigenetic alterations impart to cancer cells a set of properties that are referred to collectively** as *cancer hallmarks.* These properties produce the cellular phenotypes that dictate the natural history of cancers as well as their response to various therapies. The molecular underpinnings of each hallmark of cancer are discussed in later sections.

Basic research has elucidated many of the cellular and molecular abnormalities that give rise to cancer and govern its pernicious behavior. These insights are in turn leading to a revolution in the diagnosis and treatment of cancer, an emerging triumph of biomedical science.

NOMENCLATURE

Neoplasia literally means "new growth." Neoplastic cells are said to be transformed because they continue to replicate, apparently oblivious to the regulatory influences that control normal cells. Neoplasms therefore enjoy a degree of autonomy and tend to increase in size regardless of their local environment. Their autonomy is by no means complete, however. All neoplasms depend on the host for their nutrition and blood supply. Neoplasms derived from hormone responsive tissues often also require endocrine support, and such dependencies sometimes can be exploited therapeutically.

In common medical usage, a neoplasm often is referred to as a *tumor,* and the study of tumors is called *oncology* (from *oncos,* "tumor," and *logos,* "study of"). Among tumors, the division of neoplasms into benign and malignant categories is based on a judgment of a tumor's potential clinical behavior.

- **A tumor is said to be *benign* when its microscopic and gross characteristics are considered to be relatively innocent, implying that it will remain localized and is amenable to local surgical removal.** Affected patients generally survive. Of note, however, benign tumors can produce more than localized lumps, and sometimes they produce significant morbidity or are even lethal.
- *Malignant,* **as applied to a neoplasm, implies that the lesion can invade and destroy adjacent structures and spread to distant sites (metastasize) to cause death.** Malignant tumors are collectively referred to as *cancers,* derived from the Latin word for "crab"—that is, they adhere to any part that they seize in an obstinate manner, similar to a crab's behavior. Not all cancers pursue so deadly a course. The most aggressive are also some of the most curable, but the designation *malignant* constitutes a red flag.

All tumors, benign and malignant, have two basic components: (1) the *parenchyma,* made up of transformed or neoplastic cells, and (2) the supporting, host-derived, non-neoplastic *stroma,* made up of connective tissue, blood vessels, and host-derived inflammatory cells. The parenchyma of the neoplasm largely determines its biologic behavior, and it is this component from which the tumor derives its name. The stroma is crucial to the growth of the neoplasm, since it carries the blood supply and provides support for the growth of parenchymal cells. Although the biologic behavior of tumors largely reflects the behavior of the parenchymal cells, there has been a growing realization that stromal cells and neoplastic cells carry on a two-way conversation that influences the growth of the tumor.

Benign Tumors

In general, benign tumors are designated by attaching the suffix *-oma* to the cell type from which the tumor arises. For example, a benign tumor arising in fibrous tissue is a *fibroma;* a benign cartilaginous tumor is a *chondroma.* More varied and complex nomenclature is applied to benign epithelial tumors. The term *adenoma* is generally applied not only to benign epithelial neoplasms that produce glandlike structures, but also to benign epithelial neoplasms that are derived from glands but lack a glandular growth pattern. Thus, a benign epithelial neoplasm arising from renal tubule cells and growing in a glandlike pattern is termed an adenoma, as is a mass of benign epithelial cells that produces no glandular patterns but has its origin in the adrenal cortex. *Papillomas* are benign epithelial neoplasms, growing on any surface, that produce microscopic or macroscopic fingerlike fronds. A *polyp* is a mass that projects above a mucosal surface, as in the gut, to form a macroscopically visible structure (Fig. 6.1). Although this term commonly is used for benign tumors, some malignant tumors also may grow as polyps, whereas other polyps (such as nasal polyps) are not neoplastic but inflammatory in origin. *Cystadenomas* are hollow cystic masses that typically arise in the ovary.

Malignant Tumors

The nomenclature of malignant tumors essentially follows that of benign tumors, with certain additions and exceptions.

- Malignant neoplasms arising in "solid" mesenchymal tissues or its derivatives are called *sarcomas,* whereas those arising from the mesenchymal cells of the blood are called leukemias or lymphomas. Sarcomas are designated based on their cell-type composition, which presumably reflects their cell of origin. Thus, a malignant neoplasm comprised of fat-like cells is a *lipo*sarcoma, and a malignant neoplasm composed of chondrocyte-like cells is a *chondro*sarcoma.
- While the epithelia of the body are derived from all three germ cell layers, malignant neoplasms of epithelial cells are called *carcinomas* regardless of the tissue of origin. Thus, malignant neoplasms arising in the renal tubular epithelium (mesoderm), the skin (ectoderm), and lining epithelium of the gut (endoderm) are all considered carcinomas. Furthermore, mesoderm may give rise to carcinomas (epithelial), sarcomas (mesenchymal), and hematolymphoid tumors (leukemias and lymphomas).
- Carcinomas are subdivided further. Carcinomas that grow in a glandular pattern are called *adenocarcinomas,* and those that produce squamous cells are called *squamous cell carcinomas.* Sometimes the tissue or organ of origin can be identified, as in the designation of renal cell adenocarcinoma, but it is not uncommon for tumors

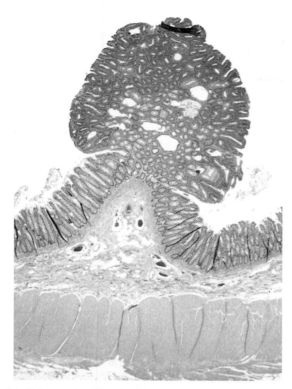

Fig. 6.1 Colonic polyp. This glandular tumor is seen projecting into the colonic lumen. The polyp is attached to the mucosa by a distinct stalk.

to show little or no differentiation. Such tumors are referred to as *poorly differentiated* or *undifferentiated carcinoma*.

The transformed cells in a neoplasm, whether benign or malignant, usually resemble each other, consistent with their origin from a single transformed progenitor cell. In some unusual instances, however, the tumor cells undergo divergent differentiation, creating so-called "mixed tumors". Mixed tumors are still of monoclonal origin, but the progenitor cell in such tumors has the capacity to differentiate down more than one lineage. The best example is mixed tumor of salivary gland. These tumors have obvious epithelial components dispersed throughout a fibromyxoid stroma, sometimes harboring islands of cartilage or bone (Fig. 6.2). All of these diverse elements are thought to derive from a single transformed epithelial progenitor cell, and the preferred designation for these neoplasms is *pleomorphic adenoma*. Fibroadenoma of the female breast is another common mixed tumor. This benign tumor contains a mixture of proliferating ductal elements (adenoma) embedded in loose fibrous tissue (fibroma). Unlike pleomorphic adenoma, only the fibrous component is neoplastic, but the term *fibroadenoma* remains in common usage.

Teratoma is a special type of mixed tumor that contains recognizable mature or immature cells or tissues derived from more than one germ cell layer, and sometimes all three. Teratomas originate from totipotential germ cells such as those that normally reside in the ovary and testis

and that are sometimes abnormally present in midline embryonic rests. Germ cells have the capacity to differentiate into any of the cell types found in the adult body; not surprisingly, therefore, they may give rise to neoplasms that contain elements resembling bone, epithelium, muscle, fat, nerve, and other tissues, all thrown together in a helter-skelter fashion.

The specific names of the more common neoplasms are presented in Table 6.1. Some glaring inconsistencies may be noted. For example, the terms *lymphoma, mesothelioma, melanoma,* and *seminoma* are used for malignant neoplasms. Unfortunately for students, these exceptions are firmly entrenched in medical terminology.

There also are other instances of confusing terminology:

- *Hamartoma* is a mass of disorganized tissue indigenous to the particular site, such as the lung or the liver. While traditionally considered developmental malformations, many hamartomas have clonal chromosomal aberrations that are acquired through somatic mutations and on this basis are now considered to be neoplastic.
- *Choristoma* is a congenital anomaly consisting of a heterotopic nest of cells. For example, a small nodule of well-developed and normally organized pancreatic tissue may be found in the submucosa of the stomach, duodenum, or small intestine. The designation -*oma*, connoting a neoplasm, imparts to these lesions an undeserved gravity, as they are usually of trivial significance.

Although the terminology of neoplasms is regrettably complex, an understanding of the nomenclature is important because it is the language by which a tumor's nature and significance is communicated among physicians in different disciplines involved in cancer care.

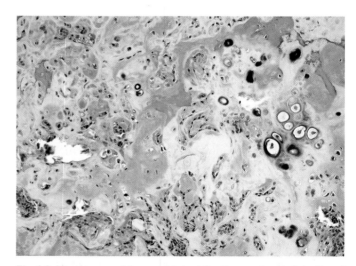

Fig. 6.2 Mixed tumor of the parotid gland. Small nests of epithelial cells and myxoid stroma forming cartilage and bone (an unusual feature) are present in this field. *(Courtesy of Dr. Vicky Jo, Department of Pathology, Brigham and Women's Hospital, Boston, Massachusetts.)*

Table 6.1 Nomenclature of Tumors

Tissue of Origin	Benign	Malignant
One Parenchymal Cell Type		
Connective tissue and derivatives	Fibroma	Fibrosarcoma
	Lipoma	Liposarcoma
	Chondroma	Chondrosarcoma
	Osteoma	Osteogenic sarcoma
Endothelium and related cell types		
Blood vessels	Hemangioma	Angiosarcoma
Lymph vessels	Lymphangioma	Lymphangiosarcoma
Mesothelium		Mesothelioma
Brain coverings	Meningioma	Invasive meningioma
Blood cells and related cell types		
Hematopoietic cells		Leukemias
Lymphoid tissue		Lymphomas
Muscle		
Smooth	Leiomyoma	Leiomyosarcoma
Striated	Rhabdomyoma	Rhabdomyosarcoma
Skin		
Stratified squamous	Squamous cell papilloma	Squamous cell or epidermoid carcinoma
Basal cells of skin or adnexa		Basal cell carcinoma
Tumors of melanocytes	Nevus	Malignant melanoma
Epithelial lining of glands or ducts	Adenoma	Adenocarcinoma
	Papilloma	Papillary carcinomas
	Cystadenoma	Cystadenocarcinoma
Lung	Bronchial adenoma	Bronchogenic carcinoma
Kidney	Renal tubular adenoma	Renal cell carcinoma
Liver	Liver cell adenoma	Hepatocellular carcinoma
Bladder	Urothelial papilloma	Urothelial carcinoma
Placenta	Hydatidiform mole	Choriocarcinoma
Testicle		Seminoma
		Embryonal carcinoma
More Than One Neoplastic Cell Type—Mixed Tumors, Usually Derived From One Germ Cell Layer		
Salivary glands	Pleomorphic adenoma (mixed tumor of salivary gland)	Malignant mixed tumor of salivary gland
Renal anlage		Wilms tumor
More Than One Neoplastic Cell Type Derived From More Than One Germ Cell Layer—Teratogenous		
Totipotential cells in gonads or in embryonic rests	Mature teratoma, dermoid cyst	Immature teratoma, teratocarcinoma

CHARACTERISTICS OF BENIGN AND MALIGNANT NEOPLASMS

There are three fundamental features by which most benign and malignant tumors can be distinguished: differentiation and anaplasia, local invasion, and metastasis. In general, rapid growth also signifies malignancy, but many malignant tumors grow slowly and as a result growth rate is not a reliable discriminator between good and bad actors. Nothing is more important to the patient with a tumor than being told: "It is benign." Although some neoplasms defy easy characterization, in most instances the determination of benign versus malignant is made with remarkable accuracy using long-established clinical and anatomic criteria.

Differentiation and Anaplasia

Differentiation refers to the extent to which neoplasms resemble their parenchymal cells of origin, both morphologically and functionally; lack of differentiation is called *anaplasia.* In general, benign neoplasms are composed of well-differentiated cells that closely resemble their normal counterparts. A lipoma is made up of mature fat cells laden with cytoplasmic lipid vacuoles, and a chondroma is made up of mature cartilage cells that synthesize their usual cartilaginous matrix—evidence of morphologic and functional differentiation. In well-differentiated benign tumors, mitoses are usually rare and are of normal configuration.

By contrast, while malignant neoplasms exhibit a wide range of parenchymal cell differentiation, most exhibit morphologic alterations that betray their malignant nature.

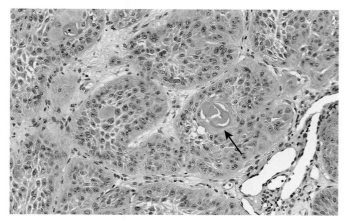

Fig. 6.3 Well-differentiated squamous cell carcinoma of the skin. The tumor cells are strikingly similar to normal squamous epithelial cells, with intercellular bridges and nests of keratin *(arrow)*. *(Courtesy of Dr. Trace Worrell, Department of Pathology, University of Texas Southwestern Medical School, Dallas, Texas.)*

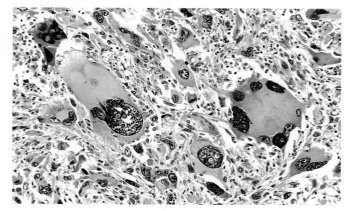

Fig. 6.4 Pleomorphic malignant tumor (rhabdomyosarcoma). Note the marked variation in cell and nuclear sizes, the hyperchromatic nuclei, and the presence of tumor giant cells. *(Courtesy of Dr. Trace Worrell, Department of Pathology, University of Texas Southwestern Medical School, Dallas, Texas.)*

In well-differentiated cancers, these features may be quite subtle (Fig. 6.3). For example, well-differentiated adenocarcinoma of the thyroid gland may contain normal-appearing follicles, its malignant potential being only revealed by invasion into adjacent tissues or metastasis. The stroma carrying the blood supply is crucial to the growth of tumors but does not aid in the separation of benign from malignant ones. The amount of stromal connective tissue does, however, determine the consistency of a neoplasm. Certain cancers induce a dense, abundant fibrous stroma (desmoplasia), making them hard, so-called "scirrhous tumors".

Tumors composed of undifferentiated cells are said to be *anaplastic*, a feature that is a reliable indicator of malignancy. The term *anaplasia* literally means "backward formation"—implying dedifferentiation, or loss of the structural and functional differentiation of normal cells. It is now known, however, that at least some cancers arise from stem cells in tissues; in these tumors, failure of differentiation of transformed stem cells, rather than dedifferentiation of specialized cells, accounts for their anaplastic appearance. Recent studies also indicate that in some cases, dedifferentiation of apparently mature cells occurs during carcinogenesis. Anaplastic cells often display the following morphologic features:

- *Pleomorphism* (i.e., variation in size and shape) (Fig. 6.4)
- *Nuclear abnormalities*, consisting of extreme hyperchromatism (dark-staining), variation in nuclear size and shape, or unusually prominent single or multiple nucleoli. Enlargement of nuclei may result in an increased nuclear-to-cytoplasmic ratio that approaches 1:1 instead of the normal 1:4 or 1:6. Nucleoli may attain astounding sizes, sometimes approaching the diameter of normal lymphocytes.
- *Tumor giant cells* may be formed. These are considerably larger than neighboring cells and may possess either one enormous nucleus or several nuclei.
- *Atypical mitoses*, which may be numerous. Anarchic multiple spindles may produce tripolar or quadripolar mitotic figures (Fig. 6.5).
- *Loss of polarity*, such that anaplastic cells lack recognizable patterns of orientation to one another. Such cells may grow in sheets, with total loss of communal

structures, such as glands or stratified squamous architecture.

Well-differentiated tumor cells are likely to retain the functional capabilities of their normal counterparts, whereas **anaplastic tumor cells are much less likely to have specialized functional activities.** For example, benign neoplasms and even well-differentiated cancers of endocrine glands frequently elaborate the hormones characteristic of their cell of origin. Similarly, well-differentiated squamous cell carcinomas produce keratin (see Fig. 6.3), just as well-differentiated hepatocellular carcinomas secrete bile. In other instances, unanticipated functions emerge. Some cancers may express fetal proteins not produced by comparable cells in the adult. Cancers of nonendocrine origin may produce so-called "ectopic hormones." For example, certain lung carcinomas may produce adrenocorticotropic hormone (ACTH), parathyroid hormone–like hormone, insulin, glucagon, and others. More is said about these so-called "paraneoplastic" phenomena later.

Also of relevance in the discussion of differentiation and anaplasia is *dysplasia*, referring to disorderly proliferation.

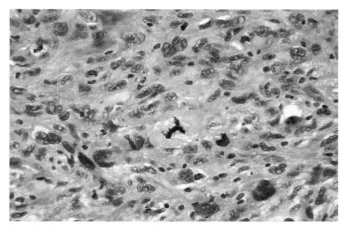

Fig. 6.5 High-power detailed view of anaplastic tumor cells shows cellular and nuclear variation in size and shape. The prominent cell in the center field has an abnormal tripolar spindle.

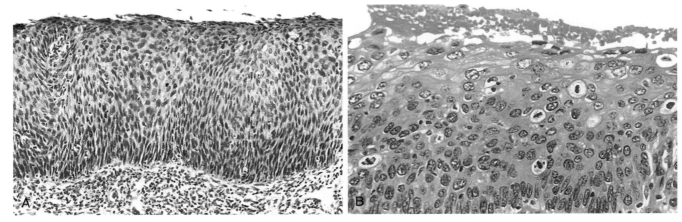

Fig. 6.6 Carcinoma in situ. (A) Low-power view shows that the entire thickness of the epithelium is replaced by atypical dysplastic cells. There is no orderly differentiation of squamous cells. The basement membrane is intact, and there is no tumor in the subepithelial stroma. (B) High-power view of another region shows failure of normal differentiation, marked nuclear and cellular pleomorphism, and numerous mitotic figures extending toward the surface. The intact basement membrane (below) is not seen in this section.

Dysplastic epithelium is recognized by a loss in the uniformity of individual cells and in their architectural orientation. Dysplastic cells exhibit considerable pleomorphism and often possess abnormally large, hyperchromatic nuclei. Mitotic figures are more abundant than usual and frequently appear in abnormal locations within the epithelium. In dysplastic stratified squamous epithelium, mitoses are not confined to the basal layers, where they normally occur, but may be seen throughout the epithelium. In addition, there is considerable architectural anarchy. For example, the usual progressive maturation of tall cells in the basal layer to flattened squames on the surface may be lost and replaced by a disordered hodgepodge of dark basal-appearing cells. When dysplastic changes are severe and involve the entire thickness of the epithelium, the lesion is referred to as *carcinoma in situ*, a preinvasive stage of cancer (Fig. 6.6).

It is important to appreciate that dysplasia is not synonymous with cancer. Mild to moderate dysplasias that do not involve the entire thickness of the epithelium sometimes regress completely, particularly if inciting causes are removed. However, dysplasia is often noted adjacent to frankly malignant neoplasms (e.g., in cigarette smokers with lung cancer), and in general the presence of dysplasia marks a tissue as being at increased risk for developing an invasive cancer.

Local Invasion

The growth of cancers is accompanied by progressive infiltration, invasion, and destruction of surrounding tissues, whereas most benign tumors grow as cohesive expansile masses that remain localized to their sites of origin. Because benign tumors grow and expand slowly, they usually develop a rim of compressed fibrous tissue (Figs. 6.7 and 6.8). This capsule consists largely of extracellular matrix that is deposited by stromal cells such as fibroblasts, which are activated by hypoxic damage to parenchymal cells resulting from compression by the expanding tumor. Encapsulation creates a tissue plane that makes the tumor discrete, moveable (non-fixed), and

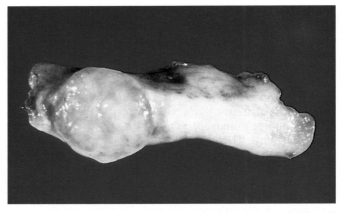

Fig. 6.7 Fibroadenoma of the breast. The tan-colored, encapsulated small tumor is sharply demarcated from the whiter breast tissue.

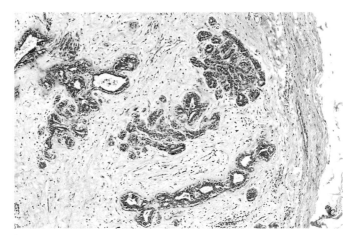

Fig. 6.8 Microscopic view of fibroadenoma of the breast seen in Fig. 6.7. The fibrous capsule *(right)* sharply delimits the tumor from the surrounding tissue. *(Courtesy of Dr. Trace Worrell, Department of Pathology, University of Texas Southwestern Medical School, Dallas, Texas.)*

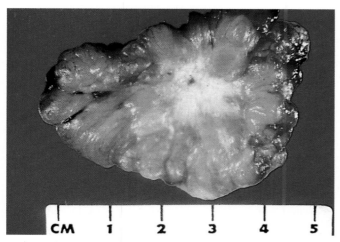

Fig. 6.9 Cut section of invasive ductal carcinoma of the breast. The lesion is retracted, infiltrating the surrounding breast substance, and was stony-hard on palpation.

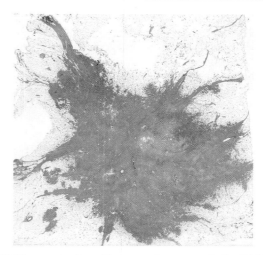

Fig. 6.10 Microscopic view of breast carcinoma seen in Fig. 6.9 illustrates the invasion of breast stroma and fat by nests and cords of tumor cells (compare with Fig. 6.8). Note the absence of a well-defined capsule. *(Courtesy of Dr. Susan Lester, Brigham and Women's Hospital, Boston, Massachusetts.)*

readily excisable by surgical enucleation. However, it is important to recognize that not all benign neoplasms are encapsulated. For example, the leiomyoma of the uterus is discretely demarcated from the surrounding smooth muscle by a zone of compressed and attenuated normal myometrium, but lacks a capsule. A few benign tumors are neither encapsulated nor discretely defined; lack of demarcation is particularly likely in benign vascular neoplasms such as hemangiomas, which understandably may be difficult to excise. These exceptions are pointed out only to emphasize that although encapsulation is the rule in benign tumors, the lack of a capsule does not mean that a tumor is malignant. Sadly, because of their uncivilized nature, tumor cells sometimes do not follow the rules set by humans. We will see such deviations many times in this chapter.

Next to the development of metastases, invasiveness is the feature that most reliably distinguishes cancers from benign tumors (Figs. 6.9 and 6.10). Cancers lack well-defined capsules. There are instances in which a slowly growing malignant tumor deceptively appears to be encased by the stroma of the surrounding host tissue, but microscopic examination reveals tiny crablike feet penetrating the margin and infiltrating adjacent structures. This infiltrative mode of growth makes it necessary to remove a wide margin of surrounding normal tissue when surgical excision of a malignant tumor is attempted. Surgical pathologists carefully examine the margins of resected tumors to ensure that they are devoid of cancer cells *(clean margins)*.

Metastasis

Metastasis is defined by the spread of a tumor to sites that are physically discontinuous with the primary tumor and unequivocally marks a tumor as malignant, as by definition benign neoplasms do not metastasize. The invasiveness of cancers permits them to penetrate into blood vessels, lymphatics, and body cavities, providing opportunities for spread (Fig. 6.11). Overall, approximately 30% of patients with newly diagnosed solid tumors (excluding skin cancers other than melanomas) present with

clinically evident metastases. An additional 20% have occult (hidden) metastases at the time of diagnosis.

In general, the more anaplastic and the larger the primary neoplasm, the more likely is metastatic spread, but as with most rules there are exceptions. Extremely small cancers have been known to metastasize; conversely, some large and ominous-looking lesions may not. While all malignant tumors can metastasize, some do so very infrequently. For example, basal cell carcinomas of the skin and most primary tumors of the central nervous system are highly locally invasive but rarely metastasize. It is evident then that the properties of local invasion and metastasis are sometimes separable.

A special circumstance involves so-called "blood cancers", the leukemias and lymphomas. These tumors are derived from blood-forming cells that normally have the capacity to enter the bloodstream and travel to distant sites; as a result, with only rare exceptions, leukemias and lymphomas are taken to be disseminated diseases at diagnosis and are always considered to be malignant.

Malignant neoplasms disseminate by one of three pathways: (1) seeding within body cavities, (2) lymphatic

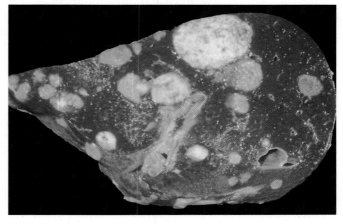

Fig. 6.11 A liver studded with metastatic cancer.

spread, or (3) hematogenous spread. *Spread by seeding* occurs when neoplasms invade a natural body cavity. This mode of dissemination is particularly characteristic of cancers of the ovary, which often cover the peritoneal surfaces widely. The implants literally may glaze all peritoneal surfaces and yet not invade the underlying tissues. Here is an instance where the ability to reimplant and grow at sites distant from the primary tumor seems to be separable from the capacity to invade. Neoplasms of the central nervous system, such as a medulloblastoma or ependymoma, may penetrate the cerebral ventricles and be carried by the cerebrospinal fluid to reimplant on the meningeal surfaces, either within the brain or in the spinal cord.

Lymphatic spread is more typical of carcinomas, whereas hematogenous spread is favored by sarcomas. There are numerous interconnections, however, between the lymphatic and vascular systems, so all forms of cancer may disseminate through either or both systems. The pattern of lymph node involvement depends principally on the site of the primary neoplasm and the natural pathways of local lymphatic drainage. Lung carcinomas arising in the respiratory passages metastasize first to the regional bronchial lymph nodes and then to the tracheobronchial and hilar nodes. Carcinoma of the breast usually arises in the upper outer quadrant and first spreads to the axillary nodes. However, medial breast lesions may drain through the chest wall to the nodes along the internal mammary artery. Thereafter, in both instances, the supraclavicular and infraclavicular nodes may be seeded. In some cases, the cancer cells seem to travel in lymphatic channels within the immediately proximate nodes to be trapped in subsequent lymph nodes, producing so-called "skip metastases." The cells may traverse all of the lymph nodes ultimately to reach the vascular compartment by way of the thoracic duct.

A "sentinel lymph node" is the first regional lymph node that receives lymph flow from a primary tumor. It can be identified by injection of blue dyes or radiolabeled tracers near the primary tumor. Biopsy of sentinel lymph nodes allows determination of the extent of spread of tumor and can be used to plan treatment.

Of note, although enlargement of nodes near a primary neoplasm should arouse concern for metastatic spread, it does not always imply cancerous involvement. The necrotic products of the neoplasm and tumor antigens often evoke immunologic responses in the nodes, such as hyperplasia of the follicles (lymphadenitis) and proliferation of macrophages in the subcapsular sinuses (sinus histiocytosis). Thus, histopathologic verification of tumor within an enlarged lymph node is required.

While hematogenous spread is the favored pathway for sarcomas, carcinomas use it as well. As might be expected, arteries are penetrated less readily than are veins. With venous invasion, the bloodborne cells follow the venous flow draining the site of the neoplasm, with tumor cells often stopping in the first capillary bed they encounter. Since all portal area drainage flows to the liver, and all caval blood flows to the lungs, the liver and lungs are the most frequently involved secondary sites in hematogenous dissemination. Cancers arising near the vertebral column often embolize through the paravertebral plexus; this pathway probably is involved in the frequent vertebral metastases of carcinomas of the thyroid and prostate glands.

Certain carcinomas have a propensity to grow within veins. Renal cell carcinoma often invades the renal vein to grow in a snakelike fashion up the inferior vena cava, sometimes reaching the right side of the heart. Hepatocellular carcinomas often penetrate and grow within the radicles of portal and hepatic veins, eventually reaching the main venous channels. Remarkably, such intravenous growth may not be accompanied by widespread dissemination.

Many observations suggest that the anatomic localization of a neoplasm and its venous drainage cannot wholly explain the systemic distributions of metastases. For example, prostatic carcinoma preferentially spreads to bone, bronchogenic carcinoma tends to involve the adrenal glands and the brain, and neuroblastoma spreads to the liver and bones. Conversely, skeletal muscles, although rich in capillaries, are rarely sites of tumor metastases. The molecular basis of such tissue-specific homing of tumor cells is discussed later.

Thus, numerous features of tumors (Fig. 6.12) usually permit the differentiation of benign and malignant neoplasms.

SUMMARY

CHARACTERISTICS OF BENIGN AND MALIGNANT TUMORS

- Benign and malignant tumors can be distinguished from one another based on the degree of differentiation, rate of growth, local invasiveness, and distant spread.
- Benign tumors resemble the tissue of origin and are well differentiated; malignant tumors are poorly or completely undifferentiated (anaplastic).
- Benign tumors tend to be slow growing, whereas malignant tumors generally grow faster.
- Benign tumors are well circumscribed and have a capsule; malignant tumors are poorly circumscribed and invade the surrounding normal tissues.
- Benign tumors remain localized to the site of origin, whereas malignant tumors are locally invasive and metastasize to distant sites.

EPIDEMIOLOGY

Study of cancer occurrence in populations has contributed substantially to knowledge about its origins. The now well-established concept that cigarette smoking is causally associated with lung cancer arose primarily from epidemiologic studies. A comparison of the incidence rates for colon cancer and dietary patterns in the Western world and in Africa led to the recognition that dietary fat and fiber content may figure importantly in the causation of this cancer. Major insights into the causes of cancer can be obtained by epidemiologic studies that relate particular environmental, racial (possibly hereditary), and cultural influences to the occurrence of specific neoplasms. Certain diseases associated with an increased risk for developing cancer also provide clues to the pathogenesis of cancer. The following discussion first summarizes the overall incidence of cancer to provide insight into the magnitude of the cancer problem and then reviews factors relating to the

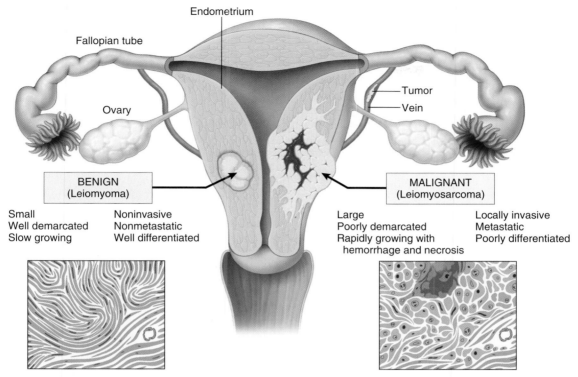

Fig. 6.12 Comparison between a benign tumor of the myometrium (leiomyoma) and a malignant tumor of similar origin (leiomyosarcoma).

patient and the environment that influence the predisposition to cancer.

Cancer Incidence

For the year 2012, the World Health Organization (WHO) estimated that there were about 14.1 million new cancer cases worldwide, leading to 8.2 million deaths (approximately 22,500 deaths per day). Moreover, due to increasing population size, by the year 2035 the WHO projects that the numbers of cancer cases and deaths worldwide will increase to 24 million and 14.6 million, respectively (based on current mortality rates). Additional perspective on the likelihood of developing a specific form of cancer can be gained from national incidence and mortality data. In the United States, it is estimated that the year 2016 will be marked by approximately 1.69 million new cases of cancer and 595,000 cancer deaths. Incidence data for the most common forms of cancer, with the major killers identified, are presented in Fig. 6.13.

Over several decades, the death rates for many forms of cancer have changed. Since 1995, the incidence of cancer in men and women in the United States has been roughly stable, but the cancer death rate has decreased by roughly 20% in men and 10% in women. Among men, 80% of the decrease is accounted for by lower death rates for cancers of the lung, prostate, and colon; among women, nearly 60% of the decrease is due to reductions in death rates from breast and colorectal cancers. Decreased use of tobacco products is responsible for the reduction in lung cancer deaths, while improved detection and treatment are responsible for the decrease in death rates for colorectal, female breast, and prostate cancers.

The last half-century has also seen a sharp decline in death rates from cervical cancer and gastric cancer in the United States. The decrease in cervical cancer is directly attributable to widespread use of the Papanicolaou (PAP) smear test for early detection of this tumor and its precursor lesions. The deployment of the human papillomavirus (HPV) vaccine may nearly eliminate this cancer in coming years. The cause of the decline in death rates for cancers of the stomach is obscure; it may be related to decreasing exposure to unknown dietary carcinogens.

Environmental Factors

Environmental exposures appear to be the dominant risk factors for many common cancers, suggesting that a high fraction of cancers are potentially preventable. This notion is supported by the geographic variation in death rates from specific forms of cancer, which is thought to stem mainly from differences in environmental exposures. For instance, death rates from breast cancer are about four to five times higher in the United States and Europe than in Japan. Conversely, the death rate for stomach carcinoma in men and women is about seven times higher in Japan than in the United States. Liver cell carcinoma is relatively infrequent in the United States but is the most lethal cancer among many African populations. Nearly all the evidence indicates that these geographic differences have environmental rather than genetic origins. For example, Nisei (second-generation Japanese living in the United States) have mortality rates for certain forms of cancer that are intermediate between those in natives of Japan and in Americans who have lived in the United States for many generations. The two rates come closer with each passing generation.

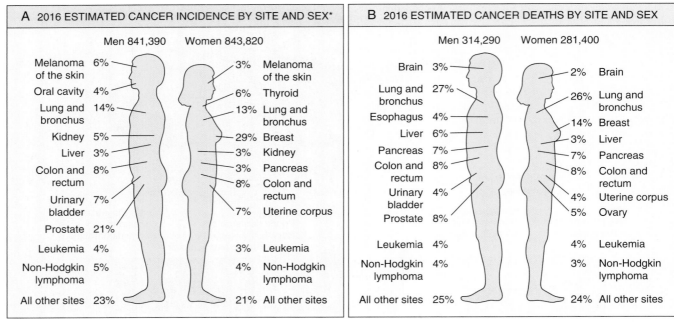

Fig. 6.13 Estimated cancer incidence and mortality by site and sex in the United States. Excludes basal cell and squamous cell skin cancers and in situ carcinomas, except urinary bladder. *(Adapted from* Cancer facts & figures 2016. *American Cancer Society. www.cancer.org/research/cancer-facts-statistics/all-cancer-facts-figures/cancer-facts-figures-2016.html.)*

There is no paucity of environmental factors that contribute to cancer. They lurk in the ambient environment, in the workplace, in food, and in personal practices. They can be as universal as sunlight or be largely restricted to urban settings (e.g., asbestos) or particular occupations (Table 6.2). The most important environmental exposures linked to cancer include the following:

• *Diet.* Certain features of diet have been implicated as predisposing influences. More broadly, obesity, currently epidemic in the United States, is associated with a modestly increased risk for developing many different cancers.

• *Smoking.* Smoking, particularly of cigarettes, has been implicated in cancer of the mouth, pharynx, larynx, esophagus, pancreas, bladder, and, most significantly, the lung, as 90% of lung cancer deaths are related to smoking.

• *Alcohol consumption.* Alcohol abuse is an independent risk factor for cancers of the oropharynx, larynx, esophagus, and (due to alcoholic cirrhosis) liver. Moreover,

Table 6.2 Occupational Cancers

Agents or Groups of Agents	Human Cancers for Which Reasonable Evidence Is Available	Typical Use or Occurrence
Arsenic and arsenic compounds	Lung carcinoma, skin carcinoma	By-product of metal smelting; component of alloys, electrical and semiconductor devices, medications and herbicides, fungicides, and animal dips
Asbestos	Lung, esophageal, gastric, and colon carcinoma; mesothelioma	Formerly used for many applications because of fire, heat, and friction resistance; still found in existing construction as well as fire-resistant textiles, friction materials (i.e., brake linings), underlayment and roofing papers, and floor tiles
Benzene	Acute myeloid leukemia	Principal component of light oil; despite known risk, many applications exist in printing and lithography, paint, rubber, dry cleaning, adhesives and coatings, and detergents; formerly widely used as solvent and fumigant
Beryllium and beryllium compounds	Lung carcinoma	Missile fuel and space vehicles; hardener for lightweight metal alloys, particularly in aerospace applications and nuclear reactors
Cadmium and cadmium compounds	Prostate carcinoma	Uses include yellow pigments and phosphors; found in solders; used in batteries and as alloy and in metal platings and coatings
Chromium compounds	Lung carcinoma	Component of metal alloys, paints, pigments, and preservatives
Nickel compounds	Lung and oropharyngeal carcinoma	Nickel plating; component of ferrous alloys, ceramics, and batteries; by-product of stainless-steel arc welding
Radon and its decay products	Lung carcinoma	From decay of minerals containing uranium; potentially serious hazard in quarries and underground mines
Vinyl chloride	Hepatic angiosarcoma	Refrigerant; monomer for vinyl polymers; adhesive for plastics; formerly inert aerosol propellant in pressurized containers

Modified from Stellman JM, Stellman SD: Cancer and the workplace, *CA Cancer J Clin* 46:70–92, 1996, with permission from Lippincott Williams & Wilkins.

alcohol and tobacco smoking synergistically increase the risk for developing cancers of the upper airways and upper digestive tract.

- *Reproductive history.* There is strong evidence that lifelong cumulative exposure to estrogen stimulation, particularly if unopposed by progesterone, increases the risk for developing cancers of the endometrium and breast, both of which are estrogen-responsive tissues.
- *Infectious agents.* It is estimated that infectious agents cause approximately 15% of cancers worldwide.

Thus, there is no escape: it seems that everything people do to earn a livelihood, to subsist, or to enjoy life turns out to be illegal, immoral, or fattening, or—most disturbing—possibly carcinogenic!

Age and Cancer

In general, the frequency of cancer increases with age. Most cancer deaths occur between 55 and 75 years of age; the rate declines, along with the population base, after 75 years of age. The rising incidence with age may be explained by the accumulation of somatic mutations that drive the emergence of malignant neoplasms (discussed later). The decline in immune competence that accompanies aging also may be a factor.

Although cancer preferentially affects older adults, it also is responsible for slightly more than 10% of all deaths among children younger than 15 years of age (Chapter 7). The major lethal cancers in children are leukemias, tumors of the central nervous system, lymphomas, and soft-tissue and bone sarcomas. As discussed later, study of several childhood tumors, such as retinoblastoma, has provided fundamental insights into the pathogenesis of malignant transformation.

Acquired Predisposing Conditions

Acquired conditions that predispose to cancer include disorders associated with chronic inflammation, immunodeficiency states, and precursor lesions. Many chronic inflammatory conditions create a fertile "soil" for the development of malignant tumors (Table 6.3). Tumors arising in the context of chronic inflammation are mostly carcinomas, but also include mesothelioma and several kinds of lymphoma. By contrast, immunodeficiency states mainly predispose to virus-induced cancers, including specific types of lymphoma and carcinoma and some sarcoma-like proliferations.

Precursor lesions are localized disturbances of epithelial differentiation that are associated with an elevated risk for developing carcinoma. They may arise secondary to chronic inflammation or hormonal disturbances (in endocrine-sensitive tissues), or may occur spontaneously. Molecular analyses have shown that precursor lesions often possess some of the genetic lesions found in their associated cancers (discussed later). However, progression to cancer is not inevitable, and it is important to recognize precursor lesions because their removal or reversal lowers cancer risk.

Many different precursor lesions have been described; among the most common are the following:

Table 6.3 Chronic Inflammatory States and Cancer

Pathologic Condition	Associated Neoplasm(s)	Etiologic Agent
Asbestosis, silicosis	Mesothelioma, lung carcinoma	Asbestos fibers, silica particles
Inflammatory bowel disease	Colorectal carcinoma	
Lichen sclerosis	Vulvar squamous cell carcinoma	
Pancreatitis	Pancreatic carcinoma	Alcoholism, germ line mutations (e.g., in the trypsinogen gene)
Chronic cholecystitis	Gallbladder cancer	Bile acids, bacteria, gallbladder stones
Reflux esophagitis, Barrett esophagus	Esophageal carcinoma	Gastric acid
Sjögren syndrome, Hashimoto thyroiditis	MALT lymphoma	
Opisthorchis, cholangitis	Cholangiocarcinoma, colon carcinoma	Liver flukes (*Opisthorchis viverrini*)
Gastritis/ulcers	Gastric adenocarcinoma, MALT lymphoma	*Helicobacter pylori*
Hepatitis	Hepatocellular carcinoma	Hepatitis B and/or C virus
Osteomyelitis	Carcinoma in draining sinuses	Bacterial infection
Chronic cervicitis	Cervical carcinoma	Human papillomavirus
Chronic cystitis	Bladder carcinoma	Schistosomiasis

Adapted from Tlsty TD, Coussens LM: Tumor stroma and regulation of cancer development, *Ann Rev Pathol Mech Dis* 1:119, 2006.

- *Squamous metaplasia and dysplasia of bronchial mucosa,* seen in in habitual smokers—a risk factor for lung carcinoma (Chapter 13)
- *Endometrial hyperplasia and dysplasia,* seen in women with unopposed estrogenic stimulation—a risk factor for endometrial carcinoma (Chapter 19)
- *Leukoplakia of the oral cavity, vulva, and penis,* which may progress to squamous cell carcinoma (Chapters 15, 18, and 19)
- *Villous adenoma of the colon,* associated with a high risk for progression to colorectal carcinoma (Chapter 15)

In this context it also may be asked, "What is the risk for malignant change in a benign neoplasm?"—or, stated differently, "Are benign tumors precancers?" In general the answer is no, but inevitably there are exceptions, and perhaps it is better to say that each type of benign tumor is associated with a particular level of risk, ranging from high to virtually nonexistent. As cited earlier, adenomas of the colon as they enlarge can undergo malignant transformation in up to 50% of cases; by contrast, malignant change is extremely rare in leiomyomas of the uterus.

Interactions Between Environmental and Genetic Factors

Cancer behaves like an inherited trait in some families, usually due to germ line mutations that affect the function of a gene that suppresses cancer (a so-called "tumor suppressor gene," discussed later). What then can be said about the influence of heredity on sporadic malignant neoplasms, which constitute roughly 95% of the cancers in the United States?

While the evidence suggests that sporadic cancers can largely be attributed to environmental factors or acquired predisposing conditions, lack of family history does not preclude an inherited component. It may in fact be difficult to tease out hereditary and genetic contributions because these factors often interact. Such interactions may be particularly complex when tumor development is affected by small contributions from multiple genes. Furthermore, genetic factors may alter the risk for developing environmentally induced cancers. Instances where this holds true often involve inherited variation in enzymes such as components of the cytochrome P-450 system that metabolize procarcinogens to active carcinogens. Conversely, environmental factors can influence the risk for developing cancer, even in individuals who inherit well-defined "cancer genes." For instance, breast cancer risk in females who inherit mutated copies of the *BRCA1* or *BRCA2* tumor suppressor genes (discussed later) is almost three-fold higher for women born after 1940 than for women born before that year, perhaps because of changes in reproductive behavior or increases in obesity in more recent times.

SUMMARY

EPIDEMIOLOGY OF CANCER

- The incidence of cancer varies with age, geographic factors, and genetic background. The geographic variation in cancer incidence results mostly from different environmental exposures. Cancer can occur at any age, but is most common in older adults.
- Environmental factors implicated in carcinogenesis include infectious agents, smoking, alcohol, diet, obesity, reproductive history, and exposure to carcinogens.
- Cancer risk rises in certain tissues in the setting of increased cellular proliferation caused by chronic inflammation or hormonal stimulation.
- Epithelial cell linings may develop morphologic changes that signify an increased risk for developing cancer; such lesions are referred to as *precursor lesions*.
- The risk for developing cancer is modified by interactions between environmental exposures and genetic variants.

CANCER GENES

It could be argued that the proliferation of literature on the molecular basis of cancer has outpaced the growth of even the most malignant of tumors. Researchers and students alike can easily get lost in the growing forest of information. But it has become eminently clear that cancer is a disease caused by mutations that alter the function of of a finite subset of the 20,000 or so human genes. For simplicity, we will refer to these genes as cancer genes. Cancer genes can be defined as genes that are recurrently affected by genetic aberrations in cancers, presumably because they contribute directly to the malignant behavior of cancer cells. Causative mutations that give rise to cancer genes may be acquired by the action of environmental agents, such as chemicals, radiation, or viruses, may occur spontaneously, or may be inherited in the germ line. If such mutations drive carcinogenesis, a key prediction is that each cell in an individual tumor should share mutations that were present in the founding cell at the time of transformation. This expectation has been realized in all tumors that have been systematically analyzed by genomic sequencing, providing strong support for the hypothesis that cancer is at its root a genetic disease.

Cancer genes number in the hundreds and new ones are still being discovered. Not only are these genes numerous, but many have unpronounceable acronyms for names that are difficult to remember, even for the aficionado. One way to try to simplify this complexity is to consider that cancer genes fall into one of four major functional classes:

- *Oncogenes* are genes that induce a transformed phenotype when expressed in cells by promoting increased cell growth. A major discovery in cancer was the realization that oncogenes are mutated or overexpressed versions of normal cellular genes, which are called *proto-oncogenes.* Most oncogenes encode transcription factors, factors that participate in pro-growth signaling pathways, or factors that enhance cell survival. They are considered dominant genes because a mutation involving a single allele is sufficient to produce a pro-oncogenic effect.
- *Tumor suppressor genes* are genes that normally prevent uncontrolled growth and, when mutated or lost from a cell, allow the transformed phenotype to develop. Often both normal alleles of tumor suppressor genes must be damaged for transformation to occur. Tumor suppressor genes can be placed into two general groups, *"governors"* that act as important brakes on cellular proliferation, and *"guardians"* that are responsible for sensing genomic damage. Some guardian genes initiate and choreograph a complex "damage control response" that leads to the cessation of proliferation or, if the damage is too great to be repaired, or induce apoptosis.
- *Genes that regulate apoptosis* primarily act by enhancing cell survival, rather than stimulating proliferation *per se.* Understandably, genes of this class that protect against apoptosis are often overexpressed in cancer cells, whereas those that promote apoptosis tend to be underexpressed or functionally inactivated by mutations.
- To this list may now be added *genes that regulate interactions between tumor cells and host cells,* as these genes are also recurrently mutated or functionally altered in certain cancers. Particularly important are genes that enhance or inhibit recognition of tumors cells by the host immune system.

In most instances, the mutations that give rise to cancer genes are acquired during life and are confined to the cancer cells. However, causative mutations sometimes are inherited in the germ line and are therefore present in

Table 6.4 Inherited Predisposition to Cancer

Inherited Predisposition	Gene(s)
Autosomal Dominant Cancer Syndromes	
Retinoblastoma	*RB*
Li-Fraumeni syndrome (various tumors)	*TP53*
Melanoma	*CDKN2A*
Familial adenomatous polyposis/colon cancer	*APC*
Neurofibromatosis 1 and 2	*NF1, NF2*
Breast and ovarian tumors	*BRCA1, BRCA2*
Multiple endocrine neoplasia 1 and 2	*MEN1, RET*
Hereditary nonpolyposis colon cancer	*MSH2, MLH1, MSH6*
Nevoid basal cell carcinoma syndrome	*PTCH1*
Autosomal Recessive Syndromes of Defective DNA Repair	
Xeroderma pigmentosum	Diverse genes involved in nucleotide excision repair
Ataxia-telangiectasia	*ATM*
Bloom syndrome	*BLM*
Fanconi anemia	Diverse genes involved in repair of DNA cross-links

every cell in the body, placing the affected individual at high risk for developing cancer. Understandably, in families in which these germ line mutations are passed from generation to generation, cancer behaves like an inherited trait (Table 6.4). We will touch on important familial cancer syndromes and associated genes and cancers later in this chapter.

Presented next is a discussion of the varied genetic lesions that underlie altered cancer gene expression and function.

GENETIC LESIONS IN CANCER

The genetic changes found in cancers vary from point mutations involving single nucleotides to abnormalities large enough to produce gross changes in chromosome structure. In certain neoplasms, genetic abnormalities are nonrandom and highly characteristic. Specific chromosomal abnormalities have been identified in most leukemias and lymphomas and in an increasing number of nonhematopoietic tumors, while other tumors are characterized by particular point mutations. It is believed that all recurrent genetic changes alter the activity of one or more cancer genes in a fashion that gives the affected cells a selective advantage, presumably by contributing to one or more of the hallmarks of cancer.

Driver and Passenger Mutations

In the following sections, we briefly review the types of mutations that are commonly found in cancers. Before doing so, however, we must first touch on the important concept of driver mutations and passenger mutations. **Driver mutations are mutations that alter the function of** cancer genes and thereby directly contribute to the development or progression of a given cancer. They are usually acquired, but as mentioned earlier, occasionally inherited. By contrast, passenger mutations are acquired mutations that are neutral in terms of fitness and do not affect cellular behavior; they just come along for the proverbial ride. Because they occur at random, passenger mutations are sprinkled throughout the genome, whereas driver mutations tend to be tightly clustered within cancer genes. It is now appreciated that particularly in cancers caused by carcinogen exposure, such as melanoma and smoking-related lung cancer, passenger mutations greatly outnumber driver mutations.

Despite their apparently innocuous nature, passenger mutations have nevertheless proven to be important in several ways:

- *In carcinogen-associated cancers, mutational analysis has provided definitive evidence that most genomic damage is directly caused by the carcinogen in question.* For example, before sequencing of melanoma genomes, the causative role of sun exposure in this cancer was debated. This is no longer so, as most melanomas have thousands of mutations of a type that is specifically linked to damage caused by ultraviolet light.
- *A second, more nefarious effect of passenger mutations is that they create genetic variants that, while initially neutral, may provide tumor cells with a selective advantage in the setting of therapy.* The evidence for this comes from DNA sequence analyses of tumors at the time of recurrence after drug therapy; in many instances, mutations that lead directly to drug resistance are found in most tumor cells. Generally, the same resistance mutations can also be found before therapy, but only in a very small fraction of cells. In such instances, it appears that the selective pressure of therapy "converts" a neutral passenger mutation into a driver mutation, to the benefit of the tumor and the detriment of the patient.

Point Mutations

Point mutations can either activate or inactivate the protein products of the affected genes depending on their precise position and consequence. Point mutations that convert proto-oncogenes into oncogenes generally produce a gain-of-function by altering amino acid residues in a domain that normally holds the protein's activity in check. A cardinal example is point mutations that convert the *RAS* gene into a cancer gene, one of the most comment events in human cancers. By contrast, point mutations (as well as larger aberrations, such as insertions and deletions) in tumor suppressor genes reduce or disable the function of the encoded protein. The tumor suppressor gene that is most commonly affected by point mutations in cancer is *TP53*, a prototypical "guardian" type tumor suppressor gene (discussed later).

Gene Rearrangements

Gene rearrangements may be produced by chromosomal translocations or inversions. Specific chromosomal translocations and inversions are highly associated with certain malignancies, particularly neoplasms derived from hematopoietic cells and other kinds of mesenchymal cells.

These rearrangements can activate proto-oncogenes in two ways:

- **Some gene rearrangements result in overexpression of proto-oncogenes by removing them from their normal regulatory elements and placing them under control of an inappropriate, highly active promoter or enhancer.** Two different kinds of B cell lymphoma provide illustrative examples of this mechanism. In more than 90% of cases of *Burkitt lymphoma,* the cells have a translocation, usually between chromosomes 8 and 14, that leads to overexpression of the *MYC* gene on chromosome 8 by juxtaposition with immunoglobulin heavy chain gene regulatory elements on chromosome 14 (Fig. 6.14). In *follicular lymphoma,* a reciprocal translocation between chromosomes 14 and 18 leads to overexpression of the anti-apoptotic gene, *BCL2,* on chromosome 18, also driven by immunoglobulin gene regulatory elements.
- **Other oncogenic gene rearrangements create fusion genes encoding novel chimeric proteins.** Most notable is the Philadelphia (Ph) chromosome in chronic myeloid leukemia, consisting of a balanced reciprocal translocation between chromosomes 9 and 22 (see Fig. 6.14). As a consequence, the derivative chromosome 22 (the Philadelphia chromosome) appears smaller than normal. This cytogenetic change is seen in more than 90% of cases of chronic myeloid leukemia and results in the fusion of portions of the *BCR* gene on chromosome 22 and the *ABL* gene on chromosome 9. The few Philadelphia chromosome–negative cases harbor a cryptic (cytogenetically silent) *BCR-ABL* fusion gene, the presence of which is the *sine qua non* of chronic myeloid leukemia. As discussed later, the *BCR-ABL* fusion gene encodes a novel tyrosine kinase with potent transforming activity.

Lymphoid tumors are most commonly associated with recurrent gene rearrangements. This relationship exists because normal lymphocytes express special enzymes that purposefully introduce DNA breaks during the processes of immunoglobulin or T cell receptor gene recombination. Repair of these DNA breaks is error-prone, and the resulting mistakes sometimes result in gene rearrangements that activate proto-oncogenes. Two other types of mesenchymal tumors, myeloid neoplasms (acute myeloid leukemias and myeloproliferative disorders) and sarcomas, also frequently possess gene rearrangements. Unlike lymphoid neoplasms, the cause of the DNA breaks that lead to gene rearrangements in myeloid neoplasms and sarcomas is unknown. In general, the rearrangements that are seen in myeloid neoplasms and sarcomas create fusion genes that encode either hyperactive tyrosine kinases (akin to BCR-ABL) or novel oncogenic transcription factors. A well-characterized example of the latter is the (11;22)(q24;q12) translocation in Ewing sarcoma. This rearrangement creates a fusion gene encoding a chimeric oncoprotein composed of portions of two different transcription factors called EWS and FLI1.

Identification of pathogenic gene rearrangements in carcinomas has lagged because karyotypically evident translocations and inversions (which point to the location of important oncogenes) are rare in carcinomas. However, advances in DNA sequencing have revealed recurrent cryptic pathogenic gene rearrangements in carcinomas as well. As with hematologic malignancies and sarcomas, gene rearrangements in solid tumors can contribute to carcinogenesis either by increasing expression of an oncogene or by generation of a novel fusion gene. Examples will be discussed along with specific cancers in other chapters. As with a fusion gene such as BCR-ABL, some of the fusion genes in solid tumors also provide drug targets (e.g., EML-ALK in lung cancer; Chapter 13).

Deletions

Deletions are another prevalent abnormality in tumor cells. Deletion of specific regions of chromosomes may result in the loss of particular tumor suppressor genes. Tumor suppressors generally require inactivation of both alleles in order for them to contribute to carcinogenesis. A common mechanism for this is an inactivating point mutation in one allele, followed by deletion of the other, non-mutated allele. As discussed later, deletions involving

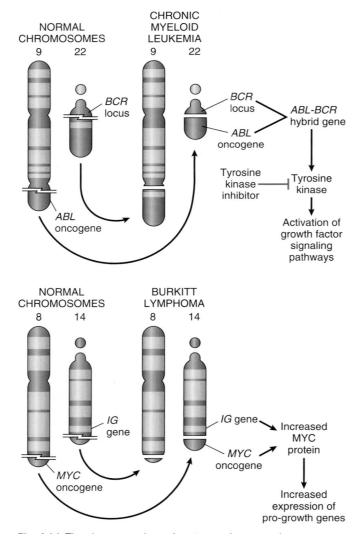

Fig. 6.14 The chromosomal translocations and associated oncogenes in chronic myelogenous leukemia and Burkitt lymphoma.

13q14, the site of the *RB* gene, are associated with retinoblastoma, and deletion of 17p is associated with loss of *TP53,* arguably the most important tumor suppressor gene.

Gene Amplifications

Proto-oncogenes may be converted to oncogenes by gene amplification, with consequent overexpression and hyperactivity of otherwise normal proteins. Such amplification may produce several hundred copies of the gene, a change in copy number that can be readily detected by molecular hybridization with appropriate DNA probes. In some cases, the amplified genes produce chromosomal changes that can be identified microscopically. Two mutually exclusive patterns are seen: multiple small, extrachromosomal structures called *double minutes*; and *homogeneously staining regions*. The latter derive from the insertion of the amplified genes into new chromosomal locations, which may be distant from the normal location of the involved genes; because regions containing amplified genes lack a normal banding pattern, they appear homogeneous in a G-banded karyotype. Two clinically important examples of amplification involve the *NMYC* gene in neuroblastoma and the *HER2* gene in breast cancers. *NMYC* is amplified in 25% to 30% of neuroblastomas, and the amplification is associated with poor prognosis (Fig. 6.15). *HER2* (also known as *ERBB2*) amplification occurs in about 20% of breast cancers, and antibody therapy directed against the receptor encoded by the *HER2* gene has proved effective in this subset of tumors.

Aneuploidy

Aneuploidy is defined as a number of chromosomes that is not a multiple of the haploid state; for humans, that is a chromosome number that is not a multiple of 23. Aneuploidy is remarkably common in cancers, particularly carcinomas, and was proposed as a cause of carcinogenesis over 100 years ago. Aneuploidy frequently results from errors of the mitotic checkpoint, the major cell cycle control mechanism that acts to prevent mistakes in chromosome segregation. The mitotic checkpoint prevents aneuploidy by inhibiting the irreversible transition to anaphase until all of the replicated chromosomes have made productive attachments to spindle microtubules. Complete absence of the mitotic checkpoint leads to rapid cell death as a consequence of abnormal chromosome segregation.

Mechanistic data establishing aneuploidy as a cause of carcinogenesis, rather than a consequence, have been difficult to generate. However, statistical approaches made possible by detailed analysis of cancer cells suggest (as might be expected) that aneuploidy tends to increase the copy number of key oncogenes and decrease the copy number of potent tumor suppressors. For example, chromosome 8, which almost never is lost and often is present in increased copies in tumor cells, is where the *MYC* oncogene is located. By contrast, portions of chromosome 17, where the *TP53* gene is located, are often lost and are infrequently gained. Thus, tumor development and progression may be molded by changes in chromosome numbers that enhance the dosage of oncogenes while restricting the activity of tumor suppressor genes.

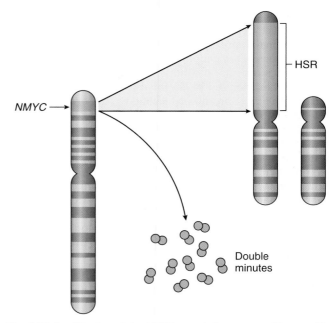

Fig. 6.15 Amplification of the *NMYC* gene in human neuroblastoma. The *NMYC* gene, present normally on chromosome 2p, becomes amplified and is seen either as extrachromosomal double minutes or as a chromosomally integrated homogeneous-staining region (HSR). The integration involves other autosomes, such as 4, 9, or 13. *(Modified from Brodeur GM, Seeger RC, Sather H, et al: Clinical implications of oncogene activation in human neuroblastomas. Cancer 58:541, 1986. Reprinted by permission of Wiley-Liss, Inc, a subsidiary of John Wiley & Sons, Inc.)*

MicroRNAs and Cancer

As discussed in Chapter 1, microRNAs (miRNAs) are noncoding, single-stranded RNAs, approximately 22 nucleotides in length, that function as negative regulators of genes. They inhibit gene expression posttranscriptionally by repressing translation or, in some cases, by messenger RNA (mRNA) cleavage. In view of their important functions in control of cell growth, differentiation, and survival, it is not surprising that accumulating evidence indicates that miRNAs also can contribute to carcinogenesis. Specifically, if the target of a miRNA is a tumor suppressor gene, then overactivity of the miRNA can reduce the tumor suppressor protein. Such miRNAs are sometimes referred to as *oncomIRs.* Conversely, if an miRNA inhibits the translation of an oncogene, a reduction in the quantity or function of that miRNA will lead to overproduction of the oncogene product. Such relationships have already been established by miRNA profiling of several human tumors. For example, downregulation or deletion of certain miRNAs in some leukemias and lymphomas results in increased expression of *BCL2,* an anti-apoptotic gene. Thus, by negatively regulating *BCL2,* such miRNAs behave as tumor suppressor genes. Dysregulation of other miRNAs that control the expression of the *RAS* and *MYC* oncogenes also has been detected in lung tumors and in certain B-cell leukemias, respectively.

Epigenetic Modifications and Cancer

You will recall from Chapter 1 that epigenetics refers to reversible, heritable changes in gene expression that occur without mutation. Such changes involve posttranslational modifications of histones and DNA methylation, both of which affect gene expression. In normal, differentiated cells, the major portion of the genome is not expressed. These regions of the genome are silenced by DNA methylation and histone modifications. On the other hand, cancer cells are characterized by a global DNA hypomethylation and selective promoter-localized hypermethylation. Indeed, it has become evident during the past several years that tumor suppressor genes are sometimes silenced by hypermethylation of promoter sequences, rather than by mutation. In addition, genome-wide hypomethylation has been shown to cause chromosomal instability and can induce tumors in mice. Thus, epigenetic changes may influence carcinogenesis in many ways. As an added wrinkle, deep sequencing of cancer genomes has identified mutations in genes that regulate epigenetic modifications in many cancers. Thus, certain genetic changes in cancers may be selected because they lead to alterations of the "epigenome" that favor cancer growth and survival.

The epigenetic state of particular cell types—a feature described as the epigenetic context—also dictates their response to signals that control growth and differentiation. As mentioned earlier, epigenetic modifications regulate gene expression, allowing cells with the same genetic makeup (e.g., a neuron and a keratinocyte) to have completely different appearances and functions. In some instances, the epigenetic state of a cell dramatically affects its response to otherwise identical signals. For example, the *NOTCH1* gene has an oncogenic role in T-cell leukemia, yet acts as a tumor suppressor in squamous cell carcinomas. As would be expected, this dichotomy exists because activated *NOTCH1* turns on pro-growth genes in T-cell progenitors and tumor suppressor genes in keratinocytes.

SUMMARY

GENETIC LESIONS IN CANCER

- Mutations in cancer cells fall into two major classes, driver (pathogenic) mutations and passenger (neutral) mutations.
- Passenger mutations may become driver mutations if selective pressure on the tumor changes, for example, in the setting of treatment with an effective therapeutic drug.
- Tumor cells may acquire driver mutations through several means, including point mutations and nonrandom chromosomal abnormalities that contribute to malignancy; these include gene rearrangements, deletions, and amplifications.
- Gene rearrangements (usually caused by translocations, but sometimes by inversions of other more complex events) contribute to carcinogenesis by overexpression of oncogenes or generation of novel fusion proteins with altered signaling capacity.
- Deletions frequently affect tumor suppressor genes, whereas gene amplification increases the expression of oncogenes.
- Overexpression of miRNAs can contribute to carcinogenesis by reducing the expression of tumor suppressors, while deletion or loss of expression of miRNAs can lead to overexpression of proto-oncogenes.
- Tumor suppressor genes and DNA repair genes also may be silenced by epigenetic changes, which involve reversible, heritable changes in gene expression that occur not by mutation but by methylation of the promoter.

CARCINOGENESIS: A MULTISTEP PROCESS

Fortunately, in most if not all instances, no single mutation is sufficient to transform a normal cell into a cancer cell. Carcinogenesis is thus a multistep process resulting from the accumulation of multiple genetic alterations that collectively give rise to the transformed phenotype and all of its associated hallmarks, discussed later. As mentioned earlier, the presence of driver mutations in some nonneoplastic precursor lesions suggest the need for additional mutations for transition to a full blown cancer and thus support this model.

Beyond tumor initiation from a single founding cell, it is important to recognize that cancers continue to undergo Darwinian selection and therefore continue to evolve (Fig. 6.16). It is well established that during their course cancers generally become more aggressive and acquire greater malignant potential, a phenomenon referred to as *tumor progression*. At the molecular level, tumor progression most likely results from mutations that accumulate independently in different cells. Some of these mutations may be lethal, but others may affect the function of cancer genes, thereby making the affected cells more adept at growth, survival, invasion, metastasis, or immune evasion. Due to this selective advantage, subclones that acquire these mutations may come to dominate one area of a tumor, either at the primary site or at sites of metastasis. **As a result of continuing mutation and Darwinian selection, even though malignant tumors are monoclonal in origin they are typically genetically heterogeneous by the time of their clinical presentation.** In advanced tumors exhibiting genetic instability, the extent of genetic heterogeneity may be enormous.

Genetic evolution shaped by darwinian selection can explain the two most pernicious properties of cancers: the tendency over time for cancers to become both more aggressive and less responsive to therapy. Thus, genetic heterogeneity has implications not only for cancer progression but also for its response to therapy. Experience has shown that when tumors recur after chemotherapy, the recurrent tumor is almost always resistant to the original drug regimen if it is given again. Experimental data suggest that this acquired resistance stems from the outgrowth of subclones that have, by chance, mutations (or epigenetic alterations) that impart drug resistance.

HALLMARKS OF CANCER

This overview serves as background for a more detailed consideration of the molecular pathogenesis of cancer. As mentioned earlier, *bona fide* cancer genes number in the hundreds, at a minimum. While it is traditional to describe the function of cancer genes one gene at a time, the blizzard of mutated genes emerging from the sequencing of cancer genomes has blanketed the landscape and revealed the limitations of trying to grasp the fundamental properties of cancer, gene by gene. A much more tractable and conceptually satisfying way to think about the biology of cancer is to consider the common phenotypic and

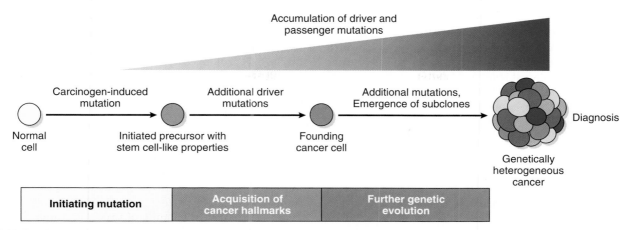

Fig. 6.16 Development of cancer through stepwise accumulation of complementary driver mutations. The order in which various driver mutations occur is usually unknown and may vary from tumor to tumor.

biological properties of cancer cells. It appears that **all cancers display eight fundamental changes in cell physiology, which are considered the hallmarks of cancer.** These changes are illustrated in Fig. 6.17 and consist of the following:

- *Self-sufficiency in growth signals*
- *Insensitivity to growth-inhibitory signals*
- *Altered cellular metabolism*
- *Evasion of apoptosis*
- *Limitless replicative potential (immortality)*
- *Sustained angiogenesis*
- *Invasion and metastasis*
- *Evasion of immune surveillance*

The acquisition of the genetic and epigenetic alterations that confer these hallmarks may be accelerated by *cancer-promoting inflammation* and by *genomic instability*. These are considered enabling characteristics because they promote cellular transformation and subsequent tumor progression.

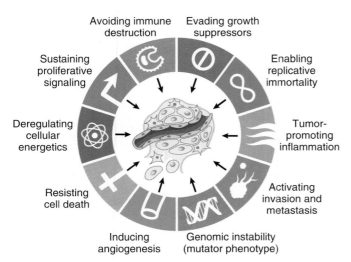

Fig. 6.17 Eight cancer hallmarks and two enabling factors (genomic instability and tumor-promoting inflammation). Most cancer cells acquire these properties during their development, typically due to mutations in critical genes. *(From Hanahan D, Weinberg RA: Hallmarks of cancer: the next generation. Cell 144:646, 2011.)*

Mutations in genes that regulate some or all of these cellular traits are seen in every cancer; accordingly, these traits form the basis of the following discussion of the molecular origins of cancer. Of note, by convention, gene symbols are italicized but their protein products are not (e.g., *RB* gene and RB protein, *TP53* and p53, *MYC* and MYC).

Self-Sufficiency in Growth Signals

The self-sufficiency in growth that characterizes cancer cells generally stems from gain-of-function mutations that convert proto-oncogenes to oncogenes. Oncogenes encode proteins called *oncoproteins* that promote cell growth, even in the absence of normal growth-promoting signals. To appreciate how oncogenes drive inappropriate cell growth, it is helpful to review briefly the sequence of events that characterize normal cell proliferation (introduced in Chapter 1). Under physiologic conditions, cell proliferation can be readily resolved into the following steps:

1. Binding of a growth factor to its specific receptor on the cell membrane
2. Transient and limited activation of the growth factor receptor, which in turn activates several signal-transducing proteins on the inner leaflet of the plasma membrane
3. Transmission of the transduced signal across the cytosol to the nucleus by second messengers or a cascade of signal transduction molecules
4. Induction and activation of nuclear regulatory factors that initiate and regulate DNA transcription and the biosynthesis of other cellular components that are needed for cell division, such as organelles, membrane components, and ribosomes
5. Entry and progression of the cell into the cell cycle, resulting ultimately in cell division

The mechanisms that endow cancer cells with the ability to proliferate can be grouped according to their role in the growth factor–induced signal transduction cascade and cell cycle regulation. Indeed, each one of the listed steps is susceptible to corruption in cancer cells.

Growth Factors

Cancers may secrete their own growth factors or induce stromal cells to produce growth factors in the tumor microenvironment. Most soluble growth factors are made by one cell type and act on a neighboring cell to stimulate proliferation (paracrine action). Normally, cells that produce the growth factor do not express the cognate receptor, preventing the formation of positive feedback loops within the same cell. This "rule" may be broken by cancer cells in several different ways.

- Some cancer cells acquire growth self-sufficiency by acquiring the ability to synthesize the same growth factors to which they are responsive. For example, many glioblastomas secrete platelet-derived growth factor (PDGF) and express the PDGF receptor, and many sarcomas make both transforming growth factor-α (TGF-α) and its receptor. Similar autocrine loops are fairly common in many types of cancer.
- Another mechanism by which cancer cells acquire growth self-sufficiency is by interaction with stroma. In some cases, tumor cells send signals to activate normal cells in the supporting stroma, which in turn produce growth factors that promote tumor growth.

Growth Factor Receptors

The next group in the sequence of signal transduction is growth factor receptors. Some growth factor receptors have an intrinsic tyrosine kinase activity that is activated by growth factor binding, while others signal by stimulating the activity of downstream proteins. **Many of the myriad growth factor receptors function as oncoproteins when they are mutated or if they overexpressed.** The best-documented examples of overexpression involve the epidermal growth factor (EGF) receptor family. ERBB1, the EGF receptor, is overexpressed in 80% of squamous cell carcinomas of the lung, 50% or more of glioblastomas, and 80% to 100% of epithelial tumors of the head and neck. As mentioned earlier, the gene encoding a related receptor, *HER2 (ERBB2),* is amplified in approximately 20% of breast cancers and in a smaller fraction of adenocarcinomas of the lung, ovary, stomach, and salivary glands. These tumors are exquisitely sensitive to the mitogenic effects of small amounts of growth factors. The significance of *HER2* in the pathogenesis of breast cancers is illustrated dramatically by the clinical benefit derived from blocking the extracellular domain of this receptor with anti-HER2 antibodies, an elegant example of "bench to bedside" medicine. In other instances, tyrosine kinase activity is stimulated by point mutations or small indels that lead to subtle but functionally important changes in protein structure, or gene rearrangements that create fusion genes encoding chimeric receptors. In each of these cases, the mutated receptors are constitutively active, delivering mitogenic signals to cells even in the absence of growth factors. These types of mutations are most common in leukemias, lymphomas, and certain forms of sarcoma.

Downstream Signal-Transducing Proteins

Cancer cells often acquire growth autonomy as a result of mutations in genes that encode components of signaling pathways downstream of growth factor receptors. The signaling proteins that couple growth factor receptors to their nuclear targets are activated by ligand binding to growth factor receptors. The signals are trasnmitted to the nucleus through various signal transduction molecules. Two important oncoproteins in the category of signaling molecules are RAS and ABL. Each of these is discussed briefly next.

RAS

RAS is the most commonly mutated oncogene in human tumors. Approximately 30% of all human tumors contain mutated *RAS* genes, and the frequency is even higher in some specific cancers (e.g., pancreatic adenocarcinoma). RAS is a member of a family of small G proteins that bind guanosine nucleotides (guanosine triphosphate [GTP] and guanosine diphosphate [GDP]). Signaling by RAS involves the following sequential steps:

- *Normally, RAS flips back and forth between an excited signal-transmitting state and a quiescent state.* RAS is inactive when bound to GDP; stimulation of cells by growth factors such as EGF and PDGF leads to exchange of GDP for GTP and subsequent conformational changes

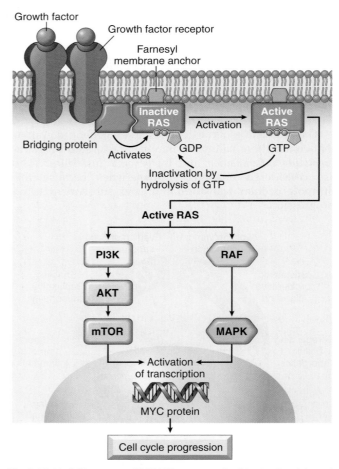

Fig. 6.18 Model for action of RAS. When a normal cell is stimulated through a growth factor receptor, inactive (GDP-bound) RAS is activated to a GTP-bound state. Activated RAS transduces proliferative signals to the nucleus along two pathways: the so-called "RAF/ERK/MAP kinase pathway" and the *PI3 kinase/AKT pathway. GDP,* Guanosine diphosphate; *GTP,* guanosine triphosphate; *MAP,* mitogen-activated protein; *PI3,* phosphatidylinositol-3.

that generate active RAS (Fig. 6.18). This excited signal-emitting state is short-lived, however, because the intrinsic guanosine triphosphatase (GTPase) activity of RAS hydrolyzes GTP to GDP, releasing a phosphate group and returning the protein to its quiescent GDP-bound state. The GTPase activity of activated RAS is magnified dramatically by a family of GTPase-activating proteins (GAPs), which act as molecular brakes that prevent uncontrolled RAS activation by favoring hydrolysis of GTP to GDP.

- *Activated RAS stimulates downstream regulators of proliferation by several interconnected pathways that converge on the nucleus and alter the expression of genes that regulate growth, such as* MYC. While details of the signaling cascades (some of which are illustrated in Fig. 6.18) downstream of RAS are not discussed here, an important point is that mutational activation of these signaling intermediates mimics the growth promoting effects of activated RAS. For example, BRAF, which lies in the so-called "RAF/ERK/MAP kinase pathway" is mutated in more than 60% of melanomas and is associated with unregulated cell proliferation. Mutations of phosphatidyl inositol-3 kinase (PI3 kinase) in the PI3K/AKT pathway also occur with high frequency in some tumor types, with similar consequences.

RAS most commonly is activated by point mutations in amino acid residues that are either within the GTP-binding pocket or in the enzymatic region that carries out GTP hydrolysis. Both kinds of mutations interfere with breakdown of GTP, which is essential to inactivate RAS. RAS is thus trapped in its activated, GTP-bound form, and the cell is forced into a continuously proliferating state. It follows from this scenario that the consequences of activating mutations in RAS should be mimicked by loss-of-function mutations in GAPs, which would lead to a failure to simulate GTP hydrolysis and thereby restrain RAS. Indeed, the GAP neurofibromin-1 (NF1) is mutated in the cancer-prone familial disorder neurofibromatosis type 1 (Chapter 22) and is a bona fide tumor suppressor. Similarly, another important tumor suppressor called PTEN is a negative inhibitor of PI3 kinase and is frequently mutated in carcinomas, certain leukemias, and other cancers as well.

ABL

Several non–receptor tyrosine kinases function as signal transduction molecules. In this group, ABL is the best defined with respect to carcinogenesis.

The ABL proto-oncoprotein has tyrosine kinase activity that is dampened by internal negative regulatory domains. As discussed earlier (see Fig. 6.14), in chronic myeloid leukemia and certain acute leukemias, a part of the *ABL* gene is translocated from its normal abode on chromosome 9 to chromosome 22, where it fuses with part of the breakpoint cluster region *(BCR)* gene. This fusion gene encodes as BCR-ABL hybrid protein that contains the ABL tyrosine kinase domain and a BCR domain that self-associates, an event that unleashes a constitutive tyrosine kinase activity. Of interest, the BCR-ABL protein activates all of the signals that are downstream of RAS, making it a potent stimulator of cell growth.

The crucial role of BCR-ABL in cancer has been confirmed by the dramatic clinical response of patients with chronic myeloid leukemia to BCR-ABL kinase inhibitors. The prototype of this kind of drug, imatinib mesylate (Gleevec), galvanized interest in design of drugs that target specific molecular lesions found in various cancers (so-called "targeted therapy"). BCR-ABL also is an example of the concept of *oncogene addiction,* wherein a tumor is profoundly dependent on a single signaling molecule. *BCR-ABL* fusion gene formation is an early, perhaps initiating, event that drives leukemogenesis. Development of leukemia probably requires other collaborating mutations, but the transformed cell continues to depend on BCR-ABL for signals that mediate growth and survival. BCR-ABL signaling can be seen as the central lodgepole around which the transformed state is "built". If the lodgepole is removed by inhibition of the BCR-ABL kinase, the structure collapses. In view of this level of dependency, it is not surprising that acquired resistance of tumors to BCR-ABL inhibitors often is due to the outgrowth of a subclone with a mutation in BCR-ABL that prevents binding of the drug to the BCR-ABL protein.

Nuclear Transcription Factors

The ultimate consequence of signaling through oncoproteins such as RAS or ABL is inappropriate and continuous stimulation of nuclear transcription factors that drive the expression of growth-promoting genes. Growth autonomy may thus be a consequence of mutations affecting genes that regulate DNA transcription. A host of oncoproteins, including products of the *MYC, MYB, JUN, FOS,* and *REL* oncogenes, function as transcription factors that regulate the expression of growth-promoting genes, such as cyclins. Of these, MYC is involved most commonly in human tumors.

Dysregulation of MYC promotes tumorigenesis by simultaneously promoting the progression of cells through the cell cycle and enhancing alterations in metabolism that support cell growth. MYC primarily functions by activating the transcription of other genes. Genes activated by MYC include several growth-promoting genes, including cyclin-dependent kinases (CDKs), whose products drive cells into the cell cycle (discussed next), and genes that control pathways that produce the building blocks (e.g., amino acids, lipids, nucleotides) that are needed for cell growth and division. As mentioned earlier (see Fig. 6.14), dysregulation of *MYC* results from a (8;14) translocation in Burkitt lymphoma, a highly aggressive B-cell tumor. *MYC* also is amplified in breast, colon, lung, and many other cancers, while the related *NMYC* and *LMYC* genes are amplified in neuroblastomas and small cell cancers of lung, respectively.

Cyclins and Cyclin-Dependent Kinases

As mentioned in Chapter 1, growth factors transduce signals that stimulate the orderly progression of cells through the various phases of the cell cycle, the process by which cells replicate their DNA in preparation for cell division. You will recall that progression of cells through the cell cycle is orchestrated by *cyclin-dependent kinases* (CDKs), which are activated by binding to *cyclins,* so called because of the cyclic nature of their production and degradation.

The CDK-cyclin complexes phosphorylate crucial target proteins that drive cells forward through the cell cycle. While cyclins arouse the CDKs, *CDK inhibitors* (CDKIs), of which there are many, silence the CDKs and exert negative control over the cell cycle. Expression of these inhibitors is downregulated by mitogenic signaling pathways, thus promoting the progression of the cell cycle.

There are two main cell cycle checkpoints, one at the G1/S transition and the other at the G2/M transition, each of which is tightly regulated by a balance of growth-promoting and growth-suppressing factors, as well as by sensors of DNA damage (Chapter 1). If activated, these DNA-damage sensors transmit signals that arrest cell cycle progression and, if cell damage cannot be repaired, initiate apoptosis. Once cells pass through the G_1/S checkpoint, they are committed to undergo cell division. Understandably, then, defects in the G_1/S checkpoint are particularly important in cancer, since these lead directly to increased cell division. Indeed, all cancers appear to have genetic lesions that disable the G_1/S checkpoint, causing cells to continually reenter the S phase. For unclear reasons, particular lesions vary widely in frequency across tumor types, but they fall into two major categories.

- *Gain-of-function mutations involving CDK4 or D cyclins.* Mishaps increasing the expression of cyclin D or CDK4 are common events in neoplastic transformation. The cyclin D genes are overexpressed in many cancers, including those affecting the breast, esophagus, liver, and a subset of lymphomas and plasma cell tumors. Amplification of the *CDK4* gene occurs in melanomas, sarcomas, and glioblastomas. Mutations affecting cyclins B and E and other CDKs also occur, but they are much less frequent than those affecting cyclin D and CDK4.
- *Loss-of-function mutations involving CDKIs.* CDKIs frequently are disabled by mutation or gene silencing in many human malignancies. For example, germline mutations of *CDKN2A*, a gene that encodes the CDK inhibitor p16, are present in 25% of melanoma-prone kindreds, and acquired deletion or inactivation of *CDKN2A* is seen in 75% of pancreatic carcinomas, 40% to 70% of glioblastomas, 50% of esophageal cancers and certain leukemias, and 20% of non–small cell lung carcinomas, soft-tissue sarcomas, and bladder cancers.

A final consideration of importance in a discussion of growth-promoting signals is that the increased production of oncoproteins does not by itself lead to sustained proliferation of cancer cells. There are two built-in mechanisms, cell senescence and apoptosis, that oppose oncogene-mediated cell growth. As discussed later, genes that regulate these two braking mechanisms must be disabled to allow the action of oncogenes to proceed unopposed.

SUMMARY

SELF-SUFFICIENCY IN GROWTH SIGNALS

- *Proto-oncogenes:* normal cellular genes whose products promote cell proliferation
- *Oncogenes:* mutant or overexpressed versions of proto-oncogenes that function autonomously without a requirement for normal growth-promoting signals

- Oncoproteins promote uncontrolled cell proliferation by several mechanisms:
  - Stimulus-independent expression of growth factor and its receptor, setting up an autocrine loop of cell proliferation (e.g., PDGF–PDGF receptor in brain tumors)
  - Mutations in genes encoding growth factor receptors or tyrosine kinases leading to constitutive signaling
  - Amplification of EGF receptor family genes such as *HER2* in breast cancer
  - Fusion of portions of the *ABL* tyrosine kinase gene and the *BCR* protein gene, creating a *BCR-ABL* fusion gene encoding a constitutively active tyrosine kinase, in certain leukemias
  - Mutations in genes encoding signaling molecules
  - RAS commonly is mutated in human cancers and normally flips between resting GDP-bound state and active GTP-bound state; mutations block hydrolysis of GTP to GDP, leading to unchecked signaling
  - Overproduction or unregulated activity of transcription factors
  - Translocation of MYC in some lymphomas leads to overexpression and unregulated expression of its target genes controlling cell cycling and survival
  - Mutations that activate cyclin genes or inactivate negative regulators of cyclins and cyclin-dependent kinases
- Complexes of cyclins with CDKs drive the cell cycle by phosphorylating various substrates and normally are controlled by CDK inhibitors. Mutations in genes encoding cyclins, CDKs, and CDK inhibitors result in uncontrolled cell cycle progression and are found in a wide variety of cancers including melanomas and brain, lung, and pancreatic cancers.

Insensitivity to Growth Inhibitory Signals: Tumor Suppressor Genes

Isaac Newton theorized that every action has an equal and opposite reaction. Although Newton was not a cancer biologist, his formulation holds true for cell growth. **Whereas oncogenes encode proteins that promote cell growth, the products of tumor suppressor genes apply brakes to cell proliferation.** Disruption of such genes renders cells refractory to growth inhibition and mimics the growth-promoting effects of oncogenes. The following discussion describes tumor suppressor genes, their products, and possible mechanisms by which loss of their function contributes to unregulated cell growth.

In principle, anti-growth signals can prevent cell proliferation by several complementary mechanisms. The signal may cause dividing cells to enter G_0 (quiescence), where they remain until external cues prod their reentry into the proliferative pool. Alternatively, the cells may enter a postmitotic, differentiated pool and lose replicative potential. Nonreplicative senescence, alluded to earlier, is another mechanism of escape from sustained cell growth. And, as a last-ditch effort, the cells may be programmed for death by apoptosis. As we will see, tumor suppressor genes have all these "tricks" in their toolbox designed to halt wayward cells from becoming malignant.

RB: Governor of the Cell Cycle

RB, a key negative regulator of the cell cycle, is directly or indirectly inactivated in most human cancers. The retinoblastoma gene *(RB)* was the first tumor suppressor gene to be discovered and is now considered the prototype of this family of cancer genes. As with many advances in medicine, the discovery of tumor suppressor genes was accomplished by the study of a rare disease—in this case, retinoblastoma, an uncommon childhood tumor. Approximately 60% of retinoblastomas are sporadic, while the remaining ones are familial, the predisposition to develop the tumor being transmitted as an autosomal dominant trait. To account for the sporadic and familial occurrence of an identical tumor, Knudson, in 1974, proposed his now famous two-hit hypothesis, which in molecular terms can be stated as follows:

- Two mutations *(hits)* are required to produce retinoblastoma. These involve the *RB* gene, which has been mapped to chromosomal locus 13q14. Both of the normal alleles of the *RB* locus must be inactivated (hence the two hits) for the development of retinoblastoma (Fig. 6.19).
- In familial cases, children inherit one defective copy of the *RB* gene in the germ line; the other copy is normal.

Retinoblastoma develops when the normal *RB* gene is lost in retinoblasts as a result of somatic mutation. Because in retinoblastoma families a single germ line mutation is sufficient to transmit disease risk, the trait has an autosomal dominant inheritance pattern.

- In sporadic cases, both normal *RB* alleles are lost by somatic mutation in one of the retinoblasts. The end result is the same: a retinal cell that has lost both of the normal copies of the *RB* gene becomes cancerous.

From the above, it is evident that although the risk for developing retinoblastoma in retinoblastoma families is inherited as a dominant trait, at the level of the cell, one intact *RB* gene is all that is needed for normal function.

Although the loss of normal *RB* genes initially was discovered in retinoblastomas, it is now evident that biallelic loss of this gene is a fairly common feature of several tumors, including breast cancer, small cell cancer of the lung, and bladder cancer. Patients with familial retinoblastoma also are at greatly increased risk for developing osteosarcomas and some soft-tissue sarcomas.

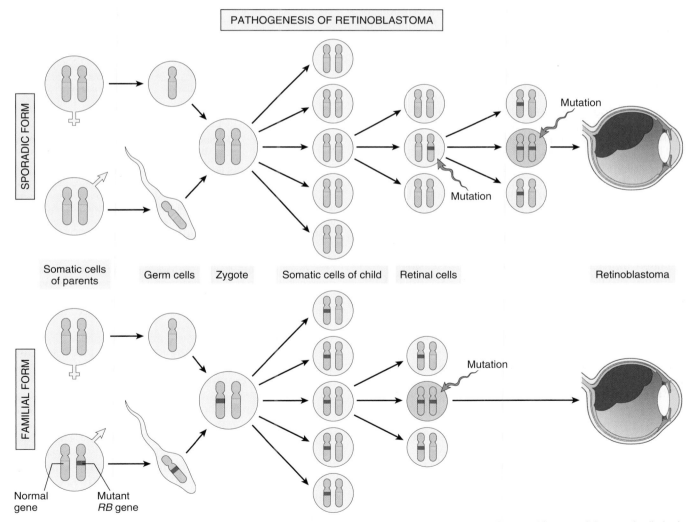

Fig. 6.19 Pathogenesis of retinoblastoma. Two mutations of the *RB* chromosomal locus, on 13q14, lead to neoplastic proliferation of the retinal cells. In the sporadic form, both *RB* mutations in the tumor-founding retinal cell are acquired. In the familial form, all somatic cells inherit one mutant *RB* gene from a carrier parent, and as a result only one additional *RB* mutation in a retinal cell is required for complete loss of *RB* function.

The function of the RB protein is to regulate the G1/S checkpoint, the portal through which cells must pass before DNA replication commences. Although each phase of the cell cycle circuitry is monitored carefully, the transition from G_1 to S is an extremely important checkpoint in the cell cycle "clock." In the G_1 phase, diverse signals are integrated to determine whether the cell should progress through the cell cycle, or exit the cell cycle and differentiate. The *RB* gene product, RB, is a DNA-binding protein that serves as a point of integration for these diverse signals, which ultimately act by altering the phosphorylation state of RB. Specifically, signals that promote cell cycle progression lead to the phosphorylation and inactivation of RB, while those that block cell cycle progression act by maintaining RB in an active hypophosphorylated state.

To appreciate this crucial role of RB in the cell cycle, it is helpful to review the mechanisms that enforce the G_1/S transition.

- The initiation of DNA replication (S phase) requires the activity of cyclin E/CDK2 complexes, and expression of cyclin E is dependent on the E2F family of transcription factors. Early in G_1, RB is in its hypophosphorylated active form, and it binds to and inhibits the E2F family of transcription factors, preventing transcription of cyclin E. Hypophosphorylated RB blocks E2F-mediated transcription in at least two ways (Fig. 6.20). First, it sequesters E2F, preventing it from interacting with other transcriptional activators. Second, RB recruits chromatin remodeling proteins, such as histone deacetylases and histone methyltransferases, which bind to the promoters of E2F-responsive genes such as cyclin E. These enzymes modify chromatin at the promoters to make DNA insensitive to transcription factors.

- This situation is changed on mitogenic signaling. Growth factor signaling leads to cyclin D expression and activation of cyclin D–CDK4/6 complexes. The level of cyclin D-CDK4/6 activity is tempered by antagonists such as p16, which is itself subject to regulation by growth inhibitors such as TGFβ that serve to set a threshold for mitogenic responses. If the stimulus is sufficiently strong, cyclin D-CDK4/6 complexes phosphorylate RB, inactivating the protein and releasing E2F to induce target genes such as cyclin E. Cyclin E/CDK complexes then stimulate DNA replication and progression through the cell cycle. When the cells enter S phase, they are committed to divide without additional growth factor stimulation. During the ensuing M phase, the phosphate groups are removed from RB by cellular phosphatases, regenerating the hypophosphorylated form of RB.

- E2F is not the sole target of RB. The versatile RB protein binds to a variety of other transcription factors that regulate cell differentiation. For example, RB stimulates myocyte-, adipocyte-, melanocyte-, and macrophage-specific transcription factors. Thus, the RB pathway couples control of cell cycle progression at G_1 with differentiation, which may explain how differentiation is associated with exit from the cell cycle.

In view of the centrality of RB to the control of the cell cycle, an interesting question is why RB is not mutated in every cancer. In fact, mutations in other genes that control

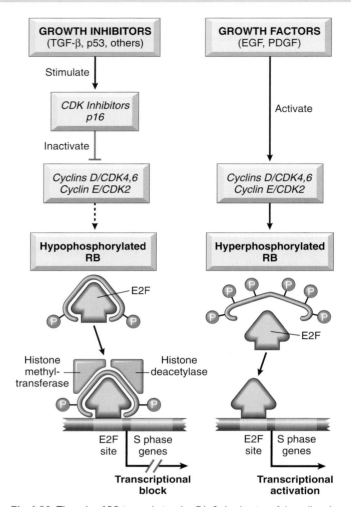

Fig. 6.20 The role of RB in regulating the G1–S checkpoint of the cell cycle. Hypophosphorylated RB in complex with the E2F transcription factors binds to DNA, recruits chromatin remodeling factors (histone deacetylases and histone methyltransferases), and inhibits transcription of genes whose products are required for the S phase of the cell cycle. When RB is phosphorylated by the cyclin D–CDK4, cyclin D–CDK6, and cyclin E–CDK2 complexes, it releases E2F. The latter then activates transcription of S-phase genes. The phosphorylation of RB is inhibited by CDKIs, because they inactivate cyclin-CDK complexes. Virtually all cancer cells show dysregulation of the G1–S checkpoint as a result of mutation in one of four genes that regulate the phosphorylation of RB; these genes are *RB, CDK4, cyclin D,* and *CDKN2A [p16]. EGF,* Epidermal growth factor; *PDGF,* platelet-derived growth factor.

RB phosphorylation can mimic the effect of RB loss and are commonly found in many cancers that have normal *RB* genes. For example, mutational activation of CDK4 and overexpression of cyclin D favor cell proliferation by facilitating RB phosphorylation and inactivation. Indeed, cyclin D is overexpressed in many tumors because of amplification or translocation of the cyclin D1 gene. Mutational inactivation of genes encoding CDKIs also can drive the cell cycle by removing important brakes on cyclin/CDK activity. As mentioned earlier, the *CDKN2A* gene, which encodes the CDK inhibitor p16, is an extremely common target of deletion or mutational inactivation in human tumors.

It is now accepted that loss of normal cell cycle control is central to malignant transformation and that at least

one of the four key regulators of the cell cycle (p16, cyclin D, CDK4, RB) is mutated in most human cancers. Notably, in cancers caused by certain oncogenic viruses (discussed later), this is achieved through direct targeting of RB by viral proteins. For example, the human papillomavirus (HPV) E7 protein binds to the hypophosphorylated form of RB, preventing it from inhibiting the E2F transcription factors. Thus, RB is functionally deleted, leading to uncontrolled growth.

SUMMARY

RB: GOVERNOR OF THE CELL CYCLE

- Like other tumor suppressor genes, both copies of RB must be dysfunctional for tumor development to occur.
- In cases of familial retinoblastoma, one defective copy of the RB gene is present in the germ line, so that only one additional somatic mutation is needed to completely eliminate RB function.
- RB exerts anti-proliferative effects by controlling the G_1-to-S transition of the cell cycle. In its active form, RB is hypophosphorylated and binds to E2F transcription factors. This interaction prevents transcription of genes like cyclin E that are needed for DNA replication, and so the cells are arrested in G_1.
- Growth factor signaling leads to cyclin D expression, activation of cyclin D–CDK4/6 complexes, inactivation of RB by phosphorylation, and thus release of E2F.
- Loss of cell cycle control is fundamental to malignant transformation. Almost all cancers have a disabled G_1 checkpoint due to mutation of either RB or genes that affect RB function, such as cyclin D, CDK4, and CDKIs.
- Many oncogenic DNA viruses, like HPV, encode proteins (e.g., E7) that bind RB and render it nonfunctional.

TP53: Guardian of the Genome

The p53-encoding tumor suppressor gene, *TP53*, is the most commonly mutated gene in human cancer. The p53 protein is a transcription factor that thwarts neoplastic transformation by three interlocking mechanisms: activation of temporary cell cycle arrest (termed *quiescence*), induction of permanent cell cycle arrest (termed *senescence*), or triggering of programmed cell death (termed *apoptosis*). If RB is a "sensor" of external signals, p53 can be viewed as a central monitor of internal stress, directing the stressed cells toward one of these pathways.

A variety of stresses trigger the p53 response pathways, including anoxia, inappropriate pro-growth stimuli (e.g., unbridled MYC or RAS activity), and DNA damage. By managing the DNA damage response, p53 plays a central role in maintaining the integrity of the genome, as discussed next.

In nonstressed, healthy cells, p53 has a short half-life (20 minutes) because of its association with MDM2, a protein that targets p53 for destruction. When the cell is stressed, for example, by an assault on its DNA, "sensors" that include protein kinases such as ATM (ataxia telangiectasia mutated) are activated. These activated sensors catalyze posttranslational modifications in p53 that release it from

MDM2, increasing its half-life and enhancing its ability to drive the transcription of target genes. Hundreds of genes whose transcription is triggered by p53 have been found. These genes suppress neoplastic transformation by three mechanisms:

- *p53-mediated cell cycle arrest may be considered the primordial response to DNA damage* (Fig. 6.21). It occurs late in the G_1 phase and is caused mainly by p53-dependent transcription of the CDKI gene *CDKN1A (p21)*. The p21 protein inhibits cyclin–CDK complexes and prevents phosphorylation of RB, thereby arresting cells in the G_1 phase. Such a pause in cell cycling is welcome, because it gives the cells "breathing time" to repair DNA damage. The p53 protein also induces expression of DNA damage repair genes. If DNA damage is repaired successfully, p53 upregulates transcription of MDM2, leading to its own destruction and relief of the cell cycle block. If the damage cannot be repaired, the cell may enter p53-induced senescence or undergo p53-directed apoptosis.
- *p53-induced senescence is a form of permanent cell cycle arrest* characterized by specific changes in morphology and gene expression that differentiate it from quiescence or reversible cell cycle arrest. Senescence requires activation of p53 and/or Rb and expression of their mediators, such as the CDKIs. The mechanisms of senescence are unclear but seem to involve global chromatin changes, which drastically and permanently alter gene expression.
- *p53-induced apoptosis of cells with irreversible DNA damage is the ultimate protective mechanism against neoplastic transformation.* It is mediated by upregulation of several pro-apoptotic genes, including *BAX* and *PUMA* (discussed later).

To summarize, p53 is activated by stresses such as DNA damage and assists in DNA repair by causing G_1 arrest and inducing the expression of DNA repair genes. A cell with damaged DNA that cannot be repaired is directed by p53 to either enter senescence or undergo apoptosis (see Fig. 6.21). In view of these activities, p53 has been rightfully called the "guardian of the genome." With loss of normal p53 function, DNA damage goes unrepaired, mutations become fixed in dividing cells, and the cell turns onto a one-way street leading to malignant transformation.

Confirming the importance of *TP53* in controlling carcinogenesis, more than 70% of human cancers have a defect in this gene, and the remaining malignant neoplasms often have defects in genes upstream or downstream of *TP53*. Biallelic abnormalities of the *TP53* gene are found in virtually every type of cancer, including carcinomas of the lung, colon, and breast—the three leading causes of cancer deaths. In most cases, mutations affecting both *TP53* alleles are acquired in somatic cells. In other tumors, such as certain sarcomas, the *TP53* gene is intact but p53 function is lost because of amplification and overexpression of the *MDM2* gene, which encodes a potent inhibitor of p53. Less commonly, patients inherit a mutant *TP53* allele; the resulting disorder is called the *Li-Fraumeni syndrome*. As in the case with familial retinoblastoma, inheritance of one mutant *TP53* allele predisposes affected

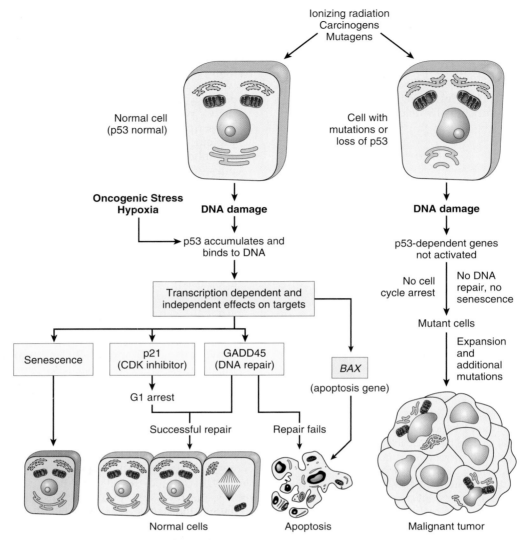

Fig. 6.21 The role of p53 in maintaining the integrity of the genome. Activation of normal p53 by DNA-damaging agents or by hypoxia leads to cell cycle arrest in G1 and induction of DNA repair, by transcriptional upregulation of the cyclin-dependent kinase inhibitor CDKN1A (p21) and the *GADD45* genes. Successful repair of DNA allows cells to proceed with the cell cycle; if DNA repair fails, p53 triggers either apoptosis or senescence. In cells with loss or mutations of TP53, DNA damage does not induce cell cycle arrest or DNA repair, and genetically damaged cells proliferate, giving rise eventually to malignant neoplasms.

individuals to develop malignant tumors because only one additional hit is needed to inactivate the second, normal allele. Patients with the Li-Fraumeni syndrome have a 25-fold greater chance of developing a malignant tumor by 50 years of age compared with the general population. In contrast to tumors developing in patients who inherit a mutant *RB* allele, the spectrum of tumors that develop in patients with the Li-Fraumeni syndrome is much more varied; the most common types are sarcomas, breast cancer, leukemia, brain tumors, and carcinomas of the adrenal cortex. Compared with individuals diagnosed with sporadic tumors, patients with Li-Fraumeni syndrome develop tumors at a younger age and may develop multiple primary tumors.

As with RB, normal p53 also can be rendered nonfunctional by certain oncogenic DNA viruses. Proteins encoded by oncogenic HPVs, certain polyoma viruses, and hepatitis

B virus bind to p53 and nullify its protective function. Thus, transforming DNA viruses subvert two of the best-understood tumor suppressors, RB and p53.

SUMMARY

TP53: GUARDIAN OF THE GENOME

- *TP53* encodes p53, the central monitor of stress in the cell, which can be activated by anoxia, inappropriate oncogene signaling, or DNA damage. Activated p53 controls the expression and activity of genes involved in cell cycle arrest, DNA repair, cellular senescence, and apoptosis.
- DNA damage leads to activation of p53 by phosphorylation. Activated p53 drives transcription of CDKN1A (p21), which prevents RB phosphorylation, thereby causing a G_1-S block in

the cell cycle. This pause allows the cells to repair DNA damage.
- If DNA damage cannot be repaired, p53 induces cellular senescence or apoptosis.
- Of human tumors, 70% demonstrate biallelic mutations in *TP53*. Patients with the rare Li-Fraumeni syndrome inherit one defective copy of *TP53* in the germ line, such that only one additional mutation is required to lose normal p53 function. Li-Fraumeni syndrome patients are prone to develop a wide variety of tumors.
- As with RB, p53 can be incapacitated when bound by proteins encoded by oncogenic DNA viruses such as HPV.

Transforming Growth Factor-β Pathway

Although much is known about the circuitry that applies brakes to the cell cycle, the molecules that transmit antiproliferative signals to cells are less well characterized. Best-known is TGF-β, a member of a family of dimeric growth factors that includes bone morphogenetic proteins and activins. In most normal epithelial, endothelial, and hematopoietic cells, TGF-β is a potent inhibitor of proliferation. It regulates cellular processes by binding to a complex composed of TGF-β receptors I and II. Dimerization of the receptor upon ligand binding leads to a cascade of events that result in the transcriptional activation of CDKIs with growth-suppressing activity, as well as repression of growth-promoting genes such as *MYC* and *CDK4*.

In many forms of cancer, the growth-inhibiting effects of the TGF-β pathways are impaired by mutations affecting TGF-β signaling. These mutations may alter the type II TGF-β receptor or SMAD molecules that serve to transduce anti-proliferative signals from the receptor to the nucleus. Mutations affecting the type II receptor are seen in cancers of the colon, stomach, and endometrium. Mutational inactivation of SMAD4, 1 of the 10 proteins known to be involved in TGF-β signaling, is common in pancreatic cancers. In other cancers, by contrast, loss of TGF-β–mediated growth control occurs at a level downstream of the core TGF-β signaling pathway; for example, there may be loss of p21 expression and/or overexpression of *MYC*. These tumor cells can then use other elements of the TGF-β–induced program, including immune system suppression or promotion of angiogenesis, to facilitate tumor progression. Thus, TGF-β can function to prevent or promote tumor growth, depending on the state of other genes in the cell. Indeed, in many late-stage tumors, TGF-β signaling activates epithelial-to-mesenchymal transition (EMT), a process that promotes migration, invasion, and metastasis, as discussed later.

Contact Inhibition, NF2, and APC

When cancer cells are grown in the laboratory, their proliferation fails to be inhibited when they come in contact with each other. This is in sharp contrast to nontransformed cells, which stop proliferating once they form confluent monolayers. The mechanisms that govern contact inhibition are only now being discovered.

Cell–cell contacts in many tissues are mediated by homodimeric interactions between transmembrane proteins called *cadherins*. E-cadherin (E for *epithelial*) mediates cell–cell contact in epithelial layers. Two mechanisms have been proposed to explain how E-cadherin maintains contact inhibition:
- One mechanism is mediated by the tumor suppressor gene *NF2*. Its product, neurofibromin-2, more commonly called *merlin,* acts downstream of E-cadherin in a signling pathway that helps fo maintain contact inhibition. Homozygous loss of *NF2* is known to cause certain neural tumors, and germ line mutations in *NF2* are associated with a tumor-prone hereditary condition called *neurofibromatosis type 2.*
- A second mechanism by which E-cadherin may regulate contact inhibition involves its ability to bind β-catenin, another signaling protein. β-catenin is a key component of the WNT signaling pathway (described below), which has broad but as of yet incompletely understood roles in regulating the morphology and organization of epithelial cells lining structures such as the gut.

A further clue to the important of E-cadherin and β-catenin in epithelial cancers is illustrated by the rare hereditary disease *adenomatous polyposis coli* (APC). This disorder is characterized by the development of numerous adenomatous polyps in the colon that have a very high incidence of transformation into colonic cancers. The polyps consistently show loss of a tumor suppressor gene called *APC* (named for the disease), which exerts anti-proliferative effects in an unusual manner. *APC* encodes a cytoplasmic protein whose dominant function is to promote the degradation of β-catenin, which has several functions. In addition to binding E-cadherin, β-catenin also is a key component of the WNT signaling pathway (illustrated in Fig. 6.22). WNTs are soluble factors that bind WNT receptors, which in turn transmit signals that prevent the APC-mediated degradation of β-catenin, allowing it to translocate to the nucleus, where it acts as a transcriptional activator. In quiescent cells that have not been exposed to WNT, cytoplasmic β-catenin is degraded by a *destruction complex*, of which APC is an integral part. With loss of APC (e.g., in colon cancers), β-catenin degradation is prevented, and the WNT signaling response is inappropriately activated even in the absence of WNT factors. In colonic epithelium this leads to increased transcription of growth-promoting genes, such as cyclin D1 and *MYC*, as well as transcriptional regulators, such as TWIST and SLUG, which repress E-cadherin expression and thus reduce contact inhibition.

APC behaves as a typical tumor suppressor gene. Individuals born with one mutated allele typically are found to have hundreds to thousands of adenomatous polyps in the colon by their teens or twenties; these polyps show loss of the other *APC* allele. Almost invariably, one or more polyps undergo malignant transformation, as discussed later. *APC* mutations are seen in 70% to 80% of sporadic colon cancers. Colonic cancers with normal *APC* genes sometimes show activating mutations of β-catenin that render them refractory to the degrading action of APC.

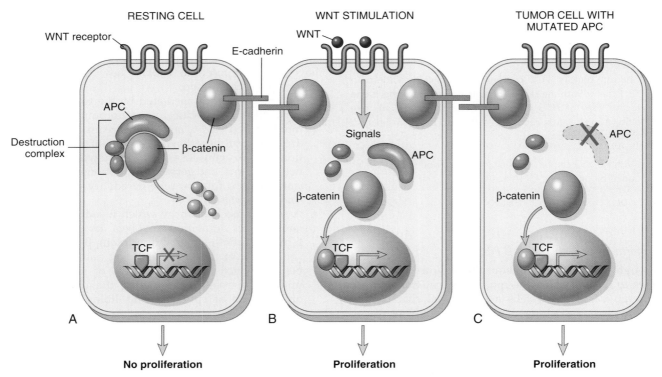

Fig. 6.22 The role of APC in regulating the stability and function of β-catenin. APC and β-catenin are components of the WNT signaling pathway. (A) In resting cells (not exposed to WNT), β-catenin forms a macromolecular complex containing the APC protein. This complex leads to the destruction of β-catenin, and intracellular levels of β-catenin are low. (B) When cells are stimulated by secreted WNT molecules, the destruction complex is deactivated, β-catenin degradation does not occur, and cytoplasmic levels increase. β-Catenin translocates to the nucleus, where it binds to TCF, a transcription factor that activates several genes involved in the cell cycle. (C) When APC is mutated or absent, the destruction of β-catenin cannot occur. β-Catenin translocates to the nucleus and coactivates genes that promote the cell cycle, and cells behave as if they are under constant stimulation by the WNT pathway.

SUMMARY

TGF-β, CONTACT INHIBITION, AND APC-β-CATENIN PATHWAYS

- TGF-β inhibits proliferation of many cell types by activation of growth-inhibiting genes such as *CDKIs* and suppression of growth-promoting genes such as *MYC* and those encoding cyclins.
- TGF-β function is compromised in many tumors by mutations in its receptors (colon, stomach, endometrium) or by mutational inactivation of *SMAD* genes that transduce TGF-β signaling (pancreas).
- E-cadherin maintains contact inhibition, which is lost in malignant cells.
- The *APC* gene exerts anti-proliferative actions by regulating the destruction of the cytoplasmic protein β-catenin. With a loss of APC, β-catenin is not destroyed, and it translocates to the nucleus, where it acts as a growth-promoting transcription factor.
- In familial adenomatous polyposis syndrome, inheritance of a germ line mutation in the *APC* gene and sporadic loss of the sole normal allele causes the development of hundreds of colonic polyps at a young age. Inevitably, one or more of these polyps evolves into a colonic cancer. Somatic loss of both alleles of the *APC* gene is seen in approximately 70% of sporadic colon cancers.

Altered Cellular Metabolism

Even in the presence of ample oxygen, cancer cells demonstrate a distinctive form of cellular metabolism characterized by high levels of glucose uptake and increased conversion of glucose to lactose (fermentation) via the glycolytic pathway. This phenomenon, called the *Warburg effect* and also known as *aerobic glycolysis,* has been recognized for many years (indeed, Otto Warburg received the Nobel Prize in 1931 for its discovery). Clinically, the "glucose-hunger" of tumors is used to visualize tumors via positron emission tomography (PET) scanning, in which patients are injected with ^{18}F-fluorodeoxyglucose, a glucose derivative that is preferentially taken up into tumor cells (as well as normal, actively dividing tissues such as the bone marrow). Most tumors are PET-positive, and rapidly growing ones are markedly so.

Warburg's discovery was largely neglected for many years, but over the past decade, metabolism has become one of the most active areas of cancer research. Metabolic pathways (like signaling pathways) in normal and cancer cells are still being elucidated, and the details are complex, but at the heart of the Warburg effect lies a simple question: why is it advantageous for a cancer cell to rely on seemingly inefficient glycolysis (which generates two molecules of ATP per molecule of glucose) instead of oxidative phosphorylation (which generates up to 36 molecules of ATP per molecule of glucose)? While pondering this question, it is important to recognize that rapidly proliferating normal cells, such as in embryonic tissues and lymphocytes during immune responses, also rely on aerobic fermentation. Thus, "Warburg metabolism" is not cancer specific, but instead is a general property of growing cells that becomes "fixed" in cancer cells.

The answer to this riddle is simple: **Aerobic glycolysis provides rapidly dividing tumor cells with metabolic intermediates that are needed for the synthesis of cellular components, whereas mitochondrial oxidative phosphorylation does not.** The reason growing cells rely on aerobic glycolysis becomes readily apparent when one considers that a growing cell has a strict biosynthetic requirement; it must duplicate all of its cellular components—DNA, RNA, proteins, lipid, and organelles—before it can divide and produce two daughter cells. While oxidative phosphorylation yields abundant ATP, it fails to produce any carbon moieties that can be used to build the cellular components needed for growth (proteins, lipids, and nucleic acids). Even cells that are not actively growing must shunt some metabolic intermediates away from oxidative phosphorylation in order to synthesize macromolecules that are needed for cellular maintenance.

By contrast, in actively growing cells only a small fraction of the cellular glucose is shunted through the oxidative phosphorylation pathway, such that on average each molecule of glucose metabolized produces approximately four molecules of ATP. Presumably, this balance (heavily biased toward aerobic fermentation, with a bit of oxidative phosphorylation) hits a metabolic "sweet spot" that is optimal for growth. It follows that growing cells do rely on mitochondrial metabolism. However, a major function of mitochondria in growing cells is not to generate ATP, but rather to carry out reactions that generate metabolic intermediates that can be shunted off and used as precursors in the synthesis of cellular building blocks. For example, lipid biosynthesis requires acetyl-CoA, and acetyl-CoA is largely synthesized in growing cells from intermediates such as citrate that are generated in mitochondria.

So how is this profound reprogramming of metabolism, the Warburg effect, triggered in growing normal and malignant cells? As might be guessed, **metabolic reprogramming is produced by signaling cascades downstream of growth factor receptors, the very same pathways that are deregulated by mutations in oncogenes and tumors suppressor genes in cancers.** Thus, whereas in rapidly dividing normal cells aerobic glycolysis ceases when the tissue is no longer growing, in cancer cells this reprogramming persists due to the action of oncogenes and the loss of tumor suppressor gene function. Some of the important points of cross-talk between pro–growth signaling factors and cellular metabolism are shown in Fig. 6.23 and include the following:

- *Growth factor receptor signaling.* In addition to transmitting growth signals to the nucleus, signals from growth factor receptors also influence metabolism by

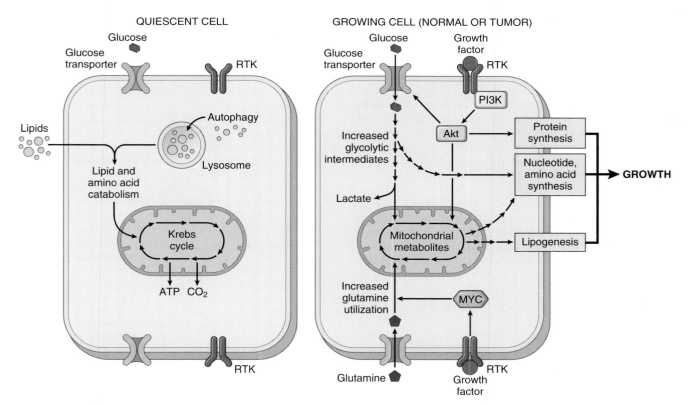

Fig. 6.23 Metabolism and cell growth. Quiescent cells rely mainly on the Krebs cycle for ATP production; if starved, autophagy (self-eating) is induced to provide a source of fuel. When stimulated by growth factors, normal cells markedly upregulate glucose and glutamine uptake, which provide carbon sources for synthesis of nucleotides, proteins, and lipids. In cancers, oncogenic mutations involving growth factor signaling pathways and other key factors such as MYC deregulate these metabolic pathways, an alteration known as the *Warburg effect.*

upregulating glucose uptake and inhibiting the activity of pyruvate kinase, which catalyzes the last step in the glycolytic pathway, the conversion of phosphoenolpyruvate to pyruvate. This creates a damming effect that leads to the buildup of upstream glycolytic intermediates, which are siphoned off for synthesis of DNA, RNA, and protein.

- *RAS signaling.* Signals downstream of RAS upregulate the activity of glucose transporters and multiple glycolytic enzymes, thus increasing glycolysis; promote shunting of mitochondrial intermediates to pathways leading to lipid biosynthesis; and stimulate factors that are required for protein synthesis.
- *MYC.* As mentioned earlier, pro-growth pathways upregulate expression of the transcription factor MYC, which drives changes in gene expression that support anabolic metabolism and cell growth. Among the MYC-regulated genes are those for several glycolytic enzymes and glutaminase, which is required for mitochondrial utilization of glutamine, a key source of carbon moieties needed for biosynthesis of cellular building blocks.

The flipside of the coin is that tumor suppressors often inhibit metabolic pathways that support growth. We have already discussed the "braking" effect of the tumor suppressors NF1 and PTEN on signals downstream of growth factor receptors and RAS, allowing them to oppose the Warburg effect. Indeed, it may be that many (and perhaps all) tumor suppressors that induce growth arrest suppress the Warburg effect. For example, p53, arguably the most important tumor suppressor, upregulates target genes that collectively inhibit glucose uptake, glycolysis, lipogenesis, and the generation of NADPH (a key cofactor needed for the biosynthesis of macromolecules). Thus, it is increasingly clear that the functions of many oncoproteins and tumor suppressors are inextricably intertwined with cellular metabolism.

Beyond the Warburg effect, there are two other links between metabolism and cancer that are of sufficient importance to merit brief mention, autophagy and an unusual set of oncogenic mutations that lead to the creation of *oncometabolites,* small molecules that appear to directly contribute to the transformed state.

Autophagy

Autophagy is a state of severe nutrient deficiency in which cells not only arrest their growth, but also cannibalize their own organelles, proteins, and membranes as carbon sources for energy production (Chapter 2). If this adaptation fails, the cells die. Tumor cells often seem to be able to grow under marginal environmental conditions without triggering autophagy, suggesting that the pathways that induce autophagy are deranged. In keeping with this, several genes that promote autophagy are tumor suppressors. Whether autophagy is always bad from the vantage point of the tumor, however, remains a matter of active investigation and debate. For example, under conditions of severe nutrient deprivation, tumor cells may use autophagy to become "dormant," a state of metabolic hibernation that allows cells to survive hard times for long periods. Such cells are believed to be resistant to therapies that kill actively dividing cells, and could therefore be

responsible for therapeutic failures. Thus, autophagy may be a tumor's friend or foe depending on how the signaling pathways that regulate it are "wired" in a given tumor.

Oncometabolism

Another surprising group of genetic alterations discovered through tumor genome sequencing studies are mutations in enzymes that participate in the Krebs cycle. Of these, mutations in isocitrate dehydrogenase (IDH) have garnered the most interest, as they have revealed a new mechanism of oncogenesis termed *oncometabolism* (Fig. 6.24).

The proposed steps in the oncogenic pathway involving IDH are as follows:

- IDH acquires a mutation that leads to a specific amino acid substitution involving residues in the active site of the enzyme. As a result, the mutated protein loses it ability to function as an isocitrate dehydrogenase and instead acquires a new enzymatic activity that catalyzes the production of 2-hydroxglutarate (2-HG).
- 2-HG in turn acts as an inhibitor of several other enzymes that are members of the TET family, including TET2.
- TET2 is one of several factors that regulate DNA methylation, which you will recall is an epigenetic modification that controls normal gene expression and often goes awry in cancer. According to the model, loss of TET2 activity leads to abnormal patterns of DNA methylation.
- Abnormal DNA methylation in turn leads to misexpression of currently unknown cancer genes, which drive cellular transformation and oncogenesis.

Thus, according to this scenario, mutated IDH acts as an oncoprotein by producing 2-HG, which is considered a prototypical *oncometabolite.* Oncogenic IDH mutations

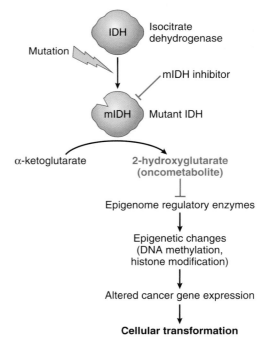

Fig. 6.24 Proposed action of the oncometabolite 2-hydroxyglutarate (2-HG) in cancer cells with mutated isocitrate dehydrogenase (mIDH).

have now been described in a diverse collection of cancers, including a sizable fraction of cholangiocarcinomas, gliomas, acute myeloid leukemias, and sarcomas. Of clinical significance, because the mutated IDH proteins have an altered structure, it has been possible to develop drugs that inhibit mutated IDH and not the normal IDH enzyme. These drugs are now being tested in cancer patients and have produced encouraging therapeutic responses. This developing story is a remarkable example of how detailed understanding of oncogenic mechanisms can yield entirely new kinds of anti-cancer drugs.

SUMMARY

ALTERED CELLULAR METABOLISM

- Warburg metabolism is a form of pro-growth metabolism favoring glycolysis over oxidative phosphorylation. It is induced in normal cells by exposure to growth factors and becomes fixed in cancer cells due to the action of certain driver mutations.
- Many oncoproteins (RAS, MYC, mutated growth factor receptors) induce or contribute to Warburg metabolism, and many tumor suppressors (PTEN, NF1, p53) oppose it.
- Stress may induce cells to consume their components in a process called *autophagy*. Cancer cells may accumulate mutations to avoid autophagy, or may corrupt the process to provide nutrients for continued growth and survival.
- Some oncoproteins such as mutated IDH act by causing the formation of high levels of "oncometabolites" that alter the epigenome, thereby leading to changes in gene expression that are oncogenic.

Evasion of Cell Death

Tumor cells frequently contain mutations in genes that regulate apoptosis, making the cells resistant to cell death. As discussed in Chapter 2, apoptosis, or regulated cell death, refers to an orderly dismantling of cells into component pieces, which are then efficiently consumed by neighboring cells and professional phagocytes without stimulating inflammation. You will recall that there are two pathways that lead to apoptosis: the extrinsic pathway, triggered by the death receptors FAS and FAS-ligand; and the intrinsic pathway (also known as the *mitochondrial pathway*), initiated by perturbations such as loss of growth factors and DNA damage. Cancer cells are subject to a number of intrinsic stresses that can initiate apoptosis, particularly DNA damage, but also metabolic disturbances stemming from dysregulated growth as well as hypoxia caused by insufficient blood supply. These stresses are enhanced manyfold when tumors are treated with chemotherapy or radiation therapy, which kill tumor cells by activating the intrinsic pathway of apoptosis. Thus, there is strong selective pressure, both before and during therapy, for cancer cells to develop resistance to intrinsic stresses that may induce apoptosis. Accordingly, **evasion of apoptosis by cancer cells occurs mainly by way of acquired mutations and changes in gene expression that disable**

key components of the intrinsic pathway, or that reset the balance of regulatory factors so as to favor cell survival in the face of intrinsic stresses (Figure 6.25).

Before delving into modes of resistance to apoptosis, a brief review of the intrinsic pathway is in order. Activation of this pathway leads to permeabilization of the mitochondrial outer membrane and release of molecules, such as cytochrome c, that initiate apoptosis. The integrity of the mitochondrial outer membrane is determined by a delicate balancing act between pro-apoptotic and anti-apoptotic members of the BCL2 protein family. The pro-apoptotic proteins BAX and BAK are required for apoptosis and directly promote mitochondrial permeabilization. Their action is inhibited by the anti-apoptotic members of this family, which are exemplified by BCL2, BCL-XL, and MCL1. A third set of proteins, the so-called "BH3-only proteins," which include BAD, BID, and PUMA, shift the balance between the pro-apoptotic and anti-apoptotic family members by neutralizing the actions of anti-apoptotic proteins like BCL2 and BCL-XL, thereby promoting apoptosis. When the sum total of all the BH3-only proteins "overwhelms" the protective BCL2/BCL-XL factors, BAX and BAK are activated and form pores in the mitochondrial membrane. These allow mitochondrial cytochrome c to

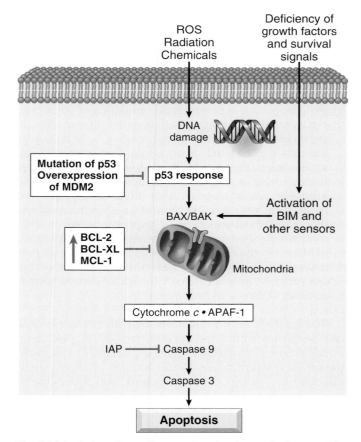

Fig. 6.25 Intrinsic pathway of apoptosis and major mechanisms used by tumor cells to evade cell death. (1) Loss of p53, either through mutation or through antagonism by MDM2. (2) Reduced egress of cytochrome c from mitochondria as a result of upregulation of anti-apoptotic factors such as BCL2, BCL-XL, and MCL-1. IAP, Inhibitor of apoptosis.

leak out into the cytosol, where it binds to APAF-1 and activates caspase-9, which in turn cleaves and activates executioner caspases such as caspase-3. Another group of factors that function as negative regulators of the intrinsic pathway is known as *inhibitor of apoptosis proteins (IAPs)*, which bind caspase-9 and prevent apoptosis.

Within this framework, it is possible to illustrate the major mechanisms by which apoptosis is evaded by cancer cells (Figure 6.25). These mainly involve loss of p53, the key component of early steps in the intrinsic pathway, and increased expression of anti-apoptotic members of the BCL2 family.

- *Loss of TP53 function.* As already discussed, *TP53* is commonly mutated in cancers at diagnosis, and the frequency of *TP53* mutations is even higher in tumors that relapse after therapy. In addition to mutation of *TP53*, other lesions in cancers impair p53 function indirectly, most notably amplification of *MDM2*, which encodes an inhibitor of p53. Loss of p53 function prevents the upregulation of PUMA, a pro-apoptotic BH3-only member of the BCL2 family that is a direct target of p53. As a result, cells survive levels of DNA damage and cell stress that otherwise would result in their death.

- *Overexpression of anti-apoptotic members of the BCL2 family.* Overexpression of BCL2 is a common event leading to the protection of tumor cells from apoptosis and occurs through several mechanisms. One of the best understood examples is found follicular lymphoma (Chapter 12), a B-cell tumor carrying a characteristic (14;18) (q32;q21) translocation that fuses the *BCL2* (located at 18q21) to the transcriptionally active immunoglobulin heavy chain gene (located at 14q32). The resulting overabundance of BCL2 protects lymphocytes from apoptosis and allows them to survive for abnormally long periods, producing a steady accumulation of B lymphocytes that results in lymphadenopathy. Because BCL2-overexpressing follicular lymphomas arise in large part through reduced cell death rather than explosive cell proliferation, they tend to be indolent (slow-growing). In other tumors such as chronic lymphocytic leukemia (Chapter 12), it appears that BCL2 is upregulated because of loss of expression of specific micro-RNAs that normally dampen BCL2 expression. Many other mechanisms leading to overexpression of anti-apoptotic members of the BCL2 family have been described, particularly in the setting of resistance to chemotherapy. For example, amplification of the *MCL1* gene is seen in a subset of lung and breast cancers.

Recognition of the mechanisms by which cancers evade cell death has stimulated several lines of targeted drug development. Restoration of p53 function in *TP53*-mutated tumors is a daunting problem (because of the inherent difficulty of "fixing" defective genes), but is possible in tumors in which p53 is inactive because of overexpression of its inhibitor, MDM2. Indeed, inhibitors of MDM2 that reactivate p53 and induce apoptosis in tumors with *MDM2* gene amplification, such as certain types of sarcoma, are being tested in clinical trials. Even more promising results are being generated with drugs that mimic the activities of BH3-only proteins and inhibit the function of anti-apoptotic members of the BCL2 family, particularly BCL2

itself. These drugs have potent activity against tumors characterized by BCL2 overexpression (such as chronic lymphocytic leukemia) and are likely to become a standard part of cancer treatment over the course of the next few years.

SUMMARY

EVASION OF APOPTOSIS

- Evasion of cell death by cancers mainly involves acquired abnormalities that interfere with the intrinsic (mitochondrial) pathway of apoptosis.
- The most common abnormalities involve loss of p53 function, either by way of *TP53* mutations or overexpression of the p53 inhibitor MDM2.
- Other cancers evade cell death by overexpressing anti-apoptotic members of the BCL2 family, such as BCL2, BCL-XL, and MCL1, which protect cells from the action of BAX and BAK, the pro-apoptotic members of the BCL2 family.
- In a large majority of follicular B-cell lymphomas, BCL2 levels are high because of a (14;18) translocation that fuses the *BCL2* gene with regulatory elements of the immunoglobulin heavy chain gene.
- Inhibitors of MDM2 (which activate p53) and inhibitors of BCL2 family members induce the death of cancer cells by stimulating the intrinsic pathway of apoptosis and are being developed as therapeutic agents.

Limitless Replicative Potential (Immortality)

Tumor cells, unlike normal cells, are capable of limitless replication. As discussed previously in the context of cellular aging (Chapter 2), most normal human cells have a capacity of at most 70 doublings. Thereafter, the cells lose the ability to divide and enter replicative senescence. This phenomenon has been ascribed to progressive shortening of telomeres at the ends of chromosomes.

Markedly eroded telomeres are recognized by the DNA repair machinery as double-stranded DNA breaks, leading to cell cycle arrest and senescence, mediated by *TP53* and *RB*. In cells in which *TP53* or *RB* mutations are disabled by mutations, the nonhomologous end-joining pathway is activated in a last-ditch effort to save the cell, joining the shortened ends of two chromosomes.

Such an inappropriately activated repair system results in dicentric chromosomes that are pulled apart at anaphase, resulting in new double-stranded DNA breaks. The resulting genomic instability from the repeated bridge–fusion–breakage cycles eventually produces mitotic catastrophe, characterized by massive apoptosis.

It follows that for tumors to acquire the ability to grow indefinitely, loss of growth restraints is not enough; both cellular senescence and mitotic catastrophe must also be avoided (Fig. 6.26). If during crisis a cell manages to reactivate telomerase, the bridge–fusion–breakage cycles cease, and the cell is able to avoid death. However, during this period of genomic instability that precedes telomerase activation, numerous mutations could accumulate, helping the

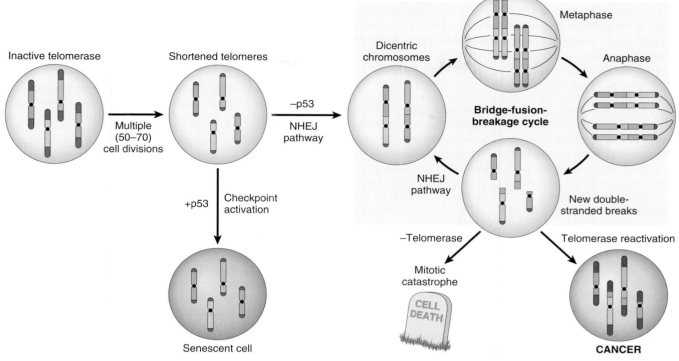

Fig. 6.26 Escape of cells from replicative senescence and mitotic catastrophe caused by telomere shortening.

cell march toward malignancy. Telomerase, active in normal stem cells, is absent from or present at very low levels in most somatic cells. By contrast, telomere maintenance is seen in virtually all types of cancers. In 85% to 95% of cancers, this is due to upregulation of the enzyme telomerase. A few tumors use other mechanisms, termed *alternative lengthening of telomeres,* which depend on DNA recombination.

Of interest, in a study of the progression from colonic adenoma to colonic adenocarcinoma, early lesions had a high degree of genomic instability with low telomerase expression, whereas malignant lesions had complex karyotypes with high levels of telomerase activity, consistent with a model of telomere-driven tumorigenesis in human cancer. Thus, it appears that unregulated proliferation in incipient tumors leads to telomere shortening, followed by chromosomal instability and the accumulation of mutations. If telomerase is then reactivated in these cells, telomeres are extended and these mutations become fixed, contributing to tumor growth.

SUMMARY

LIMITLESS REPLICATIVE POTENTIAL (IMMORTALITY)

- In normal cells, which lack expression of telomerase, the shortened telomeres generated by cell division eventually activate cell cycle checkpoints, leading to senescence and placing a limit on the number of divisions a cell may undergo.
- In cells that have disabled checkpoints, DNA repair pathways are inappropriately activated by shortened telomeres, leading to massive chromosomal instability and mitotic crisis.
- Tumor cells reactivate telomerase, thus staving off mitotic catastrophe and achieving immortality.

Sustained Angiogenesis

Even if a solid tumor possesses all of the genetic aberrations that are required for malignant transformation, it cannot enlarge beyond 1 to 2 mm in diameter unless it has the capacity to induce angiogenesis. Like normal tissues, tumors require delivery of oxygen and nutrients and removal of waste products; presumably the 1- to 2-mm zone represents the maximal distance across which oxygen, nutrients, and waste can diffuse to and from blood vessels. Growing cancers stimulate neoangiogenesis, during which vessels sprout from previously existing capillaries. Neovascularization has a dual effect on tumor growth: perfusion supplies needed nutrients and oxygen, and newly formed endothelial cells stimulate the growth of adjacent tumor cells by secreting growth factors, such as insulin-like growth factors (IGFs) and PDGF. While the resulting tumor vasculature is effective at delivering nutrients and removing wastes, it is not entirely normal; the vessels are leaky and dilated, and have a haphazard pattern of connection, features that can be appreciated on angiograms. By permitting tumor cells access to these abnormal vessels, angiogenesis also contributes to metastasis. Angiogenesis is thus an essential facet of malignancy.

How do growing tumors develop a blood supply? The current paradigm is that **angiogenesis is controlled by a balance between angiogenesis promoters and inhibitors; in angiogenic tumors this balance is skewed in favor of promoters.** Early in their development, most human tumors do not induce angiogenesis. Starved of nutrients, these tumors remain small or in situ, possibly for years, until an *angiogenic switch* terminates this stage of vascular quiescence. The molecular basis of the angiogenic switch involves increased production of angiogenic factors and/or loss of angiogenic inhibitors. These factors may be produced by the tumor cells themselves or by inflammatory cells (e.g., macrophages) or resident stromal cells (e.g., tumor-associated fibroblasts). Proteases, either elaborated by the tumor cells or by stromal cells in response to the tumor, are also involved in regulating the balance between angiogenic and anti-angiogenic factors. Many proteases can release proangiogenic basic fibroblast growth factors (bFGF) that are stored in the ECM; conversely, the angiogenesis inhibitors angiostatin and endostatin are produced by proteolytic cleavage of plasminogen and collagen, respectively.

The local balance of angiogenic and anti-angiogenic factors is influenced by several factors:

- Relative lack of oxygen due to hypoxia stabilizes HIF1α, an oxygen-sensitive transcription factor mentioned earlier, which then activates the transcription of proangiogenic cytokines such as VEGF. These factors create an angiogenic gradient that stimulates the proliferation of endothelial cells and guides the growth of new vessels toward the tumor.

- Mutations involving tumor suppressors and oncogenes in cancers also tilt the balance in favor of angiogenesis. For example, p53 stimulates expression of antiangiogenic molecules, such as thrombospondin-1, and represses expression of proangiogenic molecules, such as VEGF. Thus, loss of p53 in tumor cells provides a more permissive environment for angiogenesis.

- The transcription of VEGF also is influenced by signals from the RAS-MAP kinase pathway, and gain-of-function mutations in *RAS* or *MYC* upregulate the production of VEGF. Notably, elevated levels of VEGF can be detected in the serum and urine of a significant fraction of cancer patients.

The idea that angiogenesis is essential if solid tumors are to grow to clinically significant sizes has provided a powerful impetus for the development of therapeutic agents that block angiogenesis. These agents are now a part of the armamentarium that oncologists use against cancers; a cardinal example is bevacizumab, a monoclonal antibody that neutralizes VEGF activity and is approved for use in the treatment of multiple cancers. However, angiogenesis inhibitors have not been nearly as effective as was originally hoped; they can prolong life, but usually for only a few months and at high financial cost. The mechanisms that underlie the persistence and ultimate progression of cancers in the face of therapy with angiogenesis inhibitors are not yet clear. The modest benefit of anti-angiogenic therapy highlights the pernicious nature of advanced cancers, which can even elude therapies directed at stromal support cells such as endothelium.

Improvements are only possible with greater understanding of the "escape routes" through which tumor cells sidestep the effects of the angiogenesis inhibitors that are now in use.

SUMMARY

SUSTAINED ANGIOGENESIS

- Vascularization of tumors is essential for their growth and is controlled by the balance between angiogenic and anti-angiogenic factors that are produced by tumor and stromal cells.
- Hypoxia triggers angiogenesis through the actions of HIF-1α on the transcription of the proangiogenic factor VEGF.
- Many other factors regulate angiogenesis; for example, p53 induces synthesis of the angiogenesis inhibitor thrombospondin-1, while RAS, MYC, and MAPK signaling all upregulate VEGF expression and stimulate angiogenesis.
- VEGF inhibitors are used to treat a number of advanced cancers and prolong the clinical course, but are not curative.

Invasion and Metastasis

Invasion, and metastasis, the major causes of cancer-related morbidity and mortality, result from complex interactions involving cancer cells, stromal cells, and the extracellular matrix (ECM). These interactions can be broken down into a series of steps consisting of local invasion, intravasation into blood and lymph vessels, transit through the vasculature, extravasation from the vessels, formation of micrometastases, and growth of micrometastases into macroscopic tumors (Fig. 6.27). Predictably, this sequence of steps may be interrupted at any stage by either host-related or tumor-related factors. For the purpose of discussion, the metastatic cascade can be subdivided into two phases: (1) invasion of ECM and (2) vascular dissemination and homing of tumor cells.

Invasion of Extracellular Matrix

Human tissues are organized into a series of compartments separated from each other by two types of ECM: basement membranes and interstitial connective tissue (Chapter 1). Although organized differently, each type of ECM is composed of collagens, glycoproteins, and proteoglycans. Tumor cells must interact with the ECM at several stages in the metastatic cascade (see Fig. 6.27). A carcinoma first must breach the underlying basement membrane, then traverse the interstitial connective tissue, and ultimately gain access to the circulation by penetrating the vascular basement membrane. This process is repeated in reverse when tumor cell emboli extravasate at a distant site. Invasion of the ECM initiates the metastatic cascade and is an active process that can be resolved into several sequential steps (Fig. 6.28):

- *Loosening of intercellular connections between tumor cells.* As mentioned earlier, E-cadherins act as intercellular glues, and their cytoplasmic portions bind to β-catenin (see Fig. 6.22). Adjacent E-cadherin molecules keep the cells together; in addition, as discussed earlier, E-cadherin can transmit anti-growth signals by sequestering β-catenin. E-cadherin function is lost in almost all

plasminogen activator, have been implicated in tumor cell invasion. MMPs regulate tumor invasion not only by remodeling insoluble components of the basement membrane and interstitial matrix but also by releasing ECM-sequestered growth factors, which have chemotactic, angiogenic, and growth-promoting effects. For example, MMP-9 is a gelatinase that cleaves type IV

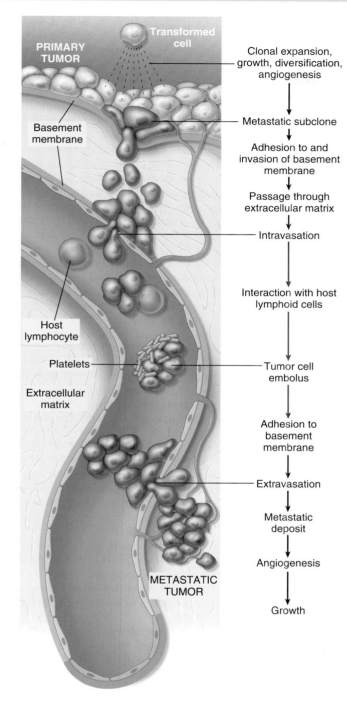

Fig. 6.27 The metastatic cascade: The sequential steps involved in the hematogenous spread of a tumor.

epithelial cancers, either by mutational inactivation of E-cadherin genes, activation of β-catenin genes, or inappropriate expression of the SNAIL and TWIST transcription factors, which suppress E-cadherin expression.

- *Local degradation of the basement membrane and interstitial connective tissue.* Tumor cells may either secrete proteolytic enzymes themselves or induce stromal cells (e.g., fibroblasts and inflammatory cells) to elaborate proteases. Multiple different proteases, such as matrix metalloproteinases (MMPs), cathepsin D, and urokinase

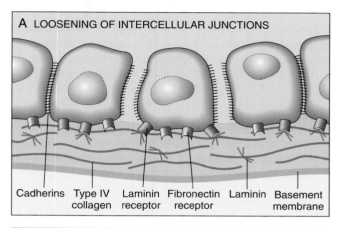

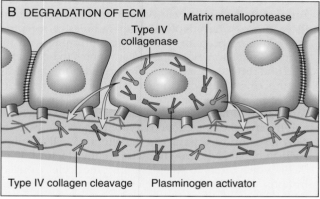

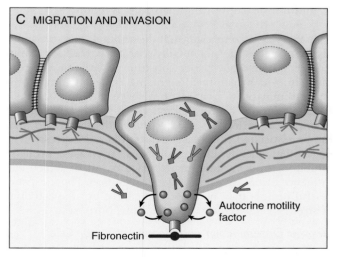

Fig. 6.28 Sequence of events in the invasion of epithelial basement membranes by tumor cells. Tumor cells detach from each other because of reduced adhesiveness and attract inflammatory cells. Proteases secreted from tumor cells and inflammatory cells degrade the basement membrane. Binding of tumor cells to proteolytically generated binding sites and tumor cell migration follow.

collagen of the epithelial and vascular basement membrane and also stimulates release of VEGF from ECM-sequestered pools. Benign tumors of the breast, colon, and stomach show little type IV collagenase activity, whereas their malignant counterparts overexpress this enzyme. Concurrently, the levels of metalloproteinase inhibitors are reduced so that the balance is tilted greatly toward tissue degradation. Indeed, overexpression of MMPs and other proteases has been reported for many malignant tumors.

- *Changes in attachment of tumor cells to ECM proteins.* Normal epithelial cells have receptors, such as integrins, for basement membrane laminin and collagens that are polarized at their basal surface; these receptors help to maintain the cells in a resting, differentiated state. Loss of adhesion in normal cells leads to induction of apoptosis, while, not surprisingly, tumor cells are resistant to this form of cell death. Additionally, the matrix itself is modified in ways that promote invasion and metastasis. For example, cleavage of the basement membrane proteins, collagen IV, and laminin by MMP-2 or MMP-9 generates novel sites that bind to receptors on tumor cells and stimulate migration.
- *Locomotion* is the final step of invasion, propelling tumor cells through the degraded basement membranes and zones of matrix proteolysis. Migration is a complex, multistep process that involves many families of receptors and signaling proteins that eventually impinge on the actin cytoskeleton. Such movement seems to be potentiated and directed by tumor cell–derived cytokines, such as autocrine motility factors. In addition, cleavage products of matrix components (e.g., collagen, laminin) and some growth factors (e.g., insulin-like growth factors I and II) have chemotactic activity for tumor cells. Stromal cells also produce paracrine effectors of cell motility, such as hepatocyte growth factor/scatter factor (HGF/SCF), which binds to receptors on tumor cells. Concentrations of HGF/SCF are elevated at the advancing edges of the highly invasive brain tumor glioblastoma multiforme, supporting their role in motility.

It also has become clear that the stromal cells surrounding tumor cells are not merely a static barrier for tumor cells to traverse but rather constitute a variable environment in which reciprocal signaling between tumor cells and stromal cells such as fibroblasts and immune cells enable multiple cancer hallmarks (discussed later). For example, a variety of studies have demonstrated that tumor-associated fibroblasts exhibit altered expression of genes that encode ECM molecules, proteases, protease inhibitors, and various growth factors, all of which can influence tumor invasion and extravasation. The most successful tumors may be those that can co-opt the activities of stromal cells to their own nefarious purposes.

Vascular Dissemination and Homing of Tumor Cells

Because of their invasive properties, tumor cells frequently escape their sites of origin and enter the circulation. It is now recognized from studies of "liquid biopsies," blood samples taken from patients with solid tumors, that millions of tumor cells are shed daily from even small cancers; hence both tumor cells and tumor-derived DNA can be detected in circulation. Most of these tumor cells circulate as single cells, while others form emboli by aggregating and adhering to circulating blood elements, particularly platelets.

Given the ease with which tumor cells access the circulation, it is apparent that the ability of cancers cells to leave the circulation, invade, and grow to clinically significant sizes at other sites in the body is (fortunately for the patient) highly inefficient.

Several factors seem to limit the metastatic potential of circulating tumor cells. While in the circulation, tumor cells are vulnerable to destruction by host immune cells (discussed later), and the process of adhesion to normal vascular beds and invasion of normal distant tissues may be much more difficult than the escape of tumor cells from the cancer. Even following extravasation, tumor cells that have been selected for growth in the originating tissue may find it difficult to grow in a second site due to lack of critical stromal support or because of recognition and suppression by resident immune cells. Indeed, the concept of tumor dormancy, referring to the prolonged survival of micrometastases without progression, is well described in melanoma and in breast and prostate carcinoma. Dormancy of tumor cells at distant sites may well be the last defense against clinically significant metastatic disease.

Despite these limiting factors, if neglected, virtually all malignant tumors will eventually produce macroscopic metastases. **The site at which metastases appear is related to two factors: the anatomic location and vascular drainage of the primary tumor, and the tropism of particular tumors for specific tissues.** As mentioned earlier, most metastases occur in the first capillary bed available to the tumor, hence the frequency of metastases to liver and lung. Many observations, however, suggest that natural pathways of drainage do not wholly explain the distribution of metastases. For example, prostatic carcinoma preferentially spreads to bone, bronchogenic carcinomas tend to involve the adrenal glands and the brain, and neuroblastomas spread to the liver and bones. Such organ tropism may be related to the following mechanisms:

- Tumor cells may have adhesion molecules whose ligands are expressed preferentially on the endothelial cells of the target organ.
- Chemokines may have an important role in determining the target tissues for metastasis. For instance, many cancers express the chemokine receptor CXCR4, which has been implicated in the extravasation of circulating tumor cells originating from tumors such as breast cancer.
- In some cases, the target tissue may be a nonpermissive environment, "unfavorable soil," so to speak, for the growth of tumor seedlings. For example, although they are well vascularized, skeletal muscle and spleen are rarely sites of metastasis.

It must be admitted, however, that although particular tumors "prefer" certain metastatic sites, the precise localization of metastases cannot be predicted in individual patients with any form of cancer. Evidently, much to the dismay of medical students, many tumors have not read the relevant chapters of pathology textbooks! Although the molecular mechanisms of colonization are still being unraveled, a consistent theme seems to be that tumor cells secrete cytokines, growth factors, and proteases that act on the resident stromal cells, which in turn make the metastatic site habitable for the cancer cell. With a better molecular understanding of the mechanisms of metastasis, the clinician's ability to target them therapeutically will be greatly enhanced.

Metastasis

Of central importance in oncology is the question, why do only some tumors metastasize? It is sobering to realize that satisfying answers are still lacking. Some variation in metastasis clearly relates to inherent differences in the behavior of particular tumors; for example, small cell carcinoma of the lung virtually always metastasizes to distant sites, whereas with some tumors, such as basal cell carcinoma, metastasis is the exception rather than the rule. In general, large tumors are more likely to metastasize than small tumors, presumably because (all other things being equal) large tumors will have been present in the patient for longer periods of time, providing additional chances for metastasis to occur. However, tumor size and type cannot adequately explain the behavior of individual cancers, and it is still open to question whether metastasis is merely probabilistic (a matter of chance multiplied by tumor cell number and time) or reflects inherent differences in metastatic potential from tumor to tumor (a deterministic model).

The deterministic model proposes that metastasis is inevitable with certain tumors because the tumor harbors cells with a specific metastatic phenotype. As discussed earlier, as tumor cells grow they randomly accumulate mutations, creating subclones with distinct combinations of mutations. One possibility is that only rare tumor cells accumulate all of the mutations necessary for metastasis, and that this accounts for the inefficiency of the process. However, identification of metastasis-specific mutations and metastasis-specific patterns of gene expression has proven to be difficult. An alternative idea is that some tumors acquire all of the mutations needed for metastasis early in their development, and that these are the tumors that are fated to be "bad actors." Metastasis, according to this view, is not dependent on the stochastic generation of metastatic subclones during tumor progression, but is an intrinsic property of the tumor that develops early on during carcinogenesis. These mechanisms are not mutually exclusive, and it could be that aggressive tumors acquire a metastasis-permissive gene expression pattern early in tumorigenesis, yet also require some additional random mutations to complete the metastatic phenotype. Nor can all blame be placed on tumor cells: as mentioned earlier, there is evidence that the makeup of the stroma, the presence of infiltrating immune cells, and the degree and quality of angiogenesis also influence metastasis.

Another open question is whether there are genes whose principal or sole contribution is to control programs of gene expression that promote metastasis. This question is of more than academic interest, because if altered forms of certain genes promote or suppress the metastatic phenotype, their detection in a primary tumor would have both prognostic and therapeutic implications. Among candidates for such metastasis oncogenes are those encoding

SNAIL and TWIST, transcription factors whose primary function is to promote epithelial-to-mesenchymal transition (EMT). In EMT, carcinoma cells downregulate certain epithelial markers (e.g., E-cadherin) and upregulate certain mesenchymal markers (e.g., vimentin, smooth muscle actin). These molecular changes are accompanied by phenotypic alterations such as morphologic change from polygonal epithelioid cell shape to a spindly mesenchymal shape, along with increased production of proteolytic enzymes that promote migration and invasion. These changes are believed to favor the development of a promigratory phenotype that is essential for metastasis. Loss of E-cadherin expression seems to be a key event in EMT, and SNAIL and TWIST are transcriptional repressors that downregulate E-cadherin expression. How expression of these master regulator transcription factors is stimulated in tumors is not clear; however, experimental models suggest that interactions of tumor cells with stromal cells are a key stimulus for this change. Thus, acquisition of a metastatic phenotype may not require a set of mutations but may be an emergent property arising from the interactions of tumor cells and stroma.

SUMMARY

INVASION AND METASTASIS

- Ability to invade tissues, a hallmark of malignancy, occurs in four steps: loosening of cell–cell contacts, degradation of ECM, attachment to novel ECM components, and migration of tumor cells.
- Cell–cell contacts are lost by the inactivation of E-cadherin through a variety of pathways.
- Basement membrane and interstitial matrix degradation is mediated by proteolytic enzymes secreted by tumor cells and stromal cells, such as MMPs and cathepsins.
- Proteolytic enzymes also release growth factors sequestered in the ECM and generate chemotactic and angiogenic fragments from cleavage of ECM glycoproteins.
- The metastatic site of many tumors can be predicted by the location of the primary tumor. Many tumors arrest in the first capillary bed they encounter (lung and liver, most commonly).
- Some tumors show organ tropism, probably due to activation of adhesion or chemokine receptors whose ligands are expressed by endothelial cells at the metastatic site.

Evasion of Immune Surveillance

Long one of the "holy grails" of oncology, the promise of therapies that enable the host immune system to recognize and destroy cancer cells is finally coming to fruition, largely due to a clearer understanding of the mechanisms by which cancer cells evade the host response. Paul Ehrlich first conceived the idea that tumor cells can be recognized as "foreign" and eliminated by the immune system. Subsequently, Lewis Thomas and Macfarlane Burnet formalized this concept by coining the term *immune surveillance*, based on the premise that a normal function of the immune system is to constantly "scan" the body for emerging malignant cells and destroy them. This idea has been supported by many observations—the direct demonstration of tumor-specific T cells and antibodies in patients; data showing that the extent and quality of immune infiltrates in cancers often correlates with outcome; the increased incidence of certain cancers in immunodeficient people and mice; and most recently and most directly, the dramatic success of immunotherapy in the treatment of several cancers.

The specific factors that govern the outcome of interactions between tumor cells and the host immune system are numerous and are still being defined. In the face of this complexity, it is helpful to consider a few overarching principles:

- Cancer cells express a variety of antigens that stimulate the host immune system, which appears to have an important role in preventing the emergence of cancers.
- Despite the antigenicity of cancer cells, the immune response to established tumors is ineffective, and in some instances may actually promote cancer growth, due to acquired changes that allow cancer cells to evade anti-tumor responses and foster pro-tumor responses.
- Defining mechanisms of immune evasion and "immuno-manipulation" by cancer cells has led to effective new immunotherapies that work by reactivating latent host immune responses.

Tumor Antigens. As we have discussed, cancer is a disorder that is caused by driver mutations in oncogenes and tumor suppressor genes, which in most instances are acquired rather than inherited. In addition to pathogenic driver mutations, cancers, due to their inherent genetic instability, also accumulate passenger mutations. These may be particularly abundant in cancers that are caused by mutagenic exposures (e.g., sunlight, smoking). All of these varied mutations may generate new protein sequences (*neoantigens*) that the immune system has not seen and therefore is not tolerant of and can react to.

In some instances, unmutated proteins expressed by tumor cells also can stimulate the host immune response.

- One such antigen is *tyrosinase*, an enzyme involved in melanin biosynthesis that is expressed only in normal melanocytes and melanomas. It may be surprising that the immune system is able to respond to this normal self-antigen. The probable explanation is that tyrosinase is normally produced in such small amounts and in so few normal cells that it is not recognized by the immune system and fails to induce tolerance.
- Another group of tumor antigens, the *cancer-testis antigens*, are encoded by genes that are silent in all adult tissues except germ cells in the testis—hence their name. Although the protein is present in the testis it is not expressed on the cell surface in a form that can be recognized by CD8+ T cells, because sperm do not express MHC class I molecules. Thus, for all practical purposes these antigens are tumor specific and are therefore capable of stimulating anti-tumor immune responses.

An additional important class of tumor antigens consists of viral proteins that are expressed in cancer cells transformed by oncogenic viruses. The most potent of these antigens are proteins produced by cells that are latently infected with DNA viruses, the most important of which are human papilloma virus (HPV) and Epstein-Barr virus (EBV). There is abundant evidence that cytotoxic T lymphocytes (CTLs) recognize viral antigens and play important roles in surveillance against virus-induced tumors through their ability to recognize and kill virus-infected cells. Most notably, multiple cancers associated with oncogenic viruses, including HPV-associated cervical carcinoma and EBV-related B cell lymphomas, occur at significantly higher rates in individuals with defective T cell immunity, such as patients infected with HIV.

Effective Immune Responses to Tumor Antigens. Assuming that the immune system is normally capable of eliminating emerging cancers, we may ask, what are the key components of an effective host immune response? It appears likely that immune reactions to cancers are initiated by the death of individual cancer cells, which occurs at some frequency in all cancers due to dysregulated growth, metabolic stresses, and hypoxia due to insufficient blood supply. When tumor cells die they release "danger signals" (damage associated molecular patterns, see Chapter 5) that stimulate innate immune cells, including resident phagocytes and antigen presenting cells. It is believed that some of the dead cells are phagocytosed by dendritic cells, which migrate to draining lymph nodes and present tumor neoantigens in the context of MHC class I molecules, a process termed cross-presentation. The displayed tumor antigens are recognized by antigen-specific CD8+ T cells, which become activated, proliferate, differentiate into active CTLs, and home to the site of the tumor, where they recognize and kill tumor cells presenting neoantigens in the context of their own MHC class I molecules (Fig. 6.29). IFN-γ-producing T helper cells of the Th1 subset, which may be induced by recognition of tumor antigens, can activate macrophages and also contribute to the destruction of tumors.

As will be discussed shortly, some the strongest evidence for the importance of CTL responses in immunosurveillance stems from the characterization of established human cancers, which often feature acquired mutations that prevent CTLs from recognizing tumor cells as "foreign". It also has been noted in large studies of a wide variety of human tumors that high levels of infiltrating CTLs and Th1 cells correlate with better clinical outcomes. While other cell types such as natural killer cells also have been implicated in anti-tumor responses, the quality and strength of CTL responses are believed to be of preeminent importance.

Immune Evasion by Cancers. Since the immune system is capable of recognizing and eliminating nascent cancers, it follows that tumors that reach clinically significant sizes must be composed of cells that are either invisible to the host immune system or that express factors that actively suppress host immunity. The term *cancer immunoediting* has been used to describe the ability of the immune system to promote the darwinian selection of the tumor subclones that are most able to avoid host immunity or even manipulate the immune system for their own malignant purposes. Since CTL responses appear to be the most important defense that the host has against tumors, it should come as

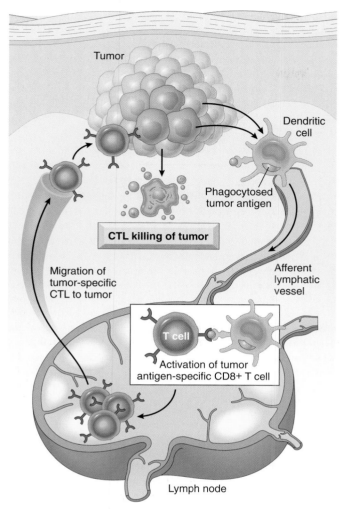

Fig. 6.29 Cross-presentation of tumor antigens and induction of CD8+ cytotoxic T cell antitumor response. *(Modified from Abbas AK, Lichtman AH, Pillai S: Cellular and molecular immunology, ed 9, Philadelphia, 2018, Elsevier.)*

block these checkpoints and release the brakes on the immune response. Current checkpoint blockade therapies have resulted in response rates of 10–30% in a variety of solid tumors (melanoma, lung cancer, bladder cancer, and others), and even higher rates in some hematologic malignancies such as Hodgkin lymphoma (Chapter 12). Because these checkpoints evolved to prevent responses to self antigens (Chapter 5), it is not surprising that patients treated with checkpoint blockade therapy develop various autoimmune manifestations, such as colitis and other types of systemic inflammation. Most of these reactions can be controlled with anti-inflammatory agents.

The remarkable response of advanced cancers to immune checkpoint inhibitors has energized other work focused on harnessing the immune system to combat cancer. These include efforts to develop personalized tumor vaccines using neoantigens identified in the tumors of individual patients, as well as new kinds of adoptive immunotherapy. The most advanced of the latter are patient-derived CTLs that are engineered to express chimeric antigen receptors (CARs). CARs have extracellular domains consisting of antibodies that bind tumor antigens and intracellular domains that delivered signals that activate CTLs following their engagement with antigen on the surface of tumor cells. CAR T cells are potent killers of tumor cells and have produced long-term remissions in patients with certain leukemias, such as B cell acute lymphoblastic leukemia (Chapter 12). However, CAR T cells also are associated with serious complications related to cytokines released from the activated CTLs, and it remains to be seen if they will become a routine part of cancer treatment.

Beyond complications of immunotherapy, it also should be recognized that the host immune response to tumors is not an unalloyed blessing. For example, tumors release incompletely characterized factors that alter the function of certain immune cells, such as macrophages and Th2 lymphocytes, in a fashion that is suspected of promoting angiogenesis, tissue fibrosis, and the accumulation of alternatively activated (M2) macrophages, which you will recall from Chapter 5 are associated with suppression of the immune response during wound healing. These types of responses may promote tumor growth, the converse of what one would expect from a protective anti-tumor immune response.

To summarize, while the future appears very bright for cancer immunotherapy, important hurdles remain to be cleared. At present, response and resistance to immune checkpoint inhibitors are unpredictable, and new biomarkers are needed to better tailor therapies for individual patients. This will entail the development of new diagnostic tests to gauge both the host immune response and the likely means of immune evasion in individual cancers. There is reason to believe that immune checkpoint inhibitors may be more effective if given before the patient receives chemotherapy (which is immunosuppressive) or in combination with certain targeted therapies directed against tumor cells, and many well-designed clinical trials will need to be conducted before these questions are answered. Currently available immunotherapies are effective in some cancers but not others. Thus, there is a need for development of safe adaptive therapies that are

no surprise that tumor cells show a variety of alterations that abrogate CTL responses. These include acquired mutations in β2-microglobulin that prevent the assembly of functional MHC class I molecules, and increased expression of a variety of proteins that inhibit CTL function. These proteins work by activating what is referred to as *immune checkpoints*, inhibitory pathways that normally are crucial for maintaining self-tolerance and controlling the size and duration of immune responses so as to minimize collateral tissue damage.

One of the best-characterized immune checkpoints involves a protein called PD-L1 (programmed cell death ligand 1), which is often expressed on the surface of tumor cells (Figure 6.30). When PD-L1 engages its receptor, PD-1, on CTLs, the CTLs become unresponsive and lose their ability to kill tumor cells. Experimental studies have identified several other immune checkpoint pathways, involving different ligands and receptors, which also have been implicated in immunoevasion by tumors. Of these, the best characterized involves CTLA4, another receptor expressed on T cells that inhibits T cell function.

The discovery of checkpoints that shut off anti-tumor immunity has led to the development of antibodies that

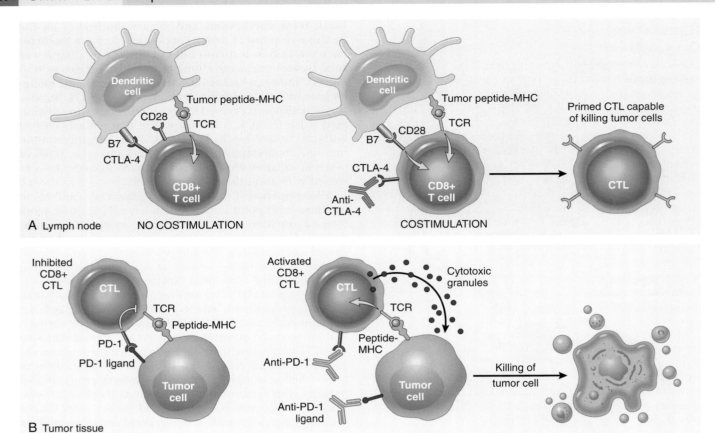

Fig. 6.30 Activation of host antitumor immunity by checkpoint inhibitors. (A) Blockade of the CTLA4 surface molecule with an inhibitor antibody allows cytolytic CD8+ T cells (CTLs) to engage B7 family coreceptors, leading to T cell activation. (B) Blockade of PD-1 receptor or PD-1 ligand by inhibitory antibodies abrogates inhibitory signals transmitted by PD-1, again leading to activation of CTLs. *(Reprinted from Abbas AK, Lichtman AH, Pillai S:* Cellular and molecular immunology, *ed 9, Philadelphia, 2018, Elsevier.)*

effective in a wide variety of cancers. With all of these caveats, it seems certain that the field of oncology is on the threshold of transformative therapeutic advances, all made possible by careful study of the normal immune response and its myriad variations in cancers.

SUMMARY

EVASION OF IMMUNE SURVEILLANCE

- Tumor cells can be recognized by the immune system as non-self and destroyed.
- Antitumor activity is mediated by predominantly cell-mediated mechanisms. Tumor antigens are presented on the cell surface by MHC class I molecules and are recognized by CD8+ CTLs.
- The different classes of tumor antigens include products of mutated genes, overexpressed or aberrantly expressed proteins, and tumor antigens produced by oncogenic viruses.
- Immunosuppressed patients have an increased risk for development of cancer, particularly types caused by oncogenic DNA viruses.
- In immunocompetent patients, tumors may avoid the immune system by several mechanisms, including selective outgrowth of antigen-negative variants, loss or reduced expression of histocompatibility molecules, and immunosuppression mediated by expression of certain factors (e.g., TGF-β, PD-1 ligands) by the tumor cells.

- Antibodies that overcome some of these mechanisms of immune evasion are now approved for treatment of patients with advanced forms of cancer.

Genomic Instability as an Enabler of Malignancy

The preceding section identified the eight defining features of malignancy, all of which appear to be produced by genetic alterations involving cancer genes. How do these mutations arise? Although humans are awash in environmental agents that are mutagenic (e.g., chemicals, radiation, sunlight), cancers are relatively rare outcomes of these encounters. This state of affairs results from the ability of normal cells to sense and repair DNA damage.

The importance of DNA repair in maintaining the integrity of the genome is highlighted by several inherited disorders in which genes that encode proteins involved in DNA repair are defective. **Individuals born with inherited defects in DNA repair genes are at greatly increased risk for the development of cancer.** Defects in three types of DNA repair systems—mismatch repair, nucleotide excision repair, and recombination repair—are presented next. While these discussions focus on inherited syndromes, a point worthy of emphasis is that sporadic cancers often incur mutations in DNA repair genes as well; this in turn enables the accumulation of mutations in cancer genes that contribute directly to development of cancer.

Hereditary Nonpolyposis Colon Cancer Syndrome

Hereditary nonpolyposis colon carcinoma (HNPCC) syndrome dramatically illustrates the role of DNA repair genes in predisposition to cancer. This disorder, characterized by familial carcinomas of the colon affecting predominantly the cecum and proximal colon (Chapter 14), results from defects in genes involved in DNA mismatch repair. When a strand of DNA is being repaired, the products of mismatch repair genes act as "spell checkers." For example, if there is an erroneous pairing of G with T, rather than the normal A with T, the mismatch repair genes correct the defect. Without these "proofreaders," errors accumulate at an increased rate. Mutations in at least four mismatch repair genes have been found to underlie HNPCC (Chapter 15). Each affected individual inherits one defective copy of one of several DNA mismatch repair genes and acquires the second "hit" in colonic epithelial cells. Thus, DNA repair genes affect cell growth only indirectly—by allowing mutations in other genes during the process of normal cell division. A characteristic finding in the genome of patients with mismatch repair defects is *microsatellite instability* (MSI). Microsatellites are tandem repeats of one to six nucleotides found throughout the genome (Chapter 1). In normal people, the length of these microsatellites remains constant. By contrast, in patients with HNPCC, these satellites are unstable and increase or decrease in length. Although HNPCC accounts for only 2% to 4% of all colonic cancers, MSI can be detected in about 15% of sporadic cancers due to acquired mutations that disrupt the function of mismatch repair genes.

Xeroderma Pigmentosum

Xeroderma pigmentosum is an autosomal recessive disorder caused by a defect in DNA repair that is associated with a greatly increased risk for cancers arising in sun-exposed skin. Ultraviolet (UV) rays in sunlight cause cross-linking of pyrimidine residues, preventing normal DNA replication. Such DNA damage is repaired by the nucleotide excision repair system. Several proteins are involved in nucleotide excision repair, and the inherited loss of any one of these can give rise to xeroderma pigmentosum.

Diseases With Defects in DNA Repair by Homologous Recombination

A group of autosomal recessive disorders comprising *Bloom syndrome*, *ataxia-telangiectasia*, and *Fanconi anemia* is characterized by hypersensitivity to DNA-damaging agents, such as ionizing radiation (in Bloom syndrome and ataxia-telangiectasia), or to DNA cross-linking agents, such as nitrogen mustard (in Fanconi anemia). Their phenotype is complex and includes, in addition to predisposition to cancer, features such as neural symptoms (in ataxia-telangiectasia), anemia (in Fanconi anemia), and developmental defects (in Bloom syndrome). The gene mutated in ataxia-telangiectasia is ATM, which encodes a protein kinase that is important in "sensing" DNA damage caused by ionizing radiation and then directing p53 to initiate the DNA damage response, as described earlier.

Evidence for the role of DNA repair genes in the origin of cancer also comes from the study of hereditary breast cancer. **Germ line mutations in two genes, BRCA1 and BRCA2, account for 50% of cases of familial breast cancer. In addition to breast cancer, women with BRCA1 mutations have a substantially higher risk for developing epithelial ovarian cancers, and men have a slightly higher risk for developing prostate cancer.** Likewise, germ line mutations in the *BRCA2* gene increase the risk for developing breast cancer in both men and women, as well as cancers originating from the ovary, prostate, pancreas, bile ducts, stomach, melanocytes, and B lymphocytes. Although the functions of BRCA1 and BRCA2 have not been elucidated fully, cells with a defective version of these genes develop chromosomal breaks and severe aneuploidy. Indeed, both genes seem to function, at least in part, in the homologous recombination DNA repair pathway. For example, BRCA1 forms a complex with other proteins in the homologous recombination pathway and also is linked to the ATM kinase pathway. BRCA2 was identified as one of several genes mutated in Fanconi anemia, and the BRCA2 protein has been shown to bind to RAD51, a protein required for homologous recombination. Similar to other tumor suppressor genes, both copies of BRCA1 and BRCA2 must be inactivated for cancer to develop. Although linkage of BRCA1 and BRCA2 to familial breast cancers is well established, these genes are rarely inactivated in sporadic cases of breast cancer. In this regard, BRCA1 and BRCA2 are different from other tumor suppressor genes, such as APC and TP53, which are frequently inactivated in sporadic cancers.

Cancers Resulting From Mutations Induced by Regulated Genomic Instability: Lymphoid Neoplasms

A special type of DNA damage plays a central role in the pathogenesis of tumors of B cells and T lymphocytes. As discussed earlier, adaptive immunity relies on the ability of B cells and T cells to diversify their antigen receptor genes. Immature B cells and T progenitors both express a pair of gene products, RAG1 and RAG2, that carry out V(D)J segment recombination, permitting the assembly of functional immunoglobulin and T-cell receptor genes. In addition, after encountering antigen, mature B cells express a specialized enzyme called *activation-induced cytosine deaminase (AID)*, which catalyzes both immunoglobulin gene class switch recombination and immunoglobulin diversification through somatic hypermutation. Errors that occur during antigen receptor gene assembly and immunoglobulin gene class switching and diversification provide fertile soil for many of the mutations that cause lymphoid neoplasms, discussed in detail in Chapter 12.

SUMMARY

GENOMIC INSTABILITY AS AN ENABLER OF MALIGNANCY

- Individuals with inherited mutations of genes involved in DNA repair systems are at greatly increased risk for the development of cancer.

- Patients with HNPCC syndrome have defects in the mismatch repair system, leading to development of carcinomas of the colon. These patients' genomes show microsatellite instability (MSI), characterized by changes in length of short tandem repeating sequences throughout the genome.
- Patients with xeroderma pigmentosum have a defect in the nucleotide excision repair pathway. They are at increased risk for the development of skin cancers in sites exposed to sunlight because of an inability to repair pyrimidine dimers induced by UV light.
- Syndromes involving defects in the homologous recombination DNA repair system constitute a group of disorders—Bloom syndrome, ataxia-telangiectasia, and Fanconi anemia—that are characterized by hypersensitivity to DNA-damaging agents, such as ionizing radiation. *BRCA1* and *BRCA2*, which are mutated in familial breast cancers, also are involved in homologous DNA repair.
- Mutations incurred in lymphocytes expressing gene products that induce genomic instability (RAG1, RAG2, AID) are important in the pathogenesis of lymphoid neoplasms.

Tumor-Promoting Inflammation as an Enabler of Malignancy

Infiltrating cancers provoke a chronic inflammatory reaction. In patients with advanced cancers, this inflammatory reaction can be so extensive as to cause systemic signs and symptoms, such as anemia (the so-called "anemia of chronic disease"), fatigue, and cachexia. However, studies carried out on cancers in animal models suggest that inflammatory cells also modify the tumor microenvironment to enable many of the hallmarks of cancer. These effects may stem from direct interactions between inflammatory cells and tumor cells, or through indirect effects of inflammatory cells on other resident stromal cells, particularly cancer-associated fibroblasts and endothelial cells. Proposed cancer-enabling effects of inflammatory cells and resident stromal cells include the following:

- *Release of factors that promote proliferation.* Infiltrating leukocytes and activated stromal cells have been shown to secrete a wide variety of growth factors, such as EGF, and proteases that can liberate growth factors from the extracellular matrix (ECM).
- *Removal of growth suppressors.* As mentioned earlier, the growth of epithelial cells is suppressed by cell–cell and cell–ECM interactions. Proteases released by inflammatory cells can degrade the adhesion molecules that mediate these interactions, removing a barrier to growth.
- *Enhanced resistance to cell death.* Detachment of epithelial cells from basement membranes and from cell–cell interactions can lead to a particular form of programmed cell death called *anoikis*. It is suspected that tumor-associated macrophages may prevent anoikis by expressing adhesion molecules such as integrins that promote direct physical interactions with tumor cells.
- *Angiogenesis.* Inflammatory cells release numerous factors, including VEGF, that stimulate angiogenesis.

- *Invasion and metastasis.* Proteases released from macrophages foster tissue invasion by remodeling the ECM, while factors such as TNF and EGF may directly stimulate tumor cell motility. As mentioned earlier, other factors released from stromal cells such as TGF-β may promote epithelial-mesenchymal transition (EMT), which may be a key event in the process of invasion and metastasis.
- *Evasion of immune destruction.* A variety of soluble factors released by macrophages and other stromal cells are believed to contribute to an immunosuppressive tumor microenvironment. The leading suspects include TGF-β and other factors that either favor the recruitment of immunosuppressive T regulatory cells or suppress the function of CD8+ cytotoxic T cells. Furthermore, there is abundant evidence in cancer models and emerging evidence in human disease that advanced cancers contain mainly alternatively activated (M2) macrophages (Chapter 3). M2 macrophages produce cytokines that promote angiogenesis, fibroblast proliferation, and collagen deposition, all of which are commonly observed in invasive cancers and in healing wounds, giving rise to the notion that cancers are like "wounds that do not heal."

A thorough understanding of how cancers "manipulate" inflammatory cells to support their growth and survival remains elusive. However, the results from animal studies are intriguing and raise the possibility of therapies directed at tumor-induced inflammation and its downstream consequences. An example of one such intervention involves aspirin and other COX-2 inhibitors, use of which is associated with a decreased risk of colorectal cancer in several epidemiological studies.

Important clinical considerations emerge from the principles presented in the foregoing discussion of the hallmarks of cancer: These hallmarks provide a road map for the development of new therapeutic agents for the treatment of cancer (Fig. 6.31).

ETIOLOGY OF CANCER: CARCINOGENIC AGENTS

Carcinogenic agents inflict genetic damage, which lies at the heart of carcinogenesis. Three classes of carcinogenic agents have been identified: (1) chemicals, (2) radiant energy, and (3) microbial products. Chemicals and radiant energy are documented causes of cancer in humans, and oncogenic viruses are involved in the pathogenesis of tumors in several animal models and some human tumors. In the following discussion, each class of agents is considered separately; of note, however, several may act in concert or sequentially to produce the multiple genetic abnormalities characteristic of neoplastic cells.

Chemical Carcinogens

More than 200 years ago, the London surgeon Sir Percival Pott correctly attributed scrotal skin cancer in chimney sweeps to chronic exposure to soot. On the basis of this observation, the Danish Chimney Sweeps Guild ruled that

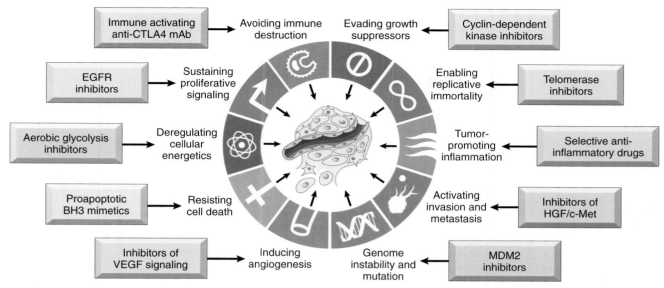

Fig. 6.31 Therapeutic targeting of the hallmarks of cancer. *(From Hanahan D, Weiberg RA: The hallmarks of cancer: the next generation. Cell 144:646, 2011.)*

its members must bathe daily. No public health measure since that time has achieved so much in the control of a form of cancer. Subsequently, hundreds of chemicals have been shown to be carcinogenic in animals.

Some of the major agents are presented in Table 6.5. A few comments on a handful of these are offered next.

Direct-Acting Agents

Direct-acting agents require no metabolic conversion to become carcinogenic. They are typically weak carcinogens but are important because some of them are cancer chemotherapy drugs (e.g., alkylating agents) used in regimens that may cure certain types of cancer (e.g., Hodgkin lymphoma), only to evoke a subsequent, second form of cancer, usually leukemia. This situation is even more tragic when the initial use of such agents has been for non-neoplastic disorders, such as rheumatoid arthritis or granulomatosis with polyangiitis. The associated risk for induced cancer is low, but its existence dictates judicious use of such agents.

Indirect-Acting Agents

The designation indirect-acting refers to chemicals that require metabolic conversion to an ultimate carcinogen. Some of the most potent indirect chemical carcinogens are polycyclic hydrocarbons that are created with burning of fossil fuels, plant, and animal material. For example, benzo[a]pyrene and other carcinogens formed during the combustion of tobacco are implicated in the causation of lung cancer, and in olden days, benzo[a]pyrene created during the burning of coal was likely responsible for the high incidence of scrotal cancer in chimney sweeps. Polycyclic hydrocarbons also may be produced from animal fats during the process of broiling meats and are present in smoked meats and fish. In the body, benzo[a]pyrene is

Table 6.5 Major Chemical Carcinogens

Direct-Acting Carcinogens

Alkylating Agents

β-Propiolactone
Dimethyl sulfate
Diepoxybutane
Anti-cancer drugs (cyclophosphamide, chlorambucil, nitrosoureas, and others)

Acylating Agents

1-Acetyl-imidazole
Dimethylcarbamyl chloride

Procarcinogens That Require Metabolic Activation

Polycyclic and Heterocyclic Aromatic Hydrocarbons

Benz(a)anthracene
Benzo(a)pyrene
Dibenz(a,h)anthracene
3-Methylcholanthrene
7, 12-Dimethylbenz(a)anthracene

Aromatic Amines, Amides, Azo Dyes

2-Naphthylamine (β-naphthylamine)
Benzidine
2-Acetylaminofluorene
Dimethylaminoazobenzene (butter yellow)

Natural Plant and Microbial Products

Aflatoxin B_1
Griseofulvin
Cycasin
Safrole
Betel nuts

Others

Nitrosamine and amides
Vinyl chloride, nickel, chromium
Insecticides, fungicides
Polychlorinated biphenyls

metabolized to epoxides, which form covalent adducts (addition products) with molecules in the cell, principally DNA, but also with RNA and proteins.

The aromatic amines and azo dyes constitute another class of indirect-acting carcinogens. Before its carcinogenicity was recognized, β-naphthylamine was responsible for a 50-fold increased incidence of bladder cancers in heavily exposed workers in the aniline dye and rubber industries. Examples of other occupational carcinogens are listed in Table 6.5. Because indirect-acting carcinogens require metabolic activation for their conversion to DNA-damaging agents, much interest is focused on the enzymatic pathways that are involved, such as that mediated by the cytochrome P-450–dependent monooxygenases. The genes that encode these enzymes are polymorphic, and enzyme activity varies among individuals. It is widely believed that the susceptibility to chemical carcinogenesis depends at least in part, on the specific allelic form of the enzyme that is inherited. Thus, it may be possible in the future to assess cancer risk in a given individual by genetic analysis of enzyme polymorphisms.

A few other agents merit brief mention. Aflatoxin B₁ is of interest because it is a naturally occurring agent produced by some strains of *Aspergillus,* a mold that grows on improperly stored grains and nuts. A strong correlation has been found between the dietary level of this food contaminant and the incidence of hepatocellular carcinoma in some parts of Africa and the Far East. Additionally, vinyl chloride, arsenic, nickel, chromium, insecticides, fungicides, and polychlorinated biphenyls are potential carcinogens in the workplace and about the house. Finally, nitrites used as food preservatives have caused concern, since they cause nitrosylation of amines contained in food. The nitrosamines thus formed are suspected to be carcinogenic.

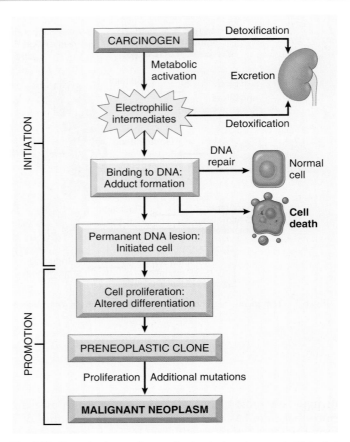

Fig. 6.32 General schema of events in chemical carcinogenesis. Note that promoters cause clonal expansion of the initiated cell, thus producing a preneoplastic clone. Further proliferation induced by the promoter or other factors causes accumulation of additional mutations and emergence of a malignant tumor.

Mechanisms of Action of Chemical Carcinogens

Because malignant transformation results from mutations, it should come as no surprise that most chemical carcinogens are mutagenic. Indeed, all direct and ultimate carcinogens contain highly reactive electrophile groups that form chemical adducts with DNA, as well as with proteins and RNA. Any gene may be the target of chemical carcinogens, but understandably it is the mutation of important cancer genes, such as *RAS* and *TP53,* that is responsible for carcinogenesis. Indeed, specific chemical carcinogens, such as aflatoxin B₁, produce characteristic mutations in *TP53,* such that detection of mutations within particular codons strongly points toward aflatoxin as the causative agent. Such specific "mutational signatures" also exist for cancers caused by UV light, tobacco smoke, and other environmental carcinogens and are proving to be useful tools in epidemiologic studies of carcinogenesis.

Carcinogenicity of some chemicals is augmented by subsequent administration of *promoters* (e.g., phorbol esters, hormones, phenols, certain drugs), which are by themselves nontumorigenic. To be effective, repeated or sustained exposure to the promoter must follow the application of the mutagenic chemical, or *initiator* (Fig. 6.32). The initiation-promotion sequence of chemical carcinogenesis

raises an important question: Since promoters are not mutagenic, how do they contribute to tumorigenesis? Although the effects of tumor promoters are pleiotropic, **induction of cell proliferation is a** *sine qua non* **of tumor promotion.** It seems most likely that while the application of an initiator may cause the mutational activation of an oncogene such as *RAS,* subsequent application of promoters leads to clonal expansion of initiated (mutated) cells. Forced to proliferate, the initiated clone of cells accumulates additional mutations, developing eventually into a malignant tumor. Indeed, the concept that sustained cell proliferation increases the risk for mutagenesis, and hence promotes neoplastic transformation, also is applicable to human carcinogenesis. For example, endometrial hyperplasia (Chapter 19) and increased regenerative activity that accompanies chronic liver cell injury are associated with the development of cancer in these organs. Were it not for the DNA repair mechanisms discussed earlier, the incidence of chemically induced cancers in all likelihood would be much higher. As mentioned previously, the rare hereditary disorders of DNA repair, including xeroderma pigmentosum, are associated with greatly increased risk for developing cancers induced by UV light and certain chemicals.

SUMMARY

CHEMICAL CARCINOGENS

- Chemical carcinogens have highly reactive electrophile groups that directly damage DNA, leading to mutations and eventually cancer.
- Direct-acting agents do not require metabolic conversion to become carcinogenic, while indirect-acting agents are not active until converted to an ultimate carcinogen by endogenous metabolic pathways. Hence, polymorphisms of endogenous enzymes such as cytochrome P-450 may influence carcinogenesis by altering the conversion of indirect-acting agents to active carcinogens.
- After exposure of a cell to a mutagen or an initiator, tumorigenesis can be enhanced by exposure to promoters, which stimulate proliferation of the mutated cells.
- Examples of human carcinogens are direct-acting agents (e.g., alkylating agents used for chemotherapy), indirect-acting agents (e.g., benzo(a)pyrene, azo dyes, aflatoxin), and tumor promoters.
- Tumor promoters act by stimulating cell proliferation. Increased proliferation may occur through direct effects of tumor promoters on target cells or may be secondary to tissue injury and regenerative repair.

Radiation Carcinogenesis

Radiation, whatever its source (UV rays of sunlight, radiographs, nuclear fission, radionuclides), is an established carcinogen. Unprotected miners of radioactive elements have a 10-fold increased incidence of lung cancers. A follow-up study of survivors of the atomic bombs dropped on Hiroshima and Nagasaki disclosed a markedly increased incidence of leukemia after an average latent period of about 7 years, as well as increased mortality rates for thyroid, breast, colon, and lung carcinomas. The nuclear power accident at Chernobyl in the former Soviet Union continues to exact its toll in the form of high cancer incidence in the surrounding areas. More recently, it is feared that radiation release from a nuclear power plant in Japan damaged by a massive earthquake and tsunami will result in significantly increased cancer incidence in the surrounding geographic areas.

Therapeutic irradiation of the head and neck can give rise to papillary thyroid cancers years later. The oncogenic properties of ionizing radiation are related to its mutagenic effects; it causes chromosome breakage, chromosomal rearrangements such as translocations and inversions, and, less frequently, point mutations. Biologically, double-stranded DNA breaks seem to be the most important form of DNA damage caused by radiation.

The oncogenic effect of UV rays merits special mention because it highlights the importance of DNA repair in carcinogenesis. Natural UV radiation derived from the sun can cause skin cancers (melanomas, squamous cell carcinomas, and basal cell carcinomas). At greatest risk are fair-skinned people who live in locales such as Australia and New Zealand that receive a great deal of sunlight. Nonmelanoma skin cancers are associated with total cumulative exposure to UV radiation, whereas melanomas are associated with intense intermittent exposure—as occurs with sunbathing. UV light has several biologic effects on cells. Of particular relevance to carcinogenesis is the ability to damage DNA by forming pyrimidine dimers. This type of DNA damage is repaired by the nucleotide excision repair pathway. With extensive exposure to UV light, the repair systems may be overwhelmed, and skin cancer results. As mentioned earlier, patients with the inherited disease *xeroderma pigmentosum* have a defect in the nucleotide excision repair pathway. As expected, there is a greatly increased predisposition to skin cancers in this disorder.

SUMMARY

RADIATION CARCINOGENESIS

- Ionizing radiation causes chromosome breakage, chromosome rearrangements, and, less frequently, point mutations, any of which may affect cancer genes and thereby drive carcinogenesis.
- UV rays in sunlight induce the formation of pyrimidine dimers within DNA, leading to mutations that can give rise to squamous cell carcinomas and melanomas of the skin.

Viral and Microbial Oncogenesis

Many DNA and RNA viruses have proved to be oncogenic in animals as disparate as frogs and primates. Despite intense scrutiny, however, only a few viruses have been linked with human cancer. The following discussion focuses on human oncogenic viruses. Also discussed is the role of the bacterium *Helicobacter pylori* in gastric cancer.

Oncogenic RNA Viruses

Although the study of animal retroviruses has provided spectacular insights into the molecular basis of cancer, only one human retrovirus, human T-cell leukemia virus type 1 (HTLV-1), is firmly implicated in the pathogenesis of cancer in humans.

HTLV-1 causes *adult T-cell leukemia/lymphoma* (ATLL), a tumor that is endemic in certain parts of Japan, the Caribbean basin, South America, and Africa, and found sporadically elsewhere, including the United States. Worldwide, it is estimated that 15 to 20 million people are infected with HTLV-1. Similar to the human immunodeficiency virus, which causes AIDS, HTLV-1 has tropism for CD4+ T cells, and hence this subset of T cells is the major target for neoplastic transformation. Human infection requires transmission of infected T cells via sexual intercourse, blood products, or breastfeeding. Leukemia develops in only 3% to 5% of the infected individuals, typically after a long latent period of 40 to 60 years.

There is little doubt that HTLV-1 infection of T lymphocytes is necessary for leukemogenesis, but the molecular mechanisms of transformation are not certain. In contrast to several murine retroviruses, HTLV-1 does not contain an oncogene, and no consistent pattern of proviral integration next to a proto-oncogene has been discovered. In leukemic cells, however, viral integration shows a clonal pattern. In other words, although the site of viral integration in host chromosomes is random (the viral DNA is found at different locations in different cancers), the site of integration is identical within all cells of a given cancer. This would not occur if HTLV-1 were merely a passenger that infects cells after transformation; rather, it means that HTLV-1 must have been present at the moment of transformation, placing it at the "scene of the crime."

The HTLV-1 genome contains the *gag, pol, env,* and long-terminal-repeat regions typical of all retroviruses, but, in contrast to other leukemia viruses, it contains another gene referred to as *tax.* **Several aspects of HTLV-1's transforming activity are attributable to Tax, the protein product of the *tax* gene.** Tax is essential for viral replication, because it stimulates transcription of viral RNA from the 5′ long-terminal repeat. However, Tax also alters the transcription of several host cell genes and interacts with certain host cell signaling proteins. By doing so, Tax contributes to the acquisition of several cancer hallmarks, including the following:

- *Increased survival and growth of infected cells.* Tax appears to interact with PI3 kinase and thereby stimulate the downstream signaling cascade, which you will recall promotes both cell survival and metabolic alterations that enhance cell growth. Tax also upregulates the expression of cyclin D and represses the expression of multiple CDK inhibitors, changes that promote cell cycle progression. Finally, Tax can activate the transcription factor NF-κB, which promotes the survival of many cell types, including lymphocytes.
- *Increased genomic instability.* Tax may also cause genomic instability by interfering with DNA-repair functions and inhibiting cell cycle checkpoints activated by DNA damage. In line with these defects, HTLV-1–associated leukemias tend to be highly aneuploid.

The precise steps that lead to the development of adult T-cell leukemia/lymphoma are still not known, but a plausible scenario is as follows. Infection by HTLV-1 causes the expansion of a nonmalignant polyclonal cell population through stimulatory effects of Tax on cell proliferation. The proliferating T cells are at increased risk for mutations and genomic instability due to the effects of Tax and possibly other viral factors as well. This instability allows the accumulation of oncogenic mutations and eventually a monoclonal neoplastic T-cell population emerges. The most common driver mutations identified thus far are predicted to enhance T cell receptor signaling and stimulate NF-κB activation.

SUMMARY

ONCOGENIC RNA VIRUSES

- HTLV-I causes a T cell leukemia that is endemic in Japan and the Caribbean.
- The HTLV-I genome encodes a viral protein called *Tax,* which stimulates proliferation, enhances cell survival, and interferes with cell cycle controls. Although this proliferation initially is polyclonal, the proliferating T cells are at increased risk for secondary mutations that may lead to the outgrowth of a monoclonal leukemia.

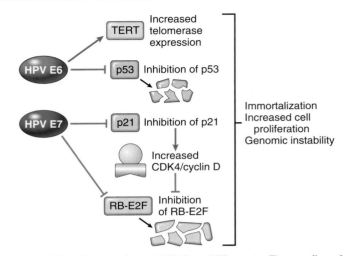

Fig. 6.33 Transforming effects of HPV E6 and E7 proteins. The net effect of HPV E6 and E7 proteins is to immortalize cells and remove the restraints on cell proliferation.

Oncogenic DNA Viruses

As with RNA viruses, several oncogenic DNA viruses that cause tumors in animals have been identified. Five DNA viruses—HPV, Epstein-Barr virus (EBV), Kaposi sarcoma herpesvirus (KSHV, also called human herpesvirus-8 [HHV-8]), a polyoma virus called Merkel cell virus, and hepatitis B virus (HBV)—are of special interest because they are strongly associated with human cancer. KSHV and Kaposi sarcoma are discussed in Chapter 5. Merkel cell virus is associated with a particular cancer, Merkel cell carcinoma, that is too rare to merit further discussion. The others are presented here. We also briefly touch on the oncogenic effects of hepatitis C virus, an RNA virus, during our discussion of HBV, since both viruses share an association with chronic liver injury and liver cancer.

Human Papillomavirus

Scores of genetically distinct types of HPV have been identified. Some types (e.g., 1, 2, 4, and 7) cause benign squamous papillomas (warts) in humans (Chapters 18 and 24). Genital warts have low malignant potential and are also associated with low-risk HPVs, predominantly HPV-6 and HPV-11. By contrast, high-risk HPVs (e.g., types 16 and 18) cause several cancers, particularly squamous cell carcinoma of the cervix and anogenital region. In addition, at least 20% of oropharyngeal cancers, particularly those arising in the tonsils, are associated with high-risk HPVs.

The oncogenic potential of HPV can be related to products of two early viral genes, E6 and E7 (Fig. 6.33), each of which has several activities that are pro-oncogenic.

- *Oncogenic activities of E6.* The E6 protein binds to and mediates the degradation of p53, and also stimulates the expression of TERT, the catalytic subunit of telomerase, which you will recall contributes to the immortalization of cells. E6 from high-risk HPV types has a higher affinity for p53 than E6 from low-risk HPV types, a property that is likely to contribute to oncogenesis.
- *Oncogenic activities of E7.* The E7 protein has effects that complement those of E6, all of which are centered on

speeding cells through the G$_1$-S cell cycle checkpoint. It binds to the RB protein and displaces the E2F transcription factors that are normally sequestered by RB, promoting progression through the cell cycle. As with E6 proteins and p53, E7 proteins from high-risk HPV types have a higher affinity for RB than do E7 proteins from low-risk HPV types. E7 also inactivates the CDK inhibitors p21 and p27, and binds and presumably activates cyclins E and A.

An additional factor that contributes to the oncogenic potential of HPVs is viral integration into the host genome. In benign warts, the HPV genome is maintained in a non-integrated episomal form, while in cancers, the HPV genome is randomly integrated into the host genome. Integration interrupts a negative regulatory region in the viral DNA, resulting in overexpression of the E6 and E7 oncoproteins. Furthermore, cells in which the viral genome has integrated show significantly more genomic instability, which may contribute to acquisition of pro-oncogenic mutations in host cancer genes.

To summarize, **high-risk HPVs encode oncogenic proteins that inactivate RB and p53, activate cyclin/CDK complexes, and combat cellular senescence.** Thus, it is evident that HPV proteins promote many of the hallmarks of cancer. The primacy of HPV infection in the causation of cervical cancer is confirmed by the effectiveness of HPV vaccines in preventing it. However, infection with HPV itself is not sufficient for carcinogenesis, and full-blown transformation requires the acquisition of mutations in host cancer genes, such as *RAS*. A high proportion of women infected with HPV clear the infection by immunologic mechanisms, but others do not, some because of acquired immune abnormalities, such as those that result from HIV infection. As might be expected, women who are coinfected with high-risk HPV types and HIV are at particularly high risk for developing cervical cancer.

Epstein-Barr Virus

EBV, a member of the herpesvirus family, was the first virus linked to a human tumor, Burkitt lymphoma. Burkitt lymphoma is an aggressive tumor that is endemic in certain parts of Africa and occurs sporadically elsewhere. In endemic areas, the tumor cells in virtually all affected patients carry the EBV genome. Since its initial discovery in Burkitt lymphoma some 50 years ago, EBV has been detected within the cells of a surprisingly diverse list of other tumors, including most nasopharyngeal carcinomas and a subset of T cell lymphomas, NK cell lymphomas, gastric carcinomas, and even, in rare instances, sarcomas, mainly in the immunosuppressed.

The manner in which EBV causes B cell tumors such as Burkitt lymphoma is complex and incompletely understood, but best appreciated by considering its effects on normal B cells. EBV uses the complement receptor CD21 to attach to and infect B cells. In vitro, such infection leads to polyclonal B cell proliferation and generation of immortal B lymphoblastoid cell lines. One EBV-encoded gene, *LMP1* (latent membrane protein 1), acts as an oncogene, as proven by its ability to induce B cell lymphomas in transgenic mice. LMP1 promotes B cell proliferation, mimicking

the effects of a key surface receptor known as CD40. CD40 is normally activated by interaction with CD40 ligands expressed mainly on T cells. By contrast, LMP1 is constitutively active and stimulates signaling through the NF-κB and JAK/STAT pathways, both of which promote B cell proliferation and survival. Thus, the virus "borrows" a normal B cell activation pathway to promote its own replication by expanding the pool of infected cells. Another EBV-encoded protein, EBNA2, transactivates several host genes, including cyclin D and the *SRC* family of proto-oncogenes. In addition, the EBV genome contains a viral cytokine, vIL-10, that was pirated from the host genome. This viral cytokine can prevent macrophages and monocytes from activating T cells and killing virally infected cells. In immunologically normal persons, the EBV-driven polyclonal B cell proliferation is readily controlled by cytotoxic T cells, and the affected patient either remains asymptomatic or experiences a self-limited episode of infectious mononucleosis. However, a small number of EBV-infected B cells downregulate expression of immunogenic viral proteins such as LMP-1 and EBNA2 and enter a long-lived pool of memory B cells that persist throughout life.

Given these observations, how then does EBV contribute to the genesis of endemic Burkitt lymphoma? One possibility is shown in Fig. 6.34. In regions of the world where

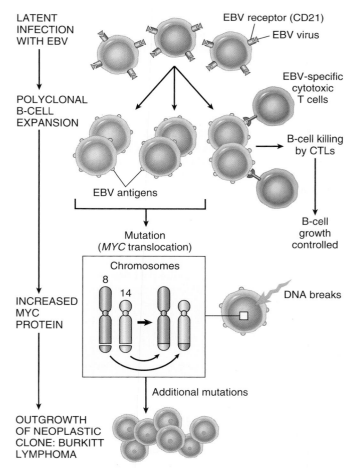

Fig. 6.34 Possible evolution of EBV-induced Burkitt lymphoma.

Burkitt lymphoma is endemic, concomitant infections such as malaria impair immune competence, allowing sustained B-cell proliferation. Eventually, cytotoxic T cells eliminate most of the EBV-infected B cells, but a small number survive. It appears that lymphoma cells emerge from this residual population only with the acquisition of specific mutations, most notably translocations that activate the *MYC* oncogene. It should be noted that in nonendemic areas 80% of these tumors are unrelated to EBV, but virtually all endemic and sporadic tumors possess the t(8;14) translocation or other translocations that dysregulate *MYC*. Thus, although sporadic Burkitt lymphomas are triggered by mechanisms other than EBV infection, they appear to develop through similar oncogenic pathways.

The oncogenic role played by EBV is more direct in EBV-positive B-cell lymphomas in immunosuppressed patients. Some individuals with AIDS or who receive immunosuppressive therapy for preventing allograft rejection develop EBV-positive B-cell tumors, often at multiple sites. These proliferations are polyclonal at the outset but can evolve into monoclonal neoplasms. In contrast to Burkitt lymphoma, the tumors in immunosuppressed patients usually lack *MYC* translocations and uniformly express LMP-1 and EBNA2, which, as discussed, are antigenic and can be recognized by cytotoxic T cells. These potentially lethal proliferations can be subdued if T cell function can be restored, as may occur with withdrawal of immunosuppressive drugs in transplant recipients.

Nasopharyngeal carcinoma also is associated with EBV infection. This tumor is endemic in southern China, in some parts of Africa, and in the Inuit population of the Arctic. In contrast to Burkitt lymphoma, 100% of nasopharyngeal carcinomas obtained from all parts of the world contain EBV. The integration site of the viral genome is identical (clonal) in all of the tumor cells within individual tumors, excluding the possibility that EBV infection occurred after tumor development. The uniform association of EBV with nasopharyngeal carcinoma suggests that EBV has a central role in the genesis of the tumor, but (as with Burkitt lymphoma) the restricted geographic distribution indicates that genetic or environmental cofactors, or both, also contribute to tumor development. Unlike Burkitt lymphoma, LMP-1 is expressed in nasopharyngeal carcinoma cells and, as in B cells, activates the NF-κB pathway. NF-κB, in turn, upregulates the expression of factors such as VEGF and matrix metalloproteases that may contribute to oncogenesis.

The relationship of EBV to the pathogenesis of Hodgkin lymphoma, yet another EBV-associated tumor, is discussed in Chapter 12.

SUMMARY

ONCOGENIC DNA VIRUSES

- HPV is associated with benign warts, as well as cervical cancer.
- The oncogenicity of HPV is related to the expression of two viral oncoproteins, E6 and E7, which bind to the p53 and RB tumor suppressors, respectively, neutralizing their function.
- E6 and E7 from high-risk strains of HPV (which give rise to cancers) have higher affinity for their targets than do E6 and E7 from low-risk strains of HPV (which give rise to benign warts).
- EBV is implicated in the pathogenesis of Burkitt lymphomas, lymphomas in immunosuppressed patients, Hodgkin lymphoma, uncommon T-cell and NK-cell tumors, nasopharyngeal carcinoma, a subset of gastric carcinoma, and rarely sarcomas.
- Certain EBV gene products contribute to oncogenesis by stimulating normal B-cell proliferation pathways. Concomitant compromise of immune competence allows sustained B-cell proliferation, leading eventually to development of lymphoma.

Hepatitis B and Hepatitis C Viruses

The epidemiologic evidence linking chronic HBV and hepatitis C virus (HCV) infection with hepatocellular carcinoma is strong (Chapter 16). **It is estimated that 70% to 85% of hepatocellular carcinomas worldwide are caused by HBV or HCV.** However, the mode of action of these viruses in tumorigenesis is not fully elucidated. The HBV and HCV genomes do not encode any viral oncoproteins, and although the HBV DNA is integrated within the human genome, there is no consistent pattern of integration in liver cells. Indeed, the oncogenic effects of HBV and HCV are multifactorial, but the dominant effect seems to be immunologically mediated chronic inflammation with hepatocyte death, leading to regeneration and genomic damage. Although the immune system generally is thought to be protective, recent work has demonstrated that in the setting of unresolved chronic inflammation, as occurs in viral hepatitis or chronic gastritis caused by *H. pylori* (see later), the immune response may become maladaptive, promoting tumorigenesis.

As with any cause of hepatocellular injury, chronic viral infection leads to the compensatory proliferation of hepatocytes. This regenerative process is aided and abetted by a plethora of growth factors, cytokines, chemokines, and other bioactive substances produced by activated immune cells that promote cell survival, tissue remodeling, and angiogenesis. The activated immune cells also produce other mediators, such as reactive oxygen species, that are genotoxic and mutagenic. A key molecular step seems to be activation of the nuclear factor-κB (NF-κB) pathway in hepatocytes caused by mediators derived from the activated immune cells. Activation of the NF-κB pathway blocks apoptosis, allowing the dividing hepatocytes to incur genotoxic stress and to accumulate mutations. Although this seems to be the dominant mechanism in the pathogenesis of virus-induced hepatocellular carcinoma, both HBV and HCV also contain proteins within their genomes that may more directly promote the development of cancer. The HBV genome contains a gene known as *HBx*, and hepatocellular cancers develop in mice engineered to have HBx transgenes. *HBx* can directly or indirectly activate a variety of transcription factors and several signal transduction pathways, and may interfere with p53 function. In addition, viral integration can cause secondary rearrangements of chromosomes, including multiple deletions that may harbor unknown tumor suppressor genes.

HCV, an RNA virus, also is strongly linked to the pathogenesis of liver cancer. The molecular mechanisms used by HCV are even less well defined than those for HBV. In addition to chronic liver cell injury and compensatory regeneration, components of the HCV genome, such as the HCV core protein, may have a direct effect on tumorigenesis, possibly by activating a variety of growth-promoting signal transduction pathways.

SUMMARY

HEPATITIS B AND HEPATITIS C VIRUSES

- Between 70% and 85% of hepatocellular carcinomas worldwide are due to infection with HBV or HCV.
- The oncogenic effects of HBV and HCV are multifactorial, but the dominant effect seems to be immunologically mediated chronic inflammation, with hepatocellular injury, stimulation of hepatocyte proliferation, and production of reactive oxygen species that can damage DNA.
- The HBx protein of HBV and the HCV core protein can activate a variety of signal transduction pathways that also may contribute to carcinogenesis.

Helicobacter pylori

H. pylori infection is implicated in the genesis of both gastric adenocarcinomas and gastric lymphomas. First incriminated as a cause of peptic ulcers, *H. pylori* now has acquired the dubious distinction of being the first bacterium classified as a carcinogen.

The scenario for the development of gastric adenocarcinoma is similar to that for HBV- and HCV-induced liver cancer. It involves increased epithelial cell proliferation on a background of chronic inflammation. As in viral hepatitis, the inflammatory milieu contains numerous genotoxic agents, such as reactive oxygen species. The sequence of histopathologic changes consists of initial development of chronic inflammation/gastritis, followed by gastric atrophy, intestinal metaplasia of the lining cells, dysplasia, and cancer. This sequence takes decades to complete and occurs in only 3% of infected patients. Like those of HBV and HCV, the *H. pylori* genome also contains genes directly implicated in oncogenesis. Strains associated with gastric adenocarcinoma have been shown to contain a "pathogenicity island" that contains cytotoxin-associated A gene (*CagA*). Although *H. pylori* is noninvasive, *CagA* is injected into gastric epithelial cells, where it has a variety of effects, including the initiation of a signaling cascade that mimics unregulated growth factor stimulation.

As mentioned earlier, *H. pylori* is associated with an increased risk for the development of gastric lymphomas as well. The gastric lymphomas are of B-cell origin, and because the transformed B cells grow in a pattern resembling that of normal mucosa-associated lymphoid tissue (MALT), they have been referred to as *MALT lymphomas* (Chapter 12). Their molecular pathogenesis is incompletely understood but seems to involve strain-specific *H. pylori* factors, as well as host genetic factors, such as polymorphisms in the promoters of inflammatory cytokines such as IL-1β and tumor necrosis factor (TNF). It is thought that *H. pylori* infection leads to the activation of *H. pylori*–reactive T cells, which in turn cause polyclonal B cell proliferation. In time, a monoclonal B cell tumor emerges from the proliferating B cells, perhaps as a result of accumulation of mutations in growth regulatory genes. In keeping with this model, early in the course of disease, eradication of *H. pylori* with antibiotics causes regression of the lymphoma by removing the antigenic stimulus for T cells. MALT lymphoma is thus a remarkable example of a tumor that depends on signals elicited by interactions with host immune cells for its continued growth and survival.

SUMMARY

HELICOBACTER PYLORI

- *H. pylori* infection has been implicated in both gastric adenocarcinoma and MALT lymphoma.
- The mechanism of *H. pylori*–induced gastric cancers is multifactorial, including immunologically mediated chronic inflammation, stimulation of gastric cell proliferation, and production of reactive oxygen species that damage DNA. *H. pylori* pathogenicity genes, such as *CagA*, also may contribute by stimulating growth factor pathways.
- It is thought that *H. pylori* infection leads to polyclonal B-cell proliferations and that eventually a monoclonal B-cell tumor (MALT lymphoma) emerges as a result of accumulation of mutations.

CLINICAL ASPECTS OF NEOPLASIA

The importance of neoplasms ultimately lies in their effects on patients. Although malignant tumors are of course more threatening than benign tumors, morbidity and mortality may be associated with any tumor, even a benign one. Indeed, both malignant and benign tumors may cause problems because of (1) location and impingement on adjacent structures, (2) functional activity such as hormone synthesis or the development of paraneoplastic syndromes, (3) bleeding and infections when the tumor ulcerates through adjacent surfaces, (4) symptoms that result from rupture or infarction, and (5) cachexia or wasting. The following discussion considers the effects of a tumor on the host, the grading and clinical staging of cancer, and the laboratory diagnosis of neoplasms.

Effects of Tumor on Host

Location is crucial in both benign and malignant tumors. A small (1-cm) pituitary adenoma can compress and destroy the surrounding normal gland, giving rise to hypopituitarism. A 0.5-cm leiomyoma in the wall of the renal artery may encroach on the blood supply, leading to renal ischemia and hypertension. A comparably small carcinoma within the common bile duct may induce fatal biliary tract obstruction.

Signs and symptoms related to hormone production are often seen in patients with benign and malignant neoplasms arising in endocrine glands. Adenomas and carcinomas arising in the beta cells of the pancreatic islets of Langerhans can produce hyperinsulinism, sometimes fatal. Similarly, some adenomas and carcinomas of the adrenal cortex disrupt homeostatic mechanisms by elaborating steroid hormones (e.g., aldosterone, which induces sodium retention, hypertension, and hypokalemia). Such hormonal activity is more likely with a well-differentiated benign tumor than with a corresponding carcinoma.

A tumor may ulcerate through a surface, with consequent bleeding or secondary infection. Benign or malignant neoplasms that protrude into the gut lumen may become caught in the peristaltic pull of the gut, causing intussusception (Chapter 15) and intestinal obstruction or infarction.

Cancer Cachexia

Many cancer patients suffer progressive loss of body fat and lean body mass, accompanied by profound weakness, anorexia, and anemia—a condition referred to as *cachexia.* There is some correlation between the size and extent of spread of the cancer and the severity of the cachexia. However, cachexia is not caused by the nutritional demands of the tumor. Although patients with cancer often are anorexic, current evidence indicates that cachexia results from the action of soluble factors such as cytokines produced by the tumor and the host, rather than reduced food intake. In patients with cancer, calorie expenditure remains high, and basal metabolic rate is increased, despite reduced food intake. This is in contrast with the lower metabolic rate that occurs as an adaptive response in starvation. The basis of these metabolic abnormalities is not fully understood. It is suspected that TNF and other cytokines produced by macrophages in response to tumor cells or by the tumor cells themselves mediate cachexia. TNF suppresses appetite and inhibits the action of lipoprotein lipase, preventing the release of free fatty acids from lipoproteins. There is no satisfactory treatment for cancer cachexia other than removal of the underlying cause, the tumor.

Paraneoplastic Syndromes

Symptom complexes that occur in patients with cancer and that cannot be readily explained by local or distant spread of the tumor or by the elaboration of hormones indigenous to the tissue of origin of the tumor are referred to as *paraneoplastic syndromes.* They appear in 10% to 15% of patients with cancer, and their clinical recognition is important for several reasons:

- Such syndromes may represent the earliest manifestation of an occult neoplasm.
- In affected patients, the pathologic changes may be associated with significant clinical illness and may even be lethal.
- The symptom complex may mimic metastatic disease, thereby confounding treatment.

The paraneoplastic syndromes are diverse and are associated with many different tumors (Table 6.6). **The most common paraneoplastic syndromes are hypercalcemia, Cushing syndrome, and nonbacterial thrombotic endocarditis**, and the neoplasms most often associated with these and other syndromes are lung and breast cancers and hematologic malignancies. Hypercalcemia in cancer patients is multifactorial, but the most important mechanism is the synthesis of a parathyroid hormone–related protein (PTHrP) by tumor cells. Also implicated are other tumor-derived factors, such as TGF-α and the active form of vitamin D. Another possible mechanism for hypercalcemia is widespread osteolytic metastatic disease of bone; of note, however, hypercalcemia resulting from skeletal metastases is not a paraneoplastic syndrome. Cushing syndrome arising as a paraneoplastic phenomenon usually is related to ectopic production of ACTH or ACTH-like polypeptides by cancer cells, as occurs in small cell carcinoma of the lung.

Paraneoplastic syndromes also may manifest as hypercoagulability, leading to venous thrombosis and nonbacterial thrombotic endocarditis (Chapter 11). Other manifestations are clubbing of the fingers and hypertrophic osteoarthropathy in patients with lung carcinomas (Chapter 13). Still others are discussed in the consideration of cancers of the various organs of the body.

Grading and Staging of Cancer

Methods to quantify the probable clinical aggressiveness of a given neoplasm and its apparent extent and spread in the individual patient are necessary for arriving at an accurate prognosis and for comparing end results of various treatment protocols. For instance, the results of treating well-differentiated thyroid adenocarcinomas localized to the thyroid gland will on average be very different from those obtained from treating highly anaplastic thyroid cancers that have invaded the neck organs. Systems have been developed to express, at least in semiquantitative terms, the level of differentiation, or *grade,* and extent of spread of a cancer within the patient, or *stage,* as parameters of the clinical gravity of the disease. Of note, **when compared with grading, staging has proved to be of greater clinical value.**

- *Grading.* Grading of a cancer is based on the degree of differentiation of the tumor cells and, in some cancers, the number of mitoses and the presence of certain architectural features. Grading schemes have evolved for each type of malignancy, and generally range from two categories (low grade and high grade) to four categories. Criteria for the individual grades vary in different types of tumors and so are not detailed here, but all attempt, in essence, to judge the extent to which the tumor cells resemble or fail to resemble their normal counterparts. Although histologic grading is useful, the correlation between histologic appearance and biologic behavior is less than perfect. In recognition of this problem and to avoid spurious quantification, it is common practice to characterize a particular neoplasm in descriptive terms, for example, well-differentiated, mucin-secreting adenocarcinoma of the stomach, or poorly differentiated pancreatic adenocarcinoma.
- *Staging.* The staging of solid cancers is based on the size of the primary lesion, its extent of spread to regional lymph nodes, and the presence or absence of blood-borne metastases. The major staging system currently in use is the American Joint Committee on Cancer Staging. This system uses a classification called the *TNM system* — T for primary tumor, N for regional lymph node involvement, and M for metastases. TNM staging varies for specific forms of cancer, but there are general principles. The primary lesion is characterized as T1 to T4 based on increasing size. T0 is used to indicate an in situ

Table 6.6 Paraneoplastic Syndromes

Clinical Syndrome	Major Forms of Neoplasia	Causal Mechanism(s)/Agent(s)
Endocrinopathies		
Cushing syndrome	Small cell carcinoma of lung Pancreatic carcinoma Neural tumors	ACTH or ACTH-like substance
Syndrome of inappropriate anti-diuretic hormone secretion	Small cell carcinoma of lung; intracranial neoplasms	Anti-diuretic hormone or atrial natriuretic hormones
Hypercalcemia	Squamous cell carcinoma of lung Breast carcinoma Renal carcinoma Adult T cell leukemia/lymphoma	Parathyroid hormone–related protein, TGF-α
Hypoglycemia	Fibrosarcoma Other mesenchymal sarcomas Ovarian carcinoma	Insulin or insulin-like substance
Polycythemia	Renal carcinoma Cerebellar hemangioma Hepatocellular carcinoma	Erythropoietin
Nerve and Muscle Syndrome		
Myasthenia	Bronchogenic carcinoma, thymoma	Immunologic
Disorders of the central and peripheral nervous systems	Breast carcinoma, teratoma	Immunologic
Dermatologic Disorders		
Acanthosis nigricans	Gastric carcinoma Lung carcinoma Uterine carcinoma	Immunologic; secretion of epidermal growth factor
Dermatomyositis	Bronchogenic and breast carcinoma	Immunologic
Osseous, Articular, and Soft-Tissue Changes		
Hypertrophic osteoarthropathy and clubbing of the fingers	Bronchogenic carcinoma	Unknown
Vascular and Hematologic Changes		
Venous thrombosis (Trousseau phenomenon)	Pancreatic carcinoma Bronchogenic carcinoma Other cancers	Tumor products (mucins that activate clotting)
Nonbacterial thrombotic endocarditis	Advanced cancers	Hypercoagulability
Anemia	Thymoma	Immunologic
Others		
Nephrotic syndrome	Various cancers	Tumor antigens, immune complexes

ACTH, Adrenocorticotropic hormone; *IL-1,* interleukin-1; *TGF-α,* transforming growth factor-α; *TNF,* tumor necrosis factor.

lesion. N0 would mean no nodal involvement, whereas N1 to N3 would denote involvement of an increasing number and range of nodes. M0 signifies no distant metastases, whereas M1 or sometimes M2 reflects the presence and estimated number of metastases.

In modern practice, grading and staging of tumors are being supplemented by molecular characterization, described later.

SUMMARY

CLINICAL ASPECTS OF TUMORS

- *Cachexia,* defined as progressive loss of body fat and lean body mass, accompanied by profound weakness, anorexia, and anemia, is caused by release of cytokines by the tumor or host.
- Paraneoplastic syndromes, defined as systemic symptoms that cannot be explained by tumor spread or by hormones appropriate to the tissue, are caused by the ectopic production and secretion of bioactive substances such as ACTH, PTHrP, or TGF-α.
- Grading of tumors is determined by cytologic appearance and is based on the idea that behavior and differentiation are related, with poorly differentiated tumors having more aggressive behavior.
- Staging (extent of tumor), determined by surgical exploration or imaging, is based on size, local and regional lymph node spread, and distant metastases. Staging is of greater clinical value than grading.

Laboratory Diagnosis of Cancer

Every year the approach to laboratory diagnosis of cancer becomes more complex, more sophisticated, and more specialized. For virtually every neoplasm mentioned in this text, the experts have characterized several subcategories;

we must walk, however, before we can run. Each of the following sections attempts to present the state of the art, avoiding details of technologies.

Morphologic Methods

In most instances, the laboratory diagnosis of cancer is not difficult. The two ends of the benign–malignant spectrum pose no problems; in the middle, however, lies a "no man's land" where the wise tread cautiously. Clinicians tend to underestimate the contributions they make to the diagnosis of a neoplasm. Clinical and radiologic data are invaluable for optimal pathologic diagnosis. Radiation-induced changes in the skin or mucosa can be similar to those of cancer. Sections taken from a healing fracture can mimic an osteosarcoma. The laboratory evaluation of a lesion can be only as good as the specimen submitted for examination. The specimen must be adequate, representative, and properly preserved.

Several sampling approaches are available, including excision or biopsy, fine-needle aspiration, and cytologic smears. When excision of a lesion is not possible, selection of an appropriate site for biopsy of a large mass requires awareness that the margins may not be representative and the center may be largely necrotic. Requesting *frozen section* diagnosis is sometimes desirable, as, for example, in determining the nature of a mass lesion or in evaluating the regional lymph nodes in a patient with cancer for metastasis. This method, in which a sample is quick-frozen and sectioned, permits histologic evaluation within minutes. In experienced, competent hands, frozen section diagnosis is accurate, but there are particular instances in which the superior histologic detail provided by more time-consuming routine methods is needed. In such instances, it is better to wait a few days, despite the drawbacks, than to perform inadequate or unnecessary surgery.

Fine-needle aspiration of tumors is another approach that is widely used. It involves aspiration of cells from a mass, followed by cytologic examination of the cells after they have been spread out on a slide. This procedure is used most commonly with readily palpable lesions affecting the breast, thyroid gland, lymph nodes, and salivary glands. Modern imaging techniques permit extension of the method to deeper structures, such as the liver, pancreas, and pelvic lymph nodes. Use of this diagnostic modality obviates surgery and its attendant risks. Although it entails some difficulties, such as small sample size and sampling errors, in experienced hands it can be reliable, rapid, and useful.

Cytologic (Papanicolaou) smears provide another method for the detection of cancer. Historically, this approach has been used widely for discovery of carcinoma of the cervix, often at an in situ stage, but now it is used to investigate many other forms of suspected malignancy, such as endometrial carcinoma, bronchogenic carcinoma, bladder and prostate tumors, and gastric carcinomas; for the identification of tumor cells in abdominal, pleural, joint, and cerebrospinal fluids; and, less commonly, for evaluation of other forms of neoplasia. Neoplastic cells are less cohesive than others and are therefore shed into fluids or secretions (Fig. 6.35). The shed cells are evaluated for features of anaplasia indicative of their origin from a tumor. The

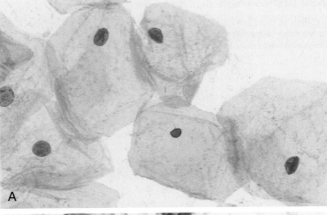

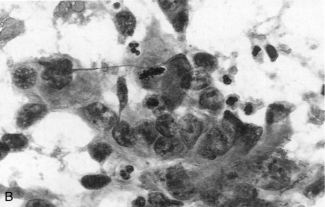

Fig. 6.35 (A) Normal Papanicolaou smear from the uterine cervix. Large, flat cells with small nuclei are typical. (B) Abnormal smear containing a sheet of malignant cells with large hyperchromatic nuclei. Nuclear pleomorphism is evident, and one cell is in mitosis. A few interspersed neutrophils, much smaller in size and with compact, lobate nuclei, are seen. *(Courtesy of Dr. Richard M. DeMay, Department of Pathology, University of Chicago, Chicago, Illinois.)*

gratifying control of cervical cancer is the best testament to the value of the cytologic method.

Immunohistochemistry offers a powerful adjunct to routine histologic examination. Detection of cytokeratin by stains performed with specific monoclonal antibodies points to a diagnosis of undifferentiated carcinoma rather than large cell lymphoma. Similarly, detection of prostate-specific antigen (PSA) in metastatic deposits by immunohistochemical staining allows definitive diagnosis of a primary tumor in the prostate gland. Immunocytochemical detection of estrogen receptors allows prognostication and directs therapeutic intervention in breast cancers.

Flow cytometry is used routinely in the classification of leukemias and lymphomas. In this method, fluorescently labeled antibodies against cell surface molecules and differentiation antigens are used to obtain the phenotype of malignant cells (Chapter 12).

Tumor Markers

Biochemical assays for tumor-associated enzymes, hormones, and other tumor markers in the blood cannot be utilized for definitive diagnosis of cancer; however, they are used with varying success as screening tests and have utility in monitoring the response to therapy or detecting disease recurrence. The application of these assays is considered with many of the specific forms of neoplasia discussed in other chapters, so only a few examples suffice here. PSA, used to screen for prostatic adenocarcinoma, is one of the most frequently used tumor markers in clinical practice. Prostatic carcinoma can be suspected when elevated levels of PSA are found in the blood. However, PSA screening also highlights problems encountered with use of virtually every tumor marker. Although PSA levels often are elevated in cancer, PSA levels also may be elevated in benign prostatic hyperplasia (Chapter 18). Furthermore, there is no PSA level that ensures that a patient does not have prostate cancer. **Thus, the PSA test suffers from both low sensitivity and low specificity, and its use as a screening tool has become quite controversial.** The PSA assay is extremely valuable, however, for detecting residual disease or recurrence following treatment for prostate cancer. Other tumor markers used in clinical practice include carcinoembryonic antigen (CEA), which is elaborated by carcinomas of the colon, pancreas, stomach, and breast, and alpha fetoprotein (AFP), which is produced by hepatocellular carcinomas, yolk sac remnants in the gonads, and occasionally teratocarcinomas and embryonal cell carcinomas. Like PSA, CEA and AFP can be elevated in a variety of non-neoplastic conditions and thus also lack the specificity and sensitivity required for the early detection of cancers, but they may be useful in monitoring disease once the diagnosis is established. With successful resection of the tumor, these markers disappear from the serum; their reappearance almost always signifies recurrence. CEA is further discussed in Chapter 15 and alpha fetoprotein in Chapter 16.

Molecular Diagnosis

An increasing number of molecular techniques are being used for the diagnosis of tumors and for predicting their behavior.

- *Diagnosis of malignancy.* Because each T cell and B cell has unique antigen receptor gene rearrangements, polymerase chain reaction (PCR)–based detection of rearranged T-cell receptor or immunoglobulin genes allows monoclonal (neoplastic) and polyclonal (reactive) proliferations to be distinguished. Many hematopoietic neoplasms, as well as a few solid tumors, are defined by particular translocations, so the diagnosis can be made by detection of such translocations. For example, fluorescence in situ hybridization (FISH) or PCR analysis (Chapter 7) can be used to detect translocations characteristic of Ewing sarcoma and several leukemias and lymphomas. PCR-based detection of *BCR-ABL* transcripts can confirm the diagnosis of chronic myeloid leukemia (Chapter 12). Finally, certain hematologic malignancies are now defined by the presence of point mutations in particular oncogenes. For example, as mentioned earlier, the diagnosis of another myeloid neoplasm called *polycythemia vera* requires the identification of specific mutations in *JAK2,* a gene that encodes a nonreceptor tyrosine kinase.
- *Prognosis and behavior.* Certain genetic alterations are associated with a poor prognosis, and thus the presence

of these alterations determines the patient's subsequent therapy. FISH and PCR methods can be used to detect amplification of oncogenes such as *HER2* and *NMYC,* which provide therapeutic and prognostic information for breast cancers and neuroblastomas, respectively. Sequencing of cancer genomes is now routine in some centers, allowing for the identification of point mutations in cancer genes such as *TP53* that predict a poor outcome in many different types of cancer. Although not yet standard of care, efforts are ongoing to develop tests that assess the host immune response to tumors, for example, by quantifying the number of infiltrating cytotoxic T cells, as this too is helpful in gauging prognosis.

- *Detection of minimal residual disease.* Another emerging use of molecular techniques is for detection of minimal residual disease after treatment. For example, detection of *BCR-ABL* transcripts by PCR assay gives a measure of residual disease in patients treated for chronic myeloid leukemia. Recognition that virtually all advanced tumors are associated with both intact circulating tumor cells and products derived from tumors (e.g., cell-free circulating tumor DNA) has led to interest in following tumor burden through sensitive blood tests designed to identify tumor-specific nucleic acid sequences.
- *Diagnosis of hereditary predisposition to cancer.* Germ line mutation of several tumor suppressor genes, such as *BRCA1,* increases a patient's risk for developing certain types of cancer. Thus, detection of these mutated alleles may allow the patient and the physician to devise an aggressive screening protocol, as well as an opportunity for prophylactic surgery. In addition, such detection allows genetic counseling of relatives who are at risk.
- *Therapeutic decision-making.* Therapies that directly target specific mutations are increasingly being developed, and thus detection of such mutations in a tumor can guide the development of targeted therapy, as discussed later. It is now becoming evident that certain targetable mutations transgress morphologic categories. One example involves a valine for glutamate substitution in amino acid 600 (V600E) of the serine/threonine kinase BRAF, which you will recall lies downstream of RAS in the growth factor signaling pathway. Melanomas with the V600E *BRAF* mutation respond well to BRAF inhibitors, whereas melanomas without this mutation show no response. Subsequently, it was realized that the same V600E mutation is also present in a subset of many other diverse cancers, including carcinomas of the colon and thyroid gland, most hairy cell leukemias, and many cases of Langerhans cell histiocytosis (Fig. 6.36). These tumors are morphologically diverse and have distinct cells of origin, but they share identical oncogenic lesions in a common pro-growth pathway.

Molecular Profiling of Tumors: The Future of Cancer Diagnostics

Until recently, molecular studies of tumors involved the analysis of individual genes. However, the past few years have seen the introduction of revolutionary technologies that can rapidly sequence an entire genome; assess

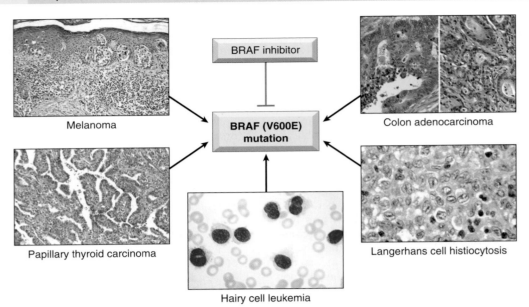

Fig. 6.36 Diverse tumor types that share a common mutation, BRAF (V600E), may be candidates for treatment with the same BRAF inhibitors.

epigenetic modifications genome-wide (the epigenome); quantify all of the RNAs expressed in a cell population (the transcriptome); measure many proteins simultaneously (the proteome); and take a snapshot of all of the cell's metabolites (the metabolome). Thus, the diagnosis, management and study of cancer has entered the age of "omics!"

The most common method for large-scale analysis of RNA expression in use in research laboratories has been based on DNA microarrays, but newer methods involving RNA sequencing that offer a more comprehensive and quantitative assessment of RNA expression are beginning to supplant older methods. However, RNA is prone to degradation and is a more difficult analyte to work with than DNA in clinical practice. Furthermore, DNA sequencing is technically simpler than RNA sequencing, permitting the development of methods that rely on massively parallel sequencing (so-called "next-generation [NextGen] sequencing") that can be readily performed on virtually any tissue specimen (Chapter 7). The increases in DNA sequencing capacity and speed that such methods have enabled over the past decade have been breathtaking, and are matched by an equally remarkable decrease in cost. The first reasonably complete draft of the sequence of the human genome, released in 2003, took 12 years of work and cost about $2,700,000,000. The cost of sequencing the whole genome has now decreased to less than $5000 in some commercial laboratories, making the test readily affordable. At present, using NextGen sequencing, the process of whole-genome of individual tumors can be completed in as little as a few weeks, which includes the time required for the extraordinarily complex task of assembling and analyzing the sequencing data.

These advances have enabled the systematic sequencing and cataloging of genomic alterations in various human cancers, an effort sponsored by the National Cancer Institute called The Cancer Genome Atlas (TCGA). The main impact of cancer genome sequencing to date has been in the area of research: identification of new mutations that

underlie various cancers; description of the full panoply of genetic lesions that are found in individual cancers; and a greater appreciation of the genetic heterogeneity that exists in individual cancers from area to area. While whole-genome sequencing to manage patients can be performed, most efforts in the clinical realm are focused on developing sequencing methods that permit identification of therapeutically "actionable" genetic lesions in a timely fashion at a reasonable cost. Such approaches seem particularly applicable to tumors, such as lung carcinomas, that are genetically diverse and require a "personalized" approach if targeted therapy is to succeed (Fig. 6.37). Thus, the current trend in molecular diagnostic laboratories is to develop methods that permit several hundred exons of key genes to be sequenced simultaneously at sufficient "depth" (fold coverage of the sequence in question) to reliably detect any mutations that might be present in as few as 5% of tumor cells. A second method that is moving into clinical practice involves the use of DNA arrays to identify changes in DNA copy number, such as amplifications and deletions. Arrays containing probes that span the entire genome at some standard spacing can detect all but the smallest copy number aberrations, providing information that is complementary to that obtained from focused DNA sequencing. Other "omics," such as proteomics and epigenomics, are currently being used mainly in the realm of clinical research, but with many drugs that target the cancer epigenome moving into the clinic, it can be anticipated that tests directed at assessing the state of the epigenome that predict response to such agents are soon to follow.

The excitement created by the development of new techniques for the global molecular analysis of tumors has led some scientists to predict that the end of histopathology is in sight. However, histopathologic inspection of tumors provides information about important characteristics of cancers, such as anaplasia, invasiveness, and tumor heterogeneity, that cannot be gleaned from DNA sequences. Histopathology coupled with in situ biomarker tests performed

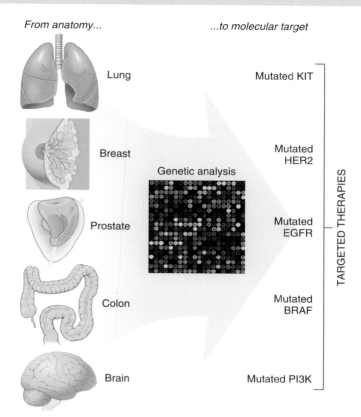

From anatomy...   ...to molecular target

Lung   Mutated KIT

Breast   Mutated HER2

Genetic analysis

Prostate   Mutated EGFR

Colon   Mutated BRAF

Brain   Mutated PI3K

TARGETED THERAPIES

Fig. 6.37 Genetic analysis of cancers is being utilized to identify mutations that can be targeted by drugs.

on tissue sections also remains the best way to assess tumor : stromal cell interactions, such as angiogenesis and host immune responses; the latter may have an increasingly important role in guiding therapeutic interventions that are designed to counteract immune evasion by tumors. Thus, what lies ahead is not the replacement of one set of techniques by another. On the contrary, for the foreseeable future the most accurate diagnosis and assessment of prognosis in cancer patients will be arrived at by a combination of morphologic and molecular techniques.

With all of the advances in genomic analyses and targeted therapies, one can safely predict that we are on the cusp of the golden age of tumor diagnosis and treatment. Those of you who are in medical school now can safely assume that the expectations for rapid advances in cancer diagnosis and therapy will be realized while you are still in practice. Get ready!

SUMMARY

LABORATORY DIAGNOSIS OF CANCER

- Several sampling approaches exist for the diagnosis of tumors, including excision, biopsy, fine-needle aspiration, and cytologic smears.
- Immunohistochemistry and flow cytometry studies help in the diagnosis and classification of tumors, because distinct protein expression patterns define different entities.

- Proteins released by tumors into the serum, such as PSA, can be used to screen populations for cancer and to monitor for recurrence after treatment.
- Molecular analyses are used to determine diagnosis and prognosis, to detect minimal residual disease, and to diagnose patients with a hereditary predisposition to cancer.
- Molecular profiling of tumors by RNA expression profiling, DNA sequencing, and DNA copy number arrays are useful in molecular stratification of otherwise identical tumors or those of distinct histogenesis that share a mutation for the purpose of targeted treatment and prognostication.
- Assays of circulating tumor cells and of DNA shed into blood, stool, sputum, and urine are under development.

SUGGESTED READINGS

Artandi SE, DePinho RA: Telomeres and telomerase in cancer, *Carcinogenesis* 31:9–18, 2010. [*A review discussing the importance of telomeres and telomerase.*]

Bai L, Wang S: Targeting apoptosis pathways for new cancer therapeutics, *Annual Rev Med* 65:139–155, 2014. [*A review of apoptosis pathways and therapeutic strategies to activate them in cancer cells.*]

Burkhart DL, Sage J: Cellular mechanisms of tumour suppression by the retinoblastoma gene, *Nat Rev Cancer* 8:671–682, 2008. [*A review of Rb function.*]

Cilloni D, Saglio G: Molecular pathways: BCR-ABL, *Clin Cancer Res* 18:930–937, 2012. [*A discussion of the functional consequences and clinical significance of aberrant tyrosine kinase activity in chronic myeloid leukemia mediated by the constitutive enzyme activity of BCR-ABL.*]

Coussens LM, Zitvogel L, Palucka AK: Neutralizing tumor-promoting chronic inflammation: a magic bullet?, *Science* 339:286–291, 2013. [*A discussion of clinical and experimental studies describing protumorigenic roles for immune cells that elicit cancer-associated inflammation.*]

Hanahan D, Coussens L: Accessories to the crime: functions of cell recruited to the tumor microenvironment, *Cancer Cell* 20:309–322, 2012. [*A review discussing the role of stroma in cancer.*]

Hanahan D, Weinberg RA: The hallmarks of cancer (2011): the next generation, *Cell* 144:646–674, 2011. [*A reexamination of the hallmarks of cancer.*]

Joerger AC, Fersht AR: The p53 pathway: Origins, inactivation in cancer, and emerging therapeutic approaches, *Annu Rev Biochem* 85:375–404, 2016. [*A wide-ranging discussion of p53 functions and dysfunction in cancer, with an eye towards development of new cancer therapies.*]

Lord C, Ashworth A: BRCAness revisited, *Nat Rev Cancer* 16:110–120, 2016. [*A discussion of how BRCAs function as tumor suppressors and how this informs therapy for tumors with evidence of BRCA dysfunction.*]

Manning AL, Dyson NJ: RB: mitotic implications of a tumour suppressor, *Nat Rev Cancer* 12:220–226, 2012. [*In addition to the well-established roles of RB in control of cell cycle progression and proliferation, this review describes other emerging tumor suppressive functions, such as maintenance of genomic stability.*]

Martinez P, Blasco MA: Telomeric and extra-telomeric roles for telomerase and the telomere-binding proteins, *Nat Rev Cancer* 11:161–176, 2011. [*A review discussing the role of telomeric proteins in immortalization of cancer cells and other emerging non-telomeric functions that may also contribute to oncogenesis.*]

Massagué J, Obenauf AC: Metastatic colonization by circulating tumour cells, *Nature* 529:298–306, 2016. [*A discussion of concepts to explain metastasis.*]

Munoz-Espin D, Serrano M: Cellular senescence: from physiology to pathology, *Nat Rev Mol Cell Biol* 15:482–496, 2014. [*A discussion of the mechanisms of senescence and their potential therapeutic relevance.*]

Nieto MA, Huang RY-J, Jackson RA, et al: EMT: 2016, *Cell* 166:21–45, 2016. *[A far-ranging discussion of the causes and consequences of epithelial-mesenchymal transition in cancer.]*

Pickup M, Novitskly S, Moses HL: The roles of TGF-β in the tumor microenvironment, *Nat Rev Cancer* 13:788–799, 2013. *[A review discussing the tumor-promoting effects of TGF-β.]*

Stine ZE, Walton ZE, Altman BJ, et al: MYC, metabolism, and cancer, *Cancer Discov* 5:1024–1039, 2015. *[A review of the connections between MYC and cancer cell metabolism.]*

Stratton MR, Campbell PJ, Futreal PA: The cancer genome, *Nature* 458:719–724, 2009. *[An excellent summary of next-generation sequencing technologies and their application to cancer.]*

van Roy F: Beyond E-cadherin: roles of other cadherin superfamily members in cancer, *Nat Rev Cancer* 14:121–134, 2014. *[A review discussing the role of members of the cadherin family in cancer.]*

Ward PS, Thompson C: Metabolic reprogramming: a cancer hallmark even Warburg did not anticipate, *Cancer Cell* 21:297–308, 2012. *[An account of the molecular pathways of reprogramming of energy metabolism in cancer and the emergence of "oncometabolites."]*

Welti J, Loges S, Dimmeler S, et al: Recent molecular discoveries in angiogenesis and anti-angiogenesis therapies in cancer, *J Clin Invest* 123:3190–3200, 2013. *[A discussion of angiogenic mechanisms and successes and challenges of anti-angiogenic therapy in cancer.]*

White E: The role of autophagy in cancer, *J Clin Invest* 125:42–46, 2016. *[A discussion of the diverse possible contributions of autophagy to cancer.]*

Genetic and Pediatric Diseases

CHAPTER OUTLINE

Genetic Diseases 243
 Nature of Genetic Abnormalities
  Contributing to Human Disease 244
 Mutations in Protein-Coding Genes 244
 Alterations in Protein-Coding Genes Other Than
  Mutations 244
 Mendelian Disorders: Diseases Caused by
  Single-Gene Defects 245
 Transmission Patterns of Single-Gene
  Disorders 246
 Diseases Caused by Mutations in Genes
  Encoding Structural Proteins 247
 Diseases Caused by Mutations in Genes
  Encoding Receptor Proteins or Channels 248
 Diseases Caused by Mutations in Genes
  Encoding Enzyme Proteins 254
 Diseases Caused by Mutations in Genes
  Encoding Proteins That Regulate Cell
  Growth 261
 Complex Multigenic Disorders 261
 Cytogenetic Disorders 262
 Numeric Abnormalities 262

Structural Abnormalities 263
General Features of Chromosomal
 Disorders 264
Cytogenetic Disorders Involving Autosomes 264
Cytogenetic Disorders Involving Sex
 Chromosomes 267
Single-Gene Disorders With Atypical
 Patterns of Inheritance 269
Triplet Repeat Mutations 269
Diseases Caused by Mutations in Mitochondrial
 Genes 271
Diseases Caused by Alterations of Imprinted
 Regions: Prader-Willi and Angelman
 Syndromes 271
Pediatric Diseases 273
 Congenital Anomalies 273
 Etiology 275
 Perinatal Infections 277
 Prematurity and Fetal Growth
  Restriction 277
 Respiratory Distress Syndrome of the
  Newborn 278

Necrotizing Enterocolitis 279
Sudden Infant Death Syndrome
 (SIDS) 280
Fetal Hydrops 282
Immune Hydrops 283
Nonimmune Hydrops 283
Tumors and Tumorlike Lesions of Infancy
 and Childhood 285
Benign Neoplasms 285
Malignant Neoplasms 286
Molecular Diagnosis of Mendelian and
 Complex Disorders 291
Indications for Genetic Analysis 292
Molecular Diagnosis of Copy Number
 Abnormalities 292
Direct Detection of DNA Mutations by
 Polymerase Chain Reaction (PCR)
 Analysis 294
Linkage Analysis and Genomewide Association
 Studies 295

Genetic Diseases

The completion of the human genome project was a landmark achievement in the study of human diseases. It established that humans have only about 25,000 protein-coding genes, far fewer than the 100,000 previously estimated and almost half the number in the lowly rice plant (*Oryza sativa*)! The unraveling of this "genetic architecture" is beginning to unlock secrets of inherited as well as acquired human disease. Powerful technologies now allow applications of the human gene sequences to the analysis of human diseases. Current high-throughput "next-generation" sequencing technologies can routinely sequence the human exome (the entire compendium of coding genes) in a couple of days for as little as $1000. The speed and reduced costs of DNA sequencing are increasingly facilitating the application of "personalized medicine" (also known as

"precision medicine") to the treatment of cancer and other diseases with a genetic component.

Because disorders of childhood are of genetic origin, developmental and pediatric diseases are discussed along with genetic diseases in this chapter. However, it must be borne in mind that not all genetic disorders manifest in infancy and childhood, and conversely, many pediatric diseases are not of genetic origin. To the latter category belong diseases resulting from immaturity of organ systems. In this context it is helpful to clarify three commonly used terms: hereditary, familial, and congenital. *Hereditary disorders,* by definition, are derived from one's parents, are transmitted in the gametes through the generations, and therefore are familial. The term *congenital* simply implies "present at birth." Of note, some congenital diseases are not genetic (e.g., congenital syphilis). On the other hand, not all genetic diseases are congenital; the expression of Huntington disease, for example, begins only after the third or fourth decade of life.

NATURE OF GENETIC ABNORMALITIES CONTRIBUTING TO HUMAN DISEASE

There are several types of genetic abnormalities that affect the structure and function of proteins, disrupting cellular homeostasis and contributing to disease.

Mutations in Protein-Coding Genes

The term *mutation* refers to permanent changes in the DNA. Those that affect germ cells are transmitted to the progeny and may give rise to inherited diseases. Mutations in somatic cells are not transmitted to the progeny but are important in the causation of cancers and some congenital malformations.

Details of specific mutations and their effects are discussed along with the relevant disorders throughout this book. Cited here are some common examples of gene mutations and their effects:

- *Point mutations* result from the substitution of a single nucleotide base by a different base, resulting in the replacement of one amino acid by another in the protein product. The mutation in the β-globin chain of hemoglobin giving rise to sickle cell anemia is an excellent example of a point mutation that alters the meaning of the genetic code. Such mutations are sometimes called missense mutations. By contrast, certain point mutations may change an amino acid codon to a chain termination codon, or a stop codon. Such *"nonsense" mutations* interrupt translation, and in most cases RNAs are rapidly degraded, a phenomenon called *nonsense mediated decay*, such that little or no protein is formed.
- *Frameshift mutations* occur when the insertion or deletion of one or two base pairs alters the reading frame of the DNA strand.
- *Trinucleotide repeat mutations* belong to a special category, because these mutations are characterized by amplification of a sequence of three nucleotides. Although the specific nucleotide sequence that undergoes amplification varies with different disorders, all affected sequences share the nucleotides guanine (G) and cytosine (C). For example, in fragile X syndrome, prototypical of this category of disorders, there are 200 to 4000 tandem repeats of the sequence CGG within a gene called *FMR1*. In normal populations, the number of repeats is small, averaging 29. The expansions of the trinucleotide sequences prevent normal expression of the *FMR1* gene, thus giving rise to mental retardation. Another distinguishing feature of trinucleotide repeat mutations is that they are dynamic (i.e., the degree of amplification increases during gametogenesis). These features, discussed in greater detail later in this chapter, influence the pattern of inheritance

and the phenotypic manifestations of the diseases caused by this class of mutations.

Alterations in Protein-Coding Genes Other Than Mutations

In addition to alterations in DNA sequence, coding genes also can undergo structural variations, such as copy number changes—*amplifications* or *deletions*—or *translocations* that result in aberrant gain or loss of protein function. As with mutations, structural changes may occur in the germline, or be acquired in somatic tissues. In many instances, pathogenic germline alterations involve a contiguous portion of a chromosome rather than a single gene, such as in the 22q microdeletion syndrome, discussed later. With the widespread availability of next-generation sequencing technology for assessing DNA copy number variation at very high resolution genome wide, pathogenic structural alterations have now been discovered in common disorders such as autism. Cancers often contain somatically acquired structural alterations, including amplifications, deletions, and translocations. The so-called "Philadelphia chromosome"—translocation t(9;22) between the *BCR* and *ABL* genes in chronic myeloid leukemia (Chapter 12)—is a classic example.

Alterations in Non-Coding RNAs

It is worth noting that until recently the major focus of gene hunting has been discovery of genes that encode proteins. Recent studies indicate, however, that a very large number of genes do not encode proteins. Instead, the non-encoded products of these genes—so-called "non-coding RNAs (ncRNAs)"—play important regulatory functions. Although many distinct families of ncRNAs exist, the two most important examples,—small RNA molecules called microRNAs (miRNAs) and long non-coding RNAs (lncRNAs)—are discussed in Chapter 1.

With this brief review of the nature of abnormalities that contribute to the pathogenesis of human diseases, we can turn our attention to the three major categories of genetic disorders:

- *Mendelian disorders resulting from mutations in single genes.* The genetic abnormalities show high penetrance, meaning that most individuals who inherit the anomaly show phenotypic effects. These diseases are hereditary and familial. They include many uncommon conditions, such as storage diseases and inborn errors of metabolism.
- *Complex disorders involving multiple genes as well as environmental influences.* These are sometimes called multifactorial diseases. They include some of the most common disorders of mankind, including hypertension, diabetes, and allergic and autoimmune diseases.
- *Diseases arising from chromosomal abnormalities*, including changes in the number or structure of chromosomes. Several rare developmental abnormalities are attributable to chromosomal alterations.
- *Other genetic diseases*, which involve single gene mutations but do not follow simple mendelian rules of inheritance. These single-gene disorders with nonclassic

inheritance patterns include those resulting from triplet repeat mutations or from mutations in mitochondrial DNA, and those in which the transmission is influenced by an epigenetic phenomenon called genomic imprinting. Each of these four categories is discussed separately.

MENDELIAN DISORDERS: DISEASES CAUSED BY SINGLE-GENE DEFECTS

Single-gene defects (mutations) follow the well-known mendelian patterns of inheritance (Tables 7.1 and 7.2). Although individually rare, together they account for approximately 1% of all adult admissions to hospitals and about 6% to 8% of all pediatric hospital admissions. Listed next are a few important tenets and caveats when considering mendelian disorders:

- **Mutations involving single genes follow one of three patterns of inheritance: autosomal dominant, autosomal recessive, or X-linked.**
- A single-gene mutation may have many phenotypic effects *(pleiotropy)* and, conversely, mutations at several genetic loci may produce the same trait *(genetic heterogeneity)*. For example, Marfan syndrome, which results from a basic defect in connective tissue, is associated with widespread effects involving the skeleton, eyes, and cardiovascular system, all of which stem from a mutation in the gene encoding fibrillin, a component of connective tissues. On the other hand, several different types of mutations can cause retinitis pigmentosa, an inherited disorder associated with abnormal retinal pigmentation and consequent visual impairment.

Recognition of genetic heterogeneity not only is important in genetic counseling but also facilitates understanding of the pathogenesis of common disorders such as diabetes mellitus (Chapter 20).

- It is now increasingly recognized that the phenotypic manifestations of mutations affecting a known single

Table 7.1 Estimated Prevalence of Selected Mendelian Disorders Among Live-Born Infants

Disorder	Estimated Prevalence
Autosomal Dominant Inheritance	
Familial hypercholesterolemia	1 in 500
Polycystic kidney disease	1 in 1000
Hereditary spherocytosis	1 in 5000 (northern Europe)
Marfan syndrome	1 in 5000
Huntington disease	1 in 10,000
Autosomal Recessive Inheritance	
Sickle cell anemia	1 in 500 (U.S. African Americans)*
Cystic fibrosis	1 in 3200 (U.S. Caucasians)
Tay-Sachs disease	1 in 3500 (U.S. Ashkenazi Jewish; French Canadians)
Phenylketonuria	1 in 10,000
MPSs—all types	1 in 25,000
Glycogen storage diseases—all types	1 in 50,000
Galactosemia	1 in 60,000
X-Linked Inheritance	
Duchenne muscular dystrophy	1 in 3500 (U.S. males)
Hemophilia	1 in 5000 (U.S. males)

*The prevalence of heterozygous sickle cell trait is 1 in 12 for U.S. African Americans.
MPS, Mucopolysaccharidosis.

Table 7.2 Biochemical Basis and Inheritance Pattern for Selected Mendelian Disorders

Disease	Abnormal Protein	Protein Type/Function
Autosomal Dominant Inheritance		
Familial hypercholesterolemia	LDL receptor	Receptor transport
Marfan syndrome	Fibrillin	Structural support: extracellular matrix
Ehler-Danlos syndrome*	Collagen	Structural support: extracellular matrix
Hereditary spherocytosis	Spectrin, ankyrin, or protein 4.1	Structural support: red blood cell membrane
Neurofibromatosis, type I	Neurofibromin-1 (NF-1)	Growth regulation
Adult polycystic kidney disease	Polycystin-1 (PKD-1)	Cell–cell and cell–matrix interactions
Autosomal Recessive Inheritance		
Cystic fibrosis	Cystic fibrosis transmembrane regulator	Ion channel
Phenylketonuria	Phenylalanine hydroxylase	Enzyme
Tay-Sachs disease	Hexosaminidase	Enzyme
Severe combined immunodeficiency	Adenosine deaminase	Enzyme
α- and β-thalassemias†	Hemoglobin	Oxygen transport
Sickle cell anemia†	Hemoglobin	Oxygen transport
X-Linked Recessive Inheritance		
Hemophilia A	Factor VIII	Coagulation
Duchenne/Becker muscular dystrophy	Dystrophin	Structural support: cell membrane
Fragile X syndrome	FMRP	RNA translation

*Some variants of Ehler-Danlos syndrome have an autosomal recessive inheritance pattern.
†Although full-blown symptoms require biallelic mutations, heterozygotes for thalassemia and sickle cell anemia may present with mild clinical disease. Thus, these disorders sometimes are categorized as "autosomal codominant" entities.

gene are influenced by other genetic loci, which are called modifier genes. As discussed later in the section on cystic fibrosis these modifier loci can affect the severity or extent of the disease.

- The use of proactive prenatal genetic screening in high-risk populations (e.g., persons of Ashkenazi Jewish descent) has significantly reduced the incidence (Table 7.1) of certain genetic disorders such as Tay-Sachs disease.

Transmission Patterns of Single-Gene Disorders

Disorders of Autosomal Dominant Inheritance

Disorders of autosomal dominant inheritance are manifested in the heterozygous state, so at least one parent in an index case usually is affected. Both males and females can be affected, and both sexes can transmit the condition. When an affected person marries an unaffected one, each child has one chance in two of having the disease. The following features also pertain to autosomal dominant diseases:

- *With any autosomal dominant disorder, some patients do not have affected parents.* Such patients owe their disorder to new mutations involving either the egg or the sperm from which they were derived. Their siblings are neither affected nor at increased risk for development of the disease.
- *Clinical features can be modified by reduced penetrance and variable expressivity.* Some persons inherit the mutant gene but are phenotypically normal, a phenomenon referred to as *reduced penetrance.* The variables that affect penetrance are not clearly understood. In contrast with penetrance, if a trait is consistently associated with a mutant gene but is expressed differently among persons carrying the gene, the phenomenon is called *variable expressivity.* For example, manifestations of neurofibromatosis 1 range from brownish spots on the skin to multiple tumors and skeletal deformities.
- *In many conditions, the age at onset is delayed, and symptoms and signs do not appear until adulthood* (as in Huntington disease).
- *In autosomal dominant disorders, a 50% reduction in the normal gene product is associated with clinical signs and symptoms.* Because a 50% loss of enzyme activity can be compensated for, involved genes in autosomal dominant disorders usually do not encode enzyme proteins, but instead fall into two other categories of proteins:
  - Those involved in regulation of complex metabolic pathways, often subject to feedback control (e.g., membrane receptors, transport proteins). An example of this pathogenic mechanism is found in familial hypercholesterolemia, which results from mutation in the low-density lipoprotein (LDL) receptor gene (discussed later).
  - Key structural proteins, such as collagen and components of the red cell membrane skeleton (e.g., spectrin, abnormalities of which result in hereditary spherocytosis).

The biochemical mechanisms by which a 50% reduction in the levels of such proteins results in an abnormal phenotype are not fully understood. In some cases, especially when the gene encodes one subunit of a multimeric protein, the product of the mutant allele can interfere with the assembly of a functionally normal multimer. For example, the collagen molecule is a trimer in which the three collagen chains are arranged in a helical configuration. The presence of mutated collagen chains reduces the assembly of the remaining normal chains, producing a marked deficiency of collagen. In this instance the mutant allele is called *dominant negative,* because it impairs the function of a normal allele. This effect is illustrated in some forms of osteogenesis imperfecta (Chapter 21).

Disorders of Autosomal Recessive Inheritance

Disorders of autosomal recessive inheritance are manifested in the homozygous state. They occur when both of the alleles at a given gene locus are mutants. Therefore, such disorders are characterized by the following features: (1) The trait does not usually affect the parents, who are carriers of one diseased allele, but multiple siblings may show the disease; (2) siblings have one chance in four of being affected (i.e., the recurrence risk is 25% for each birth); and (3) if the mutant gene occurs with a low frequency in the population, there is a strong likelihood that the affected patient (the proband) is the product of a consanguineous marriage. They make up the largest group of mendelian disorders.

In contrast with the features of autosomal dominant diseases, the following features generally apply to most autosomal recessive disorders:

- *The expression of the defect tends to be more uniform than in autosomal dominant disorders.*
- *Complete penetrance is common.*
- *Onset is frequently early in life.*
- *Although new mutations for recessive disorders do occur, they are rarely detected clinically.* Because the affected person is an asymptomatic heterozygote, several generations may pass before the descendants of such a person mate with other heterozygotes and produce affected offspring.
- *In many cases, enzymes are affected by the mutation.* In heterozygotes, equal amounts of normal and defective enzyme are synthesized. Usually the natural "margin of safety" ensures that cells with half of their complement of the enzyme function normally.

X-Linked Disorders

The Y chromosome is home to the testes-determining gene SRY, which directs male sexual differentiation, but apart from very rare instances of Y-linked familial deafness, no Y chromosome–linked mendelian disorders have ever been reported. **Thus, for the most part, sex-linked disorders are X linked.** Most X-linked disorders are X-linked recessive and are characterized by the following features:

- *Heterozygous female carriers transmit them only to sons, who of course are hemizygous for the X chromosome.*
- *Heterozygous females rarely express the full phenotypic change, because they have the paired normal allele.* Although one of the X chromosomes in females is inactivated (see further text), this process of inactivation is random, which typically allows sufficient numbers of cells with the normal expressed allele to emerge.

- *An affected male does not transmit the disorder to sons, but all daughters are carriers.* Sons of heterozygous women have one chance in two of receiving the mutant gene.

SUMMARY

TRANSMISSION PATTERNS OF SINGLE-GENE DISORDERS

- Autosomal dominant disorders are characterized by expression in heterozygous state; they affect males and females equally, and both sexes can transmit the disorder.
- Autosomal dominant disorders often invovle dysfunctional receptors and structural proteins.
- Autosomal recessive diseases occur when both copies of a gene are mutated and frequently involve enzymes. Males and females are affected equally.
- X-linked disorders are transmitted by heterozygous females to their sons, who manifest the disease. Female carriers usually are unaffected because of random inactivation of one X chromosome.

Diseases Caused by Mutations in Genes Encoding Structural Proteins

Marfan Syndrome

Marfan syndrome is an autosomal dominant disorder of connective tissues, manifested principally by changes in the skeleton, eyes, and cardiovascular system. It is caused by an inherited defect in an extracellular glycoprotein called *fibrillin-1.* This glycoprotein, secreted by fibroblasts, is the major component of microfibrils found in the extracellular matrix. Microfibrils serve as scaffolding for the deposition of tropoelastin, an integral component of elastic fibers. Although microfibrils are widely distributed in the body, they are particularly abundant in the aorta, ligaments, and the ciliary zonules that support the ocular lens, precisely the tissues that are prominently affected in Marfan syndrome.

Fibrillin is encoded by the *FBN1* gene, which maps to chromosomal locus 15q21. Mutations in *FBN1* are found in all patients with Marfan syndrome. More than 1800 distinct causative mutations in the very large *FBN1* gene have been found, a level of complexity that complicates diagnosis by DNA sequencing. As a result, the diagnosis is mainly based on clinical findings. Because heterozygotes have clinical symptoms, it is thought that the mutant fibrillin protein may act as a dominant negative, preventing the assembly of normal microfibrils. The prevalence of Marfan syndrome is estimated to be 1 in 5000. Approximately 70% to 85% of cases are familial, and the rest are sporadic, arising from de novo *FBN1* mutations in the germ cells of parents.

Although many of the abnormalities in Marfan syndrome can be explained on the basis of structural failure of connective tissues, some, such as overgrowth of bones, are difficult to relate to simple loss of fibrillin. It is now evident that loss of microfibrils gives rise to abnormal and excessive activation of transforming growth factor-β (TGF-β), because normal microfibrils sequester TGF-β, thereby controlling the bioavailability of this cytokine.

Excessive TGF-β signaling has deleterious effects on vascular smooth muscle development and the integrity of extracellular matrix. In support of this hypothesis, mutations in the TGF-β type II receptor give rise to a related syndrome, called Marfan syndrome type 2 (MFS2). Furthermore, patients with germline mutations in one isoform of TGF-β, called TGF-β3, present with an inherited predisposition to aortic aneurysm and other cardiovascular manifestations similar to those found in "classic" Marfan patients (see later). Of note, angiotensin receptor blockers, which inhibit the activity of TGF-β, improve aortic and cardiac function in mouse models of Marfan syndrome. Prevention of cardiovascular disease entails the use of beta-aderenergic blocking agents, which lower blood pressure, as well as angiotensin receptor inhibitors, which not only lower blood pressure but also interfere with TGF-β activity.

MORPHOLOGY

Skeletal abnormalities are the most obvious feature of Marfan syndrome. Patients have a slender, elongated habitus with abnormally long legs, arms, and fingers (arachnodactyly); a high-arched palate; and hyperextensibility of joints. A variety of spinal deformities, such as severe kyphoscoliosis, may be present. The chest is deformed, exhibiting either pectus excavatum (i.e., deeply depressed sternum) or a pigeon-breast deformity. The most characteristic **ocular change** is bilateral dislocation, or subluxation, of the lens secondary to weakness of its suspensory ligaments **(ectopia lentis).** Ectopia lentis, particularly if bilateral, is highly specific for Marfan syndrome and strongly suggests the diagnosis. Most serious, however, is the involvement of the **cardiovascular system.** Fragmentation of the elastic fibers in the tunica media of the aorta predisposes affected patients to aneurysmal dilation and aortic dissection (Chapter 10). These changes, called **cystic medionecrosis,** are not specific for Marfan syndrome; similar lesions occur in hypertension and with aging. Loss of medial support causes dilation of the aortic valve ring, giving rise to aortic incompetence. The cardiac valves, especially the mitral valve, may be excessively distensible and regurgitant **(floppy valve syndrome),** giving rise to mitral valve prolapse and congestive cardiac failure (Chapter 11). Aortic rupture is the most common cause of death and may occur at any age. Less frequently, cardiac failure is the terminal event.

Although the lesions described are typical of Marfan syndrome, they are not seen in all cases. There is much variation in clinical expression, and some patients may exhibit predominantly cardiovascular lesions with minimal skeletal and ocular changes. It is believed that the variable expressivity is related to different mutations in the *FBN1* gene.

SUMMARY

MARFAN SYNDROME

- Marfan syndrome is caused by a mutation in the *FBN1* gene encoding fibrillin, which is required for structural integrity of connective tissues and activation of TGF-β.
- The major tissues affected are the skeleton, eyes, and cardiovascular system.

- Clinical features may include tall stature, long fingers, bilateral subluxation of lens, mitral valve prolapse, aortic aneurysm, and aortic dissection.
- Prevention of cardiovascular disease involves the use of drugs that lower blood pressure and inhibit TGF-β signaling.

Ehlers-Danlos Syndromes

Ehlers-Danlos syndromes (EDSs) are a group of diseases characterized by defects in collagen synthesis or structure. All are single-gene disorders, but the mode of inheritance encompasses both autosomal dominant and recessive patterns. There are approximately 30 distinct types of collagen; all have characteristic tissue distributions and are the products of different genes. To some extent, the clinical heterogeneity of EDS can be explained by mutations in different collagen genes.

At least six clinical and genetic variants of EDS are recognized. Because defective collagen is the basis for these disorders, certain clinical features are common to all variants.

- *Tissues rich in collagen, such as skin, ligaments, and joints, frequently are affected in most variants of EDS.* Because the abnormal collagen fibers lack adequate tensile strength, joints are hypermobile. These features permit grotesque contortions, such as bending the thumb backward to touch the forearm and bending the knee upward to create almost a right angle. Indeed, it is believed that most contortionists have some form of EDS; however, a predisposition to joint dislocation is one of the prices paid for this virtuosity.
- *Skin fragility. The skin is extraordinarily stretchable, extremely fragile, and vulnerable to trauma.* Minor injuries produce gaping defects, and surgical repair or any surgical intervention is accomplished only with great difficulty because of the lack of normal tensile strength.
- *Structural failure of organ or tissues.* The structural defect in connective tissue may lead to *serious internal complications,* including rupture of the colon and large arteries (vascular EDS); ocular fragility, with rupture of the cornea and retinal detachment (kyphoscoliotic EDS); and diaphragmatic hernias (classical EDS), among others.

The molecular bases for three of the more common variants are as follows:

- *Deficient synthesis of type III collagen resulting from mutations affecting the COL3A1 gene.* This variant, vascular EDS, is inherited as an autosomal dominant disorder and is characterized by weakness of tissues rich in type III collagen (e.g., blood vessels, bowel wall), predisposing them to rupture.
- *Deficiency of the enzyme lysyl hydroxylase.* Decreased hydroxylation of lysyl residues in types I and III collagen interferes with the formation of crosslinks among collagen molecules. As might be expected, this variant (kyphoscoliotic EDS), resulting from an enzyme deficiency, is inherited as an autosomal recessive disorder. Patients typically manifest with congenital scoliosis and ocular fragility.

- *Deficient synthesis of type V collagen* resulting from mutations in COL5A1 and COL5A2 is inherited as an autosomal dominant disorder and results in classical EDS.

SUMMARY

EHLERS-DANLOS SYNDROMES

- There are six variants of EDS, all characterized by defects in collagen synthesis or assembly. Each of the variants is caused by a distinct mutation.
- Clinical features may include fragile, hyperextensible skin vulnerable to trauma, hypermobile joints, and ruptures involving colon, cornea, or large arteries. Wound healing is poor.

Diseases Caused by Mutations in Genes Encoding Receptor Proteins or Channels

Familial Hypercholesterolemia

Familial hypercholesterolemia is a "receptor disease" caused by loss-of-function mutations in the gene encoding the LDL receptor, which is involved in the transport and metabolism of cholesterol. As a consequence of receptor abnormalities there is a loss of feedback control that normally holds cholesterol synthesis in check. The resulting elevated levels of cholesterol induce premature atherosclerosis and greatly increase the risk of myocardial infarction. Familial hypercholesterolemia is among the most common of mendelian disorders; the frequency of the heterozygous condition is 1 in 500 in the general population. Approximately 7% of the body's cholesterol circulates in the plasma, predominantly in the form of LDL. As might be expected, the amount of plasma cholesterol is influenced by its synthesis and catabolism, and the liver plays a crucial role in both these processes, as described later. A brief review of the synthesis and transport of cholesterol follows.

Normal Cholesterol Metabolism. Cholesterol may be derived from the diet or from endogenous synthesis. Dietary triglycerides and cholesterol are incorporated into chylomicrons in the intestinal mucosa and travel by way of the gut lymphatics to the blood. These chylomicrons are hydrolyzed by an endothelial lipoprotein lipase in the capillaries of muscle and fat. The chylomicron remnants, rich in cholesterol, are then delivered to the liver. Some of the cholesterol enters the metabolic pool (to be described), and some is excreted as free cholesterol or as bile acids into the biliary tract. The endogenous synthesis of cholesterol and LDL begins in the liver (Fig. 7.1). The first step in the synthesis is the secretion of triglyceride-rich very-low-density lipoprotein (VLDL) by the liver into the blood. In the capillaries of adipose tissue and muscle, the VLDL particle undergoes lipolysis and is converted to intermediate-density lipoprotein (IDL). In comparison with VLDL, the content of triglyceride is reduced and that of cholesteryl esters is enriched in IDL, but IDL retains on its surface the VLDL-associated apolipoproteins B-100 and E. Further metabolism of IDL occurs along two pathways: Most of the

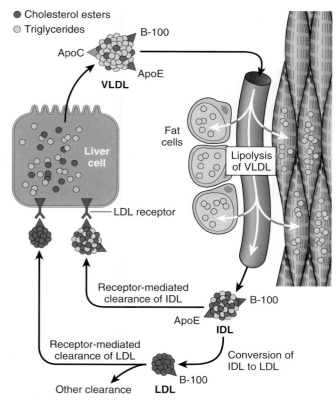

Fig. 7.1 Low-density lipoprotein (LDL) metabolism and the role of the liver in its synthesis and clearance. Lipolysis of very-low-density lipoprotein (VLDL) by lipoprotein lipase in the capillaries releases triglycerides, which are then stored in fat cells and used as a source of energy in skeletal muscles. IDL (intermediate-density lipoprotein) remains in the blood and is taken up by the liver.

IDL particles are directly taken up by the liver through the LDL receptor described later; others are converted to cholesterol-rich LDL by a further loss of triglycerides and the loss of apolipoprotein E. In the liver cells, IDL is recycled to generate VLDL.

The LDL receptor pathway metabolizes two-thirds of the resultant LDL particles, and the rest is metabolized by a receptor for oxidized LDL (scavenger receptor), to be described later. The LDL receptor binds to apolipoproteins B-100 and E and thus is involved in the transport of both LDL and IDL. Although the LDL receptors are widely distributed, approximately 75% are located on hepatocytes, so the liver plays an extremely important role in LDL metabolism. The first step in the receptor-mediated transport of LDL involves binding to the cell surface receptor, followed by endocytotic internalization inside so-called clathrin-coated pits (Fig. 7.2). Within the cell, the endocytic vesicles fuse with the lysosomes, and the LDL molecule is enzymatically degraded, resulting ultimately in the release of free cholesterol into the cytoplasm. The exit of cholesterol from the lysosomes requires the action of two proteins, called NPC1 and NPC2 (described later). The cholesterol not only is used by the cell for membrane synthesis but also takes part in intracellular cholesterol homeostasis by a sophisticated system of feedback control:

- It suppresses cholesterol synthesis by inhibiting the activity of the enzyme 3-hydroxy-3-methylglutaryl–coenzyme A reductase (HMG-CoA reductase), which is the rate-limiting enzyme in the synthetic pathway.
- It stimulates the formation of cholesterol esters for storage of excess cholesterol.
- It downregulates the synthesis of cell surface LDL receptors, thus preventing excessive accumulation of cholesterol inside cells.

The transport of LDL by the scavenger receptors, alluded to earlier, seems to occur in cells of the mononuclear-phagocyte system and possibly in other cells as well. Monocytes and macrophages have receptors for chemically modified (e.g., acetylated or oxidized) LDLs. The amount catabolized by this scavenger receptor pathway is directly related to the plasma cholesterol level.

Pathogenesis

In familial hypercholesterolemia, mutations in the LDL receptor protein impair the intracellular transport and catabolism of LDL, resulting in accumulation of LDL cholesterol in the plasma. In addition, the absence of LDL receptors on liver cells impairs the transport of IDL into the liver, so a greater proportion of plasma IDL is converted into LDL. Thus, patients with familial hypercholesterolemia develop excessive levels of serum cholesterol as a result of the combined effects of reduced catabolism and excessive biosynthesis (Fig. 7.1). This leads to a marked increase of cholesterol uptake by the monocyte-macrophages and vascular walls through the scavenger receptor. This accounts for the appearance of skin xanthomas and premature atherosclerosis.

Familial hypercholesterolemia is an autosomal dominant disease. Heterozygotes have a twofold- to threefold elevation of plasma cholesterol levels, whereas homozygotes may have in excess of a fivefold elevation. Although their cholesterol levels are elevated from birth, heterozygotes remain asymptomatic until adult life, when they develop cholesterol deposits (xanthomas) along tendon sheaths and premature atherosclerosis resulting in coronary artery disease. Homozygotes are much more severely affected, developing cutaneous xanthomas in childhood and often dying of myocardial infarction before the age of 20 years.

Analysis of the cloned LDL receptor gene has shown that more than 900 different mutations can give rise to familial hypercholesterolemia. These can be divided into five categories. Class I mutations are uncommon, and they are associated with complete loss of receptor synthesis. With class II mutations, the most prevalent type, the receptor protein is synthesized, but its transport from the endoplasmic reticulum to the Golgi apparatus is impaired because of defects in protein folding. Class III mutations produce receptors that are transported to the cell surface but fail to bind LDL normally. Class IV mutations give rise to receptors that fail to internalize within clathrin pits after binding to LDL, whereas class V mutations encode receptors that can bind LDL and are internalized but are trapped in endosomes because dissociation of receptor and bound LDL does not occur.

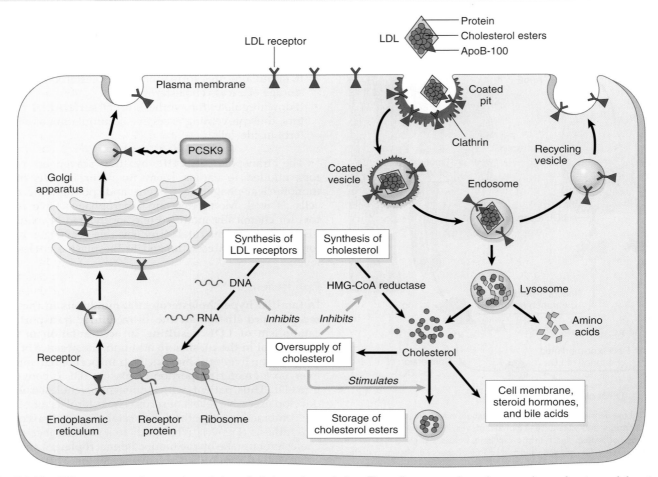

Fig. 7.2 The LDL receptor pathway and regulation of cholesterol metabolism. The *yellow arrows* show three regulatory functions of free intracellular cholesterol: (1) suppression of cholesterol synthesis by inhibition of HMG-CoA reductase, (2) stimulating the storage of excess cholesterol as esters, and (3) inhibition of synthesis of LDL receptors. PCSK9 causes intracellular degradation of LDL receptors in liver cells, reducing the level of LDL receptors on the cell membrane. *HMG-CoA reductase,* 3-Hydroxy-3-methylglutaryl–coenzyme A reductase; *LDL,* low-density lipoprotein; *PCSK9,* proprotein convertase subtilisin/kexin type 9.

In recent years, a new mechanism of posttranslational regulation of plasma LDL levels has been elucidated, wherein an enzyme referred to as PCSK9 causes intracellular degradation of LDL receptors in hepatocytes, before they reach the cell surface. With fewer LDL receptors on the cell surface, there is reduced uptake of plasma LDL, leading to hypercholesterolemia. Families with activating mutations of the gene *PCSK9*, which codes for the enzyme, have many features similar to classic familial hypercholesterolemia.

The discovery of the critical role of LDL receptors in cholesterol homeostasis has led to the rational design of the statin family of drugs that are now widely used to lower plasma cholesterol. They inhibit the activity of HMG-CoA reductase and thus promote greater synthesis of LDL receptors (Fig. 7.2). However, the upregulation of LDL receptors is accompanied by a compensatory increase in PCSK9 levels, which dampens the effects of statins. Therefore, agents that antagonize PCSK9 enzymatic function have been developed, and large clinical trials have shown the benefits using such inhibitors in patients with refractory hypercholesterolemia.

SUMMARY

FAMILIAL HYPERCHOLESTEROLEMIA

- Familial hypercholesterolemia is an autosomal dominant disorder caused by mutations in the gene encoding the LDL receptor. Activating mutations of PCSK9 (far less common), which degrades LDL receptors, also cause a similar phenotype.
- Patients develop hypercholesterolemia as a consequence of impaired transport of LDL into the cells.
- In heterozygotes, elevated serum cholesterol greatly increases the risk of atherosclerosis and resultant coronary artery disease; homozygotes have an even greater increase in serum cholesterol and a higher frequency of ischemic heart disease. Cholesterol also deposits along tendon sheaths to produce xanthomas.

Cystic Fibrosis

Cystic fibrosis (CF) is a disorder of epithelial ion transport affecting fluid secretion in exocrine glands and the epithelial linings of the respiratory, gastrointestinal, and reproductive tracts. The ion transport defects lead to abnormally viscid mucous secretions that block the airways and the pancreatic ducts which in turn are responsible for the two most important clinical manifestations: recurrent and chronic pulmonary infections and pancreatic insufficiency. In addition, although the exocrine sweat glands are structurally normal (and remain so throughout the course of this disease), *a high level of sodium chloride in the sweat is a consistent and characteristic biochemical abnormality in CF.* At the same time, it must be remembered that CF can present with a bewilderingly variable set of clinical findings. This variation in phenotype results from diverse mutations in the CF-associated gene, tissue-specific effects of loss of the CF gene's function, and the influence of disease modifier genes.

With an incidence of 1 in 2500 live births in the United States, CF is the most common lethal genetic disease that affects white populations. The carrier frequency in the United States is 1 in 20 among Caucasians but significantly lower among African Americans, Asians, and Hispanics. CF follows simple autosomal recessive transmission, although even heterozygous carriers have a predisposition toward pulmonary and pancreatic disease at higher rates than the general population.

Pathogenesis

The primary defect in CF is reduced production, or abnormal function of an epithelial chloride channel protein encoded by the CF transmembrane conductance regulator (*CFTR*) gene. Disruptive mutations in *CFTR* render the epithelial membranes relatively impermeable to chloride ions (Fig. 7.3). However, the impact of this defect on transport function is tissue specific. The major function of the CFTR protein in the sweat gland ducts is to reabsorb luminal chloride ions and augment sodium reabsorption through the epithelial sodium channel (ENaC). Therefore, in the sweat ducts, loss of CFTR function leads to decreased reabsorption of sodium chloride and production of hypertonic ("salty") sweat (Fig. 7.3, top). In contrast to sweat glands, CFTR in the respiratory and intestinal epithelium is one of the most important avenues for active luminal secretion of chloride. At these sites, CFTR mutations result in loss or reduction of chloride secretion into the lumen (Fig. 7.3, bottom). Active luminal sodium absorption through ENaCs also is increased, and both of these ion changes increase passive water reabsorption from the lumen, lowering the water content of the surface fluid layer coating mucosal cells. Thus, unlike the sweat ducts, there

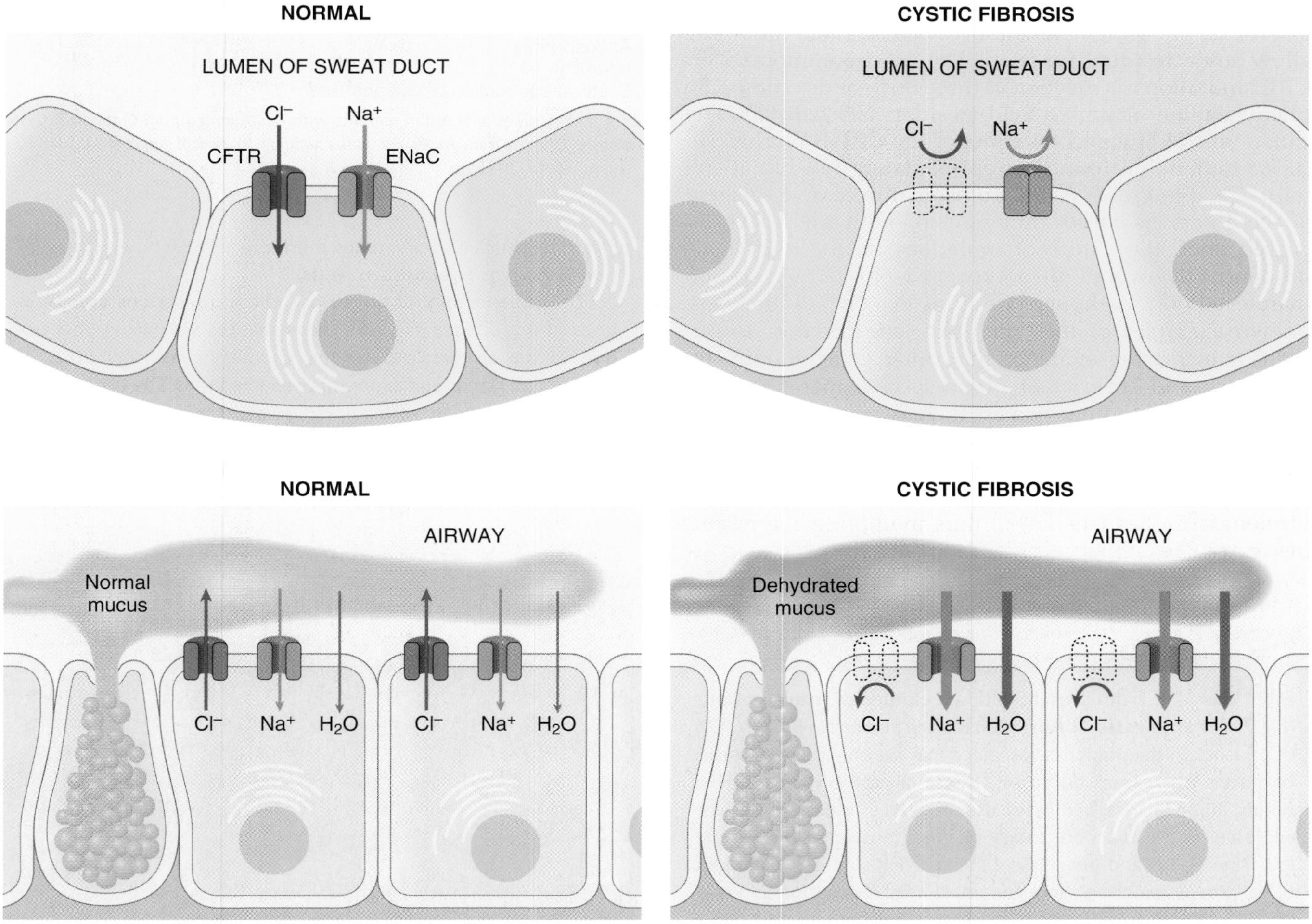

Fig. 7.3 *(Top)* In CF, a chloride channel defect in the sweat duct causes increased chloride and sodium concentration in sweat. *(Bottom)* Patients with CF have decreased chloride secretion and increased sodium and water reabsorption in the airways, leading to dehydration of the mucus layer coating epithelial cells, defective mucociliary action, and mucous plugging. *CFTR,* Cystic fibrosis transmembrane conductance regulator; *ENaC,* epithelial sodium channel responsible for intracellular sodium conduction.

is no difference in the salt concentration of the surface fluid layer coating the respiratory and intestinal mucosal cells in normal persons and in those with CF. Instead, respiratory and intestinal complications in CF seem to stem from dehydration of surface fluid layer. In the lungs, this dehydration leads to defective mucociliary action and the accumulation of concentrated, viscid secretions that obstruct the air passages and predispose to recurrent pulmonary infections. In addition to chloride, CFTR also regulates secretion of bicarbonate ions. In fact, certain CFTR variants manifest only with abnormal bicarbonate transport while chloride ion transport is largely preserved. Pancreatic insufficiency, a feature of classic CF, is virtually always present in patients who carry CFTR mutations with abnormal bicarbonate conductance.

Since the CFTR gene was cloned in 1989, more than 1800 disease-causing mutations have been identified. They can be classified on the basis of clinical course of CF or the nature of the underlying defect. Mechanistically, they may result in reduced quantity of functional CFTR that reaches the cell surface or reduced function of CFTR that reaches the cell surface. As we shall see these differences impact on the development of treatment strategies. They can also be classified as severe or mild, depending on the clinical phenotype. Severe mutations are associated with complete loss of CFTR protein function, whereas mild mutations allow some residual function. The most common severe CFTR mutation is a deletion of three nucleotides coding for phenylalanine at amino acid position 508 (*ΔF508*). This causes misfolding and total loss of the CFTR. Worldwide, *ΔF508* mutation is found in approximately 70% of patients with CF. Since CF is an autosomal recessive disease, affected persons harbor mutations on both alleles. As discussed later, the nature of mutations on the two alleles influences the overall phenotype, as well as organ-specific manifestations. Although CF remains one of the best-known examples of the "one gene–one disease" axiom, there is increasing evidence that other genes modify the frequency and severity of organ-specific manifestations. Examples of modifier genes include mannose-binding lectin 2 (MBL2) and transforming growth factor-β1 (TGF-β1). It is postulated that polymorphisms in these genes influence the ability of the lungs to tolerate infections with virulent microbes (see later), thus modifying the natural history of CF.

MORPHOLOGY

Even "classic" CF can present with a multitude of manifestations (Fig. 7.4). **Pancreatic abnormalities** are present in 85% to 90% of patients. In the milder cases, there may be only accumulations of mucus in the small ducts, with some dilation of the exocrine glands. In more advanced cases, usually seen in older children or adolescents, the ducts are totally plugged, causing atrophy of the exocrine glands and progressive fibrosis (Fig. 7.5). The total loss of pancreatic exocrine secretion impairs fat absorption and may lead to vitamin A deficiency. This may contribute to squamous metaplasia of the lining epithelium of the pancreatic ducts, which may exacerbate injury caused by the inspissated mucus secretions. Thick viscid plugs of mucus also may be found in the small

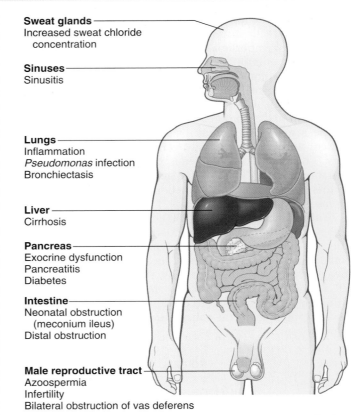

Sweat glands
Increased sweat chloride
  concentration

Sinuses
Sinusitis

Lungs
Inflammation
Pseudomonas infection
Bronchiectasis

Liver
Cirrhosis

Pancreas
Exocrine dysfunction
Pancreatitis
Diabetes

Intestine
Neonatal obstruction
  (meconium ileus)
Distal obstruction

Male reproductive tract
Azoospermia
Infertility
Bilateral obstruction of vas deferens

Fig. 7.4 Tissues affected in patients with CF. (*Adapted from Cutting GR: Cystic fibrosis genetics: from molecular understanding to clinical application.* Nat Rev Genet 16:45, 2015.)

intestine of infants. Sometimes these cause small bowel obstruction, known as **meconium ileus.**

The **pulmonary changes** are the most serious complications of this disease (Fig. 7.6). These changes stem from obstruction of the air passages by the viscous mucus secretions of submucosal glands and superimposed infections. The bronchioles often are distended with thick mucus, associated with marked hyperplasia and hypertrophy of the mucus-secreting cells. Superimposed infections give rise to severe chronic bronchitis and

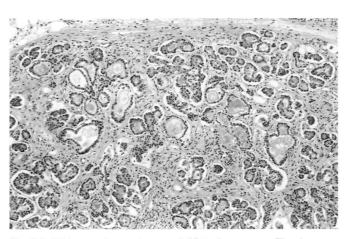

Fig. 7.5 Mild to moderate changes of CF in the pancreas. The ducts are dilated and plugged with eosinophilic mucin, and the parenchymal glands are atrophic and replaced by fibrous tissue.

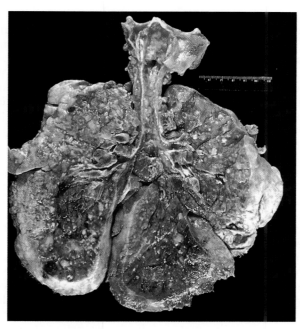

Fig. 7.6 Lungs of a patient who died of cystic fibrosis. Extensive mucous plugging and dilation of the tracheobronchial tree are apparent. The pulmonary parenchyma is consolidated by a combination of both secretions and pneumonia; the greenish discoloration is the product of *Pseudomonas* infections. *(Courtesy of Dr. Eduardo Yunis: Children's Hospital of Pittsburgh, Pittsburgh, Pennsylvania.)*

bronchiectasis. Development of lung abscesses is common. *Staphylococcus aureus*, *Haemophilus influenzae*, and *Pseudomonas aeruginosa* are the three most common organisms responsible for lung infections. Even more sinister is the increasing frequency of infection with another pseudomonad, *Burkholderia cepacia*. This opportunistic bacterium is particularly hardy, and infection with this organism has been associated with fulminant illness ("cepacia syndrome"). The **liver involvement** follows the same basic pattern. Bile canaliculi are plugged by mucinous material, accompanied by ductular proliferation and portal inflammation. Hepatic **steatosis** ("fatty liver") is a common finding in liver biopsies. With time, cirrhosis develops, resulting in diffuse hepatic nodularity. Such severe hepatic involvement is encountered in less than 10% of patients. **Azoospermia** and **infertility** are found in 95% of the affected males who survive to adulthood; **bilateral absence of the vas deferens** is a frequent finding in these patients. In some males, this may be the only feature suggesting an underlying CFTR mutation.

Clinical Course

In few childhood diseases are clinical manifestations as protean as those of CF (Fig. 7.4). Approximately 5% to 10% of the cases come to clinical attention at birth or soon after because of an attack of meconium ileus. Exocrine pancreatic insufficiency occurs in a majority (85% to 90%) of patients and is associated with "severe" *CFTR* mutations on both alleles (e.g., *ΔF508/ΔF508*). By contrast, 10% to 15% of patients, who have one "severe" and one "mild" *CFTR* mutation, or two "mild" *CFTR* mutations, retain sufficient pancreatic exocrine function that enzyme supplementation

is not required—the pancreas-sufficient phenotype. Pancreatic insufficiency is associated with malabsorption of protein and fat and increased fecal loss. Manifestations of malabsorption (e.g., large, foul-smelling stools; abdominal distention; poor weight gain) appear during the first year of life. The faulty fat absorption may induce deficiency states of the fat-soluble vitamins, resulting in manifestations of avitaminosis A, D, or K. Hypoproteinemia may be severe enough to cause generalized edema. Persistent diarrhea may result in rectal prolapse in as many as 10% of children with CF. The pancreas-sufficient phenotype usually is not associated with other gastrointestinal complications, and in general, these patients demonstrate excellent growth and development. In contrast to exocrine insufficiency, endocrine insufficiency (i.e., diabetes) is uncommon in CF and occurs late in the course of the disease especially with improved survival of patients with CF.

Cardiorespiratory complications, such as chronic cough, persistent lung infections, obstructive pulmonary disease, and cor pulmonale, constitute the most common cause of death (accounting for approximately 80% of fatalities) in patients who receive follow-up care in most CF centers in the United States. By 18 years of age, 80% of patients with classic CF harbor *P. aeruginosa*, and 3.5% harbor *B. cepacia*. With the indiscriminate use of antibiotic prophylaxis, there has been an unfortunate resurgence of resistant strains of *Pseudomonas* in many patients. Significant liver disease occurs late in the natural history of CF and is foreshadowed by pulmonary and pancreatic involvement; with increasing life expectancy, liver disease is now the third most common cause of death in patients with CF (after cardiopulmonary and transplant-related complications). More extensive DNA sequencing has shown that the spectrum of diseases caused by germline *CFTR* mutations (either biallelic or in heterozygous carriers) is broader than the "classic" multisystem disease described earlier. For example, some patients suffering from recurrent bouts of abdominal pain and pancreatitis since childhood who were previously classified as having "idiopathic" chronic pancreatitis are now known to harbor biallelic *CFTR* variants that are distinct from those seen in "classic" CF. Patients with isolated pancreatitis or bilateral absence of vas deferens (see earlier) resulting from CFTR mutations are included under the umbrella of "CFTR-opathies." Similarly, whereas CF carriers were initially thought to be asymptomatic, studies suggest that they have an increased lifetime risk for chronic lung disease (especially bronchiectasis) and recurrent sinonasal polyps. In most cases, the diagnosis of CF is based on persistently elevated sweat electrolyte concentrations (often the mother makes the diagnosis because her infant "tastes salty"), characteristic clinical findings (sinopulmonary disease and gastrointestinal manifestations), or a family history. Sequencing the *CFTR* gene is the gold standard for diagnosis of CF.

There have been major improvements in the management of acute and chronic complications of CF, including more potent anti-microbial therapies, pancreatic enzyme replacement, and bilateral lung transplantation. Importantly, two new forms of treatment aimed at increasing CFTR protein function in certain CFTR variants have been approved. For example, a group of agents known as CFTR "potentiators" are used in a minority (~3% to 5%) of CF patients who harbor a G155D mutation in the CFTR gene. In this variant, functionally defective CFTR is present in otherwise normal amounts at the cell membrane; the orally bioavailable CFTR "potentiator" partially restores the critical ion transport functions to the defective channel. Another approved drug contains a combination of two agents—one the aforementioned potentiator and the second a drug that increases the transport of the defective Δ508 CFTR protein to the cell membrane. It is too early determine the impact of the emerging molecular therapies on prognosis and survival. Overall, improved management of CF have extended the median life expectancy to close to 40 years and, is steadily changing a lethal disease of childhood into a chronic disease of adults.

SUMMARY

CYSTIC FIBROSIS

- CF is an autosomal recessive disease caused by mutations in the *CFTR* gene encoding the CF transmembrane regulator.
- The principal defect is of chloride ion transport, resulting in high salt concentrations in sweat and in viscous luminal secretions in respiratory and gastrointestinal tracts.
- CFTR mutations can be severe (ΔF508), resulting in multisystem disease, or mild, with limited disease extent and severity.
- Cardiopulmonary complications constitute the most common cause of death; pulmonary infections, especially with resistant *Pseudomonas* or *Burkholderia* species, are frequent. Bronchiectasis and right-sided heart failure are long-term sequelae.
- Pancreatic insufficiency is extremely common; infertility caused by congenital bilateral absence of vas deferens is a characteristic finding in adult patients with CF.
- Liver disease, including cirrhosis, is increasing in frequency as life expectancy increases.
- Molecular therapies that enhance the transport or stability of mutant CFTR protein are useful in patients who harbor certain CFTR alleles.

Diseases Caused by Mutations in Genes Encoding Enzyme Proteins

Phenylketonuria (PKU)

PKU results from mutations that cause a severe lack of the enzyme phenylalanine hydroxylase (PAH). It affects 1 in 10,000 live-born white infants and there are several variants of this disease. The most common form, referred to as classic phenylketonuria, is common in persons of Scandinavian descent and is distinctly uncommon in African-American and Jewish populations.

Homozygotes with this autosomal recessive disorder classically have a severe lack of PAH, leading to hyperphenylalaninemia and PKU. Affected infants are normal at birth but within a few weeks exhibit a rising plasma phenylalanine level, which impairs brain development. Usually, by 6 months of life, severe mental retardation becomes all too evident; less than 4% of untreated phenylketonuric children have intelligence quotients (IQs) greater than 60. About one-third of these children are never able to walk, and two-thirds cannot talk. Seizures, other neurologic abnormalities, decreased pigmentation of hair and skin, and eczema often accompany the mental retardation in untreated children. Hyperphenylalaninemia and the resultant mental retardation can be avoided by restricting phenylalanine intake early in life. Hence, several screening procedures are routinely performed to detect PKU in the immediate postnatal period.

Many female patients with PKU who receive dietary treatment beginning early in life reach childbearing age and are clinically normal. Most of them have marked hyperphenylalaninemia, because dietary treatment is discontinued after they reach adulthood. Between 75% and 90% of children born to such women are mentally retarded and microcephalic, and 15% have congenital heart disease, even though the infants themselves are heterozygotes. This syndrome, termed maternal PKU, results from the teratogenic effects of phenylalanine or its metabolites that cross the placenta and affect specific fetal organs during development. The presence and severity of the fetal anomalies directly correlate with the maternal phenylalanine level, so it is imperative that maternal dietary restriction of phenylalanine be initiated before conception and continued throughout pregnancy.

The biochemical abnormality in PKU is an inability to convert phenylalanine into tyrosine. In normal children, less than 50% of the dietary intake of phenylalanine is necessary for protein synthesis. The remainder is converted to tyrosine by the phenylalanine hydroxylase system (Fig. 7.7). When phenylalanine metabolism is blocked because of a lack of PAH enzyme, shunt pathways come into play, yielding several intermediates that are excreted in large amounts in the urine and in the sweat. These impart a strong musty or mousy odor to affected infants. It is believed that excess phenylalanine or its metabolites contribute to the brain damage in PKU. Concomitant lack of tyrosine (Fig. 7.7), a precursor of melanin, is responsible for the light color of hair and skin.

At the molecular level, approximately 500 mutant alleles of the *PAH* gene have been identified, only some of which cause a severe deficiency of the enzyme. Infants with mutations resulting in a severe lack of PAH activity present with the classic features of PKU, whereas those with some residual activity present with milder disease or may be asymptomatic, a condition referred to as *benign hyperphenylalaninemia*. Because the numerous disease-causing alleles of the *PAH* gene, complicate molecular diagnosis, measurement of serum phenylalanine levels is used to differentiate benign hyperphenylalaninemia from PKU; the levels in the latter disorder typically are ≥5 times higher than normal. After a biochemical diagnosis is established, the specific mutation causing PKU can be determined. With this information, carrier testing of at-risk family members can be performed. Currently, enzyme replacement therapy is being tried as a method for reducing circulating phenylalanine levels in patients with classic PKU. The replacement enzyme, known as phenylalanine ammonia lyase (or PAL), converts excess phenylalanine to ammonia and other nontoxic metabolites.

Although 98% of cases of hyperphenylalaninemia are attributable to mutations in PAH, approximately 2% arise

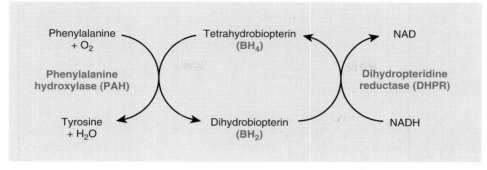

Fig. 7.7 The phenylalanine hydroxylase system. *NADH,* Nicotinamide adenine dinucleotide, reduced form.

from abnormalities in synthesis or recycling of the cofactor tetrahydrobiopterin (Fig. 7.7). Clinical recognition of these variant forms is important because these patients cannot be treated by dietary restriction of phenylalanine alone, but also require supplementation with tetrahydrobiopterin, certain neurotransmitter precursors, and folic acid.

SUMMARY

PHENYLKETONURIA

- PKU is an autosomal recessive disorder caused by a lack of the enzyme phenylalanine hydroxylase and a consequent inability to metabolize phenylalanine.
- Clinical features of untreated PKU may include severe mental retardation, seizures, and decreased pigmentation of skin, which can be avoided by restricting the intake of phenylalanine in the diet.
- Female patients with PKU who discontinue dietary treatment can give birth to children with malformations and neurologic impairment resulting from transplacental passage of phenylalanine metabolites.

Galactosemia

Galactosemia is an autosomal recessive disorder of galactose metabolism resulting from a mutation in the gene encoding the enzyme galactose-1-phosphate uridyltransferase (GALT). It affects 1 in 60,000 live-born infants. Normally, lactase splits lactose, the major carbohydrate of mammalian milk, into glucose and galactose in the intestinal microvilli. Galactose is then converted to glucose in several steps, in one of which the enzyme GALT is required. As a result of this transferase deficiency, galactose-1-phosphate and other metabolites, including galactitol, accumulate in many tissues, including the liver, spleen, lens of the eye, kidney, and cerebral cortex.

The liver, eyes, and brain bear the brunt of the damage. The early-onset hepatomegaly results largely from fatty change, but in time widespread scarring that closely resembles the cirrhosis of alcohol abuse may supervene (Chapter 16). Opacification of the lens (cataract) develops, probably because the lens absorbs water and swells as galactitol, produced by alternative metabolic pathways, accumulates and increases its tonicity. Nonspecific alterations appear in the central nervous system (CNS), including loss of nerve cells, gliosis, and edema. There is still no

clear understanding of the mechanism of injury to the brain, although elevated galactitol levels in neuronal tissues suggests that this may contribute to the damage.

Almost from birth, affected infants fail to thrive. Vomiting and diarrhea appear within a few days of milk ingestion. Jaundice and hepatomegaly usually become evident during the first week of life. Accumulation of galactose and galactose-1-phosphate in the kidney impairs amino acid transport, resulting in aminoaciduria. Fulminant *Escherichia coli* septicemia occurs with increased frequency. Newborn screening tests are widely utilized in the United States. They depend on fluorometric assay of GALT enzyme activity on a dried blood spot. A positive screening test must be confirmed by assay of GALT levels in RBC. Antenatal diagnosis is possible by assay of GALT activity in cultured amniotic fluid cells or determination of galactitol level in amniotic fluid supernatant.

Many of the clinical and morphologic changes of galactosemia can be prevented or ameliorated by removal of galactose from the diet for at least the first 2 years of life. If instituted soon after birth, this diet prevents cataracts and liver damage and permits almost normal development. Even with dietary restrictions, however, older patients frequently are affected by a speech disorder and gonadal failure (especially premature ovarian failure) and, less commonly, by an ataxic condition.

SUMMARY

GALACTOSEMIA

- Galactosemia is an autosomal recessive disorder caused by lack of the GALT enzyme, leading to the accumulation of galactose-1-phosphate and its metabolites in tissues.
- Clinical features may include jaundice, liver damage, cataracts, neural damage, vomiting and diarrhea, and *E. coli* sepsis. Dietary restriction of galactose can prevent at least some of the more severe complications.

Lysosomal Storage Diseases

Lysosomes, the digestive system of the cells, contain a variety of hydrolytic enzymes that are involved in the breakdown of complex substrates, such as sphingolipids and mucopolysaccharides, into soluble end products. These large molecules may be derived from the turnover of intracellular organelles that enter the lysosomes by *autophagy,* or they may be acquired from outside the cell by phagocytosis. With an inherited lack of a lysosomal enzyme, catabolism of its substrate remains incomplete, leading to accumulation of the partially degraded insoluble metabolites within the lysosomes (Fig. 7.8). This is called *primary storage*. Stuffed with incompletely digested macromolecules, lysosomes become large and numerous enough to interfere with normal cell functions. Because lysosomal function is also essential for autophagy, impaired autophagy gives rise to *secondary storage* of autophagic substrates such as polyubiquinated proteins and old and effete mitochondria. The absence of this quality-control mechanism causes accumulation of dysfunctional mitochondria, which can trigger the generation of free radicals and apoptosis.

Approximately 60 lysosomal storage diseases have been identified. These may result from abnormalities of

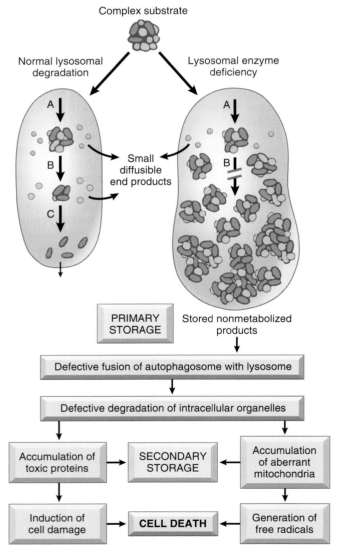

Fig. 7.8 Pathogenesis of lysosomal storage diseases. In this example, a complex substrate is normally degraded by a series of lysosomal enzymes into soluble end products (A, B and C). If there is a deficiency or malfunction of one of the enzymes (e.g., B), catabolism is incomplete, and insoluble intermediates accumulate in the lysosomes. In addition to this primary storage, secondary storage and toxic effects result from defective autophagy.

lysosomal enzymes or proteins involved in substrate degradation, endosomal sorting, or lysosomal membrane integrity. Lysosomal storage disorders are divided into categories based on the biochemical nature of the substrates and the accumulated metabolites. (Table 7.3). Within each group are several entities, each resulting from the deficiency of a specific enzyme.

Although the combined frequency of lysosomal storage disorders (LSDs) is about 1 in 5000 live births, lysosomal dysfunction may be involved in the etiology of several more-common diseases. For example, an important genetic risk factor for developing Parkinson disease is the carrier state for Gaucher disease, and virtually all Gaucher disease patients develop Parkinson disease. Niemann Pick C is another LSD connected to the risk for Alzheimer disease. Such interconnectedness stems from the multifunctionality of the lysosome. For example, lysosomes play critical roles in (i) autophagy, resulting from fusion with the autophagosome; (ii) immunity, as they fuse with phagosomes; and (iii) membrane repair, through fusion with the plasma membrane.

LSDs are typically fatal, with many displaying profound neurologic impairment that begins in childhood. Studies show that several neurodegenerative LSDs also are associated with a dysregulation of the immune system. For example, immunosuppression occurs in Gaucher disease and mucopolysaccharidoses VII, whereas in Niemann Pick disease-type-C1, hyperactivation of the immune system is seen. The mechanistic basis of linkage to immunologic changes remains to be deciphered.

Despite this complexity, certain features are common to most diseases in this group:
- Autosomal recessive transmission
- Patient population consisting of infants and young children
- Storage of insoluble intermediates in the mononuclear phagocyte system, giving rise to hepatosplenomegaly
- Frequent CNS involvement with associated neuronal damage
- Cellular dysfunction caused not only by storage of undigested material, but also by a cascade of secondary events, for example, macrophage activation and release of cytokines

Most of these conditions are very rare, and their detailed description is better relegated to specialized texts and reviews. Only a few of the more common conditions are considered here.

Tay-Sachs Disease (GM2 Gangliosidosis: Deficiency in Hexosaminidase β Subunit)

Gangliosidoses are characterized by accumulation of gangliosides, principally in the brain, as a result of a deficiency of one of the lysosomal enzymes that catabolize these glycolipids. Depending on the ganglioside involved, these disorders are subclassified into GM1 and GM2 categories. Tay-Sachs disease, by far the most common of all gangliosidoses, is caused by loss-of-function mutations of the β subunit of the enzyme *hexosaminidase A*, which is necessary for the degradation of GM2. More than 100 mutations have been described; most disrupt protein folding or intracellular transport. Tay-Sachs disease, similar to other lipid storage disorders, is most common among

Table 7.3 Lysosomal Storage Disorders

Disease	Enzyme Deficiency	Major Accumulating Metabolites
Glycogenosis, type 2-Pompe disease	α-1,4-Glucosidase (lysosomal glucosidase)	Glycogen
Sphingolipidoses GM1 gangliosidosis Type 1—infantile, generalized Type 2—juvenile	GM1 ganglioside β-galactosidase	GM1 ganglioside, galactose-containing oligosaccharides
GM2 gangliosidosis Tay-Sachs disease	Hexosaminidase, α subunit	GM2 ganglioside
Sandhoff disease	Hexosaminidase, β subunit	GM2 ganglioside, globoside
GM2 gangliosidosis variant AB	Ganglioside activator protein	GM2 ganglioside
Sulfatidoses Metachromatic leukodystrophy	Arylsulfatase A	Sulfatide
Multiple sulfatase deficiency	Arylsulfatase A, B, C; steroid sulfatase; iduronate sulfatase; heparan N-sulfatase	Sulfatide, steroid sulfate, heparan sulfate, dermatan sulfate
Krabbe disease	Galactosylceramidase	Galactocerebroside
Fabry disease	α-Galactosidase A	Ceramide trihexoside
Gaucher disease	Glucocerebrosidase	Glucocerebroside
Niemann-Pick disease: types A and B	Sphingomyelinase	Sphingomyelin
Mucopolysaccharidoses (MPSs) MPS I H (Hurler)	α-L-Iduronidase	Dermatan sulfate, heparan sulfate
MPS II (Hunter)	I-Iduronosulfate sulfatase	
Mucolipidoses (MLs) I-cell disease (ML II) and pseudo-Hurler polydystrophy	Deficiency of phosphorylating enzymes essential for the formation of mannose-6-phosphate recognition marker; acid hydrolases lacking the recognition marker cannot be targeted to the lysosomes but are secreted extracellularly	Mucopolysaccharide, glycolipid
Other diseases of complex carbohydrates Fucosidosis	α-Fucosidase	Fucose-containing sphingolipids and glycoprotein fragments
Mannosidosis	α-Mannosidase	Mannose-containing oligosaccharides
Aspartylglycosaminuria	Aspartylglycosamine amide hydrolase	Aspartyl-2-deoxy-2-acetamido-glycosylamine
Other lysosomal storage diseases Wolman disease	Acid lipase	Cholesterol esters, triglycerides
Acid phosphate deficiency	Lysosomal acid phosphatase	Phosphate esters

Ashkenazi Jews, among whom the frequency of heterozygous carriers is estimated to be 1 in 30. Heterozygote carriers can be detected by measuring the level of hexosaminidase in the serum or by DNA sequencing.

In the absence of hexosaminidase A, G_{M2} ganglioside accumulates in many tissues (e.g., heart, liver, spleen, nervous system), but the **involvement of neurons in the central and autonomic nervous systems and retina dominates the clinical picture.** The accumulation of GM2 occurs within neurons, axon cylinders of nerves, and glial cells throughout the CNS. Affected cells appear swollen and sometimes foamy (Fig. 7.9A). Electron microscopy shows whorled onionskin-like configurations within lysosomes composed of layers of membranes (Fig. 7.9B). These pathologic changes are found throughout the CNS (including the spinal cord), peripheral nerves, and autonomic nervous system. The retina usually is involved as well, where the pallor produced by swollen ganglion cells in the peripheral retina results in a contrasting "cherry red" spot in the relatively unaffected central macula.

The molecular basis for neuronal injury is not fully understood. Because in many cases the mutant protein is misfolded, it induces the so-called "unfolded protein" response (Chapter 2). If such misfolded enzymes are not stabilized by chaperones, they undergo proteasomal degradation, leading to accumulation of toxic substrates and intermediates within neurons. These findings have spurred clinical trials of molecular chaperone therapy for some variants of later-onset Tay-Sachs and other selected lysosomal storage diseases. Such therapy involves the use of synthetic chaperones that can cross the blood–brain barrier, bind to the mutated protein, and enable its proper folding. Sufficient functional enzyme can then be rescued to ameliorate the effects of the inborn error.

In the most common acute infantile variant of Tay-Sachs disease, infants appear normal at birth, but motor weakness begins at 3 to 6 months of age, followed by neurologic impairment, onset of blindness, and progressively more severe neurologic dysfunctions. Death occurs within 2 to 3 years.

Niemann-Pick Disease Types A and B

Type A and type B Niemann-Pick diseases are related entities characterized by a primary deficiency of *acid*

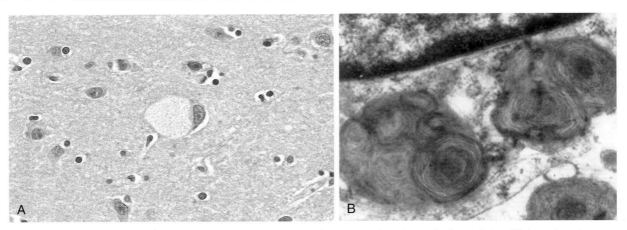

Fig. 7.9 Ganglion cells in Tay-Sachs disease. (A) Under the light microscope, a large neuron has obvious lipid vacuolation. (B) A portion of a neuron under the electron microscope shows prominent lysosomes with whorled configurations just below part of the nucleus. *(A, Courtesy of Dr. Arthur Weinberg, Department of Pathology, University of Texas Southwestern Medical Center, Dallas, Texas. B, Courtesy of Dr. Joe Rutledge, Children's Regional Medical Center, Seattle, Washington.)*

sphingomyelinase and the resultant accumulation of sphingomyelin. As with Tay-Sachs disease, Niemann-Pick disease types A and B are common in Ashkenazi Jews. The gene for acid sphingomyelinase maps to chromosome 11p15.4 and is one of the imprinted genes that is preferentially expressed from the maternal chromosome as a result of epigenetic silencing of the paternal gene (discussed later).

In type A, characterized by a severe deficiency of sphingomyelinase, the breakdown of sphingomyelin into ceramide and phosphorylcholine is impaired, and excess sphingomyelin accumulates in phagocytic cells and in neurons. Macrophages become stuffed with droplets or particles of the complex lipid, imparting a fine vacuolation or foaminess to the cytoplasm (Fig. 7.10). Electron microscopy shows engorged secondary lysosomes that often contain membranous cytoplasmic bodies resembling concentric lamellated myelin figures, sometimes called "zebra" bodies. Because of their high content of phagocytic cells, the organs most severely affected are the spleen, liver, bone marrow, lymph nodes, and lungs. The splenic enlargement may be striking. In addition, the entire CNS, including the spinal cord and ganglia, is involved in this inexorable process. The affected neurons are enlarged and vacuolated as a result of the accumulation of lipids. This variant manifests in infancy with massive organomegaly and severe neurologic deterioration. Death usually occurs within the first 3 years of life. By comparison, patients with the type B variant, which is associated with mutant sphigomyelinase with some residual activity, have organomegaly but no neurologic manifestations. Estimation of sphingomyelinase activity in the leukocytes can be used for diagnosis of suspected cases, as well as for detection of carriers. Molecular genetic tests are also available for diagnosis at specialized centers.

Niemann-Pick Disease Type C

Although previously considered to be related to type A and type B Niemann-Pick disease type C (NPC) is quite distinct at the biochemical and molecular levels and is more common than types A and B combined. Mutations in two related genes, NPC1 and NPC2, can give rise to this disorder, with NPC1 being responsible for a majority of cases. Unlike most other lysosomal storage diseases, NPC results from a primary defect in lipid transport. Affected cells accumulate cholesterol as well as gangliosides such as GM1 and GM2. Both NPC1 and NPC2 are involved in the transport of free cholesterol from the lysosomes to the cytoplasm. NPC is clinically heterogeneous. The most common form manifests in childhood and is marked by ataxia, vertical supranuclear gaze palsy, dystonia, dysarthria, and psychomotor regression.

Gaucher Disease

Gaucher disease results from mutation in the gene that encodes *glucocerebrosidase*, and the resultant deficiency of this enzyme leads to an accumulation of glucocerebroside, an intermediate in glycolipid metabolism, in the mononuclear phagocytic cells. There are three autosomal recessive variants of Gaucher disease resulting from distinct allelic mutations. Common to all is deficient activity of a glucocerebrosidase that cleaves the glucose residue from ceramide. Normally, macrophages,

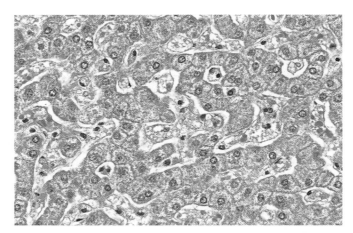

Fig. 7.10 Niemann-Pick disease in liver. The hepatocytes and Kupffer cells have a foamy, vacuolated appearance resulting from deposition of lipids. *(Courtesy of Dr. Arthur Weinberg, Department of Pathology, University of Texas Southwestern Medical Center, Dallas, Texas.)*

particularly in the liver, spleen, and bone marrow, sequentially degrade glycolipids derived from the breakdown of senescent blood cells. In Gaucher disease, the degradation stops at the level of glucocerebrosides, which accumulate in macrophages. These cells—the so-called "Gaucher cells"—become enlarged, with some reaching a diameter as great as 100 μm, because of the presence of distended lysosomes, and they acquire a pathognomonic cytoplasmic appearance characterized as "wrinkled tissue paper" (Fig. 7.11). It is evident now that Gaucher disease is caused not just by the burden of storage material but also by activation of the macrophages. High levels of macrophage-derived cytokines, such as interleukins (IL-1, IL-6) and tumor necrosis factor (TNF), are found in affected tissues.

One variant, type 1, also called the chronic nonneuronopathic form, accounts for 99% of cases of Gaucher disease. It is characterized by clinical or radiographic bone involvement (osteopenia, focal lytic lesions, and osteonecrosis) in 70% to 100% of cases. Additional features are hepatosplenomegaly and the absence of CNS involvement. The spleen often enlarges to massive proportions, filling the entire abdomen. Gaucher cells are found in the liver, spleen, lymph nodes, and bone marrow. Marrow replacement and cortical erosion may produce radiographically visible skeletal lesions, and peripheral blood cytopenias. It is believed that bone changes are caused by the aforementioned macrophage-derived cytokines. Type 1 is most common in Ashkenazi Jews; unlike other variants, it is compatible with long life. Neurologic signs and symptoms characterize types 2 and 3 variants. In type 2, these manifestations appear during infancy *(acute infantile neuronopathic form)* and are more severe, whereas in type 3, they emerge later and are milder *(chronic neuronopathic form)*. Although the liver and spleen also are involved, the clinical features in types 2 and 3 are dominated by neurologic disturbances, including convulsions and progressive mental deterioration. As mentioned earlier mutation of the glucocerebroside gene is a very important risk factor for Parkinson disease. Patients with Gaucher disease have a 20 fold higher risk of developing Parkinson disease (compared to controls) and 5–10% of patients with Parkinson disease have mutations in the gene encoding glucocerebrosidase.

There is a reciprocal relationship between the level of this enzyme and alpha synuclein. The latter is involved in the pathogenesis of Parkinson disease (Chapter 24). The level of glucocerebrosides in leukocytes or cultured fibroblasts is helpful in diagnosis and in the detection of heterozygote carriers. DNA testing is also available in select populations.

Currently, there are two approved therapies for type I Gaucher disease. The first is lifelong enzyme replacement therapy via infusion of recombinant glucocerebrosidase. The second, known as *substrate reduction therapy*, involves oral intake of an inhibitor of the enzyme glucosylceramide synthase. This leads to reduced systemic levels of glucocerebroside, the substrate for the defective enzyme in Gaucher disease. Clinical trials have confirmed that substrate reduction therapy leads to reduced spleen and liver sizes, improved blood counts, and enhanced skeletal function. Other emerging treatments include gene therapy through transplant of hematopoietic stem cells containing the corrected enzyme.

Mucopolysaccharidoses

Mucopolysaccharidoses (MPSs) are characterized by defective degradation and excessive storage of mucopolysaccharides in various tissues. Recall that mucopolysaccharides are part of the extracellular matrix and are synthesized by connective tissue fibroblasts. Most mucopolysaccharide is secreted, but a certain fraction is degraded within lysosome through a catabolic pathway involving multiple enzymes. Several clinical variants of MPS, classified numerically from MPS I to MPS VII, have been described, each resulting from the deficiency of one specific enzyme in this pathway. The mucopolysaccharides that accumulate within the tissues include dermatan sulfate, heparan sulfate, keratan sulfate, and (in some cases) chondroitin sulfate.

Hepatosplenomegaly, skeletal deformities, lesions of heart valves, subendothelial arterial deposits, particularly in the coronary arteries, and lesions in the brain, are features that are seen in all of the MPSs. In many of the more protracted syndromes, coronary subendothelial lesions lead to myocardial ischemia. Thus, myocardial infarction and cardiac decompensation are important causes of death. Most cases are associated

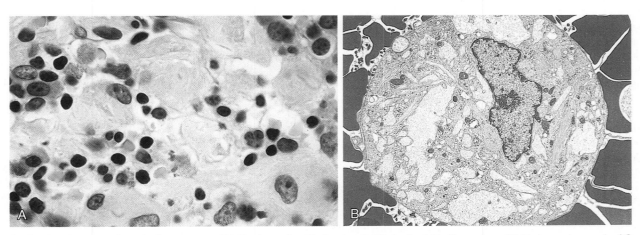

Fig. 7.11 Gaucher disease involving the bone marrow. (A) Gaucher cells with abundant lipid-laden "wrinkled" cytoplasm. (B) Electron micrograph of Gaucher cells with elongated distended lysosomes. *(Courtesy of Dr. Matthew Fries, Department of Pathology, University of Texas Southwestern Medical Center, Dallas, Texas.)*

with coarse facial features, clouding of the cornea, joint stiffness, and mental retardation. Urinary excretion of the accumulated mucopolysaccharides often is increased. With all of these disorders except one, the mode of inheritance is autosomal recessive; the exception, Hunter syndrome, is an X-linked recessive disease. Of the seven recognized variants, only two well-characterized syndromes are discussed briefly here.

- *MPS type I, also known as Hurler syndrome, is caused by a deficiency of α-L-iduronidase.* In Hurler syndrome, affected children have a life expectancy of 6 to 10 years, and death is often a result of cardiac complications. Accumulation of dermatan sulfate and heparan sulfate is seen in cells of the mononuclear phagocyte system, in fibroblasts, and within endothelium and smooth muscle cells of the vascular wall. The affected cells are swollen and have clear cytoplasm, resulting from the accumulation of material positive for periodic acid–Schiff staining within engorged, vacuolated lysosomes. Lysosomal inclusions also are found in neurons, accounting for the mental retardation.
- *MPS type II or Hunter syndrome, differs from Hurler syndrome in its mode of inheritance (X-linked), the absence of corneal clouding, and often its milder clinical course.* As in Hurler syndrome, the accumulated mucopolysaccharides in Hunter syndrome are heparan sulfate and dermatan sulfate, but this results from a deficiency of L-iduronate sulfatase. Despite the difference in enzyme deficiency, an accumulation of identical substrates occurs because breakdown of heparan sulfate and dermatan sulfate requires both α-L-iduronidase and the sulfatase; if either one is missing, further degradation is blocked. Diagnosis is made by measuring the level of enzyme in leukocytes. DNA diagnosis is not routinely employed because of the large number of alellic mutations.

SUMMARY

LYSOSOMAL STORAGE DISEASES

- Tay-Sachs disease is caused by an inability to metabolize GM2 gangliosides because of a lack of the β subunit of lysosomal hexosaminidase. GM2 gangliosides accumulate in the CNS and cause severe mental retardation, blindness, motor weakness, and death by 2 to 3 years of age.
- Niemann-Pick disease types A and B are caused by a deficiency of sphingomyelinase. In the more severe, type A variant, accumulation of sphingomyelin in the nervous system results in neuronal damage. Sphingomyelin also is stored in phagocytes within the liver, spleen, bone marrow, and lymph nodes, causing their enlargement. In type B, neuronal damage is not present.
- Niemann-Pick disease type C is caused by a defect in cholesterol transport and resultant accumulation of cholesterol and gangliosides in the nervous system. Affected children exhibit ataxia, dysarthria, and psychomotor regression.
- Gaucher disease results from lack of the lysosomal enzyme glucocerebrosidase and accumulation of glucocerebroside in mononuclear phagocytic cells. In the most common, type I variant, affected phagocytes become enlarged (Gaucher cells) and accumulate in liver, spleen, and bone marrow, causing

hepatosplenomegaly and bone erosion. Types 2 and 3 are characterized by variable neuronal involvement.
- MPSs result from accumulation of mucopolysaccharides in many tissues including liver, spleen, heart, blood vessels, brain, cornea, and joints. Affected patients in all forms have coarse facial features. Manifestations of Hurler syndrome include corneal clouding, coronary arterial and valvular deposits, and death in childhood. Hunter syndrome is associated with a milder clinical course.

Glycogen Storage Diseases (Glycogenoses)

An inherited deficiency of any one of the enzymes involved in glycogen synthesis or degradation can result in excessive accumulation of glycogen or some abnormal form of glycogen in various tissues. The type of glycogen stored, its intracellular location, and the tissue distribution of the affected cells vary depending on the specific enzyme deficiency. Regardless of the tissue or cells affected, the glycogen most often is stored within the cytoplasm, or sometimes within nuclei. One variant, Pompe disease, is a form of lysosomal storage disease, because the missing enzyme is localized to lysosomes. Most glycogenoses are inherited as autosomal recessive diseases, as is common with "missing enzyme" syndromes.

Approximately a dozen forms of glycogenoses have been described in association with specific enzyme deficiencies. Based on pathophysiologic findings, they can be grouped into three categories (Table 7.4):

- *Hepatic type.* Liver contains several enzymes that synthesize glycogen for storage and also break it down into free glucose. Hence, a deficiency of the hepatic enzymes involved in glycogen metabolism is associated with two major clinical effects: enlargement of the liver due to storage of glycogen and hypoglycemia due to a failure of glucose production (Fig. 7.12). *Von Gierke disease* (type I glycogenosis), resulting from a lack of glucose-6-phosphatase, is the most important example of the hepatic form of glycogenosis (Table 7.4).
- *Myopathic type.* In striated muscle, glycogen is an important source of energy. Not surprisingly, most forms of glycogen storage disease affect muscles. When enzymes that are involved in glycolysis are deficient, glycogen storage occurs in muscles and there is an associated muscle weakness due to impaired energy production. Typically, the myopathic forms of glycogen storage diseases are marked by muscle cramps after exercise, myoglobinuria, and failure of exercise to induce an elevation in blood lactate levels because of a block in glycolysis. *McArdle disease* (type V glycogenosis), resulting from a deficiency of muscle phosphorylase, is the prototype of myopathic glycogenoses.
- Type II glycogenosis (*Pompe disease*) is caused by a deficiency of lysosomal acid maltase and is associated with deposition of glycogen in virtually every organ, but cardiomegaly is most prominent. Most affected patients die within 2 years of onset of cardiorespiratory failure. Therapy with the missing enzyme (glucosidase) can reverse cardiac muscle damage and modestly increase longevity.

Table 7.4 Principal Subgroups of Glycogenoses

Clinicopathologic Category	Specific Type	Enzyme Deficiency	Morphologic Changes	Clinical Features
Hepatic type	Hepatorenal (von Gierke disease, type I)	Glucose-6-phosphatase	Hepatomegaly: intracytoplasmic accumulations of glycogen and small amounts of lipid; intranuclear glycogen Renomegaly: intracytoplasmic accumulations of glycogen in cortical tubular epithelial cells	In untreated patients, failure to thrive, stunted growth, hepatomegaly, and renomegaly Hypoglycemia resulting from failure of glucose mobilization, often leading to convulsions Hyperlipidemia and hyperuricemia resulting from deranged glucose metabolism; many patients develop gout and skin xanthomas Bleeding tendency caused by platelet dysfunction With treatment (providing continuous source of glucose), most patients survive and develop late complications (e.g., hepatic adenomas)
Myopathic type	McArdle disease (type V)	Muscle phosphorylase	Skeletal muscle only: accumulations of glycogen predominant in subsarcolemmal location	Painful cramps associated with strenuous exercise Myoglobinuria occurs in 50% of cases Onset in adulthood (>20 year) Muscular exercise fails to raise lactate level in venous blood Compatible with normal longevity
Miscellaneous type	Generalized glycogenosis (Pompe disease, type II)	Lysosomal glucosidase (acid maltase)	Mild hepatomegaly: ballooning of lysosomes with glycogen creating lacy cytoplasmic pattern Cardiomegaly: glycogen within sarcoplasm as well as membrane-bound Skeletal muscle: similar to heart (see earlier, under cardiomegaly)	Massive cardiomegaly, muscle hypotonia, and cardiorespiratory failure before age 2 Milder adult form with only skeletal muscle involvement manifests with chronic myopathy

SUMMARY

GLYCOGEN STORAGE DISEASES

- Inherited deficiency of enzymes involved in glycogen metabolism can result in storage of normal or abnormal forms of glycogen, predominantly in liver or muscles or in all tissues.
- In the hepatic form (von Gierke disease), liver cells store glycogen because of a lack of hepatic glucose-6-phosphatase.
- There are several myopathic forms, including McArdle disease, in which lack of muscle phosphorylase gives rise to storage in skeletal muscles and cramps after exercise.
- In Pompe disease there is lack of lysosomal acid maltase, and all organs are affected, but heart involvement is predominant.

Diseases Caused by Mutations in Genes Encoding Proteins That Regulate Cell Growth

As detailed in Chapter 6, two classes of genes, protooncogenes and tumor suppressor genes, regulate normal cell growth. Mutations affecting these genes, most often in somatic cells, are involved in the pathogenesis of tumors. In approximately 5% to 10% of all cancers, however, mutations affecting certain tumor suppressor genes are present in all cells of the body, including germ cells, and hence can

be transmitted to the offspring. These mutant genes predispose the offspring to hereditary tumors, a topic discussed in greater detail in Chapter 6. A few salient examples of familial neoplasms arising in children are discussed later in this chapter.

COMPLEX MULTIGENIC DISORDERS

Complex multigenic disorders—so-called "multifactorial or polygenic disorders"—are caused by interactions between genetic variants and environmental factors. A genetic variant that occurs in at least 1% of the population is called a polymorphism. According to the common disease–common variant hypothesis, complex multigenic disorders occur when many polymorphisms, each with a modest effect and low penetrance, are coinherited. Two additional important facts have emerged from studies of common complex disorders such as type 1 diabetes:

- Although complex disorders result from the collective inheritance of many polymorphisms, different polymorphisms vary in significance. For example, of the 20 to 30 genes implicated in type 1 diabetes, 6 or 7 are most important, and a few HLA alleles contribute more than 50% of the risk (Chapter 20).

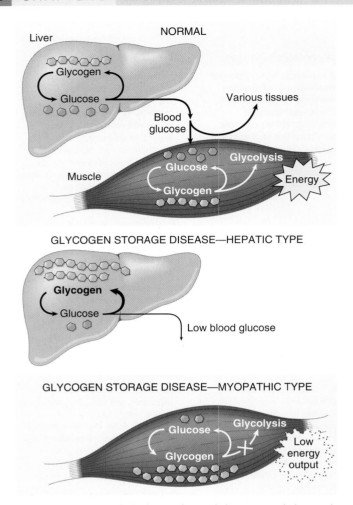

Fig. 7.12 *(Top)* A simplified scheme of normal glycogen metabolism in the liver and skeletal muscles. *(Middle)* The effects of an inherited deficiency of hepatic enzymes involved in glycogen metabolism. *(Bottom)* The consequences of a genetic deficiency in the enzymes that metabolize glycogen in skeletal muscles.

- Some polymorphisms are common to multiple diseases of the same type, whereas others are disease-specific. This observation is well illustrated in immune-mediated inflammatory diseases (Chapter 5).
- Many of the disease-associated polymorphisms are in noncoding regions so they likely affect epigenetic regulation of gene expression.

Several normal phenotypic characteristics are governed by multigenic inheritance, such as hair color, eye color, skin color, height, and intelligence. These characteristics (also known as quantitative trait loci [QTLs]) show a continuous variation within, as well as across, all population groups. Environmental influences, however, significantly modify the phenotypic expression of complex traits. For example, type 2 diabetes mellitus has many of the features of a complex multigenic disorder. It is well recognized clinically that affected persons often first exhibit clinical manifestations of this disease after weight gain. Thus, obesity, as well as other environmental influences, unmasks the diabetic genetic trait. Assigning a disease to this mode

of inheritance must be done with caution. Such attribution depends on many factors but first on familial clustering and the exclusion of mendelian and chromosomal modes of transmission. A range of levels of severity of a disease is suggestive of a complex multigenic disorder, but, as pointed out earlier, variable expressivity and reduced penetrance of single mutant genes also may account for this phenomenon. Because of these issues, it is sometimes difficult to distinguish between mendelian and multifactorial disorders.

CYTOGENETIC DISORDERS

Chromosomal abnormalities occur much more frequently than is generally appreciated. It is estimated that approximately 1 in 200 newborn infants has some form of chromosomal abnormality. The figure is much higher in fetuses that do not survive to term; in as many as 50% of first-trimester spontaneous abortions, the fetus may have a chromosomal abnormality. Cytogenetic disorders result from alterations in the number or structure of chromosomes and may affect autosomes or sex chromosomes.

Before embarking on a discussion of chromosomal aberrations, it is appropriate to review karyotyping as the basic tool of the cytogeneticist. **A karyotype is a photographic representation of a stained metaphase spread in which the chromosomes are arranged in order of decreasing length.** A variety of techniques for staining chromosomes has been developed. With the widely used Giemsa stain (G banding) technique, each chromosome set can be seen to possess a distinctive pattern of alternating light and dark bands of variable widths (Fig. 7.13). The use of banding techniques allows identification of each chromosome, and can detect and localize structural abnormalities large enough to produce changes in banding pattern (described later).

Numeric Abnormalities

In humans, the normal chromosome count is 46 (i.e., 2n = 46). Any exact multiple of the haploid number (n) is called *euploid*. Chromosome numbers such as 3n and 4n are called polyploid. Polyploidy generally results in a spontaneous abortion. Any number that is not an exact multiple of n is called *aneuploid*. The chief cause of aneuploidy is nondisjunction of a homologous pair of chromosomes at the first meiotic division or a failure of sister chromatids to separate during the second meiotic division. The latter also may occur during mitosis in somatic cells, leading to the production of two aneuploid cells. Failure of pairing of homologous chromosomes followed by random assortment (anaphase lag) also can lead to aneuploidy. When nondisjunction occurs at the time of meiosis, the gametes formed have either an extra chromosome (n + 1) or one less chromosome (n − 1). Fertilization of such gametes by normal gametes would result in two types of zygotes: trisomic, with an extra chromosome (2n + 1), or monosomic (2n − 1). Monosomy involving an autosome is incompatible with life, whereas trisomies of certain autosomes and monosomy involving sex chromosomes are compatible with life. These, as we shall see, are

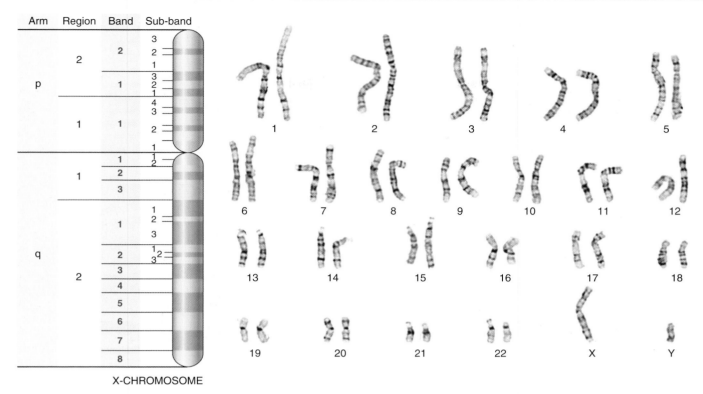

| Arm | Region | Band | Sub-band |

Fig. 7.13 G-banded karyotype from a normal male (46,XY). Also shown is the banding pattern of the X-chromosome with nomenclature of arms, regions, bands, and subbands. *(Karyotype courtesy of Dr. Stuart Schwartz, Department of Pathology, University of Chicago, Chicago, Illinois.)*

associated with variable degrees of phenotypic abnormality. *Mosaicism* is a term used to describe the presence of two or more populations of cells with different complements of chromosomes in the same individual. In the context of chromosome numbers, postzygotic mitotic nondisjunction would result in the production of a trisomic and a monosomic daughter cell; the descendants of these cells would then produce a mosaic. As discussed later, mosaicism affecting sex chromosomes is common, whereas autosomal mosaicism is not.

Structural Abnormalities

Structural changes in the chromosomes typically result from chromosomal breakage followed by loss or rearrangement of material. Such changes usually are designated using a cytogenetic shorthand in which p (French, petit) denotes the short arm of a chromosome, and q, the long arm. Each arm is then divided into numbered regions (1, 2, 3, and so on) from centromere outward, and within each region the bands are numerically ordered (Fig. 7.13). Thus, 2q34 indicates chromosome 2, long arm, region 3, band 4. The patterns of chromosomal rearrangement after breakage (Fig. 7.14) are as follows:

- *Translocation* implies transfer of a part of one chromosome to another chromosome. The process is usually reciprocal (i.e., fragments are exchanged between two chromosomes). In genetic shorthand, translocations are indicated by t followed by the involved chromosomes in numeric order—for example, 46,XX,t(2;5)(q31;p14). This notation would indicate a reciprocal translocation

involving the long arm (q) of chromosome 2 at region 3, band 1, and the short arm of chromosome 5, region 1, band 4. When the entire broken fragments are exchanged, the resulting *balanced reciprocal translocation* (Fig. 7.14) is not harmful to the carrier, who has the normal number of chromosomes and the full complement of genetic material. However, during gametogenesis, abnormal (unbalanced) gametes are formed, resulting in abnormal zygotes. A special pattern of translocation involving two acrocentric chromosomes is called *centric fusion type*, or *robertsonian, translocation*. The breaks typically occur close to the centromere, affecting the short arms of both chromosomes. Transfer of the segments leads to one very large chromosome and one extremely small one (Fig. 7.14). The short fragments are lost, and the carrier has 45 chromosomes. Because the short arms of all acrocentric chromosomes carry highly redundant genes (e.g., ribosomal RNA genes), such loss is compatible with survival. However, difficulties arise during gametogenesis, resulting in the formation of unbalanced gametes that could lead to abnormal offspring.

- *Isochromosomes* result when the centromere divides horizontally rather than vertically. One of the two arms of the chromosome is then lost, and the remaining arm is duplicated, resulting in a chromosome with only two short arms or two long arms. The most common isochromosome present in live births involves the long arm of the X chromosome and is designated i(Xq). When fertilization occurs by a gamete that contains a normal X chromosome, the result is monosomy for genes on Xp and trisomy for genes on Xq.

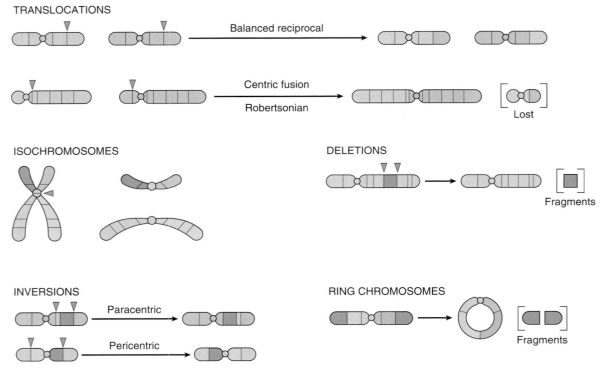

Fig. 7.14 Types of chromosomal rearrangements.

- *Deletion* involves loss of a portion of a chromosome. A single break may delete a terminal segment. Two interstitial breaks, with reunion of the proximal and distal segments, may result in loss of an internal segment. The isolated fragment, which lacks a centromere, almost never survives, and thus many genes are lost.
- *Inversions* occur when there are two interstitial breaks in a chromosome, and the segment reunites after a complete turnaround.
- A *ring chromosome* is a variant of a deletion. After loss of segments from each end of the chromosome, the arms unite to form a ring.

General Features of Chromosomal Disorders

- Chromosomal disorders may be associated with absence (deletion, monosomy), excess (trisomy), or abnormal rearrangements (translocations) of chromosomes.
- In general, a loss of chromosomal material produces more severe defects than does a gain of chromosomal material.
- Excess chromosomal material may result from a complete chromosome (as in trisomy) or from part of a chromosome (as in Robertsonian translocation).
- Imbalances of sex chromosomes (excess or loss) are tolerated much better than are similar imbalances of autosomes.
- Sex chromosomal disorders often produce subtle abnormalities, sometimes not detected at birth. Infertility, a common manifestation, cannot be diagnosed until adolescence.
- In most cases, chromosomal disorders result from de novo changes (i.e., parents are normal, and risk of

recurrence in siblings is low). The translocation form of Down syndrome (described later) exhibits an uncommon but important exception to this principle.

Some specific examples of diseases involving changes in the karyotype are presented next.

Cytogenetic Disorders Involving Autosomes

Three autosomal trisomies (21, 18, and 13) and one deletion syndrome (cri du chat syndrome), which results from partial deletion of the short arm of chromosome 5, were the first chromosomal abnormalities identified. More recently, several additional trisomies and deletion syndromes (such as those affecting 22q) have been described. Most of these disorders are quite uncommon, but their clinical features should permit ready recognition (Fig. 7.15).

Only trisomy 21 and 22q11.2 deletions occur with sufficient frequency to merit further consideration.

Trisomy 21 (Down Syndrome)

Down syndrome, characterized by extra copy of genes on chromosome 21, is the most common of the chromosomal disorders. About 95% of affected persons have trisomy 21, so their chromosome count is 47. As mentioned earlier, the most common cause of trisomy, and therefore of Down syndrome, is meiotic nondisjunction. The parents of such children are normal in all respects. Maternal age has a strong influence on the incidence of Down syndrome. It occurs in 1 in 1550 live births in women younger than 20 years, in contrast with 1 in 25 live births in women older than 45 years. The correlation with maternal age suggests

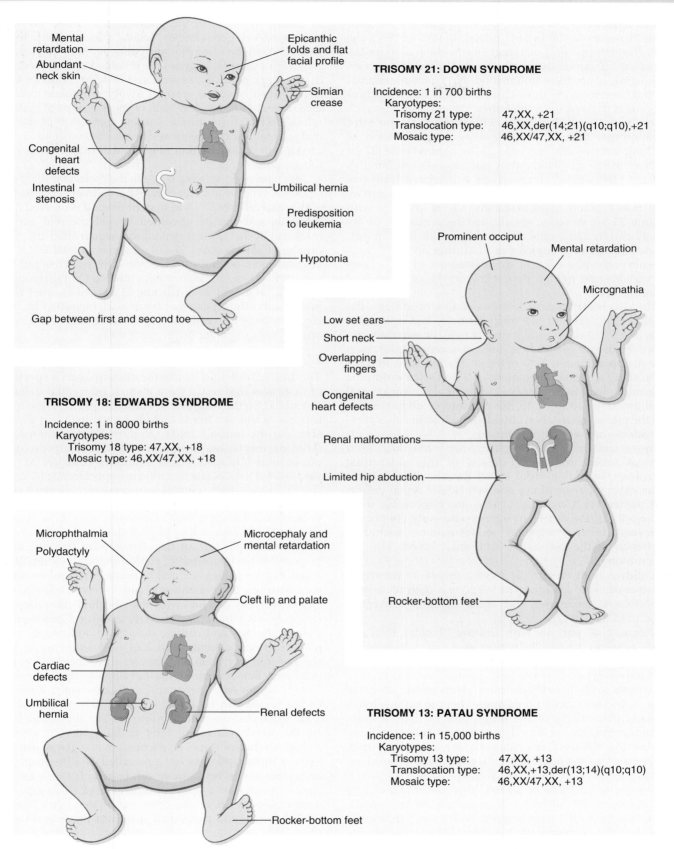

TRISOMY 21: DOWN SYNDROME

Incidence: 1 in 700 births
Karyotypes:
    Trisomy 21 type: 47,XX, +21
    Translocation type: 46,XX,der(14;21)(q10;q10),+21
    Mosaic type: 46,XX/47,XX, +21

Mental retardation
Abundant neck skin
Epicanthic folds and flat facial profile
Simian crease
Congenital heart defects
Intestinal stenosis
Umbilical hernia
Predisposition to leukemia
Hypotonia
Gap between first and second toe

TRISOMY 18: EDWARDS SYNDROME

Incidence: 1 in 8000 births
Karyotypes:
    Trisomy 18 type: 47,XX, +18
    Mosaic type: 46,XX/47,XX, +18

Prominent occiput
Mental retardation
Micrognathia
Low set ears
Short neck
Overlapping fingers
Congenital heart defects
Renal malformations
Limited hip abduction
Rocker-bottom feet

Microphthalmia
Polydactyly
Microcephaly and mental retardation
Cleft lip and palate
Cardiac defects
Umbilical hernia
Renal defects
Rocker-bottom feet

TRISOMY 13: PATAU SYNDROME

Incidence: 1 in 15,000 births
Karyotypes:
    Trisomy 13 type: 47,XX, +13
    Translocation type: 46,XX,+13,der(13;14)(q10;q10)
    Mosaic type: 46,XX/47,XX, +13

Fig. 7.15 Clinical features and karyotypes of the three most common autosomal trisomies.

that in most cases the meiotic nondisjunction of chromosome 21 occurs in the ovum. Indeed, in 95% of cases the extra chromosome is of maternal origin. The reason for the increased susceptibility of the ovum to nondisjunction with aging is not fully understood. No effect of paternal age has been found in those cases in which the extra chromosome is derived from the father.

In about 4% of all patients with trisomy 21, the extra chromosomal material is present as a translocation of the long arm of chromosome 21 to chromosome 22 or 14. Such cases frequently (but not always) are familial, and the translocated chromosome is inherited from one of the parents, who typically is a carrier of a Robertsonian translocation. Approximately 1% of patients with trisomy 21 are mosaics, usually having a mixture of 46- and 47-chromosome cells. These cases result from mitotic nondisjunction of chromosome 21 during an early stage of embryogenesis. Clinical manifestations in such cases are variable and milder, depending on the proportion of abnormal cells.

The diagnostic clinical features of this condition—flat facial profile, oblique palpebral fissures, and epicanthic folds (Fig. 7.15)—are usually readily evident, even at birth. Down syndrome is a leading cause of severe mental retardation; approximately 80% of those afflicted have an IQ of 25 to 50. By contrast, some mosaics with Down syndrome have mild phenotypic changes and normal or near-normal intelligence. In addition to the phenotypic abnormalities and the mental retardation already noted, some other clinical features are worthy of mention:

- *Approximately 40% of the patients have congenital heart disease*, most commonly defects of the endocardial cushion, including atrial septal defects, atrioventricular valve malformations, and ventricular septal defects (Chapter 11). Cardiac problems are responsible for a majority of the deaths in infancy and early childhood. Several other congenital malformations, including atresias of the esophagus and small bowel, also are common.
- Children with trisomy 21 have a *tenfold- to twentyfold increased risk of developing acute leukemia*. Both acute lymphoblastic leukemias and acute myeloid leukemias occur (Chapter 12).
- Virtually all patients with trisomy 21 older than age 40 develop *neuropathologic changes* characteristic of Alzheimer disease, a degenerative disorder of the brain (Chapter 23).
- Patients with Down syndrome demonstrate *abnormal immune responses* that predispose them to serious infections, particularly of the lungs, and to thyroid autoimmunity (Chapter 20). Although several abnormalities, affecting mainly T cell functions, have been reported, the basis for the immunologic disturbances is not clear.

Despite all of these problems, improved medical care has increased the longevity of persons with trisomy 21. Currently the median age at death is 60 years (up from 25 years in 1983). Although the karyotype of Down syndrome has been known for decades, the molecular basis for this disease remains elusive. Studies of humans with partial trisomy of chromosome 21 and mouse models of trisomy have identified the critical region of human chromosome 21 that is involved in the pathogenesis. Based on these studies, several gene clusters, each of which is predicted to participate in the same biologic pathway, have been implicated. For example, 16 genes are involved in the mitochondrial energy pathway, several are likely to influence CNS development, and one group is involved in folate metabolism. It is not known how each of these groups of genes is related to Down syndrome. Adding complexity is the fact that several miRNA genes reside on chromosome 21 that can shut down translation of genes that map elsewhere in the genome.

Much progress is being made in the molecular diagnosis of Down syndrome prenatally. Approximately 5% to 10% of the total cell free DNA in maternal blood is derived from the fetus and can be identified by polymorphic genetic markers. By using next-generation sequencing, the gene dosage of chromosome 21-linked genes in fetal DNA can be determined with great precision. This has emerged as a sensitive and specific noninvasive method ("liquid biopsy") for prenatal diagnosis of trisomy 21 as well as other trisomies. Currently, all cases of trisomy 21 identified by such liquid biopsies are confirmed by conventional cytogenetics on fetal cells obtained by amniocentesis.

22q11.2 Deletion Syndrome

The 22q11.2 deletion syndrome encompasses a spectrum of disorders that result from a small interstitial deletion of band 11 on the long arm of chromosome 22. The clinical features of this syndrome include congenital heart disease affecting the outflow tracts, abnormalities of the palate, facial dysmorphism, developmental delay, thymic hypoplasia with impaired T cell immunity (Chapter 5), and parathyroid hypoplasia resulting in hypocalcemia (Chapter 20). Previously, these clinical features were believed to represent two different disorders: DiGeorge syndrome and velocardiofacial syndrome. However, it is now known that both are caused by 22q11.2 deletion. Variations in the size and position of the deletion are thought to be responsible for the differing clinical manifestations. When T cell immunodeficiency and hypocalcemia are the dominant features, the patients are said to have *DiGeorge syndrome,* whereas patients with the so-called *velocardiofacial syndrome* have mild immunodeficiency and pronounced dysmorphology and cardiac defects. In addition to these malformations, patients with 22q11.2 deletion are at high risk for schizophrenia and bipolar disorder. In fact, it is estimated that schizophrenia develops in approximately 25% of adults with this syndrome. Conversely, deletions of the region can be found in 2% to 3% of individuals with childhood-onset schizophrenia. The molecular basis for this syndrome is not fully understood. The affected region of chromosome 11 encodes many genes. Among these, a transcription factor gene called *TBX1* is suspected to be one of the responsible candidates, because its loss seems to correlate with the occurrence of DiGeorge syndrome. Clearly there are other genes that contribute to the behavioral and psychiatric disorders that remain to be identified.

The diagnosis of this condition may be suspected on clinical grounds but can be established only by detection of the deletion, typically by fluorescence in situ hybridization (FISH) (see Fig. 7.38B).

SUMMARY

CYTOGENETIC DISORDERS INVOLVING AUTOSOMES

- Down syndrome is associated with an extra copy of genes on chromosome 21, most commonly due to trisomy 21 and less frequently from translocation of extra chromosomal material from chromosome 21 to other chromosomes or from mosaicism.
- Patients with Down syndrome have severe mental retardation, flat facial profile, epicanthic folds, cardiac malformations, higher risk of leukemia and infections, and premature development of Alzheimer disease.
- Deletion of genes at chromosomal locus 22q11.2 gives rise to malformations affecting the face, heart, thymus, and parathyroids. The resulting disorders are recognized as (1) DiGeorge syndrome (thymic hypoplasia with diminished T-cell immunity and parathyroid hypoplasia with hypocalcemia), and (2) velocardiofacial syndrome (congenital heart disease involving outflow tracts, facial dysmorphism, and developmental delay).

Cytogenetic Disorders Involving Sex Chromosomes

A number of abnormal karyotypes involving the sex chromosomes, ranging from 45,X to 49,XXXXY, are compatible with life. Indeed, phenotypically normal males with two and even three Y chromosomes have been identified. Such extreme karyotypic deviations are not encountered with the autosomes. In large part, this latitude relates to two factors: (1) lyonization of X chromosomes and (2) the small amount of genetic information carried by the Y chromosome. The consideration of lyonization must begin with Mary Lyon, who in 1962 proposed that in females, only one X chromosome is genetically active. X inactivation occurs early in fetal life, about 16 days after conception. Either the paternal or the maternal X chromosome is randomly inactivated in each cell of the developing embryo. Once inactivated, the same X chromosome remains inactive in all of the progeny of these cells. Moreover, all but one X chromosome is inactivated, and so a 48,XXXX female has only one active X chromosome. This phenomenon explains why normal females do not have a double dose (compared with males) of phenotypic attributes encoded on the X chromosome. The Lyon hypothesis also explains why normal females are in reality mosaics, containing two cell populations: one with an active maternal X, the other with an active paternal X. The molecular basis of X inactivation involves a long non–coding RNA that is encoded by the *XIST* gene. This non–coding RNA is retained in the nucleus, where it "coats" the X chromosome that it is transcribed from and silences the genes on that chromosome. The other *XIST* allele is switched off in the active X, allowing genes encoded one one X chromosome to be expressed.

Although essentially accurate, the Lyon hypothesis subsequently has been somewhat modified. Most important, the initial presumption that all of the genes on the inactive X are "switched off" has been revised, as roughly 21% of genes on Xp, and a smaller number (3%) on Xq, escape X inactivation. This observation has implications for

monosomic X chromosome disorders, or Turner syndrome, as discussed later.

Extra Y chromosomes are readily tolerated because the only information known to be carried on the Y chromosome seems to relate to male differentiation. Of note, whatever the number of X chromosomes, the presence of a Y invariably dictates the male phenotype. The gene for male differentiation (SRY, sex-determining region of Y chromosome) is located on the short arm of the Y.

Described briefly next are two disorders, Klinefelter syndrome and Turner syndrome, that result from aberrations of sex chromosomes.

Klinefelter Syndrome

Klinefelter syndrome is defined as male hypogonadism that develops when there are at least two X chromosomes and one or more Y chromosomes. It is the most common cause of hypogonadism in males. Most affected patients have a 47,XXY karyotype. This karyotype results from nondisjunction of sex chromosomes during meiosis. The extra X chromosome may be of either maternal or paternal origin. Advanced maternal age and a history of irradiation in either parent may contribute to the meiotic error resulting in this condition. Approximately 15% of the patients show mosaic patterns, including 46,XY/47,XXY, 47,XXY/48,XXXY, and variations on this theme. The presence of a 46,XY line in mosaics usually is associated with a milder clinical condition.

Klinefelter syndrome is associated with a wide range of clinical manifestations. In some persons it may be expressed only as hypogonadism, but most patients have a distinctive body habitus with an increase in length between the soles and the pubic bone, which creates the appearance of an elongated body. Also characteristic is eunuchoid body habitus. Reduced facial, body, and pubic hair and gynecomastia also are frequently seen. The testes are markedly reduced in size, sometimes to only 2 cm in greatest dimension. In keeping with the testicular atrophy, the serum testosterone levels are lower than normal, and urinary gonadotropin levels are elevated.

Only rarely are patients with the Klinefelter syndrome fertile, and presumably such persons are mosaics with a large proportion of 46,XY cells. The sterility is due to impaired spermatogenesis, sometimes to the extent of total azoospermia. Histologic examination shows hyalinization of tubules, which appear as ghostlike structures on tissue section. By contrast, Leydig cells are prominent, as a result of either hyperplasia or an apparent increase related to loss of tubules. Although Klinefelter syndrome may be associated with mental retardation, the degree of intellectual impairment typically is mild, and in some cases, no deficit is detectable. The reduction in intelligence is correlated with the number of extra X chromosomes. Klinefelter syndrome is associated with a higher frequency of several disorders, including breast cancer (seen 20 times more commonly than in normal males), extragonadal germ-cell tumors, and autoimmune diseases such as systemic lupus erythematosus.

Turner Syndrome

Turner syndrome, characterized by primary hypogonadism in phenotypic females, results from partial or

complete monosomy of the short arm of the X chromosome. With routine cytogenetic methods, the entire X chromosome is found to be missing in 57% of patients, resulting in a 45,X karyotype. These patients are the most severely affected, and the diagnosis often can be made at birth or early in childhood. *Typical clinical features associated with 45,X Turner syndrome include* growth retardation, leading to abnormally short stature (below the third percentile); swelling of the nape of the neck because of distended lymphatic channels (in infancy) that is seen as webbing of the neck in older children; low posterior hairline; cubitus valgus (an increase in the carrying angle of the arms); shieldlike chest with widely spaced nipples; high-arched palate; lymphedema of the hands and feet; and a variety of congenital malformations such as horseshoe kidney, bicuspid aortic valve, and coarctation of the aorta (Fig. 7.16). *Cardiovascular abnormalities are the most common cause of death in childhood.* In adolescence, affected girls fail to develop normal secondary sex characteristics; the genitalia remain infantile, breast development is minimal, and little pubic hair appears. *Most patients have primary amenorrhea, and morphologic examination shows transformation of the ovaries into white streaks of fibrous stroma devoid of follicles.* The mental status of these patients usually is normal, but subtle defects in visual–spatial information processing have been noted. Curiously, hypothyroidism caused by autoantibodies occurs, especially in women with isochromosome Xp. As many as 50% of these patients develop clinical hypothyroidism. In adult patients, a combination of short stature and primary amenorrhea should prompt strong suspicion for Turner syndrome. The diagnosis is established by karyotyping.

Approximately 43% of patients with Turner syndrome either are mosaics (one of the cell lines being 45,X) or have structural abnormalities of the X chromosome. The most common is deletion of the short arm, resulting in the formation of an isochromosome of the long arm, 46,X,i(X)(q10). The net effect of the associated structural abnormalities is to produce partial monosomy of the X chromosome. Combinations of deletions and mosaicism also occur. It is important to appreciate the karyotypic heterogeneity associated with Turner syndrome because it is responsible for significant variations in the phenotype. In contrast with the patients with monosomy X, those who are mosaics or have deletion variants may have an almost normal appearance and may present only with primary amenorrhea.

The molecular pathogenesis of Turner syndrome is not completely understood, but studies have begun to shed some light. As mentioned earlier, both X chromosomes are active during oogenesis and are essential for normal development of the ovaries. During normal fetal development, ovaries contain as many as 7 million oocytes. The oocytes gradually disappear so that by menarche their numbers have dwindled to a mere 400,000, and when menopause occurs fewer than 10,000 remain. In Turner syndrome, fetal ovaries develop normally early in embryogenesis, but the absence of the second X chromosome leads to an accelerated loss of oocytes, which is complete by age 2 years. In a sense, therefore, "menopause occurs before menarche," and the ovaries are reduced to atrophic fibrous strands, devoid of ova and follicles (*streak ovaries*). Because patients with Turner syndrome also have other (nongonadal) abnormalities, it follows that genes required for normal growth and development of somatic tissues also must reside on the X chromosome. Among the genes involved in the Turner phenotype is the short stature homeobox (*SHOX*) gene at Xp22.33. This is one of the genes that remain active in both X chromosomes and is unique in having an active homologue on the short arm of the Y chromosome. Thus, both normal males and females have two active copies of this gene. Loss of one copy of *SHOX* gives rise to short stature. Indeed, deletions of the *SHOX* gene are noted in 2% to 5% of otherwise normal children with short stature. Whereas loss of one copy of *SHOX* can explain the growth deficit in Turner syndrome, it cannot explain other important clinical features such as cardiac malformations and endocrine abnormalities. Clearly, several other genes located on the X chromosome also are involved.

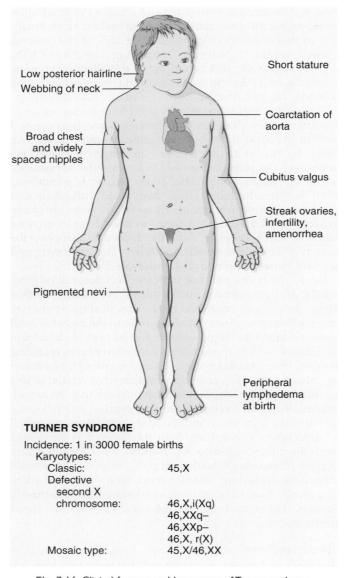

Low posterior hairline
Webbing of neck
Broad chest and widely spaced nipples
Pigmented nevi

Short stature
Coarctation of aorta
Cubitus valgus
Streak ovaries, infertility, amenorrhea
Peripheral lymphedema at birth

TURNER SYNDROME

Incidence: 1 in 3000 female births
Karyotypes:
  Classic: 45,X
  Defective
    second X
    chromosome: 46,X,i(Xq)
                   46,XXq–
                   46,XXp–
                   46,X, r(X)
  Mosaic type: 45,X/46,XX

Fig. 7.16 Clinical features and karyotypes of Turner syndrome.

SUMMARY

CYTOGENETIC DISORDERS INVOLVING SEX CHROMOSOMES

- In females, one X chromosome, maternal or paternal, is randomly inactivated during development (Lyon hypothesis).
- In Klinefelter syndrome, there are two or more X chromosomes with one Y chromosome as a result of nondisjunction of sex chromosomes. Patients have testicular atrophy, sterility, reduced body hair, gynecomastia, and eunuchoid body habitus. It is the most common cause of male sterility.
- In Turner syndrome, there is partial or complete monosomy of genes on the short arm of the X chromosome, most commonly caused by the absence of one X chromosome (45,X) and less commonly by mosaicism, or by deletions involving the short arm of the X chromosome. Short stature, webbing of the neck, cubitus valgus, cardiovascular malformations, amenorrhea, lack of secondary sex characteristics, and fibrotic ovaries are typical clinical features.

SINGLE-GENE DISORDERS WITH ATYPICAL PATTERNS OF INHERITANCE

Three groups of diseases resulting from mutations affecting single genes do not follow the mendelian rules of inheritance:
- Diseases caused by triplet repeat mutations
- Diseases caused by mutations in mitochondrial genes
- Diseases associated with alteration of imprinted regions of the genome

Triplet Repeat Mutations

Fragile X Syndrome

Fragile X syndrome is the prototype of diseases in which the causative mutation occurs in a long repeating sequence of three nucleotides. Other examples of diseases associated with trinucleotide repeat mutations are Huntington disease and myotonic dystrophy. This type of mutation is now known to cause about 40 diseases, and all disorders discovered so far are associated with neurodegenerative changes. In each of these conditions, amplification of specific sets of three nucleotides within the gene disrupts its function. Certain unique features of trinucleotide repeat mutations, described later, are responsible for the atypical pattern of inheritance of the associated diseases.

Fragile X syndrome results from a mutation in the *FMR1* gene, which maps to Xq27.3 and is the second most common genetic cause of mental retardation, after Down syndrome. It has a frequency of 1 in 1550 for males and 1 in 8000 for females. The syndrome derives its name from the karyotypic appearance of the X chromosome in the original method of diagnosis. Culturing patient cells in a folate-deficient medium typically showed a discontinuity of staining or constriction in the long arm of the X chromosome. This method has now been supplanted by DNA-based analysis of triplet repeat size, as discussed later. Clinically affected males have moderate to severe mental retardation, although the extent of impairment is highly variable. It is not unusual for some children to initially be diagnosed with autism-like symptoms. The typical physical phenotype includes a long face with a large mandible, large everted ears, and large testicles (*macroorchidism*). Although characteristic of fragile X syndrome, these abnormalities are not always present or may be quite subtle. The only distinctive physical abnormality that can be detected in at least 90% of postpubertal males with fragile X syndrome is macroorchidism.

As with all X-linked diseases, fragile X syndrome predominantly affects males. Analysis of several pedigrees, however, shows some patterns of transmission not typically associated with other X-linked recessive disorders (Fig. 7.17). These include the following:

- *Carrier males.* Approximately 20% of males who, by pedigree analysis, are known to carry a fragile X mutation do not manifest the typical neurological symptoms or physical characteristics of fragile X during childhood. As discussed below, these carrier males (also known as "transmitting males") harbor a detectable molecular abnormality at the FMR1 locus but not the full-fledged mutation observed in symptomatic children.
- *Affected females.* From 30% to 50% of carrier women with the fragile X mutation on one chromosome might show features of mild cognitive impairment or other behavioral disturbances. Approximately 20% develop features of premature reproductive failure (see below). The presence of symptoms in carrier females, albeit mild, is unusual for an X-linked recessive disease.
- *Anticipation.* This term refers to the phenomenon whereby clinical features of fragile X syndrome worsen with each successive generation, as if the mutation becomes increasingly deleterious as it is transmitted from a man to his grandsons and great-grandsons.

These unusual features have been related to the dynamic nature of the mutation. In the normal population, the number of repeats of the sequence CGG in the *FMR1* gene is small, averaging around 29, whereas affected persons have 200 to 4000 repeats. These so-called "full mutations" are believed to arise through an intermediate stage of premutations characterized by 52 to 200 CGG repeats. Carrier males and females have premutations. During oogenesis (but not spermatogenesis), the premutations can be converted to full mutations by further amplification of the CGG repeats, which can then be transmitted to both the sons and the daughters of the carrier female. These observations provide an explanation for why some carrier males are unaffected (they have premutations), and certain carrier females are affected (they inherit full mutations).

Pathogenesis

The molecular basis for fragile X syndrome is beginning to be understood and relates to silencing of the product of the *FMR1* gene, familial mental retardation protein (FMRP). The normal *FMR1* gene contains CGG repeats in its 5' untranslated region. When the number of trinucleotide repeats exceeds approximately 230, the DNA of the entire 5' region of the gene becomes abnormally methylated. Methylation also extends upstream into the promoter region of the gene, resulting in transcriptional suppression of *FMR1*. The resulting absence of FMRP is believed to cause the

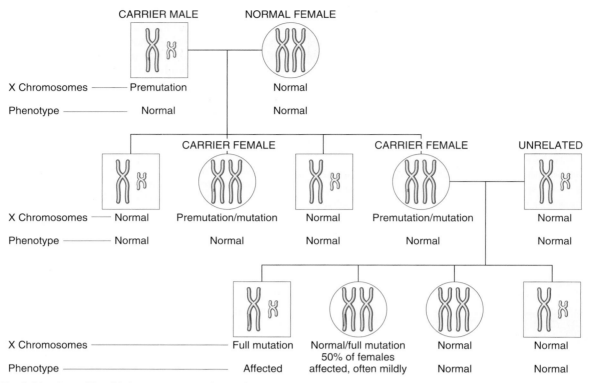

Fig. 7.17 Fragile X pedigree. X and Y chromosomes are shown. Note that in the first generation, all sons are normal and all females are carriers (harbor a premutation). During oogenesis in the carrier female, premutation expands to full mutation; hence, in the next generation, all males who inherit the X with full mutation are affected. However, only 50% of females who inherit the full mutation are affected, and often only mildly. *(Based on an original sketch courtesy of Dr. Nancy Schneider, Department of Pathology, University of Texas Southwestern Medical School, Dallas, Texas.)*

phenotypic changes. FMRP is widely expressed in normal tissues, but higher levels are found in the brain and the testis. It is an RNA-binding protein that is transported from the cytoplasm to the nucleus, where it binds specific mRNAs and transports them to the axons and dendrites (Fig. 7.18). It is in the synapses that FMRP–mRNA complexes perform critical roles in regulating the translation of specific mRNAs involved in control of synaptic functions. The absence of this finely coordinated "shuttle" function seems to underlie the fragile X syndrome.

Fragile X Tremor/Ataxia

Although initially assumed to be innocuous, CGG premutations in the *FMR1* gene can cause a disease that is phenotypically different from fragile X syndrome through a distinct mechanism involving a toxic "gain-of-function." This disease was discovered when it was noted that approximately 20% of females carrying the premutation (carrier females) have mild cognitive impairment and premature ovarian failure (before the age of 40 years), and more than 50% of premutation-carrying males (transmitting males) exhibit a progressive neurodegenerative syndrome starting in their sixth decade. This syndrome, referred to as *fragile X tremor/ataxia,* is characterized by intention tremors and cerebellar ataxia and may progress to parkinsonism.

How do premutations cause disease? In these patients, the *FMR1* gene instead of being methylated and silenced continues to be transcribed. CGG-containing *FMR1* mRNAs so formed are "toxic." They accumulate in the nucleus and form intranuclear inclusions. In this process the aggregated mRNA recruits RNA-binding proteins.

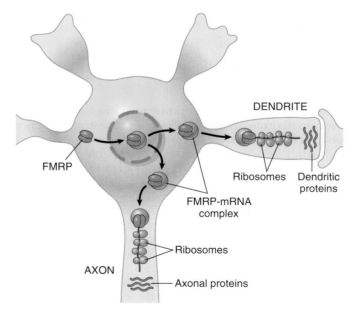

Fig. 7.18 A model for the action of familial mental retardation protein (FMRP) in neurons. FMRP plays a critical role in regulating the translation of axonal proteins from bound RNAs. These locally produced proteins, in turn, play diverse roles in the microenvironment of the synapse. *(Adapted from Hin P, Warren ST: New insights into fragile X syndrome: from molecules to neurobehavior, Trends Biochem Sci 28:152, 2003.)*

Perhaps sequestration of these proteins at abnormal locations leads to events that are toxic to the cell.

As noted, earlier many other neurodegenerative diseases related to trinucleotide repeat expansions are recognized. Some general principles follow:

- In all cases, gene functions are altered by an expansion of the repeats, but the precise threshold at which premutations are converted to full mutations differs with each disorder.
- Whereas the expansion in fragile X syndrome occurs during oogenesis, in other disorders such as Huntington disease, premutations are converted to full mutations during spermatogenesis.
- The expansion may involve any part of the gene, and the range of possibilities can be divided into two broad categories: those that affect untranslated regions (as in fragile X syndrome) and those that affect coding regions (as in Huntington disease) (Fig. 7.19). When mutations affect noncoding regions, there is "loss of function," because protein synthesis is suppressed (e.g., FMRP). By contrast, mutations involving translated parts of the gene give rise to misfolded proteins (e.g., Huntington disease). Many of these so-called "toxic gain-of-function" mutations involve CAG repeats that encode polyglutamine tracts, and the resultant diseases are sometimes referred to as polyglutamine diseases, affecting primarily the nervous system. Accumulation of misfolded proteins in aggregates within the cytoplasm is a common feature of such diseases.

SUMMARY

FRAGILE X SYNDROME AND FRAGILE X TREMOR/ATAXIA

- Pathologic amplification of trinucleotide repeats causes loss-of-function (fragile X syndrome) or gain-of-function mutations (Huntington disease). Most such mutations produce neurodegenerative disorders.
- Fragile X syndrome results from loss of *FMR1* gene function and is characterized by mental retardation, macroorchidism, and abnormal facial features.
- In the normal population, there are about 29 CGG repeats in the *FMR1* gene. The genomes of carrier males and females contain premutations with 52 to 200 CGG repeats that can expand to 4000 repeats (full mutations) during oogenesis.

- When full mutations are transmitted to progeny, fragile X syndrome occurs.
- Fragile X tremor/ataxia resulting from expression of a *FMR1* gene bearing premutation develops in some males and females. The accumulation of corresponding mRNA in the nucleus binds and sequesters certain proteins that are essential for normal neuronal functions

Diseases Caused by Mutations in Mitochondrial Genes

Mitochondria contain several genes that encode enzymes involved in oxidative phosphorylation. Inheritance of mitochondrial DNA differs from that of nuclear DNA in that the former is associated with maternal inheritance. The reason for this peculiarity is that ova contain the normal complement of mitochondria within their abundant cytoplasm, whereas spermatozoa contain few, if any, mitochondria. The mitochondrial DNA of the zygote is therefore derived entirely from the ovum. Thus, only mothers transmit mitochondrial genes to their offspring, both male and female.

Diseases caused by mutations in mitochondrial genes are rare. Because mitochondrial DNA encodes enzymes involved in oxidative phosphorylation, diseases caused by mutations in such genes affect organs most dependent on oxidative phosphorylation (CNS, skeletal muscle, cardiac muscle, liver, and kidney). *Leber hereditary optic neuropathy* is the prototypical disorder in this group. This neurodegenerative disease manifests as progressive bilateral loss of central vision that leads in due course to blindness.

Diseases Caused by Alterations of Imprinted Regions: Prader-Willi and Angelman Syndromes

All humans inherit two copies of each gene (except, of course, the sex chromosome genes in males), carried on homologous maternal and paternal chromosomes. It was long assumed that there was no difference between normal homologous genes derived from the mother and the father. Indeed, this is true for most genes. It has been established, however, that functional differences exist between the paternal and the maternal copies of some genes. **The differences arise from an epigenetic process called** *genomic imprinting,* **whereby certain homologous genes are differentially "inactivated" during paternal and maternal**

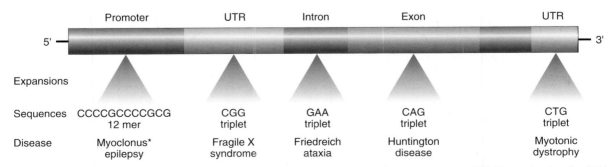

Fig. 7.19 Sites of expansion and the affected sequence in selected diseases caused by nucleotide repeat mutations. *UTR,* Untranslated region. *Although not strictly a trinucleotide-repeat disease, progressive myoclonus epilepsy is caused, like others in this group, by a heritable DNA expansion. The expanded segment is in the promoter region of the gene.

gametogenesis. Thus, maternal imprinting refers to transcriptional silencing of the maternal allele, whereas paternal imprinting implies that the paternal allele is inactivated. At the molecular level, imprinting is associated with methylation of the gene promoter, as well as related events such as modification of DNA-binding histone proteins, the sum total effect of which is to silence the gene. Imprinting occurs in ova or sperm and is then stably transmitted to all somatic cells derived from the zygote.

Genomic imprinting is best illustrated by considering two uncommon genetic disorders, Prader-Willi syndrome and Angelman syndrome.

Mental retardation, short stature, hypotonia, obesity, small hands and feet, and hypogonadism characterize Prader-Willi syndrome. In 60% to 75% of cases, an interstitial deletion of band q12 in the long arm of chromosome 15—del(15)(q11;q13)—can be detected. In many patients without a detectable cytogenetic abnormality, FISH analysis shows smaller deletions within the same region. It is striking that in all cases, the deletion affects the paternally derived chromosome 15. In contrast to Prader-Willi syndrome, patients with the phenotypically distinct Angelman syndrome are born with a deletion of the same chromosomal region derived from their mothers. **Patients with Angelman syndrome also are mentally retarded, but in addition they present with ataxic gait, seizures, and inappropriate laughter.** Because of the laughter and ataxia, this syndrome has been called the happy puppet syndrome. A comparison of these two syndromes clearly demonstrates the "parent-of-origin" effects on gene function. If all the paternal and maternal genes contained within chromosome 15 were expressed in an identical fashion, clinical features resulting from these deletions would be expected to be identical regardless of the parental origin of chromosome 15.

The molecular basis of these two syndromes can be understood in the context of imprinting (Fig. 7.20). A set of genes on the maternal chromosome at 15q12 is imprinted (and hence silenced), so the paternal chromosome provides the only functional alleles. When these are lost as a result of a deletion (in the paternal chromosome), the patient develops Prader-Willi syndrome. Among the set of genes that are deleted in Prader-Willi syndrome, the most likely culprit is believed to be a gene cluster encoding multiple distinct small nucleolar RNAs (snoRNAs), which are involved in messenger RNA processing. Conversely, a distinct gene, *UBE3A*, that also maps to the same region of chromosome 15 is imprinted on the paternal chromosome. *UBE3A* encodes for a ubiquitin ligase, a family of enzymes that targets other cellular proteins for proteasomal degradation (Chapter 1) through the addition of ubiquitin moieties. Only the maternally derived allele of the gene normally is active. Deletion of this maternal gene on chromosome 15 gives rise to the Angelman syndrome. The neurologic manifestations of Angelman are principally because of a lack of UBE3A expression in specific regions of the brain.

Molecular studies of cytogenetically normal patients with Prader-Willi syndrome have shown that in some cases, both of the structurally normal copies of chromosome 15 are derived from the mother. Inheritance of both chromosomes of a pair from one parent is called *uniparental disomy*. The net effect is the same (i.e., the patient does not have a functional set of genes from the [nonimprinted] paternal chromosome 15). Angelman syndrome, as might be expected, also can result from uniparental disomy of paternal chromosome 15.

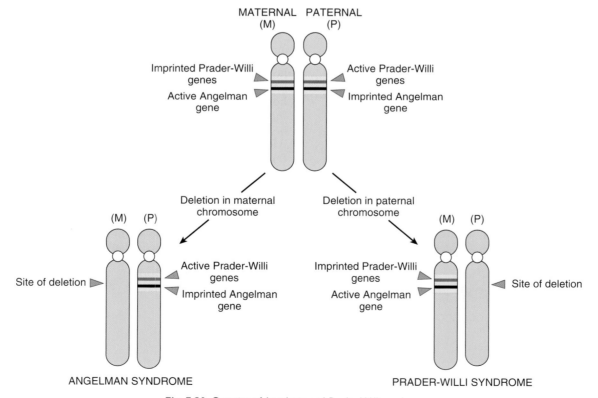

Fig. 7.20 Genetics of Angelman and Prader-Willi syndromes.

SUMMARY
GENOMIC IMPRINTING

- Imprinting involves transcriptional silencing of the paternal or maternal copies of certain genes during gametogenesis. For such genes only one functional copy exists in the individual. Loss of the functional allele (not imprinted) by deletions gives rise to diseases.

- Prader-Willi syndrome results from deletion of paternal chromosomal region 15q12 and is characterized by mental retardation, short stature, hypotonia, obesity, and hypogonadism.
- Angelman syndrome results from deletion of maternal chromosomal region 15q12 and is characterized by mental retardation, ataxia, seizures, and inappropriate laughter.

Pediatric Diseases

As mentioned earlier and as illustrated by several examples, many diseases of infancy and childhood are of genetic origin. Others, although not genetic, either are unique to children or take distinctive forms in this patient population and thus merit the designation pediatric diseases. During each stage of development, infants and children are prey to a somewhat different group of diseases (Table 7.5). Clearly, diseases of infancy (i.e., in the first year of life) pose the highest risk of death. During this phase, the neonatal period (the first 4 weeks of life) is unquestionably the most hazardous time.

After the infant survives the first year of life, the outlook brightens considerably. However, it is sobering to note that between 1 year and 14 years of age, injuries resulting from accidents are the leading cause of death. Not all conditions listed in Table 7.5 are described in this chapter; only a select few that are most common are considered here. Although general principles of neoplastic disease and specific tumors are discussed elsewhere, a few tumors of children are described, to highlight the differences between pediatric and adult neoplasms.

CONGENITAL ANOMALIES

Congenital anomalies are structural defects that are present at birth, although some, such as cardiac defects and renal anomalies, may not become clinically apparent until years later. As will be evident from the ensuing discussion, the term congenital does not imply or exclude a genetic basis. It is estimated that about 120,000 babies are born with a birth defect each year in the United States, an incidence of 1 in 33. As indicated in Table 7.5, congenital anomalies are an important cause of infant mortality. Moreover, they continue to be a significant source of illness, disability, and death throughout the early years of life.

Before considering the etiology and pathogenesis of congenital anomalies, it is essential to define some of the terms used to describe errors in morphogenesis.

- *Malformations are primary errors of morphogenesis.* In other words, there is an intrinsically abnormal developmental process. Malformations usually are multifactorial, rather than the result of a single gene or chromosomal defect.

Table 7.5 Causes of Death by Age

Causes*	Rate[†]	Causes*	Rate[†]
Younger than 1 year	**582.1**	**1–4 Years—cont'd**	**28.3**
Congenital malformations, deformations, and chromosomal anomalies		Malignant neoplasms	
Disorders related to short gestation and low birth weight		Diseases of the heart[‡]	
Sudden infant death syndrome (SIDS)		**5–9 Years**	**12.5**
Newborn affected by maternal complications of pregnancy		Accidents (unintentional injuries)	
Accidents (unintentional injuries)		Malignant neoplasms	
Newborn affected by complications of placenta, cord, and membranes		Congenital malformations, deformations, and chromosomal abnormalities	
Bacterial sepsis of newborn		Assault (homicide)	
Respiratory distress of newborn		Influenza and pneumonia	
Diseases of the circulatory system		**10–14 Years**	**15.7**
Neonatal hemorrhage		Accidents (unintentional injuries)	
1–4 Years	**24**	Malignant neoplasms	
Accidents (unintentional injuries)		Intentional self-harm (suicide)	
Congenital malformations, deformations, and chromosomal abnormalities		Assault (homicide)	
Assault (homicide)		Congenital malformations, deformations, and chromosomal anomalies	

*Causes are listed in decreasing order of frequency. All causes and rates are based on 2008 (final) and 2009 (preliminary) data.
[†]Rates are expressed per 100,000 population from all causes within each age group.
[‡]Excludes congenital heart disease.
Data source: Centers for Disease Control and Prevention/NCHS, National Vital Statistics System: mortality, 2014. www.cdc.gov/nchs/data/dvs/lcwk1_2014.pdf.

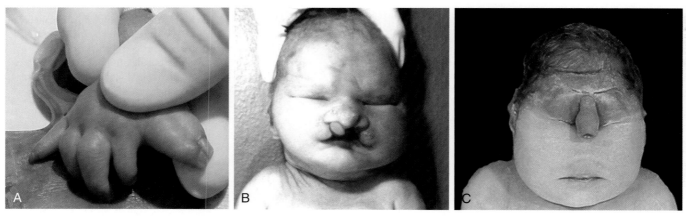

Fig. 7.21 Examples of malformations. Malformations can range in severity from the incidental to the lethal. (A) Polydactyly (one or more extra digits) and syndactyly (fusion of digits) have little functional consequence when they occur in isolation. (B) Similarly, cleft lip, with or without associated cleft palate, is compatible with life when it occurs as an isolated anomaly; in this case, however, the child had an underlying malformation syndrome (trisomy 13) and expired because of severe cardiac defects. (C) Stillbirth associated with a lethal malformation, in which the midface structures are fused or ill-formed; in almost all cases, this degree of external dysmorphogenesis is associated with severe internal anomalies such as maldevelopment of the brain and cardiac defects. *(A and C, Courtesy of Dr. Reade Quinton, Department of Pathology, University of Texas Southwestern Medical Center, Dallas, Texas. B, Courtesy of Dr. Beverly Rogers, Department of Pathology, University of Texas Southwestern Medical Center, Dallas, Texas.)*

They may manifest in any of several patterns. In some presentations, such as congenital heart diseases, single body systems may be involved, whereas in others, multiple malformations involving many organs and tissues may coexist (Fig. 7.21).

- *Disruptions result from secondary destruction of an organ or body region that was previously normal in development;* thus, in contrast with malformations, disruptions arise from an extrinsic disturbance in morphogenesis. Amniotic bands, stemming from rupture of amnion with resultant formation of "bands" that encircle, compress, or attach to parts of the developing fetus, constitute the classic example of a disruption (Fig. 7.22). A variety of environmental agents may cause disruptions (see later). Disruptions are not heritable, of course, and thus are not associated with risk of recurrence in subsequent pregnancies.

- *Deformations, like disruptions, also represent an extrinsic disturbance of development rather than an intrinsic error of morphogenesis.* Deformations are common, affecting approximately 2% of newborn infants to various degrees. They are caused by localized or generalized compression of the growing fetus by abnormal biomechanical forces, leading eventually to a variety of structural abnormalities. The most common cause of deformations is uterine constraint. Between weeks 35 and 38 of gestation, rapid increase in the size of the fetus outpaces the growth of the uterus, and the relative amount of amniotic fluid (which normally acts as a cushion) also decreases. Thus, even the normal fetus is subjected to some degree of uterine constraint. However, several variables increase the likelihood of excessive compression of the fetus, including maternal conditions such as first pregnancy, small uterus, malformed (bicornuate) uterus, and leiomyomas. Causes relating to the fetus, such as presence of multiple fetuses, oligohydramnios, and abnormal fetal presentation, also may be involved.

- *Sequence refers to multiple congenital anomalies that result from secondary effects of a single localized aberration in organogenesis.* The initiating event may be a malformation, deformation, or disruption. An excellent example is the oligohydramnios (or Potter) sequence (Fig. 7.23A). Oligohydramnios (decreased amniotic fluid) may be caused by a variety of maternal, placental, or fetal abnormalities, including chronic leakage of amniotic fluid because of rupture of the amnion; uteroplacental insufficiency resulting from maternal hypertension or severe toxemia; and renal agenesis in the fetus (because fetal urine is a major constituent of amniotic fluid). The fetal compression associated with oligohydramnios in turn results in a classic phenotype in the newborn infant consisting of flattened faces and positional abnormalities of the hands and feet (Fig. 7.23B). The hips may be dislocated. Growth of the chest wall and the lungs also is compromised, sometimes to such an extent that

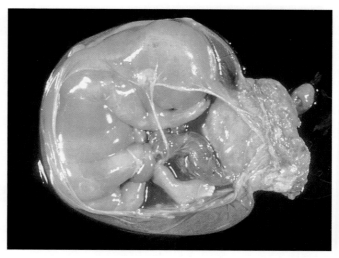

Fig. 7.22 Disruption due to amniotic bands. In the specimen shown, the placenta is at the right, and the band of amnion extends from the top portion of the amniotic sac to encircle the leg of the fetus. *(Courtesy of Dr. Theonia Boyd, Children's Hospital of Boston, Boston, Massachusetts.)*

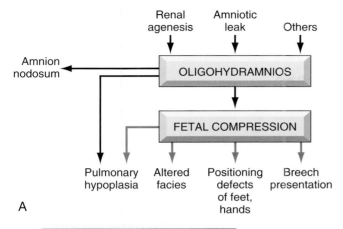

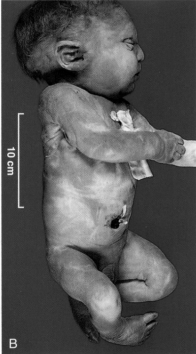

Fig. 7.23 (A) Pathogenesis of the oligohydramnios (Potter) sequence. (B) Infant with oligohydramnios (Potter) sequence. Note flattened facial features and deformed foot (talipes equinovarus).

survival is not possible. If the embryologic connection between these defects and the initiating event is not recognized, a sequence may be mistaken for a malformation syndrome.

- *Malformation syndrome refers to the presence of several defects that cannot be explained on the basis of a single localizing initiating error in morphogenesis.* Syndromes most often arise from a single causative condition (e.g., viral infection or a specific chromosomal abnormality) that simultaneously affects several tissues.

- *In addition to these global definitions, some general terms are applied to organ-specific malformations. Agenesis* refers to the complete absence of an organ or its anlage, whereas aplasia and hypoplasia indicate incomplete development and underdevelopment, respectively. *Atresia* describes the absence of an opening, usually of a hollow visceral organ or duct such as intestines and bile ducts.

Etiology

Known causes of errors in human malformations can be grouped into three major categories: genetic, environmental, and multifactorial (Table 7.6). The cause has not been identified for almost half of the reported cases.

Genetic causes of malformations include all of the previously discussed mechanisms of genetic disease. Virtually all chromosomal syndromes are associated with congenital malformations. Examples are Down syndrome and other trisomies, Turner syndrome, and Klinefelter syndrome. Most chromosomal disorders arise during gametogenesis and hence are not familial. Single-gene mutations, characterized by mendelian inheritance, may underlie major malformations. For example, holoprosencephaly is the most common developmental defect of the forebrain and midface in humans (see Chapter 23). The Hedgehog signaling pathway plays a critical role in the morphogenesis of these structures, and loss-of-function mutations of individual components within this pathway are reported in families with a history of recurrent holoprosencephaly.

Environmental influences, such as viral infections, drugs, and radiation to which the mother was exposed during pregnancy, may cause fetal malformations (the appellation of "malformation" is used loosely in this context, because technically, these anomalies represent disruptions). Among the viral infections listed in Table 7.6, rubella was a major

Table 7.6 Causes of Congenital Malformations in Humans

Cause	Frequency of Malformations* (%)
Genetic	
Chromosomal aberrations	10–15
Mendelian inheritance	2–10
Environmental	
Maternal/placental infections Rubella Toxoplasmosis Syphilis Cytomegalovirus infection Human immunodeficiency virus infection Zika virus infection	2–3
Maternal disease states Diabetes Phenylketonuria Endocrinopathies	6–8
Drugs and chemicals Alcohol Folic acid antagonists Androgens Phenytoin Thalidomide Warfarin 13-Cis-retinoic acid Others	~1
Irradiation	~1
Multifactorial	**20–25**
Unknown	**40–60**

*Live births.
Data from Stevenson RE, Hall JG, Goodman RM, editors: *Human malformations and related anomalies*, New York, 1993, Oxford University Press, p 115.

scourge of the 19th and early 20th centuries. Fortunately, *maternal rubella* and the resultant rubella embryopathy have been virtually eliminated in developed countries as a result of vaccination. As mentioned later, maternal infection with Zika Virus can give rise to severe malformations of the central nervous system. A variety of *drugs and chemicals* have been suspected to be teratogenic, but perhaps less than 1% of congenital malformations are caused by these agents. The list includes thalidomide, alcohol, anticonvulsants, warfarin (oral anti-coagulant), and 13-cis-retinoic acid, which is used in the treatment of severe acne. For example, *thalidomide,* formerly used as a tranquilizer in Europe and currently used for treatment of certain cancers, causes an extremely high incidence (50% to 80%) of limb malformations. *Alcohol,* perhaps the most widely used agent today, is an important environmental teratogen. Infants born of mothers who abuse alcohol show prenatal and postnatal growth retardation, facial anomalies (microcephaly, short palpebral fissures, maxillary hypoplasia), and psychomotor disturbances. These features in combination are designated the *fetal alcohol syndrome.* Although *cigarette smoke–derived nicotine has* not been convincingly demonstrated to be a teratogen, there is a high incidence of spontaneous abortions, premature labor, and placental abnormalities among pregnant smokers, and babies born to mothers who smoke often have a low birth weight and may be prone to the sudden infant death syndrome (SIDS). In light of these findings, it is best to avoid nicotine exposure altogether during pregnancy. Among maternal conditions listed in Table 7.6, *diabetes mellitus* is a common entity, and despite advances in antenatal obstetric monitoring and glucose control, the incidence of major malformations in infants of diabetic mothers stands between 6% and 10% in most reported series. Maternal hyperglycemia–induced fetal hyperinsulinemia results in fetal macrosomia (organomegaly and increased body fat and muscle mass); cardiac anomalies, neural tube defects, and other CNS malformations are some of the major anomalies seen in diabetic embryopathy.

Multifactorial inheritance, which implies the interaction of environmental influences with two or more genes of small effect, is the most common genetic cause of congenital malformations. Included in this category are some relatively common malformations such as cleft lip and palate and neural tube defects. The importance of environmental contributions to multifactorial inheritance is underscored by the dramatic reduction in the incidence of neural tube defects by periconceptional intake of folic acid in the diet. The recurrence risks and mode of transmission of multifactorial disorders are described earlier in this chapter.

Pathogenesis

The pathogenesis of congenital anomalies is complex and still poorly understood, but two general principles are relevant regardless of the etiologic agent:

1. *The timing of the prenatal teratogenic insult has an important impact on the occurrence and the type of anomaly produced.* The intrauterine development of humans can be divided into two phases: (1) the embryonic period, occupying the first 9 weeks of pregnancy, and (2) the fetal period, terminating at birth.

- In the *early embryonic period* (first 3 weeks after fertilization), an injurious agent damages either enough cells to cause death and abortion or only a few cells, presumably allowing the embryo to recover without developing defects. *Between the third and the ninth weeks, the embryo is extremely susceptible to teratogenesis,* with the peak sensitivity occurring between the fourth and the fifth weeks. During this period organs are being crafted out of the germ-cell layers.
- The *fetal period* that follows organogenesis is marked chiefly by the further growth and maturation of the organs, with greatly reduced susceptibility to teratogenic agents. Instead, the fetus is susceptible to growth retardation or injury to already formed organs. It is therefore possible for a given agent to produce different anomalies if exposure occurs at different times of gestation.

2. The complex interplay between environmental teratogens and intrinsic genetic defects is exemplified by the fact that features of dysmorphogenesis caused by environmental insults often can be recapitulated by genetic defects in the pathways targeted by these teratogens. Some representative examples follow:

- *Cyclopamine* is a plant teratogen. Pregnant sheep that feed on plants containing cyclopamine give birth to lambs that have severe craniofacial abnormalities including holoprosencephaly and cyclopia (single fused eye—hence the origin of the moniker cyclopamine). This compound is an inhibitor of Hedgehog signaling in the embryo, and, as stated previously, mutations of Hedgehog genes are present in subsets of fetuses with holoprosencephaly.
- *Valproic acid* is an anti-epileptic and a recognized teratogen. Valproic acid disrupts expression of a family of highly conserved developmentally critical transcription factors known as *homeobox (HOX)* proteins. In vertebrates, HOX proteins have been implicated in the patterning of limbs, vertebrae, and craniofacial structures. Not surprisingly, mutations in the *HOX* gene family are responsible for congenital anomalies that mimic features observed in *valproic acid embryopathy.*
- The vitamin A (retinol) derivative *all-trans-retinoic acid* is essential for normal development and differentiation, and its absence during embryogenesis results in a constellation of malformations affecting multiple organ systems, including the eyes, genitourinary system, cardiovascular system, diaphragm, and lungs (see Chapter 8 for vitamin A deficiency in the postnatal period). Conversely, excessive exposure to retinoic acid also is teratogenic. Infants born to mothers treated with retinoic acid for severe acne have a predictable phenotype *(retinoic acid embryopathy),* including CNS, cardiac, and craniofacial defects, such as cleft lip and cleft palate. The last entity may stem from retinoic acid–mediated deregulation of components of the transforming growth factor-β (TGF-β) signaling pathway, which is involved in palatogenesis. Mice with knockout of the *TGFB3* gene uniformly develop cleft palate, once again illustrating the functional relationship between teratogenic exposure and signaling pathways in the causation of congenital anomalies.

SUMMARY

CONGENITAL ANOMALIES

- Congenital anomalies result from intrinsic abnormalities (malformations) as well as extrinsic disturbances (deformations, disruptions).
- Congenital anomalies can result from genetic (chromosomal abnormalities, gene mutations), environmental (infections, drugs, alcohol), and multifactorial causes.
- The timing of the in utero insult has profound influence on the extent of congenital anomalies, with earlier events usually having greater impact.
- The interplay between genetic and environmental causes of anomalies is emphasized by the fact that teratogens often target signaling pathways in which mutations have been reported as a cause for the same anomalies.

PERINATAL INFECTIONS

Infections of the fetus and neonate may be acquired transcervically (ascending infections) or transplacentally (hematologic infections).

- *Transcervical, or ascending, infections* are caused by spread of microbes from the cervicovaginal canal and may be acquired in utero or during birth. Most bacterial infections (e.g., α-hemolytic streptococcal infection) and a few viral infections (e.g., herpes simplex) are acquired in this manner. In general, the fetus acquires the infection by "inhaling" infected amniotic fluid into the lungs or by passing through an infected birth canal during delivery. Fetal infection usually is associated with inflammation of the placental membranes (chorioamnionitis) and inflammation of the umbilical cord (funisitis). This mode of spread is typical for pneumonia and, in severe cases, sepsis and meningitis.

- *Transplacental infections* gain access to the fetal bloodstream by crossing the placenta via the chorionic villi, and may occur at any time during gestation or occasionally, as may be the case with hepatitis B and human immunodeficiency virus, at the time of delivery via maternal-to-fetal transfusion. Most parasitic (e.g., toxoplasma, malaria) and viral infections, and a few bacterial infections (i.e., *Listeria* and *Treponema*), follow this mode of hematogenous transmission. The clinical manifestations of these infections are highly variable, depending largely on the gestational timing and the microorganism involved. The most important transplacental infections can be conveniently remembered by the acronym *TORCH*. The elements of the TORCH complex are Toxoplasma (T), rubella virus (R), cytomegalovirus (C), herpesvirus (H), and any of a number of other (O) microbes such as *Treponema pallidum*. These agents are grouped together because they may evoke similar clinical and pathologic manifestations. TORCH infections occurring early in gestation may cause chronic sequelae in the child, including growth restriction, mental retardation, cataracts, and congenital cardiac anomalies, whereas infections later in pregnancy result primarily in tissue injury accompanied by inflammation (encephalitis, chorioretinitis, hepatosplenomegaly,

pneumonia, and myocarditis). More recently, Zika virus has emerged as another agent that can be transmitted by pregnant females to their offspring with devastating consequences such as microcephaly and brain damage.

PREMATURITY AND FETAL GROWTH RESTRICTION

Prematurity is defined by a gestational age less than 37 weeks and is the second most common cause of neonatal mortality (second only to congenital anomalies). As might be expected, infants born before completion of gestation also weigh less than normal (<2500 gm). The major risk factors for prematurity include preterm premature rupture of membranes; intrauterine infection leading to inflammation of the placental membranes (chorioamnionitis); structural abnormalities of the uterus, cervix, and placenta; and multiple gestation (e.g., twin pregnancy). Children born before completion of the full period of gestation have higher morbidity and mortality rates than full-term infants. The immaturity of organ systems in preterm infants makes them especially vulnerable to several important complications:

- Respiratory distress syndrome, also called hyaline membrane disease
- Necrotizing enterocolitis
- Sepsis
- Intraventricular and germinal matrix hemorrhage (Chapter 23)
- Long-term sequelae, including developmental delay

Although birth weight is low in preterm infants, it usually is appropriate after adjustment for gestational age. By contrast, as many as one-third of infants who weigh less than 2500 gm are born at term and are therefore undergrown rather than immature. These small-for-gestational-age (SGA) infants suffer from *fetal growth restriction*. Fetal growth restriction may result from fetal, maternal, or placental abnormalities, although in many cases the specific cause is unknown.

- *Fetal abnormalities:* This category consists of conditions that intrinsically reduce growth potential of the fetus despite an adequate supply of nutrients from the mother. Prominent among such fetal conditions are chromosomal disorders, congenital anomalies, and congenital infections. Chromosomal abnormalities may be detected in as many as 17% of fetuses evaluated for fetal growth restriction and in as many as 66% of fetuses with documented ultrasonographic malformations. Fetal infection should be considered in all growth-restricted neonates, with the TORCH group of infections (see earlier) being a common cause. When the causation is intrinsic to the fetus, fetal growth restriction is symmetric (i.e., affects all organ systems equally).

- *Placental abnormalities:* Placental causes include any factor that compromises the uteroplacental blood supply. Examples include placenta previa (low implantation of the placenta), placental abruption (separation of placenta from the decidua by a retroplacental clot), or placental infarction. With placental (and maternal) abnormalities, the fetal growth restriction is asymmetric (i.e., the brain is spared relative to visceral organs such as the liver).

- *Maternal factors:* This category comprises by far the most common causes of the growth deficit in SGA infants. Important examples are vascular diseases such as *pre-eclampsia* ("toxemia of pregnancy") (Chapter 19) and *chronic hypertension.* Another class of maternal diseases increasingly being recognized in the setting of fetal growth restriction is acquired or inherited diseases of hypercoagulability (i.e., thrombophilias) (Chapter 4). The list of other maternal conditions associated with fetal growth restriction is long, but some of the avoidable influences are maternal narcotic abuse, alcohol intake, and heavy cigarette smoking (as noted previously, many of these same causes also are involved in the pathogenesis of congenital anomalies). Drugs causing fetal growth restriction in similar fashion include teratogens, such as the commonly administered anti-convulsant phenytoin (Dilantin), as well as nonteratogenic agents. Maternal malnutrition (in particular, prolonged hypoglycemia) also may affect fetal growth.

Not only is the growth-restricted infant handicapped in the perinatal period, but the deficits persist into childhood and adult life. Affected persons are thus more likely to have cerebral dysfunction, learning disabilities, and sensory (i.e., visual and hearing) impairment.

RESPIRATORY DISTRESS SYNDROME OF THE NEWBORN

The most common cause of respiratory distress in the newborn is *respiratory distress syndrome (RDS),* also know as *hyaline membrane disease* because of the formation of "membranes" in the peripheral air spaces observed in infants who succumb to this condition. An estimated 24,000 cases of RDS are reported annually in the United States. Improvements in management of this condition have sharply decreased deaths due to respiratory insufficiency from as many as 5000 per year a decade ago to fewer than 900 cases yearly. It is primarily a disorder of premature infants. Less common causes include excessive sedation of the mother, fetal head injury during delivery, aspiration of blood or amniotic fluid, and intrauterine hypoxia secondary to compression from coiling of the umbilical cord about the neck.

Pathogenesis

RDS occurs in about 60% of infants born at less than 28 weeks' gestation, 30% of those born between 28 to 34 weeks' gestation, and less than 5% of those born after 34 weeks' gestation. There are also strong though not invariable associations with *male gender, maternal diabetes,* and delivery by *cesarean section.*

The fundamental defect in RDS is the inability of the immature lung to synthesize sufficient surfactant. Surfactant is a complex of surface-active phospholipids, principally dipalmitoylphosphatidylcholine (lecithin) and at least two groups of surfactant-associated proteins. The importance of surfactant-associated proteins in normal lung function can be gauged by the occurrence of severe

respiratory failure in neonates with congenital deficiency of surfactant caused by mutations in the corresponding genes. Surfactant is synthesized by type II pneumocytes and, with the healthy newborn's first breath, rapidly coats the surface of alveoli, reducing surface tension and thus decreasing the pressure required to keep the alveoli open. In a lung deficient in surfactant, alveoli tend to collapse, and a relatively greater inspiratory effort is required with each breath to open the alveoli. The infant rapidly tires from breathing and generalized atelectasis sets in. The resulting hypoxia sets into motion a sequence of events that leads to epithelial and endothelial damage and eventually to the formation of hyaline membranes (Fig. 7.24). As discussed later, this classical picture of surfactant deficiency is greatly modified by surfactant treatment.

Hormones regulate surfactant synthesis. Corticosteroids stimulate the formation of surfactant lipids and associated proteins. Therefore, conditions associated with intrauterine stress and fetal growth restriction, which increase corticosteroid release, lower the risk of developing RDS. Conversely, the compensatory high blood levels of insulin in infants of diabetic mothers can suppress surfactant synthesis, counteracting the effects of steroids. This may explain, in part, why infants of diabetic mothers are at higher risk for developing RDS. Labor is known to increase surfactant synthesis; accordingly, cesarean section performed before the onset of labor also may be associated with increased risk for RDS.

MORPHOLOGY

The lungs in infants with RDS are of normal size but are heavy and relatively airless. They have a mottled purple color, and on microscopic examination the tissue appears solid, with poorly developed, generally collapsed (atelectatic) alveoli. If the infant dies within the first several hours of life, only necrotic cellular debris will be present in the terminal bronchioles and alveolar ducts. Later in the course, characteristic **eosinophilic hyaline membranes** line the respiratory bronchioles, alveolar ducts, and random alveoli (Fig. 7.25). These "membranes" contain necrotic epithelial cells admixed with extravasated plasma proteins. There is a remarkable paucity of neutrophilic inflammatory reaction associated with these membranes. The lesions of hyaline membrane disease are never seen in stillborn infants or in live-born infants who die within a few hours of birth. If the infant with RDS dies after several days, evidence of reparative changes, including proliferation of type II pneumocytes and interstitial fibrosis, is seen.

Clinical Features

The classic clinical presentation before the era of treatment with exogenous surfactant was described earlier. Currently, the actual clinical course and prognosis for neonatal RDS vary, depending on the maturity and birth weight of the infant and the promptness of therapy. The control of RDS focuses on prevention, either by delaying labor until the fetal lung reaches maturity or by inducing maturation of the lung in the at-risk fetus. Critical to these objectives is the ability to assess fetal lung maturity accurately. Because pulmonary secretions are discharged into the amniotic fluid, analysis of amniotic fluid phospholipids

PREMATURITY

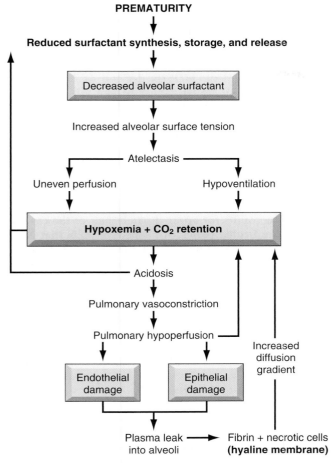

Fig. 7.24 Pathophysiology of respiratory distress syndrome (see text).

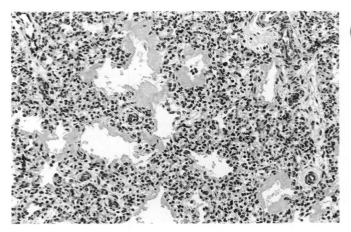

Fig. 7.25 Hyaline membrane disease (hematoxylin-eosin stain). Alternating atelectasis and dilation of the alveoli can be seen. Note the eosinophilic thick hyaline membranes lining the dilated alveoli.

provides a good estimate of the level of surfactant in the alveolar lining. Prophylactic administration at birth of exogenous surfactant to extremely premature infants (born before 28 weeks' gestational age) has proven very beneficial, such that it is now uncommon for infants to die of acute RDS.

In uncomplicated cases, recovery begins to occur within 3 or 4 days. In affected infants, oxygen is required. Use of high concentrations of ventilator-administered oxygen for prolonged periods, however, is associated with two well-known complications: retrolental fibroplasia (also called retinopathy of prematurity) in the eyes; and bronchopulmonary dysplasia. Fortunately, both complications are now significantly less common as a result of gentler ventilation techniques, antenatal glucocorticoid therapy, and prophylactic surfactant treatments. Hence they are described briefly:

- Retinopathy of prematurity has a two-phase pathogenesis. During the hyperoxic phase of RDS therapy (phase I), expression of the proangiogenic vascular endothelial growth factor (VEGF) is markedly decreased, causing endothelial cell apoptosis. VEGF levels rebound after return to relatively hypoxic room air ventilation (phase II), inducing retinal vessel proliferation (*neovascularization*) characteristic of the lesions in the retina.
- The major abnormality in bronchopulmonary dysplasia is a striking decrease in alveolar septation (manifested as large, simplified alveolar structures) and a dysmorphic capillary configuration. Multiple factors—hyperoxemia, hyperventilation, prematurity, inflammatory cytokines, and vascular maldevelopment—contribute to bronchopulmonary dysplasia and probably act additively or synergistically to promote injury.

Infants who recover from RDS also are at increased risk for developing a variety of other complications associated with preterm birth; most important among these are *patent ductus arteriosus, intraventricular hemorrhage, and necrotizing enterocolitis*. Thus, although technologic advances help save the lives of many infants with RDS, they also bring to the surface the exquisite fragility of the immature neonate.

SUMMARY

NEONATAL RESPIRATORY DISTRESS SYNDROME

- Neonatal RDS (hyaline membrane disease) is a disease of prematurity; most cases occur in neonates born before 28 weeks' gestational age.
- The fundamental abnormality in RDS is insufficient pulmonary surfactant, which results in failure of lungs to inflate after birth.
- The characteristic morphologic pattern in RDS is the presence of hyaline membranes (consisting of necrotic epithelial cells and plasma proteins) lining the airways.
- RDS can be ameliorated by prophylactic administration of steroids, surfactant therapy, and by improved ventilation techniques.
- Long-term sequelae associated with RDS therapy include retinopathy of prematurity and bronchopulmonary dysplasia; the incidence of both complications has decreased with improvements in management of RDS.

NECROTIZING ENTEROCOLITIS

Necrotizing enterocolitis (NEC) most commonly occurs in premature infants, with the incidence of the disease being inversely proportional to the gestational age. It occurs in approximately 1 of 10 very-low-birth-weight infants (<1500 gm). In addition to prematurity, most cases are associated with enteral feeding, suggesting that some postnatal insult (such as the introduction of bacteria) sets in motion the cascade culminating in tissue destruction. Although infectious agents are likely to play a role in NEC pathogenesis, no single bacterial pathogen has been linked to the disease. A large number of inflammatory mediators have been associated with pathogenesis of NEC. One particular mediator, platelet-activating factor, has been implicated in increasing mucosal permeability by promoting enterocyte apoptosis and compromising intercellular tight junctions, thereby "adding fuel to the fire."

NEC typically involves the terminal ileum, cecum, and right colon, although any part of the small or large intestine may be involved. The involved segment typically is distended, friable, and congested (Fig. 7.26), or it can be frankly gangrenous; intestinal perforation with accompanying peritonitis may be seen. On microscopic examination, mucosal or transmural coagulative necrosis, ulceration, bacterial colonization, and submucosal gas bubbles are all features associated with NEC. Evidence of reparative changes, such as granulation tissue and fibrosis, may be seen shortly after resolution of the acute episode.

The clinical course is fairly typical, with the onset of bloody stools, abdominal distention, and development of circulatory collapse. Abdominal radiographs often demonstrate gas within the intestinal wall (*pneumatosis intestinalis*). When detected early, NEC often can be managed conservatively, but many cases (20% to 60%) require operative intervention including resection of the necrotic segments of bowel. NEC is associated with high perinatal mortality; infants who survive often develop post-NEC strictures from fibrosis caused by the healing process.

SUDDEN INFANT DEATH SYNDROME (SIDS)

According to the National Institute of Child Health and Human Development, *SIDS* **is defined as "the sudden death of an infant under 1 year of age which remains unexplained after a thorough case investigation, including performance of a complete autopsy, examination of the death scene, and review of the clinical history."** It is important to emphasize that many cases of sudden death in infancy are found to have an anatomic or biochemical basis at autopsy (Table 7.7); these should not be labeled as SIDS, but rather as sudden unexpected infant death (SUID). The Centers for Disease Control and Prevention estimates that SIDS accounts for approximately half of the cases of SUID in the United States. An aspect of SIDS that is not stressed in the definition is that the infant usually dies while asleep—hence the lay terms crib death and cot death. SIDS is the leading cause of death between the ages of 1 month and 1 year in U.S. infants, and the third leading cause of death overall in this age group, after congenital anomalies and diseases of prematurity and low birth weight. In 90% of cases, the infant is younger than 6 months; most are between the ages of 2 and 4 months. SIDS in an earlier sibling is associated with a fivefold relative risk of recurrence; *traumatic child abuse must be carefully excluded under these circumstances.*

Pathogenesis

SIDS is multifactorial condition, with a mixture of contributing causes in a given case. Three interacting variables have been proposed: (1) a vulnerable infant, (2) a critical developmental period in homeostatic control, and (3) one or more exogenous stressors. According to this model, several factors make the infant vulnerable to sudden

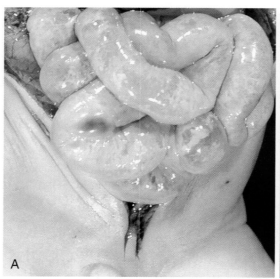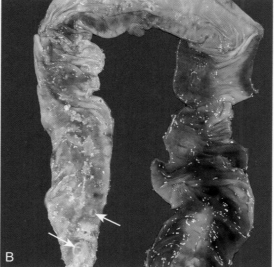

Fig. 7.26 Necrotizing enterocolitis. (A) At postmortem examination in a severe case, the entire small bowel was markedly distended and perilously thin (usually this appearance implies impending perforation). (B) The congested portion of the ileum corresponds to areas of hemorrhagic infarction and transmural necrosis. Submucosal gas bubbles (pneumatosis intestinalis) can be seen in several areas *(arrows)*.

Table 7.7 Factors Associated With Sudden Infant Death Syndrome (SIDS)

Parental

Young maternal age (age younger than 20 years)
Maternal smoking during pregnancy
Drug abuse in *either* parent, specifically paternal marijuana and maternal opiate, cocaine use
Short intergestational intervals
Late or no prenatal care
Low socioeconomic group
African-American and American Indian ethnicity (socioeconomic factors)

Infant

Brain stem abnormalities, associated with delayed development of arousal and cardiorespiratory control
Prematurity and/or low birth weight
Male sex
Product of a multiple birth
SIDS in a previous sibling
Antecedent respiratory infections
Germline polymorphisms in autonomic nervous system genes

Environment

Prone or side sleep position
Sleeping on a soft surface
Hyperthermia
Cosleeping in first 3 months of life

Postmortem Abnormalities Detected in Cases of Sudden Unexpected Infant Death (SUID)*

Infections
Viral myocarditis
Bronchopneumonia
Unsuspected congenital anomaly
Congenital aortic stenosis
Anomalous origin of the left coronary artery from the pulmonary artery
Traumatic child abuse
Intentional suffocation (filicide)
Genetic and metabolic defects
Long QT syndrome (*SCN5A* and *KCNQ1* mutations)
Fatty acid oxidation disorders (*MCAD, LCHAD, SCHAD* mutations)
Histiocytoid cardiomyopathy (*MTCYB* mutations)
Abnormal inflammatory responsiveness (partial deletions in *C4a* and *C4b*)

*SIDS is not the only cause of SUIDs, but rather is a *diagnosis of exclusion*. Therefore, performance of an autopsy may often show findings that would explain the cause of an SUID. These cases should *not*, strictly speaking, be labeled as "SIDS." *SCN5A*, Sodium channel, voltage-gated, type V, alpha polypeptide; *KCNQ1*, potassium voltage-gated channel, KQT-like subfamily, member 1; *MCAD*, medium-chain acyl coenzyme A dehydrogenase; *LCHAD*, long-chain 3-hydroxyacyl coenzyme A dehydrogenase; *SCHAD*, short-chain 3-hydroxyacyl coenzyme A dehydrogenase; *MTCYB*, mitochondrial cytochrome *b*; *C4*, complement component 4.

death during the critical developmental period (i.e., 1 month to 1 year). These vulnerability factors may be specific to the parents or the infant, whereas the exogenous stressor or stressors are attributable to the environment (Table 7.7). Although numerous factors have been proposed to account for a vulnerable infant, *the most compelling hypothesis is that SIDS reflects a delayed development of arousal and cardiorespiratory control*. The brain stem and, in particular, the medulla oblongata play a critical role in the body's "arousal" response to noxious stimuli such as episodic hypercarbia, hypoxia, and thermal stress encountered during sleep. The serotonergic (5-HT) system of the medulla is implicated in these "arousal" responses as well as regulation of other critical homeostatic functions such

as respiratory drive, blood pressure, and upper airway reflexes. Abnormalities in serotonin-dependent signaling in the brain stem may be the underlying basis for SIDS in some infants.

Among the potential *environmental causes*, prone sleeping position, sleeping on soft surfaces, and thermal stress are possibly the most important modifiable risk factors for SIDS. Many studies have clearly shown increased risk for SIDS in infants who sleep in a prone position, prompting the **American Academy of Pediatrics to recommend placing healthy infants on their backs when laying them down to sleep. This "Back to Sleep" campaign has resulted in substantial decreases in SIDS-related deaths since its inception in 1994.** The prone position increases the infant's vulnerability to one or more recognized noxious stimuli (hypoxia, hypercarbia, and thermal stress) during sleep. In addition, the prone position also is associated with decreased arousal responsiveness compared with the supine position.

Of note, SIDS is not the only cause of sudden unexpected death in infancy. *Therefore, SIDS is a diagnosis of exclusion, requiring careful examination of the death scene and a complete postmortem examination.* The latter can show an unsuspected cause of sudden death in as many as 20% or more of babies presumed to have died of SIDS (Table 7.7). Infections (e.g., viral myocarditis or bronchopneumonia) are the most common causes of SUID, followed by a congenital anomaly. As a result of advancements in molecular diagnostics, several genetic causes of SUID have emerged. For example, fatty acid oxidation disorders, characterized by defects in mitochondrial fatty acid oxidative enzymes, may be responsible for as many as 5% of sudden deaths in infancy; of these, a deficiency in medium-chain acyl-coenzyme A dehydrogenase is the most common. Retrospective analyses in cases of sudden infant death originally designated SIDS also have revealed mutations of cardiac sodium and potassium channels, which result in a form of cardiac arrhythmia characterized by prolonged QT intervals; these cases account for no more than 1% of SUIDs.

MORPHOLOGY

Anatomic studies of victims have yielded inconsistent histologic findings. **Multiple petechiae** are the most common finding in the typical SIDS autopsy (in approximately 80% of cases); these usually are present on the thymus, visceral and parietal pleura, and epicardium. The lungs usually are congested, and vascular engorgement with or without **pulmonary edema** is present in a majority of cases. Sophisticated morphometric studies have shown quantitative brain stem abnormalities such as **hypoplasia of the arcuate nucleus** or a subtle decrease in brain stem neuronal populations in several cases; these observations are not uniform, however, and the use of such studies is not feasible in most "routine" autopsy procedures.

SUMMARY

SUDDEN INFANT DEATH SYNDROME

- SIDS is a disorder of unknown cause, defined as the sudden death of an infant younger than 1 year of age that remains unexplained after a thorough case investigation including performance of an autopsy. Most SIDS deaths occur between the ages of 2 and 4 months.

- The most likely basis for SIDS is a delayed development of arousal reflexes and cardiorespiratory control.
- Numerous environmental risk factors have been proposed, of which the prone sleeping position is best recognized—hence the success of the "Back to Sleep" program in reducing the incidence of SIDS.

FETAL HYDROPS

Fetal hydrops **refers to the accumulation of edema fluid in the fetus during intrauterine growth**. The causes of fetal hydrops are manifold; the most important are listed in Table 7.8. In the past, hemolytic anemia caused by Rh blood group incompatibility between mother and fetus (immune hydrops) was the most common cause, but with the successful prophylaxis of this disorder during pregnancy, other causes of nonimmune hydrops have emerged as the principal culprits. The fluid accumulation can be quite variable, ranging in degree from progressive, generalized edema of the fetus *(hydrops fetalis)*, a usually lethal condition, to more localized and less marked edematous processes, such as isolated pleural and peritoneal effusions or postnuchal fluid collections *(cystic hygroma)*, that often are compatible with life (Fig. 7.27). The mechanism of immune hydrops is discussed first, followed by other important causes of fetal hydrops.

Table 7.8 Major Causes of Fetal Hydrops*

Cardiovascular
Malformations
Tachyarrhythmia
High-output failure

Chromosomal
Turner syndrome
Trisomy 21, trisomy 18

Thoracic Causes
Cystic adenomatoid malformation
Diaphragmatic hernia

Fetal Anemia
Homozygous α-thalassemia
Parvovirus B19
Immune hydrops (Rh and ABO)

Twin Gestation
Twin-to-twin transfusion

Infection (excluding parvovirus)
Cytomegalovirus
Syphilis
Toxoplasmosis

Genitourinary Tract Malformations

Tumors

Genetic/Metabolic Disorders

*The cause of fetal hydrops may be undetermined ("idiopathic") in up to 20% of cases.

Data from Machin GA: Hydrops, cystic hygroma, hydrothorax, pericardial effusions, and fetal ascites. In Gilbert-Barness E, et al, editors: *Potter's pathology of the fetus, infant, and child*, St. Louis, 2007, Mosby, pp 33.

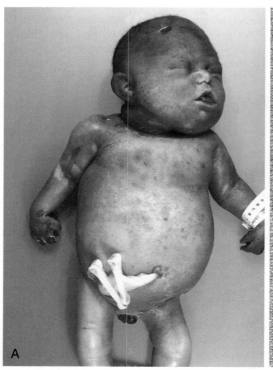 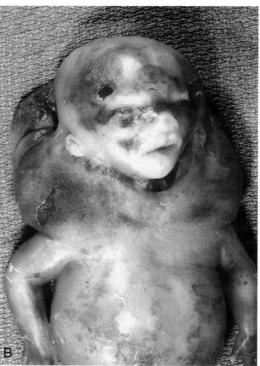

Fig. 7.27 Hydrops fetalis. (A) Generalized accumulation of fluid in the fetus. (B) Fluid accumulation particularly prominent in the soft tissues of the neck. This condition has been termed *cystic hygroma*. Cystic hygromas are characteristically seen with, but not limited to, constitutional chromosomal anomalies such as 45,X karyotypes. *(Courtesy of Dr. Beverly Rogers, Department of Pathology, University of Texas Southwestern Medical Center, Dallas, Texas.)*

Immune Hydrops

Immune hydrops results from an antibody-induced hemolytic disease in the newborn that is caused by blood group incompatibility between mother and fetus. Such an incompatibility occurs when the fetus inherits red cell antigenic determinants from the father that are foreign to the mother. The most common antigens to result in clinically significant hemolysis are the Rh and ABO blood group antigens. Of the numerous antigens included in the Rh system, only the D antigen is a major cause of Rh incompatibility. Fetal red cells may reach the maternal circulation during the last trimester of pregnancy, when the cytotrophoblast is no longer present as a barrier, or during childbirth itself (fetomaternal bleed). The mother then becomes sensitized to the foreign antigen and produces antibodies that, in future pregnancies, can freely traverse the placenta to the fetus, in which they cause red cell destruction. With initiation of immune hemolysis, progressive anemia in the fetus leads to tissue ischemia, intrauterine cardiac failure, and peripheral pooling of fluid (edema). As discussed later, cardiac failure may be the final pathway by which edema occurs in many cases of nonimmune hydrops as well.

Several factors influence the immune response to Rh-positive fetal red cells that reach the maternal circulation:

- Concurrent ABO incompatibility protects the mother against Rh immunization, because the fetal red cells are promptly coated by isohemagglutinins (preformed anti-A or anti-B antibodies) and removed from the maternal circulation.
- The antibody response depends on the dose of immunizing antigen, so hemolytic disease develops only when the mother has experienced a significant transplacental bleed (more than 1 mL of Rh-positive red cells).
- The isotype of the antibody is important, because immunoglobulin G (IgG) (but not IgM) antibodies can cross the placenta. The initial exposure to Rh antigen evokes the formation of IgM antibodies, so Rh disease is very uncommon with the first pregnancy. Subsequent exposure during the second or third pregnancy generally leads to a brisk IgG antibody response.

Appreciation of the role of previous sensitization in the pathogenesis of Rh-hemolytic disease of the newborn has led to its therapeutic control. Currently, Rh-negative mothers are given Rh immune globulin (RhIg) at 28 weeks and within 72 hours after delivery of an Rh-positive baby. The RhIg masks the antigenic sites on the fetal red cells that may have leaked into the maternal circulation during childbirth, thus preventing long-lasting sensitization to Rh antigens.

As a result of the remarkable success achieved in prevention of Rh hemolysis, fetomaternal ABO incompatibility currently is the most common cause of immune hemolytic disease of the newborn. Although ABO incompatibility occurs in approximately 20% to 25% of pregnancies, hemolysis develops in only a small fraction of infants born subsequently, and in general the disease is much milder than Rh incompatibility. In part the less severe course of disease can be attributed to the expression of A and B antigens on many cells other than red cells which act like sponge for the transferred antibody. ABO hemolytic disease occurs almost exclusively in infants of blood group A or B who are born to mothers of blood group O. The normal anti-A and anti-B isohemagglutinins in group O mothers usually are of the IgM type and therefore do not cross the placenta. However, for reasons not well understood, certain group O women possess IgG antibodies directed against group A or B antigens (or both) even without previous sensitization. Therefore, the firstborn may be affected. There is no effective method of preventing hemolytic disease resulting from ABO incompatibility.

Nonimmune Hydrops

The major causes of nonimmune hydrops include those disorders associated with cardiovascular defects, chromosomal anomalies, and fetal anemia.

- *Structural cardiovascular defects and functional abnormalities* (i.e., arrhythmias) may result in intrauterine cardiac failure and hydrops. Among the chromosomal anomalies, 45,X karyotype (Turner syndrome) and trisomies 21 and 18 are associated with fetal hydrops; the basis for this disorder usually is the presence of underlying structural cardiac anomalies, although in Turner syndrome there may be an abnormality of lymphatic drainage from the neck leading to postnuchal fluid accumulation (resulting in *cystic hygromas*).
- *Fetal anemias* resulting from causes other than Rh or ABO incompatibility also may result in hydrops. In fact, in some parts of the world (e.g., Southeast Asia), severe fetal anemia caused by homozygous α-thalassemia probably is the most common cause of fetal hydrops.
- *Transplacental infection* by parvovirus B19 is increasingly recognized as an important cause of fetal hydrops. The virus gains entry into erythroid precursors (normoblasts), where it replicates. The ensuing cellular injury leads to the death of the normoblasts and aplastic anemia. Parvoviral intranuclear inclusions can be seen within circulating and marrow erythroid precursors (Fig. 7.28).

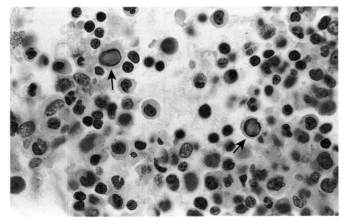

Fig. 7.28 Bone marrow from an infant infected with parvovirus B19. The *arrows* point to two erythroid precursors with large homogeneous intranuclear inclusions and a surrounding peripheral rim of residual chromatin.

The basis for hydrops in fetal anemia of immune and nonimmune causes is tissue ischemia with secondary myocardial dysfunction and circulatory failure. Additionally, secondary liver failure may occur, with loss of synthetic function contributing to hypoalbuminemia, reduced plasma osmotic pressure, and edema.

MORPHOLOGY

The anatomic findings in fetuses with intrauterine fluid accumulation vary with both the severity of the disease and the underlying etiology. As previously noted, **hydrops fetalis** represents the most severe and generalized manifestation (Fig. 7.27), and lesser degrees of edema such as isolated pleural, peritoneal, or postnuchal fluid collections can occur. Accordingly, infants may be stillborn, die within the first few days, or recover completely. The presence of dysmorphic features suggests underlying constitutional chromosomal abnormalities; postmortem examination may show a cardiac anomaly. In hydrops associated with fetal anemia, both fetus and placenta are characteristically pale; in most cases, the liver and spleen are enlarged as a consequence of **cardiac failure** and congestion. Additionally, the bone marrow shows compensatory hyperplasia of erythroid precursors (parvovirus-associated aplastic anemia being a notable exception), and **extramedullary hematopoiesis** is present in the liver, the spleen, and possibly in other tissues such as the kidneys, the lungs, the lymph nodes, and even the heart (Fig. 7.29). The increased hematopoietic activity accounts for the presence in the peripheral circulation of large numbers of normoblasts, and even more immature erythroblasts (**erythroblastosis fetalis**).

The presence of hemolysis in Rh or ABO incompatibility is associated with the added complication of increased circulating bilirubin from the red cell breakdown. The CNS may be damaged when hyperbilirubinemia is marked (usually greater than 20 mg/dL in full-term infants, but often less in premature infants). The circulating unconjugated bilirubin is taken up into the brain, on which it apparently exerts a toxic effect. The basal ganglia and brain stem are particularly prone to deposition of bilirubin pigment, which imparts a characteristic yellow hue to the parenchyma (**kernicterus**) (Fig. 7.30).

Clinical Course

Early recognition of fetal hydrops is imperative, because even severe cases can sometimes be salvaged with timely therapy. Immune hydrops that results from Rh incompatibility can be predicted with reasonable certainty, because its severity correlates well with rapidly rising Rh antibody titers in the mother during pregnancy. Antenatal identification and management of the at-risk fetus have been facilitated by amniocentesis and the advent of chorionic villus and fetal blood sampling. The direct anti-globulin test (direct Coombs test) (Chapter 12) using fetal cord blood yields a positive result if the red cells have been coated by maternal antibody. In addition, cloning of the *RHD* gene has resulted in efforts to determine fetal Rh status by sequencing cell free DNA in maternal blood. When identified, cases of severe intrauterine hemolysis may be treated by fetal intravascular transfusions via

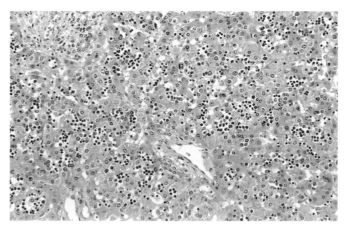

Fig. 7.29 Numerous islands of extramedullary hematopoiesis *(small blue cells)* are scattered among mature hepatocytes in this histologic preparation from an infant with nonimmune hydrops fetalis.

the umbilical cord and early delivery. Postnatally, phototherapy is helpful, because visible light converts bilirubin to readily excreted dipyrroles. As already discussed, in an overwhelming majority of cases, administration of RhIg to the mother can prevent the occurrence of immune hydrops in subsequent pregnancies. Group ABO hemolytic disease is more difficult to predict but is readily anticipated by awareness of the blood incompatibility between mother and father and by hemoglobin and bilirubin determinations in the vulnerable newborn. In fatal cases of fetal hydrops, a thorough postmortem examination is imperative to determine the cause and to exclude a potentially recurring cause such as a chromosomal abnormality.

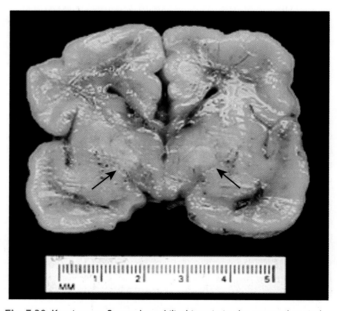

Fig. 7.30 Kernicterus. Severe hyperbilirubinemia in the neonatal period—for example, secondary to immune hydrolysis—results in deposition of bilirubin pigment *(arrows)* in the brain parenchyma. This occurs because the blood–brain barrier is less developed in the neonatal period than it is in adulthood. Infants who survive develop long-term neurologic sequelae.

SUMMARY

FETAL HYDROPS

- Fetal hydrops refers to the accumulation of edema fluid in the fetus during intrauterine growth.
- The degree of fluid accumulation is variable, from generalized hydrops fetalis to localized cystic hygromas.
- The most common causes of fetal hydrops are nonimmune (chromosomal abnormalities, cardiovascular defects, and fetal anemia), whereas immune hydrops has become less frequent as a result of Rh antibody prophylaxis.
- Erythroblastosis fetalis (circulating immature erythroid precursors) is a characteristic finding of fetal anemia-associated hydrops.
- Hemolysis-induced hyperbilirubinemia can result in bilirubin toxicity (kernicterus) in the basal ganglia and brain stem, particularly in premature infants.

TUMORS AND TUMORLIKE LESIONS OF INFANCY AND CHILDHOOD

Malignant neoplasms constitute the second most common cause of death in children between the ages of 4 and 14 years; only accidents exact a higher toll. Benign tumors are even more common than cancers.

It is sometimes difficult to segregate, on morphologic grounds, true tumors from tumorlike lesions in the infant and child. In this context, two special categories of tumorlike lesions should be recognized:

- *Heterotopia or choristoma* refers to microscopically normal cells or tissues that are present in abnormal locations. Examples are a pancreatic tissue "rest" found in the wall of the stomach or small intestine and a small mass of adrenal cells found in the kidney, lungs, ovaries, or elsewhere. Heterotopic rests usually are of little clinical significance, but on the basis of their appearance they can be confused with neoplasms.
- *Hamartoma* refers to an excessive but focal overgrowth of cells and tissues native to the organ in which it occurs. Although the cellular elements are mature and identical to those found in the remainder of the organ, they do not reproduce the normal architecture of the surrounding tissue. The line of demarcation between a hamartoma and a benign neoplasm frequently is tenuous and is variously interpreted. Hemangiomas, lymphangiomas, rhabdomyomas of the heart, and adenomas of the liver are considered by some researchers to be hamartomas and by others to be true neoplasms.

Benign Neoplasms

Virtually any neoplasm may be encountered in the pediatric age group, but three—hemangiomas, lymphangiomas, and teratomas—deserve special mention here.

Hemangiomas **are the most common neoplasms of infancy.** Both cavernous and capillary hemangiomas may be encountered (Chapter 10), although the latter often are more cellular than in adults and thus may appear deceptively worrisome. In children, most hemangiomas are located in the skin, particularly on the face and scalp, where they produce flat to elevated, irregular, red-blue masses; the flat, larger lesions are referred to as *port-wine stains.* Hemangiomas may enlarge as the child ages, but in many instances they spontaneously regress (Fig. 7.31). The vast majority of superficial hemangiomas have no more than a cosmetic significance; rarely, they may be the manifestation of a hereditary disorder associated with disease within internal organs, such as the von Hippel-Lindau syndrome (Chapter 10). A subset of CNS cavernous hemangiomas can occur in the familial setting; affected families harbor mutations in one of three *cerebral cavernous malformation* (CCM) genes.

Lymphangiomas represent the lymphatic counterpart of hemangiomas. Microscopic examination shows cystic and cavernous spaces lined by endothelial cells and surrounded by lymphoid aggregates; the spaces usually contain pale fluid. They may occur on the skin but, more importantly, they also are encountered in the deeper regions of the neck, axilla, mediastinum, and retroperitoneum. Although histologically benign, they tend to increase in size after birth and may encroach on mediastinal structures or nerve trunks in axilla.

Teratomas may occur as benign, well-differentiated cystic lesions (mature teratomas), as lesions of indeterminate potential (immature teratomas), or as unequivocally

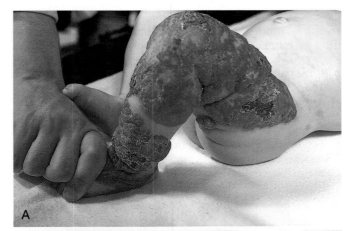

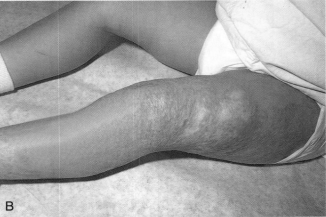

Fig. 7.31 Congenital capillary hemangioma (A) at birth and (B) at 2 years of age after the lesion had undergone spontaneous regression. *(Courtesy of Dr. Eduardo Yunis, Children's Hospital of Pittsburgh, Pittsburgh, Pennsylvania.)*

malignant teratomas (usually admixed with another germ cell tumor component such as an endodermal sinus tumor). Sacrococcygeal teratomas are the most common teratomas of childhood, accounting for 40% or more of cases (Fig. 7.32). In view of the overlap in the mechanisms underlying congenital malformations and oncogenesis, it is interesting that approximately 10% of sacrococcygeal teratomas are associated with congenital anomalies, primarily defects of the hindgut and cloacal region and other midline defects (e.g., meningocele, spina bifida) not believed to result from local effects of the tumor. Approximately 75% of these tumors are mature teratomas with a benign course, and about 12% are unmistakably malignant and lethal (Chapter 18). The remainder are designated immature teratomas, and their malignant potential correlates with the amount of immature tissue elements present. Most of the benign teratomas are encountered in younger infants (4 months of age or younger), whereas children with malignant lesions tend to be somewhat older.

Malignant Neoplasms

The organ systems involved most commonly by malignant neoplasms in infancy and childhood are the hematopoietic system, neural tissue, and soft tissues (Table 7.9). This distribution is in sharp contrast with that in adults, in whom epithelial tumors of the lung, heart, prostate, and colon are the most common forms. Malignant neoplasms of infancy and childhood differ biologically and histologically from those in adults. The main differences are as follows:

- Relatively frequent demonstration of a close relationship between abnormal development (teratogenesis) and tumor induction (oncogenesis), suggesting a common stem cell defect.
- Prevalence of genetic abnormalities or familial syndromes that predispose to cancer
- Tendency of fetal and neonatal malignancies to regress spontaneously or to undergo "differentiation" into mature elements

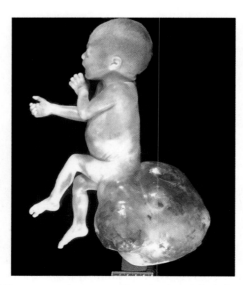

Fig. 7.32 Sacrococcygeal teratoma. Note the size of the lesion compared with that of the infant.

Table 7.9 Common Malignant Neoplasms of Infancy and Childhood

0–4 Years of Age	5–9 Years of Age	10–14 Years of Age
Leukemia	Leukemia	Hepatocellular carcinoma
Retinoblastoma	Retinoblastoma	Soft tissue sarcoma
Neuroblastoma	Neuroblastoma	Osteogenic sarcoma
Wilms tumor	Hepatocellular carcinoma	Thyroid carcinoma
Hepatoblastoma	Soft tissue sarcoma	Hodgkin disease
Soft tissue sarcoma (especially rhabdomyosarcoma)	Ewing tumor	
Teratomas	CNS tumors	
CNS tumors	Lymphoma	

CNS, Central nervous system.

- Better survival or cure of many childhood tumors, so that much attention is now paid to minimizing the adverse delayed effects of chemotherapy and radiotherapy in survivors, including the development of second malignancies

Many malignant pediatric neoplasms are histologically unique. In general, they tend to exhibit a primitive *(embryonal)* rather than pleomorphic-anaplastic microscopic appearance, and frequently they exhibit features of organogenesis specific to the site of tumor origin. **Because of their primitive histologic appearance, many childhood tumors have been collectively referred to as small, round, blue-cell tumors.** Sheets of cells with small, round nuclei characterize these tumors, which include neuroblastoma, lymphoma, rhabdomyosarcoma, Ewing sarcoma (peripheral neuroectodermal tumor), and some cases of Wilms tumor. Sufficient distinctive features usually are present to permit definitive diagnosis on the basis of histologic examination alone, but molecular studies are becoming increasingly useful, both for diagnosis and prognosis of childhood cancers. Three common tumors—neuroblastoma, retinoblastoma, and Wilms tumor—are described here to highlight the differences between pediatric tumors and those in adults.

Neuroblastoma

The term neuroblastic includes tumors of the sympathetic ganglia and adrenal medulla that are derived from primordial neural crest cells populating these sites; neuroblastoma is the most important member of this family. It is the second most common solid malignancy of childhood after brain tumors, accounting for 7% to 10% of all pediatric neoplasms, and as many as 50% of malignancies diagnosed in infancy. Neuroblastomas demonstrate several unique features in their natural history, including spontaneous regression and spontaneous or therapy-induced maturation. Most occur sporadically, but 1% to 2% are familial, with autosomal dominant transmission, and in such cases the neoplasms may involve both of the adrenals or multiple primary autonomic sites. Germline mutations in the anaplastic lymphoma kinase *(ALK)* gene have been linked to the familial predisposition to neuroblastoma. Somatic gain-of-function *ALK* mutations are also observed in 8% to 10% of sporadic neuroblastomas, and are markers of adverse prognosis. Clinical trials using inhibitors that target the mutated ALK tyrosine kinase are underway.

MORPHOLOGY

In childhood, about 40% of neuroblastomas arise in the **adrenal medulla.** The remainder occur anywhere along the sympathetic chain, with the most common locations being the paravertebral region of the abdomen (25%) and posterior mediastinum (15%). Macroscopically, neuroblastomas range in size from clinically silent minute nodules (in situ lesions) to large masses weighing more than 1 kg. In situ neuroblastomas are reported to be 40 times more frequent than tumors with clinical symptoms. The great majority of these silent lesions spontaneously regress, leaving only a focus of fibrosis or calcification in the adult. Some neuroblastomas are sharply demarcated with a fibrous pseudo-capsule, but others are infiltrative and invade surrounding structures, including the kidneys, renal vein, and vena cava, and envelop the aorta. On transection, they are composed of soft, gray-tan, brainlike tissue. Larger tumors have areas of necrosis, cystic softening, and hemorrhage.

Histologically, classic neuroblastomas are composed of small, primitive-appearing cells with dark nuclei, scant cytoplasm, and poorly defined cell borders growing in solid sheets (Fig. 7.33A). Mitotic activity, nuclear breakdown ("karyorrhexis"), and pleomorphism may be prominent. The background often demonstrates a faintly eosinophilic fibrillary material (neuropil) that corresponds to neuritic processes of the primitive neuroblasts. Typically, so-called **Homer-Wright pseudorosettes** can be found, in which the tumor cells are concentrically arranged about a central space filled with neuropil (the absence of an actual central lumen garners the designation *pseudo-*). Other helpful features include immunochemical detection of nerual markers, such as **neuron-specific enolase**, and demonstration on ultrastructural studies of small, membrane-bound, cytoplasmic catecholamine-containing secretory granules.

Some neoplasms show signs of **maturation**, either spontaneous or therapy-induced. Larger cells having more abundant cytoplasm with large vesicular nuclei and a prominent nucleolus, representing **ganglion cells** in various stages of maturation, may be found in tumors admixed with primitive neuroblasts **(ganglioneuroblastoma).** Lesions that are even better differentiated contain many more large cells resembling mature ganglion cells in the absence of residual neuroblasts; such neoplasms merit the designation *ganglioneuroma* (Fig. 7.33B). Maturation of neuroblasts into ganglion cells usually is accompanied by the appearance of Schwann cells.

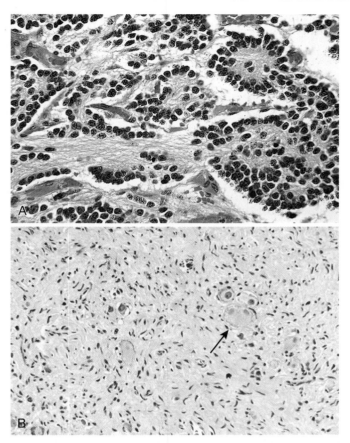

Fig. 7.33 (A) Neuroblastoma. This tumor is composed of small cells embedded in a finely fibrillar matrix (neuropil). A Homer-Wright pseudorosette (tumor cells arranged concentrically around a central core of neuropil) is seen in the upper right corner. (B) Ganglioneuromas, arising from spontaneous or therapy-induced maturation of neuroblastomas, are characterized by clusters of large ganglion cells with vesicular nuclei and abundant eosinophilic cytoplasm *(arrow)*. Spindle-shaped Schwann cells are present in the background stroma.

Clinical Course and Prognosis

Many factors influence prognosis, but the most important are the stage of the tumor and the age of the patient.

- *Staging of neuroblastomas* (Table 7.10) assumes great importance in establishing a prognosis. Special note should be taken of stage 4S (S means *special*), because the outlook for these patients is excellent, despite the spread of disease. As noted in Table 7.10, the primary tumor would be classified as stage 1 or 2 but for the presence of metastases, which are limited to liver, skin, and bone marrow, without bone involvement. Infants with 4S tumors have an excellent prognosis with minimal therapy, and it is not uncommon for the primary or metastatic tumors to undergo spontaneous regression. The biologic basis for this welcome behavior is not clear. Unfortunately, most (60% to 80%) children present with stage 3 or 4 tumors, and only 20% to 40% present with stage 1, 2A, 2B, or 4S neuroblastomas.

- *Age is the other important determinant of outcome.* The outlook for children younger than 18 months is much more favorable than for older children at a comparable stage of disease. Most neoplasms diagnosed in children during the first 18 months of life are stage 1 or 2, or stage 4S ("low" risk category in Table 7.10), whereas neoplasms in older children fall into the "intermediate" or "high" category of risk.

- *Histology* is an independent prognostic variable in neuroblastic tumors; evidence of schwannian stroma and gangliocytic differentiation is indicative of a favorable prognosis.

- *Amplification of the MYCN* oncogene has profound impact on prognosis. *MYCN* is located on the distal short arm of chromosome 2. *MYCN* amplification is present in about 25% to 30% of primary tumors, most in advanced-stage disease; the greater the number of copies, the worse the prognosis. Amplification of *MYCN* does not karyotypically manifest at the resident 2p23-p24 site, but rather as extrachromosomal double minute chromosomes or homogeneously staining regions on

Table 7.10 International Neuroblastoma Staging System

Stage I	Localized tumor completely excised, with or without microscopic residual disease; representative ipsilateral nonadherent lymph nodes negative for tumor (nodes adherent to the primary tumor may be positive for tumor)
Stage 2A	Localized tumor resected incompletely grossly; representative ipsilateral nonadherent lymph nodes negative for tumor microscopically
Stage 2B	Localized tumor with or without complete gross excision, ipsilateral nonadherent lymph nodes positive for tumor; enlarged contralateral lymph nodes, which are negative for tumor microscopically
Stage 3	Unresectable unilateral tumor infiltrating across the midline with or without regional lymph node involvement; or localized unilateral tumor with contralateral regional lymph node involvement
Stage 4	Any primary tumor with dissemination to distant lymph nodes, bone, bone marrow, liver, skin, and/or other organs (except as defined for stage 4S)
Stage 4S	Localized primary tumor (as defined for stage 1, 2A, or 2B) with dissemination limited to skin, liver, and/or bone marrow (<10% of nucleated cells are constituted by neoplastic cells; >10% involvement of bone marrow is considered as stage 4); stage 4S limited to infants younger than 1 year of age

S, Special.
Adapted from Brodeur GM, Pritchard J, Berthold F, et al: Revisions of the international neuroblastoma diagnosis, staging, and response to treatment, *J Clin Oncol* 11:1466, 1993.

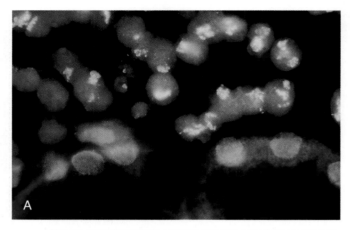

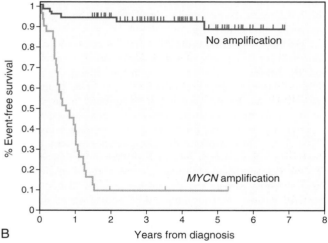

Fig. 7.34 (A) FISH using a fluorescein-labeled cosmid probe for *N-myc* on a tissue section containing neuroblastoma attached to the kidney. Note the neuroblastoma cells on the upper half of the photo with large areas of staining *(yellow-green)*; this corresponds to amplified *N-MYC* in the form of homogeneously staining regions. Renal tubular epithelial cells in the lower half of the photograph show no nuclear staining and background *(green)* cytoplasmic staining. (B) A Kaplan-Meier survival curve of infants younger than 1 year of age with metastatic neuroblastoma. The 3-year event-free survival of infants whose tumors lacked *MYCN* amplification was 93%, whereas those with tumors that had *MYCN* amplification had only a 10% event-free survival. *(A, Courtesy Dr. Timothy Triche, Children's Hospital, Los Angeles, California. B, Reproduced with permission from Brodeur GM: Neuroblastoma: biological insights into a clinical enigma, Nat Rev Cancer 3:203–216, 2003.)*

other chromosomes (Fig. 7.34). **MYCN amplification is currently the most important genetic abnormality used in risk stratification of neuroblastic tumors and automatically renders a tumor as "high" risk, irrespective of stage or age.**

- DNA ploidy is another prognostic factor, with tumors that are hyperdiploid (with whole chromosome gains) having more favorable prognosis than tumors that are near-diploid. The latter subset, although closer to diploidy on absolute number, tends to have multiple structural rearrangements between, and within, chromosomes that can result in adverse molecular events, such as *MYCN* amplification.

- Although age, stage, *MYCN* status, and ploidy are used clinically for assigning prognostication, many other "experimental" molecular aberrations have been identified that might also have prognostic bearings, or be potential candidates for targeted therapy. For example, expression of TrkA, a high-affinity receptor for nerve growth factor that is indicative of differentiation toward sympathetic ganglia lineage, is associated with favorable prognosis. Overall, besides *MYCN* amplification and *ALK* mutations (latter in ~10%), de novo neuroblastomas have few recurrent "hotspot" mutations. However, a very high frequency of relapsed neuroblastomas (>75%) have mutations in the RAS-MAP kinase signaling pathway, suggesting that relapsed tumors might be targeted with therapies against these oncogenic pathways.

Children younger than 2 years with neuroblastomas generally present with a protuberant abdomen resulting from an abdominal mass, fever, and weight loss. In older children the neuroblastomas may remain unnoticed until metastases cause hepatomegaly, ascites, and bone pain. Neuroblastomas may metastasize widely through the hematogenous and lymphatic systems, particularly to liver, lungs, bones, and the bone marrow. In neonates, disseminated neuroblastomas may manifest with multiple cutaneous metastases associated with deep blue discoloration to the skin (earning the rather unfortunate moniker of "blueberry muffin baby"). About 90% of neuroblastomas, regardless of location, produce catecholamines (similar to the catecholamines associated with pheochromocytomas), which constitutes an important diagnostic feature (i.e., elevated blood levels of catecholamines and elevated urine levels of catecholamine metabolites such as vanillylmandelic acid [VMA] and homovanillic acid [HVA]). Despite the elaboration of catecholamines, hypertension is much less frequent with these neoplasms than with pheochromocytomas (Chapter 20).

SUMMARY

NEUROBLASTOMA

- Neuroblastomas and related tumors arise from neural crest–derived cells in the sympathetic ganglia and adrenal medulla.
- Neuroblastomas are undifferentiated, whereas ganglioneuroblastomas and ganglioneuromas demonstrate evidence of differentiation (schwannian stroma and ganglion cells). Homer-Wright pseudorosettes are characteristic of neuroblastomas.
- Age, stage, and *MYCN* amplification and ploidy are the most important prognostic features; children younger than 18 months usually have a better prognosis than older children, whereas children with higher-stage tumors or *MYCN* amplification fare worse. A high frequency of relapsed neuroblastomas have mutations in the RAS-MAP kinase pathway.
- Neuroblastomas secrete catecholamines, whose metabolites (VMA/HVA) can be used for screening patients.

Retinoblastoma

Retinoblastoma is the most common primary intraocular malignancy of children. The molecular genetics of retinoblastoma has been discussed previously (Chapter 6). Approximately 40% of the tumors are associated with a germline mutation in the *RB* gene and are therefore heritable. The remaining 60% of the tumors develop sporadically, and these have somatic *RB* gene mutations. Familial cases typically are associated with development of multiple tumors that are bilateral, although they may be unifocal and unilateral. All of the sporadic, nonheritable tumors are unilateral and unifocal. Patients with familial retinoblastoma also are at increased risk for the development of osteosarcoma and other soft tissue tumors.

MORPHOLOGY

Retinoblastomas tend to be nodular masses, usually in the posterior retina, often with satellite seedings (Fig. 7.35A). On microscopic examination, undifferentiated areas of these tumors are found to be composed of small, round cells with large hyperchromatic nuclei and scant cytoplasm, resembling undifferentiated retinoblasts.

Differentiated structures are found within many retinoblastomas, the most characteristic of these being **Flexner-Wintersteiner rosettes** (Fig. 7.35B). These structures consist of clusters of cuboidal or short columnar cells arranged around a central lumen (in contrast with the pseudorosettes of neuroblastoma, which lack a central lumen). The nuclei are displaced away from the lumen, which by light microscopy appears to have a limiting membrane resembling the external limiting membrane of the retina.

Tumor cells may disseminate beyond the eye through the optic nerve or subarachnoid space. The most common sites of distant metastases are the CNS, skull, distal bones, and lymph nodes.

Clinical Features

The presenting findings include poor vision, strabismus, a whitish hue to the pupil ("cat's eye reflex"), and pain and tenderness in the eye. The median age at presentation is 2 years, although the tumor may be present at birth. Untreated, the tumors usually are fatal, but when treated with chemotherapy, radiotherapy, and (in locally advanced tumors) enucleation, survival is the rule. As noted earlier, some tumors spontaneously regress, and patients with familial retinoblastoma are at increased risk for the development of osteosarcoma and other soft tissue tumors.

Wilms Tumor

Wilms tumor, or nephroblastoma, is the most common primary tumor of the kidney in children, with most cases occurring in children between 2 and 5 years of age. This tumor illustrates several important concepts of childhood tumors: the relationship between congenital malformation and increased risk of tumors; the histologic similarity between tumor and developing organ; and finally, the remarkable success in the treatment of childhood tumors. Each of these concepts is presented in the following discussion.

Three groups of congenital malformations are associated with an increased risk for Wilms tumor. *These are WAGR syndrome (i.e., Wilms tumor, aniridia, genital abnormalities, and mental retardation); Denys-Drash syndrome (DDS), and Beckwith-Wiedemann syndrome (BWS)*. Of patients with *WAGR syndrome* approximately one in three will go on to develop this tumor. Another group of patients, those with so-called *"Denys-Drash syndrome"* (DDS), have an even higher risk (approximately 90%) of Wilms tumor. Patients with the WAGR syndrome, as the name indicates, have Wilms tumor, aniridia, genital abnormalities and mental retardation. DD syndrome is characterized by gonadal dysgenesis and early onset nephropathy leading to renal failure. Both of these conditions are associated with abnormalities of the Wilms tumor 1 *(WT1)* gene, located on 11p13. The nature of the genetic aberration differs, however: Patients with WAGR syndrome demonstrate loss of genetic material (i.e., deletions) of *WT1*, while persons with DDS harbor a dominant negative inactivating mutation in WT1 that interferes with the function of normal WT1 protein made from the other *WT1* allele. *WT1* is critical to normal renal and gonadal development; it is not surprising, therefore, that constitutional inactivation of one copy of this gene results in genitourinary abnormalities in humans.

A third group of patients, those with *Beckwith-Wiedemann syndrome* (BWS), also are at increased risk for the development of Wilms tumor. These patients exhibit enlargement of individual body organs (e.g., tongue, kidneys, or liver) or entire body segments (hemihypertrophy); enlargement of adrenal cortical cells (adrenal cytomegaly) is a characteristic microscopic feature. BWS is an example of a disorder of genomic imprinting (see earlier). The genetic locus that is involved in these patients is in band p15.5 of chromosome 11 distal to the WT1 locus. Although this locus is called "WT2" for the second Wilms tumor locus, the gene involved has not been identified. This region contains at least 10 genes that normally are expressed from only one of the two parental alleles, with

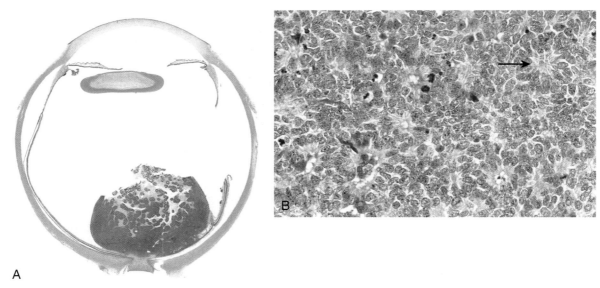

Fig. 7.35 Retinoblastoma. (A) Poorly cohesive tumor in retina is seen abutting the optic nerve. (B) Higher-power view showing Flexner-Wintersteiner rosettes *(arrow)* and numerous mitotic figures.

transcriptional silencing of the other parental homologue by methylation of the promoter region located upstream of the transcription start site. Of all candidate "WT2" genes, imprinting abnormalities of insulinlike growth factor-2 *(IGF2)* have the strongest relationship to tumor predisposition in persons with BWS. *IGF2* normally is expressed solely from the paternal allele, whereas the maternal allele is imprinted. In some Wilms tumors, loss of imprinting (i.e., reexpression of *IGF2* by the maternal allele) can be demonstrated, leading to overexpression of the IGF2 protein, which is postulated to result in both organ enlargement and tumorigenesis. Thus, these associations suggest that in some cases, congenital malformations and tumors represent related manifestations of genetic lesions affecting a single gene or closely linked genes. In addition to Wilms tumors, patients with BWS also are at increased risk for the development of hepatoblastoma, adrenocortical tumors, rhabdomyosarcomas, and pancreatic tumors.

In contrast to syndromic Wilms tumors, the molecular abnormalities underlying sporadic (i.e., nonsyndromic) tumors, which account for 90% of cases overall in children, are only recently being elucidated. Some of them are associated with specific histologic features described later. For example, gain-of-function mutations of the gene encoding β-catenin (Chapter 6) have been demonstrated in approximately 10% of sporadic Wilms tumors. Other recurrent mutations occur in genes encoding proteins involved in microRNA processing (DROSHA, DGCR8, and DICER1); these are seen in 15% to 20% of Wilms tumors with predominantly blastemal histology (see later). It is postulated that aberrations in microRNA processing lead to reduced levels of many mature microRNAs, in particular in the miR-200 family, which is involved in "mesenchymal to epithelial transformation" during renal morphogenesis. The lack of mesenchymal to epithelial transformation likely leads to persistent blastemal

"rests" in the kidney (see the following), which evolve into Wilms tumors. Finally, tumors with *TP53* mutations are associated with an especially poor prognosis and often have a distinctive anaplastic histologic appearance, described later.

MORPHOLOGY

Wilms tumor typically is a large, solitary, well-circumscribed mass, although 10% are either bilateral or multicentric at the time of diagnosis. On cut section, the tumor is soft, homogeneous, and tan to gray, with occasional foci of hemorrhage, cystic degeneration, and necrosis (Fig. 7.36).

On microscopic examination, Wilms tumors are characterized by recognizable attempts to recapitulate different stages of nephrogenesis. The classic **triphasic combination** of blastemal, stromal, and epithelial cell types is observed in most lesions, although the percentage of each component is variable (Fig. 7.37A). Sheets of small blue cells, with few distinctive features, characterize the **blastemal component**. Epithelial "differentiation" usually takes the form of **abortive tubules or glomeruli**. Stromal cells are usually fibrocytic or myxoid in nature, although skeletal muscle "differentiation" is not uncommon. Approximately 5% of tumors contain foci of **anaplasia** (cells with large, hyperchromatic, pleomorphic nuclei and abnormal mitoses) (Fig. 7.37B). The presence of anaplasia correlates with the presence of acquired *TP53* mutations and the emergence of resistance to chemotherapy. The pattern of distribution of anaplastic cells within the primary tumor (focal versus diffuse) has important implications for prognosis (see further text).

Nephrogenic rests are putative precursor lesions of Wilms tumors and are sometimes present in the renal parenchyma adjacent to the tumor. Nephrogenic rests have a spectrum of histologic appearances, from expansile masses that resemble Wilms tumors (hyperplastic rests) to sclerotic rests consisting predominantly of fibrous tissue with occasional admixed

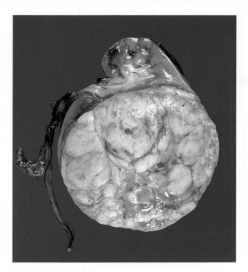

Fig. 7.36 Wilms tumor in the lower pole of the kidney with the characteristic tan to gray color and well-circumscribed margins.

immature tubules or glomeruli. It is important to document the presence of nephrogenic rests in the resected specimen, because these patients are at an increased risk for the development of Wilms tumors in the contralateral kidney.

Clinical Course

Patients typically present with a palpable abdominal mass, which may extend across the midline and down into the pelvis. Less often, the presenting features are fever and abdominal pain, hematuria or, occasionally, intestinal obstruction as a result of pressure from the tumor. The prognosis for Wilms tumor generally is very good, and excellent results are obtained with a combination of nephrectomy and chemotherapy. Anaplasia is a harbinger of adverse prognosis, but only if it is diffuse. If the anaplasia is focal and confined within the resected nephrectomy

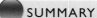

SUMMARY

WILMS TUMOR

- Wilms tumor is the most common renal neoplasm of childhood.
- Patients with three syndromes are at increased risk for Wilms tumors: Denys-Drash, Beckwith-Wiedemann, and Wilms tumor, aniridia, genital abnormalities, and mental retardation (WGAR) syndrome.
- WAGR syndrome and DDS are associated with WT1 inactivation, whereas Beckwith-Wiedemann arises through imprinting abnormalities at the WT2 locus, principally involving the *IGF2* gene.
- The morphologic components of Wilms tumor include blastema (small, round blue cells) and epithelial and stromal elements.
- Nephrogenic rests are precursor lesions of Wilms tumors.

specimen, the outcome is no different from that for tumors without evidence of anaplasia.

MOLECULAR DIAGNOSIS OF MENDELIAN AND COMPLEX DISORDERS

In the era predating the ready availability of molecular diagnostic assays, rendering the diagnosis of a genetic disorder depended on the identification of abnormal gene products (e.g., mutant hemoglobin or abnormal metabolites) or their clinical effects, such as mental retardation (e.g., in PKU). Several factors have since enabled the rapid expansion of molecular diagnostics from the realm of research to an almost ubiquitous presence in both academic and commercial pathology laboratories. These include (1) the sequencing of the human genome and the deposition of these data in publicly available databases; (2) the availability of numerous "off-the-shelf" polymerase chain

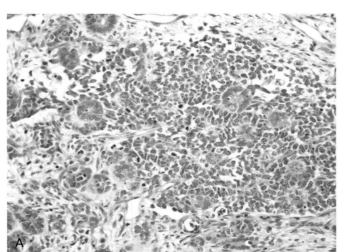
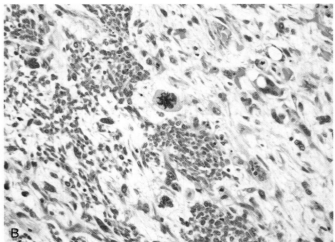

Fig. 7.37 (A) Wilms tumor with tightly packed blue cells consistent with the blastemal component and interspersed primitive tubules, representing the epithelial component. (B) Focal anaplasia was present in other areas within this Wilms tumor, characterized by cells with hyperchromatic, pleomorphic nuclei, and an abnormal mitosis (center of field). Predominance of blastemal morphology and diffuse anaplasia are associated with specific molecular lesions (see text).

reaction (PCR) kits tailor-made for the identification of specific genetic disorders; (3) the availability of high-resolution microarrays ("gene chips") that can interrogate both DNA and RNA on a genomewide scale using a single platform; and, finally, (4) the emergence of automated, high-throughput, next-generation ("NextGen") sequencing technologies. The last two advances have been especially useful in the context of new research to elucidate the genetic basis for both mendelian and complex disorders. Although a detailed discussion of molecular diagnostics is beyond the scope of this book, some of the better-known approaches are highlighted in the ensuing paragraphs. Irrespective of the technique used, the genetic aberration being queried can be either in the germline (i.e., present in each and every cell of the affected person, as with a *CFTR* mutation in a patient with CF) or somatic (i.e., restricted to specific tissue types or lesions, as with *MYCN* amplification in neuroblastoma cells). This consideration determines the nature of the sample (e.g., peripheral blood lymphocytes [PBLs], saliva, tumor tissue) used for the assay.

Indications for Genetic Analysis

In general, indications for genetic analysis can be divided into inherited conditions and acquired conditions. Within inherited conditions, genetic testing can be offered at either the prenatal or postnatal stages. It may involve conventional cytogenetics, FISH, molecular diagnostics, or a combination of these techniques.

Prenatal genetic analysis should be offered to all patients who are at risk of having cytogenetically abnormal progeny. It can be performed on cells obtained by amniocentesis, on chorionic villus biopsy material, or increasingly in "liquid biopsies" on maternal blood paired with next-generation sequencing. Some important indications are the following:

- Advanced maternal age (beyond 34 years), which is associated with greater risk of trisomies
- Confirmed carrier status for a balanced reciprocal translocation, robertsonian translocation, or inversion (in such cases, the gametes may be unbalanced, so the progeny would be at risk for chromosomal disorders)
- Fetal abnormalities observed on ultrasound, or an abnormal result on routine maternal blood screening
- A chromosomal abnormality or mendelian disorder affecting a previous child
- Determination of fetal sex when the patient or partner is a confirmed carrier of an X-linked genetic disorder

Postnatal genetic analysis usually is performed on peripheral blood lymphocytes. Indications are as follows:
- Multiple congenital anomalies
- Suspicion of a metabolic syndrome
- Unexplained mental retardation and/or developmental delay
- Suspected aneuploidy (e.g., features of Down syndrome) or other syndromic chromosomal abnormality (e.g., deletions, inversions)
- Suspected monogenic disease, whether previously described or unknown

Acquired genetic alterations, such as somatic mutations in cancer, are increasingly becoming a large focus area in molecular diagnostics laboratories, especially with the advent of targeted therapies. Although single gene tests (mutations of *EGFR* or *BRAF*, amplification of *HER2*) have been used for a while to inform treatment decisions, the advent of cost-effective next-generation sequencing approaches has now allowed interrogations of large numbers of coding genes (often in the 100s), as well as cancer-relevant translocations, in a single assay. The clinical team typically receives a "genomic report" on the patient's cancer, including potential molecularly targeted treatment recommendations. Another major focus of molecular diagnostics has been the rapid identification of infectious diseases, such as suspected tuberculosis or virulent pathogens such as Ebola, using DNA-based approaches. In general, these approaches have cut down the time required for diagnosis from weeks to a matter of days. Besides de novo identification of pathogens, molecular diagnostics laboratories can also contribute to the identification of treatment resistance (e.g., acquired mutations in influenza viruses that render them resistant to anti-virals), and to the monitoring of treatment efficacy using assays for "viral load" in the blood. Similar parameters (measuring efficacy of therapy and emergence of resistance) are also widely used in cancer patients.

Because of the rapid advances in molecular diagnostics, terms such as "personalized therapy" and "precision medicine" are being increasingly used to indicate therapy tailored to the needs of the individual patient. It is hoped that such expectations will be met in the foreseeable future. We will now discuss some of the common approaches used in molecular diagnostics laboratories for assessment of inherited and acquired indications.

Molecular Diagnosis of Copy Number Abnormalities

As already discussed in this chapter, various diseases may occur as a result of copy number abnormalities, at the level of the entire chromosome (trisomy 21), chromosomal segments (22q11 deletion syndrome), or submicroscopic intragenic deletions (WAGR syndrome). Karyotype analysis of chromosomes by G banding remains the classic approach for identifying changes at the chromosomal level; however, as might be expected, the resolution with this technique is fairly low. To identify subchromosomal alterations, both focused analysis of chromosomal regions by FISH and global genomic approaches such as comparative genomic hybridization (CGH) are commonly used.

Fluorescence in Situ Hybridization

FISH uses DNA probes that recognize sequences specific to chromosomal regions of greater than 100 kilobases in size, which defines the limit of resolution with this technique for identifying chromosomal changes. Such probes are labeled with fluorescent dyes and are applied to metaphase spreads or interphase nuclei. The probe hybridizes to its complementary sequence on the chromosome and thus labels the specific chromosomal region that can then be visualized under a fluorescence microscope. The ability of FISH to circumvent the need for dividing cells is invaluable when a rapid diagnosis is warranted (e.g., in a critically ill infant suspected of having an underlying genetic disorder). Such analysis can be performed on prenatal samples (e.g., cells obtained by amniocentesis, chorionic villus biopsy, or umbilical cord blood), peripheral blood lymphocytes, and even archival tissue sections. FISH is used for the detection of numeric abnormalities of chromosomes (aneuploidy) (Fig. 7.38A), subtle microdeletions (Fig. 7.38B) and complex translocations not indentifiable by routine karyotyping, and gene amplification (e.g., *MYCN* amplification in neuroblastomas).

Array-Based Genomic Hybridization

FISH requires previous knowledge of the one or few specific chromosomal regions suspected of being altered in the test sample. However, genomic abnormalities can also be detected without previous knowledge by using microarray technology to perform a global genomic survey. First-generation platforms were designed for comparative genomic hybridization (CGH), whereas newer platforms incorporate single nucleotide polymorphism (SNP) genotyping approaches, offering multiple benefits.

In array comparative genomic hybridization (aCGH), the test DNA and a reference (normal) DNA are labeled with two different fluorescent dyes that fluoresce red and green, respectively. The differentially labeled samples are then cohybridized to an array spotted with DNA probes that span the human genome at regularly spaced intervals, and usually cover all 22 autosomes and the sex chromosomes. At each chromosomal probe location, the binding of the labeled DNA from the two samples is compared. If the two samples are equal (i.e., the test sample is diploid), then all spots on the array will fluoresce yellow (the result of an equal admixture of green and red dyes). In contrast, if there is even a focal deletion or duplication, the probe spots corresponding to it will show skewing toward red or green (depending on gain or loss of material), allowing highly accurate determinations of copy number variants across the genome.

Newer types of "SNP chips" are based on a similar concept, but the probes are designed to identify SNP sites genomewide, which has a number of advantages over CGH. As discussed in Chapter 1, SNPs are the most common type of DNA polymorphism, occurring approximately every 1000 nucleotides throughout the genome (e.g., in exons, introns, and regulatory sequences). Thus, SNPs serve both as a physical landmark within the genome as well as a genetic marker whose transmission can be followed from parent to child. There are several testing platforms that allow SNPs to be analyzed genomewide on arrays. Like CGH probes, methods involving SNPs can be used to determine copy number variations. In addition, by discriminating between SNP alleles at each particular location, they also provide zygosity data (Fig. 7.39). This means, for example, that SNP chips can identify uniparental disomy, in which loss of heterozygosity is seen within an affected region having diploid DNA content. The current generation of SNP arrays is quite comprehensive, with the

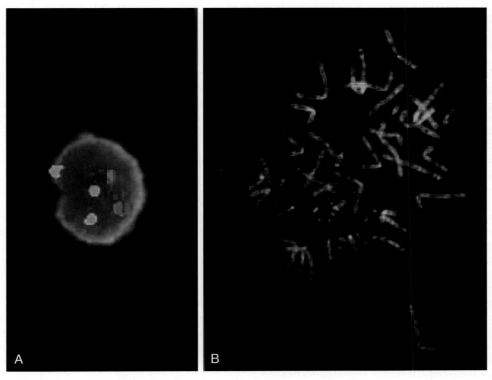

Fig. 7.38 FISH. (A) Interphase nucleus from a male patient with suspected trisomy 18. Three different fluorescent probes have been used in a "FISH cocktail"; the green probe hybridizes to the X chromosome centromere *(one copy)*, the red probe to the Y chromosome centromere *(one copy)*, and the aqua probe to the chromosome 18 centromere *(three copies)*. (B) A metaphase spread in which two fluorescent probes have been used, one hybridizing to chromosome region 22q13 *(green)* and the other hybridizing to chromosome region 22q11.2 *(red)*. There are two 22q13 signals. One of the two chromosomes does not stain with the probe for 22q11.2, indicating a microdeletion in this region. This abnormality gives rise to the 22q11.2 deletion syndrome (DiGeorge syndrome). *(Courtesy of Dr. Nancy R. Schneider and Jeff Doolittle, Cytogenetics Laboratory, University of Texas Southwestern Medical Center, Dallas, Texas.)*

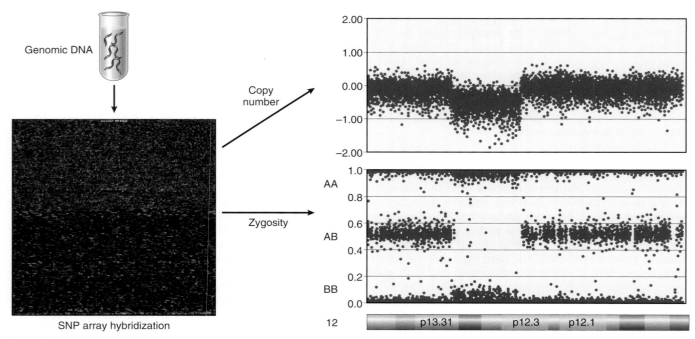

Fig. 7.39 Analysis of copy number variation via SNP cytogenomic array. Genomic DNA is labeled and hybridized to an array containing potentially millions of probe spots. Copy number is determined by overall intensity and genotype is determined by allelic ratio. The example shown is the p arm of chromosome 12 in a pediatric leukemia. Here, the normal areas *(green)* show neutral (diploid) DNA content and the zygosity plot shows the expected ratio of AA, AB, and BB SNP genotypes. The anomalous area *(red)* shows decreased overall intensity, and the zygosity plot shows loss of heterozygosity (the AB genotype); together, these findings indicate the presence of a deletion on one copy of chromosome 12p. *(Modified from Paulsson K, et al: Genetic landscape of high hyperdiploid childhood acute lymphoblastic leukemia, PNAS 107[50]:21719–21724, 2010.)*

largest containing greater than 4 million SNP probes. As a result, this technology is the mainstay of genomewide association studies (GWASs, described later).

Direct Detection of DNA Mutations by Polymerase Chain Reaction (PCR) Analysis

PCR analysis, which involves exponential amplification of DNA, is now widely used in molecular diagnosis. If RNA is used as the substrate, it is first reverse-transcribed to obtain cDNA and then amplified by PCR. This method involving *reverse transcription* (RT) often is abbreviated as RT-PCR. To amplify a DNA segment of interest, two primers that bind to the 3′ and 5′ ends of the normal sequence are designed. By using appropriate DNA polymerases and thermal cycling, the target DNA is greatly amplified, producing millions of copies of the DNA sequence between the two primer sites. The DNA sequence of the PCR product can then be analyzed in several ways:

- Sanger sequencing, named after its inventor, Nobel-laureate Frederick Sanger, has for many years been the "workhorse" of genome sequencing, including the original Human Genome Project. Here, the amplified DNA is mixed with a DNA polymerase, a DNA primer, nucleotides, and four dead-end (di-deoxy terminator) nucleotides (A, T, G, and C) labeled with different fluorescent tags. The ensuing reaction produces a series of DNA molecules of all possible lengths up to a kilobase or so, each labeled with a tag that corresponds to the base at which the reaction stopped because of the incorporation

of one of the terminator nucleotides. After size separation by capillary electrophoresis, the exact sequence can be "read" and compared with the normal sequence to detect the presence of mutations. Many applications of Sanger sequencing (and other PCR-based approaches) are starting to give way to next-generation sequencing (discussed later), particularly when the analysis of large genes or multiple genes is required. Nonetheless, even in 2016, Sanger sequencing remains the "gold standard" for many genotyping assays.

- Another approach for identifying mutations at a specific nucleotide position (say, a codon 12 mutation in the *KRAS* oncogene that converts glycine [GGT] to aspartic acid [GAT]) would be to add fluorescently labeled nucleotides C and T to the PCR mixture, which are complementary to either the wild-type (G) or mutant (A) sequence, respectively. Because these two nucleotides are labeled with different fluorophores, the fluorescence emitted by the resulting PCR product can be of one or another color, depending on whether a C or a T becomes incorporated in the process of primer extension (Fig. 7.40). The advantage of this allele-specific extension strategy is that it is more sensitive than Sanger sequencing, allowing for the identification mutated DNA sequences even if they make up a small fraction (~1%) of the total DNA (as may be the case in clinical specimens obtained from patients suspected of harboring a malignancy). An ultrasensitive variant of this assay, known as droplet digital PCR, literally separates the template DNA (or cDNA) into thousands to millions of microscopic oil "droplets," such that any given

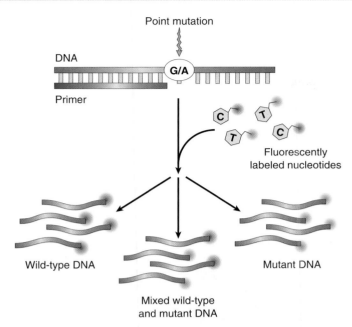

Point mutation

DNA

G/A

Primer

Fluorescently
labeled nucleotides

Wild-type DNA

Mutant DNA

Mixed wild-type
and mutant DNA

Fig. 7.40 Allele-specific polymerase chain reaction (PCR) analysis for mutation detection in a heterogeneous sample containing an admixture of normal and mutant DNA. Nucleotides complementary to the mutant and wild-type nucleotides at the queried base position are labeled with different fluorophores such that incorporation into the resulting PCR product yields fluorescent signals of variable intensity in accordance with the ratio of mutant to wild-type DNA present.

droplet contains no more than one strand of template DNA, along with requisite PCR reagents. Each such "minireactor" then generates its own PCR product, which can be digitally integrated and analyzed for the presence of mutant alleles. By assessing each template individually in parallel, rather than in a single PCR reaction, droplet digital PCR has exquisite sensitivity, being able to detect as little as 1 mutant DNA strand in 10,000 or more wild-type molecules.

Next Generation Sequencing

Increasingly, nearly all of molecular diagnostics applications requiring assessment of DNA (or RNA) are being supplanted by so-called "next-generation sequencing" (NGS) technologies, so named because the Sanger sequencing mentioned earlier is now considered "first generation." The availability of NGS technology has the potential to alter molecular diagnostics radically, by the sheer volume of sequencing data (more than 1 gigabase pairs or 1,000,000,000 base pairs of DNA per day!) at relatively low costs. The entire human genome has a little more than 3 gigabases, so true "whole genome sequencing" can be performed several times in a matter of days. In contrast with Sanger sequencing, NGS technologies use platforms in which sequencing of multiple fragments of the human genome (DNA or cDNA) can occur in parallel ("massively parallel sequencing"), significantly enhancing its speed (Fig. 7.41). Fluorescently labeled nucleotides are incorporated that are complementary to the template DNA strands, which are immobilized on a solid phase, with one nucleotide added per template per cycle. An image is captured at the end of each cycle, and the cycles are repeated until a

"read" of sufficient length is generated to map each read back to the human genome using sophisticated bioinformatics. In addition to differences of time and scale, another key difference between NGS and traditional Sanger sequencing is the ability of the former to detect variant alleles that occur at low frequency in samples that contain a heterogeneous mixture of cells. With Sanger sequencing, the lower limit of detection for variant allele frequency is 20% or more, thus requiring either homogeneous samples (such as germline DNA) or some form of enrichment, such as microdissection of tumor cells from a biopsy that also contains normal tissue. The ability of NGS to "read" the same region of the genome multiple times (from 100- to 1000-fold redundancy) allows detection of allele frequencies as low as 1%, making NGS particularly useful when searching for mutations in tissue biopsies that contain more nonneoplastic stroma than the tumor cells.

Clinical and research applications of NGS (which can be performed on either germline or somatic DNA, or both) include targeted sequencing (typically a panel of a few to several hundred genes); whole exome sequencing (WES), which interrogates all coding regions of the human genome; and whole genome sequencing (WGS), which includes the remaining 99% of the human genome, including regions that express noncoding RNAs. In addition to DNA, NGS can also be used for measuring the transcriptome (RNA-Seq) and genomewide binding sites for transcription factors or histones (chromatin immunoprecipitation and sequencing, or ChIP-Seq).

Linkage Analysis and Genomewide Association Studies

Direct diagnosis of mutations is possible only if the gene responsible for a genetic disorder is known and its sequence has been identified. In several diseases that have a genetic basis, including some common disorders, direct genetic diagnosis is not possible, either because the causal gene has not been identified or because the disease is multifactorial (polygenic) and no single gene is involved. In such cases, two types of analyses can be performed for unbiased identification of disease-associated gene(s): linkage analysis and GWASs. In both instances, surrogate markers in the genome, also known as marker loci, must be used to localize the chromosomal regions of interest, based on their linkage to one or more putative disease-causing genes. The marker loci used are naturally occurring variations in DNA sequences known as polymorphisms, typically SNPs, as described previously.

Two technologic breakthroughs have enabled the application of SNPs to high-throughput "gene hunting." First is the completion of several large genomic sequencing projects (the HapMap project and the 1000 genome project) that have provided linkage disequilibrium patterns in multiple ethnoracial groups, based on genomewide SNP mapping. The entire human genome can now be divided into blocks known as "haplotypes," which contain varying numbers of contiguous SNPs on the same chromosome that are in linkage disequilibrium and hence inherited together as a cluster. As a result, rather than querying every single SNP in the human genome, comparable information about shared DNA can be obtained simply by

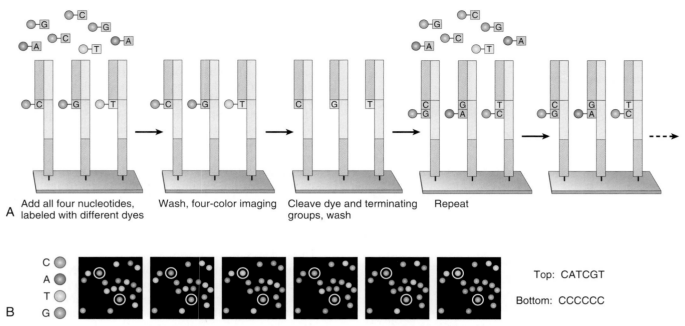

Fig. 7.41 Principle of next-generation sequencing. Several alternative approaches currently are available for "NextGen" sequencing, and one of the more commonly used platforms is illustrated. (A) Short fragments of genomic DNA ("template") between 100 and 500 base pairs in length are immobilized on a solid phase platform such as a glass slide, using universal capture primers that are complementary to adapters that have previously been added to ends of the template fragments. The addition of fluorescently labeled complementary nucleotides, one per template DNA per cycle, occurs in a "massively parallel" fashion, at millions of templates immobilized on the solid phase at the same time. A four-color imaging camera captures the fluorescence emanating from each template location (corresponding to the specific incorporated nucleotide), following which the fluorescent dye is cleaved and washed away, and the entire cycle is repeated. (B) Powerful computational programs can decipher the images to generate sequences complementary to the template DNA at the end of one "run," and these sequences are then mapped back to the reference genomic sequence, to identify alterations. *(Reproduced with permission from Metzker M: Sequencing technologies—the next generation, Nat Rev Genet 11:31–46, 2010, © Nature Publishing Group.)*

looking for shared haplotypes, using single or a small number of SNPs that "tag" or identify a specific haplotype. Second, it is now possible to genotype millions of SNPs simultaneously, in a cost-effective way, using high-density SNP arrays, as described earlier.

Linkage Analysis

Linkage analysis deals with assessing shared marker loci (i.e., SNPs) in family members exhibiting the disease or trait of interest, with the assumption that SNPs in linkage disequilibrium with the disease allele are transmitted through pedigrees. With time it becomes possible to define a "disease haplotype" based on a panel of SNPs, all of which cosegregate with the putative disease allele. Eventually, linkage analysis facilitates localization and cloning of the disease allele. Linkage analysis is most useful in mendelian disorders that are related to one gene with profound effects and high penetrance.

Genomewide Association Studies (GWASs)

It is now established that some of the most common human diseases, such as hypertension, diabetes, mental disorders, and asthma, have a polygenic basis, with multiple genetic loci contributing small independent effects, resulting in a disease phenotype. Conventional linkage analyses lack the statistical power to detect such genetic variants. In GWASs, large cohorts of patients with and without a disease (rather than families) are examined across the entire genome for variant SNPs that are overrepresented in persons with the

disease. This identifies regions of the genome that contain a variant gene or genes that confer disease susceptibility. The causal variant within the region is then provisionally identified using a "candidate gene" approach, in which genes are selected based on how tightly they are associated with the disease and whether their biologic function seems likely to be involved in the disease under study. In addition to polygenic diseases, GWASs also have led to the identification of genetic loci that modulate common quantitative traits in humans, such as height, body mass, hair and eye color, and bone density.

We end this chapter to reflect on the current genomic era of medicine. Advances in understanding the molecular basis of human disease are taking place at a breathtaking pace, as are molecular diagnostic techniques. Throughout this book we will illustrate how these changes have impacted on the management of certain diseases in the clinic. By the time this book reaches the reader we hope that many more such examples will become commonplace.

SUGGESTED READINGS

Bianchi DW, Parker RL, Wentworth J, et al: DNA sequencing versus standard prenatal aneuploidy screening, *N Engl J Med* 370:799–808, 2014. *[Seminal study that demonstrated potential superiority of maternal "liquid biopsies" paired with next-generation sequencing for prenatal diagnosis of trisomies in the fetus, when compared to conventional prenatal tests.]*

Bresler SC, Weiser DA, Huwe PJ, et al: ALK mutations confer differential oncogenic activation and sensitivity to ALK inhibition therapy in neuroblastoma, *Cancer Cell* 26(5):682–694, 2014. *[An important study demonstrating the potential for targeted therapy in neuroblastomas harboring ALK mutations, using small molecule ALK inhibitors.]*

Cutting GR: Cystic fibrosis genetics: from molecular understanding to clinical application, *Nat Rev Genet* 16:45–56, 2015. *[An outstanding review on cystic fibrosis by one of the doyens in the field, with a particular focus on genetic and environmental modifiers of the disease.]*

Eleveld TF, Oldridge DA, Bernard V, et al: Relapsed neuroblastomas show frequent RAS-MAPK pathway mutations, *Nat Genet* 47:864–871, 2015. *[A landmark study demonstrating a high frequency of alterations in the RAS-MAPK pathway in treated neuroblastomas, providing a new opportunity for targeted therapy in this lethal tumor of childhood.]*

Gudbjartsson DF, Helgason H, Gudjonsson SA, et al: Large-scale whole-genome sequencing of the Icelandic population, *Nat Genet* 47:435–444, 2015. *[A unique study that reiterates the power of modern-day next-generation sequencing, wherein the whole genomes of over 2600 Icelandic natives were sequenced for identification of genetic variants that might influence genetic diversity as well as risk for multifactorial diseases.]*

Hagerman PJ, Hagerman RJ: Fragile X-associated tremor/ataxia syndrome (FTAS), *Ann N Y Acad Sci* 1338:58–70, 2015. *[An authoritative review on FMR1 protein, and the role of premutations at the fragile X loci in causing the symptomatic neurodegenerative condition, FTAS.]*

Jameson JL, Longo DL: Precision medicine—personalized, problematic, and promising, *N Engl J Med* 372:2229–2234, 2015. *[An insightful review on the challenges and opportunities of personalized medicine, also known as precision medicine, in the modern era of genomics and high throughput sequencing.]*

Kalsner L, Chamberlain SJ: Prader-Willi, Angelman, and 15q11-q13 duplication syndromes, *Pediatr Clin North Am* 62:587–606, 2015. *[An up-to-date review on the genetics, clinical findings, and natural history of children with these two imprinting disorders.]*

Page MM, Stefanutti C, Sniderman A, et al: Recent advances in the understanding and care of familial hypercholesterolemia: significance of the biology and therapeutic regulation of proprotein convertase subtilisin/kexin type 9, *Clin Sci* 129:63–79, 2015. *[A state-of-the-art review on mechanisms of cholesterol regulation by PCSK9, and how inhibition of this protein is being leveraged in the clinic for augmenting statin effects.]*

Robinson JG, Farnier M, Krempf M, et al: Efficacy and safety of alirocumab in reducing lipids and cardiovascular events, *N Engl J Med* 372(16):1489–1499, 2015. *[Seminal study establishing the benefits of PCSK9 inhibitors in hyperlipidemia.]*

Stoltz DA, Meyerholz DK, Welsh MJ: Origins of cystic fibrosis lung disease, *N Engl J Med* 372:351–362, 2015. *[An exhaustive review on pathophysiological mechanisms that contribute to the panorama of pulmonary diseases in cystic fibrosis, with numerous excellent illustrations.]*

Trachtenberg FL, Haas EA, Kinney HC, et al: Risk factor changes for sudden infant death syndrome after initiation of Back-to-Sleep campaign, *Pediatrics* 129:630–638, 2012. *[An important study that measures the impact of the "Back to Sleep" campaign on SIDS mortality, and what additional risk factors have emerged since then.]*

Wainwright CE, TRAFFIC Study Group, TRANSPORT Study Group: Lumacaftor-Ivacaftor in patients with cystic fibrosis homozygous for Phe508del CFTR, *N Engl J Med* 373:220–231, 2015. *[Seminal study that led to FDA approval of the combination regimen of Lumacaftor and Ivacaftor, which enhance mutant Phe508del CFTR function in cystic fibrosis; Ivacaftor alone is approved for another variant of CFTR.]*

Walz AL, Ooms A, Gadd S, et al: Recurrent DGCR8, DROSHA, and SIX homeodomain mutations in favorable histology Wilms tumors, *Cancer Cell* 27(2):286–297, 2015. *[Seminal sequencing study in Wilms tumors identifying mutations of genes involved in microRNA processing and consequent microRNA deregulation.]*

Wong LC, Behr ER: Sudden unexplained death in infants and children: the role of undiagnosed inherited cardiac conditions, *Europace* 16:1706–1713, 2014. *[An insightful review on how unsuspected cardiac conditions, specifically "channelopathies," leading to sudden death in infancy might be erroneously diagnosed as SIDS.]*

Yang Y, Muzny DM, Xia F, et al: Molecular findings among patients referred for clinical whole exome sequencing, *JAMA* 312:1870–1879, 2014. *[An elegant study highlighting the prowess of next-generation techniques, wherein 2000 consecutive patients with suspected genetic disorders underwent germline whole exome sequencing, leading to the discovery of causal pathogenic mutations in as many as 25% of patients.]*

Environmental and Nutritional Diseases

8

CHAPTER OUTLINE

Health Effects of Climate Change 299
Toxicity of Chemical and Physical
 Agents 301
Environmental Pollution 302
Air Pollution 302
Metals as Environmental Pollutants 304
Industrial and Agricultural
 Exposures 306
Effects of Tobacco 307
Effects of Alcohol 310

Injury by Therapeutic Drugs and Drugs of
 Abuse 312
Injury by Therapeutic Drugs: Adverse Drug
 Reactions 312
Injury by Nontherapeutic Agents (Drug
 Abuse) 315
Injury by Physical Agents 317
Mechanical Trauma 317
Thermal Injury 318
Electrical Injury 319

Injury Produced by Ionizing Radiation 320
Nutritional Diseases 323
Malnutrition 324
Severe Acute Malnutrition 324
Anorexia Nervosa and Bulimia 326
Vitamin Deficiencies 326
Obesity 334
Diet and Systemic Diseases 337
Diet and Cancer 338

Many diseases are caused or influenced by environmental factors. Broadly defined, the term *ambient environment* encompasses the various outdoor, indoor, and occupational settings in which humans live and work. In each of these settings, the air people breathe, the food and water they consume, and the toxic agents they are exposed to are major determinants of health. Other environmental factors pertain to the individual ("personal environment") and include tobacco use, alcohol ingestion, therapeutic and "recreational" drug consumption, diet, and the like. It is generally believed that factors in the personal environment have a larger effect on human health than that of the ambient environment, but new threats related to global warming (described later) may change this equation.

The term environmental disease refers to disorders caused by exposure to chemical or physical agents in the ambient, workplace, and personal environments, including diseases of nutritional origin. Environmental diseases are surprisingly common. The International Labor Organization has estimated that work-related injuries and illnesses kill more people per year globally than do road accidents and wars combined. Most of these work-related problems are caused by illnesses rather than accidents. The burden of disease in the general population created by nonoccupational exposures to toxic agents is much more difficult to estimate, mostly because of the diversity of agents and the difficulties in measuring the dose and duration of exposures. Whatever the precise numbers, environmental diseases are major causes of disability and suffering and constitute a heavy financial burden, particularly in developing countries.

Environmental diseases are sometimes the consequence of major disasters, such as the methyl mercury contamina-tion of Minamata Bay in Japan in the 1960s, the leakage of methyl isocyanate gas in Bhopal, India, in 1984, the Chernobyl nuclear accident in 1986, the Fukushima nuclear meltdown following the tsunami in 2011, and lead poisoning resulting from contaminated drinking water in the city of Flint in the United States in 2016. Fortunately, these are unusual and infrequent occurrences. Less dramatic, but much more common, are diseases and injury produced by chronic exposure to relatively low levels of contaminants. It should be noted that a host of factors, including complex interactions between pollutants producing multiplicative effects, as well as the age, genetic predisposition, and different tissue sensitivities of exposed persons, create wide variations in individual sensitivity. Disease related to malnutrition is even more pervasive. In 2010, it was estimated that 925 million people were malnourished—one in every seven persons worldwide. Children are disproportionately affected by undernutrition, which accounts for more than 50% of childhood mortality worldwide.

In this chapter, we first consider the emerging problem of the health effects of climate change. We then discuss the mechanisms of toxicity of chemical and physical agents, and address specific environmental disorders, including those of nutritional origin.

HEALTH EFFECTS OF CLIMATE CHANGE

Global temperature measurements show that the earth has warmed significantly since the early 20th century, and especially since the mid-1960s. Record-breaking global temperatures have become common, with 2005, 2010, 2014, and 2015 each setting successive high-temperature records. Of note, 15 of the 16 warmest years since 1880 have occurred during the 21st century. During 2015, the global land temperature was 0.9° C warmer than the 20th century average. Mean global ocean temperatures also set new records in 2015, with an annual average temperature 0.74° C above the 20th century average. As of this writing, 2016 is on track to approach or exceed the records just set in 2015.

The rising atmospheric and ocean temperatures have led to a large number of effects that include changes in storm frequency, drought, and flood, as well as large-scale ice losses in Greenland, Antarctica, and the vast majority of the other glaciated regions on earth, as well as dramatic thinning or disappearance of Arctic ocean sea ice. The melting of land-based glacial ice and the thermal expansion of the warming oceans has produced approximately 80 mm of global average sea level rise since 1993, and the sea level currently is rising at a global average rate of 3.5 ± 0.4 mm/year.

Although politicians quibble, among scientists there is a general acceptance that climate change is, at least in part, man-made. The culprit is the rising atmospheric level of greenhouse gases, particularly carbon dioxide (CO_2) released through the burning of fossil fuels (Fig. 8.1A), as well as ozone (an important air pollutant, discussed later), and methane. These gases, along with water vapor, produce the so-called "greenhouse effect" by absorbing energy radiated from Earth's surface that otherwise would be lost into space. The annual average level of atmospheric CO_2 (about 401 ppm) in 2015 was higher than at any point in approximately 650,000 years and, without changes in human behavior, is expected to increase to 500 to 1200 ppm by the end of this century—levels not experienced for tens of millions of years. This increase stems not only from increased CO_2 production but also from deforestation and the attendant decrease in carbon fixation by plants. Depending on the computer model used, increased levels of greenhouse gases are projected to cause the global temperature to rise by 2°C to 5°C by the year 2100 (Fig. 8.1B). The health consequences of climate change will depend on its extent and rapidity, the severity of the ensuing consequences, and humankind's ability to mitigate the damaging effects. Even in the best-case scenario, however, climate change is expected to have a serious negative impact on human health by increasing the incidence of a number of diseases, including the following:

- *Cardiovascular, cerebrovascular, and respiratory diseases,* all of which will be exacerbated by heat waves and air pollution.
- *Gastroenteritis,* cholera, and other food- and waterborne infectious diseases, caused by contamination as a consequence of floods and disruption of clean water supplies and sewage treatment, after heavy rains and other environmental disasters.
- *Vector-borne infectious diseases,* such as malaria and dengue fever, resulting from changes in vector number and geographic distribution related to increased temperatures, crop failures, and more extreme weather variation (e.g., more frequent and severe El Niño events).
- *Malnutrition,* caused by changes in local climate that disrupt crop production. Such changes are anticipated to be most severe in tropical locations, in which average

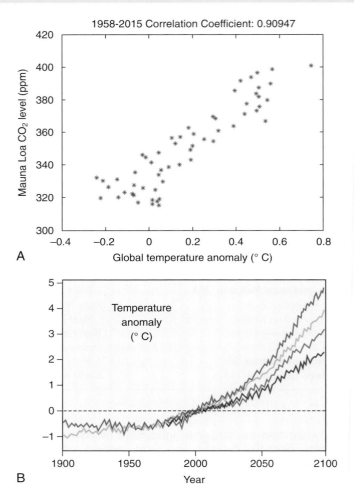

Fig. 8.1 Climate change, past and future. (A) Correlation of CO_2 levels measured at the Mauna Loa Observatory in Hawaii with average global temperature trends since the mid-1960s. "Global temperature" in any given year was deduced at the Hadley Center (United Kingdom) from measurements taken at more than 3000 weather stations located around the globe. (B) Predicted temperature increases during the 21st century. Different computer models plot anticipated rises in global temperatures of 2°C to 5°C by the year 2100. (A, Courtesy of Dr. Richard Aster, Department of Geosciences, Colorado State University, Fort Collins, Colorado.)

temperatures may already be near or above crop tolerance levels; it is estimated that by 2080, agricultural productivity may decline by 10% to 25% in some developing countries as a consequence of climate change.

Beyond these disease-specific effects, it is estimated that the melting of glacial ice, particularly in Greenland and other parts of the Northern Hemisphere, combined with the thermal expansion of warming oceans, will raise sea levels by 2 to 6 feet by 2100. Approximately 10% of the world's population—roughly 600 million people—live in low-lying areas that are at risk for flooding even if the rise in ocean levels is at the low end of these estimates. For example, a rise in sea level by 1.5 feet will submerge 70% of the land mass of Maldive islands by 2100 and a 3-foot rise will inundate 100% all of the islands by 2085. The resulting displacement of people will disrupt lives and commerce, creating conditions ripe for political unrest, war, and poverty, the "vectors" of malnutrition, sickness, and death. Worldwide recognition of the catastrophic effects of climate change led in late 2015 to a historic meeting of 196 countries in Paris, France, at which the participating countries agreed to the following objective:

Holding the increase in the global average temperature to well below 2°C above preindustrial levels and to pursue efforts to limit the temperature increase to 1.5°C above preindustrial levels, recognizing that this would significantly reduce the risks and impacts of climate change.

TOXICITY OF CHEMICAL AND PHYSICAL AGENTS

Toxicology **is defined as the science of poisons. It studies the distribution, effects, and mechanisms of action of toxic agents.** More broadly, it also includes the study of the effects of physical agents such as radiation and heat. Approximately 4 billion pounds of toxic chemicals, including 72 million pounds of known carcinogens, are produced each year in the United States. In general, however, little is known about the potential health effects of chemicals. Of the approximately 100,000 chemicals in use in the United States, less than 1% have been tested experimentally for health effects.

We now consider some basic principles regarding the toxicity of exogenous chemicals and drugs.

- The definition of a poison is not straightforward. It is a quantitative concept strictly dependent on dosage. The quote from Paracelsus in the 16th century that "all substances are poisons; the right dosage differentiates a poison from a remedy" is perhaps even more valid today, in view of the proliferation of therapeutic drugs with potentially harmful effects.
- Xenobiotics are exogenous chemicals in the environment that may be absorbed by the body through inhalation, ingestion, or skin contact (Fig. 8.2).
- Chemicals may be excreted in urine or feces or eliminated in expired air, or they may accumulate in bone, fat, brain, or other tissues.
- Chemicals may act at the site of entry, or they may be transported to other sites. Some agents are not modified on entry in the body, but most solvents and drugs are metabolized to form water-soluble products *(detoxification)* or are activated to form toxic metabolites.
- Most solvents and drugs are lipophilic, which facilitates their transport in the blood by lipoproteins and penetration through lipid components of cell membranes.
- The reactions that metabolize xenobiotics into non-toxic products, or activate xenobiotics to generate toxic compounds (Fig. 8.3; see also Fig. 8.2), occur in two phases. In phase I reactions, chemicals can undergo hydrolysis, oxidation, or reduction. Products of phase I reactions often are metabolized into water-soluble compounds through phase II reactions of glucuronidation, sulfation, methylation, and conjugation with glutathione (GSH). Water-soluble compounds are readily excreted.

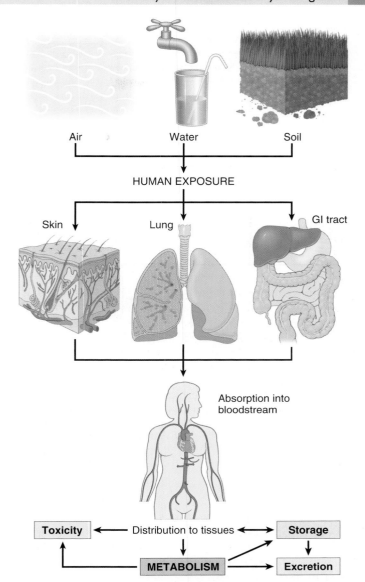

Fig. 8.2 Human exposure to pollutants. Pollutants contained in air, water, and soil are absorbed through the lungs, gastrointestinal (GI) tract, and skin. In the body, they may act at the site of absorption, but they generally are transported through the bloodstream to various organs, where they are stored or metabolized. Metabolism of xenobiotics may result in the formation of water-soluble compounds, which are excreted, or in activation of the agent, creating a toxic metabolite.

- The most important cellular enzyme system involved in phase I reactions is the cytochrome P-450 system. The P-450 system is present in organs throughout the body, but it is most active in the endoplasmic reticulum (ER) of the liver. The system catalyzes reactions that may either detoxify xenobiotics or convert xenobiotics into active compounds that cause cellular injury. Both types of reactions may produce, as a byproduct, reactive oxygen species (ROS), which can cause cellular damage (discussed in Chapter 2). Examples of metabolic activation of chemicals through the P-450 system are the conversion of carbon tetrachloride to the toxic trichloromethyl free radical, and the generation of a DNA-binding

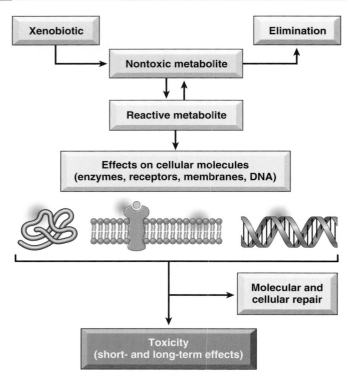

Fig. 8.3 Xenobiotic metabolism. Xenobiotics can be metabolized to non-toxic metabolites and eliminated from the body (detoxification). However, their metabolism also may result in formation of a reactive metabolite that is toxic to cellular components. If repair is not effective, short- and long-term effects develop. *(Modified from Hodgson E: A textbook of modern toxicology, ed 3, Fig. 1–1. Hoboken, NJ, 2004, John Wiley & Sons.)*

metabolite from benzo[a]pyrene, a carcinogen present in cigarette smoke. The cytochrome P-450 system also participates in the metabolism of a large number of common therapeutic drugs such as acetaminophen, barbiturates, and anti-convulsants, and in alcohol metabolism (discussed later).

- P-450 enzymes vary widely in activity among different people, owing to both polymorphisms in the genes encoding the enzymes and interactions with drugs that are metabolized through the system. The activity of the enzymes also may be decreased by fasting or starvation, and increased by alcohol consumption and smoking.

ENVIRONMENTAL POLLUTION

Air Pollution

Air pollution is a significant cause of morbidity and mortality worldwide, particularly among at-risk individuals with preexisting pulmonary or cardiac disease. The life-giving air that we breathe is also often laden with many potential causes of disease. Airborne microorganisms have long been major causes of morbidity and death. More widespread are the chemical and particulate pollutants found in the air, both in so-called "developed" and "under-developed" countries. Specific hazards have been recognized for both outdoor and indoor air.

Outdoor Air Pollution

The ambient air in industrialized nations is contaminated with an unsavory mixture of gaseous and particulate pollutants, more so in cities and in proximity to heavy industry. In the United States, the Environmental Protection Agency (EPA) monitors and sets allowable upper limits for six pollutants: sulfur dioxide, CO, ozone, nitrogen dioxide, lead, and particulate matter. Together, some of these agents produce the well-known smog that sometimes stifles major cities such as Cairo, Los Angeles, Houston, Mexico City, and São Paulo. It may seem that air pollution is a modern phenomenon. This is not the case; Seneca wrote in AD 61 that he felt an alteration of his disposition as soon as he left the "pestilential vapors, soot, and heavy air of Rome." The first environmental-control law was proclaimed by Edward I in 1306 and was straightforward in its simplicity: "Whoever should be found guilty of burning coal shall suffer the loss of his head." What has changed in modern times is the nature and sources of air pollutants, and the types of regulations that control their emission. It could be argued that modern man has lost his head to drown himself in pollution!

The lungs bear the brunt of the adverse consequences of air pollution, but air pollutants affect many organ systems (as with the effects of lead poisoning and CO, discussed later). More detailed discussion of pollutant-caused lung diseases is found in Chapter 13. Here we consider the major health effects of ozone, sulfur dioxide, particulates, and CO (Table 8.1).

Table 8.1 Health Effects of Outdoor Air Pollutants

Pollutant	Populations at Risk	Effect(s)
Ozone	Healthy adults and children	Decreased lung function Increased airway reactivity Lung inflammation
	Athletes, outdoor workers	Decreased exercise capacity
	Asthmatics	Increased hospitalizations
Nitrogen dioxide	Healthy adults	Increased airway reactivity
	Asthmatics	Decreased lung function
	Children	Increased respiratory infections
Sulfur dioxide	Healthy adults	Increased respiratory symptoms
	Patients with chronic lung disease	Increased mortality
	Asthmatics	Increased hospitalization Decreased lung function
Acid aerosols	Healthy adults	Altered mucociliary clearance
	Children	Increased respiratory infections
	Asthmatics	Decreased lung function Increased hospitalizations
Particulates	Children	Increased respiratory infections Decreased lung function
	Patients with chronic lung or heart disease	Excess mortality
	Asthmatics	Increased attacks

Data from Health Effects of Outdoor Air Pollution, Part 2. Committee of the Environmental and Occupational Health Assembly of the American Thoracic Society, *Am J Respir Crit Care Med* 153:477, 1996.

Ozone is one of the most pervasive air pollutants, with levels in many cities exceeding EPA standards. It is a gas formed by sunlight-driven reactions involving nitrogen oxides, which are released mostly by automobile exhaust. Together with oxides and fine particulate matter, ozone forms the familiar smog (from the words *smoke* and *fog*). Its toxicity stems from its participation in chemical reactions that generate free radicals, which injure the lining cells of the respiratory tract and the alveoli. Low levels of ozone may be tolerated by healthy persons but are detrimental to lung function, especially in those with asthma or emphysema, and when present along with particulate pollution. Unfortunately, pollutants rarely occur singly but combine to create a veritable "witches' brew."

Sulfur dioxide, particles, and acid aerosols are emitted by coal- and oil-fired power plants and industrial processes burning these fuels. Of these, particles appear to be the main cause of morbidity and death. Particles less than 10 μm in diameter are particularly harmful, because when inhaled they are carried by the airstream all the way to the alveoli. Here, they are phagocytosed by macrophages and neutrophils, causing the release of mediators (possibly by activating inflammasomes, Chapter 2) and inciting an inflammatory reaction. By contrast, larger particles are removed in the nose or are trapped by the mucociliary "escalator" and as a result are less dangerous.

Carbon monoxide (CO) is a nonirritating, colorless, tasteless, odorless gas. It is produced by the incomplete oxidation of carbonaceous materials. Its sources include automotive engines, industries using fossil fuels, home oil burners, and cigarette smoke. The low levels often found in ambient air may contribute to impaired respiratory function but usually are not life threatening. However, persons working in confined environments with high exposure to fumes, such as tunnel and underground garage workers, may develop chronic poisoning. CO is included here as an air pollutant, but it also is an important cause of accidental and suicidal death. In a small, closed garage, exhaust from a running car engine can induce a lethal coma within 5 minutes. CO is a systemic asphyxiant that kills by binding to hemoglobin and preventing oxygen transport. Hemoglobin has a 200-fold greater affinity for CO than for O_2. The carboxyhemoglobin, that is formed by binding of CO is incapable of carrying oxygen. Hypoxia leads to central nervous system (CNS) depression, which develops so insidiously that victims often are unaware of their plight and are unable to help themselves. Systemic hypoxia appears when the hemoglobin is 20% to 30% saturated with CO, and unconsciousness and death are probable with 60% to 70% saturation. The diagnosis of CO poisoning is based on detection of high levels of carboxyhemoglobin in the blood.

MORPHOLOGY

Chronic poisoning by CO develops because carboxyhemoglobin, once formed, is remarkably stable. As a result, with low-level persistent exposure to CO, carboxyhemoglobin may accumulate to a life-threatening concentration in the blood. The slowly developing hypoxia can evoke widespread ischemic changes in the brain, particularly in the basal ganglia and lenticular nuclei. With cessation of exposure to CO, the patient usually recovers, but there may be permanent neurologic damage.

Acute poisoning by CO generally is a consequence of accidental exposure or suicide attempt. In light-skinned people, it is marked by a characteristic **generalized cherry-red color of the skin and mucous membranes,** a color imparted by carboxyhemoglobin. If death occurs rapidly, morphologic changes may not be present; with longer survival, the brain may be slightly edematous and exhibit punctate hemorrhages and hypoxia-induced neuronal changes. These changes are not specific; they simply imply systemic hypoxia (Chapter 23). In victims who survive CO poisoning, complete recovery is possible; however, impairments of memory, vision, hearing, and speech sometimes remain.

Indoor Air Pollution

As modern homes are increasingly "buttoned up" to exclude the environment, the potential for pollution of the indoor air increases. The most common pollutant is tobacco smoke (discussed later), but additional offenders are CO, nitrogen dioxide (already mentioned as outdoor pollutants), and asbestos (discussed in Chapter 13). A few comments about some other agents are presented here.

- *Smoke from burning of organic materials,* containing various oxides of nitrogen and carbon particulates, is an irritant that predisposes exposed persons to lung infections and may contain carcinogenic polycyclic hydrocarbons. It is estimated that one-third of the world, mainly in developing areas, burn carbon-containing material such as wood, dung, or charcoal in their homes for cooking, heating, and light.
- *Radon,* a radioactive gas derived from uranium, is widely present in soil and in homes. Although radon exposure can cause lung cancer in uranium miners (particularly in those who smoke), it does not appear that low-level chronic exposures in the home increase lung cancer risk, at least for nonsmokers.
- *Bioaerosols* may contain pathogenic microbiologic agents, such as those that can cause Legionnaires' disease, viral pneumonia, and the common cold, as well as allergens derived from pet dander, dust mites, and fungi and molds, which can cause rhinitis, eye irritation, and even asthma.

SUMMARY

ENVIRONMENTAL DISEASES AND ENVIRONMENTAL POLLUTION

- Environmental diseases are conditions caused by exposure to chemical or physical agents in the ambient, workplace, and personal environments.
- Exogenous chemicals, known as xenobiotics, enter the body through inhalation, ingestion, and skin contact, and can either be eliminated or accumulate in fat, bone, brain, and other tissues.
- Xenobiotics can be converted into nontoxic products or toxic compounds through a two-phase reaction process that involves the cytochrome P-450 system.

- The most common air pollutants are ozone (which in combination with oxides and particulate matter forms smog), sulfur dioxide, acid aerosols, and particles less than 10 μm in diameter.
- CO is an air pollutant and an important cause of death from accidents and suicide; it binds hemoglobin with high affinity, leading to systemic asphyxiation resulting in CNS depression.

Metals as Environmental Pollutants

Lead, mercury, arsenic, and cadmium, the heavy metals most commonly associated with harmful effects in human populations, are considered here.

Lead

Lead is a readily absorbed metal that binds to sulfhydryl groups in proteins and interferes with calcium metabolism, leading to hematologic, skeletal, neurologic, GI, and renal toxicities. Lead exposure occurs through contaminated air, food, and water. For most of the 20th century the major sources of lead in the environment were house paints and gasoline. Although the use of lead-based paints and leaded gas has greatly diminished, many sources of lead persist in the environment, such as mines, foundries, batteries, and spray paints, all of which constitute occupational hazards. However, *flaking lead paint* in older houses and soil contamination pose the major hazards for youngsters. Blood levels of lead in children living in older homes containing lead-based paint or lead-contaminated dust often exceed 5 μg/dL, the level at which the Centers for Disease Control and Prevention (CDC) recommends that measures be taken to limit further exposure. A dramatic case of lead contamination of drinking water occurred in the U.S. city of Flint, Michigan, in 2014–2016. The so-called "Flint water crisis" occurred when the source of water supply to the city was changed from Lake Huron to the Flint River. Because water from the Flint River had a higher chloride concentration than the lake waters, it leached lead from century-old lead pipes. This caused an increase in lead levels in tap water above the acceptable limit of 15 parts per billion (ppb) in about 25% of the homes and in some cases as high as 13,200 ppb. As a result 6000 to 12,000 residents developed very high lead levels in their blood. Ingested lead is particularly harmful to children because they absorb more than 50% of lead from food, whereas adults absorb approximately 15%. A more permeable blood–brain barrier in children creates a high susceptibility to brain damage. The clinical features of lead poisoning are shown in Fig. 8.4.

Most absorbed lead (80% to 85%) is taken up into developing teeth and into bone, where it competes with calcium, binds phosphates, and has a half-life of 20 to 30 years. About 5% to 10% of the absorbed lead remains in the blood, and the remainder is distributed throughout soft tissues. Excess lead is toxic to nervous tissues in adults and children; peripheral neuropathies predominate in adults, whereas central effects are more common in children. The effects of chronic lead exposure in children may be subtle, producing mild dysfunction, or they may be massive and lethal. In young children, sensory, motor, intellectual, and psychologic impairments have been described, including reduced IQ, learning disabilities, retarded psychomotor

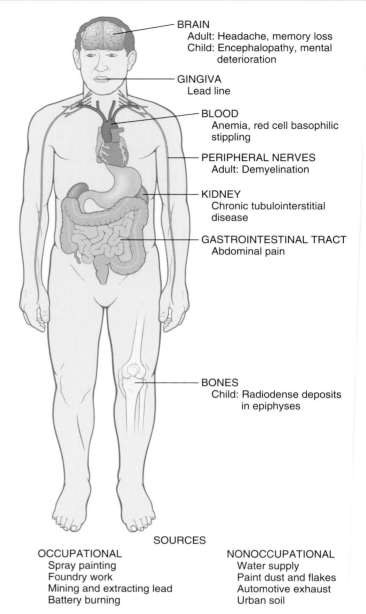

BRAIN
Adult: Headache, memory loss
Child: Encephalopathy, mental deterioration

GINGIVA
Lead line

BLOOD
Anemia, red cell basophilic stippling

PERIPHERAL NERVES
Adult: Demyelination

KIDNEY
Chronic tubulointerstitial disease

GASTROINTESTINAL TRACT
Abdominal pain

BONES
Child: Radiodense deposits in epiphyses

SOURCES

OCCUPATIONAL
Spray painting
Foundry work
Mining and extracting lead
Battery burning

NONOCCUPATIONAL
Water supply
Paint dust and flakes
Automotive exhaust
Urban soil

Fig. 8.4 Pathologic features of lead poisoning.

development, and, in more severe cases, blindness, psychoses, seizures, and coma. Lead-induced peripheral neuropathies in adults generally remit with the elimination of exposure, but both peripheral and CNS abnormalities in children usually are irreversible. Other effects of lead exposure include the following.

Excess lead interferes with the normal remodeling of calcified cartilage and primary bone trabeculae in the epiphyses in children, causing increased bone density detected as radiodense "lead lines" (Fig. 8.5). Lead lines of a different sort also may occur in the gums, where excess lead stimulates hyperpigmentation. *Lead inhibits the healing of fractures* by increasing chondrogenesis and delaying cartilage mineralization. Excretion of lead occurs by way of the kidneys, and acute exposures may cause damage to proximal tubules.

Lead has a high affinity for sulfhydryl groups and interferes with two enzymes involved in heme synthesis:

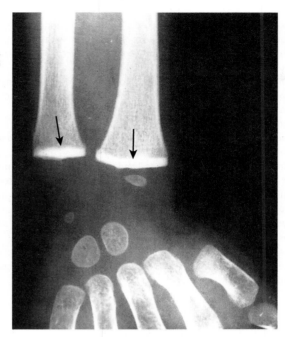

Fig. 8.5 Lead poisoning. Impaired remodeling of calcified cartilage in the epiphyses *(arrows)* of the wrist has caused a marked increase in their radiodensity, so that they are as radiopaque as the cortical bone. *(Courtesy of Dr. GW Dietz: Department of Radiology, University of Texas Southwestern Medical School, Dallas, Texas.)*

aminolevulinic acid dehydratase and delta ferrochelatase. Iron incorporation into heme is impaired, leading to *anemia.* Lead also inhibits sodium- and potassium-dependent ATPases in cell membranes, an effect that may increase the fragility of red cells, causing *hemolysis.* The diagnosis of lead poisoning requires constant vigilance. It may be suspected on the basis of neurologic changes in children or unexplained anemia with basophilic stippling in red cells in adults and children. Elevated blood lead and red cell free protoporphyrin levels (greater than 50 µg/dL) or, alternatively, zinc-protoporphyrin levels, are required for definitive diagnosis. In milder cases of lead exposure, anemia may be the only obvious abnormality.

MORPHOLOGY

The major anatomic targets of lead toxicity are the blood, bone marrow, nervous system, GI tract, and kidneys (Fig. 8.4).

Blood changes are one of the earliest signs of lead accumulation and are characteristic, consisting of a microcytic, hypochromic anemia associated with a distinctive punctate **basophilic stippling** of red cells. These changes in the blood stem from the inhibition of heme synthesis in marrow erythroid progenitors. Another consequence of this blockade is that zinc-protoporphyrin is formed instead of heme. Thus, elevated blood levels of zinc-protoporphyrin or its product, free red cell protoporphyrin, are important indicators of lead poisoning.

Brain damage is prone to occur in children. The anatomic changes underlying the more subtle functional deficits are ill defined; at the more severe end of the spectrum, changes include brain edema, demyelination of the cerebral and cerebellar white matter, and necrosis of cortical neurons accompanied by diffuse astrocytic proliferation. In adults, the CNS is less-often affected, but frequently a **peripheral demyelinating neuropathy** appears, typically involving motor neurons innervating the most commonly used muscles. Thus, the extensor muscles of the wrist and fingers are often the first to be affected, followed by paralysis of the peroneal muscles (**wristdrop** and **footdrop**).

The **GI tract** also is a site of major clinical manifestations. Lead "colic" is characterized by extremely severe, poorly localized abdominal pain.

The **kidneys** may develop proximal tubular damage with intranuclear lead inclusions. Chronic renal damage leads eventually to interstitial fibrosis and possibly renal failure and findings suggestive of gout ("saturnine gout"). Other features of lead poisoning are shown in Fig. 8.4.

Mercury

Mercury, like lead, binds to sulfhydryl groups in certain proteins with high affinity, leading to damage in the CNS and several other organs such as the GI tract and the kidneys. Humans have used mercury in many ways throughout history, including as a pigment in cave paintings, a cosmetic, a remedy for syphilis, and a component of diuretics. Poisoning from inhalation of mercury vapors has long been recognized and is associated with tremor, gingivitis, and bizarre behavior, such as that of the "Mad Hatter" in Lewis Carroll's *Alice in Wonderland* (mercury formerly was used in hat-making).

Today, the main sources of exposure to mercury are contaminated fish and dental amalgams, which release mercury vapors. In some areas of the world, mercury used in gold mining has contaminated rivers and streams. Inorganic mercury from the natural degassing of the earth's crust or from industrial contamination is converted to organic compounds such as methyl mercury by bacteria. Methyl mercury enters the food chain, and in carnivorous fish such as swordfish, shark, and bluefish, mercury levels may be 1 million times higher than in the surrounding water. Almost 90% of the ingested mercury is absorbed in the GI tract. The consumption of contaminated fish from the release of methyl mercury in Minamata Bay and the Agano River in Japan, and the consumption of bread containing grain treated with a methyl mercury–based fungicide in Iraq, caused widespread morbidity and many deaths.

The medical disorders associated with the Minamata episode became known as *"Minamata disease"* and include cerebral palsy, deafness, blindness, and major CNS defects in children exposed in utero. *The developing brain is extremely sensitive to methyl mercury;* for this reason, the CDC in the United States has recommended that pregnant women avoid the consumption of fish known to contain mercury.

Ingested mercury can injure the gut and cause ulcerations and bloody diarrhea. In the kidneys, mercury can cause acute tubular necrosis and renal failure.

Arsenic

Arsenic salts interfere with several aspects of cellular metabolism, leading to toxicities that are most prominent in the GI tract, nervous system, skin, and heart. Arsenic was poison of choice of skilled practitioners in the Borgia and Medici families in Renaissance Italy. Today, arsenic exposure is an important health problem in many areas of the world. Arsenic is found naturally in soil and water and is used in wood preservatives, herbicides, and other agricultural products. It may be released into the environment by the mining and smelting industries. Arsenic is present in Chinese and Indian herbal medicine, and arsenic trioxide is a frontline treatment for acute promyelocytic leukemia (Chapter 6). Large concentrations of inorganic arsenic are present in ground water in countries such as Bangladesh, Chile, and China. Between 35 and 77 million people in Bangladesh drink water contaminated with arsenic, constituting one of the greatest environmental cancer risks yet uncovered.

If ingested in large quantities, arsenic causes acute toxicity manifesting as severe abdominal pain, diarrhea; cardiac arrhythmias, shock and respiratory distress syndrome; and acute encephalopathy. GI, cardiovascular and CNS toxicity may be severe enough to cause death. These effects may be attributed to the interference with mitochondrial oxidative phosphorylation. Chronic exposure to arsenic causes hyperpigmentation and hyperkeratosis of the skin, which may be followed by the development of basal and squamous cell carcinomas (but not melanomas). A symmetrical sensorimotor polyneuropathy can also develop. Arsenic-induced skin tumors differ from those induced by sunlight by appearing on palms and soles, and by occurring as multiple lesions. Arsenic exposure also is associated with an increased risk of lung carcinoma. The mechanisms of arsenic carcinogenesis in the skin and the lung are uncertain.

Cadmium

Cadmium is preferentially toxic to the kidneys and the lungs through uncertain mechanisms that may involve increased production of ROS. In contrast with the metals already discussed, cadmium is a relatively modern toxic agent. It is used mainly in nickel-cadmium batteries, which generally are disposed of as household waste. Cadmium can contaminate soil and plants directly or through fertilizers and irrigation water. Food is the most important source of exposure for the general population. Excessive cadmium intake can lead to obstructive lung disease and renal toxicity, initially as tubular damage that may progress to end-stage renal disease. Cadmium exposure can also cause skeletal abnormalities associated with calcium loss. Cadmium-contaminated water used to irrigate rice fields in Japan caused a disease in postmenopausal women known as "itai-itai" (ouch-ouch), a combination of osteoporosis and osteomalacia associated with renal disease. A survey showed that 5% of persons aged 20 years and older in the U.S. population have urinary cadmium levels that, according to research data, may produce subtle kidney injury and increased calcium loss.

SUMMARY

TOXIC EFFECTS OF HEAVY METALS

- Lead, mercury, arsenic, and cadmium are the heavy metals most commonly associated with toxic effects in humans.
- Children absorb more ingested lead than adults; the main source of exposure for children is lead-containing paint.
- Excess lead causes CNS defects in children and peripheral neuropathy in adults. Excess lead competes with calcium in bones and interferes with the remodeling of cartilage; it also causes anemia.
- The major source of mercury is contaminated fish. The developing brain is highly sensitive to methyl mercury, which accumulates in the brain and blocks ion channels.
- Exposure of the fetus to high levels of mercury in utero may lead to Minamata disease, characterized by cerebral palsy, deafness, and blindness.
- Arsenic is naturally found in soil and water and is a component of some wood preservatives and herbicides. Excess arsenic interferes with mitochondrial oxidative phosphorylation and causes toxic effects in the GI tract, CNS, and cardiovascular system; long-term exposure causes polyneuropathy, skin lesions and carcinomas.
- Cadmium from nickel-cadmium batteries and chemical fertilizers can contaminate soil. Excess cadmium causes obstructive lung disease and kidney damage.

Industrial and Agricultural Exposures

More than 10 million occupational injuries occur annually in the United States, and approximately 65,000 people die as a consequence of occupational injuries and illnesses. Industrial exposures to toxic agents are as varied as the industries themselves. They range from merely annoying irritations of respiratory airways by formaldehyde or ammonia fumes, to lung cancers arising from exposure to asbestos, arsenic, or uranium. Human diseases associated with occupational exposures are listed in Table 8.2. In addition to toxic metals (already discussed), other important agents that contribute to environmental diseases include the following:

- *Organic solvents* are widely used in huge quantities worldwide. Some, such as chloroform and carbon tetrachloride, are found in degreasing and dry cleaning agents and paint removers. Acute exposure to high levels of vapors from these agents can cause dizziness and confusion, leading to CNS depression and even coma. Lower levels may cause liver and kidney toxicity. Occupational exposure of rubber workers to benzene and 1,3-butadiene increases the risk of leukemia. Benzene is oxidized to an epoxide through hepatic CYP2E1, a component of the P-450 enzyme system already mentioned. The epoxide and other metabolites disrupt progenitor cell differentiation in the bone marrow, and may lead to marrow aplasia and acute myeloid leukemia.
- *Polycyclic hydrocarbons* are released during the combustion of coal and gas, particularly at the high temperatures used in steel foundries, and also are present in tar and soot. (Pott identified soot as the cause of scrotal cancers in chimney sweeps in 1775, as mentioned in Chapter 6). Polycyclic hydrocarbons are among the most potent carcinogens, and industrial exposures have been implicated in the causation of lung and bladder cancer.
- *Organochlorines* (and halogenated organic compounds in general) are synthetic products that resist degradation and are lipophilic. Important organochlorines used

Table 8.2 Human Diseases Associated With Occupational Exposures

Organ/System	Effect(s)	Toxicant(s)
Cardiovascular system	Heart disease	CO, lead, solvents, cobalt, cadmium
Respiratory system	Nasal cancer Lung cancer Chronic obstructive lung disease Hypersensitivity Irritation Fibrosis	Isopropyl alcohol, wood dust Radon, asbestos, silica, bis(chloromethyl)ether, nickel, arsenic, chromium, mustard gas Grain dust, coal dust, cadmium Beryllium, isocyanates Ammonia, sulfur oxides, formaldehyde Silica, asbestos, cobalt
Nervous system	Peripheral neuropathies Ataxic gait CNS depression Cataracts	Solvents, acrylamide, methyl chloride, mercury, lead, arsenic, DDT Chlordane, toluene, acrylamide, mercury Alcohols, ketones, aldehydes, solvents Ultraviolet radiation
Urinary system	Toxicity Bladder cancer	Mercury, lead, glycol ethers, solvents Naphthylamines, 4-aminobiphenyl, benzidine, rubber products
Reproductive system	Male infertility Female infertility Teratogenesis	Lead, phthalate plasticizers Cadmium, lead Mercury, polychlorinated biphenyls
Hematopoietic system	Leukemia	Benzene, radon, uranium
Skin	Folliculitis and acneiform dermatosis Cancer	Polychlorinated biphenyls, dioxins, herbicides Ultraviolet radiation
GI tract	Liver angiosarcoma	Vinyl chloride

CNS, Central nervous system; *CO,* carbon monoxide; *DDT,* dichlorodiphenyltrichloroethane; *GI,* gastrointestinal.
Data from Leigh JP, Markowitz SB, Fahs M, et al: Occupational injury and illness in the United States: estimates of costs, morbidity, and mortality, *Arch Intern Med* 157:1557, 1997; Mitchell FL: Hazardous waste. In Rom WN, editor: *Environmental and occupational medicine,* ed 2, Boston, 1992, Little, Brown, pp 1275; and Levi PE: Classes of toxic chemicals. In Hodgson E, Levi PE, editors: *A textbook of modern toxicology,* Stamford, CT, 1997, Appleton & Lange, pp 229.

as pesticides are DDT (dichlorodiphenyltrichloroethane) and its metabolites, and agents such as lindane, aldrin, and dieldrin. Nonpesticide organochlorines include polychlorinated biphenyls (PCBs) and dioxin (TCDD [2,3,7,8-tetrachlorodibenzo-p-dioxin]). DDT was banned in the United States in 1973, but more than half of the population have detectable serum levels of p,p'-DDE, a long-lasting DDT metabolite, including those born after the ban on DDT went into effect. PCB and TCDD also are present in the blood of most of the U.S. population. Acute DDT poisoning in humans causes neurologic toxicity. Most organochlorines are endocrine disruptors and have anti-estrogenic or anti-androgenic activity in laboratory animals, but long-term health effects in humans have not been firmly established.

- *Nonpesticide organochlorines* include polychlorinated biphenyls (PCBs) and dioxin (TCDD [2,3,7,8-tetrachlorodibenzo-p-dioxin]). Dioxins and PCBs can cause skin disorders such as folliculitis and acneiform dermatosis known as chloracne, which consists of acne, cyst formation, hyperpigmentation, and hyperkeratosis, generally around the face and behind the ears. It can be accompanied by abnormalities in the liver and CNS. Because PCBs induce the P-450 enzyme system, workers exposed to these substances may show altered drug metabolism. Environmental disasters in Japan and China in the late 1960s caused by the consumption of rice oil contaminated by PCBs poisoned about 2000 people in each episode. The primary manifestations of the disease (yusho in Japan, yu-cheng in China) were chloracne and hyperpigmentation of the skin and nails.

- *Bisphenol A* (BPA) is used in the synthesis of polycarbonate food and water containers and of epoxy resins that line almost all food bottles and cans; as a result, exposure to BPA is virtually ubiquitous in humans. BPA has long been known as a potential endocrine disruptor. Several large retrospective studies have linked elevated urinary BPA levels to heart disease in adult populations. In addition, infants who drink from BPA-containing containers may be particularly susceptible to BPA's endocrine effects. In 2010, Canada was the first country to list BPA as a toxic substance, and the largest makers of baby bottles and "sippy" cups have stopped using BPA in the manufacturing process. The extent of the human health risks associated with BPA remains uncertain, however, and requires further study.

- *Vinyl chloride,* used in the synthesis of polyvinyl resins, can cause angiosarcoma of the liver, a rare type of liver tumor.

- Inhalation of *mineral dusts* causes chronic, nonneoplastic lung diseases called pneumoconioses. This group of disorders includes diseases induced by organic and inorganic particulates as well as chemical fume- and vapor-induced nonneoplastic lung diseases. The most common pneumoconioses are caused by exposures to coal dust (in mining of hard coal), silica (in sandblasting and stone cutting), asbestos (in mining, fabrication, and insulation work), and beryllium (in mining and fabrication). Exposure to these agents nearly always occurs in the workplace. The increased risk of cancer as a result of asbestos exposure, however, extends to family members of asbestos workers and to other persons exposed outside the workplace. Pneumoconioses and their pathogenesis are discussed in Chapter 13.

EFFECTS OF TOBACCO

Tobacco is the most common exogenous cause of human cancers, being responsible for 90% of lung cancers. The

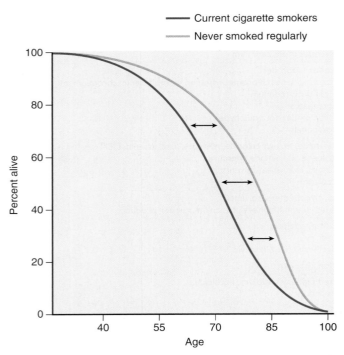

Fig. 8.6 The effects of smoking on survival. The study compared age-specific death rates for current cigarette smokers with those of individuals who never smoked regularly (British Doctors Study). The difference in survival, measured at age 75 between smokers and nonsmokers is 7.5 years. *(Modified from Stewart BW, Kleihues P, editors:* World cancer report, *Lyon, 2003, IARC Press.)*

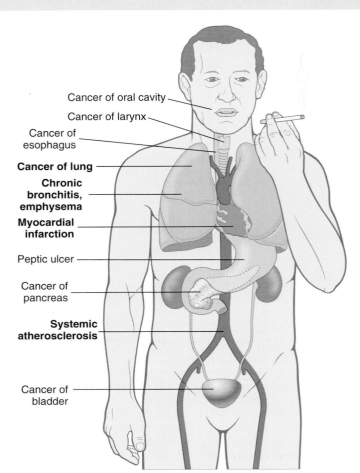

Fig. 8.7 Adverse effects of smoking. The more common are in boldface.

main culprit is cigarette smoking, but smokeless tobacco in its various forms (snuff, chewing tobacco) also is harmful to health and is an important cause of oral cancer. Not only does the use of tobacco products create personal risk, but also passive tobacco inhalation from the environment ("second-hand smoke") can cause lung cancer in nonsmokers. From 1998 to 2007 in the United States, the incidence of smoking declined modestly, but this trend failed to continue, and approximately 20% of adults remain smokers. In recent years, China has become the world's largest producer and consumer of cigarettes. China has approximately 350 million smokers who in aggregate consume about 33% of all cigarettes smoked worldwide. Cigarette smoking causes, worldwide, more than 4 million deaths annually, mostly from cardiovascular disease, various types of cancers, and chronic respiratory problems. It is expected that there will be 8 million tobacco-related deaths yearly by 2020, the major increase occurring in developing countries. Of people alive today, an estimated 500 million will die from tobacco-related illnesses. In the United States alone, tobacco is responsible for more than 400,000 deaths per year, with one-third of these attributable to lung cancer.

Smoking is the most important cause of preventable human death. It reduces overall survival in a dose-dependent fashion. Whereas 80% of nonsmokers are alive at age 70, only about 50% of smokers survive to this age (Fig. 8.6). Cessation of smoking greatly reduces the risk of death from lung cancer, and it even has an effect, albeit reduced, on people who stop smoking at age 60. Discussed

next are some of the agents contained in tobacco and diseases associated with tobacco consumption. Adverse effects of smoking in various organ systems are shown in Fig. 8.7.

The number of potentially noxious chemicals in tobacco smoke is vast; Table 8.3 presents only a partial list and includes the type of injury produced by these agents. Nicotine, an alkaloid present in tobacco leaves, is not a direct cause of tobacco-related diseases, but it is highly addictive. Nicotine binds to receptors in the brain and, through the

Table 8.3 Effects of Selected Tobacco Smoke Constituents

Substance	Effect(s)
Tar	Carcinogenesis
Polycyclic aromatic hydrocarbons	Carcinogenesis
Nicotine	Ganglionic stimulation and depression, tumor promotion
Phenol	Tumor promotion; mucosal irritation
Benzopyrene	Carcinogenesis
CO	Impaired oxygen transport and use
Formaldehyde	Toxicity to cilia; mucosal irritation
Oxides of nitrogen	Toxicity to cilia; mucosal irritation
Nitrosamine	Carcinogenesis

Table 8.4 Organ-Specific Carcinogens in Tobacco Smoke

Organ	Carcinogen(s)
Lung, larynx	Polycyclic aromatic hydrocarbons 4-(Methylnitrosoamino)-1-(3-pyridyl)-1-butanone (NNK) ^{210}Polonium
Esophagus	N'-Nitrosonornicotine (NNN)
Pancreas	NNK (?)
Bladder	4-Aminobiphenyl, 2-naphthylamine
Oral cavity: smoking	Polycyclic aromatic hydrocarbons, NNK, NNN
Oral cavity: snuff	NNK, NNN, ^{210}polonium

Data from Szczesny LB, Holbrook JH: Cigarette smoking. In Rom WH, editor: *Environmental and occupational medicine*, ed 2, Boston, 1992, Little, Brown, pp 1211.

release of catecholamines, is responsible for the acute effects of smoking, such as increased heart rate and blood pressure, and increased cardiac contractility and output.

The most common diseases caused by cigarette smoking involve the lung and include emphysema, chronic bronchitis, and lung cancer, all discussed in Chapter 13. The mechanisms responsible for some tobacco-induced diseases include the following:
- *Direct irritant effect on the tracheobronchial mucosa,* producing inflammation and increased mucus production (bronchitis). Cigarette smoke also causes the recruitment of leukocytes to the lung, increasing local elastase production and subsequent injury to lung tissue that leads to emphysema.
- *Carcinogensis.* Components of cigarette smoke, particularly polycyclic hydrocarbons and nitrosamines (Table 8.4), are potent carcinogens in animals and probably are involved in the causation of lung carcinomas in humans (see Chapter 13). The risk of developing lung cancer is related to the intensity of exposure, frequently expressed in terms of "pack years" (e.g., one pack daily for 20 years equals 20 pack years) or in cigarettes smoked per day (Fig. 8.8). In addition to lung cancers, tobacco smoke

contributes to the development of cancers of the oral cavity, esophagus, pancreas, and bladder. Table 8.4 lists organ-specific carcinogens contained in tobacco smoke. Moreover, smoking multiplies the risk of disease associated with other carcinogens; well-recognized examples are the 10-fold increased incidence of lung carcinomas in asbestos workers and uranium miners who smoke than in those who do not. The combination of tobacco (chewed or smoked) and alcohol consumption has multiplicative effects on the risks of oral, laryngeal, and esophageal cancers. An example of the carcinogenic interaction of these all-too-common vices is shown for laryngeal cancer (Fig. 8.9).
- *Atherosclerosis* and its major complication, myocardial infarction, are strongly linked to cigarette smoking. The causal mechanisms probably relate to several factors, including increased platelet aggregation, decreased myocardial oxygen supply (because of lung disease coupled with hypoxia related to CO in cigarette smoke) accompanied by increased oxygen demand, and a decreased threshold for ventricular fibrillation. Almost one-third of all heart attacks are associated with cigarette smoking. Smoking has a multiplicative effect on risk when combined with hypertension and hypercholesterolemia.
- *Maternal smoking increases the risk of spontaneous abortions and preterm births* and results in intrauterine growth retardation (Chapter 7); however, birth weights of infants born to mothers who stopped smoking before pregnancy are normal.

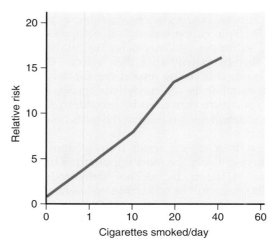

Fig. 8.8 The risk of lung cancer is determined by the number of cigarettes smoked. *(Data from Stewart BW, Kleihues P, editors: World cancer report, Lyon, 2003, IARC Press.)*

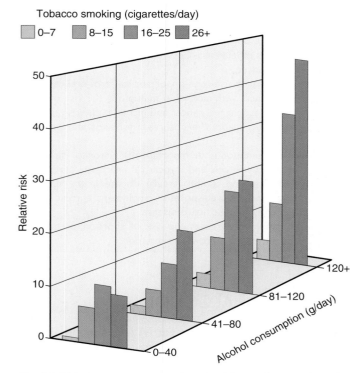

Fig. 8.9 Multiplicative increase in the risk of laryngeal cancer from the interaction between cigarette smoking and alcohol consumption. *(Data from Stewart BW, Kleihues P, editors: World cancer report, Lyon, 2003, IARC Press.)*

- *Passive smoke inhalation* is also associated with detrimental effects. It is estimated that the relative risk of lung cancer in nonsmokers exposed to environmental smoke is about 1.3 times that in nonsmokers who are not exposed to smoke. In the United States, approximately 3000 lung cancer deaths in nonsmokers older than 35 years can be attributed each year to environmental tobacco smoke. Even more striking is the increased risk of coronary atherosclerosis and fatal myocardial infarction. Studies report that 30,000 to 60,000 cardiac deaths annually in the United States are associated with passive exposure to smoke. Children living in a household with an adult who smokes have an increased frequency of respiratory illnesses and asthma. Passive smoke inhalation in nonsmokers can be estimated by measuring the blood levels of cotinine, a metabolite of nicotine. In the United States, median cotinine levels in nonsmokers have decreased by more than 60% since around 2000 because of the adoption of nonsmoking policies in public places. However, passive exposure to tobacco smoke in the home remains a major public health concern, particularly for children. It is clear that the transient pleasure a puff may provide comes with a heavy long-term price.

SUMMARY

HEALTH EFFECTS OF TOBACCO

- Smoking is the most preventable cause of human death.
- Tobacco smoke contains more than 2000 compounds. Among these are nicotine, which is responsible for tobacco addiction, and strong carcinogens—mainly, polycyclic aromatic hydrocarbons, nitrosamines, and aromatic amines.
- Approximately 90% of lung cancers occur in smokers. Smoking is also associated with an increased risk of cancers of the oral cavity, larynx, esophagus, stomach, bladder, and kidney, as well as some forms of leukemia. Cessation of smoking reduces the risk of lung cancer.
- Smokeless tobacco use is an important cause of oral cancers. Tobacco interacts with alcohol in multiplying the risk of oral, laryngeal, and esophageal cancer and increases the risk of lung cancers from occupational exposures to asbestos, uranium, and other agents.
- Tobacco consumption is an important risk factor for development of atherosclerosis and myocardial infarction, peripheral vascular disease, and cerebrovascular disease. In the lungs, in addition to cancer, it predisposes to emphysema, chronic bronchitis, and chronic obstructive disease.
- Maternal smoking increases the risk of abortion, premature birth, and intrauterine growth retardation.

EFFECTS OF ALCOHOL

Ethanol is consumed, at least partly, for its mood-altering properties, but when used in moderation its effects are socially acceptable and not injurious. When excessive amounts are used, alcohol can cause marked physical and psychologic damage. Here we describe the lesions that are directly associated with the abuse of alcohol.

Despite all the attention given to illegal drugs, alcohol abuse is a more widespread hazard and claims many more lives. Fifty percent of adults in the Western world drink alcohol, and approximately 5% to 10% have chronic alcoholism. It is estimated that *there are more than 10 million chronic alcoholics in the United States and that alcohol consumption is responsible for more than 100,000 deaths annually*. Almost 50% of these deaths result from accidents caused by drunken driving and alcohol-related homicides and suicides, and about 15% are a consequence of cirrhosis of the liver.

After consumption, ethanol is absorbed unaltered in the stomach and small intestine and then distributes to all of the tissues and fluids of the body in direct proportion to the blood level. Less than 10% is excreted unchanged in the urine, sweat, and breath. The amount exhaled is proportional to the blood level and forms the basis for the breath test used by law enforcement agencies. A concentration of 80 mg/dL in the blood constitutes the legal definition of drunk driving in most states. For an average individual, this alcohol concentration may be reached after consumption of three standard drinks, about three (12 ounce) bottles of beer, 15 ounces of wine, or 4 to 5 ounces of 80-proof distilled spirits. Drowsiness occurs at 200 mg/dL, stupor at 300 mg/dL, and coma, with possible respiratory arrest, at higher levels. The rate of metabolism affects the blood alcohol level. Chronic alcoholics develop tolerance to alcohol. They metabolize alcohol at a higher rate than normal and hence show lower peak levels of alcohol than average for the same about of alcohol consumed. Most of the alcohol in the blood is metabolized to acetaldehyde in the liver by three enzyme systems: alcohol dehydrogenase; cytochrome P-450 isoenzymes; and catalase (Fig. 8.10). Of these, *the main enzyme involved in alcohol metabolism is alcohol dehydrogenase,* located in the cytosol of hepatocytes. At high blood alcohol levels, however, the microsomal ethanol-oxidizing system also plays an important role. This system involves cytochrome P-450 enzymes, particularly the CYP2E1 isoform, located in the smooth ER. Induction of P-450 enzymes by alcohol explains the increased susceptibility of alcoholics to other compounds metabolized by the same enzyme system, which include drugs (acetaminophen, cocaine), anesthetics, carcinogens, and industrial solvents. Of note, however, when alcohol is present in the blood at high concentrations, it competes with other CYP2E1 substrates and may delay the catabolism of other drugs, thereby potentiating their effects. Catalase is of minor importance, being responsible for only about 5% of alcohol metabolism. Acetaldehyde produced by these systems is in turn converted by acetaldehyde dehydrogenase to acetate, which is used in the mitochondrial respiratory chain.

Several toxic effects result from ethanol metabolism. Listed here are only the most important of these:

- *Alcohol oxidation* by alcohol dehydrogenase causes a decrease in nicotinamide adenine dinucleotide (NAD^+) and an increase in NADH (the reduced form of NAD^+). NAD^+ is required for fatty acid oxidation in the liver. Its deficiency is a main cause of fat accumulation in the liver of alcoholics. The increase in the $NADH/NAD^+$ ratio in alcoholics also causes lactic acidosis.

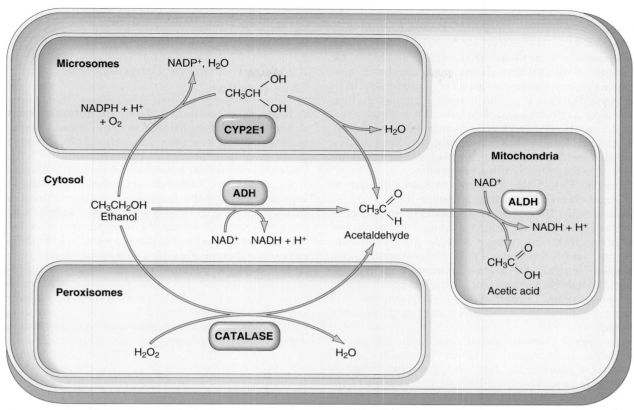

Fig. 8.10 Metabolism of ethanol: oxidation of ethanol to acetaldehyde by three different routes, and the generation of acetic acid. Note that oxidation by alcohol dehydrogenase (ADH) takes place in the cytosol; the cytochrome P-450 system and its CYP2E1 isoform are located in the ER (microsomes), and catalase is located in peroxisomes. Oxidation of acetaldehyde by aldehyde dehydrogenase (ALDH) occurs in mitochondria. *(Data from Parkinson A: Biotransformation of xenobiotics. In Klassen CD, editor:* Casarett and Doull's toxicology: The basic science of poisons, *ed 6, New York, 2001, McGraw-Hill, pp 133.)*

- *Acetaldehyde toxicity* may be responsible for some of the acute effects of alcohol. Acetaldehyde metabolism differs between populations because of genetic variation. Most notably, about 50% of Asians express a defective form of acetaldehyde dehydrogenase. After ingesting alcohol, such persons experience flushing, tachycardia, and hyperventilation owing to the accumulation of acetaldehyde.
- *ROS generation.* Metabolism of ethanol in the liver by CYP2E1 produces ROS and causes lipid peroxidation of cell membranes. Nevertheless, the precise mechanisms that account for alcohol-induced cellular injury have not been well defined.
- *Endotoxin release.* Alcohol may cause the release of endotoxin (lipopolysaccharide), a product of gram-negative bacteria, from the intestinal flora. Endotoxin stimulates the release of tumor necrosis factor (TNF) and other cytokines from circulating macrophages and from Kupffer cells in the liver, causing cell injury.

Acute alcoholism exerts its effects mainly on the CNS but also may induce reversible hepatic and gastric injuries. Even with moderate intake of alcohol, multiple fat droplets accumulate in the cytoplasm of hepatocytes *(fatty change* or *hepatic steatosis).* Gastric damage occurs in the form of acute *gastritis and ulceration.* In the CNS, alcohol is a depressant, first affecting subcortical structures that

modulate cerebral cortical activity. Consequently there is stimulation and disordered cortical, motor, and intellectual behavior. At progressively higher blood levels, cortical neurons and then lower medullary centers are depressed, including those that regulate respiration. Respiratory arrest may follow.

Chronic alcoholism affects not only the liver and stomach but virtually all other organs and tissues as well. Chronic alcoholics suffer significant morbidity and have a shortened life span, related principally to damage to the liver, GI tract, CNS, cardiovascular system, and pancreas.

- *The liver* is the main site of chronic injury. In addition to fatty change, mentioned earlier, chronic alcoholism causes alcoholic hepatitis and cirrhosis (described in Chapter 16). Cirrhosis is associated with portal hypertension and an increased risk of hepatocellular carcinoma.
- *In the GI tract,* chronic alcoholism can cause massive bleeding from gastritis, gastric ulcer, or esophageal varices (associated with cirrhosis), which may prove fatal.
- *Neurologic effects.* Thiamine deficiency is common in chronic alcoholics; the principal lesions resulting from this deficiency are peripheral neuropathies and the Wernicke-Korsakoff syndrome (see Table 8.9 and Chapter 23). Cerebral atrophy, cerebellar degeneration, and optic neuropathy may also occur.

- *Cardiovascular effects.* Alcohol has diverse effects on the cardiovascular system. Injury to the myocardium may produce dilated congestive cardiomyopathy *(alcoholic cardiomyopathy)*, discussed in Chapter 11. Moderate amounts of alcohol (one drink per day) have been reported to increase serum levels of high-density lipoproteins (HDLs) and inhibit platelet aggregation, thus protecting against coronary artery disease. However, heavy consumption, with attendant liver injury, results in decreased levels of HDL, increasing the likelihood of heart disease. Chronic alcoholism also is associated with an increased incidence of hypertension.
- *Pancreatitis.* Excess alcohol intake increases the risk of acute and chronic pancreatitis (Chapter 16).
- *Effects on fetus.* The use of ethanol during pregnancy—reportedly even in low amounts—can cause fetal alcohol syndrome. It consists of microcephaly, growth retardation and facial abnormalities in the newborn, and a reduction of mental functions in older children. It is difficult to establish the amount of alcohol consumption that can cause fetal alcohol syndrome, but consumption during the first trimester of pregnancy is particularly harmful.
- *Carcinogenesis.* Chronic alcohol consumption is associated with an increased incidence of cancers of the oral cavity, esophagus, liver, and, possibly, breast in females. The mechanisms of the carcinogenic effect are uncertain.
- *Malnutrition.* Ethanol is a substantial source of energy, but is often consumed at the expense of food (empty calories). Chronic alcoholism is thus associated with malnutrition and deficiencies, particularly of the B vitamins.

SUMMARY

ALCOHOL—METABOLISM AND HEALTH EFFECTS

- Acute alcohol abuse causes drowsiness at blood levels of approximately 200 mg/dL. Stupor and coma develop at higher levels.
- Alcohol is oxidized to acetaldehyde in the liver primarily by alcohol dehydrogenase, and to a lesser extent by the cytochrome P-450 system, and by catalase. Acetaldehyde is converted to acetate in mitochondria and is used in the respiratory chain.
- Alcohol oxidation by alcohol dehydrogenase depletes NAD, leading to accumulation of fat in the liver and to metabolic acidosis.
- The main effects of chronic alcoholism are fatty liver, alcoholic hepatitis, and cirrhosis, which leads to portal hypertension and increases the risk for development of hepatocellular carcinoma.
- Chronic alcoholism can cause bleeding from gastritis and gastric ulcers, peripheral neuropathy associated with thiamine deficiency, and alcoholic cardiomyopathy, and it increases the risk for development of acute and chronic pancreatitis.
- Chronic alcoholism is a major risk factor for cancers of the oral cavity, larynx, and esophagus. The risk is greatly increased by concurrent smoking or the use of smokeless tobacco.

INJURY BY THERAPEUTIC DRUGS AND DRUGS OF ABUSE

Injury by Therapeutic Drugs: Adverse Drug Reactions

Adverse drug reactions (ADRs) are untoward effects of drugs that are administered in conventional therapeutic settings. These reactions are extremely common in the practice of medicine and are believed to affect 7% to 8% of patients admitted to a hospital. About 10% of such reactions prove fatal. Table 8.5 lists common pathologic findings in ADRs and the drugs most frequently involved. As can be seen, many of the drugs involved in ADRs, such as the anti-neoplastic agents, are highly potent, and the ADR is a calculated risk for the dosage assumed to achieve the maximum therapeutic effect. Commonly used drugs such as long-acting tetracyclines, which are used to treat diverse conditions, including acne, may produce localized or systemic reactions (Fig. 8.11). Because they are widely used, estrogens and oral contraceptives (OCs) are discussed next in more detail. In addition, acetaminophen and aspirin, which are nonprescription drugs but are important

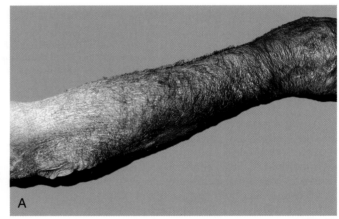

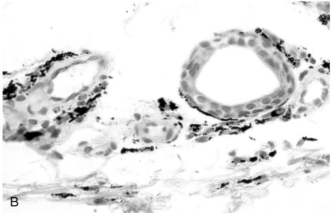

Fig. 8.11 Adverse reaction to minocycline, a long-acting tetracycline derivative. (A) Diffuse blue-gray pigmentation of the forearm, secondary to minocycline administration. (B) Deposition of drug metabolite/iron/melanin pigment particles in the dermis. *(A and B, Courtesy of Dr. Zsolt Argenyi, Department of Pathology, University of Washington, Seattle, Washington.)*

Table 8.5 Some Common Adverse Drug Reactions and Their Agents

Reaction	Major Offenders
Blood Dyscrasias*	
Granulocytopenia, aplastic anemia, pancytopenia	Anti-neoplastic agents, immunosuppressives, and chloramphenicol
Hemolytic anemia, thrombocytopenia	Penicillin, methyldopa, quinidine
Cutaneous	
Urticaria, macules, papules, vesicles, petechiae, exfoliative dermatitis, fixed drug eruptions, abnormal pigmentation	Anti-neoplastic agents, sulfonamides, hydantoins, some antibiotics, and many other agents
Cardiac	
Arrhythmias	Theophylline, hydantoins
Cardiomyopathy	Doxorubicin, daunorubicin
Renal	
Glomerulonephritis	Penicillamine
Acute tubular necrosis	Aminoglycoside antibiotics, cyclosporine, amphotericin B
Tubulointerstitial disease with papillary necrosis	Phenacetin, salicylates
Pulmonary	
Asthma	Salicylates
Acute pneumonitis	Nitrofurantoin
Interstitial fibrosis	Busulfan, nitrofurantoin, bleomycin
Hepatic	
Fatty change	Tetracycline
Diffuse hepatocellular damage	Halothane, isoniazid, acetaminophen
Cholestasis	Chlorpromazine, estrogens, contraceptive agents
Systemic	
Anaphylaxis	Penicillin
Lupus erythematosus syndrome (drug-induced lupus)	Hydralazine, procainamide
CNS	
Tinnitus and dizziness	Salicylates
Acute dystonic reactions and parkinsonian syndrome	Phenothiazine anti-psychotics
Respiratory depression	Sedatives

*Feature in almost half of all drug-related deaths.

causes of accidental or intentional overdose, merit special comment.

Exogenous Estrogens and Oral Contraceptives
Menopausal Hormone Therapy (MHT)

The most common type of MHT (previously referred to as hormone replacement therapy, or HRT) consists of the administration of estrogens together with a progestogen. Because of the risk of uterine cancer, estrogen therapy alone is used only in hysterectomized women. Initially used to counteract "hot flashes" and other symptoms of menopause, early clinical studies suggested that MHT use in postmenopausal women could prevent or slow the progression of osteoporosis (Chapter 21) and reduce the likelihood of myocardial infarction. However, subsequent randomized clinical trials have produced decidedly mixed results. According to these, although MHT did reduce the number of fractures in women on treatment, it was also reported that after 5 years of treatment, combination MHT increased the risk of breast cancer (Chapter 19), stroke, and venous thromboembolism and had no effect on the incidence of coronary heart disease. But during the past few

years there has been a reappraisal of the risks and benefits of MHT. These newer analyses showed that **MHT effects depend on the type of hormone therapy regimen used (combination estrogen-progestin versus estrogen alone), the age and risk factor status of the woman at the start of treatment, the duration of the treatment, and possibly the hormone dose, formulation, and route of administration**. The current risk:benefit consensus can be summarized as follows:

- *Combination estrogen-progestin* increases the risk of breast cancer after a median time of 5 to 6 years. In contrast, estrogen alone in women with hysterectomy is associated with a borderline reduction in the risk of breast cancer.
- *MHT may have a protective effect on the development of atherosclerosis and coronary disease* in women younger than 60 years of age, but there is no protection in women who started MHT at an older age. These data support the notion that there may be a critical therapeutic window for MHT effects on the cardiovascular system. Protective effects in younger women depend in part on the response of estrogen receptors in healthy vascular endothelium. However, MHT should not be used for the

prevention of cardiovascular disease or other chronic diseases.

- *MHT increases the risk of stroke and venous thromboembolism* (VTE), including deep vein thrombosis and pulmonary embolism. The increase in VTE is more pronounced during the first 2 years of treatment and in women who have other risk factors, such as immobilization and hypercoagulable states caused by prothrombin or factor V Leiden mutations (Chapter 4). Whether risks of VTE and stroke are lower with transdermal than oral routes of estrogen administration warrants further study.

As can be appreciated from these associations, assessment of risks and benefits when considering the use of MHT in women is complex. The current feeling is that these agents have a role in the management of menopausal symptoms in early menopause but should not be used long term for chronic disease prevention.

Oral Contraceptives

Although OCs have been used for several decades, disagreement continues about their safety and adverse effects. They nearly always contain a synthetic estradiol and a variable amount of a progestin ("combination OCs"), but a few preparations contain only progestins. Currently prescribed OCs contain a smaller amount of estrogens (less than 50 µg/day) and clearly have fewer side effects than those reported for earlier formulations. Hence, the results of epidemiologic studies must be interpreted in the context of the dosage. Nevertheless, there is reasonable evidence to support the following conclusions:

- *Breast carcinoma:* The prevailing opinion is that OCs do not cause an increase in breast cancer risk.
- *Endometrial cancer and ovarian cancers:* OCs have a protective effect against these tumors.
- *Cervical cancer:* OCs may increase the risk of cervical carcinomas in women infected with human papillomavirus.
- *Thromboembolism:* Most studies indicate that OCs, including the newer low-dose (less than 50 µg of estrogen) preparations, are associated with a threefold to sixfold increased risk of venous thrombosis and pulmonary thromboembolism resulting from increased hepatic synthesis of coagulation factors. This risk may be even higher with newer "third-generation" OCs that contain synthetic progestins, particularly in women who are carriers of the factor V Leiden mutation. To put this complication into context, however, the risk of thromboembolism associated with OC use is two to six times lower than the risk of thromboembolism associated with pregnancy.
- *Cardiovascular disease:* There is considerable uncertainty about the risk of atherosclerosis and myocardial infarction in users of OCs. It seems that OCs do not increase the risk of coronary artery disease in women younger than 30 years or in older women who are nonsmokers, but the risk approximately doubles in women older than 35 years who smoke.
- *Hepatic adenoma:* There is a well-defined association between the use of OCs and this rare benign hepatic tumor, especially in older women who have used OCs for prolonged periods (Chapter 14).

Obviously, the pros and cons of OCs must be viewed in the context of their wide applicability and acceptance as a form of contraception that protects against unwanted pregnancies.

Acetaminophen

At therapeutic doses, acetaminophen, a widely used nonprescription analgesic and anti-pyretic, is mostly conjugated in the liver with glucuronide or sulfate. About 5% or less is metabolized to NAPQI (*N*-acetyl-*p*-benzoquinoneimine) through the hepatic P-450 system. With very large doses, however, *NAPQI accumulates, leading to centriloblar hepatic necrosis.* The mechanisms of injury produced by NAPQI include (1) covalent binding to hepatic proteins and (2) depletion of reduced GSH. The depletion of GSH makes the hepatocytes more susceptible to cell death caused by ROS. The window between the usual therapeutic dose (0.5 g) and the toxic dose (15 to 25 g) is large, and the drug ordinarily is very safe. Nevertheless, accidental overdoses occur in children, and suicide attempts using acetaminophen are not uncommon, particularly in the United Kingdom. In the United States, acetaminophen toxicity is causes about 50% of acute liver failure. Toxicity begins with nausea, vomiting, diarrhea, and sometimes shock, followed in a few days by the appearance of jaundice. Overdoses of acetaminophen can be treated in early stages by the administration of *N*-acetylcysteine, which restores GSH. With serious overdoses, liver failure ensues, and centrilobular necrosis may extend to involve entire lobules; such patients often require liver transplantation. Some patients also show evidence of concurrent renal damage.

Aspirin (Acetylsalicylic Acid)

Aspirin overdose may result from accidental ingestion in young children or suicide attempts in adults. The major untoward consequences are metabolic, with few morphologic changes. At first, *respiratory alkalosis develops, followed by a metabolic acidosis* that often proves fatal. Fatal doses may be as little as 2 to 4 g in children and 10 to 30 g in adults, but survival has been reported after doses five times larger.

Chronic aspirin toxicity (salicylism) may develop in persons who take 3 gm or more daily (the dose used to treat chronic inflammatory conditions). Chronic salicylism is manifested by headache, dizziness, ringing in the ears (tinnitus), difficulty in hearing, mental confusion, drowsiness, nausea, vomiting, and diarrhea. The CNS changes may progress to convulsions and coma. The morphologic consequences of chronic salicylism are varied. Most often, there is an acute erosive gastritis (Chapter 15), which may produce overt or covert GI bleeding and lead to gastric ulceration. A bleeding tendency may appear concurrently with chronic toxicity because aspirin irreversibly inhibits platelet cyclooxygenase and blocks the ability to make thromboxane A_2, an activator of platelet aggregation (Chapter 4). Petechial hemorrhages may appear in the skin and internal viscera, and bleeding from gastric ulcerations may be exaggerated.

Proprietary analgesic mixtures of aspirin and phenacetin or its active metabolite, acetaminophen, when taken throughout several years, can cause tubulointerstitial

Table 8.6 Common Drugs of Abuse

Class	Molecular Target	Examples
Opioid narcotics	Mu opioid receptor (agonist)	Heroin, hydromorphone (Dilaudid) Oxycodone Methadone (Dolophine)
Sedative-hypnotics	GABA receptor (agonist)	Barbiturates Ethanol Methaqualone ("Quaalude") Glutethimide (Doriden) Ethchlorvynol (Placidyl)
Psychomotor stimulants	Dopamine transporter (antagonist) Serotonin receptors (toxicity)	Cocaine Amphetamine 3,4-methylenedioxymethamphetamine (MDMA) (i.e., "ecstasy")
Phencyclidine-like drugs	NMDA glutamate receptor channel (antagonist)	Phencyclidine (PCP) (i.e., "angel dust") Ketamine
Cannabinoids	CB1 cannabinoid receptors (agonist)	Marijuana Hashish
Nicotine	Nicotine acetylcholine receptor (agonist)	Tobacco products
Hallucinogens	Serotonin 5-HT2 receptors (agonist)	Lysergic acid diethylamide (LSD) Mescaline Psilocybin

CB1, Cannabinoid receptor type 1; *GABA*, γ-aminobutyric acid; *5-HT2*, 5-hydroxytryptamine; *NMDA*, N-methyl-D-aspartate; *PCP*, 1-(1-phenylcyclohexyl)piperidine. Data from Hyman SE: A 28-year-old man addicted to cocaine, *JAMA* 286:2586, 2001.

nephritis with renal papillary necrosis. This clinical entity is referred to as *analgesic nephropathy* (Chapter 14).

Injury by Nontherapeutic Agents (Drug Abuse)

Drug abuse generally involves the use of mind-altering substances beyond therapeutic or social norms. Drug addiction and overdose are serious public health problems. Common drugs of abuse are listed in Table 8.6. Considered here are cocaine, opiates, and marijuana, with a brief mention of a few other drugs.

Cocaine

In 2014, it was estimated that there were 1.5 million users of cocaine in the United States, of which approximately 15% to 20% were users of "crack" cocaine. Use is highest among adults 18 to 25 years of age, of whom 1.4% reported taking cocaine within the past month. Extracted from the leaves of the coca plant, cocaine usually is prepared as a water-soluble powder, cocaine hydrochloride, but when sold on the street it is liberally diluted with talcum powder, lactose, or other look-alikes. Crystallization of the pure alkaloid from cocaine hydrochloride yields nuggets of crack (so called because of the popping sound it makes when heated). The pharmacologic actions of cocaine and crack are identical, but crack is far more potent. Both forms can be snorted, smoked after mixing with tobacco, ingested, or injected subcutaneously or intravenously.

Cocaine produces a sense of intense euphoria and mental alertness, making it one of the most addictive of all drugs. Experimental animals will press a lever more than 1000 times and will forgo food and drink to obtain the drug. In cocaine users, although physical dependence seems not to occur, the psychologic dependence is profound. Intense cravings are particularly severe in the first several months after abstinence and can recur for years.

Acute overdose produces seizures, cardiac arrhythmias, and respiratory arrest. The following are the important manifestations of cocaine toxicity:

- *Cardiovascular effects.* The most serious physical effects of cocaine relate to its acute action on the cardiovascular system. Cocaine is a sympathomimetic agent (Fig. 8.12), both in the CNS, where it blocks the reuptake of dopamine, and at adrenergic nerve endings, where it blocks the reuptake of both epinephrine and norepinephrine while stimulating the presynaptic release of norepinephrine. The net effect is the accumulation of these neurotransmitters in synapses and excessive stimulation, manifested by tachycardia, hypertension, and peripheral vasoconstriction. Cocaine also induces myocardial ischemia, the basis for which is multifactorial. It causes coronary artery vasoconstriction and promotes thrombus formation by facilitating platelet aggregation. Cigarette smoking potentiates cocaine-induced coronary vasospasm. Thus, by increasing myocardial oxygen demand by its sympathomimetic action and, at the same time, reducing coronary blood flow, cocaine often triggers myocardial ischemia, which may lead to myocardial infarction. Cocaine also can precipitate lethal arrhythmias by enhanced sympathetic activity as well as by disrupting normal ion (K+, Ca2+, Na+) transport in the myocardium. These toxic effects are not necessarily dose related, and a fatal event may occur in a first-time user with what is a typical mood-altering dose.
- *CNS effects.* The most common CNS findings are hyperpyrexia (thought to be caused by aberrations of the dopaminergic pathways that control body temperature) and seizures.
- *Effects on the fetus.* In pregnant women, cocaine may cause decreased blood flow to the placenta, resulting in fetal hypoxia and spontaneous abortion. Neurologic development may be impaired in the fetuses of pregnant women who are chronic drug users.

CENTRAL NERVOUS SYSTEM SYNAPSE

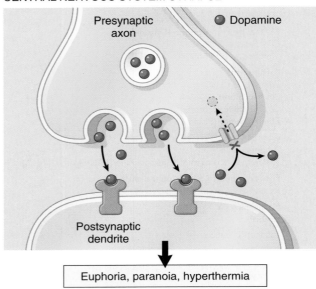

Euphoria, paranoia, hyperthermia

SYMPATHETIC NEURON–TARGET CELL INTERFACE

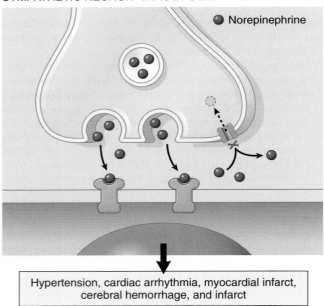

Hypertension, cardiac arrhythmia, myocardial infarct, cerebral hemorrhage, and infarct

Fig. 8.12 The effect of cocaine on neurotransmission. The drug inhibits reuptake of the neurotransmitters dopamine and norepinephrine in the central and peripheral nervous systems.

- *Chronic cocaine use.* Chronic use may cause (1) perforation of the nasal septum in snorters, (2) decrease in lung diffusing capacity in users who inhale the smoke, and (3) the development of dilated cardiomyopathy.

Heroin and Other Opioids

Heroin is an addictive opioid derived from the poppy plant and is closely related to morphine. Its effects are even more harmful than those of cocaine. Nevertheless, it is estimated that almost 4 million people in the United States have used heroin at least once, and that in 2012 more than 650,000 people used the drug at some time during the year. As sold

on the street, it is cut (diluted) with an agent (often talc or quinine); thus, the size of the dose not only is variable but also usually is unknown to the buyer. Heroin, along with any contaminating substances, usually is self-administered intravenously or subcutaneously. Effects are varied and include euphoria, hallucinations, somnolence, and sedation. Heroin has a wide range of adverse physical effects that can be categorized etiologically according to (1) the pharmacologic action of the agent, (2) reactions to the cutting agents or contaminants, (3) hypersensitivity reactions to the drug or its adulterants, and (4) diseases contracted through the sharing of needles. Some of the most important adverse effects of heroin are the following:

- *Sudden death.* Sudden death, usually related to overdose, is an ever-present risk, because drug purity generally is unknown and may range from 2% to 90%. The yearly incidence of sudden death among chronic users in the United States is estimated to be between 1% and 3%. Sudden death sometimes is due to a loss of tolerance for the drug, such as after a period of incarceration. The mechanisms of death include profound respiratory depression, arrhythmia and cardiac arrest, and pulmonary edema.

- *Pulmonary disease.* Pulmonary complications include edema, septic embolism, lung abscess, opportunistic infections, and foreign body granulomas from talc and other adulterants. Although granulomas occur principally in the lung, they also are sometimes found in the spleen, liver, and lymph nodes that drain the upper extremities. Examination under polarized light often highlights trapped talc crystals, sometimes enclosed within foreign body giant cells.

- *Infections.* Infectious complications are common. The sites most commonly affected are the skin and subcutaneous tissue, heart valves, liver, and lungs. In a series of addicted patients admitted to the hospital, more than 10% had endocarditis, which often takes a distinctive form involving right-sided heart valves, particularly the tricuspid. Most cases are caused by *Staphylococcus aureus,* but fungi and a multitude of other organisms have also been implicated. Viral hepatitis is the most common infection among addicts and is acquired by the sharing of dirty needles. In the United States, this practice has also led to a very high incidence of human immunodeficiency virus (HIV) infection in intravenous drug abusers.

- *Skin lesions.* Cutaneous lesions probably are the most frequent telltale sign of heroin addiction. Acute changes include abscesses, cellulitis, and ulcerations resulting from subcutaneous injections. Scarring at injection sites, hyperpigmentation over commonly used veins, and thrombosed veins are the usual sequelae of repeated intravenous inoculations.

- *Renal problems.* Kidney disease is a relatively common hazard. The two forms most frequently encountered are amyloidosis (generally secondary to skin infections) and focal glomerulosclerosis; both induce heavy proteinuria and the nephrotic syndrome.

Tragically, more widespread availability of prescription opiates, such as hydrocodone and oxycodone, has fueled an epidemic of opioid abuse that surpasses that associated with heroin. In 2014, it was estimated that 4.3 million Americans engaged in non-medical use of prescription opioids, and that prescription opioid overdoses led to approximately 19,000 deaths, mainly from respiratory failure. Moreover, an increasing number of heroin users start with prescription opioids, then switch to heroin because it is a substantially less expensive habit. This trend underlies a near doubling of heroin use in the United States between 2005 and 2012. Current efforts are focused on making opioid antagonists widely available to first responders, which has prevented many deaths, and tightening the use of prescription opioids to limit their potential for abuse.

Marijuana

Marijuana, or "pot," is the most widely used illegal drug. As of 2014 in the United States, 22.2 million people (7.0% of the population) admitted use during the previous month. Several states in the United States have legalized the "recreational" use of marijuana, and more states appear poised to follow; thus, its status as an illicit drug is undergoing reevaluation.

Marijuana is made from the leaves of the *Cannabis sativa* plant, which contain the psychoactive substance Δ^9-tetrahydrocannabinol (THC). When marijuana is smoked, about 5% to 10% of the THC content is absorbed. Despite numerous studies, whether the drug includes persistent adverse physical and functional effects remains unresolved. Some of the untoward anecdotal effects may be allergic or idiosyncratic reactions or are possibly related to contaminants in the preparations, rather than to marijuana's pharmacologic effects. On the other hand, beneficial effects of THC include its capacity to decrease intraocular pressure in glaucoma and to combat intractable nausea secondary to cancer chemotherapy.

The functional and organic CNS consequences of marijuana have received great scrutiny. Marijuana use is well recognized to distort sensory perception and impair motor coordination, but these acute effects generally clear in 4 to 5 hours. With continued use, these changes may progress to cognitive and psychomotor impairments, such as the inability to judge time, speed, and distance. Among adolescents, such impairment often leads to automobile accidents. Marijuana increases the heart rate and sometimes blood pressure and it may cause angina in a person with coronary artery disease.

The lungs are affected by chronic marijuana smoking; laryngitis, pharyngitis, bronchitis, cough, hoarseness, and asthmalike symptoms all have been described, along with mild but significant airway obstruction. Smoking a marijuana cigarette, compared with a tobacco cigarette, is associated with a 3-fold increase in the amount of tar inhaled and retained in the lungs, as a consequence of deeper inhalation and longer breath holding.

Other Illicit Drugs

The variety of drugs that have been tried by those seeking "new experiences" (highs, lows, "out-of-body experiences") defies belief. These drugs include various stimulants, depressants, analgesics, and hallucinogens. Among these are PCP (1-(1-phenylcyclohexyl) piperidine), or phencyclidine, and ketamine (related anesthetic agents); lysergic acid diethylamide (LSD), the most potent hallucinogen known; "ecstasy" (3,4-methylenedioxymethamphetamine [MDMA]); and "bath salts", synthetic cathinones that are chemically related to khat, a widely used stimulant in East Africa. Not much is known about the long-term deleterious effects of any of these agents. Acutely, LSD has unpredictable effects on mood, affect, and thought, sometimes leading to bizarre and dangerous behaviors. Chronic use of ecstasy may deplete the CNS of serotonin, potentially leading to sleep disorders, depression, anxiety, and aggressive behavior.

SUMMARY

DRUG INJURY

- Therapeutic drugs (ADRs) or nontherapeutic agents (drug abuse) might cause drug injury.
- Anti-neoplastic agents, long-acting tetracyclines, and other antibiotics, HRT preparations and OCs, acetaminophen, and aspirin are the drugs most frequently involved.
- HRT increases the risk of endometrial and breast cancers and thromboembolism but does not appear to protect against ischemic heart disease. OCs have a protective effect against endometrial and ovarian cancers but increase the risk of thromboembolism and hepatic adenomas.
- Overdose of acetaminophen may cause centrilobular liver necrosis, leading to liver failure. Early treatment with agents that restore GSH levels may limit toxicity. Aspirin blocks the production of thromboxane A2, which may produce gastric ulceration and bleeding.
- The common drugs of abuse include sedative-hypnotics (barbiturates, ethanol), psychomotor stimulants (cocaine, amphetamine, ecstasy), opioid narcotics (heroin, methadone, oxycodone), hallucinogens (LSD, mescaline), and cannabinoids (marijuana, hashish). They have diverse effects on various organs.

INJURY BY PHYSICAL AGENTS

Injury induced by physical agents is divided into the following categories: mechanical trauma, thermal injury, electrical injury, and injury produced by ionizing radiation. Each type is considered separately.

Mechanical Trauma

Mechanical forces may inflict a variety of forms of damage. The type of injury depends on the shape of the colliding object, the amount of energy discharged at impact, and the tissues or organs that bear the impact. Bone and head injuries result in unique damage and are discussed elsewhere (Chapter 23). All soft tissues react similarly to mechanical forces, and the patterns of injury can be divided into abrasions, contusions, lacerations, incised wounds, and puncture wounds (Fig. 8.13).

MORPHOLOGY

An **abrasion** is a wound produced by scraping or rubbing the skin surface, which damages the superficial layer. Typical skin abrasions remove only the epidermal layer. A **contusion,** or bruise, is a wound usually produced by a blunt trauma and is characterized by damage to a vessel and extravasation of blood

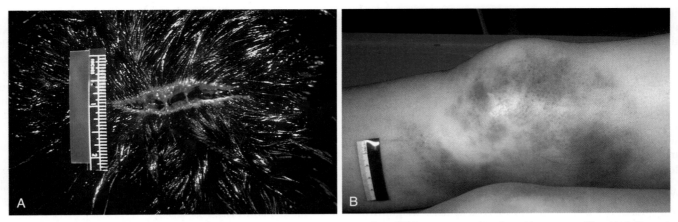

Fig. 8.13 (A) Laceration of the scalp: The bridging strands of fibrous tissues are evident. (B) Contusion resulting from blunt trauma. The skin is intact, but hemorrhage of subcutaneous vessels has produced extensive discoloration. *(A and B, From the teaching collection of the Department of Pathology, University of Texas Southwestern Medical School, Dallas, Texas.)*

into tissues. A **laceration** is a tear or disruptive stretching of tissue caused by the application of force by a blunt object. In contrast with an incision, most lacerations have intact bridging blood vessels and jagged, irregular edges. An **incised wound** is one inflicted by a sharp instrument. The bridging blood vessels are severed. A **puncture wound** is typically caused by a long, narrow instrument and is termed **penetrating** when the instrument pierces the tissue and **perforating** when it traverses a tissue to also create an exit wound. Gunshot wounds are special forms of puncture wounds that demonstrate distinctive features important to the forensic pathologist. For example, a wound from a bullet fired at close range leaves powder burns, whereas one fired from more than 4 or 5 feet away does not.

One of the most common causes of mechanical injury is **vehicular accident.** Injuries typically sustained result from (1) hitting a part of the interior of the vehicle or being hit by objects that enter the passenger compartment during the crash, such as engine parts; (2) being thrown from the vehicle; or (3) being trapped in a burning vehicle. The pattern of injury relates to whether one or all three of these mechanisms are operative. For example, in a head-on collision, a common pattern of injury sustained by a driver who is not wearing a seat belt includes trauma to the head (windshield impact), chest (steering column impact), and knees (dashboard impact). Common chest injuries stemming from such accidents include sternal and rib fractures, heart contusions, aortic lacerations, and (less commonly) lacerations of the spleen and liver. Thus, in caring for an automobile injury victim, it is essential to recognize that internal wounds often accompany superficial abrasions, contusions, and lacerations. Indeed, in many cases, external evidence of serious internal damage is completely absent.

Thermal Injury

Both excess heat and excess cold are important causes of injury. Burns are all too common and are discussed first; a brief discussion of hyperthermia and hypothermia follows.

Thermal Burns

In the United States, burns cause 3500 deaths per year and result in the hospitalization of more than 10 times that

many persons. Many victims are children, in whom the cause of injury often is scalding by hot liquids. Fortunately, since the 1970s marked decreases have been seen in both mortality rates and the length of hospitalizations. These improvements have been achieved through better understanding of the systemic effects of massive burns and the discovery of better ways to prevent wound infection and to facilitate the healing of skin surfaces.

The clinical severity of burns depends on the following important variables:
- Depth
- Percentage of body surface involved
- Whether internal injuries from the inhalation of hot and toxic fumes are present
- Promptness and efficacy of therapy, especially fluid and electrolyte management and prevention or control of wound infections

A *full-thickness* burn produces total destruction of the epidermis and dermis, including the dermal appendages that harbor cells needed for epithelial regeneration. Both third- and fourth-degree burns are in this category. In *partial-thickness* burns, at least the deeper portions of the dermal appendages are spared. Partial-thickness burns include first-degree burns (epithelial involvement only) and second-degree burns (involving both the epidermis and the superficial dermis).

MORPHOLOGY

On gross inspection, **full-thickness burns** are white or charred, dry, and anesthetic (as a result of the destruction of nerve endings), whereas **partial-thickness burns,** depending on the depth, are pink or mottled, blistered, and painful. Histologic examination of devitalized tissue shows coagulative necrosis adjacent to vital tissue, which quickly accumulates inflammatory cells and marked exudation.

Despite continuous improvement in therapy, any burn exceeding 50% of the total body surface, whether superficial or deep, is grave and potentially fatal. With burns of more than 20% of the body surface, there is a rapid shift of body fluids into the interstitial compartments, both at the burn site and systemically, which can result in **hypovolemic shock** (Chapter 4). Because protein from the blood is lost into interstitial tissue, generalized edema, including **pulmonary edema,** may become severe.

Another important consideration is the degree of injury to the airways and lungs. **Inhalation injury** is frequent in persons trapped in burning buildings and may result from the direct effect of heat on the mouth, nose, and upper airways or from the inhalation of heated air and gases in the smoke. Water-soluble gases, such as chlorine, sulfur oxides, and ammonia, may react with water to form acids or alkalis, particularly in the upper airways, resulting in inflammation and swelling, which may lead to partial or complete airway obstruction. Lipid-soluble gases, such as nitrous oxide and products of burning plastics, are more likely to reach deeper airways, producing pneumonitis. Unlike in shock, which develops within hours, pulmonary manifestations may not develop for 24 to 48 hours.

Organ system failure resulting from **sepsis** continues to be the leading cause of death in burned patients. The burn site is ideal for the growth of microorganisms; the serum and debris provide nutrients, and the burn injury compromises blood flow, blocking effective inflammatory responses. The most common offender is the opportunist *Pseudomonas aeruginosa,* but antibiotic-resistant strains of other common hospital-acquired bacteria, such as *S. aureus* and fungi, particularly *Candida* spp., also may be involved. Furthermore, cellular and humoral defenses against infections are compromised, and both lymphocyte and phagocyte functions are impaired. Direct bacteremic spread and release of toxic substances such as endotoxin from the local site have dire consequences. **Pneumonia** or **septic shock,** accompanied by **renal failure** and/or the acute respiratory distress syndrome (ARDS) (Chapter 13), are the most common serious sequelae.

Another very important pathophysiologic effect of burns is the development of a hypermetabolic state, with excess heat loss and an increased need for nutritional support. It is estimated that when more than 40% of the body surface is burned, the resting metabolic rate may approach twice normal.

Hyperthermia

Prolonged exposure to elevated ambient temperatures can result in heat cramps, heat exhaustion, or heat stroke.

- *Heat cramps* result from loss of electrolytes through sweating. Cramping of voluntary muscles, usually in association with vigorous exercise, is the hallmark sign. Heat-dissipating mechanisms are able to maintain normal core body temperature.
- *Heat exhaustion* is probably the most common hyperthermic syndrome. Its onset is sudden, with prostration and collapse, and it results from a failure of the cardiovascular system to compensate for hypovolemia, secondary to water depletion. After a period of collapse, which is usually brief, equilibrium is spontaneously reestablished if the victim is able to rehydrate.
- *Heat stroke* is associated with high ambient temperatures and high humidity. Thermoregulatory mechanisms fail, sweating ceases, and core body temperature rises. In the clinical setting, a rectal temperature of 106°F or higher is considered a grave prognostic sign, and the mortality rate for such patients exceeds 50%. The underlying mechanism is marked generalized peripheral vasodilation with peripheral pooling of blood and a decreased effective circulating blood volume. Necrosis of the muscles and myocardium may occur. Arrhythmias, disseminated intravascular coagulation, and other systemic effects are common. Elderly people, persons with cardiovascular disease, and otherwise healthy people undergoing physical stress (such as young athletes and military recruits) are prime candidates for heat stroke.
- *Malignant hyperthermia,* although similar sounding, is not caused by exposure to high temperatures. It is a genetic condition resulting from mutations in genes such as *RYR1* that control calcium levels in skeletal muscle cells. In affected individuals, exposure to certain anesthetics during surgery may trigger a rapid rise in calcium levels in skeletal muscle, which in turn leads to muscle rigidity and increased heat production. The resulting hyperthermia has a mortality rate of approximately 80% if untreated, but this falls to less than 5% if the condition is recognized and muscle relaxants are administered promptly.

Hypothermia

Prolonged exposure to low ambient temperature leads to hypothermia. The condition is seen all too frequently in homeless alcoholics, in whom wet or inadequate clothing and dilation of superficial blood vessels, occurring as a result of the ingestion of alcohol, hasten the lowering of body temperature. At about 90°F, loss of consciousness occurs, followed by bradycardia and atrial fibrillation at lower core temperatures.

Chilling or freezing of cells and tissues causes injury by two mechanisms:

- *Direct effects* probably are mediated by physical disruptions within cells and high salt concentrations incident to the crystallization of the intra- and extracellular water.
- *Indirect effects* are the result of circulatory changes, which vary depending on the rate and the duration of the temperature drop. Slowly developing, prolonged chilling may induce vasoconstriction and increased permeability, leading to edema. Such changes are typical of "trench foot." This condition developed in soldiers who spent long periods of time in waterlogged trenches during the First World War (1914–1918), frequently causing gangrene that necessitated amputation. Alternatively, with sudden sharp drops in temperature, the vasoconstriction and increased viscosity of the blood in the local area may cause ischemic injury and degenerative changes in peripheral nerves. In this situation, the vascular injury and increased permeability with exudation only become evident with rewarming. If the period of ischemia is prolonged, hypoxic changes and infarction of the affected tissues (e.g., gangrene of toes or feet) may result.

Electrical Injury

Electrical injuries, which may be fatal, can arise from low-voltage currents (i.e., in the home and workplace) or from high-voltage currents carried in power lines or by lightning. Injuries are of two types: (1) burns and (2) ventricular fibrillation or cardiac and respiratory center failure resulting from disruption of normal electrical impulses. The type of injury and the severity and extent of burning depend on the amperage of the electric current and its path within the body.

Voltage in the household and the workplace (120 or 220 V) is high enough that with low resistance at the site of contact (as when the skin is wet), sufficient current can pass through the body to cause serious injury, including ventricular fibrillation. If current flow continues long enough, it generates enough heat to produce burns at the site of entry and exit as well as in internal organs. An important characteristic of alternating current, the type available in most homes, is that it induces tetanic muscle spasm, so that when a live wire or switch is grasped, irreversible clutching is likely to occur, prolonging the period of current flow. This results in a greater likelihood of extensive electrical burns and, in some cases, spasm of the chest wall muscles, producing death from asphyxia. Currents generated from high-voltage sources cause similar damage; however, because of the large current flows generated, these injuries are more likely to produce paralysis of medullary centers and extensive burns. Lightning is a classic cause of high-voltage electrical injury.

Injury Produced by Ionizing Radiation

Radiation is energy that travels in the form of waves or high-speed particles. It has a wide range of energies that span the electromagnetic spectrum; it can be divided into nonionizing and ionizing radiation. The energy of nonionizing radiation, such as ultraviolet (UV) and infrared light, microwaves, and sound waves, can move atoms in a molecule or cause them to vibrate but is not sufficient to displace electrons from atoms. By contrast, ionizing radiation has sufficient energy to remove tightly bound electrons. Collision of these free electrons with other atoms releases additional electrons, in a reaction cascade referred to as ionization. The main sources of ionizing radiation are (1) x-rays and *gamma* rays, which are electromagnetic waves of very high frequencies, and (2) high-energy neutrons, alpha particles (composed of two protons and two neutrons), and beta particles, which are essentially electrons. At equivalent amounts of energy, alpha particles induce heavy damage in a restricted area, whereas x-rays and gamma rays dissipate energy over a longer, deeper course, and produce considerably less damage per unit of tissue. Some of the total dose of ionizing radiation received by the U.S. population is human-made, mostly originating from medical devices and radioisotopes. In fact, the exposure of patients to ionizing radiation during radiologic imaging tests roughly doubled between the early 1980s and 2006, mainly because of much more widespread use of CT scans.

Ionizing radiation is indispensable in medical practice, but this application constitutes a two-edged sword. Radiation in this form is used in the treatment of cancer, in diagnostic imaging, and as therapeutic or diagnostic radioisotopes. However, it also is *mutagenic, carcinogenic,* and *teratogenic.*

The following terms are used to express exposure, absorption, and dose of ionizing radiation:

- *Curie* (Ci) represents the disintegrations per second of a spontaneously disintegrating radionuclide (radioiso-

tope). One Ci is equal to 3.7×10^{10} disintegrations per second.
- *Gray* (Gy) is a unit that expresses the energy absorbed by a target tissue. It corresponds to the absorption of 10^4 ergs per gram of tissue. A centigray (cGy), which is the absorption of 100 ergs per gram of tissue, is equivalent to the exposure of tissue to 100 rads (R) ("radiation absorbed dose"). The cGy nomenclature has now replaced the rad in medical parlance.
- *Sievert* (Sv) is a unit of equivalent dose that depends on the biologic rather than the physical effects of radiation (it replaced a unit called the rem). For the same absorbed dose, various types of radiation differ in the extent of damage they produce. The equivalent dose controls for this variation and provides a uniform measuring unit. The equivalent dose (expressed in sieverts) corresponds to the absorbed dose (expressed in grays) multiplied by the relative biologic effectiveness of the radiation. The relative biologic effectiveness depends on the type of radiation, the type and volume of the exposed tissue, and the duration of the exposure, as well as other biologic factors (discussed next). The effective dose of x-rays, computed tomography (CT), and other imaging and nuclear medicine procedures are commonly expressed in millisieverts (mSv). For x-radiation, 1 mSv = 1 mGy.

Main Determinants of the Biologic Effects of Ionizing Radiation

In addition to the physical properties of the radiation, its biologic effects depend heavily on the following variables:

- *Rate of delivery.* The rate of delivery significantly modifies the biologic effect. Although the effect of radiant energy is cumulative, delivery in divided doses may allow cells to repair some of the damage in the intervals. Thus, fractional doses of radiant energy have a cumulative effect only to the extent that repair during the intervals is incomplete. Radiotherapy of tumors exploits the capability of normal cells to repair themselves and to recover more rapidly than tumor cells.
- *Field size.* The size of the field exposed to radiation has a great influence on its consequences. The body can sustain relatively high doses of radiation when they are delivered to small, carefully shielded fields, whereas smaller doses delivered to larger fields may be lethal.
- *Cell proliferation.* Because ionizing radiation damages DNA, rapidly dividing cells are more vulnerable to injury than are quiescent cells. Except at extremely high doses that impair DNA transcription, DNA damage is compatible with survival in nondividing cells, such as neurons and muscle cells. However, as discussed in Chapter 6, in dividing cells DNA damage is detected by sensors that produce signals leading to the upregulation of p53, the "guardian of the genome." p53 in turn upregulates the expression of genes that initially lead to cell-cycle arrest and, if the DNA damage is too great to repair, genes that cause cell death through apoptosis. Understandably, therefore, tissues with a high rate of cell turnover, such as gonads, bone marrow, lymphoid tissue, and the mucosa of the GI tract, are extremely vulnerable to radiation, and the injury is manifested early after exposure.

- *Hypoxia.* The production of ROS by the radiolysis of water is the most important mechanism of DNA damage by ionizing radiation. Tissue hypoxia, such as may exist in the center of rapidly growing, poorly vascularized tumors, may thus reduce the extent of damage and the effectiveness of radiotherapy directed against tumors.
- *Vascular damage.* Damage to endothelial cells, which are moderately sensitive to radiation, may cause narrowing or occlusion of blood vessels, leading to impaired healing, fibrosis, and chronic ischemic atrophy. These changes may appear months or years after exposure. Despite the low sensitivity of brain cells to radiation, vascular damage after irradiation can lead to late manifestations of radiation injury in this tissue.

DNA Damage and Carcinogenesis

The most important cellular target of ionizing radiation is DNA (Fig. 8.14). Damage to DNA caused by ionizing radiation that is not precisely repaired leads to mutations, which can manifest years or decades later as cancer. Ionizing radiation can cause many types of damage in DNA, including single-base damage, single- and double-strand breaks, and crosslinks between DNA and protein. In surviving cells, simple defects may be reparable by various enzyme repair systems contained in mammalian cells (see Chapter 6). These repair systems are linked to cell-cycle regulation through proteins such as ATM (ataxia-telangiectasia mutated) that initiate signal transduction after the damage, and p53, which can transiently arrest the cell cycle to allow for DNA repair or to trigger apoptosis of cells that are irreparable. However, double-strand breaks may persist without repair, or the repair of lesions may be imprecise (error prone), creating mutations. If cell-cycle checkpoints are not functioning (for instance, because of mutations in *TP53*), cells with abnormal and unstable genomes survive

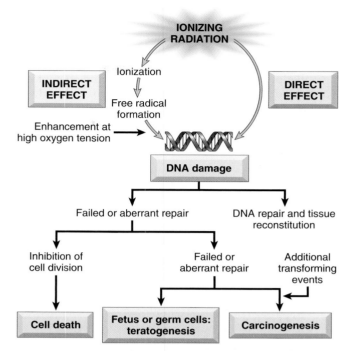

Fig. 8.14 Effects of ionizing radiation on DNA and their consequences. The effects on DNA can be direct or, most important, indirect, through free radical formation.

and may expand as abnormal clones to form tumors eventually.

Fibrosis

A common consequence of cancer radiotherapy is the development of fibrosis in the irradiated field (Fig. 8.15). Fibrosis may occur weeks or months after irradiation,

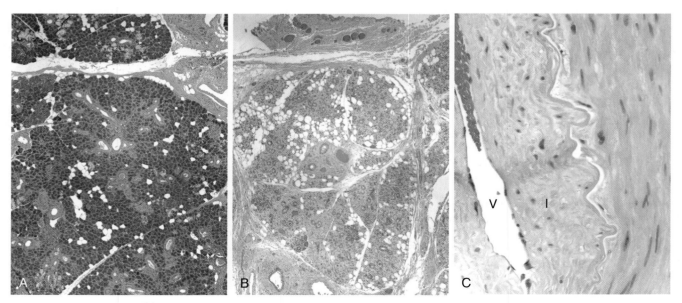

Fig. 8.15 Vascular changes and fibrosis of salivary glands produced by radiation therapy of the neck region. (A) Normal salivary gland; (B) fibrosis caused by radiation; (C) fibrosis and vascular changes consisting of fibrointimal thickening and arteriolar sclerosis. *V*, Vessel lumen; *I*, thickened intima. *(A–C, Courtesy of Dr. Melissa Upton, Department of Pathology, University of Washington, Seattle, Washington.)*

leading to the replacement of dead parenchymal cells by connective tissue and the formation of scars and adhesions (see Chapter 3). As already mentioned, ionizing radiation causes vascular damage and consequent tissue ischemia. Vascular damage, the killing of tissue stem cells by ionizing radiation, and the release of cytokines and chemokines that promote an inflammatory reaction all contribute to fibroblast activation and the development of radiation-induced fibrosis.

MORPHOLOGY

Cells surviving radiant energy damage show a wide range of structural **changes in chromosomes,** including deletions, breaks, translocations, and fragmentation. The mitotic spindle often becomes disorderly, and polyploidy and aneuploidy may be encountered. **Nuclear swelling** and condensation and clumping of chromatin may appear; breaks in the nuclear membrane also may be noted. **Apoptosis** may occur. Cells with abnormal nuclear morphology may be produced and persist for years, including giant cells with pleomorphic nuclei or more than one nucleus. At extremely high dose levels of radiant energy, features that foretell impending cell death, such as nuclear pyknosis, appear quickly.

In addition to affecting DNA and nuclei, radiant energy may induce a variety of **cytoplasmic changes,** including cytoplasmic swelling, mitochondrial distortion, and degeneration of the ER. Plasma membrane breaks and focal defects may appear. The histologic constellation of cellular pleomorphism, giant cell formation, changes in nuclei, and mitotic figures creates a more than passing similarity between radiation-injured cells and cancer cells, a problem that plagues the pathologist when evaluating postirradiation tissues for persistence or recurrence of cancer.

At the light microscopic level, vascular changes and interstitial fibrosis are prominent in irradiated tissues (Fig. 8.15). During the immediate postirradiation period, vessels may show only dilation. Later, or with higher doses, a variety of degenerative changes appear, including endothelial cell swelling and vacuolation, or even necrosis of the walls of small vessels such as capillaries and venules. Affected vessels may rupture or undergo thrombosis. Still later, endothelial cell proliferation and collagenous hyalinization with thickening of the media layer are seen in irradiated vessels, resulting in marked narrowing or obliteration of the vascular lumina. At this time, an increase in interstitial collagen in the irradiated field, leading to scarring and contractions, usually becomes evident.

Effects on Organ Systems

Fig. 8.16 depicts the main consequences of radiation injury. As already mentioned, *the most sensitive organs and tissues are the gonads, the hematopoietic and lymphoid systems, and the lining of the GI tract.* Estimated threshold doses for the effects of acute exposure to radiation in various organs are shown in Table 8.7. The changes in the hematopoietic and lymphoid systems, along with cancers induced by environmental or occupational exposure to ionizing radiation, are summarized as follows:

- *Hematopoietic and lymphoid systems.* The hematopoietic and lymphoid systems are extremely susceptible to radiation injury and deserve special mention. With high

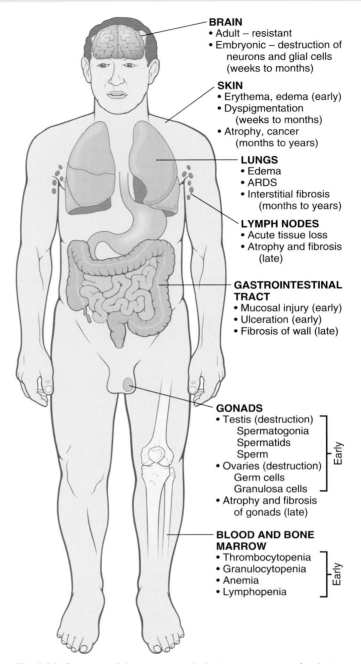

BRAIN
- Adult – resistant
- Embryonic – destruction of neurons and glial cells (weeks to months)

SKIN
- Erythema, edema (early)
- Dyspigmentation (weeks to months)
- Atrophy, cancer (months to years)

LUNGS
- Edema
- ARDS
- Interstitial fibrosis (months to years)

LYMPH NODES
- Acute tissue loss
- Atrophy and fibrosis (late)

GASTROINTESTINAL TRACT
- Mucosal injury (early)
- Ulceration (early)
- Fibrosis of wall (late)

GONADS
- Testis (destruction) Spermatogonia Spermatids Sperm
- Ovaries (destruction) Germ cells Granulosa cells — Early
- Atrophy and fibrosis of gonads (late)

BLOOD AND BONE MARROW
- Thrombocytopenia
- Granulocytopenia
- Anemia
- Lymphopenia — Early

Fig. 8.16 Overview of the major morphologic consequences of radiation injury. Early changes occur in hours to weeks; late changes occur in months to years. *ARDS,* Acute respiratory distress syndrome.

Table 8.7 Estimated Threshold Doses for Acute Radiation Effects on Specific Organs

Health Effect	Organ/Structure	Dose (Sv)
Temporary sterility	Testes	0.15
Depression of hematopoiesis	Bone marrow	0.50
Reversible skin effects (e.g., erythema)	Skin	1.0–2.0
Permanent sterility	Ovaries	2.5–6.0
Temporary hair loss	Skin	3.0–5.0
Permanent sterility	Testis	3.5
Cataract	Lens of eye	5.0

dose levels and large exposure fields, severe lymphopenia may appear within hours of irradiation, along with shrinkage of the lymph nodes and spleen. Radiation directly destroys lymphocytes, both in the circulating blood and in tissues (nodes, spleen, thymus, gut). With sublethal doses of radiation, regeneration from viable progenitors is prompt, leading to restoration of a normal lymphocyte count. Hematopoietic precursors in the bone marrow are also quite sensitive to radiant energy, which produces a dose-dependent *marrow aplasia*. The acute effects of marrow irradiation on peripheral blood counts reflects the kinetics of turnover of the formed elements—the granulocytes, platelets, and red cells, which have half-lives of less than 1 day, 10 days, and 120 days, respectively. After a brief rise in the circulating neutrophil count, *neutropenia* appears within several days. Neutrophil counts reach their nadir, often at counts near zero, during the second week. If the patient survives, full recovery of granulocytes may require 2 to 3 months. *Thrombocytopenia* appears by the end of the first week, with the platelet count nadir occurring somewhat later than that of granulocytes; recovery is similarly delayed. *Anemia* appears after 2 to 3 weeks and may persist for months. Understandably, higher doses of radiation produce more severe cytopenias and more prolonged periods of recovery. Very high doses kill marrow stem cells and induce permanent aplasia *(aplastic anemia)* marked by a failure of blood count recovery, whereas with lower doses the aplasia is transient.

- *Environmental exposure and cancer development.* Any cell capable of division that has sustained mutations has the potential to become cancerous. Thus, an increased incidence of neoplasms may occur in any organ after exposure to ionizing radiation. The level of radiation required to increase the risk of cancer development is difficult to determine, but there is little doubt that acute or prolonged exposures that result in doses of 100 mSv cause serious consequences, including cancer. This is documented by the increased incidence of leukemias and tumors at various sites (such as thyroid, breast, and lung) in survivors of the atomic bombings of Hiroshima and Nagasaki, the increase in thyroid cancers in survivors of the Chernobyl accident, and the development of "second cancers," such as acute myeloid leukemia, myelodysplastic syndrome, and solid tumors, in individuals who received radiation therapy for cancers such as Hodgkin lymphoma. It is believed that the risk of secondary cancers following irradiation is greatest in children. This is based in part on a large-scale epidemiologic study showing that children who receive at least two CT scans have very small but measurable increased risks for leukemia and malignant brain

tumors, and on older studies showing that radiation therapy to the chest is particularly likely to produce breast cancers when administered to adolescent females.

- *Occupational exposure and cancer development.* Radon is a ubiquitous product of the spontaneous decay of uranium. The carcinogenic agents are two radon decay byproducts (polonium-214 and polonium-218, or "radon daughters"), which emit alpha particles and have a short half-life. These particulates are deposited in the lung, and chronic exposure in uranium miners may give rise to lung carcinomas. Risks also are present in those homes in which the levels of radon are very high, comparable to those found in mines. However, there is little or no evidence to suggest that radon contributes to the risk of lung cancer in the average household.

Total-Body Irradiation

Exposure of large areas of the body to even small doses of radiation may have devastating effects. Dosages less than 1 Sv produce minimal or no symptoms. Greater exposures, however, cause health effects known as acute radiation syndromes, which at progressively higher doses involve the hematopoietic system, GI system, and CNS. The syndromes associated with total-body exposure to ionizing radiation are summarized in Table 8.8.

SUMMARY

RADIATION INJURY

- Ionizing radiation may injure cells directly or indirectly by generating free radicals from water or molecular oxygen.
- Ionizing radiation damages DNA; therefore, rapidly dividing cells such as germ cells, and those in the bone marrow and GI tract are very sensitive to radiation injury.
- DNA damage that is not adequately repaired may result in mutations that predispose affected cells to neoplastic transformation.
- Ionizing radiation may cause vascular damage and sclerosis, resulting in ischemic necrosis of parenchymal cells and their replacement by fibrous tissue.

NUTRITIONAL DISEASES

Millions of people in developing nations starve or live on the cruel edge of starvation, whereas those in the developed world, and more recently in the developing world, struggle to avoid calories and the attendant obesity or fear that what they eat may contribute to atherosclerosis and

Table 8.8 Effects of Whole-Body Ionizing Radiation

	0–1 Sv	1–2 Sv	2–10 Sv	10–20 Sv	>50 Sv
Main site of injury	None	Lymphocytes	Bone marrow	Small bowel	Brain
Main signs and symptoms	—	Moderate leukopenia	Leukopenia, hemorrhage, epilation, vomiting	Diarrhea, fever, electrolyte imbalance, vomiting	Ataxia, coma, convulsions, vomiting
Timing	—	1 day–1 week	4–6 weeks	5–14 days	1–4 hours
Lethality	—	None	Variable (0%–80%)	100%	100%

hypertension. So both the lack of nutrition and overnutrition are major health concerns.

Malnutrition

A healthy diet provides (1) sufficient energy, in the form of carbohydrates, fats, and proteins, for the body's daily metabolic needs; (2) essential (as well as nonessential) amino acids and fatty acids, used as building blocks for synthesis of structural and functional proteins and lipids; and (3) vitamins and minerals, which function as co-enzymes or hormones in vital metabolic pathways or, as in the case of calcium and phosphate, as important structural components. In *primary malnutrition,* one or all of these components are missing from the diet. By contrast, in *secondary, or conditional, malnutrition,* the dietary intake of nutrients is adequate, and malnutrition results from nutrient malabsorption, impaired use or storage, excess losses, or increased requirements. The causes of secondary malnutrition can be grouped into three general but overlapping categories: GI diseases, chronic wasting diseases, and acute critical illness.

Malnutrition is widespread and may be gross or subtle. Some common causes of dietary insufficiencies are listed here.

- *Poverty.* Homeless people, elderly persons, and children of the poor often suffer from severe malnutrition as well as trace nutrient deficiencies. In poor countries, poverty, together with droughts, crop failure, and livestock deaths, creates the setting for malnourishment of children and adults.
- *Ignorance.* Even the affluent may fail to recognize that infants, adolescents, and pregnant women have increased nutritional needs. Ignorance about the nutritional content of various foods also contributes to malnutrition, as follows: (1) iron deficiency often develops in infants exclusively fed artificial milk diets; (2) polished rice used as the mainstay of a diet may lack adequate amounts of thiamine; and (3) iodine often is lacking in food and water in regions removed from the oceans, unless supplementation is provided.
- *Chronic alcoholism.* Alcoholic persons may sometimes suffer from malnutrition but are more frequently lacking in several vitamins, especially thiamine, pyridoxine, folate, and vitamin A, as a result of dietary deficiency, defective GI absorption, abnormal nutrient utilization and storage, increased metabolic needs, and an increased rate of loss. A failure to recognize thiamine deficiency in patients with chronic alcoholism may result in irreversible brain damage (e.g., Korsakoff psychosis, discussed in Chapter 23).
- *Acute and chronic illnesses.* The basal metabolic rate becomes accelerated in many illnesses (in patients with extensive burns, it may double), resulting in increased daily requirements for all nutrients. Failure to recognize these nutritional needs may delay recovery. Malnutrition is often present in patients with advanced cancer and AIDS.
- *Self-imposed dietary restriction.* Anorexia nervosa, bulimia, and less overt eating disorders affect a large population of persons who are concerned about body image or suffer from an unreasonable fear of cardiovascular

disease (anorexia and bulimia are discussed in a separate section in this chapter).
- *Other causes.* Additional causes of malnutrition include GI diseases, acquired and inherited malabsorption syndromes, specific drug therapies (which block uptake or use of particular nutrients), and total parenteral nutrition.

The remainder of this section presents a general overview of nutritional disorders. Particular attention is devoted to severe acute malnutrition, anorexia nervosa and bulimia, deficiencies of vitamins and trace minerals, and obesity, with a brief consideration of the relationships of diet to atherosclerosis and cancer. Other nutrients and nutritional issues are discussed in the context of specific diseases throughout the text.

Severe Acute Malnutrition

The World Health Organization defines severe acute malnutrition (SAM) as a state characterized by a greatly reduced weight for height ratio that is below 3 standard deviation of WHO standards. Worldwide about 16 million children under the age of 5 years are affected by it. It is common in poor countries, where as many as 25% of children may be affected and where it is a major contributor to the high death rates among the very young. In addition to loss of life, wars also exact a heavy toll on refugees who live in abject poverty. In camps set up for refugees from Syria, as many as 20% of the children are severely or moderately malnourished.

SAM previously called protein energy malnutrition (PEM) manifests as a range of clinical syndromes, all resulting from a dietary intake of protein and calories that is inadequate to meet the body's needs. The two ends of the spectrum of SAM are known as *marasmus* and *kwashiorkor.* It should be noted that from a functional standpoint, there are two protein compartments in the body: the somatic compartment, represented by proteins in skeletal muscles, and the visceral compartment, represented by protein stores in the visceral organs, primarily the liver. These two compartments are regulated differently, as detailed subsequently. The somatic compartment is affected more severely in marasmus and the visceral compartment is depleted more severely in kwashiorkor. Clinical assessment of undernutrition is discussed next, followed by descriptions of marasmus and kwashiorkor.

The diagnosis of SAM is obvious in its most severe forms. In mild to moderate forms, the usual approach is to compare the body weight for a given height against standard tables; other helpful parameters are fat stores, muscle mass, and levels of certain serum proteins. With a loss of fat, measured skinfold thickness (which includes skin and subcutaneous tissue) is reduced. If the somatic protein compartment is catabolized, the resultant reduction in muscle mass is reflected by reduced circumference of the midarm. Measurement of serum proteins (albumin, transferrin, and others) provides an estimate of the adequacy of the visceral protein compartment. Recent studies suggest a role for the gut microbiome in the pathogenesis of SAM. There is a substantial difference in the microbial flora of children with SAM when compared with the gut

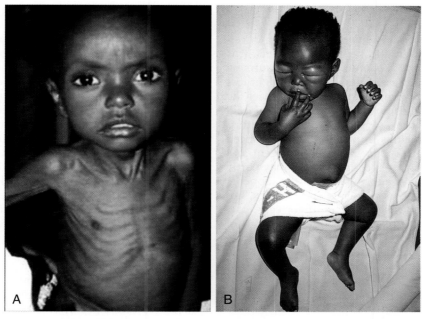

Fig. 8.17 Childhood malnutrition. (A) Marasmus. Note the loss of muscle mass and subcutaneous fat; the head appears to be too large for the emaciated body. (B) Kwashiorkor. The infant shows generalized edema, seen as ascites and puffiness of the face, hands, and legs. *(A, From Clinic Barak, Reisebericht Kenya.)*

microbiome of normal children. It seems that the alterations in the microbiome are not merely the consequences of SAM but play a role in their causation.

Marasmus

Marasmus develops when the diet is severely lacking in calories (Fig. 8.17A). A marasmic child suffers growth retardation and loss of muscle mass as a result of catabolism and depletion of the somatic protein compartment. This seems to be an adaptive response that provides the body with amino acids as a source of energy. Of interest, the visceral protein compartment, which presumably is more critical for survival, is depleted only marginally, so *serum albumin levels are either normal or only slightly reduced.* In addition to muscle proteins, subcutaneous fat is also mobilized and used as fuel. Leptin (discussed later under "Obesity") production is low, which may stimulate the hypothalamic-pituitary-adrenal axis to produce the high levels of cortisol that contribute to lipolysis. With such losses of muscle and subcutaneous fat, the *extremities are emaciated;* by comparison, the head appears too large for the body. Anemia and manifestations of multivitamin deficiencies are present, and there is evidence of *immune deficiency,* particularly of T-cell–mediated immunity. Hence, concurrent infections are usually present, which impose an additional stress on an already weakened body.

Kwashiorkor

Kwashiorkor occurs when protein deprivation is relatively greater than the reduction in total calories (Fig. 8.17B). This is the most common form of SAM seen in African children who have been weaned too early and subsequently fed, almost exclusively, a carbohydrate diet (the name kwashiorkor, from the Ga language in Ghana, describes the illness in a baby that appears after the arrival of another child). The prevalence of kwashiorkor also is high in impoverished countries of Southeast Asia. Less severe forms may occur worldwide in persons with chronic diarrheal states, in which protein is not absorbed, or in those with chronic protein loss (e.g., protein-losing enteropathies, the nephrotic syndrome, or the aftermath of extensive burns). Rare cases of kwashiorkor resulting from fad diets or replacement of milk by rice-based beverages have been reported in the United States.

In kwashiorkor, unlike in marasmus, marked protein deprivation is associated with severe loss of the visceral protein compartment, and the resultant hypoalbuminemia gives rise to *generalized or dependent edema* (Fig. 8.17). The weight of children with severe kwashiorkor typically is 60% to 80% of normal. However, the true loss of weight is masked by the increased fluid retention (edema). In further contrast with marasmus, there is relative sparing of subcutaneous fat and muscle mass. The modest loss of these compartments may also be masked by edema.

Children with kwashiorkor have characteristic *skin lesions* with alternating zones of hyperpigmentation, desquamation, and hypopigmentation, giving a "flaky paint" appearance. *Hair changes* include loss of color or alternating bands of pale and darker color, straightening, fine texture, and loss of firm attachment to the scalp. Other features that distinguish kwashiorkor from marasmus include an enlarged, *fatty liver* (resulting from reduced synthesis of the carrier protein component of lipoproteins) and the development of apathy, listlessness, and loss of appetite. As in marasmus, vitamin deficiencies are likely to be present, as are *defects in immunity* and *secondary infections.* In kwashiorkor, the inflammation caused by infection produces a catabolic state that aggravates the malnutrition. As already mentioned, marasmus and kwashiorkor represent two ends of a spectrum, and considerable overlap exists.

Secondary Malnutrition

In the United States, secondary malnutrition often develops in chronically ill, older, and bedridden patients. It is estimated that more than 50% of older residents in nursing homes in the United States are malnourished. Weight loss of more than 5% resulting from malnutrition increases the risk of mortality in nursing home patients by almost 5-fold. A particularly severe form of secondary malnutrition, called *cachexia*, often develops in patients with advanced cancer (Chapter 6). The wasting is all too apparent and often presages death. Although loss of appetite may partly explain it, cachexia may appear before the appetite decreases. The underlying mechanisms are complex, but appear to involve cytokines secreted by tumor cells, particularly TNF, which are released as part of the host response to advanced tumors. These factors directly stimulate the degradation of skeletal muscle proteins, and also stimulate fat mobilization from lipid stores.

MORPHOLOGY

The hallmark anatomic changes in SAM are (1) growth failure, (2) peripheral edema in kwashiorkor, and (3) loss of body fat and atrophy of muscle, more marked in marasmus.

The **liver** in kwashiorkor, but not in marasmus, is enlarged and fatty; superimposed cirrhosis is rare.

In kwashiorkor (rarely in marasmus) the **small bowel** shows a decrease in the mitotic index in the crypts of the glands, associated with mucosal atrophy and loss of villi and microvilli. In such cases concurrent loss of small intestinal enzymes occurs, most often manifested as disaccharidase deficiency. Hence, infants with kwashiorkor are lactate intolerant initially and may not respond well to full-strength, milk-based diets. With treatment, the mucosal changes are reversible.

The **bone marrow** in both kwashiorkor and marasmus may be hypoplastic, mainly as a result of decreased numbers of red cell precursors. Thus, anemia is usually present, most often hypochromic, microcytic due to iron deficiency, but a concurrent deficiency of folate may lead to a mixed microcytic-macrocytic anemia.

The **brain** in infants who are born to malnourished mothers and who suffer from SAM during the first 1 or 2 years of life has been reported by some investigators to show cerebral atrophy, a reduced number of neurons, and impaired myelination of white matter.

Many other changes may be present, including (1) thymic and lymphoid atrophy (more marked in kwashiorkor than in marasmus), (2) anatomic alterations induced by intercurrent infections, particularly with endemic helminths and other parasites, and (3) deficiencies of other required nutrients such as iodine and vitamins.

Anorexia Nervosa and Bulimia

Anorexia nervosa is a state of self-induced starvation resulting in marked weight loss; bulimia is a condition in which the patient binges on food and then induces vomiting. Bulimia is more common than anorexia nervosa and carries a better prognosis. It is estimated to occur in 1% to 2% of women and 0.1% of men, with an average age

at onset of 20 years. These disorders occur primarily in previously healthy young women who have acquired an obsession with attaining or maintaining thinness.

The clinical findings in anorexia nervosa generally are similar to those in SAM. In addition, effects on the endocrine system are prominent. *Amenorrhea*, resulting from decreased secretion of gonadotropin-releasing hormone (and consequent decreased secretion of luteinizing and follicle-stimulating hormones), is so common that its presence is almost a diagnostic feature. Other common findings, related to *decreased thyroid hormone* release, include cold intolerance, bradycardia, constipation, and changes in the skin and hair. In addition, dehydration and electrolyte abnormalities are frequent findings. Body hair may be increased but usually is fine and pale (lanugo). *Bone density is decreased,* most likely because of low estrogen levels, which mimics the postmenopausal acceleration of osteoporosis. As expected with severe malnutrition, anemia, lymphopenia, and hypoalbuminemia may be present. A major complication of anorexia nervosa is an increased susceptibility to *cardiac arrhythmia and sudden death,* both resulting from hypokalemia.

In bulimia, *binge eating* is the norm. Huge amounts of food, principally carbohydrates, are ingested, only to be followed by induced vomiting. Although menstrual irregularities are common, amenorrhea occurs in less than 50% of bulimic patients, probably because weight and gonadotropin levels are maintained near normal. The major medical complications are related to continual induced vomiting and chronic use of laxatives and diuretics. These include (1) electrolyte imbalances (hypokalemia), which predispose the patient to cardiac arrhythmias; (2) pulmonary aspiration of gastric contents; and (3) esophageal and stomach rupture. Nevertheless, there are no specific signs and symptoms for this syndrome, and the diagnosis must rely on a comprehensive psychologic assessment of the patient.

Vitamin Deficiencies

Before we summarize the functions of individual vitamins and the consequence of their deficiency, some general comments are in order.

- *Thirteen vitamins are necessary for health; four—A, D, E, and K—are fat-soluble and the remainder are water-soluble.* The distinction between fat- and water-soluble vitamins is important; although the former are more readily stored in the body, they may be poorly absorbed in fat malabsorption disorders, caused by disturbances of digestive functions (discussed in Chapter 15).
- *Certain vitamins can be synthesized endogenously*—vitamin D from precursor steroids, vitamin K and biotin by the intestinal microflora, and niacin from tryptophan, an essential amino acid. Notwithstanding this endogenous synthesis, a dietary supply of all vitamins is essential for health.
- Deficiency of a single vitamin is uncommon, and single- or multiple-vitamin deficiencies may accompany concurrent SAM.

In the following sections, vitamins A, D, and C are presented in some detail because of their wide-ranging functions and the morphologic changes of deficient states. This is followed by a summary in tabular form of the main consequences of deficiencies of the remaining vitamins—E, K, and the B complex—and some essential minerals.

Vitamin A

The major functions of vitamin A are maintenance of normal vision, regulation of cell growth and differentiation, and regulation of lipid metabolism. Vitamin A is a generic name for a group of related fat-soluble compounds that include *retinol, retinal, and retinoic acid,* which have similar biologic activities. Retinol is the chemical name for vitamin A. It is the transport form and, as retinol ester, also the storage form. A widely used term, *retinoids,* refers to both natural and synthetic chemicals that are structurally related to vitamin A but may not necessarily have vitamin A activity. Animal-derived foods such as liver, fish, eggs, milk, and butter are important dietary sources of preformed vitamin A. Yellow and leafy green vegetables such as carrots, squash, and spinach supply large amounts of carotenoids, many of which are provitamins that are metabolized to active vitamin A in the body. Carotenoids contribute approximately 30% of the vitamin A in human diets; the most important of these is β-carotene, which is efficiently converted to vitamin A. The recommended dietary allowance for vitamin A is expressed in retinol equivalents, to take into account both preformed vitamin A and β-carotene.

Vitamin A is a fat-soluble vitamin, and its absorption requires bile, pancreatic enzymes, and some level of anti-oxidant activity in the food. Retinol (generally ingested as retinol ester) and β-carotene are absorbed through the intestinal wall, where β-carotene is converted to retinol (Fig. 8.18). Retinol is then transported in chylomicrons, where it is taken up into liver cells through the apolipoprotein E receptor. More than 90% of the body's vitamin A reserves are stored in the liver, predominantly in the perisinusoidal stellate (Ito) cells. In healthy persons who consume an adequate diet, these reserves are sufficient to support the body's needs for at least 6 months. Retinol esters stored in the liver can be mobilized; before release, retinol binds to a specific retinol-binding protein (RBP), synthesized in the liver. The uptake of retinol and RBP in peripheral tissues is dependent on cell surface RBP receptors. After uptake by cells, retinol is released, and the RBP is recycled back into the blood. Retinol may be stored in peripheral tissues as retinyl ester or may be oxidized to form retinoic acid.

Function. In humans, the best-defined functions of vitamin A are the following:

- *Maintaining normal vision in reduced light.* The *visual process* involves four forms of vitamin A–containing pigments: rhodopsin, located in rod cells, the most light-sensitive pigment and therefore important in reduced light; and three iodopsins, located in cone cells, each responsive to a specific color in bright light. The synthesis of rhodopsin from retinol involves (1) oxidation to all-trans-retinal, (2) isomerization to 11-cis-retinal, and (3) interaction with opsin to form rhodopsin. A photon of light causes the isomerization of 11-cis-retinal to all-trans-retinal, and a sequence of configuration changes

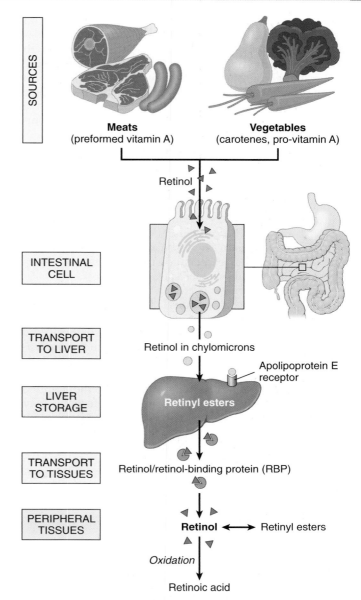

Fig. 8.18 Vitamin A metabolism.

SOURCES

Meats (preformed vitamin A)   Vegetables (carotenes, pro-vitamin A)

Retinol

INTESTINAL CELL

TRANSPORT TO LIVER   Retinol in chylomicrons

Apolipoprotein E receptor

LIVER STORAGE   Retinyl esters

TRANSPORT TO TISSUES   Retinol/retinol-binding protein (RBP)

PERIPHERAL TISSUES   **Retinol** ⟷ Retinyl esters

Oxidation

Retinoic acid

in rhodopsin, which produce a visual signal. In the process, a nerve impulse is generated (by changes in membrane potential) and transmitted by means of neurons from the retina to the brain. During dark adaptation, some of the all-trans-retinal is reconverted to 11-cis-retinal, but most is reduced to retinol and lost to the retina, explaining the need for a continuous supply of retinol.

- *Potentiating the differentiation of specialized epithelial cells.* Vitamin A and retinoids play an important role in the orderly differentiation of mucus-secreting columnar epithelium; when a deficiency state exists, the epithelium undergoes *squamous metaplasia,* differentiating into a keratinizing epithelium. Activation of retinoic acid receptors (RARs) by their ligands causes the release of corepressors and the obligatory formation of heterodimers with another retinoid receptor, known as the *retinoic X receptor* (RXR). Both RAR and RXR have three isoforms, α, β, and γ. The RAR/RXR heterodimers bind to retinoic acid response elements located in the regulatory regions of genes that encode receptors for growth factors, tumor suppressor genes, and secreted proteins. Through these effects, retinoids regulate cell growth and differentiation, cell-cycle control, and other biologic responses. *All-trans-retinoic acid*, a potent acid derivative of vitamin A, has the highest affinity for RARs compared with other retinoids.

- *Metabolic effects of retinoids.* The RXR, believed to be activated by 9-*cis* retinoic acid, can form heterodimers with other nuclear receptors, such as receptors involved in drug metabolism, the peroxisome proliferator-activated receptors (PPARs), and vitamin D receptors. PPARs are key regulators of fatty acid metabolism, including fatty acid oxidation in fat and muscle, adipogenesis, and lipoprotein metabolism. The association between RXR and PPARγ provides an explanation for the metabolic effects of retinoids on adipogenesis.
- *Enhancing immunity to infections.* Vitamin A supplementation can reduce morbidity and mortality rates for some forms of diarrhea. Similarly, supplementation in preschool children with measles, particularly those who are malnourished, can reduce mortality and complications of the disease, including eye damage and blindness. The effects of vitamin A on infections probably derive in part from its ability to stimulate the immune system through unclear mechanisms. Infections may reduce the bioavailability of vitamin A, possibly by inducing the acute phase response, which appears to inhibit RBP synthesis in the liver. The drop in hepatic RBP causes a decrease in circulating retinol, which reduces the tissue availability of vitamin A. The beneficial effect of vitamin A in diarrheal diseases may be related to the maintenance and restoration of the integrity of the epithelium of the gut.

In addition, the retinoids, β-carotene, and some related carotenoids can function as photoprotective and antioxidant agents. Retinoids have broad biologic effects, including effects on embryonic development, cellular differentiation and proliferation, and lipid metabolism.

Retinoids are used clinically to treat skin disorders such as severe acne and certain forms of psoriasis, and also to treat acute promyelocytic leukemia. As discussed in Chapter 6, all-*trans*-retinoic acid induces the differentiation and subsequent apoptosis of acute promyelocytic leukemia cells through its ability to bind to a PML-RARα fusion protein that characterizes this form of cancer.

Deficiency States. Vitamin A deficiency occurs worldwide as a consequence of either poor nutrition or fat malabsorption. In children, stores of vitamin A are depleted by infections, and the absorption of the vitamin is poor in newborn infants. In adults, vitamin A deficiency, in conjunction with depletion of other fat-soluble vitamins, may develop in patients with malabsorption syndromes, such as celiac disease, Crohn disease, and colitis. Bariatric surgery and the continuous use of mineral oil laxatives also may lead to deficiency. The multiple effects of vitamin A deficiency are as follows:

- As was already discussed, vitamin A is a component of rhodopsin and other visual pigments. Not surprisingly, one of the earliest manifestations of vitamin A deficiency is impaired vision, particularly in reduced light (*night blindness*).
- Other effects of vitamin A deficiency are related to its role in maintaining the differentiation of epithelial cells (Fig. 8.19). Persistent deficiency gives rise to a series of changes involving epithelial metaplasia and keratization. The most devastating changes occur in the eyes and result in the clinical entity referred to as xerophthalmia (dry eye). First, there is dryness of the conjunctiva (xerosis conjunctivae) as the normal lachrymal and

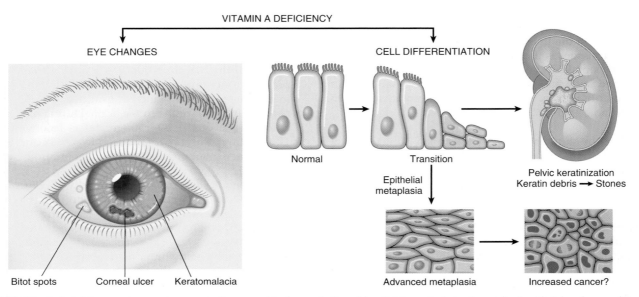

Fig. 8.19 Vitamin A deficiency: major consequences in the eye and in the production of keratinizing metaplasia of specialized epithelial surfaces, and its possible role in epithelial metaplasia. Not depicted are night blindness and immune deficiency.

mucus-secreting epithelium are replaced by keratinized epithelium. This is followed by a buildup of keratin debris in small opaque plaques *(Bitot spots)* and, eventually, the erosion of the roughened corneal surface, leading to softening and destruction of the cornea *(keratomalacia)* and total *blindness.*

- Vitamin A deficiency also leads to replacement of the epithelium lining the upper respiratory passage and urinary tract by keratinizing squamous cells (squamous metaplasia). Loss of the mucociliary epithelium of the airways predisposes affected patients to pulmonary infections, and desquamation of keratin debris in the urinary tract predisposes to renal and bladder stones. Hyperplasia and hyperkeratinization of the epidermis with plugging of the ducts of the adnexal glands may produce *follicular* or *papular dermatosis.*
- Another serious consequence of the lack of vitamin A is *immune deficiency.* This impairment of immunity leads to higher mortality rates from common infections such as measles, pneumonia, and infectious diarrhea. In parts of the world with a high prevalence of vitamin A deficiency, dietary supplements reduce mortality rates for infectious disorders by 20% to 30%.

Vitamin A Toxicity. Both short- and long-term excesses of vitamin A may produce toxic manifestations—a point of concern because of the megadoses being touted by certain sellers of supplements. The consequences of acute hypervitaminosis A were first described in 1597 by Gerrit de Veer, a ship's carpenter stranded in the Arctic, who recounted in his diary the serious symptoms that he and other crew members developed after eating polar bear liver. With this cautionary tale in mind, the adventurous eater should note that acute vitamin A toxicity also has been described in "hepatoaficionados" who feasted on the livers of whales, sharks, and even tuna!

The signs and symptoms of acute toxicity include headache, dizziness, vomiting, stupor, and blurred vision—all of which may be confused with those of a brain tumor. Chronic toxicity is associated with weight loss, anorexia, nausea, vomiting, and bone and joint pain. Retinoic acid stimulates the production and function of osteoclasts, leading to increased bone resorption and a consequent high risk of fractures. Although synthetic retinoids used for the treatment of acne are not associated with these complications, their use in pregnancy must be avoided because of the well-established teratogenic effect of retinoids.

Vitamin D

The major function of the fat-soluble vitamin D is the maintenance of adequate plasma levels of calcium and phosphorus to support metabolic functions, bone mineralization, and neuromuscular transmission. In this capacity, the vitamin is required for the prevention of bone diseases known as *rickets* (in children whose epiphyses have not already closed), *osteomalacia* (in adults), and hypocalcemic tetany. With respect to tetany, vitamin D maintains the correct concentration of ionized calcium in the extracellular fluid compartment. When deficiency develops, the drop in ionized calcium in the extracellular fluid results in continuous excitation of muscle (tetany). It should be noted, however, that any reduction in the level of serum calcium is rapidly corrected by excess secretion of parathyroid hormone. Hence tetany is quite uncommon. Our attention here is focused on the function of vitamin D in the regulation of serum calcium levels.

Metabolism. The major source of vitamin D for humans is its endogenous synthesis in the skin by photochemical conversion of a precursor, 7-dehydrocholesterol, powered by the energy of solar or artificial UV light. Irradiation of this compound forms *cholecalciferol,* known as vitamin D_3; in the following discussion, for the sake of simplicity, the term *vitamin D* is used to refer to this compound. Under usual conditions of sun exposure, approximately 90% of the vitamin D needed is endogenously derived from 7-dehydrocholesterol present in the skin. However, blacks may have a lower level of vitamin D production in the skin because of melanin pigmentation (perhaps a small price to pay for protection against UV-induced cancers). The small remainder comes from dietary sources, such as deep-sea fish, plants, and grains. In plant sources, vitamin D is present in a precursor form, ergosterol, which is converted to vitamin D in the body.

The metabolism of vitamin D can be outlined as follows (Fig. 8.20):

1. Absorption of vitamin D along with other fats in the gut or synthesis from precursors in the skin
2. Binding to plasma α_1-globulin (vitamin D–binding protein) and transport to liver
3. Conversion to 25-hydroxyvitamin D (25-OH-D) by 25-hydroxylase in the liver
4. Conversion of 25-OH-D to 1,25-dihydroxyvitamin D [1,25-$(OH)_2$-D] (biologically the most active form of vitamin D) by α1-hydroxylase in the kidney

Renal production of 1,25-$(OH)_2$-D is regulated by three mechanisms:

- *Hypocalcemia stimulates secretion of parathyroid hormone (PTH),* which in turn augments the conversion of 25-OH-D to 1,25-$(OH)_2$-D by activating α1-hydroxylase.
- *Hypophosphatemia directly activates α1-hydroxylase,* thereby increasing the formation of 1,25$(OH)_2$-D.
- In a feedback loop, increased levels of 1,25-$(OH)_2$-D downregulate the synthesis of this metabolite by inhibiting the action of α1-hydroxylase (decreases in 1,25-$(OH)_2$-D have the opposite effect).

Functions. Like retinoids and steroid hormones, 1,25-$(OH)_2$-D acts by binding to a high-affinity nuclear receptor that in turn binds to regulatory DNA sequences, thereby inducing transcription of specific target genes. The receptors for 1,25-$(OH)_2$-D are present in most nucleated cells of the body, and they transduce signals that result in various biologic activities, beyond those involved in calcium and phosphorus homeostasis. Nevertheless, the best-understood functions of vitamin D relate to the maintenance of normal plasma levels of calcium and phosphorus, through action on the intestines, bones, and kidneys (Fig. 8.20).

The active form of vitamin D:

- *Stimulates intestinal absorption of calcium* through upregulation of calcium transport, in enterocytes

NORMAL VITAMIN D METABOLISM

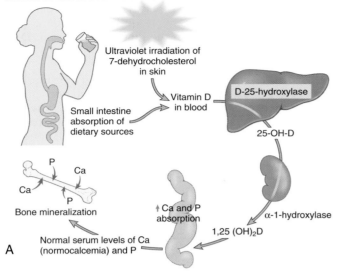

A

VITAMIN D DEFICIENCY

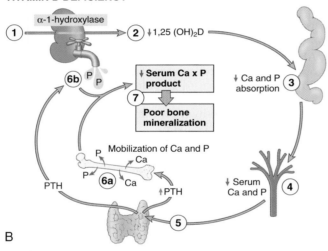

B

Fig. 8.20 (A) Normal vitamin D metabolism. (B) Vitamin D deficiency. There is inadequate substrate for the renal hydroxylase (*1*), yielding a deficiency of 1,25-(OH)₂D (*2*), and deficient absorption of calcium and phosphorus from the gut (*3*), with consequent depressed serum levels of both (*4*). The hypocalcemia activates the parathyroid glands (*5*), causing mobilization of calcium and phosphorus from bone (*6a*). Simultaneously, parathyroid hormone (PTH) induces wasting of phosphate in the urine (*6b*) and calcium retention. Consequently, the serum levels of calcium are normal or nearly normal, but the phosphate is low; hence, mineralization is impaired (*7*).

- *Stimulates calcium resorption in renal distal tubules.*
- *Collaborates with PTH to regulate blood calcium.* This occurs in part through upregulation of RANK ligand on osteoblasts, which in turn activates RANK receptors on osteoclast precursors. RANK activation produces signals that increase osteoclast differentiation and bone resorptive activities (Chapter 21).
- *Promotes the mineralization of bone.* Vitamin D is needed for the mineralization of osteoid matrix and epiphyseal cartilage during the formation of flat and long bones. It stimulates osteoblasts to synthesize the calcium-binding protein osteocalcin, which promotes calcium deposition.

Of note, effects of vitamin D on bone depend on the plasma levels of calcium: On the one hand, in hypocalcemic states 1,25-(OH)₂-D together with PTH increases the resorption of calcium and phosphorus from bone to support blood levels. On the other hand, in normocalcemic states, vitamin D is required for calcium deposition in epiphyseal cartilage and osteoid matrix.

Deficiency States

Vitamin D deficiency causes rickets in growing children and osteomalacia in adults; these skeletal diseases have worldwide distribution. They may result from diets deficient in calcium and vitamin D, but probably more important is limited exposure to sunlight (for instance, in heavily veiled women; children born to mothers who have frequent pregnancies followed by lactation, which leads to vitamin D deficiency; and inhabitants of northern climates with scant sunlight). Other, less common causes of rickets and osteomalacia include renal disorders causing decreased synthesis of 1,25-(OH)₂-D or phosphate depletion, and malabsorption disorders. Although rickets and osteomalacia rarely occur outside high-risk groups, milder forms of vitamin D deficiency (also called vitamin D insufficiency) leading to bone loss and hip fractures are common among elderly persons. Studies also suggest that vitamin D may be important for preventing demineralization of bones. It appears that certain genetically determined variants of the vitamin D receptor are associated with an accelerated loss of bone minerals with aging and certain familial forms of osteoporosis (Chapter 21).

Whatever the basis, a deficiency of vitamin D tends to cause hypocalcemia. This in turn stimulates PTH production, which (1) activates renal α₁-hydroxylase, increasing the amount of active vitamin D and calcium absorption; (2) mobilizes calcium from bone; (3) decreases renal calcium excretion; and (4) increases renal excretion of phosphate. Thus, the serum level of calcium is restored to near normal, but hypophosphatemia persists, so mineralization of bone is impaired or there is high bone turnover.

An understanding of the morphologic changes in rickets and osteomalacia is facilitated by a brief summary of normal bone development and maintenance. The development of flat bones in the skeleton involves intramembranous ossification, whereas the formation of long tubular bones proceeds by endochondral ossification. With intramembranous bone formation, mesenchymal cells differentiate directly into osteoblasts, which synthesize the collagenous osteoid matrix on which calcium is deposited. By contrast, with endochondral ossification, growing cartilage at the epiphyseal plates is provisionally mineralized and then progressively resorbed and replaced by osteoid matrix, which undergoes mineralization to create bone (Fig. 8.21A).

● MORPHOLOGY

The basic derangement in both rickets and osteomalacia is an excess of unmineralized bone matrix. The changes that occur in the growing bones of children with rickets, however, are complicated by inadequate provisional calcification

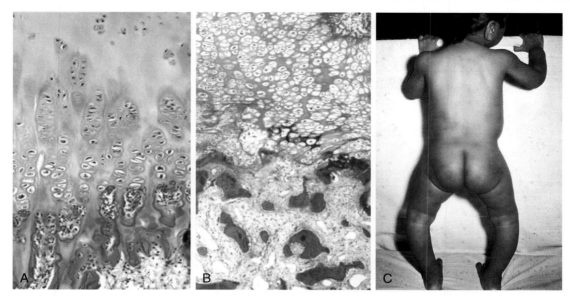

Fig. 8.21 Rickets. (A) Normal costochondral junction of a young child. Note cartilage palisade formation and orderly transition from cartilage to new bone. (B) Rachitic costochondral junction in which the palisade of cartilage is absent. Darker trabeculae are well-formed bone; paler trabeculae consist of uncalcified osteoid. (C) Note bowing of legs as a consequence of the formation of poorly mineralized bone in a child with rickets. (B, Courtesy of Dr. Andrew E. Rosenberg, Massachusetts General Hospital, Boston, Massachusetts.)

of epiphyseal cartilage, deranging endochondral bone growth. The following sequence ensues in rickets:

- Overgrowth of epiphyseal cartilage caused by inadequate provisional calcification and failure of the cartilage cells to mature and disintegrate
- Persistence of distorted, irregular masses of cartilage, many of which project into the marrow cavity
- Deposition of osteoid matrix on inadequately mineralized cartilaginous remnants
- Disruption of the orderly replacement of cartilage by osteoid matrix, with enlargement and lateral expansion of the osteochondral junction (Fig. 8.21B)
- Abnormal overgrowth of capillaries and fibroblasts in the disorganized zone resulting from microfractures and stresses on the inadequately mineralized, weak, poorly formed bone
- Deformation of the skeleton resulting from the loss of structural rigidity of the developing bones

The gross skeletal changes depend on the severity of the rachitic process; its duration; and, in particular, the stresses to which individual bones are subjected. During the nonambulatory stage of infancy, the head and chest sustain the greatest stresses. The softened occipital bones may become flattened, and the parietal bones can be buckled inward by pressure; with the release of the pressure, elastic recoil snaps the bones back into their original positions **(craniotabes).** An excess of osteoid produces **frontal bossing** and a squared appearance to the head. Deformation of the chest results from overgrowth of cartilage or osteoid tissue at the costochondral junction, producing the **"rachitic rosary."** The weakened metaphyseal areas of the ribs are subject to the pull of the respiratory muscles, causing them to bend inward creating anterior protrusion of the sternum **(pigeon breast deformity).** The inward pull at the margin of the diaphragm creates the **Harrison groove,** girdling the thoracic cavity at the lower margin of the rib cage. The pelvis may

become deformed. When an ambulating child develops rickets, deformities are likely to affect the spine, pelvis, and long bones (e.g., tibia), causing, most notably, **lumbar lordosis** and **bowing of the legs** (Fig. 8.21C).

In adults with **osteomalacia,** the lack of vitamin D deranges the normal bone remodeling that occurs throughout life. The newly formed osteoid matrix laid down by osteoblasts is inadequately mineralized, producing the excess of persistent osteoid that is characteristic of osteomalacia. Although the contours of the bone are not affected, the bone is weak and vulnerable to gross fractures or microfractures, which are most likely to affect vertebral bodies and femoral necks. On histologic examination, the unmineralized osteoid can be visualized as a thickened layer of matrix (which stains pink in hematoxylin and eosin preparations) arranged about the more basophilic, normally mineralized trabeculae.

Nonskeletal Effects of Vitamin D. As mentioned earlier, the vitamin D receptor is present in various cells and tissues that do not participate in calcium and phosphorus homeostasis. In addition, macrophages, keratinocytes, and tissues such as breast, prostate, and colon can produce 1,25-dihydroxyvitamin D. It appears that pathogen-induced activation of Toll-like receptors in macrophages causes increased expression of vitamin D receptor as well as increased local synthesis of 1,25-dihydroxyvitamin D. This causes activation of vitamin-D-dependent gene expression in macrophages and other neighboring immune cells. The net effect of these changes on the immune response remains to be determined. It appears that in some patients with tuberculosis, vitamin D supplements increase lymphocyte counts and enhance the clearance of *Mycobacterium tuberculosis.* It has also been reported that low levels

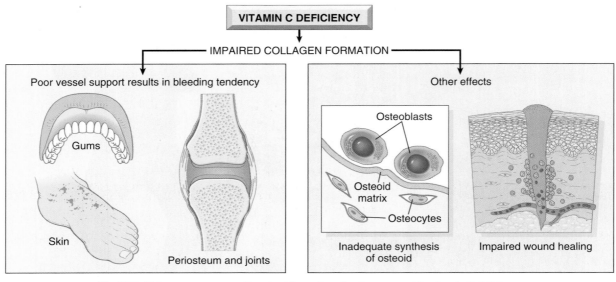

Fig. 8.22 Major consequences of impaired formation of collagen caused by vitamin C deficiency.

of 1,25-dihydroxyvitamin D (<20 ng/mL) are associated with a 30% to 50% increase in the incidence of colon, prostate, and breast cancers, but whether or not vitamin D supplementation can reduce cancer risk has not been firmly established.

Toxicity. Prolonged exposure to sunlight may cause sunburns but it does not produce an excess of vitamin D, but megadoses of orally administered vitamin can lead to hypervitaminosis. In children, hypervitaminosis D may take the form of metastatic calcifications of soft tissues such as the kidney; in adults, it causes bone pain and hypercalcemia. As a point of some interest, the toxic potential of this vitamin is so great that in sufficiently large doses it is a potent rodenticide!

Vitamin C (Ascorbic Acid)

A deficiency of water-soluble vitamin C leads to the development of scurvy, characterized principally by bone disease in growing children and by hemorrhages and healing defects in both children and adults. Sailors of the British Royal Navy were nicknamed "limeys" because at the end of the 18th century the Navy began to provide lime and lemon juice to them to prevent scurvy during their long sojourns at sea. It was not until 1932 that ascorbic acid was identified and synthesized. Unlike vitamin D, ascorbic acid is not synthesized endogenously in humans, who therefore are entirely dependent on the diet for this nutrient. Vitamin C is present in milk and some animal products (liver, fish) and is abundant in a variety of fruits and vegetables. All but the most restricted diets provide adequate amounts of vitamin C.

Function. **Ascorbic acid acts in a variety of biosynthetic pathways by accelerating hydroxylation and amidation reactions.** The most clearly established function of vitamin C is the activation of prolyl and lysyl hydroxylases from inactive precursors, allowing for hydroxylation

of procollagen. Inadequately hydroxylated procollagen cannot acquire a stable helical configuration or be adequately crosslinked, so it is poorly secreted from the fibroblasts. Those molecules that are secreted lack tensile strength, are more soluble, and are more vulnerable to enzymatic degradation. Collagen, which normally has the highest content of hydroxyproline, is most affected, particularly in blood vessels, accounting for the predisposition to hemorrhages in scurvy. In addition, a deficiency of vitamin C suppresses the synthesis of collagen polypeptides, independent of effects on proline hydroxylation. Vitamin C also has *anti-oxidant properties*. These include an ability to scavenge free radicals directly and the participation in metabolic reactions that regenerate the anti-oxidant form of vitamin E.

Deficiency States. Consequences of vitamin C deficiency are illustrated in Fig. 8.22. Fortunately, because of the abundance of ascorbic acid in foods, scurvy has ceased to be a global problem. It is sometimes encountered in affluent populations as a secondary deficiency, particularly among elderly persons, people who live alone, and chronic alcoholics—groups often characterized by erratic and inadequate eating patterns. Occasionally, scurvy appears in patients undergoing peritoneal dialysis and hemodialysis and among food faddists.

Toxicity. The popular notion that megadoses of vitamin C protect against the common cold or at least allay the symptoms has not been borne out by controlled clinical studies. Such slight relief as may be experienced probably is a result of the mild antihistamine action of ascorbic acid. The large excess of vitamin C is promptly excreted in the urine but may cause uricosuria and increased absorption of iron, with the potential for iron overload.

Other vitamins and some essential minerals are listed and briefly described in Tables 8.9 and 8.10. Folic acid and vitamin B$_{12}$ are discussed in Chapter 12.

Table 8.9 Vitamins: Major Functions and Deficiency Syndromes

Vitamin	Functions	Deficiency Syndromes
Fat-Soluble		
Vitamin A	A component of visual pigment Maintenance of specialized epithelia Maintenance of resistance to infection	Night blindness, xerophthalmia, blindness Squamous metaplasia Vulnerability to infection, particularly measles
Vitamin D	Facilitates intestinal absorption of calcium and phosphorus and mineralization of bone	Rickets in children Osteomalacia in adults
Vitamin E	Major anti-oxidant; scavenges free radicals	Spinocerebellar degeneration
Vitamin K	Cofactor in hepatic carboxylation of procoagulants—factors II (prothrombin), VII, IX, and X; and protein C and protein S	Bleeding diathesis
Water-Soluble		
Vitamin B_1 (thiamine)	As pyrophosphate, is coenzyme in decarboxylation reactions	Dry and wet beriberi, Wernicke syndrome, Korsakoff syndrome
Vitamin B_2 (riboflavin)	Converted to coenzymes flavin mononucleotide and flavin adenine dinucleotide, cofactors for many enzymes in intermediary metabolism	Cheilosis, stomatitis, glossitis, dermatitis, corneal vascularization
Niacin	Incorporated into nicotinamide adenine dinucleotide (NAD) and NAD phosphate; involved in a variety of oxidation-reduction (redox) reactions	Pellagra—"three Ds": dementia, dermatitis, diarrhea
Vitamin B_6 (pyridoxine)	Derivatives serve as coenzymes in many intermediary reactions	Cheilosis, glossitis, dermatitis, peripheral neuropathy
Vitamin B_{12}*	Required for normal folate metabolism and DNA synthesis Maintenance of myelinization of spinal cord tracts	Combined system disease (megaloblastic anemia and degeneration of posterolateral spinal cord tracts)
Vitamin C	Serves in many redox reactions and hydroxylation of collagen	Scurvy
Folate*	Essential for transfer and use of one-carbon units in DNA synthesis	Megaloblastic anemia, neural tube defects
Pantothenic acid	Incorporated in coenzyme A	No nonexperimental syndrome recognized
Biotin	Cofactor in carboxylation reactions	No clearly defined clinical syndrome

*See also Chapter 12.

Table 8.10 Selected Trace Elements and Deficiency Syndromes

Element	Function	Basis of Deficiency	Clinical Features
Zinc	Component of enzymes, principally oxidases	Inadequate supplementation in artificial diets Interference with absorption by other dietary constituents Inborn error of metabolism	Rash around eyes, mouth, nose, and anus called *acrodermatitis enteropathica* Anorexia and diarrhea Growth retardation in children Depressed mental function Depressed wound healing and immune response Impaired night vision Infertility
Iron	Essential component of hemoglobin as well as several iron-containing metalloenzymes	Inadequate diet Chronic blood loss	Hypochromic, microcytic anemia
Iodine	Component of thyroid hormone	Inadequate supply in food and water	Goiter and hypothyroidism
Copper	Component of cytochrome c oxidase, dopamine β-hydroxylase, tyrosinase, and lysyl oxidase (involved in crosslinking collagen)	Inadequate supplementation in artificial diet Interference with absorption	Muscle weakness Neurologic defects Abnormal collagen crosslinking
Fluoride	Replaces calcium during remineralization of teeth, producing fluorapatite, which is more resistant to acids	Inadequate supply in soil and water Inadequate supplementation	Dental caries
Selenium	Component of GSH peroxidase Anti-oxidant with vitamin E	Inadequate amounts in soil and water	Myopathy Cardiomyopathy (Keshan disease)

SUMMARY

NUTRITIONAL DISEASES

- Primary SAM is a common cause of childhood deaths in poor countries. The two main primary SAM syndromes are marasmus and kwashiorkor. Secondary SAM occurs in the chronically ill and in patients with advanced cancer (as a result of cachexia).
- Kwashiorkor is characterized by hypoalbuminemia, generalized edema, fatty liver, skin changes, and defects in immunity. It is caused by diets low in protein but normal in calories.
- Marasmus is characterized by emaciation resulting from loss of muscle mass and fat with relative preservation of serum albumin. It is caused by diets severely lacking in calories—both protein and nonprotein.
- Anorexia nervosa is self-induced starvation; it is characterized by amenorrhea and multiple manifestations of low thyroid hormone levels. Bulimia is a condition in which food binges alternate with induced vomiting.
- Vitamins A and D are fat-soluble vitamins with a wide range of activities. Vitamin C and members of the vitamin B family are water-soluble (Table 8.9 lists vitamin functions and deficiency syndromes).

Obesity

Excess adiposity (obesity) and excess body weight are associated with increased incidence of several of the most important diseases of humans, including type 2 diabetes, dyslipidemias, cardiovascular disease, hypertension, and cancer. It is a major public health problem in developed countries and an emerging health problem in developing nations, such as India. In the United States, obesity has reached epidemic proportions. The prevalence of obesity increased from 13% to 34% between 1960 and 2008, and as of 2015, 68.6% of Americans between 20 and 75 years of age were overweight as were 17% of the children. Globally, the World Health Organization (WHO) estimates that in 2015, 700 million adults were obese. The causes of this epidemic are complex but undoubtedly are related to societal changes in diet and levels of physical activity. **Obesity is defined as a state of increased body weight, caused by adipose tissue accumulation, that is of sufficient magnitude to produce adverse health effects.** How does one measure fat accumulation? Several high-tech methods have been devised, but for practical purposes the body mass index (BMI) is most commonly used. BMI is calculated as (weight in kilograms)/(height in meters)^2, or kg/m^2.

The BMI is closely correlated with body fat. BMIs in the range 18.5 to 25 kg/m^2 are considered normal, whereas BMIs between 25 and 30 kg/m^2 identify the overweight, and BMIs greater than 30 kg/m^2, the obese. It is generally agreed that a BMI greater than 30 kg/m^2 imparts a health risk. In the following discussion, for the sake of simplicity, the term obesity is applied to both the overweight and the truly obese.

The untoward effects of obesity are related not only to the total body weight but also to the distribution of the stored fat. *Central, or visceral, obesity,* in which fat accumulates in the trunk and in the abdominal cavity (in the mesentery and around viscera), is associated with a much higher risk for several diseases than is a condition of excess accumulation of fat in a diffuse distribution in subcutaneous tissue.

The etiology of obesity is complex and incompletely understood. Involved are genetic, environmental, and psychologic factors. However, simply put, *obesity is a disorder of energy balance.* The two sides of the energy equation, intake and expenditure, are finely regulated by neural and hormonal mechanisms, so that body weight is maintained within a narrow range for many years. Apparently, this fine balance is controlled by an internal set point, or "lipostat," that senses the quantity of energy stores (adipose tissue) and appropriately regulates food intake as well as energy expenditure. Several "obesity genes" have been identified. As might be expected, they encode the molecular components of the physiologic system that regulates energy balance. A key player in energy homeostasis is the *LEP* gene and its product, *leptin.* This unique member of the cytokine family, secreted by adipocytes, regulates both sides of the energy equation—intake of food and expenditure of energy. As discussed later, *the net effect of leptin is to reduce food intake and to enhance the expenditure of energy.*

In a simplified way, the neurohumoral mechanisms that regulate energy balance and body weight may be divided into three components (Fig. 8.23):
- *The peripheral or afferent system* generates signals from various sites. Its main components are leptin and adiponectin produced by fat cells, insulin from the pancreas, ghrelin from the stomach, and peptide YY from the ileum and colon. Leptin reduces food intake and is discussed in further detail later. Ghrelin secretion stimulates appetite, and it may function as a "meal-initiating" signal. Peptide YY, which is released postprandially by endocrine cells in the ileum and colon, is a satiety signal.
- *The arcuate nucleus in the hypothalamus,* processes and integrates the peripheral signals and generates new signals that are transmitted by (1) POMC (proopiomelanocortin) and CART (cocaine- and amphetamine-regulated transcript) neurons; and (2) NPY (neuropeptide Y) and AgRP (agouti-related peptide) neurons.
- *The efferent system,* which consists of hypothalamic neurons regulated by the arcuate nucleus, is organized along two pathways, anabolic and catabolic, which control food intake and energy expenditure, respectively.
- POMC/CART neurons activate efferent neurons that enhance energy expenditure and weight loss through the production of molecules such as α-melanocyte stimulating hormone (MSH) that reduce food intake (anorexigenic effect). MSH signals through melanocortin receptor (MC4R). By contrast NPY/AgRP neurons activate efferent neurons that promote food intake (orexigenic effect) and weight gain. Signals transmitted by efferent neurons also communicate with forebrain and midbrain centers that control the autonomic nervous system.

Discussed next are two important components of the afferent system that regulate appetite and satiety: leptin and gut hormones, and adiponectin that regulates fat consumption.

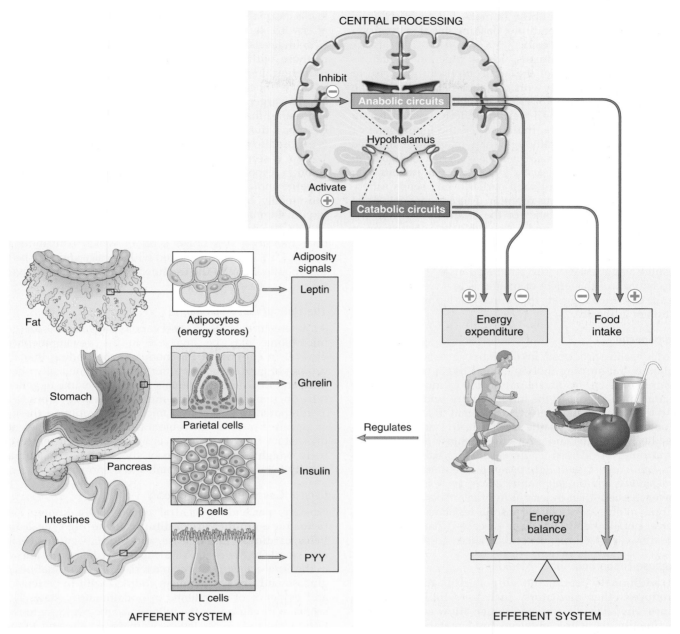

Fig. 8.23 Energy balance regulatory circuitry. When sufficient energy is stored in adipose tissue and the individual is well fed, afferent adiposity signals (insulin, leptin, ghrelin, peptide YY) are delivered to the central neuronal processing units, in the hypothalamus. Here the adiposity signals inhibit anabolic circuits and activate catabolic circuits. The effector arms of these central circuits then influence energy balance by inhibiting food intake and promoting energy expenditure. This in turn reduces the energy stores, and proadiposity signals are blunted. Conversely, when energy stores are low, the available anabolic circuits take over, at the expense of catabolic circuits, to generate energy stores in the form of adipose tissue.

Leptin

Leptin is secreted by fat cells, and its output is regulated by the adequacy of fat stores. BMI and body fat stores are directly related to leptin secretion. With abundant adipose tissue, leptin secretion is stimulated, and the hormone crosses the blood–brain barrier and travels to the hypothalamus, where it *reduces food intake by stimulating POMC/ CART neurons and inhibiting NPY/AgRP neurons.* The opposite sequence of events occurs when there are inadequate stores of body fat: Leptin secretion is diminished and food intake is increased. In persons of stable weight, the

activities of these pathways are balanced. Leptin also increases energy expenditure by stimulating physical activity, energy expenditure, and *thermogenesis,* and these may be the most important catabolic effects mediated by leptin through the hypothalamus. Although the effects of leptin on food intake and energy expenditure can be readily demonstrated in nonobese mice and humans, the anorexigenic response of leptin is blunted in states of obesity despite high levels of circulating leptin. Such leptin resistance in obese mice can be bypassed by intraventricular injection of leptin. In keeping with this observation, injections of leptin in obese humans fail to affect food intake and energy expenditure, dashing initial enthusiasm of leptin therapy for obesity.

In rodents and humans, loss-of-function mutations affecting components of the leptin pathway give rise to massive obesity. Mice with mutations that disable the leptin gene or its receptor fail to sense the adequacy of fat stores, so they behave as if they are undernourished, eating ravenously. As in mice, mutations of the leptin gene or receptor in humans, although rare, may cause massive obesity. *More common are mutations in the melanocortin receptor-4 gene (MC4R), found in 4% to 5% of patients with massive obesity.* As mentioned earlier, MSH sends satiety signals by binding to this receptor. These monogenic traits underscore the importance of the leptin pathway in the control of body weight, and it is possible that more common types of defects in this pathway will be discovered in the obese. In closing it should be mentioned that, like leptin, insulin also exerts anorexigenic responses. However, the mechanism of this effect of insulin is less clear, and most of the evidence suggests the primacy of leptin in the regulation of adiposity.

Adiponectin

Adiponectin, produced in the adipose tissue, has been called a "fat-burning molecule" and the "guardian angel against obesity." It directs fatty acids to muscle for their oxidation. It decreases the influx of fatty acids to the liver and the total hepatic triglyceride content. It also decreases glucose production in the liver, causing an increase in insulin sensitivity and protecting against the metabolic syndrome. *In addition to its metabolic effects, adiponectin has anti-diabetic, anti-inflammatory, anti-atherogenic, anti-proliferative, and cardioprotective effects.* Its serum levels are lower in obese than in lean individuals. These effects contribute to obesity-associated insulin resistance, type 2 diabetes, nonalcoholic fatty liver disease (Chapter 14), and possibly increased risk of certain cancers, discussed later.

Adipose Tissue and Other Mediators

In addition to leptin and adiponectin, adipose tissue produces other mediators, such as cytokines, chemokines, and steroid hormones, which allow adipose tissue to function as a link between lipid metabolism, nutrition, and inflammatory responses. The total number of adipocytes is established by the time of adolescence and is higher in people who were obese as children, providing another reason for concern about childhood obesity. Although in adults approximately 10% of adipocytes turn over annually, the number of adipocytes remains constant, regardless of individual body mass. Diets fail in part because the loss of fat from adipocytes causes leptin levels to fall, stimulating the appetite and diminishing energy expenditure.

Gut Hormones

Gut hormones are rapidly acting initiators and terminators of volitional eating. Prototypical examples are ghrelin and peptide YY (PYY). *Ghrelin* is produced in the stomach and the arcuate nucleus of the hypothalamus. It increases food intake, acting most likely by stimulating the NPY/AgRP neurons in the hypothalamus. Ghrelin levels normally rise before meals and fall 1 to 2 hours afterward, but this drop is attenuated in obese persons. Ghrelin levels are lower in obese individuals as compared to those with normal weight, and they increase with a reduction in obesity. Interestingly, the rise in ghrelin levels is much reduced in individuals in whom gastric bypass surgery is performed for the treatment of obesity, suggesting that the beneficial effects of such surgery may be in part due to a reduced surface of gastric mucosa that is exposed to food.

PYY is secreted from endocrine cells in the ileum and colon in response to the consumption of food. It decreases appetite and augments a sense of fullness (satiety). It acts, presumably, by stimulating POMC/CART neurons in the hypothalamus, thereby decreasing food intake.

PYY also reduces the rate of gastric emptying and intestinal motility ("ilea brake"), all of which contribute to satiety. PYY levels are reduced with obesity and may be of therapeutic value in the treatment of those who are overweight or obese.

The Role of Gut Microbiome

An interesting series of observations suggest that the gut microbiome may be involved in the development of obesity. In support of this notion is the finding that the profiles of gut microbiota differ between genetically obese mice and their lean littermates. The microbiome of genetically obese mice can harvest much more energy from food as compared to that of lean mice. Colonization of the gut of germfree mice by microbiota from obese mice (but not microbiota from lean mice) is associated with increased body weight. The relevance of these models to human obesity is tantalizing but remains to be proven.

Clinical Consequences of Obesity

Obesity, particularly central obesity, is a known risk factor for a number of conditions, including type 2 diabetes, cardiovascular disease, and cancer. Central obesity also stands at the center of a cluster of alterations known as the *metabolic syndrome*, characterized by abnormalities of glucose and lipid metabolism coupled with hypertension and evidence of a systemic proinflammatory state. This seems to be caused by the inflammasome response to free fatty acids and excess levels of lipids in cells and tissue. The inflammasome stimulates secretion of IL-1, which induces insulin resistance. The following associations are worthy of note:

- *Obesity is associated with insulin resistance and hyperinsulinemia,* important features of type 2 diabetes (Chapter 20). Excess insulin, in turn, may play a role in the retention of sodium, expansion of blood volume, production of excess norepinephrine, and smooth muscle proliferation that are the hallmarks of hypertension. Whatever the mechanism, the risk of developing hypertension among previously normotensive persons increases proportionately with weight.
- *Obese persons generally have hypertriglyceridemia and low HDL cholesterol levels,* factors that increase the risk of coronary artery disease. The association between obesity and heart disease is not straightforward, however, and such linkage as there is relates more to the associated diabetes and hypertension than to weight per se.

- *Nonalcoholic fatty liver disease* is commonly associated with obesity and type 2 diabetes. It can progress to fibrosis and cirrhosis (Chapter 16).

- *Cholelithiasis (gallstones)* is six times more common in obese than in lean subjects. The mechanism is mainly an increase in total body cholesterol, increased cholesterol turnover, and augmented biliary excretion of cholesterol in the bile, which in turn predisposes affected persons to the formation of cholesterol-rich gallstones (Chapter 16).

- *Hypoventilation syndrome* is a constellation of respiratory abnormalities in very obese persons. It has been called the pickwickian syndrome, after the fat lad who was constantly falling asleep in Charles Dickens' *The Pickwick Papers.* Hypersomnolence, both at night and during the day, is characteristic and is often associated with apneic pauses during sleep (sleep apnea), polycythemia, and eventual right-sided heart failure.

- *Marked adiposity is a predisposing factor for the development of degenerative joint disease* (osteoarthritis). This form of arthritis, which typically appears in older persons, is attributed in large part to the cumulative effects of wear and tear on joints. The greater the body burden of fat, the greater the trauma to joints with the passage of time.

- Markers of inflammation, such as C-reactive protein (CRP) and proinflammatory cytokines like TNF, are often elevated in obese persons. The basis for the inflammation is uncertain; both a direct proinflammatory effect of excess circulating lipids and increased release of cytokines from fat-laden adipocytes have been proposed. Whatever the cause, it is thought that chronic inflammation may contribute to many of the complications of obesity, including insulin resistance, metabolic abnormalities, thrombosis, cardiovascular disease, and cancer.

Obesity and Cancer

There is an increased incidence of certain cancers in the overweight, including cancers of the esophagus, thyroid, colon, and kidney in men and cancers of the esophagus, endometrium, gallbladder, and kidney in women. Overall, obesity is associated with approximately 20% of cancer deaths in women and 14% of deaths in men. The underlying mechanisms are unknown and are likely to be multiple.

- *Elevated insulin levels.* Insulin resistance leads to hyperinsulinemia, which includes multiple effects that may directly or indirectly contribute to cancer. For example, hyperinsulinemia causes a rise in levels of free insulin-like growth factor-1 (IGF-1). IGF-1 is a mitogen, and its receptor, IGFR-1, is highly expressed in many human cancers. IGFR-1 activates the RAS and PI3K/AKT pathways, which promote the growth of both normal and neoplastic cells (Chapter 6).

- Obesity has effects on *steroid hormones* that regulate cell growth and differentiation in the breast, uterus, and other tissues. Specifically, obesity increases the synthesis of estrogen from androgen precursors, increases androgen synthesis in ovaries and adrenals, and enhances estrogen availability in obese persons by inhibiting the production of sex-hormone–binding globulin (SHBG) in the liver.

- As discussed earlier, *adiponectin* secretion from adipose tissue is reduced in obese individuals. Adiponectin suppresses cell proliferation and promotes apoptosis. It also counteracts the actions of p53 and p21. In obese individuals these anti-neoplastic actions of adiponectin may be compromised.

- The *proinflammatory state* that is associated with obesity may itself be carcinogenic, through mechanisms discussed in Chapter 6.

SUMMARY

OBESITY

- Obesity is a disorder of energy regulation. It increases the risk for a number of important conditions such as insulin resistance, type 2 diabetes, hypertension, and hypertriglyceridemia, which are associated with the development of coronary artery disease.

- The regulation of energy balance is very complex. It has three main components: (1) afferent signals, provided mostly by insulin, leptin, ghrelin, and peptide YY; (2) the central hypothalamic system, which integrates afferent signals and triggers the efferent signals; and (3) efferent signals, which control energy balance.

- Leptin plays a key role in energy balance. Its output from adipose tissues is regulated by the abundance of fat stores. Leptin binding to its receptors in the hypothalamus reduces food intake by stimulating POMC/CART neurons and inhibiting NPY/AgRP neurons.

- In addition to diabetes and cardiovascular disease, obesity also is associated with increased risk for certain cancers, nonalcoholic fatty liver disease, and gallstones.

Diet and Systemic Diseases

The problems of under- and overnutrition, as well as specific nutrient deficiencies, have been discussed; however, the composition of the diet, even in the absence of any of these problems, may make a significant contribution to the causation and progression of a number of diseases. A few examples suffice here.

Currently, one of the most important and controversial issues is the contribution of diet to atherogenesis. The central question is whether dietary modification—specifically, reduction in the consumption of foods high in cholesterol and saturated animal fats (e.g., eggs, butter, beef)—can reduce serum cholesterol levels and prevent or retard the development of atherosclerosis (of most importance, coronary heart disease) in those with no previous episode of cardiovascular disease. This is called "primary prevention". We know some but not all the answers. The average adult in the United States consumes a large amount of fat and cholesterol daily, with a ratio of saturated fatty acids to polyunsaturated fatty acids of about 3:1. Lowering the level of saturates to the level of the polyunsaturates causes a 10% to 15% reduction in serum cholesterol within a few weeks. Vegetable oils (e.g., corn and safflower oils) and fish oils contain polyunsaturated fatty acids and are good sources of such cholesterol-lowering lipids. Fish oil fatty acids belonging to the omega-3, or *n*-3, family have more double bonds than do the omega-6, or *n*-6, fatty acids found in vegetable oils. A corollary of this idea is that supplementation of diet with fish oils might protect against atherosclerosis. One study of Dutch men whose usual daily diet contained 30 g of fish showed a substantially lower frequency of death from coronary heart disease than that among comparable control subjects. However, other studies have shown that omega-3 fatty acid supplements do not reduce the risk of cardiovascular diseases, suggesting that yet unknown components of fish may be required for cardioprotection.

Other specific effects of diet on disease have been recognized:

- Restricting sodium intake reduces hypertension.
- Dietary fiber, or roughage, resulting in increased fecal bulk, is thought by some investigators to provide a preventive effect against diverticulosis of the colon.
- Caloric restriction has been convincingly demonstrated to increase life span in experimental animals, including monkeys. The basis for this striking observation is not clear (Chapter 2).
- Even lowly garlic has been touted to protect against heart disease (and also, alas, against kisses—and the devil), although research has yet to prove this effect unequivocally.

Diet and Cancer

With respect to carcinogenesis, three aspects of the diet are of concern: (1) the content of exogenous carcinogens, (2) the endogenous synthesis of carcinogens from dietary components, and (3) the lack of protective factors.

- An example of an exogenous carcinogen is *aflatoxin*, which is an important factor in the development of hepatocellular carcinomas in parts of Asia and Africa. Exposure to aflatoxin causes a specific mutation (codon 249) in the *TP53* gene in tumor cells. The mutation can be used as a molecular signature for aflatoxin exposure in epidemiologic studies.
- The concern about *endogenous* synthesis of carcinogens or promoters from components of the diet relates principally to gastric carcinomas. *Nitrosamines and nitrosamides* are suspected to generate these tumors in humans, as they induce gastric cancer in animals. These compounds are formed in the body from nitrites and amines or amides derived from digested proteins. Sources of nitrites include sodium nitrite, added to foods as a preservative, and nitrates, present in common vegetables, which are reduced in the gut by bacterial flora. There is, then, the potential for endogenous production of carcinogenic agents from dietary components, which might well have an effect on the stomach.
- *High animal fat intake combined with low fiber intake has been implicated in the causation of colon cancer.* The most convincing explanation for this association is as follows: High fat intake increases the level of bile acids in the gut, which in turn modifies intestinal flora, favoring the growth of microaerophilic bacteria. The bile acids or bile acid metabolites produced by these bacteria might serve as carcinogens or promoters. The protective effect of a high-fiber diet might relate to (1) increased stool bulk and decreased transit time, which decreases the exposure of mucosa to putative offenders, and (2) the capacity of certain fibers to bind carcinogens and thereby protect the mucosa. Attempts to document these

theories in clinical and experimental studies have, on the whole, led to contradictory results.

- Vitamins C and E, β-carotenes, and selenium have been assumed to have anti-carcinogenic effects because of their anti-oxidant properties. To date, however, no convincing evidence has emerged to show that these antioxidants act as chemopreventive agents. As already mentioned, retinoic acid promotes epithelial differentiation and is believed to reverse squamous metaplasia.

Thus, despite many tantalizing trends and proclamations by "diet gurus," to date there is no definite proof that diet in general can cause or protect against cancer. Nonetheless, concern persists that carcinogens lurk in things as pleasurable as a juicy steak and rich ice cream.

SUGGESTED READINGS

Bellinger DC: Lead, *Pediatrics* 113:1016, 2004. *[An excellent overview of the subject.]*

Boffetta P, Hecht S, Gray N, et al: Smokeless tobacco and cancer, *Lancet Oncol* 9:667, 2009. *[A review of cancer risks associated with smokeless tobacco worldwide.]*

Casals-Casas C, Desvergne B: Endocrine disruptors: from endocrine to metabolic disruption, *Annu Rev Phys* 73:135, 2011. *[An update discussing the scope and possible consequences of human exposure to this class of chemical.]*

Global Burden of Disease Study 2010: *Lancet*, epublished December 13, 2012. *[An entire issue of this journal devoted to a detailed summary of the latest global disease data from the GBD project.]*

Graham C, Mullen A, Whelan K: Obesity and gastrointestinal microbiota: a review of associations and mechanisms, *Nutr Rev* 73:376, 2016. *[A review of the emerging data on the role of the microbiome in obesity.]*

Gregor MF, Hotamisligil GS: Inflammatory mechanisms in obesity, *Annu Rev Immunol* 29:445, 2011. *[A concise discussion of current views of the proinflammatory state associated with obesity.]*

Hanna-Attisha M, LaChance J, Sadler RC, et al: Elevated blood lead levels in children associated with the Flint drinking water crisis: a spatial analysis of risk and public health response, *Am J Public Health* 106:283, 2016. *[An article that discusses public health issues resulting from water pollution with lead in Flint, Michigan, USA.]*

Hollick MF: Vitamin D deficiency, *N Engl J Med* 357:266, 2007. *[A comprehensive review of vitamin D deficiency.]*

McCreanor J, Cullinan P, Nieuwenhuijsen MJ, et al: Respiratory effects of exposure to diesel traffic in persons with asthma, *N Engl J Med* 357:2348, 2007. *[A paper discussing the danger of particulates in diesel exhaust to patients with asthma.]*

Matthew JD, Forsythe AV, Brady Z, et al: Cancer risk in 680,000 people exposed to computed tomography scans in childhood or adolescence: data linkage study of 11 million Australians, *BMJ* 346:f2360, 2013. *[A paper showing that children who have undergone CT scans have a 24% increased risk of cancer, adding to accruing evidence that CT scans increase the risk of secondary cancers in children and adolescents.]*

Manson JE, Hsia J, Johnson KC, et al: Estrogen plus progestin and the risk of coronary heart disease, *N Engl J Med* 349:523, 2003. *[A landmark study from the Women's Health Initiative.]*

Nigro E, Scudiero O, Monaco ML, et al: New insights into adiponectin role in obesity and obesity-related diseases, *Biomed Res Int* 2014:658913, 2014. doi: 10.1155/2014/658913. Epub July 7, 2014. *[Role of adiponectin in fat utilization and other systemic effects.]*

Pope CA, Ezzati M, Dockery DW: Fine-particulate air pollution and life expectancy in the United States, *N Engl J Med* 360:376, 2009. *[A* paper correlating increases in life expectancy in major U.S. cities with decreases in fine-particulate air pollution.]

Ravdin PM, Cronin KA, Howlader N, et al: The decrease in breast cancer incidence in 2003 in the United States, *N Engl J Med* 356:1670, 2007. [*A paper documenting the decrease in breast cancer that followed its linkage to menopausal hormone therapy.*]

Rice KM, Walker EM Jr, Wu M, et al: Environmental mercury and its toxic effects, *J Prev Med Public Health* 47:74, 2014. [*Mercury toxicity review.*]

Roberts DL, Dive C, Renehan AG: Biological mechanisms linking obesity and cancer risk: new perspectives, *Annu Rev Med* 61:301, 2010. [*A discussion of the possible interactions between obesity and cancer.*]

Seitz HK, Stickel F: Molecular mechanisms of alcohol-mediated carcinogenesis, *Nat Rev Cancer* 7:599, 2007. [*A review of the multifactorial effects of alcohol that may contribute to cancer development.*]

Tang X-H, Gudas LJ: Retinoids, retinoic acid receptors, and cancer, *Annu Rev Pathol* 6:345, 2011. [*A review of the role of retinoids in cancer, with a focus on solid tumors.*]

van der Klaauw AA, Farooqi IS: The hunger genes: pathways to obesity, *Cell* 161:119, 2015. [*A succinct review of the afferent pathways to obesity.*]

Wilson J, Enriori PJ: A talk between fat tissue, gut, pancreas, and brain to control body weight, *Mol Cell Endocrinol* 418:108, 2015. [*Excellent discussion of the various afferent pathways in obesity.*]

General Pathology of Infectious Diseases

9

CHAPTER OUTLINE

General Principles of Microbial
  Pathogenesis 341
Categories of Infectious Agents 341
The Microbiome 346
Techniques for Identifying Infectious
  Agents 346
Newly Emerging and
  Reemerging Infectious
  Diseases 347
Agents of Bioterrorism 348

Transmission and Dissemination of
  Microbes 349
Routes of Entry of Microbes 349
*Spread and Dissemination of Microbes Within
  the Body 351*
Transmission of Microbes 352
How Microorganisms Cause Disease 352
Mechanisms of Viral Injury 353
Mechanisms of Bacterial Injury 353
Injurious Effects of Host Immune Responses 355

Immune Evasion by Microbes 355
Spectrum of Inflammatory Responses to
  Infection 357
*Mononuclear and Granulomatous
  Inflammation 357*
Cytopathic-Cytoproliferative Reaction 357
Tissue Necrosis 358
Chronic Inflammation and Scarring 358
*Infections in Individuals With
  Immunodeficiencies 358*

Humans are prey to thousands of infectious agents ranging from submicroscopic viruses to several meters long tape worms. This chapter reviews the general principles of the pathogenesis of infectious disease and describes the characteristic histopathologic changes caused by different types of microbes. Infections that involve specific organs are discussed in other chapters of this book.

GENERAL PRINCIPLES OF MICROBIAL PATHOGENESIS

Infectious diseases are an important health problem in the United States and worldwide despite the availability of effective vaccines and antibiotics for many types of infections. Influenza and pneumonia combined are the eighth leading cause of death in the United States. In low-income countries, limited access to healthcare, unsanitary living conditions, and malnutrition contribute to a massive burden of infectious diseases. Lower-respiratory infections, HIV/AIDS, and diarrheal diseases are the top three causes of death in developing countries, and malaria and tuberculosis are among the top ten. Infectious diseases are particularly important causes of death among children, older adults, individuals with chronic debilitating diseases and inherited or acquired immunodeficiency states (e.g., AIDS), and in patients receiving immunosuppressive drugs.

Categories of Infectious Agents

Infectious agents belong to a wide range of classes and vary greatly in size, ranging from prion protein aggregates of under 20 nm to tapeworms 10 meters in length (Table 9.1).

Prions

Prions are composed of abnormal forms of a host protein termed *prion protein (PrP)*. These agents cause transmissible spongiform encephalopathies, including kuru (associated with human cannibalism), hereditary or sporadic Creutzfeldt-Jakob disease (CJD), bovine spongiform encephalopathy (BSE) (better known as *mad cow disease*), and variant Creutzfeldt-Jakob disease (vCJD) (probably transmitted to humans through consumption of meat from BSE-infected cattle). PrP is found normally in neurons. Diseases occur when the PrP undergoes a conformational change that confers resistance to proteases. The protease-resistant PrP promotes conversion of the normal protease-sensitive PrP to the abnormal form, explaining the transmissable nature of these diseases. CJD can be transmitted from person to person iatrogenically, by surgery, organ transplantation, or blood transfusion. These diseases are discussed in detail in Chapter 23.

Viruses

Viruses are obligate intracellular parasites that depend on the host cell's metabolic machinery for their replication. They consist of a nucleic acid genome surrounded by a protein coat (called a *capsid*) that is sometimes encased in a lipid membrane. Viruses are classified by their nucleic acid genome (DNA or RNA, but not both), the shape of the capsid (icosahedral or helical), the presence or absence of a lipid envelope, their mode of replication, their preferred cell type for replication (called *tropism*), or the type of

Table 9.1 Classes of Human Pathogens

Taxonomic Category	Size	Propagation Site(s)	Example(s)	Disease(s)
Prions	<20 nm	Intracellular	Prion protein	Creutzfeldt-Jacob disease
Viruses	20–400 nm	Obligate intracellular	Poliovirus	Poliomyelitis
Bacteria	0.2–15 μm	Obligate intracellular Extracellular Facultative intracellular	*Chlamydia trachomatis* *Streptococcus pneumoniae* *Mycobacterium tuberculosis*	Trachoma, urethritis Pneumonia Tuberculosis
Fungi	2–200 μm	Extracellular Facultative intracellular	*Candida albicans* *Histoplasma capsulatum*	Thrush Histoplasmosis
Protozoa	1–50 μm	Extracellular Facultative intracellular Obligate intracellular	*Trypanosoma brucei* *Trypanosoma cruzi* *Leishmania donovani*	Sleeping sickness Chagas disease Kala-azar
Helminths	3 mm–10 m	Extracellular Intracellular	*Wuchereria bancrofti* *Trichinella spiralis*	Filariasis Trichinosis

pathology they cause. Some viral components and particles aggregate within infected cells and form characteristic *inclusion bodies,* which may be seen with the light microscope and are useful for diagnosis (Fig. 9.1). For example, cytomegalovirus (CMV)-infected cells are enlarged and show a large eosinophilic nuclear inclusion and smaller basophilic cytoplasmic inclusions; herpesviruses form a large nuclear inclusion surrounded by a clear halo; and both smallpox and rabies viruses form characteristic cytoplasmic inclusions. However, many viruses (e.g., poliovirus) do not produce inclusions.

Accounting for a large share of human infections, viruses can cause disease in several ways (Table 9.2). Many viruses cause transient illnesses (e.g., colds, influenza). Other viruses are not eliminated from the body and persist within cells of the host for years, either continuing to multiply (e.g., chronic infection with hepatitis B virus [HBV]) or survive in some latent nonreplicating form, with the potential to be reactivated later. For example, herpes zoster virus, the cause of chickenpox, can enter dorsal root ganglia and establish latency at the site, with periodic reactivation at later times to cause shingles, a painful skin condition. Some viruses are involved in transformation of a host cell into a benign or malignant tumor (e.g., human papillomavirus [HPV]-induced benign warts and cervical carcinoma). Different species of viruses can produce the same clinical picture (e.g., adenovirus and rhinovirus

causing upper respiratory infection); conversely, a single virus can cause different clinical manifestations depending on the age or immune status of the host (e.g., CMV causing congenital neurologic damage or gastroenteritis in the immunocompromised).

Bacteria

Bacteria are *prokaryotes,* meaning that they have a cell membrane but lack membrane-bound nuclei and other membrane-enclosed organelles. Most bacteria are bounded by a cell wall consisting of peptidoglycan, a polymer of long sugar chains linked by peptide bridges surrounding the cell membrane. There are two common forms of cell wall structure: a thick wall that retains crystal-violet stain (gram-positive bacteria) and a thin cell wall surrounded by an outer membrane (gram-negative bacteria) (Fig. 9.2). Bacteria are classified by Gram staining (positive or negative), shape (spherical, called *cocci,* or rod-shaped, called *bacilli*) (Fig. 9.3), and their requirement for oxygen (aerobic or anaerobic). Motile bacteria have flagella, long helical filaments extending from the cell surface that rotate and move the bacteria. Some bacteria possess pili, another kind of surface projection that can attach bacteria to host cells or extracellular matrix. Bacteria synthesize their own DNA, RNA, and proteins, but they depend on the host for favorable growth conditions. Many bacteria remain extracellular when they grow in the host, while

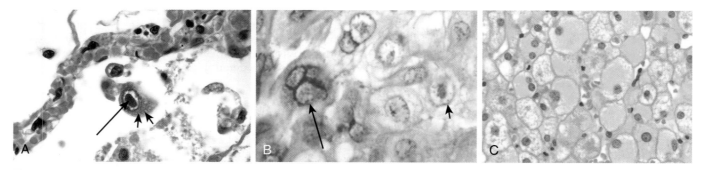

Fig. 9.1 Examples of viral inclusions. (A) Cytomegalovirus infection in the lung. Infected cells show distinct nuclear *(long arrow)* and ill-defined cytoplasmic *(short arrows)* inclusions. (B) Varicella-zoster virus infection in the skin. Herpes simplex virus and varicella-zoster virus both cause characteristic cytopathologic changes, including fusion of epithelial cells, which produces multinucleate cells with molding of nuclei to one another *(long arrow)*, and eosinophilic haloed nuclear inclusions *(short arrow)*. (C) Hepatitis B viral infection in liver. In chronic infections, infected hepatocytes show diffuse granular ("ground-glass") cytoplasm, reflecting accumulated hepatitis B surface antigen (HBsAg).

Table 9.2 Selected Human Viral Diseases and Their Pathogens

Organ System	Pathogen	Disease(s)
Respiratory	Adenovirus	Upper- and lower-respiratory tract infections, conjunctivitis
	Rhinovirus	Upper-respiratory tract infection
	Influenza viruses A, B	Influenza
	Respiratory syncytial virus	Bronchiolitis, pneumonia
Digestive	Mumps virus	Mumps, pancreatitis, orchitis
	Rotavirus	Childhood gastroenteritis
	Norovirus	Gastroenteritis
	Hepatitis A virus	Acute viral hepatitis
	Hepatitis B virus	Acute or chronic hepatitis
	Hepatitis D virus	*With hepatitis B virus infection:* acute or chronic hepatitis
	Hepatitis C virus	Acute or chronic hepatitis
	Hepatitis E virus	Acute viral hepatitis
Systemic		
With skin eruptions	Measles virus	Measles (rubeola)
	Rubella virus	German measles (rubella)
	Varicella-zoster virus	Chickenpox, shingles
	Herpes simplex virus type 1	Oral herpes ("cold sore")
	Herpes simplex virus type 2	Genital herpes
With hematopoietic disorders	Cytomegalovirus	Cytomegalic inclusion disease in the newborn, gastroenteritis in transplant patients
	Epstein-Barr virus	Infectious mononucleosis
	HIV-1 and HIV-2	AIDS
Skin/genital warts	Papillomavirus	Condyloma; cervical carcinoma
Central nervous system	Poliovirus	Poliomyelitis
	JC virus	Progressive multifocal leukoencephalopathy (opportunistic)
	Zika virus	Congenital microcephaly

AIDS, Acquired immunodeficiency syndrome; *HIV*, human immunodeficiency virus.

others can survive and replicate both outside and inside of host cells (*facultative intracellular* bacteria such as mycobacteria), and some grow only inside host cells (*obligate intracellular* bacteria, such as rickettsia).

Bacteria cause a range of infections from common pharyngitis and urinary tract infections to rare diseases such as leprosy (Table 9.3). *Chlamydia* and *Rickettsia* are obligate intracellular bacteria that replicate inside membrane-bound vacuoles in epithelial and endothelial cells, respectively. These bacteria get most or all of their energy source, ATP, from the host cell. *Chlamydia trachomatis* is a frequent infectious cause of female sterility (by scarring and narrowing of the fallopian tubes) and blindness (by chronic inflammation of the conjunctiva that eventually causes scarring and opacification of the cornea). *Rickettsiae* injure the endothelial cells in which they grow, causing a hemorrhagic vasculitis, often visible as a rash, but they also may injure the central nervous system (CNS), with potentially fatal outcome, as in Rocky Mountain spotted fever and epidemic typhus. *Rickettsiae* are transmitted by arthropod vectors, including lice (in epidemic typhus), ticks (in Rocky Mountain spotted fever and ehrlichiosis), and mites (in scrub typhus).

Mycoplasma and the related genus *Ureaplasma* are unique among extracellular bacterial pathogens in that they do not have a cell wall. These are the tiniest free-living organisms known (125 to 300 nm).

Fungi

Fungi are eukaryotes with thick cell walls composed of complex carbohydrates such as beta-glucans, chitin, and mannosylated glycoproteins. Calcofluor-white, a

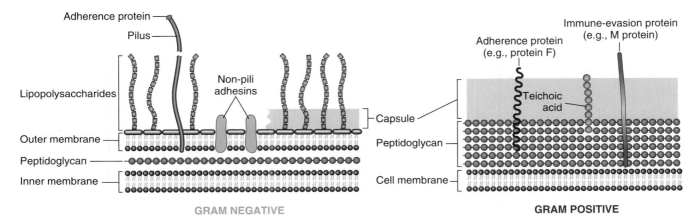

Fig. 9.2 Molecules on the surface of gram-negative and gram-positive bacteria involved in the pathogenesis of infection.

Table 9.3 Selected Human Bacterial Diseases and Their Pathogens

Microbiologic Category / Clinical Category	Species	Frequent Disease Presentation(s)
Infections by pyogenic cocci	*Staphylococcus aureus, Staphylococcus epidermidis*	Abscess, cellulitis, pneumonia, sepsis
	Streptococcus pyogenes	Pharyngitis, erysipelas, scarlet fever
	Streptococcus pneumoniae	Lobar pneumonia, meningitis
	Neisseria meningitidis	Meningitis
	Neisseria gonorrhoeae	Gonorrhea
Gram-negative infections	*Escherichia coli, Klebsiella pneumoniae, Enterobacter aerogenes, Proteus mirabilis, Serratia marcescens, Pseudomonas aeruginosa, Bacteroides fragilis*	Urinary tract infection, wound infection, abscess, pneumonia, sepsis, shock, endocarditis
	Legionella pneumophila	Legionnaires' disease
Clostridial infections	*Clostridium tetani*	Tetanus (lockjaw)
	Clostridium botulinum	Botulism (paralytic food poisoning)
	Clostridium perfringens, Clostridium septicum	Gas gangrene, necrotizing cellulitis
	Clostridium difficile	Pseudomembranous colitis
Zoonotic bacterial infections	*Bacillus anthracis*	Anthrax
	Yersinia pestis	Bubonic plague
	Francisella tularensis	Tularemia
	Brucella melitensis, Brucella suis, Brucella abortus	Brucellosis (undulant fever)
	Borrelia recurrentis	Relapsing fever
	Borrelia burgdorferi	Lyme disease
Treponemal infections	*Treponema pallidum*	Syphilis
Mycobacterial infections	*Mycobacterium tuberculosis, M. bovis*	Tuberculosis
	Mycobacterium leprae	Leprosy
	Mycobacterium kansasii, Mycobacterium avium complex	Pulmonary disease, lymphadenitis, disseminated disease
Actinomycetal infections	*Nocardia asteroides complex*	Pulmonary disease, brain abscess
	Actinomyces israelii	Head and neck abscess
Contagious childhood bacterial diseases	*Haemophilus influenzae*	Meningitis, upper- and lower-respiratory tract infections
	Bordetella pertussis	Whooping cough
	Corynebacterium diphtheriae	Diphtheria
Enteric infections	Enteropathogenic *E. coli, Shigella* spp., *Vibrio cholera, Campylobacter jejuni, Campylobacter coli, Yersinia enterocolitica, Salmonella* spp.	Invasive or noninvasive gastroenterocolitis
	Salmonella enterica serotype Typhi	Typhoid fever

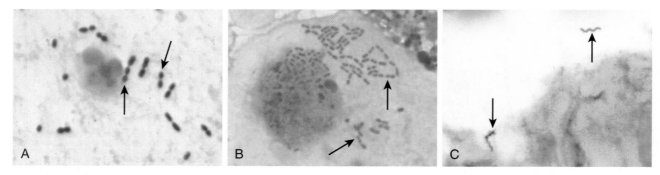

Fig. 9.3 Bacterial morphologies. The bacteria are indicated by arrows. (A) Gram stain preparation of sputum from a patient with pneumonia. Gram-positive, elongated cocci in pairs and short chains *(Streptococcus pneumoniae)* and a neutrophil are evident. (B) Gram stain preparation of a bronchoalveolar lavage specimen showing gram-negative intracellular rods typical of members of *Enterobacteriaceae* such as *Klebsiella pneumoniae* or *Escherichia coli*. (C) Silver stain preparation of brain tissue from a patient with Lyme disease meningoencephalitis. Two helical spirochetes *(Borrelia burgdorferi)* are shown *(arrows)*. (A), (B), and (C) are at different magnifications. *(A and C, Courtesy of Dr. Kenneth Van Horn, Focus Diagnostics, Cypress, California. B, Courtesy of Dr. Karen Krisher, Clinical Microbiology Institute, Wilsonville, Oregon.)*

fluorescent stain that binds chitin, provides a useful way to identify fungi in patient specimens. Assays for beta-glucans in blood are used to diagnose disseminated fungal infections. Fungi can grow either as rounded yeast cells or as slender, filamentous hyphae. An important distinguishing characteristic is whether hyphae are septate (with cell walls separating individual cells) or aseptate. Some of the most important pathogenic fungi exhibit thermal dimorphism; that is, they grow as hyphal forms at room temperature but as yeast forms at body temperature. Fungi may produce sexual spores or, more commonly, asexual spores called *conidia*. The latter are produced on specialized structures or fruiting bodies arising along the hyphal filament.

Fungi may cause superficial or deep infections.

- *Superficial infections* involve the skin, hair, and nails. Fungal species that cause superficial infections are called *dermatophytes*. Infection of the skin is called *tinea*; thus, *tinea pedis* is "athlete's foot" and *tinea capitis* is scalp ringworm. Certain fungi invade the subcutaneous tissue, causing abscesses or granulomas. Chronic infections, often in the foot, are called *mycetomas*.
- *Deep fungal infections* can spread systemically and invade tissues, destroying vital organs in immunocompromised hosts, but usually resolve or remain latent in otherwise normal hosts.

Fungi are divided into endemic and opportunistic species.

- *Endemic fungi* are invasive species that are usually limited to particular geographic regions (e.g., *Coccidioides* in the southwestern United States, *Histoplasma* in the Ohio River Valley).
- *Opportunistic fungi* (e.g., *Candida, Aspergillus, Mucor, Cryptococcus*), by contrast, are ubiquitous organisms that either colonize individuals or are encountered from environmental sources but do not cause severe disease in healthy individuals. In immunodeficient individuals, opportunistic fungi give rise to life-threatening invasive infections characterized by vascular occlusion, hemorrhage, and tissue necrosis, with little or no inflammatory response (Fig. 9.4). Patients with AIDS are very susceptible to infection with the opportunistic fungus *Pneumocystis jiroveci* (previously called *Pneumocystis carinii*).

Protozoa

Protozoa are single-celled eukaryotes that are major causes of disease and death in developing countries. Protozoa can replicate intracellularly within a variety of cells (e.g., *Plasmodium* in red cells, *Leishmania* in macrophages) or extracellularly in the urogenital system, intestine, or blood. *Trichomonas vaginalis* organisms are sexually transmitted flagellated protozoal parasites that often colonize the vagina and male urethra. The most prevalent pathogenic intestinal protozoans, *Entamoeba histolytica* and *Giardia lamblia*, are ingested as nonmotile *cysts* in contaminated food or water and become motile *trophozoites* that attach to intestinal epithelial cells. Bloodborne protozoa (e.g., *Plasmodium, Trypanosoma, Leishmania*) are transmitted by insect vectors, in which they replicate before being

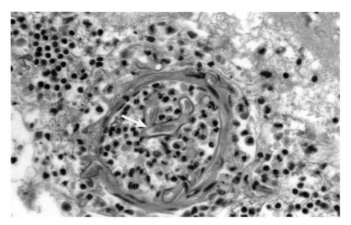

Fig. 9.4 Meningeal blood vessels with angioinvasive *Mucor* species. Note the irregular width and near right-angle branching of the hyphae *(arrow)*. *(Courtesy of Dr. Dan Milner, Department of Pathology, Brigham and Women's Hospital, Boston, Massachusetts.)*

passed to new human hosts. *Toxoplasma gondii* is acquired either through contact with oocyst-shedding cats or by eating cyst-ridden, undercooked meat.

Helminths

Parasitic worms are highly differentiated multicellular organisms. Their life cycles are complex; most alternate between sexual reproduction in the definitive host and asexual multiplication in an intermediate host or vector. Thus, depending on the species, humans may harbor adult worms (e.g., *Ascaris lumbricoides*), immature stages (e.g., *Toxocara canis*), or asexual larval forms (e.g., *Echinococcus* spp.). Once adult worms take up residence in humans, they usually do not multiply but they produce eggs or larvae that typically are passed in stool. Often, the severity of disease is proportional to the number of infecting organisms. For example, a burden of 10 hookworms is associated with mild or no clinical disease, whereas 1000 hookworms consume enough blood to cause severe anemia. In some helminthic infections, such as schistosomiasis, disease is caused by inflammatory responses to the eggs or larvae rather than the adult worms.

Helminths comprise three groups:

- *Roundworms (nematodes)* are circular in cross-section and nonsegmented. Intestinal nematodes include *A. lumbricoides, Strongyloides stercoralis,* and hookworms. Nematodes that invade tissues include the filariae, such as *Wuchereria bancrofti* and *Trichinella spiralis* (Fig. 9.5).
- *Tapeworms (cestodes)* have a head (scolex) and a ribbon of multiple flat segments (proglottids). They adsorb nutrition through their tegument and do not have a digestive tract. They include the fish, beef, and pork tapeworms that make their home in the human intestine. The larvae that develop after ingestion of eggs of certain tapeworms can cause cystic disease within tissues (*Echinococcus granulosus* larvae cause *hydatid* cysts; pork tapeworm larvae produce cysts called *cysticerci* in many organs).
- *Flukes (trematodes)* are leaf-shaped flatworms with prominent suckers that are used to attach to the host. They include liver and lung flukes and schistosomes.

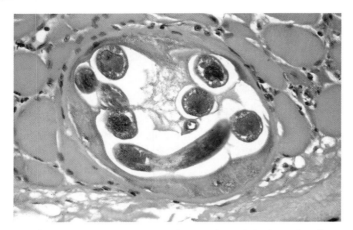

Fig. 9.5 Coiled *Trichinella spiralis* larva within a skeletal muscle cell.

Ectoparasites

Ectoparasites are insects (e.g., lice, bedbugs, fleas) or arachnids (e.g., mites, ticks, spiders) that cause disease by biting or by attaching to and living on or in the skin. Infestation of the skin by arthropods is characterized by itching and excoriations, such as pediculosis caused by lice attached to hairs, or scabies caused by mites burrowing into the stratum corneum. At the site of bites, mouth parts may be found associated with a mixed infiltrate of lymphocytes, macrophages, and eosinophils. Arthropods also can serve as vectors for other pathogens, such as *Borrelia burgdorferi*, the agent of Lyme disease, which is transmitted by deer ticks.

THE MICROBIOME

The microbiome is the diverse microbial population of bacteria, fungi, and viruses found in or on the human body (e.g., in the intestinal tract, skin, upper airway, and vagina). While most of these organisms do not harm the healthy host, a few cause diseases such as skin and soft-tissue infections (*Staphylococcus aureus* and *Streptococcus pyogenes*), acne (*Propionibacterium acnes*), and tooth decay (*Streptococcus mitus*). The microbiome has important roles in normal health and development. In the intestinal tract, the normal flora are responsible for absorption of digested foods, for maintaining the integrity of the epithelium and the normal functioning of the intestinal immune system, and for competitively inhibiting invasion and colonization by potentially pathogenic microbes. The gut microbiome is also emerging as a regulator of nutritional status.

New techniques of bacterial identification relying on ribosomal RNA sequencing have dramatically improved our understanding of the microbiome:

- In healthy individuals, the microbiome is very diverse. For example, there are estimated to be over 1000 species of bacteria in the normal intestinal flora of an individual. In a healthy person, a part of the bacterial population at various body sites is relatively stable over time, but may be altered by diet and environment.
- The diversity of bacteria is greatest in the oral cavity and the stool, intermediate on the skin, and least in the vagina.
- The bacterial microbiomes at various body sites are partially similar in different individuals.

Dysbiosis refers to changes in composition of the microbiome that are associated with disease. These changes may result from therapies or various pathophysiologic conditions, including the following:

- Use of some antibiotics is an important risk factor for intestinal infections caused by toxin-producing *Clostridium difficile*. These antibiotics kill or inhibit normal commensal bacteria, allowing overgrowth of *C. difficile*. Restoration of the microbiome by duodenal infusion of stool containing commensal flora from healthy donors successfully treats *C. difficile* infection in many individuals who have relapsed after antibiotic therapy.
- The microbiome in the stool of obese individuals is less diverse than that of lean individuals, and the proportions of bacterial phyla differ as well. The proportions of these phyla in obese individuals who change their diet and lose weight shifts to resemble that of lean individuals. Experimental animals gain more weight when colonized with bacterial populations associated with a high-fat diet than when colonized with bacterial populations associated with a normal diet.
- The intestinal bacterial populations in individuals with inflammatory bowel disease are altered, with reduced diversity and changes in the proportions of bacterial phyla, compared to individuals without inflammatory bowel disease. Interestingly, inflammatory bowel disease also is associated with changes in the viral populations in stool. The specific roles of different viruses and bacteria in gastrointestinal dysbiosis is an area of very active investigation.

TECHNIQUES FOR IDENTIFYING INFECTIOUS AGENTS

There are several methods for identifying microorganisms in tissue and body fluids:

- *Culture.* Bacterial and fungal cultures remain essential for diagnostic testing, in conjunction with additional methods, but culture of viruses has been replaced to a great extent by alternative methods.
- *Histology.* Some infectious agents can be seen in hematoxylin and eosin (H&E)–stained sections (e.g., the inclusion bodies formed by CMV and herpes simplex virus (HSV); bacterial clumps, which usually stain blue; *Candida* and *Mucor* among the fungi; most protozoans; all helminths). Many infectious agents, however, are better visualized by special stains that identify organisms on the basis of particular characteristics of their cell wall or coat—Gram, acid-fast, silver, mucicarmine, and Giemsa stains—or after labeling with specific antibodies (Table 9.4). Organisms are usually best visualized at the advancing edge of a lesion rather than at its center, particularly if there is necrosis.
- *Serology.* Acute infections can be diagnosed serologically by detecting pathogen-specific antibodies in the serum. The presence of specific immunoglobulin M (IgM) antibody shortly after the onset of symptoms is often diagnostic. Alternatively, specific antibody titers

Table 9.4 Techniques for Identifying Infectious Agents

Technique	Infectious Agent(s)
Gram stain	Most bacteria
Wet Mount/Calcofluor-white/ Fungi-fluor	Fungi
Acid-fast stain	Mycobacteria, nocardiae (modified)
Silver stain	Fungi, legionellae, *Pneumocystis*
Periodic acid–Schiff stain	Fungi, amebae
Mucicarmine stain	Cryptococci
Giemsa stain	Leishmaniae, *Plasmodium*
Antibodies	All classes
Culture	All classes
DNA probes and polymerase chain reaction	All classes
Proteomic methods/mass spectrometry	Bacteria, mycobacteria, fungi

can be measured early ("acute") and again at 4 to 6 weeks ("convalescent") after infection; a 4-fold rise in titer usually is considered diagnostic. Assays for serum antibodies are very useful for the diagnosis of viral hepatitis. Antibodies that are not pathogen-specific are produced by patients with syphilis or infectious mononucleosis, and assays for these cross-reacting antibodies are used in diagnosis.

- *Molecular diagnostics.* Nucleic acid amplification techniques, such as polymerase chain reaction (PCR) and transcription-mediated amplification, are used for diagnosis of gonorrhea, chlamydial infection, tuberculosis, and herpes encephalitis. Molecular assays are much more sensitive than conventional testing for some pathogens. PCR testing of cerebrospinal fluid (CSF) for HSV encephalitis has a sensitivity of about 80%, whereas viral culture of CSF has a sensitivity of less than 10%. Similarly, nucleic acid tests for genital *Chlamydia* detect 10% to 30% more cases than conventional *Chlamydia* culture does. For other infections, such as gonorrhea, the sensitivity of nucleic acid testing is similar to that of culture. Quantitative PCR for BK virus, CMV, and Epstein-Barr virus (EBV) is used to assess viral loads in transplant recipients. Molecular panels for detection of 20 or more pathogens are now routinely used to diagnose respiratory bacterial and viral infections, as well as gastrointestinal bacterial, viral and parasitic infections. Quantitative assays for viral nucleic acids are used to guide the medical management of patients infected with human immunodeficiency virus (HIV), HBV, and hepatitis C virus (HCV). Next-generation sequencing, with or without initial PCR amplification, is being used for the detection of novel or rare pathogens, and for epidemiologic investigations.
- *Proteomics.* Mass spectrometry can be used to identify microorganisms based on protein content and has been introduced into routine clinical laboratories. It has the advantage of rapid identification of the bacterial species but is not useful for antibiotic sensitivity. That still requires culture.

NEWLY EMERGING AND REEMERGING INFECTIOUS DISEASES

A surprising number of new infectious agents continue to be discovered, and there are several reasons for this:

- Some pathogens were discovered due to improved methods of detection, although they have likely been present in humans for centuries. For example, *Helicobacter pylori*, which causes gastritis and peptic ulcer disease, was only discovered in the 1980s. More recently, a new cause of leprosy was discovered, *Mycobacterium lepromatosis*. This agent, identified by sequencing bacterial DNA from biopsy material of patients who died of leprosy, is a close relative of the previously known *Mycobacterium leprae*.
- Animals are a source of new pathogens that infect humans. Two coronaviruses that cause severe respiratory tract infections in humans, Middle East respiratory syndrome coronavirus (MERS CoV) and the severe acute respiratory syndrome (SARS) virus, likely spread to humans from animals and were first detected in 2003 and 2012, respectively. Other examples of pathogens that emerged in humans after being transmitted from animals include HIV and *B. burgdorferi*.
- Microorganisms can acquire genes that enhance virulence or overcome host defense. In 2011, almost 4000 individuals in Germany were infected with a new strain of highly virulent shiga-toxin producing *Escherichia coli* that spread in sprout seeds. The new strain was derived from a different type of *E. coli* that acquired a gene for the shiga-toxin from a bacteriophage.
- Other pathogens have become much more common because of immunosuppression caused by AIDS, or therapy to prevent transplant rejection or treat cancers (e.g., human herpes virus 8, *Mycobacterium avium* complex, *P. jirovecii*).

Additional clinical syndromes may be recognized after the pathogen has been known for some time, possibly due to new contributing factors. Although Zika virus was discovered in 1947 in Uganda, very few human cases were reported for many years, until the virus more recently spread through additional countries, expanding the range from Africa, Asia, and the Pacific to the Americas, causing newly recognized clinical cases. The virus is contracted primarily via the Aedes species mosquito but also via sexual transmission and possibly blood transfusion. Although many individuals infected have no or mild nonspecific symptoms, infection may be associated with Guillain-Barre syndrome, a form of rapid-onset muscle weakness caused by immune system damage to the nervous system. Infection with Zika virus during pregnancy is associated with birth defects, including microcephaly. Many more congenital cases were diagnosed in the 2015 outbreak beginning in Brazil compared to earlier outbreaks, creating a Public Health Emergency of International Concern. Further investigation is ongoing to determine if other variables may be contributing to the CNS effects such as genetics, co-infections, immunity from past infections, or yet to be defined environmental factors.

Several factors contribute to the emergence of infectious diseases:

- Human behavior affects the spread and demographics of infections. AIDS was first recognized in the United States as predominantly a disease of homosexual men and drug abusers, but heterosexual transmission is now more common. In sub-Saharan Africa, the area of the world with the highest number of AIDS cases, it is predominantly a heterosexual disease. The Ebola virus epidemic of 2014 spread to more countries than previous Ebola outbreaks due in part to the frequent movement of people across borders in West Africa, as well as burial practices that involved contact with the bodies of the deceased. SARS, mentioned earlier, spread very quickly to 24 countries due to human air travel before it was contained.
- Changes in the environment occasionally increase the incidence of infectious diseases. Regrowth of forests in the eastern United States with cessation of farming has led to massive increases in deer and mice, which carry the ticks that transmit Lyme disease, babesiosis, and ehrlichiosis. Global warming also has had an impact on the spread of infections. For example, the mosquitoes that carry Dengue fever and Zika viruses, which used to be confined to the U.S.-Mexican border, are now found in more than half of the states. Chikungunya virus transmitted by mosquitoes, which causes fever and joint pain that can be severe for some, was first seen in the Americas in 2013, and transmission of Dengue and Zika viruses has recently been reported in Florida.
- Infectious diseases that are common in one geographic area may be introduced into a new area due to increased travel or movement of infected animals, invertebrates, or birds. For example, West Nile virus has been common in Europe, Asia, and Africa for years but was first described in the United States in 1999, possibly transported by an infected mosquito or bird. Highly pathogenic H5 influenza viruses, which have led to death of some patients in Asia, have spread throughout the world during the last 2 decades in bird populations, due to their natural migration and transport of domestic birds.
- Pathogens adapt rapidly to selective pressures exerted by widespread use of antibiotics. Antibiotic resistance has developed and is now common in *Mycobacterium tuberculosis*, *Neisseria gonorrhoeae*, *Klebsiella pneumoniae*, and *S. aureus*. Similarly, development of drug-resistant parasites has dramatically increased the morbidity and mortality associated with *Plasmodium falciparum* infection in Asia, Africa, and Latin America.

AGENTS OF BIOTERRORISM

Sadly, the anthrax attacks in the United States in 2001 transformed the theoretical threat of bioterrorism into reality. The Centers for Disease Control and Prevention (CDC) has evaluated the danger microorganisms pose as weapons on the basis of the efficiency with which disease can be transmitted, how difficult the microorganisms are to produce and distribute, what can be done to defend against them, and the extent to which they are likely to

Table 9.5 Potential Agents of Bioterrorism

Category A Diseases and Agents
Anthrax: *Bacillus anthracis*
Botulism: *Clostridium botulinum* toxin
Plague: *Yersinia pestis*
Smallpox: *Variola major* virus
Tularemia: *Francisella tularensis*
Viral hemorrhagic fevers: Ebola, Marburg, Lassa, others
Category B Diseases and Agents
Brucellosis: *Brucella* spp.
Epsilon toxin of *Clostridium perfringens*
Food safety threats: *Salmonella* spp., *Escherichia coli* O157:H7, *Shigella*, others
Glanders: *Burkholderia mallei*
Melioidosis: *Burkholderia pseudomallei*
Psittacosis: *Chlamydia psittaci*
Q fever: *Coxiella burnetii*
Ricin toxin from castor beans (*Ricinus communis*)
Staphylococcal enterotoxin B
Typhus fever: *Rickettsia prowazekii*
Mosquito-borne encephalitis viruses: Venezuelan equine encephalitis, Eastern equine encephalitis, Western equine encephalitis, others
Water safety threats: *Vibrio cholerae*, *Cryptosporidium parvum*, others
Category C Diseases and Agents
Emerging infectious disease threats: Nipah virus, hantavirus, others

Adapted from Centers for Disease Control and Prevention Information (http://emergency.cdc.gov).

alarm the public and produce widespread fear. Based on these criteria, **the CDC has ranked bioweapons into three categories, designated A, B, and C** (Table 9.5).

The agents in the highest-risk category A can be readily disseminated or transmitted from person to person, typically cause diseases that carry a high mortality rate with potential for major public health impact, may cause pandemics leading to widespread panic and social disruption, and are likely to require special action for public health preparedness. For example, the smallpox virus is a category A agent because of its high transmissibility, case mortality rates of 30% or greater, and the lack of effective therapy. Smallpox readily spreads from person to person, mainly through respiratory secretions and by direct contact with virus in skin lesions. Since routine smallpox vaccination ended in the United States in 1972, immunity has waned, leaving the population highly susceptible. Concern that smallpox could be used for bioterrorism has led to reinstitution of vaccination for some medical and military personnel.

Category B agents are less easy to disseminate, cause disease associated with moderate morbidity but low mortality, and require specific diagnostic and disease surveillance. Many of these agents can be spread in food or water. Category C agents include emerging pathogens that could be engineered for mass dissemination because of ease of availability, production, and dissemination; the potential for high morbidity and mortality; and great impact on health.

TRANSMISSION AND DISSEMINATION OF MICROBES

Microbes can enter the host through several body surfaces and, once in the host, can disseminate by different routes.

Routes of Entry of Microbes

Microbes can enter the host through breaches in the skin, by inhalation or ingestion, or by sexual transmission. The first defenses against infection are intact skin and mucosal surfaces, which provide physical barriers and produce anti-microbial substances. In general, respiratory, gastrointestinal, or genitourinary tract infections that occur in otherwise healthy individuals are caused by relatively virulent microorganisms that are capable of damaging or penetrating intact epithelial barriers. By contrast, most skin infections in healthy individuals are caused by less virulent organisms that breach the skin through damaged sites (Table 9.6).

Skin

The dense, keratinized outer layer of skin is a natural barrier to infection; furthermore, the low pH of the skin (less than 5.5) combined with the presence of fatty acids inhibit growth of microorganisms other than the normal bacteria and fungi. Included among these normal flora are potential opportunists, such as *S. aureus* and *Candida albicans*.

Cutaneous infections are typically acquired by entry of microbes through breaks in the skin, including wounds or surgical incisions *(Staphylococci)*, burns *(Pseudomonas aeruginosa)*, and diabetic and pressure-related foot sores (multibacterial infections). Intravenous catheters in hospitalized patients provide portals for local or systemic infection. Needle sticks can expose the recipient to infected blood and transmit HBV, HCV, or HIV. Some pathogens penetrate the skin via an insect or animal bite. Bites by fleas, ticks, mosquitoes, mites, and lice break the skin and transmit arboviruses (causes of yellow fever and encephalitis), bacteria (plague, Lyme disease, Rocky Mountain spotted fever), protozoa (malaria, leishmaniasis), and helminths (filariasis). Animal bites can lead to infections with bacteria, such as *Pasteurella,* or viruses, such as rabies. Only a few microorganisms are able to cross the skin barrier directly. For example, *Schistosoma* larvae released from freshwater snails penetrate swimmers' skin by releasing enzymes that dissolve the extracellular matrix, traversing unbroken skin. Similarly, certain fungi (dermatophytes) can infect intact stratum corneum of the skin, hair, and nails.

Gastrointestinal Tract

Gastrointestinal pathogens are transmitted by food or drink contaminated with fecal material. When hygiene fails, as may occur with natural disasters such as floods and earthquakes, diarrheal disease becomes rampant. Acidic gastric secretions are important defenses and are lethal for many gastrointestinal pathogens. Healthy volunteers do not become infected by *Vibrio cholerae* unless they are fed 10^{11} organisms, but neutralizing the stomach acid reduces the infectious dose by 10,000-fold. By contrast, some

Table 9.6 Routes of Microbial Infection

Site	Major Local Defense(s)	Basis for Failure of Local Defense	Pathogen/Disease (Examples)
Skin	Epidermal barrier	Mechanical defects (punctures, burns, ulcers)	*Staphylococcus aureus, Candida albicans, Pseudomonas aeruginosa*
		Needle sticks	HIV, hepatitis viruses
		Arthropod and animal bites	Yellow fever, plague, Lyme disease, malaria, rabies, Zika virus
		Direct penetration	*Schistosoma*
Gastrointestinal tract	Epithelial barrier	Attachment and local proliferation of microbes	*Vibrio chloerae, Giardia*
		Attachment and local invasion of microbes	*Shigella, Salmonella, Campylobacter*
		Uptake through M cells	Poliovirus, certain pathogenic bacteria
	Acidic secretions	Acid-resistant cysts and eggs	Many protozoa and helminths
	Bile and pancreatic enzymes	Resistant microbial external coats	Hepatitis A, Rotavirus, Norovirus
	Normal protective flora	Broad-spectrum antibiotic use	*Clostridium difficile*
Respiratory tract	Mucociliary clearance	Attachment and local proliferation of microbes	Influenza viruses
		Ciliary paralysis by toxins	*Haemophilus influenzae, M. pneumoniae, Bordetella pertussis*
	Resident alveolar macrophages	Resistance to killing by phagocytes	*M. tuberculosis*
Urogenital tract	Urination	Obstruction, microbial attachment, and local proliferation	*E. coli*
	Normal vaginal flora	Antibiotic use	*Candida albicans*
	Intact epidermal/epithelial barrier	Microbial attachment and local proliferation	*Neisseria gonorrhoeae*
		Direct infection/local invasion	Herpes viruses, Zika virus, *Treponema pallidum*
		Local trauma	Various sexually transmitted diseases (e.g., human papilloma virus)

ingested agents, such as *Shigella* and *Giardia* cysts, are relatively resistant to gastric acid, so fewer than 100 organisms can cause illness.

Other normal defenses within the gastrointestinal tract include (1) the layer of viscous mucus covering the intestinal epithelium, (2) lytic pancreatic enzymes and bile detergents, (3) mucosal anti-microbial peptides called defensins, (4) normal flora, and (5) secreted IgA antibodies. IgA antibodies are made by plasma cells located in mucosa-associated lymphoid tissue (MALT). These lymphoid aggregates are covered by a single layer of specialized epithelial cells called *M cells,* which are important for transport of antigens to MALT. Numerous gut pathogens use M cells to enter the host from the intestinal lumen, including poliovirus, enteropathic *E. coli, V. cholerae, Salmonella enterica* serotype Typhi, and *Shigella flexneri.*

Infection via the gastrointestinal tract occurs when local defenses are weakened or the organisms develop strategies to overcome these defenses. Host defenses are weakened by low gastric acidity, by antibiotics that alter the normal bacterial flora (e.g., in pseudomembranous colitis due to *C. difficile*), or when there is stalled peristalsis or mechanical obstruction. Viruses that can enter the body through the intestinal tract (e.g., hepatitis A, rotavirus) are those that lack envelopes, because enveloped viruses are inactivated by bile and digestive enzymes.

Enteropathogenic bacteria cause gastrointestinal disease in several ways:

- *Toxin production in food. S. aureus* and *Bacillus cereus* can contaminate and grow in food, where they release powerful enterotoxins that, when ingested, cause food poisoning without any bacterial growth in the gut.
- *Adhesion, local proliferation, and toxin production in the host. V. cholerae* and enterotoxigenic *E. coli* bind to the intestinal epithelium and multiply in the overlying mucous layer, where they release exotoxins that cause epithelial cells to secrete large volumes of fluid, resulting in watery diarrhea.
- *Invasion. Shigella, Salmonella,* and *Campylobacter* invade locally and damage the intestinal mucosa and lamina propria, causing ulceration, inflammation, and hemorrhage—changes manifested clinically as bloody diarrhea (dysentery). *S. enterica* serotype Typhi passes from the damaged mucosa through Peyer patches and mesenteric lymph nodes and into the bloodstream, resulting in a systemic infection.

Fungal infections of the gastrointestinal tract occur in immunologically compromised individuals. *Candida,* part of the normal gastrointestinal flora, shows a predilection for stratified squamous epithelium, causing oral thrush or membranous esophagitis, but also may spread to the stomach, lower gastrointestinal tract, and other organs.

Most *intestinal parasites* enter the body by being ingested as cysts, eggs, or meat-borne larvae, but a few enter by penetrating the skin and finding their way to the intestine. Once in the intestine, these pathogens cause damage in several ways:

- *G. lamblia* attaches to the epithelial brush border, but does not invade into cells or tissue. Attachment of the organisms leads to blunting of villi, loss of brush border,

malabsorption, and chronic inflammation through mechanisms that are poorly understood.
- Cryptosporidia are taken up by enterocytes, in which they replicate, leading to extensive mucosal damage, villous atrophy, and inflammation.
- *E. histolytica* kills host cells by contact-mediated cytolysis through a channel-forming pore protein, with consequent ulceration and invasion of the colonic mucosa.
- Intestinal helminths cause disease when they are present in large numbers or travel to ectopic sites. Large numbers of *A. lumbricoides* can obstruct the gut, and this organism can invade and damage the bile ducts as well.
- Helminths also cause disease by depriving the host of nutrients. Hookworms cause iron-deficiency anemia by sucking blood from intestinal villi; *Diphyllobothrium*, the fish tapeworm, causes anemia by depriving the host of vitamin B_{12}.

Respiratory Tract

A large number of microorganisms, including viruses, bacteria, and fungi, are inhaled daily by every individual. In many cases, the microbes are inhaled in dust or aerosol particles. The distance these particles travel into the respiratory system is inversely proportional to their size. Large particles are trapped in the mucociliary blanket that lines the nose and the upper respiratory tract. Microorganisms trapped in the mucus secreted by goblet cells are transported by ciliary action to the back of the throat, where they are swallowed or coughed out. Particles smaller than 5 μm travel directly to the alveoli, where they are phagocytosed by alveolar macrophages or by neutrophils recruited to the lung by cytokines.

Microorganisms that invade the normal healthy respiratory tract have developed specific mechanisms to overcome mucociliary defenses or to avoid destruction by alveolar macrophages. Some successful respiratory viruses evade these defenses by attaching to and entering epithelial cells in the lower respiratory tract and pharynx. For example, influenza viruses possess hemagglutinin proteins that project from the surface of the virus and bind to sialic acid on the surface of epithelial cells. This attachment induces the host cell to engulf the virus, leading to viral entry and replication within the host cell.

Certain bacterial respiratory pathogens release toxins that paralyze cilia. Examples include *Haemophilus influenzae, Mycoplasma pneumoniae,* and *Bordetella pertussis.* Some bacteria lack the ability to overcome the defenses of the healthy lung and can cause respiratory infections only in compromised hosts. *Streptococcus pneumoniae* and *S. aureus* can cause pneumonia subsequent to influenza because the viral infection leads to the loss of the protective ciliated epithelium. Chronic damage to mucociliary defense mechanisms occurs in smokers and individuals with cystic fibrosis, while acute injury occurs in intubated patients and in those who aspirate gastric acid.

Some respiratory pathogens avoid phagocytosis or destruction after phagocytosis. *M. tuberculosis,* for example, gains a foothold in alveoli because it escapes killing within the phagolysosomes of macrophages. Opportunistic fungi infect the lungs when cellular immunity is depressed or when leukocytes are reduced in number (e.g., *P. jiroveci* in patients with AIDS, *Aspergillus* spp. after chemotherapy).

Urogenital Tract

The urinary tract is almost always invaded from the exterior by way of the urethra. The regular flushing of the urinary tract with urine serves as a defense against invading microorganisms. Urine in the bladder is normally sterile or contains only small numbers of fastidious bacteria; however, successful pathogens (e.g., *N. gonorrhoeae, E. coli*) adhere to the urinary epithelium, overcoming the host defense of regular flushing. Anatomy plays an important role in infection. Women have many more urinary tract infections than men because the distance between the urinary bladder and skin (i.e., the length of the urethra) is 5 cm in women, in contrast with 20 cm in men. Obstruction of urinary flow, as in benign prostatic hyperplasia, or reflux can compromise normal defenses and increase susceptibility to urinary tract infections. Urinary tract infections can spread further up from the bladder to the kidney and cause acute and chronic pyelonephritis.

From puberty until menopause, the vagina is protected from pathogens by a low pH resulting from catabolism of glycogen in the normal epithelium by lactobacilli. Antibiotics can kill the lactobacilli, allowing overgrowth of yeast, with resultant vaginal candidiasis.

Spread and Dissemination of Microbes Within the Body

Some microorganisms proliferate locally, at the site of initial infection, whereas others penetrate the epithelial barrier and spread to distant sites by way of the lymphatics, the blood, or nerves (Fig. 9.6). In contrast to those that disseminate, pathogens that cause superficial infections stay confined to the lumen of hollow viscera (e.g., *V. cholerae*) or interact exclusively with epithelial cells (e.g., papillomaviruses, dermatophytes).

Microbes can spread within the body in several ways:

- *Lysis and invasion.* Some extracellular bacteria, fungi, and helminths secrete lytic enzymes that destroy tissue and allow direct invasion. For example, *S. aureus* secretes hyaluronidase, which degrades the extracellular matrix between host cells. Invasive microbes initially follow tissue planes of least resistance and drain to regional lymphatics. *S. aureus* may travel from a localized abscess to the draining lymph nodes. This can sometimes lead to bacteremia and spread to deep organs (heart, bone).
- *Through blood and lymph.* Microorganisms may be spread either in extracellular fluid or within host cells. Some viruses (e.g., poliovirus, HBV), most bacteria and fungi, some protozoa (e.g., African trypanosomes), and all helminths are transported in the plasma. Leukocytes can carry herpesviruses, HIV, mycobacteria, *Leishmania,* and *Toxoplasma.* The parasites *Plasmodium* and *Babesia* are found within red cells.
- *Cell-to-cell transmission.* Most viruses spread locally from cell to cell by replication and release of infectious virions, but others may propagate from cell to cell by causing fusion of host cells, or by transport within nerves (as with rabies virus and varicella-zoster virus).

The consequences of bloodborne spread of pathogens vary widely depending on the virulence of the organism,

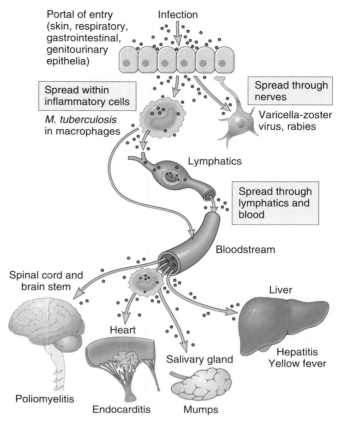

Fig. 9.6 Routes of entry and dissemination of microbes. To enter the body, microbes penetrate epithelial or mucosal barriers. Infection may remain localized at the site of entry or spread to other sites in the body. Most common microbes (selected examples are shown) spread through the lymphatics or bloodstream (either freely or within inflammatory cells). However, certain viruses and bacterial toxins also may travel through nerves. *(Adapted from Mims CA: The pathogenesis of infectious disease, ed 4, San Diego, 1996, Academic Press.)*

the magnitude of the infection, the pattern of seeding, and host factors such as immune status. Sporadic bloodstream invasion by low-virulence or nonvirulent microbes (e.g., during brushing of teeth) is common but is quickly controlled by normal host defenses. By contrast, disseminated viremia, bacteremia, fungemia, or parasitemia by virulent pathogens poses a serious danger and manifests as fever, hypotension, and multiple other systemic signs and symptoms of sepsis. Massive bloodstream invasion by bacteria can be rapidly fatal, even in previously healthy individuals.

The major manifestations of infectious disease may appear at sites distant from the point of microbe entry. For example, varicella-zoster and measles viruses enter through the airways but cause rashes in the skin; poliovirus enters through the intestine but kills motor neurons to cause paralysis. *Schistosoma mansoni* parasites penetrate the skin but eventually localize in blood vessels of the portal system and mesentery, damaging the liver and intestine. *Schistosoma hematobium* also penetrates the skin, but localizes to the urinary bladder and causes cystitis. The rabies virus travels from the site of a bite by a rabid animal to the brain by retrograde transport in sensory neurons, where it then causes encephalitis and death.

Transmission of Microbes

Transmission depends on the hardiness of the microbe. Some microbes can survive for extended periods in dust, food, or water. Bacterial spores, protozoan cysts, and thick-shelled helminth eggs can survive in a cool and dry environment. Less hardy microorganisms must be quickly passed from person to person, often by direct contact.

For transmission of disease, the mode of exit of a microorganism from the host's body is as important as entry into it. Every fluid or tissue that is normally secreted, excreted, or shed is used by microorganisms to leave the host for transmission to new victims.

- *Skin.* Skin flora, such as *S. aureus* and dermatophytes (fungi), are shed in the desquamated skin. Some sexually transmitted pathogens are transmitted from genital skin lesions, such as HSV and *Treponema pallidum* (causing syphilis).
- *Oral secretions.* Viruses that replicate in the salivary glands and are spread in saliva include mumps virus, CMV, and rabies virus.
- *Respiratory secretions.* Viruses and bacteria can be shed in respiratory secretions during talking, coughing, and sneezing. Most respiratory pathogens, including influenza viruses, spread in large respiratory droplets, which travel no more than 3 feet. However, a few organisms, including *M. tuberculosis* and varicella-zoster virus, are spread from the respiratory tract in small respiratory droplets or within dust particles that can travel long distances in the air. These properties determine the type of isolation precautions that are used to prevent the spread of infection.
- *Stool.* Organisms shed in stool include many pathogens that replicate in the lumen or epithelium of the gut, such as *Shigella, G. lamblia,* and rotavirus. Pathogens that replicate in the liver (hepatitis A virus) or gallbladder (*S. enterica* serotype Typhi) enter the intestine in bile and are shed in stool.
- *Blood.* Pathogens spread via blood may be transmitted by invertebrate vectors, medical practices (blood transfusion, reuse of equipment), or sharing of needles by intravenous drug abusers. Bloodborne parasites, including *Plasmodium* spp. and arboviruses, are transmitted by biting insects.
- *Urine.* Urine is the usual mode of exodus from the human host for only a few organisms, including *S. haematobium,* which grows in the veins of the bladder and releases eggs that reach the urine.
- *Genital tract.* Sexually transmitted infections (STIs) spread from the urethra, vagina, cervix, rectum, or oral pharynx. Organisms that cause STIs depend on direct contact for person-to-person spread because these pathogens cannot survive in the environment. Transmission of STIs often is by asymptomatic individuals who do not realize that they are infected. Infection with one STI increases the risk for additional STIs, mainly because the risk factors are the same for all STIs. STIs are described in Chapters 18 and 19.
- *Vertical transmission.* Transmission of infectious agents from mother to fetus or newborn child is a common mode of transmission for some pathogens, and may occur through several different routes. Placental-fetal transmission is most likely to occur when the mother is infected with a pathogen during pregnancy. Some of the resulting infections interfere with fetal development, and the degree and type of damage depend on the age of the fetus at the time of infection. For example, rubella infection during the first trimester can lead to heart malformations, mental retardation, cataracts, or deafness, while rubella infection during the third trimester has little effect. Congenital microcephaly and other CNS complications have been associated with Zika virus infection during pregnancy. Much is still unknown about timing of infection relative to the trimester of pregnancy. Transmission during birth is caused by contact with infectious agents during passage through the birth canal. Examples include gonococcal and chlamydial conjunctivitis. Postnatal transmission in maternal milk can transmit CMV, HIV, and HBV.

Microbes also can be transmitted from animal to human resulting in *zoonotic infections,* either through direct contact with or consumption of animal products or indirectly by an invertebrate vector.

SUMMARY

TRANSMISSION OF MICROBES

- Transmission of infections can occur via:
  - Contact (direct and indirect)
  - Respiratory droplets
  - Fecal-oral route
  - Sexual transmission
  - Vertical transmission from mother to fetus or newborn
  - Insect/arthropod vectors.
- A pathogen can establish infection if it possesses virulence factors that overcome normal host defenses or if the host defenses are compromised.
- Host defenses against infection include:
  - Skin: tough keratinized barrier, low pH, fatty acids, normal microbiota
  - Respiratory system: alveolar macrophages and mucociliary clearance by bronchial epithelium, IgA
  - Gastrointestinal system: acidic gastric pH, viscous mucus, pancreatic enzymes and bile, defensins, IgA, and normal flora
  - Urogenital tract: repeated flushing and acidic environment created by commensal vaginal flora

HOW MICROORGANISMS CAUSE DISEASE

Infectious agents establish infection and damage tissues by any of three mechanisms:

- They can contact or enter host cells and directly cause *death of infected cells.*
- They can release *toxins* that kill cells at a distance, release enzymes that degrade tissue components, or damage blood vessels and cause ischemic necrosis.

- They can induce *host immune responses* that, although directed against the invader, cause additional tissue damage. Thus, the defensive responses of the host can be a mixed blessing, helping to overcome the infection but also contributing to tissue damage.

Described next are some of the mechanisms whereby viruses and bacteria damage host tissues.

Mechanisms of Viral Injury

Viruses can directly damage host cells by entering them and replicating at the host's expense. The manifestations of viral infection are largely determined by the tropism of the virus for specific tissues and cell types. Tropism is influenced by a number of factors.

- *Host receptors for viruses.* Viruses are coated with surface proteins that bind with high specificity to particular host cell surface proteins. Entry of many viruses into cells commences with binding to normal host cell receptors. For example, HIV glycoprotein gp120 binds to CD4 and CXCR4 and CCR5 on T cells and macrophages (Chapter 5). Host proteases may be needed to enable binding of virus to host cells; for instance, a host protease cleaves and activates the influenza virus hemagglutinin.
- *Specificity of transcription factors.* The ability of the virus to replicate inside particular cell types depends on the presence of lineage-specific transcription factors that recognize viral enhancer and promoter elements. For example, the JC virus, which causes leukoencephalopathy (Chapter 23), replicates only in oligodendroglia in the CNS because the promoter and enhancer DNA sequences regulating viral gene expression are active in glial cells, but not in neurons or endothelial cells.
- *Physical characteristics of tissues.* Host environment and temperature can contribute to tissue tropism. For example, enteroviruses replicate in the intestine in part because they can resist inactivation by acids, bile, and digestive enzymes. Rhinoviruses infect cells only within the upper-respiratory tract because they replicate optimally at the lower temperatures characteristic of this site.

Once viruses are inside host cells, they can damage or kill the cells by a number of mechanisms (Fig. 9.7):

- *Direct cytopathic effects.* Viruses can kill cells by preventing synthesis of critical host macromolecules, by producing degradative enzymes and toxic proteins, or by inducing apoptosis. For example, poliovirus blocks synthesis of host proteins by inactivating cap-binding protein. HSV produces proteins that inhibit synthesis of cellular DNA and mRNA and other proteins that degrade host DNA. Viral replication also can trigger apoptosis of host cells by cell-intrinsic mechanisms, such as perturbations of the endoplasmic reticulum during virus assembly, which can activate caspases that mediate apoptosis.
- *Anti-viral immune responses.* Viral proteins on the surface of host cells may be recognized by the immune system, and lymphocytes may attack virus-infected cells. Cytotoxic T lymphocytes (CTLs) are important for defense against viral infections, but CTLs also can be responsible for tissue injury. Hepatitis B infection causes CTL-

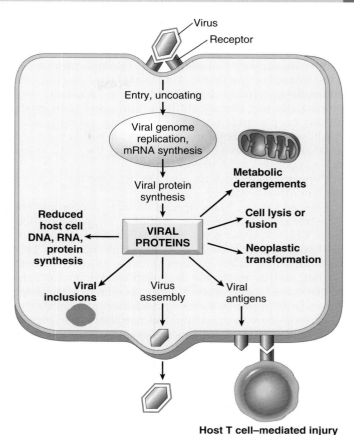

Fig. 9.7 Mechanisms by which viruses cause injury to cells.

mediated destruction of infected hepatocytes, a normal response that is attempting to clear the infection.
- *Transformation of infected cells.* Different oncogenic viruses (e.g., HPV, EBV) can stimulate cell growth and survival by a variety of mechanisms, including hijacking the control of cell cycle machinery, anti-apoptotic strategies, and insertional mutagenesis (in which the insertion of viral DNA into the host genome alters the expression of nearby host genes). Mechanisms of viral transformation are discussed in Chapter 6.

Mechanisms of Bacterial Injury

Bacterial Virulence

Bacterial damage to host tissues depends on the ability of the bacteria to adhere to host cells, invade cells and tissues, or deliver toxins. Pathogenic bacteria have virulence genes that are frequently found grouped together in clusters called *pathogenicity islands*. A small number of virulence genes can determine whether a bacterium is harmful. The *Salmonella* strains that infect humans are so closely related that they are a single species, but only a few virulence genes determine whether an isolate of *Salmonella* causes life-threatening typhoid fever or self-limited gastroenteritis.

Plasmids (small independently replicating circular DNAs) and bacteriophages (viruses) are genetic elements that spread between bacteria and can carry virulence factors, including toxins or enzymes that confer antibiotic resistance. Exchange of these elements between bacteria can endow the recipient bacteria with a survival advantage and/or the capacity to cause disease. Plasmids or transposons encoding antibiotic resistance can convert an antibiotic-susceptible bacterium into a resistant one, making effective therapy difficult. Carbapenemase genes carried on plasmids have spread among gram-negative bacilli worldwide, resulting in strains for which there are no available effective antibiotics, causing the CDC to list these organisms as an urgent threat.

Populations of bacteria also can act together in ways that alter their virulence.

- *Quorum sensing.* Many species of bacteria coordinately regulate gene expression within a large population in which specific genes, such as virulence genes, are expressed after bacteria reach high concentrations. This in turn may allow bacteria growing in discrete host sites, such as an abscess or consolidated pneumonia, to overcome host defenses. *S. aureus* coordinately regulates virulence factors by secreting *autoinducer peptides.* As the bacteria grow to increasing concentrations, the level of the autoinducer peptide increases, stimulating exotoxin production.
- *Biofilms.* Communities of bacteria can live within a viscous layer of extracellular polysaccharides that adhere to host tissues or devices such as intravascular catheters and artificial joints. Biofilms make bacteria inaccessible to immune effector mechanisms and increase their resistance to anti-microbial drugs. Biofilm formation seems to be important in the persistence and relapse of infections such as bacterial endocarditis, artificial joint infections, and respiratory infections in individuals with cystic fibrosis.

Bacterial Adherence to Host Cells

Bacterial surface molecules that bind to host cells or extracellular matrix are called *adhesins.* Diverse surface structures are involved in adhesion of various bacteria (see Fig. 9.2). *S. pyogenes* has protein F and teichoic acid projecting from its cell wall that bind to fibronectin on the surface of host cells and in the extracellular matrix. Other bacteria have filamentous proteins called *pili* on their surfaces. Stalks of pili are structurally conserved, whereas amino acids on the tips of the pili vary and determine the binding specificity of the bacteria. Strains of *E. coli* that cause urinary tract infections uniquely express a specific P pilus that binds to a Gal(α1–4)Gal moiety expressed on uroepithelial cells. Pili on *N. gonorrhoeae* bacteria mediate adherence of the bacteria to host cells and also are targets of the host antibody response. Antigenic variation affecting the antigens expressed in the pili is an important mechanism by which *N. gonorrhoeae* escapes the immune response.

Bacterial Toxins

Any bacterial substance that contributes to illness can be considered a toxin. Toxins are subclassified as endotoxins, which are components of the bacterial cell, or exotoxins, which are proteins that are secreted by the bacterium.

Bacterial endotoxin is a lipopolysaccharide (LPS) that is a component of the outer membrane of gram-negative bacteria (see Fig. 9.2). LPS is composed of a long-chain fatty acid anchor, termed *lipid A,* connected to a core sugar chain, both of which are very similar in all gram-negative bacteria. Attached to the core sugar is a variable carbohydrate chain (O antigen), which is used to serotype strains of bacteria to aid in diagnosis. Lipid A binds to CD14 on the surface of host leukocytes, and the complex then binds to Toll-like receptor 4, a pattern recognition receptor of the innate immune system that transmits signals to promote cell activation and inflammatory responses. Responses to LPS can be both beneficial and harmful to the host. The response is beneficial in that LPS activates protective immunity through induction of important cytokines and chemoattractants (chemokines), as well as increased expression of costimulatory molecules, which enhance T-lymphocyte activation. However, high levels of LPS play an important role in septic shock, disseminated intravascular coagulation, and acute respiratory distress syndrome, mainly through induction of excessive levels of cytokines such as tumor necrosis factor (Chapter 4).

Exotoxins are secreted proteins that cause cellular injury and disease. They can be classified into broad categories by their mechanism and site of action.

- *Enzymes.* Bacteria secrete enzymes (proteases, hyaluronidases, coagulases, fibrinolysins) that act on their respective substrates *in vitro,* but their role in disease is understood in only a few cases. For example, exfoliative toxins are proteases produced by *S. aureus* that cleave proteins known to hold keratinocytes together, causing the epidermis to detach from the deeper skin.
- *A-B toxins: Toxins that alter intracellular signaling or regulatory pathways.* The two-component toxins have an active (A) component with enzymatic activity and a binding (B) component that binds cell surface receptors and delivers the A protein into the cell cytoplasm. The effect of these toxins depends on the binding specificity of the B domain and the cellular pathways affected by the A domain. A-B toxins are made by many bacteria including *Bacillus anthracis, V. cholerae,* and *Corynebacterium diphtheriae.* The mechanism of action of the A-B anthrax toxin is well understood (Fig. 9.8). Anthrax toxin has two alternate A components, edema factor (EF) and lethal factor (LF), which enter cells following binding to the B component, and each A component mediates specific pathologic effects.
- *Superantigens* stimulate very large numbers of T lymphocytes by binding to conserved portions of the T cell receptor, leading to massive T lymphocyte proliferation and cytokine release. The high levels of cytokines lead to capillary leak and the systemic inflammatory response syndrome (Chapter 4). Superantigens made by *S. aureus* and *S. pyogenes* cause toxic shock syndrome.
- *Neurotoxins* produced by *Clostridium botulinum* and *Clostridium tetani* inhibit release of neurotransmitters, resulting in paralysis. These toxins do not kill neurons; instead, the A domains cleave proteins involved in secretion of neurotransmitters at the synaptic junction. Tetanus and botulism can result in death from respiratory failure due to paralysis of the chest and diaphragm muscles.
- *Enterotoxins* affect the gastrointestinal tract causing varied effects, including nausea and vomiting *(S. aureus),* voluminous watery diarrhea *(V. cholerae),* and bloody diarrhea *(C. difficile).*

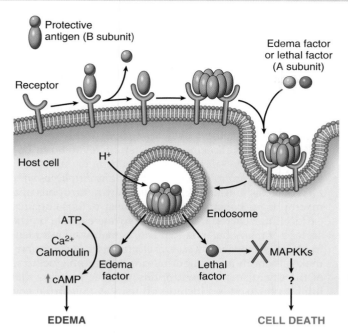

Fig. 9.8 Mechanism of anthrax exotoxin action. The B subunit, also called *protective antigen*, binds a cell-surface receptor, is cleaved by a host protease, and forms a heptamer. Three A subunits of edema factor (EF) or lethal factor (LF) bind to the B heptamer, enter the cell, and are released into the cytoplasm. EF binds calcium and calmodulin to form an adenylate cyclase that increases intracellular cAMP, which causes efflux of water and interstitial edema. LF is a protease that destroys mitogen-activated protein kinase kinases (MAPKKs), leading to cell death. cAMP, cyclic adenosine monophosphate. Note that each B subunit binds either EF or LF, but not both (as shown for simplicity). *(Adapted from Mourez M, Lacy DB, Cunningham, K, et al: 2011: A year of major advances in anthrax toxin research.* Trends Microbiol *10:287, 2002.)*

Injurious Effects of Host Immune Responses

As mentioned earlier, the host immune response to microbes can sometimes be the cause of tissue injury. A few examples of types and mechanisms of injury are as follows:

- *Granulomatous inflammation.* Infection with *M. tuberculosis* results in a delayed hypersensitivity response and the formation of granulomas, which sequester the bacilli and prevent its spread, but also produce tissue damage (caseous necrosis) and fibrosis.
- *T-cell–mediated inflammation.* Damage from HBV and HCV infection of hepatocytes is due mainly to the immune response to the infected liver cells and not to cytopathic effects of the virus.
- *Innate immune inflammation.* Pattern recognition receptors bind to pathogen-associated molecular patterns (PAMPS) and to damage-associated molecular patterns (DAMPS) released from damaged host cells, activating the immune system and leading to inflammation (discussed in Chapter 5).
- *Humoral immunity.* Poststreptococcal glomerulonephritis can develop after infection with *S. pyogenes.* It is caused by antibodies that bind to streptococcal antigens and form immune complexes, which deposit in renal glomeruli and produce nephritis.

- *Chronic inflammatory diseases.* In the development of inflammatory bowel disease (Chapter 15), an important early event may be compromise of the intestinal epithelial barrier, which enables the entry of both pathogenic and commensal microbes and their interactions with local immune cells, resulting in inflammation. The cycle of inflammation and epithelial injury may be an important component of the disease, with microbes playing the central role.
- *Cancer.* Viruses, such as HBV and HCV, and bacteria, such as *H. pylori,* that are not known to carry or to activate oncogenes are associated with cancers, presumably because these microbes trigger chronic inflammation with subsequent tissue regeneration, which provides fertile ground for the development of cancer (Chapter 6).

SUMMARY

HOW MICROORGANISMS CAUSE DISEASE

- Diseases caused by microbes involve an interplay of microbial virulence and host responses.
- Infectious agents can cause cell death or dysfunction by directly interacting with the cell.
- Injury may be due to local or systemic release of bacterial products, including endotoxins (LPS), exotoxins, or superantigens, combined with the immune response.
- Absence of an immune response may reduce the damage induced by some infections; conversely, immunocompromise can allow uncontrolled expansion of opportunistic infections that can directly cause injury.
- Chronic immunological and inflammatory diseases and cancer have been associated with specific microorgansims.

IMMUNE EVASION BY MICROBES

Humoral and cellular immune responses that protect the host from most infections are discussed in Chapter 5. Not surprisingly, microorganisms have developed many means to resist and evade the immune system (Fig. 9.9). These mechanisms of escaping the immune response are important determinants of microbial virulence and pathogenicity.

- *Antigenic variation.* Neutralizing antibodies against microbial antigens block the ability of microbes to infect cells and recruit immune cells to kill pathogens. To escape recognition, microbes use many strategies that involve genetic mechanisms for generating antigenic variation. The low fidelity of viral RNA polymerases (HIV and influenza virus) and reassortment of viral genomes (influenza viruses) create viral antigenic variation (Table 9.7). *Borrelia* species switch their surface antigens via gene rearrangement. *Trypanosoma* species have many genes for their major surface antigen, VSG, and vary the expression of this surface protein. There are more than 90 different serotypes of *S. pneumoniae,* each with a different capsular polysaccharide.
- *Modification of surface proteins.* Host cationic antimicrobial peptides, including defensins, cathelicidins,

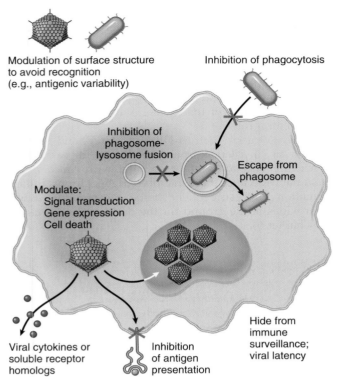

Modulation of surface structure to avoid recognition (e.g., antigenic variability)

Inhibition of phagocytosis

Inhibition of phagosome-lysosome fusion

Escape from phagosome

Modulate:
Signal transduction
Gene expression
Cell death

Hide from immune surveillance; viral latency

Viral cytokines or soluble receptor homologs

Inhibition of antigen presentation

Fig. 9.9 An overview of mechanisms used by viral and bacterial pathogens to evade innate and adaptive immunity. *(Modified with permission from Finlay B, McFadden G: Anti-immunology: evasion of the host immune system by bacterial and viral pathogens. Cell 124:767–782, 2006.)*

and thrombocidins, provide important initial defenses against invading microbes. These peptides bind the bacterial membrane and form pores, killing the bacterium by osmotic lysis. Bacterial pathogens (*Shigella* spp., *S. aureus*) avoid killing by making surface molecules that resist binding of anti-microbial peptides, or that inactivate or downregulate anti-microbial peptides.

- *Overcoming antibodies and complement.* Host defense includes coating of bacteria with antibodies or the complement protein C3b (opsonization) to facilitate phagocytosis by macrophages. However, the facultative intracellular pathogen *M. tuberculosis* subverts the complement response by activating the alternative

Table 9.7 Mechanisms of Anti-genic Variation

Mechanism	Example	
	Agent(s)	**Disease**
High mutation rate	HIV	AIDS
	Influenza virus	Influenza
Genetic reassortment	Influenza virus	Influenza
	Rotavirus	Diarrhea
Genetic rearrangement (e.g., gene recombination, gene conversion, site-specific inversion)	*Borrelia burgdorferi*	Lyme disease
	Neisseria gonorrhoeae	Gonorrhea
	Trypanosoma spp.	African sleeping sickness
	Plasmodium spp.	Malaria
Large diversity of serotypes	Rhinoviruses	Colds
	Streptococcus pneumoniae	Pneumonia, meningitis

complement pathway in the extracellular environment, and complement products coat the bacteria, resulting in uptake of the organism by monocytes; by this means, the organism reaches its site of replication. Many bacteria (such as *Shigella*, enteroinvasive *E. coli*, *M. tuberculosis*, *M. leprae*, *S. enterica* serotype Typhi) use the inside of cells as a "hideout" that allows them to escape from antibodies and complement. *Listeria monocytogenes* can manipulate the cell cytoskeleton to spread directly from cell to cell, thus allowing the bacteria to evade immune defenses.

- *Resisting phagocytosis and bacterial killing in phagosomes.* Phagocytosis and killing of bacteria by neutrophils and macrophages constitute a critical host defense against extracellular bacteria. The carbohydrate capsule on the surface of many bacteria that cause pneumonia or meningitis (*S. pneumoniae, Neisseria meningitidis, H. influenzae*) makes them more virulent by preventing phagocytosis of the organisms by neutrophils. Surface proteins that inhibit phagocytosis include proteins A (*S. aureus*) and M (*S. pyogenes*). Macrophages usually kill bacteria by fusion of the phagosome with the lysosome to form a phagolysosome. *M. tuberculosis* blocks fusion of the lysosome with the phagosome, allowing the bacteria to proliferate unchecked within the macrophage. *Legionella* produces a pore-forming protein called *listeriolysin O* and two phospholipases that degrade the phagosome membrane, allowing the bacteria to escape into the cytoplasm and avoid destruction in the macrophage. *Legionella* also secretes proteins that modulate small GTPases, master regulators of intracellular signaling to modify trafficking. Also, many bacteria make proteins that kill phagocytes, prevent their migration, or diminish their oxidative burst.

- *Escaping the inflammasome.* The activation of the cytosolic inflammasome is one pathway of innate immune responses to microbes. It is stimulated by microbial products and culminates in the activation of caspases, which induce the secretion of the pro-inflammatory cytokines IL-1 and IL-18 and induce a form of cell death called pyroptosis (Chapter 5). Both inflammation and cell death limit microbial virulence and replication. Some bacteria, such as *Yersinia* and *Salmonella*, express virulence proteins that inhibit the formation of the mature inflammasome, suppress caspase activation, block signaling pathways that are required for inflammasome activation, or limit the access of other bacterial proteins to the inflammasome. All these mechanisms serve to disable various components of this host antimicrobial defense reaction.

- *Disruption of interferon pathways.* Viruses have developed a large number of strategies to combat interferons (IFNs), which are mediators of early antiviral defense. Some viruses produce soluble homologues of IFN receptors that bind to and block the actions of secreted IFNs, or produce proteins that inhibit intracellular JAK/STAT signaling downstream of IFN receptors. RIG-I (RNA helicase retinoic acid inducible gene I protein) is a host cytoplasmic pattern recognition receptor for intracellular double-stranded RNA viruses. RIG-I inhibits signaling by this receptor, thus blocking the downstream IFN pathway and overcoming this host defense. Some viruses encode within their genomes homologs of cytokines, chemokines, or their receptors that act as competitive antagonists to inhibit immune responses. Finally, viruses have developed strategies to block apoptosis, which may give the viruses time to replicate, persist, or transform the infected host cell.

- *Decreased T-cell recognition:* DNA viruses (e.g., HSV, CMV, and EBV) can bind to or alter the localization of major histocompatibility complex (MHC) class I proteins, impairing peptide presentation to CD8+ cytotoxic T cells. Although downregulation of MHC class I molecules might cause virus-infected cells to be targets for NK cells, herpesviruses also express MHC class I homoloquess that act as decoys that engage inhibitory receptors of NK cells. Herpesviruses can target MHC class II molecules for degradation, impairing antigen presentation to CD4+ helper T cells. Viruses also can infect leukocytes to directly compromise their function (e.g., HIV infects CD4+ T cells, macrophages, and dendritic cells).

SUMMARY

IMMUNE EVASION BY MICROBES

After bypassing host tissue barriers, infectious microorganisms must also evade host innate and adaptive immunity mechanisms to successfully proliferate and be transmitted to the next host. Strategies include the following:
- Anti-genic variation
- Inactivating antibodies or complement
- Resisting phagocytosis (e.g., by producing a capsule)
- Escaping the phagosome
- Viral latency
- Suppressing the host adaptive immune response (e.g., by inhibiting antigen presentation and disrupting interferon pathways)

SPECTRUM OF INFLAMMATORY RESPONSES TO INFECTION

In contrast with the vast molecular diversity of microbes, the morphologic patterns of tissue responses to microbes are limited, as are the mechanisms directing these responses. Therefore, many pathogens produce similar reaction patterns, and few features are unique to or pathognomonic for a particular microorganism, adding to the challenge in histopathologic diagnosis.

The interaction between the microbe and the host determines the histologic features of the response to the microbes. There are five major histologic patterns of tissue reaction in infections: suppurative, mononuclear/granulomatous, cytopathic-cytoproliferative, necrosis, and chronic inflammation/scarring. Suppurative inflammation is discussed in Chapter 3.

Mononuclear and Granulomatous Inflammation

Diffuse, predominantly mononuclear, interstitial infiltrates are a common feature of all chronic inflammatory processes, but sometimes they appear acutely in response to viruses, intracellular bacteria, or intracellular parasites. In addition, spirochetes and some helminths also provoke chronic inflammation. Eosinophilia can be prominent with some helminthic infections.

MORPHOLOGY

Which mononuclear cell predominates within the inflammatory lesion depends on the host immune response to the organism. Thus, lymphocytes predominate in HBV infection (Fig. 9.10A), whereas plasma cells are common in the primary and secondary lesions of syphilis (see Fig. 9.10B). The presence of these lymphoid cells reflects cell-mediated immune responses against the pathogen or pathogen-infected cells. Granulomatous inflammation is a distinctive form of mononuclear inflammation usually evoked by infectious agents that resist eradication, but nevertheless are capable of stimulating strong T-cell–mediated immunity (e.g., *M. tuberculosis*, *Histoplasma capsulatum*, schistosome eggs). Granulomatous inflammation (Chapter 3) is characterized by accumulation of activated macrophages called epithelioid cells, which may fuse to form giant cells. In some cases, there is a central area of caseous necrosis (see Fig. 9.10C).

Cytopathic-Cytoproliferative Reaction

Cytopathic-cytoproliferative reactions usually are produced by viruses. The lesions are characterized by cell necrosis or cellular proliferation, usually with sparse inflammatory cells.

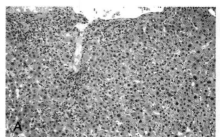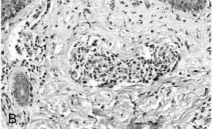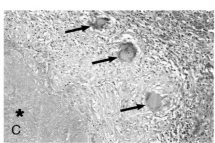

Fig. 9.10 Mononuclear and granulomatous inflammation. (A) Acute viral hepatitis characterized by a predominantly lymphocytic infiltrate. (B) Secondary syphilis in the dermis with perivascular lymphoplasmacytic infiltrate and endothelial proliferation. (C) Granulomatous inflammation in response to tuberculosis. Note the zone of caseation *(asterisk)*, which normally forms the center of the granuloma, with a surrounding rim of activated epithelioid macrophages, some of which have fused to form giant cells *(arrows)*; this in turn is surrounded by a zone of activated T lymphocytes. This high-magnification view highlights the histologic features; the granulomatous response typically takes the form of a three-dimensional sphere with the offending organism in the central area.

MORPHOLOGY

Some viruses replicate within cells and make viral aggregates that are visible as inclusion bodies (e.g., herpesviruses or adenovirus) or induce cells to fuse and form multinucleated cells called *polykaryons* (e.g., measles virus or herpesviruses) (see Fig. 9.1). Focal cell damage in the skin may cause epithelial cells to become detached, forming blisters. Some viruses can cause epithelial cells to proliferate (e.g., venereal warts caused by HPV or the umbilicated papules of molluscum contagiosum caused by poxviruses). Finally, viruses can contribute to the development of malignant neoplasms (Chapter 6).

Tissue Necrosis

Clostridium perfringens and other organisms that secrete powerful toxins can cause such rapid and severe necrosis that tissue damage is the dominant feature.

MORPHOLOGY

Because few inflammatory cells are present, necrotic lesions resemble infarcts with disruption or loss of basophilic nuclear staining and preservation of cellular outlines. *Clostridia* often are opportunistic pathogens that are introduced into muscle tissue by penetrating trauma or infection of the bowel in a neutropenic host. Similarly, the parasite *E. histolytica* causes colonic ulcers and liver abscesses characterized by extensive tissue destruction and liquefactive necrosis without a prominent inflammatory infiltrate. By entirely different mechanisms, viruses can cause widespread necrosis of host cells associated with inflammation, as exemplified by destruction of the temporal lobes of the brain by HSV or the liver by HBV. The powerful exotoxins of *C. diphtheriae* cause necrosis of laryngeal epithelium giving rise to a pseudomembrane comprised of necrotic cells enmeshed in a fibrinous exudate. This can cause asphyxia.

Chronic Inflammation and Scarring

Many infections elicit chronic inflammation, which can either resolve with complete healing or lead to extensive scarring.

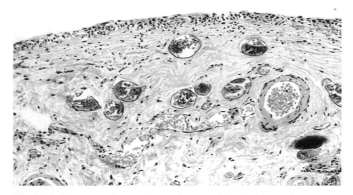

Fig. 9.11 *Schistosoma haematobium* infection of the bladder with numerous calcified eggs and extensive scarring.

MORPHOLOGY

Sometimes an exuberant scarring response is the major cause of dysfunction. For example, schistosome eggs cause "pipestem" fibrosis of the liver or fibrosis of the bladder wall (Fig. 9.11). *M. tuberculosis* causes constrictive fibrous pericarditis. Chronic HBV infection may cause cirrhosis of the liver, in which dense fibrous septa surround nodules of regenerating hepatocytes.

The patterns of tissue reactions described above are useful guidelines for analyzing microscopic features of infectious processes, but in practice it must be remembered that different types of host reactions often occur at the same time. For example, the lung of a patient with AIDS may be infected with CMV, which causes cytolytic changes, and, at the same time, by *Pneumocystis,* which causes interstitial inflammation. Similar patterns of inflammation also can be seen in tissue responses to physical or chemical agents and in other inflammatory conditions of unknown cause. Finally, in immunocompromised individuals, the absence of a host inflammatory response frequently eliminates some of the histologic clues about the potential nature of infecting microorganism(s). Because of this potential for mixed infections and/or lack of host response, other diagnostic tests for infection in addition to pathologic examination are essential to make a definitive diagnosis.

Infections in Individuals With Immunodeficiencies

Inherited or acquired defects in immunity (Chapter 5) often impair only part of the immune system, rendering the affected individuals susceptible to specific types of infections.

- Patients with antibody deficiency, as in X-linked agammaglobulinemia, contract severe bacterial infections by extracellular bacteria and a few viral infections (rotavirus and enteroviruses).
- Patients with T-cell defects are susceptible to infections with intracellular pathogens, notably viruses and some parasites.
- Patients with deficiencies in early complement components are particularly susceptible to infections by encapsulated bacteria, such as *S. pneumoniae,* whereas deficiencies of the late components of complement are associated with *Neisseria* infections.
- Deficiencies in neutrophil function lead to increased infections with *S. aureus,* some gram-negative bacteria, and fungi.
- Individuals with inherited deficiencies in specific components of innate and adaptive immunity sometimes show selective susceptibility to particular infections. These patterns reveal the essential roles of different molecules in mediating protective immunity to specific microorganisms. For example, patients with mutations in signaling molecules downstream of several TLRs are prone to pyogenic bacterial diseases, particularly with *S. pneumoniae* infections. Impaired TLR3 responses are associated with childhood HSV encephalitis. Inherited defects in IL-17 immunity (such as mutations in STAT3, a transcription factor needed for Th17 cell generation) are associated with chronic mucocutaneous candidiasis.

Acquired immunodeficiencies have a variety of causes, the most widely known being infection with HIV, which causes AIDS (Chapter 5). HIV infects and kills CD4+ helper T lymphocytes, leading to profound immunosuppression and a multitude of infections. Other causes of acquired immunodeficiency include infiltrative processes that suppress bone marrow function (e.g., leukemia), immunosuppressive drugs (such as those used to treat certain autoimmune diseases), and hemopoietic stem cell transplantation. Diseases of organ systems other than the immune system also can make patients susceptible to disease due to specific microorganisms. Individuals with cystic fibrosis and impaired respiratory clearance commonly get infections dominated by *Pseudomonas aeruginosa*. Lack of splenic function in individuals with sickle cell disease makes them susceptible to infection with encapsulated bacteria such as *S. pneumoniae*. Burns destroy skin, removing this barrier to microbes, allowing infection with pathogens such as *P. aeruginosa*. Finally, malnutrition impairs immune defenses.

MORPHOLOGY

Patients with antibody, complement, or neutrophil defects may acquire severe local bacterial infections that do not elicit any significant neutrophilic infiltrate. In these patients, the identity of the causative organism determined by culture or special stains may not have been predicted from histology. Although many viral cytopathic effects (e.g., cell fusion or inclusions) (see Fig. 9.1) may still be present, viral infections in immunocompromised hosts may not engender the anticipated mononuclear inflammatory response. In patients with AIDS who have no helper T cells and cannot mount normal cellular responses, organisms that would otherwise cause granulomatous inflammation (e.g., *M. avium* complex) fail to do so (Fig. 9.12).

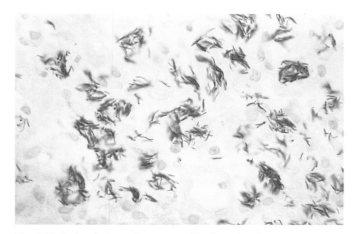

Fig. 9.12 In the absence of appropriate T-cell–mediated immunity, granulomatous host response does not occur. *Mycobacterium avium* infection in a duodenal biopsy from a patient with AIDS, showing massive intracellular macrophage infection with acid-fast organisms (filamentous and pink in this acid-fast stain preparation). The intracellular bacteria persist and even proliferate within macrophages, because there are inadequate T cells to mount a granulomatous response. AIDS, acquired immunodeficiency syndrome. *(Courtesy of Dr. Arlene Sharpe, Department of Microbiology and Immunology, Harvard Medical School, Boston, Massachusetts.)*

SUMMARY

PATTERNS OF HOST RESPONSES TO MICROBES

- In normal (immunocompetent) individuals, the patterns of host responses are fairly stereotypical for different classes of microbes; these response patterns can be used to infer possible causal organisms.
- Neutrophil-rich acute suppurative inflammation is typical of infections with many bacteria ("pyogenic" bacteria) and some fungi.
- Mononuclear cell infiltrates are common in many chronic infections and some acute viral infections.
- Granulomatous inflammation is the hallmark of infection with *M. tuberculosis* and certain fungi.
- Cytopathic and proliferative lesions are caused by some viruses.
- Necrosis results from tissue-damaging toxins produced by microbes such as *C. perfringens*.
- Chronic inflammation and scarring represent the final common pathway of many infections.

SUGGESTED READINGS

Arvanitis M, Anagnostou T, Fuchs BB, et al: Molecular and nonmolecular diagnostic methods for invasive fungal infections, *Clin Microbiol Rev* 27:490, 2014. [A very useful review of the many methods available for laboratory detection of fungal infections.]

Belkaid Y, Segre JA: Dialogue between skin microbiota and immunity, *Science* 346:954, 2014. [An excellent review of interactions between the microbiome of the skin and the immune system.]

Bennett E, Dolan R, Blaser MJ: *Mandell, Douglas, and Bennett's principles and practice of infectious diseases*, ed 8, Philadelphia, 2014, Elsevier Saunders. [A comprehensive reference for infectious diseases, including very good sections on microbial pathogenesis.]

Bergsbaken T, Fink SL, Cookson BT: Pyroptosis: host cell death and inflammation, *Nat Rev Microbiol* 7:99, 2010. [A good introduction to the inflammasome and pyroptosis, including their role in the response to infections.]

Blair JM, Webber MA, Baylay AJ, et al: Molecular mechanisms of antibiotic resistance, *Nat Rev Microbiol* 13:42, 2015. [An accessible, well-written review at the introductory level.]

Buchan BW, Ledeboer NA: Emerging technologies for the clinical microbiology laboratory, *Clin Microbiol Rev* 27:783, 2014. [A timely review of emerging technologies in clinical microbiology.]

Cadwell K: The virome in host health and disease, *Immunity* 42:805, 2015. [A good introduction to this emerging area, including a discussion of the interactions between the virome and other components of the microbiome.]

Dantas G, Sommer MO, Degnan PH, et al: Experimental approaches for defining functional roles of microbes in the human gut, *Annu Rev Microbiol* 67:459, 2013. [A thoughtful and short review of experimental methods for microbiology research.]

Galán JE, Lara-Tejero M, Marlovits TC, et al: Bacterial type III secretion systems: specialized nanomachines for protein delivery into target cells, *Annu Rev Microbiol* 68:415, 2014. [A review of the structure and mechanism of type III secretion systems.]

Geno KA, Gilbert GL, Song JY, et al: Pneumococcal capsules and their types: past, present, and future, *Clin Microbiol Rev* 28:871, 2015. [Includes the significance of capsule in pathogenesis and vaccines, as well as methods for capsule typing.]

Goo E, An JH, Kang Y, et al: Control of bacterial metabolism by quorum sensing, *Trends Microbiol* 23:567, 2015. [A review of this emerging area of study, with focus on non-enteric gram-negative bacilli.]

Hobley L, Harkins C, MacPhee CE, et al: Giving structure to the biofilm matrix: an overview of individual strategies and emerging common themes, *FEMS Microbiol Rev* 39:649, 2015. *[An exhaustive review of biofilm structure.]*

Jorgensen JH, Pfaller MA: *Manual of clinical microbiology*, ed 11, Washington, DC, 2015, ASM Press. *[A comprehensive textbook of clinical microbiology at an advanced level.]*

Jucker M, Walker LC: Self-propagation of pathogenic protein aggregates in neurodegenerative diseases, *Nature* 501:45, 2013. *[A short review of prions and other self-propagating proteins.]*

Keeney KM, Yurist-Doutsch S, Arrieta MC, et al: Effects of antibiotics on human microbiota and subsequent disease, *Annu Rev Microbiol* 68:217, 2014. *[A timely review of how antibiotics can increase vulnerability to some diseases.]*

Khabbaz RF, Moseley RR, Steiner RJ, et al: Challenges of infectious diseases in the USA, *Lancet* 384:53, 2014. *[A comprehensive but short review of current infectious disease challenges in the United States.]*

Lagier JC, Edouard S, Pagnier I, et al: Current and past strategies for bacterial culture in clinical microbiology, *Clin Microbiol Rev* 28:208, 2015. *[An exhaustive review of the utility of bacterial culture.]*

Mackey TK, Liang BA, Cuomo R, et al: Emerging and reemerging neglected tropical diseases: a review of key characteristics, risk factors, and the policy and innovation environment, *Clin Microbiol Rev* 27:949, 2014. *[A review of current challenges of emerging and neglected diseases in developing nations.]*

Nash AA, Dalziel RG, Fitzgerald JR: *Mims' pathogenesis of infectious disease*, ed 6, San Diego, 2015, Academic Press. *[A beautifully written timely and comprehensive classic text.]*

Okumura CY, Nizet V: Subterfuge and sabotage: evasion of host innate defenses by invasive gram-positive bacterial pathogens, *Annu Rev Microbiol* 68:439, 2014. *[A very good review of this complex area.]*

Panchaud A, Stojanov M, Ammerdorffer A, et al: Emerging role of Zika v irus in adverse fetal and neonatal outcomes, *Clin Microbiol Rev* 29:659, 2016. *[Review of emerging role of Zika virus in congenital brain defects.]*

Safronetz D, Feldmann H, de Wit E: Birth and pathogenesis of rogue respiratory viruses, *Annu Rev Pathol* 10:449, 2015. *[Introduces zoonotic respiratory review, with a good emphasis on pathogenesis.]*

Sommer F, Backhed F: The gut microbiota—masters of host development and physiology, *Nat Rev Microbiol* 11:227, 2013. *[An excellent introduction to intestinal microbiome and the role it plays in development of the immune response.]*

Wlodarska M, Johnston JC, Gardy JL, et al: A microbiological revolution meets an ancient disease: improving the management of tuberculosis with genomics, *Clin Microbiol Rev* 28:523, 2015. *[A good example of the important trend toward whole-bacterial genome sequencing in clinical diagnostics.]*

Blood Vessels 10

CHAPTER OUTLINE

Structure and Function of Blood Vessels 361
Vascular Organization 362
Endothelial Cells 363
Vascular Smooth Muscle Cells 364
Congenital Anomalies 364
Blood Pressure Regulation 364
Hypertensive Vascular Disease 366
Epidemiology of Hypertension 366
Mechanisms of Essential Hypertension 367
Vascular Wall Response to Injury 368
Intimal Thickening: A Stereotypical Response to Vascular Injury 368
Arteriosclerosis 369

Atherosclerosis 369
Epidemiology of Atherosclerosis 370
Clinicopathologic Consequences of Atherosclerosis 376
Aneurysms and Dissections 378
Abdominal Aortic Aneurysm 379
Thoracic Aortic Aneurysm 380
Aortic Dissection 380
Vasculitis 382
Noninfectious Vasculitis 382
Infectious Vasculitis 389
Disorders of Blood Vessel Hyperreactivity 390
Raynaud Phenomenon 390

Myocardial Vessel Vasospasm 390
Veins and Lymphatics 390
Varicose Veins of the Extremities 390
Varicosities of Other Sites 390
Thrombophlebitis and Phlebothrombosis 391
Superior and Inferior Vena Cava Syndromes 391
Lymphangitis and Lymphedema 391
Tumors 391
Benign Tumors and Tumor-Like Conditions 392
Intermediate-Grade (Borderline) Tumors 394
Malignant Tumors 396
Pathology of Vascular Intervention 397
Endovascular Stenting 397
Vascular Replacement 397

Vascular diseases are responsible for some of the most common and lethal conditions afflicting mankind. Although most clinically significant disorders involve arterial lesions, venous pathologies also can wreak havoc. Vascular disease develops through two principal mechanisms:
- *Narrowing* or *complete obstruction of* vessel lumina, occurring either progressively (e.g., by atherosclerosis) or acutely (e.g., by thrombosis or embolism)
- *Weakening* of vessel walls, causing dilation and/or rupture

We start with an overview of vascular structure and function, as background for the diseases of blood vessels discussed in the chapter.

STRUCTURE AND FUNCTION OF BLOOD VESSELS

Blood vessels are fundamentally all tubes composed of smooth muscle cells (SMCs) and extracellular matrix (ECM), with an inner luminal face covered by a continuous lining of endothelial cells (ECs). However, the relative amounts of SMCs and ECM, and the properties of the ECs, vary throughout the vasculature depending on unique functional needs (Fig. 10.1). To accommodate pulsatile flow and higher blood pressures, *arterial* walls are thicker than veins and invested with several reinforcing layers of

SMCs. As arteries narrow to *arterioles*, the ratio of wall thickness to lumen diameter increases to allow more precise regulation of intravascular pressure. *Veins*, on the other hand, are distensible thin-walled vessels with high capacitance. To facilitate maximal diffusion, *capillaries* are essentially single-cell linings of ECs lying on a basement membrane.

Since various vessels have unique structural features, it is not surprising that certain lesions characteristically involve only specific regions of the vasculature. For example, atherosclerosis occurs mainly in larger, muscular arteries, while hypertension affects small arterioles, and specific forms of vasculitis selectively involve vessels of only a certain caliber.

Vessel walls are organized into three concentric layers: *intima, media,* and *adventitia* (see Fig. 10.1). These layers are present in all vessels but are most apparent in larger vessels and particularly arteries. The intima consists of an EC monolayer on a basement membrane with minimal underlying ECM; it is separated from the media by a dense elastic membrane called the *internal elastic lamina*. The media is composed predominantly of SMCs and ECM, surrounded by loose connective tissue, nerve fibers, and smaller vessels of the adventitia. An *external elastic lamina* is present in some arteries and defines the transition between media and adventitia. Diffusion of oxygen and nutrients from the lumen is adequate to sustain thin-walled vessels and the innermost SMCs of all vessels. In large and medium-sized

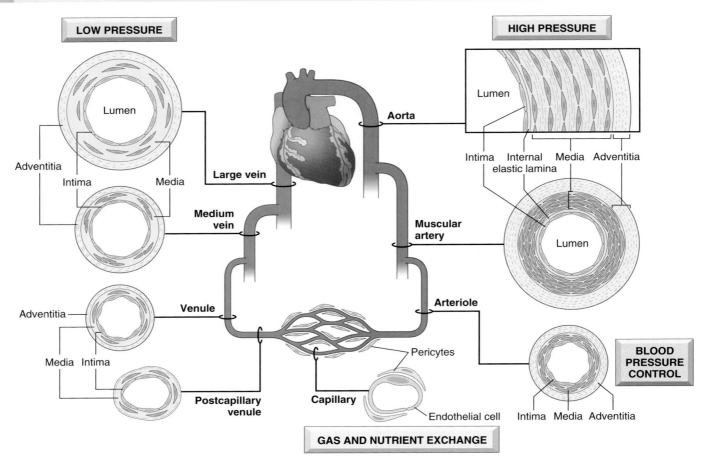

Fig. 10.1 Regional vascular specializations. Although all vessels share the same general constituents, the thickness and composition of the various layers differ as a function of hemodynamic forces and tissue requirements.

vessels, however, small arterioles within the adventitia (called *vasa vasorum* — literally, "vessels of the vessels") perfuse the outer half to two-thirds of the media.

Vascular Organization

Arteries are divided into three types based on their size and structure:

- *Large elastic arteries* (e.g., aorta, arch vessels, iliac and pulmonary arteries). In these vessels, elastic fibers alternate with SMCs throughout the media, which expands during systole (storing some of the energy of each cardiac contraction), and recoils during diastole to propel blood distally. With age and/or diseases, such as diabetes and hypertension, the elasticity is lost; the vessels become "stiff pipes" that transmit high arterial pressures to distal organs, or become dilated and tortuous (*ectatic*) and prone to rupture.
- *Medium-sized muscular arteries* (e.g., coronary and renal arteries). Here, the media is composed primarily of SMCs, with elastin limited to the internal and external elastic lamina. The medial SMCs are circularly or spirally arranged around the lumen, and regional blood flow is regulated by SMC contraction (*vasoconstriction*) and relaxation (*vasodilation*) controlled by the autonomic nervous system and local metabolic factors (e.g., acidosis). ECs also modulate arterial SMC tone, for example,

by releasing nitric oxide (NO, causing vasodilation) or endothelin (causing vasoconstriction).
- *Small arteries* (2 mm or less in diameter) *and arterioles* (20 to 100 μm in diameter) lie within the connective tissue of organs. The media in these vessels is mostly composed of SMCs. Arterioles are where blood flow resistance is regulated. As pressures drop during passage through arterioles, the velocity of blood flow is sharply reduced, and flow becomes steady rather than pulsatile. Because the resistance to fluid flow is inversely proportional to the fourth power of the diameter (i.e., halving the diameter increases resistance 16-fold), small changes in arteriolar lumen size have profound effects on blood pressure.

Capillaries have lumen diameters slightly smaller than those of red blood cells (7 to 8 μm). These vessels are lined by ECs and partially surrounded by SMC-like cells called *pericytes*. Collectively, capillary beds have a very large total cross-sectional area and a low rate of blood flow. With their thin walls and slow flow, capillaries are ideally suited to the rapid exchange of diffusible substances between blood and tissue. The capillary network of most tissues is necessarily very rich, because diffusion of oxygen and nutrients is not efficient beyond 100 μm; metabolically active tissues (e.g., heart) have the highest capillary density.

Veins receive blood from the capillary beds as postcapillary venules, which anastomose to form collecting venules and progressively larger veins. The vascular leakage (edema) and leukocyte emigration characteristic of inflammation occurs preferentially in postcapillary venules (Chapter 3).

Compared with arteries at the same level of branching, veins have larger diameters, larger lumina, and thinner walls with less distinct layers, all adaptations to the low pressures found on the venous side of the circulation (see Fig. 10.1). Thus, veins are more prone to dilation, external compression, and penetration by tumors or inflammatory processes. In veins where blood flows against gravity (e.g., in the lower extremities), backflow is prevented by valves. Collectively, the venous system has a huge *capacitance* and normally contains approximately two thirds of the blood.

Lymphatics are thin-walled, endothelium-lined channels that drain lymph (water, electrolytes, glucose, fat, proteins, and inflammatory cells) from the interstitium of tissues, eventually reconnecting with the blood stream via the *thoracic duct*. Lymphatics transport interstitial fluid and inflammatory cells from the periphery to lymph nodes, thereby facilitating antigen presentation and cell activation in the nodal tissues—and enabling continuous monitoring of peripheral tissues for infection. This can be a double-edged sword, however, as these channels can also disseminate disease by transporting microbes or tumor cells to distant sites.

Endothelial Cells

Endothelium is a continuous sheet of cells lining the entire vascular tree that regulates many aspects of blood and blood vessel function (Table 10.1). Resting ECs maintain a non-thrombogenic blood-tissue interface (Chapter 4), modulate inflammation (Chapter 3), and influence the growth and behavior of other cell types, particularly SMCs.

Table 10.1 Endothelial Cell Properties and Functions

Property/Function	Mediators/Products
Maintenance of permeability barrier	
Elaboration of anti-coagulant, anti-thrombotic, and fibrinolytic regulators	Prostacyclin Thrombomodulin Heparin-like molecules Plasminogen activator
Elaboration of prothrombotic molecules	Von Willebrand factor Tissue factor Plasminogen activator inhibitor
Production of extracellular matrix	Collagen, proteoglycans
Modulation of blood flow and vascular reactivity	*Vasoconstrictors:* endothelin, ACE *Vasodilators:* NO, prostacyclin
Regulation of inflammation and immunity	IL-1, IL-6, chemokines Adhesion molecules: VCAM-1, ICAM, E-selectin, P-selectin Histocompatibility antigens
Regulation of cell growth	*Growth stimulators:* PDGF, CSF, FGF *Growth inhibitors:* heparin, TGF-β
Oxidation of LDL	

ACE, Angiotensin-converting enzyme; *CSF,* colony-stimulating factor; *FGF,* fibroblast growth factor; *ICAM,* intercellular adhesion molecule; *IL,* interleukin; *LDL,* low-density lipoprotein; *NO,* nitric oxide; *PDGF,* platelet-derived growth factor; *TGF-β,* transforming growth factor-β; *VCAM,* vascular cell adhesion molecule.

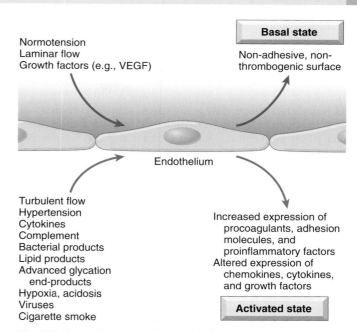

Fig. 10.2 Basal and activated endothelial cell states. Normal blood pressure, laminar flow, and stable growth factor levels promote a basal endothelial cell state that maintains a nonthrombotic surface and appropriate vascular wall smooth muscle tone. Injury or exposure to certain mediators results in endothelial activation, a state in which endothelial cells develop adhesive, procoagulant surfaces and release factors that lead to smooth muscle contraction and/or proliferation and matrix synthesis.

In most regions, the interendothelial junctions normally are impermeable. However, these junctions open under the influence of hemodynamic stress (e.g., high blood pressure) and/or vasoactive agents (e.g., histamine in inflammation), flooding the adjacent tissues with electrolytes and protein. Vacuolar transcytosis also permits the movement of large amounts of solutes across intact endothelium. Relevant to pathologic processes, ECs also are active participants in the egress of leukocytes during inflammatory cell recruitment (Chapter 3), and EC dysfunction underlies development of atherosclerosis (discussed later).

Although ECs throughout the vasculature share many attributes, they also show phenotypic variability and adaptations depending on the anatomic site and local environmental cues. Thus, EC populations from different parts of the vasculature (e.g., large vessels versus capillaries, or arteries versus veins) have distinct transcriptional programs and behaviors. *Fenestrations* (holes) in ECs lining hepatocyte cords, renal glomeruli, and choroid plexus are specializations that facilitate filtration. Conversely, in the central nervous system, ECs—in conjunction with astrocytes—collaborate to generate an impermeable *blood-brain barrier*.

Maintenance of a "normal," nonthrombogenic EC lining requires laminar flow, certain growth factors (e.g., vascular endothelial growth factor [VEGF]), and firm adhesion to the underlying basement membrane (Fig. 10.2). Trauma or other injuries that denude vessel walls of ECs tip the scales toward thrombosis and vasoconstriction. However, ECs also respond to various physiologic and pathologic stimuli by modulating their usual (constitutive) functions and by expressing new (inducible) properties—a process called *endothelial activation*.

Inducers of endothelial activation include bacterial products, inflammatory cytokines, hemodynamic stresses and lipid products (relevant to atherosclerosis, discussed later), advanced glycation end products (important in diabetic vascular injury), viruses, complement, and various metabolic insults (e.g., hypoxia) (see Fig. 10.2). Activated ECs undergo shape changes, express adhesion molecules, and produce cytokines, chemokines, growth factors, procoagulant and anti-coagulant factors, and a host of other biologically active products—all presumably intended to respond to the original stimulus.

Some of these responses are rapid (occurring within minutes), reversible, and independent of new protein synthesis (e.g., endothelial contraction induced by histamine); others involve alterations in gene and protein expression, and may take days to develop or abate. Exposure of ECs to high levels of stimuli for sustained periods can result in *endothelial dysfunction*, characterized by impaired endothelium-dependent vasodilation, hypercoagulable states, and increased oxygen free radical production. Dysfunctional endothelium can initiate thrombosis, promote atherosclerosis, or contribute to formation of the vascular lesions of hypertension and diabetes.

Vascular Smooth Muscle Cells

SMCs participate in both normal vascular repair and pathologic processes such as atherosclerosis. When stimulated by various factors, SMCs can do the following:
- Proliferate
- Upregulate ECM collagen, elastin, and proteoglycan production
- Elaborate growth factors and cytokines

SMCs also mediate the vasoconstriction or vasodilation that occurs in response to physiologic or pharmacologic stimuli.

The migratory and proliferative activities of SMCs are regulated by numerous factors. Among the most important pro–growth factors are platelet-derived growth factor (PDGF), endothelin, thrombin, fibroblast growth factors, and inflammatory mediators such as interferon-γ (IFN-γ) and interleukin-1 (IL-1). Factors that maintain SMCs in a quiescent state include heparan sulfate, NO, and transforming growth factor-α (TGF-α).

SUMMARY

VASCULAR STRUCTURE AND FUNCTION

- All vessels are lined by endothelium; although all ECs share certain homeostatic properties, ECs in specific vascular beds have special features that allow for tissue-specific functions (e.g., fenestrated ECs in renal glomeruli).
- The relative SMC and ECM content of vessel walls (e.g., in arteries, veins, and capillaries) varies according to hemodynamic demands (e.g., pressure, pulsatility) and functional requirements.
- EC function is tightly regulated in both the basal and activated states. Various physiologic and pathophysiologic stimuli induce endothelial activation and dysfunction that alter the EC phenotype (e.g., procoagulative versus anti-coagulative, proinflammatory versus anti-inflammatory, nonadhesive versus adhesive).

CONGENITAL ANOMALIES

Although rarely symptomatic, unusual anatomic variants of blood vessels can cause complications during surgery, as may occur when a vessel in an unexpected location is injured. Cardiac surgeons and interventional cardiologists also must be familiar with coronary artery variants that can occur in up to 1% to 5% of patients. Among the other congenital vascular anomalies, three deserve further mention:
- *Berry aneurysms* are thin-walled arterial outpouchings in cerebral vessels, classically at branch points around the circle of Willis; they occur where the arterial media is congenitally attenuated and can spontaneously rupture causing fatal intracerebral hemorrhage (Chapter 23).
- *Arteriovenous (AV) fistulas* are abnormal connections between arteries and veins without an intervening capillary bed. They occur most commonly as developmental defects but can also result from rupture of arterial aneurysms into adjacent veins, from penetrating injuries that pierce arteries and veins, or from inflammatory necrosis of adjacent vessels. AV fistulas can be created surgically to provide vascular access for hemodialysis. Extensive AV fistulas can cause high-output cardiac failure by shunting large volumes of blood from the arterial to the venous circulation.
- *Fibromuscular dysplasia* is a focal irregular thickening of the walls of medium- and large-sized muscular arteries due to a combination of medial and intimal hyperplasia and fibrosis. It can manifest at any age but occurs most frequently in young women. The focal wall thickening results in luminal stenosis or can be associated with vessel spasm that reduces vascular flow; in the renal arteries, it can lead to renovascular hypertension. Between the focal segments of thickened wall, the artery often exhibits medial attenuation; vascular outpouchings can develop in these portions of the vessel and sometimes rupture.

BLOOD PRESSURE REGULATION

Systemic and local blood pressure must be maintained within a narrow range to maintain health. Low blood pressure *(hypotension)* results in inadequate organ perfusion, organ dysfunction, and sometimes tissue death. Conversely, high blood pressure *(hypertension)* causes vessel and end-organ damage and is one of the major risk factors for atherosclerosis (see later).

Blood pressure is a function of cardiac output and peripheral vascular resistance, both of which are influenced by multiple genetic and environmental factors (Fig. 10.3). The integration of the various inputs ensures adequate systemic perfusion, despite regional demand differences.
- *Cardiac output is a function of stroke volume and heart rate.* The most important determinant of stroke volume is the filling pressure, which is regulated through sodium homeostasis and its effect on blood volume. Heart rate and myocardial contractility (a second factor affecting stroke volume) are both regulated by the α- and β-adrenergic systems (in addition to their effects on vascular tone).

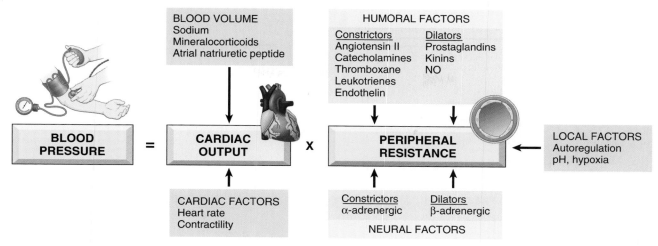

Fig. 10.3 Blood pressure regulation.

- *Peripheral resistance is regulated predominantly at the level of the arterioles* by neural and humoral inputs. Vascular tone reflects a balance between the actions of vasoconstrictors (including angiotensin II, catecholamines, and endothelin) and vasodilators (including kinins, prostaglandins, and NO). Resistance vessels also exhibit autoregulation, whereby increased blood flow induces vasoconstriction to protect tissues against hyperperfusion. Finally, blood pressure is fine-tuned by tissue pH and hypoxia to accommodate local metabolic demands.

Factors released from the kidneys, adrenal glands, and myocardium interact to influence vascular tone and to regulate blood volume by adjusting sodium balance (Fig. 10.4). Each day, the kidneys on average filter 170 liters of plasma containing 23 moles of salt. Thus, with a typical diet containing 100 mEq of sodium, 99.5% of the filtered salt must be reabsorbed to maintain total body sodium levels. About 98% of the filtered sodium is reabsorbed by several constitutively active transporters. Recovery of the remaining 2% of sodium occurs by way of the epithelial sodium channel (ENaC), which is tightly regulated by aldosterone, a downstream effector of the renin-angiotensin system; it is this pathway that determines net sodium balance.

Kidneys influence peripheral resistance and sodium excretion/retention primarily through the renin-angiotensin system. The kidneys and heart contain cells that sense changes in blood pressure and/or blood volume. In response, these cells release several important regulators that act in concert to maintain normal blood pressure:

- *Renin* is a proteolytic enzyme produced by renal juxtaglomerular cells—myoepithelial cells that surround the glomerular afferent arterioles. It is released in response to low blood pressure in afferent arterioles, elevated levels of circulating catecholamines, or low sodium levels in the distal convoluted renal tubules. The latter occurs when the glomerular filtration rate falls (e.g., when the cardiac output is low) because a higher fraction of the filtered sodium is resorbed in the proximal tubules.
- *Angiotensin.* Renin cleaves plasma angiotensinogen to angiotensin I, which in turn is converted to *angiotensin*

II by angiotensin-converting enzyme (ACE) in the periphery. Angiotensin II raises blood pressure by (1) inducing vascular SMC contraction, (2) stimulating aldosterone secretion by the adrenal gland, and (3) increasing tubular sodium resorption.
- *Vasodilators.* The kidney also produces a variety of vascular relaxing substances (including prostaglandins and NO) *that presumably counterbalance the vasopressor effects of angiotensin.*
- *Aldosterone.* Adrenal aldosterone increases blood pressure by its effect on blood volume; aldosterone increases sodium resorption (and thus water) in the distal convoluted and collecting tubules while also driving potassium excretion into the urine.
- *Natriuretic peptides.* Myocardial natriuretic peptides are released from atrial and ventricular myocardium in response to volume expansion; these inhibit sodium resorption in the distal renal tubules, thus leading to sodium excretion and diuresis. They also induce systemic vasodilation.

SUMMARY

BLOOD PRESSURE REGULATION

- Blood pressure is determined by vascular resistance and cardiac output.
- Vascular resistance is regulated at the level of the arterioles, influenced by neural and hormonal inputs.
- Cardiac output is determined by heart rate and stroke volume, the latter of which is strongly influenced by blood volume. Blood volume in turn is regulated mainly by renal sodium excretion or resorption.
- Renin, a major regulator of blood pressure, is secreted by the kidneys in response to decreased blood pressure in afferent arterioles. In turn, renin cleaves angiotensinogen to angiotensin I; subsequent peripheral catabolism produces angiotensin II, which regulates blood pressure by increasing vascular SMC tone and by increasing adrenal aldosterone secretion, which consequently increases renal sodium resorption.

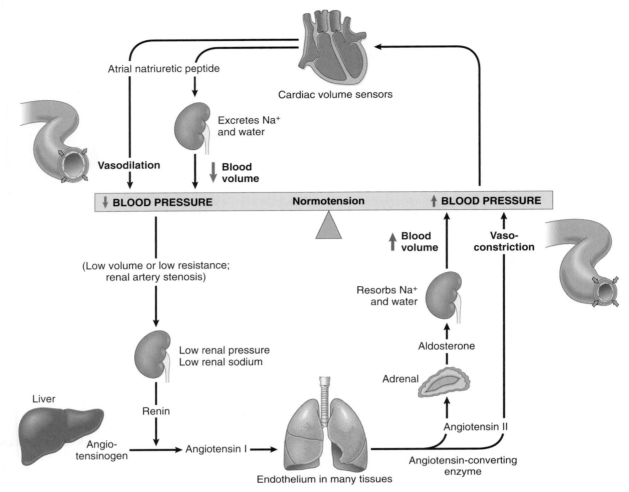

Fig. 10.4 Interplay of renin, angiotensin, aldosterone, and atrial natriuretic peptide in blood pressure regulation (see text).

HYPERTENSIVE VASCULAR DISEASE

Hypertension is a major health problem in the developed world. Although it occasionally manifests in an acute aggressive form, high blood pressure is typically asymptomatic for many years. This insidious condition has been dubbed *essential hypertension,* so called because the gradual age-associated rise in blood pressure was considered "essential" for normal perfusion of endorgans such as the brain. However, such increases are neither essential nor benign; besides increasing the risk for stroke and atherosclerotic coronary heart disease, hypertension can lead to cardiac hypertrophy and heart failure (*hypertensive heart disease;* see Chapter 11), aortic dissection, multi-infarct dementia, and renal failure. While the molecular pathways of blood pressure regulation are reasonably well understood, the mechanisms leading to hypertension in the vast majority of affected individuals remain unknown. The accepted wisdom is that **"essential hypertension" results from the interplay of several genetic polymorphisms (which individually might be inconsequential) and environmental factors, which conspire to increase blood volume and/or peripheral resistance.**

Epidemiology of Hypertension

Like height and weight, blood pressure is a continuously distributed variable; moreover, detrimental consequences increase continuously as the pressure rises, with no rigidly defined threshold dependably predicting total safety. Nevertheless, **sustained diastolic pressures greater than 90 mm Hg or sustained systolic pressures in excess of 140 mm Hg are reliably associated with an increased risk for atherosclerosis and are therefore used as cutoffs in diagnosing hypertension in clinical practice.** By these criteria, over 25% of individuals in the general population are hypertensive. As noted however, these values are somewhat arbitrary, and in patients with other cardiovascular risk factors (e.g., diabetes), lower thresholds may be applicable.

The prevalence of pathologic effects of high blood pressure increases with age and is also higher in African Americans. Without appropriate treatment, some 50% of hypertensive patients die of ischemic heart disease (IHD) or congestive heart failure, and another third succumb to stroke. Reduction of blood pressure dramatically reduces the incidence and clinical sequelae (including death) of all forms of hypertension-related disease. Indeed, treatment of asymptomatic hypertension constitutes one of the few instances in which "preventive medicine" has a major demonstrated health benefit.

A small percentage of hypertensive patients (approximately 5%) present with a rapidly rising blood pressure that, if untreated, leads to death in within 1 to 2 years. Such *malignant hypertension* usually is severe (i.e., systolic pressures over 200 mm Hg or diastolic pressures over 120 mm Hg) and frequently is associated with renal failure and retinal hemorrhages, with or without papilledema. It can arise de novo but most commonly is superimposed on preexisting benign hypertension.

Pathogenesis

Hypertension may be primary (idiopathic) or less commonly secondary to an identifiable underlying condition. In close to 95% of cases hypertension is idiopathic or "essential". Most of the remaining cases (secondary hypertension) are due to primary renal disease, renal artery narrowing (renovascular hypertension), or adrenal disorders (Table 10.2). Essential hypertension is compatible with long life unless a myocardial infarction, stroke, or other complication supervenes. Prognosis of secondary hypertension depends on adequate treatment of the underlying cause. Several relatively rare single-gene disorders cause hypertension (and hypotension) by affecting renal sodium resorption. Such disorders include the following:

- *Gene defects in enzymes involved in aldosterone metabolism* (e.g., aldosterone synthase, 11β-hydroxylase, 17α-hydroxylase), leading to increased aldosterone secretion, increased salt and water resorption, and plasma volume expansion
- *Mutations in proteins that affect sodium resorption* (as in *Liddle syndrome,* which is caused by mutations that prevent the normal degradation of the ENaC sodium channel, leading to increased distal tubular resorption of sodium)

Mechanisms of Essential Hypertension

Although the specific triggers are unknown, it appears that both altered renal sodium handling and increased vascular resistance contribute to essential hypertension.

- *Reduced renal sodium excretion* in the presence of normal arterial pressure probably is a key pathogenic feature; indeed, this is a common etiologic factor in most forms of hypertension. Decreased sodium excretion causes an obligatory increase in fluid volume and increased cardiac output, thereby elevating blood pressure (see Fig. 10.3). At the new higher blood pressure, the kidneys excrete additional sodium. Thus, a new steady state of sodium excretion is achieved, but at the expense of an elevated blood pressure.
- *Increased vascular resistance may stem from vasoconstriction or structural changes in vessel walls.* These are not necessarily independent factors, as chronic vasoconstriction may result in permanent thickening of the walls of affected vessels.
- *Genetic factors* play an important role in determining blood pressure, as shown by familial clustering of hypertension and by studies of monozygotic and dizygotic twins. In a small proportion of cases of essential hypertension there is linkage to specific angiotensinogen polymorphisms and angiotensin II receptor variants; polymorphisms of the renin-angiotensin system also may contribute to the known racial differences in blood pressure regulation. Susceptibility genes for essential hypertension in the vast majority of cases are currently unknown but probably include those that influence renal sodium resorption, the production of endogenous pressors, and SMC growth.
- *Environmental factors,* such as stress, obesity, smoking, physical inactivity, and high levels of salt consumption, modify the impact of genetic determinants. Evidence linking dietary sodium intake with the prevalence of hypertension is particularly strong.

Table 10.2 Types and Causes of Hypertension (Systolic and Diastolic)

Essential Hypertension
Accounts for 90% to 95% of all cases

Secondary Hypertension

Renal
Acute glomerulonephritis
Chronic renal disease
Polycystic disease
Renal artery stenosis
Renal vasculitis
Renin-producing tumors

Endocrine
Adrenocortical hyperfunction (Cushing syndrome, primary aldosteronism, congenital adrenal hyperplasia, licorice ingestion)
Exogenous hormones (glucocorticoids, estrogen [including pregnancy-induced and oral contraceptives], sympathomimetics and tyramine-containing foods, monoamine oxidase inhibitors)
Pheochromocytoma
Acromegaly
Hypothyroidism (myxedema)
Hyperthyroidism (thyrotoxicosis)
Pregnancy-induced (pre-eclampsia)

Cardiovascular
Coarctation of the aorta
Polyarteritis nodosa
Increased intravascular volume
Increased cardiac output
Rigidity of the aorta

Neurologic
Psychogenic
Increased intracranial pressure
Sleep apnea
Acute stress, including surgery

MORPHOLOGY

Hypertension not only accelerates atherogenesis but also causes degenerative changes in the walls of large- and medium-sized arteries that can lead to aortic dissection and cerebrovascular hemorrhage. Three forms of small blood vessel disease are hypertension-related (Fig. 10.5):

- **Hyaline arteriolosclerosis** is associated with benign hypertension. It is marked by homogeneous, pink hyaline thickening of the arteriolar walls, with loss of underlying structural detail, and luminal narrowing (see Fig. 10.5A). The lesions stem from leakage of plasma components across injured ECs into vessel

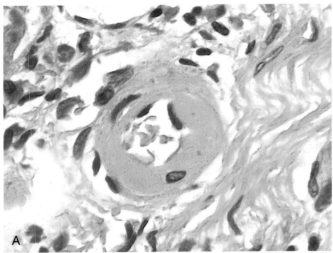

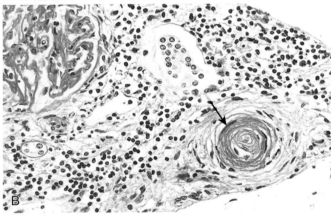

Fig. 10.5 Hypertensive vascular disease. (A) Hyaline arteriolosclerosis. The arteriolar wall is thickened with the deposition of amorphous proteinaceous material (hyalinized), and the lumen is markedly narrowed. (B) Hyperplastic arteriolosclerosis ("onion-skinning") *(arrow)* causing luminal obliteration (periodic acid–Schiff stain). *(B, Courtesy of Helmut Rennke, MD, Brigham and Women's Hospital, Boston, Massachusetts.)*

walls, and increased ECM production by SMCs in response to chronic hemodynamic stress. In the kidneys, the arteriolar narrowing caused by hyaline arteriosclerosis leads to diffuse vascular compromise and **nephrosclerosis** (glomerular scarring). Although the vessels of older adult patients (normotensive or hypertensive) show the same changes, hyaline arteriolosclerosis is more generalized and severe in patients with hypertension. The same lesions also are common in diabetic microangiopathy; in this disorder, the underlying etiology is hyperglycemia-associated EC dysfunction.

* **Hyperplastic arteriolosclerosis** is more typical of severe hypertension. Vessels exhibit "onion skin," concentric, laminated thickening of arteriolar walls and luminal narrowing (see Fig. 10.5B). The laminations consist of SMCs and thickened, reduplicated basement membrane. In malignant hypertension, these changes are accompanied by fibrinoid deposits and vessel wall necrosis **(necrotizing arteriolitis),** which are particularly prominent in the kidney.

● SUMMARY

HYPERTENSION

* Hypertension is a common disorder affecting 25% of the population; it is a major risk factor for atherosclerosis, congestive heart failure, and renal failure.
* Hypertension may be primary (idiopathic) or less commonly secondary to an identifiable underlying condition. In close to 95% of cases hypertension is idiopathic or "essential." The remaining cases (secondary hypertension) are due to primary renal disease, renal artery narrowing (renovascular hypertension), or adrenal disorders.
* Essential hypertension represents 95% of cases and is a complex, multifactorial disorder, involving both environmental influences and genetic polymorphisms that may influence sodium resorption, aldosterone pathways, the adrenergic nervous system, and the renin-angiotensin system.
* Hypertension occasionally is caused by single-gene disorders or is secondary to diseases of the renal arteries, kidneys, adrenal glands, or other endocrine organs.

VASCULAR WALL RESPONSE TO INJURY

Injury to the vessel wall — and in particular to ECs — is the fundamental basis for the vast majority of vascular disorders. Such injurious stimuli may be biochemical, immunologic, or hemodynamic. The integrated function of ECs — and the underlying SMCs — is critical for the vasculature to respond to various stimuli; such responses can be adaptive or may lead to pathologic lesions. Thus, EC injury or dysfunction (as discussed earlier) contributes to a host of pathologic processes including thrombosis, atherosclerosis, and hypertensive vascular lesions. Ensuing SMC proliferation and matrix synthesis can help to repair a damaged vessel wall, but also can eventually lead to luminal occlusion.

Intimal Thickening: A Stereotypical Response to Vascular Injury

Vascular injury leading to EC loss or dysfunction stimulates SMC growth, ECM synthesis, and thickening of the vascular wall. Healing of injured vessels involves the migration of SMCs or SMC precursor cells into the intima. These cells then proliferate and synthesize ECM in much the same way that fibroblasts fill in a wound elsewhere in the body (Fig. 10.6), forming a neointima that typically is covered by an intact EC layer. This neointimal response occurs with any form of vascular damage or dysfunction, including infection, inflammation, immune injury, physical trauma (e.g., from a balloon catheter or hypertension), or toxic exposure (e.g. oxidized lipids or cigarette smoke). Thus, intimal thickening is a stereotypical response of the vessel wall to any insult.

Of note, the phenotype of neointimal SMCs is distinct from medial SMCs. Thus, neointimal SMCs are not contractile like medial SMCs, but do have the capacity to divide and have a considerably greater synthetic capacity

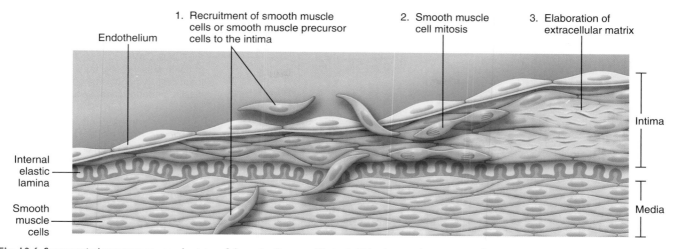

Fig. 10.6 Stereotypical response to vascular injury. Schematic diagram of intimal thickening, emphasizing intimal smooth muscle cell migration and proliferation associated with extracellular matrix synthesis. Intimal smooth muscle cells may derive from the underlying media or may be recruited from circulating precursors; they are depicted in a color different from that of the medial smooth muscle cells, to emphasize their distinct phenotype.

than their sleepy colleagues in the media. Although neo-intimal cells were previously thought to arise exclusively from dedifferentiated medial SMCs, at least a subset is derived from circulating precursor cells. The migratory, proliferative, and synthetic activities of the intimal SMCs are regulated by growth factors and cytokines produced by platelets, ECs, and macrophages, as well as by activated coagulation and complement factors (as discussed earlier).

With restoration and/or normalization of the EC layer, intimal SMCs can return to a nonproliferative state, but not before the healing response has produced intimal thickening. With persistent or recurrent insults, further thickening can occur that leads to the stenosis of small- and medium-sized blood vessels (e.g., as in *atherosclerosis*, discussed later). As a final note, it is also important to recognize that gradual ongoing intimal thickening appears to be a part of "normal aging." Fortunately, such age-related intimal change typically is of no consequence, in part because compensatory outward remodeling of the vessel wall results in little net change in the luminal diameter.

ARTERIOSCLEROSIS

Arteriosclerosis literally means "hardening of the arteries"; it is a generic term reflecting arterial wall thickening and loss of elasticity. Four distinct types are recognized, each with different clinical and pathologic causes and consequences:

- *Arteriolosclerosis* affects small arteries and arterioles and may cause downstream ischemic injury. The two variants, hyaline and hyperplastic arteriolosclerosis, were discussed earlier in relation to hypertension.
- *Mönckeberg medial sclerosis* is characterized by the presence of calcific deposits in muscular arteries, usually centered on the internal elastic lamina, and typically in individuals older than 50 years of age. The lesions do not encroach on the vessel lumen and usually are not clinically significant.
- *Fibromuscular intimal hyperplasia* is a non-atherosclerotic process that occurs in muscular arteries larger than

arterioles. This is predominantly an SMC- and ECM-rich lesion driven by inflammation (as in a healed arteritis or transplant-associated arteriopathy; see Chapter 11), or by mechanical injury (e.g., associated with stents or balloon angioplasty, see later). Such a healing response can cause substantial stenosis of the vessel; indeed such intimal hyperplasia underlies in-stent restenosis and is the major long-term limitation of solid organ transplants.

- *Atherosclerosis*, from Greek root words for "gruel" and "hardening," is the most frequent and clinically important pattern and is the subject of the next section.

ATHEROSCLEROSIS

Atherosclerosis is characterized by intimal lesions called *atheromas* (or *atheromatous* or *atherosclerotic plaques*) that impinge on the vascular lumen and can rupture to cause sudden occlusion. It underlies the pathogenesis of coronary, cerebral, and peripheral vascular disease, and causes more morbidity and mortality (roughly half of all deaths) in the Western world than any other disorder. Atheromatous plaques are raised lesions composed of soft friable (grumous) lipid cores (mainly cholesterol and cholesterol esters, with necrotic debris) covered by fibrous caps (Fig. 10.7). As they enlarged, atherosclerotic plaques may mechanically obstruct vascular lumina, leading to stenosis. Of greater concern, however, atherosclerotic plaques also are prone to rupture, an event that may result in thrombosis and sudden occlusion of the vessel. The thickness of the intimal lesions also may be sufficient to impede the perfusion of the underlying media, which may be weakened by ischemia and by changes in the ECM caused by subsequent inflammation. Together, these two factors weaken the media, setting the stage for the formation of aneurysms.

With better treatment of infectious disorders and increased access to Western dietary behaviors, atherosclerosis is also becoming increasingly prevalent in developing countries. Because coronary artery disease is an important manifestation of atherosclerosis, epidemiologic data related

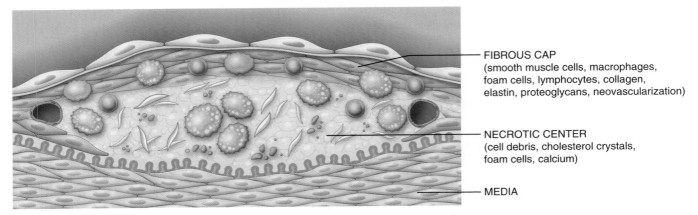

FIBROUS CAP
(smooth muscle cells, macrophages,
foam cells, lymphocytes, collagen,
elastin, proteoglycans, neovascularization)

NECROTIC CENTER
(cell debris, cholesterol crystals,
foam cells, calcium)

MEDIA

Fig. 10.7 The basic structure of an atheromatous plaque.

to atherosclerosis-related mortality typically reflect deaths caused by ischemic heart disease (IHD) (Chapter 11); indeed, myocardial infarction is responsible for roughly one quarter of all deaths in the United States.

Epidemiology of Atherosclerosis

Atherosclerosis is virtually ubiquitous among most developed nations, with prevalence increasing at an alarming pace in developing countries. The mortality rate for IHD in the United States is among the highest in the world, approximately five times higher than that in Japan. However, IHD is increasing in Japan, where it is now the second leading cause of death. Furthermore, Japanese emigrants who come to the United States and adopt American lifestyles and dietary customs acquire the same atherosclerosis risk as U.S.-born individuals, emphasizing the important etiologic role of environmental factors.

The prevalence and severity of atherosclerosis and IHD have been correlated with a number of risk factors in several prospective analyses including the landmark Framingham Heart Study; some of these risk factors are constitutional (and therefore less controllable), but others are acquired or related to modifiable behaviors (Table 10.3). *These risk factors have roughly multiplicative effects.* Thus, two factors increase the risk for myocardial infarction approximately 4-fold, and three (i.e., hyperlipidemia, hypertension, and smoking) increase the rate by a factor of 7 (Fig. 10.8).

Constitutional Risk Factors

- *Genetics.* Family history is the most important independent risk factor for atherosclerosis. Certain mendelian disorders are strongly associated with atherosclerosis (e.g., familial hypercholesterolemia) (Chapter 7), but these account for only a small percentage of cases. Most

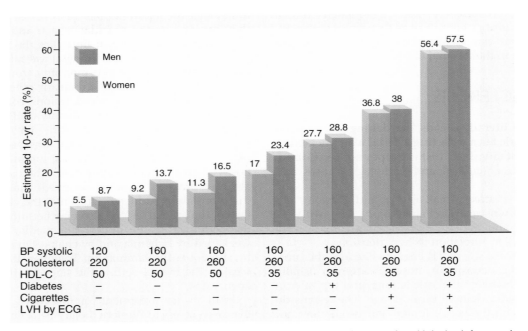

BP systolic	120	160	160	160	160	160	160
Cholesterol	220	220	260	260	260	260	260
HDL-C	50	50	50	35	35	35	35
Diabetes	–	–	–	–	+	+	+
Cigarettes	–	–	–	–	–	+	+
LVH by ECG	–	–	–	–	–	–	+

Fig. 10.8 Estimated 10-year risk for coronary artery disease in 55-year-old men and women as a function of established risk factors—hyperlipidemia, hypertension, smoking, and diabetes. BP, blood pressure; ECG, electrocardiogram; HDL-C, high-density lipoprotein cholesterol; LVH, left ventricular hypertrophy. *(Data from O'Donnell CJ, Kannel WB: Cardiovascular risks of hypertension: lessons from observational studies, J Hypertension 16[Suppl 6]:3, 1998.)*

Table 10.3 Major Risk Factors for Atherosclerosis

Nonmodifiable (Constitutional)
Genetic abnormalities
Family history
Increasing age
Male gender

Modifiable
Hyperlipidemia
Hypertension
Cigarette smoking
Diabetes
Inflammation

familial risk is related to multifactorial traits that go hand-in-hand with atherosclerosis, including hypertension, and, diabetes.

- *Age.* Atherosclerosis usually remains clinically silent until lesions reach a critical threshold in middle age or later. Thus, the incidence of myocardial infarction increases 5-fold between 40 and 60 years of age. Death rates from IHD continue to rise with each successive decade.
- *Gender.* All other factors being equal, premenopausal women are relatively protected against atherosclerosis (and its consequences) compared with age-matched men. Thus, myocardial infarction and other complications of atherosclerosis are uncommon in premenopausal women in the absence of other predisposing factors such as diabetes, hyperlipidemia, or severe hypertension. After menopause, however, the incidence of atherosclerosis-related disease increases and can even exceed that in men. Although a salutary effect of estrogen has long been proposed to explain this gender difference, clinical trials have shown no benefit of hormonal therapy for prevention of vascular disease. Indeed, estrogen replacement after 65 years of age appears to actually increase cardiovascular risk. In addition to atherosclerosis, gender also influences other factors that can affect outcome in patients with IHD, such as hemostasis, infarct healing, and myocardial remodeling.

Modifiable Major Risk Factors

- **Hyperlipidemia—and, more specifically, hypercholesterolemia—is a major risk factor for development of atherosclerosis and is sufficient to induce lesions in the absence of other risk factors.** The main cholesterol component associated with increased risk is low-density lipoprotein (LDL) cholesterol ("bad cholesterol"); LDL distributes cholesterol to peripheral tissues. By contrast, high-density lipoprotein (HDL) cholesterol ("good cholesterol") mobilizes cholesterol from developing and existing vascular plaques and transports it to the liver for biliary excretion. Consequently, higher levels of HDL correlate with reduced risk. Recognition of these relationships has spurred the development of dietary and pharmacologic interventions that lower total serum cholesterol or LDL and/or raise serum HDL, as follows:
  - *High dietary intake of cholesterol* and saturated fats (e.g., present in egg yolks, animal fats, and butter) raises plasma cholesterol levels. Conversely, diets low in cholesterol and/or containing higher ratios of polyunsaturated fats, lower plasma cholesterol levels.
  - *Omega-3 fatty acids* (abundant in fish oils) are beneficial, whereas (trans)-unsaturated fats produced by artificial hydrogenation of polyunsaturated oils (used in baked goods and margarine) adversely affect cholesterol profiles.
  - *Exercise* and moderate consumption of ethanol raise HDL levels, whereas obesity and smoking lower them.
  - *Statins* are a widely used class of drugs that lower circulating cholesterol levels by inhibiting hydroxymethylglutaryl coenzyme A (HMG-CoA) reductase, the rate-limiting enzyme in hepatic cholesterol biosynthesis (Chapter 7).
- *Hypertension* (see earlier discussion) is another major risk factor for development of atherosclerosis. On its own, hypertension can increase the risk for IHD by approximately 60% (see Fig. 10.8). Hypertension also is the major cause of left ventricular hypertrophy (LVH), which also can contribute to myocardial ischemia (see Fig. 10.8).
- *Cigarette smoking* is a well-established risk factor in men and probably accounts for the increasing incidence and severity of atherosclerosis in women. Prolonged (years) smoking of one or more packs of cigarettes per day doubles the rate of IHD-related mortality, while smoking cessation reduces the risk.
- *Diabetes mellitus* is associated with raised circulating cholesterol levels and markedly increases the risk for atherosclerosis. Other factors being equal, the incidence of myocardial infarction is twice as high in diabetics as in non-diabetics. In addition, this disorder is associated with an increased risk for stroke and a 100-fold increase in atherosclerosis-induced gangrene of the lower extremities.

Additional Risk Factors

Roughly 20% of cardiovascular events occur in the *absence of identifiable risk factors.* For example, in previously healthy women, more than 75% of cardiovascular events occur in those with LDL cholesterol levels below 130 mg/dL (a cutoff value considered to connote only borderline risk). Other factors that contribute to risk include the following:

- *Inflammation.* Inflammatory cells are present during all stages of atheromatous plaque formation and are intimately linked with plaque progression and rupture (see the following discussion). There is some evidence that a systemic pro-inflammatory state is associated with the development of atherosclerosis and hence measures of systemic inflammation have been used in risk stratification. Of various systemic markers of inflammation, determination of *C-reactive protein (CRP)* has emerged as one of the simplest and most sensitive. CRP is an acute-phase reactant synthesized primarily by the liver in response to a variety of inflammatory cytokines. In some studies, *CRP levels independently predict the risk for myocardial infarction, stroke, peripheral arterial disease, and sudden cardiac death, even among apparently healthy individuals* (Fig. 10.9). However, such studies are confounded by lack of precise definition of "healthy individuals" because clinically asymptomatic individuals may harbor

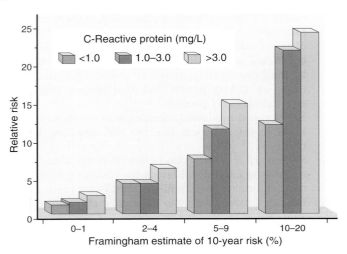

Fig. 10.9 Prognostic value of C-reactive protein (CRP) in coronary artery disease. Relative risk (y-axis) reflects the risk for a cardiovascular event (e.g., myocardial infarction). The x-axis shows the 10-year risk for a cardiovascular event calculated from the traditional risk factors identified in the Framingham Study. In each risk group, CRP levels further stratify the patients. *(Data from Ridker PM, et al: Comparison of C-reactive protein and low-density lipoprotein cholesterol levels in the prediction of first cardiovascular events.* N Engl J Med *347:1557, 2002.)*

significant atherosclerotic lesions with associated inflammation. Thus elevated CRP levels may be a marker of underlying asymptomatic atherosclerosis. Furthermore, there is no direct evidence that lowering CRP diminishes cardiovascular risk or that CRP is involved in the formation of atheromas. It is of interest that CRP is reduced by smoking cessation, weight loss, and exercise, all of which could reduce the risk of atherosclerosis independently. Thus, whether elevated CRP is a marker of or a consequence of plaque inflammation remains to be resolved.

- *Hyperhomocysteinemia.* Serum homocysteine levels correlate with coronary atherosclerosis, peripheral vascular disease, stroke, and venous thrombosis. *Homocystinuria,* due to rare inborn errors of metabolism, causes elevated circulating homocysteine (greater than 100 µmol/L) and is associated with early-onset vascular disease. Although low folate and vitamin B_{12} levels can increase homocysteine levels, supplemental vitamin ingestion does not affect the incidence of cardiovascular disease.
- *Metabolic syndrome.* Associated with central obesity (Chapter 8), this clinical entity is characterized by insulin resistance, hypertension, dyslipidemia (elevated triglycerides and depressed HDL), hypercoagulability, and a pro-inflammatory state, which may be triggered by cytokines released from adipocytes. The dyslipidemia, hyperglycemia, and hypertension are all cardiac risk factors, while the systemic hypercoagulabgramle and pro-inflammatory state may contribute to endothelial dysfunction and/or thrombosis.
- *Lipoprotein(a) levels.* Lipoprotein(a) is an LDL-like particle that contains apolipoprotein B-100 linked to apolipoprotein(a). Lipoprotein(a) levels are correlated with risk of coronary and cerebrovascular disease, independent of total cholesterol or LDL levels.

Apolipoprotein(a) is homologous to plasminogen, suggesting a potential link between thrombogenesis and circulating molecules that can drive atherosclerosis.

- *Elevated levels of procoagulants* are potent predictors of risk for major cardiovascular events including myocardial infarction and stroke. Excessive activation of thrombin, which you may recall can initiate inflammation through cleavage of protease-activated receptors (PARs; Chapter 4) on leukocytes, endothelium, and other cells, may be particularly atherogenic.
- *Clonal hematopoiesis.* It is now recognized that a surprisingly high fraction of older individuals have clonal hematopoiesis (Chapter 12), defined by the presence of a major clone of cells in the bone marrow that have acquired somatic driver mutations in one or more well-characterized oncogenes or tumor suppressor genes. Despite the presence of these mutations, such patients typically have normal blood counts. Unexpectedly, epidemiologic studies have found that clonal hematopoiesis is strongly associated with an increased risk of death from cardiovascular disease, possibly because of alterations in the function of innate immune cells derived from mutated hematopoietic stem cells. Work is ongoing to further confirm this association and determine its mechanistic basis.
- *Other factors* associated with difficult-to-quantify risks include lack of exercise and living a competitive, stressful lifestyle ("type A personality").

Pathogenesis

The currently held view of pathogenesis is embodied in the *response-to-injury hypothesis*. This model views atherosclerosis as a chronic inflammatory response of the arterial wall to endothelial injury. Lesion progression involves interaction of modified lipoproteins, monocyte-derived macrophages, T lymphocytes, and the cellular constituents of the arterial wall (Fig. 10.10). According to this model, atherosclerosis results from the following pathogenic events:

- *EC injury* – and resultant endothelial dysfunction – leading to increased permeability, leukocyte adhesion, and thrombosis
- *Accumulation of lipoproteins* (mainly oxidized LDL and cholesterol crystals) in the vessel wall
- *Platelet adhesion*
- *Monocyte adhesion to the endothelium, migration into the intima, and differentiation into macrophages and foam cells*
- *Lipid accumulation within macrophages,* which respond by releasing inflammatory cytokines
- *SMC recruitment* due to factors released from activated platelets, macrophages, and vascular wall cells
- *SMC proliferation and ECM production*

Some details of these steps are presented next.

Endothelial Injury

EC injury is the cornerstone of the response to injury hypothesis. EC loss due to any kind of injury – induced experimentally by mechanical denudation, hemodynamic forces, immune complex deposition, irradiation, or chemicals – results in intimal thickening; in the presence of high-lipid diets, typical atheromas ensue. However, early

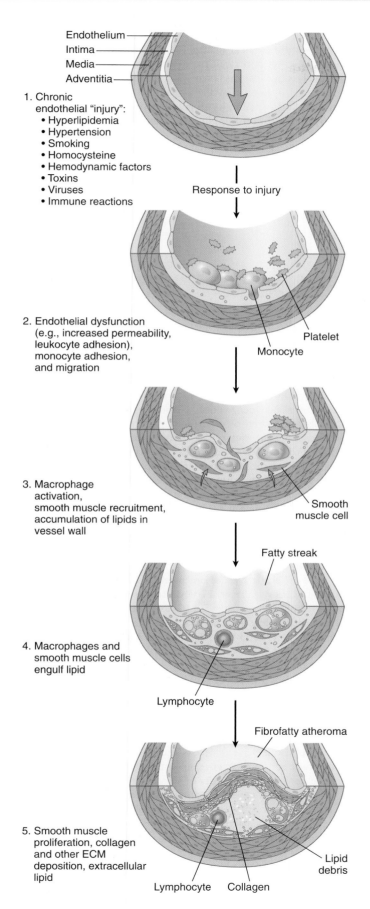

Endothelium
Intima
Media
Adventitia

1. Chronic
   endothelial "injury":
   • Hyperlipidemia
   • Hypertension
   • Smoking
   • Homocysteine
   • Hemodynamic factors
   • Toxins
   • Viruses
   • Immune reactions

Response to injury

2. Endothelial dysfunction
   (e.g., increased permeability,
   leukocyte adhesion),
   monocyte adhesion,
   and migration

Platelet
Monocyte

3. Macrophage
   activation,
   smooth muscle recruitment,
   accumulation of lipids in
   vessel wall

Smooth
muscle cell

Fatty streak

4. Macrophages and
   smooth muscle cells
   engulf lipid

Lymphocyte

Fibrofatty atheroma

5. Smooth muscle
   proliferation, collagen
   and other ECM
   deposition, extracellular
   lipid

Lipid
debris

Lymphocyte   Collagen

human atherosclerotic lesions begin at sites of intact, but dysfunctional, endothelium. These dysfunctional ECs exhibit increased permeability, enhanced leukocyte adhesion, and altered gene expression, all of which may contribute to the development of atherosclerosis.

Suspected triggers of early atheromatous lesions include hypertension, hyperlipidemia, toxins from cigarette smoke, and homocysteinemia. Inflammatory cytokines (e.g., tumor necrosis factor [TNF]) also can stimulate proatherogenic patterns of EC gene expression. Nevertheless, the two most important causes of endothelial dysfunction are hemodynamic disturbances and hypercholesterolemia.

Hemodynamic Disturbances

The importance of hemodynamic factors in atherogenesis is illustrated by the observation that plaques tend to occur at ostia of exiting vessels, at branch points, and along the posterior wall of the abdominal aorta, where there is turbulent blood flow. *In vitro* studies further demonstrate that nonturbulent laminar flow leads to the induction of endothelial genes whose products protect against atherosclerosis. Such "atheroprotective" genes may explain the nonrandom localization of early atherosclerotic lesions.

Lipids

Lipids typically are transported in the bloodstream bound to specific apoproteins (forming lipoprotein complexes). *Dyslipoproteinemias* can result from mutations in genes that encode apoproteins or lipoprotein receptors, or from disorders that derange lipid metabolism, e.g., nephrotic syndrome, alcoholism, hypothyroidism, or diabetes mellitus. Common lipoprotein abnormalities in the general population (and indeed, present in many myocardial infarction survivors) include (1) increased LDL cholesterol levels, (2) decreased HDL cholesterol levels, and 3) increased levels of lipoprotein(a).

Several lines of evidence implicate hypercholesterolemia in atherogenesis:

- The dominant lipids in atheromatous plaques are cholesterol and cholesterol esters.
- Genetic defects in lipoprotein uptake and metabolism that cause hyperlipoproteinemia are associated with accelerated atherosclerosis. Thus, homozygous familial hypercholesterolemia, caused by defective LDL receptors and inadequate hepatic LDL uptake, can lead to myocardial infarction by 20 years of age.
- Other genetic or acquired disorders (e.g., diabetes mellitus, hypothyroidism) that cause hypercholesterolemia lead to premature atherosclerosis.
- Epidemiologic analyses (e.g., the Framingham study) demonstrate a significant correlation between the levels

Fig. 10.10 Response to injury in atherogenesis: *1*, Normal. *2*, Endothelial injury with monocyte and platelet adhesion. *3*, Monocyte and smooth muscle cell migration into the intima, with macrophage activation. *4*, Macrophage and smooth muscle cell uptake of modified lipids and further activation. *5*, Intimal smooth muscle cell proliferation and extracellular matrix elaboration, forming a well-developed plaque.

of total plasma cholesterol or LDL and the severity of atherosclerosis.

- Lowering serum cholesterol by diet or drugs slows the rate of progression of atherosclerosis, causes regression of some plaques, and reduces the risk for cardiovascular events.

The mechanisms by which dyslipidemia contributes to atherogenesis include the following:

- Chronic hyperlipidemia, particularly hypercholesterolemia, can directly impair EC function by increasing local oxygen free radical production; among other things, oxygen free radicals accelerate NO decay, damping its vasodilator activity.
- With chronic hyperlipidemia, lipoproteins accumulate within the intima, where they are hypothesized to generate two pathogenic derivatives, *oxidized LDL and cholesterol crystals.* LDL is oxidized through the action of oxygen free radicals generated locally by macrophages or ECs and ingested by macrophages through the *scavenger receptor,* resulting in *foam cell* formation. Oxidized LDL stimulates the local release of growth factors, cytokines, and chemokines, increasing monocyte recruitment, and also is cytotoxic to ECs and SMCs. More recently, it has been shown that minute extracellular cholesterol crystals found in early atherosclerotic lesions serve as "danger" signals that can activate innate immune cells such as monocytes and macrophages to produce IL-1 and other pro-inflammatory mediators.

Inflammation

Inflammation contributes to the initiation, progression, and complications of atherosclerotic lesions. Normal vessels do not bind inflammatory cells. Early in atherogenesis, however, dysfunctional ECs express adhesion molecules that promote leukocyte adhesion, in particular, monocytes and T cells which migrate into the intima under the influence of locally produced chemokines.

- *Monocytes differentiate into macrophages* and avidly engulf lipoproteins, including oxidized LDL and small cholesterol crystals. Cholesterol crystals appear to be particularly important instigators of inflammation through activation of the inflammasome and subsequent release of IL-1 (Chapter 5). Activated macrophages also produce toxic oxygen species that drive LDL oxidation and elaborate growth factors that stimulate SMC proliferation.
- *T lymphocytes* recruited to the intima interact with the macrophages and also contribute to chronic inflammation. It is not clear whether the T cells are responding to specific antigens (e.g., bacterial or viral antigens, heat-shock proteins [see later], or modified arterial wall constituents and lipoproteins) or are nonspecifically activated by the local inflammatory milieu. Nevertheless, activated T cells in the growing intimal lesions elaborate inflammatory cytokines (e.g., IFN-γ), which stimulate macrophages, ECs, and SMCs.
- As a consequence of the chronic inflammatory state, activated leukocytes and vascular wall cells release growth factors that promote SMC proliferation and matrix synthesis.

SMC Proliferation and Matrix Synthesis

Intimal SMC proliferation and ECM deposition lead to conversion of the earliest lesion, a fatty streak, into a mature atheroma, thus contributing to the progressive growth of atherosclerotic lesions (see Fig. 10.10). Several growth factors are implicated in SMC proliferation and matrix synthesis, including platelet-derived growth factor (released by locally adherent platelets, macrophages, ECs, and SMCs), fibroblast growth factor, and TGF-α. The recruited SMCs synthesize ECM (most notably collagen), which stabilizes atherosclerotic plaques. However, activated inflammatory cells in atheromas also can cause intimal SMC apoptosis and breakdown of matrix, leading to the development of unstable plaques (see later).

MORPHOLOGY

The development of atherosclerosis tends to follow a series of morphologic changes described below.

Fatty Streaks. Fatty streaks begin as minute yellow, flat macules that coalesce into elongated lesions, 1 cm or more in length (Fig. 10.11). They are composed of lipid-filled foamy macrophages but are only minimally raised and do not cause any significant flow disturbance. Fatty streaks can appear in the aortas of infants younger than 1 year of age and are present in virtually all children older than 10 years of age, regardless of genetic, clinical, or dietary risk factors. Not all fatty streaks are destined to progress to atherosclerotic plaques. Nevertheless, it is notable that coronary fatty streaks form during adolescence at the same anatomic sites that are prone to plaques later in life.

Atherosclerotic Plaque. The key features of these lesions are intimal thickening and lipid accumulation (see Fig. 10.7). Atheromatous plaques are white to yellow raised lesions; they range from 0.3 to 1.5 cm in diameter but can coalesce to form larger masses. Thrombus superimposed on ulcerated plaques imparts a red-brown color (Fig. 10.12).

Atherosclerotic plaques are patchy, usually involving only a portion of any given arterial wall; on cross-section, therefore, the lesions appear "eccentric" (Fig. 10.13A). The focal nature of atherosclerotic lesions may be related to the vagaries of vascular hemodynamics. Local flow disturbances, such as turbulence at branch points, make certain parts of a vessel wall especially susceptible to plaque formation.

In descending order of severity, atherosclerosis involves the infrarenal abdominal aorta, the coronary arteries, the popliteal arteries, the internal carotid arteries, and the vessels of the circle of Willis. Even in the same patient, atherosclerosis typically is more severe in the abdominal aorta than in the thoracic aorta. Vessels of the upper extremities usually are spared, as are the mesenteric and renal arteries, except at their ostia. It is important to note that the severity of atherosclerosis in one vascular location does not necessarily predict its severity in another (e.g., aorta versus coronary arteries); nevertheless, any given patient tends to show comparable severity of disease throughout his or her vasculature. Finally, in any given vessel, lesions at various stages of severity often coexist.

Atherosclerotic plaques have three principal components: (1) cells, including SMCs, macrophages, and T cells;

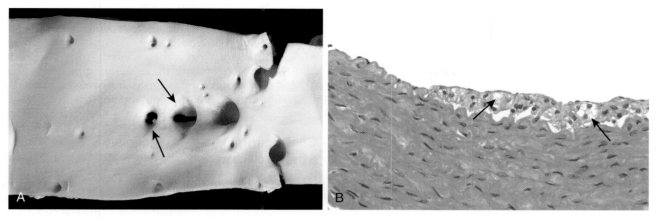

Fig. 10.11 Fatty streaks. (A) Aorta with fatty streaks *(arrows)*, mainly near the ostia of branch vessels. (B) Fatty streak in an experimental hypercholesterolemic rabbit, demonstrating intimal, macrophage-derived foam cells *(arrows). (B, Courtesy of Myron I. Cybulsky, MD, University of Toronto, Toronto, Ontario, Canada.)*

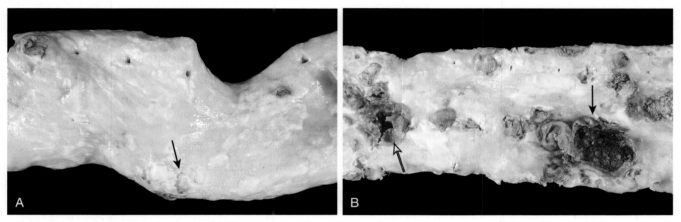

Fig. 10.12 Atherosclerotic lesions. (A) Aorta with mild atherosclerosis composed of fibrous plaques, one denoted by the *arrow*. (B) Aorta with severe diffuse complicated lesions, including an ulcerated plaque *(open arrow),* and a lesion with overlying thrombus *(closed arrow).*

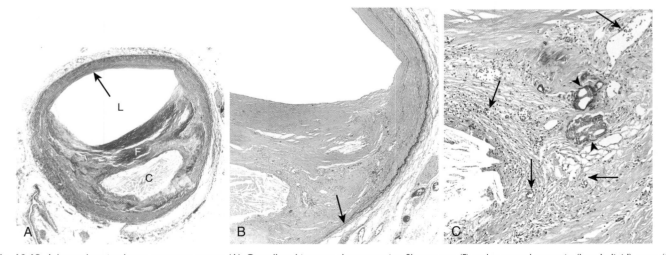

Fig. 10.13 Atherosclerotic plaque, coronary artery. (A) Overall architecture demonstrating fibrous cap *(F)* and a central necrotic (largely lipid) core *(C);* collagen *(blue)* is stained with Masson trichrome. The lumen *(L)* is moderately narrowed by this eccentric lesion, which leaves part of the vessel wall unaffected *(arrow).* (B) Moderate-power view of the plaque shown in A, stained for elastin *(black);* the internal and external elastic membranes are attenuated, and the media of the artery is thinned under the most advanced plaque *(arrow).* (C) High-power view of the junction of the fibrous cap and core, showing scattered inflammatory cells, calcification *(arrowheads),* and neovascularization *(small arrows).*

(2) ECM, including collagen, elastic fibers, and proteoglycans; and (3) intracellular and extracellular lipid (see Fig. 10.13A and B). The proportion and configuration of each component varies from lesion to lesion. Most commonly, plaques have a superficial fibrous cap composed of SMCs and relatively dense collagen. Where the cap meets the vessel wall (the "shoulder") is a more cellular area containing macrophages, T cells, and SMCs. Deep to the fibrous cap is a necrotic core, containing lipid (primarily cholesterol and cholesterol esters), necrotic debris, lipid-laden macrophages and SMCs **(foam cells)**, fibrin, variably organized thrombus, and other plasma proteins. The extracellular cholesterol frequently takes the forms of crystalline aggregates that are washed out during routine tissue processing, leaving behind empty "cholesterol clefts." The periphery of the lesions shows **neovascularization** (proliferating small blood vessels) (see Fig. 10.13C). The media deep to the plaque may be attenuated and exhibit fibrosis secondary to smooth muscle atrophy and loss. Typical atheromas contain relatively abundant lipid, but some so-called **fibrous plaques** are composed almost exclusively of SMCs and fibrous tissue.

Plaques generally progressively enlarge over time through cell death and degeneration, synthesis and degradation of ECM (remodeling), and thrombus organization. Atheromas also often undergo calcification (see Fig. 10.13C).

Atherosclerotic plaques are susceptible to several clinically important changes:

- *Rupture, ulceration, or erosion* of the luminal surface of atheromatous plaques exposes highly thrombogenic substances and induces **thrombus formation.** Thrombi may partially or completely occlude the lumen, leading to tissue ischemia (e.g., in the heart) (Chapter 11) (Fig. 10.14). If the patient survives, thrombi become organized and incorporated into the growing plaque.
- *Hemorrhage into a plaque.* Rupture of the overlying fibrous cap or of the thin-walled vessels in the areas of neovascularization can cause intra-plaque hemorrhage; the resulting hematoma may cause rapid plaque expansion or plaque rupture.

- *Atheroembolism.* Ruptured plaque can discharge debris into the blood, producing microemboli composed of plaque contents.
- *Aneurysm formation.* Atherosclerosis-induced pressure or ischemic atrophy of the underlying media, with loss of elastic tissue, causes structural weakening that can lead to aneurysmal dilation and rupture.

Clinicopathologic Consequences of Atherosclerosis

Large elastic arteries (e.g., aorta, carotid, and iliac arteries) and large- and medium-sized muscular arteries (e.g., coronary, renal, and popliteal arteries) are the vessels most commonly involved by atherosclerosis. Accordingly, atherosclerosis is most likely to present with signs and symptoms related to ischemia of the heart, brain, kidneys, and lower extremities. **Myocardial infarction (heart attack), cerebral infarction (stroke), aortic aneurysm, and peripheral vascular disease (gangrene of extremities) are the major clinical consequences of atherosclerosis.**

The natural history, morphologic features, and main pathogenic events are schematized in Figure 10.15. The principal pathophysiologic outcome stemming from atherosclerotic lesions vary depending on the size of the affected vessel, the size and stability of the plaques, and the degree to which plaques disrupt the vessel wall. We next describe the features of atherosclerotic lesions that are typically responsible for the clinical manifestations.

Atherosclerotic Stenosis

At early stages, remodeling of the media tends to preserve the luminal diameter by increasing the overall vessel circumference. Owing to limits on remodeling, however, eventually the expanding atheroma may impinge on blood flow. Although this most commonly happens as a consequence of acute plaque change (described next), it can also occur gradually, with *critical stenosis* being the tipping point at which chronic occlusion limits flow so severely

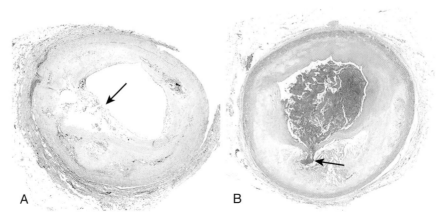

A   B

Fig. 10.14 Atherosclerotic plaque rupture. (A) Plaque rupture without superimposed thrombus, in a patient who died suddenly. (B) Acute coronary thrombosis superimposed on an atherosclerotic plaque with focal disruption of the fibrous cap, triggering fatal myocardial infarction. In both A and B, an arrow points to the site of plaque rupture. *(B, Reproduced from Schoen FJ: Interventional and surgical cardiovascular pathology: clinical correlations and basic principles, Philadelphia, 1989, Saunders, p 61.)*

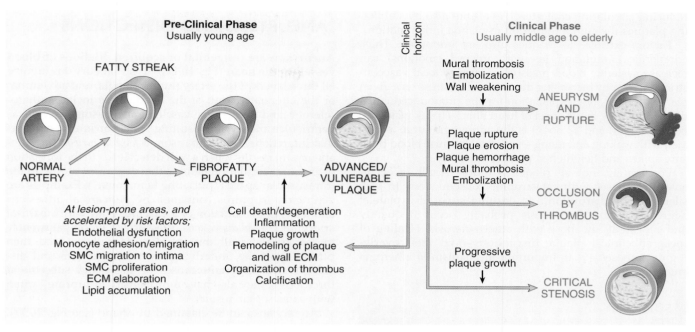

Fig. 10.15 Summary of the natural history, morphologic features, main pathogenic events, and clinical complications of atherosclerosis.

that tissue demand exceeds supply. In the coronary artery (and other) circulations, this typically occurs when the vessel is approximately 70% occluded. At rest, affected patients have adequate cardiac perfusion; but with even modest exertion, demand exceeds supply, and chest pain develops because of cardiac ischemia *(stable angina)* (Chapter 11). The toll of chronic arterial hypoperfusion due to atherosclerosis in various vascular beds includes *bowel ischemia, sudden cardiac death, chronic IHD, ischemic encephalopathy,* and *intermittent claudication* (ischemic leg pain).

Acute Plaque Change

Plaque erosion or rupture typically triggers thrombosis, leading to partial or complete vascular obstruction and often tissue infarction (Fig. 10.15). Plaque changes fall into three general categories:

- *Rupture/fissuring,* exposing highly thrombogenic plaque constituents
- *Erosion/ulceration,* exposing the thrombogenic subendothelial basement membrane to blood
- *Hemorrhage into the atheroma,* expanding its volume

It is now recognized that plaques responsible for myocardial infarctions and other acute coronary syndromes often are asymptomatic before the acute event; symptoms are triggered by thrombosis on a lesion that previously did not produce significant luminal occlusion. The worrisome conclusion is that large numbers of asymptomatic individuals are at risk for a catastrophic coronary event. The causes of acute plaque change are complex and include both intrinsic factors (e.g., plaque structure and composition) and extrinsic factors (e.g., blood pressure). These factors combine to weaken the integrity of the plaque, making it unable to withstand vascular shear forces.

Certain types of plaques are believed to be at particularly high risk of rupturing. These include plaques that contain large

numbers of foam cells and abundant extracellular lipid, plaques that have thin fibrous caps containing few SMCs, and plaques that contain clusters of inflammatory cells. Plaques at high risk for rupture are referred to as *vulnerable plaques* (Fig. 10.16). The fibrous cap also undergoes continuous remodeling; its mechanical strength and stability are proportional to its collagen content, so the balance of collagen synthesis and degradation affects cap integrity. Collagen in atherosclerotic plaques is synthesized primarily by SMCs, and loss of SMCs understandably results in cap weakening.

In general, **plaque inflammation increases collagen degradation and reduces collagen synthesis, thereby destabilizing the mechanical integrity of the cap.** Of interest, statins may have a beneficial effect not only by

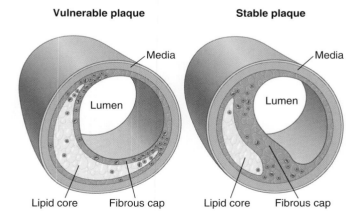

Fig. 10.16 Vulnerable and stable atherosclerotic plaque. Stable plaques have densely collagenized and thickened fibrous caps with minimal inflammation and negligible underlying atheromatous cores, whereas vulnerable plaques have thin fibrous caps, large lipid cores, and increased inflammation. *(Adapted from Libby P: Molecular bases of the acute coronary syndromes, Circulation 91:2844, 1995.)*

reducing circulating cholesterol levels but also by stabilizing plaques through a reduction in plaque inflammation.

Factors extrinsic to plaques also are important. Thus, adrenergic stimulation (as with intense emotions) can increase systemic blood pressure or induce local vasoconstriction, thereby increasing the mechanical stress on a given plaque. Indeed, one explanation for the pronounced circadian periodicity in the onset of heart attacks (peak incidence between 6 AM and 12 noon) is the adrenergic surge associated with waking and rising—sufficient to cause blood pressure spikes and heightened platelet reactivity.

Fortunately, not all plaque ruptures result in occlusive thromboses with catastrophic consequences. In fact, silent plaque disruption and ensuing superficial platelet aggregation and thrombosis probably occur frequently and repeatedly in those with atherosclerosis. Healing of these subclinical plaque disruptions—and their overlying thromboses—is an important mechanism of atheroma enlargement.

SUMMARY

ATHEROSCLEROSIS

- Atherosclerosis is an intima-based lesion composed of a fibrous cap and an atheromatous (literally, "gruel-like") core; the constituents of the plaque include SMCs, ECM, inflammatory cells, lipids, and necrotic debris.
- Atherogenesis is driven by an interplay of vessel wall injury and inflammation. The multiple risk factors for atherosclerosis all cause EC dysfunction and influence SMC recruitment and stimulation.
- Major modifiable risk factors for atherosclerosis are hypercholesterolemia, hypertension, cigarette smoking, and diabetes mellitus.
- Atherosclerotic plaques develop and grow slowly over decades. Stable plaques can produce symptoms related to chronic ischemia by narrowing vessels, whereas unstable plaques can cause dramatic and potentially fatal ischemic complications related to acute plaque rupture, thrombosis, or embolization.
- Stable plaques tend to have a dense fibrous cap, minimal lipid accumulation, and little inflammation, whereas "vulnerable" unstable plaques have thin caps, large lipid cores, and relatively dense inflammatory infiltrates.

ANEURYSMS AND DISSECTIONS

Aneurysms are congenital or acquired dilations of blood vessels or the heart (Fig. 10.17). "True" aneurysms involve all three layers of the artery (intima, media, and adventitia) or the attenuated wall of the heart; these include atherosclerotic and congenital vascular aneurysms, as well as ventricular aneurysms resulting from transmural myocardial infarctions. By comparison, a *false aneurysm* (pseudoaneurysm) results when a wall defect leads to the formation of an extravascular hematoma that communicates with the intravascular space ("pulsating hematoma"). Examples are ventricular ruptures contained by pericardial adhesions and leaks at the junction of a vascular graft with a natural artery. In *arterial dissections,* pressurized blood gains entry to the arterial wall through a surface defect and then pushes apart the underlying layers. Aneurysms and dissections are important causes of stasis and subsequent thrombosis; they also have a propensity to rupture—often with catastrophic results.

Aneurysms can be classified by shape (see Fig. 10.17). *Saccular aneurysms* are discrete outpouchings ranging from 5 to 20 cm in diameter, often with a contained thrombus. *Fusiform aneurysms* are circumferential dilations up to 20 cm in diameter; these most commonly involve the aortic arch, the abdominal aorta, or the iliac arteries.

Pathogenesis

Arteries are dynamic tissues that must withstand the constant mechanical stress of pulsatile blood flow. Aneurysms occur when alterations in SMCs or ECM compromise the structural integrity of the arterial media. Among the implicated factors in aneurysm formation are the following:

- *Inadequate or abnormal connective tissue synthesis.* Several rare inherited diseases provide insight into the types of abnormalities that can lead to aneurysm formation. As discussed earlier, TGF-β regulates SMC proliferation and matrix synthesis. Thus, mutations in TGF-β receptors or downstream signaling pathways result in defective elastin and collagen synthesis; aneurysms in affected

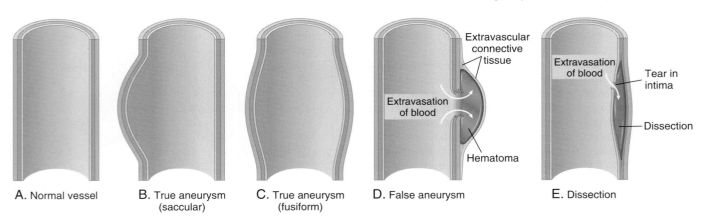

A. Normal vessel   B. True aneurysm (saccular)   C. True aneurysm (fusiform)   D. False aneurysm   E. Dissection

Fig. 10.17 Aneurysms. (A) Normal vessel. (B) True aneurysm, saccular type. The wall bulges outward and may be attenuated but is otherwise intact. (C) True aneurysm, fusiform type. There is circumferential dilation of the vessel. (D) False aneurysm. The wall is ruptured, creating a collection of blood (hematoma) bounded externally by adherent extravascular tissues. (E) Dissection. Blood has entered the wall of the vessel and separated (dissected) the layers.

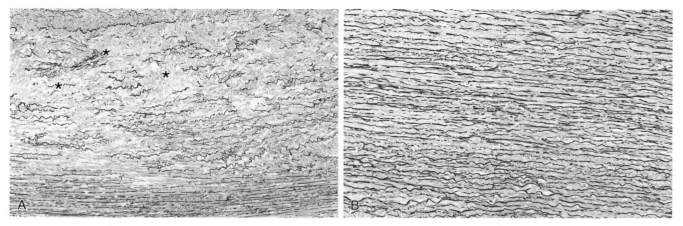

Fig. 10.18 Cystic medial degeneration. (A) Cross-section of aortic media from a patient with Marfan syndrome, showing marked elastin fragmentation and areas devoid of elastin that resemble cystic spaces *(asterisks)*. (B) Normal media for comparison, showing the regular layered pattern of elastic tissue. In both (A) and (B), elastin is stained black.

individuals often rupture, even when small. In *Marfan syndrome* (Chapter 7), defective synthesis of the scaffolding protein *fibrillin* leads to increased bioavailability of TGF-β in the aortic wall, with subsequent dilation due to dysregulated signaling and progressive loss of elastic tissue. Defective type III collagen synthesis leading to aneurysm formation is a hallmark of type IV *Ehlers-Danlos syndrome* (Chapter 7).

- *Excessive connective tissue degradation.* Increased matrix metalloprotease expression by macrophages in atherosclerotic plaque can contribute to aneurysm development by degrading arterial ECM in the arterial wall; similarly, decreased tissue inhibitors of metalloprotease expression can also tip the balance toward net ECM degradation. A genetic predisposition to aneurysm formation in the setting of inflammation may be related to polymorphisms in these factors.
- *Loss of SMCs or change in the SMC synthetic phenotype.* Atherosclerotic thickening of the intima can cause ischemia of the inner media by increasing the diffusion distance from the lumen. Conversely, systemic hypertension can cause luminal narrowing of the aortic vasa vasorum, leading to ischemia of the outer media. Such ischemia results in SMC loss as well as aortic "degenerative changes," which include fibrosis (replacing distensible elastic tissue), inadequate ECM synthesis, and accumulation of increasing amounts of amorphous proteoglycans. Histologically, these changes are collectively called *cystic medial degeneration* (Fig. 10.18), although no true cysts are formed. Such changes are nonspecific; they can occur whenever ECM synthesis is defective, including in inherited disorders such as Marfan syndrome and acquired conditions such as scurvy.

The two most important predisposing conditions for aortic aneurysms are atherosclerosis and hypertension. Atherosclerosis is the dominant factor in abdominal aortic aneurysms, while hypertension is associated with ascending aortic aneurysms. Other conditions that weaken vessel walls and lead to aneurysms include trauma, vasculitis (see later), congenital defects, and infections, giving rise to so-called "mycotic aneurysms." Mycotic aneurysms may result from (1) embolization of a septic embolus, usually as a complication of infective endocarditis; (2) extension of an adjacent suppurative process; or (3) direct infection of an arterial wall by circulating organisms. Tertiary syphilis is a rare cause of aortic aneurysms. A predilection of the spirochetes for the vasa vasorum of the ascending thoracic aorta—and the subsequent immune response to them—results in an *obliterative endarteritis* that compromises blood flow to the media; the ensuing ischemic injury leads to aneurysmal dilation that occasionally also can involve the aortic valve annulus.

Abdominal Aortic Aneurysm

Aneurysms occurring as a consequence of atherosclerosis form most commonly in the abdominal aorta and common iliac arteries, and may also involve the aortic arch and descending thoracic aorta. Abdominal aortic aneurysms (AAAs) occur more frequently in men and in smokers and rarely develop before 50 years of age. Atherosclerosis is a major cause of AAA, but other factors clearly contribute, since the incidence is less than 5% in men older than 60 years of age despite the almost universal presence of abdominal aortic atherosclerosis in this population.

In the majority of cases, AAA results from ECM degradation mediated by proteolytic enzymes released from inflammatory infiltrates in atherosclerotic lesions. Atherosclerotic plaques also compromise the diffusion of nutrients and wastes between the vascular lumen and the arterial wall, alternations that have deleterious effects on SMCs in the media. Due to this combination of effects, the media undergoes degeneration and necrosis, which results in arterial wall thinning. A familial predisposition to AAA, independent of genetic predilections to atherosclerosis or hypertension, appears to be a factor in some individuals. Of note, smokers who develop AAA tend to have more severe chronic obstructive pulmonary disease, particularly emphysema, suggesting that such patients are constitutionally predisposed to develop disorders associated with ECM degradation.

MORPHOLOGY

Abdominal aortic aneurysms typically occur between the renal arteries and the aortic bifurcation; they can be saccular or fusiform and up to 15 cm in diameter and 25 cm in length (Fig. 10.19). In the vast majority of cases, extensive atherosclerosis is present, with thinning and focal destruction of the underlying media. The aneurysm sac usually contains bland, laminated, poorly organized mural thrombus, which can fill much of the dilated segment. Not infrequently, AAAs are accompanied by smaller iliac artery aneurysms. Next we describe some of the less common forms of aortic aneurysms:

• **Inflammatory AAAs** are a distinct subtype characterized by dense periaortic fibrosis containing abundant lymphoplasmacytic inflammation with many macrophages and giant cells.

• A subset of inflammatory AAAs may be a vascular manifestation of a recently recognized entity called **immunoglobulin G4 (IgG4)-related disease.** This disorder is marked by tissue fibrosis associated with frequent infiltrating IgG4-expressing plasma cells. As discussed in Chapter 5, IgG4-related diseases can also affect a variety of tissues, including the pancreas, biliary system, thyroid gland, and salivary gland. Affected individuals have aortitis and periaortitis that weaken the wall sufficiently in some cases to give rise to aneurysms. Recognition of this entity is important since it responds well to steroid therapy.

• **Mycotic AAAs** occur when circulating microorganisms (as in bacteremia from infective endocarditis) seed the aneurysm wall or the associated thrombus; the resulting suppuration accelerates the medial destruction and may lead to rapid dilation and rupture.

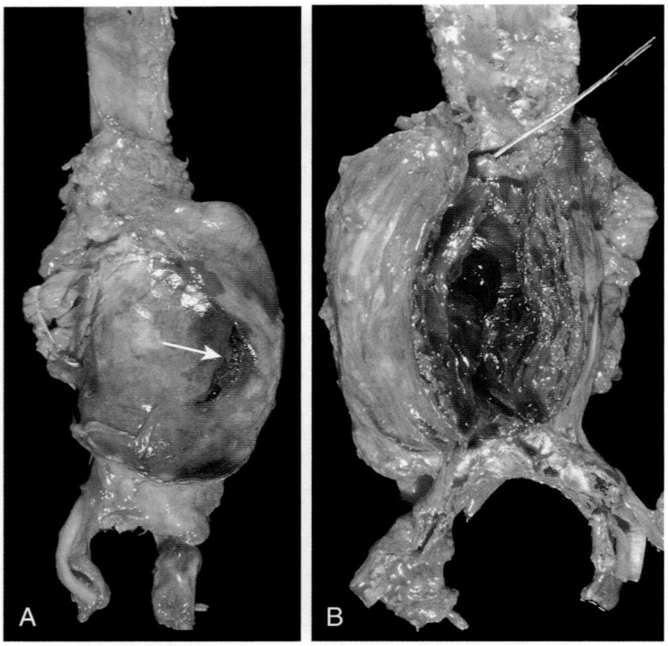

Clinical Consequences

The clinical consequences of AAA include the following:
• *Obstruction* of a vessel branching off the aorta (e.g., the renal, iliac, vertebral, or mesenteric arteries), resulting in ischemia of the kidneys, legs, spinal cord, or gastrointestinal tract, respectively
• *Embolism* of atheromatous material (e.g., cholesterol crystals) or mural thrombus
• *Impingement on adjacent structures* (e.g., compression of a ureter or erosion of vertebrae by the expanding aneurysm)
• *An abdominal mass* (often palpably pulsating) that simulates a tumor
• *Rupture* into the peritoneal cavity or retroperitoneal tissues, leading to massive, often fatal hemorrhage

The risk for rupture is related to the size of AAAs. Those 4 cm or less in diameter almost never burst, while those between 4 and 5 cm do so at a rate of 1% per year. The risk rises to 11% per year for AAAs 5 to 6 cm in diameter, and to 25% per year for aneurysms greater than 6 cm in diameter. Thus, aneurysms 5 cm in diameter or larger are managed surgically, either by open placement of tubular prosthetic grafts or with endoluminal insertion of stented grafts (expandable wire frames covered by a cloth sleeve). Timely intervention is critical, because the mortality rate for elective procedures is approximately 5%, whereas the rate for emergency surgery after rupture is roughly 50%.

A point worthy of emphasis is that because atherosclerosis is a systemic disease, a patient with AAA also is very likely to have atherosclerosis in other vascular beds and is at a significantly increased risk for ischemic heart disease and stroke.

Thoracic Aortic Aneurysm

Thoracic aortic aneurysms most commonly are associated with hypertension, bicuspid aortic valves, and Marfan syndrome. Less commonly, disorders caused by mutations in the TGF-β signaling pathway are causative. These aneurysms manifest with the following signs and symptoms:
• *Respiratory or feeding difficulties* due to airway or esophageal compression, respectively, because of encroachment on mediastinal structures
• *Persistent cough* from irritation of the recurrent laryngeal nerves
• *Pain* caused by erosion of bone (i.e., ribs and vertebral bodies)
• *Cardiac disease* due to valvular insufficiency or narrowing of the coronary ostia; heart failure induced by aortic valvular incompetence
• *Aortic dissection* or rupture

Aortic Dissection

Aortic dissection occurs when blood splays apart the laminar planes of the media to form a blood-filled channel within the aortic wall (Fig. 10.20). This development can be catastrophic if the dissecting blood ruptures through the adventitia and escapes into adjacent spaces.

Fig. 10.19 Abdominal aortic aneurysm. (A) External site of rupture of a large aortic aneurysm is indicated by the *arrow*. (B) Opened aorta, with the location of the rupture tract indicated by a *probe*. The wall of the aneurysm is attenuated, and the lumen is filled by a large, layered thrombus.

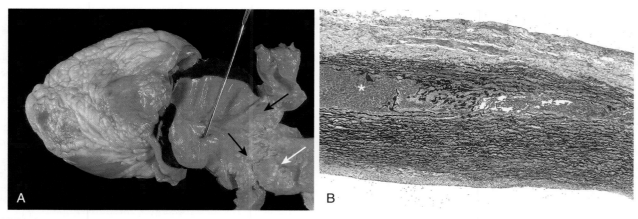

Fig. 10.20 Aortic dissection. (A) An opened aorta with a proximal dissection originating from a small, oblique intimal tear *(identified by the probe)* associated with an intramural hematoma. Note that the intimal tear occurred in a region largely free of atherosclerotic plaque. The distal edge of the intramural hematoma *(black arrows)* lies at the edge of a large area of atherosclerosis *(white arrow)*, which arrested the propagation of the dissection. (B) Histologic preparation showing the dissection and intramural hematoma *(asterisk)*. Aortic elastic layers are *black,* and blood is *red* in this section, stained with Movat stain.

Aortic dissection need not be associated with aortic dilation, and the older term *dissecting aneurysm* should be avoided. Aortic dissection occurs mainly in two age groups: (1) men 40 to 60 years of age with antecedent hypertension (more than 90% of cases); and (2) younger patients with connective tissue abnormalities that affect the aorta (e.g., Marfan syndrome). Dissections also can be iatrogenic (e.g., complicating arterial cannulation during diagnostic catheterization or cardiopulmonary bypass).

Rarely, pregnancy is associated with aortic (or other vessel) dissection (roughly 10 to 20 cases per 1 million births). This typically occurs during or after the third trimester, and may be related to hormone-induced vascular remodeling and the hemodynamic stresses of the perinatal period. Dissection is unusual in the presence of substantial atherosclerosis or other causes of medial scarring, presumably because the medial fibrosis inhibits propagation of the dissecting hematoma (see Fig. 10.20).

Pathogenesis

Hypertension is the major risk factor for aortic dissection. Aortas in hypertensive patients show narrowing of the vasa vasorum associated with degenerative changes in ECM and variable loss of medial SMCs, suggesting that diminished flow through the vasa vasorum is contributory. Abrupt , transient increase in blood pressure, as may occur with cocaine abuse, is also known to cause aortic dissection. Most other dissections are related to heritable or acquired connective tissue disorders that give rise to abnormal aortic ECM, including Marfan syndrome, Ehlers-Danlos syndrome type IV, and defects in copper metabolism.

The trigger for the intimal tear and subsequent intramural hemorrhage is not known in most cases. Nevertheless, once the tear has occurred, blood under systemic pressure dissects through the media along laminar planes. Accordingly, aggressive pressure-reducing therapy may be effective in limiting an evolving dissection. In rare cases, disruption of the vasa vasorum can give rise to an intramural hematoma without an intimal tear.

MORPHOLOGY

In most dissections, the intimal tear marking the point of origin is found in the ascending aorta within 10 cm of the aortic valve (see Fig. 10.20A). Such tears usually are transverse or oblique in orientation and 1 to 5 cm long, with sharp, jagged edges. The dissection plane can extend retrograde toward the heart or distally, occasionally as far as the iliac and femoral arteries, and usually lies between the middle and outer thirds of the media (see Fig. 10.20B).

External rupture causes massive hemorrhage, or results in cardiac tamponade if it occurs into the pericardial sac. In some (fortunate) instances, the dissecting hematoma reenters the lumen of the aorta through a second distal intimal tear, creating a second vascular channel within the media (so-called "double-barreled aorta"). Over time, such a false channel becomes endothelialized forming a chronic dissection.

In most instances, no specific underlying causal defect is identified in the aortic wall. The most frequent histologically detectable lesion is the **cystic medial degeneration** discussed earlier; this is characterized by SMC dropout and necrosis, elastic tissue fragmentation, and accumulations of amorphous proteoglycan-rich ECM (see Fig. 10.18). Inflammation is characteristically absent. Recognizable medial damage appears to be neither a prerequisite for dissection nor a guarantee that dissection is imminent. Occasionally, dissections occur in the setting of seemingly trivial medial degeneration, while marked degenerative changes may be seen at autopsy in individuals without dissection.

Clinical Consequences

The clinical manifestations of dissection depend primarily on the portion of the aorta affected; the most serious complications occur with dissections involving the proximal aorta and arch. Thus, aortic dissections generally are classified into two types (Fig. 10.21):

- *Proximal lesions (type A dissections),* involving the ascending aorta, with or without involvement of the descending aorta (DeBakey type I or II, respectively)

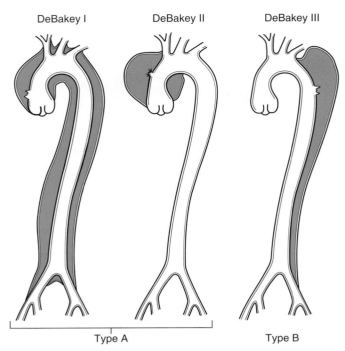

DeBakey I　　　DeBakey II　　　DeBakey III

Type A　　　　　　　　　Type B

Fig. 10.21 Classification of dissections. Type A dissections (proximal) involve the ascending aorta, either as part of a more extensive dissection (DeBakey type I), or in isolation (DeBakey type II). Type B dissections (distal, or DeBakey type III) arise after the takeoff of the great vessels. Type A dissections typically have the most serious complications and the greatest associated mortality.

- *Distal lesions (type B dissections),* usually beginning beyond the subclavian artery (DeBakey type III)

The classic clinical symptom of aortic dissection is the sudden onset of excruciating tearing or stabbing pain, usually beginning in the anterior chest, radiating to the back between the scapulae, and moving downward as the dissection progresses. The most common cause of death is rupture of the dissection into the pericardial, pleural, or peritoneal cavity. Retrograde dissection into the aortic root also can cause fatal disruption of the aortic valvular apparatus or compression of the coronary arteries. Common clinical presentations stemming from cardiac involvement include tamponade, aortic insufficiency, and myocardial infarction. Other complications are related to extension of the dissection to the great arteries of the neck and the renal, mesenteric, or iliac arteries, any of which may become obstructed. Similarly, compression of spinal arteries can cause transverse myelitis.

In type A dissections, rapid diagnosis and institution of intensive anti-hypertensive therapy coupled with surgical plication of the aortic intimal tear can save 65% to 85% of the patients. However, the mortality rate approaches 70% in patients who present with hemorrhage or symptoms related to distal ischemia, and the overall 10-year survival rate is only 40% to 60%. Most type B dissections can be managed conservatively; patients have a 75% survival rate whether they are treated with surgery or with anti-hypertensive medication only.

SUMMARY

ANEURYSMS AND DISSECTIONS

- Aneurysms are congenital or acquired dilations of the heart or blood vessels that involve the entire wall thickness. Complications are related to rupture, thrombosis, and embolization.
- Dissections occur when blood enters the wall of a vessel and separates the various layers. Complications arise as a result of rupture or obstruction of vessels branching off the aorta.
- Aneurysms and dissections result from structural weakness of the vessel wall caused by loss of SMCs or weakening of the ECM, which can be a consequence of ischemia, genetic defects, or defective matrix remodeling.

VASCULITIS

Vasculitis is a general term for vessel wall inflammation. The two most common pathogenic mechanisms of vasculitis are immune-mediated inflammation and direct vascular invasion by infectious pathogens. Infections also can indirectly precipitate immune-mediated vasculitis (e.g., by generating immune complexes or triggering cross-reactivity). In any given patient, it is critical to distinguish between infectious and immunologic mechanisms because immunosuppressive therapy is appropriate for immune-mediated vasculitis but could exacerbate infectious vasculitis. Physical and chemical injury, including that due to radiation, mechanical trauma, and toxins, also can cause vasculitis.

Some 20 primary forms of vasculitis are recognized, and classification schemes attempt (with variable success) to group them according to vessel diameter, role of immune complexes, presence of specific autoantibodies, granuloma formation, organ specificity, and even population demographics (Table 10.4 and Fig. 10.22).

The possible clinical manifestations are protean, but they largely depend on the specific vascular bed that is affected. Besides findings referable to the affected tissue(s), there are usually also signs and symptoms of systemic inflammation, such as fever, myalgia, arthralgias, and malaise. There is considerable clinical and pathologic overlap among these entities, as will be evident from the discussion of individual forms below.

Noninfectious Vasculitis

The main immunologic mechanisms underlying noninfectious vasculitis are as follows:
- Immune complex deposition
- Anti-neutrophil cytoplasmic antibodies
- Anti-EC antibodies
- Autoreactive T cells

Immune Complex–Associated Vasculitis

This form of vasculitis is seen in immunologic disorders such as systemic lupus erythematosus (Chapter 5) that are associated with autoantibody production. The vascular lesions resemble those found in experimental immune

Table 10.4 Primary Forms of Vasculitis

	Giant Cell Arteritis	Granulomatosis With Polyangiitis	Churg-Strauss Syndrome	Polyarteritis Nodosa	Leukocytoclastic Vasculitis	Buerger Disease	Behçet Disease
Sites of Involvement							
Aorta	+	−	−	−	−	−	−
Medium-sized arteries	+	+	+	+	−	+	+
Small-sized arteries	−	+	+	+	+	+	+
Capillaries	−	−	−	−	+	−	+
Veins	−	−	−	−	+	+	+
Inflammatory Cells Present							
Lymphocytes	+	+	+	±	±	±	±
Macrophages	+	+	+	±	±	±	±
Neutrophils	Rare	+	+	±	±	±	Required
Eosinophils	Very rare	±	Required	±	±	±	±
Other Features							
Granulomas	±*	Required*	±	−	−	−	−
Giant cells	Often; not required	±	−	−	−	−	−
Thrombosis	±	±	±	±	±	Required	±
Serum ANCA positivity	−	+	+	±	−	−	−
Clinical history	>40 years of age, ± polymyalgia rheumatica	Any	Asthma, atopy	Any	Any	Young male smoker	Orogenital ulcers

*The granulomas of giant cell arteritis are found within the vessel wall as part of the inflammation comprising the vasculitis, but need not be present to render the diagnosis. The granulomas of granulomatosis with polyangiitis are larger, spanning between vessels, and associated with areas of tissue necrosis.
ANCA, Anti-neutrophil cytoplasmic antibodies.
From Seidman MA, Mitchell RN: Surgical pathology of small-and medium-sized vessels. In Winters, GL, ed., *Current concepts in cardiovascular pathology*, Philadelphia, 2012, Saunders.

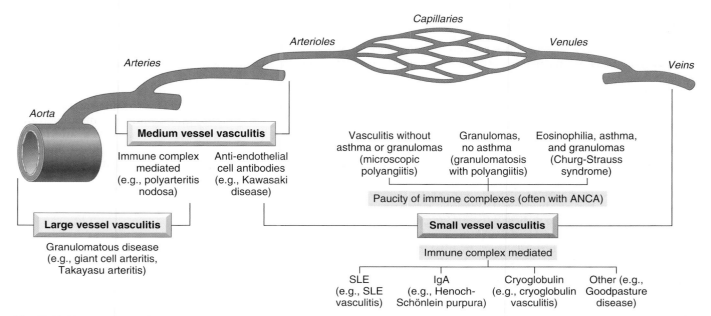

Fig. 10.22 Vascular sites involved in the more common vasculitides and their presumptive etiology. Note the considerable overlap in distributions. ANCA, anti-neutrophil cytoplasmic antibody; IgA, immunoglobulin A; SLE, systemic lupus erythematosus. *(Data from Jennette JC, Falk RJ: Nosology of primary vasculitis, Curr Opin Rheumatol 19:17, 2007.)*

complex–mediated disorders, such as the Arthus phenomenon and serum sickness, and in some cases contain readily identifiable antibody and complement. Often, however, this type of vasculitis is a diagnostic challenge. Only rarely is the specific antigen responsible for immune complex formation known, and in most instances it is not clear whether the pathogenic antigen-antibody complexes are deposited into the vessel wall from the circulation or form *in situ*. In fact, in many suspected cases, even the antigen-antibody deposits are scarce, perhaps because the immune complexes have been degraded by the time of biopsy.

Immune complex deposition is also implicated in the following vasculitides:

- *Drug hypersensitivity vasculitis.* In some cases, drugs (e.g., penicillin) appear to act as haptens by binding to host proteins; other agents are themselves foreign proteins (e.g., streptokinase). In either case, antibodies directed against the drug-modified proteins or foreign molecules result in immune complex formation. The clinical manifestations can be mild and self-limiting, or severe and even fatal; skin lesions are most common. It is always important to consider drug hypersensitivity as a cause of vasculitis, since discontinuation of the offending agent usually leads to resolution.
- *Vasculitis secondary to infections.* Antibodies to microbial constituents can form immune complexes that circulate and deposit in vascular lesions. For example, in up to 30% of patients with *polyarteritis nodosa* (discussed in greater detail later), the vasculitis can be ascribed to immune complexes composed of hepatitis B surface antigen (HBsAg) and anti-HBsAg antibody.

Anti-Neutrophil Cytoplasmic Antibodies

Many patients with vasculitis have circulating antibodies that react with neutrophil cytoplasmic antigens, so-called "anti-neutrophil cytoplasmic antibodies (ANCAs)." ANCAs are a heterogeneous group of autoantibodies directed against constituents (mainly enzymes) of neutrophil primary granules, monocyte lysosomes, and ECs. ANCAs are very useful diagnostic markers; their titers generally mirror clinical severity, and a rise in titers after periods of quiescence is predictive of disease recurrence. Although a number of ANCAs have been described, two are most important. These are classified according to their antigen specificity:

- *Anti-proteinase-3 (PR3-ANCA),* previously called *c-ANCA.* PR3 is a neutrophil azurophilic granule constituent that shares homology with numerous microbial peptides, possibly explaining the generation of PR3-ANCAs. PR3-ANCAs are associated with *granulomatosis with polyangiitis* (see later).
- *Anti-myeloperoxidase (MPO-ANCA),* previously called *p-ANCA.* MPO is a lysosomal granule constituent involved in oxygen free radical generation (Chapter 3). MPO-ANCAs are induced by several therapeutic agents, particularly propylthiouracil (used to treat hyperthyroidism). MPO-ANCAs are associated with *microscopic polyangiitis* and *Churg-Strauss syndrome* (see later).

The close association between ANCA titers and disease activity suggests a pathogenic role for these antibodies. Of note, ANCAs can directly activate neutrophils, stimulating the release of reactive oxygen species and proteolytic enzymes; in vascular beds, this may lead to EC injury. While the antigenic targets of ANCA are primarily intracellular (and therefore not usually accessible to circulating antibodies), it is now clear that ANCA antigens (especially PR3) either are constitutively expressed at low levels on the plasma membrane or are translocated to the cell surface in activated and apoptotic leukocytes.

A plausible pathogenic sequence for the development of ANCA vasculitis involves the following:

- Drugs or cross-reactive microbial antigens induce ANCA formation; alternatively, leukocyte surface expression or release of PR3 and MPO (in the setting of infection) incites ANCA development in a susceptible individual.
- Subsequent inflammatory stimuli elicit the release of cytokines such as TNF that upregulate the surface expression of PR3 and MPO on neutrophils and other cell types.
- ANCAs bind to these cytokine-activated cells, causing further neutrophil activation.
- ANCA-activated neutrophils cause EC injury by releasing granule contents and elaborating reactive oxygen species.

The ANCA auto-antibodies are directed against cellular constituents and do not form circulating immune complexes, nor do the vascular lesions typically contain demonstrable antibody and complement; therefore ANCA-associated vasculitides often are described as "pauci-immune." Of interest, ANCAs directed against proteins other than PR3 and MPO are sometimes seen in patients with non-vasculitic inflammatory disorders (e.g., inflammatory bowel disease, sclerosing cholangitis, and rheumatoid arthritis).

Anti-Endothelial Cell Antibodies and Autoreactive T Cells

Antibodies to ECs underlie certain vasculitides, such as Kawasaki disease (discussed later). Autoreactive T cells cause injury in some forms of vasculitides characterized by formation of granulomas.

Presented next is a brief overview of several of the best-characterized vasculitides. Although each is presented as a distinct entity, it must be acknowledged that many cases of vasculitis lack a classic constellation finding or have overlapping features that may render classification difficult.

Giant Cell (Temporal) Arteritis

Giant cell (temporal) arteritis is a chronic inflammatory disorder, typically with granulomatous inflammation, that principally affects large- to small-sized arteries in the head. The temporal arteries are not more vulnerable than other arteries, but have leant their name to the disorder because the diagnosis is typically established by biopsy of these vessels. Vertebral and ophthalmic arteries, as well as the aorta (*giant cell aortitis*), are other common sites of involvement. Because ophthalmic artery vasculitis can lead to sudden and permanent blindness, affected individuals must be promptly diagnosed and treated promptly. It is the most common form of vasculitis among older adults in developed countries.

Pathogenesis

Giant cell arteritis likely occurs as a result of a T-cell–mediated immune response to an as-yet uncharacterized vessel wall antigen. Pro-inflammatory cytokines (especially TNF) and anti-EC antibodies also contribute. The characteristic granulomatous inflammation, an association with certain MHC class II haplotypes, and the excellent therapeutic response to steroids, all strongly support an immune etiology. The predilection for vessels of the head remains unexplained, although one hypothesis is that vessels in various parts of the body develop from distinct anlagen and may, therefore, express unique antigens.

Clinical Features

Temporal arteritis is rare before 50 years of age. Signs and symptoms may be vague and constitutional (e.g., fever, fatigue, weight loss) or take the form of facial pain or headache, most intense along the course of the superficial temporal artery, which is painful to palpation. Ocular symptoms (associated with involvement of the ophthalmic artery) abruptly appear in about 50% of patients; these range from diplopia to complete vision loss. Diagnosis depends on biopsy and histology; however, because the vascular inflammation is patchy, a negative biopsy result does not exclude the diagnosis. Corticosteroid or anti-TNF therapies are effective treatments.

> ## MORPHOLOGY
>
> In giant cell arteritis, the pathologic changes are notoriously patchy along the length of affected vessels. Involved arterial segments exhibit nodular intimal thickening (and occasional thromboses) that reduce the vessel diameter and cause distal ischemia. The vast majority of lesions exhibit **granulomatous inflam-** **mation** within the inner media centered on the internal elastic membrane; there is an infiltrate of lymphocytes and macrophages, with multinucleate giant cells, and **fragmentation of the internal elastic lamina** (Fig. 10.23). In up to 25% of cases, granulomas and giant cells are absent, and lesions exhibit only a nonspecific panarteritis with a mixed infiltrate of acute and chronic inflammation. Healing is marked by intimal thickening, medial thinning and scarring, and adventitial fibrosis. Characteristically, lesions at different stages of development are seen within the same artery.

Takayasu Arteritis

Takayasu arteritis is a granulomatous vasculitis of medium- and large-sized arteries characterized principally by ocular disturbances and marked weakening of the pulses in the upper extremities (hence the alternate name, *pulseless disease*). This disorder manifests with transmural scarring and thickening of the aorta—particularly the aortic arch and great vessels—with severe luminal narrowing of the major branch vessels (Fig. 10.24). Aortic lesions share many of the clinical and histologic features of giant cell aortitis. Indeed, the distinction between the two entities is made largely on the basis of a patient's age; in those older than 50 years of age are said to have *giant cell aortitis,* and lesions that occur in those younger than 50 years of age are designated *Takayasu aortitis.* Although historically associated with Japanese ethnicity and certain HLA haplotypes, Takayasu aortitis has a global distribution. An autoimmune etiology is likely.

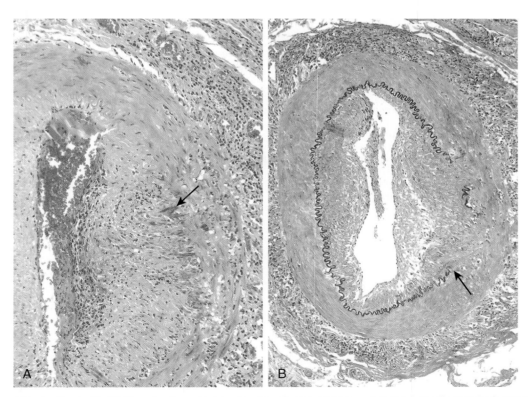

Fig. 10.23 Temporal (giant cell) arteritis. (A) Hematoxylin-eosin-stained section of a temporal artery showing giant cells near the fragmented internal elastic membrane *(arrow),* along with medial and adventitial inflammation. (B) Elastic tissue stain demonstrating focal destruction of the internal elastic membrane *(arrow)* and medial attenuation and scarring.

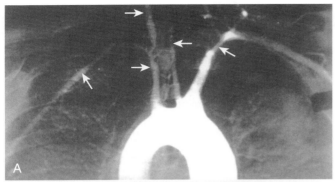

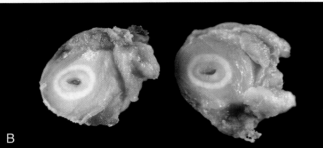

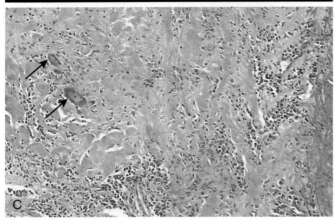

Fig. 10.24 Takayasu arteritis. (A) Aortic arch angiogram showing reduced flow of contrast material into the great vessels and narrowing of the brachiocephalic, carotid, and subclavian arteries *(arrows)*. (B) Cross-sections of the right carotid artery from the patient shown in A demonstrating marked intimal thickening and luminal narrowing. The white circles correspond to the original vessel wall; the inner core of tan tissue is the area of intimal hyperplasia. (C) Histologic appearance in active Takayasu aortitis illustrating destruction and fibrosis of the arterial media associated with mononuclear infiltrates and giant cells *(arrows)*.

MORPHOLOGY

Takayasu arteritis classically affects the aortic arch and arch vessels; one third of cases also involve the remainder of the aorta and its branches. Occasionally, aortic root involvement causes dilation and aortic valve insufficiency. Pulmonary arteries are involved in 50% of patients, and renal and coronary arteries also can be affected. The takeoffs of the great vessels can be markedly narrowed and even obliterated (see Fig. 10.24A and B), explaining the upper-extremity weakness and faint

carotid pulses. The histologic picture (see Fig. 10.24C) encompasses a spectrum ranging from adventitial mononuclear infiltrates and perivascular cuffing of the vasa vasorum, to intense transmural mononuclear inflammation, to granulomatous inflammation, replete with giant cells and patchy medial necrosis. The inflammation is associated with irregular thickening of the vessel wall, intimal hyperplasia, and adventitial fibrosis.

Clinical Features

Initial signs and symptoms usually are nonspecific, including fatigue, weight loss, and fever. With progression, vascular signs and symptoms appear and dominate the clinical picture. These include reduced upper-extremity blood pressure and pulse strength; neurologic deficits; and ocular disturbances, including visual field defects, retinal hemorrhages, and total blindness. Distal aorta disease can manifest as leg claudication, and pulmonary artery involvement can cause pulmonary hypertension. Narrowing of the coronary ostia can lead to myocardial infarction, and involvement of the renal arteries causes systemic hypertension in roughly one half of patients. The evolution of the disease is variable. Some cases rapidly progress, while others become quiescent after 1 to 2 years. In the latter scenario, long-term survival, albeit with visual or neurologic deficits, is possible.

Polyarteritis Nodosa

Polyarteritis nodosa (PAN) is a systemic vasculitis of small- or medium-sized muscular arteries; it typically involves the renal and visceral vessels and spares the pulmonary circulation. There is no association with ANCAs, but one third of patients have chronic hepatitis B infection, which leads to the formation of immune complexes containing hepatitis B antigens that deposit in affected vessels. The cause is unknown in the remaining cases.

MORPHOLOGY

Classic PAN is a **segmental transmural necrotizing inflammation** of small- to medium-sized arteries, often with superimposed thrombosis. Kidney, heart, liver, and gastrointestinal tract vessels are affected in descending order of frequency. Lesions usually involve only part of the vessel circumference and have a predilection for branch points. **Impaired perfusion** may lead to ulcerations, infarcts, ischemic atrophy, or hemorrhages in the distribution of affected vessels. The inflammatory process also **weakens the arterial wall,** leading to aneurysms and rupture.

In the acute phase, there is transmural mixed inflammatory infiltrate composed of neutrophils and mononuclear cells, frequently accompanied by **fibrinoid necrosis** and luminal thrombosis (Fig. 10.25). Older lesions show fibrous thickening of the vessel wall extending into the adventitia. Characteristically, all stages of activity (from early to late) coexist in different vessels or even within the same vessel, suggesting ongoing and recurrent pathogenic insults.

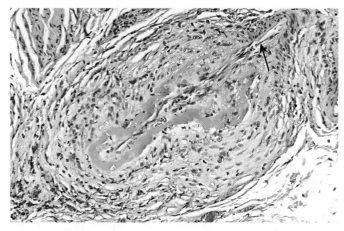

Fig. 10.25 Polyarteritis nodosa, associated with segmental fibrinoid necrosis and thrombotic occlusion of a small artery. Note that part of the vessel *(upper-right, arrow)* is uninvolved. *(Courtesy of Sidney Murphree, MD, Department of Pathology, University of Texas Southwestern Medical School, Dallas, Texas.)*

Clinical Features

PAN is primarily a disease of young adults but can occur in all age groups. The clinical course typically is episodic, with long symptom-free intervals. The systemic findings—malaise, fever, and weight loss—are nonspecific, and the vascular involvement is widely scattered, so that the clinical manifestations can be varied and puzzling. A "classic" presentation involves involve some combination of rapidly accelerating hypertension due to renal artery involvement; abdominal pain and bloody stools caused by gastrointestinal lesions; diffuse muscular aches and pains; and peripheral neuritis, predominantly affecting motor nerves. Renal involvement often is prominent and is a major cause of death. Untreated, PAN typically is fatal; however, with immunosuppression, 5-year survival is close to 80%. Relapse occurs in up to 25% of the cases, more often in non–HBV-associated cases than those that follow HBV infection. The latter have a better long-term prognosis.

Kawasaki Disease

Kawasaki disease is an acute, febrile, usually self-limited illness of infancy and childhood associated with an arteritis of mainly large- to medium-sized vessels. Approximately 80% of patients are younger than 4 years of age. Its clinical significance stems from the involvement of coronary arteries. Coronary arteritis can result in aneurysms that rupture or thrombose, causing myocardial infarction. Originally described in Japan, the disease is now recognized in the United States and elsewhere.

In genetically susceptible individuals, a variety of infectious agents (mostly viral) have been posited to trigger the disease. The vasculitis may result from a delayed-type hypersensitivity response directed against cross-reactive or newly uncovered vascular antigen(s). Subsequent cytokine production and polyclonal B cell activation result in auto-antibodies to ECs and SMCs that precipitate the vasculitis.

MORPHOLOGY

The vasculitis resembles that seen in polyarteritis nodosa. There is a dense transmural inflammatory infiltrate, although fibrinoid necrosis usually is less prominent than in polyarteritis nodosa. The vasculitis typically subsides spontaneously or in response to treatment, but aneurysm formation due to wall damage may supervene. As with other arteritides, healing may be accompanied by the development of obstructive intimal thickening. Pathologic changes outside the cardiovascular system are rarely significant.

Clinical Features

Kawasaki disease typically manifests with conjunctival and oral erythema and blistering, edema of the hands and feet, erythema of the palms and soles, a desquamative rash, and cervical lymph node enlargement (hence its other name, *mucocutaneous lymph node syndrome*). Approximately 20% of untreated patients develop cardiovascular sequelae, ranging from asymptomatic coronary arteritis, to coronary artery ectasia, to large coronary artery aneurysms (7 to 8 mm in diameter); the latter may be associated with rupture, thrombosis, myocardial infarction, and/or sudden death. Treatment consists of intravenous immunoglobulin infusions (which suppress inflammation through unclear mechanisms) and aspirin, which when given together markedly decrease the incidence of symptomatic coronary artery disease.

Microscopic Polyangiitis

Microscopic polyangiitis is a necrotizing vasculitis that generally affects capillaries, as well as small arterioles and venules. It also is called *hypersensitivity vasculitis* or *leukocytoclastic vasculitis.* Unlike in PAN, all lesions of microscopic polyangiitis tend to be of the same age in any given patient. The skin, mucous membranes, lungs, brain, heart, gastrointestinal tract, kidneys, and muscle all can be involved; *necrotizing glomerulonephritis* (seen in 90% of patients) and *pulmonary capillaritis* are particularly common. Microscopic angiitis can be a feature of a number of immune disorders, such as *Henoch-Schönlein purpura, essential mixed cryoglobulinemia,* or the vasculitis associated with connective tissue disorders.

In some cases, antibody responses to antigens such as drugs (e.g., penicillin), microorganisms (e.g., streptococci), heterologous proteins, or tumor proteins have been implicated. These reactions can either lead to immune complex deposition or trigger secondary immune responses (e.g., the development of ANCAs) that are pathogenic. Indeed, most cases of microscopic polyangiitis are associated with MPO-ANCA. Recruitment and activation of neutrophils within affected vascular beds is probably responsible for the disease manifestations.

Clinical Features

Depending on the vascular bed involved, major features include hemoptysis, hematuria, proteinuria, abdominal pain or bleeding, muscle pain or weakness, and palpable cutaneous purpura. With the exception of patients with

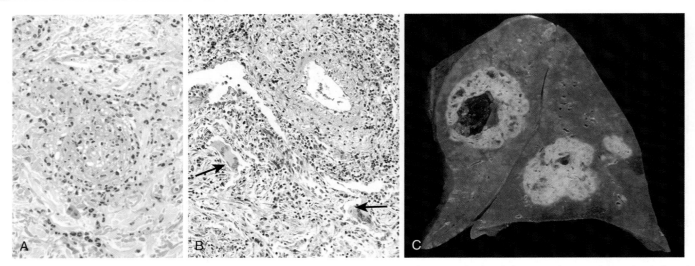

Fig. 10.26 ANCA-associated small vessel vasculitis. (A) Microscopic polyangiitis (leukocytoclastic vasculitis) with fragmented neutrophils in the thickened vessel wall. (B and C) Granulomatosis with polyangiitis. (B) Vasculitis of a small artery with adjacent granulomatous inflammation including giant cells *(arrows).* (C) Lung from a patient with granulomatosis with polyangiitis, demonstrating large nodular cavitating lesions. *(A, Courtesy of Scott Granter, MD, Brigham and Women's Hospital, Boston, Massachusetts. C, Courtesy of Sidney Murphree, MD, Department of Pathology, University of Texas Southwestern Medical School, Dallas, Texas.)*

widespread renal or CNS involvement, immunosuppression and removal of the offending agent induce durable remissions.

MORPHOLOGY

Microscopic polyangiitis is characterized by segmental fibrinoid necrosis of the media with focal transmural necrotizing lesions; granulomatous inflammation is absent. These lesions resemble those of polyarteritis nodosa but spare medium- and large-sized arteries, so that macroscopic infarcts are uncommon. In some areas (typically postcapillary venules), only infiltrating neutrophils undergoing fragmentation are seen, giving rise to the term *leukocytoclastic vasculitis* (Fig. 10.26A). Although immunoglobulins and complement components can be demonstrated in early skin lesions, most lesions are "pauci-immune" (i.e., show little or no antibody).

Granulomatosis With Polyangiitis

Previously called *Wegener granulomatosis,* granulomatosis with polyangiitis (GPA) is a necrotizing vasculitis characterized by a triad of the following:
- *Necrotizing granulomas* of the upper-respiratory tract (ear, nose, sinuses, throat) or the lower-respiratory tract (lung) or both
- *Necrotizing or granulomatous vasculitis* affecting small- to medium-sized vessels (e.g., capillaries, venules, arterioles, and arteries), most prominently the lungs and upper airways but other sites as well
- *Focal necrotizing, often crescentic, glomerulonephritis*

"Limited" forms of disease can be restricted to the respiratory tract. Conversely, when widespread the disease may affect the eyes, skin, and other organs, most notably the heart; clinically, widespread GPA resembles PAN with the additional feature of respiratory involvement.

GPA is likely initiated as a cell-mediated hypersensitivity response to inhaled infectious or environmental antigens. PR3-ANCAs are present in almost 95% of cases and probably drive the tissue injury. The ANCA level also is a useful marker of disease activity, as antibody titers fall dramatically with effective immunosuppressive therapy and rise prior to disease relapse.

MORPHOLOGY

Upper respiratory tract lesions range from **granulomatous sinusitis to ulcerative lesions** of the nose, palate, or pharynx; lung findings also vary, ranging from diffuse parenchymal infiltrates to granulomatous nodules. There is multifocal necrotizing **granulomatous vasculitis** with a surrounding fibroblastic proliferation (Fig. 10.26B). Multiple granulomata can coalesce to produce radiographically visible nodules with central cavitation (Fig. 10.26BC). Destruction of vessels can lead to hemorrhage and hemoptysis. Lesions can ultimately undergo progressive fibrosis and organization.

The **renal lesions** range from mild, focal glomerular necrosis associated with thrombosis of isolated glomerular capillary loops **(focal and segmental necrotizing glomerulonephritis)** to more advanced glomerular lesions with diffuse necrosis and parietal cell proliferation forming epithelial crescents **(crescentic glomerulonephritis)** (Chapter 14).

Clinical Features

The typical patient is a middle aged man, although women and individuals of other ages can be affected. Classic presentations include bilateral pneumonitis with nodules and cavitary lesions (95%), chronic sinusitis (90%), mucosal ulcerations of the nasopharynx (75%), and renal disease (80%). Patients with mild renal involvement may demonstrate only hematuria and proteinuria, whereas more severe disease may portend rapidly progressive renal failure. Rash, myalgias, articular involvement, neuritis, and fever also may occur. If untreated, the mortality rate at 1 year is 80%. Treatment with steroids, cyclophosphamide, TNF inhibitors, and anti–B-cell antibodies (rituximab) has improved this picture considerably. Most patients with GPA now survive, but remain at high risk for relapses that may ultimately lead to renal failure.

Churg-Strauss Syndrome

Churg-Strauss syndrome (also called *allergic granulomatosis* and *angiitis*) is a small-vessel necrotizing vasculitis classically associated with asthma, allergic rhinitis, lung infiltrates, peripheral eosinophilia, extravascular necrotizing granulomas, and a striking infiltration of vessels and perivascular tissues by eosinophils. It is a rare disorder, affecting 1 in 1 million individuals. Cutaneous involvement (with palpable purpura), gastrointestinal bleeding, and renal disease (primarily as focal and segmental glomerulosclerosis) are the major associations. Cytotoxicity produced by the myocardial eosinophilic infiltrates often leads to cardiomyopathy. Cardiac involvement is seen in 60% of patients and is a major cause of morbidity and death.

Churg-Strauss syndrome may stem from "hyperresponsiveness" to some normally innocuous allergic stimulus. MPO-ANCAs are present in a minority of cases, suggesting that the disorder is pathogenically heterogeneous. The vascular lesions differ from those of PAN or microscopic polyangiitis by virtue of the presence of granulomas and eosinophils.

Thromboangiitis Obliterans (Buerger Disease)

Thromboangiitis obliterans (Buerger disease) is characterized by segmental, thrombosing, acute and chronic inflammation of medium- and small-sized arteries, principally the tibial and radial arteries, with occasional secondary extension into the veins and nerves of the extremities. Buerger disease occurs almost exclusively in heavy tobacco smokers and usually develops before 35 years of age. Direct EC toxicity caused by some component of tobacco is suspected; alternatively, a reactive compound in tobacco may modify vessel wall components and induce an immune response. Indeed, most patients with Buerger disease are hypersensitive to tobacco extracts. A genetic predilection is suggested by an increased prevalence in certain ethnic groups (Israeli, Indian subcontinent, Japanese) and an association with certain HLA haplotypes.

> ### MORPHOLOGY
>
> In thromboangiitis obliterans, there is a **sharply segmental acute and chronic transmural vasculitis of medium- and small-sized arteries,** predominantly those of the extremities. In the early stages, mixed inflammatory infiltrates are accompanied by luminal thrombosis; small microabscesses, occasionally rimmed by granulomatous inflammation, also may be present (Fig. 10.27). The inflammation often extends into contiguous veins and nerves (a feature that is rare in other forms of vasculitis). With time, thrombi can organize and recanalize, and eventually the artery and adjacent structures become encased in fibrous tissue.

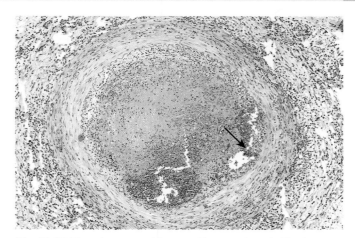

Fig. 10.27 Thromboangiitis obliterans (Buerger disease). The lumen is occluded by thrombus containing a sterile abscess *(arrow)*, and the vessel wall is infiltrated with leukocytes.

Clinical Features

Early manifestations include cold-induced Raynaud phenomenon (see later), instep foot pain induced by exercise *(instep claudication),* and superficial nodular phlebitis (venous inflammation). The vascular insufficiency of Buerger disease tends to be accompanied by severe pain—even at rest—undoubtedly from the neural involvement. Chronic extremity ulcerations may develop, progressing over time (occasionally precipitously) to frank gangrene. Smoking abstinence in the early stages of the disease often ameliorates further attacks; however, once established, the vascular lesions do not respond to smoking abstinence.

Vasculitis Associated With Other Noninfectious Disorders

Vasculitis resembling hypersensitivity angiitis or classic PAN may be seen in association with many other diseases, including malignancies and immunologic disorders such as rheumatoid arthritis, systemic lupus erythematosus, anti-phospholipid antibody syndrome, and Henoch-Schönlein purpura. *Rheumatoid vasculitis* may occur in patients with severe, long-standing rheumatoid arthritis; it can cause a clinically significant aortitis but more typically affects small- and medium-sized arteries, leading to visceral infarction. Linking vasculitis to specific disorders may have important therapeutic implications. For example, although classic immune complex *lupus vasculitis* and anti-phospholipid antibody syndrome share certain morphologic features, the former requires anti-inflammatory therapy while anticoagulation is indicated in the latter.

Infectious Vasculitis

Localized arteritis may be caused by the direct invasion of arteries by infectious agents, usually bacteria or fungi, and in particular *Aspergillus* and *Mucor* spp. Vascular invasion may be part of a nearby local tissue infection (e.g., bacterial pneumonia or an adjacent abscesses), or—less commonly—may arise from hematogenous spread of bacteria or embolization from infective endocarditis.

Vascular infections may weaken arterial walls and culminate in *mycotic aneurysms* described earlier, or may induce thrombosis and infarction. Thus, inflammation of vessels in bacterial meningitis can cause thrombosis and infarction, leading ultimately to extension of a subarachnoid infection into the brain parenchyma.

SUMMARY

VASCULITIS

- Vasculitis is defined as inflammation of vessel walls; it frequently is associated with systemic manifestations (including fever, malaise, myalgias, and arthralgias) and organ dysfunction that depends on the pattern of vascular involvement.
- Vasculitis can result from infections but more commonly has an immunologic basis such as immune complex deposition, anti-neutrophil antibodies (ANCAs), or anti-EC antibodies.
- Different forms of vasculitis tend to specifically affect vessels of a particular caliber and location (see Fig. 10.22 and Table 10.4).

DISORDERS OF BLOOD VESSEL HYPERREACTIVITY

Several disorders are characterized by inappropriate or exaggerated vasoconstriction of blood vessels.

Raynaud Phenomenon

Raynaud phenomenon results from vasoconstriction of arteries and arterioles in the extremities, particularly the fingers and toes, but also sometimes the nose, earlobes, or lips. The restricted blood flow induces paroxysmal pallor or cyanosis; involved digits characteristically show "red-white-and-blue" color changes from most proximal to most distal, reflecting proximal vasodilation, central vasoconstriction, and more distal cyanosis, respectively. Raynaud phenomenon can be a primary entity or may be secondary to other disorders.

Primary Raynaud phenomenon (previously called *Raynaud disease*) is caused by exaggerated central and local vasomotor responses to cold or emotion; it affects 3% to 5% of the general population and has a predilection for young women. Structural changes in the arterial walls are absent except late in the course, when intimal thickening may appear. The course usually is benign, but in chronic cases, atrophy of the skin, subcutaneous tissues, and muscles may occur. Ulceration and ischemic gangrene are rare.

Secondary Raynaud phenomenon refers to vascular insufficiency due to arterial disease caused by other entities including systemic lupus erythematosus, scleroderma, Buerger disease, or even atherosclerosis. Indeed, since Raynaud phenomenon may be the first manifestation of such conditions, every patient with Raynaud phenomenon should be evaluated for these secondary causes.

Myocardial Vessel Vasospasm

Vasospasm of cardiac arterial or arteriolar beds has been called *cardiac Raynaud and in a subset of cases leads to*

Prinzmetal angina (angina due to vasospasm). If such spasm is of sufficient duration (20 to 30 minutes), myocardial infarction can result. Elevated levels of catechols also increase heart rate and myocardial contractility, exacerbating ischemia caused by the vasospasm. The outcome can be sudden cardiac death (caused by a fatal arrhythmia) or an ischemic dilated cardiomyopathy—so-called "Takotsubo cardiomyopathy" (also called "broken heart syndrome," because of the association with emotional duress). Histologic findings in acute cases may include microscopic areas of necrosis characterized by myocyte hypercontraction (contraction band necrosis) (Chapter 11); in subacute and chronic cases, microscopic foci of granulation tissue and/or scar may be present.

VEINS AND LYMPHATICS

Varicose veins and phlebothrombosis/thrombophlebitis account for at least 90% of cases of clinically relevant venous disease.

Varicose Veins of the Extremities

Varicose veins are abnormally dilated tortuous veins produced by chronically increased intraluminal pressures and weakened vessel wall support. The superficial veins of the upper and lower leg typically are involved. Up to one fifth of men and one third of women develop lower-extremity varicose veins. Obesity increases the risk, and the higher incidence in women probably reflects the prolonged elevation in venous pressure caused by compression of the inferior vena cava by the gravid uterus during pregnancy. There is also a familial tendency toward premature varicosities.

Clinical Features

Varicose dilation renders the venous valves incompetent and leads to lower-extremity stasis, congestion, edema, pain, and thrombosis. The most disabling sequelae include persistent edema in the extremity and secondary ischemic skin changes, including stasis dermatitis and ulcerations. The latter can become chronic *varicose ulcers* as a consequence of poor wound healing and superimposed infections. Of note, embolism from these superficial veins is very rare, in contrast with the relatively frequent emboli that arise from thrombosed deep veins (Chapter 4).

Varicosities of Other Sites

Venous dilations in two other sites merit special attention:
- *Esophageal varices.* Liver cirrhosis (and less frequently, portal vein obstruction or hepatic vein thrombosis) causes portal venous hypertension (Chapter 16). This, in turn, leads to the opening of porto-systemic shunts and increased blood flow into veins at the (1) gastroesophageal junction (forming esophageal varices); (2) rectum (forming hemorrhoids); and (3) periumbilical veins of the abdominal wall (forming a caput medusae). Esophageal varices are most important since they are prone to ruptures that can lead to massive (even fatal) upper gastrointestinal hemorrhage.

- *Hemorrhoids* are varicose dilations of the venous plexus at the anorectal junction that result from prolonged pelvic vascular congestion associated with pregnancy or straining to defecate. Hemorrhoids are a source of bleeding and are prone to thrombosis and painful ulceration.

Thrombophlebitis and Phlebothrombosis

Thrombosis of deep leg veins accounts for more than 90% of cases of thrombophlebitis and phlebothrombosis. These two terms are largely interchangeable designations for venous thrombosis accompanied by inflammation. Other sites where venous thrombi may form are the periprostatic venous plexus in males and the pelvic venous plexus in females, as well as the large veins in the skull and the dural sinuses (especially in the setting of infection or inflammation). Peritoneal infections, including peritonitis, appendicitis, salpingitis, and pelvic abscesses, as well as certain conditions associated with hypercoagulability (e.g., polycythemia vera) (Chapter 12) can lead to portal vein thrombosis.

In deep venous thrombosis (DVT) of the legs, prolonged immobilization resulting in venous stasis is the most important risk factor. This can occur with extended bed rest or even just sitting during long plane or automobile trips. The postoperative state is another independent risk factor for DVT, as are congestive heart failure, pregnancy, oral contraceptive use, malignancy, obesity, male sex, and age over 50 years. Inherited defects in coagulation factors (Chapter 4) often predispose affected individuals to development of thrombophlebitis. Venous thrombi also can result from elaboration of procoagulant factors from cancers (Chapter 6); the resulting hypercoagulable state can manifest as evanescent thromboses in different vascular beds at different times, so-called "migratory thrombophlebitis" or "Trousseau syndrome."

Thrombi in legs tend to produce few, if any, reliable signs or symptoms. When present, local manifestations include distal edema, cyanosis, superficial vein dilation, heat, tenderness, redness, swelling, and pain. In some cases, pain is elicited by pressure over affected veins, squeezing the calf muscles, or forced dorsiflexion of the foot *(Homan sign)*. However, many DVTs are asymptomatic, especially in bedridden patients, and the absence of findings does not exclude their presence.

Pulmonary embolism is a common and serious clinical complication of DVT, resulting from fragmentation or detachment of the venous thrombus. In many cases, the first manifestation of thrombophlebitis is a pulmonary embolus. Depending on the size and number of emboli, the outcome can range from resolution with no symptoms to death.

Superior and Inferior Vena Cava Syndromes

The *superior vena cava syndrome* usually is caused by neoplasms that compress or invade the superior vena cava, such as bronchogenic carcinoma or mediastinal lymphoma. The resulting obstruction produces a characteristic clinical complex consisting of marked dilation of the veins of the head, neck, and arms associated with cyanosis. Pulmonary vessels also can be compressed, causing respiratory distress.

The *inferior vena cava syndrome* can be caused by neoplasms that compress or invade the inferior vena cava or by a thrombus from the hepatic, renal, or lower-extremity veins that propagates cephalad. Certain neoplasms—particularly hepatocellular carcinoma and renal cell carcinoma—show a striking tendency to grow within veins, and these tumors may ultimately occlude the inferior vena cava. Obstruction of the inferior vena cava induces marked lower-extremity edema, distention of the superficial collateral veins of the lower abdomen, and—with renal vein involvement—marked proteinuria.

Lymphangitis and Lymphedema

Primary disorders of lymphatic vessels are extremely uncommon. Much more commonly, lymphatic vessels are secondarily involved by inflammatory, infectious, or malignant processes.

Lymphangitis refers to an acute inflammation caused by bacterial seeding of the lymphatic vessels (Chapter 3). Clinically, the inflamed lymphatics appear as *red, painful subcutaneous streaks,* usually associated with tender enlargement of draining lymph nodes *(acute lymphadenitis)*. If bacteria are not contained within the lymph nodes, they can pass into the venous circulation and cause bacteremia or sepsis.

Primary lymphedema may occur as an isolated congenital defect (simple congenital lymphedema) or as the familial *Milroy disease (heredofamilial congenital lymphedema),* resulting from agenesis or hypoplasia of lymphatics. Secondary or obstructive lymphedema stems from the accumulation of interstitial fluid behind an obstructed, previously normal lymphatic; such obstruction can result from the following disorders or conditions:

- Tumors involving either the lymphatic channels or the regional lymph nodes
- Surgical procedures that sever lymphatic connections (e.g., axillary lymph nodes in radical mastectomy)
- Postradiation fibrosis
- Filariasis
- Postinflammatory thrombosis and scarring

Regardless of the cause, lymphedema increases the hydrostatic pressure in the lymphatics distal to the obstruction and causes edema. Chronic edema in turn may lead to deposition of ECM and fibrosis, producing brawny induration or a *peau d'orange* appearance of the overlying skin (as may occur in the skin overlying a breast carcinoma). Eventually, inadequate tissue perfusion may lead to skin ulceration. Rupture of dilated lymphatics, typically following obstruction by an infiltrating tumor mass, can lead to milky accumulations of lymph in various spaces designated *chylous ascites* (abdomen), *chylothorax,* and *chylopericardium.*

TUMORS

Tumors of blood vessels and lymphatics include benign hemangiomas (extremely common), locally aggressive

Table 10.5 Classification of Vascular Tumors and Tumor-Like Conditions

Benign Neoplasms: Developmental and Acquired Conditions
Hemangioma
Capillary hemangioma
Cavernous hemangioma
Pyogenic granuloma
Lymphangioma
Simple (capillary) lymphangioma
Cavernous lymphangioma (cystic hygroma)
Glomus tumor
Vascular ectasias
Nevus flammeus
Spider telangiectasia (arterial spider)
Hereditary hemorrhagic telangiectasis (Osler-Weber-Rendu disease)
Reactive vascular proliferations
Bacillary angiomatosis
Intermediate-Grade Neoplasms
Kaposi sarcoma
Hemangioendothelioma
Malignant Neoplasms
Angiosarcoma

neoplasms that metastasize infrequently, and rare, highly malignant angiosarcomas (Table 10.5).

Vascular neoplasms arise either from endothelium (e.g., hemangioma, lymphangioma, angiosarcoma) or cells that support or surround blood vessels (e.g., glomus tumor). Primary tumors of large vessels (aorta, pulmonary artery, and vena cava) occur infrequently and are mostly sarcomas. Although a benign hemangioma cannot by confused with an anaplastic angiosarcoma, "gray-zone" lesions of uncertain malignancy are sometimes observed. Congenital or developmental malformations and non-neoplastic reactive vascular proliferations (e.g., *bacillary angiomatosis*) can also manifest as tumor-like lesions that may present diagnostic challenges. In general, benign and malignant vascular neoplasms are distinguished by the following features:

- Benign tumors usually are composed of vascular channels filled with blood cells or lymph that are lined by a monolayer of normal-appearing ECs.
- Malignant tumors are more cellular, show cytologic atypia, are proliferative, and usually do not form well-organized vessels; confirmation of the endothelial derivation of such proliferations may require immunohistochemical detection of EC-specific markers.

Benign Tumors and Tumor-Like Conditions

Vascular Ectasias

Ectasia is a generic term for any local dilation of a structure, while *telangiectasia* is used to describe a permanent dilation of preexisting small vessels (capillaries, venules, and arterioles, usually in the skin or mucous membranes) that forms a discrete red lesion. These lesions can be congenital or acquired and are not true neoplasms.

- *Nevus flammeus* (a "birthmark"), the most common form of vascular ectasia, is a light pink to deep purple flat lesion on the head or neck composed of dilated vessels. Most ultimately regress spontaneously.
- The so-called "port wine stain" is a special form of nevus flammeus. These lesions tend to grow during childhood, thicken the skin surface, and do not fade with time. Such lesions occurring in the distribution of the trigeminal nerve are associated with the *Sturge-Weber syndrome* (also called encephalotrigeminal angiomatosis). This uncommon congenital disorder is associated with facial port wine nevi, ipsilateral venous angiomas in the cortical leptomeninges, mental retardation, seizures, hemiplegia, and radiologic opacities of the skull. Thus, a large facial telangiectasia in a child with mental deficiencies may indicate the presence of additional vascular malformations.
- *Spider telangiectasias* are non-neoplastic vascular lesions. These lesions manifest as radial, often pulsatile arrays of dilated subcutaneous arteries or arterioles (the "legs" of the spider) about a central core (the spider's "body") that blanch with pressure. Spider telangiectasias commonly occur on the face, neck, or upper chest and most frequently are associated with hyperestrogenic states (e.g., in pregnant women or patients with cirrhosis).
- *Hereditary hemorrhagic telangiectasia (Osler-Weber-Rendu disease)* is an autosomal dominant disorder caused by mutations in genes that encode components of the TGF-β signaling pathway in ECs. The telangiectasias are malformations composed of dilated capillaries and veins that are present at birth. They are widely distributed over the skin and oral mucous membranes, as well as in the respiratory, gastrointestinal, and urinary tracts. The lesions can spontaneously rupture, causing serious epistaxis (nosebleed), gastrointestinal bleeding, or hematuria.

Hemangiomas

Hemangiomas are very common tumors composed of blood-filled vessels These lesions constitute 7% of all benign tumors of infancy and childhood; most are present from birth and initially increase in size, but many eventually regress spontaneously (Fig. 10.28). While hemangiomas typically are localized lesions confined to the head and neck, they occasionally may be more extensive (*angiomatosis*) and can arise internally. Nearly one third of these internal lesions are found in the liver. Malignant transformation is rare. Several histologic and clinical variants have been described:

- *Capillary hemangiomas* are the most common type; these occur in the skin, subcutaneous tissues, and mucous membranes of the oral cavities and lips, as well as in the liver, spleen, and kidneys (Fig. 10.28A). Histologically, they are composed of thin-walled capillaries with scant stroma (Fig. 10.28B).
- *Juvenile hemangiomas* (so-called "strawberry hemangiomas") of the newborn skin are extremely common (1 in 200 births) and can be multiple. These grow rapidly for a few months but then fade by 1 to 3 years of age, with complete regression by 7 years of age in the vast majority of cases.
- *Pyogenic granulomas* are capillary hemangiomas that manifest as rapidly growing red pedunculated lesions on the skin, gingival, or oral mucosa. Microscopically they resemble exuberant granulation tissue. They bleed

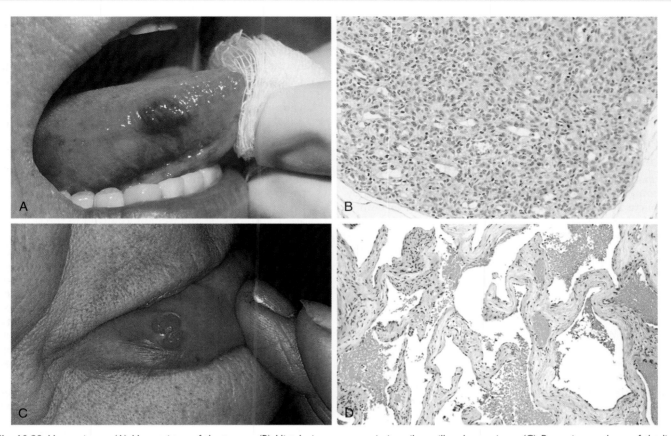

Fig. 10.28 Hemangiomas. (A) Hemangioma of the tongue. (B) Histologic appearance in juvenile capillary hemangioma. (C) Pyogenic granuloma of the lip. (D) Histologic appearance in cavernous hemangioma. *(A and D, Courtesy of John Sexton, MD, Beth Israel Hospital, Boston, Massachusetts. B, Courtesy of Christopher D.M. Fletcher, MD, Brigham and Women's Hospital, Boston, Massachusetts. C, Courtesy of Thomas Rogers, MD, University of Texas Southwestern Medical School, Dallas, Texas.)*

easily and often ulcerate (Fig. 10.28C). Roughly one fourth of the lesions develop after trauma, reaching a size of 1 to 2 cm within a few weeks. Curettage and cautery usually are curative. *Pregnancy tumor* (granuloma gravidarum) is a pyogenic granuloma that occurs infrequently in the gingiva of pregnant women. These lesions may spontaneously regress (especially after pregnancy) or undergo fibrosis, but occasionally require surgical excision.

- *Cavernous hemangiomas* are composed of large, dilated vascular channels. Compared with capillary hemangiomas, cavernous hemangiomas are more infiltrative, frequently involve deep structures, and do not spontaneously regress. On histologic examination, the mass is sharply defined but unencapsulated and is composed of large blood-filled vascular spaces separated by connective tissue stroma (Fig. 10.28D). Intravascular thrombosis and dystrophic calcification are common. These lesions may be locally destructive, and surgical excision is required in some cases. More often the tumors are of little clinical significance, but they can be cosmetically troublesome and are vulnerable to traumatic ulceration and bleeding. Brain hemangiomas are problematic, because they may cause symptoms related to compression of adjacent tissue or may rupture. Cavernous hemangiomas constitute one component of *von Hippel-Lindau disease* (Chapter 23), in which vascular lesions are commonly found in the cerebellum, brain stem, retina, pancreas, and liver. In some cases cerebral cavernous hemangiomas are familial, caused by mutations in one of three tumor suppressor genes called *CCM1, CCM2,* or *CCM3*

Lymphangiomas

Lymphangiomas are the benign lymphatic counterpart of hemangiomas.

- *Simple (capillary) lymphangiomas* are slightly elevated or sometimes pedunculated lesions up to 1 to 2 cm in diameter that occur predominantly in the head, neck, and axillary subcutaneous tissues. Histologically, lymphangiomas are composed of networks of endothelium-lined spaces that are distinguished from capillary channels only by the absence of blood cells.
- *Cavernous lymphangiomas (cystic hygromas)* typically are found in the neck or axilla of children, and more rarely in the retroperitoneum. Cavernous lymphangiomas can be large (up to 15 cm), filling the axilla or producing gross deformities of the neck. These lesions are composed of massively dilated lymphatic spaces lined by ECs and separated by intervening connective tissue stroma containing lymphoid aggregates. The tumor margins are indistinct and unencapsulated, making definitive resection difficult. Of note, cavernous lymphangiomas of the neck are common in Turner syndrome.

Glomus Tumors (Glomangiomas)

Glomus tumors are benign, exquisitely painful tumors arising from specialized SMCs of glomus bodies, arteriovenous structures involved in thermoregulation. Distinction from cavernous hemangiomas is based on clinical features and immunohistochemical staining for smooth muscle markers. They most commonly are found in the distal portion of the digits, especially under the fingernails. Excision is curative.

Bacillary Angiomatosis

Bacillary angiomatosis is a vascular proliferation in immunocompromised hosts (e.g., patients with AIDS) caused by opportunistic gram-negative bacilli of the *Bartonella* family. The lesions can involve the skin, bone, brain, and other organs. Two species have been implicated:

- *Bartonella henselae,* whose principal reservoir is the domestic cat; this organism causes cat-scratch disease (a necrotizing granulomatous inflammation of lymph nodes) in immunocompetent hosts.
- *Bartonella quintana,* which is transmitted by human body lice; this microbe was the cause of "trench fever" in World War I.

Skin lesions take the form of red papules and nodules, or rounded subcutaneous masses. Histologically, there is a proliferation of capillaries lined by prominent epithelioid ECs, which exhibit nuclear atypia and mitoses (Fig. 10.29). Other features include infiltrating neutrophils, nuclear debris, and purplish granular collections of the causative bacteria.

The bacteria induce host tissues to produce hypoxia-inducible factor-1α (HIF-1α), which drives VEGF production and vascular proliferation. The infections (and lesions) are cured by antibiotic treatment.

Intermediate-Grade (Borderline) Tumors

Kaposi Sarcoma

Kaposi sarcoma (KS) is a vascular neoplasm caused by Kaposi sarcoma herpesvirus (KSHV, also known as human herpesvirus-8, or HHV-8). Although it occurs in a number of contexts, it is most common in patients with AIDS; indeed, its presence is used as a criterion for the diagnosis. Four forms of KS, based on population demographics and risks, are recognized:

- *Classic KS* is a disorder of older men of Mediterranean, Middle Eastern, or Eastern European descent (especially Ashkenazi Jews); it is uncommon in the United States. It can be associated with malignancy or altered immunity but is not associated with HIV infection. Classic KS manifests as multiple red-purple skin plaques or nodules, usually on the distal lower extremities; these progressively increase in size and number and spread proximally. Although persistent, the tumors typically are asymptomatic and remain localized to the skin and subcutaneous tissue.
- *Endemic African KS* typically occurs in younger (under 40 years of age) HIV-seronegative individuals and can follow an indolent or aggressive course; it involves lymph nodes much more frequently than in the classic variant. In combination with AIDS-associated KS (see later), KS is now the most common tumor in central Africa. A particularly severe form, with prominent lymph node and visceral involvement, occurs in prepubertal children; the prognosis is poor, with an almost 100% mortality within 3 years.
- *Transplantation-associated KS* occurs in solid organ transplant recipients in the setting of T-cell immunosuppression. In these patients, the risk for KS is increased 100-fold. It pursues an aggressive course and often involves lymph nodes, mucosa, and viscera; cutaneous lesions may be absent. Lesions often regress with attenuation of immunosuppression, but at the risk for organ rejection.
- *AIDS-associated (epidemic) KS* is an AIDS-defining illness; worldwide it represents the most common HIV-related malignancy (Chapter 5). Although the incidence of KS has fallen more than 80% with the advent of antiretroviral therapy, it still occurs in HIV-infected individuals with a 1000-fold higher incidence than in the general population, and afflicts 2% to 3% of the HIV-infected U.S. population. AIDS-associated KS often involves

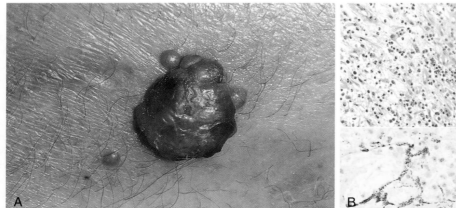
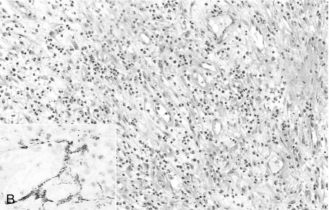

Fig. 10.29 Bacillary angiomatosis. (A) Characteristic cutaneous lesion. (B) Histologic features are those of acute inflammation and capillary proliferation. **Inset,** Modified silver (Warthin-Starry) stain demonstrates clusters of tangled bacilli *(black). (A, Courtesy of Richard Johnson, MD, Beth Israel Deaconess Medical Center, Boston, Massachusetts. B and inset, courtesy of Scott Granter, MD, Brigham and Women's Hospital, Boston, Massachusetts.)*

lymph nodes and disseminates widely to viscera early in its course. Most patients eventually die of opportunistic infections rather than from KS.

Pathogenesis

Virtually all KS lesions are infected by KSHV (HHV-8). Like Epstein-Barr virus, KSHV is a γ-herpesvirus. It is transmitted both through sexual contact and potentially via oral secretions and cutaneous exposures (of note, the prevalence of endemic African KS is inversely related to the wearing of shoes). KSHV and altered T-cell immunity probably are required for KS development; in older adults, diminished T-cell immunity may be related to aging. It also is probable that acquired somatic mutations in the cells of origin contribute to tumor development and progression.

KSHV causes lytic and latent infections in ECs, both of which probably are important in KS pathogenesis. A virally encoded G protein induces VEGF production, stimulating endothelial growth, and cytokines produced by inflammatory cells recruited to sites of lytic infection also create a local proliferative milieu. In latently infected cells, KSHV-encoded proteins disrupt normal cellular proliferation controls (e.g., through synthesis of a viral homologue of cyclin D) and prevent apoptosis by inhibiting p53. Thus, the local inflammatory environment favors cellular proliferation, and latently infected cells have a growth advantage. In its early stages, only a few cells are KSHV-infected, but with time, virtually all of the proliferating cells carry the virus. As with EBV infection, early lesions are polyclonal but with accumulation of mutations the tumors become monoclonal.

MORPHOLOGY

In classic Kaposi sarcoma (and sometimes in other variants), the cutaneous lesions progress through three stages: patch, plaque, and nodule.

- **Patches** are pink, red, or purple macules, typically confined to the distal lower extremities (Fig. 10.30A). Microscopic examination reveals dilated, irregular, and angulated blood vessels lined by ECs and an interspersed infiltrate of chronic inflammatory cells, sometimes containing hemosiderin. These lesions can be difficult to distinguish from granulation tissue.
- With time, lesions spread proximally and become larger, **violaceous, raised plaques** (Fig. 10.30A) composed of dilated, jagged dermal vascular channels lined and surrounded by plump spindle cells. Other prominent features include extravasated red cells, hemosiderin-laden macrophages, and other mononuclear cells.
- Eventually **nodular,** more overtly neoplastic, lesions appear. These are composed of plump, proliferating spindle cells, mostly located in the dermis or subcutaneous tissues (Fig. 10.30B), often with interspersed slitlike spaces. The spindle cells express both EC and SMC markers. Hemorrhage and hemosiderin deposition are more pronounced, and mitotic figures are common. The nodular stage often is accompanied by nodal and visceral involvement, particularly in the African and AIDS-associated variants.

Clinical Features

The course of disease varies widely according to the clinical setting. Most primary KSHV infections are asymptomatic. Classic KS is—at least initially—largely restricted to the surface of the body, and surgical resection usually is adequate for an excellent prognosis. Radiation therapy can be used for multiple lesions in a restricted area, and chemotherapy yields satisfactory results for more disseminated disease, including nodal involvement. In KS associated with immunosuppression, withdrawal of therapy (with or without adjunct chemotherapy or radiotherapy) often is effective. For AIDS-associated KS, HIV anti-retroviral therapy generally is beneficial, with or without additional therapy. IFN-γ and angiogenesis inhibitors also have proved variably effective.

Hemangioendotheliomas

Hemangioendotheliomas comprise a wide spectrum of borderline vascular neoplasms with clinical behaviors intermediate between those of benign, well-differentiated hemangiomas and aggressively malignant angiosarcomas

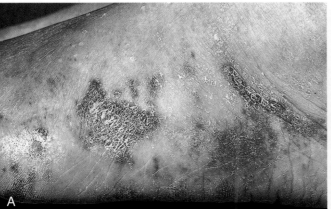
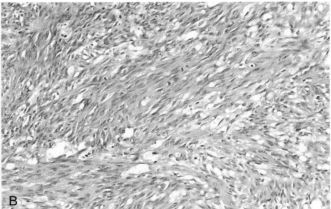

Fig. 10.30 Kaposi sarcoma. (A) Characteristic coalescent cutaneous red-purple macules and plaques. (B) Histologic view of the nodular stage, demonstrating sheets of plump, proliferating spindle cells and slitlike vascular spaces. *(Courtesy of Christopher D.M. Fletcher, MD, Brigham and Women's Hospital, Boston, Massachusetts.)*

Epithelioid hemangioendothelioma is a tumor of adults arising in association with medium- to large-sized veins. The clinical course is highly variable. While excision is curative in a majority of the cases, up to 40% of the tumors recur; 20% to 30% eventually metastasize, and 15% of patients die of their tumors.

Malignant Tumors

Angiosarcomas

Angiosarcomas are malignant endothelial neoplasms ranging from highly differentiated tumors resembling hemangiomas to wildly anaplastic lesions. Older adults are more commonly affected, without gender predilection; lesions can occur at any site, but most often involve the skin, soft tissue, breast, and liver. Clinically, angiosarcomas are aggressive tumors that invade locally and metastasize. Current 5-year survival rates are only about 30%.

Angiosarcomas can arise in the setting of lymphedema, classically in the ipsilateral upper extremity several years after radical mastectomy (i.e., with lymph node resection) for breast cancer. In such instances, the tumor presumably arises from lymphatic vessels *(lymphangiosarcoma)*. Angiosarcomas can also be induced by radiation and rarely are associated with long-term (years) indwelling foreign bodies (e.g., catheters).

Hepatic angiosarcomas are associated with certain carcinogens, including arsenical pesticides and polyvinyl chloride (one of the best known examples of human chemical carcinogenesis). Multiple years typically transpire between exposure and subsequent tumor development.

● MORPHOLOGY

In the skin, angiosarcomas begin as small, sharply demarcated, asymptomatic red nodules. More advanced lesions are large, fleshy red-tan to gray-white masses (Fig. 10.31A) with margins that blend imperceptibly with surrounding structures. Necrosis and hemorrhage are common.

On microscopic examination, the extent of differentiation is extremely variable, ranging from plump atypical ECs that form vascular channels (Fig. 10.31B) to undifferentiated spindle cell tumors without discernible blood vessels. The EC origin can be demonstrated in the poorly differentiated tumors by staining for the EC markers CD31 and von Willebrand factor (Fig. 10.31C).

● SUMMARY

VASCULAR TUMORS

- Vascular ectasias are not neoplasms, but rather dilations of existing vessels.
- Vascular neoplasms can derive from either blood vessels or lymphatics, and can be composed of ECs (e.g., hemangioma, lymphangioma, angiosarcoma) or other cells of the vascular wall (e.g., glomus tumor).
- Most vascular tumors are benign (e.g., hemangioma); some have an intermediate, locally aggressive behavior (e.g., Kaposi sarcoma); and others are highly malignant (e.g., angiosarcoma).
- Benign tumors typically form obvious vascular channels lined by normal-appearing ECs. Malignant tumors more often are solid and cellular, exhibit cytologic atypia, and lack well-defined vessels.

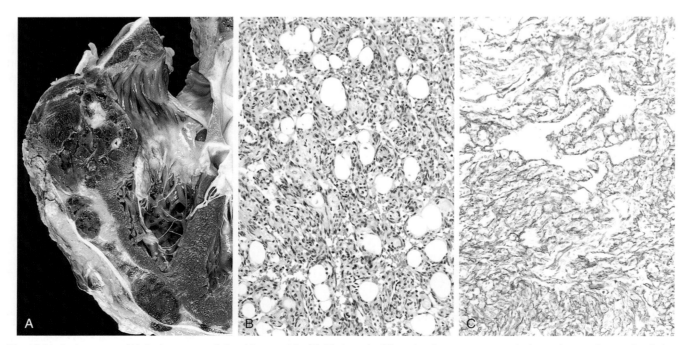

Fig. 10.31 Angiosarcoma. (A) Angiosarcoma of the right ventricle. (B) Moderately differentiated angiosarcoma with dense clumps of atypical cells lining distinct vascular lumina. (C) Immunohistochemical staining of angiosarcoma for the endothelial cell marker CD31.

PATHOLOGY OF VASCULAR INTERVENTION

The morphologic changes that occur in vessels following therapeutic intervention—balloon angioplasty, stenting, or bypass surgery—recapitulate many of the changes that occur in the setting of other forms of vascular injury. Local trauma (due to stenting), vascular thrombosis (after angioplasty), and abnormal mechanical forces (e.g., a saphenous vein inserted into the arterial circulation as a coronary artery bypass graft) all induce the same stereotypical healing responses—fibromuscular intimal hyperplastic lesions composed of SMCs and ECM. Thus, just as with atherosclerosis, interventions that injure the endothelium also tend to induce intimal thickening by recruiting SMCs and promoting ECM deposition.

Endovascular Stenting

Arterial stenoses (especially those in coronary and carotid arteries) can be dilated by transiently inflating a balloon catheter to pressures sufficient to rupture the occluding plaque *(balloon angioplasty)*; in doing so, a limited *arterial dissection* also is induced. Angioplasty can be complicated by *abrupt reclosure* resulting from compression of the lumen by an extensive circumferential or longitudinal dissection, or by thrombosis. In view of this well over 90% of endovascular coronary procedures involve both angioplasty and concurrent *coronary stent* placement.

Coronary stents are expandable tubes of metallic mesh. They provide a larger and more regular lumen, "tack down" the intimal flaps and dissections that occur during angioplasty, and mechanically limit vascular spasm. Nevertheless, as a consequence of endothelial injury, *thrombosis* is an important immediate post-stenting complication; patients must receive potent anti-thrombotic agents (primarily platelet antagonists) to prevent acute catastrophic thrombotic occlusions until the stented region becomes endothelialized. The long-term success of angioplasty is limited by the development of *proliferative in-stent restenosis*. Such intimal thickening results in clinically significant luminal occlusion in up to one third of patients within 6 to 12 months of stenting (Fig. 10.32). The newest generation of *drug-eluting stents* is designed to avoid this complication by releasing anti-proliferative drugs (e.g., paclitaxel, sirolimus) into the adjacent vessel wall that block SMC activation. Use of such stents reduces the incidence of restenosis at 1 year by 50% to 80%.

Vascular Replacement

Synthetic or autologous vascular grafts commonly are used to replace damaged vessels or bypass diseased arteries. Of the synthetic grafts, large-bore (12- to 18-mm–diameter) conduits function well in high-flow locations such as the aorta, while small-bore artificial grafts (8 mm or less in diameter) generally fail as a result of acute thrombosis or late intimal hyperplasia, primarily at the junction of the graft and the native vasculature.

Consequently, when small-bore vessel replacement is needed (e.g., for coronary artery bypass surgeries), the grafts are fashioned either from autologous saphenous vein (taken from the patient's own leg) or left internal mammary artery. The long-term patency of saphenous vein grafts is only 50% at 10 years; these grafts occlude through thrombosis (typically early), intimal thickening (months to years postoperatively), and vein graft atherosclerosis. By contrast, more than 90% of internal mammary artery grafts are patent after 10 years.

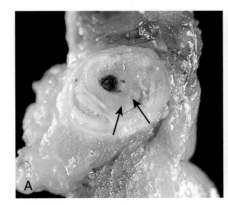 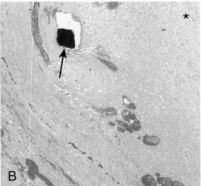

Fig. 10.32 Restenosis after angioplasty and stenting. (A) Gross view demonstrating residual atherosclerotic plaque *(arrows)* and a new, glistening intimal proliferative lesion. (B) Histologic view shows a thickened neointima overlying the stent wires *(black diamond indicated by the arrow)*, which encroaches on the lumen *(asterisk)*. *(B, Reproduced from Schoen FJ, Edwards WD: Pathology of cardiovascular interventions, including endovascular therapies, revascularization, vascular replacement, cardiac assist/replacement, arrhythmia control, and repaired congenital heart disease. In Silver MD, et al., editors: Cardiovascular pathology, ed 3, Philadelphia, 2001, Churchill Livingstone.)*

SUGGESTED READINGS

Bhutani M, Polizzotto MN, Uldrick TS, et al: Kaposi sarcoma-associated herpesvirus-associated malignancies: epidemiology, pathogenesis, and advances in treatment, *Semin Oncol* 42:247, 2015. *[A solid and thorough review.]*

Coffman TM: Under pressure: the search for the essential mechanisms of hypertension, *Nat Med* 17:1402, 2011. *[A well-written review of the current state of the field including recent translational advances.]*

Fishbein MC, Fishbein GA: Arteriosclerosis: facts and fancy, *Cardiovasc Pathol* 24:335, 2015. *[A fun and thought-provoking revisit to topics of cardiovascular "conventional wisdom."]*

Gillis E, Van Laer L, Loeys BL: Genetics of thoracic aortic aneurysm: at the crossroad of transforming growth factor-β signaling and vascular smooth muscle cell contractility, *Circ Res* 113:327, 2013. *[An up-to-date discussion of the molecular and cellular basis for thoracic aneurysms and dissections.]*

Gimbrone MA Jr, Garcia-Cardeña G: Vascular endothelium, hemodynamics, and the pathobiology of atherosclerosis, *Cardiovasc Pathol* 22:9, 2013. *[A well-written review on endothelial responses to mechanical forces from one of the leading groups in the field.]*

Grebe A, Latz E: Cholesterol crystals and inflammation, *Curr Rheumatol Rep* 15:313, 2013. *[A review of the activation of the inflammasome by cholesterol crystals, and its role in atherosclerosis.]*

Hansson GK, Libby P, Tabas I: Inflammation and plaque vulnerability, *J Intern Med* 278:483, 2015. *[An up-to-date review of the current concepts linking inflammation and plaque vulnerability.]*

Inoue T, Croce K, Morooka T, et al: Vascular inflammation and repair: implications for re-endothelialization, restenosis, and stent thrombosis, *JACC Cardiovasc Interv* 4:1057, 2011. *[An excellent overview of the inflammatory pathways that influence the outcomes of percutaneous vessel interventions.]*

Jaffe R, Strauss B: Late and very late thrombosis of drug-eluting stents: evolving concepts and perspectives, *J Am Coll Cardiol* 50:119, 2007. *[An even-handed discussion of the complications following coronary artery stent placement.]*

Jennette J, Falk R: Nosology of primary vasculitis, *Curr Opin Rheumatol* 19:10, 2007. *[A classification of vasculitis based on pathogenic pathways and the vessels involved; provides a good organization to a complex and potentially confusing aspect of vascular pathology.]*

Jennette JC, Falk RJ: Pathogenesis of antineutrophil cytoplasmic autoantibody-mediated disease, *Nat Rev Rheumatol* 10:463, 2014. *[A well-written and well-organized overview of the big picture in ANCA vasculitis.]*

Kim FY, Marhefka G, Ruggiero NJ, et al: Saphenous vein graft disease: review of pathophysiology, prevention, and treatment, *Cardiol Rev* 21:101, 2013. *[A good overview of the pathogenesis and clinical issues of saphenous vein graft acute occlusion and chronic stenosis.]*

Libby P, Lichtman AH, Hansson GK: Immune effector mechanisms implicated in atherosclerosis: from mice to humans, *Immunity* 38:1092, 2013. *[A superb review of the experimental and clinical literature describing the role of specific and adaptive immunity in atherosclerosis pathogenesis.]*

MacAlpin RN: Some observations on and controversies about coronary arterial spasm, *Int J Cardiol* 181:389, 2015. *[A good clinical overview of coronary spasm and its sequelae.]*

Michel JB, Martin-Ventura JL, Egido J, et al: Novel aspects of the pathogenesis of aneurysms of the abdominal aorta in humans, *Cardiovasc Res* 90:18, 2011. *[A good discussion of the molecular pathways underlying human abdominal aortic aneurysm formation.]*

Monahan-Earley R, Dvorak AM, Aird WC: Evolutionary origins of the blood vascular system and endothelium, *J Thromb Haemost* 11(Suppl 1):46, 2013. *[An interesting discussion of the evolutionary basis for vascular development, including cogent explanations for endothelial heterogeneity.]*

Penel N, Marréaud S, Robin YM, et al: Angiosarcoma: state of the art and perspectives, *Crit Rev Oncol Hematol* 22:1266, 2011. *[An extensive clinical summary of this aggressively malignant vascular tumor.]*

Ridker P: From C-reactive protein to interleukin-6 to interleukin-1: moving upstream to identify novel targets for atheroprotection, *Circ Res* 118:145, 2016. *[A well-written opinion piece regarding how CRP links to other inflammatory mediators, and potentially identifies therapeutic targets.]*

Heart

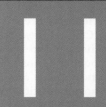

11

CHAPTER OUTLINE

Overview of Heart Disease 399
Heart Failure 400
Left-Sided Heart Failure 401
Right-Sided Heart Failure 402
Congenital Heart Disease 403
Malformations Associated With Left-to-Right Shunts 404
Malformations Associated With Right-to-Left Shunts 406
Malformations Associated With Obstructive Lesions 407
Ischemic Heart Disease 408
Angina Pectoris 411
Myocardial Infarction 411
Chronic Ischemic Heart Disease 419
Cardiac Stem Cells 419

Arrhythmias 419
Sudden Cardiac Death 420
Hypertensive Heart Disease 420
Systemic (Left-Sided) Hypertensive Heart Disease 421
Pulmonary Hypertensive Heart Disease—Cor Pulmonale 422
Valvular Heart Disease 422
Degenerative Valve Disease 423
Rheumatic Valvular Disease 425
Infective Endocarditis 427
Noninfected Vegetations 428
Cardiomyopathies and Myocarditis 429
Dilated Cardiomyopathy 429
Arrhythmogenic Right Ventricular Cardiomyopathy 432

Hypertrophic Cardiomyopathy 432
Restrictive Cardiomyopathy 433
Myocarditis 434
Other Causes of Myocardial Disease 435
Pericardial Disease 436
Pericardial Effusion and Hemopericardium 436
Pericarditis 436
Cardiac Tumors 437
Primary Neoplasms 437
Cardiac Effects of Noncardiac Neoplasms 438
Cardiac Transplantation 439

The heart is a truly remarkable organ, beating more than 40 million times per year and pumping over 7500 liters of blood a day; in a typical lifespan, its cumulative output would fill three supertankers. The cardiovascular system is the first organ system to become functional in utero (at approximately 8 weeks of gestation); without a beating heart and vascular supply, development cannot proceed, and the embryo dies. When the heart fails during postnatal life, the results are equally catastrophic. Indeed, cardiovascular disease is the leading cause of mortality worldwide and accounts for one in four of all deaths in the United States—approximately 1 death every minute, or 610,000 deaths each year (a greater mortality rate than for all forms of cancer combined). The annual economic impact of cardiac disease exceeds $200 billion, with ischemic heart disease contributing well over half. Moreover, roughly one third of these deaths are "premature," occurring in individuals younger than 75 years of age; thus, an additional economic burden is imposed through lost years of productivity.

OVERVIEW OF HEART DISEASE

Although a wide range of diseases can affect the cardiovascular system, the pathophysiologic pathways that result in a "broken" heart distill down to six principal mechanisms:

- *Failure of the pump.* In the most common situation, the cardiac muscle contracts weakly and the chambers cannot empty properly—so-called "systolic dysfunction." In some cases, the muscle cannot relax sufficiently to permit ventricular filling, resulting in *diastolic dysfunction.*
- *Obstruction to flow.* Lesions that prevent valve opening (e.g., calcific aortic valve stenosis) or cause increased ventricular chamber pressures (e.g., systemic hypertension or aortic coarctation) can overwork the myocardium, which has to pump against the obstruction.
- *Regurgitant flow.* Valve pathology that allows backward flow of blood results in increased volume workload and may overwhelm the pumping capacity of the affected chambers.
- *Shunted flow.* Defects (congenital or acquired) that divert blood inappropriately from one chamber to another, or from one vessel to another, lead to pressure and volume overloads.
- *Disorders of cardiac conduction.* Uncoordinated cardiac impulses or blocked conduction pathways can cause arrhythmias that slow contractions or prevent effective pumping altogether.
- *Rupture of the heart or major vessel.* Loss of circulatory continuity (e.g., a gunshot wound through the thoracic aorta) may lead to massive blood loss, hypotensive shock, and death.

HEART FAILURE

Heart failure, often referred to as *congestive heart failure (CHF)*, is the common end point for many forms of cardiac disease and typically is a progressive condition with a poor prognosis. In the United States alone, over 5 million individuals are affected, resulting in well over 1 million hospitalizations annually, and a financial burden in excess of $32 billion. Roughly one half of patients die within 5 years of receiving a diagnosis of CHF, and 1 in 9 deaths in the United States include heart failure as a contributory cause.

CHF occurs when the heart cannot generate sufficient output to meet the metabolic demands of the tissues, or can only do so at higher-than-normal filling pressures; in a minority of cases, heart failure is a consequence of greatly increased tissue demands, as in hyperthyroidism, or decreased oxygen carrying capacity, as in anemia *(high-output failure)*. The onset of CHF is sometimes abrupt, as in the setting of a large myocardial infarct or acute valve dysfunction. In most cases, however, CHF develops gradually and insidiously owing to the cumulative effects of chronic work overload or progressive loss of myocardium.

Heart failure may result from systolic or diastolic dysfunction. Systolic dysfunction results from inadequate myocardial contractile function, usually as a consequence of ischemic heart disease or hypertension. Diastolic dysfunction refers to an inability of the heart to adequately relax and fill, which may be a consequence of massive left ventricular hypertrophy, myocardial fibrosis, amyloid deposition, or constrictive pericarditis. Approximately one half of CHF cases are attributable to diastolic dysfunction, with a greater frequency seen in older adults, diabetic patients, and women. Heart failure may also be caused by valve dysfunction (e.g., due to endocarditis), or may occur following rapid increases in blood volume or blood pressure, even if the heart is normal.

When, the failing heart can no longer efficiently pump blood, there is an increase in end-diastolic ventricular volumes, increased end-diastolic pressures, and elevated venous pressures. Thus, inadequate cardiac output—called *forward failure*—is almost always accompanied by increased congestion of the venous circulation—that is, *backward failure*. Although the root problem in CHF typically is deficient cardiac function, virtually every other organ is eventually affected by some combination of forward and backward failure.

The cardiovascular system attempts to compensate for reduced myocardial contractility or increased hemodynamic burden through several homeostatic mechanisms:

- *The Frank-Starling mechanism.* Increased end-diastolic filling volumes dilate the heart and cause increased cardiac myofiber stretching; these lengthened fibers contract more forcibly, thereby increasing cardiac output. If the dilated ventricle is able to maintain cardiac output by this means, the patient is said to be in *compensated heart failure.* However, ventricular dilation comes at the expense of increased wall tension and magnifies the oxygen requirements of an already-compromised myocardium. With time, the failing muscle is no longer able to propel sufficient blood to meet the needs of the body, and the patient develops *decompensated heart failure.*
- *Activation of neurohumoral systems:*
  - Release of the neurotransmitter norepinephrine by the autonomic nervous system increases heart rate and augments myocardial contractility and vascular resistance.
  - Activation of the renin-angiotensin-aldosterone system spurs water and salt retention (augmenting circulatory volume) and increases vascular tone.
  - Release of atrial natriuretic peptide acts to balance the renin-angiotensin-aldosterone system through diuresis and vascular smooth muscle relaxation.
- *Myocardial structural changes, including augmented muscle mass.* Cardiac myocytes adapt to increased workload by assembling new sarcomeres, a change that is accompanied by myocyte enlargement (hypertrophy) (Fig. 11.1).
  - In *pressure overload states* (e.g., hypertension or valvular stenosis), new sarcomeres tend to be added parallel to the long axis of the myocytes, adjacent to existing sarcomeres. The growing muscle fiber diameter thus results in *concentric hypertrophy*—the ventricular wall thickness increases without an increase in the size of the chamber.
  - In *volume overload states* (e.g., valvular regurgitation or shunts), the new sarcomeres are added in series with existing sarcomeres, so that the muscle fiber length increases. Consequently, the ventricle tends to dilate, and the resulting wall thickness can be increased, normal, or decreased; thus, heart weight—rather than wall thickness—is the best measure of hypertrophy in volume-overloaded hearts.

Compensatory hypertrophy comes at a cost. The oxygen requirements of hypertrophic myocardium are amplified owing to increased myocardial cell mass. Because the myocardial capillary bed does not expand in step with the increased myocardial oxygen demands, the myocardium becomes vulnerable to ischemic injury. Hypertrophy also typically is associated with altered patterns of gene expression reminiscent of fetal myocytes, such as changes in the dominant form of myosin heavy chain produced. Altered gene expression may contribute to changes in myocyte function that lead to increases in heart rate and force of contraction, both of which improve cardiac output, but which also lead to higher cardiac oxygen consumption. In the face of ischemia and chronic increases in workload, other pathologic changes eventually supervene, including myocyte apoptosis, cytoskeletal alterations, and increased extracellular matrix (ECM) deposition.

Pathologic compensatory cardiac hypertrophy is correlated with increased mortality; indeed, cardiac hypertrophy is an independent risk factor for sudden cardiac death. By contrast, the volume-loaded hypertrophy induced by regular aerobic exercise (physiologic hypertrophy) typically is accompanied by an increase in capillary density, with decreased resting heart rate and blood

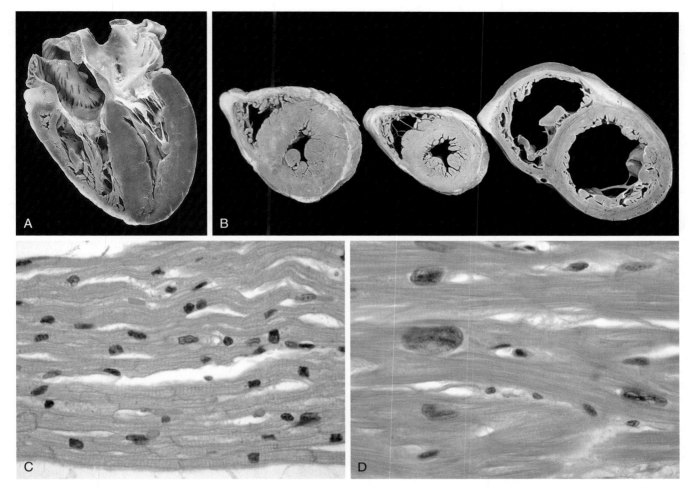

Fig. 11.1 Left ventricular hypertrophy. (A) Pressure hypertrophy due to left ventricular outflow obstruction. The left ventricle is on the *lower right* in this apical four-chamber view of the heart. (B) Left ventricular hypertrophy with and without dilation, viewed in transverse heart sections. Compared with a normal heart *(center)*, the pressure-hypertrophied hearts *(left and in A)* have increased mass and a thick left ventricular wall, while the hypertrophied, dilated heart *(right)* has increased mass and a normal wall thickness. (C) Normal myocardium. (D) Hypertrophied myocardium (panels *C* and *D* are photomicrographs at the same magnification). Note the increases in both cell size and nuclear size in the hypertrophied myocytes. *(A and B, Reproduced with permission from Edwards WD: Cardiac anatomy and examination of cardiac specimens. In Emmanouilides GC, et al, editors: Moss and Adams heart disease in infants, children, and adolescents: including the fetus and young adults, ed 5, Philadelphia, 1995, Williams & Wilkins, p 86.)*

pressure. These physiologic adaptations reduce overall cardiovascular morbidity and mortality. In comparison, static exercise (e.g., weight lifting) is associated with pressure hypertrophy and may not have the same beneficial effects.

Left-Sided Heart Failure

Heart failure can affect predominantly the left or the right side of the heart or may involve both sides. The most common causes of left-sided cardiac failure are ischemic heart disease (IHD), systemic hypertension, mitral or aortic valve disease, and primary diseases of the myocardium (e.g., amyloidosis). The morphologic and clinical effects of left-sided CHF stem from diminished systemic perfusion and elevated back-pressures within the pulmonary circulation.

MORPHOLOGY

Heart. The **gross** cardiac findings depend on the underlying disease process, for example, myocardial infarction or valvular deformities may be present. With the exception of failure due to mitral valve stenosis or restrictive cardiomyopathies (described later), the left ventricle usually is hypertrophied and can be dilated, sometimes massively. Left ventricular dilation can result in mitral insufficiency and left atrial enlargement, which is associated with an increased incidence of atrial fibrillation. The **microscopic** changes in heart failure are nonspecific, consisting primarily of myocyte hypertrophy with interstitial fibrosis of variable severity. Superimposed on this background may be other lesions that contribute to the development of heart failure (e.g., recent or old myocardial infarction).

Lungs. In acute left-sided heart failure, rising pressure in the pulmonary veins is ultimately transmitted back to the capillaries and arteries of the lungs, resulting in congestion and edema as well as pleural effusion due to an increase in hydrostatic pressure in the venules of the visceral pleura. The lungs are heavy and boggy, and microscopically show perivascular and interstitial transudates, alveolar septal edema, and **accumulation of edema fluid in the alveolar spaces**. In chronic heart failure, variable numbers of red cells extravasate from the leaky capillaries into alveolar spaces, where they are phagocytosed by macrophages. The subsequent breakdown of red cells and hemoglobin leads to the appearance of hemosiderin-laden alveolar macrophages—so-called **heart failure cells**—that reflect previous episodes of pulmonary edema.

Clinical Features

Dyspnea (shortness of breath) on exertion is usually the earliest and most significant symptom of left-sided heart failure; cough is also common as a consequence of fluid transudation into air spaces. As failure progresses, patients experience dyspnea when recumbent (*orthopnea*); this occurs because the supine position increases venous return from the lower extremities and also elevates the diaphragm. Orthopnea typically is relieved by sitting or standing, so patients usually sleep in a semi-seated position. *Paroxysmal nocturnal dyspnea* is a particularly dramatic form of breathlessness, awakening patients from sleep with extreme dyspnea bordering on feelings of suffocation.

Other manifestations of left ventricular failure include an enlarged heart (cardiomegaly), tachycardia, a third heart sound (S_3), and fine ráles at the lung bases, caused by the opening of edematous pulmonary alveoli. With progressive ventricular dilation, the papillary muscles are displaced outward, causing mitral regurgitation and a systolic murmur. Subsequent chronic dilation of the left atrium can cause *atrial fibrillation,* manifested by an "irregularly irregular" heartbeat. Such uncoordinated, chaotic atrial contractions reduce the atrial contribution to ventricular filling, thus reducing the ventricular stroke volume. Atrial fibrillation also causes stasis of the blood (particularly in the atrial appendage), frequently leading to the formation of thrombi that can shed emboli and cause strokes and manifestations of infarction in other organs.

Diminished cardiac output leads to decreased renal perfusion that in turn triggers the renin-angiotensin-aldosterone axis, increasing intravascular volume and pressures (Chapters 4 and 10). Unfortunately, with a failing heart, these compensatory effects exacerbate the pulmonary edema. With further progression of CHF, *prerenal azotemia* may supervene, with impaired excretion of nitrogenous wastes and increasing metabolic derangement. In severe CHF, diminished cerebral perfusion may manifest as *hypoxic encephalopathy* marked by irritability, diminished cognition, and restlessness that can progress to stupor and coma.

Treatment for CHF is typically focused—at least initially—on correcting the underlying cause, for example a valvular defect or inadequate cardiac perfusion. In lieu of such options, the clinical approach includes salt restriction or pharmacologic agents that variously reduce volume overload (e.g., diuretics), increase myocardial contractility (so-called "positive inotropes"), or reduce afterload (adrenergic blockade or inhibitors of angiotensin-converting enzymes). Angiotensin-converting enzyme inhibitors appear to benefit patients not only by opposing aldosterone-mediated salt and water retention, but also by limiting cardiomyocyte hypertrophy and remodeling through uncertain mechanisms. Although cardiac resynchronization therapy (exogenous pacing of both the right and left ventricles) and cardiac contractility modulation (exogenous stimulation of cardiac muscle) have recently augmented the cardiologist's armamentarium, CHF remains a serious cause of human morbidity and mortality.

Right-Sided Heart Failure

Right-sided heart failure is usually the consequence of left-sided heart failure, since any pressure increase in the pulmonary circulation inevitably produces an increased burden on the right side of the heart. Consequently, the causes of right-sided heart failure include all of those that induce left-sided heart failure. Isolated right-sided heart failure is infrequent and typically occurs in patients with one of a variety of disorders affecting the lungs; hence it is often referred to as *cor pulmonale*. Besides parenchymal lung diseases, cor pulmonale also may arise secondary to disorders that affect the pulmonary vasculature, for example, primary pulmonary hypertension (Chapter 13), recurrent pulmonary thromboembolism, or conditions that cause pulmonary vasoconstriction (obstructive sleep apnea). *The common feature of these disorders is pulmonary hypertension* (discussed later), which results in hypertrophy and dilation of the right side of the heart. In cor pulmonale, myocardial hypertrophy and dilation generally are confined to the right ventricle and atrium, although bulging of the ventricular septum to the left can reduce cardiac output by causing outflow tract obstruction.

The major morphologic and clinical effects of pure right-sided heart failure differ from those of left-sided heart failure in that engorgement of the systemic and portal venous systems typically is pronounced and pulmonary congestion is minimal.

MORPHOLOGY

Liver and Portal System. The liver usually is increased in size and weight **(congestive hepatomegaly).** A cut section displays prominent **passive congestion,** a pattern referred to as **nutmeg liver** (Chapter 4); congested centrilobular areas are surrounded by peripheral paler, noncongested parenchyma. When left-sided heart failure is also present, severe central hypoxia produces **centrilobular necrosis** in addition to the sinusoidal congestion. With long-standing severe right-sided heart failure, the central areas can become fibrotic, creating so-called **cardiac cirrhosis.**

Right-sided heart failure can also lead to elevated pressure in the portal vein and its tributaries **(portal hypertension),** with vascular congestion producing a tense, enlarged spleen **(congestive splenomegaly).** If severe, chronic passive congestion and attendant edema of the bowel wall may interfere with absorption of nutrients and medications.

Pleural, Pericardial, and Peritoneal Spaces. Systemic venous congestion due to right-sided heart failure can lead to **transudates (effusions)** in the pleural and pericardial spaces, but usually does not cause pulmonary parenchymal edema. Pleural effusions are most pronounced when there is combined right-sided and left-sided heart failure leading to elevated pulmonary and systemic venous pressures. A combination of hepatic congestion (with or without diminished albumin synthesis) and portal hypertension can lead to peritoneal transudates **(ascites).** If uncomplicated, effusions associated with right-sided CHF are trasudates with a low protein content and lack of inflammatory cells.

Subcutaneous Tissues. Edema of dependent portions of the body, especially the feet and lower legs, is a hallmark of right-sided CHF. In chronically bedridden patients, the edema may be primarily presacral.

Clinical Features

Unlike left-sided heart failure, pure right-sided heart failure typically is not associated with respiratory symptoms. Instead, the clinical manifestations are related to systemic and portal venous congestion and include hepatic and splenic enlargement, peripheral edema, pleural effusion, and ascites. Venous congestion and hypoxia of the kidneys and brain due to right-sided heart failure can produce deficits comparable to those caused by the hypoperfusion of left-sided heart failure.

Of note, cardiac decompensation is often marked by the appearance of biventricular CHF, encompassing features of both right-sided and left-sided heart failure. As CHF progresses, patients may become frankly cyanotic and acidotic, as a consequence of decreased tissue perfusion resulting from both diminished cardiac output and increasing congestion.

● SUMMARY

HEART FAILURE

- CHF occurs when the heart is unable to provide adequate perfusion to meet the metabolic demands of peripheral tissues; inadequate cardiac output usually is accompanied by congestion of the venous circulation.
- Left-sided heart failure is most commonly secondary to ischemic heart disease, systemic hypertension, mitral or aortic valve disease, or primary diseases of the myocardium; symptoms are mainly a consequence of pulmonary congestion and edema, although systemic hypoperfusion can cause renal and cerebral dysfunction.
- Right-sided heart failure is due most often to left-sided heart failure and, less commonly, to primary pulmonary disorders; signs and symptoms are related chiefly to peripheral edema and visceral congestion.

CONGENITAL HEART DISEASE

Congenital heart diseases are abnormalities of the heart or great vessels that are present at birth. They account for 20% to 30% of all birth defects and include a broad

Table 11.1 Frequency of Congenital Cardiac Malformations*

Malformation	Incidence per 1 Million Live Births	%
Ventricular septal defect	4482	42
Atrial septal defect	1043	10
Pulmonary stenosis	836	8
Patent ductus arteriosus	781	7
Tetralogy of Fallot	577	5
Coarctation of aorta	492	5
Atrioventricular septal defect	396	4
Aortic stenosis	388	4
Transposition of great arteries	388	4
Truncus arteriosus	136	1
Total anomalous pulmonary venous connection	120	1
Tricuspid atresia	118	1
TOTAL	9757	

*Summary of 44 published studies. Percentages do not add to 100% because of rounding. Data from Hoffman JI, Kaplan S: The incidence of congenital heart disease, *J Am Coll Cardiol* 39:1890, 2002.

spectrum of malformations, ranging from severe anomalies incompatible with intrauterine or perinatal survival, to lesions that produce few or no symptoms, some of which go completely unrecognized during life. Congenital heart disease affects nearly 1% of newborns (or roughly 40,000 infants per year in the United States). The incidence is higher in premature infants and in stillborns, approximately one fourth of which have significant cardiac malformations. Defects that permit live birth usually involve only single chambers or regions of the heart. Twelve entities account for 85% of congenital heart disease; their frequencies are shown in Table 11.1.

Thanks to surgical advances, the number of patients surviving with congenital heart disease is increasing rapidly and is currently estimated at over 2 million individuals in the United States alone. Although surgery may correct the hemodynamic abnormalities, the repaired heart may not be completely normal, since the myocardial hypertrophy and cardiac remodeling brought about by the congenital defect may be irreversible; in addition, virtually all cardiac surgery results in some degree of myocardial scarring. Such changes can lead secondarily to arrhythmias and myocardial dysfunction, which occasionally appear many years after surgical correction.

Pathogenesis

Congenital heart disease most commonly arises from faulty embryogenesis during gestational weeks 3 through 8, when major cardiovascular structures develop. The cause is unknown in almost 90% of cases. Of the accepted etiologic factors, environmental exposures, including congenital rubella infection, teratogens, and maternal diabetes, and genetic factors are best characterized. Genetic factors include specific loci implicated in familial forms of congenital heart disease and certain chromosomal abnormalities (e.g., trisomies 13, 15, 18, and 21, and Turner syndrome).

Cardiac morphogenesis involves multiple genes that work together to choreograph a complex series of tightly regulated events. Key steps include commitment of progenitor cells to the myocardial lineage, formation and looping of the heart tube, segmentation and growth of the cardiac chambers, cardiac valve formation, and connection of the great vessels to the heart. Proper orchestration of these remarkable transformations depends on networks of transcription factors and several signaling pathways and molecules, including the Wnt, vascular endothelial growth factor (VEGF), bone morphogenetic protein (BMP), transforming growth factor-β (TGF-β), fibroblast growth factor, and Notch pathways. Also essential for cardiac morphogenesis is the mechanical force imparted by flowing pulsatile blood, which is sensed by the cells of the developing heart and vessels.

Since crafting a normal heart involves many steps, even subtle perturbations can adversely influence the outcome. Most of the known genetic defects are autosomal dominant mutations causing loss (or sometimes gain) of function of a particular factor. Several mutations involve transcription factors. For example, atrial septal defects (ASDs) and ventricular septal defects (VSDs) and/or conduction defects may be caused by transcription factor mutations, such as *TBX5* mutations in the Holt-Oram syndrome. Other disorders (e.g., Noonan syndrome) are associated with mutations in intracellular signaling cascades that cause constitutive activation. MicroRNAs, as well as epigenetic changes (e.g., DNA methylation), also are increasingly recognized as important contributors. It is likely that even transient environmental stresses at critical junctures early in pregnancy can cause subtle changes in transcription factor activity that may recapitulate defects produced by heritable mutations.

Clinical Features

The various structural anomalies in congenital heart disease can be assigned to three major groups based on their hemodynamic and clinical consequences: (1) malformations causing a left-to-right shunt; (2) malformations causing a right-to-left shunt (cyanotic congenital heart diseases); and (3) malformations causing obstruction.

A *shunt* is an abnormal communication between chambers or blood vessels. Depending on pressure relationships, shunts permit the flow of blood from the left to the right side of the heart (or vice versa).

- With *right-to-left shunt,* a dusky blueness of the skin (cyanosis) results because the pulmonary circulation is bypassed and poorly oxygenated blood collected from the venous system enters the systemic arterial circulation.
- By contrast, *left-to-right shunts* increase blood flow into the pulmonary circulation and are not associated (at least initially) with cyanosis. However, they expose the low-pressure, low-resistance pulmonary circulation to high pressures and increased volumes; these alterations lead to adaptive changes that increase lung vascular resistance to protect the pulmonary bed, resulting in right ventricular hypertrophy and—eventually right-sided—failure. With time, increased pulmonary resistance also can cause shunt reversal (right to left) and late-onset cyanosis.

- Some congenital anomalies *obstruct vascular flow* by narrowing the chambers, valves, or major blood vessels. A malformation characterized by complete obstruction is called an *atresia.* In some disorders (e.g., tetralogy of Fallot), an obstruction (pulmonary stenosis) also is associated with a shunt (right-to-left, through a VSD).

The altered hemodynamics of congenital heart disease usually lead to chamber dilation or wall hypertrophy. However, some defects result in a reduced muscle mass or chamber size; this is called *hypoplasia* if it occurs before birth and *atrophy* if it develops postnatally.

Malformations Associated With Left-to-Right Shunts

Disorders associated with Left-to-right shunts are the most common types of congenital cardiac malformations. They include **atrial septal defects (ASDs)**, **ventricular septal defects (VSDs)**, and **patent ductus arteriosus (PDA)** (Fig. 11.2). ASDs typically increase only right ventricular and pulmonary outflow volumes, while VSDs and PDAs cause both increased pulmonary blood flow and pressure. Manifestations of these shunts range from completely asymptomatic to fulminant heart failure.

Cyanosis is not an early feature of these defects. However, as discussed earlier, prolonged left-to-right

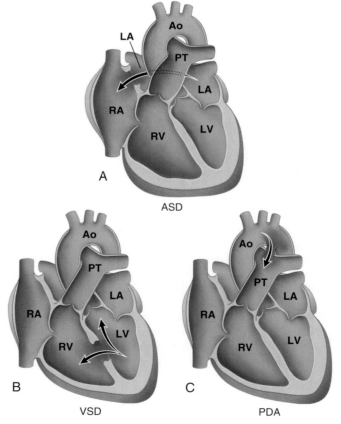

Fig. 11.2 Common congenital causes of left-to-right shunts (*arrows* indicate direction of blood flow). (A) Atrial septal defect (ASD). (B) Ventricular septal defect (VSD). (C) Patent ductus arteriosus (PDA). *Ao,* Aorta; *LA,* left atrium; *LV,* left ventricle; *PT,* pulmonary trunk; *RA,* right atrium; *RV,* right ventricle.

shunting may eventually give rise to pulmonary hypertension and right-to-left shunting of unoxygenated blood into the systemic circulation, a change marked by the appearance of cyanosis *(Eisenmenger syndrome)*. Once significant pulmonary hypertension develops, the structural defects of congenital heart disease are considered irreversible. This is the rationale for early intervention, in most cases surgically.

Atrial Septal Defects and Patent Foramen Ovale

During normal cardiac development, patency is maintained between the right and left atria by a series of fenestrations (*ostium primum* and *ostium secundum*) that eventually become the *foramen ovale*. This arrangement allows oxygenated blood from the maternal circulation to flow from the right to the left atrium, thereby sustaining fetal development. At later stages of intrauterine development, tissue flaps (*septum primum* and *septum secundum*) grow to occlude the foramen ovale, and in 80% of cases, the higher left-sided pressures in the heart that occur at birth permanently fuse the septa against the foramen ovale. In the remaining 20% of cases, a *patent foramen ovale* results; although the flap is of adequate size to cover the foramen, the unsealed septa can allow transient right-to-left blood flow, such as with a *Valsalva maneuver* during sneezing or straining during bowel movements. Although this typically has little significance, it occasionally manifests as *paradoxical embolism,* defined as venous emboli (e.g., from deep leg veins) that enter the systemic arterial circulation via a foramen ovale defect.

In contrast to patent foramen ovale, an ASD is an abnormal fixed opening in the atrial septum that allows unrestricted blood flow between the atrial chambers. A majority (90%) of ASDs are so-called "ostium secundum" defects in which growth of the septum secundum is insufficient to occlude the second ostium.

MORPHOLOGY

Ostium secundum ASDs (90% of ASDs) are smooth-walled defects near the foramen ovale, typically without other associated cardiac abnormalities. Hemodynamically significant lesions are accompanied by right atrial and ventricular dilation, right ventricular hypertrophy, and dilation of the pulmonary artery, reflecting the effects of a chronically increased volume load.

Ostium primum ASDs (accounting for 5% of these defects) occur at the lowest part of the atrial septum and can be associated with mitral and tricuspid valve abnormalities, reflecting the close relationship between development of the septum primum and the endocardial cushions. In more severe cases, additional defects may include a VSD and a **common atrioventricular canal.**

Sinus venosus ASDs (accounting for another 5% of the cases) are located high in the atrial septum and often are accompanied by anomalous drainage of the pulmonary veins into the right atrium or superior vena cava.

Clinical Features

ASDs usually are asymptomatic until adulthood. Although VSDs are more common, many close spontaneously. Consequently, ASDs—which are less likely to spontaneously close—are the most common defects to be first diagnosed in adults. ASDs initially cause left-to-right shunts, due to lower pressures in the pulmonary circulation and the right side of the heart. In general, these defects are well tolerated, especially if they are less than 1 cm in diameter; even larger lesions do not usually produce any symptoms in childhood. Over time, however, chronic volume and pressure overloads can cause pulmonary hypertension. Surgical or intravascular ASD closure is thus performed to preempt the development of heart failure, paradoxical embolization, and irreversible pulmonary vascular disease. Mortality is low, and postoperative survival is comparable to that for an unaffected population.

Ventricular Septal Defects

Defects in the ventricular septum allow left-to-right shunting and constitute the most common congenital cardiac anomaly at birth (see Table 11.1 and Fig. 11.3). The ventricular septum normally is formed by a muscular ridge that grows upward from the heart apex fusing with a thinner membranous partition that grows downward from the endocardial cushions. The basal (membranous) region is the last part of the septum to develop and is the site of approximately 90% of VSDs. Most VSDs close spontaneously in childhood, but only 20% to 30% of VSDs occur in isolation; the remainder are associated with other cardiac malformations.

MORPHOLOGY

The size and location of VSDs are variable (see Fig. 11.3), ranging from minute defects in the membranous septum to large defects involving virtually the entire interventricular wall. In defects associated with a significant left-to-right shunt, the right ventricle is hypertrophied and often dilated. The diameter of the pulmonary artery is increased, owing to the increased right ventricular output and higher right sided pressures. Vascular changes typical of pulmonary hypertension are common (Chapter 13).

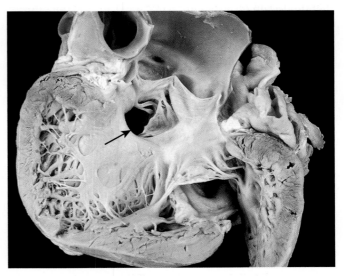

Fig. 11.3 Ventricular septal defect of the membranous type *(arrow). (Courtesy of William D. Edwards, MD, Mayo Clinic, Rochester, Minnesota.)*

Clinical Features

Small VSDs may be asymptomatic; half of those in the muscular portion of the septum close spontaneously during infancy or childhood. Larger defects, however, result in chronic left-to-right shunting, often complicated by pulmonary hypertension and CHF. Progressive pulmonary hypertension, with resultant reversal of the shunt and cyanosis, occurs earlier and more frequently with VSDs than with ASDs. Early surgical correction is therefore indicated for such lesions. Small- or medium-sized defects that produce jet lesions in the right ventricle cause endothelial damage and increase the risk for infective endocarditis.

Patent Ductus Arteriosus

The *ductus arteriosus* arises from the left pulmonary artery and joins the aorta just distal to the origin of the left subclavian artery. During intrauterine life, it permits blood to flow from the pulmonary artery to the aorta, bypassing the unoxygenated lungs. Within 1 to 2 days of birth in healthy term infants, the ductus constricts and closes; these changes occur in response to increased arterial oxygenation, decreased pulmonary vascular resistance, and declining local levels of prostaglandin E_2. Complete obliteration occurs within the first few months of extrauterine life, leaving only a strand of residual fibrous tissue known as the *ligamentum arteriosum*. Ductal closure can be delayed (or even absent) in infants with hypoxia (related to respiratory distress or heart disease). PDAs account for about 7% of congenital heart lesions (see Table 11.1 and Fig. 11.2); the great majority of these (90%) are isolated defects.

Clinical Features

PDAs are high-pressure left-to-right shunts that produce harsh, "machinery-like" murmurs. A small PDA generally causes no symptoms, although larger defects eventually can lead to Eisenmenger syndrome with cyanosis and congestive heart failure. High-pressure shunts also predispose patients to developing infective endocarditis. While isolated PDAs should be closed as early in life as is feasible, preservation of ductal patency (by administering prostaglandin E) can be lifesaving when a PDA is the only means to sustain systemic or pulmonary blood flow (e.g., in infants with aortic or pulmonic atresia).

Malformations Associated With Right-to-Left Shunts

Cardiac malformations associated with right-to-left shunts are distinguished by early cyanosis. This occurs because poorly oxygenated blood from the right side of the heart flows directly into the arterial circulation. Two of the most important conditions associated with cyanotic congenital heart disease are tetralogy of Fallot and transposition of the great vessels (Fig. 11.4). Clinical consequences of severe, systemic cyanosis include clubbing of the tips of the fingers and toes (hypertrophic osteoarthropathy), polycythemia, and paradoxical embolization.

Tetralogy of Fallot

Tetralogy of Fallot is the most common cause of cyanotic congenital heart disease. It accounts for about 5% of all

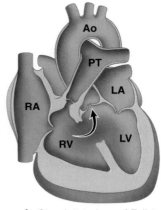

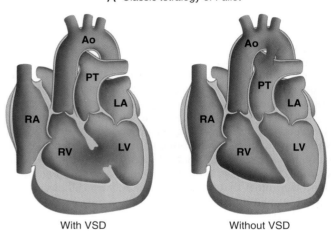

A Classic tetralogy of Fallot

With VSD   Without VSD

B Complete transposition

Fig. 11.4 Common congenital right-to-left shunts (cyanotic congenital heart disease). (A) Tetralogy of Fallot (*arrow* indicates direction of blood flow). (B) Transposition of the great vessels with and without VSD. *Ao,* Aorta; *LA,* left atrium; *LV,* left ventricle; *PT,* pulmonary trunk; *RA,* right atrium; *RV,* right ventricle.

congenital cardiac malformations (see Table 11.1). The four cardinal features are (Fig. 11.4A):

- VSD
- Right ventricular outflow tract obstruction (subpulmonic stenosis)
- Overriding of the VSD by the aorta
- Right ventricular hypertrophy

All of the features of tetralogy of Fallot result from anterosuperior displacement of the infundibular septum leading to abnormal septation between the pulmonary trunk and the aortic root.

MORPHOLOGY

The heart is enlarged and "boot-shaped" as a consequence of **right ventricular hypertrophy;** the proximal aorta is dilated, while the pulmonary trunk is hypoplastic. The left-sided cardiac chambers are of normal size, while the right ventricular wall is markedly hypertrophied, sometimes even exceeding the thickness of the left ventricle. The **VSD** usually is large and lies in the vicinity of the membranous portion of the interventricular septum; the aortic valve lies immediately over the VSD **(over-riding aorta)** and is the major site of egress for blood flow from both ventricles. The obstruction of the right ventricular outflow most often is due to narrowing of the infundibulum **(subpulmonic stenosis)** but also can be caused by pulmonary valve stenosis or complete atresia of the valve and the proximal pulmonary arteries. In such cases, a persistent PDA or dilated bronchial arteries are the only route for blood to reach the lungs.

Clinical Features

The hemodynamic consequences of tetralogy of Fallot are right-to-left shunting, decreased pulmonary blood flow, and increased aortic volumes. The clinical severity largely depends on the degree of the pulmonary outflow obstruction; even untreated, some patients can survive into adult life. Thus, if the pulmonic obstruction is mild, the condition resembles an isolated VSD because the high left-sided pressure causes only a left-to-right shunt with no cyanosis. More commonly, more severe degrees of pulmonic stenosis cause early cyanosis. Moreover, as the child grows and the heart increases in size, the pulmonic orifice does not expand proportionately, leading to progressive worsening of the stenosis. Fortuitously, the pulmonic outflow stenosis protects the pulmonary vasculature from pressure and volume overloads, so that pulmonary hypertension does not develop, and right ventricular failure is rare. Nevertheless, patients develop the typical sequelae of cyanotic heart disease, such as hypertrophic osteoarthropathy and polycythemia (due to hypoxia) with attendant hyperviscosity; right-to-left shunting also increases the risk for infective endocarditis and systemic embolization. Complete surgical repair is possible with classic tetralogy of Fallot but is more complicated in the setting of pulmonary atresia.

Transposition of the Great Arteries

Transposition of the great arteries is a discordant connection of the ventricles to their vascular outflow. The embryologic defect is an abnormal formation of the truncal and aortopulmonary septa so that the aorta arises from the right ventricle and the pulmonary artery emanates from the left ventricle (Fig. 11.4B). The atrium-to-ventricle connections, however, are normal (concordant), with the right atrium joining the right ventricle and the left atrium emptying into the left ventricle.

The functional outcome is separation of the systemic and pulmonary circulations, a condition incompatible with postnatal life unless a shunt (such as a VSD) allows delivery of oxygenated blood to the aorta. Indeed, VSDs occur in one third of cases (see Fig. 11.4, *B*). There is marked right ventricular hypertrophy, since that chamber functions as the systemic ventricle; the left ventricle is hypoplastic, since it pumps only to the low-resistance pulmonary circulation. Some newborns with transposition of the great arteries have a patent foramen ovale or PDA that allows oxygenated blood to reach the aorta, but these tend to close; such infants typically require emergent surgical intervention within the first few days of life.

Clinical Features

The dominant manifestation is cyanosis, with the prognosis depending on the magnitude of shunting, the degree of tissue hypoxia, and the ability of the right ventricle to maintain systemic pressures. Without surgery (even with stable shunting), most patients with uncorrected transposition of the great arteries die within the first months of life. However, improved surgical techniques now permit definitive repair, and such patients often survive into adulthood.

Malformations Associated With Obstructive Lesions

Congenital obstruction of blood flow can occur at the level of the heart valves or more distally within a great vessel. Obstruction can also occur proximal to the valve, as with subpulmonic stenosis in tetralogy of Fallot. Relatively common examples of congenital obstructions are pulmonic valve stenosis, aortic valve stenosis or atresia, and coarctation of the aorta.

Aortic Coarctation

Coarctation (narrowing, or constriction) of the aorta is a common form of obstructive congenital heart disease (see Table 11.1). Males are affected twice as often as females, although females with Turner syndrome frequently have coarctation. There are two classic forms (Fig. 11.5):

- An "infantile" preductal form featuring hypoplasia of the aortic arch proximal to a PDA
- An "adult" postductal form consisting of a discrete ridgelike infolding of the aorta, adjacent to the ligamentum arteriosum

Coarctation can occur as a solitary defect, but in more than half of the cases is accompanied by a bicuspid aortic valve. Aortic valve stenosis, ASD, VSD, or mitral regurgitation also can be present.

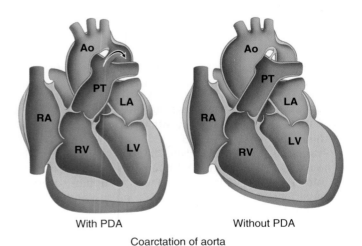

With PDA   Without PDA

Coarctation of aorta

Fig. 11.5 Coarctation of the aorta with ("infantile" or preductal form) and without a patent ductus arteriosus (PDA) ("adult" or postductal form); *arrow* indicates direction of blood flow. *Ao,* Aorta; *LA,* left atrium; *LV,* left ventricle; *PT,* pulmonary trunk; *RA,* right atrium; *RV,* right ventricle.

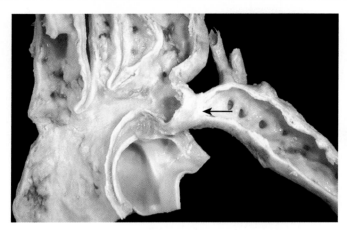

Fig. 11.6 Coarctation of the aorta, postductal type. The coarctation is a segmental narrowing of the aorta *(arrow)*. Such lesions typically manifest later in life than preductal coarctations. The dilated ascending aorta and major branch vessels are to the left of the coarctation. The lower extremities are perfused predominantly by way of dilated, tortuous collateral channels. *(Courtesy of Sid Murphree, MD, Department of Pathology, University of Texas Southwestern Medical School, Dallas, Texas.)*

MORPHOLOGY

Preductal coarctation is characterized by circumferential narrowing of the aortic segment between the left subclavian artery and the ductus arteriosus; the ductus typically is patent and is the main source of (unoxygenated) blood delivered to the distal aorta. The pulmonary trunk is dilated to accommodate the increased blood flow; because the right side of the heart now perfuses the body distal to the narrowed segment ("coarct"), the right ventricle typically is hypertrophied.

In the more common **"adult" postductal coarctation,** the aorta is sharply constricted by a tissue ridge adjacent to the nonpatent ligamentum arteriosum (Fig. 11.6). The constricted segment is made up of smooth muscle and elastic fibers derived from the aortic media. Proximal to the coarctation, the aortic arch and its branch vessels are dilated and the left ventricle is hypertrophied.

Clinical Features

Clinical manifestations depend on the severity of the narrowing and the patency of the ductus arteriosus.

- *Preductal coarctation with a PDA* usually presents early in life, classically as cyanosis localized to the lower half of the body; without intervention, most affected infants die in the neonatal period.
- *Postductal coarctation without a PDA* usually is asymptomatic, and the disease may remain unrecognized well into adult life. Classically, there is upper-extremity hypertension paired with weak pulses and relative hypotension in the lower extremities, associated with symptoms of claudication and coldness. Exuberant collateral circulation "around" the coarctation often develops through markedly enlarged intercostal and internal mammary arteries; expansion of the flow through these vessels can lead to radiographically visible "notching" of the ribs.

In most cases, significant coarctations are associated with systolic murmurs and occasionally palpable thrills. Balloon dilation and stent placement or surgical resection with end-to-end anastomosis (or replacement of the affected aortic segment by a prosthetic graft) yields excellent results.

SUMMARY

CONGENITAL HEART DISEASE

- Congenital heart disease represents defects of cardiac chambers or the great vessels; these either result in shunting of blood between the right- and left-sided circulation or cause outflow obstructions. Lesions range from relatively asymptomatic to rapidly fatal. Environmental (toxic or infectious) and genetic causes both contribute.
- Malformations associated with Left-to-right shunts are the most common and include ASDs, VSDs, and PDA. Shunting results in right-sided volume overload that eventually causes pulmonary hypertension and, with reversal of flow and right-to-left shunting, cyanosis *(Eisenmenger syndrome)*.
- Malformations associated with Right-to-left shunts include tetralogy of Fallot and transposition of the great arteries. These lesions cause early-onset cyanosis and are associated with polycythemia, hypertrophic osteoarthropathy, and paradoxical embolization.
- Obstructive lesions include forms of aortic coarctation; the clinical severity of these lesions depends on the degree of stenosis and the patency of the ductus arteriosus.

ISCHEMIC HEART DISEASE

Ischemic heart disease (IHD) is a broad term encompassing several closely related syndromes caused by myocardial ischemia—an imbalance between cardiac blood supply (perfusion) and myocardial oxygen and nutritional requirements. Since cardiac myocytes generate energy almost exclusively through mitochondrial oxidative phosphorylation, cardiac function is strictly dependent upon the continuous flow of oxygenated blood through the coronary arteries. Despite dramatic improvements in therapy in the past quarter century, IHD in its various forms remains the leading cause of mortality in the United States and other developed nations, accounting for 7.5 million deaths worldwide each year.

In more than 90% of cases, IHD is a consequence of reduced coronary blood flow secondary to obstructive atherosclerotic vascular disease (Chapter 10). Thus, unless otherwise specified, IHD usually is synonymous with coronary artery disease (CAD). In most cases, the various syndromes of IHD are consequences of coronary atherosclerosis that has been gradually progressing for decades (beginning even in childhood or adolescence). In the remaining cases, cardiac ischemia may be the result of *increased demand* (e.g., with increased heart rate or hypertension); *diminished blood volume* (e.g., with hypotension or shock); *diminished oxygenation* (e.g., due to pneumonia or CHF); or *diminished oxygen-carrying capacity* (e.g., due to anemia or carbon monoxide poisoning).

The manifestations of IHD are a direct consequence of the insufficient blood supply to the heart. The clinical presentation may include one or more of the following *cardiac syndromes:*

- *Angina pectoris* (literally, "chest pain"). Ischemia induces pain but is insufficient to cause myocyte death. Angina can be *stable* (occurring predictably at certain levels of exertion), can be caused by vessel spasm *(Prinzmetal angina),* or can be *unstable* (occurring with progressively less exertion or even at rest).
- *Myocardial infarction (MI).* This occurs when the severity or duration of ischemia is sufficient to cause cardiomyocyte death.
- *Chronic IHD with CHF.* This progressive cardiac decompensation, which occurs after acute MI or secondary to accumulated small ischemic insults, eventually precipitates mechanical pump failure.
- *Sudden cardiac death (SCD).* This can occur as a consequence of tissue damage from MI, but most commonly results from a lethal *arrhythmia* without myocyte necrosis (see "Arrhythmias" later in the chapter).

The term *acute coronary syndrome* is applied to any of the three catastrophic manifestations of IHD—unstable angina, MI, and SCD.

Epidemiology

More than 700,000 Americans experience a MI each year, and roughly half of those affected die. As troubling as this toll is, it represents a spectacular advance; since peaking in 1963, the mortality related to IHD in the United States has declined by 50%. The improvement is largely attributed to interventions that have diminished *cardiac risk factors* (behaviors or conditions that promote atherosclerosis; (Chapter 10), in particular smoking cessation programs, hypertension and diabetes treatment, and use of cholesterol-lowering agents. To a lesser extent, diagnostic and therapeutic advances also have contributed; these include aspirin prophylaxis, better arrhythmia control, establishment of coronary care units, thrombolysis for MI, angioplasty and endovascular stenting, and coronary artery bypass graft surgery. Maintaining this downward trend in mortality will be particularly challenging given the predicted longevity of "baby boomers," as well as the epidemic of obesity that is sweeping the United States and other parts of the world.

Pathogenesis

IHD is a consequence of inadequate coronary perfusion relative to myocardial demand, usually as a consequence of a preexisting ("fixed") atherosclerotic occlusion of the coronary arteries and new, superimposed thrombosis and/or vasospasm. Atherosclerotic narrowing can affect any of the coronary arteries—left anterior descending (LAD), left circumflex (LCX), and right coronary artery (RCA)—singly or in combination. Clinically significant plaques tend to occur within the first several centimeters of the LAD and LCX takeoff from the aorta, and along the entire length of the RCA. Sometimes, secondary branches also are involved (i.e., diagonal branches of the LAD, obtuse marginal branches of the LCX, or posterior descending branch of the RCA).

Fixed obstructions that occlude less than 70% of a coronary vessel lumen typically are asymptomatic, even with exertion. In comparison, lesions that occlude more than 70% of a vessel lumen—resulting in so-called "critical stenosis"—generally cause symptoms in the setting of increased demand; with critical stenosis, certain levels of exertion predictably cause chest pain, and the patient is said to have *stable angina.* A fixed stenosis that occludes 90% or more of a vascular lumen can lead to inadequate coronary blood flow with symptoms even at rest—one of the forms of *unstable angina* (see "Angina Pectoris" later in the chapter).

Of importance, if an atherosclerotic lesion progressively occludes a coronary artery at a sufficiently slow rate over years, other coronary vessels may undergo remodeling and provide compensatory blood flow to the area at risk; such *collateral perfusion* can subsequently protect against MI, even if the original vessel becomes completely occluded. Unfortunately, with acute coronary blockage, there is no time for collateral flow to develop and infarction results.

The following elements contribute to the development and consequences of coronary atherosclerosis:

- *Inflammation plays an essential role at all stages of atherosclerosis,* from inception to plaque rupture (Chapter 10). It begins with the interaction of endothelial cells and circulating leukocytes, resulting in T-cell and macrophage recruitment and activation. These cells drive subsequent smooth muscle cell accumulation and proliferation, with associated matrix production, superimposed on an atheromatous core of lipid, cholesterol, calcification, and necrotic debris. At later stages, destabilization of atherosclerotic plaque can occur through macrophage metalloproteinase secretion.
- *Thrombosis associated with an eroded or ruptured plaque triggers the acute coronary syndromes.* Partial vascular occlusion by a newly formed thrombus on a disrupted atherosclerotic plaque can wax and wane with time and lead to unstable angina or sudden death; alternatively, even partial luminal occlusion by a thrombus can compromise blood flow sufficiently to cause a infarction of the innermost zone of the myocardium *(subendocardial infarct).* Organizing thrombi produce potent activators of smooth muscle proliferation, which can contribute to the growth of atherosclerotic lesions. Mural thrombi in a coronary artery can also embolize; indeed, small emboli can be found in the distal intramyocardial circulation (along with associated microinfarcts) at autopsy of patients with unstable angina. In the most serious case, completely obstructive thrombus over a disrupted plaque can cause massive MI.
- *Vasoconstriction* directly compromises lumen diameter; moreover, by increasing local mechanical shear forces, vessel spasm can potentiate plaque disruption. Vasoconstriction in atherosclerotic plaques can be stimulated by the following:
  - Circulating adrenergic agonists
  - Locally released platelet contents
  - Imbalance between endothelial cell–relaxing factors (e.g., nitric oxide) and –contracting factors (e.g., endothelin) due to endothelial dysfunction
  - Mediators released from perivascular inflammatory cells

Acute Plaque Change

Onset of myocardial ischemia depends not only on the extent and severity of fixed atherosclerotic disease but also on dynamic changes in coronary plaque morphology. **In most patients, unstable angina, infarction, and sudden cardiac death occur because of abrupt plaque change followed by thrombosis—hence the term** *acute coronary syndrome* (Fig. 11.7).

The initiating event is typically a sudden disruption (ranging from erosion to rupture) of a partially occlusive plaque. More than one mechanism of injury may be involved: *rupture, fissuring, or ulceration* of plaques expose highly thrombogenic constituents or underlying subendothelial basement membrane, leading to rapid thrombosis. In addition, hemorrhage into the core of plaques can expand plaque volume, thereby acutely exacerbating the degree of luminal occlusion.

Factors that trigger plaque erosion include endothelial injury and apoptosis, likely attributable to some combination of inflammatory and toxic exposures. Acute plaque rupture, on the other hand, involves factors that influence plaque susceptibility to disruption by mechanical stress. These include intrinsic aspects of plaque composition and structure (Chapter 10) and extrinsic factors, such as blood pressure and platelet reactivity:

- *Plaques that contain large atheromatous cores or have thin overlying fibrous caps are more likely to rupture and are therefore termed vulnerable.* Fissures frequently occur at the junction of the fibrous cap and the adjacent normal plaque-free arterial segment, where the mechanical stresses are highest and the fibrous cap is thinnest. Fibrous caps also are continuously remodeling; their overall balance of collagen synthesis versus degradation determines mechanical strength and plaque stability. Collagen is produced by smooth muscle cells and degraded by the action of metalloproteases elaborated by macrophages. Consequently, atherosclerotic lesions with a paucity of smooth muscle cells or large numbers of inflammatory cells are vulnerable to rupture. Of interest, statins (inhibitors of hydroxymethylglutaryl Co-A reductase, a key enzyme in cholesterol synthesis) can provide additional benefit in CAD and IHD by reducing plaque inflammation and increasing plaque stability, effects distinct from and their primary cholesterol-lowering activity.

- *Influences extrinsic to the plaque also are important.* Adrenergic stimulation can put physical stress on the plaque by causing hypertension or local vasospasm. Indeed, the surge in adrenergic stimulation associated with awakening and rising may underlie the observation that the incidence of acute MI is highest between 6 AM and 12 noon. Intense emotional stress also leads to adrenergic stimulation, explaining the association of natural catastrophes such as earthquakes and floods with secondary waves of MIs in susceptible individuals.

In a majority of cases, the "culprit lesion" in patients who suffer an MI was not critically stenotic or even symptomatic before its rupture. As noted previously, anginal symptoms typically occur with fixed lesions exhibiting greater than 70% chronic occlusion. Pathologic and clinical studies show that two thirds of ruptured plaques are less than or equal to 50% stenotic before plaque rupture, and 85% exhibit initial stenotic occlusion of less than or equal to 70%. Thus, the worrisome conclusion is that a large number of asymptomatic adults are at significant risk for a catastrophic coronary event. At present, it is impossible to predict plaque rupture in any given patient.

Plaque disruption and ensuing non-occlusive thrombosis also are common, repetitive, and often clinically silent complications of atheromas. The healing of such subclinical plaque disruption and overlying thrombosis is an important mechanism by which atherosclerotic lesions progressively enlarge (Fig. 11.7).

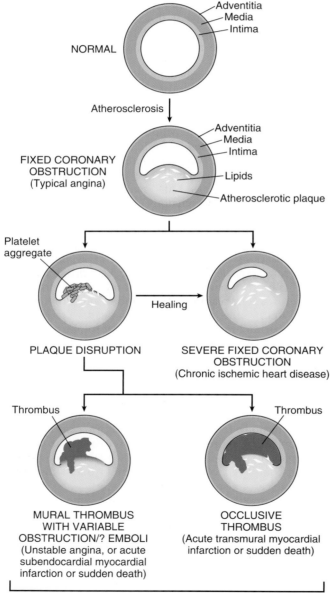

Fig. 11.7 Diagram of sequential progression of coronary artery lesions leading to various acute coronary syndromes. *(Modified and redrawn from Schoen FJ: Interventional and surgical cardiovascular pathology: clinical correlations and basic principles, Philadelphia, 1989, Saunders, p 63.)*

Angina Pectoris

Angina pectoris is an intermittent chest pain caused by transient, reversible myocardial ischemia. The pain is a consequence of the ischemia-induced release of adenosine, bradykinin, and other molecules that stimulate autonomic nerves. The following three variants are recognized:

- *Typical* or *stable angina* is predictable episodic chest pain associated with particular levels of exertion or some other increased demand (e.g., tachycardia). The pain is described as a crushing or squeezing substernal sensation that often radiates down the left arm or to the left jaw (referred pain). The pain usually is relieved by rest (reducing demand) or by drugs such as nitroglycerin, a vasodilator that increases coronary perfusion.

- *Prinzmetal* or *variant angina* occurs at rest and is caused by coronary artery spasm. Although such spasms typically occur on or near existing atherosclerotic plaques, a completely normal vessel can be affected. Prinzmetal angina typically responds promptly to vasodilators such as nitroglycerin and calcium channel blockers.

- *Unstable angina* (also called *crescendo angina*) is characterized by increasingly frequent pain, precipitated by progressively less exertion or even occurring at rest. Unstable angina is associated with plaque disruption and superimposed thrombosis, distal embolization of the thrombus, and/or vasospasm; it can be a harbinger of MI, portending complete vascular occlusion.

Myocardial Infarction

Myocardial infarction (MI), also commonly referred to as "heart attack," is necrosis of the heart muscle resulting from ischemia. The major underlying cause of IHD is atherosclerosis; while MIs can occur at virtually any age, the frequency rises progressively with aging and with increasing risk factors for atherosclerosis (Chapter 10). Nevertheless, approximately 10% of MIs occur before 40 years of age, and 45% occur before 65 years of age. Blacks and whites are equally affected. Men are at greater risk than women, although the gap progressively narrows with age. In general, women tend to be protected against MI during their reproductive years. However, menopause—with declining estrogen production—is associated with exacerbation of coronary artery disease, and IHD is the most common cause of death in older adult women.

Pathogenesis

The vast majority of MIs are caused by acute thrombosis within coronary arteries (Fig. 11.7). In most instances, disruption or erosion of preexisting atherosclerotic plaque serves as the nidus for thrombus generation, vascular occlusion, and subsequent infarction of the perfused myocardium. In 10% of MIs, however, transmural infarction occurs in the absence of occlusive atherosclerotic vascular disease; such infarcts are mostly ascribed to coronary artery vasospasm or to embolization from mural thrombi (e.g., in the setting of atrial fibrillation) or from valve vegetations. Occasionally, especially with infarcts limited to the innermost (subendocardial) myocardium, thrombi or emboli are absent. In such cases, severe fixed coronary atherosclerosis leads to marginal perfusion of the heart. In this setting, a prolonged period of increased demand (e.g., due to tachycardia or hypertension) can lead to ischemic necrosis of endomyocardium, the portion of the heart that is most distal to the epicardial vessels. Finally, ischemia without detectable atherosclerosis or thromboembolic disease can be caused by disorders of small intramyocardial arterioles, including vasculitis, amyloid deposition, or stasis, as in sickle cell disease.

Coronary Artery Occlusion

In a typical MI, the following sequence of events takes place:

- *An atheromatous plaque is eroded* or suddenly disrupted by endothelial injury, intraplaque hemorrhage, or mechanical forces, exposing subendothelial collagen and necrotic plaque contents to the blood.

- *Platelets adhere, aggregate, and are* activated, releasing thromboxane A_2, adenosine diphosphate (ADP), and serotonin—causing further platelet aggregation and vasospasm (Chapter 4).

- *Activation of coagulation* by exposure of tissue factor and other mechanisms adds to the growing thrombus.

- Within minutes, the thrombus can evolve to completely occlude the coronary artery lumen.

The evidence for this scenario derives from autopsy studies of patients dying of acute MI, as well as imaging studies demonstrating a high frequency of thrombotic occlusion early after MI. Angiography performed within 4 hours of the onset of MI demonstrates coronary thrombosis in almost 90% of cases. When angiography is performed 12 to 24 hours after onset of symptoms, however, evidence of thrombosis is seen in only 60% of patients, even without intervention. Thus, at least some occlusions clear spontaneously through lysis of the thrombus or relaxation of spasm. This sequence of events in a typical MI also has therapeutic implications: early thrombolysis and/or angioplasty can be highly successful in limiting the extent of myocardial necrosis.

Myocardial Response to Ischemia

Loss of blood supply has profound functional, biochemical, and morphologic consequences for the myocardium. Within seconds of vascular obstruction, aerobic metabolism ceases, leading to a drop in adenosine triphosphate (ATP) and accumulation of potentially noxious metabolites (e.g., lactic acid) in the cardiac myocytes. The functional consequence is a rapid loss of contractility, occurring within a minute or so of the onset of ischemia. Ultrastructural changes (including myofibrillar relaxation, glycogen depletion, cellular and mitochondrial swelling) are also seen. These early changes are reversible. Only prolonged ischemia lasting at least 20 to 40 minutes causes irreversible damage and coagulative necrosis of myocytes (Chapter 2). With longer periods of ischemia, vessel injury ensues, leading to superimposed microvascular thrombosis.

Thus, if blood flow is restored before irreversible injury occurs, myocardium can be preserved; this is the goal of early diagnosis and prompt intervention by thrombolysis or angioplasty. However, as discussed later, reperfusion can have deleterious effects. Even if reperfusion is timely,

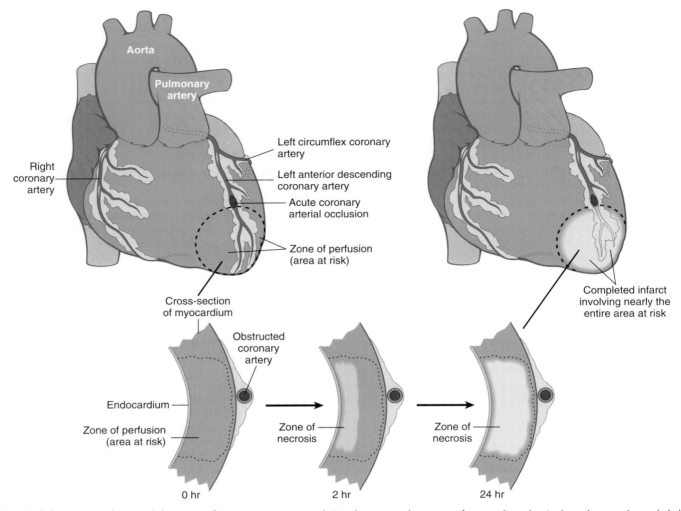

Fig. 11.8 Progression of myocardial necrosis after coronary artery occlusion. A transmural segment of myocardium that is dependent on the occluded vessel for perfusion constitutes the area at risk (*outlined*). Necrosis begins in the subendocardial region in the center of the ischemic zone and with time expands to involve the entire wall thickness. Note that a very narrow zone of myocardium immediately beneath the endocardium is spared from necrosis because it can be oxygenated by diffusion from the ventricle.

postischemic myocardium can be profoundly dysfunctional for a number of days due to persistent abnormalities in cellular biochemistry that result in a noncontractile state (stunned myocardium). Such stunning can be severe enough to produce transient but reversible cardiac failure.

Myocardial ischemia also contributes to arrhythmias, probably by causing electrical instability (irritability) of ischemic regions of the heart. Although massive myocardial damage can cause a fatal mechanical failure, sudden cardiac death in the setting of myocardial ischemia most often (in 80% to 90% of cases) is due to ventricular fibrillation caused by myocardial irritability.

Irreversible injury of ischemic myocytes first occurs in the subendocardial zone (Fig. 11.8). As already mentioned, this region is especially susceptible to ischemia because it is the last area to receive blood delivered by the epicardial vessels, and also because it is exposed to relatively high intramural pressures, which act to impede the inflow of blood. With more prolonged ischemia, a wavefront of cell death moves through other regions of the myocardium,

driven by progressive tissue edema and myocardial-derived reactive oxygen species and inflammatory mediators. An infarct usually achieves its full extent within 3 to 6 hours; in the absence of intervention, an infarct caused by occlusion of an epicardial vessel can involve the entire wall thickness (transmural infarct). Clinical intervention within this critical window of time can lessen the size of the infarct within the "territory at risk."

Patterns of Infarction

The location, size, and morphologic features of an acute myocardial infarct depend on multiple factors:

- *Size and distribution* of the involved vessel (Fig. 11.9)
- *Rate of development* and duration of the occlusion
- *Metabolic demands* of the myocardium (affected, for example, by blood pressure and heart rate)
- *Extent of collateral supply*

Acute occlusion of the proximal left anterior descending (LAD) artery is the cause of 40% to 50% of all MIs and

TRANSMURAL INFARCTS   **NON-TRANSMURAL INFARCTS**

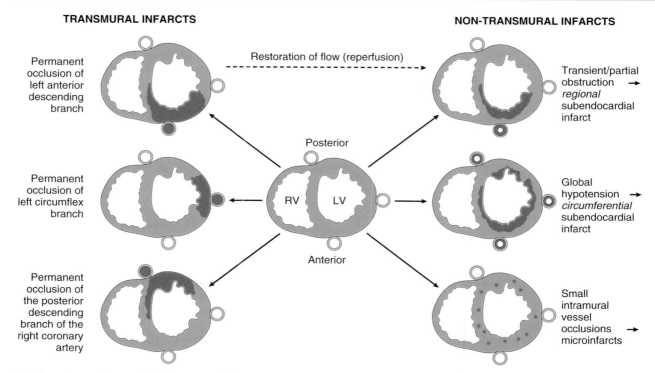

Permanent occlusion of left anterior descending branch

Restoration of flow (reperfusion)

Transient/partial obstruction → *regional* subendocardial infarct

Posterior

Permanent occlusion of left circumflex branch

RV   LV

Global hypotension → *circumferential* subendocardial infarct

Anterior

Permanent occlusion of the posterior descending branch of the right coronary artery

Small intramural vessel occlusions → microinfarcts

Fig. 11.9 Dependence of myocardial infarction on the location and nature of the diminished perfusion. *Left,* Patterns of transmural infarction resulting from major coronary artery occlusion. The right ventricle may be involved with occlusion of the right main coronary artery *(not depicted). Right,* Patterns of infarction resulting from partial or transient occlusion *(top),* global hypotension superimposed on fixed three-vessel disease *(middle),* or occlusion of small intramyocardial vessels *(bottom).*

typically results in infarction of the anterior wall of the left ventricle, the anterior two thirds of the ventricular septum, and most of the heart apex; more distal occlusion of the same vessel may affect only the apex. Similarly, acute occlusion of the proximal left circumflex (LCX) artery (seen in 15% to 20% of MIs) causes necrosis of the lateral left ventricle, and proximal right coronary artery (RCA) occlusion (30% to 40% of MIs) affects much of the right ventricle. Coronary occlusion in the proximal left anterior descending artery has been dubbed the "widow maker" because so much myocardial territory is perfused by that vessel, and acute obstructions are often fatal.

The posterior third of the septum and the posterior left ventricle are perfused by the posterior descending artery. The posterior descending artery can arise from either the RCA (in 90% of individuals) or the LCX. By convention, the coronary artery—either RCA or LCX—that gives rise to the posterior descending artery and thereby perfuses portions of the inferior/posterior left ventricle and the posterior third of the septum is considered the dominant vessel. Thus, in a right dominant heart, occlusion of the RCA can lead to posterior septal and posterior wall ischemic injury. In comparison, in a left dominant heart, where the posterior descending artery arises from the circumflex artery, occlusion of the LCX generally affects the left lateral wall as well as the posterior third of the septum, and the inferior and posterior wall of the left ventricle.

Occlusions also can occur within secondary branches, such as the diagonal branches of the LAD artery or marginal branches of the LCX artery. Interestingly, atherosclerosis is primarily a disease of epicardial vessels; significant

atherosclerosis or thrombosis of penetrating intramyocardial branches of coronary arteries is rare—although these can be affected by vasculitis or vasospasm, and can be occluded by embolization.

Even though the three major coronary arteries are end arteries, these epicardial vessels are interconnected by numerous intercoronary anastomoses (collateral circulation). Although these channels are normally closed, gradual narrowing of one artery allows blood to flow from high- to low-pressure areas through the collateral channels. In this manner, gradual collateral dilation can provide adequate perfusion to areas of the myocardium despite occlusion of an epicardial vessel. Based on the size of the involved vessel and the degree of collateral circulation, myocardial infarcts may take one of the following patterns:

- *Transmural infarctions* involve the full thickness of the ventricle and are caused by epicardial vessel occlusion through a combination of chronic atherosclerosis and acute thrombosis; such transmural MIs typically yield ST segment elevations on the electrocardiogram (ECG) and can have negative Q waves with loss of R wave amplitude. These infarcts are also called *ST-segment elevated MIs (STEMIs).*
- *Subendocardial infarctions* are MIs limited to the inner third of the myocardium; these infarcts typically do not exhibit ST segment elevations or Q waves on the ECG tracing (so-called "non–ST-segment elevated MIs" or "NSTEMIs"), although they can have ST-segment depressions or T wave abnormalities. As mentioned earlier, the subendocardial region is most vulnerable to hypoperfusion and hypoxia. Thus, in the setting of

severe coronary artery disease, transient decreases in oxygen delivery (as from hypotension, anemia, or pneumonia) or increases in oxygen demand (as with tachycardia or hypertension) can cause subendocardial ischemic injury. This pattern also can occur when an occlusive thrombus lyses before a full-thickness infarction can develop.

- *Microscopic infarcts* occur in the setting of small-vessel occlusions and may not show any diagnostic ECG changes. These can occur in the setting of vasculitis, embolization of valve vegetations or mural thrombi, or vessel spasm due to elevated catecholamines, as may occur in extreme emotional stress, with certain tumors (e.g., pheochromocytoma), or as a consequence of cocaine use.

MORPHOLOGY

Nearly all transmural infarcts (involving 50% or more of the ventricle thickness) affect at least a portion of the left ventricle and/or interventricular septum. Roughly 15% to 30% of MIs that involve the posterior or posteroseptal wall also extend into the right ventricle. Isolated right ventricle infarcts occur in only 1% to 3% of cases. Even in transmural infarcts, a narrow rim (approximately 0.1 mm) of viable subendocardial myocardium is preserved by diffusion of oxygen and nutrients from the ventricular lumen.

The gross and microscopic appearance of an MI depends on the age of the injury. Areas of damage progress through a highly characteristic sequence of morphologic changes from coagulative necrosis, to acute and then chronic inflammation, to fibrosis (Table 11.2). Myocardial necrosis proceeds invariably to scar formation without any significant regeneration; studies looking at whether tissue stem cells can be used to regenerate functional myocardium are ongoing but have yet to bear fruit.

Gross and/or microscopic recognition of very recent myocardial infarcts can be challenging, particularly when death occurs within a few hours. **Myocardial infarcts less than 12 hours old usually are not grossly apparent.** However, infarcts more than 3 hours old can be visualized by exposing myocardium to vital stains, such as triphenyltetrazolium chloride, a substrate for lactate dehydrogenase. Because this enzyme is depleted in the area of ischemic necrosis (it leaks out of the damaged cells), the infarcted area is unstained (pale), while old scars appear white and glistening (Fig. 11.10). **By 12 to 24 hours after MI, an infarct usually can be grossly identified by a red-blue discoloration caused by stagnated, trapped blood.** Thereafter, infarcts become progressively better delineated as soft, yellow-tan areas; by 10 to 14 days, infarcts are rimmed by hyperemic (highly vascularized) granulation tissue. Over the succeeding weeks, the infarcted tissue evolves to a fibrous scar.

The microscopic appearance also undergoes a characteristic sequence of changes (see Table 11.2 and Fig. 11.11). Typical features of coagulative necrosis (Chapter 2) become detectable within 4 to 12 hours of infarction. "Wavy fibers" also can be present at the edges of an infarct; these reflect the stretching and buckling of noncontractile dead fibers. Sublethal ischemia can also induce intracellular **myocyte vacuolization;** such myocytes are viable but frequently contract poorly.

Necrotic myocardium elicits acute inflammation (typically most prominent 1 to 3 days after MI), followed by a wave of macrophages that remove necrotic myocytes and neutrophil

Table 11.2 Evolution of Morphologic Changes in Myocardial Infarction

Time Frame	Gross Features	Light Microscopic Findings	Electron Microscopic Findings
Reversible Injury			
0–½ hour	None	None	Relaxation of myofibrils; glycogen loss; mitochondrial swelling
Irreversible Injury			
½–4 hours	None	Usually none; variable waviness of fibers at border	Sarcolemmal disruption; mitochondrial amorphous densities
4–12 hours	Occasionally dark mottling	Beginning coagulation necrosis; edema; hemorrhage	
12–24 hours	Dark mottling	Ongoing coagulation necrosis; pyknosis of nuclei; hypereosinophilic appearance of myocytes; marginal contraction band necrosis; beginning neutrophilic infiltrate	
1–3 days	Mottling with yellow-tan infarct center	Coagulation necrosis with loss of nuclei and striations; interstitial infiltrate of neutrophils	
3–7 days	Hyperemic border; central yellow-tan softening	Beginning disintegration of dead myofibers, with dying neutrophils; early phagocytosis of dead cells by macrophages at infarct border	
7–10 days	Maximally yellow-tan and soft, with depressed red-tan margins	Well-developed phagocytosis of dead cells; early formation of fibrovascular granulation tissue at margins	
10–14 days	Red-gray depressed infarct borders	Well-established granulation tissue with new blood vessels and collagen deposition	
2–8 weeks	Gray-white scar, progressive from border toward core of infarct	Increased collagen deposition, with decreased cellularity	
>2 months	Scarring complete	Dense collagenous scar	

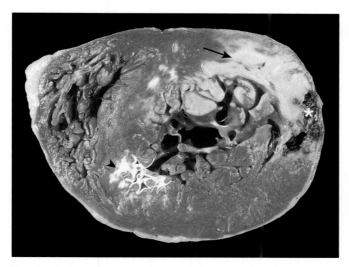

Fig. 11.10 Acute myocardial infarct of the posterolateral left ventricle demonstrated by a lack of triphenyltetrazolium chloride staining in areas of necrosis *(arrow)*; the absence of staining is due to enzyme leakage after cell death. Note the anterior scar *(arrowhead)*, indicative of remote infarction. The myocardial hemorrhage at the right edge of the infarct *(asterisk)* is due to ventricular rupture, and was the acute cause of death in this patient (specimen is oriented with the posterior wall at the *top*).

fragments (most pronounced 5 to 10 days after MI). The infarcted zone is progressively replaced by granulation tissue (most prominent 1 to 2 weeks after MI), which in turn forms the provisional scaffolding upon which dense collagenous scar forms. In most instances, scarring is well advanced by the end of the sixth week, but the efficiency of repair depends on the size of the original lesion and the ability of the host tissues to heal. Healing requires the migration of inflammatory cells and ingrowth of new vessels from the infarct margins. Thus, an MI heals from its borders toward the center, and a large infarct may not heal as fast or as completely as a small one. Moreover, malnutrition, poor vasculature, or exogenous anti-inflammatory steroids can impede infarct scarring (Chapter 3). Once an MI is completely healed, it is impossible to distinguish its age: whether present for 8 weeks or 10 years, fibrous scars look the same.

Infarct Modification by Reperfusion

The therapeutic goal in acute MI is restoration of tissue perfusion as quickly as possible (hence the adage "time is myocardium"). Such reperfusion is achieved by thrombolysis (dissolution of thrombus by tissue plasminogen activator), angioplasty, or coronary arterial bypass graft.

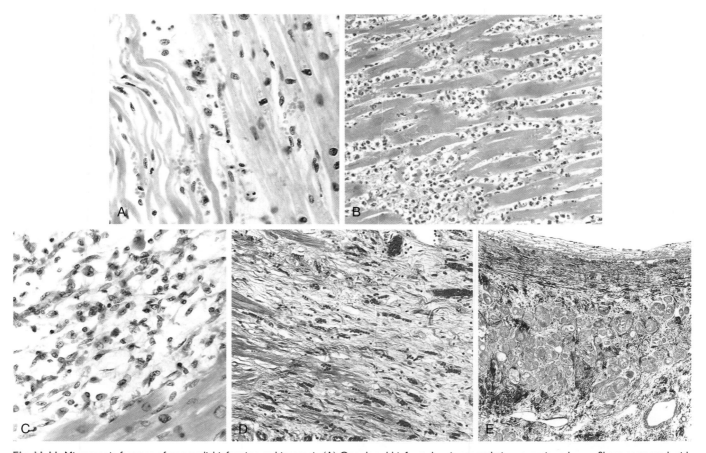

Fig. 11.11 Microscopic features of myocardial infarction and its repair. (A) One-day-old infarct showing coagulative necrosis and wavy fibers, compared with adjacent normal fibers *(right)*. Necrotic cells are separated by edema fluid. (B) Dense neutrophilic infiltrate in the area of a 2- to 3-day-old infarct. (C) Nearly complete removal of necrotic myocytes by phagocytic macrophages (7 to 10 days). (D) Granulation tissue characterized by loose connective tissue and abundant capillaries. (E) Healed myocardial infarct consisting of a dense collagenous scar. A few residual cardiac muscle cells are present. (D) and (E) are Masson's trichrome stain, which stains collagen blue.

Unfortunately, while preservation of a viable (but at-risk) heart can improve both short- and long-term outcomes, reperfusion is not an unalloyed blessing. Indeed, late restoration of blood flow into ischemic tissues can incite greater local damage than might otherwise have occurred — so-called "reperfusion injury".

The factors that contribute to reperfusion injury include the following:

- *Mitochondrial dysfunction.* Ischemia alters the mitochondrial membrane permeability, which allows proteins to move into the mitochondria. This leads to swelling and rupture of the outer membrane, releasing mitochondrial contents that promote apoptosis.
- *Myocyte hypercontracture.* During periods of ischemia, the intracellular levels of calcium are increased as a result of impaired calcium cycling and sarcolemmal damage. After reperfusion, the contraction of myofibrils is augmented and uncontrolled, causing cytoskeletal damage and cell death.
- *Free radicals,* including superoxide anion ($\bullet O_2^-$), hydrogen peroxide (H_2O_2), hypochlorous acid (HOCl), nitric oxide–derived peroxynitrite, and hydroxyl radicals ($\bullet$OH). These are produced within minutes of reperfusion and cause damage to the myocytes by altering membrane proteins and phospholipids.
- *Leukocyte aggregation* may occlude the microvasculature and contribute to the "no-reflow" phenomenon. Further, leukocytes elaborate proteases and elastases that cause cell death.
- *Platelet and complement activation* also contribute to microvascular injury. Complement activation is thought to play a role in the no-reflow phenomenon by injuring the endothelium.

The typical appearance of reperfused myocardium in the setting of an acute MI is shown in Figure 11.12. Such infarcts are hemorrhagic as a consequence of vascular injury and leakiness. Microscopically, irreversibly damaged myocytes after reperfusion develop *contraction band necrosis;* in this pathologic process, intense eosinophilic bands of hypercontracted sarcomeres are created by an influx of calcium across plasma membranes that heightens actin-myosin interactions. In the absence of ATP, the sarcomeres cannot relax and get stuck in an agonal tetanic state. Thus, while reperfusion can salvage reversibly injured cells, it also alters the morphology of irreversibly injured cells.

Clinical Features

The classic MI is heralded by severe, crushing substernal chest pain (or pressure) that can radiate to the neck, jaw, epigastrium, or left arm. In contrast to angina pectoris, the associated pain typically lasts several minutes to hours, and is not relieved by nitroglycerin or rest. However, in a substantial minority of patients (10% to 15%), MIs present with the atypical signs and symptoms, and may even be entirely asymptomatic. Such "silent" infarcts are particularly common in patients with underlying diabetes mellitus (in which autonomic neuropathy may prevent perception of pain) and in older adults.

The pulse generally is rapid and weak, and patients are often diaphoretic (sweating) and nauseous (particularly with posterior wall MIs). Dyspnea is common, resulting from impaired myocardial contractility and dysfunction of the mitral valve apparatus, with resultant acute pulmonary congestion and edema. With massive MIs (involving more than 40% of the left ventricle), cardiogenic shock develops.

Electrocardiographic abnormalities are important for the diagnosis of MI; these include Q waves, ST segment changes, and T wave inversions (the latter two representing abnormalities in myocardial repolarization). Arrhythmias caused by electrical abnormalities in the ischemic myocardium and conduction system are common; indeed, sudden cardiac death from a lethal arrhythmia accounts for the vast majority of MI-related deaths occurring before hospitalization.

The laboratory evaluation of MI is based on measuring blood levels of macromolecules that leak out of injured myocardial cells through damaged cell membranes (Fig. 11.13). These molecules include myoglobin, cardiac troponins T and I (TnT, TnI), creatine kinase (CK;

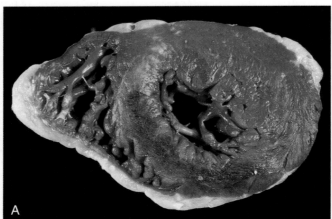 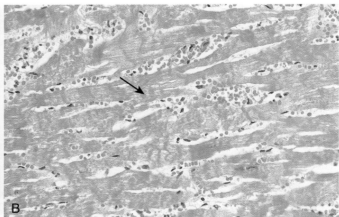

Fig. 11.12 Reperfused myocardial infarction. (A) The transverse heart slice (stained with triphenyl tetrazolium chloride) exhibits a large anterior wall myocardial infarction that is hemorrhagic because of bleeding from damaged vessels. The posterior wall is at the *top.* (B) Hemorrhage and contraction bands, visible as prominent hypereosinophilic cross-striations spanning myofibers *(arrow),* are seen microscopically.

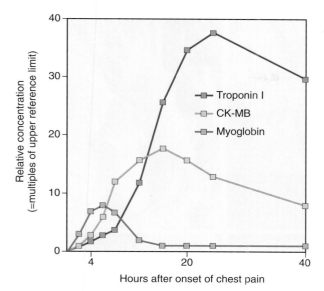

Fig. 11.13 Acute increases in myocardium-derived troponin I, myocardial creatine kinase (CK-MB), and myoglobin followling myocardial infarction. The kinetics of enzyme elevations can be used to estimate the timing of the MI. Myoglobin can also be measured, but is substantially less sensitive and specific for myocardial injury.

specifically the myocardial isoform, CK-MB), and lactate dehydrogenase. Troponins (and to a lesser extent CK-MB) have high specificity and sensitivity for myocardial damage.

- *CK-MB* has long been the biomarker of myocardial injury, but is now tested for less frequently in favor of the more sensitive cardiac-specific troponins. Total CK activity is not a reliable marker of cardiac injury since various isoforms of CK are found in non-cardiac tissues. However, the CK-MB isoform—principally derived from myocardium, but also present at low levels in skeletal muscle—is a more specific indicator of heart damage. CK-MB activity begins to rise within 2 to 4 hours of MI, peaks at 24 to 48 hours, and returns to normal within approximately 72 hours.

- *TnI and TnT* normally are not found in the circulation; however, after acute MI, both are detectable within 2 to 4 hours, with levels peaking at 48 hours and remaining elevated for 7 to 10 days. Persistence of elevated troponin levels allows the diagnosis of an acute MI to be made long after CK-MB levels have returned to normal. With reperfusion, both troponin and CK-MB levels may peak earlier owing to more rapid washout of the enzyme from the necrotic tissue.

Consequences and Complications of Myocardial Infarction

Extraordinary progress has been made in improving patient outcomes after acute MI; the overall in-hospital death rate for MI is approximately 7% to 8%, with MI associated with ST segment elevations (approximately 10% mortality) experiencing higher mortality rates than those without (approximately 6%). Unfortunately, out-of-hospital mortality is substantially poorer: one third of individuals with STEMIs die, usually of an arrhythmia within

1 hour of symptom onset, before they receive appropriate medical attention. Such statistics make the rising rate of coronary artery disease in developing countries with scarce hospital facilities all the more worrisome.

Nearly three fourths of patients experience one or more of the following complications after an acute MI (Fig. 11.14):

- *Contractile dysfunction.* In general, MIs affect left ventricular pump function in proportion to the volume of damage. In most cases, there is some degree of left ventricular failure manifested as hypotension, pulmonary congestion, and pulmonary edema. Severe "pump failure" *(cardiogenic shock)* occurs in roughly 10% of patients with transmural MIs and typically is associated with infarcts that damage 40% or more of the left ventricle.

- *Papillary muscle dysfunction.* Although papillary muscles rupture infrequently after MI, they often are dysfunctional and can be poorly contractile as a result of ischemia, leading to postinfarct mitral regurgitation. Much later, papillary muscle fibrosis and shortening or global ventricular dilation also can cause mitral valve insufficiency.

- *Right ventricular infarction.* Although isolated right ventricular infarction occurs in only 1% to 3% of MIs, the right ventricle is affected by RCA occlusions leading to posterior septal or left ventricular infarction. In either case, right-sided heart failure is a common outcome, leading to pooling of blood in the venous circulation and systemic hypotension.

- *Myocardial rupture.* Rupture complicates only 1% to 5% of MIs but is frequently fatal when it occurs. Left ventricular free wall rupture is most common, usually resulting in rapidly fatal hemopericardium and cardiac tamponade (Fig. 11.14A). Ventricular septal rupture creates a VSD with left-to-right shunting (Fig. 11.14B), and papillary muscle rupture leads to severe mitral regurgitation (Fig. 11.14C). Rupture occurs most commonly within 3 to 7 days after infarction—the time in the healing process when lysis of necrotic myocardium is maximal and when much of the infarct has been converted to soft, friable granulation tissue. Risk factors for free wall rupture include age older than 60 years, anterior or lateral wall infarctions, female gender, lack of left ventricular hypertrophy, and first MI (since scarring associated with prior MIs tends to limit the risk for myocardial tearing).

- *Arrhythmias.* MIs lead to myocardial irritability and conduction disturbances that can cause sudden death. Approximately 90% of patients develop some form of rhythm disturbance, with the incidence being higher in STEMIs versus NSTEMIs. MI-associated arrhythmias include heart block of variable degree (including asystole), bradycardia, supraventricular tachyarrhythmias, ventricular premature contractions or ventricular tachycardia, and ventricular fibrillation. The risk for serious arrhythmias (e.g., ventricular fibrillation) is greatest in the first hour and declines thereafter.

- *Pericarditis.* Transmural MIs can elicit a fibrinohemorrhagic pericarditis; this is an epicardial manifestation of the underlying myocardial inflammation (Fig. 11.14D). Heralded by anterior chest pain and a pericardial

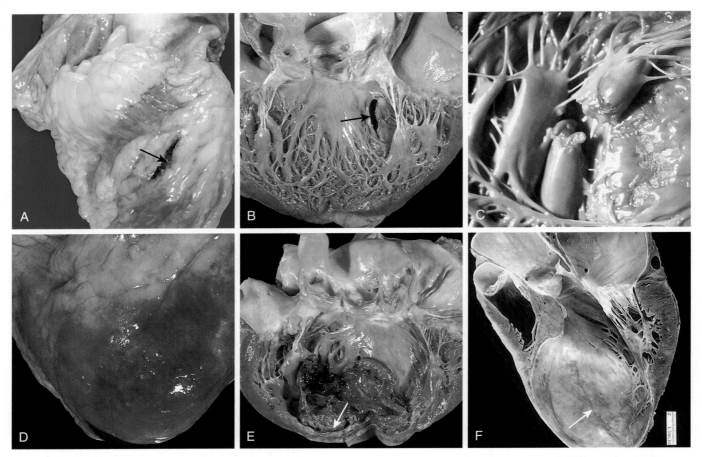

Fig. 11.14 Complications of myocardial infarction. (A to C) Cardiac rupture. (A) Anterior free wall myocardial rupture *(arrow)*. (B) Ventricular septal rupture *(arrow)*. (C) Papillary muscle rupture. (D) Fibrinous pericarditis, with a hemorrhagic, roughened epicardial surface overlying an acute infarct. (E) Recent expansion of an anteroapical infarct with wall stretching and thinning *(arrow)* and mural thrombus. (F) Large apical left ventricular aneurysm *(arrow)*. *(A to E, Reproduced by permission from Schoen FJ: Interventional and surgical cardiovascular pathology: clinical correlations and basic principles, Philadelphia, 1989, Saunders; F, Courtesy of William D. Edwards, MD, Mayo Clinic, Rochester, Minnesota.)*

friction rub, pericarditis typically appears 2 to 3 days after infarction and then gradually resolves over the next few days. Extensive infarcts or severe pericardial inflammation occasionally can lead to large effusions or can organize to form dense adhesions that eventually manifest as a constrictive lesion.

- *Chamber dilation.* Because of the weakening of necrotic muscle, there may be disproportionate stretching, thinning, and dilation of the infarcted region (especially with anteroseptal infarcts).
- *Mural thrombus.* With any infarct, the combination of attenuated myocardial contractility (causing stasis), chamber dilation, and endocardial damage (causing a thrombogenic surface) can foster *mural thrombosis* (Fig. 11.14E), eventually leading to left-sided *thromboembolism.*
- *Ventricular aneurysm.* A late complication, aneurysms of the ventricle most commonly result from a large transmural anteroseptal infarct that heals with the formation of a thinned wall of scar tissue (Fig. 11.14F). Although ventricular aneurysms frequently give rise to formation of mural thrombi, arrhythmias, and heart failure, they do not rupture.
- *Progressive heart failure.* This is discussed under "Chronic Ischemic Heart Disease" next.

The risk for complications and the overall prognosis depends on infarct size, site, and type (subendocardial versus transmural infarct). Thus, large transmural infarcts are associated with a higher probability of cardiogenic shock, arrhythmias, and late CHF, and patients with anterior transmural MIs are at greatest risk for free wall rupture, expansion, aneurysm formation, and formation of mural thrombi. By contrast, posterior transmural infarcts are more likely to be complicated by conduction blocks, right ventricular involvement, or both; when ventricular septal ruptures occur in this area, they are more difficult to manage. Overall, patients with anterior infarcts have a much more guarded prognosis than those with posterior infarcts. With subendocardial infarcts, thrombi may form on the endocardial surface, but pericarditis, rupture, and aneurysms rarely occur.

In addition to the aforementioned scarring, the remaining viable myocardium attempts to compensate for the loss of contractile mass. Noninfarcted regions undergo hypertrophy and dilation; in combination with the scarring and thinning of the infarcted zones, the changes are collectively termed *ventricular remodeling.* The initial compensatory hypertrophy of noninfarcted myocardium is hemodynamically beneficial. The adaptive effect of remodeling can be overwhelmed, however, and ventricular function may decline in the setting of ventricular aneurysm formation.

The long-term prognosis after MI depends on many factors, the most important of which are the quality of left ventricular function and the severity of atherosclerotic narrowing of vessels perfusing the remaining viable myocardium. The overall mortality rate within the first year is about 30%, including deaths occurring before the patient reaches the hospital. Thereafter, the annual mortality rate for patients who have suffered an MI is 3% to 4%.

Chronic Ischemic Heart Disease

Chronic IHD, also called ischemic cardiomyopathy, is progressive heart failure secondary to ischemic myocardial damage. In most instances, there is a known clinical history of previous MI. After prior infarction(s), chronic IHD appears when the compensatory mechanisms (e.g., hypertrophy) of residual myocardium begin to fail. In other cases, severe CAD can cause diffuse myocardial dysfunction, and even micro-infarction and replacement fibrosis, without any clinically evident episode of frank infarction.

The heart failure of chronic IHD is typically severe and is occasionally punctuated by new episodes of angina or infarction. Arrhythmias, CHF, and intercurrent MI account for most of the associated morbidity and mortality.

MORPHOLOGY

Patients with chronic IHD typically exhibit left ventricular dilation and hypertrophy, often with discrete areas of gray-white scarring from previous healed infarcts. Invariably, there is moderate to severe atherosclerosis of the coronary arteries, sometimes with total occlusion. The endocardium generally shows patchy, fibrous thickening, and mural thrombi may be present. Microscopic findings include myocardial hypertrophy, diffuse subendocardial myocyte vacuolization, and fibrosis from previous infarction.

Cardiac Stem Cells

Because of the serious morbidity associated with IHD, there is much interest in exploring the possibility of using cardiac stem cells to replace damaged myocardium. Although cardiac regeneration in metazoans (such as newts and zebrafish) is well described, cardiac myocytes of higher-order animals are classically considered a postmitotic cell population without replicative potential. Increasing evidence, however, points to the presence of bone marrow–derived precursors—as well as a small resident stem cell population within the myocardium—capable of repopulating the mammalian heart. These cells express a cluster of cell surface markers that allow their isolation and purification, and like all other tissue stem cells, they occur in very low frequency.

Besides self-renewal, these cardiac stem cells can generate all cell lineages seen within the myocardium. They have a slow intrinsic rate of proliferation, which is greatest in neonates and decreases with age. Of interest, stem cell numbers and progeny also increase after myocardial injury or hypertrophy, albeit to a limited extent, since hearts that suffer an MI clearly do not recover any significant function in the necrotic zone. Nevertheless, the potential for stimulating the proliferation of these cells *in vivo* is tantalizing because it could facilitate recovery of myocardial function after acute MI or chronic IHD. Ex vivo expansion and subsequent administration of such cells after an MI is another area of vigorous investigation. Unfortunately, results thus far have been less than exciting.

SUMMARY

ISCHEMIC HEART DISEASE

- In the vast majority of cases, cardiac ischemia is due to coronary artery atherosclerosis; vasospasm, vasculitis, and embolism are less common causes.
- Cardiac ischemia results from a mismatch between coronary supply and myocardial demand and manifests as different, albeit overlapping syndromes:
  - *Angina pectoris* is exertional chest pain due to inadequate perfusion, and is typically due to atherosclerotic disease causing greater than 70% fixed stenosis (so-called "critical stenosis").
  - *Unstable angina* is characterized by increasingly frequent pain, precipitated by progressively less exertion or even occurring at rest. It results from an erosion or rupture of atherosclerotic plaque triggering platelet aggregation, vasoconstriction, and formation of a mural thrombus that need not necessarily be occlusive.
  - *Acute myocardial infarction* typically results from acute thrombosis after plaque disruption; a majority occur in plaques that did not previously exhibit critical stenosis.
  - *Sudden cardiac death* usually results from a fatal arrhythmia, typically without significant acute myocardial damage.
  - *Ischemic cardiomyopathy* is progressive heart failure due to ischemic injury, either from previous infarction(s) or chronic ischemia.
- Myocardial ischemia leads to loss of myocyte function within 1 to 2 minutes but causes death after only 30 to 40 minutes. Myocardial infarction is diagnosed on the basis of symptoms, electrocardiographic changes, and measurement of serum biomarkers such as cardiac-specific troponins. Gross and histologic changes of infarction require hours to days to develop.
- Infarction can be modified by therapeutic intervention (e.g., thrombolysis or stenting), which salvages myocardium at risk but may also induce reperfusion-related injury.
- Complications of infarction include ventricular rupture, papillary muscle rupture, aneurysm formation, mural thrombus, arrhythmia, pericarditis, and CHF.

ARRHYTHMIAS

Aberrant rhythms can be initiated anywhere in the conduction system, from the sinoatrial (SA) node down to the level of an individual myocyte; they are typically designated as originating from the atrium (*supraventricular*) or within the ventricular myocardium. Abnormalities in myocardial conduction can be sustained or sporadic *(paroxysmal)*. They can manifest as *tachycardia* (fast heart rate), *bradycardia* (slow heart rate), an irregular rhythm with normal ventricular contraction, chaotic depolarization without functional ventricular contraction *(ventricular fibrillation)*, or no electrical activity at all *(asystole)*. Patients may be unaware of a rhythm disorder, or may note a "racing heart" or *palpitations* (irregular rhythm); loss of adequate cardiac output due to sustained arrhythmia can produce lightheadedness (near syncope), loss of consciousness *(syncope)*, or *sudden cardiac death* (see later).

Ischemic injury is the most common cause of rhythm disorders, either through direct damage or through the dilation of heart chambers that alters signal conduction.

- If the SA node is damaged (e.g., *sick sinus syndrome*), other fibers or even the atrioventricular (AV) node can take over pacemaker function, albeit at a much slower intrinsic rate (causing bradycardia).
- If the atrial myocytes become "irritable" and depolarize independently and sporadically (as occurs with atrial dilation), the signals are variably transmitted through the AV node leading to the random "irregularly irregular" heart rate of *atrial fibrillation*.
- If the AV node is dysfunctional, varying degrees of *heart block* occur, ranging from simple prolongation of the P-R interval on the ECG *(first-degree heart block)*, to intermittent transmission of the signal *(second-degree heart block)*, to complete failure *(third-degree heart block)*.

Certain heritable conditions (fortunately rare) can also cause arrhythmias. They are important to recognize because they may alert physicians to the need for intervention to prevent sudden cardiac death (discussed later) in the proband and their family members. Some of these disorders are associated with recognizable anatomic abnormalities (e.g., congenital anomalies, hypertrophic cardiomyopathy, mitral valve prolapse). However, other heritable disorders precipitate arrythmias and sudden death in the absence of structural cardiac pathology (so-called "primary electrical disorders"). These syndromes can only be diagnosed by genetic testing, which is performed in those with a positive family history or an unexplained nonlethal arrhythmia. The most important of these are the *channelopathies*, which are caused by mutations in genes that are required for normal function of Na^+, K^+, and Ca^+ channels. Since ion channels are responsible for conducting the electrical currents that mediate contraction of the heart, it is not surprising that defects in these channels may provoke arrythmias. The prototype is the *long QT syndrome*, characterized by prolongation of the QT segment in ECGs and susceptibility to malignant ventricular arrhythmias. Mutations in several different genes account for the cases of long QT syndrome, with *KCNQ1* being the most common; it results in decreased potassium currents.

Sudden Cardiac Death

Sudden cardiac death (SCD) is defined as unexpected death due to a lethal arrhythmia such as asystole or sustained ventricular fibrillation. Roughly 400,000 individuals are victims of SCD each year in the United States. Coronary artery disease is the leading cause of SCD, being responsible for 80% to 90% of cases. Unfortunately, SCD

may be the first manifestation of IHD. Of interest, autopsy typically shows severe atherosclerotic disease without evidence of acute plaque disruption. Thus, in the vast majority of cases, there is no associated myocardial infarction; 80% to 90% of patients who suffer SCD but are successfully resuscitated do not show any enzymatic or ECG evidence of myocardial necrosis—even if the cause is IHD! Healed remote MIs are present in about 40% of cases.

In younger victims of SCD, nonatherosclerotic causes are more common, including the following:

- Hereditary (channelopathies) or acquired abnormalities of the cardiac conduction system
- Congenital coronary arterial abnormalities
- Mitral valve prolapse
- Myocarditis or sarcoidosis
- Dilated or hypertrophic cardiomyopathy
- Pulmonary hypertension
- Myocardial hypertrophy. Increased cardiac mass is an independent risk factor for SCD; thus, in some young individuals who die suddenly, including athletes, hypertensive hypertrophy or unexplained increased cardiac mass is the only pathologic finding.

Although ischemic injury (and other pathologic conditions) can directly affect the major components of the conduction system, most cases of fatal arrhythmia are triggered by electrical irritability of myocardium distant from the conduction system.

The prognosis of many patients at risk for SCD, including those with chronic IHD, is markedly improved by implantation of a pacemaker or an automatic cardioverter defibrillator, which senses and electrically counteracts an episode of ventricular fibrillation.

The relationship of coronary artery disease to the various clinical end points discussed earlier is depicted in Fig. 11.15.

⬤ SUMMARY

ARRHYTHMIAS

- Arrhythmias can be caused by ischemic or structural changes in the conduction system or by myocyte electrical instability. In structurally normal hearts, arrhythmias more often are due to mutations in ion channels that cause aberrant repolarization or depolarization.
- SCD most frequently is due to coronary artery disease leading to ischemia. Myocardial irritability typically results from nonlethal ischemia or from preexisting fibrosis from previous myocardial injury. SCD less often is due to acute plaque rupture with thrombosis that induces a rapidly fatal arrhythmia.

HYPERTENSIVE HEART DISEASE

Hypertensive heart disease (HHD) is a consequence of the increased demands placed on the heart by hypertension, causing pressure overload and ventricular hypertrophy. As discussed in Chapter 10, hypertension is a common disorder associated with considerable morbidity and affecting many organs, including the heart, brain, and kidneys. The comments here will focus specifically on the major cardiac

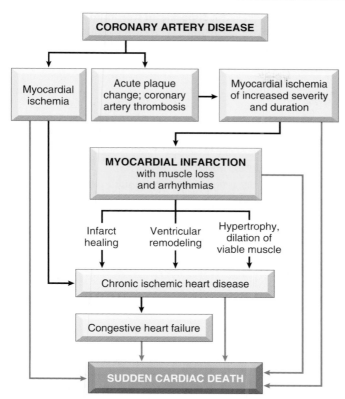

CORONARY ARTERY DISEASE

Myocardial ischemia

Acute plaque change; coronary artery thrombosis

Myocardial ischemia of increased severity and duration

MYOCARDIAL INFARCTION with muscle loss and arrhythmias

Infarct healing

Ventricular remodeling

Hypertrophy, dilation of viable muscle

Chronic ischemic heart disease

Congestive heart failure

SUDDEN CARDIAC DEATH

Fig. 11.15 Pathways in the progression of ischemic heart disease showing the relationships among coronary artery disease and its major sequelae.

complications of hypertension, which result from pressure overload and ventricular hypertrophy. Myocyte hypertrophy is an adaptive response to pressure overload; there are limits to myocardial adaptive capacity, however, and persistent hypertension eventually can culminate in dysfunction, cardiac dilation, CHF, and even sudden death. Although hypertensive heart disease most commonly affects the left

side of the heart secondary to systemic hypertension, pulmonary hypertension also can cause right-sided hypertensive changes—so-called "cor pulmonale."

Systemic (Left-Sided) Hypertensive Heart Disease

The criteria for the diagnosis of systemic hypertensive heart disease are (1) left ventricular hypertrophy in the absence of other cardiovascular pathology (e.g., valvular stenosis), and (2) a history or pathologic evidence of hypertension. The Framingham Heart Study established unequivocally that even mild hypertension (above 140/90 mm Hg), if sufficiently prolonged, induces left ventricular hypertrophy. Roughly 25% of the U.S. population suffers from at least this degree of hypertension.

MORPHOLOGY

As discussed earlier, systemic hypertension imposes pressure overload on the heart and is associated with gross and microscopic changes somewhat distinct from those caused by volume overload. The essential feature of hypertensive heart disease is left ventricular hypertrophy, typically without ventricular dilation until very late in the process (Fig. 11.16A). The heart weight can exceed 500 g (normal for a 60- to 70-kg individual is 320 to 360 g), and the left ventricular wall thickness can exceed 2.0 cm (normal is 1.2 to 1.4 cm). With time, the increased left ventricular wall thickness imparts a stiffness that impairs diastolic filling and can result in left atrial dilation. In long-standing systemic hypertensive heart disease leading to congestive failure, the hypertrophic left ventricle typically is dilated.

Microscopically, the transverse diameter of myocytes is increased and there is prominent nuclear enlargement and hyperchromasia ("boxcar nuclei"), as well as intercellular fibrosis (see also Fig. 11.1D).

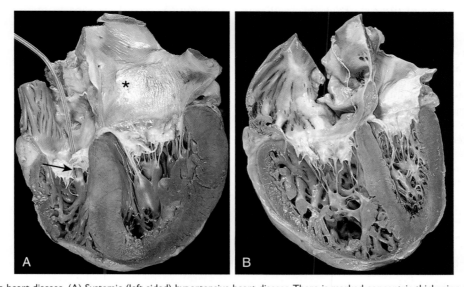

Fig. 11.16 Hypertensive heart disease. (A) Systemic (left-sided) hypertensive heart disease. There is marked concentric thickening of the left ventricular wall causing reduction in lumen size. The left ventricle and left atrium are shown on the *right* in this four-chamber view of the heart. A pacemaker is present incidentally in the right ventricle *(arrow)*. Note also the left atrial dilation *(asterisk)* due to stiffening of the left ventricle and impaired diastolic relaxation, leading to atrial volume overload. (B) Chronic cor pulmonale. The right ventricle *(shown on the left)* is markedly dilated and hypertrophied with a thickened free wall and hypertrophied trabeculae. The shape and volume of the left ventricle have been distorted by the enlarged right ventricle.

Clinical Features

Compensated HHD typically is asymptomatic and is suspected only from discovery of elevated blood pressure on routine physical examination, or from ECG or echocardiographic findings of left ventricular hypertrophy. In some patients, the disease comes to attention with the onset of atrial fibrillation (secondary to left atrial enlargement) and/or CHF. The mechanisms by which hypertension leads to heart failure are incompletely understood; presumably the hypertrophic myocytes fail to contract efficiently, possibly due to structural abnormalities in newly assembled sarcomeres and because the vascular supply is inadequate to meet the demands of the increased muscle mass. Depending on the severity and duration of the condition, the underlying cause of hypertension, and the adequacy of therapeutic control, patients can (1) enjoy normal longevity and die of unrelated causes, (2) develop IHD owing to the effects of hypertension in potentiating coronary atherosclerosis, (3) suffer renal damage or cerebrovascular stroke, or (4) experience congestive heart failure. The risk for SCD also is increased. Effective hypertension control can prevent or lead to the regression of cardiac hypertrophy and its attendant risks.

Pulmonary Hypertensive Heart Disease—Cor Pulmonale

Cor pulmonale consists of right ventricular hypertrophy and dilation—frequently accompanied by right-sided heart failure—caused by pulmonary hypertension attributable to primary disorders of the lung parenchyma or pulmonary vasculature (Table 11.3). Right ventricular dilation and hypertrophy caused by left ventricular failure (or by congenital heart disease) is substantially more common but is excluded by this definition.

Cor pulmonale can be acute in onset, as with pulmonary embolism, or can have a slow and insidious onset when due to prolonged pressure overload in the setting of chronic lung and pulmonary vascular disease (see Table 11.3).

MORPHOLOGY

In **acute cor pulmonale,** the right ventricle usually shows only dilation; if an embolism causes sudden death, the heart may even be of normal size. **Chronic cor pulmonale** is characterized by right ventricular (and often right atrial) hypertrophy. In extreme cases, the thickness of the right ventricular wall may be comparable to or even exceed that of the left ventricle (Fig. 11.16B). When ventricular failure develops, the right ventricle and atrium often are dilated. Because chronic cor pulmonale occurs in the setting of pulmonary hypertension, the pulmonary arteries often contain atheromatous plaques and other lesions, reflecting long-standing pressure elevations.

VALVULAR HEART DISEASE

Valvular disease may result in stenosis, insufficiency (regurgitation or incompetence), or both.

- *Stenosis* is the failure of a valve to open completely, obstructing forward flow. Valvular stenosis is almost

Table 11.3 Disorders Predisposing to Cor Pulmonale

Diseases of the Pulmonary Parenchyma
Chronic obstructive pulmonary disease
Diffuse pulmonary interstitial fibrosis
Pneumoconiosis
Cystic fibrosis
Bronchiectasis
Diseases of the Pulmonary Vessels
Recurrent pulmonary thromboembolism
Primary pulmonary hypertension
Extensive pulmonary arteritis (e.g., Granulomatosis with polyangiitis)
Drug-, toxin-, or radiation-induced vascular obstruction
Extensive pulmonary tumor microembolism
Disorders Affecting Chest Movement
Kyphoscoliosis
Marked obesity (Pickwickian syndrome)
Neuromuscular diseases
Disorders Inducing Pulmonary Arterial Constriction
Metabolic acidosis
Hypoxemia
Obstructive sleep apnea
Idiopathic alveolar hypoventilation

SUMMARY

HYPERTENSIVE HEART DISEASE

- Hypertensive heart disease can affect either the left ventricle or the right ventricle; in the latter case, the disorder is most often due to primary pulmonary disease and is called *cor pulmonale.* Elevated pressures induce myocyte hypertrophy and interstitial fibrosis that increases wall thickness and stiffness.
- The chronic pressure overload of systemic hypertension causes left ventricular concentric hypertrophy, often associated with left atrial dilation due to impaired diastolic filling of the ventricle. Persistently elevated pressure overload can cause ventricular failure with dilation.
- Cor pulmonale results from pulmonary hypertension due to primary lung parenchymal or vascular disorders. Hypertrophy of both the right ventricle and the right atrium is characteristic; dilation also may be seen when failure supervenes.

always due to a primary cuspal abnormality stemming from a chronic process (e.g., calcification or valve scarring).

- *Insufficiency* results from failure of a valve to close completely, thereby allowing regurgitation (backflow) of blood. Valvular insufficiency can result from either intrinsic disease of the valve cusps (e.g., endocarditis) or disruption of the supporting structures (e.g., the aorta, mitral annulus, tendinous cords, papillary muscles, or ventricular free wall) without primary cuspal injury. It can appear abruptly, as with chordal rupture, or insidiously as a consequence of leaflet scarring and retraction.

Stenosis or regurgitation may occur alone or together in the same valve. Valvular disease can involve only one valve (the mitral valve being the most common target), or more than one valve. Turbulent flow through diseased valves typically produces abnormal heart sounds called *murmurs*; severe lesions can even be externally palpated as *thrills*. Depending on the valve involved, murmurs are best heard at different locations on the chest wall; moreover, the nature (regurgitation versus stenosis) and severity of the valvular disease determines the quality and timing of the murmur (e.g., harsh systolic or soft diastolic murmurs).

The outcome of valvular disease depends on the valve involved, the degree of impairment, the tempo of its development, and the effectiveness of compensatory mechanisms. For example, rapid destruction of an aortic valve cusp by infection can cause massive regurgitation and the abrupt onset of cardiac failure. By contrast, rheumatic mitral stenosis usually progresses over years, and its clinical effects are well tolerated until late in the course.

Valvular abnormalities can be congenital or acquired. By far the most common congenital valvular lesion is a *bicuspid aortic valve*, containing only two functional cusps instead of the normal three; this malformation occurs with a frequency of 1% to 2% of all live births, and has been associated with a number of mutations, including those affecting proteins of the Notch signaling pathway. The two cusps are of unequal size, with the larger cusp exhibiting a midline *raphe* resulting from incomplete cuspal separation (Fig. 11.17B). Bicuspid aortic valves are generally neither stenotic nor incompetent through early life; however, they are more prone to early and progressive degenerative calcification that gives rise to stenosis (see later).

The most important causes of acquired valvular diseases are summarized in Table 11.4; acquired stenoses of the aortic and mitral valves account for approximately two thirds of all valve disease.

Degenerative Valve Disease

Degenerative valve disease is a term used to describe changes that affect the integrity of valvular ECM. Degenerative changes include the following:
- *Calcifications*, which can be cuspal (typically in the aortic valve) (Fig. 11.17A and B) or annular (in the mitral valve) (Fig. 11.17C and D). Mitral annular calcification is usually asymptomatic unless it encroaches on the adjacent conduction system.
- *Alterations in the ECM*. In some cases, changes consist of increased proteoglycan and diminished fibrillar collagen and elastin (*myxomatous degeneration*); in other cases, the valve becomes fibrotic and scarred.
- *Changes in the production of matrix metalloproteinases or their inhibitors*
- *Degenerative changes in the cardiac valves* are probably an inevitable aspect of aging related to the repetitive mechanical stresses to which valves are subjected—40 million beats per year, with each normal opening and closing requiring substantial valve deformation.

Calcific Aortic Stenosis

Calcific aortic degeneration is the most common cause of aortic stenosis. In most cases, calcific degeneration is asymptomatic and is discovered only incidentally by viewing

Table 11.4 Etiology of Acquired Heart Valve Disease

Mitral Valve Disease	Aortic Valve Disease
Mitral Stenosis	**Aortic Stenosis**
Postinflammatory scarring (rheumatic heart disease)	Postinflammatory scarring (rheumatic heart disease)
	Senile calcific aortic stenosis
	Calcification of congenitally deformed valve
Mitral Regurgitation	**Aortic Regurgitation**
Abnormalities of leaflets and commissures	Intrinsic valvular disease
Postinflammatory scarring	Postinflammatory scarring (rheumatic heart disease)
Infective endocarditis	Infective endocarditis
Mitral valve prolapse	Aortic disease
"Fen-phen"–induced valvular fibrosis	Degenerative aortic dilation
Abnormalities of tensor apparatus	Syphilitic aortitis
Rupture of papillary muscle	Ankylosing spondylitis
Papillary muscle dysfunction (fibrosis)	Rheumatoid arthritis
Rupture of chordae tendineae	Marfan syndrome
Abnormalities of left ventricular cavity and/or annulus	
Left ventricular enlargement (myocarditis, dilated cardiomyopathy)	
Calcification of mitral ring	

Fen-phen, Fenfluramine-phentermine.
Data from Schoen FJ: Surgical pathology of removed natural and prosthetic valves, *Hum Pathol* 18:558, 1987.

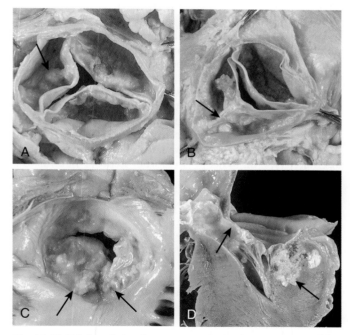

Fig. 11.17 Calcific valvular degeneration. (A) Calcific aortic stenosis of a previously normal valve (viewed from above the valve). Nodular masses of calcium are heaped up within the sinuses of Valsalva *(arrow)*. Note that the commissures are not fused, as in rheumatic aortic valve stenosis (see Fig. 11.19C). (B) Calcific aortic stenosis occurring on a congenitally bicuspid valve. One cusp has a partial fusion at its center, called a raphe *(arrow)*. (C and D) Mitral calcification, with calcific nodules within the annulus (attachment margin) of the mitral leaflets *(arrows)*. (C) Left atrial view. (D) Section demonstrating the extension of calcification into the underlying myocardium. Such involvement of adjacent structures near the interventricular septum can impinge on the conduction system.

calcifications on a routine chest radiograph or at autopsy. In other patients, valvular sclerosis and/or calcification can be severe enough to cause stenosis, necessitating surgical intervention. The incidence of calcific aortic stenosis is increasing in pace with longevity. In anatomically normal valves, it typically begins to manifest when patients reach their 70s and 80s; onset with bicuspid aortic valves is at a much earlier age (often 40 to 50 years of age).

Although simple progressive age-associated "wear and tear" is often invoked to explain the process, cuspal fibrosis and calcification also can be viewed as the valvular counterparts to age-related arteriosclerosis. Thus, chronic injury due to hyperlipidemia, hypertension, inflammation, and other factors implicated in atherosclerosis have been proposed as contributors to valvular degenerative changes, but firm evidence is lacking.

MORPHOLOGY

The hallmark of calcific aortic stenosis is heaped-up calcified masses on the outflow side of the cusps; these protrude into the sinuses of Valsalva and mechanically impede valve opening (Fig. 11.17A and B); commissural fusion (usually a sign of previous inflammation) is not a typical feature of degenerative aortic stenosis, although the cusps may become secondarily fibrosed and thickened. An earlier, hemodynamically inconsequential stage of the calcification process is called *aortic valve sclerosis*.

Clinical Features

In severe disease, valve orifices can be compromised by as much as 70% to 80% (from a normal area of approximately 4 cm²). Cardiac output is maintained only by virtue of concentric left ventricular hypertrophy; the chronic outflow obstruction can drive left ventricular pressures to 200 mm Hg or more. The hypertrophied myocardium is prone to ischemia, and angina may develop. Systolic and diastolic dysfunction collude to cause CHF, and cardiac decompensation eventually ensues. The development of angina, CHF, or syncope in aortic stenosis heralds the exhaustion of compensatory cardiac hyperfunction and carries a poor prognosis; without surgical intervention, 50% to 80% of patients die within 2 to 3 years.

Myxomatous Mitral Valve

In *myxomatous degeneration of the mitral valve,* one or both mitral leaflets are "floppy" and prolapse—they balloon back into the left atrium during systole. Primary *mitral valve prolapse* is a form of myxomatous mitral degeneration affecting some 0.5% to 2.4% of adults; thus, it is one of the most common forms of valvular heart disease, with women affected almost 7-fold more often than men. Conversely, secondary myxomatous mitral degeneration affects men and women equally, and can occur in any one of a number of settings in which mitral regurgitation is caused by some other underlying cause (e.g., IHD).

Pathogenesis

The basis for primary myxomatous degeneration of the mitral valve is unknown. Nevertheless, an underlying (possibly systemic) intrinsic defect of connective tissue

synthesis or remodeling is likely. Thus, myxomatous degeneration of the mitral valve is a common feature of Marfan syndrome (due to *fibrillin-1* mutations, Chapter 7) and occasionally occurs in other connective tissue disorders. In some patients with primary disease, additional hints of systemic structural abnormalities in connective tissue, including scoliosis and high-arched palate, may be found. Subtle defects in structural proteins (or the cells that make them) may cause hemodynamically stressed connective tissues rich in microfibrils and elastin (e.g., cardiac valves) to elaborate defective ECM. Secondary myxomatous change presumably results from injury to the valve myofibroblasts, imposed by chronically aberrant hemodynamic forces.

MORPHOLOGY

Myxomatous degeneration of the mitral valve is characterized by ballooning (hooding) of the mitral leaflets (Fig. 11.18). The affected leaflets are enlarged, redundant, thick, and rubbery; the tendinous cords also tend to be elongated, thinned, and occasionally rupture. In those with primary mitral disease, concomitant tricuspid valve involvement is frequent (20% to 40% of cases); less commonly, aortic and pulmonic valves also may be affected. On histologic examination, the essential change is thinning of the valve layer known as the **fibrosa** layer of the valve, on which the structural integrity of the leaflet depends, accompanied by expansion of the middle **spongiosa** layer owing to increased deposition of myxomatous (mucoid) material. The same changes occur whether the myxomatous degeneration is due to an intrinsic ECM defect (primary), or is caused by regurgitation secondary to another etiologic process (e.g., ischemic dysfunction).

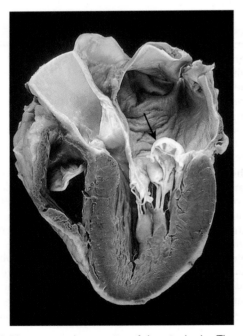

Fig. 11.18 Myxomatous degeneration of the mitral valve. There is prominent hooding with prolapse of the posterior mitral leaflet *(arrow)* into the left atrium; the atrium also is dilated, reflecting long-standing valvular insufficiency and volume overload. The left ventricle is shown on the *right* in this four-chamber view. *(Courtesy of William D. Edwards, MD, Mayo Clinic, Rochester, Minnesota.)*

Clinical Features

Most patients are asymptomatic, and the valvular abnormality is discovered incidentally. In a minority of cases, patients complain of palpitations, dyspnea, or atypical chest pain. Auscultation discloses a midsystolic click, caused by abrupt tension on the redundant valve leaflets and chordae tendineae as the valve attempts to close; there is sometimes an associated regurgitant murmur. Although in most instances the natural history and clinical course are benign, approximately 3% of patients develop complications such as hemodynamically significant mitral regurgitation and CHF, particularly if the chordae or valve leaflets rupture. Patients with primary myxomatous degeneration also are at increased risk for the development of infective endocarditis (see later), as well as SCD due to ventricular arrhythmias. Stroke or other systemic infarctions may rarely occur from embolism of thrombi formed in the left atrium.

Rheumatic Valvular Disease

Rheumatic fever is an acute, immunologically mediated, multisystem inflammatory disease that occurs after group A β-hemolytic streptococcal infections (usually pharyngitis, but also occasionally infections at other sites, such as skin). *Rheumatic heart disease* is the cardiac manifestation of rheumatic fever. It is associated with inflammation of all parts of the heart, but valvular inflammation and scarring produce the most important clinical features.

The valvular disease principally takes the form of deforming fibrotic mitral stenosis; indeed rheumatic heart disease is essentially the *only* cause of acquired mitral stenosis. The incidence of rheumatic fever (and thus rheumatic heart disease) has declined remarkably in many parts of the Western world over the past several decades due to a combination of improved socioeconomic conditions, rapid diagnosis and treatment of streptococcal pharyngitis, and a fortuitous (and unexplained) decline in the virulence of many strains of group A streptococci. Nevertheless, in developing countries and economically depressed urban areas in the United States, rheumatic fever and rheumatic heart disease remain important public health problems.

Pathogenesis

Acute rheumatic fever is a hypersensitivity reaction classically attributed to antibodies directed against group A streptococcal molecules that cross-react with host myocardial antigens (see also Chapter 5). In particular, antibodies against M proteins of certain streptococcal strains bind to proteins in the myocardium and cardiac valves and cause injury through the activation of complement and Fc receptor–bearing cells (including macrophages). CD4+ T cells that recognize streptococcal peptides can cross-react with host antigens and elicit cytokine-mediated inflammatory responses. The characteristic 2- to 3-week delay in symptom onset after infection is explained by the time needed to generate an immune response; streptococci are completely absent from the lesions. Since only a small minority of infected patients develop rheumatic fever (estimated at 3%), genetic susceptibility to the development of the cross-reactive immune responses is likely in those

affected. The deforming fibrotic lesions are the predictable consequence of healing and scarring associated with the resolution of the acute inflammation.

MORPHOLOGY

Acute rheumatic fever is characterized by discrete inflammatory foci within a variety of tissues. The myocardial inflammatory lesions—called **Aschoff bodies** (Fig. 11.19B); these are collections of lymphocytes (primarily T cells), scattered plasma cells, and plump activated macrophages called **Anitschkow cells** associated with zones of fibrinoid necrosis. The Anitschkow cells have abundant cytoplasm and nuclei with chromatin that is centrally condensed into a slender, wavy ribbon (so-called "caterpillar cells"). During acute rheumatic fever, Aschoff bodies can be found in any of the three layers of the heart—pericardium, myocardium, or endocardium (including valves). Hence, rheumatic fever is said to cause pancarditis, with the following salient features:

- The pericardium may exhibit a fibrinous exudate, which generally resolves without sequelae.
- The myocardial involvement—myocarditis—takes the form of scattered Aschoff bodies within the interstitial connective tissue.
- Valve involvement results in fibrinoid necrosis and fibrin deposition along the lines of closure (Fig. 11.19A) forming 1- to 2-mm vegetations—**verrucae**—that cause little disturbance in cardiac function.

Chronic rheumatic heart disease is characterized by organization of acute inflammation and subsequent scarring. Aschoff bodies are replaced by fibrous scar so that these lesions are rarely seen in chronic disease. Most characteristically, valve cusps and leaflets become permanently thickened and retracted. Classically, the mitral valves exhibit **leaflet thickening, commissural fusion and shortening, and thickening and fusion of the chordae tendineae** (Fig. 11.19C to E). Fibrous bridging across the valvular commissures and calcification create "fish-mouth" or "buttonhole" stenoses (Fig. 11.19C). Microscopic examination shows neovascularization (visibly evident in Fig. 11.19D) and diffuse fibrosis that obliterates the normal leaflet architecture.

The most important functional consequence of rheumatic heart disease is **valvular stenosis and regurgitation;** stenosis tends to predominate. The mitral valve alone is involved in 70% of cases, and combined mitral and aortic disease in seen in another 25%; the tricuspid valve is less frequently (and less severely) involved; and the pulmonic valve almost always escapes injury. With tight mitral stenosis, the left atrium progressively dilates owing to pressure overload, precipitating atrial fibrillation. The combination of dilation and fibrillation is a fertile substrate for thrombosis, and formation of large mural thrombi is common. Long-standing passive venous congestion gives rise to pulmonary vascular and parenchymal changes typical of left-sided heart failure. In time, this leads to right ventricular hypertrophy and failure. With pure mitral stenosis, the left ventricle generally is normal.

Clinical Features

Acute rheumatic fever occurs most often in children; the principal clinical manifestation is carditis. Nevertheless,

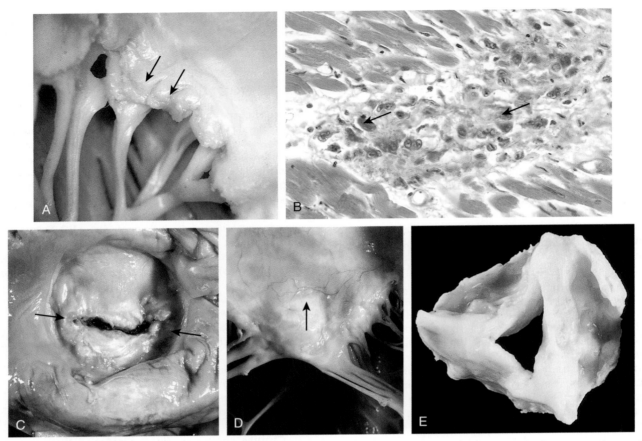

Fig. 11.19 Rheumatic heart disease. (A) Acute rheumatic mitral valvulitis superimposed on chronic rheumatic heart disease. Small vegetations (verrucae) are visible along the line of closure of the mitral valve leaflet *(arrows)*. Previous episodes of rheumatic valvulitis have caused fibrous thickening and fusion of the chordae tendineae. (B) Microscopic appearance of an Aschoff body in acute rheumatic carditis; there is central necrosis associated with a circumscribed collection of mononuclear inflammatory cells, including some activated macrophages with prominent nucleoli and central wavy (caterpillar) chromatin *(arrows)*. (C and D) Mitral stenosis with diffuse fibrous thickening and distortion of the valve leaflets, commissural fusion *(arrows)*, and thickening and shortening of the chordae tendineae. There is marked left atrial dilation as seen from above the valve (C). (D) Anterior leaflet of an opened rheumatic mitral valve; note the neovascularization *(arrow)*. (E) Surgically removed specimen of rheumatic aortic stenosis, demonstrating thickening and distortion of the cusps with commissural fusion. *(E, From Schoen FJ, St John-Sutton M: Contemporary issues in the pathology of valvular heart disease,* Hum Pathol *18:568, 1967.)*

about 20% of first attacks occur in adults, with arthritis being the predominant feature. Symptoms in all age groups typically begin 2 to 3 weeks after streptococcal infection and are heralded by fever and migratory polyarthritis—one large joint after another becomes painful and swollen for a period of days, followed by spontaneous resolution with no residual disability. Although cultures are negative for streptococci at the time of symptom onset, serum titers of antibodies against one or more streptococcal antigens (e.g., streptolysin O or DNAase) usually are elevated. The clinical signs of carditis include pericardial friction rubs and arrhythmias; myocarditis may be sufficiently severe to cause cardiac dilation and resultant functional mitral insufficiency and CHF. Nevertheless, less than 1% of patients die of acute rheumatic fever.

The diagnosis of acute rheumatic fever is made based on serologic evidence of previous streptococcal infection in conjunction with two or more of the *Jones criteria:* (1) carditis; (2) migratory polyarthritis of large joints; (3) subcutaneous nodules; (4) erythematous annular rash (erythema marginatum) in the skin; and (5) Sydenham chorea, a neurologic disorder characterized by involuntary

purposeless, rapid movements (also called *St. Vitus dance*). Minor criteria such as fever, arthralgias, EKG changes, or elevated acute phase reactants also can help support the diagnosis.

After an initial attack and the generation of immunologic memory, patients are increasingly vulnerable to disease reactivation with any subsequent streptococcal infections. Carditis is likely to worsen with each recurrence, and the damage is cumulative. However, *chronic rheumatic carditis* usually is not clinically evident until years or even decades after the initial episode of rheumatic fever. At that time, the signs and symptoms of valvular disease depend on which cardiac valve(s) is involved. In addition to various cardiac murmurs, cardiac hypertrophy and dilation, and CHF, patients with chronic rheumatic heart disease often have arrhythmias (particularly atrial fibrillation in the setting of mitral stenosis), and thromboembolic complications due to atrial mural thrombi. In addition, scarred and deformed valves are more susceptible to infective endocarditis. The long-term prognosis is highly variable. In some cases, a relentless cycle of valvular deformity ensues, yielding hemodynamic abnormality, which begets further deforming fibrosis. Surgical repair or replacement of diseased valves—mitral valvuloplasty—has greatly improved the outlook for patients with rheumatic heart disease.

Infective Endocarditis

Infective endocarditis (IE) is a microbial infection of the heart valves or the mural endocardium that leads to the formation of *vegetations* composed of thrombotic debris and organisms, often associated with destruction of the underlying cardiac tissues. The aorta, aneurysmal sacs, other blood vessels, and prosthetic devices also may become infected. Although fungi, rickettsiae (agents of Q fever), and chlamydial species can cause endocarditis, the vast majority of cases are caused by extracellular bacteria.

Infective endocarditis is classified into *acute* and *subacute* forms based on the tempo and severity of the clinical course; the distinctions are related to the virulence of the responsible microbe and whether underlying cardiac disease is present. Of note, a clear delineation between acute and subacute endocarditis is not always possible, and many cases fall somewhere along the spectrum between the two forms.

- *Acute endocarditis* refers to tumultuous, destructive infections, frequently involving a highly virulent organism attacking a previously normal valve. It is associated with of substantial morbidity and mortality, even with appropriate antibiotic therapy and/or surgery.
- *Subacute endocarditis* refers to infections by organisms of low virulence affecting a previously abnormal heart, especially scarred or deformed valves. The disease typically appears insidiously and—even if untreated—follows a protracted course of weeks to months; most patients recover after appropriate antibiotic therapy.

Pathogenesis

Infective endocarditis can develop on previously normal valves, but cardiac abnormalities predispose to such infections; rheumatic heart disease, mitral valve prolapse, bicuspid aortic valves, and calcific valvular stenosis are all common substrates. Prosthetic heart valves (discussed later) now account for 10% to 20% of all cases of IE. Sterile platelet-fibrin deposits at sites of pacemaker lines, indwelling vascular catheters, or endocardium damage by flow "jets" stemming from preexisting cardiac disease all can be foci for bacterial seeding and development of endocarditis. Host factors such as neutropenia, immunodeficiency, malignancy, diabetes mellitus, and alcohol or intravenous drug abuse also increase the risk for IE and adversely affect outcomes.

The causative organisms differ depending on the underlying risk factors; 50% to 60% of cases occurring on damaged or deformed valves are caused by *Streptococcus viridans*, a relatively banal group of normal oral flora. By contrast, the more virulent *S. aureus* (common to skin) can attack healthy as well as deformed valves and is responsible for 10% to 20% of cases overall; it also is the major offender in infections occurring in intravenous drug abusers. Additional bacterial agents include enterococci and the so-called "HACEK group" (*Haemophilus, Actinobacillus, Cardiobacterium, Eikenella,* and *Kingella*), all commensal in the oral cavity. More rarely, gram-negative bacilli and fungi are involved. In about 10% of all cases of endocarditis, no organism is isolated from the blood ("culture-negative" endocarditis) because of previous antibiotic therapy, difficulty in isolating the offending agent, or because deeply embedded organisms within the enlarging vegetation are not readily released into the blood.

Foremost among the factors predisposing to endocarditis is seeding of the blood with microbes. The mechanism or portal of entry of the agent into the bloodstream may be an obvious infection elsewhere, a dental or surgical procedure that causes a transient bacteremia, injection of contaminated material directly into the bloodstream by intravenous drug abusers, an occult source from the gut, or oral cavity, or trivial injuries. Recognition of predisposing anatomic substrates and clinical conditions causing bacteremia allows appropriate antibiotic prophylaxis.

MORPHOLOGY

In both acute and subacute forms of the disease, friable, bulky, and potentially destructive vegetations containing fibrin, inflammatory cells, and microorganisms are present on the heart valves (Figs. 11.20 and 11.21). **The aortic and mitral valves are the most common sites of infection, although the tricuspid valve is a frequent target in the setting of intravenous drug abuse.** Vegetations may be single or multiple and may involve more than one valve; they can sometimes erode into the underlying myocardium to produce an abscess cavity (**ring abscess**) (Fig. 11.21B). Shedding of **emboli** is common because of the friable nature of the vegetations. Since the fragmented vegetations contain large numbers of organisms, abscesses often develop at the sites where emboli lodge, leading to development of **septic infarcts** and aneurysms resulting from bacterial infection of the arterial wall (**mycotic aneurysms**).

Subacute endocarditis typically causes less valvular destruction than acute endocarditis. On microscopic examination, the vegetations of subacute endocarditis often have granulation tissue at their bases (suggesting chronicity), promoting development of chronic inflammatory infiltrates, fibrosis, and calcification over time.

Clinical Features

Fever is the most consistent sign of infective endocarditis. However, in subacute disease (particularly in older adults), fever may be absent, and the only manifestations may be nonspecific fatigue, weight loss, and a flulike syndrome; splenomegaly also is common in subacute cases. By contrast, acute endocarditis often manifests with rapidly developing fever, chills, weakness, and lassitude. Murmurs are present in 90% of patients with left-sided lesions. In those who are not treated promptly, microemboli are formed, which can give rise to petechia, nail bed *(splinter)* hemorrhages, retinal hemorrhages *(Roth spots)*, painless palm or sole erythematous lesions *(Janeway lesions)*, or painful fingertip nodules *(Osler nodes)*; diagnosis is confirmed by positive blood cultures and echocardiographic findings.

Prognosis depends on the infecting organism and the development of complications. Adverse sequelae generally begin within the first weeks after onset of the infectious process and can include glomerulonephritis due to glomerular trapping of antigen-antibody complexes, with

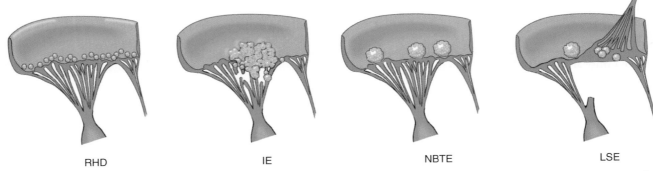

| RHD | IE | NBTE | LSE |

Fig. 11.20 Major forms of vegetative endocarditis. The acute rheumatic fever phase of rheumatic heart disease (RHD) is marked by the appearance of small, warty, inflammatory vegetations along the lines of valve closure; as the inflammation resolves, substantial scarring can result. Infective endocarditis (IE) is characterized by large, irregular, often destructive masses that can extend from valve leaflets onto adjacent structures (e.g., chordae or myocardium). Non-bacterial thrombotic endocarditis (NBTE) typically manifests with small- to medium-sized, bland, nondestructive vegetations at the line of valve closure. Libman-Sacks endocarditis (LSE) is characterized by small- to medium-sized inflammatory vegetations that can be attached on either side of the valve leaflets; these heal with scarring.

hematuria, albuminuria, or renal failure (Chapter 14). Clinical features of septicemia, arrhythmias (suggesting extension to underlying myocardium and conduction system), and systemic embolization bode ill for the patient. Left untreated, IE generally is fatal. However, with appropriate long-term (6 weeks or more) antibiotic therapy and/or valve replacement, mortality is reduced. For infections with low-virulence organisms (e.g., *Streptococcus viridans* or *Streptococcus bovis*), the cure rate is 98%, and for enterococci and *Staphylococcus aureus* infections, cure rates range from 60% to 90%; however, infections with aerobic gram-negative bacilli or fungi are associated with fatality rate of approximately 50%.

Noninfected Vegetations

Nonbacterial Thrombotic Endocarditis

Nonbacterial thrombotic endocarditis (NBTE) is characterized by the deposition of sterile thrombi on cardiac valves, typically in those with an underlying hypercoagulable state. Although NBTE can occur in otherwise healthy individuals, a wide variety of diseases associated with general debility or wasting are associated with an increased risk for NBTE—hence the alternate term *marantic endocarditis*. In contrast to infective endocarditis, the sterile valvular lesions of NBTE are nondestructive (Fig. 11.22).

The vegetations in NBTE are typically small (1 to 5 mm in diameter) and valvular damage is not a prerequisite. Indeed, the condition usually occurs on previously normal valves. Rather, hypercoagulable states are the usual precursor to NBTE; such conditions include chronic disseminated intravascular coagulation, hyperestrogenic states, and those associated with underlying malignancy, particularly mucinous adenocarcinomas. This last association probably relates to the procoagulant effect of circulating mucin and/or tissue factor elaborated by these tumors. Endocardial trauma, such as from an indwelling catheter, also is a well-recognized predisposing condition.

Although the local effect on the valve usually is trivial, NBTE lesions can become clinically significant by giving rise to emboli that can cause infarcts in the brain, heart, and other organs. NBTE also can serve as a potential nidus for bacterial colonization and the consequent development of infective endocarditis.

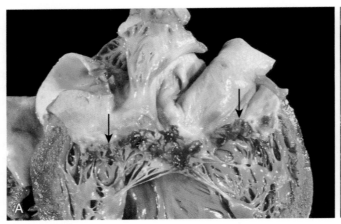
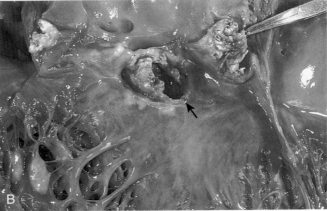

Fig. 11.21 Infective endocarditis. (A) Subacute endocarditis caused by *Streptococcus viridans* on a previously myxomatous mitral valve. The large, friable vegetations are denoted by *arrows*. (B) Acute endocarditis caused by *Staphylococcus aureus* on a congenitally bicuspid aortic valve with extensive cuspal destruction and ring abscess *(arrow)*.

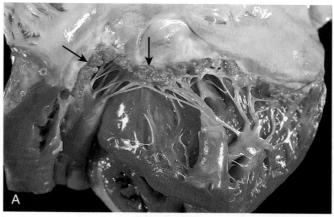

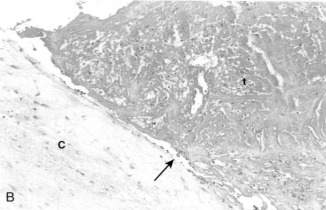

Fig. 11.22 Nonbacterial thrombotic endocarditis (NBTE). (A) Small thrombotic vegetations along the line of closure of the mitral valve leaflets (arrows). (B) Photomicrograph of NBTE lesion, showing bland thrombus, with virtually no inflammation in the valve cusp (C) or the thrombotic deposit (t). The thrombus is only loosely attached to the cusp (arrow).

Endocarditis in Systemic Lupus Erythematosus: Libman-Sacks Endocarditis

Libman-Sacks endocarditis is characterized by the presence of sterile vegetations on the valves of patients with systemic lupus erythematosus. It occurs in about 10% of patients with SLE. The lesions probably develop as a consequence of immune complex deposition and thus exhibit associated inflammation, often with fibrinoid necrosis of the valve adjacent to the vegetation; subsequent fibrosis and serious deformity can result in lesions that resemble chronic rheumatic heart disease. These can occur anywhere on the valve surface, on the cords, or even on the atrial or ventricular endocardium (see Fig. 11.20). Similar lesions can occur in the setting of anti-phospholipid antibody syndrome (Chapter 4).

SUMMARY

VALVULAR HEART DISEASE

- Valve pathology can lead to occlusion (stenosis) and/or regurgitation (insufficiency); acquired aortic or mitral valve stenosis accounts for approximately two thirds of all valve disease.

- Valve calcification typically results in stenosis; abnormal matrix synthesis and turnover leads to myxomatous degeneration and insufficiency.
- Inflammatory valve diseases cause postinflammatory neovascularization and scarring. Rheumatic heart disease results from anti-streptococcal antibodies that cross-react with cardiac tissues; it most commonly affects the mitral valve and is responsible for almost all cases of acquired mitral stenosis.
- Infective endocarditis can rapidly destroy normal valves, or can be indolent and minimally destructive of previously abnormal valves. Systemic embolization can produce septic infarcts.
- Nonbacterial thrombotic endocarditis occurs on previously normal valves as a result of hypercoagulable states; embolization is an important complication.

CARDIOMYOPATHIES AND MYOCARDITIS

Cardiac diseases due to intrinsic myocardial dysfunction are termed *cardiomyopathies* (literally, "heart muscle diseases"); these can be primary—that is, principally confined to the myocardium—or secondary presenting as the cardiac manifestation of a systemic disorder. Cardiomyopathies are thus a diverse group that includes inflammatory disorders (e.g., myocarditis), immunologic diseases (e.g., sarcoidosis), systemic metabolic disorders (e.g., hemochromatosis), muscular dystrophies, and genetic disorders of myocardial fibers. In many cases, the cardiomyopathy is of unknown etiology and thus is termed idiopathic; however, a number of previously "idiopathic" cardiomyopathies have been shown to be the consequence of specific genetic abnormalities in cardiac energy metabolism or in structural and contractile proteins.

Cardiomyopathies can be classified according to a variety of criteria, including the underlying genetic basis of dysfunction; indeed, some of the arrhythmia-inducing channelopathies that are included in some classifications of cardiomyopathy were alluded to earlier. For purposes of general diagnosis and therapy, however, three time-honored clinical, functional, and pathologic patterns are recognized (Fig. 11.23 and Table 11.5):
- Dilated cardiomyopathy (DCM) (including arrhythmogenic right ventricular cardiomyopathy)
- Hypertrophic cardiomyopathy (HCM)
- Restrictive cardiomyopathy

Of the three major patterns, DCM is most common (90% of cases), and restrictive cardiomyopathy is the least frequent. Within each pattern, there is a spectrum of clinical severity, and in some cases clinical features overlap among the groups. In addition, each of these patterns can be caused by a specific identifiable cause, or can be idiopathic (see Table 11.5).

Dilated Cardiomyopathy

Dilated cardiomyopathy (DCM) is characterized by progressive cardiac dilation and contractile (systolic) dysfunction, usually with concurrent hypertrophy; regardless of the cause, the clinicopathologic patterns are similar.

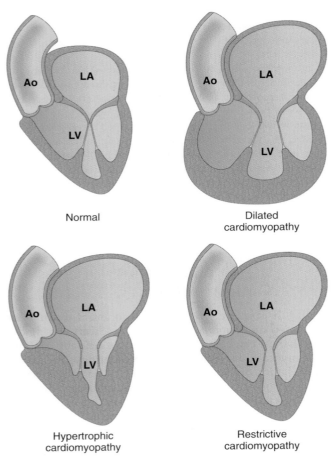

Normal

Dilated
cardiomyopathy

Hypertrophic
cardiomyopathy

Restrictive
cardiomyopathy

Fig. II.23 The three major forms of cardiomyopathy. Dilated cardiomyopathy leads primarily to systolic dysfunction, whereas restrictive and hypertrophic cardiomyopathies result in diastolic dysfunction. Note the changes in atrial and/or ventricular dilation and in ventricular wall thickness. *Ao,* Aorta; *LA,* left atrium; *LV,* left ventricle.

Pathogenesis

Although many individuals with DCM have a familial (genetic) form, DCM can also result from various acquired myocardial insults. These include the following:

- *Myocarditis* (an inflammatory disorder that precedes the development of cardiomyopathy in at least some cases, and is sometimes caused by viral infections)

- *Toxicities,* including adverse effects of chemotherapeutic agents and chronic alcoholism, a history of which can be elicited in 10% to 20% of patients
- *Pregnancy,* so-called "peripartum cardiomyopathy"
- *Stress-provoked*
- *Tachycardia-induced*

By the time it is diagnosed, DCM has frequently already progressed to end-stage disease; the heart is dilated and poorly contractile, and at autopsy or cardiac transplant, fails to reveal any specific pathologic features. Nevertheless, genetic and epidemiologic studies suggest that at least five general pathways can lead to end-stage DCM (Fig. 11.24):

- *Genetic causes.* DCM has a hereditary basis in 20% to 50% of cases. Over 50 genes are known to be mutated in this form of cardiomyopathy, with autosomal dominant inheritance being the predominant pattern; mutations affecting cytoskeletal proteins or proteins that link the sarcomere to the cytoskeleton (e.g., α-cardiac actin) are most commonly involved. X-linked DCM is most frequently associated with mutatons in dystrophin, a cell membrane protein that physically couples the intracellular cytoskeleton to the ECM (Chapter 22). Uncommon forms of DCM are caused by mutations of mitochondrial proteins involved in oxidative phosphorylation or fatty acid β-oxidation, presumably leading to defective ATP generation. Other genetic forms of DCM include those with mutations in cytoskeletal proteins such as desmin (the principal intermediate filament protein in cardiac myocytes), and the nuclear lamins A and C. Since contractile myocytes and conduction fibers share a common developmental pathway, congenital conduction abnormalities also can be a feature of inherited forms of DCM.
- *Infection.* The nucleic acid "footprints" of coxsackievirus B and other enteroviruses can occasionally be detected in the myocardium from late-stage DCM patients. Moreover, sequential endomyocardial biopsies have documented instances in which infectious myocarditis progressed to DCM. Simply finding viral transcripts or demonstrating elevated anti-viral antibody titers may be sufficient to invoke a myocarditis that was "missed" in its early stages. Consequently, many cases of DCM are attributed to viral infections, even though inflammation is absent from the end-stage heart.
- *Alcohol or other toxic exposure.* Alcohol abuse is strongly associated with the development of DCM. Alcohol and

Table II.5 Cardiomyopathies: Functional Patterns, Causes

Functional Pattern	Left Ventricular Ejection Fraction*	Mechanisms of Heart Failure	Causes	Secondary Myocardial Dysfunction (Mimicking Cardiomyopathy)
Dilated	<40%	Impairment of contractility (systolic dysfunction)	Genetic; alcohol; peripartum; myocarditis; hemochromatosis; chronic anemia; doxorubicin (Adriamycin); sarcoidosis; idiopathic	Ischemic heart disease; valvular heart disease; hypertensive heart disease; congenital heart disease
Hypertrophic	50%–80%	Impairment of compliance (diastolic dysfunction)	Genetic; Friedreich ataxia; storage diseases; infants of diabetic mothers	Hypertensive heart disease; aortic stenosis
Restrictive	45%–90%	Impairment of compliance (diastolic dysfunction)	Amyloidosis; radiation-induced fibrosis; idiopathic	Pericardial constriction

*Range of normal values is approximately 50% to 65%.

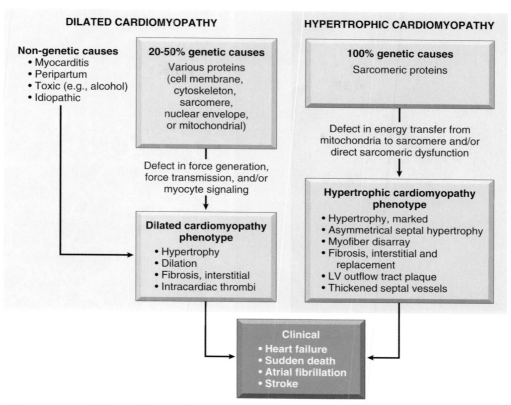

DILATED CARDIOMYOPATHY

Non-genetic causes
- Myocarditis
- Peripartum
- Toxic (e.g., alcohol)
- Idiopathic

20-50% genetic causes
Various proteins (cell membrane, cytoskeleton, sarcomere, nuclear envelope, or mitochondrial)

Defect in force generation, force transmission, and/or myocyte signaling

Dilated cardiomyopathy phenotype
- Hypertrophy
- Dilation
- Fibrosis, interstitial
- Intracardiac thrombi

HYPERTROPHIC CARDIOMYOPATHY

100% genetic causes
Sarcomeric proteins

Defect in energy transfer from mitochondria to sarcomere and/or direct sarcomeric dysfunction

Hypertrophic cardiomyopathy phenotype
- Hypertrophy, marked
- Asymmetrical septal hypertrophy
- Myofiber disarray
- Fibrosis, interstitial and replacement
- LV outflow tract plaque
- Thickened septal vessels

Clinical
- Heart failure
- Sudden death
- Atrial fibrillation
- Stroke

Fig. 11.24 Causes and consequences of dilated and hypertrophic cardiomyopathy. A significant fraction of dilated cardiomyopathies—and virtually all hypertrophic cardiomyopathies—have a genetic origin. Dilated cardiomyopathies can be caused by mutations in cytoskeletal, sarcomeric, nuclear envelope, or mitochondrial proteins; hypertrophic cardiomyopathies typically are caused by sarcomeric protein mutations. Although the two forms of cardiomyopathy differ in cause and morphology, they have common clinical end points. *LV,* Left ventricle.

its metabolites (especially acetaldehyde) have a direct toxic effect on the myocardium. Moreover, chronic alcoholism can be associated with thiamine deficiency, introducing an element of beriberi heart disease (Chapter 8). DCM also can develop after exposure to other toxic agents, such as cobalt, and particularly doxorubicin (Adriamycin), a chemotherapeutic drug.

- *Peripartum cardiomyopathy* occurs late in gestation or several weeks to months postpartum. The etiology is multifactorial, including pregnancy-associated hypertension, volume overload, nutritional deficiency, metabolic derangements (e.g., gestational diabetes), and/or immunologic responses. Recent work suggests that the primary defect is impaired angiogenesis within the myocardium leading to ischemic injury. Antiangiogenic cleavage products of the hormone prolactin (which rises late in pregnancy) and placental-derived antagonists to the VEGF have been implicated. Fortunately, approximately one half of these patients spontaneously recover normal function.

- *Iron overload* in the heart can result either from hereditary hemochromatosis (Chapter 16) or from multiple transfusions. Iron overload also can cause restrictive cardiomyopathy due to interstitial fibrosis, but DCM is the most common manifestation; it has been attributed to interference with metal-dependent enzyme systems or to injury caused by iron-mediated production of reactive oxygen species.

MORPHOLOGY

The heart in DCM characteristically is enlarged (up to two to three times the normal weight) and **flabby,** with dilation of all chambers (Fig. 11.25). Because of the wall thinning that accompanies dilation, the ventricular thickness may be less than, equal to, or greater than normal. **Mural thrombi** are often present and may be a source of thromboemboli. By definition, valvular and vascular lesions (e.g., atherosclerotic coronary artery disease) that can cause cardiac dilation secondarily are absent.

The characteristic histologic abnormalities in DCM are nonspecific. Most myocytes exhibit **hypertrophy** with enlarged nuclei, but many are attenuated, stretched, and irregular. There is also variable interstitial and endocardial fibrosis, with scattered areas of replacement fibrosis; the latter mark previous myocyte ischemic necrosis caused by hypoperfusion, or they may be the footprints of a previous "missed" myocarditis.

In DCM secondary to iron overload, there is a marked accumulation of intramyocardial hemosiderin, which is demonstrable by staining with Prussian blue.

Clinical Features

The fundamental defect in DCM is ineffective contraction. Thus, in end-stage DCM, the cardiac ejection fraction typically is less than 25% (normal is 50% to 65%). Secondary mitral regurgitation and abnormal cardiac rhythms are

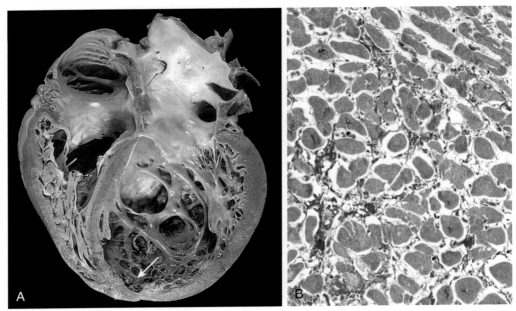

Fig. 11.25 Dilated cardiomyopathy (DCM). (A) Four-chamber dilation and hypertrophy are evident. A small mural thrombus can be seen at the apex of the left ventricle *(arrow)*. (B) The nonspecific histologic picture in typical DCM, with myocyte hypertrophy and interstitial fibrosis. (Collagen is *blue* in this Masson trichrome–stained preparation.)

common, and embolism from intracardiac (mural) thrombi can occur. DCM most commonly is diagnosed between 20 and 50 years of age. It typically manifests with signs of slowly progressive CHF, including dyspnea, easy fatigability, and poor exertional capacity. One half of patients die within 2 years and only 25% survive longer than 5 years; death is usually due to progressive cardiac failure or arrhythmia. Cardiac transplantation is the only definitive treatment, although implantation of long-term ventricular assist devices is increasingly utilized; in some patients, a course of mechanical assistance can produce durable regression of cardiac dysfunction.

Arrhythmogenic Right Ventricular Cardiomyopathy

Arrhythmogenic right ventricular cardiomyopathy is an autosomal dominant disorder that classically manifests with right-sided heart failure and rhythm disturbances, which can cause sudden cardiac death. Its prevalence in the general adult population is close to 1 in 5000 in a study from Italy. Similar prevalence is likely in the US where it seems to be under reported. Almost 10% of cases of sudden deaths in athletes have been ascribed to this entity. Morphologically, the right ventricular wall is severely thinned owing to myocyte replacement by fatty infiltration and lesser amounts of fibrosis (Fig. 11.26). Many of the causative mutations involve genes encoding desmosomal junctional proteins at the intercalated disk (e.g., plakoglobin), as well as proteins that interact with the desmosome (e.g., the intermediate filament desmin). It's thought that myocyte death is caused by desmosomal detachment, particularly during strenuous exercise.

Hypertrophic Cardiomyopathy

Hypertrophic cardiomyopathy (HCM) is characterized by myocardial hypertrophy, defective diastolic filling, and — in one third of cases — ventricular outflow obstruction. The heart is thick-walled, heavy, and hypercontractile, in striking contrast to the flabby, poorly contractile heart in DCM. Systolic function usually is preserved in HCM, but the myocardium does not relax and therefore exhibits primary diastolic dysfunction. HCM needs to be distinguished clinically from disorders causing ventricular stiffness (e.g., amyloid deposition) and ventricular hypertrophy (e.g., aortic stenosis and hypertension).

Pathogenesis

Most cases of HCM are caused by missense mutations in one of several genes encoding proteins that form the contractile apparatus. The usual pattern of transmission is autosomal dominant, with variable expression. Although more than 400 causative mutations in nine different genes have been identified, all have one unifying feature: they all affect sarcomeric proteins and increase myofilament function. This results in myocyte hypercontractility, increased energy use, and a net negative energy balance. Of the various sarcomeric proteins, β-myosin heavy chain is most frequently involved, followed by myosin-binding protein C and troponin T. Mutations in these three genes account for 70% to 80% of all cases of HCM.

Some of the genes mutated in HCM also are mutated in DCM (e.g., beta-myosin), but in DCM the mutations depress motor function as opposed to the gain of function seen in HCM.

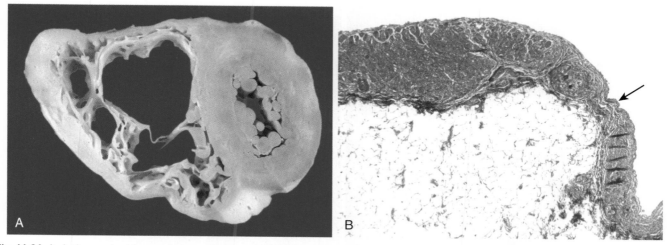

Fig. 11.26 Arrhythmogenic right ventricular cardiomyopathy. (A) The right ventricle is markedly dilated with focal, almost transmural replacement of the free wall by adipose tissue and fibrosis. The left ventricle has a grossly normal appearance in this heart; it can be involved (albeit to a lesser extent) in some instances. (B) The right ventricular myocardium *(red)* is focally replaced by fibrous connective tissue *(blue, arrow)* and fat (Masson trichrome stain).

MORPHOLOGY

Hypertrophic cardiomyopathy is marked by massive myocardial hypertrophy without ventricular dilation (Fig. 11.27A). Classically, there is disproportionate thickening of the ventricular septum relative to the left ventricle free wall (so-called **asymmetric septal hypertrophy**); nevertheless, in about 10% of cases of HCM, concentric hypertrophy is seen. On longitudinal sectioning, the ventricular cavity loses its usual round-to-ovoid shape and is compressed into a "banana-like" configuration. The anterior mitral leaflet contacts the septum during ventricular systole, producing a plaque in the left ventricular outflow tract and thickening of the mitral leaflet; these changes correlate with functional left ventricular outflow tract obstruction due to systolic anterior motion of the mitral valve.

The characteristic histologic features in HCM are marked myocyte hypertrophy, haphazard **myocyte** (and myofiber) **disarray**, and interstitial fibrosis (Fig. 11.27B).

Clinical Features

Although HCM can present at any age, it typically manifests during the postpubertal growth spurt. The clinical symptoms can be best understood in the context of the functional abnormalities. It is characterized by massive left ventricular hypertorphy associated with (paradoxically) a markedly reduced stroke volume. This latter occurs as a consequence of impaired diastolic filling and overall smaller chamber size. In addition, roughly 25% of patients have dynamic obstruction to the left ventricular outflow by the anterior leaflet of the mitral valve. Reduced cardiac output and a secondary increase in pulmonary venous pressure cause exertional dyspnea, with a *harsh systolic ejection murmur*. A combination of massive hypertrophy, high left ventricular pressures, and compromised intramural arteries frequently leads to myocardial ischemia (with angina), even in the absence of concomitant CAD. Major clinical problems include atrial fibrillation with mural thrombus formation, ventricular fibrillation leading to sudden cardiac death, infectious endocarditis of the mitral valve, and CHF. Most patients' symptoms are improved by therapy that promotes ventricular relaxation; partial surgical excision or controlled alcohol-induced infarction of septal muscle also can relieve the outflow tract obstruction. As mentioned earlier, HCM is an important cause of sudden cardiac death. In almost one third of cases of sudden cardiac death in athletes younger than 35 years of age, the underlying cause is HCM.

Restrictive Cardiomyopathy

Restrictive cardiomyopathy is characterized by a primary decrease in ventricular compliance, resulting in impaired ventricular filling during diastole (simply put, the wall is *stiffer*). This form of cardiomyopathy may be idiopathic or may be associated with systemic diseases that affect the myocardium, for example, radiation fibrosis, amyloidosis, sarcoidosis, or products of inborn errors of metabolism.

Three forms of restrictive cardiomyopathy merit brief mention:

- *Amyloidosis* is caused by the deposition of extracellular proteins with a predilection for forming insoluble β-pleated sheets (Chapter 5). Cardiac amyloidosis can occur in the setting of systemic amyloidosis (e.g., multiple myeloma) or can be predominantly restricted to the heart (e.g., senile cardiac amyloidosis). In the latter case, deposition of normal (or mutant) forms of transthyretin (a liver-synthesized circulating protein that transports thyroxine and retinol) in the hearts of older adult patients results in a restrictive cardiomyopathy. Four percent of African Americans carry a specific mutation of transthyretin that increases the risk of cardiac amyloidosis in that population over fourfold. Besides depositing as amyloid, immunoglobulin light-chains in AL-type amyloid also are directly cardiotoxic and can induce myocardial dysfunction.

- *Endomyocardial fibrosis* is principally a disease of children and young adults in Africa and other tropical areas. It is

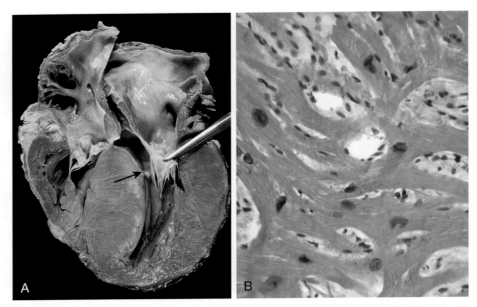

Fig. 11.27 Hypertrophic cardiomyopathy with asymmetric septal hypertrophy. (A) The septal muscle bulges into the left ventricular outflow tract, giving rise to a "banana-shaped" ventricular lumen, and the left atrium is enlarged. The anterior mitral leaflet has been moved away from the septum to reveal a fibrous endocardial plaque *(arrow)* (see text). (B) Histologic appearance demonstrating disarray, extreme hypertrophy, and characteristic branching of myocytes, as well as interstitial fibrosis.

characterized by dense diffuse fibrosis of the ventricular endocardium and subendocardium, often involving the tricuspid and mitral valves. The fibrous tissue markedly diminishes the volume and compliance of affected chambers, resulting in a restrictive physiology. Endomyocardial fibrosis has been linked to nutritional deficiencies and/or inflammation related to helminthic infections (e.g., hypereosinophilia); worldwide, it is the most common form of restrictive cardiomyopathy.

- *Loeffler endomyocarditis* also exhibits endocardial fibrosis, typically associated with formation of large mural thrombi. It has no geographic or population predilection. It is characterized by peripheral hypereosinophilia and eosinophilic tissue infiltrates; release of eosinophil granule contents, especially major basic protein, probably engenders endocardial and myocardial necrosis, followed by scarring, layering of the endocardium by thrombus, and finally thrombus organization. Of interest, some patients have an underlying hypereosinophilic myeloproliferative neoplasm driven by gene rearrangements that lead to expression of constitutively active tyrosine kinases (Chapter 12). Treatment of such patients with tyrosine kinase inhibitors can result in hematologic remission and reversal of the endomyocardial lesions.

MORPHOLOGY

In restrictive cardiomyopathy, the ventricles are of approximately normal size or only slightly enlarged, the cavities are not dilated, and the myocardium is firm. However, both atria are typically dilated as a consequence of restricted ventricular filling and pressure overloads. Microscopic examination reveals variable degrees of interstitial fibrosis. Although gross morphologic findings are similar for restrictive cardiomyopathy of disparate causes, endomyocardial biopsy often can reveal a specific etiology.

Myocarditis

Myocarditis encompasses a diverse group of clinical entities in which infectious agents and/or inflammatory processes target the myocardium. It is important to distinguish myocarditis from conditions such as IHD, where the inflammatory process is secondary to some other cause of myocardial injury.

Pathogenesis

In the United States, viral infections are the most common cause of myocarditis, with coxsackieviruses A and B and other enteroviruses accounting for a majority of the cases. Cytomegalovirus (CMV), human immunodeficiency virus (HIV), influenza virus, and others are less common pathogens. Offending agents can be identified by serologic studies that show rising antibody titers or through molecular diagnostic techniques using infected tissues. While some viruses cause direct cell death, in most cases the injury results from an immune response directed against virally infected cells; this is analogous to the damage inflicted by virus-specific T cells on hepatitis virus–infected liver cells (Chapter 16). In some cases, viruses trigger a reaction against cross-reacting proteins such as myosin heavy chain.

The nonviral infectious causes of myocarditis run the entire gamut of the microbial world. The protozoan *Trypanosoma cruzi* is the agent of Chagas disease. Although uncommon in the northern hemisphere, Chagas disease affects up to one half of the population in endemic areas of South America, with myocardial involvement in the vast majority. About 10% of the patients die during an acute attack; others can enter a chronic immune-mediated phase with development of progressive signs of CHF and arrhythmia 10 to 20 years later. *Toxoplasma gondii* (household cats are the most common vector) also can cause myocarditis, particularly in immunocompromised individuals.

Trichinosis is the most common helminthic disease associated with cardiac involvement.

Myocarditis occurs in approximately 5% of patients with Lyme disease, a systemic illness caused by the bacterial spirochete *Borrelia burgdorferi* (Chapter 9). Lyme myocarditis manifests primarily as self-limited conduction system disease, frequently requiring temporary pacemaker insertion.

Noninfectious causes of myocarditis include systemic diseases of immune origin, such as systemic lupus erythematosus and polymyositis. Drug hypersensitivity reactions affecting the heart (hypersensitivity myocarditis) may occur with exposure to a wide range of agents; such reactions typically are benign and only in rare circumstances lead to CHF or sudden death.

MORPHOLOGY

In acute myocarditis, the heart may appear normal or dilated; in advanced stages, the myocardium typically is flabby and often mottled with pale and hemorrhagic areas. Mural thrombi may be present.

Microscopically, myocarditis is characterized by edema, interstitial inflammatory infiltrates, and myocyte injury (Fig. 11.28). A diffuse lymphocytic infiltrate is most common (see Fig. 11.28A), although the inflammatory involvement is often patchy and can be "missed" on endomyocardial biopsy. If the patient survives the acute phase of myocarditis, lesions may resolve without significant sequelae or heal by progressive fibrosis.

In **hypersensitivity myocarditis,** interstitial and perivascular infiltrates are composed of lymphocytes, macrophages, and a high proportion of eosinophils (Fig. 11.28B). **Giant cell myocarditis** is a morphologically distinctive entity characterized by widespread inflammatory cell infiltrates containing multinucleate giant cells (formed by macrophage fusion). Giant cell myocarditis probably represents the aggressive end of the spectrum of lymphocytic myocarditis, and there is at least focal—and frequently extensive—necrosis (Fig. 11.28C). This variant carries a poor prognosis.

Chagas myocarditis is characterized by the parasitization of scattered myofibers by trypanosomes accompanied by an inflammatory infiltrate of neutrophils, lymphocytes, macrophages, and occasional eosinophils (Fig. 11.28D).

Clinical Features

The clinical spectrum of myocarditis is broad; at one end, the disease is asymptomatic, and patients recover without sequelae. At the other extreme is the precipitous onset of heart failure or arrhythmias, occasionally with sudden death. Between these extremes are many levels of involvement associated with a variety of signs and symptoms, including fatigue, dyspnea, palpitations, pain, and fever. The clinical features of myocarditis can mimic those of acute MI. Clinical progression from myocarditis to DCM occasionally is seen.

Other Causes of Myocardial Disease

Cardiotoxic Drugs

Cardiac complications of cancer therapy are an important clinical problem. Cardiotoxicity can be associated with conventional chemotherapeutic agents, targeted drugs such as tyrosine kinase inhibitors, and certain forms of immunotherapy (e.g., immune checkpoint blockade for cancer). The anthracyclines doxorubicin and daunorubicin are the chemotherapeutic agents that are most frequently associated with toxic myocardial injury, which often takes the form of a dilated cardiomyopathy and heart failure. Anthracycline toxicity is dose-dependent (cardiotoxicity becomes progressively more frequent above a total dose of 500 mg/m^2) and is attributed primarily to peroxidation of lipids in myocyte membranes.

Many other agents, such as lithium, phenothiazines, and chloroquine, have been implicated in myocardial injury and sometimes sudden death. Common findings in hearts injured by many of these chemicals and drugs (including diphtheria exotoxin and doxorubicin) are myofiber swelling, cytoplasmic vacuolization, and fatty change. Discontinuing such agents can lead to complete resolution, with no apparent sequelae. Sometimes, however, more extensive damage produces myocyte necrosis and leads to a dilated cardiomyopathy.

Catecholamines

Foci of myocardial necrosis with contraction bands, often associated with a sparse mononuclear inflammatory infiltrate (mostly macrophages), can occur in individuals with pheochromocytoma, a tumor that elaborates catecholamines (Chapter 20). Similar changes can occur with a variety of agents—endogenous or exogenous—under the rubric of "catecholamine effect." These include cocaine, high doses of ephedrine (an adrenergic agent in many cold and allergy formulations), intense autonomic stimulation secondary to intracranial lesions, or vasopressor agents such as dopamine. The mechanism of catecholamine cardiotoxicity is uncertain, but seems to relate either to a direct toxicity of catecholamines on cardiac myocytes via calcium overload or to vasoconstriction in the face of an increased heart rate. The mononuclear cell infiltrate is probably a reaction to microscopic foci of myocyte cell death.

SUMMARY

CARDIOMYOPATHIES AND MYOCARDITIS

- *Cardiomyopathy* refers to intrinsic cardiac muscle disease; there may be specific causes, or it may be idiopathic.
- The three general pathophysiologic categories of cardiomyopathy are *dilated* (accounting for 90% of the cases), *hypertrophic*, and *restrictive* (least common).
- DCM results in systolic (contractile) dysfunction. Causes include myocarditis, toxic exposures (e.g., alcohol), and pregnancy. In 20% to 50% of cases, mutations affecting cytoskeletal proteins are responsible.
- HCM results in diastolic (relaxation) dysfunction. Virtually all cases are due to autosomal dominant mutations in the proteins that make up the contractile apparatus, in particular β-myosin heavy chain.
- Restrictive cardiomyopathy results in a stiff, noncompliant myocardium and can be due to depositions (e.g., amyloid), increased interstitial fibrosis (e.g., due to radiation), or endomyocardial scarring.

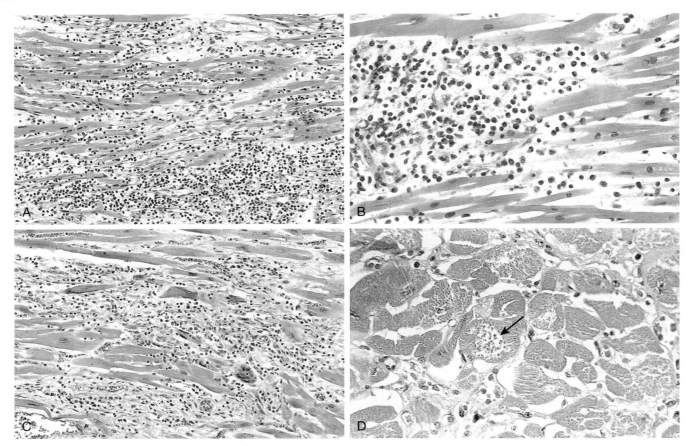

Fig. 11.28 Myocarditis. (A) Lymphocytic myocarditis, with edema and associated myocyte injury. (B) Hypersensitivity myocarditis, characterized by perivascular eosinophil-rich inflammatory infiltrates. (C) Giant cell myocarditis, with lymphocyte and macrophage infiltrates, extensive myocyte damage, and multinucleate giant cells. (D) Chagas myocarditis. A myofiber distended with trypanosomes *(arrow)* is present, along with mononuclear inflammation and myofiber necrosis.

- Arrhythmogenic right ventricular cardiomyopathy is an autosomal dominant disorder of cardiac muscle that manifests with right-sided heart failure and rhythm disturbances that can cause sudden cardiac death in athletes.
- Myocarditis is an inflammatory disorder caused by infections or immune reactions. Coxsackieviruses A and B are the most common pathogens in the United States. Clinically, myocarditis may be asymptomatic, give rise to acute heart failure, or evolve to DCM.

PERICARDIAL DISEASE

Pericardial lesions typically are associated with a pathologic process elsewhere in the heart or surrounding structures, or are secondary to a systemic disorder. Pericardial disorders include effusions and inflammatory conditions, sometimes resulting in fibrous constriction.

Pericardial Effusion and Hemopericardium

Normally, the pericardial sac contains less than 50 cc of thin, clear, straw-colored fluid. Under various circumstances, the pericardial sac may be distended by accumulations of serous fluid *(pericardial effusion)*, blood *(hemopericardium)*, or pus *(purulent pericarditis)*.

Pericardial effusions and their causes include the following:
- *Serous:* Congestive heart failure, hypoalbuminemia of any cause
- *Serosanguineous:* Blunt chest trauma, malignancy, ruptured MI, or aortic dissection
- *Chylous:* Mediastinal lymphatic obstruction

With long-standing cardiac enlargement or with slowly accumulating fluid, the pericardium has time to dilate. This permits chronic pericardial effusions to become quite large without interfering with cardiac function. Thus, with chronic effusions of less than 500 cc in volume, the only clinical significance is a characteristic globular enlargement of the heart shadow on chest radiograph. In contrast, rapidly developing fluid collections of as little as 200 to 300 cc (e.g., due to hemopericardium caused by a ruptured MI or aortic dissection) can produce clinically devastating compression of the thin-walled atria and venae cavae, or the ventricles themselves; cardiac filling is thereby restricted, producing potentially fatal *cardiac tamponade.*

Pericarditis

Primary pericarditis is uncommon. It is typically due to viral infection (often with concurrent myocarditis),

although bacteria, fungi, or parasites may also be involved. In most cases, pericarditis is secondary to acute MI or cardiac surgery (so-called "Dressler's syndrome"), radiation to the mediastinum, or processes involving other thoracic structures (e.g., pneumonia or pleuritis). *Uremia* is the most common systemic disorder associated with pericarditis. Less common secondary causes include rheumatic fever, systemic lupus erythematosus, and metastatic malignancies. Pericarditis can (1) cause immediate hemodynamic complications if it elicits a large effusion (resulting in cardiac *tamponade*), (2) resolve without significant sequelae, or 3) progress to a chronic fibrosing process.

MORPHOLOGY

In patients with acute viral pericarditis or uremia, the exudate typically is fibrinous, imparting an irregular, shaggy appearance to the pericardial surface (so-called "bread and butter" pericarditis). In acute bacterial pericarditis, the exudate is fibrinopurulent (suppurative), often with areas of frank pus (Fig. 11.29); tuberculous pericarditis can exhibit areas of caseation. Pericarditis due to malignancy often is associated with an exuberant, shaggy fibrinous exudate and a bloody effusion; metastases can be grossly evident as irregular excrescences or may be grossly inapparent, especially in the case of leukemia. In most cases, acute fibrinous or fibrinopurulent pericarditis resolves without any sequelae. With extensive suppuration or caseation, however, healing can result in fibrosis (chronic pericarditis).

Chronic pericarditis may be associated with delicate adhesions or dense, fibrotic scars that obliterate the pericardial space. In extreme cases, the heart is so completely encased by dense fibrosis that it cannot expand normally during diastole—resulting in the condition known as **constrictive pericarditis.**

Clinical Features

Pericarditis classically manifests with atypical chest pain (not related to exertion and worse in recumbency), and a prominent friction rub. When associated with significant fluid accumulation, acute pericarditis can cause cardiac *tamponade,* which leads to declining cardiac output and consequent shock. Chronic constrictive pericarditis produces a combination of right-sided venous distention and low cardiac output, similar to the clinical picture in restrictive cardiomyopathy.

CARDIAC TUMORS

Primary Neoplasms

Primary cardiac tumors are uncommon; moreover, most also are (fortunately) benign. The five most common have no malignant potential and account for 80% to 90% of all primary heart tumors. In descending order of frequency, these are myxomas, fibromas, lipomas, papillary fibroelastomas, and rhabdomyomas. Angiosarcomas constitute the most common primary *malignant* tumor of the heart. Only the myxomas and rhabdomyomas merit further mention here.

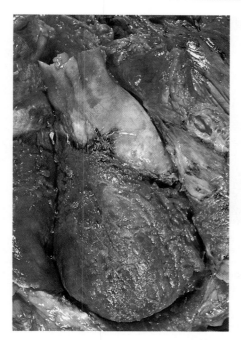

Fig. 11.29 Acute suppurative (purulent, exudative) pericarditis, caused by extension from a pneumonia.

Myxomas are the most common primary tumors of the adult heart (Fig. 11.30). Roughly 90% are atrial, with the left atrium accounting for 80% of those.

Rhabdomyomas are the most frequent primary tumors of the heart in infants and children; they frequently are discovered owing to valvular or outflow obstruction. Cardiac rhabdomyomas occur with high frequency in patients with tuberous sclerosis caused by mutations in the *TSC1* or *TSC2* tumor suppressor genes; loss of TSC-1 and TSC-2 activity leads to myocyte overgrowth. Because they often regress spontaneously (for unknown reasons), rhabdomyomas are sometimes considered to be hamartomas rather than true neoplasms. In keeping with this not all cardiac rhabdomyomas that occur in patients with tuberous sclerosis are clonal.

MORPHOLOGY

Myxomas are almost always single, classically arising in the region of the fossa ovalis (atrial septum). They can be small (less than 1 cm in diameter) or massive (up to 10 cm across), sessile or pedunculated masses (Fig. 11.30A), most often manifesting as soft, translucent, villous lesions with a gelatinous appearance. Pedunculated forms often are sufficiently mobile to swing into the mitral or tricuspid valve during systole, causing intermittent obstruction or exerting a "wrecking ball" effect that damages the valve leaflets.

Histologically, myxomas are composed of stellate, frequently multinucleated myxoma cells (typically with hyperchromatic nuclei), admixed with cells showing endothelial, smooth muscle, and/or fibroblastic differentiation; all of the cell types arise from differentiation of multipotential mesenchymal tumor cells. The cells are embedded in an abundant acid mucopolysaccharide ground substance (Fig. 11.30B). Hemorrhage, poorly organizing thrombus, and mononuclear inflammation also are usually present.

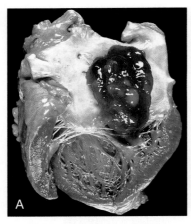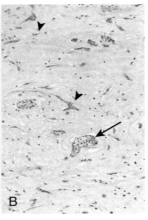

Fig. 11.30 Atrial myxoma. (A) A large pedunculated lesion arises from the region of the fossa ovalis and extends into the mitral valve orifice. (B) Abundant amorphous extracellular matrix contains scattered multinucleate myxoma cells *(arrowheads)* in various groupings, including abnormal vascular formations *(arrow)*.

Rhabdomyomas are gray-white masses up to several centimeters in diameter that protrude into the ventricular chambers. Histologic examination shows a mixed population of cells; most characteristic, however, are large, rounded, or polygonal cells containing numerous glycogen-laden vacuoles separated by strands of cytoplasm running from the plasma membrane to the centrally located nucleus, so-called "spider cells".

Clinical Features

The major clinical manifestations of myxomas are due to valvular "ball-valve" obstruction, embolization, or a syndrome of constitutional signs and symptoms including fever and malaise. This syndrome is caused by elaboration of the cytokine interleukin-6 by the tumor cells, a major mediator of the acute-phase response. Echocardiography is the diagnostic modality of choice, and surgical resection is almost uniformly curative.

Cardiac Effects of Noncardiac Neoplasms

With enhanced patient survival due to diagnostic and therapeutic advances, significant cardiovascular effects of noncardiac neoplasms and their therapy are increasingly encountered (Table 11.6). The pathologic consequences include direct tumor metastasis or infiltration, effects of circulating mediators, and therapeutic complications.

The most frequent metastatic tumors involving the heart are carcinomas of the lung and breast, melanomas, leukemias, and lymphomas. Metastases can reach the heart and pericardium by retrograde lymphatic extension (carcinomas), by hematogenous seeding (many tumors), by direct contiguous extension (primary carcinoma of the lung, breast, or esophagus), or by venous extension (tumors of the kidney or liver). Clinical symptoms are most often associated with pericardial spread, which can cause symptomatic pericardial effusions or a mass-effect that is sufficient to restrict cardiac filling. Bronchogenic carcinoma or malignant lymphoma may infiltrate the mediastinum

extensively, causing encasement, compression, or invasion of the superior vena cava and obstruction to blood flow from the head and upper extremities *(superior vena cava syndrome)*. Renal cell carcinoma often invades the renal vein and may grow as a continuous column of tumor up the inferior vena cava and into the right atrium, blocking venous return to the heart.

Noncardiac tumors also may affect cardiac function indirectly, sometimes via circulating tumor-derived substances. The consequences include nonbacterial thrombotic endocarditis, carcinoid heart disease, pheochromocytoma-associated myocardial damage, and myeloma-associated AL-type amyloidosis.

Complications of chemotherapy were discussed earlier in this chapter. Radiation used to treat breast, lung, or mediastinal neoplasms can cause pericarditis, pericardial effusion, myocardial fibrosis, and chronic pericardial disorders. Other cardiac effects of radiation therapy include accelerated coronary artery disease and mural and valvular endocardial fibrosis.

Carcinoid Heart Disease

The carcinoid syndrome results from bioactive compounds such as serotonin released by carcinoid tumors (Chapter 15); systemic manifestations include flushing, diarrhea, dermatitis, and bronchoconstriction. *Carcinoid heart disease* refers to the cardiac manifestation caused by the bioactive compounds and occurs in one half of patients in whom the systemic syndrome develops. Cardiac lesions typically do not occur until there is a massive hepatic metastatic burden, since the liver normally inactivates circulating mediators before they can affect the heart. Classically, endocardium and valves of the right heart are primarily affected since they are the first cardiac tissues bathed by the mediators released by gastrointestinal carcinoid tumors. The left side of the heart is afforded some measure of protection because the pulmonary vascular bed degrades the mediators. However, left-sided heart carcinoid lesions can occur in the setting of atrial or ventricular septal defects and right-to-left flow, or they can arise in association with primary pulmonary carcinoid tumors.

Table 11.6 Cardiovascular Effects of Noncardiac Neoplasms

Direct Consequences of Tumor
Pericardial and myocardial metastases
Large vessel obstruction
Pulmonary tumor emboli
Indirect Consequences of Tumor (Complications of Circulating Mediators)
Nonbacterial thrombotic endocarditis
Carcinoid heart disease
Pheochromocytoma-associated heart disease
Myeloma-associated amyloidosis
Effects of Tumor Therapy
Chemotherapy
Radiation therapy

Modified from Schoen FJ, et al: Cardiac effects of non-cardiac neoplasms, *Cardiol Clin* 2:657, 1984.

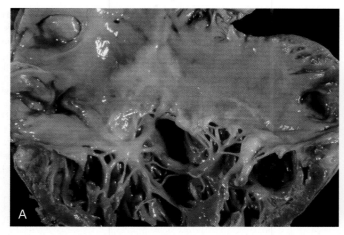
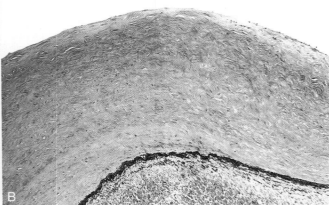

Fig. 11.31 Carcinoid heart disease. (A) Characteristic endocardial fibrotic *(light gray)* lesion "coating" the right ventricle and tricuspid valve, and extending onto the chordae tendineae. (B) Microscopic appearance of the thickened endocardium, which contains smooth muscle cells and abundant acid mucopolysaccharides (blue-green in this Movat stain, which colors the underlying endocardial elastic tissue black).

Pathogenesis

The mediators elaborated by carcinoid tumors include serotonin (5-hydroxytryptamine), kallikrein, bradykinin, histamine, prostaglandins, and tachykinins. Although it is not clear which of these is causative, plasma levels of serotonin and urinary excretion of the serotonin metabolite 5-hydroxyindoleacetic acid correlate with the severity of right-sided heart lesions. The valvular plaques in carcinoid syndrome also are similar to lesions that occur with the administration of fenfluramine (an appetite suppressant) or ergot alkaloids (for migraine headaches); of interest, these agents either affect systemic serotonin metabolism or directly bind to hydroxytryptamine receptors on heart valves.

MORPHOLOGY

The cardiovascular lesions associated with the carcinoid syndrome are distinctive, glistening white, intimal, plaquelike thickenings on the endocardial surfaces of the cardiac chambers and valve leaflets (Fig. 11.31). The lesions are composed of smooth muscle cells and sparse collagen fibers embedded in an acid mucopolysaccharide–rich matrix. Underlying structures are intact. With right-sided involvement, typical findings are tricuspid insufficiency and pulmonic stenosis.

CARDIAC TRANSPLANTATION

Although permanent ventricular assist device implantation is increasingly an option for management of end-stage heart disease, cardiac transplantation remains the treatment of choice for patients with intractable heart failure. Without transplantation, medically managed end-stage heart failure carries a 50% 1-year mortality rate, and less than 10% of patients survive 5 years. Over 5000 heart transplantation procedures are performed annually worldwide, mostly for DCM and IHD.

The major complications of cardiac transplantation are acute cardiac rejection and allograft arteriopathy.

The immunosuppression required for allograft survival also increases the risk for opportunistic infections and certain malignancies (e.g., Epstein-Barr virus–associated lymphoma).

- *Rejection* is characterized by interstitial lymphocytic inflammation, myocyte damage and a histologic pattern similar to that seen in viral myocarditis. Both T cell- and antibody responses to the allograft are involved in the rejection reaction.
- *Allograft arteriopathy* is the single most important long-term limitation for cardiac transplantation. It is marked by late, progressive, diffusely stenosing intimal proliferation in the coronary arteries, leading to ischemic injury.

Despite these problems, the outlook for transplant recipients generally is good, with a 1-year survival rate of 90% and a 5-year survival rate of more than 70%.

SUGGESTED READINGS

Azaouagh A, Churzidse S, Konorza T, et al: Arrhythmogenic right ventricular cardiomyopathy/dysplasia: a review and update, *Clin Res Cardiol* 100:383, 2011. [*An excellent look at this entity and its genetic causes.*]

Bruneau BG: The developmental genetics of congenital heart disease, *Nature* 451:943, 2008. [*A succinct overview of the relationships between cardiac development and congenital heart disease.*]

Cerrone M, Priori SG: Genetics of sudden death: focus on inherited channelopathies, *Eur Heart J* 32:2109, 2011. [*A well-organized description of the known ion channel disorders that cause sudden cardiac death.*]

Cooper LT Jr: Myocarditis, *N Engl J Med* 360:1526, 2009. [*A nice review of etiology, pathogenesis, and clinical features.*]

Grozinsky-Glasberg S, Grossman AB, Gross DJ: Carcinoid heart disease: from pathophysiology to treatment—"something in the way it moves" *Neuroendocrinology* 101:263, 2015. [*A good review of the pathophysiology, diagnosis, and treatment of this entity.*]

Guilherme L, Köhler KF, Kalil J: Rheumatic heart disease: mediation by complex immune events, *Adv Clin Chem* 53:31, 2011. [*A well-written and scholarly discussion of the pathogenic mechanisms regarding rheumatic heart disease.*]

Hausenloy DJ, Yellon DM: Myocardial ischemia-reperfusion injury: a neglected therapeutic target, *J Clin Invest* 123:92, 2013. [*A nice* discussion of the mechanisms and possible therapeutic approaches in ischemia-reperfusion injury.]

Heusch G, Libby P, Gersh B, et al: Cardiovascular remodelling in coronary artery disease and heart failure, *Lancet* 383:1933, 2014. *[An excellent review of the pathophysiologic changes that occur as ischemic hearts develop CHF.]*

Hill EE, Herijgers P, Herregods MC, et al: Evolving trends in infective endocarditis, *Clin Microbiol Infect* 12:5, 2006. *[A good, clinically oriented overview of the developments in microorganisms, diagnosis, and therapies for infective endocarditis.]*

Huang JB, Liu YL, Sun PW, et al: Molecular mechanisms of congenital heart disease, *Cardiovasc Pathol* 19:e183, 2010. *[A comprehensive review of the genes and pathways underlying congenital heart disease.]*

Li C, Xu S, Gotlieb AI: The response to valve injury. A paradigm to understand the pathogenesis of heart valve disease, *Cardiovasc Pathol* 20:183, 2011. *[A nice overview of pathologic concepts in valvular disease.]*

Mann DL, Zipes DP, Libby P, et al, editors: *Braunwald's heart disease: a textbook of cardiovascular medicine*, ed 10, Philadelphia, 2015, Elsevier. *[An outstanding and authoritative text, with excellent sections on heart failure and atherosclerotic cardiovascular disease.]*

Maron BJ, Towbin JA, Thiene G, et al: Contemporary definitions and classification of the cardiomyopathies: an American Heart Association Scientific Statement from the Council on Clinical Cardiology, Heart Failure and Transplantation Committee; Quality of Care and Outcomes Research and Functional Genomics and Translational Biology Interdisciplinary Working Groups; and Council on Epidemiology and Prevention, *Circulation* 113:1807, 2006. *[A consensus document regarding an updated classification of cardiomyopathies, heavily weighted to genetic etiologies rather than pathophysiologic manifestations.]*

Mitchell RN: Graft vascular disease: immune response meets the vessel wall, *Annu Rev Pathol* 4:19, 2009. *[A comprehensive overview of allograft arteriopathy, including animal models, pathogenic mechanisms, clinical diagnosis, and therapy.]*

New SE, Aikawa E: Molecular imaging insights into early inflammatory stages of arterial and aortic valve calcification, *Circ Res* 108:1381, 2011. *[A good overview of the mechanisms leading to degenerative calcification on valves and vessels.]*

Ovize M, Baxter GF, Di Lisa F, et al: Postconditioning and protection from reperfusion injury: where do we stand? Position paper from the Working Group of Cellular Biology of the Heart of the European Society of Cardiology, *Cardiovasc Res* 87:406, 2010. *[A good overview of the mechanisms and potential therapeutic interventions for ischemia-reperfusion injury and for ischemic pre-conditioning in limiting infarct size.]*

Patten IS, Rana S, Shahul S, et al: Cardiac angiogenic imbalance leads to peripartum cardiomyopathy, *Nature* 485:333, 2012. *[A new perspective on the mechanisms underlying pregnancy-associated cardiomyopathy.]*

Rasmussen TL, Raveendran G, Zhang J, et al: Getting to the heart of myocardial stem cells and cell therapy, *Circulation* 123:1771, 2011. *[A well-written overview of the challenges and current state of the art regarding stem cell therapies in heart disease.]*

Seidman CE, Seidman JG: Identifying sarcomere gene mutations in hypertrophic cardiomyopathy: a personal history, *Circ Res* 108:743, 2011. *[A well-written and authoritative overview of the genetics and pathophysiology of hypertrophic cardiomyopathy from one of the leading groups in the world.]*

Watkins H, Houman A, Redwood C: Inherited cardiomyopathies, *N Engl J Med* 364:1643, 2011. *[An excellent review of the molecular basis of cardiomyopathies.]*

Wu JC, Child JS: Common congenital heart disorders in adults, *Curr Probl Cardiol* 29:641, 2004. *[A thorough overview of the congenital heart disorders seen in the adult population, often as a consequence of improved pediatric therapies.]*

Hematopoietic and Lymphoid Systems

12

CHAPTER OUTLINE

Red Cell Disorders 442
Anemia of Blood Loss: Hemorrhage 443
Hemolytic Anemia 443
Hereditary Spherocytosis 444
Sickle Cell Anemia 445
Thalassemia 447
*Glucose-6-Phosphate Dehydrogenase
  Deficiency 450*
Paroxysmal Nocturnal Hemoglobinuria 450
Immunohemolytic Anemia 451
*Hemolytic Anemia Resulting From Mechanical
  Trauma to Red Cells 451*
Malaria 452
Anemia of Diminished Erythropoiesis 453
Iron Deficiency Anemia 453
Anemia of Chronic Inflammation 455
Megaloblastic Anemias 456
Aplastic Anemia 458
Myelophthisic Anemia 458
Polycythemia 459

White Cell Disorders 459
**Nonneoplastic Disorders of White
  Cells 459**
Leukopenia 459
Reactive Leukocytosis 460
Reactive Lymphadenitis 461
**Neoplastic Proliferations of White
  Cells 463**
Lymphoid Neoplasms 463
Myeloid Neoplasms 478
Histiocytic Neoplasms 484
Bleeding Disorders 485
**Disseminated Intravascular Coagulation
  (DIC) 486**
Thrombocytopenia 488
Immune Thrombocytopenic Purpura 488
Heparin-Induced Thrombocytopenia 488
*Thrombotic Microangiopathies: Thrombotic
  Thrombocytopenic Purpura and Hemolytic
  Uremic Syndrome 489*

Coagulation Disorders 489
*Deficiencies of Factor VIII–von Willebrand Factor
  Complex 489*
Complications of Transfusion 491
Allergic Reactions 491
Hemolytic Reactions 491
**Transfusion-Related Acute Lung
  Injury 492**
Infectious Complications 492
**Disorders of the Spleen and
  Thymus 492**
Splenomegaly 492
Disorders of the Thymus 493
Thymic Hyperplasia 493
Thymoma 493

The hematopoietic and lymphoid systems are affected by a wide spectrum of diseases. One useful way to organize these disorders is based on whether they primarily affect red cells, white cells, or the coagulation system, which includes platelets and clotting factors. The most common red cell disorders are those that lead to *anemia,* a state of red cell deficiency. White cell disorders, by contrast, are most often associated with excessive proliferation resulting from malignant transformation. Derangements in blood coagulation may result in hemorrhagic diatheses (bleeding disorders). Finally, splenomegaly, a feature of numerous diseases, is discussed at the end of the chapter, as are tumors of the thymus.

Although these divisions are useful, in reality the production, function, and destruction of red cells, white cells, and components of the hemostatic system are closely linked, and derangements primarily affecting one cell type or component of the system often lead to alterations in others. For example, in certain conditions B cells make autoantibodies against components of the red cell membrane. The opsonized red cells are recognized and destroyed by phagocytes in the spleen, which becomes enlarged. The increased red cell destruction causes anemia, which in turn drives a compensatory hyperplasia of red cell progenitors in the bone marrow.

Other levels of interplay and complexity stem from the anatomically dispersed nature of the hematolymphoid system and the capacity of both normal and malignant white cells to "traffic" between various compartments. Hence, a patient who is diagnosed with lymphoma by lymph node biopsy also may be found to have neoplastic lymphoid cells in the bone marrow and blood. The malignant clone of lymphoid cells in the marrow may suppress hematopoiesis, giving rise to low blood cell counts (cytopenias), and the dissemination of tumor cells to the liver and spleen may lead to organomegaly. Thus, in both benign and malignant hematolymphoid disorders, a single underlying abnormality can result in diverse systemic manifestations. Keeping these complexities in mind, we will use the time-honored classification of hematolymphoid disorders based on predominant involvement of red cells, white cells, and the hemostatic system.

Red Cell Disorders

Disorders of red cells can result in anemia or, less commonly, polycythemia (an increase in red cells also known as erythrocytosis). *Anemia* is defined as a reduction in the oxygen-transporting capacity of blood, resulting from a decrease in the red cell mass to subnormal levels.

Anemia can stem from bleeding, increased red cell destruction, or decreased red cell production. These mechanisms serve as one basis for classifying anemia (Table 12.1). In some entities overlap occurs, for example in thalassemia, where both reduced red cell production and early destruction contribute to anemia. With the exception of anemia caused by chronic renal failure or chronic inflammation (described

Table 12.1 Classification of Anemia According to Underlying Mechanism

Blood Loss

Acute: trauma
Chronic: gastrointestinal tract lesions, gynecologic disturbances

Increased Destruction (Hemolytic Anemias)

Intrinsic (Intracorpuscular) Abnormalities

Hereditary
Membrane abnormalities
   Membrane skeleton proteins: spherocytosis, elliptocytosis
   Membrane lipids: abetalipoproteinemia
Enzyme deficiencies
   Enzymes of hexose monophosphate shunt: glucose-6-phosphate dehydrogenase, glutathione synthetase
   Glycolytic enzymes: pyruvate kinase, hexokinase
Disorders of hemoglobin synthesis
   Structurally abnormal globin synthesis (hemoglobinopathies): sickle cell anemia, unstable hemoglobins
   Deficient globin synthesis: thalassemia syndromes
Acquired
Membrane defect: paroxysmal nocturnal hemoglobinuria

Extrinsic (Extracorpuscular) Abnormalities

Antibody-mediated
   Isohemagglutinins: transfusion reactions, immune hydrops (Rh disease of the newborn)
   Autoantibodies: idiopathic (primary), drug-associated, systemic lupus erythematosus
Mechanical trauma to red cells
   Microangiopathic hemolytic anemias: thrombotic thrombocytopenic purpura, disseminated intravascular coagulation
   Defective cardiac valves
Infections: malaria

Impaired Red Cell Production

Disturbed proliferation and differentiation of stem cells: aplastic anemia, pure red cell aplasia
Disturbed proliferation and maturation of erythroblasts
   Defective DNA synthesis: deficiency or impaired use of vitamin B_{12} and folic acid (megaloblastic anemias)
   Anemia of renal failure (erythropoietin deficiency)
   Anemia of chronic disease (iron sequestration, relative erythropoietin deficiency)
   Anemia of endocrine disorders
   Defective hemoglobin synthesis
      Deficient heme synthesis: iron deficiency, sideroblastic anemias
      Deficient globin synthesis: thalassemias
Marrow replacement: primary hematopoietic neoplasms (acute leukemia, myelodysplastic syndromes)
Marrow infiltration (myelophthisic anemia): metastatic neoplasms, granulomatous disease

later), the decrease in tissue oxygen tension that accompanies anemia triggers increased production of the growth factor *erythropoietin* from specialized cells in the kidney. This in turn drives a compensatory hyperplasia of erythroid precursors in the bone marrow and, in severe anemia, the appearance of *extramedullary hematopoiesis* within the secondary hematopoietic organs (the liver, spleen, and lymph nodes). In well-nourished persons who become anemic because of acute bleeding or increased red cell destruction (hemolysis), the compensatory response can increase the production of red cells fivefold to eightfold. The rise in marrow output is signaled by the appearance of increased numbers of newly formed red cells *(reticulocytes)* in the peripheral blood. By contrast, anemia caused by decreased red cell production (aregenerative anemia) is associated with subnormal reticulocyte counts (reticulocytopenia).

Anemia also can be classified on the basis of red cell morphology, which often points to particular causes. Features that provide etiologic clues include the size, color, and shape of the red cells. These are judged subjectively by visual inspection of peripheral smears and also are expressed quantitatively using the following indices:

- *Mean cell volume* (MCV): the average volume per red cell, expressed in femtoliters (cubic microns)
- *Mean cell hemoglobin* (MCH): the average mass of hemoglobin per red cell, expressed in picograms
- *Mean cell hemoglobin concentration* (MCHC): the average concentration of hemoglobin in a given volume of packed red cells, expressed in grams per deciliter
- *Red cell distribution width* (RDW): the coefficient of variation of red cell volume

Red cell indices are directly measured or automatically calculated by specialized instruments in clinical laboratories. The same instruments also determine the *reticulocyte count,* a simple measure that distinguishes between hemolytic and aregenerative anemia. Adult reference ranges for these tests are shown in Table 12.2. Depending on the differential diagnosis, a number of other blood tests also may be performed to evaluate anemia, including (1) *serum iron indices* (iron levels, iron-binding capacity, transferrin saturation, and ferritin concentrations), which help distinguish among microcytic anemia caused by iron deficiency, chronic inflammation, and thalassemia; (2) *plasma unconjugated bilirubin, haptoglobin, and lactate dehydrogenase levels,* which are abnormal in hemolytic anemia; (3) *serum and red cell folate and vitamin B_{12} concentrations,* which are low in megaloblastic anemia; (4) *hemoglobin electrophoresis,* which is used to detect abnormal hemoglobin; and (5) the *Coombs test,* which is used to detect antibodies or complement bound to red cells in suspected cases of antibody-mediated hemolytic anemia. In isolated anemia, tests performed on the peripheral blood usually suffice to establish the cause. By contrast, when anemia occurs along with thrombocytopenia and/or granulocytopenia, it is much more likely to be associated with marrow aplasia or infiltration; in such instances a marrow examination usually is warranted.

As discussed later, the clinical consequences of anemia are determined by its severity, rapidity of onset, and underlying

Table 12.2 Adult Reference Ranges for Red Blood Cells[a]

	Units	Men	Women
Hemoglobin (Hb)	g/dL	13.2–16.7	11.9–15.0
Hematocrit (Hct)	%	38–48	35–44
Red cell count	×10⁶/μL	4.2–5.6	3.8–5.0
Reticulocyte count	%	0.5–1.5	0.5–1.5
Mean cell volume (MCV)	fL	81–97	81–97
Mean cell Hb (MCH)	pg	28–34	28–34
Mean cell Hb concentration (MCHC)	g/dL	33–35	33–35
Red cell distribution width (RDW)		11.5–14.8	

[a]Reference ranges vary among laboratories. The reference ranges for the laboratory providing the result should always be used in interpreting a laboratory test.

pathogenic mechanism. If the onset is slow, the deficit in O_2-carrying capacity is compensated for by increases in cardiac output, respiratory rate, and red cell 2,3-diphosphoglycerate (DPG), a glycolytic pathway intermediate that enhances the release of O_2 from hemoglobin. These adaptive changes mitigate the effects of mild to moderate anemia in otherwise healthy persons but are less effective in those with compromised pulmonary or cardiac function. Pallor, fatigue, and lassitude are common to all forms of anemia. Anemia caused by the premature destruction of red cells *(hemolytic anemia)* is associated with hyperbilirubinemia, jaundice, and pigment gallstones (if hemolysis is chronic), all related to increases in the turnover of hemoglobin. Anemia that stems from *ineffective hematopoiesis* (the premature death of marrow erythroid progenitors) is associated with inappropriate increases in iron absorption from the gut, which can lead to iron overload *(secondary hemochromatosis)* with consequent damage to endocrine organs and the heart. If left untreated, a severe congenital anemia such as β-thalassemia major inevitably results in growth retardation, skeletal abnormalities, and cachexia.

SUMMARY

PATHOLOGY OF ANEMIA

Causes

- Blood loss (hemorrhage)
- Increased red cell destruction (hemolysis)
- Decreased red cell production

Morphology

- Microcytic (iron deficiency, thalassemia)
- Macrocytic (folate or vitamin B_{12} deficiency)
- Normocytic but with abnormal shapes (hereditary spherocytosis, sickle cell disease)

Clinical Manifestations

- **Acute:** shortness of breath, organ failure, shock
- **Chronic**
  - Pallor, fatigue, lassitude
  - With hemolysis: jaundice and gallstones
  - With ineffective erythropoiesis: iron overload, heart and endocrine failure
  - If severe and congenital: growth retardation, bone deformities due to reactive marrow hyperplasia

ANEMIA OF BLOOD LOSS: HEMORRHAGE

Anemia of blood loss can be divided into anemia caused by acute bleeding (hemorrhage) and anemia caused by chronic blood loss (described later). **The effects of acute bleeding are mainly due to the loss of intravascular volume, which if massive can lead to cardiovascular collapse, shock, and death.** If blood loss exceeds 20% of blood volume, the immediate threat is hypovolemic shock rather than anemia. If the patient survives, hemodilution begins at once and achieves its full effect within 2 to 3 days; only then is the full extent of the red cell loss revealed. The anemia is normocytic and normochromic. Recovery from blood loss anemia is enhanced by a compensatory rise in the erythropoietin level, which stimulates increased red cell production and reticulocytosis within a period of 5 to 7 days.

With chronic blood loss, iron stores are gradually depleted. Iron is essential for hemoglobin synthesis and erythropoiesis, and its deficiency leads to a chronic anemia of underproduction. Iron deficiency anemia can occur in other clinical settings as well; it is described later along with other forms of anemia caused by decreased red cell production.

HEMOLYTIC ANEMIA

Hemolytic anemias are a diverse group of disorders that have as a common feature accelerated red cell destruction (hemolysis). By definition, the red cell life span is shortened to less than its normal 120 days, often markedly so. Regardless of cause, low tissue O_2 levels trigger increased erythropoietin release from the kidney, which in turn stimulates the growth of erythroid elements and increased release of reticulocytes from the bone marrow. Thus, *erythroid hyperplasia* and *reticulocytosis* are hallmarks of all hemolytic anemias. In severe hemolytic anemias, the erythropoietic drive may be so pronounced that *extramedullary hematopoiesis* appears in the liver, spleen, and lymph nodes.

There are several ways to organize hemolytic anemias. One approach groups them according to whether the pathogenic red cell defect is *intrinsic (intracorpuscular)* or *extrinsic (extracorpuscular)* (see Table 12.1). A second more clinically useful approach groups hemolytic anemias according to whether hemolysis is primarily extravascular or intravascular. *Extravascular hemolysis* **is caused by defects that increase the destruction of red cells by phagocytes, particularly in the spleen.** The spleen contains large numbers of macrophages, the principal cell responsible for the removal of damaged or antibody-coated red cells from the circulation. Because extreme alterations of shape are necessary for red cells to navigate the splenic sinusoids, any reduction in red cell deformability makes this passage difficult, and red cells that become "stuck" are recognized and phagocytosed by resident splenic macrophages. As described later in the chapter, diminished deformability is a major cause of red cell destruction in several hemolytic anemias. Findings that are relatively specific for extravascular hemolysis

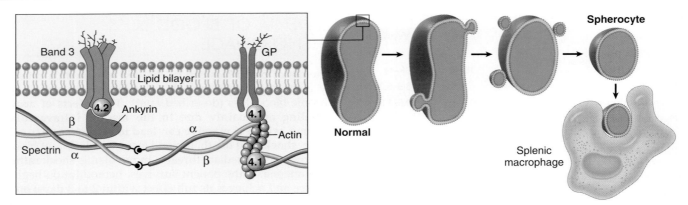

Fig. 12.1 Pathogenesis of hereditary spherocytosis. *(Left panel)* Normal organization of the major red cell membrane skeleton proteins. Mutations in α-spectrin, β-spectrin, ankyrin, band 4.2, and band 3 that weaken the association of the membrane skeleton with the overlying plasma membrane cause red cells to shed membrane vesicles and transform into spherocytes *(right panel).* The nondeformable spherocytes are trapped in the splenic cords and phagocytosed by macrophages. *GP,* Glycophorin.

(as compared to intravascular hemolysis) include the following:

- *Hyperbilirubinemia* and *jaundice,* stemming from degradation of hemoglobin in macrophages
- Varying degrees of *splenomegaly* due to "work hyperplasia" of phagocytes in the spleen
- If long-standing, formation of *bilirubin-rich gallstones* (pigment stones) and an increased risk of *cholelithiasis*

***Intravascular hemolysis,* by contrast, is characterized by injuries so severe that red cells literally burst within the circulation**. Intravascular hemolysis may result from mechanical forces (e.g., turbulence created by a defective heart valve) or biochemical or physical agents that severely damage the red cell membrane (e.g., fixation of complement, or exposure to clostridial toxins or heat). Findings that distinguish intravascular hemolysis from extravascular hemolysis include the presence of the following:

- *Hemoglobinemia, hemoglobinuria,* and *hemosiderinuria.* Hemoglobin released into the circulation is small enough to pass into the urinary space. Here, it is partially resorbed by renal tubular cells and processed into hemosiderin, which is then lost in the urine when renal tubular cells are sloughed.
- *Loss of iron,* which may lead to iron deficiency if hemolysis is persistent. By contrast, iron recycling by phagocytes is very efficient, and so iron deficiency is not a feature of extravascular hemolytic anemias.

A final feature of both intravascular and extravascular hemolysis is decreased serum levels of *haptoglobin,* a plasma protein that binds free hemoglobin and is then removed from the circulation. Apparently macrophages "regurgitate" sufficient hemoglobin during consumption of red cells to cause haptoglobin levels to fall, even when hemolysis is entirely extravascular.

We now turn to some of the common hemolytic anemias.

Hereditary Spherocytosis

This disorder stems from inherited (intrinsic) defects in the red cell membrane that lead to the formation of spherocytes, nondeformable cells that are highly vulnerable to sequestration and destruction in the spleen. Hereditary spherocytosis is usually transmitted as an autosomal dominant trait; a more severe, autosomal recessive form of the disease affects a small minority of patients.

Pathogenesis

Hereditary spherocytosis is caused by inherited defects in the membrane skeleton, a network of proteins that stabilizes the lipid bilayer of the red cell (Fig. 12.1). The major membrane skeleton protein is spectrin, a long, flexible heterodimer that self-associates at one end and binds short actin filaments at its other end. These contacts create a two-dimensional meshwork that is connected to the transmembrane proteins band 3 and glycophorin via the linker proteins ankyrin, band 4.2, and band 4.1.

Mutations that cause hereditary spherocytosis most frequently involve ankyrin, band 3, or spectrin. **The common feature of the pathogenic mutations is that they weaken vertical interactions between the membrane skeleton and intrinsic red cell membrane proteins**. This defect destabilizes the lipid bilayer of red cells, which shed membrane vesicles into the circulation as they age. Little cytoplasm is lost in the process and as a result the surface area-to-volume ratio decreases progressively with time until the cells become spherical (Fig. 12.1).

The critical role of the spleen in hereditary spherocytosis is illustrated by the beneficial effect of splenectomy; although the red cell defect and spherocytes persist, the anemia is corrected. Red cells must undergo extreme degrees of deformation to pass through the splenic cords. The floppy discoid shape of normal red cells allows considerable latitude for shape changes. By contrast, spherocytes have limited deformability and are sequestered in the splenic cords, where they are destroyed by the plentiful resident macrophages.

MORPHOLOGY

On smears, **spherocytes** are dark red and lack central pallor (Fig. 12.2). The excessive red cell destruction and resultant anemia lead to a compensatory hyperplasia of red cell progenitors in the marrow and an increase in red cell production

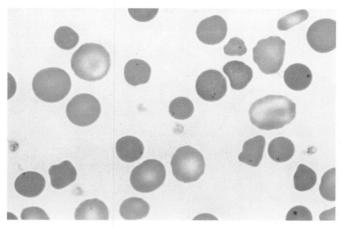

Fig. 12.2 Hereditary spherocytosis—peripheral blood smear. Note the anisocytosis and several hyperchromic spherocytes. Howell-Jolly bodies (small nuclear remnants) are also present in the red cells of this asplenic patient. *(Courtesy of Dr. Robert W. McKenna, Department of Pathology, University of Texas Southwestern Medical School, Dallas, Texas.)*

---

marked by reticulocytosis. **Splenomegaly** is more common and prominent in hereditary spherocytosis than in any other form of hemolytic anemia. The splenic weight usually is between 500 and 1000 g. The enlargement results from marked congestion of the splenic cords and increases in the numbers of macrophages. Phagocytosed red cells are seen within macrophages lining the sinusoids and, in particular, within the cords. The other general features of hemolytic anemia also are present, including **cholelithiasis,** which occurs in 40% to 50% of patients with hereditary spherocytosis.

Clinical Features. The characteristic features are anemia, splenomegaly, and jaundice. The anemia is variable in severity, ranging from subclinical to profound; most commonly it is moderate in degree. Because of their spherical shape, red cells in hereditary spherocytosis show increased *osmotic fragility* when placed in hypotonic salt solutions, a characteristic that can help establish the diagnosis.

The course is generally stable but may be punctuated by *aplastic crises,* the most severe of which are triggered by *parvovirus B19 infection.* This virus has a marked tropism for erythroblasts, which undergo apoptosis during viral replication. Until the immune response controls the infection (usually in 10–14 days), the marrow may be virtually devoid of red cell progenitors. Because of the shortened life span of red cells in hereditary spherocytosis, a lack of red cell production, even for a few days, results in rapid worsening of the anemia. Blood transfusions may be needed to support patients until the infection is cleared.

There is no specific treatment. Splenectomy improves the anemia by removing the major site of red cell destruction. The benefits of splenectomy must be weighed against the increased risk of serious bacterial infections, particularly in children. Partial splenectomy is gaining favor in children because this approach produces hematologic improvement while maintaining protection against sepsis. The downside is that because the partially resected spleen eventually regains its size, many patients will need a second resection.

The hope is that this can be delayed until adulthood, when the risk of serious infection is lower.

Sickle Cell Anemia

Hemoglobinopathies **are a group of hereditary disorders caused by inherited mutations that lead to structural abnormalities in hemoglobin.** Sickle cell anemia, the prototypic hemoglobinopathy, is caused by a mutation in β-globin that creates sickle hemoglobin (HbS). Numerous other hemoglobinopathies have been described, but these are infrequent and beyond the scope of this discussion.

Sickle cell anemia is the most common familial hemolytic anemia. In parts of Africa where malaria is endemic, the gene frequency approaches 30% as a result of a protective effect against *Plasmodium falciparum* malaria. In the United States, approximately 8% of blacks are heterozygous HbS carriers and about 1 in 600 have sickle cell anemia.

Pathogenesis

Sickle cell anemia is caused by a single amino acid substitution in β-globin that results in a tendency for deoxygenated HbS to self-associate into polymers. Normal hemoglobins are tetramers composed of two pairs of similar chains. On average, the normal adult red cell contains 96% HbA (α2β2), 3% HbA2 (α2δ2), and 1% fetal Hb (HbF, α2γ2). In patients with sickle cell anemia, HbA is completely replaced by HbS, whereas in heterozygous carriers, only about half is replaced. HbS differs from HbA by having a valine residue instead of a glutamate residue at the 6th amino acid position in β-globin. On deoxygenation HbS molecules undergo a conformational change that allows polymers to form via intermolecular contacts involving the abnormal valine residue. These polymers distort the red cell, which assumes an elongated crescentic, or sickle, shape (Fig. 12.3).

The sickling of red cells initially is reversible on reoxygenation. However, membrane distortion produced by each sickling episode leads to an influx of calcium, which causes the loss of potassium and water and also damages the membrane skeleton. With time, this cumulative damage creates *irreversibly sickled cells* that rapidly undergo hemolysis.

Three factors are particularly important in determining whether clinically significant polymerization of HbS occurs in patients:

- *The intracellular levels of hemoglobins other than HbS.* In heterozygotes approximately 40% of Hb is HbS and the remainder is HbA, which interacts only weakly with deoxygenated HbS. Because HbA greatly retards HbS polymerization, the red cells of HbS heterozygotes have little tendency to sickle in vivo. Such persons are said to have *sickle cell trait.* Similarly, because fetal hemoglobin (HbF) interacts weakly with HbS, newborns with sickle cell anemia do not manifest the disease until HbF falls to adult levels, generally around the age of 5 to 6 months. Hemoglobin C (HbC), another mutant β-globin, has a lysine residue instead of the normal glutamic acid residue at position 6. About 2.3% of American blacks are heterozygous carriers of HbC and about 1 in 1250 newborns are compound HbC/HbS heterozygotes. HbC has a greater tendency to aggregate with HbS than does

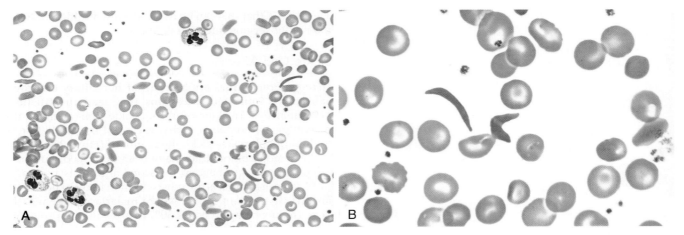

Fig. 12.3 Sickle cell anemia—peripheral blood smear. (A) Low magnification shows sickle cells, anisocytosis, poikilocytosis, and target cells. (B) Higher magnification shows an irreversibly sickled cell in the center. *(Courtesy of Dr. Robert W. McKenna, Department of Pathology, University of Texas Southwestern Medical School, Dallas, Texas.)*

HbA, and as a result HbS/HbC compound heterozygotes have a symptomatic sickling disorder called *HbSC disease.*

- *The intracellular concentration of HbS.* The polymerization of deoxygenated HbS is strongly concentration-dependent. Thus, red cell dehydration, which increases the Hb concentration, facilitates sickling. Conversely, the coexistence of α-thalassemia (described later), which decreases the Hb concentration, reduces sickling.

- *The time required for red cells to pass through the microvasculature.* The normal transit times of red cells through capillary beds are too short for significant polymerization of deoxygenated HbS to occur. Hence, the tissues that are most susceptible to obstruction by sickling are those in which blood flow is normally sluggish, such as the spleen and the bone marrow. However, sickling may occur in other microvascular beds in the face of factors that retard the passage of red cells, particularly inflammation. Recall that inflammation slows blood flow by increasing the adhesion of leukocytes and red cells to endothelium and by inducing the exudation of fluid through leaky vessels (Chapter 4). In addition, sickle red cells have a greater tendency than normal red cells to adhere to endothelial cells, apparently because repeated bouts of sickling cause membrane damage that makes the red cells sticky. These factors conspire to prolong the transit times of sickle red cells, increasing the probability of clinically significant sickling.

The sickling of red cells has two major pathologic consequences: chronic moderately severe hemolytic anemia, produced by red cell membrane damage, and vascular obstructions, which result in ischemic tissue damage and pain crises (Fig. 12.4). The mean life span of red cells in sickle cell anemia averages only 20 days (one-sixth of normal), and the severity of the hemolysis correlates with the fraction of irreversibly sickled cells that are present in the blood. Vasoocclusion, by contrast, does not correlate with the number of irreversibly sickled cells and instead appears to result from superimposed factors such as infection, inflammation, dehydration, and acidosis, all

of which enhance the tendency of red cells to sickle within the microvasculature.

● MORPHOLOGY

The anatomic alterations in sickle cell anemia stem from (1) severe chronic hemolytic anemia, (2) increased breakdown of heme to bilirubin, and (3) microvascular obstructions, which provoke tissue ischemia and infarction. In peripheral smears, elongated, spindled, or boat-shaped **irreversibly sickled red cells** are evident (Fig. 12.3). Both the anemia and the vascular stasis lead to hypoxia-induced fatty changes in the heart, liver, and renal tubules. There is a compensatory **hyperplasia of erythroid progenitors** in the marrow. The cellular proliferation in the marrow often causes bone resorption and secondary new bone formation, resulting in prominent cheekbones and changes in the skull resembling a "crewcut" in radiographs. Extramedullary hematopoiesis may appear in the liver and spleen.

In children there is moderate **splenomegaly** (splenic weight up to 500 g) due to red pulp congestion caused by entrapment of sickled red cells. However, chronic splenic erythrostasis produces hypoxic damage and infarcts, which with time reduce the spleen to a useless nubbin of fibrous tissue. This process, referred to as **autosplenectomy,** is complete by adulthood.

Vascular congestion, thrombosis, and infarction can affect any organ, including the bones, liver, kidney, retina, brain, lung, and skin. The bone marrow is particularly prone to ischemia because of its sluggish blood flow and high rate of metabolism. Priapism, another frequent problem, can lead to penile fibrosis and erectile dysfunction. As with the other hemolytic anemias, **hemosiderosis** and **pigment gallstones** are common.

Clinical Features. From its onset, the disease runs an unremitting course punctuated by sudden crises. Homozygous sickle cell disease usually is asymptomatic until 6 months of age when the shift from HbF to HbS is complete. The anemia is moderate to severe; most patients have hematocrits of 18% to 30% (normal range, 38%–48%). The

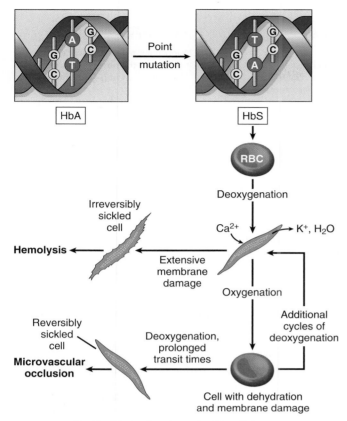

Fig. 12.4 Pathophysiology of sickle cell disease.

chronic hemolysis is associated with hyperbilirubinemia and compensatory reticulocytosis.

Much more serious are vasoocclusive crises, which are characteristically associated with pain and often lead to tissue damage and significant morbidity and mortality. Among the most common and serious of these vasoocclusive crises are the following:

- *Hand-foot syndrome*, resulting from infarction of bones in the hands and feet, is the most common presenting symptom in young children.
- *Acute chest syndrome*, in which sluggish blood flow in inflamed lung (e.g., an area of pneumonia) leads to sickling within hypoxemic pulmonary beds. This exacerbates pulmonary dysfunction, creating a vicious circle of worsening pulmonary and systemic hypoxemia, sickling, and vasoocclusion. Acute chest syndrome may also be triggered by fat emboli emanating from infarcted bone.
- *Stroke*, which sometimes occurs in the setting of the acute chest syndrome. Stroke and the acute chest syndrome are the two leading causes of ischemia-related death.
- *Proliferative retinopathy*, a consequence of vasoocclusions in the eye that can lead to loss of visual acuity and blindness.

Another acute event, *aplastic crisis,* is caused by a sudden decrease in red cell production. As in hereditary spherocytosis, this usually is triggered by the infection of erythroblasts by parvovirus B19 and, although severe, is self-limited.

In addition to these crises, patients with sickle cell disease are prone to infections. Both children and adults with sickle cell disease are functionally asplenic, making them susceptible to infections caused by encapsulated bacteria, such as pneumococci. In adults the basis for "hyposplenism" is autoinfarction. In the earlier childhood phase of splenic enlargement, congestion caused by trapped sickled red cells apparently interferes with bacterial sequestration and killing; hence, even children with enlarged spleens are at risk for the development of fatal septicemia. Patients with sickle cell disease also are predisposed to *Salmonella* osteomyelitis, possibly in part because of poorly understood acquired defects in complement function.

In homozygous sickle cell disease, irreversibly sickled red cells are seen in routine peripheral blood smears. In sickle cell trait, sickling can be induced in vitro by exposing cells to marked hypoxia. The diagnosis is confirmed by electrophoretic demonstration of HbS. Prenatal diagnosis of sickle cell anemia can be performed by analyzing fetal DNA obtained by amniocentesis or biopsy of chorionic villi.

The clinical course of sickle cell disease is highly variable. As a result of improvements in supportive care, an increasing number of patients are surviving into adulthood. Approximately 50% of patients now survive beyond the fifth decade. Of particular importance is prophylactic treatment with penicillin to prevent pneumococcal infections, especially in children younger than age 5.

A mainstay of therapy is hydroxyurea, a "gentle" inhibitor of DNA synthesis. Hydroxyurea reduces pain crises and lessens the anemia through several effects, including (1) an increase in levels of HbF; (2) an anti-inflammatory effect because of the inhibition of white cell production; (3) an increase in red cell size, which lowers the intracellular hemoglobin concentration; and (4) its metabolism to NO, a potent vasodilator and inhibitor of platelet aggregation. Encouraging results also have been obtained with allogeneic bone marrow transplantation, which is potentially curative.

Thalassemia

Thalassemias are inherited disorders caused by mutations in globin genes that decrease the synthesis of α- or β-globin. Decreased synthesis of one globin results not only in a deficiency of Hb, but also in red cell damage that is caused by precipitates formed from excess unpaired "normal" globin chains. The mutations that cause thalassemia are particularly common in Mediterranean, African, and Asian regions in which malaria is endemic. As with HbS, it is hypothesized that globin mutations associated with thalassemia protect against falciparum malaria.

Pathogenesis

A diverse collection of α-globin and β-globin mutations underlies the thalassemias, which are autosomal codominant conditions. As described previously, adult hemoglobin, or HbA, is a tetramer composed of two α chains and two β chains. The α chains are encoded by two α-globin

Table 12.3 Clinical and Genetic Classification of Thalassemias

Clinical Syndrome	Genotype	Clinical Features	Molecular Genetics
β-Thalassemias			Mainly point mutations that lead to defects in the transcription, splicing, or translation of β-globin mRNA
β-Thalassemia major	Homozygous β-thalassemia (β^0/β^0, β^+/β^+, β^0/β^+)	Severe anemia; regular blood transfusions required	
β-Thalassemia intermedia	Variable (β^0/β^+, β^+/β^+, β^0/β, β^+/β)	Moderately severe anemia; regular blood transfusions not required	
β-Thalassemia minor	Heterozygous β-thalassemia (β^0/β, β^+/β)	Asymptomatic with mild or absent anemia; red cell abnormalities seen	
α-Thalassemias			Mainly gene deletions
Silent carrier	$-/\alpha$, α/α	Asymptomatic; no red cell abnormality	
α-Thalassemia trait	$-/-$, α/α (Asian) $-/\alpha$, $-/\alpha$ (black African, Asian)	Asymptomatic, like β-thalassemia minor	
HbH disease	$-/-$, $-/\alpha$	Severe; resembles β-thalassemia intermedia	
Hydrops fetalis	$-/-$, $-/-$	Lethal in utero without transfusions	

HgH, Hemoglobin H; *mRNA*, messenger ribonucleic acid.

genes lying in tandem on chromosome 16, whereas the β chains are encoded by a single β-globin gene located on chromosome 11. The clinical features vary widely depending on the specific combination of mutated alleles that are inherited by the patient (Table 12.3), as described next.

β-Thalassemia

Mutations associated with β-thalassemia fall into two categories: (1) β^0, in which no β-globin chains are produced; and (2) β^+, in which there is reduced (but detectable) β-globin synthesis. Sequencing of β-thalassemia genes has shown more than 100 different causative mutations, a majority consisting of single-base changes. Persons inheriting one abnormal allele have *β-thalassemia minor* (also known as *β-thalassemia trait*), which is asymptomatic or mildly symptomatic. Most people inheriting any two β^0 and β^+ alleles have *β-thalassemia major*; occasionally, persons inheriting at least one β^+ allele have a milder disease termed *β-thalassemia intermedia*. In contrast with α-thalassemia (described later), gene deletions rarely underlie β-thalassemia (Table 12.3).

The mutations responsible for β-thalassemia are diverse and disrupt β-globin synthesis in several different ways. The most common mutations lead to abnormal RNA splicing, whereas others fall in the β-globin gene promoter or coding regions. The specific nature of the mutation determines whether the outcome is a β^+ or β^0 allele.

Defective synthesis of β-globin in β-thalassemia contributes to anemia through two mechanisms: (1) inadequate HbA formation, resulting in small (microcytic), poorly hemoglobinized (hypochromic) red cells; and (2) by allowing the accumulation of unpaired α-globin chains, which form toxic precipitates that severely damage the membranes of red cells and erythroid precursors. A high fraction of erythroid precursors are so badly damaged that they die by apoptosis (Fig. 12.5), a phenomenon termed *ineffective erythropoiesis*, and the few red cells that are produced have a shortened life span. Ineffective hematopoiesis has another untoward effect; it is associated with an inappropriate increase in the absorption of dietary iron, which without medical intervention inevitably leads to *iron overload*. The increased iron absorption is caused by

inappropriately low hepcidin, which is a negative regulator of iron absorption (see later).

α-Thalassemia

Unlike β-thalassemia, **α-thalassemia is caused mainly by deletions involving one or more of the α-globin genes.** The severity of the disease is proportional to the number of α-globin genes that are deleted (Table 12.3). For example, loss of a single α-globin gene produces a silent-carrier state, whereas deletion of all four α-globin genes is lethal in utero because the red cells have virtually no oxygen-delivering capacity. With loss of three α-globin genes there is a relative excess of β-globin or (early in life) γ-globin chains. Excess β-globin and γ-globin chains form relatively stable β4 and γ4 tetramers known as *HbH* and *Hb Bart*, respectively, which cause less membrane damage than the free α-globin chains that are found in β-thalassemia; as a result, ineffective erythropoiesis is less pronounced in α-thalassemia. Unfortunately, both HbH and Hb Bart have an abnormally high affinity for oxygen, which renders them ineffective at delivering oxygen to the tissues.

MORPHOLOGY

A range of morphologies is seen, depending on the specific underlying molecular lesion. On one end of the spectrum is β-thalassemia minor and α-thalassemia trait, in which abnormalities are confined to the peripheral blood. In smears the red cells are small (microcytic) and pale (hypochromic), but regular in shape. Often seen are **target cells,** cells with an increased surface area-to-volume ratio that allows the cytoplasm to collect in a central, dark-red "puddle." On the other end of the spectrum, in β-thalassemia major peripheral blood smears show marked **microcytosis, hypochromia, poikilocytosis** (variation in cell shape), and **anisocytosis** (variation in cell size). Nucleated red cells (normoblasts) are also seen that reflect the underlying erythropoietic drive. β-Thalassemia intermedia and

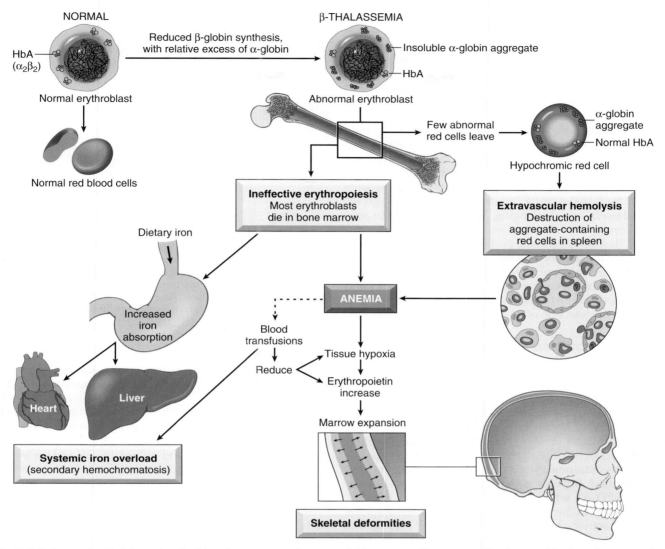

Fig. 12.5 Pathogenesis of β-thalassemia major. Note that aggregates of excess α-globin are not visible on routine blood smears. Blood transfusions constitute a double-edged sword, diminishing the anemia and its attendant complications but also adding to the systemic iron overload.

HbH disease are associated with peripheral smear findings that lie between these two extremes.

The anatomic changes in β-thalassemia major are similar in kind to those seen in other hemolytic anemias but are profound in degree. Ineffective erythropoiesis and hemolysis result in a striking hyperplasia of erythroid progenitors, with a shift toward early forms. The expanded erythropoietic marrow may completely fill the intramedullary space of the skeleton, invade the bony cortex, impair bone growth, and produce **skeletal deformities.** Extramedullary hematopoiesis and hyperplasia of mononuclear phagocytes result in prominent **splenomegaly,** hepatomegaly, and lymphadenopathy. The ineffective erythropoietic precursors consume nutrients and produce growth retardation and a degree of **cachexia** reminiscent of that seen in cancer patients. Unless steps are taken to prevent iron overload, during the span of years severe **hemosiderosis** develops (Fig. 12.5). HbH disease and β-thalassemia intermedia are also associated with splenomegaly, erythroid hyperplasia, and growth retardation related to anemia, but these are less severe than in β-thalassemia major.

Clinical Features. β-*Thalassemia trait* and α-*thalassemia trait* are typically asymptomatic. There is usually only a mild microcytic hypochromic anemia; generally, these patients have a normal life expectancy. Iron deficiency anemia is associated with a similar red cell appearance and must be excluded by appropriate laboratory tests (described later).

β-*Thalassemia major* manifests postnatally as HbF synthesis diminishes. Affected children suffer from growth retardation that commences in infancy. They are sustained by blood transfusions, which improve the anemia and reduce the skeletal deformities associated with excessive erythropoiesis. With transfusions alone, survival into the second or third decade is possible, but systemic iron overload gradually develops owing to inappropriate uptake of iron from the gut and the iron load in transfused red cells. Unless patients are treated aggressively with iron chelators, cardiac dysfunction from *secondary hemochromatosis* inevitably develops and often is fatal in the second or third decade of life. When feasible, hematopoietic stem cell transplantation at an early age is the treatment of choice. *HbH disease* and *β-thalassemia intermedia* are not as severe as β-thalassemia major, because the imbalance in α- and β-globin chain synthesis is not as great and hematopoiesis is more effective. Anemia is of moderate severity and patients usually do not require transfusions. Thus, the iron overload that is so common in β-thalassemia major is rarely seen.

The diagnosis of β-thalassemia major can be strongly suspected on clinical grounds. Hb electrophoresis shows a profound reduction or absence of HbA and increased levels of HbF. The HbA2 level may be normal or increased. Similar but less severe changes are noted in patients affected by β-thalassemia intermedia. Prenatal diagnosis of β-thalassemia is challenging, but can be made in specialized centers by DNA analysis. In fact, thalassemia was the first disease diagnosed by DNA-based tests, opening the way for the field of molecular diagnostics. The diagnosis of β-thalassemia minor is made by Hb electrophoresis, which typically shows a reduced level of HbA ($\alpha 2\beta 2$) and an increased level of HbA2 ($\alpha 2\delta 2$). HbH disease can be diagnosed by detection of $\beta 4$ tetramers by electrophoresis.

Glucose-6-Phosphate Dehydrogenase Deficiency

Red cells are constantly exposed to both endogenous and exogenous oxidants, which are normally inactivated by reduced glutathione (GSH). Abnormalities affecting enzymes responsible for the synthesis of GSH leave red cells vulnerable to oxidative injury and hemolysis. By far the most common of these conditions is glucose-6-phosphate dehydrogenase (G6PD) deficiency. The G6PD gene is on the X chromosome. More than 400 G6PD variants have been identified, but only a few are associated with disease. One is G6PD A⁻, which is carried by approximately 10% of black males in the United States. G6PD A⁻ has a normal enzymatic activity but a decreased half-life. Because red cells do not synthesize proteins, older G6PD A⁻ red cells become progressively deficient in enzyme activity and GSH. This in turn renders older red cells more sensitive to oxidant damage.

Pathogenesis

G6PD deficiency is associated with transient episodes of intravascular hemolysis caused by exposure to an environmental factor (usually infectious agents or drugs) that produces oxidant stress. Incriminated drugs include antimalarials (e.g., primaquine), sulfonamides, nitrofurantoin, phenacetin, aspirin (in large doses), and vitamin K derivatives. More commonly episodes of hemolysis are triggered by infection, which induce phagocytes to generate oxidants as part of the host response. These oxidants, such as hydrogen peroxide, are normally sopped up by GSH, which is converted to oxidized GSH in the process. Because regeneration of GSH is impaired in G6PD-deficient cells, oxidants are free to "attack" other red cell components including globin chains. Oxidized hemoglobin denatures and precipitates, forming intracellular inclusions called *Heinz bodies*, which can damage the red cell membrane so severely that intravascular hemolysis results. Other cells with lesser damage lose their deformability and suffer further injury when splenic phagocytes attempt to "pluck

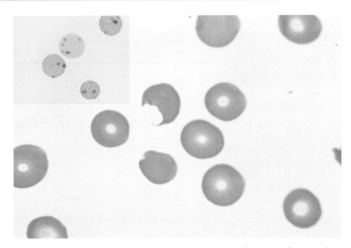

Fig. 12.6 Glucose-6-phosphate dehydrogenase deficiency after oxidant drug exposure—peripheral blood smear. (Inset) Red cells with precipitates of denatured globin (Heinz bodies) shown by supravital staining. As the splenic macrophages pluck out these inclusions, "bite cells" similar to the one in this smear are produced. *(Courtesy of Dr. Robert W. McKenna, Department of Pathology, University of Texas Southwestern Medical School, Dallas, Texas.)*

out" the Heinz bodies, creating *bite cells* (Fig. 12.6). Such cells become trapped on recirculation to the spleen and are destroyed by phagocytes (extravascular hemolysis).

Clinical Features. Hemolysis typically develops 2 or 3 days after drug exposure and is of variable severity. Because G6PD is X-linked, the red cells of affected males are uniformly deficient and vulnerable to oxidant injury. By contrast, random inactivation of one X chromosome in heterozygous females (Chapter 7) creates two populations of red cells, one normal and the other G6PD-deficient. Most carrier females are unaffected except for those with a large proportion of deficient red cells (a chance situation known as *unfavorable lyonization*). In the case of the G6PD A⁻ variant, it is mainly older red cells that are susceptible to lysis. Because the marrow compensates for the anemia by increasing its production of new red cells with adequate levels of G6PD, the hemolysis abates even if the drug exposure continues. In other variants such as G6PD Mediterranean, found mainly in the Middle East, the enzyme deficiency and the hemolysis that occur on exposure to oxidants are more severe.

Paroxysmal Nocturnal Hemoglobinuria

Paroxysmal nocturnal hemoglobinuria (PNH) is a hemolytic anemia that stems from acquired mutations in *PIGA*, a gene required for the synthesis of phosphatidylinositol glycan (PIG), which serves as a membrane anchor for many proteins. Because *PIGA* is X-linked, normal cells have only one active *PIGA* gene, a mutation of which is sufficient to cause PIGA deficiency. The pathogenic mutations in PNH occur in an early hematopoietic progenitor that is capable of giving rise to red cells, leukocytes, and platelets. Progeny of the *PIGA*-mutated clone lack the ability to make "PIG-tailed" proteins, including several that limit the activity of complement; as a result, red cells derived from *PIGA*-deficient precursors are inordinately sensitive to lysis by the complement C5b-C9 membrane attack complex. Leukocytes share the same deficiency but are less sensitive to complement than are red cells, and so red cells take the brunt of the attack. The nocturnal hemolysis that gives PNH its name occurs because complement fixation is enhanced by the decrease in blood pH that accompanies sleep (owing to CO_2 retention). However, most patients present less dramatically with anemia and iron deficiency resulting from chronic intravascular hemolysis.

The most feared complication of PNH is thrombosis, which often occurs within abdominal vessels such as the portal vein and the hepatic vein. The prothrombotic state also is somehow related to excessive complement activity, as Eculizimab, an antibody that binds C5 and inhibits the assembly of the C5b–C9 membrane attack complex, greatly lessens the incidence of thrombosis as well as the degree of intravascular hemolysis. Eculizimab has no effect on early stages of complement fixation, and treated patients continue to have varying degrees of extravascular hemolysis because of the deposition of C3b on red cell surfaces. Loss of C5b-C9 activity in patients receiving Eculizimab poses a risk for *Neisseria* infections, particularly meningococcal sepsis; thus, all treated patients must be vaccinated against *N. meningococcus*.

Immunohemolytic Anemia

Immunohemolytic anemia is caused by antibodies that bind to determinants on red cell membranes. These antibodies may arise spontaneously or be induced by exogenous agents such as drugs or chemicals. Immunohemolytic anemia is uncommon and is classified based on (1) the nature of the antibody and (2) the presence of predisposing conditions (summarized in Table 12.4).

The diagnosis depends on the detection of antibodies and/or complement on red cells. This is done with the *direct Coombs test,* in which the patient's red cells are incubated with antibodies against human immunoglobulin or complement. In a positive test result, these antibodies cause the patient's red cells to clump (agglutinate). The *indirect Coombs test,* which assesses the ability of the patient's serum to agglutinate test red cells bearing defined surface determinants, can then be used to characterize the target of the antibody.

Warm Antibody Immunohemolytic Anemia

In this entity, hemolysis results from the binding of high-affinity autoantibodies to red cells, which are then removed from the circulation by phagocytes in the

spleen and elsewhere. In addition to frank erythrophagocytosis, incomplete consumption ("nibbling") of antibody-coated red cells by macrophages removes membrane and transforms red cells into *spherocytes,* which are rapidly destroyed in the spleen, just as in hereditary spherocytosis (described earlier). Warm antibody immunohemolytic anemia is caused by immunoglobulin G (IgG) or (rarely) IgA antibodies that are active at 37°C. More than 60% of cases are idiopathic (primary), whereas another 25% are secondary to an underlying immunologic disorder (e.g., systemic lupus erythematosus) or are induced by drugs. The clinical severity is variable, but most patients have chronic mild anemia and moderate splenomegaly and require no treatment.

The mechanisms of hemolysis induced by drugs are varied and in some instances poorly understood. Drugs such as α-methyldopa induce autoantibodies against intrinsic red cell constituents, in particular Rh blood group antigens. Presumably, the drug somehow alters the immunogenicity of native epitopes and thereby circumvents T cell tolerance (Chapter 5). Other drugs such as penicillin act as haptens, which induce an antibody response by binding covalently to red cell membrane proteins. Sometimes antibodies recognize a drug in the circulation and form immune complexes that are deposited on red cells. Here they may fix complement or act as opsonins, either of which can lead to hemolysis.

Cold Antibody Immunohemolytic Anemia

Cold antibody immunohemolytic anemia usually is caused by low-affinity IgM antibodies that bind to red cell membranes only at temperatures below 30°C, such as occur in distal parts of the body (e.g., ears, hands, and toes) in cold weather. Although bound IgM fixes complement, the latter steps of the complement cascade occur inefficiently at temperatures lower than 37°C. As a result, most cells with bound IgM pick up some C3b but are not lysed intravascularly. When these cells travel to warmer areas, the weakly bound IgM antibody is released, but the coating of C3b remains. Because C3b is an opsonin (Chapter 2), the cells are phagocytosed by macrophages, mainly in the spleen and liver; hence, in most cases the hemolysis is mainly extravascular. Binding of pentavalent IgM also crosslinks red cells and causes them to clump (*agglutinate*). Sludging of blood in capillaries because of agglutination often produces *Raynaud phenomenon* in the extremities of affected individuals. Cold agglutinins sometimes also appear transiently during recovery from pneumonia caused by *Mycoplasma* spp. and infectious mononucleosis, producing a mild anemia of little clinical importance. More important, chronic forms of cold agglutinin hemolytic anemia occur in association with certain B cell neoplasms or as an idiopathic condition.

Hemolytic Anemia Resulting From Mechanical Trauma to Red Cells

Hemolysis of red cells due to their exposure to abnormal mechanical forces occurs in two major settings. Clinically significant *traumatic hemolysis* is sometimes produced by defective cardiac valve prostheses, which may create sufficiently turbulent blood flow to shear red cells (the blender

Table 12.4 Classification of Immunohemolytic Anemias

Warm Antibody Type
Primary (idiopathic)
Secondary: B cell neoplasms (e.g., chronic lymphocytic leukemia), autoimmune disorders (e.g., systemic lupus erythematosus), drugs (e.g., α-methyldopa, penicillin, quinidine)

Cold Antibody Type
Acute: Mycoplasma infection, infectious mononucleosis
Chronic: idiopathic, B cell lymphoid neoplasms (e.g., lymphoplasmacytic lymphoma)

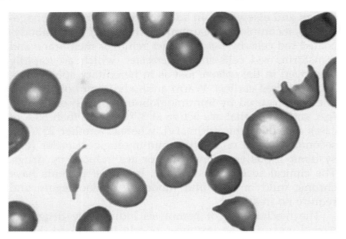

Fig. 12.7 Microangiopathic hemolytic anemia—peripheral blood smear. This specimen from a patient with hemolytic uremic syndrome contains several fragmented red cells. *(Courtesy of Dr. Robert W. McKenna, Department of Pathology, University of Texas Southwestern Medical School, Dallas, Texas.)*

effect). More commonly, it occurs incidentally during an activity involving repeated physical pounding of one or more body parts (e.g., marathon racing, karate chopping, bongo drumming). *Microangiopathic hemolytic anemia* is observed in pathologic states in which small vessels become partially obstructed or narrowed by lesions that predispose passing red cells to mechanical damage. The most frequent of these conditions is disseminated intravascular coagulation (DIC) (see later), in which vessels are narrowed by the intravascular deposition of fibrin. Other causes of microangiopathic hemolytic anemia include malignant hypertension, systemic lupus erythematosus, thrombotic thrombocytopenic purpura (TTP), hemolytic uremic syndrome (HUS), and disseminated cancer. Mechanical fragmentation of red cells (*schistocytosis*) leads to the appearance of characteristic "burr cells," "helmet cells," and "triangle cells" in peripheral blood smears (Fig. 12.7). Although microangiopathic hemolysis is not usually a major clinical problem in and of itself, it often points to a serious underlying condition.

Malaria

It is estimated that malaria affects 500 million and kills more than 1 million people per year, making it one of the most serious afflictions of humans. Malaria is endemic in Asia and Africa, but with widespread jet travel cases are now seen all over the world. It is caused by one of five types of protozoa. Of these, the most important is *Plasmodium falciparum*, which causes tertian malaria (falciparum malaria), a disorder with a high fatality rate. The other four species of *Plasmodium* that infect humans—*Plasmodium malariae, Plasmodium vivax, Plasmodium knowlesi*, and *Plasmodium ovale*—cause relatively benign disease. All forms are transmitted by the bite of female *Anopheles* mosquitoes, and humans are the only natural reservoir.

Pathogenesis

The life cycle of plasmodia is complex (Fig. 12.8). As mosquitoes feed on human blood, *sporozoites* are introduced from the saliva and within a few minutes infect liver cells. Here the parasites multiply rapidly to form a schizont containing thousands of *merozoites*. After a period of days to several weeks that varies with the *Plasmodium* species, the infected hepatocytes release the merozoites, which quickly infect red cells. Intraerythrocytic parasites either continue asexual reproduction to produce more merozoites or give rise to *gametocytes* capable of infecting the next hungry mosquito. During their asexual reproduction in red cells, each of the four forms of malaria develops into *trophozoites*. The asexual phase is completed when the trophozoites give rise to new merozoites, which escape by lysing the red cells.

Fatal falciparum malaria often involves the small vessels of the brain, a complication known as cerebral malaria. Normally, red cells bear negatively charged surfaces that interact poorly with endothelial cells. Infection of red cells with *P. falciparum* induces the appearance of positively charged surface knobs containing parasite-encoded proteins, which bind to adhesion molecules expressed on activated endothelium. Several endothelial cell adhesion molecules, including intercellular adhesion molecule-1 (ICAM-1), appear to mediate this interaction, which leads to the trapping of red cells in postcapillary venules. In an unfortunate minority of patients, mainly children, this process involves cerebral vessels, which become engorged and occluded.

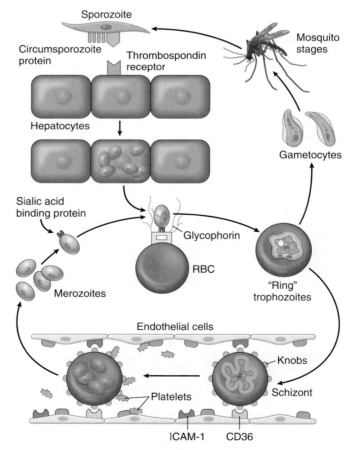

Fig. 12.8 Life cycle of *Plasmodium falciparum*. *ICAM-1*, Intercellular adhesion molecule-1; *RBC*, red blood cell. *(Drawn by Dr. Jeffrey Joseph, Department of Pathology, Beth Israel Deaconess Hospital, Boston, Massachusetts.)*

MORPHOLOGY

Red cell trophozoites from each *Plasmodium* species have a somewhat distinctive appearance, allowing expert observers to determine which species is responsible for an infection from examination of appropriately stained thick smears of peripheral blood. The destruction of red cells leads to **hemolytic anemia**, with its attendant features and laboratory findings. A characteristic brown malarial pigment derived from hemoglobin called **hematin** is released from the ruptured red cells and produces discoloration of the spleen, liver, lymph nodes, and bone marrow. Activation of defense mechanisms in the host leads to a marked hyperplasia of mononuclear phagocytes, producing **massive splenomegaly** and occasional hepatomegaly.

Clinical Features

Showers of new merozoites are released from the red cells at intervals of approximately 24 hours for *P. knowlesi*, 48 hours for *P. vivax*, *P. ovale*, and *P. falciparum*, and 72 hours for *P. malariae*. Episodic shaking, chills, and fever coincide with this release. Hemolytic anemia of varying severity is a constant feature. *Cerebral malaria* associated with *P. falciparum* is rapidly progressive; convulsions, coma, and death usually occur within days to weeks. Fortunately, falciparum malaria more often pursues a chronic course that may be punctuated at any time by *blackwater fever*. The trigger is obscure for this uncommon complication, which is associated with massive intravascular hemolysis, hemoglobinemia, hemoglobinuria, and jaundice.

With appropriate chemotherapy, the prognosis for patients with most forms of malaria is good; however, falciparum malaria is becoming more difficult to treat due to the emergence of drug-resistant strains. Because of the potentially serious consequences of the disease, early diagnosis and treatment are important. The ultimate solution is an effective vaccine, which is long sought but still elusive.

SUMMARY

HEMOLYTIC ANEMIA

Hereditary Spherocytosis

- Autosomal dominant disorder caused by mutations that affect the red cell membrane skeleton, leading to loss of membrane and eventual conversion of red cells to spherocytes, which are phagocytosed and removed in the spleen
- Manifested by anemia, splenomegaly

Sickle Cell Anemia

- Autosomal recessive disorder resulting from a mutation in β-globin that causes deoxygenated hemoglobin to self-associate into long polymers that distort the red cell
- Blockage of vessels by sickled cells causes pain crises and tissue infarction, particularly of the marrow and spleen
- Red cell membrane damage caused by repeated bouts of sickling results in a moderate to severe hemolytic anemia
- Patients are at high risk for bacterial infections and stroke

Thalassemia

- Autosomal codominant disorders caused by mutations in α- or β-globin that reduce hemoglobin synthesis, resulting in a microcytic, hypochromic anemia. In β-thalassemia, unpaired α-globin chains form aggregates that damage red cell precursors and further impair erythropoiesis.

Glucose-6-Phosphate Dehydrogenase (G6PD) Deficiency

- X-linked disorder caused by mutations that destabilize G6PD, making red cells susceptible to oxidant damage

Immunohemolytic Anemia

- Caused by antibodies against either normal red cell constituents or antigens modified by haptens (such as drugs)
- Antibody binding results in either red cell opsonization and extravascular hemolysis or (uncommonly) complement fixation and intravascular hemolysis

Malaria

- Intracellular red cell parasite that causes chronic hemolysis of variable severity
- Falciparum malaria may be fatal because of the propensity of infected red cells to adhere to small vessels in the brain (cerebral malaria)

ANEMIA OF DIMINISHED ERYTHROPOIESIS

Anemias of diminished erythropoiesis include those caused by an inadequate dietary supply of nutrients, particularly iron, folic acid, and vitamin B_{12}. Other anemias of this type are associated with bone marrow failure (aplastic anemia), systemic inflammation (anemia of chronic inflammation), or bone marrow infiltration by tumor or inflammatory cells (myelophthisic anemia). In this section, some common examples of anemias of these types are discussed individually.

Iron Deficiency Anemia

Deficiency of iron is the most common nutritional deficiency in the world and results in clinical signs and symptoms that are mostly related to anemia. About 10% of people living in developed countries and 25% to 50% of those in developing countries are anemic, and in both settings the most frequent cause is iron deficiency. The factors responsible for iron deficiency differ in various populations and are best understood in the context of normal iron metabolism.

The normal total body iron mass is about 2.5 g for women and 3.5 g for men. Approximately 80% of functional body iron is present in hemoglobin, with the remainder located in myoglobin and iron-containing enzymes (e.g., catalase, cytochromes). The iron storage pool, consisting of hemosiderin and ferritin-bound iron in the liver, spleen, bone marrow, and skeletal muscle, contains on average 15% to 20% of total body iron. Because *serum ferritin* is largely derived from this storage pool, the serum ferritin level is a good measure of iron stores. *Assessment of bone marrow iron is another reliable but more invasive method for estimating iron stores.* Iron is transported in the plasma bound to the protein *transferrin*. In normal persons, transferrin is about 33% saturated with iron, yielding serum iron levels that average 120 µg/dL in men and 100 µg/dL in women. Thus, the normal total iron-binding capacity of serum is 300 to 350 µg/dL.

In keeping with the high prevalence of iron deficiency, evolutionary pressures have yielded metabolic pathways that are strongly biased toward iron retention. Iron is lost at a rate of 1 to 2 mg/day through the shedding of mucosal and skin epithelial cells, and this loss must be balanced by the absorption of dietary iron, which is tightly regulated (described later). The normal daily Western diet contains 10 to 20 mg of iron. Most is found in heme within meat and poultry, with the remainder present as inorganic iron in vegetables. About 20% of heme and 1% to 2% of nonheme iron are absorbable; hence, the average Western diet contains sufficient iron to balance fixed daily losses.

Regulation of iron absorption occurs within the duodenum (Fig. 12.9). After reduction by ferric reductase, ferrous

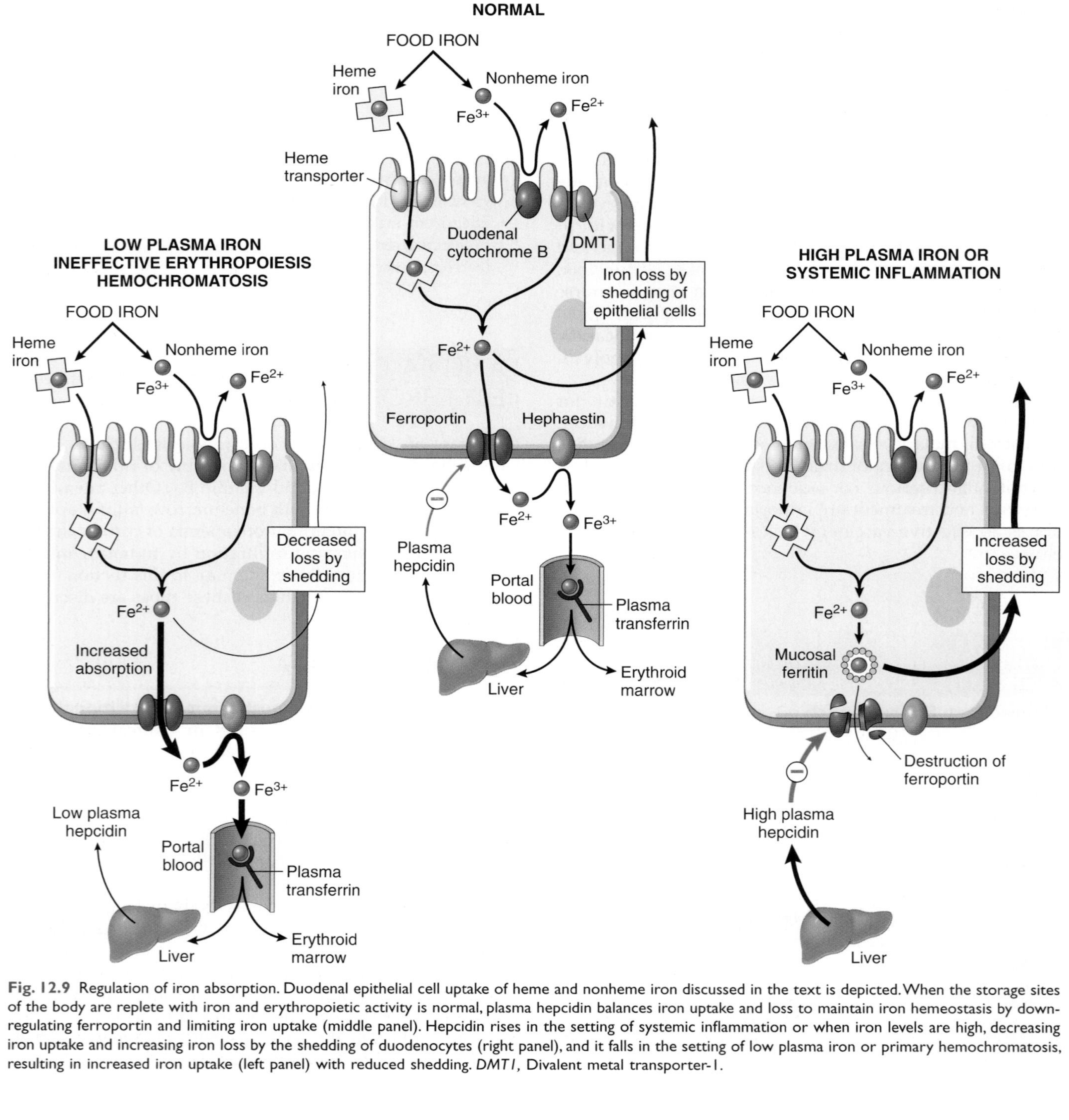

Fig. 12.9 Regulation of iron absorption. Duodenal epithelial cell uptake of heme and nonheme iron discussed in the text is depicted. When the storage sites of the body are replete with iron and erythropoietic activity is normal, plasma hepcidin balances iron uptake and loss to maintain iron hemeostasis by down-regulating ferroportin and limiting iron uptake (middle panel). Hepcidin rises in the setting of systemic inflammation or when iron levels are high, decreasing iron uptake and increasing iron loss by the shedding of duodenocytes (right panel), and it falls in the setting of low plasma iron or primary hemochromatosis, resulting in increased iron uptake (left panel) with reduced shedding. *DMT1,* Divalent metal transporter-1.

iron (Fe^{2+}) is transported across the apical membrane by divalent metal transporter-1 (DMT1). A second transporter, ferroportin, then moves iron from the cytoplasm to the plasma across the basolateral membrane. The newly absorbed iron is next oxidized by hephaestin and ceruloplasmin to ferric iron (Fe^{3+}), the form of iron that binds to transferrin. Both DMT1 and ferroportin are widely distributed in the body and are involved in iron transport in other tissues as well. As depicted in Fig. 12.9 (middle panel), part of the iron that enters enterocytes is delivered to transferrin by ferroportin, whereas the remainder is incorporated into cytoplasmic ferritin and is lost through the exfoliation of mucosal cells.

The fraction of iron that is absorbed is regulated by hepcidin, a small peptide that is synthesized and secreted from the liver in an iron-dependent fashion. In general, high iron levels in the plasma enhance hepcidin production, whereas low iron levels suppress it. However, hepcidin production also is sensitive to inflammation and to factors released from erythroblasts in the bone marrow. Specifically, hepcidin levels rise in the face of systemic inflammation because of the direct effects of inflammatory mediators such as IL-6 on hepatocytes, and in the setting of ineffective hematopoiesis, which is marked by increased numbers of erythroblasts in the bone marrow. Hepcidin circulates to the duodenum, where it binds ferroportin and induces its internalization and degradation. Thus, when hepcidin concentrations are elevated (Fig. 12.9, right panel), such as when serum iron levels are high or there is systemic inflammation, ferroportin levels fall and more iron is incorporated into cytoplasmic ferritin and is lost by excretion. Conversely, when hepcidin levels are low (Fig. 12.9, left panel), such as when there is iron deficiency, ineffective hematopoiesis, or the genetic defects that lead to primary hemochromatosis (Chapter 16), the basolateral transport of iron is increased. In iron deficiency, the suppression of hepcidin is beneficial as it serves to help to correct the deficiency, but inappropriately low levels of hepcidin, as in primary hemochromatosis, eventually lead to systemic iron overload.

Pathogenesis

Iron deficiency arises in a variety of settings:
- **Chronic blood loss is the most important cause of iron deficiency anemia in the Western world.** The most common sources of bleeding are the gastrointestinal tract (e.g., peptic ulcers, colon cancer, hemorrhoids) and the female genital tract (e.g., menorrhagia, metrorrhagia, endometrial cancer).
- **In the developing world, low intake and poor bioavailability because of predominantly vegetarian diets are the most common causes of iron deficiency.** In the United States, low dietary intake is an infrequent culprit but is sometimes culpable in infants fed exclusively milk, in the impoverished, in the elderly, and in teenagers subsisting predominantly on junk food.
- Increased demands not met by normal dietary intake occur worldwide during pregnancy and infancy.
- Malabsorption can occur with celiac disease or after gastrectomy (Chapter 15).

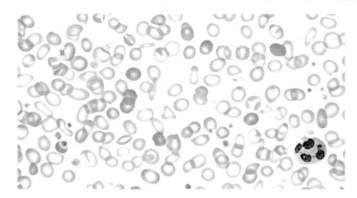

Fig. 12.10 Iron deficiency anemia—peripheral blood smear. Note the increased central pallor of most of the red cells. Scattered, fully hemoglobinized cells, from a recent blood transfusion, stand out in contrast. *(Courtesy of Dr. Robert W. McKenna, Department of Pathology, University of Texas Southwestern Medical School, Dallas, Texas.)*

Regardless of the cause, iron deficiency develops insidiously. Iron stores are depleted first, marked by a decline in serum ferritin and the absence of stainable iron in the bone marrow. These changes are followed by a decrease in serum iron and a rise in the serum transferrin. Ultimately, the capacity to synthesize hemoglobin, myoglobin, and other iron-containing proteins is diminished, leading to microcytic anemia, impaired work and cognitive performance, and even reduced immunocompetence.

Clinical Features. In most instances iron deficiency anemia is mild and asymptomatic. Nonspecific manifestations, such as weakness, listlessness, and pallor, may be present in severe cases. With long-standing anemia, abnormalities of the fingernails, including thinning, flattening, and "spooning," may appear. A curious but characteristic neurobehavioral complication is *pica,* the compunction to consume nonfoodstuffs such as dirt or clay.

In peripheral smears, red cells are *microcytic* and *hypochromic* (Fig. 12.10). Diagnostic criteria include anemia, hypochromic and microcytic red cell indices, low serum ferritin and iron levels, low transferrin saturation, increased total iron-binding capacity, and, ultimately, response to iron therapy. For unclear reasons, the platelet count often is elevated. Erythropoietin levels are elevated, but the marrow response is blunted by the iron deficiency; thus, marrow cellularity usually is only slightly increased.

Persons often die with iron deficiency anemia, but virtually never of it. An important point is that in well-nourished persons, microcytic hypochromic anemia is not a disease but rather a symptom of some underlying disorder.

Anemia of Chronic Inflammation

Often referred to as the anemia of chronic disease, anemia associated with chronic inflammation is the most common form of anemia in hospitalized patients. It superficially resembles the anemia of iron deficiency but arises instead from the suppression of erythropoiesis by systemic inflammation. It occurs in a variety of disorders associated with sustained inflammation:
- Chronic microbial infections, such as osteomyelitis, bacterial endocarditis, and lung abscess

- Chronic immune disorders, such as rheumatoid arthritis and regional enteritis
- Neoplasms, such as Hodgkin lymphoma and carcinomas of the lung and breast

Pathogenesis

The anemia of chronic inflammation stems from high levels of plasma hepcidin, which blocks the transfer of iron to erythroid precursors by downregulating ferroportin in macrophages. The elevated hepcidin levels are caused by proinflammatory cytokines such as IL-6, which increase hepatic hepcidin synthesis. In addition, chronic inflammation blunts erythropoietin synthesis by the kidney, lowering red cell production by the marrow. The functional advantages of these adaptations in the face of systemic inflammation are unclear; they may serve to inhibit the growth of iron-dependent microorganisms or to augment certain aspects of host immunity.

Clinical Features. As in anemia of iron deficiency, the serum iron levels usually are low in the anemia of chronic disease, and the red cells may be slightly hypochromic and microcytic. Unlike iron deficiency anemia, however, storage iron in the bone marrow and serum ferritin are increased and the total iron-binding capacity is reduced. Administration of erythropoietin and iron can improve the anemia, but only effective treatment of the underlying condition is curative.

Megaloblastic Anemias

The two principal causes of megaloblastic anemia are folate deficiency and vitamin B_{12} deficiency. Both vitamins are required for DNA synthesis and the effects of their deficiency on hematopoiesis are essentially identical. However, the causes and consequences of folate and vitamin B_{12} deficiency differ in important ways. We will first review some of the common features and then touch on those that are specific to folate and vitamin B_{12} deficiency.

Pathogenesis

Megaloblastic anemia stems from metabolic defects that lead to inadequate biosynthesis of thymidine, one of the building blocks of DNA. As we will discuss, folate and vitamin B_{12} are both essential factors for the synthesis of thymidylate, which is required for DNA replication. Thymidine deficiency causes abnormalities in rapidly dividing cells throughout the body, but the hematopoietic marrow is most severely affected. Because the synthesis of RNA and cytoplasmic elements proceeds at a normal rate and thus outpaces that of the nucleus, the hematopoietic precursors show *nuclear-cytoplasmic asynchrony* (described later). This maturational derangement contributes to the anemia in several ways. Many red cell progenitors are so defective in DNA synthesis that they undergo apoptosis in the marrow *(ineffective hematopoiesis)*. Others mature into red cells but do so after fewer cell divisions, further diminishing the output of red cells. Granulocyte and platelet precursors also are affected (although not as severely) and most patients present with pancytopenia (anemia, thrombocytopenia, and granulocytopenia).

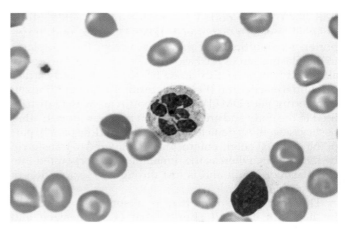

Fig. 12.11 Megaloblastic anemia. A peripheral blood smear shows a hypersegmented neutrophil with a six-lobed nucleus. *(Courtesy of Dr. Robert W. McKenna, Department of Pathology, University of Texas Southwestern Medical School, Dallas, Texas.)*

MORPHOLOGY

Certain morphologic features are common to all forms of megaloblastic anemia. The bone marrow is markedly hypercellular and contains numerous megaloblastic erythroid progenitors. **Megaloblasts** are larger than normal erythroid progenitors (normoblasts) and have delicate, finely reticulated nuclear chromatin (indicative of nuclear immaturity). As megaloblasts differentiate and acquire hemoglobin, the nucleus retains its finely distributed chromatin and fails to undergo the chromatin clumping typical of normoblasts, a classic example of nuclear-cytoplasmic asynchrony. The granulocytic precursors also demonstrate nuclear-cytoplasmic asynchrony, yielding **giant metamyelocytes.** Megakaryocytes may also be abnormally large and have bizarre multilobed nuclei.

In the peripheral blood the earliest change is the appearance of **hypersegmented neutrophils** (Fig. 12.11), which appear before the onset of anemia. Normal neutrophils have three or four nuclear lobes, but in megaloblastic anemias they often have five or more. The red cells typically include large, **egg-shaped macroovalocytes;** the MCV often is greater than 110 fL (normal, 82–96 fL). Although macrocytes appear hyperchromic, in reality their hemoglobin content is normal. Large, misshapen platelets also may be seen. Morphologic changes in other systems, especially the gastrointestinal tract, also occur, giving rise to some of the clinical manifestations.

Folate (Folic Acid) Deficiency Anemia

Folate deficiency is usually the result of inadequate dietary intake, sometimes complicated by increased metabolic demands. Although folate is present in nearly all foods, it is destroyed by 10 to 15 minutes of cooking, and as a result folate stores are marginal in a surprising number of healthy persons. The risk of overt folate deficiency is highest in those with a poor diet (the economically deprived, the indigent, and the elderly) or those with increased metabolic needs (pregnant women and patients with chronic hemolytic anemias, such as sickle cell disease).

Deficiency may also stem from problems with absorption or metabolism. Food folates are predominantly in polyglutamate form and must be split into monoglutamates for absorption, a conversion that is inhibited by acidic foods and substances found in beans and other legumes. Some drugs, such as phenytoin (dilantin), also interfere with folate absorption, whereas others, such as methotrexate, inhibit folate metabolism. Malabsorptive disorders, such as *celiac disease* and *tropical sprue*, that affect the upper third of the small intestine where folate is absorbed, may also impair folate uptake.

Pathogenesis

The metabolism and functions of folate are complex. Here it is sufficient to note that its conversion within cells from dihydrofolate to tetrahydrofolate by *dihydrofolate reductase* is particularly important. Tetrahydrofolate acts as an acceptor and donor of one-carbon units in several reactions that are required for the synthesis of deoxythymidine monophosphate (dTMP). If intracellular stores of folate fall, insufficient dTMP is synthesized and DNA replication is blocked, leading to megaloblastic anemia.

Clinical Features. The onset of the anemia of folate deficiency is insidious, being associated with nonspecific symptoms such as weakness and easy fatigability. The clinical picture may be complicated by the coexistent deficiency of other vitamins, especially in alcoholics. Because the cells lining the gastrointestinal tract, like the hematopoietic system, turn over rapidly, symptoms referable to the alimentary tract, such as sore tongue, are common. Unlike in vitamin B_{12} deficiency (described later), neurologic abnormalities do not occur.

The diagnosis of a megaloblastic anemia is readily made from the examination of smears of peripheral blood and bone marrow. The anemia of folate deficiency is best distinguished from that of vitamin B_{12} deficiency by measuring serum and red cell folate and vitamin B_{12} levels.

Vitamin B_{12} (Cobalamin) Deficiency Anemia

Vitamin B_{12} is widely present in foods, is resistant to cooking and boiling, and is even synthesized by gut flora. Thus, unlike folate, vitamin B_{12} deficiency is virtually never caused by inadequate intake except in vegetarians who scrupulously avoid milk and eggs. Instead, deficiencies typically arise from some abnormality that interferes with vitamin B_{12} absorption, a complex process involving the following steps:

1. Peptic digestion releases dietary vitamin B_{12}, allowing it to bind a salivary protein called *haptocorrin*.
2. On entering the duodenum, haptocorrin–B_{12} complexes are processed by pancreatic proteases; this releases B_{12}, which attaches to *intrinsic factor* secreted from the parietal cells of the gastric fundic mucosa.
3. The intrinsic factor–B_{12} complexes pass to the distal ileum and attach to cubilin, a receptor for intrinsic factor, and are taken up into enterocytes.
4. The absorbed vitamin B_{12} is transferred across the basolateral membranes of enterocytes to plasma *transcobalamin*, which delivers vitamin B_{12} to the liver and other cells of the body.

After absorption, the body handles vitamin B_{12} very efficiently. It is stored in the liver, which normally contains reserves sufficient to support bodily needs for 5 to 20 years. Because of these large liver stores, clinical presentations of vitamin B_{12} deficiency typically follow years of unrecognized malabsorption.

Pathogenesis

The most frequent cause vitamin B_{12} deficiency is *pernicious anemia*, which is believed to result from an autoimmune attack on the gastric mucosa that suppresses the production of intrinsic factor. Histologically, there is a *chronic atrophic gastritis* marked by a loss of parietal cells, a prominent infiltrate of lymphocytes and plasma cells, and megaloblastic changes in mucosal cells similar to those found in erythroid precursors. The serum of most affected patients contains several types of *autoantibodies* that block the binding of vitamin B_{12} to intrinsic factor or prevent binding of the intrinsic factor–vitamin B_{12} complex to cubilin. Autoantibodies are of diagnostic use, but they are not thought to be the primary cause of the gastric pathology; rather, it seems that an *autoreactive T cell response* initiates gastric mucosal injury and triggers the formation of autoantibodies. When the mass of intrinsic factor-secreting cells falls below a threshold (and reserves of stored vitamin B_{12} are depleted), anemia develops.

Other causes of vitamin B_{12} malabsorption include *gastrectomy* (leading to loss of intrinsic factor–producing cells), *ileal resection* (resulting in loss of intrinsic factor–B_{12} complex–absorbing cells), and disorders that disrupt the function of the distal ileum (such as *Crohn disease, tropical sprue,* and *Whipple disease*). Particularly in older persons, *gastric atrophy* and *achlorhydria* may interfere with the production of acid and pepsin, which are needed to release the vitamin B_{12} from its bound form in food.

The metabolic defects responsible for the anemia of vitamin B_{12} deficiency are intertwined with folate metabolism. Vitamin B_{12} is required for recycling tetrahydrofolate, which, as described previously, is the form of folate that is needed for DNA synthesis. In keeping with this relationship, the anemia of vitamin B_{12} deficiency is reversed with the administration of folate.

By contrast, folate administration does not prevent and may in fact worsen certain neurologic symptoms that are specific to vitamin B_{12} deficiency. The main neurologic lesions associated with vitamin B_{12} deficiency are demyelination of the posterior and lateral columns of the spinal cord, sometimes beginning in the peripheral nerves. In time, axonal degeneration may supervene. The severity of the neurologic manifestations is not related to the degree of anemia. Indeed, neurologic disease may occur in the absence of overt megaloblastic anemia.

Clinical Features. The manifestations of vitamin B_{12} deficiency are nonspecific. As with all anemias, findings include pallor, easy fatigability, and, in severe cases, dyspnea and even congestive heart failure. The increased destruction of erythroid progenitors because of ineffective erythropoiesis may give rise to *mild jaundice*, and megaloblastic changes in the oropharyngeal epithelium may produce a *beefy red tongue*. The *spinal cord disease* begins with symmetric numbness, tingling, and burning in the feet or hands, followed by unsteadiness of gait and loss of position sense, particularly in the toes. Although the anemia responds dramatically to parenteral vitamin B_{12}, the neurologic manifestations often fail to resolve. As discussed in Chapter 15, patients with pernicious anemia have an increased risk for the development of gastric carcinoma.

Findings supporting the diagnosis of vitamin B_{12} deficiency are (1) low serum vitamin B_{12} levels, (2) normal or elevated serum folate levels, (3) moderate to severe macrocytic anemia, (4) leukopenia with hypersegmented granulocytes, and (5) a dramatic reticulocytic response (within 2 to 3 days) to parenteral administration of vitamin B_{12}. Pernicious anemia is associated with all of these findings plus the presence of serum antibodies to intrinsic factor.

Aplastic Anemia

Aplastic anemia is a disorder in which multipotent myeloid stem cells are suppressed, leading to bone marrow failure and pancytopenia. The marrow often is virtually devoid of recognizable hematopoietic elements. It must be distinguished from pure red cell aplasia, in which only erythroid progenitors are affected and anemia is the only manifestation.

Pathogenesis

The pathogenesis of aplastic anemia is not fully understood, but two major etiologies have been invoked: an extrinsic, immune-mediated suppression of marrow progenitors, and an intrinsic abnormality of stem cells. Experimental studies have focused on a model in which activated T cells suppress hematopoietic stem cells. It is hypothesized that stem cells are first antigenically altered by exposure to drugs, infectious agents, or other unidentified environmental insults. This provokes a cellular immune response, during which activated T_H1 cells produce cytokines such as interferon-γ (IFN-γ) and TNF that suppress and kill hematopoietic progenitors. This scenario is supported by experience with immunosuppressive therapy directed against T cells, which restores hematopoiesis in 60% to 70% of patients.

Alternatively, **the notion that aplastic anemia results from an intrinsic stem cell abnormality is supported by observations showing that from 5% to 10% of patients have inherited defects in telomerase**, which, as mentioned earlier, is needed for the maintenance and stability of chromosomes. It is hypothesized that the defect in telomerase leads to premature senescence of hematopoietic stem cells. Of further interest, the bone marrow cells in an additional 50% of cases have unusually short telomeres, possibly stemming from as-yet undiscovered defects in telomerase or excessive replication of hematopoietic stem cells. These two mechanisms are not mutually exclusive, because genetically altered stem cells (e.g., those with abnormal telomeres) also might express "neoantigens" that serve as targets for a T cell attack.

Clinical Features. Aplastic anemia affects persons of all ages and both sexes. The slowly progressive anemia causes the insidious development of weakness, pallor, and dyspnea. Thrombocytopenia often manifests with petechiae and ecchymoses. Neutropenia may set the stage for serious infections.

It is important to separate aplastic anemia from anemia caused by marrow infiltration (myelophthisic anemia), "aleukemic leukemia," and granulomatous diseases, which may have similar clinical presentations but are easily distinguished by examination of the bone marrow. Aplastic anemia does not cause splenomegaly; if present, another diagnosis should be sought.

The prognosis is unpredictable. Withdrawal of an inciting drug sometimes leads to remission, but this is the exception. Hematopoietic stem cell transplantation often is curative, particularly in nontransfused patients younger than 40 years of age. Transfusion sensitizes patients to alloantigens, producing a high rate of engraftment failure; thus, it must be minimized in persons eligible for transplantation. Successful transplantation requires "conditioning" with immunosuppressive radiation or chemotherapy, reinforcing the notion that autoimmunity has an important role in the disease. As mentioned earlier, patients who are poor transplantation candidates often benefit from immunosuppressive therapy.

Myelophthisic Anemia

Myelophthisic anemia is caused by extensive infiltration of the marrow by tumors or other lesions. It most commonly is associated with metastatic breast, lung, or prostate cancer. Other tumors, advanced tuberculosis, lipid storage disorders, and osteosclerosis may produce a similar clinical picture. The principal manifestations include anemia and thrombocytopenia; in general, the white cell series is less affected. Characteristically misshapen red cells, some resembling teardrops, are seen in the peripheral blood. Immature granulocytic and erythrocytic precursors also may be present (*leukoerythroblastosis*) along with mild leukocytosis. Treatment is directed at the underlying condition.

● SUMMARY

ANEMIA OF DIMINISHED ERYTHROPOIESIS

Iron Deficiency Anemia

- Caused by chronic bleeding or inadequate iron intake; results in insufficient hemoglobin synthesis and hypochromic, microcytic red cells

Anemia of Chronic Inflammation

- Caused by inflammatory cytokines, which increase hepcidin levels and thereby sequester iron in macrophages, and also suppress erythropoietin production

Megaloblastic Anemia

- Caused by deficiencies of folate or vitamin B_{12} that lead to inadequate synthesis of thymidine and defective DNA replication
- Results in enlarged abnormal hematopoietic precursors (megaloblasts), ineffective hematopoiesis, macrocytic anemia, and (in most cases) pancytopenia

Aplastic Anemia

- Caused by bone marrow failure (hypocellularity) resulting from diverse causes, including exposures to toxins and radiation, idiosyncratic reactions to drugs and viruses, and inherited defects in telomerase and DNA repair

Myelophthisic Anemia

- Caused by replacement of the bone marrow by infiltrative processes such as metastatic carcinoma and granulomatous disease
- Leads to the appearance of early erythroid and granulocytic precursors (leukoerythroblastosis) and teardrop-shaped red cells in the peripheral blood

Table 12.5 Pathophysiologic Classification of Polycythemia

Relative
Reduced plasma volume (hemoconcentration)

Absolute
Primary
Abnormal proliferation of myeloid stem cells, normal or low erythropoietin levels (polycythemia vera); inherited activating mutations in the erythropoietin receptor (rare)
Secondary
Increased erythropoietin levels
Adaptive: Lung disease, high-altitude living, cyanotic heart disease
Paraneoplastic: Erythropoietin-secreting tumors (e.g., renal cell carcinoma, hepatomacellular carcinoma, cerebellar hemangioblastoma)
Surreptitious: Endurance athletes

POLYCYTHEMIA

Polycythemia, or *erythrocytosis,* denotes an increase in red cells per unit volume of peripheral blood. It may be *absolute* (defined as an increase in total red cell mass) or *relative.* Relative polycythemia results from dehydration, such as occurs with water deprivation, prolonged vomiting, diarrhea, or the excessive use of diuretics. Absolute polycythemia is described as *primary* when the increased red cell mass results from an autonomous proliferation of erythroid progenitors, and *secondary* when the excessive proliferation stems from elevated levels of erythropoietin. Primary polycythemia (polycythemia vera) is a clonal myeloid neoplasm considered later in this chapter. The increases in erythropoietin that cause secondary forms of absolute polycythemia include a variety of causes (Table 12.5).

White Cell Disorders

Disorders of white cells include deficiencies (leukopenias) and proliferations, which may be reactive or neoplastic. Reactive proliferation in response to a primary, often microbial, disease is common. Neoplastic disorders, although less common, are more ominous: They cause approximately 9% of all cancer deaths in adults and a staggering 40% in children younger than 15 years of age.

Presented next are brief descriptions of some nonneoplastic conditions, followed by more detailed considerations of the malignant proliferations of white cells.

NONNEOPLASTIC DISORDERS OF WHITE CELLS

Leukopenia

Leukopenia results most commonly from a decrease in granulocytes, the most numerous circulating white cells. Lymphopenia is much less common; it is associated with rare congenital immunodeficiency diseases, advanced human immunodeficiency virus (HIV) infection, and treatment with high doses of corticosteroids. Only the more common leukopenias of granulocytes are discussed here.

Neutropenia/Agranulocytosis

A reduction in the number of granulocytes in blood is known as *neutropenia* or, when severe, agranulocytosis. Neutropenic persons are susceptible to severe, potentially fatal bacterial and fungal infections. The risk of infection rises sharply as the neutrophil count falls below 500 cells/μL.

Pathogenesis

The mechanisms underlying neutropenia can be divided into two broad categories:

- *Decreased granulocyte production.* Clinically important reductions in granulopoiesis are most often caused by marrow hypoplasia (as occurs transiently with cancer chemotherapy and chronically with aplastic anemia) or extensive replacement of the marrow by tumor (such as with leukemia). Alternatively, neutrophil production may be suppressed while other blood lineages are unaffected. This is most often caused by certain drugs or by neoplastic proliferations of cytotoxic T cells and natural killer (NK) cells (so-called "large granular lymphocytic leukemia").
- *Increased granulocyte destruction.* This can be encountered with immune-mediated injury (triggered in some cases by drugs) or in overwhelming bacterial, fungal, or rickettsial infections resulting from increased peripheral use. Splenomegaly also can lead to the sequestration and accelerated removal of neutrophils.

MORPHOLOGY

The alterations in the bone marrow depend on the underlying cause. Compensatory marrow hypercellularity is seen when there is excessive neutrophil destruction or ineffective granulopoiesis, such as occurs in megaloblastic anemia. Drugs that selectively suppress granulocytopoiesis are associated with decreased numbers of granulocytic precursors and preservation of erythroid elements and megakaryocytes, while myelotoxic chemotherapy drugs reduce the number of elements from all lineages.

Clinical Features. Infections constitute the major problem. They commonly take the form of ulcerating, necrotizing lesions of the gingiva, floor of the mouth, buccal mucosa, pharynx, or other sites within the oral cavity *(agranulocytic angina)*. Owing to the lack of leukocytes, such lesions often contain large masses or sheets of microorganisms. In addition to local inflammation, systemic symptoms usually are present consisting of malaise, chills, and fever. Because of the danger of sepsis, patients are started on broad-spectrum antibiotics covering both bacterial and fungal infections at the first sign of infection. Depending on the clinical context, patients also may be treated with granulocyte colony-stimulating factor (G-CSF), a growth factor that speeds recovery of neutrophil counts.

Reactive Leukocytosis

An increase in the number of white cells in the blood is common in a variety of inflammatory states caused by microbial and nonmicrobial stimuli. Leukocytoses are relatively nonspecific and are classified according to the particular white cell series that is affected (Table 12.6). As discussed later, in some cases reactive leukocytosis may mimic leukemia. Such *"leukemoid reactions"* must be distinguished

Table 12.6 Causes of Leukocytosis

Neutrophilic Leukocytosis
Acute bacterial infections (especially those caused by pyogenic organisms); sterile inflammation caused by, e.g., tissue necrosis (myocardial infarction, burns)
Eosinophilic Leukocytosis (Eosinophilia)
Allergic disorders such as asthma, hay fever, allergic skin diseases (e.g., pemphigus, dermatitis herpetiformis); parasitic infestations; drug reactions; certain malignancies (e.g., Hodgkin lymphoma and some non-Hodgkin lymphomas); collagen-vascular disorders and some vasculitides; atheroembolic disease (transient)
Basophilic Leukocytosis (Basophilia)
Rare, often indicative of a myeloproliferative neoplasm (e.g., chronic myeloid leukemia)
Monocytosis
Chronic infections (e.g., tuberculosis), bacterial endocarditis, rickettsiosis, and malaria; collagen vascular diseases (e.g., systemic lupus erythematosus); and inflammatory bowel diseases (e.g., ulcerative colitis)
Lymphocytosis
Accompanies monocytosis in many disorders associated with chronic immunologic stimulation (e.g., tuberculosis, brucellosis); viral infections (e.g., hepatitis A, cytomegalovirus, Epstein-Barr virus); *Bordetella pertussis* infection

from true white cell malignancies. Infectious mononucleosis merits separate consideration because it gives rise to a distinctive syndrome associated with lymphocytosis.

Infectious Mononucleosis

Infectious mononucleosis is an acute, self-limited disease of adolescents and young adults that is caused by Epstein-Barr virus (EBV), a member of the herpesvirus family. The infection is characterized by (1) fever, sore throat, and generalized lymphadenitis and (2) a lymphocytosis of activated, CD8+ T cells. Of note, cytomegalovirus infection induces a similar syndrome that can be differentiated only by serologic methods.

EBV is ubiquitous in all human populations. In the developing world, EBV infection in early childhood is nearly universal. Even though infected children mount an immune response (described later), most remain asymptomatic and more than half continue to shed virus, usually for life. By contrast, in developed countries with better standards of hygiene, infection typically is delayed until adolescence or young adulthood and symptomatic infection is much more common. For unclear reasons, only about 20% of healthy seropositive persons in developed countries shed the virus, and only about 50% of those exposed to the virus acquire the infection.

Pathogenesis

Transmission to a seronegative "kissing cousin" usually involves direct oral contact. It is hypothesized that the virus initially infects oropharyngeal epithelial cells and then spreads to underlying lymphoid tissue (tonsils and adenoids), where mature B cells are infected. The infection of B cells takes one of two forms. In a minority of cells, the infection is lytic, leading to viral replication and release of virions. More commonly, the infection is nonproductive and the virus persists in latent form as an extrachromosomal episome.

B cells that are latently infected with EBV become "activated" and proliferate as a result of the action of several viral proteins (Chapter 6). These cells disseminate in the circulation and secrete antibodies with unusual specificities, including the antibodies that recognize sheep red cells that are detected in diagnostic tests for mononucleosis. During acute infections, EBV is shed in the saliva; it is not known whether the source of these virions is oropharyngeal epithelial cells or B cells.

The host T cell response controls the proliferation of EBV-infected B cells and the spread of the virus. Early in the course of the infection, IgM antibodies are formed against viral capsid antigens. Later the serologic response shifts to IgG antibodies, which persist for life. More important in the control of the EBV-positive B cell proliferation are cytotoxic CD8+ T cells. Virus-specific CD8+ T cells appear in the circulation as atypical lymphocytes, a finding that is characteristic of mononucleosis. In otherwise healthy persons, the fully developed humoral and cellular responses to EBV act as brakes on viral shedding. In most cases, however, a small number of latently infected EBV-positive B cells escape the immune response and persist for the life of the patient. As described later, **impaired T cell immunity places patients at high risk for EBV-driven B cell proliferations.**

MORPHOLOGY

The major alterations involve the blood, lymph nodes, spleen, liver, and occasionally other organs. There is peripheral blood **leukocytosis**; the white cell count is usually between 12,000 and 18,000 cells/µL. Typically more than half of these cells are large **atypical lymphocytes,** 12 to 16 µm in diameter, with an oval, indented, or folded nucleus and abundant cytoplasm with a few azurophilic granules (Fig. 12.12). These atypical lymphocytes, which are sufficiently distinctive to suggest the diagnosis, are mainly CD8+ T cells.

Lymphadenopathy is common and is most prominent in the posterior cervical, axillary, and groin regions. On histologic examination, the enlarged nodes are flooded by atypical lymphocytes, which occupy the paracortical (T cell) areas. A few cells resembling Reed-Sternberg (RS) cells, the hallmark of Hodgkin lymphoma, often are seen. Because of these atypical features, special tests are sometimes needed to distinguish the reactive changes of mononucleosis from lymphoma.

The **spleen** is enlarged in most cases, weighing between 300 and 500 g, and exhibits a heavy infiltration of atypical lymphocytes. As a result of the rapid increase in splenic size and the infiltration of the trabeculae and capsule by the lymphocytes, such spleens are fragile and are prone to rupture after even minor trauma.

Atypical lymphocytes usually also infiltrate the portal areas and sinusoids of the liver. Scattered apoptotic cells or foci of parenchymal necrosis associated with a lymphocytic infiltrate also may be present—a picture that can be difficult to distinguish from that in other forms of viral hepatitis.

Clinical Features. Infectious mononucleosis classically manifests with fever, sore throat, and lymphadenitis, but atypical presentations are not unusual. Sometimes there is little or no fever and only fatigue and lymphadenopathy exist, raising the specter of lymphoma; fever of unknown origin, unassociated with lymphadenopathy or other localized findings; hepatitis that is difficult to differentiate from one of the hepatotropic viral syndromes (Chapter 16); or a febrile rash resembling rubella. Ultimately, the diagnosis depends on the following, in increasing order of specificity: (1) the presence of atypical lymphocytes in the peripheral blood; (2) a positive heterophil reaction (Monospot test);

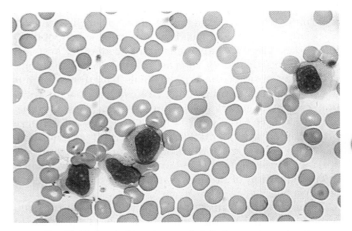

Fig. 12.12 Atypical lymphocytes in infectious mononucleosis.

and (3) a rising titer of antibodies specific for EBV antigens. In most patients, mononucleosis resolves within 4 to 6 weeks, but sometimes the fatigue lasts longer. Occasionally, one or more complications supervene. Perhaps the most common of these is hepatic dysfunction, associated with jaundice, elevated liver enzyme levels, disturbed appetite, and, rarely, even liver failure. Other complications involve the nervous system, kidneys, bone marrow, lungs, eyes, heart, and spleen (including fatal splenic rupture).

EBV is a potent transforming virus that plays a role in the pathogenesis of a number of human malignancies, including several types of B cell lymphoma (Chapter 6). A serious complication in those lacking T cell immunity is unimpeded EBV-driven B cell proliferation. This process can be initiated by an acute infection or by the reactivation of a latent B cell infection and generally begins as a polyclonal proliferation that transforms to overt monoclonal B cell lymphoma over time. Reconstitution of immunity (e.g., by cessation of immunosuppressive drugs) is sometimes sufficient to cause complete regression of the B cell proliferation, which is uniformly fatal if left untreated.

The importance of the cellular immune response in controlling EBV infection also is driven home by *X-linked lymphoproliferative syndrome (XLP)*, a rare inherited immunodeficiency characterized by an ineffective response to EBV. Most affected boys have mutations in the *SH2D1A* gene, which encodes a signaling protein that participates in the activation of T and NK cells. In more than 50% of cases, EBV causes an acute overwhelming infection, often complicated by hemophagocytic lymphohistiocytosis (HLH, described later), whereas other patients succumb to EBV-driven lymphoma or secondary infections related to hypogammaglobulinemia, the basis of which is not understood.

Reactive Lymphadenitis

Infections and nonmicrobial inflammatory stimuli often activate immune cells residing in lymph nodes, which act as defensive barriers. Any immune response against foreign antigens can lead to lymph node enlargement (lymphadenopathy). Infections causing lymphadenitis are varied and numerous, and may be acute or chronic. In most instances the histologic appearance of the lymph node reaction is nonspecific. A somewhat distinctive form of lymphadenitis that occurs with cat-scratch disease is described separately later.

Acute Nonspecific Lymphadenitis

This form of lymphadenitis may be isolated to a group of nodes draining a local infection, or be generalized, as in systemic infectious and inflammatory conditions.

MORPHOLOGY

Inflamed nodes in acute nonspecific lymphadenitis are swollen, gray-red, and engorged. Histologically, there are **large germinal centers** containing numerous mitotic figures. When the cause is a pyogenic organism, a neutrophilic infiltrate is seen around the follicles and within the lymphoid sinuses. With severe infections, the centers of follicles can undergo necrosis, leading to the formation of an abscess.

Affected nodes are tender and may become fluctuant if abscess formation is extensive. The overlying skin is frequently red and may develop draining sinuses. With control of the infection the lymph nodes may revert to a normal "resting" appearance or, if damaged, undergo scarring.

Chronic Nonspecific Lymphadenitis

Depending on the causative agent, chronic nonspecific lymphadenitis can assume one of three patterns: follicular hyperplasia, paracortical hyperplasia, or sinus histiocytosis.

MORPHOLOGY

Follicular Hyperplasia. This pattern occurs with infections or inflammatory processes that activate B cells, which migrate into B cell follicles and create the **follicular (or germinal center) reaction.** Reactive follicles contain numerous activated B cells, scattered T cells, phagocytic macrophages containing nuclear debris (tingible body macrophages), and a meshwork of antigen-presenting follicular dendritic cells. Causes of follicular hyperplasia include **rheumatoid arthritis, toxoplasmosis,** and early **HIV infection.** This form of lymphadenitis must be distinguished from follicular lymphoma (discussed later). Findings that favor follicular hyperplasia are (1) the preservation of the lymph node architecture; (2) variation in the shape and size of the germinal centers; (3) the presence of a mixture of germinal center lymphocytes of varying shapes and sizes; and (4) prominent phagocytic and mitotic activity in germinal centers.

Paracortical Hyperplasia. This pattern is caused by immune reactions involving the **T cell regions** of the lymph node. When activated, parafollicular T cells transform into large proliferating immunoblasts that can efface the B cell follicles. Paracortical hyperplasia is encountered in **viral infections** (such as EBV), after certain **vaccinations** (e.g., smallpox), and in immune reactions induced by **drugs** (especially phenytoin).

Sinus Histiocytosis. This reactive pattern is characterized by distention and prominence of the lymphatic sinusoids, owing to a marked **hypertrophy of lining endothelial cells** and an **infiltrate of macrophages (histiocytes).** It often is encountered in lymph nodes draining cancers and may represent an immune response to the tumor or its products

Cat-Scratch Disease

Cat-scratch disease is a self-limited lymphadenitis caused by the bacterium *Bartonella henselae*. It is primarily a disease of childhood; 90% of the patients are younger than 18 years of age. It manifests with regional lymphadenopathy, most frequently in the axilla and the neck. The nodal enlargement appears approximately 2 weeks after a feline scratch or, less commonly, after a splinter or thorn injury. An inflammatory nodule, vesicle, or eschar is sometimes visible at the site of the skin injury. In most patients the lymph node enlargement regresses during a period of 2 to 4 months. Rarely, encephalitis, osteomyelitis, or thrombocytopenia may develop in patients.

MORPHOLOGY

The nodal changes in cat-scratch disease are quite characteristic. Initially sarcoidlike granulomas form, but these then undergo central necrosis associated with an infiltrate of neutrophils. These **irregular stellate necrotizing granulomas** are similar in appearance to those seen in a limited number of other infections, such as lymphogranuloma venereum. The microbe is extracellular and can be visualized with silver stains. The diagnosis is based on a history of exposure to cats, the characteristic clinical findings, a positive result on serologic testing for antibodies to *Bartonella*, and the distinctive morphologic changes in the lymph nodes.

Hemophagocytic Lymphohistiocytosis (HLH)

HLH is an uncommon disorder in which a viral infection or other proinflammatory exposures trigger activation of macrophages throughout the body, leading to phagocytosis of blood cells and their precursors, cytopenias, and symptoms related to systemic inflammation and organ dysfunction. Inherited defects in several genes that regulate the function of immune cells are associated with a greatly elevated risk of HLH. The involved genes and proteins are diverse, but they share a common feature in that they are required for the cytolytic function of CD8+ T cells and NK cells. Owing to this defect in "killer lymphocytes," cytotoxic lymphocytes are unable to kill their targets (e.g. virus infected cells) and remain engaged with targeted cells for longer than normal periods of time, leading to excessive release of cytokines, such as interferon gamma, that activate macrophages. The unbridled macrophage activation results in the release of toxic levels of additional proinflammatory cytokines, such as TNF and IL-6, producing signs and symptoms that closely resemble those associated with sepsis and other conditions that lead to the systemic inflammatory response syndrome (SIRS) (Chapter 4).

HLH occurs in several distinct settings. It is most common in infants and young children with homozygous defects in genes that are required for cytotoxic lymphocyte function, such the gene *PRF1*, which encodes perforin, an essential component of cytotoxic granules. In this setting the trigger may be some normally trivial childhood viral infection. Other times, HLH arises in older male children and adolescents with X-linked lymphoproliferative disorder, in which the trigger is EBV infection. In those affected, inherited defects in a signaling molecule called SLAM-associated protein (SAP) leads to inefficient killing of EBV-infected B cells. HLH also may complicate other systemic inflammatory disorders, such as rheumatologic conditions. At least a subset of these individuals have heterozygous defects in genes required for cytotoxic lymphocyte function, creating a genetic background that increases the likelihood of HLH. Finally, HLH may be seen as a secondary phenomenon in patients with peripheral T cell lymphomas. The precise mechanism in this context is uncertain; aberrant cytokine production by malignant T cells leading to dysregulation of non-neoplastic cytotoxic lymphocytes is suspected.

Regardless of cause, patients with HLH typically present with fever, splenomegaly, and pancytopenia. In severe cases, DIC and organ failure may supervene. An examination of the bone marrow shows macrophages phagocytosing red cells, platelets, and nucleated marrow cells. Laboratory abnormalities typically include a very high ferritin level (>10,000 μg/L), hypertriglyceridemia, high serum levels of soluble IL2 receptor, and low levels of circulating NK cells and cytotoxic T lymphocytes. In concert, these findings are quite sensitive and specific for HLH. Treatment varies depending on the underlying cause, but it is generally poor. In those with HLH stemming from inherited defects, hematopoietic stem cell transplantation offers a chance for cure.

NEOPLASTIC PROLIFERATIONS OF WHITE CELLS

The most important disorders of white cells are neoplasms. Virtually all of these tumors are considered to be malignant, but they demonstrate a wide range of behaviors, ranging from some of the most aggressive cancers of man to tumors that are so indolent that they were only recognized recently as true neoplasms. Hematologic malignancies occur at all ages and include disorders that preferentially affect infants, children, and young adults, as well as the very old. As a group they are quite common; in aggregate, there are about 150,000 new hematologic malignancies diagnosed each year in the United States.

Current systems of classifying white cell neoplasms rely on a mixture of morphologic and molecular criteria, including lineage-specific protein markers and genetic findings. We will organize our discussion by dividing the white cell neoplasms into four broad categories based on the origin and differentiation state of the tumor cells, as follows:

- *Lymphoid neoplasms*, which include certain leukemias and the non-Hodgkin and Hodgkin lymphomas. In many instances these tumors are composed of cells resembling some normal stage of lymphocyte differentiation, a feature that serves as one of the bases for their classification. A special group of lymphoid neoplasms are the plasma cell neoplasms and related entities, in which many of the clinical manifestations stem from abnormal immunoglobulins that are synthesized and secreted from the neoplastic cells.
- *Myeloid neoplasms*, which include certain leukemias, myelodysplastic syndromes (MDSs), and myeloproliferative neoplasms. These tumors have in common an origin from a hematopoietic stem cell or some other very early hematopoietic progenitor, and they typically involve the bone marrow.
- *Histiocytic neoplasms*, which include proliferative lesions of macrophages and dendritic cells. Of special interest is a spectrum of proliferations of Langerhans cells (*Langerhans cell histiocytoses*).

Lymphoid Neoplasms

The numerous lymphoid neoplasms vary widely in their clinical presentation and behavior, and thus present challenges to students and clinicians alike. Some characteristically manifest as *leukemias*, with involvement of the bone marrow and the peripheral blood. Others tend to present as *lymphomas*, tumors that produce masses in lymph nodes or other tissues. *Plasma cell tumors* usually arise within the bones and manifest as discrete masses, causing systemic symptoms related to the production of a complete or partial monoclonal immunoglobulin. Although these tendencies are reflected in the names given to particular entities, in reality all lymphoid neoplasms have the potential to spread to lymph nodes and other tissues, especially the liver, spleen, bone marrow, and peripheral blood. Because of their overlapping clinical behavior, the diagnosis of lymphoid neoplasms is based on the morphologic and molecular characteristics of the tumor cells. Stated another way, for purposes of diagnosis and prognostication, it is most important to focus on what kind of cell the tumor is made up of, not where the tumor resides in the patient.

Two groups of lymphomas are recognized: *Hodgkin lymphomas* and *non-Hodgkin lymphomas*. Although both arise most commonly in lymphoid tissues, Hodgkin lymphoma is set apart by the presence of distinctive neoplastic RS giant cells (see later), which usually are greatly outnumbered by nonneoplastic inflammatory cells. The biologic behavior and clinical treatment of Hodgkin lymphoma also are different from those of NHLs, making the distinction of practical importance.

An international group of pathologists, molecular biologists, and clinicians working on behalf of the World Health Organization (WHO) has formulated a widely accepted classification scheme for lymphoid neoplasms and myeloid neoplasms (discussed later) that relies on a combination of morphologic, phenotypic, genotypic, and clinical features. As background for the subsequent discussion of this classification, certain important principles warrant consideration:

- **B and T cell tumors often are composed of cells that are arrested at or derived from a specific stage of normal lymphocyte differentiation** (Fig. 12.13). The diagnosis and classification of these tumors rely heavily on tests (either immunohistochemistry or flow cytometry) that detect lineage-specific antigens (e.g., B cell, T cell, and NK cell markers) and markers of maturity. By convention, many such markers are identified by their cluster of differentiation (CD) number.
- **Class switching and somatic hypermutation are mistake-prone forms of regulated genomic instability that place germinal center B cells at relatively high risk for potentially transforming mutations.** The most common lymphomas are derived from B cells that have migrated into germinal centers following antigen stimulation. This conclusion is drawn from analyses showing that most B cell lymphomas have undergone somatic hypermutation, an event confined to germinal center B cells. Normal germinal center B cells also undergo immunoglobulin class switching, which allows B cells to express immunoglobulins other than IgM. Many of the recurrent chromosomal translocations found in mature B cell malignancies involve the immunoglobulin loci and appear to stem from "accidents" during attempted diversification of the immunoglobulin genes. By contrast, mature T cells, which are genomically stable, give rise to lymphoma infrequently and only very rarely have chromosomal translocations involving the T cell receptor loci.

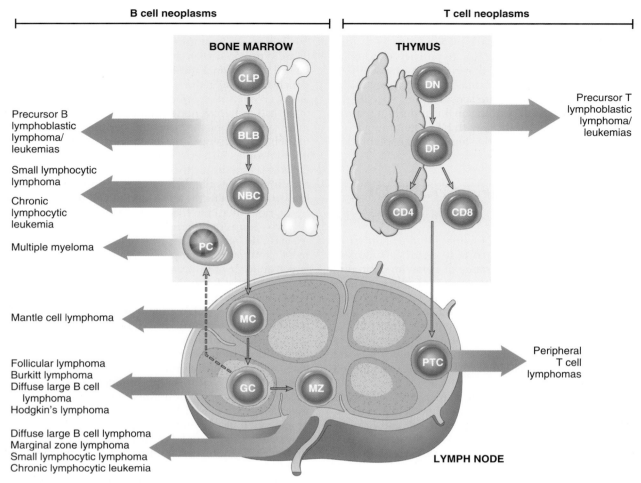

Fig. 12.13 Origin of lymphoid neoplasms. Stages of B and T cell differentiation from which specific lymphoid and tumors emerge are shown. *BLB,* Pre-B lymphoblast; *CLP,* common lymphoid progenitor; *DN,* CD4−/CD8− (double-negative) pro-T cell; *DP,* CD4+/CD8+ (double-positive) pre-T cell; *GC,* germinal center B cell; *MC,* mantle zone B cell; *MZ,* marginal zone B cell; *NBC,* naive B cell; *PC,* plasma cell; *PTC,* peripheral T cell.

- **Like other cancers, lymphoid neoplasms are derived from a single transformed cell and are therefore clonal.** As described in Chapter 5, precursor B and T cells rearrange their antigen receptor genes through a mechanism that ensures that each lymphocyte makes a single, unique antigen receptor. Because antigen receptor gene rearrangement virtually always precedes transformation, the daughter cells derived from a given malignant progenitor share the same antigen receptor gene configuration and synthesize identical antigen receptor proteins (either immunoglobulins or T cell receptors). Thus, analyses of antigen receptor genes and their protein products can be used to differentiate lymphoid neoplasms (which are clonal) from immune reactions (which are polyclonal).
- **Lymphoid neoplasms often disrupt normal immune function.** Both immunodeficiency (made evident by increased susceptibility to infection) and autoimmunity may be seen, sometimes in the same patient. Ironically, patients with inherited or acquired immunodeficiencies are at high risk for the development of certain lymphoid neoplasms, particularly those associated with EBV infection.

- **Although NHLs often manifest at a particular tissue site, sensitive molecular assays usually show that the tumor is widely disseminated at diagnosis.** As a result, with few exceptions, only systemic therapies are curative for those with NHL. By contrast, Hodgkin lymphoma often arises at a single site and spreads in a predictable fashion to contiguous lymph node groups.

The WHO classification of lymphoid neoplasms (Table 12.7) considers the morphology, cell of origin (determined by immunophenotyping), clinical features, and genotype (e.g., karyotype, presence of viral genomes) of each entity. As is evident, the diagnostic entities are numerous. We will focus our discussion on a subset that are particularly clinically important or pathogenically illustrative:
- Precursor B and T cell lymphoblastic lymphoma/leukemia—commonly called acute lymphoblastic leukemia (ALL)
- Chronic lymphocytic leukemia/small lymphocytic lymphoma
- Follicular lymphoma
- Mantle cell lymphoma

Table 12.7 WHO Classification of Lymphoid Neoplasms[a]

Precursor B Cell Neoplasms
Precursor B cell leukemia/lymphoma (B-ALL)

Peripheral B Cell Neoplasms
B cell chronic lymphocytic leukemia (CLL)/small lymphocytic lymphoma (SLL)
B cell prolymphocytic leukemia
Lymphoplasmacytic lymphoma
Mantle cell lymphoma
Follicular lymphoma
Extranodal marginal zone lymphoma
Splenic and nodal marginal zone lymphoma
Hairy cell leukemia
Plasmacytoma/plasma cell myeloma
Diffuse large B cell lymphoma (multiple subtypes)
Burkitt lymphoma

Precursor T Cell Neoplasms
Precursor T cell leukemia/lymphoma (T-ALL)

Peripheral T/NK Cell Neoplasms
T cell prolymphocytic leukemia
T cell granular lymphocytic leukemia
Mycosis fungoides/Sézary syndrome
Peripheral T cell lymphoma, unspecified
Angioimmunoblastic T cell lymphoma
Anaplastic large cell lymphoma
Enteropathy-type T cell lymphoma
Panniculitis-like T cell lymphoma
Hepatosplenic γδ T cell lymphoma
Adult T cell lymphoma/leukemia
Extranodal NK/T cell lymphoma
Aggressive NK cell leukemia

Hodgkin Lymphoma
Nodular sclerosis
Mixed cellularity
Lymphocyte-rich
Lymphocyte-depleted
Lymphocyte predominant

NK, Natural killer; *WHO*, World Health Organization.
[a]Entries in *italics* are among the most common lymphoid tumors.

- Extranodal marginal zone lymphoma
- Diffuse large B cell lymphomas
- Burkitt lymphoma
- Multiple myeloma and related entities
- Hodgkin lymphoma

Together these neoplasms constitute more than 90% of the lymphoid tumors seen in the United States.

The salient features of the more common lymphoid leukemias, non-Hodgkin lymphomas, and plasma cell tumors are summarized in Table 12.8 and are discussed in the following sections. We will then cover Hodgkin lymphoma and finish by briefly mentioning a few uncommon entities with distinctive clinicopathologic features.

Precursor B and T Cell Neoplasms
Acute Lymphoblastic Leukemia/Lymphoma

Acute lymphoblastic leukemia/lymphomas (ALLs) are neoplasms composed of immature B (pre-B) or T (pre-T) cells, which are referred to as *lymphoblasts*. About 85% are B-ALLs, which typically manifest as childhood acute "leukemias." The less common T-ALLs tend to present in adolescent males as thymic "lymphomas." There is,

however, considerable overlap in the clinical behavior of B- and T-ALL; for example, many T-ALLs present with or evolve to a leukemic picture. Because of their morphologic and clinical similarities, the various forms of ALL will be considered here together.

ALL is the most common cancer of children. Approximately 2500 new cases are diagnosed each year in the United States, most occurring in individuals younger than 15 years of age. ALL is almost three times as common in whites as in blacks and is slightly more frequent in boys than in girls. Hispanics have the highest incidence of any ethnic group. B-ALL peaks in incidence at about the age of 3, perhaps because the number of normal bone marrow pre-B cells (the cell of origin) is greatest very early in life. Similarly the peak incidence of T-ALL is in adolescence, the age when the thymus reaches its maximum size.

Pathogenesis

Many chromosomal aberrations seen in ALL dysregulate the expression and function of transcription factors that are required for the normal differentiation of B and T cell progenitors. Up to 70% of T-ALLs have gain-of-function mutations in *NOTCH1*, a gene that is essential for T cell differentiation, whereas a high fraction of B-ALLs has loss-of-function mutations in genes that are required for B cell differentiation, such as *PAX5*. These varied mutations appear to promote maturation arrest and increased self-renewal, a feature of immortalized cells, which, as mentioned, is one of the hallmarks of cancers.

In keeping with the multistep origins of cancer, mutations in transcription factor genes are not sufficient to produce ALL, and aberrations that drive cell growth, such as mutations that increase tyrosine kinase activity and RAS signaling, also are common. Ongoing deep sequencing of ALL genomes is rapidly filling in the remaining gaps. Early returns suggest that fewer than 10 mutations are sufficient to produce full-blown ALL; hence, compared to solid tumors, ALL is a genetically simple tumor.

MORPHOLOGY

In leukemic presentations, **the marrow is hypercellular and packed with lymphoblasts,** which replace normal marrow elements. **Mediastinal masses** occur in 50% to 70% of T-ALLs, which are also more likely to be associated with lymphadenopathy and splenomegaly. In both B- and T-ALL, the tumor cells have scant basophilic cytoplasm and nuclei with delicate, finely stippled chromatin and small nucleoli (Fig. 12.14A). In keeping with the aggressive clinical behavior, the mitotic rate is high. The appearance of the blasts is identical in pre-B and pre-T ALLs and is not sufficiently characteristic to exclude the other major subtype of acute leukemia, acute myeloid leukemia (AML, discussed later). For this reason, definitive diagnosis relies on stains performed with antibodies specific for B and T cell antigens (Fig. 12.14B–C). Histochemical stains are also helpful, in that (in contrast to myeloblasts) lymphoblasts are myeloperoxidase-negative and often contain periodic acid-Schiff–positive glycogen granules.

Table 12.8 Characteristics of the More Common Lymphoid Leukemias, Non-Hodgkin Lymphomas, and Plasma Cell Tumors

Clinical Entity	Frequency	Salient Morphology	Cell of Origin	Comments
Precursor B cell lymphoblastic leukemia/lymphoma	85% of childhood acute leukemias	Lymphoblasts with irregular nuclear contours, condensed chromatin, small nucleoli, and scant, agranular cytoplasm	TdT+ precursor B cell	Usually manifests as acute leukemia; less common in adults; prognosis is predicted by karyotype
Precursor T cell leukemia/lymphoma	15% of childhood acute leukemias; 40% of childhood lymphomas	Identical to precursor B cell lymphoblastic leukemia/lymphoma	TdT+ precursor T cell	Most common in adolescent males; often manifests as a mediastinal mass associated with NOTCH1 mutations
Small lymphocytic lymphoma/chronic lymphocytic leukemia	3%–4% of adult lymphomas; 30% of all leukemias	Small resting lymphocytes mixed with variable numbers of large activated cells; lymph nodes diffusely effaced	CD5+ B cell	Occurs in older adults; usually involves nodes, marrow, spleen; and peripheral blood; indolent
Follicular lymphoma	40% of adult lymphomas	Frequent small "cleaved" cells mixed with large cells; nodular (follicular) growth pattern	Germinal center B cell	Associated with t(14;18); indolent
Mantle cell lymphoma	6% of adult lymphomas	Small to intermediate-sized irregular lymphocytes; diffuse growth pattern	CD5+ B cell overexpressing cyclin D1	Associated with t(11;14); moderately aggressive
Extranodal marginal zone lymphoma	~5% of adult lymphomas	Tumor cells often home to epithelium, creating "lymphoepithelial lesions"	CD5−, CD10−B cell	Associated with chronic inflammation; indolent
Diffuse large B cell lymphoma	40%–50% of adult lymphomas	Variable; most resemble large germinal center B cells; diffuse growth pattern	Germinal center or postgerminal center B cell	Heterogeneous, may arise at extranodal sites; aggressive
Burkitt lymphoma	<1% of lymphomas in the United States	Intermediate-sized cells with several nucleoli; diffuse growth pattern; frequent apoptotic cells ("starry sky" appearance)	Germinal center B cell	Associated with t(8;14) and EBV (subset); highly aggressive
Plasmacytoma/plasma cell myeloma	Most common lymphoid neoplasm in older adults	Plasma cells in sheets, sometimes with prominent nucleoli or inclusions containing immunoglobulin	Postgerminal center B cell	CRAB (hypercalcemia, renal failure, anemia, bone fractures)

EBV, Epstein-Barr virus; *TdT,* terminal deoxynucleotidyl transferase.

The peripheral blood findings are highly variable. The white cell count may be greater than 100,000 cells/μL but in about half of the patients is less than 10,000 cells/μL. A few patients have no circulating blasts (aleukemic leukemia). Anemia almost always is present, and the platelet count usually is below 100,000/μL. Neutropenia is another common finding.

Genetics. Approximately 90% of ALLs have nonrandom karyotypic abnormalities. Most common in childhood pre–B cell tumors are hyperdiploidy (more than 50 chromosomes/cell) and a (12;21) translocation involving the *ETV6* and *RUNX1* genes, creating a fusion gene encoding an aberrant transcription factor, whereas about 25% of adult pre–B cell tumors have a (9;22) translocation involving the *ABL* and *BCR* genes. Pre–T cell tumors are associated with diverse chromosomal aberrations, including frequent translocations involving the T cell receptor loci and certain transcription factor genes, as well as mutations that inactivate tumors suppressor genes such as *PTEN* (leading to increased pro-growth signaling) and *CDKN2A,* which encodes a negative regulator of the cell cycle and a positive regulator of p53.

Immunophenotype. As mentioned, immunophenotyping is very useful in subtyping ALLs and distinguishing them from AML. Terminal deoxynucleotidyl transferase (TdT),

an enzyme specifically expressed in pre–B and pre–T cells, is present in more than 95% of cases. Further subtyping of ALL into pre–B and pre–T cell types relies on stains for lineage-specific markers, such as the B cell marker CD19 and the T cell marker CD3.

Clinical Features. ALL is an aggressive disease, and most patients present within a few weeks of the onset of symptoms. Among the most important signs and symptoms are the following:

* *Symptoms related to depression of marrow function,* including fatigue resulting from anemia; fever, reflecting infections secondary to neutropenia; and bleeding due to thrombocytopenia
* *Mass effects caused by neoplastic infiltration,* including bone pain resulting from marrow expansion and infiltration of the subperiosteum; generalized lymphadenopathy, splenomegaly, and hepatomegaly; and in T-ALL, complications related to compression of large vessels and airways in the mediastinum
* *Central nervous system manifestations* resulting from meningeal spread, such as headache, vomiting, and nerve palsies

Despite its highly malignant natural history, pediatric ALL is one of the great success stories of oncology. With aggressive chemotherapy, about 95% of children with ALL obtain a remission, and 75% to 85% are cured. It is sobering

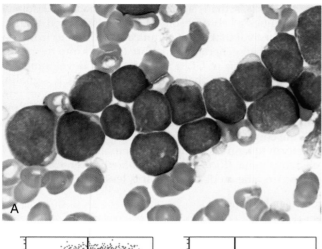

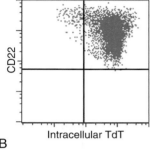 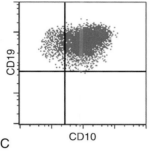

B   Intracellular TdT   C   CD10

Fig. 12.14 Acute lymphoblastic leukemia (ALL). (A) Lymphoblasts with condensed nuclear chromatin, small nucleoli, and scant agranular cytoplasm. (B) and (C) show flow cytometry results for the ALL shown in (A). The tumor cells are positive for the B cell markers CD19 and CD22; CD10 (a marker expressed on a subset of ALLs), and TdT (a specialized DNA polymerase that is expressed in pre-B and pre-T cells). (A, *Courtesy of Dr. Robert W. McKenna, Department of Pathology, University of Texas Southwestern Medical School, Dallas, Texas. B and C, Courtesy of Dr. Louis Picker, Oregon Health Science Center, Portland, Oregon.*)

to consider, however, that ALL remains the leading cause of cancer deaths in children, and that only 35% to 40% of affected adults are cured. Several factors are associated with a worse prognosis: (1) age younger than 2 years, largely because these tumors are genetically distinct, often being associated with translocations involving the *MLL* gene; (2) presentation in adolescence or adulthood; and (3) peripheral blood blast counts greater than 100,000. Favorable prognostic markers include (1) age between 2 and 10 years, (2) a low white cell count, and (3) hyperdiploidy. The molecular detection of residual disease after therapy also is predictive of a worse outcome in both B- and T-ALL and is being used to guide therapy.

Although most chromosomal aberrations in ALL alter the function of transcription factors, the t(9;22) instead creates a fusion gene encoding a constitutively active BCR-ABL tyrosine kinase (described later under chronic myeloid leukemia). Treatment of t(9;22)-positive ALLs with BCR-ABL kinase inhibitors in combination with conventional chemotherapy is highly effective and has improved the outcome for this subtype of B-ALL in both children and adults. Tests to identify other "targetable" mutated tyrosine kinases in ALLs lacking BCR-ABL are under development. The outlook for adults with ALL remains guarded, in part

because of differences in the molecular pathogenesis of adult and childhood ALL, and also because older adults cannot tolerate the intensive chemotherapy regimens that are curative in children.

Chronic Lymphocytic Leukemia/Small Lymphocytic Lymphoma

Chronic lymphocytic leukemia (CLL) and small lymphocytic lymphoma (SLL) are essentially identical, differing only in the extent of peripheral blood involvement. Somewhat arbitrarily, if the peripheral blood lymphocyte count exceeds 5000 cells/μL, the patient is diagnosed with CLL. Most cases fit the diagnostic criteria for CLL, which is the most common leukemia of adults in the Western world. By contrast, SLL constitutes only 4% of NHLs. For unclear reasons, CLL/SLL is much less common in Asia.

Pathogenesis

CLL/SLL is an indolent, slowly growing tumor in which increased tumor cell survival appears to be more important than tumor cell proliferation per se. In line with this idea, CLL/SLL cells contain high levels of BCL2, a protein that inhibits apoptosis (Chapters 1 and 6). One mechanism of *BCL2* overexpression appears to be chromosomal deletions that lead to the loss of genes encoding micro-RNAs that are negative regulators of *BCL2*. *Also of critical importance are signals generated by surface immunoglobulin (the so-called B cell receptor, or BCR).* BCR signals flow through an intermediary called *Bruton tyrosine kinase (BTK)* that ultimately contributes to the expression of genes that promote the survival of CLL/SLL cells.

CLL/SLL also causes immune dysregulation, particularly of normal B cells. Through unclear mechanisms, the accumulation of CLL/SLL cells suppresses normal B cell function, often resulting in *hypogammaglobulinemia.* Paradoxically, approximately 15% of patients develop autoantibodies against their own red cells or platelets. When present, the autoantibodies are made by nonmalignant bystander B cells, indicating that CLL/SLL cells somehow impair immune tolerance.

MORPHOLOGY

Involved lymph nodes are effaced by sheets of small lymphocytes and by scattered ill-defined foci of larger, actively dividing cells (Fig. 12.15A). The predominant cells are small, resting lymphocytes with dark, round nuclei, and scanty cytoplasm (Fig. 12.15B). The foci of mitotically active cells are called **proliferation centers,** which are pathognomonic for CLL/SLL. In addition to the lymph nodes, the bone marrow, spleen, and liver are involved in almost all cases. In most patients there is an absolute **lymphocytosis** featuring small, mature-looking lymphocytes. These circulating cells are fragile and during the preparation of smears many are disrupted, producing characteristic **smudge cells.** Variable numbers of larger activated lymphocytes also are usually present in blood smears.

Immunophenotype and Genetics. CLL/SLL is a neoplasm of mature B cells expressing the CD20 and surface immunoglobulins. The tumor cells also express CD5. This

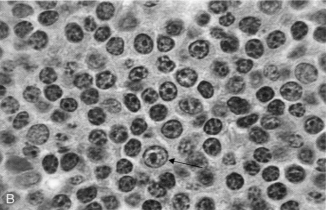

Fig. 12.15 Small lymphocytic lymphoma/chronic lymphocytic leukemia—lymph node. (A) Low-power view shows diffuse effacement of nodal architecture. (B) At high power, a majority of the tumor cells have the appearance of small, round lymphocytes. A "prolymphocyte," a larger cell with a centrally placed nucleolus, also is present in this field *(arrow)*. (A, *Courtesy of Dr. José Hernandez, Department of Pathology, University of Texas Southwestern Medical School, Dallas, Texas.)*

is a helpful diagnostic clue, since among B cell lymphomas only CLL/SLL and mantle cell lymphoma (discussed later) commonly express CD5. Approximately 50% of tumors have karyotypic abnormalities, the most common of which are trisomy 12 and deletions involving portions of chromosomes 11, 13, and 17. *Unlike in other B cell neoplasms, chromosomal translocations are rare.*

Clinical Features. When first detected, CLL/SLL often is asymptomatic. The most common signs and symptoms are nonspecific and include easy fatigability, weight loss, and anorexia. Generalized lymphadenopathy and hepatosplenomegaly are present in 50% to 60% of patients. The leukocyte count may be increased only slightly (in SLL) or may exceed 200,000 cells/μL. Hypogammaglobulinemia develops in more than 50% of the patients, usually late in the course, and leads to an increased susceptibility to bacterial infections. Less commonly, autoimmune hemolytic anemia and thrombocytopenia are seen.

The course and prognosis of CLL/SLL are highly variable and depend on the disease stage and genetic findings. For example, the presence of abnormalities in the *TP53* tumor suppressor gene is associated with an overall

survival of less than 30% at 10 years, whereas isolated abnormalities of chromosome 13q are associated with an overall survival that is not significantly different from that of the matched general population. Insights into the molecular pathogenesis of CLL/SLL has led to development of effective new drugs that variously inhibit BCR signaling (e.g., by targeting BTK) or BCL2 function. However, cure may only be achieved with hematopoietic stem cell transplantation, which is reserved for relatively young patients who fail conventional therapies. A small fraction of tumors transform to aggressive tumors resembling diffuse large B cell lymphoma *(Richter transformation)*; after transformation occurs, the median survival is less than 1 year.

Follicular Lymphoma

This relatively common tumor constitutes 40% of the adult NHLs in the United States. Like CLL/SLL, it occurs much less frequently in Asian populations.

Pathogenesis

Greater than 85% of follicular lymphomas have a characteristic (14;18) translocation that fuses the *BCL2* gene on chromosome 18 to the *IgH* locus on chromosome 14. This chromosomal rearrangement results in the inappropriate "overexpression" of BCL2 protein, which you will recall is an inhibitor of apoptosis that contributes to cell survival (Chapters 1 and 6). Whole genome sequencing of follicular lymphomas has identified additional mutations in genes encoding histone-modifying proteins in about one-third of cases, suggesting that epigenetic changes also contribute to the genesis of these tumors.

MORPHOLOGY

Lymph nodes usually are effaced by a distinctly **nodular proliferation** (Fig. 12.16A). Most commonly, the predominant neoplastic cells are so-called "**centrocytes**", cells slightly larger than resting lymphocytes that have angular "cleaved" nuclei with prominent indentations and linear infoldings (Fig. 12.16B). The nuclear chromatin is coarse and condensed, and nucleoli are indistinct. These centrocytes are mixed with variable numbers of **centroblasts**, larger cells with vesicular chromatin, several nucleoli, and modest amounts of cytoplasm. In most tumors, centroblasts are a minor component of the overall cellularity, mitoses are infrequent, and single necrotic cells (cells undergoing apoptosis) are not seen. These features help to distinguish follicular lymphoma from follicular hyperplasia, in which mitoses and apoptosis are prominent. Uncommonly, large cells predominate, a histologic pattern that correlates with a more aggressive clinical behavior.

Immunophenotype. These tumors express B cell markers such as CD20 and the germinal center B cell markers CD10 and BCL6; of note, BCL6 is a transcription factor that is required for the generation of germinal center B cells.

Clinical Features. Follicular lymphoma mainly occurs in adults older than 50 years of age and affects males and females equally. It usually manifests as painless, generalized lymphadenopathy. The bone marrow is involved at diagnosis in approximately 80% of cases. Although the

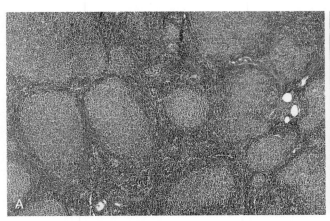
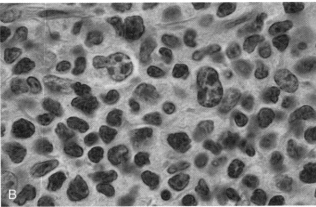

Fig. 12.16 Follicular lymphoma—lymph node. (A) Nodular aggregates of lymphoma cells are present throughout. (B) At high magnification, small lymphoid cells with condensed chromatin and irregular or cleaved nuclear outlines (centrocytes) are mixed with a population of larger cells with nucleoli (centroblasts). (A, *Courtesy of Dr. Robert W. McKenna, Department of Pathology, University of Texas Southwestern Medical School, Dallas, Texas.*)

natural history is prolonged (overall median survival, approximately 10 years), follicular lymphoma is not curable, an unfortunate feature shared with most other relatively indolent lymphoid malignancies. As a result, therapy with cytotoxic drugs and rituximab (anti-CD20 antibody) is reserved for those with bulky, symptomatic disease. BTK and BCL2 inhibitors are also active in this disease and are being evaluated in clinical trials. In about 30% to 40% of patients, follicular lymphoma progresses to diffuse large B cell lymphoma. This transformation is an ominous event, as tumors arising from such conversions are much less curable than de novo diffuse large B cell lymphomas, described later.

Mantle Cell Lymphoma

Mantle cell lymphoma is composed of cells resembling the naive B cells found in the mantle zones of normal lymphoid follicles. It constitutes approximately 6% of all NHLs and occurs mainly in men older than 50 years of age.

Pathogenesis

Almost all tumors have an (11;14) translocation that fuses the cyclin D1 gene to the IgH locus. This translocation leads to overexpression of cyclin D1, which you will recall stimulates growth by promoting the progression of cells from the G_1 phase to the S phase of the cell cycle (Chapter 6).

MORPHOLOGY

Mantle cell lymphoma may involve lymph nodes in a diffuse or vaguely nodular pattern. Proliferation centers are absent, a feature that helps to distinguish mantle cell lymphoma from CLL/SLL. The tumor cells usually are slightly larger than normal lymphocytes and have an irregular nucleus, inconspicuous nucleoli, and scant cytoplasm. Less commonly, the cells are larger and morphologically resemble lymphoblasts. The bone marrow is involved in most cases and the peripheral blood in about 20% of cases. The tumor sometimes arises in the gastrointestinal tract, often manifesting as multifocal submucosal nodules that grossly resemble polyps (lymphomatoid polyposis).

Immunophenotype. The tumor cells express surface IgM and IgD, the B cell antigen CD20, and CD5, and they contain high levels of cyclin D1 protein.

Clinical Features. Most patients present with fatigue and lymphadenopathy and are found to have generalized disease involving the bone marrow, spleen, liver, and (often) the gastrointestinal tract. These tumors are moderately aggressive and incurable. The median survival is 4 to 6 years. Like CLL/SLL cells, mantle cell lymphoma cells depend on signals generated through BTK for survival, and it is hoped that newly available BTK inhibitors will improve clinical outcomes.

Extranodal Marginal Zone Lymphoma

This indolent B cell tumor arises most commonly in epithelial tissues such as the stomach, salivary glands, small and large bowel, lungs, orbit, and breast.

Pathogenesis

Extranodal marginal zone lymphoma is an example of a cancer that arises within and is sustained by chronic inflammation. It tends to develop within tissues that are involved by chronic inflammation triggered by autoimmune disorders (such as the salivary gland in Sjögren syndrome and the thyroid gland in Hashimoto thyroiditis) or that are the sites of chronic infection (such as *H. pylori* gastritis). In the case of *H. pylori*–associated gastric marginal zone lymphoma, eradication of *H. pylori* with antibiotic therapy often leads to regression of the tumor cells, which depend on inflammatory cytokines secreted by *H. pylori*–specific T cells for their growth and survival. Based on these observations, it is supposed that the disease is initiated within the context of a polyclonal immune reaction. With the acquisition of still-unknown initiating mutations, a B cell clone emerges that depends on antigen-stimulated T-helper cells for signals that drive growth and survival. At this stage, withdrawal of the responsible antigen causes tumor involution. As further clonal evolution leads to greater tumor cell autonomy, spread to distant sites may occur. This theme of polyclonal to monoclonal transition during lymphomagenesis is also applicable to the pathogenesis of EBV-induced lymphoma (discussed in Chapter 6).

Immunophenotype. This is a tumor of mature B cells expressing CD20 and surface immunoglobulin, usually IgM.

Clinical Features. These tumors often present as swelling of the salivary gland, thyroid or orbit or are discovered incidentally in the setting of *H. pylori*–induced gastritis or an imaging procedure. When localized, they are often cured by simple excision followed by radiotherapy.

Diffuse Large B Cell Lymphoma

Diffuse large B cell lymphoma is the most common type of lymphoma in adults, accounting for approximately 35% of adult NHLs. It includes several subtypes that share an aggressive natural history.

Pathogenesis

About one-third of diffuse large B cell lymphomas have rearrangements of the *BCL6* gene, located on 3q27, and an even higher fraction of tumors have activating point mutations in the *BCL6* promoter. Both aberrations result in increased levels of BCL6 protein, an important transcriptional regulator of gene expression in germinal center B cells. Another 30% of tumors have a (14;18) translocation involving the *BCL2* gene that results in overexpression of BCL2 protein. Some of these tumors may represent "transformed" follicular lymphomas. The remaining tumors have other diverse driver mutations, such as translocations involving the *MYC* gene.

MORPHOLOGY

The neoplastic B cells are large (at least three to four times the size of resting lymphocytes) and vary in appearance from tumor to tumor. In many tumors, cells with round or oval nuclear contours, dispersed chromatin, several distinct nucleoli, and modest amounts of pale cytoplasm predominate (Fig. 12.17). In other tumors the cells have a round or multilobate vesicular nucleus, one or two prominent centrally placed nucleoli, and abundant pale or basophilic cytoplasm. Occasionally, the tumor cells are highly anaplastic and include tumor giant cells resembling RS cells, the malignant cells of Hodgkin lymphoma.

Immunophenotype. These tumors express the B cell antigen CD20. Many also express surface IgM and/or IgG. Other antigens (e.g., CD10, BCL2) are variably expressed.

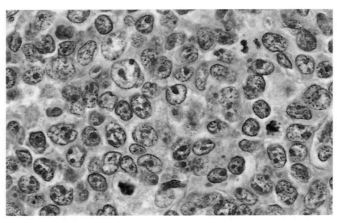

Fig. 12.17 Diffuse large B cell lymphoma—lymph node. The tumor cells have large nuclei with open chromatin and prominent nucleoli. *(Courtesy of Dr. Robert W. McKenna, Department of Pathology, University of Texas Southwestern Medical School, Dallas, Texas.)*

Special Subtypes. Several distinctive clinicopathologic subtypes are included in the category of diffuse large B cell lymphoma.

• *EBV-associated diffuse large B cell lymphomas* arise in the setting of AIDS, iatrogenic immunosuppression (e.g., in transplant recipients), and the elderly. In the posttransplantation setting, these tumors often begin as EBV-driven polyclonal B cell proliferations that may regress if immune function is restored.

• *Kaposi sarcoma herpesvirus* (KSHV), also called *human herpesvirus type 8* (HHV-8), is associated with rare *primary effusion lymphomas,* which may arise within the pleural cavity, pericardium, or peritoneum. These tumors are latently infected with KSHV, which encodes proteins homologous to several known oncoproteins, including cyclin D1. As with EBV-related lymphomas, most affected patients are immunosuppressed.

• *Mediastinal large B cell lymphoma* occurs most often in young women and shows a predilection for spread to abdominal viscera and the central nervous system.

Clinical Features. Although the median age at presentation is about 60 years, diffuse large B cell lymphoma can occur at any age; it constitutes about 15% of childhood lymphomas. Patients typically present with a rapidly enlarging, often symptomatic mass at one or several sites. Extranodal presentations are common. The gastrointestinal tract is the most common extranodal site, but tumors can appear in virtually any organ or tissue. Unlike the more indolent lymphomas (e.g., follicular lymphoma), involvement of the liver, spleen, and bone marrow is not common at diagnosis.

Without treatment, diffuse large cell B lymphomas are aggressive and rapidly fatal. With intensive combination chemotherapy and anti-CD20 immunotherapy, complete remissions are achieved in 60% to 80% of the patients; of these, approximately 50% remain free of disease and appear to be cured. For those not so fortunate, other aggressive treatments (e.g., high-dose chemotherapy and hematopoietic stem cell transplantation) offer some hope.

Burkitt Lymphoma

Burkitt lymphoma is endemic in parts of Africa and occurs sporadically in other geographic areas, including the United States. Histologically, the African and nonendemic diseases are identical, although there are clinical and virologic differences.

Pathogenesis

Burkitt lymphoma is highly associated with translocations involving the *MYC* gene on chromosome 8 that result in overexpression of the MYC transcription factor. As mentioned in Chapter 6, MYC is a master regulator of Warburg metabolism (aerobic glycolysis), a cancer hallmark that is associated with rapid cell growth. In keeping with this association, Burkitt lymphoma is said to be the fastest growing human tumor. Most translocations fuse *MYC* with the IgH gene on chromosome 14, but variant translocations involving the κ or λ light chain loci also are observed. The net result of each is the same—the dysregulation and overexpression of *MYC*. In most endemic cases and about 20% of sporadic cases, the tumor cells are latently infected with EBV, a relationship also discussed in Chapter 6.

MORPHOLOGY

The tumor cells are intermediate in size and typically have round or oval nuclei and two to five distinct nucleoli (Fig. 12.18). There is a moderate amount of basophilic or amphophilic cytoplasm that often contains small, lipid-filled vacuoles (a feature appreciated on smears). Very high rates of proliferation and apoptosis are characteristic, the latter accounting for the presence of numerous tissue macrophages containing ingested nuclear debris. These benign macrophages often are surrounded by a clear space, creating a **"starry sky" pattern.**

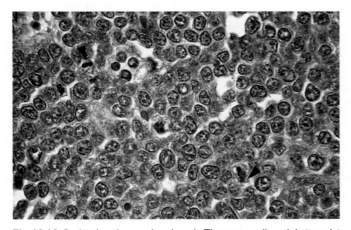

Fig. 12.18 Burkitt lymphoma—lymph node. The tumor cells and their nuclei are fairly uniform, giving a monotonous appearance. Note the high level of mitotic activity *(arrowheads)* and prominent nucleoli. The "starry sky" pattern produced by interspersed, lightly staining, normal macrophages is better appreciated at a lower magnification. *(Courtesy of Dr. Robert W. McKenna, Department of Pathology, University of Texas Southwestern Medical School, Dallas, Texas.)*

Immunophenotype. These tumors express surface IgM, the B cell marker CD20, and the germinal center B cell markers CD10 and BCL6.

Clinical Features. Both the endemic and nonendemic sporadic forms affect mainly children and young adults. Burkitt lymphoma accounts for approximately 30% of childhood NHLs in the United States. The disease usually arises at extranodal sites. Endemic tumors often manifest as maxillary or mandibular masses, whereas abdominal tumors involving the bowel, retroperitoneum, and ovaries are more common in North America. Leukemic presentations sometimes occur and must be distinguished from ALL, which is treated with different drug regimens. Burkitt lymphoma is highly aggressive; however, with very intensive chemotherapy regimens, a majority of patients can be cured.

Plasma Cell Neoplasms and Related Entities

These B cell proliferations contain neoplastic plasma cells that virtually always secrete a monoclonal immunoglobulin or immunoglobulin fragment, which serve as tumor markers and often have pathologic consequences. Collectively, plasma cell neoplasms and related disorders account for about 15% of the deaths caused by lymphoid neoplasms. The most common and deadly of these neoplasms is multiple myeloma, of which there are about 15,000 new cases per year in the United States.

A monoclonal immunoglobulin identified in the blood is referred to as an *M protein*, in reference to myeloma. Because complete M proteins have molecular weights of 160,000 or higher, they are restricted to the plasma and extracellular fluid and excluded from the urine in the absence of glomerular damage. However, *neoplastic plasma cells often synthesize excess immunoglobulin light chains along with complete immunoglobulins*. In unusual cases, tumors may produce only light chains, which are detected and quantified in the blood and the urine by highly sensitive tests.

Terms used to describe the abnormal immunoglobulins associated with plasma cell neoplasms include *monoclonal gammopathy, dysproteinemia,* and *paraproteinemia*. These abnormal proteins are associated with several clinicopathologic entities:

- *Multiple myeloma (plasma cell myeloma)*, the most important plasma cell neoplasm, usually presents as tumorous masses scattered throughout the skeletal system. *Solitary plasmacytoma* is an infrequent variant that presents as a single mass in bone or soft tissue. *Smoldering myeloma* is another uncommon variant defined by a lack of symptoms and a high plasma M component.
- *Monoclonal gammopathy of undetermined significance (MGUS)* is applied to patients without signs or symptoms who have small to moderately large M components in their blood. MGUS is very common in older adults and has a low but constant rate of transformation to a symptomatic monoclonal gammopathy, most often multiple myeloma.
- *Primary or immunocyte-associated amyloidosis* results from a monoclonal proliferation of plasma cells secreting light chains that are deposited as amyloid. Some

patients have overt multiple myeloma, but others have only a minor clonal population of plasma cells in the marrow.

- *Waldenström macroglobulinemia* is a syndrome in which high levels of IgM lead to symptoms related to hyperviscosity of the blood. It occurs in older adults, most commonly in association with lymphoplasmacytic lymphoma (described later).

With this background, we now turn to some of the specific clinicopathologic entities. Primary amyloidosis was discussed along with other disorders of the immune system in Chapter 5.

Multiple Myeloma

Multiple myeloma is one of the most common lymphoid malignancies; approximately 20,000 new cases are diagnosed in the United States each year. The median age at diagnosis is 70 years, and it is more common in males and in people of African origin. It principally involves the bone marrow and usually is associated with lytic lesions throughout the skeletal system.

The most frequent M protein produced by myeloma cells is IgG (60%), followed by IgA (20%–25%); only rarely are IgM, IgD, or IgE M proteins observed. In the remaining cases, the plasma cells produce only κ or λ light chains. Because free light chains are small in size, they are also excreted in the urine, where they are referred to as *Bence Jones proteins*. In many cases, the malignant plasma cells secrete both complete immunoglobulins and free light chains and thus produce both M proteins and Bence Jones proteins. As described later, the excess light chains have important pathogenic effects.

Pathogenesis

As with most other B cell malignancies, **myeloma often has chromosomal translocations that fuse the IgH locus on chromosome 14 to oncogenes such as the cyclin D1 and cyclin D3 genes.** As might be surmised from this, dysregulation of D cyclins is common in multiple myeloma and is believed to contribute to increases in cell proliferation. Proliferation of myeloma cells also is supported by the cytokine interleukin 6 (IL-6), which is produced by fibroblasts and macrophages in the bone marrow stroma. Late in the course, translocations involving *MYC* are sometimes observed, particularly in patients with aggressive disease.

Multiple myeloma has a number of untoward effects on the skeleton, the immune system, and the kidney, all of which contribute to morbidity and mortality:

- **Factors produced by neoplastic plasma cells mediate bone destruction, the major pathologic feature of multiple myeloma.** Of particular importance, myeloma-derived factors upregulate the expression of the receptor activator of NF-κB ligand (RANKL) by bone marrow stromal cells, which in turn activate osteoclasts. Other factors released from tumor cells are potent inhibitors of osteoblast function. The net effect is increased bone resorption, leading to hypercalcemia and pathologic fractures.
- **Myeloma causes defects in humoral immunity.** Through still-uncertain mechanisms, myeloma cells compromise the function of normal B cells. Ironically,

although the plasma has elevated levels of immunoglobulin owing to the presence of an M protein, the production of functional antibodies often is profoundly depressed. As a result, patients are at high risk for bacterial infections.

- **Renal dysfunction** stems from several pathologic effects of myeloma that may occur alone or in combination. Most important are *obstructive proteinaceous casts*, which often form in the distal convoluted tubules and the collecting ducts. The casts consist mostly of Bence Jones proteins along with variable amounts of complete immunoglobulin, Tamm-Horsfall protein, and albumin. *Light chain deposition* in the glomeruli or the interstitium, either as amyloid or linear deposits, also may contribute to renal damage. Completing the assault is *hypercalcemia*, which may lead to dehydration and renal stones, and frequent bouts of *bacterial pyelonephritis*, which stem in part from the hypogammaglobulinemia.

MORPHOLOGY

Multiple myeloma usually manifests with **multifocal destructive skeletal lesions** that most commonly involve the vertebral column, ribs, skull, pelvis, femur, clavicle, and scapula. The lesions arise in the medullary cavity, erode cancellous bone, and progressively destroy the bone cortex. Bone destruction often leads to **pathologic fractures,** most frequently in the vertebral column or femur. The bone lesions usually appear as **punched-out defects** 1 to 4 cm in diameter (Fig. 12.19A). Microscopic examination of the marrow shows increased numbers of plasma cells, which usually constitute greater than 30% of the cellularity. Myeloma cells may resemble normal plasma cells but more often show abnormal features such as prominent nucleoli or abnormal cytoplasmic inclusions containing immunoglobulin (Fig. 12.19B). With disease progression, myeloma cells may spread to the viscera and other soft tissue sites, and in terminal stages a leukemic picture may emerge.

Renal involvement **(myeloma nephrosis)** is associated with proteinaceous casts consisting mostly of Bence Jones proteins that obstruct the distal convoluted tubules and the collecting ducts. Multinucleate giant cells derived from macrophages usually surround the casts. Very often the **epithelial cells adjacent to the casts become necrotic or atrophic** owing to the toxic effects of Bence Jones proteins. Other common pathologic processes involving the kidney include **metastatic calcification,** stemming from bone resorption and hypercalcemia; **light chain (AL) amyloidosis,** involving the renal glomeruli and vessel walls; and **bacterial pyelonephritis,** secondary to the increased susceptibility to bacterial infections. Rarely, infiltrates of neoplastic plasma cells are seen in the renal interstitium.

Clinical Features. Clinical findings stem mainly from (1) the effects of plasma cells on the skeleton; (2) the production of excessive immunoglobulins, which often have abnormal physicochemical properties; and (3) the suppression of humoral immunity.

Bone resorption often leads to *pathologic fractures* and *chronic pain*. The attendant *hypercalcemia* can give rise to neurologic manifestations, such as confusion, weakness, and lethargy, and contributes to renal dysfunction. Decreased

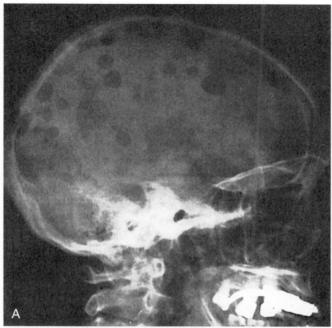

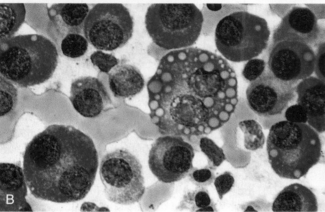

Fig. 12.19 Multiple myeloma. (A) Radiograph of the skull, lateral view. The sharply punched-out bone defects are most obvious in the calvaria. (B) Bone marrow aspirate. Normal marrow cells are largely replaced by plasma cells, including atypical forms with multiple nuclei, prominent nucleoli, and cytoplasmic droplets containing immunoglobulin.

production of normal immunoglobulins sets the stage for *recurrent bacterial infections*. Of great significance is *renal insufficiency,* which trails only infections as a cause of death. Renal failure occurs in up to 50% of patients and is associated strongly with the presence and level of *Bence Jones proteinuria,* highlighting the importance of free light chains in renal disease. Certain light chains also are prone to cause *amyloidosis* of the AL type (Chapter 5), which can exacerbate renal dysfunction and deposit in other tissues as well.

Laboratory analyses typically show increased levels of immunoglobulins in the blood and/or Bence Jones proteins in the urine. Free light chains and an M protein component are observed together in 60% to 70% of cases, whereas in about 20% of patients only free light chains are present. Around 1% of myelomas are nonsecretory; hence, the absence of detectable M component does not completely exclude the diagnosis.

The diagnosis rests on radiologic and laboratory findings. It can be strongly suspected when imaging studies show typical bone lesions, but definitive diagnosis requires a bone marrow examination. Marrow involvement often gives rise to a normocytic normochromic anemia, sometimes accompanied by moderate leukopenia and thrombocytopenia.

The prognosis is variable. Patients with multiple bony lesions, if untreated, rarely survive for more than 6 to 12 months, whereas patients with "smoldering myeloma" may be asymptomatic for many years. The median survival is 4 to 7 years. Although cures have yet to be achieved, new therapies offer hope. Myeloma cells are sensitive to inhibitors of the proteasome, a cellular organelle that degrades unwanted and misfolded proteins. As discussed in Chapter 2, misfolded proteins activate apoptotic pathways, and myeloma cells are prone to the accumulation of misfolded, unpaired immunoglobulin chains. Proteasome inhibitors likely induce myeloma cell death by exacerbating this inherent tendency. The thalidomide-like compound lenalidomide also is effective in treating myeloma, but through a different mechanism that involves its ability to stimulate the degradation of specific proteins with oncogenic activities. Biphosphonates, drugs that inhibit bone resorption, reduce pathologic fractures and limit the hypercalcemia. Hematopoietic stem cell transplantation prolongs life but has not yet proven to be curative.

Lymphoplasmacytic Lymphoma

Lymphoplasmacytic lymphoma is a B cell neoplasm of older adults that usually presents in the sixth or seventh decade of life. Although bearing a superficial resemblance to CLL/SLL, it differs in that a substantial fraction of the tumor cells undergo terminal differentiation to plasma cells. Most commonly, the plasma cell component secretes monoclonal IgM, often in amounts sufficient to cause a hyperviscosity syndrome known as *Waldenström macroglobulinemia.* Unlike multiple myeloma, complications stemming from the secretion of free light chains (e.g., renal failure and amyloidosis) are relatively rare and bone destruction does not occur.

Pathogenesis

Virtually all cases of lymphoplasmacytic lymphoma are associated with acquired mutations in *MYD88*. The *MYD88* gene encodes an adaptor protein that participates in signaling events that activate NF-κB and also augment signals downstream of the BCR (Ig) complex, both of which may promote the growth and survival of the tumor cells.

MORPHOLOGY

Typically, the marrow contains an infiltrate of lymphocytes, plasma cells, and plasmacytoid lymphocytes in varying proportions, often accompanied by mast cell hyperplasia. Some tumors also contain a population of larger lymphoid cells with more vesicular nuclear chromatin and prominent nucleoli. Periodic acid-Schiff-positive inclusions containing immunoglobulin are frequently seen in the cytoplasm (**Russell bodies**) or the nucleus (**Dutcher bodies**) of some of the plasma cells. At diagnosis the tumor has usually disseminated to the lymph nodes, spleen, and liver. Infiltration of the nerve roots, meninges, and more rarely the brain can also occur with disease progression.

Immunophenotype. The lymphoid component expresses B cell markers such as CD20 and surface immunoglobulin, whereas the plasma cell component secretes the same immunoglobulin that is expressed on the surface of the lymphoid cells. In almost all tumors, the secreted immunoglobulin is an IgM.

Clinical Features. The dominant presenting complaints are nonspecific and include weakness, fatigue, and weight loss. Approximately half the patients have lymphadenopathy, hepatomegaly, and splenomegaly. Anemia caused by marrow infiltration is common. About 10% of patients have *autoimmune hemolysis* caused by *cold agglutinins*, IgM antibodies that bind to red cells at temperatures of less than 37°C.

Patients with IgM-secreting tumors have additional signs and symptoms stemming from the physicochemical properties of IgM. Because of its large size, at high concentrations IgM greatly increases the viscosity of the blood, giving rise to a *hyperviscosity syndrome* characterized by the following:

- *Visual impairment* associated with venous congestion, which is reflected by striking tortuosity and distention of retinal veins; retinal hemorrhages and exudates may also contribute to problems with vision
- *Neurologic problems* such as headaches, dizziness, deafness, and stupor, all stemming from sluggish venous blood flow
- *Bleeding* related to the formation of complexes between macroglobulins and clotting factors as well as interference with platelet function
- *Cryoglobulinemia* resulting from the precipitation of macroglobulins at low temperatures, which produces symptoms such as Raynaud phenomenon and cold urticaria

Lymphoplasmacytic lymphoma is an incurable progressive disease. Because most IgM is intravascular, symptoms caused by the high IgM levels (e.g., hyperviscosity and hemolysis) can be alleviated temporarily by plasmapheresis. Tumor growth can be controlled with low doses of chemotherapeutic drugs and immunotherapy with anti-CD20 antibody, and recent work has shown that BTK inhibitors are also effective. Transformation to large-cell lymphoma occurs but is uncommon. Median survival is about 4 years.

Hodgkin Lymphoma

Hodgkin lymphoma encompasses a distinctive group of neoplasms that are characterized by the presence of *a tumor giant cell, the RS cell*. Unlike most NHLs, Hodgkin lymphomas arise in a single lymph node or chain of lymph nodes and typically spread in a stepwise fashion to anatomically contiguous nodes. Although the Hodgkin

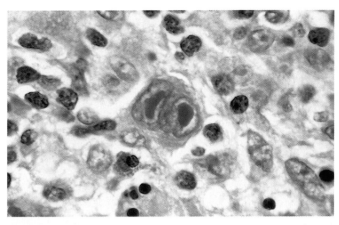

Fig. 12.20 Hodgkin lymphoma—lymph node. A binucleate Reed-Sternberg cell with large, inclusion-like nucleoli and abundant cytoplasm is surrounded by lymphocytes, macrophages, and an eosinophil. *(Courtesy of Dr. Robert W. McKenna, Department of Pathology, University of Texas Southwestern Medical School, Dallas, Texas.)*

lymphomas are now understood to be unusual tumors of B cell origin, they are distinguished from the NHLs by their unusual pathologic and clinical features.

Classification. Five subtypes of Hodgkin lymphoma are recognized: (1) nodular sclerosis, (2) mixed cellularity, (3) lymphocyte rich, (4) lymphocyte depletion, and (5) lymphocyte predominant. In the first four subtypes the RS cells share certain morphologic and immunophenotypic features (described later), leading some researchers to lump together these entities under the rubric *classical Hodgkin lymphoma*. The lymphocyte predominant type is set apart by the expression of germinal center B cell markers by the RS cells. This subtype and the two most common forms of classical Hodgkin lymphoma, the nodular sclerosis and mixed-cellularity types, are discussed next.

MORPHOLOGY

The sine qua non of Hodgkin lymphoma is the **Reed-Sternberg (RS) cell** (Fig. 12.20), a very large cell (15 to 45 μm in diameter) with an enormous multilobate nucleus, exceptionally prominent nucleoli, and abundant, usually slightly eosinophilic, cytoplasm. Particularly characteristic are cells with **two mirror-image nuclei or nuclear lobes, each containing a large (inclusion-like) acidophilic nucleolus surrounded by a clear zone**, features that impart an owl-eye appearance. Typical RS cells and variants have a characteristic immunophenotype, as they express CD15 and CD30 and fail to express CD45 (leukocyte common antigen), B cell antigens, and T cell antigens. As we shall see, "classic" RS cells are common in the mixed-cellularity subtype, uncommon in the nodular sclerosis subtype, and rare in the lymphocyte-predominance subtype; in these latter two subtypes, other characteristic RS cell variants predominate.

Nodular sclerosis Hodgkin lymphoma is the most common form. It is equally frequent in men and in women and has a striking propensity to involve the lower cervical, supraclavicular, and mediastinal lymph nodes. Most patients are

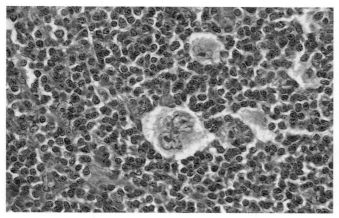

Fig. 12.21 Hodgkin lymphoma, nodular sclerosis type—lymph node. A distinctive "lacunar cell" with a multilobed nucleus containing many small nucleoli is seen lying within a clear space created by retraction of its cytoplasm. It is surrounded by lymphocytes. *(Courtesy of Dr. Robert W. McKenna, Department of Pathology, University of Texas Southwestern Medical School, Dallas, Texas.)*

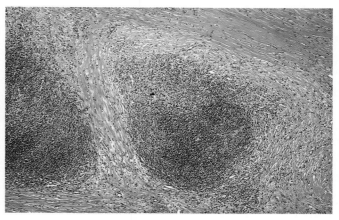

Fig. 12.22 Hodgkin lymphoma, nodular sclerosis type—lymph node. A low-power view shows well-defined bands of pink, acellular collagen that have subdivided the tumor cells into nodules. *(Courtesy of Dr. Robert W. McKenna, Department of Pathology, University of Texas Southwestern Medical School, Dallas, Texas.)*

adolescents or young adults, and the overall prognosis is excellent. It is characterized morphologically by the following:

- **Lacunar cells** (Fig. 12.21), a particular RS cell variant that has a single multilobate nucleus, multiple small nucleoli, and abundant, pale-staining cytoplasm. In sections of formalin-fixed tissue, the cytoplasm often is torn away, leaving the nucleus lying in an empty space (a lacune). The immunophenotype of lacunar variants is identical to that of other RS cells found in classical subtypes.
- **Collagen bands**, which divide the involved lymphoid tissue into circumscribed nodules (Fig. 12.22). The fibrosis may be scant or abundant and the cellular infiltrate contains varying proportions of lymphocytes, eosinophils, histiocytes, and lacunar cells.

Mixed-cellularity Hodgkin lymphoma is the most common form of Hodgkin lymphoma in patients older than 50 years of age and comprises about 25% of cases overall. There is a male predominance. **Classic RS cells are plentiful** within a heterogeneous inflammatory infiltrate containing small lymphocytes, eosinophils, plasma cells, and macrophages (Fig. 12.23). This subtype is more likely to be disseminated and to be associated with systemic manifestations than the nodular sclerosis subtype.

Lymphocyte-predominant Hodgkin lymphoma, accounting for about 5% of cases, is characterized by the presence of **lymphohistiocytic (L&H) variant RS cells** that have a delicate multilobed, puffy nucleus resembling popped corn ("popcorn cell"). L&H variants usually are found within large nodules containing mainly small B cells admixed with variable numbers of macrophages (Fig. 12.24). Other reactive cells, such as eosinophils, are scanty or absent, and typical RS cells are rare. Unlike the RS variants in "classical" Hodgkin lymphoma, L&H variants express B cell markers (e.g., CD20) and usually fail to express CD15 and CD30. Most patients present with isolated cervical or axillary lymphadenopathy, and the prognosis typically is excellent.

It is apparent that Hodgkin lymphoma spans a wide range of histologic patterns that often simulate a reactive inflammatory

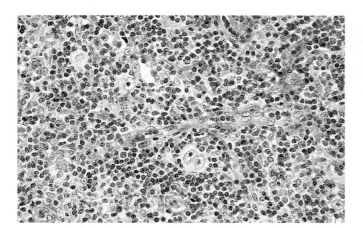

Fig. 12.23 Hodgkin lymphoma, mixed-cellularity type—lymph node. A diagnostic, binucleate Reed-Sternberg cell is surrounded by eosinophils, lymphocytes, and histiocytes. *(Courtesy of Dr. Robert W. McKenna, Department of Pathology, University of Texas Southwestern Medical School, Dallas, Texas.)*

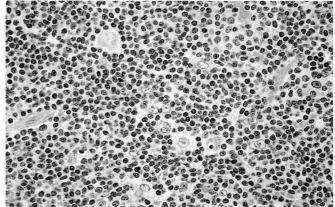

Fig. 12.24 Hodgkin lymphoma, nodular lymphocyte-predominant type—lymph node. Numerous mature-looking lymphocytes surround scattered, large, pale-staining lymphocytic and histiocytic variants ("popcorn" cells). *(Courtesy of Dr. Robert W. McKenna, Department of Pathology, University of Texas Southwestern Medical School, Dallas, Texas.)*

process. Regardless of subtype, **the diagnosis rests on the definitive identification of RS cells or variants in the appropriate background of reactive cells.** Immunophenotyping plays an important role in distinguishing Hodgkin lymphoma from reactive conditions and other forms of lymphoma. In all subtypes, involvement of the spleen, liver, bone marrow, and other organs may appear in due course and takes the form of irregular nodules composed of a mixture of RS cells and reactive cells, similar to what is observed in lymph nodes.

Pathogenesis

The origin of RS cells remained mysterious through most of the 20th century, but was finally solved by elegant studies performed on single microdissected RS cells. These showed that every RS cell from any given case possesses the same immunoglobulin gene rearrangements and that these rearranged immunoglobulin genes have undergone somatic hypermutation. As a result, it is now agreed that **Hodgkin lymphoma is a neoplasm that arises from germinal center B cells.**

Another clue into the etiology of Hodgkin lymphoma stems from the frequent involvement of EBV. EBV is present in the RS cells in as many as 70% of cases of the mixed-cellularity subtype and a smaller fraction of other "classical" forms of Hodgkin lymphoma. The structure of the EBV genome is identical in all RS cells in a given case, indicating that infection precedes (and therefore may be related to) transformation and clonal expansion. Thus, EBV infection probably is one of several steps contributing to tumor development, particularly of the mixed-cellularity subtype.

The characteristic nonneoplastic, inflammatory cell infiltrate is generated by a number of cytokines. Some of these are secreted by RS cells, including IL-5, a chemoattractant for eosinophils; transforming growth factor-β, a fibrogenic factor; and IL-13, which may stimulate RS cell growth through an autocrine mechanism. Conversely, the responding inflammatory cells, rather than being innocent bystanders, produce additional factors that aid the growth and survival of RS cells and contribute further to the tissue reaction.

Hodgkin lymphoma is a cardinal example of a tumor that escapes from the host immune response by expressing proteins that inhibit T cell function. The RS cells of classical Hodgkin lymphoma express high levels of PD ligands, factors that antagonize T cell responses. In many tumors the region on chromosome 9 containing the genes encoding the two PD ligands, PD-L1 and PD-L2, is amplified, an alteration that appears to contribute to their overexpression. The importance of PD ligand expression has been proven in clinical trials of antibodies that block PD-1, which is the T cell receptor for PD ligands (Chapter 6). Most tumors, even those that are resistant to all other therapies, are responsive to PD-1 antibodies, presumably because of the reactivation of a latent host response that was stifled by the PD ligand/ PD-1 signaling axis.

Clinical Features. Hodgkin lymphoma, like NHL, usually manifests as painless lymphadenopathy. Although a definitive distinction from NHL can be made only by

Table 12.9 Clinical Differences Between Hodgkin and Non-Hodgkin Lymphomas

Hodgkin Lymphoma	Non-Hodgkin Lymphoma
More often localized to a single axial group of nodes (cervical, mediastinal, paraaortic)	More frequent involvement of multiple peripheral nodes
Orderly spread by contiguity	Noncontiguous spread
Mesenteric nodes and Waldeyer ring rarely involved	Mesenteric nodes and Waldeyer ring commonly involved
Extranodal involvement uncommon	Extranodal involvement common

examination of a tissue biopsy, several clinical features favor the diagnosis of Hodgkin lymphoma (Table 12.9). After the diagnosis is established, staging is used to guide therapy and determine prognosis (Table 12.10). Younger patients with more favorable subtypes tend to present with stage I or stage II disease and usually are free of so-called "B symptoms" (fever, weight loss, night sweats). Patients with advanced disease (stages III and IV) are more likely to exhibit B symptoms as well as pruritus and anemia. Because of the long-term complications of radiotherapy, even patients with stage I disease are now treated with systemic chemotherapy. More advanced disease is generally also treated with chemotherapy, sometimes together with involved field radiotherapy.

The outlook, even for those with advanced disease, is very good. The 5-year survival rate for patients with stage I-A or II-A disease is more than 90%. Even with advanced disease (stage IV-A or IV-B), the overall 5-year disease-free survival rate is around 50%. Among long-term survivors treated with radiotherapy, a higher risk of certain malignancies, including lung cancer and breast cancer, as well as cardiovascular disease, has been reported. These sobering results have spurred development of new regimens that minimize the use of radiotherapy and use less toxic chemotherapy. As already mentioned, anti-PD-1 antibodies have produced excellent responses in patients with relapsed,

Table 12.10 Clinical Staging of Hodgkin and Non-Hodgkin Lymphomas (Ann Arbor Classification)[a]

Stage	Distribution of Disease
I	Involvement of a single lymph node region (I) or involvement of a single extralymphatic organ or tissue (I_E)
II	Involvement of two or more lymph node regions on the same side of the diaphragm alone (II) or with involvement of limited contiguous extralymphatic organs or tissue (II_E)
III	Involvement of lymph node regions on both sides of the diaphragm (III), which may include the spleen (III_S), limited contiguous extralymphatic organ or site (III_E), or both (III_{ES})
IV	Multiple or disseminated foci of involvement of one or more extralymphatic organs or tissues with or without lymphatic involvement

[a]All stages are further divided based on the absence (A) or presence (B) of the following systemic symptoms and signs: significant fever, night sweats, unexplained loss of more than 10% of normal body weight.
From Carbone PT, et al: Symposium (Ann Arbor): staging in Hodgkin disease. *Cancer Res* 31:1707, 1971.

refractory disease and represent a promising immune-based therapy.

Miscellaneous Lymphoid Neoplasms

Among the many other forms of lymphoid neoplasia in the WHO classification, several with distinctive or clinically important features merit brief discussion.

Hairy Cell Leukemia. Hairy cell leukemia is an uncommon, indolent B cell neoplasm characterized by the presence of fine, hairlike cytoplasmic projections. The tumor cells express B cell markers (CD20), surface immunoglobulin, and CD11c and CD103; the latter two antigens are not present on most other B cell tumors, making them diagnostically useful. Virtually all cases are associated with activating mutations in the serine/threonine kinase BRAF, which is also mutated in diverse other cancers (Chapter 6).

Hairy cell leukemia occurs mainly in older males, and its manifestations result from infiltration of bone marrow and spleen. *Splenomegaly,* often massive, is the most common and sometimes only physical finding. *Pancytopenia,* resulting from marrow infiltration and splenic sequestration, is seen in more than half of cases. Lymph node involvement is rare. Leukocytosis is uncommon, being present only in 15% to 20% of patients, but scattered "hairy cells" can be identified in the peripheral blood smear in most cases. The disease is indolent but progressive if untreated; pancytopenia and infections are the major clinical problems. Unlike most other indolent lymphoid neoplasms, hairy cell leukemia is extremely sensitive to chemotherapeutic agents, particularly purine nucleosides. Complete durable responses are the rule and the overall prognosis is excellent. Tumors that fail conventional therapy have excellent responses to BRAF inhibitors, which ultimately may become the treatment of choice.

Mycosis Fungoides and Sézary Syndrome. These tumors of neoplastic CD4+ T cells home to the skin; as a result, they often are referred to as cutaneous T cell lymphoma. Mycosis fungoides usually manifests as a nonspecific erythrodermic rash that progresses with time to a plaque phase and then to a tumor phase. Histologically, neoplastic T cells, often with a cerebriform appearance produced by marked infolding of the nuclear membranes, infiltrate the epidermis and upper dermis. With disease progression, both nodal and visceral dissemination appear. Sézary syndrome is a clinical variant characterized by (1) a generalized exfoliative erythroderma and (2) tumor cells (Sézary cells) in the peripheral blood. Circulating tumor cells also are present in as many as 25% of cases of plaque- or tumor-phase mycosis fungoides. Patients diagnosed with early-phase mycosis fungoides often survive for many years, whereas patients with tumor-phase disease, visceral disease, or Sézary syndrome survive on average for 1 to 3 years.

Adult T Cell Leukemia/Lymphoma. **This neoplasm of CD4+ T cells is caused by a retrovirus, human T cell leukemia virus type 1 (HTLV-1).** HTLV-1 infection is endemic in southern Japan, the Caribbean basin, and West Africa, and occurs sporadically elsewhere, including in the southeastern United States. The pathogenesis of this tumor is discussed in Chapter 6. In addition to lymphoid

malignancies, HTLV-1 infection also can cause tropical spastic paraparesis, a progressive demyelinating disease affecting the central nervous system and the spinal cord.

Adult T cell leukemia/lymphoma commonly is associated with skin lesions, lymphadenopathy, hepatosplenomegaly, hypercalcemia, and variable lymphocytosis. In addition to CD4, the leukemic cells express high levels of CD25, the IL-2 receptor α chain. In most cases the tumor is very aggressive and responds poorly to treatment. The median survival time is about 8 months.

Peripheral T Cell Lymphoma. This heterogeneous group of tumors makes up about 10% of adult NHLs. Although several rare distinctive subtypes fall under this heading, most tumors in this group are unclassifiable. In general, these are aggressive tumors that respond poorly to therapy. Moreover, because these are tumors of functional T cells, patients often suffer from symptoms related to tumor-derived inflammatory products, even when the tumor burden is relatively low.

Before ending our review of lymphoid neoplasms, it is worthwhile pausing to summarize the manner in which common driver mutations in specific entities produce changes in cellular behavior that exemplify particular hallmarks of cancer (Fig. 12.25). Such alterations not only highlight important pathogenic principles, but are increasingly the targets of effective therapies, such as antibodies that block PD-1 (Hodgkin lymphoma) and drugs that antagonize BCL2 (follicular lymphoma and other B cell tumors).

SUMMARY

LYMPHOID NEOPLASMS

- Classification is based on cell of origin and stage of differentiation
- Most common types in children are ALLs/lymphoblastic lymphomas derived from precursor B and T cells
- Most common types in adults are non-Hodgkin lymphomas derived from germinal center B cells

Acute Lymphoblastic Leukemia/Lymphoma

- Highly aggressive tumors that manifest with signs and symptoms of bone marrow failure, or as rapidly growing masses
- Tumor cells contain genetic lesions that block differentiation, leading to the accumulation of immature, nonfunctional blasts

Small Lymphocytic Lymphoma/Chronic Lymphocytic Leukemia

- Mature B cell tumor that usually manifests with bone marrow and lymph node involvement
- Indolent course, commonly associated with immune abnormalities, including an increased susceptibility to infection and autoimmune disorders

Follicular Lymphoma

- Tumor cells recapitulate the growth pattern of normal germinal center B cells; most cases are associated with a (14;18) translocation that results in the overexpression of BCL2

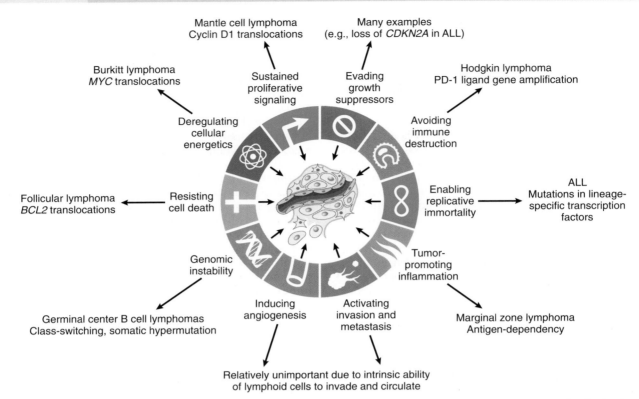

Fig. 12.25 Cancer hallmarks exemplified by particular lymphoid neoplasms. Some of the best characterized pathogenic mechanisms in lymphoid malignancies are summarized here, including dysregulation of MYC in Burkitt lymphoma (leading to Warburg metabolisms and rapid cell growth); dysregulation of BCL2 in follicular lymphoma (leading to resistance to apoptosis); PD-1 ligand gene amplification in Hodgkin lymphoma (leading to evasion of host immunity); events leading to loss of cell cycle control (cyclin D1 rearrangements in mantle cell lymphoma and loss of the *CDKN2A* gene in acute lymphoblastic leukemia [ALL]); mutations in various transcription factors, particularly in ALL, that block differentiation and enhance "leukemia stem cell" self-renewal; and chronic immune stimulation, in marginal zone lymphoma. By contrast, because lymphoid cells normally circulate throughout the body, there is relatively little selective pressure in lymphoid malignancies for aberrations that increase angiogenesis or activate invasion and metastasis.

Mantle Cell Lymphoma

- Mature B cell tumor that usually manifests with advanced disease involving lymph nodes, bone marrow, and extranodal sites such as the gut
- Associated with an (11;14) translocation that results in over-expression of cyclin D1, a regulator of cell cycle progression

Extranodal Marginal Zone Lymphoma

- Mature B cell tumor arising at extranodal sites involved by chronic inflammation resulting from autoimmunity or infection (e.g., *H. pylori*)
- Remains localized for long periods and may regress if the inflammatory stimulus is removed

Diffuse Large B Cell Lymphoma

- Heterogeneous group of mature B cell tumors that shares large cell morphology and aggressive clinical behavior and is the most common type of lymphoma
- Rearrangements or mutations of *BCL6* gene are recognized associations; one-third carry a (14;18) translocation involving *BCL2*

Burkitt Lymphoma

- Very aggressive mature B tumor that usually arises at extra-nodal sites

- Nearly always associated with translocations involving the *MYC* protooncogene
- Tumor cells often are latently infected by EBV

Multiple Myeloma

- Plasma cell tumor often manifesting with multiple lytic bone lesions associated with pathologic fractures and hypercalcemia
- Neoplastic plasma cells suppress normal humoral immunity and secrete partial immunoglobulins that are nephrotoxic (Bence Jones proteins)

Hodgkin Lymphoma

- Unusual B cell tumor consisting mostly of reactive lympho-cytes, macrophages, and stromal cells
- Malignant RS cells make up a minor part of the tumor mass.

Myeloid Neoplasms

Myeloid neoplasms arise from hematopoietic progenitors and typically give rise to proliferations that involve the bone marrow and replace normal marrow elements. There are three broad categories of myeloid neoplasia:

- In *acute myeloid leukemia (AML)*, the neoplastic cells are blocked at an early stage of myeloid cell development. Immature myeloid cells (blasts) accumulate in the marrow and replace normal elements, and frequently circulate in the peripheral blood.

- In *myeloproliferative neoplasms,* the neoplastic clone continues to undergo terminal differentiation but exhibits increased or dysregulated growth. Commonly, these are associated with an increase in one or more of the formed elements (red cells, platelets, and/or granulocytes) in the peripheral blood.
- In *myelodysplastic syndromes (MDS),* terminal differentiation occurs but in a disordered and ineffective fashion, leading to the appearance of dysplastic marrow precursors and peripheral blood cytopenias.

Although these three categories provide a useful starting point, the divisions between the myeloid neoplasms sometimes blur. Both MDS and myeloproliferative neoplasms often transform to AML, and some neoplasms have features of both myelodysplasia and myeloproliferative neoplasms. Because all myeloid neoplasms arise from early multipotent progenitors, the close relationship among these disorders is not surprising.

It also is now recognized that AML and MDS often arise from an asymptomatic precursor referred to as clonal hematopoieis of indeterminant prognosis (CHIP) CHIP is characterized by normal blood counts despite the presence of one of more clonal acquired "driver" mutations in myeloid cells in the blood and the marrow. CHIP progresses to an overt white cell neoplasm at a frequency of about 1% per year and appears to be an important risk factor for cardiovascular disease (Chapter 10).

Acute Myeloid Leukemia

AML primarily affects older adults; the median age is 50 years. It is very heterogeneous, as discussed later. The clinical signs and symptoms closely resemble those produced by ALL and usually are related to the replacement of normal marrow elements by leukemic blasts. Fatigue, pallor, abnormal bleeding, and infections are common in newly diagnosed patients, who typically present within a few weeks of the onset of symptoms. Splenomegaly and lymphadenopathy generally are less prominent than in ALL, but on rare occasions AML mimics a lymphoma by manifesting as a discrete tissue mass (a so-called "granulocytic sarcoma"). The diagnosis and classification of AML are based on morphologic, histochemical, immunophenotypic, and karyotypic findings. Of these, the karyotype is most predictive of outcome.

Pathogenesis

Most AMLs harbor mutations in genes encoding transcription factors that are required for normal myeloid cell differentiation. These mutations interfere with the differentiation of early myeloid cells, leading to the accumulation of myeloid precursors (blasts) in the marrow. Of particular interest is the (15;17) translocation in acute promyelocytic leukemia, which results in the fusion of the retinoic acid receptor α *(RARA)* gene on chromosome 17 and the *PML* gene on chromosome 15. The chimeric gene produces a PML/RARA fusion protein that blocks myeloid differentiation at the promyelocytic stage, probably in part by inhibiting the function of normal retinoic acid receptors. Remarkably, pharmacologic doses of all-*trans* retinoic acid (ATRA), an

analogue of vitamin A (Chapter 7), overcome this block and induce the neoplastic promyelocytes to differentiate into neutrophils rapidly. Because neutrophils die after an average life span of 6 hours, ATRA treatment rapidly clears the tumor. The effect is very specific; AMLs without translocations involving *RARA* do not respond to ATRA. More recently, it has been noted that the combination of ATRA and arsenic trioxide, a salt that induces the degradation of the PML/RARA fusion protein, is even more effective than ATRA alone, producing cures in more than 80% of patients. This is an important example of a highly effective therapy targeted at a tumor-specific molecular defect.

Other work using mice has shown that the mutations in transcription factors found in AML are not sufficient to cause the disease. Putative collaborating mutations in several other tyrosine kinase genes and in the *RAS* gene have been detected.

Sequencing of the AML genomes also has identified frequent mutations in genes that directly impact the epigenome, suggesting that epigenetic alterations have a central role in AML. For example, about 15% to 20% of AMLs are associated with mutations in isocitrate dehydrogenase (IDH). In such tumors, an "oncometabolite" synthesized by the mutated IDH protein blocks the function of enzymes that regulate the epigenome and interferes with myeloid cell differentiation (discussed in Chapter 6). Inhibitors of mutant IDH prevent the production of the oncometabolite and often produce remissions in this particular molecular subtype of AML.

MORPHOLOGY

By definition, in AML myeloid blasts or promyelocytes make up more than 20% of the bone marrow cellularity. **Myeloblasts** (precursors of granulocytes) have delicate nuclear chromatin, three to five nucleoli, and fine azurophilic cytoplasmic granules (Fig. 12.26). **Auer rods,** distinctive red-staining rodlike structures, may be present in myeloblasts or more differentiated cells; they are particularly numerous in acute promyelocytic leukemia (Fig. 12.27). Auer rods are specific for neoplastic myeloblasts and thus are a helpful diagnostic clue when present. In other subtypes of AML, monoblasts, erythroblasts, or megakaryoblasts predominate.

Classification. AMLs are diverse in terms of genetics, cellular lineage, and degree of maturation. The WHO classification relies on all of these features to divide AML into four categories (Table 12.11): (1) AMLs associated with specific genetic aberrations, which are important because they predict outcome and they guide therapy; (2) AMLs with dysplasia, many of which arise from MDSs; (3) AMLs occurring after genotoxic chemotherapy; and (4) AMLs lacking any of the foregoing features. AMLs in the last category are subclassified based on the predominant line of differentiation that the tumor exhibits.

Immunophenotype. The expression of immunologic markers is heterogeneous in AML. Most tumors express some combination of myeloid-associated antigens, such as CD13, CD14, CD15, CD64, or CD117 (KIT). CD34, a marker of hematopoietic stem cells, is often present on myeloblasts. Such markers are helpful in distinguishing AML

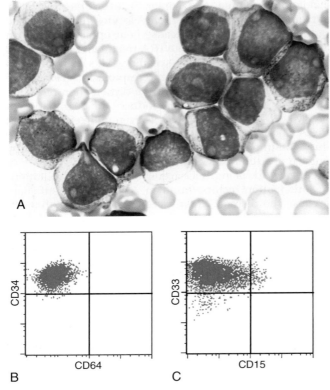

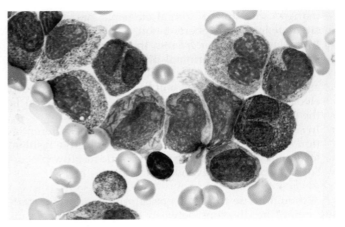

Fig. 12.27 Acute promyelocytic leukemia—bone marrow aspirate. The neoplastic promyelocytes have abnormally coarse and numerous azurophilic granules. Other characteristic findings include a cell in the center of the field with multiple needlelike Auer rods. *(Courtesy of Dr. Robert W. McKenna, Department of Pathology, University of Texas Southwestern Medical School, Dallas, Texas.)*

Fig. 12.26 Acute myeloid leukemia (AML). (A) Myeloblasts with delicate nuclear chromatin, prominent nucleoli, and fine azurophilic cytoplasmic granules. (B) and (C) show flow cytometry results for the AML shown in (A). The tumor cells are positive for the stem cell marker CD34 and the myeloid lineage specific markers CD33 and CD15 (subset). *(A, Courtesy of Dr. Robert W. McKenna, Department of Pathology, University of Texas Southwestern Medical School, Dallas, Texas. B and C, Courtesy of Dr. Louis Picker, Oregon Health Science Center, Portland, Oregon.)*

from ALL and in identifying AMLs with only minimal differentiation.

Clinical Features. Most patients present within weeks or a few months of the onset of symptoms with complaints related to anemia, neutropenia, and thrombocytopenia, most notably fatigue, fever, and spontaneous mucosal and cutaneous bleeding. As mentioned earlier, these findings are very similar to those produced by ALL. Thrombocytopenia results in a bleeding diathesis. Cutaneous petechiae and ecchymoses, serosal hemorrhages into the linings of the body cavities and viscera, and mucosal hemorrhages into the gingivae and urinary tract are common. Procoagulants and fibrinolytic factors released by leukemic cells, especially in AML with the t(15;17), exacerbate the bleeding tendency. Infections are frequent and are often caused by opportunists such as fungi, *Pseudomonas,* and commensals. Signs and symptoms related to the involvement of soft tissues are usually less striking in AML than in ALL, but tumors with monocytic differentiation often infiltrate the skin (leukemia cutis) and the gingiva. Central nervous system spread occurs but also is less common than in ALL.

AML remains a devastating disease. Tumors with "good-risk" karyotypic abnormalities (t[8;21], inv[16]) are associated with a 50% chance of long-term disease-free

survival, but the overall survival in all patients is only 15% to 30% with conventional chemotherapy. AML associated with *TP53* mutations has emerged as a subtype with a particularly poor prognosis. A bright spot is the improvement in outcomes in acute promyelocytic leukemia brought about by targeted treatment with ATRA and arsenic salts. IDH inhibitors also have produced encouraging results, apparently (like ATRA) by inducing the differentiation of AML blasts. An increasing number of patients with AML are being treated with more aggressive approaches, such as allogeneic hematopoietic stem cell transplantation, which can be curative in some patients.

Myelodysplastic Syndromes

The term *myelodysplastic syndrome* (MDS) refers to a group of clonal stem cell disorders characterized by

Table 12.11 WHO Classification of AML

Class	Prognosis
I. AML With Recurrent Chromosomal Translocations	
AML with t(8;21)(q22;q22); *RUNXT1/RUNX1* fusion gene	Favorable
AML with inv(16)(p13;q22); *CBFB/MYH11* fusion gene	Favorable
AML with t(15;17)(q22;q21.1); *PML/RARA* fusion gene	Favorable
AML with t(11q23;variant); *MLL* fusion genes	Poor
AML with mutated *NPM1*	Variable
II. AML With Multilineage Dysplasia	
With previous MDS	Very poor
Without previous MDS	Poor
III. AML, Therapy-Related	
Alkylating agent–related	Very poor
Epipodophyllotoxin-related	Very poor
IV. AML, Not Otherwise Classified	
Subclasses defined by extent and type of differentiation (e.g., myelocytic, monocytic)	Intermediate

AML, Acute myeloid leukemia; *MDS,* myelodysplastic syndrome; *NPM1,* nucleophosmin 1; *WHO,* World Health Organization.

maturation defects that are associated with ineffective hematopoiesis and a high risk of transformation to AML. In MDSs, the bone marrow is partly or wholly replaced by the clonal progeny of a transformed multipotent stem cell that retains the capacity to differentiate into red cells, granulocytes, and platelets, but in a manner that is both ineffective and disordered. As a result, the marrow usually is hypercellular or normocellular, but the peripheral blood shows one or more cytopenias. The abnormal stem cell clone in the bone marrow is genetically unstable and prone to the acquisition of additional mutations and the eventual transformation to AML. Most cases are idiopathic, but some develop after chemotherapy with alkylating agents or exposure to ionizing radiation therapy.

Pathogenesis

Important new insights have come from deep sequencing of MDS genomes, which has identified a number of recurrently mutated genes. These genes can be lumped into three major functional categories, as follows:

- *Epigenetic factors.* Frequent mutations are seen involving many of the same epigenetic factors that are mutated in AML, including factors that regulate DNA methylation and histone modifications; thus, like AML, dysregulation of the epigenome appears to be important in the genesis of MDS.
- *RNA splicing factors.* A subset of tumors has mutations involving the RNA splicing machinery that are proposed to drive transformation by altering RNA processing, They are commonly associated with *ring sideroblasts,* a classic form of dysplasia that is seen in a subset of MDS.
- *Transcription factors.* These mutations affect transcription factors that are required for normal myelopoiesis and may contribute to the deranged differentiation that characterizes MDS.

In addition, roughly 10% of MDS cases have loss-of-function mutations in the tumor suppressor gene *TP53,* which correlate with the presence of a complex karyotype and particularly poor clinical outcomes. Both primary MDS and therapy-related MDS are associated with similar *recurrent chromosomal abnormalities, including monosomies 5 and 7, deletions of 5q, 7q, and 20q, and trisomy 8.*

MORPHOLOGY

In MDS, the marrow is populated by abnormal-appearing hematopoietic precursors. Some of the more common abnormalities include **megaloblastoid erythroid precursors** resembling those seen in the megaloblastic anemias, erythroid forms with iron deposits within their mitochondria **(ring sideroblasts)**, granulocyte precursors with **abnormal granules** or nuclear maturation, and small megakaryocytes with single small nuclei or multiple separate nuclei.

Clinical Features. MDS often is described as rare, but actually is about as common as AML, affecting up to 15,000 patients per year in the United States. Most patients present between the ages of 50 and 70. As a result of cytopenias, many suffer from infections, symptoms related to anemia,

and hemorrhages. The response to conventional chemotherapy usually is poor, perhaps because MDS arises in a background of stem cell damage. Transformation to AML occurs in 10% to 40% of patients. The prognosis is variable; the median survival time ranges from 9 to 29 months and is worse in cases associated with increased marrow blasts, cytogenetic abnormalities, or *TP53* mutations.

Myeloproliferative Neoplasms

The common pathogenic feature of myeloproliferative neoplasms is the presence of mutated, constitutively activated tyrosine kinases or other acquired aberrations in signaling pathways that lead to growth factor independence. This insight provides a satisfying explanation for the observed overproduction of blood cells and is important therapeutically because of the availability of tyrosine kinase inhibitors. The neoplastic progenitors tend to seed secondary hematopoietic organs (the spleen, liver, and lymph nodes), resulting in hepatosplenomegaly (caused by neoplastic extramedullary hematopoiesis).

Four major diagnostic entities are recognized: chronic myeloid leukemia (CML), polycythemia vera, primary myelofibrosis, and essential thrombocythemia. Their distinctive features are listed below:

- CML is separated from the others by its association with a characteristic abnormality, the BCR-ABL fusion gene, which produces a constitutively active BCR-ABL tyrosine kinase.
- The most common genetic abnormalities in the "BCR-ABL–negative" myeloproliferative neoplasms are activating mutations in the tyrosine kinase JAK2, which occur in virtually all cases of polycythemia vera and about 50% of cases of primary myelofibrosis and essential thrombocythemia
- Some rare myeloproliferative neoplasms are associated with activating mutations in other tyrosine kinases, such as platelet-derived growth factor receptor-α and platelet-derived growth factor receptor-β.

In addition, all myeloproliferative neoplasms have variable propensities to transform to a "spent phase" resembling primary myelofibrosis or to a "blast crisis" identical to acute leukemia, both presumably triggered by the acquisition of other somatic mutations. Only CML, polycythemia vera, and primary myelofibrosis are presented here, as other myeloproliferative neoplasms are too infrequent to merit discussion.

Chronic Myeloid Leukemia

CML principally affects adults between 25 and 60 years of age. The peak incidence is in the fourth and fifth decades of life. About 4500 new cases are diagnosed per year in the United States.

Pathogenesis

CML is distinguished from other myeloproliferative neoplasms by the presence of a chimeric *BCR-ABL* gene derived from portions of the *BCR* gene on chromosome 22 and the *ABL* gene on chromosome 9. In about 95% of cases, the *BCR-ABL* gene is the product of a balanced (9;22) translocation that moves *ABL* from chromosome 9 to a position on chromosome 22 adjacent to *BCR.* In the remaining

5% of cases, a *BCR-ABL* fusion gene is created by cytogenetically cryptic or complex rearrangements involving more than two chromosomes. The *BCR-ABL* fusion gene is present in granulocytic, erythroid, megakaryocytic, and B cell precursors, and in some cases T cell precursors as well, indicating that the tumor arises from a transformed hematopoietic stem cell. Although the Ph chromosome is highly characteristic of CML, it also is present in 25% of adult B cell–ALLs and a small subset of AMLs.

As described in Chapter 6, the *BCR-ABL* gene encodes a fusion protein consisting of portions of BCR and the tyrosine kinase domain of ABL. Normal myeloid progenitors depend on signals generated by growth factors and their receptors for growth and survival. **The growth factor dependence of CML progenitors is greatly decreased by constitutive signals generated by BCR-ABL that mimic the effects of growth factor receptor activation.** Importantly, because BCR-ABL does not inhibit differentiation, the early disease course is marked by excessive production of relatively normal blood cells, particularly granulocytes and platelets.

MORPHOLOGY

The peripheral blood findings are highly characteristic. The leukocyte count is elevated, often exceeding 100,000 cells/μL. **The circulating cells are predominantly neutrophils, metamyelocytes, and myelocytes** (Fig. 12.28), but **basophils** and **eosinophils** are also prominent and platelets are usually increased. The bone marrow is hypercellular owing to increased numbers of maturing granulocytic and megakaryocytic precursors. The red pulp of the enlarged spleen resembles bone marrow because of the presence of extensive **extramedullary hematopoiesis**. This burgeoning proliferation often compromises the local blood supply, leading to **splenic infarcts.**

Clinical Features

The onset of CML is insidious, as the initial symptoms usually are nonspecific (e.g., easy fatigability, weakness,

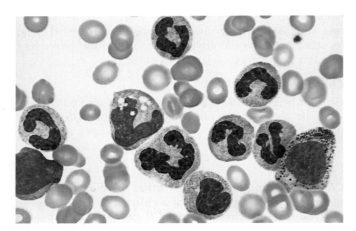

Fig. 12.28 CML—peripheral blood smear. Granulocytic forms at various stages of differentiation are present. *(Courtesy of Dr. Robert W. McKenna, Department of Pathology, University of Texas Southwestern Medical School, Dallas, Texas.)*

weight loss). Sometimes the first symptom is a dragging sensation in the abdomen caused by splenomegaly. On occasion it may be necessary to distinguish CML from a *lekemoid reaction* a dramatic elevation of the granulocyte count in response to infection, stress, chronic inflammation, and certain neoplasms. This distinction can be achieved definitively by testing for the presence of the BCR-ABL fusion gene, which can be done by karyotyping, fluorescence in situ hybridization, or PCR assay.

The natural history of CML initially is one of slow progression. Even without treatment, the median survival is 3 years. After a variable (and unpredictable) period, approximately half of CML cases enter an accelerated phase marked by increasing anemia and new thrombocytopenia, the appearance of additional cytogenetic abnormalities, and finally transformation into a picture resembling acute leukemia (blast crisis). In the remaining 50% of cases, blast crisis occurs abruptly, without an accelerated phase. Of note, in 30% of cases the blast crisis resembles precursor-B cell ALL, further attesting to the origin of CML from hematopoietic stem cells. In the remaining 70% of cases, the blast crisis resembles AML. Less commonly, CML progresses to a phase of extensive bone marrow fibrosis resembling primary myelofibrosis.

Fortunately for those affected, the natural history of CML has been altered dramatically by the emergence of targeted therapy. Treatment with tyrosine kinase inhibitors, particularly in patients with early disease, induces sustained remissions with manageable toxicity and prevents progression to blast crisis, apparently by suppressing the proliferative drive that leads to the acquisition of additional mutations. When patients on tyrosine kinase inhibitors relapse, their tumors frequently are found to have acquired mutations in the kinase domain of BCR-ABL that prevent the drugs from binding. The selective outgrowth of these cells is explained by the powerful antitumor effects of BCR-ABL inhibitors, and indicates that many resistant tumors are still "addicted" to the progrowth signals created by BCR-ABL. In some instances resistant tumors can be treated with "third-generation" BCR-ABL inhibitors. For others, hematopoietic stem cell transplantation offers a chance of cure, but carries with it substantial risks, particularly in the aged.

Polycythemia Vera

Polycythemia vera is strongly associated with activating point mutations in the tyrosine kinase JAK2. JAK2 normally acts in the signaling pathways downstream of the erythropoietin receptor and other growth factor receptors. The most common JAK2 mutation, sharply lowers the dependence of hematopoietic cells on growth factors for growth and survival. This produces excessive proliferation of erythroid, granulocytic, and megakaryocytic elements (panmyelosis), but most clinical signs and symptoms are related to an absolute increase in red cell mass. Polycythemia vera must be distinguished from relative polycythemia, which results from hemoconcentration. Unlike reactive forms of absolute polycythemia, polycythemia vera is associated with low levels of serum erythropoietin, which is a reflection of the growth factor–independent growth of the neoplastic clone.

MORPHOLOGY

The major anatomic changes in polycythemia vera stem from increases in blood volume and viscosity brought about by the polycythemia. **Congestion** of many tissues is characteristic. The liver is enlarged and often contains small foci of extramedullary hematopoiesis. The spleen usually is slightly enlarged (250 to 300 g) because of vascular congestion. As a result of the increased viscosity and vascular stasis, **thromboses and infarctions are common,** particularly in the heart, spleen, and kidneys. Hemorrhages also occur in about a third of the patients. These most often affect the gastrointestinal tract, oropharynx, or brain and may occur spontaneously or following some minor trauma or surgical procedure. Platelets produced from the neoplastic clone often are dysfunctional, a derangement that contributes to the elevated risk of thrombosis and bleeding. As in CML, the peripheral blood often shows **basophilia.**

The bone marrow is hypercellular owing to increased numbers of erythroid, myeloid, and megakaryocytic forms. In addition, some degree of marrow fibrosis is present in 10% of patients at the time of diagnosis. In a subset of patients, this progresses to a spent phase where the marrow is largely replaced by fibroblasts and collagen.

Clinical Features

Polycythemia vera appears insidiously, usually in late middle age. Patients are plethoric and often somewhat cyanotic. Histamine released from the neoplastic basophils may contribute to pruritus and also may account for the increased incidence of peptic ulceration. Other complaints are referable to the thrombotic and hemorrhagic tendencies and to hypertension. Headache, dizziness, gastrointestinal symptoms, hematemesis, and melena are common. Because of the high rate of cell turnover, symptomatic gout is seen in 5% to 10% of cases.

The diagnosis usually is made in the laboratory. Red cell counts range from 6 to 10 million/μL, and the hematocrit is often 60% or greater. The granulocyte count can be as high as 50,000 cells/μL, and the platelet count is often more than 400,000/μL. Basophilia is common. The platelets are functionally abnormal in most cases, and giant platelets and megakaryocyte fragments are often seen in the blood. About 30% of patients develop thrombotic complications, usually affecting the brain or heart. Hepatic vein thrombosis giving rise to *Budd-Chiari syndrome* (Chapter 15) is an uncommon but grave complication. Minor hemorrhages (e.g., epistaxis and bleeding from gums) are common and life-threatening hemorrhages that occur in 5% to 10% of patients. In those receiving no treatment, death occurs from vascular complications within months; however, the median survival is increased to about 10 years by lowering the red cell count to near normal through repeated phlebotomy.

Unfortunately, prolonged survival has shown a propensity for polycythemia vera to evolve to a "spent phase" resembling primary myelofibrosis. After an average interval of 10 years, 15% to 20% of cases undergo such a transformation. Owing to the extensive marrow fibrosis, hematopoiesis shifts to the spleen, which enlarges markedly. Inhibitors that target JAK2 have been approved for treatment of the spent phase of polycythemia vera and lead to some improvement in most patients. Transformation to a "blast crisis" identical to AML also occurs, but much less frequently than in CML.

Primary Myelofibrosis

The hallmark of primary myelofibrosis is the development of obliterative marrow fibrosis, which reduces bone marrow hematopoiesis and leads to cytopenias and extensive extramedullary hematopoiesis. Histologically, the appearance is identical to the spent phase that occurs occasionally late in the course of other myeloproliferative disorders. This similarity also extends to the underlying pathogenesis.

JAK-STAT signaling seems to be the underlying driver in almost all cases. Thus, JAK2 mutations are present in 50% to 60% of cases and activating mutations in MPL, the thrombopoietin receptor, are seen in an additional 1% to 5% of cases. Most of the remaining cases have other mutations, which also are hypothesized to stimulate increased JAK-STAT signaling. Why JAK2 mutations are associated with polycythemia vera in some patients and primary myelofibrosis in others is not understood; differences in the cell of origin and the genetic backgrounds that give rise to these two disorders are suspected.

It is believed that the characteristic marrow fibrosis is caused by the inappropriate release of fibrogenic factors from neoplastic megakaryocytes. Two factors synthesized by megakaryocytes have been implicated: *platelet-derived growth factor* and *TGF-β*. As you recall, platelet-derived growth factor and TGF-β are fibroblast mitogens. In addition, TGF-β promotes collagen deposition and causes angiogenesis, both of which are observed in myelofibrosis.

As marrow fibrosis progresses, displaced hematopoietic stem cells take up residence in niches in secondary hematopoietic organs, such as the spleen, the liver, and the lymph nodes, leading to the appearance of extramedullary hematopoiesis. For incompletely understood reasons, red cell production at extramedullary sites is disordered. This factor and the concomitant suppression of marrow function result in moderate to severe anemia.

MORPHOLOGY

The peripheral blood smear is markedly abnormal (Fig. 12.29). Red cells often exhibit bizarre shapes **(poikilocytes, teardrop cells)**, and nucleated erythroid precursors are commonly seen along with immature white cells (myelocytes and metamyelocytes), a combination of findings referred to as **leukoerythroblastosis.** Abnormally large platelets often are present as well. The bone marrow in advanced cases is hypocellular and diffusely fibrotic, whereas early in the course it may be hypercellular and have only focal areas of fibrosis. Throughout the course, marrow megakaryocytes are present in clusters and have characteristic hyperchromatic nuclei with "cloudlike" outlines. Marked **splenomegaly** resulting from extensive extramedullary hematopoiesis, often associated with **subcapsular infarcts,** also is typical. The spleen may weigh as much as 4000 g, roughly twenty times its normal weight. Moderate **hepatomegaly**, also due to extramedullary hematopoiesis, is commonplace. Lymph nodes also are involved by extramedullary hematopoiesis, but not to a degree sufficient to cause appreciable enlargement.

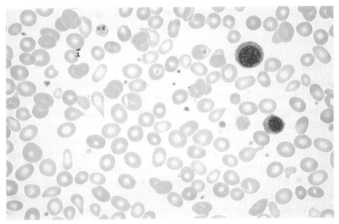

Fig. 12.29 Primary myelofibrosis—peripheral blood smear. Two nucleated erythroid precursors and several teardrop-shaped red cells (dacryocytes) are evident. Immature myeloid cells were present in other fields. An identical histologic picture can be seen in other diseases producing marrow distortion and fibrosis.

Clinical Features

Primary myelofibrosis usually occurs in individuals older than 60 years who come to attention because of progressive anemia and splenomegaly. Nonspecific symptoms such as fatigue, weight loss, and night sweats are common. Hyperuricemia and secondary gout resulting from a high rate of cell turnover also are frequently seen.

Laboratory studies typically show a moderate to severe normochromic normocytic anemia accompanied by *leukoerythroblastosis*. The white cell count is usually normal or mildly reduced, but can be elevated early in the course. The platelet count is usually normal or elevated at diagnosis, but thrombocytopenia often supervenes as the disease progresses. These blood findings are not specific, and bone marrow biopsy is essential for diagnosis.

Primary myelofibrosis is more difficult to treat than polycythemia vera and CML. The median survival is in the range of 4 to 5 years. Threats to life include infection, thrombosis and bleeding related to platelet abnormalities, and transformation to AML, which occurs in 5% to 20% of cases. JAK2 inhibitors are effective at decreasing the splenomegaly and constitutional symptoms, even in those without JAK2 mutations, presumably because increased JAK/STAT signaling is common to all molecular subtypes. Hematopoietic stem cell transplantation may be curative in those young and fit enough to withstand the procedure.

SUMMARY

MYELOID NEOPLASMS

Myeloid tumors occur mainly in adults and fall into three major groups:
- **AML**
  - Aggressive tumors comprised of immature myeloid lineage blasts, which replace the marrow and suppress normal hematopoiesis

- Associated with diverse acquired mutations that lead to expression of abnormal transcription factors, which interfere with myeloid differentiation
- **MDS**
  - Myeloid tumors characterized by disordered and ineffective hematopoiesis
  - Manifest with one or more cytopenias and progress in 10% to 40% of cases to AML
- **Myeloproliferative neoplasms**
  - Myeloid tumors in which production of formed myeloid elements is initially increased, leading to high blood counts and extramedullary hematopoiesis
  - Commonly associated with acquired mutations that lead to constitutive activation of tyrosine kinases, which mimic signals from normal growth factors. The most common pathogenic kinases are BCR-ABL (associated with CML) and mutated JAK2 (associated with polycythemia vera and primary myelofibrosis).
  - All can transform to acute leukemia and to a spent phase of marrow fibrosis associated with anemia, thrombocytopenia, and splenomegaly.

Histiocytic Neoplasms

Langerhans Cell Histiocytoses

The term *histiocytosis* is an "umbrella" designation for a variety of proliferative disorders of dendritic cells or macrophages. Some, such as very rare histiocytic lymphomas, are highly malignant neoplasms. Others, such as most histiocytic proliferations in lymph nodes, are completely benign and reactive. Between these two extremes lie a group of relatively rare tumors comprised of Langerhans cells, the *Langerhans cell histiocytoses*. As described in Chapter 5, Langerhans cells are immature dendritic cells found in the epidermis; similar cells are found in many other organs, and they function to capture antigens and display them to T cells.

Langerhans cell proliferations take on different clinical forms, but all are believed to be variations of the same basic disorder. The proliferating Langerhans cells express MHC class II antigens, CD1a, and langerin. Langerin is a transmembrane protein found in *Birbeck granules,* cytoplasmic pentalaminar rodlike tubular structures that in electron micrographs have a characteristic periodicity and sometimes a dilated terminal end ("tennis racket" appearance). Under the light microscope, the proliferating Langerhans cells do not resemble their normal dendritic counterparts. Instead, they have abundant, often vacuolated cytoplasm and vesicular nuclei, an appearance more akin to that of tissue macrophages (called histiocytes by morphologists)—hence the term *Langerhans cell histiocytosis*.

Langerhans cell histiocytoses can be grouped into two major relatively distinctive clinicopathologic entities.
- *Multisystem Langerhans cell histiocytosis (Letterer-Siwe disease)* usually occurs in children younger than 2 years of age. It typically manifests with multifocal cutaneous lesions that grossly resemble seborrheic skin eruptions and are composed of Langerhans cells. Most affected patients have hepatosplenomegaly, lymphadenopathy, pulmonary lesions, and (later in the course) destructive

osteolytic bone lesions. Extensive marrow infiltration often leads to pancytopenia and predisposes the patient to recurrent bacterial infections. The disease is rapidly fatal if untreated. With intensive chemotherapy, 50% of patients survive 5 years.

- *Unisystem Langerhans cell histiocytosis (eosinophilic granuloma)* may be unifocal or multifocal. It is characterized by expanding accumulations of Langerhans cells, usually within the medullary cavities of bones or less commonly in the skin, lungs, or stomach. The Langerhans cells are admixed with variable numbers of lymphocytes, plasma cells, neutrophils, and eosinophils, which are usually prominent. Virtually any bone may be involved; the calvaria, ribs, and femur are most commonly affected. *Unifocal disease* most often involves a single bone. It may be asymptomatic or cause pain, tenderness, and pathologic fracture. It is an indolent disorder that may heal spontaneously or be cured by local excision or irradiation. *Multifocal unisystem disease* usually affects children and typically manifests with multiple erosive bony masses that sometimes extend into soft tissues. In about 50% of cases, involvement of the posterior pituitary stalk of the hypothalamus leads to diabetes insipidus. The combination of calvarial bone defects, diabetes insipidus, and exophthalmos is referred to as the *Hand-Schüller-Christian triad*. Many patients experience spontaneous regressions; others are treated effectively with chemotherapy.

A clue to the pathogenesis of Langerhans cell tumors lies in the discovery that the different clinical forms are frequently associated with an acquired mutation in the serine/threonine kinase BRAF, that leads to hyperactivity of the kinase. This same mutation is found in a variety of other tumors, including hairy cell leukemia (described earlier), benign nevi, malignant melanoma, papillary thyroid carcinoma, and some colon cancers (Chapter 6). BRAF is a component of the RAS signaling pathway that drives cellular proliferation and survival, effects that likely contribute to the growth of neoplastic Langerhans cells.

Bleeding Disorders

Bleeding disorders are characterized clinically by abnormal bleeding, which can appear spontaneously or follow some inciting event (e.g., trauma or surgery). As described in Chapter 4, normal clotting involves the vessel wall, the platelets, and the clotting factors. It follows that abnormalities in any of these components can lead to clinically significant bleeding. A review of the laboratory tests used in the evaluation of patients with a suspected bleeding disorder, along with the principles involved, is presented next, followed by consideration of specific disorders of coagulation. We finish with a discussion of a few clinically important complications of blood product transfusion.

The most important tests for investigation of suspected coagulopathies include the following:

- *Prothrombin time* (PT). This test assesses the extrinsic and common coagulation pathways. It measures the time (in seconds) needed for plasma to clot after addition of tissue thromboplastin (e.g., brain extract) and Ca^{2+} ions. A prolonged PT can result from a deficiency of factor V, VII, or X; prothrombin; or fibrinogen or the presence of an acquired inhibitor (typically an antibody) that interferes with the extrinsic pathway.
- *Partial thromboplastin time* (PTT). This test assesses the intrinsic and common coagulation pathways. It measures the time (in seconds) needed for the plasma to clot after the addition of kaolin, cephalin, and Ca^{2+}. Kaolin activates the contact-dependent factor XII and cephalin substitutes for platelet phospholipids. Prolongation of PTT can be caused by a deficiency of factor V, VIII, IX, X, XI, or XII; prothrombin; or fibrinogen or the presence of an acquired inhibitor that interferes with the intrinsic pathway.
- *Platelet count.* This is obtained on anti-coagulated blood using an electronic particle counter. The reference range is 150,000 to 450,000/µL. Counts outside this range must be confirmed by a visual inspection of a peripheral blood smear.
- *Tests of platelet function.* At present no single test provides an adequate assessment of the complex functions of platelets. Aggregation tests that measure the response of platelets to certain agonists and qualitative and quantitative tests of von Willebrand factor (vWF) (which you will recall is required for platelet adherence to subvascular collagen) are both commonly used in clinical practice. An old test, the bleeding time, has some value but is time-consuming and difficult to standardize and is therefore performed only rarely. Newer instrument-based assays that provide quantitative measures of platelet function are being evaluated but are not yet available for routine use in the clinic.

In addition, more specialized tests are available that measure the levels of specific clotting factors and fibrin split products or assess the presence of circulating anti-coagulants.

Bleeding disorders may stem from abnormalities of vessels, platelets, or coagulation factors, alone or in combination. Bleeding resulting from *vascular fragility* is seen with vitamin C deficiency (scurvy) (Chapter 8), systemic amyloidosis (Chapter 5), chronic glucocorticoid use, rare inherited conditions affecting the connective tissues, and a large number of infectious and hypersensitivity vasculitides. Some of these conditions are discussed in other chapters; others are beyond the scope of this book. Bleeding that results purely from vascular fragility is characterized by the "spontaneous" appearance of petechiae and ecchymoses in the skin and mucous membranes (probably resulting from minor trauma). In most instances laboratory tests of coagulation are normal.

Bleeding also can be triggered by systemic conditions that inflame or damage endothelial cells. If severe enough, such insults convert the vascular lining to a pro-thrombotic surface that activates coagulation throughout the circulatory system, a condition known as *disseminated intravascular coagulation* (DIC) (discussed in the next section). Paradoxically, in DIC, platelets and coagulation factors often are used up faster than they can be replaced, resulting in deficiencies that may lead to severe bleeding (a condition referred to as *consumptive coagulopathy*).

Deficiencies of platelets (thrombocytopenia) also are an important cause of bleeding. These occur in a variety of clinical settings that are discussed later. Other bleeding disorders stem from qualitative defects in platelet function. Such defects may be acquired, as in uremia and certain myeloproliferative disorders and after aspirin ingestion; or inherited, as in von Willebrand disease and other rare congenital disorders. The clinical signs of inadequate platelet function include easy bruising, nosebleeds, excessive bleeding from minor trauma, and menorrhagia.

In bleeding disorders stemming from defects in one or more coagulation factors, the PT, PTT, or both are prolonged. Unlike platelet defects, petechiae and mucosal bleeding are usually absent. Instead, hemorrhages tend to occur in parts of the body that are subject to trauma, such as the joints of the lower extremities. Massive hemorrhage may occur after surgery, dental procedures, or severe trauma. This category includes the hemophilias, an important group of inherited coagulation disorders.

It is not uncommon for bleeding to occur as a consequence of a mixture of defects. This is the case in DIC, in which both thrombocytopenia and coagulation factor deficiencies contribute to bleeding, and in von Willebrand disease, a fairly common inherited disorder in which both platelet function and (to a lesser degree) coagulation factor function are abnormal.

With the foregoing overview as background, we now turn to specific bleeding disorders.

DISSEMINATED INTRAVASCULAR COAGULATION (DIC)

DIC occurs as a complication of a wide variety of disorders; it is caused by the systemic activation of coagulation and results in the formation of thrombi throughout the microcirculation. As a consequence, platelets and coagulation factors are consumed and, secondarily, fibrinolysis is activated. Thus, DIC can give rise either to tissue hypoxia and microinfarcts caused by myriad microthrombi or to a bleeding disorder related to pathologic activation of fibrinolysis and the depletion of the elements required for hemostasis (hence the term *consumptive coagulopathy*). This entity probably causes bleeding more commonly than all of the congenital coagulation disorders combined.

Pathogenesis

Before discussing specific disorders associated with DIC, we must first consider in a general way the pathogenic mechanisms by which intravascular clotting occurs. Reference to earlier comments on normal blood coagulation (Chapter 4) may be helpful at this point. It suffices to recall that clotting can be initiated by either the extrinsic pathway, which is triggered by the release of tissue factor

(tissue thromboplastin); or the intrinsic pathway, which involves the activation of factor XII by surface contact, collagen, or other negatively charged substances. Both pathways lead to the generation of thrombin. Clotting normally is limited by the rapid clearance of activated clotting factors by the macrophages and the liver, endogenous anticoagulants (e.g., protein C), and the concomitant activation of fibrinolysis.

DIC usually is triggered by either (1) the release of tissue factor or thromboplastic substances into the circulation or (2) widespread endothelial cell damage (Fig. 12.30). Thromboplastic substances can be released into the circulation from a variety of sources—for example, the placenta in obstetric complications or certain types of cancer cells, particularly those of acute promyelocytic leukemia and adenocarcinomas. Cancer cells may also provoke coagulation in other ways, such as by releasing proteolytic enzymes and by expressing tissue factor. In gram-negative and gram-positive sepsis (important causes of DIC), endotoxins or exotoxins stimulate the release of tissue factor from monocytes. Activated monocytes also release IL-1 and tumor necrosis factor, both of which stimulate the expression of tissue factor on endothelial cells and simultaneously decrease the expression of thrombomodulin. The latter, as discussed, activates protein C, an anticoagulant (Chapter 4). The net result of these alterations is the enhanced generation of thrombin and the blunting of inhibitory pathways that limit coagulation.

Severe endothelial cell injury can initiate DIC by causing the release of tissue factor and by exposing subendothelial collagen and vWF. However, even subtle forms of endothelial damage can unleash procoagulant activity by stimulating tissue factor expression on endothelial cell surfaces. Widespread endothelial injury can be produced by the deposition of antigen-antibody complexes (e.g., in systemic lupus erythematosus), by temperature extremes (e.g., after heat stroke or burn injury), or by infections (e.g., resulting from meningococci or rickettsiae). As discussed in Chapter 4, endothelial injury is an important consequence of systemic inflammatory response syndrome (SIRS) triggered by sepsis and other systemic insults, and, not surprisingly, DIC is a frequent complication of SIRS.

Disorders associated with DIC are listed in Table 12.12. Of these, *DIC is most often associated with sepsis, obstetric complications, malignancy, and major trauma (especially to the brain)*. The initiating events in these conditions are multiple and often interrelated. For example, in obstetric conditions, tissue factor derived from the placenta, retained dead fetus, or amniotic fluid enters the circulation; however, shock, hypoxia, and acidosis often coexist and can lead to widespread endothelial injury. Trauma to the brain releases fat and phospholipids, which act as contact factors and thereby activate the intrinsic arm of the coagulation cascade.

Whatever the pathogenic mechanism, DIC has two consequences. First, there is widespread fibrin deposition within the microcirculation. The associated obstruction leads to ischemia in the more severely affected or vulnerable organs and hemolysis as red cells are traumatized while passing through vessels narrowed by fibrin thrombi (*microangiopathic hemolytic anemia*). Second, because of the depletion of platelets and clotting factors and the secondary

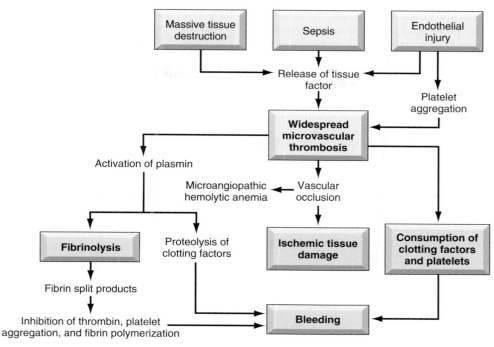

Fig. 12.30 Pathophysiology of disseminated intravascular coagulation.

release of plasminogen activators, there is a superimposed bleeding tendency. Plasmin cleaves not only to fibrin (fibrinolysis) but also to factors V and VIII, thereby reducing their concentration further. In addition, fibrinolysis creates fibrin degradation products. These inhibit platelet aggregation, have anti-thrombin activity, and impair fibrin polymerization, all of which contribute to the hemostatic failure (Fig. 12.30).

Table 12.12 Major Disorders Associated With Disseminated Intravascular Coagulation

Obstetric Complications
Abruptio placentae
Retained dead fetus
Septic abortion
Amniotic fluid embolism
Toxemia

Infections
Sepsis (gram-negative and gram-positive)
Meningococcemia
Rocky Mountain spotted fever
Histoplasmosis
Aspergillosis
Malaria

Neoplasms
Carcinomas of pancreas, prostate, lung, and stomach
Acute promyelocytic leukemia

Massive Tissue Injury
Trauma
Burns
Extensive surgery

Miscellaneous
Acute intravascular hemolysis, snakebite, giant hemangioma, shock, heat stroke, vasculitis, aortic aneurysm, liver disease

MORPHOLOGY

In DIC, **microthrombi** are most often found in the arterioles and capillaries of the kidneys, adrenals, brain, and heart, but no organ is spared. The glomeruli contain small fibrin thrombi. These may be associated with only a subtle, reactive swelling of the endothelial cells or varying degrees of focal glomerulitis. The microvascular occlusions give rise to small infarcts in the renal cortex. In severe cases the ischemia can destroy the entire cortex and cause bilateral renal cortical necrosis. Involvement of the adrenal glands can produce the **Waterhouse-Friderichsen syndrome** (Chapter 20). Microinfarcts also are commonly encountered in the brain and are often surrounded by microscopic or gross foci of hemorrhage. These can give rise to bizarre neurologic signs. Similar changes are seen in the heart and often in the anterior pituitary. DIC may contribute to the development of **Sheehan postpartum pituitary necrosis** (Chapter 19). The bleeding tendency associated with DIC is manifested not only by larger-than-expected hemorrhages near foci of infarction but also by diffuse petechiae and ecchymoses on the skin, serosal linings of the body cavities, epicardium, endocardium, lungs, and mucosal lining of the urinary tract.

Clinical Features

As might be imagined, depending on the balance between clotting and bleeding tendencies, the range of possible clinical manifestations is enormous. In general, acute DIC (e.g., that associated with obstetric complications) is dominated by bleeding, whereas chronic DIC (e.g., as occurs in those with cancer) tends to manifest with signs and symptoms related to thrombosis. The abnormal clotting usually is confined to the microcirculation, but large vessels are involved on occasion. The manifestations may be minimal, or there may be shock, acute renal failure, dyspnea, cyanosis, convulsions, and coma. Most often, the onset of DIC is announced by prolonged and copious postpartum bleeding or the presence of petechiae and ecchymoses on the skin. These may be the only manifestations, or there may be severe hemorrhage into the gut or urinary tract. Laboratory evaluation shows thrombocytopenia and prolongation of the PT and the PTT (from depletion of platelets, clotting factors, and fibrinogen). Fibrin split products are increased in the plasma.

The prognosis varies widely depending on the nature of the underlying disorder and the severity of the intravascular clotting and fibrinolysis. Acute DIC can be life threatening and must be treated aggressively with anticoagulants such as heparin or the coagulants contained in fresh frozen plasma. Conversely, chronic DIC is sometimes identified unexpectedly by laboratory testing. In either circumstance, definitive treatment must be directed at the underlying cause.

THROMBOCYTOPENIA

Isolated thrombocytopenia is associated with a bleeding tendency and *normal coagulation tests*. A count less than 150,000 platelets/μL generally is considered thrombocytopenia. However, only when platelet counts fall to 20,000 to 50,000 platelets/μL is there an increased risk of posttraumatic bleeding, and spontaneous bleeding is unlikely until counts fall below 5000 platelets/μL. Most bleeding occurs from small, superficial blood vessels and produces *petechiae* or large *ecchymoses* in the skin, the mucous membranes of the gastrointestinal and urinary tracts, and other sites. Larger hemorrhages into the central nervous system are a major hazard in those with markedly depressed platelet counts.

The major causes of thrombocytopenia are listed in Table 12.13. Clinically important thrombocytopenia is confined to disorders with reduced production or increased destruction of platelets. When the cause is the accelerated destruction of platelets, the bone marrow usually shows a compensatory increase in the number of megakaryocytes. Also of note, thrombocytopenia is one of the most common hematologic manifestations of AIDS. It can occur early in the course of HIV infection and has a multifactorial basis, including immune complex–mediated platelet destruction, anti-platelet autoantibodies, and HIV-mediated suppression of megakaryocyte development and survival.

Immune Thrombocytopenic Purpura

Immune thrombocytopenic purpura (ITP) includes two clinical subtypes. *Chronic ITP* is a relatively common disorder that tends to affect women between the ages of 20 and 40 years. *Acute ITP* is a self-limited form seen mostly in children after viral infections.

Antibodies directed against platelet membrane glycoproteins IIb/IIIa or Ib/IX complexes can be detected in roughly 80% of cases of chronic ITP. The spleen is an important site of anti-platelet antibody production and the major site of destruction of the IgG-coated platelets. Although splenomegaly is not a feature of uncomplicated chronic ITP, the importance of the spleen in the premature

Table 12.13 Causes of Thrombocytopenia

Decreased Production of Platelets
Generalized Bone Marrow Dysfunction
Aplastic anemia: congenital and acquired
Marrow infiltration: leukemia, disseminated cancer
Selective Impairment of Platelet Production
Drug-induced: alcohol, thiazides, cytotoxic drugs
Infections: measles, HIV infection
Ineffective Megakaryopoiesis
Megaloblastic anemia
Paroxysmal nocturnal hemoglobinuria
Decreased Platelet Survival
Immunologic Destruction
Autoimmune: ITP, systemic lupus erythematosus
Isoimmune: posttransfusion and neonatal
Drug-associated: quinidine, heparin, sulfa compounds
Infections: infectious mononucleosis, HIV infection, cytomegalovirus infection
Nonimmunologic Destruction
Disseminated intravascular coagulation
TTP
Giant hemangiomas
Microangiopathic hemolytic anemias
Sequestration
Hypersplenism
Dilutional
Multiple transfusions (e.g., for massive blood loss)

DIC, Disseminated intravascular coagulation; *HIV,* human immunodeficiency virus; *ITP,* immune thrombocytopenic purpura; *TTP,* thrombotic thrombocytopenic purpura.

destruction of platelets is proved by the benefits of splenectomy, which normalizes the platelet count and induces a complete remission in more than two-thirds of patients. The bone marrow usually contains increased numbers of megakaryocytes, a finding common to all forms of thrombocytopenia caused by accelerated platelet destruction.

The onset of chronic ITP is insidious. Common findings include petechiae, easy bruising, epistaxis, gum bleeding, and hemorrhages after minor trauma. Fortunately, more serious intracerebral or subarachnoid hemorrhages are uncommon. The diagnosis rests on the clinical features, the presence of thrombocytopenia, examination of the marrow, and the exclusion of secondary ITP. Reliable clinical tests for anti-platelet antibodies are not available. Treatment usually involves the use of immunosuppressive agents and, in some cases, splenectomy.

Heparin-Induced Thrombocytopenia

This special type of drug-induced thrombocytopenia (discussed in more detail in Chapter 4) merits brief mention because of its clinical importance. Moderate to severe thrombocytopenia develops in 3% to 5% of patients after 1 to 2 weeks of treatment with unfractionated heparin. The disorder is caused by IgG antibodies that bind to platelet factor 4 on platelet membranes in a heparin-dependent fashion. Resultant activation of the platelets induces their aggregation, thereby exacerbating the condition that heparin is used to treat—thrombosis. Both venous and arterial thromboses occur, even in the setting of marked thrombocytopenia, and may cause severe morbidity (e.g., loss of limbs) and death. Cessation of heparin therapy breaks the cycle of platelet activation and consumption. The risk of this complication is lowered (but not prevented entirely) by use of low-molecular-weight heparin preparations.

Thrombotic Microangiopathies: Thrombotic Thrombocytopenic Purpura and Hemolytic Uremic Syndrome

The term *thrombotic microangiopathies* encompasses a spectrum of clinical syndromes that include thrombotic thrombocytopenic purpura (TTP) and hemolytic uremic syndrome (HUS). As originally defined, TTP is associated with the pentad of fever, thrombocytopenia, microangiopathic hemolytic anemia, transient neurologic deficits, and renal failure. HUS also is associated with microangiopathic hemolytic anemia and thrombocytopenia but is distinguished from TTP by the absence of neurologic symptoms, the dominance of acute renal failure, and frequent occurrence in children (Chapter 14). Clinical experience has blurred these distinctions, as many adults with TTP lack one or more of the five criteria, and some patients with HUS have fever and neurologic dysfunction. Fundamental to both conditions is the widespread formation of platelet-rich thrombi in the microcirculation. The consumption of platelets leads to thrombocytopenia, and the narrowing of blood vessels by the platelet-rich thrombi results in a microangiopathic hemolytic anemia. All of the thrombotic microangiopathies produce renal damage of variable severity, and their pathogenesis is discussed in greater detail in Chapter 14.

It is important to note that although DIC and the thrombotic microangiopathies share features such as microvascular occlusion and microangiopathic hemolytic anemia, they are pathogenically distinct. Furthermore, unlike in DIC, in TTP and HUS activation of the coagulation cascade is not of primary importance, and so the results of laboratory tests of coagulation (e.g., the PT and PTT tests) usually are normal.

COAGULATION DISORDERS

Coagulation disorders result from either congenital or acquired deficiencies of clotting factors. Acquired deficiencies are most common and often involve several factors simultaneously. As discussed in Chapter 8, vitamin K is required for the synthesis of prothrombin and clotting factors VII, IX, and X, and its deficiency causes a severe coagulation defect. The liver synthesizes several coagulation factors and also removes many activated coagulation factors from the circulation; thus, hepatic parenchymal diseases are common causes of complex hemorrhagic diatheses. As already discussed, DIC also may lead to multiple concomitant factor deficiencies. Rarely, autoantibodies may cause acquired deficiencies limited to a single factor.

Hereditary deficiencies of many coagulation factors also have been identified. Hemophilia A (a deficiency of factor VIII) and hemophilia B (Christmas disease, a deficiency of factor IX) are X-linked traits, whereas other deficiencies are autosomal recessive disorders. Of the inherited deficiencies, only von Willebrand disease, hemophilia A, and hemophilia B are sufficiently common to warrant further consideration.

Deficiencies of Factor VIII–von Willebrand Factor Complex

Hemophilia A and von Willebrand disease are caused by qualitative or quantitative defects involving the factor VIII–vWF complex. As background for subsequent discussion of these disorders, it is useful to review the structure and function of these two proteins (Fig. 12.31).

As described earlier, factor VIII is an essential cofactor for factor IX, which activates factor X in the intrinsic coagulation pathway. Circulating factor VIII binds noncovalently to vWF, which exists as large multimers of up to

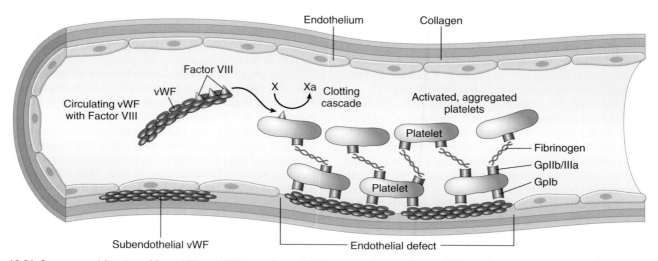

Fig. 12.31 Structure and function of factor VIII–von Willebrand factor (vWF) complex. Factor VIII and vWF circulate as a complex. vWF also is present in the subendothelial matrix of normal blood vessels. Factor VIII takes part in the coagulation cascade by activating factor X by means of factor IX *(not shown)*. vWF causes adhesion of platelets to subendothelial collagen, primarily through the glycoprotein Ib (GpIb) platelet receptor.

20 Megadaltons in weight. Endothelial cells are the major source of plasma vWF, whereas most factor VIII is synthesized in the liver. vWF is found in the plasma (in association with factor VIII), in platelet granules, in endothelial cells within cytoplasmic vesicles called Weibel-Palade bodies, and in the subendothelium, where it binds to collagen.

When endothelial cells are stripped away by trauma or injury, subendothelial vWF is exposed and binds platelets, mainly through glycoprotein Ib and to a lesser degree through glycoprotein IIb/IIIa (Fig. 12.31). The most important function of vWF is to facilitate the adhesion of platelets to damaged blood vessel walls, a crucial early event in the formation of a hemostatic plug. Inadequate platelet adhesion is believed to underlie the bleeding tendency in von Willebrand disease. In addition to its role in platelet adhesion, vWF also stabilizes factor VIII; thus, vWF deficiency leads to a secondary deficiency of factor VIII.

The various forms of von Willebrand disease are diagnosed by measuring the quantity, size, and function of vWF. vWF function is assessed using the *ristocetin platelet agglutination test*. Ristocetin somehow "activates" the bivalent binding of vWF and platelet membrane glycoprotein Ib, creating interplatelet "bridges" that cause platelets to clump (agglutination), an event that can be measured easily. Thus, ristocetin-dependent platelet agglutination serves as a useful bioassay for vWF.

With this background we now turn to the discussion of diseases resulting from deficiencies of factor VIII–vWF complex.

von Willebrand Disease

von Willebrand disease is transmitted as an autosomal dominant disorder. It usually presents as spontaneous bleeding from mucous membranes, excessive bleeding from wounds, and menorrhagia. It is underrecognized, as the diagnosis requires sophisticated tests and the clinical manifestations often are quite mild. Actually, this disease is surprisingly prevalent, particularly in persons of European descent. **It is estimated that approximately 1% of people in the United States have von Willebrand disease, making it the most common inherited bleeding disorder.**

People with von Willebrand disease have compound defects in platelet function and coagulation, but in most cases only the platelet defect produces clinical findings. The exceptions are rare in patients with homozygous von Willebrand disease, in whom there is a concomitant deficiency of factor VIII severe enough to produce features resembling those of hemophilia (described later).

The effects of the causative mutations vary, allowing von Willebrand disease to be divided into several subtypes

- *Type 1* is the classic and most common variant of von Willebrand disease. It is an autosomal dominant disorder in which the quantity of circulating vWF is reduced. There is also a measurable but clinically insignificant decrease in factor VIII levels.
- *Type II* is divided into several subtypes characterized by the selective loss of high–molecular-weight multimers of vWF. Because these large multimers are the most active form, there is a functional deficiency of vWF. In type IIA, the high-molecular-weight multimers are not synthesized, leading to a true deficiency. In type IIB, abnormal "hyperfunctional" high-molecular-weight multimers

are synthesized that are rapidly removed from the circulation. These high-molecular-weight multimers cause spontaneous platelet aggregation (a situation reminiscent of the very-high–molecular-weight multimer aggregates seen in TTP); indeed, some people with type IIB von Willebrand disease have mild chronic thrombocytopenia, presumably resulting from platelet consumption.

Hemophilia A—Factor VIII Deficiency

Hemophilia A is the most common hereditary cause of serious bleeding. It is an X-linked recessive disorder caused by reduced factor VIII activity. It primarily affects males. Much less commonly, excessive bleeding occurs in heterozygous females, presumably due to preferential inactivation of the X chromosome carrying the normal factor VIII gene (unfavorable lyonization). Approximately 30% of cases are caused by new mutations; in the remainder, there is a positive family history. Severe hemophilia A is observed in people with marked deficiencies of factor VIII (activity levels < 1% of normal). Milder deficiencies may only become apparent in the face of trauma or other hemostatic stressses. The varying degrees of factor VIII deficiency are explained by the existence of many different causative mutations, including deletions, inversions, and splice junction mutations. In about 10% of patients, the factor VIII concentration is normal by immunoassay, but the coagulant activity is low because of a mutation in factor VIII that causes a loss of function.

In symptomatic cases there is a tendency toward easy bruising and massive hemorrhage after trauma or operative procedures. In addition, "spontaneous" hemorrhages frequently are encountered in tissues that normally are subject to mechanical stress, particularly the joints, where recurrent bleeds (*hemarthroses*) lead to progressive deformities that can be crippling. Petechiae are characteristically absent. Specific assays for factor VIII are used to confirm the diagnosis of hemophilia A. Typically, patients with hemophilia A have a prolonged PTT that is corrected by mixing the patient's plasma with normal plasma. Specific factor assays are then used to confirm the deficiency of factor VIII. In approximately 15% of those with severe hemophilia A, replacement therapy is complicated by the development of neutralizing antibodies against factor VIII, probably because factor VIII is seen by the immune system as a "foreign" antigen. In these persons, the PTT fails to correct in mixing studies.

Hemophilia A is treated with factor VIII infusions. Historically, factor VIII was prepared from human plasma, carrying with it the risk of transmission of viral diseases. As mentioned in Chapter 5, before 1985 thousands of hemophiliacs received factor VIII preparations contaminated with HIV and subsequently developed AIDS. The availability and widespread use of recombinant factor VIII and more highly purified factor VIII concentrates have now eliminated the infectious risk of factor VIII replacement therapy.

Hemophilia B—Factor IX Deficiency

Severe factor IX deficiency is an X-linked disorder that is indistinguishable clinically from hemophilia A but is much less common. The PTT is prolonged. The diagnosis is made using specific assays of factor IX. It is treated by infusion of recombinant factor IX.

SUMMARY

BLEEDING DISORDERS

Disseminated Intravascular Coagulation

- Syndrome in which systemic activation of the coagulation leads to consumption of coagulation factors and platelets
- Can be dominated by bleeding, vascular occlusion and tissue hypoxemia, or both
- Common triggers: sepsis, major trauma, certain cancers, obstetric complications

Immune Thrombocytopenic Purpura

- Caused by autoantibodies against platelet antigens
- May be triggered by drugs, infections, or lymphomas, or may be idiopathic

Thrombotic Thrombocytopenic Purpura and Hemolytic Uremic Syndrome

- Both manifest with thrombocytopenia, microangiopathic hemolytic anemia, and renal failure; fever and CNS involvement are more typical of TTP.
- *TTP*: Caused by acquired or inherited deficiencies of ADAMTS 13, a plasma metalloprotease that cleaves very-high-molecular-weight multimers of vWF. Deficiency of ADAMTS 13 results in abnormally large vWF multimers that activate platelets.
- *Hemolytic uremic syndrome*: Caused by deficiencies of complement regulatory proteins or agents that damage endothelial cells, such as a Shiga-like toxin elaborated by *E. coli* strain O157:H7. The endothelial injury initiates platelet activation, platelet aggregation, and microvascular thrombosis.

von Willebrand Disease

- Autosomal dominant disorder caused by mutations in vWF, a large protein that promotes the adhesion of platelets to subendothelial collagen.
- Typically causes a mild to moderate bleeding disorder resembling that associated with thrombocytopenia.

Hemophilia

- *Hemophilia A*: X-linked disorder caused by mutations in factor VIII. Affected males typically present with severe bleeding into soft tissues and joints and have a PTT.
- *Hemophilia B*: X-linked disorder caused by mutations in coagulation factor IX. It is clinically identical to hemophilia A.

Complications of Transfusion

Blood products often are rightly called "the gift of life," permitting people to survive traumatic injuries and procedures such as hematopoietic stem cell transplantation and complex surgical procedures that would otherwise prove fatal. Over 5 million red cell transfusions are given in U.S. hospitals each year. Thanks to improved screening of donors, blood products (packed red blood cells, platelets, and fresh-frozen plasma) are safer than ever before.

Nevertheless, complications still occur. Most are minor and transient. The most common is referred to as a *febrile nonhemolytic reaction*, which takes the form of fever and chills, sometimes with mild dyspnea, within 6 hours of a transfusion of red cells or platelets. It is thought that these reactions are caused by inflammatory mediators derived from donor leukocytes. The frequency of these reactions increases with the storage age of the product and is decreased by measures that limit donor leukocyte contamination. Symptoms respond to anti-pyretics and are short-lived.

Other transfusion reactions are uncommon or rare, but can have severe and sometimes fatal consequences, and therefore merit brief discussion.

ALLERGIC REACTIONS

Severe, potentially fatal allergic reactions may occur when blood products containing certain antigens are given to previously sensitized recipients. These are most likely to occur in patients with IgA deficiency, which has a frequency of 1:300 to 1:500 people. The reaction is triggered by IgG antibodies that recognize IgA in the infused blood product. Fortunately, most patients with IgA deficiency do not develop such antibodies, and these severe reactions are rare, occurring in 1 in 20,000 to 1 in 50,000 transfusions. *Urticarial allergic reactions* may be triggered by the presence of an allergen in the donated blood product that is recognized by IgE antibodies in the recipient. These are more common, occurring in 1% to 3% of transfusions, but they are generally mild.

HEMOLYTIC REACTIONS

Acute hemolytic reactions **usually are caused by preformed IgM antibodies against donor red cells that fix complement.** They most commonly stem from an error in patient identification or tube labeling that allows a patient to receive an ABO incompatible unit of blood. Preexisting "natural" IgM antibodies, usually against blood group antigens A or B, bind to red cells and rapidly induce complement-mediated lysis, intravascular hemolysis, and hemoglobinuria associated with fever, shaking chills, and flank pain. The direct Coombs test is positive unless all of the donor red cells have lysed. The signs and symptoms are due to complement activation rather than hemolysis per se, as osmotic lysis of red cells (e.g., by mistakenly infusing red cells and 5% dextrose in water simultaneously) produces hemoglobinuria without any other symptoms. In severe cases the process may rapidly progress to DIC, shock, renal failure, and death.

Delayed hemolytic reactions **are caused by antibodies that recognize red cell antigens that the recipient was sensitized to previously, for example, through a**

previous blood transfusion. These are typically caused by IgG antibodies and are associated with a positive direct Coombs test and laboratory features of hemolysis (e.g., low haptoglobin and elevated LDH). Antibodies to antigens such as Rh, Kell, and Kidd sometimes fix complement, resulting in severe and potentially fatal reactions identical to those seen with ABO mismatches. Other antibodies that do not fix complement typically result in extravascular hemolysis and relatively minor signs and symptoms.

TRANSFUSION-RELATED ACUTE LUNG INJURY

Transfusion-related acute lung injury (**TRALI**) **is a severe, frequently fatal complication in which factors in a transfused blood product trigger the activation of neutrophils in the lung microvasculature.** The incidence is low, probably less than 1 per 10,000 transfusions. Current thinking about TRALI favors a "two hit" hypothesis. The first hit is an exposure that activates endothelial cells in pulmonary capillaries. This "priming" event has diverse causes, including smoking, sepsis, and shock, and leads to sequestration of neutrophils. The primed neutrophils are then activated by a factor present in the transfused blood product, which constitutes the second hit.

The leading "second hit" candidate is an antibody in the transfused blood product that recognizes antigens expressed on neutrophils. By far the most common antibodies associated with TRALI are those that bind major histocompatibility complex (MHC) class I antigens. These antibodies are often found in multiparous women, in whom they are generated in response to foreign MHC antigens expressed by the fetus. Indeed, measures to exclude multiparous women from plasma donation have resulted in the incidence of TRALI being cut in half. The presentation is dramatic, with sudden onset of respiratory failure associated with diffuse bilateral pulmonary infiltrates during or soon after a transfusion. The treatment is largely supportive and the outcome is guarded; mortality is 5% in uncomplicated cases and up to 67% in those who are severely ill.

INFECTIOUS COMPLICATIONS

Virtually any infectious agent can be transmitted through blood products, but bacterial and viral infections are most likely to be so. Significant bacterial contamination (sufficient to produce symptoms) is much more common in platelet preparations than red cell preparations, because of the fact that platelets (unlike red cells) must be stored at room temperature, which favors growth of bacterial contaminants. Rates of bacterial infection secondary to platelet transfusion can be as high as 1 in 5000. Many of the symptoms (fever, chills, hypotension) resemble those of transfusion reactions, and it may be necessary to start broad-spectrum antibiotics prospectively in symptomatic patients while awaiting laboratory results.

Advances in donor selection, donor screening, and infectious disease testing have dramatically decreased the incidence of viral transmission by blood products. However on rare occasions when the donor is acutely infected, there can still be transfusion-related transmission of viruses. Rates of transmission of HIV, hepatitis C, and hepatitis B are estimated to be 1 in 2 million, 1 in 1 million, and 1 in 500,000, respectively. There also remains a low risk of "exotic" infectious agents such as West Nile virus, trypanosomiasis, and babesiosis.

Disorders of the Spleen and Thymus

SPLENOMEGALY

The spleen is frequently involved in a wide variety of systemic diseases. In virtually all instances the spleen responds by enlarging (splenomegaly), an alteration that produces a set of stereotypical signs and symptoms. Evaluation of splenic enlargement is aided by recognition of the usual limits of splenomegaly produced by specific disorders. It would be erroneous to attribute an enlarged spleen pushing into the pelvis to vitamin B_{12} deficiency, or to entertain a diagnosis of CML in the absence of splenomegaly. Disorders may be grouped according to the degree of splenomegaly that they characteristically produce:

* *Massive splenomegaly* (weight > 1000 g)
    Myeloproliferative neoplasms (CML, primary myelofibrosis); certain indolent leukemias (CLL and hairy cell leukemia); many lymphomas; infectious diseases (e.g., malaria); Gaucher disease
* *Moderate splenomegaly* (weight 500–1000 g)
    Chronic congestive splenomegaly (portal hypertension or splenic vein obstruction); acute leukemias; disorders with extravascular hemolysis (hereditary spherocytosis, thalassemia major, autoimmune hemolytic anemia; amyloidosis; Niemann-Pick disease; many infections, including infective endocarditis, tuberculosis, and typhoid; sarcoidosis; metastatic carcinoma or sarcoma
* *Mild splenomegaly* (weight < 500 g)
    Acute splenitis; acute splenic congestion; infectious mononucleosis; miscellaneous disorders, including septicemia, systemic lupus erythematosus, and intraabdominal infections

The microscopic changes associated with these diseases are discussed in the relevant sections of this and other chapters.

A chronically enlarged spleen often removes excessive numbers of one or more of the formed elements of blood, resulting in anemia, leukopenia, or thrombocytopenia. This is referred to as *hypersplenism,* a state that can be associated with many of the diseases listed previously. In addition, platelets are particularly susceptible to sequestration in the interstices of the red pulp; as a result, *thrombocytopenia* is more prevalent and severe in persons with splenomegaly than is anemia or neutropenia.

DISORDERS OF THE THYMUS

As is well known, the thymus has a crucial role in T cell differentiation. It is not surprising, therefore, that the thymus can be involved by lymphomas, particularly those of T cell lineage (discussed earlier in this chapter). The focus here is on the two most frequent (albeit still uncommon) disorders of the thymus: thymic hyperplasia and thymoma.

Thymic Hyperplasia

Thymic enlargement often is associated with the presence of lymphoid follicles, or germinal centers, within the medulla. These germinal centers contain reactive B cells, which are only present in small numbers in normal thymuses. Thymic follicular hyperplasia is found in most patients with *myasthenia gravis* and sometimes also occurs in other autoimmune diseases, such as systemic lupus erythematosus and rheumatoid arthritis. The relationship between the thymus and myasthenia gravis is discussed in Chapter 22. Of significance, removal of the hyperplastic thymus is often beneficial early in the disease.

Thymoma

Thymomas are tumors of thymic epithelial cells. Several classification systems for thymoma based on cytologic and biologic criteria have been proposed. One simple and clinically useful classification is as follows:

- Benign or encapsulated thymoma: cytologically and biologically benign
- Malignant thymoma
  - *Type I*: cytologically benign but infiltrative and locally aggressive
  - *Type II* (thymic carcinoma): cytologically and biologically malignant

MORPHOLOGY

Macroscopically, thymomas are lobulated, firm, gray-white masses up to 15 to 20 cm in dimension. Most appear encapsulated, but 20% to 25% penetrate the capsule and infiltrate perithymic tissues. Microscopically, virtually all thymomas are composed of a mixture of epithelial tumor cells and nonneoplastic thymocytes (immature T cells). In **benign thymomas,** the epithelial cells are spindled or elongated and resemble those that normally populate the medulla. As a result, these are sometimes referred to as **medullary thymomas.** In other tumors, there is an admixture of the plumper, rounder, cortical-type epithelial cells; this pattern is sometimes referred to as a mixed thymoma. The medullary and mixed patterns account for 60% to 70% of all thymomas.

Malignant thymoma type I is cytologically bland but locally invasive; it accounts for 20% to 25% of all thymomas. These tumors also occasionally (and unpredictably) metastasize. They are composed of varying proportions of epithelial cells and reactive thymocytes. The epithelial cells usually have abundant cytoplasm and rounded vesicular nuclei, an appearance similar to normal thymic cortical epithelial cells; spindled epithelial cells are sometimes present as well. The epithelial cells often palisade around blood vessels. The critical distinguishing feature is the penetration of the capsule with the invasion of surrounding structures.

Malignant thymoma type II is perhaps better thought of as a form of thymic carcinoma. These tumors account for about 5% of thymomas. Macroscopically, they usually are fleshy, obviously invasive masses that often metastasize to such sites as the lungs. Microscopically, most resemble squamous cell carcinoma.

Clinical Features

Thymomas are rare. They may arise at any age, but most occur in middle-aged adults. In a large series about 30% were asymptomatic; 30% to 40% produced local manifestations such as cough, dyspnea, and superior vena cava syndrome; and the remainder were associated with a systemic disease, most commonly myasthenia gravis, in which a concomitant thymoma is discovered in 15% to 20% of patients. Removal of the tumor often leads to improvement of the neuromuscular disorder. In addition to myasthenia gravis , thymomas may be associated with several other pareneoplastic syndromes. These include in rough order of frequency , pure red cell aplasia, hypogammaglobulinemia, and multi organ autoimmunity. The latter bears resemblance with graft versus host disease.

SUGGESTED READINGS

Red Cell Disorders

Brodsky RA: Paroxysmal nocturnal hemoglobinuria, *Blood* 124:2804, 2014. [*A concise current review.*]

Da Cost L, Galimand J, Fenneteau O, et al: Hereditary spherocytosis, elliptocytosis, and other red cell membrane disorders, *Blood Rev* 27:167, 2013. [*An excellent overview of inherited red cell membrane defects.*]

Ganz T: Systemic iron homeostasis, *Physiol Rev* 93:1721, 2013. [*A review of iron metabolism in health and disease.*]

Platt OS: Hydroxyurea for the treatment of sickle cell disease, *N Engl J Med* 358:1362, 2008. [*A review focused on the beneficial effects of hydroxyurea in sickle cell disease.*]

Wassmer SC, Taylor TE, Rathod PK, et al: Investigating the pathogenesis of severe malaria: a multidisciplinary and cross-geographical approach, *Am J Trop Med Hyg* 93(Suppl):42, 2015. [*A review of the proposed pathophysiology of severe forms of malaria.*]

Wong TE, Brandow AM, Lim W, et al: Update on the use of hydroxyurea therapy in sickle cell disease, *Blood* 124:3850, 2014. [*A review focused on the beneficial effects of hydroxyurea in sickle cell disease.*]

Young NS, Bacigalupo A, Marsh JC: Aplastic anemia: pathophysiology and treatment, *Biol Blood Marrow Transplant* 16:S119, 2010. [*Discussion of the role of the immune system and telomerase mutations in aplastic anemia.*]

White Cell Disorders

Anderson KC, Carrasco RD: Pathogenesis of myeloma, *Annu Rev Pathol* 6:249, 2011. [*A review of advances in understanding the molecular pathogenesis of multiple myeloma.*]

Arber DA, Orazi A, Hasserjian R, et al: The 2016 revision to the World Health Organization classification of myeloid neoplasms and acute leukemia, *Blood* 127:2391, 2016. [*A report providing the rationale for revision of the WHO classification of myeloid neoplasms.*]

Inaba H, Greaves M, Mullighan CG: Acute lymphoblastic leukemia, *Lancet* 381:1943, 2013. *[A review of the pathogenesis, diagnosis, and treatment of ALL.]*

Mathas S, Hartmann S, Kuppers R: Hodgkin lymphoma: Pathology and biology, *Semin Hematol* 53:139, 2016. *[A concise review of Hodgkin lymphoma pathogenesis.]*

Swerdlow SH, Campo E, Pileri SA, et al: The 2016 revision of the World Health Organization classification of lymphoid neoplasms, *Blood* 127:2375, 2016. *[An overview of the most recent WHO classification of lymphoid neoplasms.]*

The Cancer Genome Atlas Research Network: Genomic and epigenomic networks landscapes in adult de novo acute myeloid leukemia, *N Engl J Med* 368:2059, 2013. *[Landmark paper that uses next-generation sequencing and other genome-wide approaches to systematically describe genomic alterations in AML.]*

Young RM, Staudt LM: Targeting pathological B cell receptor signaling in lymphoid malignancies, *Nat Rev Drug Discov* 12:229, 2013. *[An excellent review of the role of B cell receptor signaling in non-Hodgkin lymphoma and its potential as a therapeutic target.]*

Bleeding Disorders

Arepally GM, Ortel TL: Heparin-induced thrombocytopenia, *Annu Rev Med* 61:77, 2010. *[A discussion of pathogenesis, clinical features, diagnostic criteria, and therapeutic approaches in HIT.]*

Ng C, Motto DG, Di Paola J: Diagnostic approach to von Willebrand disease, *Blood* 125:2029, 2015. *[A review on the molecular pathogenesis and diagnosis of vWD.]*

Noris M, Mescia F, Remuzzi G: STEC-HUS, atypical HUS and TTP are all diseases of complement activation, *Nat Rev Nephrol* 8:622, 2013. *[An article focused on the possible role of excessive activation of the alternative complement pathway in HUS and TTP.]*

Pawlinski R, Mackman N: Cellular sources of tissue factor in endotoxemia and sepsis, *Thromb Res* 125(S1):S70, 2010. *[An overview of the role of cellular procoagulants in DIC associated with bacterial infection.]*

Zhou Z, Nguyen TC, Guchhait P, et al: Von Willebrand factor, ADAMTS-13, and thrombotic thrombocytopenia purpura, *Semin Thromb Hemost* 36:71, 2010. *[A review focused on the role of vWF deregulation and ADAMTS 13 deficiency in TTP.]*

Disorders That Affect the Spleen and Thymus

Choi SS, Kim KD, Chung KY: Prognostic and clinical relevance of the World Health Organization schema for the classification of thymic epithelial tumors: a clinicopathologic study of 108 patients and literature review, *Chest* 127:755, 2005. *[A large clinicopathologic series that shows that stage is the best predictor of outcome in thymoma.]*

CHAPTER

Lung 13

Atelectasis (Collapse) 495
Acute Respiratory Distress
  Syndrome 496
Obstructive Versus Restrictive
  Pulmonary Diseases 498
Obstructive Lung (Airway)
  Diseases 498
Emphysema 498
Chronic Bronchitis 502
Asthma 503
Bronchiectasis 505
Chronic Interstitial (Restrictive,
  Infiltrative) Lung Diseases 506
Fibrosing Diseases 507
Granulomatous Diseases 512
Pulmonary Eosinophilia 515
Smoking-Related Interstitial
  Diseases 515

Pulmonary Diseases of Vascular
  Origin 515
Pulmonary Embolism, Hemorrhage, and
  Infarction 515
Pulmonary Hypertension 517
Diffuse Alveolar Hemorrhage Syndromes 519
Pulmonary Infections 519
Community-Acquired Bacterial Pneumonias 520
Community-Acquired Viral Pneumonias 523
Hospital-Acquired Pneumonias 524
Aspiration Pneumonia 525
Lung Abscess 525
Chronic Pneumonias 525
Tuberculosis 526
Histoplasmosis, Coccidioidomycosis, and
  Blastomycosis 532
Pneumonia in the Immunocompromised
  Host 533

Opportunistic Fungal Infections 535
Pulmonary Disease in Human Immunodeficiency
  Virus Infection 537
Lung Tumors 537
Carcinomas 537
Carcinoid Tumors 543
Pleural Lesions 544
Pleural Effusion and Pleuritis 544
Pneumothorax, Hemothorax, and
  Chylothorax 544
Malignant Mesothelioma 544
Lesions of the Upper Respiratory
  Tract 545
Acute Infections 545
Nasopharyngeal Carcinoma 546
Laryngeal Tumors 546

The major function of the lung is to replenish oxygen and remove carbon dioxide from blood. Developmentally, the respiratory system is an outgrowth from the ventral wall of the foregut. The midline trachea develops two lateral outpouchings, the lung buds. The right lung bud eventually divides into three main bronchi, and the left into two main bronchi, thus giving rise to three lobes on the right and two on the left. The main bronchi branch dichotomously, giving rise to progressively smaller airways, termed *bronchioles*, which are distinguished from bronchi by the lack of cartilage and submucosal glands within their walls. Additional branching of bronchioles leads to *terminal bronchioles*; the part of the lung distal to the terminal bronchiole is called an *acinus*. Pulmonary acini are composed of *respiratory bronchioles* (emanating from the terminal bronchiole) that proceed into *alveolar ducts*, which immediately branch into *alveolar sacs*, the blind ends of the respiratory passages, whose walls are formed entirely of *alveoli*, the ultimate site of gas exchange. The alveolar walls (or alveolar septa) consist of the following components, proceeding from blood to air (Fig. 13.1):

- *The capillary endothelium and basement membrane.*
- *The pulmonary interstitium*, composed of fine elastic fibers, small bundles of collagen, a few fibroblast-like cells, smooth muscle cells, mast cells, and rare mononuclear cells.

- *Alveolar epithelium*, consisting of a continuous layer of two principal cell types: flattened, plate-like type I pneumocytes covering 95% of the alveolar surface; and rounded type II pneumocytes. The latter synthesize pulmonary surfactant and are the main cell type involved in repair of alveolar epithelium after damage to type I pneumocytes.

A few alveolar macrophages usually lie free within the alveolar space. In the city dwellers, these macrophages often contain phagocytosed carbon particles.

Lung diseases can broadly be divided into those affecting (1) the airways, (2) the interstitium, and (3) the pulmonary vascular system. This division into discrete compartments is, of course, deceptively simple. In reality, disease in one compartment often causes secondary alterations of morphology and function in others.

ATELECTASIS (COLLAPSE)

Atelectasis, also known as collapse, is loss of lung volume caused by inadequate expansion of air spaces. It results in shunting of inadequately oxygenated blood from pulmonary arteries into veins, thus giving rise to a ventilation-perfusion imbalance and hypoxia. On the basis of the

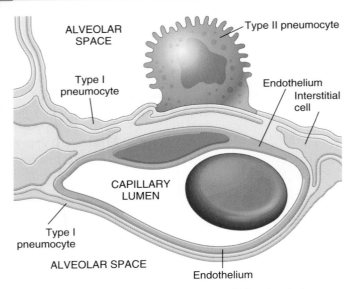

Fig. 13.1 Microscopic structure of the alveolar wall. Note that the basement membrane *(yellow)* is thin on one side and widened where it is continuous with the interstitial space.

underlying mechanism and the distribution of alveolar collapse, atelectasis is classified into three forms

- *Resorption atelectasis* occurs when an obstruction prevents air from reaching distal airways. Any air present gradually becomes absorbed, and alveolar collapse follows. The most common cause of resorption collapse is obstruction of a bronchus. Resorption atelectasis most frequently occurs postoperatively due to intrabronchial mucous or mucopurulent plugs, but also may result from foreign body aspiration (particularly in children), bronchial asthma, bronchiectasis, chronic bronchitis, or intrabronchial tumor, in which it may be the first sign of malignancy.
- *Compression atelectasis* is usually associated with accumulation of fluid, blood, or air within the pleural cavity. A frequent cause is pleural effusions occurring in the setting of congestive heart failure. Leakage of air into the pleural cavity (pneumothorax) also leads to compression atelectasis. Basal atelectasis resulting from a failure to breath deeply commonly occurs in bedridden patients, in patients with ascites, and during and after surgery.
- *Contraction atelectasis* (or cicatrization atelectasis) occurs when local or diffuse fibrosis affecting the lung or the pleura hamper lung expansion.

Atelectasis (except when caused by contraction) is potentially reversible and should be treated promptly to prevent hypoxemia and superimposed infection of the collapsed lung.

ACUTE RESPIRATORY DISTRESS SYNDROME

The epidemiology and definition of acute respiratory distress syndrome (ARDS) are evolving. Formerly considered to be the severe end of a spectrum of acute lung injury, it is now defined as respiratory failure occurring within 1 week of a known clinical insult with bilateral opacities on chest imaging, not fully explained by effusions, atelectasis, cardiac failure, or fluid overload. It is graded based on the severity of the changes in arterial blood oxygenation. Causes are diverse; the shared feature is that all lead to extensive bilateral injury to alveoli.

Severe ARDS is characterized by rapid onset of life-threatening respiratory insufficiency, cyanosis, and severe arterial hypoxemia that is refractory to oxygen therapy. The histologic manifestation of ARDS in the lungs is known as *diffuse alveolar damage (DAD)*. ARDS may occur in a multitude of clinical settings and is associated with primary pulmonary diseases and severe systemic inflammatory disorders such as sepsis. The most frequent triggers of ARDS are pneumonia (35%–45%) and sepsis (30%–35%), followed by aspiration, trauma (including brain injury, abdominal surgery, and multiple fractures), pancreatitis, and transfusion reactions. ARDS should not be confused with respiratory distress syndrome of the newborn; the latter is caused by a deficiency of surfactant caused by prematurity.

Pathogenesis

In ARDS, the integrity of the alveolar-capillary membrane is compromised by endothelial and epithelial injury. Most work suggests that ARDS stems from an inflammatory reaction initiated by a variety of pro-inflammatory mediators (Fig. 13.2). As early as 30 minutes after an acute insult, there is increased synthesis of interleukin 8 (IL-8), a potent neutrophil chemotactic and activating agent, by pulmonary macrophages. Release of IL-8 and other factors, such as IL-1 and tumor necrosis factor (TNF), leads to endothelial activation and sequestration and activation of neutrophils in pulmonary capillaries. Neutrophils are thought to have an important role in the pathogenesis of ARDS. Histologic examination of lungs early in the disease process shows increased numbers of neutrophils within the vascular space, the interstitium, and the alveoli. Activated neutrophils release a variety of products (e.g., reactive oxygen species, proteases) that damage the alveolar epithelium and endothelium. The assault on the endothelium and epithelium causes vascular leakiness and loss of surfactant that render the alveolar unit unable to expand. Of note, the destructive forces unleashed by neutrophils can be counteracted by an array of endogenous anti-proteases and anti-oxidants that are upregulated by proinflammatory cytokines. In the end, it is the balance between the destructive and protective factors that determines the degree of tissue injury and clinical severity of the ARDS.

MORPHOLOGY

In the **acute phase of ARDS,** the lungs are dark red, firm, airless, and heavy. Microscopic examination reveals capillary congestion, necrosis of alveolar epithelial cells, interstitial and intra-alveolar edema and hemorrhage, and (particularly with sepsis) collections of neutrophils in capillaries. The most characteristic finding is the presence of **hyaline membranes,** particularly

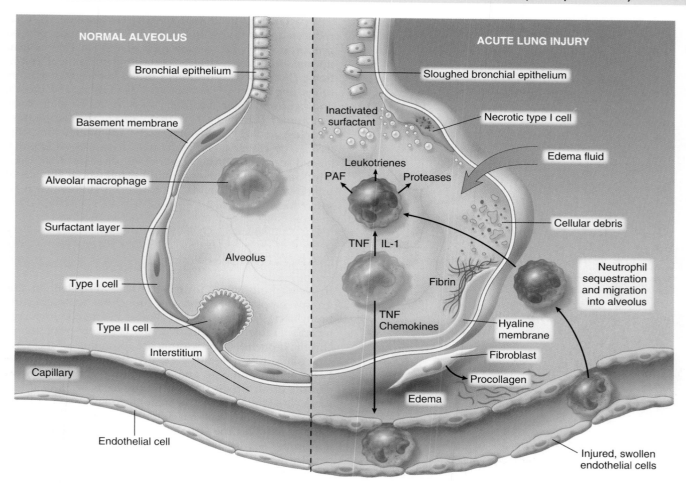

Fig. 13.2 The normal alveolus *(left)* and the injured alveolus in the early phase of acute lung injury and the acute respiratory distress syndrome. Under the influence of proinflammatory cytokines such as interleukins IL-8 and IL-1 and tumor necrosis factor (TNF) (released by macrophages), neutrophils are sequestered in the pulmonary microvasculature and then egress into the alveolar space, where they undergo activation. Activated neutrophils release leukotrienes, oxidants, proteases, and platelet-activating factor (PAF), which contribute to local tissue damage, accumulation of edema fluid, surfactant inactivation, and hyaline membrane formation. Subsequently, the release of macrophage-derived fibrogenic cytokines such as transforming growth factor-β (TGF-β) and platelet-derived growth factor (PGDF) stimulate fibroblast growth and collagen deposition associated with the healing phase of injury. *(Modified from Ware LB: Pathophysiology of acute lung injury and the acute respiratory distress syndrome, Semin Respir Crit Care Med 27:337, 2006.)*

lining the distended alveolar ducts (Fig. 13.3). Such membranes consist of fibrin-rich edema fluid admixed with remnants of necrotic epithelial cells. Overall, the picture is remarkably similar to that seen in respiratory distress syndrome of the newborn (Chapter 6). In the **organizing stage,** type II pneumocytes proliferate vigorously in an attempt to regenerate the alveolar lining. Resolution is unusual; more commonly, the fibrin-rich exudates organize into intraalveolar fibrosis. Marked thickening of the alveolar septa ensues due to proliferation of interstitial cells and deposition of collagen.

Clinical Features

The clinical syndrome of acute lung injury or ARDS affects approximately 190,000 patients per year in the United States. In 85% of cases, it develops within 72 hours of the initial insult. The overall hospital mortality rate is 38.5% (27%, 32%, and 45% for mild, moderate, and severe ARDS, respectively). Predictors of poor prognosis include

advanced age, bacteremia (sepsis), and the development of multiorgan failure. Most patients who survive the acute insult recover normal respiratory function within 6 to 12 months, but the rest develop diffuse interstitial fibrosis leading to chronic respiratory insufficiency.

SUMMARY

ACUTE RESPIRATORY DISTRESS SYNDROME

- ARDS is a clinical syndrome of progressive respiratory insufficiency caused by diffuse alveolar damage in the setting of sepsis, severe trauma, or diffuse pulmonary infection.
- Neutrophils and their products have a crucial role in the pathogenesis of ARDS by causing endothelial and epithelial injury.
- The characteristic histologic picture is that of alveolar edema, epithelial necrosis, accumulation of neutrophils, and presence of hyaline membranes lining the alveolar wall and ducts.

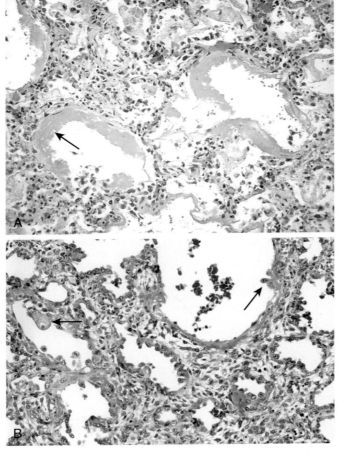

Fig. 13.3 Acute lung injury and acute respiratory distress syndrome. (A) Diffuse alveolar damage in the acute phase. Some alveoli are collapsed, while others are distended; many are lined by bright pink hyaline membranes *(arrow)*. (B) The healing stage is marked by resorption of hyaline membranes and thickening of alveolar septa by inflammatory cells, fibroblasts, and collagen. Numerous reactive type II pneumocytes also are seen at this stage *(arrows)*, associated with regeneration and repair.

OBSTRUCTIVE VERSUS RESTRICTIVE PULMONARY DISEASES

Diffuse pulmonary diseases can be classified into two categories: (1) obstructive (airway) disease, characterized by an increase in resistance to air flow caused by partial or complete obstruction at any level; and (2) restrictive disease, characterized by reduced expansion of lung parenchyma and decreased total lung capacity.

The major diffuse obstructive disorders are emphysema, chronic bronchitis, bronchiectasis, and asthma. In patients with these diseases, forced vital capacity (FVC) is either normal or slightly decreased, while the expiratory flow rate, usually measured as the forced expiratory volume at 1 second (FEV$_1$), is significantly decreased. Thus, the ratio of FEV to FVC is characteristically decreased. Expiratory obstruction may result from anatomic airway narrowing, classically observed in asthma, or from loss of elastic recoil, characteristic of emphysema.

By contrast, in diffuse restrictive diseases, FVC is reduced and the expiratory flow rate is normal or reduced proportionately. Hence, the ratio of FEV to FVC is near normal. Restrictive defects occur in two general conditions: (1) chest wall disorders in the presence of normal lungs (e.g., with severe obesity, diseases of the pleura, and neuromuscular disorders, such as the Guillain-Barré syndrome [Chapter 22], that affect the respiratory muscles) and (2) acute or chronic interstitial lung diseases. The classic acute restrictive disease is ARDS, discussed earlier. Chronic restrictive diseases (discussed later) include the pneumoconioses, interstitial fibrosis of unknown etiology, and infiltrative conditions such as sarcoidosis.

OBSTRUCTIVE LUNG (AIRWAY) DISEASES

In their prototypical forms, the four disorders in this group—emphysema, chronic bronchitis, asthma, and bronchiectasis—have distinct clinical and anatomic characteristics (Table 13.1), but overlaps between emphysema, chronic bronchitis, and asthma are common.

It should be noted that emphysema is defined on the basis of morphologic and radiologic features, whereas chronic bronchitis is defined on the basis of clinical features (described later). The anatomic distribution of these disorders also is somewhat different, as chronic bronchitis initially involves the large airways, whereas emphysema affects the acinus. In severe or advanced cases of both, small airway disease (chronic bronchiolitis) is also present. Although emphysema may exist without chronic bronchitis (particularly in inherited α1-anti-trypsin deficiency, discussed later) and vice versa, the two diseases usually coexist. This is almost certainly because cigarette smoking is the major underlying cause of both. In view of their propensity to coexist, emphysema and chronic bronchitis often are grouped together under the rubric of *chronic obstructive pulmonary disease (COPD)*. COPD affects more than 10% of the U.S. adult population and is the fourth leading cause of death in this country. The largely irreversible airflow obstruction of COPD distinguishes it from asthma, which, as discussed later, is characterized by reversible airflow obstruction (Fig. 13.4).

Emphysema

Emphysema is characterized by permanent enlargement of the air spaces distal to the terminal bronchioles, accompanied by destruction of their walls without significant fibrosis. It is classified according to its anatomic distribution. As discussed earlier, the acinus is the structure distal to terminal bronchioles, and a cluster of three to five acini is called a *lobule* (Fig. 13.5A). There are four major types of emphysema: (1) centriacinar, (2) panacinar, (3) distal acinar, and (4) irregular. Only the first two types cause significant airway obstruction, with centriacinar emphysema being about 20 times more common than panacinar disease.

- *Centriacinar (centrilobular) emphysema.* **The distinctive feature of centriacinar emphysema is that the central or proximal parts of the acini, formed by respiratory**

Table 13.1 Disorders Associated With Airflow Obstruction: The Spectrum of Chronic Obstructive Pulmonary Disease

Clinical Entity	Anatomic Site	Major Pathologic Changes	Etiology	Signs/Symptoms
Chronic bronchitis	Bronchus	Mucous gland hypertrophy and hyperplasia, hypersecretion	Tobacco smoke, air pollutants	Cough, sputum production
Bronchiectasis	Bronchus	Airway dilation and scarring	Persistent or severe infections	Cough, purulent sputum, fever
Asthma	Bronchus	Smooth muscle hypertrophy and hyperplasia, excessive mucus, inflammation	Immunologic or undefined causes	Episodic wheezing, cough, dyspnea
Emphysema	Acinus	Air space enlargement, wall destruction	Tobacco smoke	Dyspnea
Small airway disease, bronchiolitis*	Bronchiole	Inflammatory scarring, partial obliteration of bronchioles	Tobacco smoke, air pollutants	Cough, dyspnea

*Can be present in all forms of obstructive lung disease or by itself.

bronchioles, are affected, while distal alveoli are spared. Thus, both emphysematous and normal air spaces exist within the same acinus and lobule (see Fig. 13.5B). The lesions are more common and severe in the upper lobes, particularly in the apical segments. In severe centriacinar emphysema, the distal acinus also becomes involved, and thus, the differentiation from panacinar emphysema becomes difficult. This type of emphysema is most common in cigarette smokers, often in association with chronic bronchitis.

- *Panacinar (panlobular) emphysema.* **In panacinar (panlobular) emphysema, the acini are uniformly enlarged,** from the level of the respiratory bronchiole to the terminal blind **alveoli** (see Fig. 13.5C). In contrast to centriacinar emphysema, panacinar emphysema occurs more commonly in the lower lung zones and is associated with α1-anti-trypsin deficiency.
- *Distal acinar (paraseptal) emphysema.* **In this form of emphysema, the proximal portion of the acinus is normal but the distal part is primarily involved.** The emphysema is more striking adjacent to the pleura, along the lobular connective tissue septa, and at the

margins of the lobules. It occurs adjacent to areas of fibrosis, scarring, or atelectasis and is usually more severe in the upper half of the lungs. The characteristic finding is the presence of multiple, contiguous, enlarged air spaces ranging in diameter from less than 0.5 mm to more than 2.0 cm, sometimes forming cystic structures that, with progressive enlargement, give rise to *bullae.* The cause of this type of emphysema is unknown; it comes to attention most often in young adults who present with spontaneous pneumothorax.

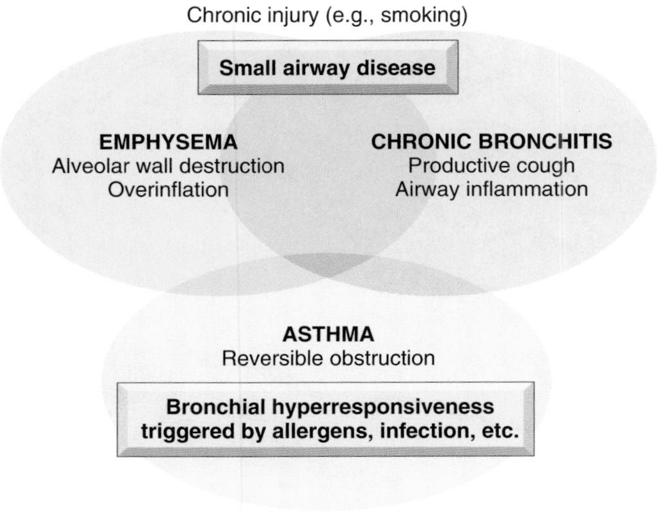

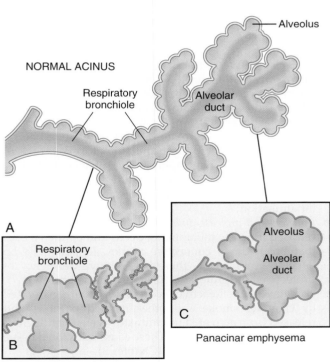

Fig. 13.5 Major patterns of emphysema. (A) Diagram of normal structure of the acinus, the fundamental unit of the lung. (B) Centriacinar emphysema with dilation that initially affects the respiratory bronchioles. (C) Panacinar emphysema with initial distention of all the peripheral structures (i.e., the alveolus and alveolar duct); the disease later extends to affect the respiratory bronchioles.

Chronic injury (e.g., smoking)

Small airway disease

EMPHYSEMA
Alveolar wall destruction
Overinflation

CHRONIC BRONCHITIS
Productive cough
Airway inflammation

ASTHMA
Reversible obstruction

Bronchial hyperresponsiveness triggered by allergens, infection, etc.

Fig. 13.4 Schematic representation of overlap between chronic obstructive lung diseases.

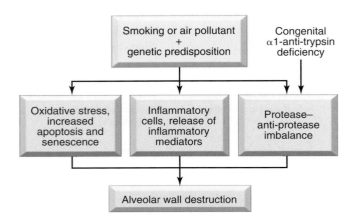

Fig. 13.6 Pathogenesis of emphysema. See text for details.

to develop pulmonary emphysema, which is compounded by smoking. About 1% of all patients with emphysema have this defect. α1-anti-trypsin, normally present in serum, tissue fluids, and macrophages, is a major inhibitor of proteases (particularly elastase) secreted by neutrophils during inflammation. α1-anti-trypsin is encoded by a gene in the proteinase inhibitor *(Pi)* locus on chromosome 14. The *Pi* locus is polymorphic, and approximately 0.012% of the U.S. population is homozygous for the Z allele, a genotype that is associated with markedly decreased serum levels of α1-anti-trypsin. More than 80% of these individuals develop symptomatic panacinar emphysema, which occurs at an earlier age and is of greater severity if the individual smokes.

Protease-mediated damage of extracellular matrix has a central role in the airway obstruction seen in emphysema. Small airways are normally held open by the elastic recoil of the lung parenchyma, and the loss of elastic tissue in the walls of alveoli that surround respiratory bronchioles reduces radial traction and thus causes the respiratory bronchioles to collapse during expiration. This leads to functional airflow obstruction despite the absence of mechanical obstruction.

- *Irregular emphysema.* **Irregular emphysema, so named because the acinus is irregularly involved, is almost invariably associated with scarring,** such as that resulting from healed inflammatory diseases. Although clinically asymptomatic, this may be the most common form of emphysema.

Pathogenesis

Inhaled cigarette smoke and other noxious particles cause lung damage and inflammation, which, particularly in patients with a genetic predisposition, result in parenchymal destruction (emphysema) and airway disease (bronchiolitis and chronic bronchitis). Factors that influence the development of emphysema include the following (Fig. 13.6):

- *Inflammatory cells and mediators:* A wide variety of inflammatory mediators have been shown to be increased (including leukotriene B$_4$, IL-8, TNF, and others) that attract more inflammatory cells from the circulation (chemotactic factors), amplify the inflammatory process (proinflammatory cytokines), and induce structural changes (growth factors). The inflammatory cells present in lesions include neutrophils, macrophages, and CD4+ and CD8+ T cells. It is not known if the T cells are specific for a particular antigen or are recruited as part of inflammation.
- *Protease–anti-protease imbalance:* Several proteases are released from the inflammatory cells and epithelial cells that break down connective tissues. In patients who develop emphysema, there is a relative deficiency of protective anti-proteases (further discussed below).
- *Oxidative stress:* Reactive oxygen species are generated by cigarette smoke and other inhaled particles and released from activated inflammatory cells such as macrophages and neutrophils. These cause additional tissue damage and inflammation (Chapter 3).
- *Airway infection:* Although infection is not thought to play a role in the initiation of tissue destruction, bacterial and/or viral infections cause acute exacerbations.

The idea that proteases are important is based in part on the observation that patients with a genetic deficiency of the anti-protease α1-anti-trypsin have a predisposition

MORPHOLOGY

The diagnosis and classification of emphysema depend largely on the macroscopic appearance of the lung. Typical **panacinar emphysema** produces pale, voluminous lungs that often obscure the heart when the anterior chest wall is removed at autopsy. The macroscopic features of **centriacinar emphysema** are less impressive. Until late stages, the lungs are a deeper pink than in panacinar emphysema and less voluminous, and the upper two-thirds of the lungs are more severely affected than the lower lungs. Histologic examination reveals **destruction of alveolar walls without fibrosis, leading to enlarged air spaces** (Fig. 13.7). In addition to alveolar loss, the number of alveolar capillaries is diminished. Terminal and respiratory bronchioles may be deformed because of the loss of septa that help

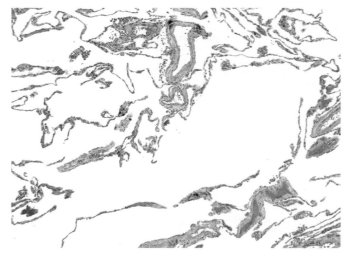

Fig. 13.7 Pulmonary emphysema. There is marked enlargement of the air spaces, with destruction of alveolar septa but without fibrosis. Note the presence of black anthracotic pigment.

tether these structures in the parenchyma. With the **loss of elastic tissue** in the surrounding alveolar septa, radial traction on the small airways is reduced. As a result, they tend to collapse during expiration—an important cause of chronic airflow obstruction in severe emphysema. Bronchiolar inflammation and submucosal fibrosis are consistently present in advanced disease.

Clinical Features

Dyspnea usually is the first symptom; it begins insidiously but is steadily progressive. In patients with underlying chronic bronchitis or chronic asthmatic bronchitis, cough and wheezing may be the initial complaints. Weight loss is common and may be severe enough to suggest an occult malignant tumor. Pulmonary function tests reveal reduced FEV_1 with normal or near-normal FVC. Hence, the FEV_1 to FVC ratio is reduced.

The classic presentation of emphysema with no "bronchitic" component is one in which the patient is barrel-chested and dyspneic, with obviously prolonged expiration, sitting forward in a hunched-over position. In these patients, air space enlargement is severe and diffusing capacity is low. Dyspnea and hyperventilation are prominent, so that until very late in the disease, gas exchange is adequate and blood gas values are relatively normal. Because of prominent dyspnea and adequate oxygenation of hemoglobin, these patients sometimes are sometimes called "pink puffers."

At the other end of the clinical spectrum is a patient with emphysema who also has pronounced chronic bronchitis and a history of recurrent infections. Dyspnea usually is less prominent, and in the absence of increased respiratory drive the patient retains carbon dioxide, becoming hypoxic and often cyanotic. For unclear reasons, such patients tend to be obese—hence the designation "blue bloaters."

In most patients with COPD the symptoms fall in between these two extremes. Hypoxia-induced pulmonary vascular spasm and loss of pulmonary capillary surface area from alveolar destruction causes the gradual development of *secondary pulmonary hypertension*, which in 20% to 30% of patients leads to right-sided congestive heart failure (cor pulmonale, Chapter 11). Death from emphysema is related to either respiratory failure or right-sided heart failure.

Conditions Related to Emphysema

Several conditions involving abnormal airspaces or accumulations of air within the lungs or other tissues also are recognized:

- *Compensatory emphysema* describes the dilation of residual alveoli in response to loss of lung substance elsewhere, such as occurs after surgical removal of a diseased lung or lobe.
- *Obstructive overinflation* refers to expansion of the lung due to air trapping. A common cause is subtotal obstruction of an airway by a tumor or foreign object. Obstructive overinflation can be life-threatening if expansion of the affected portion produces compression of the remaining normal lung.
- *Bullous emphysema* refers to any form of emphysema that produces large subpleural blebs or bullae (spaces >1 cm

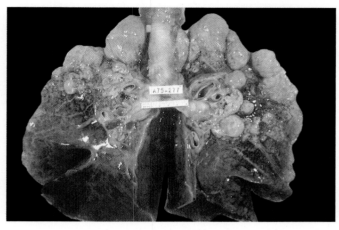

Fig. 13.8 Bullous emphysema with large apical and subpleural bullae. *(From the Teaching Collection of the Department of Pathology, University of Texas Southwestern Medical School, Dallas, Texas.)*

in diameter in the distended state) (Fig. 13.8). Such blebs represent localized accentuations of one of the four forms of emphysema; most often the blebs are subpleural, and on occasion they may rupture, leading to pneumothorax.

- *Mediastinal (interstitial) emphysema* is caused by entry of air into the interstitium of the lung, from where it may track to the mediastinum and sometimes the subcutaneous tissue. It may occur spontaneously if a sudden increase in intraalveolar pressure (as with vomiting or violent coughing) produces alveolar rupture, which allows air to dissect into the interstitium. Sometimes it develops in children with whooping cough. It may also occur in patients on respirators who have partial bronchiolar obstruction or in individuals with a perforating injury (e.g., a fractured rib). When the interstitial air gets into the subcutaneous tissue, the patient may literally blow up like a balloon, with marked swelling of the head and neck and crackling crepitation over the chest (subcutaneous emphysema). In most instances the air is resorbed spontaneously after the site of entry seals.

SUMMARY

EMPHYSEMA

- Emphysema is a chronic obstructive airway disease characterized by enlargement of air spaces distal to terminal bronchioles.
- Subtypes include centriacinar (most common: smoking-related), panacinar (seen in α_1-anti-trypsin deficiency), distal acinar, and irregular.
- Smoking and inhaled pollutants cause ongoing accumulation of inflammatory cells, which are the source of proteases such as elastases that irreversibly damage alveolar walls.
- Patients with uncomplicated emphysema present with increased chest volumes, dyspnea, and relatively normal blood oxygenation at rest ("pink puffers").
- Most patients with emphysema also have signs and symptoms of concurrent chronic bronchitis, since cigarette smoking is a risk factor for both.

Chronic Bronchitis

Chronic bronchitis is diagnosed on clinical grounds: it is defined by the presence of a persistent productive cough for at least 3 consecutive months in at least 2 consecutive years. It is common among cigarette smokers and urban dwellers in smog-ridden cities; some studies indicate that 20% to 25% of men in the 40- to 65-year-old age group have the disease. In early stages of the disease, the cough raises mucoid sputum, but airflow is not obstructed. Some patients with chronic bronchitis have evidence of hyperresponsive airways, with intermittent bronchospasm and wheezing (asthmatic bronchitis), while other bronchitic patients, especially heavy smokers, develop chronic outflow obstruction, usually with associated emphysema (COPD).

Pathogenesis

The distinctive feature of chronic bronchitis is hypersecretion of mucus, beginning in the large airways. Although the most important cause is cigarette smoking, other air pollutants, such as sulfur dioxide and nitrogen dioxide, may contribute. These environmental irritants induce hypertrophy of mucous glands in the trachea and bronchi as well as an increase in mucin-secreting goblet cells in the epithelial surfaces of smaller bronchi and bronchioles. These irritants also cause inflammation marked by the infiltration of macrophages, neutrophils, and lymphocytes. In contrast with asthma, eosinophils are not seen in chronic bronchitis. Whereas the defining mucus hypersecretion is primarily a reflection of involvement of large bronchi, the airflow obstruction in chronic bronchitis results from (1) small airway disease, induced by mucous plugging of the bronchiolar lumen, inflammation, and bronchiolar wall fibrosis, and (2) coexistent emphysema. In general, while small airway disease (*chronic bronchiolitis*) is an important component of early, mild airflow obstruction, chronic bronchitis with significant airflow obstruction almost always is complicated by emphysema.

It is postulated that many of the effects of environmental irritants on respiratory epithelium are mediated by local release of cytokines such as IL-13 from T cells and innate lymphoid cells. The transcription of the mucin gene in bronchial epithelium and the production of neutrophil elastase are increased as a consequence of exposure to tobacco smoke. Microbial infection often is present but has a secondary role, chiefly by maintaining inflammation and exacerbating symptoms.

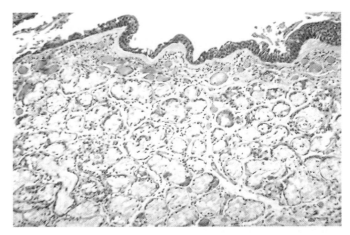

Fig. 13.9 Chronic bronchitis. The lumen of the bronchus is above. Note the marked thickening of the mucous gland layer (approximately twice-normal) and squamous metaplasia of lung epithelium. *(From the Teaching Collection of the Department of Pathology, University of Texas, Southwestern Medical School, Dallas, Texas.)*

lymphocytes and macrophages but sometimes also admixed neutrophils, are frequently seen in the bronchial mucosa. **Chronic bronchiolitis** (small airway disease), characterized by goblet cell metaplasia, mucous plugging, inflammation, and fibrosis, also is seen. In severe cases, there may be complete obliteration of the lumen as a consequence of fibrosis **(bronchiolitis obliterans).** It is the submucosal fibrosis that leads to luminal narrowing and airway obstruction. Emphysematous changes often coexist.

Clinical Features

The course of chronic bronchitis is quite variable. In some patients, cough and sputum production persist indefinitely without ventilatory dysfunction, while others develop COPD with significant outflow obstruction marked by hypercapnia, hypoxemia, and cyanosis. Patients with chronic bronchitis and COPD have frequent exacerbations, more rapid disease progression, and poorer outcomes than those with emphysema alone. Progressive disease is marked by the development of pulmonary hypertension, sometimes leading to cardiac failure (Chapter 11); recurrent infections; and ultimately respiratory failure.

MORPHOLOGY

As seen in gross specimens, the mucosal lining of the larger airways usually is **hyperemic and swollen** by edema fluid and is covered by a layer of mucinous or mucopurulent **secretions.** The smaller bronchi and bronchioles also may be filled with secretions. The diagnostic feature of chronic bronchitis in the trachea and larger bronchi is **enlargement of the mucus-secreting glands** (Fig. 13.9). The magnitude of the increase in size is assessed by the ratio of the thickness of the submucosal gland layer to that of the bronchial wall (the Reid index— normally 0.4). Variable numbers of inflammatory cells, largely

SUMMARY

CHRONIC BRONCHITIS

- Chronic bronchitis is defined as persistent productive cough for at least 3 consecutive months in at least 2 consecutive years.
- Cigarette smoking is the most important underlying risk factor; air pollutants also contribute.
- Chronic airway obstruction largely results from small airway disease (chronic bronchiolitis) and coexistent emphysema.
- Histologic examination demonstrates enlargement of mucus-secreting glands, goblet cell metaplasia, and bronchiolar wall fibrosis.

Asthma

Asthma is a chronic inflammatory disorder of the airways that causes recurrent episodes of wheezing, breathlessness, chest tightness, and cough, particularly at night and/or early in the morning. The hallmarks of asthma are intermittent, reversible airway obstruction; chronic bronchial inflammation with eosinophils; bronchial smooth muscle cell hypertrophy and hyperreactivity; and increased mucus secretion. Sometimes trivial stimuli are sufficient to trigger attacks in patients, because of airway hyperreactivity. Many cells play a role in the inflammatory response, in particular eosinophils, mast cells, macrophages, lymphocytes, neutrophils, and epithelial cells. Of note, asthma has increased in incidence significantly in the Western world over the past 4 decades. One explanation for this troubling trend is the *hygiene hypothesis,* according to which a lack of exposure to infectious organisms (and possibly nonpathogenic microorganisms as well) in early childhood results in defects in immune tolerance and subsequent hyperreactivity to immune stimuli later in life.

Pathogenesis

Major factors contributing to the development of asthma include genetic predisposition to type I hypersensitivity (atopy), acute and chronic airway inflammation, and bronchial hyperresponsiveness to a variety of stimuli. Asthma may be subclassified as *atopic* (evidence of allergen sensitization) or *nonatopic*. In both types, episodes of bronchospasm may be triggered by diverse exposures, such as respiratory infections (especially viral), airborne irritants (e.g., smoke, fumes), cold air, stress, and exercise. There also are varying patterns of inflammation—eosinophilic (most common), neutrophilic, mixed inflammatory, and pauci-granulocytic—that are associated with differing etiologies, immunopathologies, and responses to treatment.

The classic atopic form is associated with excessive type 2 helper T (T_H2) cell activation. Cytokines produced by T_H2 cells account for most of the features of atopic asthma— IL-4 and IL-13 stimulate IgE production, IL-5 activates eosinophils, and IL-13 also stimulates mucus production. IgE coats submucosal mast cells, which on exposure to allergen release their granule contents and secrete cytokines and other mediators. Mast cell–derived mediators produce two waves of reaction: an early (immediate) phase and a late phase (Fig. 13.10):

- The *early-phase reaction* is dominated by bronchoconstriction, increased mucus production, and vasodilation. Bronchoconstriction is triggered by mediators released from mast cells, including histamine, prostaglandin D2, and leukotrienes LTC4, D4, and E4, and also by reflex neural pathways.
- The *late-phase reaction* is inflammatory in nature. Inflammatory mediators stimulate epithelial cells to produce chemokines (including eotaxin, a potent chemoattractant and activator of eosinophils) that promote the recruitment of T_H2 cells, eosinophils, and other leukocytes, thus amplifying an inflammatory reaction that is initiated by resident immune cells.

- Repeated bouts of inflammation lead to structural changes in the bronchial wall that are collectively referred to as *airway remodeling*. These changes include hypertrophy of bronchial smooth muscle and mucus glands and increased vascularity and deposition of sub-epithelial collagen, which may occur as early as several years before initiation of symptoms.

Asthma tends to "run" in families, but the role of genetics in asthma is complex. Genome-wide association studies have identified a number of genetic variants associated with asthma risk, some in genes enocding factors like the IL-4 receptor that are clearly involved in asthma pathogenesis. However, the precise contribution of asthma-associated genetic variants to the development of disease remains to be determined.

Atopic Asthma

This is the most common type of asthma and is a classic example of type I IgE–mediated hypersensitivity reaction (Chapter 5). It usually begins in childhood. A positive family history of atopy and/or asthma is common, and the onset of asthmatic attacks is often preceded by allergic rhinitis, urticaria, or eczema. Attacks may be triggered by allergens in dust, pollen, animal dander, or food, or by infections. A skin test with the offending antigen results in an immediate wheal-and-flare reaction. Atopic asthma also can be diagnosed based on serum radioallergosorbent tests (RASTs) that identify the presence of IgEs that recognize specific allergens.

Non-Atopic Asthma

Patients with nonatopic forms of asthma do not have evidence of allergen sensitization, and skin test results usually are negative. A positive family history of asthma is less common. Respiratory infections due to viruses (e.g., rhinovirus, parainfluenza virus) and inhaled air pollutants (e.g., sulfur dioxide, ozone, nitrogen dioxide) are common triggers. It is thought that virus-induced inflammation of the respiratory mucosa lowers the threshold of the subepithelial vagal receptors to irritants. Although the connections are not well understood, the ultimate humoral and cellular mediators of airway obstruction (e.g., eosinophils) are common to both atopic and nonatopic variants of asthma, so they are treated in a similar way.

Drug-Induced Asthma

Several pharmacologic agents provoke asthma, aspirin being the most striking example. Patients with aspirin sensitivity present with recurrent rhinitis, nasal polyps, urticaria, and bronchospasm. The precise pathogenesis is unknown but is likely to involve some abnormality in prostaglandin metabolism stemming from inhibition of cyclooxygenase by aspirin.

Occupational Asthma

Occupational asthma may be triggered by fumes (epoxy resins, plastics), organic and chemical dusts (wood, cotton, platinum), gases (toluene), and other chemicals. Asthma attacks usually develop after repeated exposure to the inciting antigen(s).

A NORMAL AIRWAY

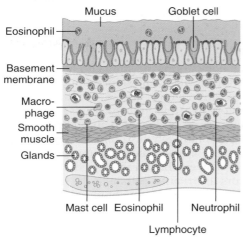

B AIRWAY IN ASTHMA

C TRIGGERING OF ASTHMA

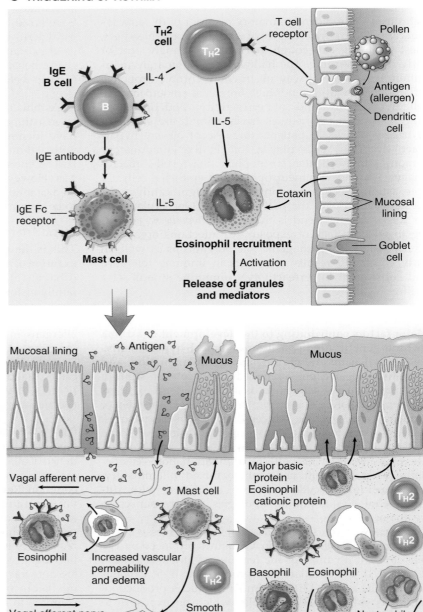

D IMMEDIATE PHASE (MINUTES)

E LATE PHASE (HOURS)

Fig. 13.10 (A and B) Comparison of a normal airway and an airway involved by asthma. The asthmatic airway is marked by accumulation of mucus in the bronchial lumen secondary to an increase in the number of mucus-secreting goblet cells in the mucosa and hypertrophy of submucosal glands; intense chronic inflammation due to recruitment of eosinophils, macrophages, and other inflammatory cells; thickened basement membrane; and hypertrophy and hyperplasia of smooth muscle cells. (C) Inhaled allergens (antigen) elicit a T_H2-dominated response favoring IgE production and eosinophil recruitment. (D) On reexposure to antigen (Ag), the immediate reaction is triggered by Ag-induced cross-linking of IgE bound to Fc receptors on mast cells. These cells release preformed mediators that directly and via neuronal reflexes induce bronchospasm, increased vascular permeability, mucus production, and recruitment of leukocytes. (E) Leukocytes recruited to the site of reaction (neutrophils, eosinophils, and basophils; lymphocytes and monocytes) release additional mediators that initiate the late phase of asthma. Several factors released from eosinophils (e.g., major basic protein, eosinophil cationic protein) also cause damage to the epithelium.

MORPHOLOGY

The morphologic changes in asthma have been described in individuals who die of prolonged severe attacks (status asthmaticus) and in mucosal biopsy specimens of individuals challenged with allergens. In fatal cases, the lungs are distended due to air trapping (overinflation), and there may be small areas of atelectasis. The most striking finding is occlusion of bronchi and bronchioles by thick, tenacious **mucous plugs** containing whorls of shed epithelium **(Curschmann spirals).** Numerous eosinophils and **Charcot-Leyden crystals** (crystalloids made up of the eosinophil protein galectin-10) also are present. Other characteristic morphologic changes in asthma (Fig. 13.10B), collectively called airway remodeling, include

- Thickening of airway wall
- Sub-basement membrane fibrosis (Fig. 13.11)
- Increased submucosal vascularity
- An increase in size of the submucosal glands and goblet cell metaplasia of the airway epithelium
- Hypertrophy and/or hyperplasia of the bronchial muscle

Clinical Features

An attack of asthma is characterized by severe dyspnea and wheezing due to bronchoconstriction and mucus plugging, which leads to trapping of air in distal airspaces and progressive hyperinflation of the lungs. In the usual case, attacks last from 1 to several hours and subside either spontaneously or with therapy. Intervals between attacks are characteristically free from overt respiratory difficulties, but persistent, subtle deficits can be detected by pulmonary function tests. Occasionally a severe paroxysm occurs that does not respond to therapy and persists for days and even weeks (*status asthmaticus*). The associated hypercapnia, acidosis, and severe hypoxia may be fatal, although in most cases the condition is more disabling than lethal. Standard therapies include anti-inflammatory drugs, particularly glucocorticoids, and bronchodilators such as beta-adrenergic drugs and leukotriene inhibitors (recall that leukotrienes are potent bronchoconstrictors). Agents that block specific immune mediators, such as IL-4 and IL-5, are of modest benefit in some patients but are not broadly efficacious, perhaps because of disease heterogeneity. Another approach called *bronchial thermoplasty*, which involves controlled delivery of thermal energy during bronchoscopy to reduce the mass of smooth muscle and airway responsiveness, is being evaluated in patients with severe, poorly controlled asthma.

SUMMARY

ASTHMA

- Asthma is characterized by reversible bronchoconstriction caused by airway hyperresponsiveness to a variety of stimuli.
- Atopic asthma most often is caused by a T_H2 and IgE-mediated immunologic reaction to environmental allergens and is characterized by early-phase (immediate) and late-phase reactions. The T_H2 cytokines IL-4, IL-5, and IL-13 are important mediators. Non-T_H2 inflammation also has roles in atopic asthma that are being defined.
- Triggers for nonatopic asthma are less clear but include viral infections and inhaled air pollutants, which also can trigger atopic asthma.
- Eosinophils are key inflammatory cells found in almost all subtypes of asthma; eosinophil products (such as major basic protein) are responsible for airway damage.
- Airway remodeling (sub-basement membrane thickening and hypertrophy of bronchial glands and smooth muscle) adds an irreversible component to the obstructive disease.

Bronchiectasis

Bronchiectasis is the permanent dilation of bronchi and bronchioles caused by destruction of smooth muscle and the supporting elastic tissue; it typically results from or is associated with chronic necrotizing infections. It is not a primary disorder, as it always occurs secondary to persistent infection or obstruction caused by a variety of conditions. Bronchiectasis gives rise to a characteristic symptom complex dominated by cough and expectoration of copious amounts of purulent sputum. Diagnosis depends on an appropriate history and radiographic demonstration of bronchial dilation. The conditions that most commonly predispose to bronchiectasis include:

- *Bronchial obstruction.* Common causes are tumors, foreign bodies, and impaction of mucus. In these conditions, bronchiectasis is localized to the obstructed lung segment. Bronchiectasis also may complicate atopic asthma and chronic bronchitis.
- *Congenital or hereditary conditions*—for example:
  - *Cystic fibrosis,* in which widespread severe bronchiectasis results from obstruction caused by abnormally viscid mucus and secondary infections (Chapter 7).
  - *Immunodeficiency states,* particularly immunoglobulin deficiencies, in which localized or diffuse bronchiectasis often develops because of recurrent bacterial infections.

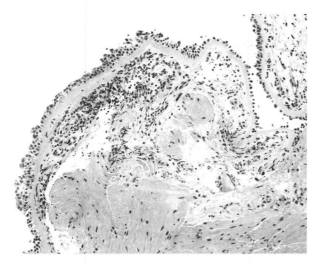

Fig. 13.11 Bronchial biopsy specimen from an asthmatic patient showing sub–basement membrane fibrosis, eosinophilic inflammation, and smooth muscle hyperplasia.

- *Primary ciliary dyskinesia* (also called the immotile cilia syndrome). This is a rare autosomal recessive disorder that is frequently associated with bronchiectasis and with sterility in males. It is caused by inherited abnormalities of cilia that impair mucociliary clearance of the airways, leading to persistent infections.
- *Necrotizing, or suppurative, pneumonia,* particularly with virulent organisms such as *Staphylococcus aureus* or *Klebsiella spp.,* predispose affected patients to development of bronchiectasis. Posttuberculosis bronchiectasis continues to be a significant cause of morbidity in endemic areas.

Pathogenesis

Two intertwined processes contribute to bronchiectasis: obstruction and chronic infection. Either may be the initiator. For example, obstruction caused by a foreign body impairs clearance of secretions, providing a favorable substrate for superimposed infection. The resultant inflammatory damage to the bronchial wall and the accumulating exudate further distend the airways, leading to irreversible dilation. Conversely, a persistent necrotizing infection in the bronchi or bronchioles may lead to poor clearance of secretions, obstruction, and inflammation with peribronchial fibrosis and traction on the bronchi, culminating again in full-blown bronchiectasis.

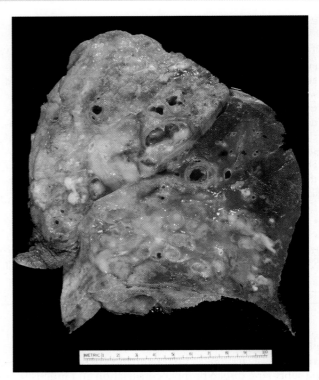

Fig. 13.12 Bronchiectasis in a patient with cystic fibrosis who underwent lung resection for transplantation. Cut surface of lung shows markedly dilated bronchi filled with purulent mucus that extend to subpleural regions.

MORPHOLOGY

Bronchiectasis usually affects the lower lobes bilaterally, particularly those air passages that are most vertical. When caused by tumors or aspiration of foreign bodies, the involvement may be sharply localized to a single segment of the lungs. Usually, the most severe involvement is found in the more distal bronchi and bronchioles. **The airways may be dilated to as much as four times their usual diameter** and can be seen on gross examination almost out to the pleural surface (Fig. 13.12). By contrast, in normal lungs, the bronchioles cannot be followed by eye beyond a point 2 to 3 cm from the pleura.

The histologic findings vary with the activity and chronicity of the disease. In full-blown active cases, an intense acute and chronic inflammatory exudate within the walls of the bronchi and bronchioles leads to desquamation of lining epithelium and extensive areas of ulceration. Typically, mixed flora are cultured from the sputum. The usual organisms include staphylococci, streptococci, pneumococci, enteric organisms, anaerobic and microaerophilic bacteria, and (particularly in children) *Haemophilus influenzae* and *Pseudomonas aeruginosa.*

When healing occurs, the lining epithelium may regenerate completely; however, the injury usually cannot be repaired and abnormal dilation and scarring persist. Fibrosis of the bronchial and bronchiolar walls and peribronchiolar fibrosis develop in more chronic cases. In some instances the necrosis destroys the bronchial or bronchiolar walls, producing an abscess cavity.

Clinical Features

Bronchiectasis is characterized by severe, persistent cough associated with expectoration of mucopurulent, sometimes fetid, sputum. Other common symptoms include dyspnea, rhinosinusitis, and hemoptysis. Symptoms often are episodic and are precipitated by upper-respiratory tract infections or the introduction of new pathogenic agents. Severe, widespread bronchiectasis may lead to significant obstructive ventilatory defects, with hypoxemia, hypercapnia, pulmonary hypertension, and cor pulmonale. However, with current treatment outcomes have improved and severe complications of bronchiectasis, such as brain abscess, amyloidosis (Chapter 5), and cor pulmonale, occur less frequently now than in the past.

CHRONIC INTERSTITIAL (RESTRICTIVE, INFILTRATIVE) LUNG DISEASES

Chronic interstitial diseases are a heterogeneous group of disorders characterized by bilateral, often patchy, pulmonary fibrosis mainly affecting the walls of the alveoli (see Fig. 13.1). Many of the entities in this group are of unknown cause and pathogenesis; some have an intraalveolar and an interstitial component. Chronic interstitial lung diseases are categorized based on clinicopathologic features and characteristic histology (Table 13.2). However, it must be acknowledged that there is frequent overlap in histologic features among the different conditions. The shared histologic features and the similarity in clinical signs, symptoms, radiographic alterations, and pathophysiologic changes justify their consideration as a

Table 13.2 Major Categories of Chronic Interstitial Lung Disease

Fibrosing
Usual interstitial pneumonia (idiopathic pulmonary fibrosis)
Nonspecific interstitial pneumonia
Cryptogenic organizing pneumonia
Collagen vascular disease-associated
Pneumoconiosis
Therapy-associated (drugs, radiation)

Granulomatous
Sarcoidosis
Hypersensitivity pneumonia

Eosinophilic
Loeffler syndrome
Drug allergy–related
Idiopathic chronic eosinophilic pneumonia

Smoking-Related
Desquamative interstitial pneumonia
Respiratory bronchiolitis

group. The hallmark of these disorders is reduced compliance (stiff lungs), which in turn necessitates increased effort to breathe (dyspnea). Furthermore, damage to the alveolar epithelium and interstitial vasculature produces abnormalities in the ventilation–perfusion ratio, leading to hypoxia. Chest radiographs show small nodules, irregular lines, or "ground-glass shadows." With progression, patients may develop respiratory failure, pulmonary hypertension, and cor pulmonale (Chapter 11). When advanced, the etiology of the underlying diseases may be difficult to determine because they all result in diffuse scarring and gross destruction of the lung, referred to as *end-stage* or *"honeycomb" lung*.

Fibrosing Diseases

Idiopathic Pulmonary Fibrosis

Idiopathic pulmonary fibrosis (IPF) refers to a pulmonary disorder of unknown etiology that is characterized by patchy, progressive bilateral interstitial fibrosis. Because its etiology is unknown, it is also known as *cryptogenic fibrosing alveolitis*. Males are affected more often than females, and it is a disease of aging, virtually never occurring before 50 years of age. The radiologic and histologic pattern of fibrosis is referred to as *usual interstitial pneumonia (UIP)*, which is required for the diagnosis of IPF. Of note, similar pathologic changes in the lung may be present in entities such as asbestosis, collagen vascular diseases, and other conditions. Therefore, IPF is a diagnosis of exclusion.

Pathogenesis

The interstitial fibrosis that characterizes IPF is believed to result from repeated injury and defective repair of alveolar epithelium, often in a genetically predisposed individual (Fig. 13.13). The cause of the injury is obscure, and a variety of sources have been proposed, including chronic gastroesophageal reflux. However, only a small fraction of individuals suffering from reflux or exposed to other proposed environmental triggers develop IPF; thus, other factors must have a predominant role. The clearest

etiologic clues come from genetic studies. Germ line mutations leading to loss of telomerase are associated with increased risk, suggesting that cellular senescence contributes to a profibrotic phenotype. The link to cellular aging also is in line with the observation that IPF is a disorder of older adults, rarely occurring before the age of 55 years. Other genetic associations also point to the primary defect residing in epithelial cells. Specifically, approximately 35% of affected individuals have a genetic variant in the *MUC5B* gene that alters the production of mucin, while a smaller number of affected patients have germ line mutations in surfactant genes. These genes are only expressed in lung epithelial cells, indicating that epithelial cell abnormalities can be the primary initiators of IPF. It is hypothesized that abnormal epithelial repair at the sites of chronic injury and inflammation gives rise to exuberant fibroblastic or myofibroblastic proliferation, leading to the characteristic fibroblastic foci. Although the mechanisms of fibrosis are incompletely understood, recent data point to excessive activation of profibrotic factors such as TGF-β.

MORPHOLOGY

Grossly, the pleural surfaces of the lung are cobblestoned due to retraction of scars along the interlobular septa. The cut surface shows firm, rubbery white areas of fibrosis, which occurs preferentially within the lower lobe, the subpleural regions, and along the interlobular septa. Histologically, the hallmark is **patchy interstitial fibrosis,** which varies in intensity (Fig. 13.14) and

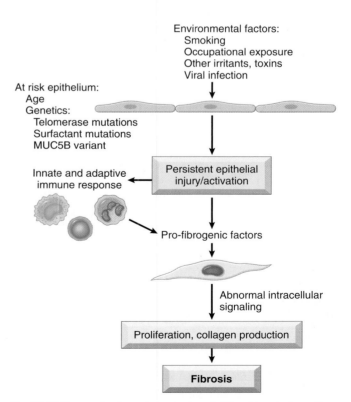

Fig. 13.13 Proposed pathogenic mechanisms in idiopathic pulmonary fibrosis. See text for details.

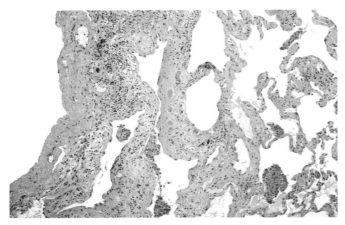

Fig. 13.14 Usual interstitial pneumonia. The fibrosis, which varies in intensity, is more pronounced in the subpleural region.

worsens with time. The earliest lesions demonstrate exuberant fibroblastic proliferation (**fibroblastic foci**) (Fig. 13.15). Over time these areas become more collagenous and less cellular. Quite typical is the existence of both early and late lesions. The dense fibrosis causes collapse of alveolar walls and formation of cystic spaces lined by hyperplastic type II pneumocytes or bronchiolar epithelium (**honeycomb fibrosis**). The interstitial inflammation usually is patchy and consists of an alveolar septal infiltrate of mostly lymphocytes and occasional plasma cells, mast cells, and eosinophils. Secondary pulmonary hypertensive changes (intimal fibrosis and medial thickening of pulmonary arteries) are often present.

Clinical Features

IPF usually presents with the gradual onset of a nonproductive cough and progressive dyspnea. On physical examination, most patients have characteristic "dry" or "Velcrolike" crackles during inspiration. Cyanosis, cor pulmonale, and peripheral edema may develop in later stages of the disease. The characteristic clinical and radiologic

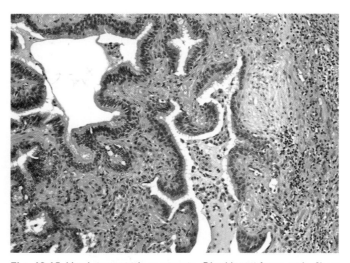

Fig. 13.15 Usual interstitial pneumonia. Fibroblastic focus with fibers running parallel to surface and bluish myxoid extracellular matrix. Honeycombing is present to the left.

findings (subpleural and basilar fibrosis, reticular abnormalities, and "honeycombing") often are diagnostic. Anti-inflammatory therapies have proven to be of little use, in line with the idea that inflammation is of secondary pathogenic importance. By contrast, anti-fibrotic therapies such as nintedanib, a tyrosine kinase inhibitor, and pirfenidone, an inhibitor of TGF-β, have produced positive outcomes in clinical trials and are now approved for use in patients with IPF. The overall prognosis remains poor, however; survival is only 3 to 5 years, and lung transplantation is the only definitive treatment.

Other Fibrosing Diseases

Other rare pulmonary diseases associated with fibrosis need to be considered in the differential diagnosis of IPF, several of which are worthy of brief mention. One is *nonspecific interstitial pneumonia* (NSIP). NSIP is a chronic bilateral interstitial lung disease of unknown etiology, which (despite its name) has distinct radiologic, histologic, and clinical features, including a frequent association with collagen vascular disorders such as rheumatoid arthritis. It is important to recognize NSIP because it has a much better prognosis than IPF. It is characterized by mild to moderate interstitial chronic inflammation and/or fibrosis that is patchy but uniform in the areas involved. A second uncommon entity associated with fibrosis is *cryptogenic organizing pneumonia*. It presents with cough and dyspnea, and chest radiographs demonstrate subpleural or peribronchial patchy areas of airspace consolidation which are due to intraalveolar plugs of loose organizing connective tissue. Some patients recover spontaneously while most require treatment, usually with oral steroids. Also in the differential diagnosis of fibrosing pulmonary disorders are several rheumatologic entitiies, such as systemic sclerosis, rheumatoid arthritis and systemic lupus erythematosus, which may be complicated by diffuse pulmonary fibrosis.

SUMMARY

CHRONIC INTERSTITIAL LUNG DISEASES

- Diffuse interstitial fibrosis of the lung gives rise to restrictive lung diseases characterized by reduced lung compliance and reduced forced vital capacity (FVC). The ratio of FEV to FVC is normal.
- Diseases that cause diffuse interstitial fibrosis are heterogeneous. The unifying pathogenic factor is injury to the alveoli leading to activation of macrophages and release of fibrogenic cytokines such as TGF-β.
- Idiopathic pulmonary fibrosis is prototypic of restrictive lung diseases. It is characterized by patchy interstitial fibrosis, fibroblastic foci, and formation of cystic spaces (honeycomb lung). This histologic pattern is known as usual interstitial pneumonia (UIP).

Pneumoconioses

Pneumoconiosis is a term originally coined to describe lung disorders caused by inhalation of mineral dusts. The term has been broadened to include diseases induced by organic and inorganic particulates, and some experts also regard

Table 13.3 Mineral Dust–Induced Lung Disease

Agent	Disease	Exposure
Coal dust	Simple coal worker's pneumoconiosis: macules and nodules Complicated coal worker's pneumoconiosis: PMF	Coal mining
Silica	Silicosis	Sandblasting, quarrying, mining, stone cutting, foundry work, ceramics
Asbestos	Asbestosis, pleural effusions, pleural plaques, or diffuse fibrosis; mesothelioma; carcinoma of the lung and larynx	Mining, milling, and fabrication of ores and materials; installation and removal of insulation

PMF, Progressive massive fibrosis.

chemical fume- and vapor-induced lung diseases as pneumoconioses. The mineral dust pneumoconioses—the three most common of which are caused by inhalation of coal dust, silica, and asbestos—usually stem from exposure in the workplace. Asbestos is the exception, as with this mineral the increased risk for cancer extends to family members of asbestos workers and to individuals exposed outside of the workplace. Table 13.3 indicates the pathologic conditions associated with each mineral dust and the major industries in which the dust exposure may produce disease.

Pathogenesis

The reaction of the lung to mineral dusts depends on many variables, including the size, shape, solubility, and reactivity of the particles. For example, particles greater than 5 to 10 μm are unlikely to reach distal airways, whereas particles smaller than 0.5 μm move into and out of alveoli, often without substantial deposition and injury. Particles that are 1 to 5 μm in diameter are the most dangerous, because they get lodged at the bifurcation of the distal airways. Coal dust is relatively inert, and large amounts must be deposited in the lungs before lung disease is clinically detectable. Silica, asbestos, and beryllium are more reactive than coal dust, resulting in fibrotic reactions at lower concentrations. Most inhaled dust is entrapped in the mucus blanket and rapidly removed from the lung by ciliary movement. However, some of the particles become impacted at alveolar duct bifurcations, where macrophages accumulate and engulf the trapped particulates.

The pulmonary alveolar macrophage is a key cellular element in the initiation and perpetuation of inflammation, lung injury and fibrosis. Following phagocytosis by macrophages, many particles activate the inflammasome and induce production of the pro-inflammatory cytokine IL-1 as well as the release of other factors, which initiates an inflammatory response that leads to fibroblast proliferation and collagen deposition. Some of the inhaled particles may reach the lymphatics either by direct drainage or within migrating macrophages and thereby initiate an immune response to components of the particulates and/or to self-proteins that are modified by the particles. This then leads to an amplification and extension of the local reaction. Tobacco smoking worsens the effects of all inhaled mineral dusts, more so with asbestos than other particles.

Coal Worker's Pneumoconiosis

Worldwide dust reduction in coal mines has greatly reduced the incidence of coal dust–induced disease. The spectrum of lung findings in coal workers is wide, ranging from *asymptomatic anthracosis,* in which pigment deposits without a perceptible cellular reaction; to *simple coal worker's pneumoconiosis (CWP),* in which macrophages accumulate with little to no pulmonary dysfunction; to *complicated CWP* or *progressive massive fibrosis (PMF),* in which fibrosis is extensive and lung function is compromised (see Table 13.3). Although statistics vary, it seems that less than 10% of cases of simple CWP progress to PMF. Of note, PMF is a generic term that applies to a confluent fibrosing reaction in the lung; this can be a complication of any of the pneumoconioses discussed here.

Although coal is mainly carbon, coal mine dust contains a variety of trace metals, inorganic minerals, and crystalline silica. The ratio of carbon to contaminating chemicals and minerals ("coal rank") increases from bituminous to anthracite coal; in general, anthracite mining has been associated with a higher risk for CWP.

MORPHOLOGY

Pulmonary anthracosis is the most innocuous coal-induced pulmonary lesion in coal miners and also is commonly seen in urban dwellers and tobacco smokers. Inhaled carbon pigment is engulfed by alveolar or interstitial macrophages, which then accumulate in the connective tissue along the pulmonary and pleural lymphatics and in draining lymph nodes.

Simple CWP is characterized by the presence of **coal macules** and larger **coal nodules.** The coal macule consists of dust-laden macrophages and small amounts of collagen fibers arrayed in a delicate network. Although these lesions are scattered throughout the lung, the upper lobes and upper zones of the lower lobes are more heavily involved. In due course, **centrilobular emphysema** may occur. Functionally significant emphysema is more common in the United Kingdom and Europe, probably because in these locales the coal rank is higher than in the United States.

Complicated CWP (PMF) occurs on a background of simple CWP by coalescence of coal nodules and generally develops over many years. It is characterized by multiple, dark black scars larger than 2 cm and sometimes up to 10 cm in greatest diameter that consist of dense collagen and pigment (Fig. 13.16).

Clinical Features

CWP usually is a benign disease that produces little decrement in lung function. In those in whom PMF develops, there is increasing pulmonary dysfunction, pulmonary hypertension, and cor pulmonale. Progression from CWP to PMF has been linked to a variety of variables including

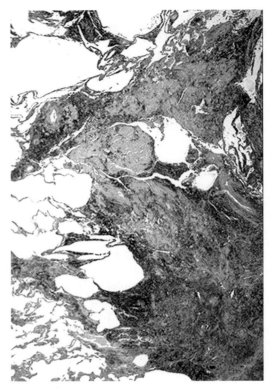

Fig. 13.16 Progressive massive fibrosis in a coal worker. A large amount of black pigment is associated with fibrosis. *(From Klatt EC: Robbins and Cotran atlas of pathology, ed 2, Elsevier, Philadelphia, p 121.)*

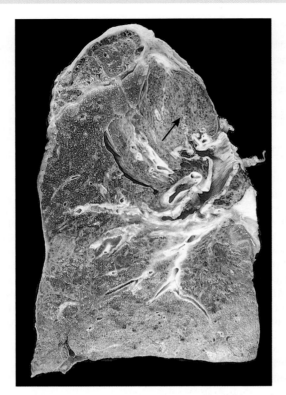

Fig. 13.17 Advanced silicosis, seen in a transected lung. Scarring has contracted the upper lobe into a small dark mass *(arrow)*. Note the dense pleural thickening. *(Courtesy of Dr. John Godleski, Brigham and Women's Hospital, Boston, Massachusetts.)*

higher coal dust exposure levels and total dust burden. Unfortunately, once established PMF has a tendency to progress even in the absence of further exposure. After taking smoking-related risk into account, there is no increased frequency of lung carcinoma in coal miners, a feature that distinguishes CWP from both silica and asbestos exposures (discussed next).

Silicosis

Silicosis is currently the most prevalent chronic occupational disease in the world. It is caused by inhalation of crystalline silica, mostly in occupational settings. Workers involved in sandblasting and hard-rock mining are at particularly high risk. Silica occurs in both crystalline and amorphous forms, but crystalline forms (including quartz, cristobalite, and tridymite) are by far the most toxic and fibrogenic. Of these, quartz is most commonly implicated in silicosis. After inhalation, the particles interact with epithelial cells and macrophages. Ingested silica particles cause activation of the inflammasome and the subsequent release of inflammatory mediators by pulmonary macrophages, including IL-1, TNF, fibronectin, lipid mediators, oxygen-derived free radicals, and fibrogenic cytokines. When mixed with other minerals, the fibrogenic effect of quartz is reduced. This fortuitous situation is commonplace, as quartz in the workplace is rarely pure. Thus, for example, miners of the iron-containing ore hematite may have abundant quartz in their lungs yet have relatively mild lung disease because of the protective effect of hematite.

MORPHOLOGY

Silicotic nodules in their early stages are tiny, barely palpable, discrete, pale-to-black (if coal dust is present) nodules in the upper zones of the lungs (Fig. 13.17). Microscopically, the silicotic nodule demonstrates **concentrically arranged hyalinized collagen fibers** surrounding an amorphous center. The "whorled" appearance of the collagen fibers is quite distinctive for silicosis (Fig. 13.18). Examination of the nodules by **polarized**

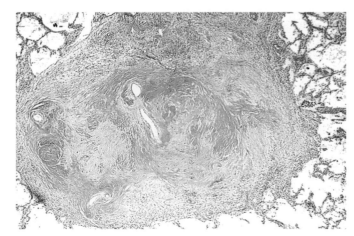

Fig. 13.18 Coalescent collagenous silicotic nodules. *(Courtesy of Dr. John Godleski, Brigham and Women's Hospital, Boston, Massachusetts.)*

microscopy reveals weakly birefringent silica particles, primarily in the center of the nodules. As the disease progresses, individual nodules may coalesce into hard, collagenous scars, with eventual progression to PMF. The intervening lung parenchyma may be compressed or overexpanded, and a honeycomb pattern may develop. Fibrotic lesions also may occur in hilar lymph nodes and the pleura.

Clinical Features

Silicosis usually is detected in asymptomatic workers on routine chest radiographs, which typically show a fine nodularity in the upper zones of the lung. Most patients do not develop shortness of breath until late in the course, after PMF is present. Many patients with PMF develop pulmonary hypertension and cor pulmonale as a result of chronic hypoxia–induced vasoconstriction and parenchymal destruction. The disease is slowly progressive, often impairing pulmonary function to such a degree that physical activity is severely limited. Silicosis is associated with an increased susceptibility to tuberculosis. It is postulated that silicosis depresses cell-mediated immunity, and crystalline silica may inhibit the ability of pulmonary macrophages to kill phagocytosed mycobacteria. Nodules of silicotuberculosis often contain a central zone of caseation. The relationship between silica and lung cancer is unsettled, but most studies suggest that silica exposure is associated with some increase in risk.

Asbestosis and Asbestos-Related Diseases

Asbestos is a family of crystalline hydrated silicates with a fibrous geometry. On the basis of epidemiologic studies, occupational exposure to asbestos is linked to (1) parenchymal interstitial fibrosis *(asbestosis);* (2) localized fibrous plaques, or, rarely, diffuse fibrosis in the pleura; (3) pleural effusions; (4) lung carcinoma; (5) malignant pleural and peritoneal mesothelioma; and (6) laryngeal carcinoma. An increased incidence of asbestos-related cancers in family members of asbestos workers has alerted the general public to the potential hazards of asbestos in the environment.

Pathogenesis

As with silica crystals, once phagocytosed by macrophages, asbestos fibers activate the inflammasome and damage phagolysosomal membranes, stimulating the release of proinflammatory factors and fibrogenic mediators. In addition to cellular and fibrotic lung reactions, asbestos probably also functions as both a tumor initiator and a promoter. Some of the oncogenic effects of asbestos on the mesothelium are mediated by reactive free radicals generated by asbestos fibers, which preferentially localize in the distal lung close to the mesothelial layer. However, potentially toxic chemicals adsorbed onto the asbestos fibers also undoubtedly contribute to the pathogenicity of the fibers. For example, the adsorption of carcinogens in tobacco smoke onto asbestos fibers may be the basis for the remarkable synergy between tobacco smoking and the development of lung carcinoma in asbestos workers.

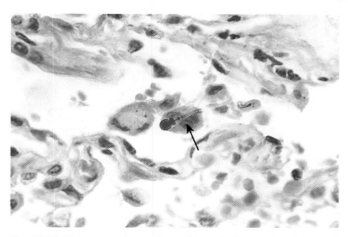

Fig. 13.19 High-power detail of an asbestos body, revealing the typical beading and knobbed ends *(arrow).*

MORPHOLOGY

Asbestosis is marked by **diffuse pulmonary interstitial fibrosis**, characterized by the presence of **asbestos bodies,** which are seen as golden brown, fusiform or beaded rods with a translucent center. They consist of asbestos fibers coated with an iron-containing proteinaceous material (Fig. 13.19). Asbestos bodies apparently are formed when macrophages attempt to phagocytose asbestos fibers; the iron "crust" is derived from phagocyte ferritin.

In contrast with CWP and silicosis, asbestosis begins in the lower lobes and subpleurally, spreading to the middle and upper lobes of the lungs as the fibrosis progresses. Contraction of the fibrous tissue distorts the normal architecture, creating enlarged air spaces enclosed within thick fibrous walls; eventually, the affected regions become honeycombed. Simultaneously, fibrosis develops in the visceral pleura, causing adhesions between the lungs and the chest wall. The scarring may trap and narrow pulmonary arteries and arterioles, causing pulmonary hypertension and cor pulmonale.

Pleural plaques are the most common manifestation of asbestos exposure and are well-circumscribed plaques of dense collagen (Fig. 13.20), often containing calcium. They develop most frequently on the anterior and posterolateral aspects of the **parietal pleura** and over the domes of the diaphragm. Uncommonly, asbestos exposure induces pleural effusion or diffuse pleural fibrosis.

Clinical Features

The clinical findings in asbestosis are indistinguishable from those of any other chronic interstitial lung disease. Progressively worsening dyspnea appears 10 to 20 years after exposure. It is usually accompanied by a cough and production of sputum. The disease may remain static or progress to congestive heart failure, cor pulmonale, and death. Pleural plaques are usually asymptomatic and are detected on radiographs as circumscribed densities.

Both lung carcinoma and malignant mesothelioma develop in workers exposed to asbestos. The risk for developing lung carcinoma is increased about 5-fold for asbestos workers; the relative risk for mesothelioma, normally a very

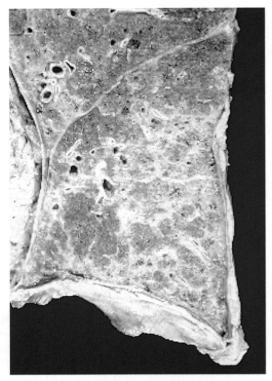

Fig. 13.20 Asbestosis. Markedly thickened visceral pleura covers the lateral and diaphragmatic surface of the lung. Note also severe interstitial fibrosis diffusely affecting the lower lobe of the lung.

rare tumor (2–17 cases per 1 million individuals), is more than 1000 times greater. Concomitant cigarette smoking greatly increases the risk for lung carcinoma but not for mesothelioma. Lung or pleural cancer associated with asbestos exposure carries a particularly poor prognosis.

SUMMARY

PNEUMOCONIOSES

- Pneumoconioses encompass a group of chronic fibrosing diseases of the lung resulting from exposure to organic and inorganic particulates, most commonly mineral dust.
- Pulmonary alveolar macrophages play a central role in the pathogenesis of lung injury by promoting inflammation and producing reactive oxygen species and fibrogenic cytokines.
- Coal dust–induced disease varies from asymptomatic anthracosis, to simple coal worker's pneumoconiosis (coal macules or nodules, and centrilobular emphysema), to progressive massive fibrosis (PMF), manifested by increasing pulmonary dysfunction, pulmonary hypertension, and cor pulmonale.
- Silicosis is the most common pneumoconiosis in the world, and crystalline silica (e.g., quartz) is the usual culprit.
- The manifestations of silicosis range from asymptomatic silicotic nodules to PMF; individuals with silicosis also have an increased susceptibility to tuberculosis. The relationship between silica exposure and subsequent lung cancer is controversial.
- Asbestos exposure is linked with six disease processes: (1) parenchymal interstitial fibrosis (asbestosis); (2) localized

fibrous plaques or, rarely, diffuse pleural fibrosis; (3) pleural effusions; (4) lung cancer; (5) malignant pleural and peritoneal mesothelioma; and (6) laryngeal cancer.
- Cigarette smoking increases the risk for lung cancer in the setting of asbestos exposure; moreover, even family members of workers exposed to asbestos are at increased risk for cancer.

Drug- and Radiation-Induced Pulmonary Disease

Drugs can cause a variety of acute and chronic alterations in respiratory structure and function. For example, *bleomycin,* an anti-cancer agent, causes pneumonitis and interstitial fibrosis as a result of direct toxicity of the drug and by stimulating the influx of inflammatory cells into the alveoli. *Amiodarone,* an anti-arrhythmic agent, also is associated with risk for pneumonitis and fibrosis. *Radiation pneumonitis* is a well-known complication of irradiation of pulmonary and other thoracic tumors. *Acute radiation pneumonitis,* which typically occurs 1 to 6 months after therapy in as many as 20% of the patients, is manifested by fever, dyspnea out of proportion to the volume of irradiated lung, pleural effusion, and pulmonary infiltrates in the irradiated lung bed. These signs and symptoms may resolve with corticosteroid therapy or progress to *chronic radiation pneumonitis,* associated with pulmonary fibrosis.

Granulomatous Diseases

Sarcoidosis

Sarcoidosis is a multisystem disease of unknown etiology characterized by noncaseating granulomatous inflammation in many tissues and organs. We discuss it here because one presentation of sarcoidosis is as a restrictive lung disease. Other diseases, including mycobacterial or fungal infections and berylliosis, sometimes also produce noncaseating granulomas; therefore, the histologic diagnosis of sarcoidosis is one of exclusion. Although sarcoidosis can manifest in many different ways, bilateral hilar lymphadenopathy or lung involvement (or both), visible on chest radiographs, is the major finding at presentation in most cases. Eye and skin involvement each occurs in about 25% of cases, and either may occasionally be the presenting feature of the disease.

Epidemiology

Sarcoidosis occurs throughout the world, affecting both genders and all races and age groups. There are, however, certain interesting epidemiologic trends:
- A consistent predilection for adults younger than 40 years of age.
- A high incidence in Danish and Swedish populations, and in the United States among African Americans (in whom the frequency is 10 times higher than in whites).
- A higher prevalence among nonsmokers, an association that is virtually unique to sarcoidosis among pulmonary diseases.

Etiology and Pathogenesis

Although the etiology of sarcoidosis remains unknown, several lines of evidence suggest that it is a disease of

disordered immune regulation in genetically predisposed individuals exposed to certain environmental agents. The role of each of these contributory influences is summarized in the following discussion.

Several immunologic abnormalities in sarcoidosis suggest the development of a cell-mediated response to an unidentified antigen. The process is driven by CD4+ helper T cells. These immunologic "clues" include the following:

- Intraalveolar and interstitial accumulation of CD4+ T_H1 cells, with peripheral T cell cytopenia
- Oligoclonal expansion of CD4+ T_H1 T cells within the lung as determined by analysis of T cell receptor rearrangements
- Increases in T_H1 cytokines such as IL-2 and IFN-γ, resulting in T cell proliferation and macrophage activation, respectively
- Increases in several cytokines in the local environment (IL-8, TNF, macrophage inflammatory protein-1α) that favor recruitment of additional T cells and monocytes and contribute to the formation of granulomas
- Anergy to common skin test antigens such as *Candida* or purified protein derivative (PPD)
- Polyclonal hypergammaglobulinemia
- Familial and racial clustering of cases, suggesting the involvement of genetic factors

After lung transplantation, sarcoidosis recurs in the new lungs in at least one-third of patients, but without any effect on survival. Finally, several putative "antigens" have been proposed as the inciting agent for sarcoidosis (e.g., viruses, mycobacteria, *Borrelia,* pollen), but there is no "smoking gun" linking sarcoidosis to any specific antigen or infectious agent.

MORPHOLOGY

The cardinal histopathologic feature of sarcoidosis, irrespective of the organ involved, is the **nonnecrotizing epithelioid granuloma** (Fig. 13.21). This is a discrete, compact collection of epithelioid cells rimmed by an outer zone rich in CD4+ T cells. It is not uncommon to see intermixed multinucleate giant cells formed by fusion of macrophages. Early on, a thin layer of laminated fibroblasts is found peripheral to the granuloma; over time, these proliferate and lay down collagen that replaces the entire granuloma with a hyalinized scar. Two other microscopic features are sometimes seen in the granulomas: (1) **Schaumann bodies,** laminated concretions composed of calcium and proteins; and (2) **asteroid bodies,** stellate inclusions enclosed within giant cells. Their presence is not required for diagnosis of sarcoidosis, and they may also occur in granulomas of other origins. Rarely, foci of central necrosis may be present in sarcoid granulomas, especially in the nodular form.

The **lungs** are involved at some stage of the disease in 90% of patients. The granulomas predominantly involve the interstitium rather than air spaces, with some tendency to localize in the connective tissue around bronchioles and pulmonary venules and in the pleura ("lymphangitic" distribution). The bronchoalveolar lavage fluid contains abundant CD4+ T cells. In 5% to 15% of patients, the granulomas eventually are replaced by **diffuse interstitial fibrosis,** resulting in a so-called "honeycomb lung".

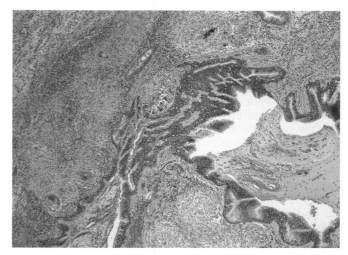

Fig. 13.21 Sarcoid. Characteristic peribronchial noncaseating granulomas with many giant cells are present.

Intrathoracic **hilar and paratracheal lymph nodes** are enlarged in 75% to 90% of patients, while one-third present with peripheral lymphadenopathy. The nodes are characteristically painless and have a firm, rubbery texture. Unlike in tuberculosis, lymph nodes in sarcoidosis are "nonmatted" (nonadherent) and do not ulcerate.

Skin lesions are encountered in approximately 25% of patients. **Erythema nodosum,** the hallmark of acute sarcoidosis, consists of raised, red, tender nodules on the anterior aspects of the legs. Sarcoidal granulomas are uncommon in these lesions. By contrast, discrete painless subcutaneous nodules can also occur in sarcoidosis, and these usually reveal abundant noncaseating granulomas.

Involvement of the eye and lacrimal glands occurs in about one-fifth to one-half of patients. The ocular involvement takes the form of **iritis** or **iridocyclitis** and may be unilateral or bilateral. As a consequence, corneal opacities, glaucoma, and (less commonly) total loss of vision may develop. The posterior uveal tract also is affected, with resultant **choroiditis, retinitis,** and **optic nerve involvement.** These ocular lesions are frequently accompanied by inflammation in the lacrimal glands, with suppression of lacrimation **(sicca syndrome). Unilateral or bilateral parotitis with painful enlargement of the parotid glands** occurs in less than 10% of patients with sarcoidosis; some go on to develop xerostomia (dry mouth). Combined uveoparotid involvement is designated **Mikulicz syndrome.**

The spleen may appear unaffected grossly, but in about three-fourths of cases, it contains granulomas. In approximately 10%, it becomes clinically enlarged. **The liver** demonstrates microscopic granulomatous lesions, usually in the portal triads, about as often as the spleen, but only about one-third of patients demonstrate hepatomegaly or abnormal liver function. Sarcoid involvement of **bone marrow** is reported in as many as 40% of patients, although it rarely causes severe manifestations. Other findings may include hypercalcemia and hypercalciuria. These changes are not related to bone destruction but rather are caused by increased calcium absorption secondary to production of active vitamin D by the macrophages that form the granulomas.

Clinical Features

In many affected individuals, the disease is entirely asymptomatic, discovered on routine chest films as bilateral hilar adenopathy or as an incidental finding at autopsy. In others, peripheral lymphadenopathy, cutaneous lesions, eye involvement, splenomegaly, or hepatomegaly may be presenting manifestations. In about two-thirds of symptomatic cases, there is gradual appearance of respiratory symptoms (shortness of breath, dry cough, or vague substernal discomfort) or constitutional signs and symptoms (fever, fatigue, weight loss, anorexia, night sweats). A definitive diagnostic test for sarcoidosis does not exist, and establishing a diagnosis requires the presence of clinical and radiologic findings that are consistent with the disease, the exclusion of other disorders with similar presentations, and the identification of noncaseating granulomas in involved tissues. In particular, tuberculosis must be excluded.

Sarcoidosis follows an unpredictable course characterized by either progressive chronicity or periods of activity interspersed with remissions. The remissions may be spontaneous or initiated by steroid therapy and often are permanent. Overall, 65% to 70% of affected individuals recover with minimal or no residual manifestations. Another 20% develop permanent lung dysfunction or visual impairment. Of the remaining 10% to 15%, most succumb to progressive pulmonary fibrosis and cor pulmonale.

SUMMARY

SARCOIDOSIS

- Sarcoidosis is a multisystem disease of unknown etiology; the diagnostic histopathologic feature is the presence of noncaseating granulomas in various tissues.
- Immunologic abnormalities include high levels of CD4+ T_H1 cells in the lung that secrete cytokines such as IFN-γ.
- Clinical manifestations include lymph node enlargement, eye involvement (sicca syndrome [dry eyes], iritis, or iridocyclitis), skin lesions (erythema nodosum, painless subcutaneous nodules), and visceral involvement (liver, skin, bone marrow). Lung involvement occurs in 90% of cases, with formation of granulomas and interstitial fibrosis.

Hypersensitivity Pneumonitis

Hypersensitivity pneumonitis is an immunologically mediated inflammatory lung disease that primarily affects the alveoli and is therefore often called *allergic alveolitis.* Most often it is an occupational disease that results from heightened sensitivity to inhaled antigens such as those found in moldy hay (Table 13.4). Unlike bronchial asthma, in which bronchi are the focus of immunologically mediated injury, the damage in hypersensitivity pneumonitis occurs at the level of alveoli. Hence, it manifests predominantly as a restrictive lung disease with the typical decreases in diffusion capacity, lung compliance, and total lung volume. The responsible occupational and household exposures are diverse, but the syndromes share common clinical and pathologic findings and probably have a very similar pathophysiologic basis.

Table 13.4 Sources of Antigens Causing Hypersensitivity Pneumonitis

Source of Antigen	Types of Exposures
Mushrooms, fungi, yeasts	Contaminated wood, humidifiers, central hot air heating ducts, peat moss plants
Bacteria	Dairy barns (farmer's lung)
Mycobacteria	Metalworking fluids, sauna, hot tub
Birds	Pigeons, dove feathers, ducks, parakeets
Chemicals	Isocyanates (auto painters), zinc, dyes

From Lacasse Y, Girard M, Cormier Y: Recent advances in hypersensitivity pneumonitis, *Chest* 142:208, 2012.

Several lines of evidence suggest that hypersensitivity pneumonitis is an immunologically mediated disease:
- Bronchoalveolar lavage specimens consistently show increased numbers of CD4+ and CD8+ T lymphocytes.
- Most affected patients have specific antibodies against the offending antigen in their serum.
- Complement and immunoglobulins have been demonstrated within vessel walls by immunofluorescence.
- Noncaseating granulomas are found in the lungs of two-thirds of affected patients.

MORPHOLOGY

The histopathologic picture in both acute and chronic forms of hypersensitivity pneumonitis includes patchy mononuclear cell infiltrates in the pulmonary interstitium, with a characteristic peribronchiolar accentuation. Lymphocytes predominate, but plasma cells and epithelioid macrophages also are present. In acute forms of the disease, variable numbers of neutrophils also may be seen. **"Loose," poorly formed granulomas,** without necrosis, are present in more than two-thirds of cases, usually in a peribronchiolar location (Fig. 13.22). In advanced chronic cases, bilateral, upper-lobe–dominant interstitial fibrosis (UIP pattern) occurs.

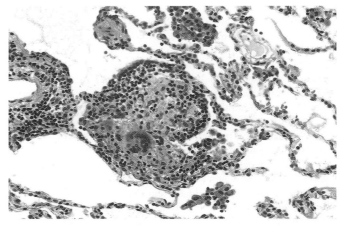

Fig. 13.22 Hypersensitivity pneumonitis, histologic appearance. Loosely formed interstitial granulomas and chronic inflammation are characteristic.

Clinical Features

Hypersensitivity pneumonitis may manifest either as an acute reaction, with fever, cough, dyspnea, and constitutional signs and symptoms arising 4 to 8 hours after exposure, or as a chronic disease characterized by insidious onset of cough, dyspnea, malaise, and weight loss. With the acute form, the diagnosis is usually obvious because of the temporal relationship of symptom onset and exposure to the incriminating antigen. If antigenic exposure is terminated after acute attacks of the disease, complete resolution of pulmonary symptoms occurs within days. Failure to remove the inciting agent from the environment eventually results in an irreversible chronic interstitial pulmonary disease.

Pulmonary Eosinophilia

A number of disorders are characterized by pulmonary infiltrates rich in eosinophils, which are recruited to the lung by local release of chemotactic factors. These diverse diseases generally are of immunologic origin, but the etiology is not understood. Pulmonary eosinophilia is divided into the following categories:

- *Acute eosinophilic pneumonia with respiratory failure,* characterized by rapid onset of fever, dyspnea, hypoxia, and diffuse pulmonary infiltrates on chest radiographs. The bronchoalveolar lavage fluid typically contains more than 25% eosinophils. There is prompt response to corticosteroids.
- *Simple pulmonary eosinophilia (Loeffler syndrome),* characterized by transient pulmonary lesions, eosinophilia in the blood, and a benign clinical course. The alveolar septa are thickened by an infiltrate containing eosinophils and occasional giant cells.
- *Tropical eosinophilia,* caused by infection with microfilariae and helminthic parasites
- *Secondary eosinophilia,* seen, for example, in association with asthma, drug allergies, and certain forms of vasculitis
- *Idiopathic chronic eosinophilic pneumonia,* characterized by aggregates of lymphocytes and eosinophils within the septal walls and the alveolar spaces, typically in the periphery of the lung fields, and accompanied by high fever, night sweats, and dyspnea. This is a disease of exclusion, once other causes of pulmonary eosinophilia have been ruled out.

Smoking-Related Interstitial Diseases

In addition to obstructive lung disease (COPD), smoking is also is associated with restrictive or interstitial lung diseases. *Desquamative interstitial pneumonia (DIP)* and *respiratory bronchiolitis* are two related examples of smoking-associated interstitial lung disease. The most striking histologic feature of DIP is the accumulation of large numbers of macrophages containing dusty-brown pigment *(smoker's macrophages)* in the air spaces (Fig. 13.23). The alveolar septa are thickened by a sparse inflammatory infiltrate (usually lymphocytes); interstitial fibrosis, when present, is mild. Pulmonary function tests usually show a mild restrictive abnormality. Overall,

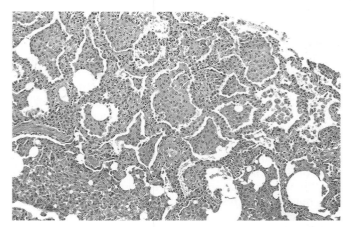

Fig. 13.23 Desquamative interstitial pneumonia. There is accumulation of large numbers of macrophages within the alveolar spaces with only slight fibrous thickening of the alveolar walls.

patients with DIP have a good prognosis and an excellent response to steroids and smoking cessation; however, some patients progress despite therapy. Respiratory bronchiolitis is a common lesion found in smokers that is characterized by the presence of pigmented intraluminal macrophages akin to those in DIP, but in a "bronchiolocentric" distribution (first- and second-order respiratory bronchioles). Mild peribronchiolar fibrosis also is seen. As with DIP, affected patients present with gradual onset of dyspnea and dry cough, and the symptoms recede with smoking cessation.

PULMONARY DISEASES OF VASCULAR ORIGIN

Pulmonary Embolism, Hemorrhage, and Infarction

Thromboembolism causes approximately 50,000 deaths per year in the United States and even when not directly fatal often complicates the course of other diseases. The true incidence of nonfatal pulmonary embolism is not known. Some cases undoubtedly occur outside the hospital in ambulatory patients, in whom the emboli are small and clinically silent. Even among hospitalized patients, no more than one-third are diagnosed before death. Autopsy data on the incidence of pulmonary embolism vary widely, ranging from 1% in the general hospitalized population, to 30% in individuals dying after severe burns, trauma, or fractures.

Blood clots that occlude the large pulmonary arteries are almost always embolic in origin. More than 95% of all pulmonary emboli arise from thrombi within the large deep veins of the legs, most often those that have propagated to involve the popliteal vein and larger veins above it. The influences that predispose to venous thrombosis in the legs are discussed in Chapter 4, but the following risk factors are paramount: (1) prolonged bed rest (particularly with immobilization of the legs); (2) surgery, especially orthopedic surgery on the knee or hip; (3) severe trauma (including burns or multiple fractures); (4) congestive heart failure; (5) in women, the period around parturition or the use of oral contraception pills with high estrogen content; (6) disseminated cancer; and (7) primary disorders of hypercoagulability (e.g., factor V Leiden) (Chapter 4).

The pathophysiologic consequences of pulmonary thromboembolism depend largely on the size of the embolus, which in turn dictates the size of the occluded pulmonary artery, and the cardiopulmonary status of the patient. There are two important consequences of pulmonary arterial occlusion: (1) an increase in pulmonary artery pressure from blockage of flow and, possibly, vasospasm caused by neurogenic mechanisms and/or release of mediators (e.g., thromboxane A_2, serotonin); and (2) ischemia of the downstream pulmonary parenchyma. Thus, occlusion of a major vessel results in an abrupt increase in pulmonary artery pressure, diminished cardiac output, right-sided heart failure (*acute cor pulmonale),* and sometimes sudden death. If smaller vessels are occluded, the result is less catastrophic and may even be clinically silent. Hypoxemia develops as a result of multiple mechanisms:

- *Perfusion of atelectatic lung zones.* Alveolar collapse occurs in ischemic areas because of a reduction in surfactant production and because pain associated with embolism leads to reduced movement of the chest wall.
- The decrease in cardiac output causes a *widening of the difference in arterial-venous oxygen saturation.*
- *Right-to-left shunting* of blood may occur through a patent foramen ovale, present in 30% of normal individuals.

Recall that the lungs are oxygenated not only by the pulmonary arteries but also by bronchial arteries and directly from air in the alveoli. Thus, ischemic necrosis (infarction) is the exception rather than the rule, occurring in as few as 10% of patients with thromboemboli. It occurs only if there is compromise in cardiac function or bronchial circulation, or if the region of the lung at risk is underventilated as a result of underlying pulmonary disease.

● MORPHOLOGY

The consequences of pulmonary embolism, as noted, depend on the size of the embolic mass and the general state of the circulation. A large embolus may embed in the main pulmonary artery or its major branches or lodge astride the bifurcation as a **saddle embolus** (Fig. 13.24). Death usually follows so suddenly from hypoxia or acute failure of the right side of the heart (acute cor pulmonale) that there is no time for morphologic alterations in the lung. Smaller emboli become impacted in medium-sized and small-sized pulmonary arteries. With adequate circulation and bronchial arterial flow, the vitality of the lung parenchyma is maintained, but alveolar hemorrhage may occur as a result of ischemic damage to the endothelial cells.

With compromised cardiovascular status, as may occur with congestive heart failure, **infarction** results. The more peripheral the embolic occlusion, the higher the risk for infarction. About three-fourths of all infarcts affect the lower lobes, and more than one-half are multiple. Characteristically, they are wedge-shaped, with their base at the pleural surface and the apex pointing toward the hilus of the lung. Pulmonary infarcts typically are

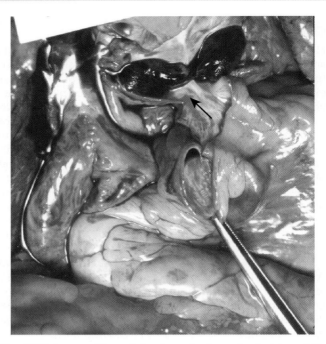

Fig. 13.24 Large saddle embolus from the femoral vein lying astride the main left and right pulmonary arteries. *(Courtesy of Dr. Linda Margraf, Department of Pathology, University of Texas Southwestern Medical School, Dallas, Texas.)*

hemorrhagic and appear as raised, red-blue areas of coagulative necrosis in the early stages (Fig. 13.25). The adjacent pleural surface often is covered by a fibrinous exudate. The occluded vessel is usually located near the apex of the infarcted area. The red cells begin to lyse within 48 hours, and the infarct gradually becomes red-brown as hemosiderin is produced. In time, fibrous replacement begins at the margins as a gray-white peripheral zone and eventually converts the infarct into a scar.

Clinical Features

The clinical consequences of pulmonary thromboembolism are summarized as follows:

- Most (60% to 80%) are clinically silent because they are small; the bronchial circulation sustains the viability of

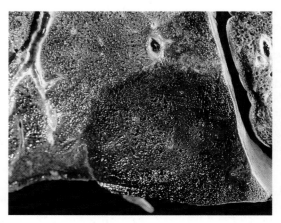

Fig. 13.25 A small, roughly wedge-shaped hemorrhagic pulmonary infarct of recent occurrence.

the affected lung parenchyma, and the embolic mass is rapidly removed by fibrinolytic activity.

- In 5% of cases, death, acute right-sided heart failure, or cardiovascular collapse (shock) occurs suddenly. Massive pulmonary embolism is one of the few causes of virtually instantaneous death. These severe consequences typically happen when more than 60% of the total pulmonary vasculature is obstructed by a large embolus or multiple simultaneous small emboli.
- Obstruction of small to medium pulmonary branches (10% to 15% of cases) causes pulmonary infarction if some element of circulatory insufficiency also is present. Typically, individuals who sustain infarctions present with dyspnea.
- In a small but significant subset of patients (accounting for <3% of cases), recurrent "showers" of emboli lead to pulmonary hypertension, chronic right-sided heart failure, and, in time, pulmonary vascular sclerosis with progressively worsening of dyspnea.

Emboli usually resolve after the initial acute event, as endogenous fibrinolytic activity often leads to their complete dissolution. However, in the presence of an underlying predisposing factor, a small, innocuous embolus may presage a larger one, and patients who have experienced one pulmonary embolism have a 30% chance of developing a second. Prophylactic therapy may include anticoagulation, early ambulation for postoperative and postparturient patients, application of elastic stockings, intermittent pneumatic calf compression, and isometric leg exercises for bedridden patients. Those who develop pulmonary embolism are given anti-coagulation therapy. Patients with massive pulmonary embolism who are hemodynamically unstable (shock, acute right heart failure) are candidates for thrombolytic therapy.

Nonthrombotic pulmonary emboli come in several uncommon but potentially lethal forms, such as air, fat, and amniotic fluid embolism (Chapter 4). Intravenous drug abuse often is associated with foreign body embolism in the pulmonary microvasculature; the presence of magnesium trisilicate (talc) in the intravenous mixture elicits a granulomatous response within the interstitium or pulmonary arteries. Involvement of the interstitium may lead to fibrosis, while vascular involvement leads to pulmonary hypertension. Residual talc crystals can be demonstrated within the granulomas using polarized light. Bone marrow embolism (denoted by the presence of hematopoietic and fat elements within a pulmonary artery) can occur after massive trauma and in patients with bone infarction secondary to sickle cell anemia.

SUMMARY

PULMONARY EMBOLISM

- Almost all large pulmonary artery thrombi are embolic in origin, usually arising from the deep veins of the lower leg.
- Risk factors include prolonged bed rest, knee or hip surgery, severe trauma, congestive heart failure, use of oral contraceptives (especially those with high estrogen content), disseminated cancer, and genetic causes of hypercoagulability.

- Most emboli (60% to 80%) are clinically silent; a minority (5%, typically large "saddle emboli") cause acute right-sided heart failure, shock, or sudden death; and the remainder cause pulmonary infarction.
- Risk for recurrence is high.

Pulmonary Hypertension

The pulmonary circulation normally is one of low resistance, and pulmonary blood pressures are only about one-eighth of systemic pressures. **Pulmonary hypertension (defined as pressures of 25 mm Hg or more at rest) may be caused by a decrease in the cross-sectional area of the pulmonary vascular bed or, less commonly, by increased pulmonary vascular blood flow.** Based on shared features, the World Health Organization has classified pulmonary hypertension into the following five groups:

- *Pulmonary arterial hypertension,* a diverse collection of disorders that includes heritable forms of pulmonary hypertension and diseases that cause pulmonary hypertension by affecting small pulmonary muscular arterioles; these include connective tissue diseases, human immunodeficiency virus, and congenital heart disease with left to right shunts
- *Pulmonary hypertension due to left-sided heart disease,* including systolic and diastolic dysfunction and valvular disease
- *Pulmonary hypertension due to lung diseases and/or hypoxia,* including COPD and interstitial lung disease
- *Chronic thromboembolic pulmonary hypertension*
- *Pulmonary hypertension with unclear or multifactorial mechanisms*

Pathogenesis

As can be gathered from this classification, pulmonary hypertension has diverse causes. Some of the more common causes are the following:

- *Chronic obstructive or interstitial lung diseases* (group 3). These diseases obliterate alveolar capillaries, increasing pulmonary resistance to blood flow and, secondarily, pulmonary blood pressure.
- *Antecedent congenital or acquired heart disease* (group 2). Mitral stenosis, for example, causes an increase in left atrial pressure and pulmonary venous pressure that is eventually transmitted to the arterial side of the pulmonary vasculature, leading to hypertension.
- *Recurrent thromboemboli* (group 4). Recurrent pulmonary emboli may cause pulmonary hypertension by reducing the functional cross-sectional area of the pulmonary vascular bed, which in turn leads to an increase in pulmonary vascular resistance.
- *Autoimmune diseases* (group 1). Several of these diseases (most notably systemic sclerosis) involve the pulmonary vasculature and/or the interstitium, leading to increased vascular resistance and pulmonary hypertension.
- *Obstructive sleep apnea* (also group 3) is a common disorder that is associated with obesity and hypoxemia. It is now recognized to be a significant contributor to the development of pulmonary hypertension and cor pulmonale.

Uncommonly, pulmonary hypertension is encountered in patients in whom all known causes are excluded; this is referred to as *idiopathic pulmonary arterial hypertension*. This name is a misnomer, however, as up to 80% of "idiopathic" pulmonary hypertension (sometimes referred to as *primary pulmonary hypertension*) has a genetic basis, sometimes being inherited in families as an autosomal dominant trait. Within these families, there is incomplete penetrance, and only 10% to 20% of the family members develop overt disease. As is often the case, investigating the molecular basis of an uncommon familial form of the disease has provided new pathogenic insights, in this instance by shining a spotlight on the role of the bone morphogenetic protein (BMP)–signaling pathway. Inactivating germ line mutations in the gene encoding bone morphogenetic protein receptor 2 (BMPR2) are found in 75% of the familial cases of pulmonary hypertension and 25% of sporadic cases. More recently, mutations in other genes that are involved in the BMPR2 pathway also have been identified in affected patients. Details remain to be worked out, but it appears that defects in BMPR2 signaling leads to dysfunction of endothelium and proliferation of vascular smooth muscle cells in the pulmonary vasculature. Because only 10% to 20% of individuals with *BMPR2* mutations develop disease, it is likely that modifier genes and/or environmental triggers also contribute to the pathogenesis of the disorder.

MORPHOLOGY

Regardless of their etiology, all forms of pulmonary hypertension are associated with **medial hypertrophy of the pulmonary muscular and elastic arteries, pulmonary arterial atherosclerosis, and right ventricular hypertrophy.** The presence of organizing or recanalized thrombi favors recurrent pulmonary emboli as the cause, and the coexistence of diffuse pulmonary fibrosis, or severe emphysema and chronic bronchitis, points to chronic hypoxia as the initiating event. The vessel changes can involve the entire arterial tree, from the main pulmonary arteries down to the arterioles (Fig. 13.26). In severe cases, atheromatous deposits form in the pulmonary artery and its major branches. The arterioles and small arteries are most prominently affected by medial hypertrophy and intimal fibrosis, sometimes narrowing the lumens to pinpoint channels. An uncommon but characteristic pathologic change is the **plexiform lesion,** so called because a tuft of capillary formations is present, producing a network, or web, that spans the lumens of dilated thin-walled, small arteries and may extend outside the vessel.

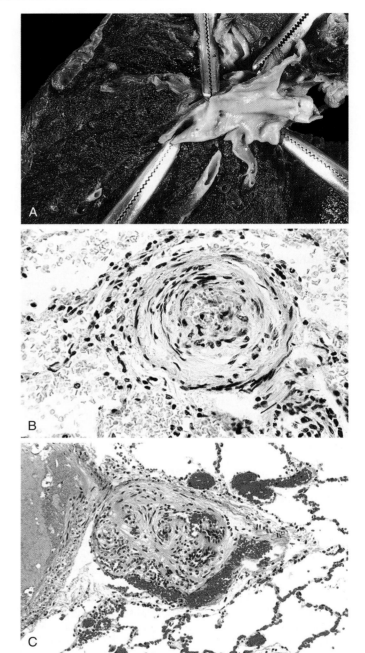

Fig. 13.26 Vascular changes in pulmonary hypertension. (A) Atheroma formation, a change usually limited to large pulmonary arteries. (B) Marked medial hypertrophy. (C) Plexiform lesion characteristic of advanced pulmonary hypertension seen in small arteries.

Clinical Features

Pulmonary hypertension produces symptoms when the disease is advanced. Idiopathic pulmonary hypertension is most common in women 20 to 40 years of age and occurs occasionally in young children. The presenting features are usually dyspnea and fatigue, but some patients have anginal chest pain. Over time, respiratory distress, cyanosis, and right ventricular hypertrophy appear, and death from decompensated cor pulmonale, often with superimposed thromboembolism and pneumonia, ensues within 2 to 5 years in 80% of patients.

Treatment choices depend on the underlying cause. For those with secondary disease, therapy is directed at the trigger (e.g., thromboembolic disease or hypoxemia). A variety of vasodilators have been used with varying success in those with group 1 disease or refractory disease belonging to other groups. Lung transplantation is the definitive treatment for selected patients.

Diffuse Alveolar Hemorrhage Syndromes

Pulmonary hemorrhage is a dramatic complication of some interstitial lung disorders. Among these so-called "pulmonary hemorrhage syndromes" are (1) Goodpasture syndrome, (2) idiopathic pulmonary hemosiderosis, and (3) granulomatosis with polyangiitis.

Goodpasture Syndrome

Goodpasture syndrome is an uncommon autoimmune disease in which lung and kidney injury are caused by circulating autoantibodies against certain domains of type IV collagen that are intrinsic to the basement membranes of renal glomeruli and pulmonary alveoli. The antibodies trigger destruction and inflammation of the basement membranes in pulmonary alveoli and renal glomeruli, giving rise to *necrotizing hemorrhagic interstitial pneumonitis* and *rapidly progressive glomerulonephritis.*

MORPHOLOGY

The lungs are heavy and have areas of red-brown consolidation due to **diffuse alveolar hemorrhage.** Microscopic examination shows focal necrosis of alveolar walls associated with intra-alveolar hemorrhage, fibrous thickening of septa, and hypertrophic type II pneumocytes. There is abundant **hemosiderin** due to earlier episodes of hemorrhage (Fig. 13.27). The characteristic **linear pattern of immunoglobulin deposition** (usually IgG, sometimes IgA or IgM) that is the hallmark diagnostic finding in renal biopsy specimens (Chapter 14) also may be seen along the alveolar septa.

Most cases of Goodpasture syndrome occur in patients in their teens or twenties. In contrast to many other autoimmune diseases, there is a male preponderance. The majority of patients are active smokers. Plasmapheresis and immunosuppressive therapy have markedly improved a once-dismal prognosis. Plasma exchange removes offending antibodies, and immunosuppressive drugs inhibit antibody production. With severe renal disease, renal transplantation is eventually required.

Granulomatosis and Polyangiitis

More than 80% of patients with granulomatosis and polyangiitis (GPA; formerly *Wegener granulomatosis*) develop upper-respiratory or pulmonary manifestations at some time in their course. This is discussed in Chapter 10. Here we list the salient pulmonary features. The lung lesions are characterized by a combination of necrotizing vasculitis ("angiitis") and parenchymal necrotizing granulomatous inflammation. The signs and symptoms stem from involvement of the upper-respiratory tract (chronic sinusitis, epistaxis, nasal perforation) and the lungs (cough, hemoptysis, chest pain). Anti-neutrophil cytoplasmic antibodies (PR3-ANCAs) are present in close to 95% of cases (Chapter 10).

PULMONARY INFECTIONS

Pulmonary infections in the form of pneumonia are responsible for one sixth of all deaths in the United States. Pneumonia can be broadly defined as any infection in the lung. Normally, the lung parenchyma remains sterile because of a number of highly effective immune and nonimmune defense mechanisms that extend throughout the respiratory system from the nasopharynx to the alveolar air spaces (Fig. 13.28). The vulnerability of the lung to infection dsepite these defenses is not surprising because (1) many microbes are airborne and readily inhaled into the lungs; (2) nasopharyngeal flora are regularly aspirated during sleep, even by healthy individuals; and (3) lung diseases often lower local immune defenses.

The importance of immune defenses in preventing pulmonary infections is emphasized by patients with inherited or acquired defects in innate immunity (including neutrophil and complement defects) or adaptive immunity (e.g., humoral immunodeficiency), all of which lead to an

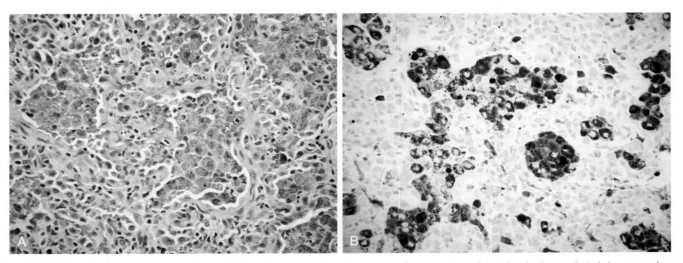

Fig. 13.27 Diffuse alveolar hemorrhage syndrome. (A) Lung biopsy specimen demonstrates large numbers of intraalveolar hemosiderin-laden macrophages on a background of thickened fibrous septa. (B) The tissue has been stained with Prussian blue, an iron stain that highlights the abundant intracellular hemosiderin. *(From the Teaching Collection of the Department of Pathology, Children's Medical Center, Dallas, Texas.)*

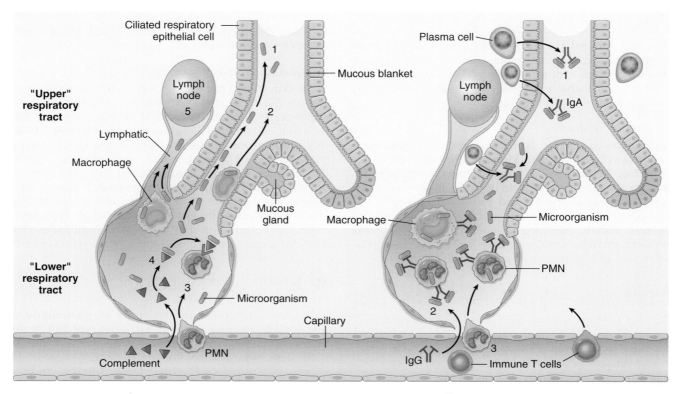

A INNATE IMMUNE DEFENSES   B ADAPTIVE IMMUNE DEFENSES

Fig. 13.28 Lung defense mechanisms. (A) Innate defenses against infection: *1*, In the normal lung, removal of microbial organisms depends on entrapment in the mucous blanket and removal by means of the mucociliary elevator; *2*, Phagocytosis by alveolar macrophages can kill and degrade organisms and remove them from the air spaces by migrating onto the mucociliary elevator; or *3*, phagocytosis and killing by neutrophils recruited by macrophage factors; *4*, Complement may enter the alveoli and be activated by the alternative pathway to produce the opsonin C3b, which enhances phagocytosis; *5*, Organisms, including those ingested by phagocytes, may reach the draining lymph nodes to initiate immune responses. (B) Additional mechanisms operate after development of adaptive immunity: *1*, Secreted IgA can block attachment of the microorganism to epithelium in the upper-respiratory tract; *2*, In the lower-respiratory tract, serum antibodies (IgM, IgG) are present in the alveolar lining fluid and activate complement more efficiently by the classic pathway, yielding C3b *(not shown)*; In addition, IgG is an opsonin; *3*, The accumulation of immune T cells is important for controlling infections by viruses and other intracellular microorganisms. *PMN*, neutrophil.

increased incidence of infections with pyogenic bacteria. For example, patients with mutations in MYD88, an adaptor protein required for signaling by Toll-like receptors, are extremely susceptible to severe necrotizing pneumococcal infections, while patients with congenital defects in IgA production (the major immunoglobulin in airways secretions) are at increased risk for pneumonias caused by encapsulated organisms such as pneumococcus and *H. influenzae*. On the other hand, defects in T_H1 cell–mediated immunity lead mainly to increased infections with intracellular microbes such as atypical mycobacteria. Much more commonly, lifestyle choices interfere with host immune defense mechanisms and facilitate infections. For example, cigarette smoke compromises mucociliary clearance and pulmonary macrophage activity, and alcohol impairs neutrophile function as well as cough and epiglottic reflexes (thereby increasing the risk for aspiration).

Bacterial pneumonias are classified according to the specific etiologic agent or, if no pathogen can be isolated, by the clinical setting in which the infection occurs. Altogether, seven distinct clinical settings are recognized, each associated with a fairly distinct group of pathogens (summarized in Table 13.5). Thus, consideration of the clinical

setting can be a helpful guide when anti-microbial therapy has to be given empirically.

Community-Acquired Bacterial Pneumonias

Bacterial pneumonias often follow a viral upper-respiratory tract infection. *S. pneumoniae* (i.e., the pneumococcus) is the most common cause of community-acquired acute pneumonia and is discussed first, followed by other relative common pathogens.

Streptococcus pneumoniae

Pneumococcal infections occur with increased frequency in two clinical settings: (1) chronic diseases such as CHF, COPD, or diabetes; and (2) congenital or acquired defects in immunoglobulin production (e.g., acquired immune deficiency syndrome [AIDS]). In addition, decreased or absent splenic function (e.g., sickle cell disease or after splenectomy) greatly increases the risk for overwhelming pneumococcal sepsis. You will recall that the spleen contains the largest collection of phagocytes in the body and is the major organ responsible for removing pneumococci from the blood. The spleen also is an important site for

Table 13.5 The Pneumonia Syndromes and Implicated Pathogens

Community-Acquired Bacterial Pneumonia

Streptococcus pneumoniae
Haemophilus influenzae
Moraxella catarrhalis
Staphylococcus aureus
Legionella pneumophila
Enterobacteriaceae (Klebsiella pneumoniae) and Pseudomonas spp.
Mycoplasma pneumoniae
Chlamydia pneumoniae
Coxiella burnetii (Q fever)

Community-Acquired Viral Pneumonia

Respiratory syncytial virus, human metapneumovirus, parainfluenza virus (children); influenza A and B (adults); adenovirus (military recruits)

Nosocomial Pneumonia

Gram-negative rods belonging to Enterobacteriaceae (Klebsiella spp., Serratia marcescens, Escherichia coli) and Pseudomonas spp.
S. aureus (usually methicillin-resistant)

Aspiration Pneumonia

Anaerobic oral flora (Bacteroides, Prevotella, Fusobacterium, Peptostreptococcus), admixed with aerobic bacteria (S. pneumoniae, S. aureus, H. influenzae, and Pseudomonas aeruginosa)

Chronic Pneumonia

Nocardia
Actinomyces
Granulomatous: Mycobacterium tuberculosis and atypical mycobacteria, Histoplasma capsulatum, Coccidioides immitis, Blastomyces dermatitidis

Necrotizing Pneumonia and Lung Abscess

Anaerobic bacteria (extremely common), with or without mixed aerobic infection
S. aureus, K. pneumoniae, Streptococcus pyogenes, and type 3 pneumococcus (uncommon)

Pneumonia in the Immunocompromised Host

Cytomegalovirus
Pneumocystis jiroveci
Mycobacterium avium complex (MAC)
Invasive aspergillosis
Invasive candidiasis
"Usual" bacterial, viral, and fungal organisms (listed above)

---

production of antibodies against polysaccharides, which are the dominant protective antibodies against encapsulated bacteria.

The presence of numerous neutrophils in sputum containing the typical gram-positive, lancet-shaped diplococci supports the diagnosis of pneumococcal pneumonia, but it must be remembered that *S. pneumoniae* is a part of the endogenous flora in 20% of adults, and therefore false-positive results may be obtained. Isolation of pneumococci from blood cultures is more specific but less sensitive (in the early phase of illness, only 20% to 30% of patients have positive blood cultures). Pneumococcal vaccines containing capsular polysaccharides from the common serotypes are used in individuals at high risk for pneumococcal sepsis.

Haemophilus influenzae

Both encapsulated and unencapsulated forms of *H. influenzae* are important causes of community-acquired pneumonias. The former can cause a particularly life-threatening form of pneumonia in children, often after a respiratory viral infection. Adults at risk for developing infections include those with chronic pulmonary diseases such as chronic bronchitis, cystic fibrosis, and bronchiectasis. *H. influenzae* is the most common bacterial cause of acute exacerbations of COPD. Encapsulated *H. influenzae* type b was formerly an important cause of epiglottitis and suppurative meningitis in children, but vaccination against this organism in infancy has significantly reduced the risk.

Moraxella catarrhalis

M. catarrhalis is being increasingly recognized as a cause of bacterial pneumonia, especially in older adults. It is the second most common bacterial cause of acute exacerbation of COPD in adults. Along with *S. pneumoniae* and *H. influenzae*, *M. catarrhalis* is one of the three most frequent causes of otitis media (infection of the middle ear) in children.

Staphylococcus aureus

S. aureus is an important cause of secondary bacterial pneumonia in children and healthy adults after viral respiratory illnesses (e.g., measles in children and influenza in both children and adults). Staphylococcal pneumonia is associated with a high incidence of complications, such as lung abscess and empyema. Staphylococcal pneumonia occurring in association with right-sided staphylococcal endocarditis is a serious complication of intravenous drug abuse. It is also an important cause of nosocomial pneumonia (discussed later).

Klebsiella pneumoniae

K. pneumoniae is the most frequent cause of gram-negative bacterial pneumonia. *Klebsiella*-related pneumonia frequently afflicts debilitated and malnourished individuals, particularly *chronic alcoholics*. Thick and gelatinous sputum is characteristic, because the organism produces an abundant viscid capsular polysaccharide, which the patient may have difficulty coughing up.

Pseudomonas aeruginosa

Although discussed here with community-acquired pathogens because of its association with infections in cystic fibrosis, *P. aeruginosa* infection is most commonly is seen in nosocomial settings (discussed later). *Pseudomonas* pneumonia also is common in individuals who are neutropenic, usually secondary to chemotherapy; in victims of extensive burns; and in patients requiring mechanical ventilation. *P. aeruginosa* has a propensity to invade blood vessels at the site of infection, with consequent extrapulmonary spread. *Pseudomonas* bacteremia is a fulminant disease, with death often occurring within a matter of days. Histologic examination reveals organisms invading the walls of necrotic blood vessels (*Pseudomonas vasculitis*), leading to secondary coagulative necrosis of the pulmonary parenchyma.

Legionella pneumophila

L. pneumophila is the agent of Legionnaire disease, an eponym for the epidemic and sporadic forms of pneumonia caused by this organism. Pontiac fever is a related self-limited upper-respiratory tract infection caused by *L. pneumophila*, without pneumonic symptoms. *L. pneumophila* flourishes in artificial aquatic environments, such as water-cooling towers and within the tubing system of domestic (potable) water supplies. The mode of transmission is thought to be either inhalation of aerosolized organisms or aspiration of contaminated drinking water. *Legionella* pneumonia is common in individuals with some predisposing condition such as cardiac, renal, immunologic, or hematologic disease. Organ transplant recipients are particularly susceptible. *Legionella* pneumonia may be quite severe, frequently requiring hospitalization and producing a fatality rate of 30% to 50% in immunosuppressed individuals. Rapid diagnosis is facilitated by demonstration of *Legionella* antigens in the urine or by a positive fluorescent antibody test on sputum samples; culture remains the standard diagnostic modality. PCR-based tests can be used on bronchial secretions in atypical cases.

Mycoplasma pneumoniae

Mycoplasma infections are particularly common among children and young adults. They occur sporadically or as local epidemics in closed communities (schools, military camps, prisons). Tests for *Mycoplasma* antigens and polymerase chain reaction (PCR) testing for *Mycoplasma* DNA are available.

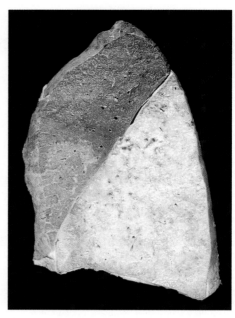

Fig. 13.30 Lobar pneumonia with gray hepatization. The lower lobe is uniformly consolidated.

MORPHOLOGY

Bacterial pneumonia has two patterns of anatomic distribution: lobular bronchopneumonia and lobar pneumonia (Fig. 13.29). In the context of pneumonias, the term "consolidation," used frequently, refers to "solidification" of the lung due to replacement of the air by exudate in the alveoli. Patchy consolidation of the lung is the dominant characteristic of **bronchopneumonia**, while consolidation of a large portion of a lobe or of an entire lobe defines **lobar pneumonia** (Fig. 13.30). These anatomic categorizations may be difficult to apply in individual cases because patterns overlap, and patchy involvement may evolve to become

confluent over time, producing complete lobar consolidation. Moreover, the same organisms may produce either pattern depending on patient susceptibility. Most important from the clinical standpoint are identification of the causative agent and determination of the extent of disease.

In **lobar pneumonia**, four stages of the inflammatory response have classically been described. In the first stage of **congestion,** the lung is heavy, boggy, and red. It is characterized by vascular engorgement, intraalveolar fluid with few neutrophils, and often the presence of numerous bacteria. The stage of **red hepatization** that follows is characterized by massive confluent exudation, as neutrophils, red cells, and fibrin fill the alveolar spaces (Fig. 13.31A). On gross examination, the lobe is red, firm, and airless, with a liver-like consistency, hence the term hepatization. The stage of **gray hepatization** that follows is marked by progressive disintegration of red cells and the persistence of a fibrinosuppurative exudate (see Fig. 13.31B), resulting in a color change to grayish-brown. In the final stage of **resolution,** the exudate within the alveolar spaces is broken down by enzymatic digestion to produce granular, semifluid debris that is resorbed, ingested by macrophages, expectorated, or organized by fibroblasts growing into it (Fig. 13.31C). Pleural fibrinous reaction to the underlying inflammation is often present in the early stages if the consolidation extends to the surface **(pleuritis).** It may resolve or undergo organization, leaving fibrous thickening or permanent adhesions.

Foci of **bronchopneumonia** are consolidated areas of acute suppurative inflammation. The consolidation may be confined to one lobe but is more often multilobar and frequently bilateral and basal because of the tendency of secretions to gravitate to the lower lobes. Well-developed lesions are slightly elevated, dry, granular, gray-red to yellow, and poorly delimited at their margins. Histologically, a neutrophil-rich exudate fills the bronchi, bronchioles, and adjacent alveolar spaces (see Fig. 13.31A).

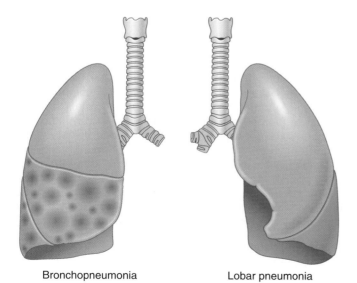

Bronchopneumonia   Lobar pneumonia

Fig. 13.29 The anatomic distribution of bronchopneumonia and lobar pneumonia affecting the lower lobes of the lung.

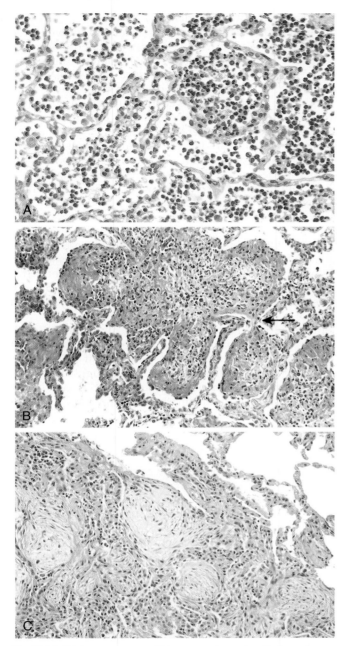

Fig. 13.31 (A) Acute pneumonia. The congested septal capillaries and extensive neutrophil exudation into alveoli correspond to early red hepatization. Fibrin nets have not yet formed. (B) Early organization of intraalveolar exudates, seen in areas to be streaming through the pores of Kohn *(arrow)*. (C) Advanced organizing pneumonia, featuring transformation of exudates to fibromyxoid masses richly infiltrated by macrophages and fibroblasts.

Complications of pneumonia include (1) tissue destruction and necrosis, causing **abscess formation**; (2) spread of infection to the pleural cavity, causing the intrapleural fibrinosuppurative reaction known as **empyema**; and (3) **bacteremic dissemination** to the heart valves, pericardium, brain, kidneys, spleen, or joints, causing metastatic abscesses, endocarditis, meningitis, or suppurative arthritis.

Clinical Features

The major symptoms of typical community-acquired acute bacterial pneumonia are abrupt onset of high fever, shaking chills, and cough producing mucopurulent sputum; occasional patients have hemoptysis. When pleuritis is present, it is accompanied by pleuritic pain and pleural friction rub. The whole lobe is radiopaque in lobar pneumonia, whereas there are focal opacities in bronchopneumonia.

The clinical picture is markedly modified by the administration of effective antibiotics. Treated patients may be relatively afebrile with few clinical signs 48 to 72 hours after the initiation of antibiotics. The identification of the organism and the determination of its antibiotic sensitivity are the keystones of therapy. Less than 10% of patients with pneumonia severe enough to merit hospitalization now succumb, and in most such instances death results from a complication, such as empyema, meningitis, endocarditis, or pericarditis, or to some predisposing influence, such as debility or chronic alcoholism.

Community-Acquired Viral Pneumonias

The most common causes of community-acquired viral pneumonias are influenza types A and B, the respiratory syncytial viruses, human metapneumovirus, adenovirus, rhinoviruses, rubeola virus, and varicella virus (see Table 13.5). Nearly all of these agents also cause upper-respiratory tract infections ("common cold").

These pathologic viruses share a propensity to infect and damage resspiratory epithelium, producing an inflammatory response. When the process extends to alveoli, there is usually interstitial inflammation, but some outpouring of fluid into alveolar spaces may also occur, so that on chest films the changes may mimic those of bacterial pneumonia. As a result, it is not possible to distinguish bacterial and viral pneumonia based on radiologic appearance alone. Moreover, damage leading to necrosis of the respiratory epithelium inhibits mucociliary clearance and predisposes to secondary bacterial infections. Such serious complications of viral infection are more likely in infants, older adults, malnourished patients, alcoholics, and immunosuppressed individuals.

MORPHOLOGY

The morphologic patterns in viral pneumonias are similar. The process may be patchy, or it may involve whole lobes bilaterally or unilaterally. Macroscopically, the affected areas are red-blue, congested, and subcrepitant. On histologic examination, the **inflammatory reaction is largely confined to the walls of the alveoli** (Fig. 13.32). The septa are widened and edematous; they usually contain a mononuclear inflammatory infiltrate of lymphocytes, macrophages and, occasionally, plasma cells. In the classic case, alveolar spaces in viral pneumonias are free of cellular exudate. In severe cases, however, full-blown diffuse alveolar damage with hyaline membranes may develop. In less severe, uncomplicated cases, subsidence of the disease is followed by reconstitution of the normal architecture. Superimposed bacterial infection, as expected, results in a mixed histologic picture.

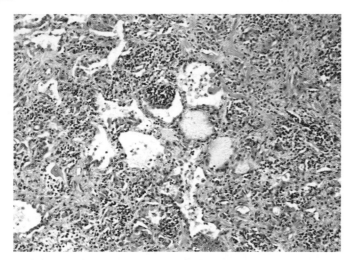

Fig. 13.32 Viral pneumonia. The thickened alveolar walls are infiltrated with lymphocytes and some plasma cells, which are spilling over into alveolar spaces. Note the focal alveolar edema *(center)* and early fibrosis *(upper right)*.

Clinical Features

The clinical course of viral pneumonia is extremely varied. It may masquerade as a severe upper-respiratory tract infection or "chest cold" that goes undiagnosed, or manifest as a fulminant, life-threatening infection in immunocompromised patients. The initial presentation usually is that of an acute, nonspecific febrile illness characterized by fever, headache, and malaise and, later, cough with minimal sputum. The localization of the inflammatory exudate to the alveolar walls, prevents oxygenation of blood flowing through the affected air spaces which in turn causes mismatch of ventilation and perfusion. As a result, the degree of respiratory distress often seems out of proportion to the physical and radiographic findings. Identifying the causative agent can be difficult.

Influenza Infections

Perhaps no other communicable disorder causes as much public concern in the developed world as the threat of an influenza epidemic. The influenza virus is a single-stranded RNA virus, bound by a nucleoprotein that determines the virus type—A, B, or C. The viral surface has a lipid bilayer containing the viral hemagglutinin and neuraminidase, which determine the subtype (e.g., H1N1, H3N2). Host antibodies to the hemagglutinin and neuraminidase prevent and ameliorate, respectively, future infection with the influenza virus. The type A viruses infect humans, pigs, horses, and birds and are the major cause of *pandemic* and *epidemic* influenza infections. Epidemics of influenza occur through mutations of the hemagglutinin and neuraminidase antigens that allow the virus to escape most host antibodies *(antigenic drift)*. Pandemics, which last longer and are more widespread than epidemics, may occur when both the hemagglutinin and neuraminidase are replaced through recombination of RNA segments with those of animal viruses, making all animals susceptible to the new influenza virus *(antigenic shift)*. Commercially available influenza vaccines provide reasonable protection against the disease, especially in vulnerable infants and in older adults.

Insight into future pandemics has come from studying those past. DNA analysis of viral genomes retrieved from the lungs of a soldier who died in the great 1918 influenza pandemic that killed 20 million to 40 million individuals worldwide identified swine influenza sequences, consistent with this virus having its origin in an antigenic shift. The first flu pandemic of this century, in 2009, also resulted from an antigenic shift involving a virus of swine origin. It caused particularly severe infections in young adults, apparently because older adults had antibodies against past influenza strains that conveyed partial protection. Comorbidities such as diabetes, heart disease, lung disease, and immunosuppression also were associated with a higher risk for severe infection.

What then might be the source of the next great pandemic? One concern is centered on avian influenza, which normally infects birds. One avian strain, type H5N1, has spread throughout the world in wild and domestic birds. As of September 2015, approximately 700 H5N1 influenza virus infections and 400 deaths in humans (from 15 countries) have been reported to the World Health Organization (WHO). Nearly all cases have been acquired by close contact with domestic birds; most deaths resulted from pneumonia. Fortunately, the transmission of the current H5N1 avian virus is inefficient. However, if H5N1 influenza recombines with an influenza that is highly infectious for humans, a strain might emerge that is capable of sustained human-to-human transmission (and, thus, of causing the next great pandemic).

SUMMARY

ACUTE PNEUMONIAS

- *S. pneumoniae* (the pneumococcus) is the most common cause of community-acquired bacterial pneumonia and usually has a lobar pattern of involvement.
- Morphologically, lobar pneumonias evolve through four stages: congestion, red hepatization, gray hepatization, and resolution.
- Other common causes of bacterial pneumonias in the community include *H. influenzae* and *M. catarrhalis* (both associated with acute exacerbations of COPD), *S. aureus* (usually secondary to viral respiratory infections), *K. pneumoniae* (observed in chronic alcoholics), *P. aeruginosa* (seen in individuals with cystic fibrosis, in burn victims, and in patients with neutropenia), and *L. pneumophila*, seen particularly in organ transplant recipients.
- *Viral pneumonias* are characterized by respiratory distress out of proportion to the clinical and radiologic signs, and by inflammation that is predominantly confined to alveolar septa, with generally clear alveoli.
- Common causes of viral pneumonia include influenza A and B, respiratory syncytial virus, human metapneumovirus, parainfluenza virus, and adenovirus.

Hospital-Acquired Pneumonias

Nosocomial, or hospital-acquired, pneumonias are defined as pulmonary infections acquired in the course of a hospital stay. These infections not only have an adverse impact on the clinical course of ill patients, but also add considerably to the burgeoning costs of health care. Nosocomial infections are common in hospitalized individuals with severe underlying disease, those who are immunosuppressed, or those on prolonged antibiotic regimens. Patients on mechanical ventilation are a particularly high-risk group, and infections acquired in this setting are given the designation *ventilator-associated pneumonia*. Gram-negative rods (members of *Enterobacteriaceae* and *Pseudomonas* spp.) and *S. aureus* are the most common isolates; unlike community-acquired pneumonias, *S. pneumoniae* is not a common pathogen in the hospital setting.

Aspiration Pneumonia

Aspiration pneumonia occurs in debilitated patients or those who aspirate gastric contents while unconscious (e.g., after a stroke) or during repeated vomiting. Those affected have abnormal gag and swallowing reflexes that facilitate aspiration. The resultant pneumonia is partly chemical, due to the extremely irritating effects of the gastric acid, and partly bacterial. Typically, more than one organism is recovered on culture, aerobes being more common than anaerobes (see Table 13.5). Aspiration pneumonia is often necrotizing, pursues a fulminant clinical course, and is a frequent cause of death in individuals predisposed to aspiration. In those who survive, abscess formation is a common complication. Microaspiration, by contrast, occurs in many individuals, especially those with gastroesophageal reflux, and may exacerbate other lung diseases but does not lead to pneumonia.

Lung Abscess

Lung abscess **refers to a localized area of suppurative necrosis within the pulmonary parenchyma, resulting in the formation of one or more large cavities.** The causative organism may be introduced into the lung by any of the following mechanisms:

- *Aspiration of infective material* from carious teeth or infected sinuses or tonsils. This may occur during oral surgery, anesthesia, coma, or alcoholic intoxication, and in debilitated patients with depressed cough reflexes.
- *Aspiration of gastric contents,* usually accompanied by infectious organisms originating in the oropharynx.
- *As a complication of necrotizing bacterial pneumonias,* particularly those caused by *S. aureus, Streptococcus pyogenes, K. pneumoniae, Pseudomonas* spp., and, rarely, type 3 pneumococci. Mycotic infections and bronchiectasis also may lead to lung abscesses.
- *Bronchial obstruction,* particularly with bronchogenic carcinoma obstructing a bronchus or bronchiole. Impaired drainage, distal atelectasis, and aspiration of blood and tumor fragments all contribute to the development of abscesses. An abscess also may form within an excavated necrotic portion of a tumor.
- *Septic embolism,* from infective endocarditis of the right side of the heart.
- In addition, lung abscesses may result from *hematogenous spread of bacteria* in disseminated pyogenic infection. This occurs most characteristically in staphylococcal bacteremia and often results in multiple lung abscesses.

Anaerobic bacteria are present in almost all lung abscesses, and they are the exclusive isolates in one-third to two-thirds of cases. The most frequently encountered anaerobes are commensals normally found in the oral cavity, principally species of *Prevotella, Fusobacterium, Bacteroides, Peptostreptococcus,* and microaerophilic streptococci.

MORPHOLOGY

Abscesses range in diameter from a few millimeters to large cavities 5 to 6 cm across. The localization and number of abscesses depend on their mode of development. Pulmonary abscesses resulting from aspiration of infective material are **more common on the right side** (with its more vertical airways) than on the left, and most are single. On the right side, they tend to occur in the posterior segment of the upper lobe and in the apical segments of the lower lobe, because these locations reflect the probable course of aspirated material when the patient is recumbent. Abscesses that develop in the course of pneumonia or bronchiectasis commonly are multiple, basal, and diffusely scattered. Septic emboli and abscesses arising from hematogenous seeding are commonly multiple and may affect any region of the lungs.

As the focus of suppuration enlarges, it almost inevitably ruptures into airways. Thus, the contained exudate may be partially drained, producing an air-fluid level on radiographic examination. Occasionally, abscesses rupture into the pleural cavity and produce bronchopleural fistulas, the consequence of which is **pneumothorax** or **empyema.** Other complications arise from embolization of septic material to the brain, giving rise to meningitis or brain abscess. On histologic examination, as expected with any abscess, the suppurative focus is surrounded by variable amounts of fibrous scarring and mononuclear infiltration (lymphocytes, plasma cells, macrophages), depending on the chronicity of the lesion.

Clinical Features

The manifestations of a lung abscess are much like those of bronchiectasis and include a prominent cough that usually yields copious amounts of foul-smelling, purulent, or sanguineous sputum; occasionally, hemoptysis occurs. Spiking fever and malaise are common. Clubbing of the fingers, weight loss, and anemia may all occur. Abscesses occur in 10% to 15% of patients with bronchogenic carcinoma; thus, when a lung abscess is suspected in an older adult, underlying carcinoma must be considered. Secondary amyloidosis (Chapter 5) may develop in chronic cases. Treatment includes antibiotic therapy and, if needed, surgical drainage. Overall, the mortality rate is in the range of 10%.

Chronic Pneumonias

Chronic pneumonia most often is a localized lesion in an immunocompetent individual, with or without regional lymph node involvement. There is typically granulomatous inflammation, which may be due to bacteria (e.g., *M. tuberculosis*) or fungi. In immunocompromised patients, such as those with debilitating illness, on immunosuppressive regimens, or with human immunodeficiency virus (HIV) infection (see later), the usual presentation is widespread disease due to systemic dissemination of the causative organism. Tuberculosis is by far the most important entity within the spectrum of chronic pneumonias.

Tuberculosis

Tuberculosis is a communicable chronic granulomatous disease caused by *Mycobacterium tuberculosis*. It usually involves the lungs but may affect any organ or tissue in the body.

Epidemiology

The World Health Organization (WHO) considers tuberculosis to be the most common cause of death resulting from a single infectious agent. It is estimated that 1.7 billion individuals are infected worldwide, with 8 to 10 million new cases and 1.5 million deaths per year. In the Western world, deaths from tuberculosis peaked in 1800 and steadily declined throughout the 1800s and 1900s. However, in 1984 the decline in new cases stopped abruptly, a change that resulted from the increased incidence of tuberculosis in HIV-infected individuals. As a consequence of intensive public health surveillance and tuberculosis prophylaxis among immunosuppressed individuals, the incidence of tuberculosis in U.S.-born individuals has declined since 1992. In 2014, there were approximately 9400 new cases of active tuberculosis in the United States, with nearly 60% of these occurring in immigrants from countries where tuberculosis is endemic.

Tuberculosis flourishes under conditions of poverty, crowding, and chronic debilitating illness. In the United States, tuberculosis is a disease of older adults, the urban poor, patients with AIDS, and members of minority communities. African Americans, Native Americans, the Inuit (from Alaska), Hispanics, and immigrants from Southeast Asia have higher rates of disease than other segments of the population. Certain disease states also increase the risk, such as diabetes mellitus, Hodgkin lymphoma, chronic lung disease (particularly silicosis), chronic renal failure, malnutrition, alcoholism, and immunosuppression. In areas of the world where HIV infection is prevalent, HIV infection is the dominant risk factor for the development of tuberculosis.

It is important that *infection* be differentiated from *disease*. Infection implies seeding of a focus with organisms, which may or may not cause clinically significant tissue damage (i.e., disease). Although other routes may be involved, most infections are acquired by direct person-to-person transmission of airborne droplets of organisms from an active case to a susceptible host. In most individuals, an asymptomatic focus of pulmonary infection appears that is self-limited, although uncommonly, primary tuberculosis may result in the development of fever and pleural effusions. Generally, the only evidence of infection, if any remains, is a tiny, telltale fibrocalcific nodule at the site of the infection. Viable organisms may remain dormant in such loci for decades, and possibly for the life of the host. Such individuals are infected but do not have active disease and therefore cannot transmit organisms to others. Yet, if their immune defenses are lowered, the infection may reac-

tivate to produce communicable and potentially life-threatening disease.

Infection with *M. tuberculosis* typically leads to the development of delayed hypersensitivity, which can be detected by the tuberculin (Mantoux) test. About 2 to 4 weeks after the infection has begun, intracutaneous injection of 0.1 mL of sterile purified protein derivative (PPD) induces a visible and palpable induration (at least 5 mm in diameter) that peaks in 48 to 72 hours. Sometimes, more PPD is required to elicit the reaction, and unfortunately, in some responders, the standard dose may produce a large, necrotizing lesion. A positive tuberculin skin test result signifies cell-mediated hypersensitivity to tubercular antigens, but does not differentiate between infection and disease. A well-recognized limitation of this test is that false-negative reactions (or skin test anergy) may be produced by certain viral infections, sarcoidosis, malnutrition, Hodgkin lymphoma, immunosuppression, and (notably) overwhelming active tuberculous disease. False-positive reactions may result from infection by atypical mycobacteria.

About 80% of the population in certain Asian and African countries is tuberculin-positive. In contrast, in 2012, approximately, 5% to 10% of the U.S. population was positive, indicating the marked difference in rates of exposure to the tubercle bacillus. In general, 3% to 4% of previously unexposed individuals acquire active tuberculosis during the first year after "tuberculin conversion," and no more than 15% do so thereafter. Thus, only a small fraction of those who contract an infection develop active disease.

Etiology and Pathogenesis

Mycobacteria are slender rods that are acid-fast (i.e., they have a high content of complex lipids that readily bind the Ziehl-Neelsen [carbol fuchsin] stain and subsequently stubbornly resist decolorization). *M. tuberculosis hominis* is responsible for most cases of tuberculosis; the reservoir of infection typically is found in individuals with active pulmonary disease. Transmission usually is direct, by inhalation of airborne organisms in aerosols generated by expectoration or by exposure to contaminated secretions of infected individuals. Oropharyngeal and intestinal tuberculosis contracted by drinking milk contaminated with *Mycobacterium bovis* infection is now rare except in those countries with tuberculous dairy cows and sales of unpasteurized milk. Other mycobacteria, particularly *Mycobacterium avium complex*, are much less virulent than *M. tuberculosis* and rarely cause disease in immunocompetent individuals. However, they cause disease in 10% to 30% of patients with AIDS.

Pathogenesis

The pathogenesis of tuberculosis in the previously unexposed immunocompetent individual is centered on the development of cell-mediated immunity, which confers resistance to the organism and results in development of tissue hypersensitivity to tubercular antigens. The pathologic features of tuberculosis, such as caseating granulomas and cavitation, are the result of the destructive tissue hypersensitivity that is part and parcel of the host immune response. Because the effector cells for both protective

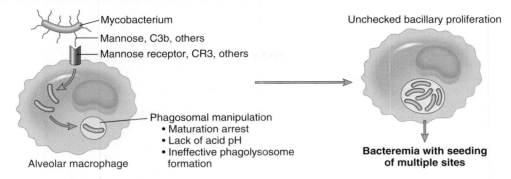

A INFECTION BEFORE ACTIVATION OF CELL MEDIATED IMMUNITY

Mycobacterium
Mannose, C3b, others
Mannose receptor, CR3, others

Unchecked bacillary proliferation

Phagosomal manipulation
• Maturation arrest
• Lack of acid pH
• Ineffective phagolysosome formation

Alveolar macrophage

Bacteremia with seeding of multiple sites

B INITIATION AND CONSEQUENCES OF CELL MEDIATED IMMUNITY

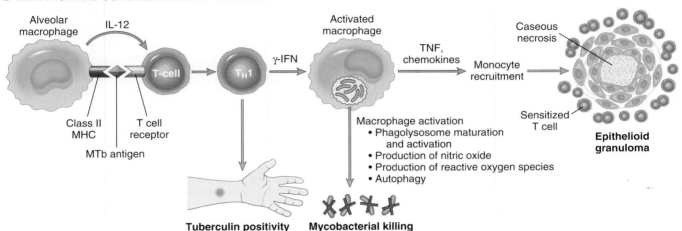

Alveolar macrophage
IL-12
T-cell
T_H1
γ-IFN
Activated macrophage
TNF, chemokines
Monocyte recruitment
Caseous necrosis

Class II MHC
T cell receptor
MTb antigen

Macrophage activation
• Phagolysosome maturation and activation
• Production of nitric oxide
• Production of reactive oxygen species
• Autophagy

Sensitized T cell

Epithelioid granuloma

Tuberculin positivity **Mycobacterial killing**

Fig. 13.33 Sequence of events in the natural history of primary pulmonary tuberculosis. This sequence commences with inhalation of virulent strains of *Mycobacterium* and culminates in the development of immunity and delayed hypersensitivity to the organism. (A) Events occurring in the first 3 weeks after exposure. (B) Events thereafter. The development of resistance to the organism is accompanied by conversion to a positive result on tuberculin skin testing. Cells and bacteria are not drawn to scale. *IFN-γ*, Interferon γ; *iNOS*, inducible nitric oxide synthase; *MHC*, major histocompatibility complex; *MTb*, Mycobacterium tuberculosis; *TNF*, tumor necrosis factor.

immunity and damaging hypersensitivity are the same, the appearance of tissue hypersensitivity also signals the acquisition of immunity to the organism. The sequence of events from inhalation of the infectious inoculum to containment of the primary focus is illustrated in Fig. 13.33 and can be outlined as follows:

• *Entry into macrophages.* A virulent strain of mycobacteria gains entry to macrophage endosomes, a process mediated by several macrophage receptors, including the macrophage mannose receptor and complement receptors that recognize several components of the mycobacterial cell walls.

• *Replication in macrophages.* Once internalized, the organisms inhibit normal microbicidal responses by preventing the fusion of the lysosomes with the phagocytic vacuole, allowing the mycobacterium to persist and proliferate. Thus, the earliest phase of primary tuberculosis (the first 3 weeks) in the nonsensitized patient is characterized by bacillary proliferation within the pulmonary alveolar macrophages and air spaces, eventually resulting in bacteremia and seeding of the organisms to multiple sites. Despite the bacteremia, most individuals at this stage are asymptomatic or have a mild flulike illness.

• *Development of cell-mediated immunity.* This occurs approximately 3 weeks after exposure. Processed mycobacterial antigens reach the draining lymph nodes and are presented to CD4 T cells by dendritic cells and macrophages. Under the influence of macrophage-secreted IL-12, CD4+ T cells of the T_H1 subset are generated that are capable of secreting IFN-γ.

• *T cell–mediated macrophage activation and killing of bacteria.* IFN-γ released by the CD4+ T cells of the T_H1 subset is crucial in activating macrophages. Activated macrophages, in turn, release a variety of mediators and upregulate expression of genes with important downstream effects, including: (1) TNF, which is responsible for recruitment of monocytes, which in turn undergo activation and differentiation into the "epithelioid histiocytes" that characterize the granulomatous response; (2) inducible nitric oxide synthase (iNOS), which raises nitric oxide (NO) levels, helping to create reactive nitrogen intermediates that appear to be particularly important in killing of mycobacteria; and (3) anti-microbial peptides (defensins) that are also toxic to mycobacterial organisms.

• *Granulomatous inflammation and tissue damage.* **In addition to stimulating macrophages to kill mycobacteria,** the T$_H$1 response orchestrates the formation of granulomas and caseous necrosis. Macrophages activated by IFN-γ differentiate into the "epithelioid histiocytes" that aggregate to form granulomas; some epithelioid cells may fuse to form giant cells. In many individuals, this response halts the infection before significant tissue destruction or illness occur. In other individuals with immune deficits due to age or immunosuppression, the infection progresses and the ongoing immune response results in caseation necrosis. Activated macrophages also secrete TNF and chemokines, which promote recruitment of more monocytes. The importance of TNF is underscored by the fact that patients with rheumatoid arthritis who are treated with a TNF antagonist have an increased risk for tuberculosis reactivation.

In summary, immunity to a tubercular infection is primarily mediated by T$_H$1 cells, which stimulate macrophages to kill mycobacteria. This immune response, while largely effective, comes at the cost of hypersensitivity and the accompanying tissue destruction. Defects in any of the steps of a T$_H$1 T cell response (including IL-12, IFN-γ, TNF, or nitric oxide production) result in poorly formed granulomas, absence of resistance, and disease progression. Individuals with inherited mutations in any component of the T$_H$1 pathway are extremely susceptible to infections with mycobacteria. Reactivation of the infection or reexposure to the bacilli in a previously sensitized host results in rapid mobilization of a defensive reaction but also increased tissue necrosis. Just as hypersensitivity and resistance appear in parallel, so, too, the loss of hypersensitivity (indicated by tuberculin negativity in a *M. tuberculosis*-infected patient) is an ominous sign of fading resistance to the organism.

Primary Tuberculosis

Primary tuberculosis is the form of disease that develops in a previously unexposed and therefore unsensitized patient. About 5% of those newly infected acquire significant disease.

In the large majority of otherwise healthy individuals, the only consequence of primary tuberculosis are the foci of scarring discussed earlier. However, these foci may harbor viable bacilli and thus serve as a nidus for disease reactivation at a later time if host defenses wane. Uncommonly, new infection leads to *progressive primary tuberculosis*. This complication occurs in patients who are overtly immunocompromised or who have more subtle defects in host defenses, as is characteristic of malnourished individuals. Certain racial groups, such as the Inuit, also are more prone to the development of progressive primary tuberculosis. The incidence of progressive primary tuberculosis is particularly high in HIV-positive patients with significant immunosuppression (i.e., CD4+ T cell counts below 200 cells/μL). Immunosuppression results in an inability to mount a CD4+ T cell–mediated response that would contain the primary focus; because hypersensitivity and resistance are most often concomitant factors, the lack of a tissue hypersensitivity reaction results in the absence of the characteristic caseating granulomas (*nonreactive tuberculosis*) (see Fig. 13.35D).

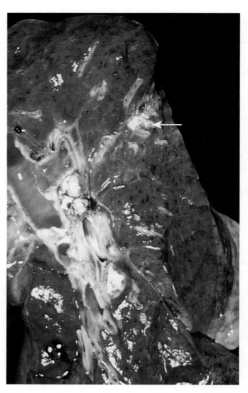

Fig. 13.34 Primary pulmonary tuberculosis, Ghon complex. The gray-white parenchymal focus (*arrow*) is under the pleura in the lower part of the upper lobe. Hilar lymph nodes with caseation are seen (*left*).

MORPHOLOGY

In countries in which bovine tuberculosis and infected milk have largely disappeared, primary tuberculosis almost always begins in the lungs. The inhaled bacilli usually implant in the distal air spaces of the lower part of the upper lobe or in the upper part of the lower lobe. They are typically close to the pleura. During the development of sensitization, a 1-cm to 1.5-cm area of gray-white inflammatory consolidation emerges. This is called the **Ghon focus.** In the majority of cases, the center of this focus undergoes caseous necrosis. Tubercle bacilli, either free or within phagocytes, travel via the lymphatic vessels to the regional lymph nodes, which also often caseate. This combination of parenchymal and nodal lesions is called the **Ghon complex** (Fig. 13.34). Lymphatic and hematogenous dissemination to other parts of the body also occurs during the first few weeks. Development of cell-mediated immunity controls the infection in approximately 95% of cases. Therefore, the Ghon complex undergoes progressive fibrosis, and calcification often follows (detectable as a **Ranke complex** on radiograph). Despite seeding of other organs, no lesions develop. Histologically, sites of infection are involved by a characteristic inflammatory reaction marked by the presence of caseating and noncaseating granulomas, which consist of epithelioid histiocytes and multinucleate giant cells (Fig. 13.35A to C).

Secondary Tuberculosis (Reactivation Tuberculosis)

Secondary tuberculosis is the pattern of disease that arises in a previously sensitized host. It may appear shortly after primary tuberculosis, but more commonly arises from reactivation of dormant primary lesions many decades

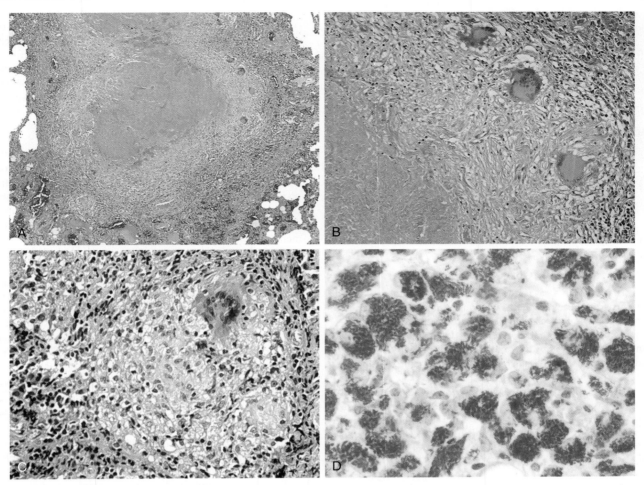

Fig. 13.35 The morphologic spectrum of tuberculosis. A characteristic tubercle at low magnification (A) and at higher power (B) shows central granular caseation surrounded by epithelioid and multinucleate giant cells. This is the usual response in individuals who develop cell-mediated immunity to the organism. (C) Occasionally, even in immunocompetent patients, tubercular granulomas may not show central caseation; hence, irrespective of the presence or absence of caseous necrosis, use of special stains for acid-fast organisms is indicated when granulomas are present. (D) In this specimen from an immunosuppressed patient, sheets of macrophages packed with mycobacteria are seen (acid-fast stain).

after initial infection, particularly when host resistance is weakened. It also may result from reinfection, which may occur either because the protection afforded by the primary disease has waned or because of exposure to a large inoculum of virulent bacilli. Whatever the source of the organism, only a few patients (<5%) with primary disease subsequently develop secondary tuberculosis.

Secondary pulmonary tuberculosis is classically localized to the apex of one or both upper lobes. The reason is obscure but may relate to high oxygen tension in the apices. Because of the preexistence of hypersensitivity, the bacilli excite a prompt and marked tissue response that tends to wall off the focus. As a result of this localization, the regional lymph nodes are less prominently involved early in the disease than they are in primary tuberculosis. On the other hand, cavitation occurs readily in the secondary form, leading to erosion into and dissemination along airways. Such changes become an important source of infectivity, because the patient now produces sputum containing bacilli.

Secondary tuberculosis should always be an important consideration in HIV-positive patients who present with pulmonary disease. Of note, although an increased risk for tuberculosis exists at all stages of HIV disease, the manifestations differ depending on the degree of immunosuppression. For example, patients with less severe immunosuppression (CD4+ T cell counts >300 cells/μL) present with "usual" secondary tuberculosis (apical disease with cavitation) while those with more advanced immunosuppression (CD4+ T cell counts below 200 cells/μL) present with a clinical picture that resembles progressive primary tuberculosis (lower and middle lobe consolidation, hilar lymphadenopathy, and noncavitary disease). The extent of immunosuppression also determines the frequency of extrapulmonary involvement, rising from 10% to 15% in mildly immunosuppressed patients to greater than 50% in those with severe immune deficiency.

MORPHOLOGY

The initial lesion usually is a small focus of consolidation, less than 2 cm in diameter, within 1 to 2 cm of the **apical pleura.** Such foci are sharply circumscribed, firm, gray-white to yellow areas that have a variable amount of central caseation and peripheral

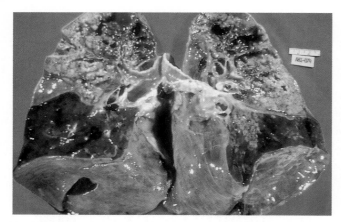

Fig. 13.36 Secondary pulmonary tuberculosis. The upper parts of both lungs are riddled with gray-white areas of caseation and multiple areas of softening and cavitation.

fibrosis. In favorable cases, the initial parenchymal focus undergoes progressive fibrous encapsulation, leaving only fibrocalcific scars. Histologically, the active lesions show characteristic coalescent tubercles with central caseation. Although tubercle bacilli can be demonstrated by appropriate methods in early exudative and caseous phases of granuloma formation, it is usually impossible to find them in the late, fibrocalcific stages.

Localized, apical, secondary pulmonary tuberculosis may heal with fibrosis either spontaneously or after therapy, or the disease may progress and extend along several different pathways. In **progressive pulmonary tuberculosis,** the apical lesion enlarges and the area of caseation expands. Erosion into a bronchus evacuates the caseous center, creating a ragged, **irregular cavity lined by caseous material** that is poorly walled off by fibrous tissue (Fig. 13.36). Erosion of blood vessels results in hemoptysis. With adequate treatment, the process may be arrested, although healing by fibrosis often distorts the pulmonary architecture. Irregular cavities, now free of caseous necrosis, may remain intact or collapse and become fibrotic. If the treatment is inadequate or host defenses are impaired, the infection may spread by direct extension and by dissemination through airways, lymphatic channels, and the vascular system. **Miliary pulmonary disease** occurs when organisms reach the bloodstream through lymphatic vessels and then recirculate to the lung via the pulmonary arteries. The lesions appear as small (2-mm) foci of yellow-white consolidation scattered through the lung parenchyma (the word *miliary* is derived from the resemblance of these foci to millet seeds). With progressive pulmonary tuberculosis, the pleural cavity is invariably involved and serous **pleural effusions, tuberculous empyema,** or **obliterative fibrous pleuritis** may develop.

Endobronchial, endotracheal, and **laryngeal tuberculosis** may develop when infective material is spread either through lymphatic channels or from expectorated infectious material. The mucosal lining may be studded with minute granulomatous lesions, sometimes apparent only on microscopic examination.

Systemic miliary tuberculosis ensues when the organisms disseminate hematogenously throughout the body. Systemic miliary tuberculosis is most prominent in the liver, bone marrow, spleen, adrenal glands, meninges, kidneys, fallopian tubes, and epididymis (Fig. 13.37).

Isolated-organ tuberculosis may appear in any one of the organs or tissues seeded hematogenously and may be the presenting manifestation of tuberculosis. Organs typically involved include the meninges (tuberculous meningitis), kidneys (renal tuberculosis), adrenal glands, bones (osteomyelitis), and fallopian tubes (salpingitis). When the vertebrae are affected, the condition is referred to as **Pott disease.** Paraspinal "cold" abscesses containing necrotic tissues may track along the tissue planes to present as an abdominal or pelvic mass.

Lymphadenitis is the most frequent form of extrapulmonary tuberculosis, usually occurring in the cervical region ("scrofula"). Lymphadenopathy tends to be unifocal, and most patients do not have concurrent extranodal disease. HIV-positive patients, on the other hand, almost always have multifocal disease, systemic symptoms, and either pulmonary or other organ involvement by active tuberculosis.

In years past, **intestinal tuberculosis** contracted by the drinking of contaminated milk was fairly common as a primary focus of tuberculosis. In developed countries today, intestinal tuberculosis is more often a complication of protracted advanced secondary tuberculosis, secondary to the swallowing of coughed-up infective material. Typically, the organisms are trapped in mucosal lymphoid aggregates of the small and large bowel, which then undergo inflammatory enlargement with ulceration of the overlying mucosa, particularly in the ileum.

The many patterns of tuberculosis are depicted in Fig. 13.38.

Clinical Features

Localized secondary tuberculosis may be asymptomatic. When manifestations appear, they are usually insidious in onset, with gradual development of both systemic and localizing symptoms and signs. Systemic manifestations, probably related to the release of cytokines by activated macrophages (e.g., TNF and IL-1), often appear early in the disease course and include malaise, anorexia, weight loss, and fever. Commonly, the fever is low grade and remittent (appearing late each afternoon and then subsiding), and night sweats occur. With progressive pulmonary involvement, increasing amounts of sputum, at first mucoid and later purulent, appear. When cavitation is present, the sputum contains tubercle bacilli. Some degree of hemoptysis

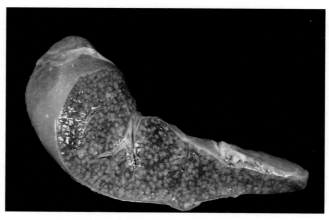

Fig. 13.37 Miliary tuberculosis of the spleen. The cut surface shows numerous gray-white granulomas.

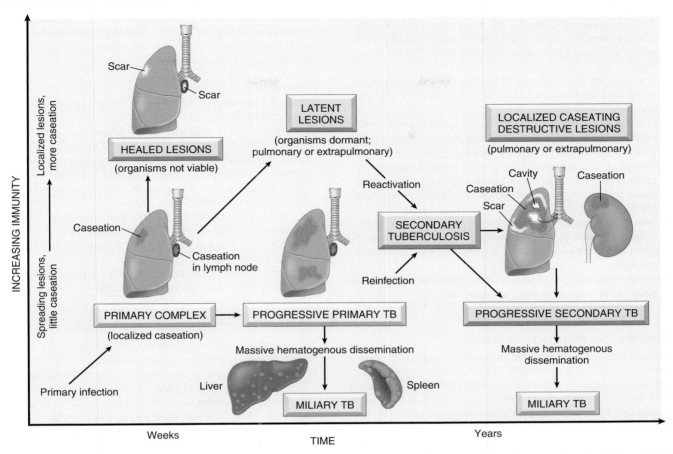

Fig. 13.38 The natural history and spectrum of tuberculosis. *(Adapted from a sketch provided by Dr. R.K. Kumar, The University of New South Wales, School of Pathology, Sydney, Australia.)*

is present in about half of all cases of pulmonary tuberculosis. Pleuritic pain may result from extension of the infection to the pleural surfaces. Extrapulmonary manifestations of tuberculosis are legion and depend on the organ system involved (e.g., tuberculous salpingitis may present as infertility, tuberculous meningitis with headache and neurologic deficits, Pott disease with back pain and paraplegia). The diagnosis of pulmonary disease is based in part on the history and on physical and radiographic findings of consolidation or cavitation in the apices of the lungs. Ultimately, however, tubercle bacilli must be identified.

The most common methodology for diagnosis of tuberculosis remains demonstration of acid-fast organisms in sputum by staining or by use of fluorescent auramine rhodamine. Conventional cultures for mycobacteria require up to 10 weeks, but liquid media–based radiometric assays that detect mycobacterial metabolism are able to provide an answer within 2 weeks. PCR amplification can be performed on liquid media with growth, as well as on tissue sections, to identify the mycobacterium. However, culture remains the standard diagnostic modality because it can identify the occasional PCR-negative case and also allows testing of drug susceptibility. Of concern, multidrug resistance (MDR), defined as resistance of mycobacteria to two or more of the primary drugs used for treatment of tuberculosis, is becoming more common, and the WHO estimated that 500,000 individuals were newly infected with

multidrug-resistant tuberculosis in 2014. This represents approximately 3% of new cases and 20% of previously treated cases. The epicenter of this troubling epidemic lies in Eastern Europe and Russia, where in some locales up to 20% of new infections are with multidrug-resistant strains. Of even greater concern, approximately 5% to 10% of such cases exhibit extensive multidrug resistance, defined by resistance to a broad spectrum of antibiotics in current use against tuberculosis.

The prognosis is determined by the extent of the infection (localized versus widespread), the immune status of the host, and the antibiotic sensitivity of the organism. Understandably, the prognosis is guarded in those with multidrug-resistant tuberculosis. Amyloidosis may develop in persistent cases.

SUMMARY

TUBERCULOSIS

- Tuberculosis is a chronic granulomatous disease caused by *M. tuberculosis*, usually affecting the lungs, but virtually any extrapulmonary organ can be involved.
- Initial exposure to mycobacteria results in development of a cellular immune response that confers resistance and leads to hypersensitivity (as determined by a positive result on the tuberculin skin test).

- The T_H1 subset of CD4+ T cells has a crucial role in cell-mediated immunity against mycobacteria; mediators of inflammation and bacterial containment include IFN-γ, TNF, and nitric oxide.
- The histopathologic hallmark of host reaction to tuberculosis in immunocompetent individuals is the presence of granulomas, usually with caseous necrosis.
- Primary pulmonary tuberculosis in immunocompetent individuals is asymptomatic and results only in healed lesions, typically in a sub-pleural focus and a draining lymph node.
- Secondary (reactivation) tuberculosis arises in previously exposed individuals when host immune defenses are compromised, and usually manifests as cavitary lesions in the lung apices.
- Both progressive primary tuberculosis and secondary tuberculosis can result in systemic seeding, causing life-threatening forms of disease such as miliary tuberculosis and tuberculous meningitis.
- HIV-seropositive status is an important risk factor for development or recrudescence of active tuberculosis.

Nontuberculous Mycobacterial Disease

Nontuberculous mycobacteria most commonly cause chronic, localized pulmonary disease in immunocompetent individuals. In the United States, strains implicated most frequently include *Mycobacterium avium-intracellulare* (also called *M. avium* complex), *Mycobacterium kansasii,* and *Mycobacterium abscessus.* It is not uncommon for nontuberculous mycobacterial infection to manifest as upper-lobe cavitary disease, mimicking tuberculosis, especially in patients with a long history of smoking or alcohol abuse. Concomitant chronic pulmonary disease (COPD, cystic fibrosis, pneumoconiosis) is often present.

In immunosuppressed individuals (primarily HIV-seropositive patients), *M. avium* complex infection manifests as a disseminated disease associated with systemic signs and symptoms (fever, night sweats, weight loss). Hepatosplenomegaly and lymphadenopathy, signifying involvement of the mononuclear phagocyte system by the opportunistic pathogen, is common, as are gastrointestinal symptoms such as diarrhea and malabsorption. Pulmonary involvement is often indistinguishable from tuberculosis in patients with AIDS. Disseminated *M. avium* complex infection in patients with AIDS tends to occur late in the clinical course, when CD4+ T cell counts have fallen below 100 cells/μL. Hence, tissue examination usually does not reveal granulomas; instead, foamy macrophages "stuffed" with atypical mycobacteria typically are seen.

Histoplasmosis, Coccidioidomycosis, and Blastomycosis

Infections caused by dimorphic fungi, which include *Histoplasma capsulatum, Coccidioides immitis,* and *Blastomyces dermatitidis,* manifest either with isolated pulmonary involvement, as commonly seen in infected immunocompetent individuals, or with disseminated disease in immunocompromised individuals. T cell–mediated immune responses are critical for containing the infection, so individuals with compromised cell-mediated immunity,

such as those with HIV, are prone to systemic disease. In part because of the overlap in clinical presentations, infectious diseases due to all three dimorphic fungi are considered together in this section.

Epidemiology

Each of the dimorphic fungi has a typical geographic distribution, as follows:

- *H. capsulatum* is endemic in the Ohio and central Mississippi River valleys and along the Appalachian Mountains in the southeastern United States. Warm, moist soil containing droppings from bats and birds provides an ideal medium for the growth of the mycelial form, which produces infectious spores.
- *C. immitis* is endemic in the southwestern and far western regions of the United States, particularly in California's San Joaquin Valley, where coccidial infection is known as "valley fever."
- *B. dermatitidis* has a distribution in the United States that overlaps with those in which histoplasmosis is found.

MORPHOLOGY

The yeast forms are fairly distinctive, which helps in the identification of individual fungi in tissue sections:
- *H. capsulatum:* round to oval, small yeast forms measuring 2 to 5 μm in diameter (Fig. 13.39A)
- *C. immitis:* thick-walled, nonbudding spherules, 20 to 60 μm in diameter, often filled with small endospores (see Fig. 13.39B)
- *B. dermatitidis:* round to oval and larger yeast forms than *Histoplasma* (5 to 25 μm in diameter) that reproduce by characteristic broad-based budding (see Fig. 13.39C and D)

Clinical Features

Clinical manifestations may take the form of (1) *acute (primary) pulmonary infection,* (2) *chronic (granulomatous) pulmonary disease,* or (3) *disseminated miliary disease.* The primary pulmonary nodules, composed of aggregates of macrophages filled with organisms, are associated with similar lesions in the regional lymph nodes. These lesions evolve into small granulomas complete with giant cells and may develop central necrosis and later fibrosis and calcification. The similarity to primary tuberculosis is striking, and differentiation requires identification of the yeast forms (best seen with silver stains). The clinical symptoms and signs resemble those of a "flulike" syndrome and are most often self-limited. In the vulnerable host, chronic cavitary pulmonary disease develops, with a predilection for the upper lobe, resembling the secondary form of tuberculosis. It is not uncommon for these fungi to give rise to perihilar mass lesions that resemble bronchogenic carcinoma radiologically. At this stage, manifestations may include cough, hemoptysis, and even dyspnea and chest pain.

In infants or immunocompromised adults, particularly those with HIV infection, disseminated disease (analogous to miliary tuberculosis) may develop. Under these circumstances, there are no well-formed granulomas. Instead, focal collections of phagocytes containing yeast forms are seen within the liver, spleen, lymph nodes, lymphoid tissue of the gastrointestinal tract, and bone marrow. The adrenal glands and meninges also may be involved, and in

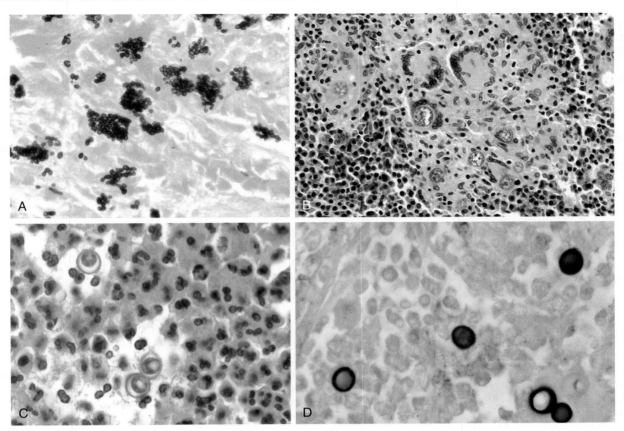

Fig. 13.39 (A) *Histoplasma capsulatum* yeast forms fill phagocytes in a lymph node of a patient with disseminated histoplasmosis (silver stain). (B) Coccidioidomycosis with intact spherules within multinucleated giant cells. (C) Blastomycosis, with rounded budding yeasts, larger than neutrophils. Note the characteristic thick wall and nuclei (not seen in other fungi). (D) Silver stain highlights the broad-based budding seen in *Blastomyces immitis* organisms.

a minority of cases, ulcers form in the nose and mouth, on the tongue, or in the larynx. Disseminated disease produces a febrile illness marked by hepatosplenomegaly, anemia, leukopenia, and thrombocytopenia. Cutaneous infections with disseminated *Blastomyces* organisms frequently induce striking epithelial hyperplasia, which may be mistaken for squamous cell carcinoma.

Pneumonia in the Immunocompromised Host

The appearance of a pulmonary infiltrate and signs of infection (e.g., fever) are some of the most common and serious complications in individuals with immune systems that are suppressed by disease, immunosuppressive drugs, or therapeutic irradiation. A wide variety of "opportunistic" pathogens, many of which rarely cause infection in normal individuals, can cause infections in these settings, and often more than one agent is involved. The more common pulmonary pathogens include (1) bacteria *(P. aeruginosa, Mycobacterium* spp., *L. pneumophila,* and *Listeria monocytogenes);* (2) viruses (cytomegalovirus and herpesvirus); and (3) fungi *(P. jiroveci, Candida* spp., *Aspergillus* spp., and *Cryptococcus neoformans).*

Cytomegalovirus Infection

Infection by cytomegalovirus (CMV), a member of the herpesvirus family, may manifest in various forms, depending partly on the age and the immune status of the host. Cells infected by the virus exhibit gigantism of both the cytoplasm and the nucleus. The nucleus typically contains a large inclusion surrounded by a clear halo ("owl's eye"), which gives the name to the classic form of symptomatic disease that occurs in neonates—*cytomegalic inclusion disease.* Although classic cytomegalic inclusion disease involves many organs, CMV infections are discussed here because in immunosuppressed adults, particularly patients with AIDS and recipients of allogeneic hematopoietic stem cell transplants, CMV pneumonitis is a serious problem.

Transmission of CMV can occur by several mechanisms, depending on the age group:

- A fetus can be infected transplacentally from a newly acquired or reactivated infection in the mother (*congenital* CMV infection).
- The virus can be transmitted to the infant through cervical or vaginal secretions at birth, or later through the breast milk of a mother with an active infection (*perinatal* CMV infection).
- Preschool children, especially in day care centers, can acquire it through saliva. Toddlers so infected readily transmit the virus to their parents.
- In patients older than 15 years of age, the venereal route is the dominant mode of transmission, but spread also may occur through contact with respiratory secretions and by the fecal-oral route.
- Iatrogenic transmission can occur at any age through organ transplantation or blood transfusion.

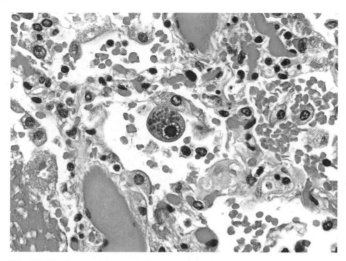

Fig. 13.40 Cytomegalovirus infection of the lung. A distinct nuclear inclusion and multiple cytoplasmic inclusions are seen in an enlarged cell.

MORPHOLOGY

Histologically, the characteristic enlargement of CMV-infected cells is readily appreciated. In the glandular organs, the parenchymal epithelial cells are affected; in the brain, the neurons; in the lungs, the alveolar macrophages and epithelial and endothelial cells; and in the kidneys, the tubular epithelial and glomerular endothelial cells. **Infected cells are strikingly enlarged, often to a diameter of 40 μm, and exhibit cellular and nuclear pleiomorphism.** Prominent intranuclear basophilic inclusions spanning half the nuclear diameter are usually set off from the nuclear membrane by a clear halo (Fig. 13.40). Within the cytoplasm of these cells, smaller basophilic inclusions also may be seen.

Cytomegalovirus Mononucleosis

In healthy young children and adults, the disease is nearly always asymptomatic. In surveys around the world, 50% to 100% of adults demonstrate anti-CMV antibodies in the serum, indicating previous exposure. The most common clinical manifestation of CMV infection in immunocompetent hosts beyond the neonatal period is an infectious mononucleosis–like illness marked by fever, atypical lymphocytosis, lymphadenopathy, and hepatomegaly accompanied by abnormal liver function test results, suggesting mild hepatitis. Most patients recover from CMV mononucleosis without any sequelae, although excretion of the virus may occur in body fluids for months to years. Irrespective of the presence or absence of symptoms after infection, an individual who is once infected becomes seropositive for life. The virus remains latent within leukocytes, which are the major reservoirs.

Cytomegalovirus Infection in Immunosuppressed Individuals

Immunosuppression-related CMV infection occurs most commonly in recipients of transplants (such as heart, liver, kidney, lung, or hematopoietic stem cell) and in patients with AIDS. This can be either primary infection or reactivation of a latent infection. CMV is the most common opportunistic viral pathogen in AIDS.

In all of these settings, serious disseminated CMV infections primarily affect the lungs (pneumonitis), gastrointestinal tract (colitis), and retina (retinitis); the central nervous system usually is spared. In the lung, infection is associated with typical cytomegalic changes, mononuclear infiltrates, and foci of necrosis, which may progress to acute respiratory distress syndrome. Intestinal necrosis and ulceration can develop and may be extensive, leading to the formation of "pseudomembranes" (Chapter 15) and debilitating diarrhea. CMV retinitis, by far the most common form of opportunistic CMV disease, can occur either alone or in combination with involvement of the lungs and intestinal tract. Diagnosis of CMV infection is made by demonstration of characteristic viral inclusions in tissue sections, successful viral culture, rising anti-viral antibody titer, and qualitative or quantitative PCR assay–based detection of CMV DNA. The latter has revolutionized the approach to monitoring patients after transplantation.

Pneumocystis

P. jiroveci (previously *P. carinii*), an opportunistic infectious agent formerly considered to be a protozoan, is now classified as a fungus. Serologic evidence indicates that virtually all individuals are exposed to *Pneumocystis* during the first few years of life, but in most the infection remains latent. Reactivation with development of clinical disease occurs almost exclusively in immunocompromised individuals. Indeed, patients with AIDS are extremely susceptible to infection with *P. jiroveci*, and it also may infect severely malnourished infants and immunosuppressed individuals (especially after organ transplantation or in individuals receiving cytotoxic chemotherapy or corticosteroids). In patients with AIDS, the risk for acquiring *P. jiroveci* infections increases in inverse proportion to the CD4+ T cell count, with counts less than 200 cells/μL having a strong predictive value. *Pneumocystis* infection is largely confined to the lung, where it produces an interstitial pneumonitis.

MORPHOLOGY

Involved areas of the lung contain a characteristic **intraalveolar foamy, pink-staining exudate** with hematoxylin-eosin (H&E) stain ("cotton candy" exudate) (Fig. 13.41A). The septa are thickened by edema and a minimal mononuclear infiltrate. Special stains are required to visualize the organism. Silver stain of tissue sections reveals **round- to cup-shaped cysts** (4 to 10 μm in diameter) within the alveolar exudates (see Fig. 13.41B).

The diagnosis of *Pneumocystis* pneumonia should be considered in any immunocompromised patient with respiratory symptoms and abnormal findings on chest radiograph. Fever, dry cough, and dyspnea occur in 90% to 95% of patients, in whom radiographic evidence of bilateral perihilar and basilar infiltrates is typical. Hypoxia is frequent; pulmonary function studies show a restrictive lung defect. The most sensitive and effective method of diagnosis is to identify the organism in induced sputum or bronchoalveolar lavage fluid using immunofluorescence. If

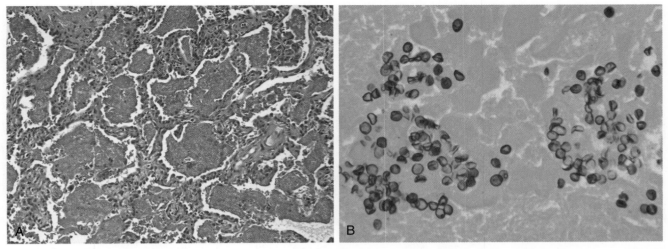

Fig. 13.41 Pneumocystis pneumonia. (A) The alveoli are filled with a characteristic foamy acellular exudate. (B) Silver stain demonstrates cup-shaped and round cysts within the exudate.

treatment is initiated before widespread involvement, the outlook for recovery is good; however, because residual organisms are likely to persist, particularly in patients with AIDS, relapses are common unless the underlying immunodeficiency is corrected or prophylactic therapy is given.

Opportunistic Fungal Infections

Candidiasis

Candida albicans is the most common disease-causing fungus. It is a normal inhabitant of the oral cavity, gastrointestinal tract, and vagina in many individuals. Systemic candidiasis (with associated pneumonia) is a disease restricted to immunocompromised patients that has protean manifestations.

MORPHOLOGY

In tissue sections, *C. albicans* demonstrates yeastlike forms (blastoconidia), pseudohyphae, and true hyphae (Fig. 13.42A). Pseudohyphae are an important diagnostic clue and represent budding yeast cells joined end to end at constrictions, thus simulating true fungal hyphae. The organisms may be visible with routine H&E stains, but a variety of special "fungal" stains (Gomori methenamine-silver, periodic acid–Schiff) commonly are used to better highlight the pathogens.

Clinical Features

Candidiasis can involve the mucous membranes, skin, and deep organs (invasive candidiasis). Among these varied presentations, the following merit brief mention:

- *Superficial infection on mucosal surfaces of the oral cavity (thrush).* This is the most common presentation. Florid proliferation of the fungi creates gray-white, dirty-looking pseudomembranes composed of matted organisms and inflammatory cells and tissue debris. Deep to

the surface, there is mucosal hyperemia and inflammation. Thrush is seen in newborns, debilitated patients, and children receiving oral corticosteroids for asthma, and after a course of broad-spectrum antibiotics that destroy competing normal bacterial flora. The other major risk group includes HIV-positive patients; patients with oral thrush not associated with an obvious underlying condition should be evaluated for HIV infection.

- *Vaginitis* is extremely common in women, especially those who are diabetic or pregnant or on oral contraceptive pills.

- *Esophagitis* is common in patients with AIDS and in those with hematolymphoid malignancies. These patients present with dysphagia (painful swallowing) and retrosternal pain; endoscopy demonstrates white plaques and pseudomembranes resembling those found on other mucosal surfaces.

- *Skin infection* can manifest in many different forms, including infection of the nail (*onychomycosis*), nail folds (*paronychia*), hair follicles (*folliculitis*), moist, intertriginous skin such as armpits or webs of the fingers and toes (*intertrigo*), and penile skin (*balanitis*). *Diaper rash* is a cutaneous candidal infection seen in the perineum of infants, in the region of contact with wet diapers.

- *Chronic mucocutaneous candidiasis* is a chronic refractory disease afflicting the mucous membranes, skin, hair, and nails; it is associated with a variety of underlying T cell defects. These in include *Job syndrome,* an inherited condition with a variety of abnormalitles including an defect in Th17 T cell responses, which are important in controlling fungal infections (Chapter 5).

- *Invasive candidiasis* implies blood-borne dissemination of organisms to various tissues or organs. Common patterns include (1) renal abscess, (2) myocardial abscess and endocarditis, (3) brain involvement (most commonly meningitis, but parenchymal microabscesses occur), (4) endophthalmitis (virtually any eye structure can be involved), (5) hepatic abscesses, and (6) *Candida* pneumonia, usually presenting with bilateral nodular infiltrates, resembling *Pneumocystis* pneumonia (see

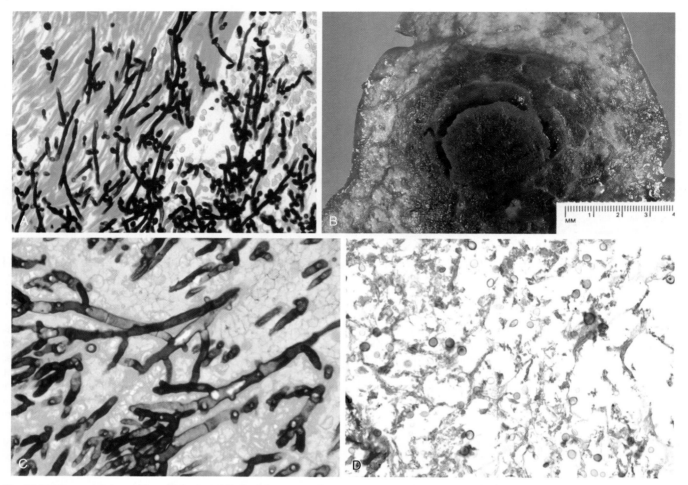

Fig. 13.42 The morphology of fungal infections. (A) Candida organism has pseudohyphae and budding yeasts (silver stain). (B) Invasive aspergillosis (gross appearance) of the lung in a hematopoietic stem cell transplant recipient. (C) Gomori methenamine-silver (GMS) stain shows septate hyphae with acute-angle branching, consistent with Aspergillus. (D) Cryptococcosis of the lung in a patient with AIDS. The organisms are somewhat variable in size. (B, *Courtesy of Dr. Dominick Cavuoti, Department of Pathology, University of Texas Southwestern Medical School, Dallas, Texas.*)

earlier). Patients with acute leukemias who are profoundly neutropenic after chemotherapy are particularly prone to the development of systemic disease. *Candida* endocarditis is the most common fungal endocarditis, usually occurring in patients with prosthetic heart valves or in intravenous drug abusers.

Cryptococcosis

Cryptococcosis, caused by *C. neoformans,* almost exclusively manifests as an opportunistic infection in immunocompromised hosts, particularly patients with AIDS or hematolymphoid malignancies.

MORPHOLOGY

The fungus, a 5- to 10-μm yeast, has a thick, gelatinous capsule and reproduces by budding (see Fig. 13.42D). Unlike in *Candida* infections, however, pseudohyphal or true hyphal forms are not seen. Identification of the capsule is a key diagnostic clue. In routine H&E stains, the capsule is not directly visible, but often a clear "halo" representing the area occupied by the capsule can be seen surrounding the individual fungi. India ink or periodic acid–Schiff staining effectively highlights the fungus. The capsular polysaccharide antigen is the substrate for the cryptococcal latex agglutination assay, which is positive in more than 95% of patients infected with the organism.

Clinical Features

Cryptococcosis usually manifests as pulmonary, central nervous system, or disseminated disease. Cryptococcus is most likely to be acquired by inhalation of aerosolized contaminated soil or bird droppings. The fungus initially localizes in the lungs and then disseminates to other sites, particularly the meninges. Sites of involvement are marked by a variable tissue response, which ranges from florid proliferation of gelatinous organisms with a minimal or absent inflammatory cell infiltrate (in immunodeficient hosts) to a granulomatous reaction (in the more reactive host). In the central nervous system these fungi grow in gelatinous masses within the meninges or expand the perivascular Virchow-Robin spaces, producing so-called "soap-bubble lesions."

The Opportunistic Molds

Mucormycosis and *invasive aspergillosis* are uncommon infections that are almost always limited to immunocompromised hosts, particularly those with hematolymphoid malignancies and profound neutropenia, those undergoing corticosteroid therapy, or following hematopoietic stem cell transplant recipients.

> ## MORPHOLOGY
>
> Mucormycosis is caused by the class of fungi known as *Zygomycetes*. *Rhizopus* and *Mucor* are the two fungi of medical importance within the Zygomycetes class. Their hyphae are **nonseptate** and branch at right angles; by contrast, the hyphae of *Aspergillus* organisms are **septate** and branch at more acute angles (see Fig. 13.42C). Both zygomycetes and *Aspergillus* cause a nondistinctive, suppurative, sometimes granulomatous reaction with a **predilection for invading blood vessel walls, causing hemorrhage, vascular necrosis and infarction** (see Fig. 13.42B).

Clinical Features

In *rhinocerebral* and *pulmonary mucormycosis,* zygomycetes have a propensity to colonize the nasal cavity or sinuses and then spread by direct extension into the brain, orbit, and other head and neck structures. Patients with diabetic ketoacidosis are most likely to develop a fulminant invasive form of rhinocerebral mucormycosis. Pulmonary disease can be localized (e.g., cavitary lesions) or may manifest radiologically with diffuse "miliary" involvement.

Invasive aspergillosis preferentially localizes to the lungs, and infection most often manifests as a necrotizing pneumonia (see Fig. 13.42B). Systemic dissemination, especially to the brain, is a complication that is often fatal.

Allergic bronchopulmonary aspergillosis occurs in patients with asthma who develop an exacerbation of symptoms caused by a type I hypersensitivity against the fungus growing in the bronchi. Such patients often have circulating IgE antibodies against *Aspergillus* and peripheral eosinophilia.

Aspergilloma ("fungus ball") formation occurs by fungal colonization of preexisting pulmonary cavities (e.g., dilated bronchi or lung cysts, posttuberculosis cavitary lesions). These masses may act as ball valves to occlude the cavity, thereby predisposing the patient to infection and hemoptysis.

Pulmonary Disease in Human Immunodeficiency Virus Infection

Pulmonary disease continues to be the leading contributor to morbidity and mortality in HIV-infected individuals. Although the use of potent anti-retroviral agents and effective chemoprophylaxis has markedly decreased the incidence and has improved outcomes, the plethora of entities involved makes diagnosis and treatment a distinct challenge.

- Despite the emphasis on "opportunistic" infections, it should be recognized that bacterial lower-respiratory tract infection caused by the "usual" pathogens is exceedingly common in HIV infection. The implicated organisms include *S. pneumoniae, S. aureus, H. influenzae,* and gram-negative rods. Bacterial pneumonias in HIV-infected individuals are more common, more severe, and more often associated with bacteremia than in those without HIV infection.
- Not all pulmonary infiltrates in HIV-infected individuals are infectious. A host of noninfectious diseases, including Kaposi sarcoma (Chapters 5 and 10), pulmonary non-Hodgkin lymphoma (Chapter 12), and primary lung cancer, occur with increased frequency and must be excluded.
- The CD4+ T cell count often is useful in narrowing the differential diagnosis. As a rule of thumb, bacterial and tubercular infections occur with mildly suppressed CD4+ counts (more than 200 cells/μL); *Pneumocystis* pneumonia usually occurs at CD4+ T cell counts below 200 cells/μL, while CMV and *M. avium* complex infections are uncommon until the very late stages of the disease (CD4+ T cell counts below 50 cells/μL).

Finally, an important point is that pulmonary disease in HIV-infected individuals may result from more than one cause, and that even common pathogens may be responsible for disease with atypical manifestations.

LUNG TUMORS

Roughly 95% of primary lung tumors are carcinomas; the remaining 5% span a miscellaneous group that includes carcinoids, mesenchymal malignancies (e.g., fibrosarcomas, leiomyomas), lymphomas, and a few benign lesions. The most common benign tumor is a spherical, small (1 to 4 cm), discrete "hamartoma" that often shows up as a so-called "coin lesion" on chest imaging. It consists mainly of mature cartilage admixed with fat, fibrous tissue, and blood vessels in various proportions. Clonal cytogenetic abnormalities have been demonstrated, indicating that it is actually a benign neoplasm and that the name hamartoma (which implies a developmental anomaly) is a misnomer.

Carcinomas

Carcinoma of the lung is the most important cause of cancer-related deaths in industrialized countries. It has long held this position among males in the United States, accounting for about one-third of cancer deaths in men, and has become the leading cause of cancer deaths in women as well. American Cancer Society estimates for 2016 include approximately 221,200 new cases of lung cancer and 158,040 deaths. The incidence among males is gradually decreasing, but it continues to increase among females, with more women dying each year from lung cancer than from breast cancers since 1987. These sobering

Table 13.6 Histologic Classification of Malignant Epithelial Lung Tumors (2015 WHO Classification, Simplified Version)

Adenocarcinoma
  Acinar, papillary, micropapillary, solid, lepidic predominant, mucinous subtypes
Squamous cell carcinoma
Large cell carcinoma
Neuroendocrine carcinoma
  Small cell carcinoma
  Large cell neuroendocrine carcinoma
  Carcinoid tumor
Mixed carcinomas
  Adenosquamous carcinoma
  Combined small cell carcinoma
Other unusual morphologic variants
  Sarcomatoid carcinoma
  Spindle cell carcinoma
  Giant cell carcinoma

statistics reflect the fact that the incidence of smoking in women increased markedly over the past half century. The peak incidence of lung cancer is in individuals in their fifties and sixties. At diagnosis, more than 50% of patients already have distant metastases, while an additional one-fourth have disease in the regional lymph nodes. The prognosis remains dismal: the 5-year survival rate for all stages of lung cancer combined is about 16%, a figure that has not changed much over the last 35 years; even with disease localized to the lung, the 5-year survival rate is only 45%.

The four major histologic types of carcinomas of the lung are adenocarcinoma, squamous cell carcinoma, small cell carcinoma (a subtype of neuroendocrine carcinoma), and large cell carcinoma (Table 13.6). In some cases, there is a combination of histologic patterns (e.g., small cell carcinoma and adenocarcinoma). Squamous cell and small cell carcinomas have the strongest association with smoking, but there is also an association with adenocarcinoma. In fact, possibly because of changes in smoking patterns in the United States, adenocarcinoma has replaced squamous cell carcinoma as the most common primary lung tumor in recent years. Adenocarcinomas also are by far the most common primary tumors arising in women, in never-smokers, and in individuals younger than 45 years of age.

Until recently, carcinomas of the lung were classified into two broad groups: small cell lung cancer (SCLC) and non–small cell lung cancer (NSCLC), the latter including adenocarcinoma, squamous and large cell carcinoma, and large cell neuroendocrine carcinomas. This classification has been recently replaced by a 2015 World Health Organization classification (a simplified version of which is shown in Table 13.6). The reason for this historic division is that virtually all SCLCs have metastasized by the time of diagnosis. Therefore, they are best treated with systemic chemotherapy, with or without radiation therapy. By contrast, NSCLCs are more likely to be resectable and usually respond poorly to conventional chemotherapy. However, therapies are now available that target specific oncoproteins that are found in a subset of NSCLC, mainly adenocarcinomas but also squamous cell carcinomas. Thus, if adequate tissue is available, NSCLC is subjected to molecular analysis to determine if targeted therapy is warranted. In addition, new immunotherapy approaches (checkpoint blockade, discussed in Chapter 6) are now approved for a subset of NSCLC and are being tested in SCLC.

Etiology and Pathogenesis

Like other cancers, smoking-related carcinomas of the lung arise by a stepwise accumulation of driver mutations that result in transformation of benign progenitor cells in the lung into neoplastic cells possessing all of the hallmarks of cancer. The sequence of molecular changes is not random but tends to follow a sequence that parallels the histologic progression toward cancer. Thus, inactivation of the putative tumor suppressor genes located on the short arm of chromosome 3 (3p) is a very common early event, whereas mutations in the *TP53* tumor suppressor gene and the *KRAS* oncogene occur relatively late. Certain genetic changes, such as loss of chromosomal material on 3p, are found even in benign bronchial epithelium of smokers without lung cancer, suggesting that large areas of the respiratory mucosa are mutagenized by exposure to carcinogens ("field effect"). On this fertile soil, those cells that accumulate additional mutations ultimately develop into cancer.

A subset of adenocarcinomas (about 10% in whites and 30% in Asians), particularly those arising in nonsmoking women, harbor mutations that activate the *epidermal growth factor receptor (EGFR)*, a receptor tyrosine kinase that stimulates downstream pro-growth pathways involving RAS, PI3K, and other signaling molecules. Of note, these tumors are sensitive to drugs that inhibit EGFR signaling, although the response is often short-lived. EGFR and KRAS mutations (in 30% of adenocarcinomas) are mutually exclusive, as might be expected since KRAS lies downstream of EGFR. Other "targetable" mutations have been described in a low frequency of adenocarcinomas (4% to 6% overall), including mutations that activate other tyrosine kinases, including ALK, ROS1, HER2, or c-MET. Each of these kinases is optimally targeted by a different drug, which has spurred a new era of "personalized" lung cancer treatment, in which the genetics of the tumor guide therapy.

With regard to carcinogenic influences, **there is strong evidence that cigarette smoking and, to a much lesser extent, other environmental carcinogens are the main culprits responsible for the mutations that give rise to lung cancers.** About 90% of lung cancers occur in active smokers or those who stopped recently. Moreover, there is a nearly linear correlation between the frequency of lung cancer and pack-years of cigarette smoking. The increased risk is 60 times greater among habitual heavy smokers (two packs a day for 20 years) than among nonsmokers. For unclear reasons, women are more susceptibile to carcinogens in tobacco smoke than men. Although cessation of smoking decreases the risk for developing lung cancer over time, it never returns to baseline levels, and genetic changes that predate the full development of lung cancer can persist for many years in the bronchial epithelium of former smokers. Passive smoking (proximity to cigarette smokers) also increases the risk for developing lung cancer, as does smoking of pipes and cigars, albeit only modestly.

Other carcinogenic influences associated with occupational exposures act in concert with smoking and may sometimes be responsible for lung cancer all by themselves; examples include work in uranium mines, work with asbestos, and inhalation of dusts containing arsenic, chromium, nickel, or vinyl chloride. A cardinal example of a synergistic interaction between two carcinogens is found in asbestos and tobacco smoking. Exposure to asbestos in nonsmokers increases the risk for developing lung cancer 5-fold, whereas in heavy smokers exposed to asbestos the risk is elevated approximately 55-fold.

Even though smoking and other environmental influences are paramount in the causation of lung cancer, not all individuals exposed to tobacco smoke develop cancer (about 11% of heavy smokers do). It is very likely that the mutagenic effect of carcinogens is modified by hereditary (genetic) factors. Recall that many chemicals require metabolic activation via the P-450 monooxygenase enzyme system for conversion into ultimate carcinogens (Chapter 6). Individuals with certain polymorphisms involving the P-450 genes have an increased capacity to activate procarcinogens found cigarette smoke, and are thus exposed to larger doses of carcinogens and incur a greater risk of developing lung cancer. Similarly, individuals whose peripheral blood lymphocytes undergo chromosomal breakages after exposure to tobacco-related carcinogens (mutagen sensitive genotype) have a greater than 10-fold increased risk for developing lung cancer over control subjects.

By analogy to the adenoma–carcinoma sequence in the colon, it is proposed that some invasive adenocarcinomas of the lung arise through an atypical adenomatous hyperplasia–adenocarcinoma in situ–invasive adenocarcinoma sequence. Studies of lung injury models in mice have identified a population of multipotent cells at the bronchioloalveolar duct junction, termed *bronchioalveolar stem cells (BASCs)*. After lung injury, multipotent BASCs proliferate and replenish the normal cell types (bronchiolar Clara cells and alveolar cells) found in this location, thereby facilitating epithelial regeneration. It is postulated that BASCs incur the initiating hit (for example, a somatic *KRAS* mutation) that enables these cells to escape normal "checkpoint" mechanisms and results in pulmonary adenocarcinomas.

The sequential changes leading development of squamous cell carcinomas are well documented; there is a linear correlation between the intensity of exposure to cigarette smoke and the appearance of ever more worrisome epithelial changes that begin with rather innocuous basal cell hyperplasia and squamous metaplasia and progress to squamous dysplasia and carcinoma in situ, before culminating in invasive cancer.

MORPHOLOGY

Carcinomas of the lung begin as small lesions that typically are firm and gray-white. They may arise as intraluminal masses, invade the bronchial mucosa, or form large bulky masses pushing into adjacent lung parenchyma. **Adenocarcinomas** are usually **peripherally located,** but also may occur closer to the hilum. In general, adenocarcinomas grow slowly and form smaller masses than do the other subtypes, but they tend to metastasize widely

at an early stage. They may assume a variety of growth patterns, including **acinar (gland-forming)** (Fig. 13.43C); **papillary; mucinous** which is often multifocal and may manifest as pneumonia-like consolidation); and **solid types.** The solid variant often requires demonstration of intracellular mucin by special stains to establish its adenocarcinomatous differentiation.

The putative precursor of adenocarcinoma is **atypical adenomatous hyperplasia** (AAH) (see Fig. 13.43A), which is thought to progress in a stepwise fashion to adenocarcinoma in situ, minimally invasive adenocarcinoma (<3 cm in diameter with an invasive component of <5 mm), and invasive adenocarcinoma (a tumor of any size with an area of invasion >5 mm). AAH appears as a well-demarcated focus of epithelial proliferation (with a diameter of 5 mm or less) composed of cuboidal to low-columnar cells that demonstrate nuclear hyperchromasia, pleomorphism, and prominent nucleoli. Genetic analyses have shown that AAH is monoclonal and shares many molecular aberrations with adenocarcinomas (e.g., *KRAS* mutations).

Adenocarcinoma in situ (AIS) (formerly bronchioloalveolar carcinoma), often involves peripheral parts of the lung as a single nodule. The key features of AIS are diameter of 3 cm or less, growth along preexisting structures, and preservation of alveolar architecture (see Fig. 13.43B). The tumor cells, which may be nonmucinous, mucinous, or mixed, grow in a monolayer along the alveolar septa, which serve as a scaffold. By definition, AIS does not demonstrate destruction of alveolar architecture or stromal invasion with desmoplasia, features that would merit the diagnosis of invasive adenocarcinoma.

Squamous cell carcinomas are more common in men than in women and are closely correlated with a smoking history; they tend to **arise centrally in major bronchi** and eventually spread to local hilar nodes, but they disseminate outside the thorax later than do other histologic types. Large lesions may undergo central necrosis, giving rise to **cavitation.** The preneoplastic lesions that antedate, and usually accompany, invasive squamous cell carcinoma are well characterized. Squamous cell carcinomas often are preceded by the development, over years, of **squamous metaplasia or dysplasia** in the bronchial epithelium, which then transforms to **carcinoma in situ,** a phase that may last for several years (Fig. 13.44). By this time, atypical cells may be identified in cytologic smears of sputum or in bronchial lavage fluids or brushings, although the lesion is asymptomatic and undetectable on radiographs. Eventually, the small neoplasm reaches a symptomatic stage, when a well-defined tumor mass begins to obstruct the lumen of a major bronchus, often producing distal atelectasis and infection. Simultaneously, the lesion invades surrounding pulmonary substance (Fig. 13.45A). On histologic examination, these tumors range from well-differentiated squamous cell neoplasms showing keratin pearls (see Fig. 13.45B) and intercellular bridges to poorly differentiated neoplasms exhibiting only minimal squamous cell features.

Large cell carcinomas are undifferentiated malignant epithelial tumors that lack the cytologic features of neuroendocrine carcinoma and show no evidence of glandular or squamous differentiation. The cells typically have large nuclei, prominent nucleoli, and moderate amounts of cytoplasm.

Small cell lung carcinomas (SCLCs) generally appear as pale gray, **centrally located masses** that extend into the lung parenchyma. These cancers are composed of relatively small tumor cells with a round to fusiform shape, scant cytoplasm, and finely granular chromatin with a salt and pepper

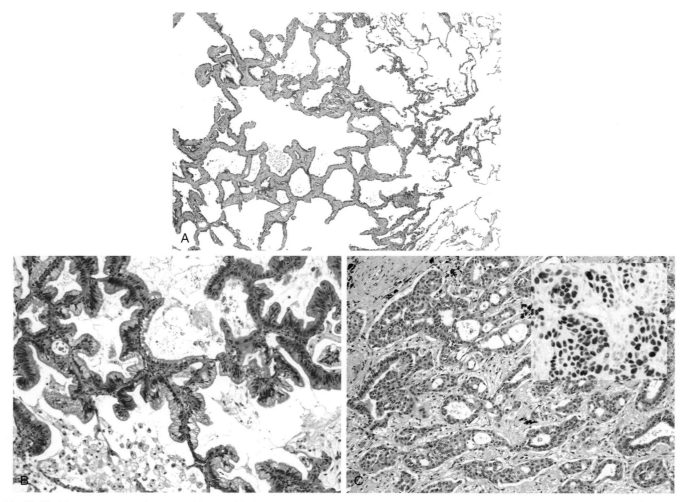

Fig. 13.43 Adenocarcinoma and associated lesions. (A) Atypical adenomatous hyperplasia with cuboidal epithelium and mild interstitial fibrosis. (B) Adenocarcinoma in situ, mucinous subtype, with characteristic growth along preexisting alveolar septa, without invasion. (C) Gland-forming adenocarcinoma; inset shows thyroid transcription factor 1 (TTF-1) positivity, which is seen in a majority of pulmonary adenocarcinomas.

appearance. Numerous mitotic figures are present (Fig. 13.46). Necrosis is invariably present and may be extensive. The tumor cells are fragile and often show fragmentation and "crush artifact" in small biopsy specimens. Another feature, best appreciated in cytologic specimens, is nuclear molding resulting from close apposition of tumor cells that have scant cytoplasm. These tumors express a variety of neuroendocrine markers (Table 13.7) and may secrete a host of polypeptide hormones that may result in paraneoplastic syndromes (see later). By the time of diagnosis, most will have metastasized to hilar and mediastinal lymph nodes. In the 2015 WHO Classification, SCLC is grouped together with large cell neuroendocrine carcinoma, another very aggressive tumor that exhibits neuroendocrine morphology and expresses neuroendocrine markers (synaptophysin, chromogranin, and CD56). **Mixed patterns** (e.g., adenosquamous carcinoma, mixed adenocarcinoma, small cell carcinoma) are seen in 10% or less of lung carcinomas.

Each of these lung cancer subtypes tends to spread to lymph nodes in the carina, the mediastinum, and the neck (scalene nodes) and clavicular regions, and, sooner or later, to distant sites. Involvement of the left supraclavicular node (Virchow node) is

particularly characteristic and sometimes calls attention to an occult primary tumor. These cancers, when advanced, often extend into the pleural or pericardial space, leading to inflammation and effusions. They may compress or infiltrate the superior vena cava to cause venous congestion or the vena caval syndrome. Apical neoplasms may invade the brachial or cervical sympathetic plexus, causing severe pain in the distribution of the ulnar nerve or Horner syndrome (ipsilateral enophthalmos, ptosis, miosis, and anhidrosis). Such apical neoplasms are sometimes called **Pancoast tumors,** and the combination of clinical findings is known as **Pancoast syndrome.** Pancoast tumor is often accompanied by destruction of the first and second ribs and sometimes the thoracic vertebrae. As with other cancers, tumor-node-metastasis (TNM) categories are used to indicate the size and spread of the primary neoplasm.

Clinical Features

Carcinomas of the lung are insidious lesions that in many cases have spread so as to be unresectable before they produce symptoms. In some instances chronic cough and

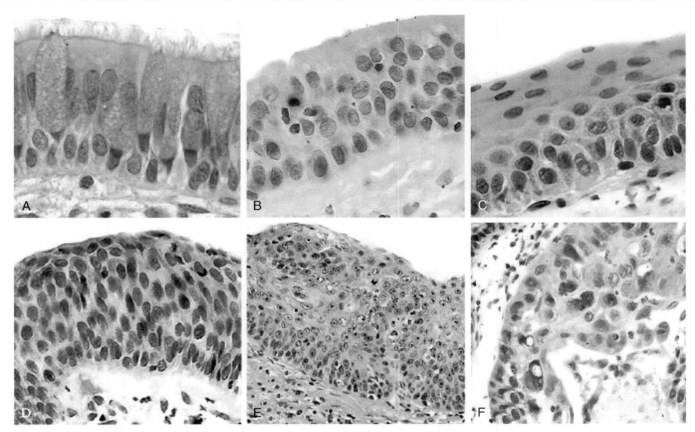

Fig. 13.44 Precursor lesions of squamous cell carcinomas. (A to C) Some of the earliest (and "mild") changes in smoking-damaged respiratory epithelium include goblet cell hyperplasia (A), basal cell (or reserve cell) hyperplasia (B), and squamous metaplasia (C). (D) More ominous changes include the appearance of squamous dysplasia, characterized by the presence of disordered squamous epithelium, with loss of nuclear polarity, nuclear hyperchromasia, pleomorphism, and mitotic figures. (E and F) Squamous dysplasia may, in turn, progress through the stages of mild, moderate, and severe dysplasia. Carcinoma in situ (CIS) (E) is the stage that immediately precedes invasive squamous cell carcinoma (F). Apart from the lack of basement membrane disruption in CIS, the cytologic features of CIS are similar to those in frank carcinoma. *(A to E, Courtesy of Dr. Adi Gazdar, Department of Pathology, University of Texas Southwestern Medical School, Dallas, Texas. F, Reproduced with permission from Travis WD, Colby TV, Corrin B, et al, editors:* World Health Organization histological typing of lung and pleural tumors, *Heidelberg, 1999, Springer.)*

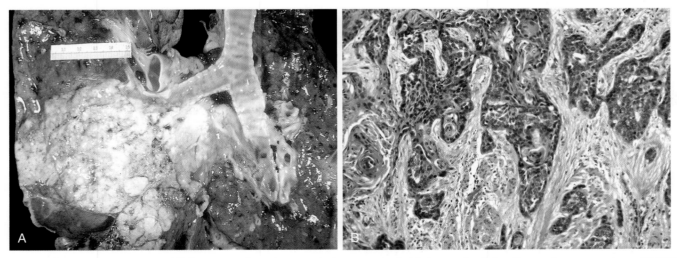

Fig. 13.45 Squamous cell carcinoma. (A) Squamous cell carcinoma appearing as a central (hilar) mass that is invading contiguous parenchyma. (B) Well-differentiated squamous cell carcinoma, showing keratinization and pearls.

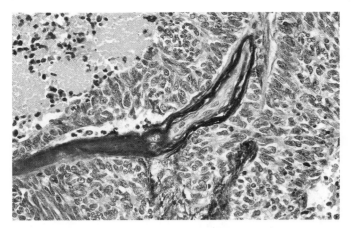

Fig. 13.46 Small cell carcinoma with small deeply basophilic cells and areas of necrosis *(top left)*. Note basophilic staining of vascular walls due to encrustation by DNA from necrotic tumor cells (Azzopardi effect).

expectoration call attention to localized, resectable disease. By the time other symptoms, such as hoarseness, chest pain, superior vena cava syndrome, pericardial or pleural effusion, or persistent segmental atelectasis or pneumonitis make their appearance, the prognosis is poor. Too often, the tumor presents with symptoms caused by metastatic spread to sites such as the brain (mental or neurologic changes), liver (hepatomegaly), or bones (pain). Although the adrenal glands may be nearly obliterated by metastatic disease, adrenal insufficiency (Addison disease) is uncommon, because islands of cortical cells sufficient to maintain adrenal function usually persist.

Overall, squamous cell carcinoma and adenocarcinoma carry a more favorable prognosis than SCLC. When squamous cell carcinomas or adenocarcinomas are detected before metastasis or local spread (as in high-risk patients undergoing surveillance imaging), cure is possible by lobectomy or pneumonectomy. Unresectable adenocarcinomas associated with targetable mutations in tyrosine kinases such as EGFR may show remarkable responses to specific inhibitors. A few of these patients have long-term remissions on the order of years, but relapse within months to a year or so is typical. Inevitably, resistant tumors are found to have new mutations that either alter the drug target themselves (e.g., an additional mutation in *EGFR* that prevents drug binding) or circumvent tumor dependence on the drug target. Much effort is currently being devoted to understanding the mechanisms of targeted drug resistance in order to develop strategies that prevent it from occurring. Immune checkpoint inhibitors produce responses in a subset of tumors, particularly those that are smoking related (perhaps because of a high burden of tumor

Table 13.7 Comparison of Small Cell Lung Carcinoma and Non–Small Cell Lung Carcinoma (Adenocarcinoma and Squamous Cell Carcinoma)

Feature	Small Cell Lung Carcinoma	Non–Small Cell Lung Carcinoma
Histology		
	Scant cytoplasm; small, hyperchromatic nuclei with fine chromatin pattern; nucleoli indistinct; diffuse sheets of cells	Abundant cytoplasm; pleomorphic nuclei with coarse chromatin pattern; nucleoli often prominent; glandular or squamous architecture
Neuroendocrine Markers		
For example, dense core granules on electron microscopy; expression of chromogranin, synaptophysin, and CD56	Present	Absent
Epithelial Markers		
Epithelial membrane antigen, carcinoembryonic antigen, and cytokeratin intermediate filaments	Present	Present
Mucin	Absent	Present in adenocarcinomas
Peptide hormone production	Adrenocorticotropic hormone, anti-diuretic hormone, gastrin-releasing peptide, calcitonin	Parathyroid hormone–related peptide (PTH-rp) in squamous cell carcinoma
Tumor Suppressor Gene Abnormalities		
3p deletions	>90%	>80%
RB mutations	~90%	~20%
p16/CDKN2A mutations	~10%	>50%
TP53 mutations	>90%	>50%
Dominant Oncogene Abnormalities		
KRAS mutations	Rare	~30% (adenocarcinomas)
EGFR mutations	Absent	~20% (adenocarcinomas, nonsmokers, women)
ALK rearrangements	Absent	4%–6% adenocarcinomas, nonsmokers, often have signet ring morphology
Response to chemotherapy and radiotherapy	Often complete response but recur invariably	Incomplete

neoantigens), and represent a hopeful new avenue for therapy.

By contrast, the picture for SCLC unfortunately has changed little. SCLCs have invariably spread by the time they are detected, even if the primary tumor appears to be small and localized; thus, surgical resection is not a viable option. SCLCs are very sensitive to chemotherapy but invariably recur, and as of yet targeted therapies are unavailable. The median survival even with treatment remains only 1 year, and only 5% are alive at 10 years. Because these tumors have a very high mutation burden, they are likely to be immunogenic. Accordingly, immune checkpoint therapies have produced encouraging responses in patients with advanced SCLC.

In addition to the direct effects of the tumor cells, it is estimated that 3% to 10% of patients with lung cancer develop *paraneoplastic syndromes* (Chapter 6). These include (1) hypercalcemia caused by secretion of a parathyroid hormone–related peptide; (2) Cushing syndrome (from increased production of adrenocorticotropic hormone); (3) syndrome of inappropriate secretion of anti-diuretic hormone; (4) neuromuscular syndromes, including a myasthenic syndrome, peripheral neuropathy, and polymyositis; (5) clubbing of the fingers and hypertrophic pulmonary osteoarthropathy; and (6) coagulation abnormalities, including migratory thrombophlebitis, nonbacterial endocarditis, and disseminated intravascular coagulation. Hypercalcemia most often is encountered with squamous cell neoplasms, the hematologic syndromes with adenocarcinomas, and the neurologic syndromes with small cell neoplasms, but exceptions abound.

- Smoking is the most important risk factor for lung cancer.
- Precursor lesions include atypical adenomatous hyperplasia and adenocarcinoma in situ for adenocarcinomas and squamous dysplasia for squamous cancer.
- Tumors 3 cm or less in diameter characterized by pure growth along preexisting structures without stromal invasion are called adenocarcinoma in situ.
- SCLCs are best treated with chemotherapy, because almost all are metastatic at presentation. The other carcinomas may be curable by surgery if limited to the lung. Targeted therapies, such as EGFR inhibitor therapy for adenocarcinomas with EGFR mutations, can be effective, an excellent example of personalized cancer therapy. Immunotherapies are under development and show promise.
- Lung cancers commonly cause a variety of paraneoplastic syndromes.

Carcinoid Tumors

Carcinoid tumors are malignant tumors composed of cells that contain dense-core neurosecretory granules in their cytoplasm and, rarely, may secrete hormonally active polypeptides. They are best thought of a low-grade neuroendocrine carcinomas and are subclassified as typical or atypical; both are often resectable and curable. They occasionally occur as part of the multiple endocrine neoplasia syndrome (Chapter 20). Bronchial carcinoids occur in young adults (mean 40 years) and represent about 5% of all pulmonary neoplasms.

SUMMARY

CARCINOMA OF THE LUNG

- The three major histologic subtypes are adenocarcinoma (most common), squamous cell carcinoma, and small cell carcinoma, each of which is clinically and genetically distinct. Adenocarcinomas are the most common cancers overall and are especially common in women and in nonsmokers.

MORPHOLOGY

Most carcinoids originate in main bronchi and grow in one of two patterns: (1) an obstructing polypoid, spherical, intraluminal mass (Fig. 13.47A); or (2) a mucosal plaque penetrating the bronchial wall to fan out in the peribronchial tissue—the so-called **collar-button lesion.** Even penetrating lesions push into the lung substance along a broad front and are well demarcated. Peripheral carcinoids are less common. Although 5% to

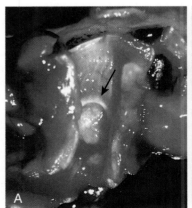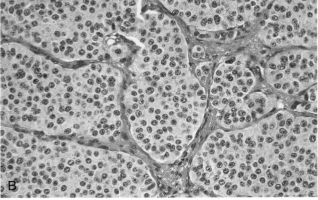

Fig. 13.47 Bronchial carcinoid. (A) Carcinoid growing as a spherical, pale mass *(arrow)* protruding into the lumen of the bronchus. (B) Histologic appearance demonstrating small, rounded, uniform nuclei and moderate cytoplasm. *(Courtesy of Dr. Thomas Krausz, Department of Pathology, University of Chicago Pritzker School of Medicine, Chicago, Illinois.)*

15% of carcinoids have metastasized to the hilar nodes at presentation, distant metastases are rare. Histologically, **typical carcinoids,** like their counterparts in the intestinal tract, are composed of nests of uniform cells that have regular round nuclei with "salt-and-pepper" chromatin, absent or rare mitoses and little pleomorphism (see Fig. 13.47B). **Atypical carcinoid** tumors display a higher mitotic rate and small foci of necrosis. These tumors have a higher incidence of lymph node and distant metastasis than typical carcinoids. Unlike typical carcinoids, the atypical tumors have *TP53* mutations in 20% to 40% of cases. Typical carcinoid, atypical carcinoid, and large cell neuroendocrine and small cell carcinoma can be viewed as a continuum of increasing histologic aggressiveness and malignant potential within the spectrum of pulmonary neuroendocrine neoplasms.

Most carcinoid tumors manifest with signs and symptoms related to their intraluminal growth, including cough, hemoptysis, and recurrent bronchial and pulmonary infections. Peripheral tumors are often asymptomatic and are discovered incidentally on chest radiographs. Only rarely do pulmonary carcinoids induce the *carcinoid syndrome,* characterized by intermittent attacks of diarrhea, flushing, and cyanosis. The reported 5- and 10-year survival rates for typical carcinoids are above 85%, while these rates drop to 56% and 35%, respectively, for atypical carcinoids.

PLEURAL LESIONS

Disease of the pleura usually is a complication of an underlying pulmonary disease. Secondary infections and pleural adhesions are common findings at autopsy. Important primary disorders are (1) primary intrapleural bacterial infections and (2) *malignant mesothelioma,* a primary neoplasm of the pleura.

Pleural Effusion and Pleuritis

Pleural effusions (fluids in the pleural space) can be either transudates or exudates. When the effusion is a transudate, the condition is termed *hydrothorax.* Congestive heart failure is the most common cause of bilateral hydrothorax. An exudate, characterized by protein content greater than 30 g/L and, often, inflammatory cells, suggests pleuritis. The four principal causes of *pleural exudate* formation are (1) microbial invasion through either direct extension of a pulmonary infection or blood-borne seeding (*suppurative pleuritis* or *empyema*); (2) cancer (lung carcinoma, metastatic neoplasms to the lung or pleural surface, mesothelioma); (3) pulmonary infarction; and (4) viral pleuritis. Other, less common causes of exudative pleural effusions are systemic lupus erythematosus, rheumatoid arthritis, and uremia, as well as previous thoracic surgery. Malignant effusions characteristically are large and frequently bloody (*hemorrhagic pleuritis*). Cytologic examination may reveal the malignant cells.

Whatever the cause, transudates and serous exudates usually are resorbed without residual effects if the inciting cause is controlled or remits. By contrast, fibrinous, hemorrhagic, and suppurative exudates may lead to fibrous organization, yielding adhesions or fibrous pleural thickenings that sometimes undergo calcification.

Pneumothorax, Hemothorax, and Chylothorax

Pneumothorax refers to presence of air or other gas in the pleural sac. It may occur in young, apparently healthy adults, usually men without any known pulmonary disease (simple or spontaneous pneumothorax), or as a result of some thoracic or lung disorder (secondary pneumothorax), such as emphysema or a fractured rib. Secondary pneumothorax is the consequence of rupture of any pulmonary lesion situated close to the pleural surface that allows inspired air to gain access to the pleural cavity. Responsible pulmonary lesions include emphysema, lung abscess, tuberculosis, carcinoma, and many other, less common processes. Mechanical ventilatory support with high pressure also may trigger secondary pneumothorax.

There are several possible complications of pneumothorax. A ball-valve leak may create a tension pneumothorax that shifts the mediastinum. Compromise of the pulmonary circulation may follow and may even be fatal. If the leak seals and the lung is not reexpanded within a few weeks (either spontaneously or through medical or surgical intervention), so much scarring may occur that it can never be fully reexpanded. In these cases, serous fluid collects in the pleural cavity, creating hydropneumothorax. With prolonged collapse, the lung becomes vulnerable to infection, as does the pleural cavity when communication between it and the lung persists. Empyema is thus an important complication of pneumothorax (pyopneumothorax).

Hemothorax, the collection of whole blood (in contrast with bloody effusion) in the pleural cavity, may be a complication of a ruptured intrathoracic aortic aneurysm, an event that is almost always fatal. With hemothorax, in contrast with bloody pleural effusions, the blood clots within the pleural cavity.

Chylothorax is a pleural collection of a milky lymphatic fluid containing microglobules of lipid. The total volume of fluid may not be large, but chylothorax is always significant because it implies obstruction of the major lymph ducts, usually by an intrathoracic cancer (e.g., a primary or secondary mediastinal neoplasm, such as a lymphoma).

Malignant Mesothelioma

Malignant mesothelioma has assumed great importance because it is highly related to exposure to airborne asbestos. It is a rare cancer of mesothelial cells, usually arising in the parietal or visceral pleura; it also occurs much less commonly in the peritoneum and pericardium. Approximately 80% to 90% of individuals with this cancer have a history of exposure to asbestos. Those who work directly with asbestos (shipyard workers, miners, insulators) are at greatest risk, but malignant mesotheliomas have appeared in individuals whose only exposure was living in proximity to an asbestos factory or being a relative of an asbestos worker. The latent period for developing malignant mesothelioma after the initial exposure is long, often 25 to 40 years, suggesting that causative driver mutations are acquired slowly, over a long period of time. As stated earlier, the combination of cigarette smoking and asbestos exposure greatly increases the risk for developing lung carcinoma, but it does not increase the risk for developing malignant mesothelioma.

Once inhaled, asbestos fibers remain in the body for life. Thus, the lifetime risk after exposure does not diminish over time (unlike with smoking, in which the risk decreases after cessation). It has been hypothesized that asbestos fibers preferentially gather near the mesothelial cell layer, where they generate reactive oxygen species that cause DNA damage and mutations. Sequencing of mesothelioma genomes has revealed multiple driver mutations, many of which cluster in pathways involved in DNA repair, cell cycle control, and growth factor signaling. Of interest, one of the most commonly mutated genes in sporadic mesothelioma, *BAP1*, encodes a tumor suppressor involved in DNA repair that also is affected by germ line mutations in families showing a high incidence of mesothelioma.

MORPHOLOGY

Malignant mesotheliomas are often preceded by extensive **pleural fibrosis and plaque formation,** readily seen on computed tomography scans. These tumors begin in a localized area and over time spread widely, either by contiguous growth or by diffuse seeding of pleural surfaces. At autopsy, the affected lung **typically is ensheathed by a layer of yellow-white, firm, variably gelatinous tumor** that obliterates the pleural space (Fig. 13.48). The neoplasm may directly invade the thoracic wall or the subpleural lung tissue, but distant metastases are uncommon. Normal mesothelial cells are biphasic, giving rise to pleural lining cells as well as the underlying fibrous tissue. In line with this potential, mesotheliomas conform to one of three morphologic appearances: (1) **epithelial,** in which cuboidal cells with small papillary buds line tubular and microcystic spaces (this is the most common pattern and also the one most likely to be confused with a pulmonary adenocarcinoma); (2) **sarcomatous,** in which spindled, occasionally fibroblastic-appearing cells grow in sheets; and (3) **biphasic,** having both sarcomatous and epithelial areas.

LESIONS OF THE UPPER RESPIRATORY TRACT

Acute Infections

Acute infections of the upper respiratory tract are among the most common afflictions of humans, most frequently manifesting as the "common cold." The clinical features are well known: nasal congestion accompanied by watery discharge; sneezing; scratchy, dry sore throat; and a slight increase in temperature that is more pronounced in young children. The most common pathogens are rhinoviruses, but coronaviruses, respiratory syncytial viruses, parainfluenza and influenza viruses, adenoviruses, enteroviruses, and sometimes even group A β-hemolytic streptococci have been implicated. In a significant number of cases (around 40%), the cause cannot be determined; perhaps new viruses will be discovered. Most of these infections occur in the fall and winter and are self-limiting (usually lasting for 1 week or less). In a minority of cases, colds may be complicated by the development of bacterial otitis media or sinusitis.

In addition to the common cold, infections of the upper-respiratory tract may produce signs and symptoms localized to the pharynx, epiglottis, or larynx. *Acute pharyngitis,* manifesting as a sore throat, may be caused by a host of agents. Mild pharyngitis with minimal physical findings frequently accompanies a cold and is the most common form of pharyngitis. More severe forms with tonsillitis, associated with marked hyperemia and exudates, occur with β-hemolytic streptococcal and adenovirus infections. Streptococcal tonsillitis is important to recognize and treat early, because of the associated potential for development of peritonsillar abscesses ("quinsy") or for progression to poststreptococcal glomerulonephritis and acute rheumatic fever. Coxsackievirus A infection may produce pharyngeal vesicles and ulcers (herpangina). Infectious mononucleosis, caused by Epstein-Barr virus (EBV), is an important cause of pharyngitis and bears the moniker of "kissing disease"—reflecting a common mode of transmission in previously nonexposed individuals.

Acute *bacterial epiglottitis* is a syndrome predominantly affecting young children who have an infection of the epiglottis caused by *H. influenzae,* in which pain and airway obstruction are the major findings. The onset is abrupt. Failure to appreciate the need to maintain an open airway for a child with this condition can have fatal consequences. The advent of vaccination against *H. influenzae* has greatly decreased the incidence of this disease.

Acute laryngitis can result from inhalation of irritants or may be caused by allergic reactions. It also may be caused

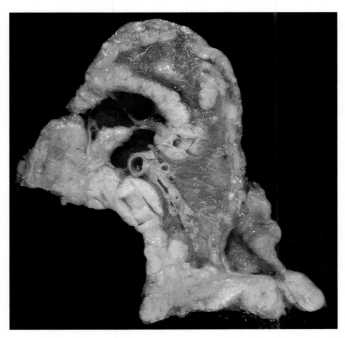

Fig. 13.48 Malignant mesothelioma. Note the thick, firm, white pleural tumor that ensheathes this bisected lung.

by agents that produce the common cold and usually involve the pharynx and nasal passages as well as the larynx. Brief mention should be made of two uncommon but important forms of laryngitis: *tuberculous* and *diphtheritic*. The former is almost always a consequence of protracted active tuberculosis, during which infected sputum is coughed up. Diphtheritic laryngitis has fortunately become uncommon because of the widespread immunization of young children against diphtheria toxin. After it is inhaled, *Corynebacterium diphtheriae* implants on the mucosa of the upper airways, where it elaborates a powerful exotoxin that causes necrosis of the mucosal epithelium, accompanied by a dense fibrinopurulent exudate, to create the classic superficial, dirty-gray pseudomembrane of diphtheria. The major hazards of this infection are sloughing and aspiration of the pseudomembrane (causing obstruction of major airways) and absorption of bacterial exotoxins (producing myocarditis, peripheral neuropathy, or other tissue injury).

In children, parainfluenza virus is the most common cause of laryngotracheobronchitis, more commonly known as *croup,* but other agents such as respiratory syncytial virus also may precipitate this condition. Although self-limited, croup may cause frightening inspiratory stridor and harsh, persistent cough. In occasional cases, the laryngeal inflammatory reaction may narrow the airway sufficiently to result in respiratory failure. Viral infections in the upper-respiratory tract predispose the patient to secondary bacterial infection, particularly by staphylococci, streptococci, and *H. influenzae.*

Nasopharyngeal Carcinoma

Nasopharyngeal carcinoma is a rare neoplasm that merits comment because of (1) the strong epidemiologic links to EBV and (2) the high frequency of this cancer among the Chinese, which raises the possibility of viral oncogenesis on a background of genetic susceptibility. It is thought that EBV infects the host by first replicating in the nasopharyngeal epithelium and then infecting nearby tonsillar B lymphocytes. In some individuals, this leads to transformation of the epithelial cells. Unlike the case with Burkitt lymphoma (Chapter 12), another EBV-associated tumor, the EBV genome is found in virtually all nasopharyngeal carcinomas, including those that occur outside the endemic areas in Asia.

The three histologic variants are keratinizing squamous cell carcinoma, nonkeratinizing squamous cell carcinoma, and undifferentiated carcinoma; the last-mentioned is the most common and the one most closely linked with EBV. The undifferentiated neoplasm is characterized by large epithelial cells with indistinct cell borders (reflecting "syncytial" growth) and prominent eosinophilic nucleoli. In nasopharyngeal carcinomas, the tumor cells are often accompanied by a striking influx of T cells, which are believed to be responding to viral antigens. Nasopharyngeal carcinomas invade locally, spread to cervical lymph nodes, and then metastasize to distant sites. They tend to be radiosensitive, and 5-year survival rates of 50% are reported, even for patients with advanced cancers. Responses to immune checkpoint inhibitors also have been reported, providing a new therapeutic strategy for tumors that do not respond to conventional therapy.

Laryngeal Tumors

A variety of nonneoplastic, benign, and malignant neoplasms of epithelial and mesenchymal origin may arise in the larynx, but only vocal cord nodules, papillomas, and squamous cell carcinomas are sufficiently common to merit comment. In all of these conditions, the most common presenting feature is hoarseness.

Nonmalignant Lesions

Vocal cord nodules ("polyps") are smooth, hemispherical protrusions (usually <0.5 cm in diameter) located, most often, on the true vocal cords. The nodules are composed of fibrous tissue and covered by stratified squamous mucosa that usually is intact but can be ulcerated from contact trauma with the other vocal cord. These lesions occur chiefly in heavy smokers or singers (singer's nodes), suggesting that they are the result of chronic irritation or over use.

Laryngeal papilloma or *squamous papilloma* of the larynx is a benign neoplasm, usually located on the true vocal cords, that forms a soft, raspberry like excrescence rarely more than 1 cm in diameter. Histologically, it consists of multiple slender, fingerlike projections supported by central fibrovascular cores and covered by an orderly, typical, stratified squamous epithelium. When the papilloma is on the free edge of the vocal cord, trauma may lead to ulceration that can be accompanied by hemoptysis.

Papillomas usually are single in adults but often are multiple in children, in whom the condition is referred to as *recurrent respiratory papillomatosis (RRP)*, since they typically tend to recur after excision. These lesions are caused by human papillomavirus (HPV) types 6 and 11 and often spontaneously regress at puberty. Cancerous transformation is rare. The most likely cause for their occurrence in children is vertical transmission from an infected mother during delivery. Therefore, the recent availability of an HPV vaccine that can protect women of reproductive age against infection with types 6 and 11 provides an opportunity for prevention of RRP in children.

Carcinoma of the Larynx

Carcinoma of the larynx represents only 2% of all cancers. It most commonly occurs after 40 years of age and is more common in men than in women (with a gender ratio of 7:1). Environmental influences are very important in its causation; nearly all cases occur in smokers, and alcohol and asbestos exposure also may play roles. Human papillomavirus sequences have been detected in about 15% of tumors, which tend to have a better prognosis than other carcinomas.

About 95% of laryngeal cancers are typical squamous cell carcinomas. Rarely, adenocarcinomas are seen, presumably arising from mucous glands. The tumor develops directly on the vocal cords (glottic tumors) in 60% to 75% of cases, but it also may arise above the cords (supraglottic; 25% to 40%) or below the cords (subglottic; <5%). Squamous cell carcinomas of the larynx begin as in situ lesions that later appear as pearly gray, wrinkled plaques on the

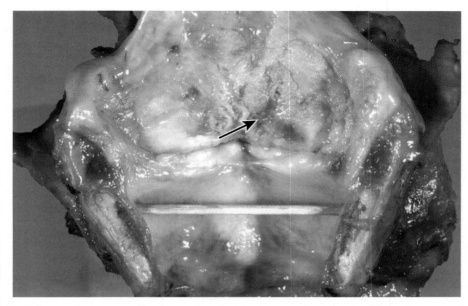

Fig. 13.49 Laryngeal squamous cell carcinoma *(arrow)* arising in a supraglottic location (above the true vocal cord).

mucosal surface, ultimately ulcerating and fungating (Fig. 13.49). The glottic tumors are usually keratinizing, well to moderately differentiated squamous cell carcinomas. As expected with lesions arising from recurrent exposure to environmental carcinogens, adjacent mucosa may demonstrate squamous cell hyperplasia with foci of dysplasia, or even carcinoma in situ.

Carcinoma of the larynx manifests clinically with persistent hoarseness. The location of the tumor within the larynx has a significant bearing on prognosis. For example, about 90% of glottic tumors are confined to the larynx at diagnosis. First, as a result of interference with vocal cord mobility, they develop symptoms early in the course of disease; second, the glottic region has a sparse lymphatic supply, and spread beyond the larynx is uncommon. By contrast, the supraglottic larynx is rich in lymphatic spaces, and nearly one-third of these tumors metastasize to regional (cervical) lymph nodes. The subglottic tumors tend to remain clinically quiescent, usually manifesting as advanced disease. With surgery, radiation therapy, or combination treatment, many patients can be cured, but about one-third die of the disease. The usual cause of death is widespread metastases and cachexia, sometimes complicated by pulmonary infection.

SUGGESTED READINGS

Armanios M, Blackburn EH: The telomere syndromes, *Nat Rev Genet* 13:693, 2013. [*A review of the role of telomere dysfunction in idiopathic pulmonary fibrosis and other diseases.*]

Ashley V, Harris CC: Biomarker development in the precision medicine era: lung cancer as a case study, *Nat Rev Cancer* 16:525, 2016. [*A discussion of the impact of targeted therapy on the diagnosis and treatment of lung cancer.*]

Best DH, Austin ED, Chung WK, et al: Genetics of pulmonary hypertension, *Curr Opin Cardiol* 29:520, 2014. [*A description of recent advances in genetic and molecular mechanisms in pulmonary hypertension.*]

Bittar HET, Yousem SA, Wenzel SE: Pathobiology of severe asthma, *Annu Rev Pathol* 10:511, 2015. [*A review addressing the pathobiology of severe asthma, inflammatory cells and pathways, the structural and remodeling changes, and targeted therapy.*]

Boyton RJ, Altmann DM: Bronchiectasis: current concepts in pathogenesis, immunology, and microbiology, *Annu Rev Pathol* 11:523, 2016. [*A review of bronchiectasis pathogenesis, focusing on interactions between host immunity and microorganisms.*]

Carmona EM, Kalra S, Ryu JH: Pulmonary sarcoidosis: diagnosis and treatment, *Mayo Clin Proc* 91:1946, 2016. [*A concise current review of a still enigmatic disorder.*]

Hogg JC, Timens W: The pathology of chronic obstructive pulmonary disease, *Annu Rev Pathol* 4:435, 2009. [*A still relevant review on the pathogenesis of COPD, stressing the roles of inflammation, tissue repair and remodeling, and small airway disease in COPD.*]

Lacasse Y, Girard M, Cormier Y: Recent advances in hypersensitivity pneumonitis, *Chest* 142:208, 2012. [*This review summarizes clinical and pathophysiologic aspects of hypersensitivity pneumonitis.*]

Leung CC, Yu ITS, Chen W: Silicosis, *Lancet* 379:2008, 2012. [*A review the pathogenesis of silicosis and its relationship to tuberculosis and lung cancer.*]

Meyers DA, Bleecker ER, Holloway JW, et al: Asthma genetics and personalized medicine, Lancet, *Respir Med* 2:405, 2014. [*A review of genetic markers that reveal possible triggers and treatment strategies for asthma.*]

Orme IM, Robinson RT, Cooper AM: The balance between protective and pathogenic immune responses in the TB-infected lung, *Nat Immunol* 16:57, 2015. [*A discussion of the delicate balance between host response, TB, immunity, and tissue damage.*]

Postma DS, Rabe KF: The asthma-COPD overlap syndrome, *N Engl J Med* 373:1241, 2015. [*A review comparing and contrasting COPD and asthma, highlighting shared and distinctive features.*]

Semenova EA, Nagel R, Berns A: Origins, genetic landscape, and emerging therapies of small cell lung cancer, *Genes Dev* 29:1447, 2015. [*A review of the pathobiology and new treatment strategies in small cell lung cancer.*]

Simonneau G, Gatzoulis MA, Adatia I, et al: Updated clinical classification of pulmonary hypertension, *J Am Coll Cardiol* 62(SupplD):34, 2013. [*A clinical classification based on pathologic and hemodynamic characteristics and therapeutic approaches.*]

Swanton C, Govinan R: Clinical implications of genomic discoveries in lung cancer, *N Engl J Med* 374:1864, 2016. [*A review focused on how* genomic insights into the pathogenesis of each major subtype of lung cancer have changed the clinical approach to patients with the disease.]

Sweatt AJ, Levitt JE: Evolving epidemiology and definitions of the acute respiratory distress syndrome and early acute lung injury, *Clin Chest Med* 35:609, 2014. [*A discussion of the impact of classification of ARDS into mild, moderate, and severe, with better definitions, prediction of mortality, and prevention and treatment strategies.*]

Travis WD, Brambilla E, Nicholson AG, et al: The 2015 World Health Organization Classification of Lung Tumors: impact of genetic, clinical and radiologic advances since the 2004 classification, *J Thorac Oncol* 6:244, 2011. [*The latest classification of lung tumors that incorporates updated clinical, radiologic, histologic, molecular, and prognostic features.*]

Travis WD, Costabel U, Hansell DM, et al: ATS/ERS Committee on Idiopathic Interstitial Pneumonias. An official American Thoracic Society/European Respiratory Society statement: update of the international multidisciplinary classification of the idiopathic interstitial pneumonias, *Am J Respir Crit Care Med* 188:733, 2013. [*An updated classification of interstitial lung diseases, which is used widely by clinicians, radiologists, and pathologists.*]

Kidney and Its Collecting System

14

Clinical Manifestations of Renal
 Diseases 549
Glomerular Diseases 550
Mechanisms of Glomerular Injury and
 Disease 552
Diseases Affecting Tubules and
 Interstitium 564
Tubulointerstitial Nephritis 564
Acute Tubular Injury/Necrosis 567
Diseases Involving Blood Vessels 569

Nephrosclerosis 569
Malignant Hypertension 570
Thrombotic Microangiopathies 571
Chronic Kidney Disease 572
Cystic Diseases of the Kidney 573
Simple Cysts 573
Autosomal Dominant (Adult) Polycystic Kidney
 Disease 574
Autosomal Recessive (Childhood) Polycystic
 Kidney Disease 575

Medullary Diseases With Cysts 575
Urinary Outflow Obstruction 576
Renal Stones (Urolithiasis) 576
Hydronephrosis 577
Congenital and Developmental
 Anomalies 578
Neoplasms 578
Neoplasms of the Kidney 578

The kidney is a structurally complex organ that has evolved to carry out a number of important functions: excretion of the waste products of metabolism, regulation of body water and salt, maintenance of acid balance, and secretion of a variety of hormones and prostaglandins. Diseases of the kidney are as complex as its structure, but their study is facilitated by dividing them into those that affect its four components: glomeruli, tubules, interstitium, and blood vessels. This traditional approach is useful because the early manifestations of diseases that affect each of these compartments tend to be distinctive. Furthermore, some structures seem to be more vulnerable to specific forms of renal injury; for example, glomerular diseases are often immunologically mediated, whereas tubular and interstitial disorders are more likely to be caused by toxic or infectious agents. However, some disorders affect more than one structure, and functional interdependence of structures in the kidney means that damage to one component almost always affects the others. Thus, severe glomerular damage impairs blood flow through the peritubular vascular system; conversely, tubular destruction, by increasing intraglomerular pressure and inducing the production of cytokines and chemokines, may lead to glomerular sclerosis. When chronic kidney disease progresses to its most advanced stage, so-called end-stage renal disease, all four compartments of the kidney are usually damaged. Due to the large functional reserve capacity of the kidney, early signs of kidney disease are often missed, and much renal damage may occur before renal dysfunction becomes clinically apparent. Before discussing individual diseases of the kidney, we describe clinical manifestations of kidney diseases shared by several disorders.

CLINICAL MANIFESTATIONS OF RENAL DISEASES

The clinical manifestations of renal disease can be grouped into reasonably well-defined syndromes. Some are peculiar to glomerular diseases, and others are shared by several renal disorders. Before we list the syndromes, a few terms must be defined.

- *Azotemia* is an elevation of blood urea nitrogen and creatinine levels and usually reflects a decreased glomerular filtration rate (GFR). GFR may be decreased as a consequence of intrinsic renal disease or extrarenal causes. *Prerenal azotemia* is encountered when there is hypoperfusion of the kidneys (usually due to reduced extracellular fluid volume). This decreases GFR in the absence of renal parenchymal damage and is usually reversible if the hypoperfusion is corrected in time. *Postrenal azotemia* results when urine outflow is obstructed. Relief of the obstruction is followed by correction of the azotemia.
- When azotemia gives rise to clinical manifestations and systemic biochemical abnormalities, it is termed *uremia*. Uremia is characterized not only by failure of renal excretory function but also by a host of metabolic and endocrine alterations incident to renal damage. In addition, there is secondary gastrointestinal (e.g., uremic gastroenteritis); neuromuscular (e.g., peripheral

neuropathy); and cardiovascular (e.g., uremic fibrinous pericarditis) involvement.

Below is a brief summary of the various clinical manifestations and syndromes of renal diseases with their defining features. The two most common syndromes associated with glomerular diseases, nephrotic and nephritic, are discussed in detail.

- *Nephrotic syndrome* is characterized by the following:
  - *Proteinuria,* with daily protein loss in the urine of 3.5 g or more in adults (said to be in the "nephrotic range")
  - *Hypoalbuminemia,* with plasma albumin levels less than 3 g/dL
  - *Generalized edema,* the most obvious clinical manifestation
  - *Hyperlipidemia* and lipiduria

    The nephrotic syndrome has diverse causes that share a common pathophysiology, a derangement in the capillary walls of the glomeruli that results in increased permeability to plasma proteins. Increased permeability of the glomerular basement membrane (GBM) may result from structural or physicochemical alterations in the GBM. With long-standing or heavy proteinuria, serum albumin is decreased, giving rise to hypoalbuminemia and a drop in plasma colloid osmotic pressure, which in turn leads to leakage of fluid from the blood into extravascular spaces. As discussed in Chapter 4, the resulting decrease in intravascular volume and renal blood flow triggers increased release of renin from renal juxtaglomerular cells. Renin in turn stimulates the angiotensin-aldosterone axis, which promotes the retention of salt and water by the kidney. This tendency is exacerbated by reductions in the cardiac secretion of natriuretic factors attributed to decreased intravascular volume. In the face of continuing proteinuria, salt and water retention further aggravates the edema and if unchecked may lead to the development of generalized edema (termed *anasarca*). At the onset, there is little or no azotemia, hematuria, or hypertension.

    The genesis of the hyperlipidemia is more obscure. Presumably, hypoalbuminemia triggers increased synthesis of lipoproteins in the liver, or massive proteinuria causes loss of an inhibitor of their synthesis. There also is abnormal transport of circulating lipid particles and impairment of peripheral breakdown of lipoproteins. The associated lipiduria reflects the increased permeability of the GBM to lipoproteins.

    The most important of the primary glomerular lesions that characteristically lead to the nephrotic syndrome are focal segmental glomerulosclerosis and minimal-change disease. The latter is more important in children; the former is more important in adults. The nephrotic syndrome is also commonly seen in two other primary kidney diseases, membranous nephropathy and membranoproliferative glomerulonephritis, and as a complication of the systemic disease diabetes mellitus.

- By contrast, *nephritic syndrome* is characterized by the following:
  - *Hematuria* (red cells and red cell casts in urine)
  - *Proteinuria* (usually in the subnephrotic range) with or without edema

  - *Azotemia*
  - *Hypertension*

    The nephritic syndrome usually has an acute onset and is caused by inflammatory lesions of glomeruli. The lesions that cause the nephritic syndrome have in common proliferation of the cells within the glomeruli, often accompanied by an infiltrate of leukocytes. The inflammatory reaction injures the capillary walls, permitting blood to pass into the urine, and induces hemodynamic changes that lead to a reduction in the GFR. The reduced GFR is manifested clinically by oliguria, fluid retention, and azotemia. Hypertension probably is a result of both the fluid retention and augmented renin release from the ischemic kidneys. The acute nephritic syndrome may be caused by primary glomerular diseases, such as postinfectious glomerulonephritis (GN) and various forms of crescentic GN, or as a result of systemic disorders such as systemic lupus erythematosus.

- *Asymptomatic hematuria* or nonnephrotic proteinuria or a combination of the two is the typical clinical presentation of IgA nephropathy, Alport syndrome, or mild forms or early presentations of other glomerular diseases.
- *Rapidly progressive glomerulonephritis (RPGN)* results in rapid loss of renal function in a few days or weeks, typically in the setting of nephritic syndrome. The characteristic histologic finding associated with RPGN is the presence of crescents (crescentic GN). Rapidly progressive glomerulonephritis is a clinical syndrome and not a specific etiologic form of GN. If untreated, it leads to death from renal failure within a period of weeks to months.
- *Acute kidney injury* refers to abrupt onset of renal dysfunction characterized by an acute increase in serum creatinine often associated with oliguria or anuria (decreased or no urine flow). It can result from glomerular injury (such as rapidly progressive GN), interstitial injury, vascular injury (such as thrombotic microangiopathy), or acute tubular epithelial cell injury.
- *Chronic kidney disease* results from progressive scarring in the kidney of any cause. It is characterized by various metabolic and electrolyte abnormalities such as hyperphosphatemia, dyslipidemia, and metabolic acidosis. However, it is often asymptomatic until the most advanced stages, when symptoms of uremia develop.
- *End-stage renal disease (ESRD)* is irreversible loss of renal function requiring dialysis or transplantation typically due to severe progressive scarring in the kidney from any cause.
- *Urinary tract infection (UTI)* is characterized by bacteriuria and pyuria (bacteria and leukocytes in the urine). It may be symptomatic or asymptomatic, and may affect the kidney (pyelonephritis) or the bladder (cystitis) only.
- *Nephrolithiasis* refers to formation of stones in the collecting system and is manifested by renal colic and hematuria (without red cell casts).

GLOMERULAR DISEASES

The glomerulus consists of an anastomosing network of capillaries invested by two layers of epithelium. The visceral epithelium (composed of podocytes) is part of the

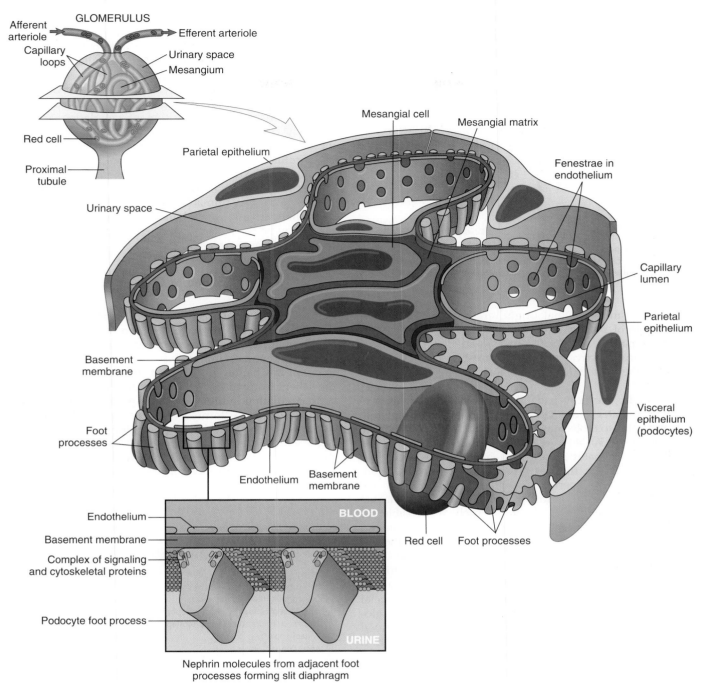

Fig. 14.1 Schematic diagram of a portion of a normal glomerulus.

capillary wall, whereas the parietal epithelium encircles Bowman space (urinary space), the cavity in which filtrate of plasma collects. The glomerular capillary is the filtration unit and consists of the following components (Figs. 14.1 and 14.2):

- Fenestrated *endothelial cells,* with each fenestra being 70 to 100 nm in diameter.
- The *glomerular basement membrane* (GBM), which has a thick, electron-dense central layer called the *lamina densa,* and two thinner, electron-lucent peripheral layers, the *lamina rara interna* and *lamina rara externa.* The GBM

consists of collagen (mostly type IV), laminin, polyanionic proteoglycans, fibronectin, and several other glycoproteins.

- *Podocytes,* cells that possess interdigitating foot processes that are embedded in and adherent to the lamina rara externa. Adjacent foot processes are separated by 20- to 30-nm–wide *filtration slits,* which are bridged by a thin slit diaphragm composed mainly of the protein nephrin (see later).
- *Mesangial cells,* which lie in a mesangial matrix between the capillaries that supports the glomerular tuft. These

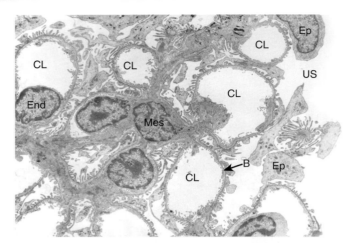

Fig. 14.2 Low-power electron micrograph of rat glomerulus. *B*, Basement membrane; *CL*, capillary lumen; *End*, endothelium; *Ep*, visceral epithelial cells (podocytes) with foot processes; *Mes*, mesangium; *US*, urinary space.

cells, of mesenchymal origin, are contractile and are capable of proliferation, of laying down collagen and other matrix components, and of secreting a number of biologically active mediators in response to cytokines and other factors (described later).

Normally, the glomerular filtration system is highly permeable to water and small solutes and almost completely impermeable to molecules of the size and molecular charge of albumin (a 70,000-kDa protein). This selective permeability discriminates among protein molecules according to size (the larger, the less permeable), charge (the more cationic, the more permeable), and shape. Podocyte slit diaphragms are important diffusion barriers for plasma proteins, and podocytes are also largely responsible for synthesis of GBM components. *Nephrin*, a transmembrane glycoprotein, is the major component of the slit diaphragms between adjacent foot processes. The intracellular part of nephrin interacts with several cytoskeletal and signaling proteins (see Fig. 14.1). Nephrin and its associated proteins, including *podocin*, have a crucial role in maintaining the selective permeability of the glomerular filtration barrier. This is dramatically illustrated by rare hereditary diseases in which mutations of nephrin or its partner proteins lead to abnormal leakage of plasma proteins into the urine and the nephrotic syndrome. As might be expected, acquired defects in podocytes and slit diaphragms, which are seen in a number of renal diseases, also are associated with proteinuria of varying severity.

Mechanisms of Glomerular Injury and Disease

Glomeruli may be injured by diverse mechanisms in the course of a number of systemic diseases (Table 14.1). These are termed *secondary glomerular diseases* to differentiate them from those in which the kidney is the only or predominant organ involved. The latter constitute the various types of *primary glomerular diseases,* which are discussed later in this section. The glomerular alterations in systemic diseases are discussed elsewhere.

Immune mechanisms underlie most types of primary glomerular diseases and many of the secondary glomerular diseases. Under experimental conditions, GN can be readily induced by antibodies, and glomerular deposits of immunoglobulins, often with various components of complement, are found frequently in patients with GN. Two mechanisms of antibody deposition in the glomerulus have been established: (1) deposition of circulating antigen-antibody complexes in the glomerular capillary wall or mesangium, and (2) antibodies reacting in situ within the glomerulus, either with fixed (intrinsic) glomerular antigens or with extrinsic molecules that are planted in the glomerulus (Fig. 14.3). These pathways are not mutually exclusive, and in humans all may contribute to injury. Abnormal activation and glomerular deposition of complement may be the sole culprit in some forms of GN. Cell-mediated immune mechanisms also may play a role in certain glomerular diseases.

Glomerulonephritis Caused by Circulating Immune Complexes

Deposition of circulating immune complexes in the glomerulus initiates complement (and/or Fc receptor) mediated leukocyte activation, resulting in glomerular injury. The pathogenesis of immune complex diseases is discussed in detail in Chapter 5. Presented here is a brief review of the salient features that relate to glomerular injury in GN.

In circulating immune complex–mediated diseases, the complexes may be formed with endogenous antigens, as in the GN associated with systemic lupus erythematosus, or the antigens may be exogenous, as is probable in the GN that follows certain bacterial (streptococcal), viral (hepatitis B), parasitic (*Plasmodium falciparum* malaria), and spirochetal (*Treponema pallidum*) infections. Often the inciting

Table 14.1 Glomerular Diseases

Primary Glomerular Diseases
Minimal-change disease
Focal segmental glomerulosclerosis
Membranous nephropathy
Acute postinfectious glomerulonephritis
Membranoproliferative glomerulonephritis
IgA nephropathy
Dense deposit disease
C3 glomerulonephritis

Glomerulopathies Secondary to Systemic Diseases
Lupus nephritis (systemic lupus erythematosus)
Diabetic nephropathy
Amyloidosis
Glomerulopathy secondary to multiple myeloma
Goodpasture syndrome
Microscopic polyangiitis
Granulomatosis with polyangiitis
Henoch-Schönlein purpura
Bacterial endocarditis–related glomerulonephritis
Thrombotic microangiopathy

Hereditary Disorders
Alport syndrome
Fabry disease
Podocyte/slit-diaphragm protein mutations

IgA, Immunoglobulin A.

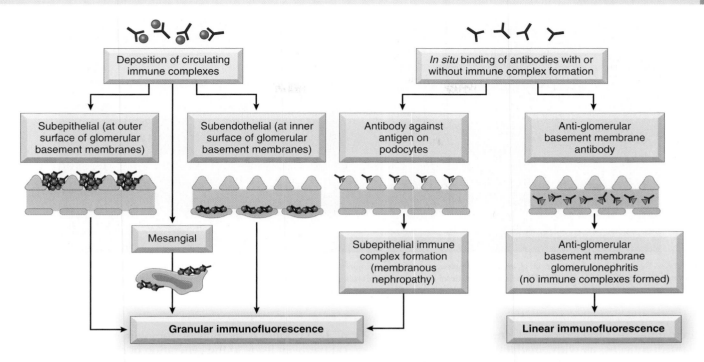

Fig. 14.3 Antibody-mediated glomerular injury. Injury can result either from the deposition of circulating immune complexes or from antibody-binding to glomerular components followed by formation of complexes in situ. Deposition of circulating immune complexes gives a granular immunofluorescence pattern. Anti-glomerular basement membrane (anti-GBM) antibody glomerulonephritis is characterized by a linear immunofluorescence pattern; there is no immune deposit formation in this disease.

antigen is unknown, as in most cases of membranoproliferative GN.

Once antigen-antibody complexes are deposited or formed in the glomeruli, they produce injury by activating complement and recruiting leukocytes. Binding of immune complexes to Fc receptors on leukocytes also may contribute to activation of the cells and injury. Morphologically, affected glomeruli exhibit leukocytic infiltrates and variable proliferation of mesangial and parietal epithelial cells. Electron microscopy reveals electron-dense immune deposits in one or more of three locations: between the endothelial cells and the GBM (subendothelial deposits), between the outer surface of the GBM and the podocytes (subepithelial deposits), or in the mesangium. The localization of antigen, antibody, or immune complexes determines the glomerular injury response. Studies in experimental models have shown that complexes deposited in the endothelium or subendothelium elicit an inflammatory reaction in the glomerulus with infiltration of leukocytes and exuberant proliferation of glomerular resident cells. By contrast, antibodies directed to the subepithelial region of glomerular capillaries are often noninflammatory, as seen in primary membranous nephropathy (discussed later). The presence of immunoglobulins and complement in these deposits can be demonstrated by immunofluorescence microscopy. **The pattern of immune complex deposition by immunofluorescence microscopy is granular**, given the rather picturesque description of "lumpy-bumpy" by pathologists (Fig. 14.4A).

Once deposited in the kidney, immune complexes may eventually be cleared by degradation or phagocytosis, mostly by infiltrating leukocytes and mesangial cells. The

inflammatory reaction may then subside if the exposure to the inciting antigen is short-lived and limited, as in most cases of poststreptococcal or acute infection–related GN. However, if exposure to antigen is sustained, repeated cycles of immune complex formation, deposition, and injury occur, leading to chronic GN. In some cases, the source of chronic antigenic exposure is clear, such as in hepatitis B virus infection and self nuclear antigens in systemic lupus erythematosus, but more often the antigen is unknown. Although immune complex deposition is a common mechanism of injury, circulating complexes are almost never identified in human disease, likely because of technical limitations.

Glomerulonephritis Caused by Immune Complexes Formed in Situ

Deposition of antibodies specific for fixed (intrinsic) or planted (from outside) antigens in the glomerulus is another major pathway of glomerular injury. Antigens expressed by podocytes have been implicated in membranous nephropathy. Antibodies also may react in situ with previously "planted" nonglomerular antigens, which deposit and become concentrated in the kidney through interaction with various glomerular components. Planted antigens include nucleosomal complexes, mainly derived from breakdown of apoptotic cells, in patients with systemic lupus erythematosus; bacterial products, such as endostreptosin, a protein expressed by group A streptococci; and large aggregated proteins (e.g., aggregated immunoglobulin G [IgG]), which tend to deposit in the mesangium. Locally formed immune complexes may also grow in size through additional interactions with

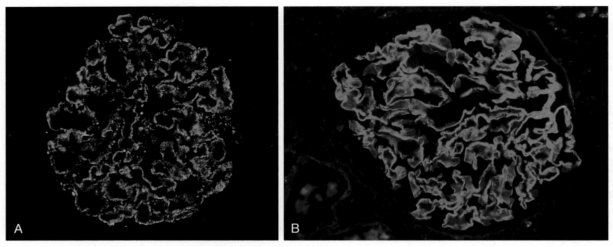

Fig. 14.4 Two patterns of deposition of immune complexes as seen by immunofluorescence microscopy. (A) Granular, characteristic of circulating and in situ immune complex deposition. (B) Linear, characteristic of classic anti-glomerular basement membrane (anti-GBM) antibody glomerulonephritis. *(A, Courtesy of Dr. J. Kowalewska, Department of Pathology, University of Washington, Seattle, Washington.)*

circulating free antibodies and antigens. Most of these planted antigens, as with circulating immune complexes deposited on the GBM, show a granular pattern of deposition by immunofluorescence microscopy.

Anti-Glomerular Basement Membrane Antibody–Mediated Glomerulonephritis

Antibody-mediated GN results from the glomerular deposition of autoantibodies directed against protein components of the GBM. The best-characterized disease in this group is anti-GBM antibody–mediated crescentic GN (see Fig. 14.3), also known as *Goodpasture disease*. In this type of injury, antibodies are directed against fixed antigens in the GBM, creating a linear pattern of staining when visualized with immunofluorescence microscopy (Fig. 14.4B). This pattern is useful in the diagnosis of glomerular disease. A known antigen that is the target of anti-GBM antibodies is the α3 chain of the type IV collagen of the GBM. Sometimes the anti-GBM antibodies cross-react with basement membranes of lung alveoli, resulting in simultaneous lung and kidney lesions (Goodpasture syndrome, Chapter 13).

Glomerular Diseases Caused by Complement Activation

The primary cause of these diseases is unregulated activation of the alternative complement pathway, which may be triggered by acquired autoantibodies against complement components or inherited abnormalities of complement regulatory proteins. Ensuing complement-mediated injury may result in renal and systemic disease. Two forms of GN (dense deposit disease and C3 GN) and one form of a systemic disease with significant renal manifestations (complement-mediated thrombotic microangiopathy [TMA] or atypical hemolytic uremic syndrome) belong to this category. Although complement-mediated thrombotic microangiopathy is a systemic condition, renal manifestation represents the major morbidity of the disease.

Mediators of Immune Injury

A major pathway of antibody-initiated glomerular injury involves complement activation and recruitment

of leukocytes. Activation of complement via the classical pathway leads to the generation of chemotactic agents (mainly C5a) for *neutrophils and monocytes.* Neutrophils release proteases, which cause GBM degradation; oxygen-derived free radicals, which cause cell damage; and arachidonic acid metabolites, which contribute to reduction in GFR. In other types of GN in which neutrophils are not prominent, complement-dependent injury may occur through assembly of the C5b-C9 membrane attack complex. There is evidence that the membrane attack complex injures epithelial cells, inducing them to secrete various inflammatory mediators. The alternative and lectin pathways of complement can be activated by cell injury or apoptosis, and also perhaps by deposited IgA.

In addition to neutrophils and monocytes, which are recruited by antibodies and complement, *T lymphocytes* activated during the immune reaction also have been implicated in glomerular injury. *Platelets* may aggregate and release mediators, including prostaglandins. Resident *glomerular cells* (epithelial, mesangial, and endothelial) can be stimulated to secrete mediators such as cytokines (interleukin-1), arachidonic acid metabolites, growth factors, and nitric oxide.

Thus, virtually all of the mediators described in the discussion of inflammation in Chapter 3 may contribute to glomerular injury.

Non-immune Mechanisms of Glomerular Injury

Mechanisms other than inflammation contribute to glomerular abnormalities in certain primary renal disorders. Two that deserve special mention are podocyte injury and nephron loss.

Podocyte Injury

Podocyte injury can be induced by antibodies to podocyte antigens; by toxins; conceivably by certain cytokines; or by still poorly characterized circulating factors, as in some cases of focal segmental glomerulosclerosis (discussed later). Podocyte injury produces morphologic changes including effacement of foot processes, vacuolization, and retraction and detachment of cells from the GBM, and often results in the development of proteinuria. Of these changes, it is the loss of normal slit diaphragms that is most highly associated with proteinuria. Germline mutations in the structural components of slit diaphragms, such as nephrin and podocin, also are associated with functional alterations that lead to rare hereditary forms of the nephrotic syndrome.

Nephron Loss

Once renal disease, glomerular or otherwise, destroys sufficient nephrons to reduce the GFR to 30% to 50% of normal, symptoms appear and progression to end-stage renal disease proceeds at varying rates. Affected individuals have proteinuria, and their glomeruli show widespread scarring, called *glomerulosclerosis*. Such progressive sclerosis is exacerbated by adaptive changes that occur in response to the loss of nephrons. Specifically, intact glomeruli undergo hypertrophy to maintain renal function, an alteration that is associated with hemodynamic changes, including increases in single-nephron GFR, blood flow, and transcapillary pressure (capillary hypertension). These alterations are ultimately "maladaptive" and lead to further endothelial and podocyte injury, increased glomerular permeability to proteins, and accumulation of proteins and lipids in the mesangial matrix. This is followed by capillary obliteration, increased deposition of mesangial matrix and plasma proteins, and finally segmental (affecting a portion) or global (complete) sclerosis of glomeruli. The latter results in further reduction of nephron mass, initiating a vicious cycle of progressive glomerulosclerosis.

SUMMARY

CLINICAL SYNDROMES AND GLOMERULAR INJURY

- The clinical manifestations of renal disease include nephrotic syndrome, nephritic syndrome, asymptomatic hematuria, rapidly progressive glomerulonephritis, acute kidney injury, chronic kidney disease, and end-stage renal disease.
- The dominant feature of nephrotic syndrome is significant (i.e., "nephrotic range") proteinuria, while nephritic syndrome is characterized by proteinuria and hematuria often in association with functional impairment.
- Glomerular injury is most often caused by depositon of antibodies or immune complexes, activation of complement and leukocyte recruitment and activation.
  - The most common forms of glomerulonephritis (GN) are caused by the formation of immune complexes, which may be deposited from the circulation or form in situ. Immune complexes show a granular pattern of deposition.
  - Autoantibodies against components of the GBM are the cause of anti-GBM-antibody–mediated disease, often associated with severe injury. The pattern of antibody deposition is linear.
- Less frequently, complement may be activated in the absence of antibody, because of acquired or hereditary defects in its regulation.

We now turn to a consideration of specific types of GN and the syndromes they produce (Table 14.2). Many primary glomerular disease cause the nephrotic syndrome, but in adults this syndrome is most often secondary to diabetes, amyloidosis, and systemic lupus erythematosus (Table 14.3). The renal lesions produced by lupus and amyloidosis are discussed in Chapter 5, and those caused by diabetes in Chapter 20.

Minimal-Change Disease

Minimal-change disease, a relatively benign disorder, is the most frequent cause of the nephrotic syndrome in children and is characterized by glomeruli that have a normal appearance by light microscopy. Diffuse effacement of podocyte foot processes is seen with electron microscopy. It may develop at any age, but is most common between 1 and 7 years of age.

Pathogenesis

A popular hypothesis for the pathogenesis of minimal-change disease is that some circulating molecules injure podocytes and cause proteinuria with effacement of foot processes. Although there are numerous reports of candidate serum "factors" produced by lymphocytes and other cells, none has been characterized biochemically or definitively established as being causative in the disease. Thus, the pathogenesis of minimal-change disease remains unknown.

MORPHOLOGY

Under the light microscope, the glomeruli appear normal, thus giving rise to the name (Fig. 14.5A). The cells of the proximal convoluted tubules often are heavily laden with protein droplets and lipids due to tubular reabsorption of the lipoproteins passing through the diseased glomeruli. The only obvious glomerular abnormality is the **diffuse effacement of the foot processes of the podocytes** (see Fig. 14.5B). The cytoplasm of the podocytes appears flattened over the external aspect of the GBM, obliterating the network of arcades between the podocytes and the GBM. Other changes in podocytes include vacuolization, microvillus formation, and occasional focal detachments, suggesting some form of podocyte injury. With reversal of the changes in the podocytes in response to corticosteroids, the proteinuria remits.

Clinical Features

The disease typically manifests with *abrupt development of the nephrotic syndrome* in an otherwise healthy child. There is no hypertension, and renal function is preserved in most of these patients. The protein loss usually is confined to smaller plasma proteins, chiefly albumin (selective proteinuria). The prognosis for children with this disorder is favorable. More than 90% of children respond to a short course of corticosteroid therapy; however, proteinuria recurs in more than two-thirds of the initial responders, some of whom become steroid-dependent with proteinuria recurring when steroids are withdrawn. Less than 5% develop chronic kidney disease after 25 years, and it is likely that most individuals in this subgroup had nephrotic syndrome caused by focal segmental glomerulosclerosis

Table 14.2 Summary of Major Primary Glomerular Diseases

Disease	Most Frequent Clinical Presentation	Pathogenesis	Glomerular Pathology		
			Light Microscopy	Fluorescence Microscopy	Electron Microscopy
Minimal-change disease	Nephrotic syndrome	Unknown; podocyte injury	Normal	Negative	Effacement of foot processes; no deposits
Focal segmental glomerulosclerosis	Nephrotic syndrome; nonnephrotic range proteinuria	Unknown: reaction to loss of renal mass; plasma factor?	Focal and segmental sclerosis and hyalinosis	Usually negative; IgM and C3 may be present in areas of scarring	Effacement of foot processes; epithelial denudation
Membranous nephropathy	Nephrotic syndrome	In situ immune complex formation; PLA2R antigen in most cases of primary disease	Diffuse capillary wall thickening and subepithelial "spike" formation	Granular IgG and C3 along GBM	Subepithelial deposits
Membranoproliferative glomerulonephritis (MPGN) type I	Nephrotic/nephritic syndrome	Immune complex	Membranoproliferative pattern; GBM splitting	Granular IgG, C3, C1q and C4 along GBM and mesangium	Subendothelial deposits
C3 glomerulopathy (dense deposit disease and C3 glomerulonephritis)	Nephrotic/nephritic syndrome; nonnephrotic proteinuria	Activation of alternative complement pathway; antibody-mediated or hereditary defect in regulation	Mesangial proliferative or membranoproliferative patterns	C3	Mesangial, intramembranous and subendothelial electron-dense or "waxy" deposits
Acute postinfectious glomerulonephritis	Nephritic syndrome	Immune complex mediated; circulating or planted antigen	Diffuse endocapillary proliferation; leukocytic infiltration	Granular IgG and C3 along GBM and mesangium	Primarily subepithelial humps
IgA nephropathy	Recurrent hematuria or proteinuria	Immune complexes containing IgA	Mesangial or focal endocapillary proliferative glomerulonephritis	IgA ± IgG, IgM, and C3 in mesangium	Mesangial and paramesangial dense deposits
Anti-GBM disease (e.g. Goodpasture syndrome)	Rapidly progressive glomerulonephritis	Autoantibodies against collagen type IV α3 chain	Extracapillary proliferation with crescents; necrosis	Linear IgG and C3; fibrin in crescents	No deposits; GBM disruptions; fibrin
Pauci-immune glomerulonephritis	Rapidly progressive glomerulonephritis	Anti-neutrophil cytoplasmic antibody	Extracapillary proliferation with crescents; necrosis	Fibrin in crescents	No deposits; GBM disruptions; fibrin

GBM, Glomerular basement membrane; *IgA*, immunoglobulin A; *IgG*, immunoglobulin G; *IgM*, immunoglobulin M.

not detected by biopsy. Because of its responsiveness to therapy in children, minimal-change disease must be differentiated from other causes of the nephrotic syndrome in nonresponders. Adults with this disease also respond to steroid therapy, but the response is slower and relapses are more common.

Focal Segmental Glomerulosclerosis

Focal segmental glomerulosclerosis (FSGS) is characterized by sclerosis of some (but not all) glomeruli that involves only a part of each affected glomerulus. FSGS may be primary (idiopathic) or secondary to one of the following conditions:

- *HIV infection* (HIV nephropathy). FSGS is seen in 5–10% of patients infected with HIV, but the incidence is decreasing with improved antiviral therapy.
- *Heroin abuse* (heroin nephropathy)
- Secondary to other forms of GN (e.g., IgA nephropathy)
- As a maladaptation to nephron loss (as discussed earlier)

- Inherited forms, including autosomal dominant forms associated with mutations in cytoskeletal proteins and podocin, both of which are required for the integrity of podocytes.

Primary FSGS accounts for approximately 20% to 30% of all cases of the nephrotic syndrome. It is an increasingly common cause of nephrotic syndrome in adults and remains a frequent cause in children.

Pathogenesis

Injury to podocytes is thought to represent the initiating event of primary FSGS. However, what causes this injury remains unknown. Some investigators have suggested that FSGS and minimal-change disease are part of a continuum and that minimal-change disease may transform into FSGS, but others believe them to be distinct clinicopathologic entities from the outset. As with minimal-change disease, permeability-increasing factors produced

Table 14.3 Causes of Nephrotic Syndrome

Cause	Prevalence (%)*	
	Children	**Adults**
Primary Glomerular Disease		
Minimal-change disease	65	10
Focal segmental glomerulosclerosis	10	35
Membranous nephropathy	5	30
Membranoproliferative glomerulonephritis	10	10
IgA nephropathy and others	10	15
Systemic Diseases With Renal Manifestations		
Diabetes mellitus		
Amyloidosis		
Systemic lupus erythematosus		
Ingestion of drugs (gold, penicillamine, "street heroin")		
Infections (malaria, syphilis, hepatitis B, HIV)		
Malignancy (carcinoma, melanoma)		
Miscellaneous (bee sting allergy, hereditary nephritis)		

HIV, Human immunodeficiency virus.
*Approximate prevalence of primary disease is 95% of the cases in children and 60% in adults. Approximate prevalence of systemic disease is 5% of the cases in children and 40% in adults.

by lymphocytes are suspected but remain unproven. The deposition of hyaline in the glomeruli is caused by the entrapment of plasma proteins and lipids in foci of injury where sclerosis develops. The recurrence of proteinuria in patients underoing renal transplantion for FSGS, sometimes within 24 hours of transplantation, supports the idea that a circulating mediator leads to podocyte damage in some cases.

⬤ MORPHOLOGY

Primary FSGS initially affects only the juxtamedullary glomeruli. With progression, eventually all levels of the cortex are affected. The lesions occur in some tufts within a glomerulus while sparing others (Fig. 14.6). The affected glomeruli exhibit **increased mesangial matrix, obliterated capillary lumina, deposition of hyaline (hyalinosis) and foamy (lipid-laden) macrophages.** In affected glomeruli, immunofluorescence microscopy often reveals nonspecific trapping of immunoglobulins, usually IgM, and complement in the areas of hyalinosis. On electron microscopy, the podocytes exhibit **effacement of foot processes,** as in minimal-change disease.

With time, progression leads to global sclerosis of the glomeruli, pronounced tubular atrophy, and interstitial fibrosis. This advanced picture is difficult to differentiate from other forms of chronic glomerular disease, discussed later.

A morphologic variant called **collapsing glomerulopathy** is characterized by collapse of the glomerular tuft and epithelial cell hyperplasia. This more severe manifestation of FSGS may be idiopathic or may be associated with HIV infection, drug-induced toxicities, and some microvascular injuries. It carries a particularly poor prognosis.

Clinical Course

It is important to distinguish FSGS from minimal-change disease, because the clinical courses and responses to therapy are markedly different. Both are associated with nephrotic syndrome, but the incidence of hematuria and hypertension is higher in individuals with FSGS. Also, unlike minimal change disease, FSGS-associated proteinuria is nonselective, and in general the response to corticosteroid therapy is poor. At least 50% of patients with FSGS develop end-stage renal disease within 10 years of diagnosis.

Membranous Nephropathy

Membranous nephropathy is characterized by subepithelial immunoglobulin-containing deposits along the GBM. Early in the disease, the glomeruli may appear normal by light microscopy, but well-developed cases show *diffuse thickening of the capillary wall.* It usually presents in adults between the ages of 30 and 60 years and follows an indolent and slowly progressive course.

Up to 80% of cases of membranous nephropathy are primary, caused by autoantibodies against podocyte

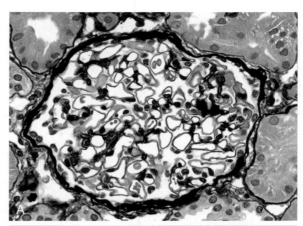

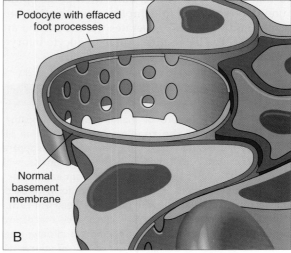

Podocyte with effaced foot processes

Normal basement membrane

B

Fig. 14.5 Minimal-change disease. (A) When viewed with a light microscope, the silver methenamine–stained glomerulus appears normal, with a delicate basement membrane. (B) Schematic diagram illustrating diffuse effacement of foot processes of podocytes with no immune deposits.

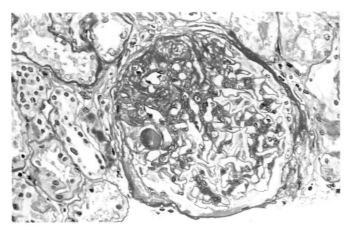

Fig. 14.6 Focal and segmental glomerulosclerosis (periodic acid–Schiff stain), seen as a collection of scarred, obliterated capillaries and accumulations of matrix material in part of the affected glomerulus. *(Courtesy of Dr. H. Rennke, Department of Pathology, Brigham and Women's Hospital, Boston, Massachusetts.)*

antigens. In the remainder, it occurs secondary to other conditions, including the following:

- *Infections* (chronic hepatitis B, syphilis, schistosomiasis, malaria)
- *Malignant neoplasms*, particularly carcinoma of the lung and colon and melanoma
- *Autoimmune diseases*, particularly systemic lupus erythematosus
- *Exposure to inorganic salts* (gold, mercury)
- *Drugs* (penicillamine, captopril, nonsteroidal anti-inflammatory agents)

Pathogenesis

Membranous nephropathy is a form of chronic immune complex glomerulonephritis induced by antibodies reacting in situ to endogenous or planted glomerular antigens. Antibodies against the podocyte antigen phospholipase A_2 receptor (PLA2R) are frequently present but it is not established that they are causative. Formation of subepithelial immune deposits leads to complement activation on the surface of podocytes and generates the membrane attack complex (C5-C9). This in turn causes podocyte injury and proteinuria.

MORPHOLOGY

The main histologic feature of membranous nephropathy is **diffuse thickening of the capillary wall** on routine H&E stains (Fig. 14.7A). Electron microscopy reveals that this apparent thickening is caused in part by **subepithelial deposits,** which nestle against the GBM and are separated from each other by small, spikelike protrusions of GBM matrix that form in reaction to the deposits **(spike and dome pattern)** (see Fig. 14.7B). As the disease progresses, these spikes close over the deposits, incorporating them into the GBM. In addition, as in other causes of nephrotic syndrome, the podocytes show **effacement of foot processes.** Later in the disease, the incorporated deposits may be broken down and eventually disappear, leaving cavities within the GBM. Continued deposition of basement membrane

matrix leads to progressive thickening of basement membranes. With further progression, glomeruli may become sclerosed. Immunofluorescence microscopy shows typical **granular deposits** of immunoglobulins and complement along the GBM (see Fig. 14.4A).

Clinical Features

Most cases of membranous nephropathy are sudden in onset and present as *full-blown nephrotic syndrome,* usually without antecedent illness; other individuals have lesser degrees of proteinuria. In contrast to minimal-change disease, the proteinuria is nonselective, and usually fails to respond to corticosteroid therapy. Secondary causes of

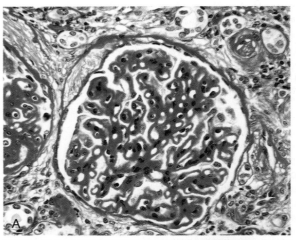

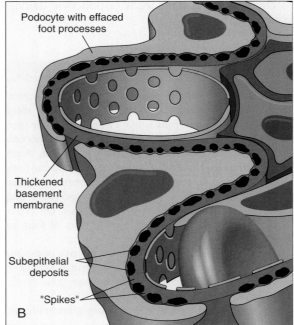

Fig. 14.7 Membranous nephropathy. (A) Diffuse thickening of the glomerular basement membrane (periodic acid–Schiff stain). (B) Schematic diagram illustrating subepithelial deposits, effacement of foot processes, and the presence of spikes of basement membrane material between the immune deposits.

Podocyte with effaced foot processes

Thickened basement membrane

Subepithelial deposits

"Spikes"

membranous nephropathy should be ruled out. Membranous nephropathy follows a notoriously variable and often indolent course. Overall, although proteinuria persists in greater than 60% of patients, only about 40% progress to renal failure over a period of 2 to 20 years. An additional 10% to 30% of cases have a more benign course with partial or complete remission of proteinuria.

Membranoproliferative Glomerulonephritis

MPGN is manifested histologically by alterations in the GBM and mesangium and by proliferation of glomerular cells. It accounts for 5% to 10% of cases of idiopathic nephrotic syndrome in children and adults. Some patients present only with hematuria or proteinuria in the nonnephrotic range; others exhibit a combined nephrotic-nephritic picture. In the past, MPGN was subclassified into two types (I and II) on the basis of distinct ultrastructural, immunofluorescence, light microscopic, and pathogenic findings. These are now recognized to be distinct entities, termed *MPGN type I* and *dense deposit disease* (formerly *MPGN type II*). Of the two types of disease, MPGN type I is far more common (about 80% of cases) and is discussed here. Dense deposit disease will be discussed later along with the related condition of C3 glomerulonephritis.

Pathogenesis

Type I MPGN may be caused by deposition of circulating immune complexes or by in situ immune complex formation with a planted antigen. The inciting antigen is not known.

By light microscopy the glomeruli are large, have an accentuated lobular appearance, and show **proliferation of mesangial and endothelial cells as well as infiltrating leukocytes** (Fig. 14.8A). The GBM is thickened, and the glomerular capillary wall often shows a double contour, or "tram track," appearance, especially evident with use of silver or periodic acid–Schiff (PAS) stains. This "splitting" of the GBM is due to extension of processes of mesangial and inflammatory cells into the peripheral capillary loops and deposition of mesangial matrix as well as subepithelial immune complexes (see Fig. 14.8B). The characteristic light microscopic glomerular manifestations are often referred to as *membranoproliferative pattern of glomerular injury*.

By electron microscopy, type I MPGN is characterized by **discrete subendothelial deposits** (see Fig. 14.8B). By immunofluorescence microscopy, C3 is deposited in an irregular granular pattern, and IgG and early complement components (C1q and C4) also often are present, indicative of an immune complex pathogenesis.

Clinical Features

The mode of presentation in approximately 50% of cases is the nephrotic syndrome, although it may begin as acute nephritis or mild proteinuria. The prognosis generally is poor. In one study, none of the 60 patients followed for 1 to 20 years showed complete remission; 40% progressed to end-stage renal failure, 30% had variable degrees of renal insufficiency, and the remaining 30% had persistent

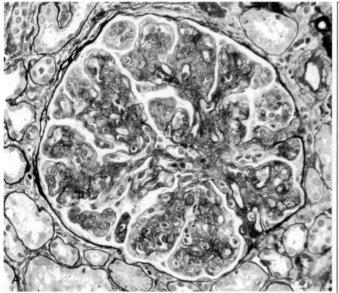

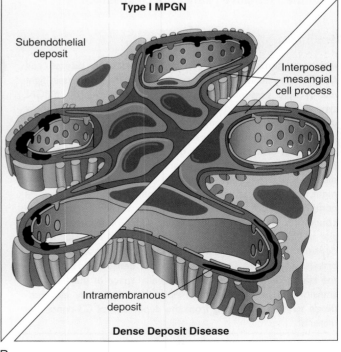

Fig. 14.8 (A) Membranoproliferative glomerulonephritis (MPGN), showing mesangial cell proliferation, basement membrane duplication, leukocyte infiltration, and accentuation of lobular architecture. (B) Schematic representation of the two patterns of MPGN. In type I, there are subendothelial deposits; in type II, now called *dense deposit disease*, intramembranous characteristically dense deposits are seen. In both types, mesangial interposition gives the appearance of split basement membranes when viewed by light microscopy.

nephrotic syndrome without renal failure. MPGN type I also may occur in association with other disorders (secondary MPGN), such as systemic lupus erythematosus, hepatitis B and C, chronic liver disease, and chronic bacterial infections. Indeed, many so-called "idiopathic" cases are believed to be associated with hepatitis C and related cryoglobulinemia.

C3 Glomerulopathy

The term *C3 glomerulopathy* encompasses two conditions, *dense deposit disease* (formerly *MPGN, type II*) and *C3 glomerulonephritis*. These are relatively rare diseases with certain shared clinical, morphologic, and pathogenic features that may be part of a spectrum of injury. They are set apart by differences in the electron microscopic appearance. Patients may present with nephrotic or nephritic syndrome, however, cases with only mild proteinuria also occur. Patients with dense deposit disease are usually younger and more likely to have low serum C3 levels than patients with C3 GN, although these distinctions are subtle.

Pathogenesis

Complement dysregulation due to acquired or hereditary abnormalities of the alternative pathway of complement activation is the underlying cause of dense deposit disease and C3 GN. Some patients have an autoantibody against C3 convertase, called *C3 nephritic factor (C3NeF),* that causes uncontrolled cleavage of C3 by the alternative complement pathway. In other patients, mutations in various complement regulatory proteins, such as Factor H, Factor I, and membrane cofactor protein (MCP), or autoantibodies to Factor H, are the cause of unregulated activation of the alternative pathway of complement.

MORPHOLOGY

Although glomerular changes in dense deposit disease and C3 GN vary from relatively subtle to severe, the classic light microscopic presentation is similar to that seen in MPGN, type I. The glomeruli are hypercellular, the capillary walls show duplicated basement membranes, and the mesangial matrix is increased. By immunofluorescence microscopy, there is **bright mesangial and glomerular capillary wall staining for C3** in both dense deposit disease and C3 GN. In dense deposit disease, C3 staining also may be seen along the tubular basement membranes. IgG and the early components of the classical complement pathway (C1q and C4) are usually absent in both conditions. By electron microscopy, C3 GN features mesangial and subendothelial electron-dense "waxy" deposits; similar deposits also may be seen along the tubular basement membranes. By contrast, in the aptly named dense deposit disease, the lamina densa and the subendothelial space of the GBM are transformed into an irregular, ribbonlike, extremely electron-dense structure, resulting from the deposition of C3-containing material.

Clinical Features

Both dense deposit disease and C3 GN carry a relatively poor prognosis and both tend to recur posttransplantation at a rate of up to 85%. In a recent study of 70 patients with dense deposit disease or C3 GN, 29% of patients progressed to end-stage renal failure after a median of 28 months.

Acute Postinfectious (Poststreptococcal) Glomerulonephritis

Acute postinfectious GN is caused by glomerular deposition of immune complexes resulting in proliferation of and damage to glomerular cells and infiltration of leukocytes, especially neutrophils. The classic pattern is seen in poststreptococcal GN. Infections by organisms other than streptococci also may be associated with postinfectious GN. These include certain pneumococcal and staphylococcal infections as well as several common viral diseases such as mumps, measles, chickenpox, and hepatitis B and C.

The typical case of poststreptococcal GN develops in a child 1 to 4 weeks after he or she recovers from a group A streptococcal infection. Only certain "nephritogenic" strains of β-hemolytic streptococci evoke glomerular disease. In most cases, the initial infection is localized to the pharynx or skin. In rare cases, the disease can develop during the infection.

Pathogenesis

Poststreptococcal GN is an immune complex disease in which tissue injury is primarily caused by complement activation by the classical pathway. Typical features of immune complex disease, such as hypocomplementemia and granular deposits of IgG and complement on the GBM, are seen. The relevant antigens probably are streptococcal proteins. Specific antigens implicated in pathogenesis include streptococcal exotoxin B (Spe B) and streptococcal glyceraldehyde-3-phosphate dehydrogenase (GAPDH). Both have an affinity for glomerular proteins and plasmin. It is not clear if immune complexes are formed mainly in the circulation or in situ (the latter by binding of antibodies to bacterial antigens "planted" in the GBM).

MORPHOLOGY

By light microscopy, the most characteristic change in postinfectious GN is **increased cellularity** of the glomerular tufts that affects nearly all glomeruli—hence the term *diffuse GN* (Fig. 14.9A). The increased cellularity is caused both by proliferation and swelling of endothelial and mesangial cells and by infiltrating neutrophils and monocytes. Sometimes there is necrosis of the capillary walls. In a few cases, "crescents" (discussed later) may be observed within the urinary space, formed in response to the severe injury. Electron microscopy shows deposited immune complexes arrayed as subendothelial, intramembranous, or, most often, **subepithelial "humps"** nestled against the GBM (see Fig. 14.9B). Mesangial deposits also are occasionally present. Immunofluorescence studies reveal scattered **granular deposits of IgG and complement** within the capillary walls and some mesangial areas, corresponding to the deposits visualized by electron microscopy. These deposits usually are cleared over a period of about 2 months.

Clinical Features

The most common clinical presentation is *acute nephritic syndrome.* Edema and hypertension are common, with mild to moderate azotemia. Characteristically, there is gross

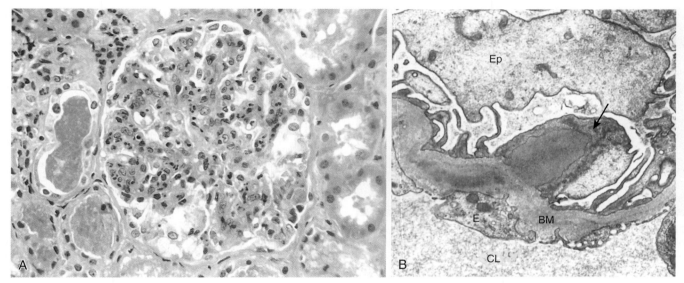

Fig. 14.9 Poststreptococcal glomerulonephritis. (A) Glomerular hypercellularity is caused by intracapillary leukocytes and proliferation of intrinsic glomerular cells. Note the red blood cell casts in the tubules. (B) Typical electron-dense subepithelial "hump" *(arrow)* and intramembranous deposits. *BM*, Basement membrane; *CL*, capillary lumen; *E*, endothelial cell; *Ep*, visceral epithelial cells (podocytes).

hematuria, the urine appearing smoky brown rather than bright red due to oxidation of hemoglobin to methemoglobin. Some degree of proteinuria is a constant feature, and, as mentioned earlier, it occasionally may be severe enough to produce the nephrotic syndrome. Serum complement levels are low during the active phase of the disease, and serum anti–streptolysin O antibody titers are elevated in poststreptococcal cases.

Recovery occurs in most children with poststreptococcal disease, but some develop rapidly progressive GN owing to severe injury with formation of crescents, or chronic renal disease from secondary scarring. The prognosis in sporadic cases is less clear. In adults, 15% to 50% of affected individuals develop end-stage renal disease over a few years or 1 to 2 decades, depending on the clinical and histologic severity. By contrast, in children with sporadic cases of acute postinfectious GN, the progression to chronicity is much lower.

IgA Nephropathy

IgA nephropathy is one of the most common causes of recurrent microscopic or gross hematuria and is the most common glomerular disease revealed by renal biopsy worldwide. This condition usually affects children and young adults and begins as an episode of gross hematuria that occurs within 1 or 2 days of a nonspecific upper-respiratory tract infection. Typically, the hematuria lasts several days and then subsides, but it recurs periodically, usually in the setting of a viral infection. It may be associated with local pain.

The hallmark of the disease is the deposition of IgA in the mesangium. Some experts have considered IgA nephropathy to be a localized variant of *Henoch-Schönlein purpura,* also characterized by IgA deposition in the mesangium. In contrast with IgA nephropathy, which is confined to the kidney, Henoch-Schönlein purpura is a systemic syndrome also involving the skin (purpuric rash), gastrointestinal tract (abdominal pain), and joints (arthritis).

Pathogenesis

An abnormally glycosylated IgA1 (i.e., galactose-deficient IgA1 [Gd-IgA1]) immunoglobulin is thought to play a central role in the pathogenesis. This abnormal IgA may elicit an autoimmune response, and autoantibodies may form large immune complexes with circulating IgA. These complexes deposit in the glomerular mesangium; this unusual location may be related to physicochemical features of the IgA and may be facilitated by an IgA1 receptor (CD71) on mesangial cells. The presence of C3 in the mesangium and the absence of C1q and C4 points to activation of the alternative complement pathway in the pathogenesis. A genetic influence is suggested by the occurrence of IgA nephropathy in families and in HLA-identical siblings, and increased frequency of certain HLA and complement genotypes in some populations. Taken together, these data suggest that in genetically susceptible individuals, respiratory or gastrointestinal exposure to microbial or other antigens (e.g., viruses, bacteria, food proteins) may lead to increased IgA synthesis, some of which is abnormally glycosylated, and deposition of IgA and IgA-containing immune complexes in the mesangium, where they activate the alternative complement pathway and initiate glomerular injury. In support of this scenario, IgA nephropathy occurs with increased frequency in individuals with celiac disease, in whom intestinal mucosal defects are seen, and in liver disease, in which there is defective hepatobiliary clearance of IgA complexes *(secondary IgA nephropathy).*

MORPHOLOGY

Histologically, the lesions in IgA nephropathy vary considerably. The glomeruli may be normal or may show mesangial widening and segmental inflammation confined to some glomeruli (focal

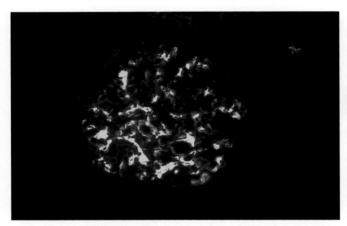

Fig. 14.10 IgA nephropathy. Characteristic immunofluorescence deposition of IgA, principally in mesangial regions, is evident. *IgA*, Immunoglobulin A.

proliferative GN); diffuse mesangial proliferation (mesangioproliferative GN); or (rarely) overt crescentic GN. The characteristic immunofluorescence picture is of **mesangial deposition of IgA,** often with C3 and properdin and smaller amounts of IgG or IgM (Fig. 14.10). Early components of the classical complement pathway usually are absent. Electron microscopy confirms the presence of electron-dense deposits in the mesangium.

Clinical Features

IgA nephropathy most often affects children and young adults. More than half of those affected present with *gross hematuria* after an infection of the respiratory or, less commonly, gastrointestinal or urinary tract; 30% to 40% have only microscopic hematuria, with or without proteinuria, and 5% to 10% develop a typical acute nephritic syndrome. The hematuria typically lasts for several days and initially subsides, but then recurs periodically, usually in the setting of a viral infection. The course is highly variable. Many patients maintain normal renal function for decades. Slow progression to end-stage renal disease occurs in 25% to 50% of cases over a period of 20 years. Renal biopsy findings may help identify those with a poorer prognosis, as indicated by diffuse mesangial proliferation, segmental sclerosis, endocapillary proliferation, or tubulointerstitial fibrosis.

Hereditary Nephritis

Hereditary nephritis refers to a group of glomerular diseases caused by mutations in genes encoding GBM proteins. The most common of these rare diseases are *Alport syndrome* and *thin basement membrane disease.* In Alport syndrome, nephritis is accompanied by sensorineural deafness and various eye disorders, including lens dislocation, posterior cataracts, and corneal dystrophy. Thin basement membrane disease is the most common cause of benign familial hematuria with no systemic manifestations.

Pathogenesis

The GBM is composed largely of type IV collagen, which is made up of heterotrimers of α3, α4, and α5 type IV collagen.

This form of type IV collagen is crucial for normal function of the lens, cochlea, and glomerulus. Mutation of any one of the α chains results in defective heterotrimer assembly and, consequently, the manifestations of Alport syndrome.

MORPHOLOGY

On histologic examination, glomeruli in hereditary nephritis appear unremarkable until late in the course. With progression, increasing glomerulosclerosis, vascular sclerosis, tubular atrophy, and interstitial fibrosis are typical changes. Under the electron microscope, the **GBM is thin** and attenuated early in the course, but over time develops irregular foci of thickening or attenuation with pronounced splitting and lamination of the lamina densa, yielding a **"basketweave"** appearance. In contrast to Alport syndrome, diffuse and uniform thinning of the glomerular basement membranes is the only morphologic finding in thin basement membrane disease.

Clinical Features

The majority of Alport syndrome patients have X-linked disease as a result of mutation of the gene on the X chromosome encoding the α5 chain of type IV collagen. Males therefore are affected more frequently and more severely than females and are more likely to develop end-stage renal disease and deafness. Rare autosomal recessive or dominant cases are linked to defects in the genes that encode α3 or α4 type IV collagen. Individuals with hereditary nephritis present at 5 to 20 years of age with gross or microscopic *hematuria and proteinuria*, and progress to overt renal failure by the ages of 20 to 50 years. Female carriers of X-linked Alport syndrome or carriers of either gender of the autosomal forms usually present with persistent asymptomatic hematuria and follow a benign nonprogressive clinical course. Heterozygous mutations in the genes encoding the α3 and α4 chains of type IV collagen are found in 40% of patients with thin basement membrane disease.

Rapidly Progressive Glomerulonephritis

RPGN is characterized by the presence of crescents (crescentic GN) and in most cases appears to be immunologically mediated. It is a clinical syndrome and not a specific etiologic form of GN. RPGN is characterized by rapid loss of renal function, laboratory findings typical of the nephritic syndrome, and often severe oliguria. If untreated, it can rapidly lead to renal failure within a period of weeks to months.

Pathogenesis

Crescentic GN may be caused by a number of different diseases, some restricted to the kidney and others systemic. RPGN may be associated with a number of diseases, as follows:

- *Anti-GBM antibody–mediated crescentic GN* (Goodpasture disease) is characterized by linear deposits of IgG and, in many cases, C3 in the GBM. In some patients, the anti-GBM antibodies also bind to pulmonary alveolar capillary basement membranes to produce the clinical picture of pulmonary hemorrhages associated with renal failure. These patients are said to have *Goodpasture syndrome*. Anti-GBM antibodies are present in the serum and are helpful in diagnosis. It is important to recognize anti-GBM antibody–mediated crescentic GN, because affected individuals benefit from plasmapheresis, which removes pathogenic antibodies from the circulation.

- *Immune complex–mediated crescentic GN* may complicate any of the immune complex nephritides, including post-streptococcal GN, systemic lupus erythematosus, IgA nephropathy, and Henoch-Schönlein purpura. In other cases, immune complexes are demonstrated but the underlying cause is undetermined. This type of RPGN frequently shows cellular proliferation and influx of leukocytes within the glomerular tuft, in addition to crescent formation. A consistent finding is the characteristic granular pattern of staining of the GBM and/or mesangium for immunoglobulin and/or complement on immunofluorescence studies. This disorder usually does not respond to plasmapheresis.
- *Pauci-immune type crescentic GN* is defined by the lack of anti-GBM antibodies or significant immune complex deposition. Anti-neutrophil cytoplasmic antibodies (ANCA) typically are found in the serum, which, as discussed in Chapter 10, have a pathogenic role in some vasculitides. In some instances, therefore, crescentic GN is a component of a systemic vasculitis such as microscopic polyangiitis or granulomatosis with polyangiitis. In many cases, however, pauci-immune crescentic GN is limited to the kidney.

MORPHOLOGY

The light microscopic changes are similar although not identical in various forms of crescentic glomerulonephritis. The glomeruli show cellular proliferation outside the capillary loops, sometimes in association with segmental capillary necrosis, breaks in GBM, and deposition of fibrin in Bowman's space. These distinctive proliferative lesions outside the capillary loops are called **crescents** owing to their shape as they fill Bowman's space. Crescents are formed both by proliferation of epithelial cells and by migration of monocytes/macrophages into Bowman's space (Fig. 14.11). Smaller numbers of other types of leukocytes also may be present. In addition to crescents, cellular proliferation also is seen within the capillary loops and/or in the mesangial areas in cases with immune complex-mediated pathogenesis, such as postinfectious GN, lupus nephritis, or IgA nephropathy. In contrast, in cases with anti-GBM antibody–mediated or pauci-immune crescentic GN, there is no endocapillary hypercellularity. Immunofluorescence studies reveal the characteristic strong **linear staining** with IgG and C3 along the GBM in anti-GBM antibody-mediated disease, a **granular pattern** of glomerular staining in immune complex-mediated GN, while in pauci-immune GN the stains are negative. Electron microscopy shows electron-dense immune complex deposits within the glomeruli in immune complex–mediated GN, but not in biopsies from those with anti-GBM and pauci-immune crescentic GN. Electron microscopy may show distinct **ruptures in the GBM,** signifying severe glomerular injury that is characteristic of this form of GN. The crescents eventually obliterate Bowman's space and compress the glomeruli. In time, crescents may undergo scarring, and glomerulosclerosis develops.

Clinical Features

The onset of RPGN is much like that of the nephritic syndrome, except that the *oliguria and azotemia* are more pronounced. Proteinuria sometimes approaching the nephrotic range may occur. Some affected individuals become anuric and require long-term dialysis or transplantation. The prognosis is roughly predicted by the fraction of involved glomeruli, as patients in whom crescents are present in less than 80% of the glomeruli have a more favorable prognosis than those in whom the percentage of crescents is higher. Plasma exchange may be of benefit in those with anti-GBM antibody GN and in some cases of ANCA-related pauci-immune crescentic GN.

SUMMARY

GLOMERULAR DISEASES

Diseases That Present Mostly With Nephrotic Syndrome

- *Minimal-change disease* is the most frequent cause of nephrotic syndrome in children. It is manifested by proteinuria and effacement of glomerular foot processes without antibody deposits.
- *Focal segmental glomerulosclerosis* (FSGS) may be primary or secondary (e.g., as a consequence of previous glomerulonephritis, hypertension, or infection such as HIV). Glomeruli show focal and segmental obliteration of capillary lumina and loss of foot processes.
- *Membranous nephropathy* is caused by an autoimmune response, most often directed against the PLA2R on podocytes. It is characterized by granular subepithelial deposits of antibodies with GBM "spike" formation, thickening and loss of foot processes but little or no inflammation.
- *Membranoproliferative glomerulonephritis type I* is an immune complex–mediated disease with immune deposits in the subendothelial location.

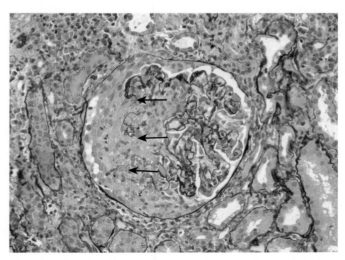

Fig. 14.11 Crescentic glomerulonephritis (silver stain). Arrows indicate areas of necrosis and crescent formation. The segmental distribution in this case is typical of ANCA (anti-neutrophil cytoplasmic antibody)–associated crescentic glomerulonephritis.

- *Dense deposit disease* and *C3 glomerulonephritis* are caused by unregulated activation of the alternative complement pathway. Immunofluorescence is positive for C3 in both conditions.

Glomerulonephritis That Presents With Nephritic Syndrome

- *Acute postinfectious glomerulonephritis* typically occurs after streptococcal infection in children and young adults but may occur following infection with many other organisms. It is caused by deposition of immune complexes, mainly in the subepithelial spaces, with abundant neutrophils and proliferation of glomerular cells.

Diseases That Present Mostly With Asymptomatic Hematuria

- *IgA nephropathy*, characterized by mesangial deposits of IgA-containing immune complexes, is the most common form of glomerulonephritis worldwide. Recurrent asymptomatic hematuria is the most common clinical presentation. It commonly affects children and young adults and has a variable course.
- *Hereditary nephritis (Alport syndrome)* is caused by mutations in genes encoding GBM collagen. It manifests as hematuria and slowly progressing proteinuria and declining renal function. Thin basement membrane disease is also caused by mutations encoding the GBM collagen, however, unlike Alport syndrome, this is usually a benign nonprogressive disorder.

Rapidly Progressive Glomerulonephritis

- RPGN is a clinical entity with features of the nephritic syndrome and rapid loss of renal function.
- It is commonly associated with severe glomerular injury with necrosis and GBM breaks and subsequent proliferation of parietal epithelium (crescents).
- RPGN may be mediated by autoantibodies to the GBM (anti-GBM antibody disease), by immune complex deposition, or it can be pauci-immune often associated with anti-neutrophil cytoplasmic antibodies (pauci-immune GN).

DISEASES AFFECTING TUBULES AND INTERSTITIUM

Most forms of tubular injury also involve the interstitium, so the two are discussed together. Presented under this heading are diseases characterized by (1) inflammatory involvement of the tubules and interstitium *(tubulointerstitial nephritis)* and (2) ischemic or toxic tubular injury, leading to *acute tubular injury* and the clinical syndrome of *acute kidney injury.*

Tubulointerstitial Nephritis

Tubulointerstitial nephritis (TIN) refers to a group of inflammatory kidney diseases that primarily involve the interstitium and tubules. The glomeruli may be spared altogether or affected only late in the course. In cases of TIN caused by bacterial infection, the renal pelvis is prominently involved—hence the more descriptive term *pyelonephritis* (from *pyelo,* "pelvis"). The term *interstitial nephritis* generally is reserved for cases of TIN that are nonbacterial in origin. These include tubular injury resulting from drugs, metabolic disorders such as hypokalemia, irradiation, viral infections, and immune reactions. On the basis of clinical features and the character of the inflammatory exudate, TIN can be divided into acute and chronic categories. Discussed next is acute pyelonephritis followed by consideration of other forms of interstitial nephritis.

Acute Pyelonephritis

Acute pyelonephritis, a common suppurative inflammation of the kidney and the renal pelvis, is caused by bacterial infection. It is an important manifestation of urinary tract infection (UTI), which can involve the lower (cystitis, prostatitis, urethritis) or upper (pyelonephritis) urinary tract, or both. As we will see, the great majority of cases of pyelonephritis are associated with infections of the lower urinary tract, which are very common. Fortunately, most infections of the lower urinary tract remain localized and do not spread to the kidney.

Pathogenesis

The principal causative organisms in acute pyelonephritis are enteric gram-negative bacilli. *Escherichia coli* is by far the most common. Other important organisms are *Proteus, Klebsiella, Enterobacter,* and *Pseudomonas;* these usually are associated with recurrent infections, especially in individuals who undergo urinary tract manipulations or have congenital or acquired anomalies of the lower urinary tract (see later). Staphylococci and *Streptococcus faecalis* also may cause pyelonephritis, but they are uncommon pathogens in this setting.

Bacteria can reach the kidneys from the lower urinary tract (ascending infection) or through the bloodstream (hematogenous infection) (Fig. 14.12). **Ascending infection from the lower urinary tract is the most important and frequent route by which bacteria reach the kidney.** Adhesion of bacteria to mucosal surfaces is followed by colonization of the distal urethra (and the introitus in females). Genetically determined properties of both the urothelium and the bacterial pathogens may facilitate adhesion to the urothelial lining by bacterial fimbriae (proteins that attach to receptors on the surface of urothelial cells), conferring susceptibility to infection. The organisms then reach the bladder, by expansive growth of the colonies and by moving against the flow of urine. This may occur during urethral instrumentation, including catheterization and cystoscopy.

In the absence of instrumentation, UTI most commonly affects females. Because of the close proximity of the female urethra to the rectum, colonization by enteric bacteria can occur more readily in females. Furthermore, the short urethra and trauma to the urethra during sexual intercourse facilitate the entry of bacteria into the urinary bladder. Normally, bladder urine is sterile, because of the anti-microbial properties of the bladder mucosa and the flushing mechanism associated with periodic voiding of urine. With outflow obstruction or bladder dysfunction, however, the natural defense mechanisms of the bladder are overwhelmed, setting the stage for UTI. In the presence of stasis, bacteria introduced into the bladder can multiply undisturbed, without being flushed out or

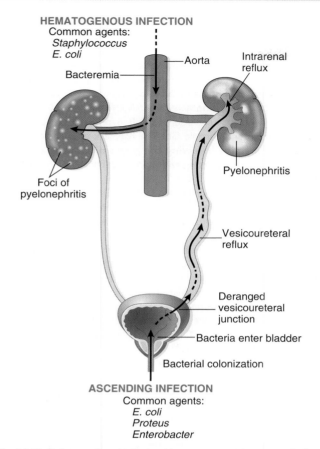

HEMATOGENOUS INFECTION
Common agents:
Staphylococcus
E. coli

Aorta

Bacteremia

Intrarenal reflux

Foci of pyelonephritis

Pyelonephritis

Vesicoureteral reflux

Deranged vesicoureteral junction

Bacteria enter bladder

Bacterial colonization

ASCENDING INFECTION
Common agents:
E. coli
Proteus
Enterobacter

Fig. 14.12 Pathways of renal infection. Hematogenous infection results from bacteremic spread. More common is ascending infection, which results from a combination of urinary bladder infection, vesicoureteral reflux, and intrarenal reflux.

destroyed by the bladder wall. Accordingly, UTI is particularly frequent among patients with urinary tract obstruction, as may occur with benign prostatic hyperplasia and uterine prolapse. From the contaminated bladder urine, the bacteria ascend along the ureters to infect the renal pelvis and parenchyma. The frequency of UTI also is increased in diabetes because of the increased susceptibility to infection and neurogenic bladder dysfunction, which predispose to urine stasis. Increased incidence of UTI during pregnancy is attributed to urine stasis due to pressure on the bladder and ureters from the growing uterus.

Incompetence of the vesicoureteral orifice, resulting in vesicoureteral reflux (VUR), is an important cause of ascending infection. The reflux allows bacteria to ascend the ureter into the pelvis. VUR is present in 20% to 40% of young children with UTI, usually as a consequence of a congenital defect that results in incompetence of the ureterovesical valve. VUR also can be acquired in individuals with a flaccid bladder resulting from spinal cord injury or with bladder dysfunction secondary to diabetes. VUR results in residual urine after voiding in the urinary tract, which favors bacterial growth. Furthermore, VUR affords a ready mechanism by which the infected bladder urine can be propelled up to the renal pelvis and further into the renal parenchyma through

open ducts at the tips of the papillae (intrarenal reflux). Additional risk factors for UTI include preexisting renal conditions with renal scarring and intraparenchymal obstruction and also immunosuppressive therapy and immunodeficiency.

Although *hematogenous spread* is far less common than ascending infection, acute pyelonephritis may result from seeding of the kidneys by bacteria in the course of septicemia or infective endocarditis.

MORPHOLOGY

One or both kidneys may be involved. The affected kidney may be normal in size or enlarged. Characteristically, **discrete, yellowish, raised abscesses are grossly apparent on the renal surface** (Fig. 14.13). They may be widely scattered or limited to one region of the kidney, or they may coalesce to form a single large area of suppuration.

The characteristic histologic feature of acute pyelonephritis is liquefactive necrosis and abscess formation within the renal parenchyma. In the early stages, pus formation (suppuration) is limited to the tubular lumina, but later abscesses rupture into the interstitial tissue. Large masses of intratubular neutrophils frequently extend within involved nephrons into the collecting ducts, giving rise to characteristic white blood cell casts in the urine. Typically, the glomeruli are not affected.

When obstruction is prominent, the pus does not drain and may fill the renal pelvis, calyces, and ureter, producing **pyonephrosis.**

A second (rare) form of pyelonephritis is **papillary necrosis,** which has three predisposing conditions: diabetes, urinary tract obstruction, and sickle cell anemia. This lesion is marked by ischemic and suppurative necrosis of the tips of the renal pyramids (renal papillae). The pathognomonic gross feature is sharply defined gray-white to yellow necrosis of the apical two-thirds of

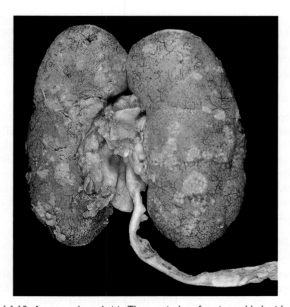

Fig. 14.13 Acute pyelonephritis. The cortical surface is studded with focal pale abscesses, more numerous in the upper pole and middle region of the kidney; the lower pole is relatively unaffected. Between the abscesses, there is dark congestion of the renal surface.

the pyramids. One papilla or several or all papillae may be affected. Microscopically, the papillary tips show coagulative necrosis surrounded by a neutrophilic infiltrate.

Involvement of the prostate can give rise to acute or chronic prostatitis, particularly in older males with benign prostatic hyperplasia.

Clinical Features

Acute pyelonephritis often is associated with predisposing conditions, as described earlier in the discussion of pathogenetic mechanisms. After the first year of life (an age by which congenital anomalies in males commonly become evident) and up to approximately 40 years of age, infections are much more frequent in females. Up to 6% of pregnant women develop bacteriuria some time during pregnancy, and 20% to 40% of these eventually develop symptomatic urinary infection if not treated. With increasing age, the incidence in males rises as a result of the development of prostatic hyperplasia, which causes urinary outflow obstruction.

The onset of uncomplicated acute pyelonephritis usually is sudden, with pain at the costovertebral angle and systemic evidence of infection, such as chills, fever, nausea, malaise, and localizing urinary tract signs of dysuria, frequency, and urgency. The urine appears turbid due to the contained pus (*pyuria*). The disease usually is unilateral, and affected individuals thus do not develop renal failure. In cases in which predisposing factors are present, the disease may become recurrent or chronic and is more likely to be bilateral. The development of papillary necrosis is associated with a much poorer prognosis.

Chronic Pyelonephritis and Reflux Nephropathy

Chronic pyelonephritis is a clinicopathologic entity in which interstitial inflammation and scarring of the renal parenchyma are associated with grossly visible scarring and deformity of the pelvicalyceal system in patients with a history of UTI. Chronic pyelonephritis is an important cause of chronic kidney disease. It can be divided into two forms: chronic obstructive pyelonephritis and chronic reflux–associated pyelonephritis.

Chronic Obstructive Pyelonephritis

As noted, obstruction predisposes the kidney to infection. Recurrent infections superimposed on diffuse or localized obstructive lesions lead to recurrent bouts of renal inflammation and scarring, which eventually cause chronic pyelonephritis. The disease can be bilateral, as with congenital anomalies of the urethra (e.g., posterior urethral valves), or unilateral, such as occurs with calculi and unilateral obstructive lesions of the ureter.

Chronic Reflux–Associated Pyelonephritis (Reflux Nephropathy)

Chronic reflux–associated pyelonephritis is the most common cause of chronic pyelonephritis. It results from superimposition of a UTI on congenital vesicoureteral reflux and intrarenal reflux. Both the reflux and the attendant renal damage may be unilateral or bilateral, the latter potentially leading to chronic renal insufficiency.

MORPHOLOGY

One or both kidneys may be involved, either diffusely or in patches. Even when involvement is bilateral, the kidneys are not equally damaged and therefore are not equally contracted. This **uneven scarring** is useful in differentiating chronic pyelonephritis from the more symmetrically contracted kidneys associated with vascular sclerosis (often referred to as *benign nephrosclerosis*) and chronic GN. The hallmark of chronic pyelonephritis is **scarring involving the pelvis or calyces,** or both, leading to papillary blunting and marked **calyceal deformities** (Fig. 14.14).

The microscopic changes are largely nonspecific, and similar alterations may be seen with other chronic tubulointerstitial disorders such as analgesic nephropathy. The parenchyma shows the following features:

- Uneven interstitial fibrosis and an inflammatory infiltrate of lymphocytes, plasma cells, and occasionally neutrophils
- Dilation or contraction of tubules, with atrophy of the epithelial lining. Many of the dilated tubules contain pink to blue, glassy-appearing PAS-positive casts, known as *colloid casts*, that suggest the appearance of thyroid tissue—hence the descriptive term *thyroidization*. Often, neutrophils are seen within the tubules
- Chronic inflammatory cell infiltration and fibrosis involving the calyceal mucosa and wall
- Arteriolosclerosis may be caused by associated hypertension
- Glomerulosclerosis that usually develops as a secondary process caused by nephron loss (a maladaptation discussed earlier)

Clinical Features

Many patients with chronic pyelonephritis come to medical attention relatively late in the course of the disease, because of the gradual onset of renal insufficiency or because signs of kidney disease are noticed on routine laboratory tests. In other cases, the renal disease is heralded by the development of hypertension. The radiologic image is characteristic: affected kidneys are asymmetrically contracted, with

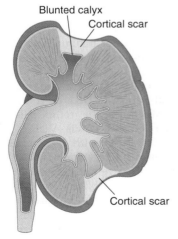

Blunted calyx
Cortical scar

Cortical scar

Fig. 14.14 Typical coarse scars of chronic pyelonephritis associated with vesicoureteral reflux. The scars are usually located at the upper or lower poles of the kidney and are associated with underlying blunted calyces.

some degree of blunting and deformity of the calyceal system (caliectasis). The presence or absence of significant bacteriuria is not particularly helpful, as its absence does not rule out chronic pyelonephritis. If the disease is bilateral and progressive, tubular dysfunction leads to an inability to concentrate the urine *(hyposthenuria)*, manifested by polyuria and nocturia.

As noted earlier, some individuals with chronic pyelonephritis or reflux nephropathy ultimately develop secondary glomerulosclerosis, associated with proteinuria; eventually, these injuries all contribute to progressive chronic kidney disease.

Drug-Induced Tubulointerstitial Nephritis

Acute drug-induced TIN occurs as an adverse reaction to any one of an increasing number of drugs. It is associated most frequently with penicillins (methicillin, ampicillin), other antibiotics (rifampin), diuretics (furosemide), proton pump inhibitors (omeprazole), nonsteroidal antiinflammatory agents, and numerous other drugs (phenindione, cimetidine, immune checkpoint inhibitors).

Pathogenesis

Many features of the disease suggest an immune mechanism. Clinical features consistent with a hypersensitivity reaction include latent period between drug exposure and development of lesions, eosinophilia and rash, the idiosyncratic nature of the drug reaction (i.e., the lack of dose dependence), and the recurrence of the reaction following reexposure to the same drug or others of similar structure. Serum IgE levels are increased in some individuals, suggesting immediate (type I) hypersensitivity. In other cases, the nature of the inflammatory infiltrate and the presence of positive skin tests to drugs suggest a T cell–mediated (type IV) hypersensitivity reaction.

The most likely sequence of pathogenic events is that the drugs act as haptens that, during secretion by tubules, covalently bind to some cytoplasmic or extracellular component of tubular cells and become immunogenic. The resultant tubulointerstitial injury is then caused by IgE- or T cell–mediated immune reactions to tubular cells or their basement membranes.

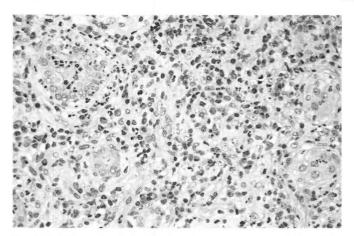

Fig. 14.15 Drug-induced interstitial nephritis, with prominent eosinophilic and mononuclear infiltrate. *(Courtesy of Dr. H. Rennke, Department of Pathology, Brigham and Women's Hospital, Boston, Massachusetts.)*

abnormalities. Urinary findings include hematuria, minimal or no proteinuria, and leukocyturia (sometimes including eosinophils). A rising serum creatinine or acute kidney injury with oliguria develops in about 50% of cases, particularly in older patients. Clinical recognition of drug-induced kidney injury is imperative, because withdrawal of the offending drug is followed by recovery, although it may take several months for renal function to return to normal.

> ## ◗ MORPHOLOGY
>
> The abnormalities in acute drug-induced nephritis are in the interstitium, which shows pronounced edema and infiltration by mononuclear cells, principally lymphocytes and macrophages (Fig. 14.15). Eosinophils and neutrophils may be present, often in large numbers. With some drugs (e.g., methicillin, thiazides, rifampin), T cell mediated reaction may give rise to interstitial nonnecrotizing granulomas with giant cells. The glomeruli are normal except in some cases caused by nonsteroidal antiinflammatory agents, in which the hypersensitivity reaction also leads to podocyte foot process effacement and the nephrotic syndrome.

Clinical Features

The disease begins about 15 days after exposure to the drug and is characterized by *fever, eosinophilia* (which may be transient), *rash* (in about 25% of individuals), and *renal*

> ## ◗ SUMMARY
>
> ### TUBULOINTERSTITIAL NEPHRITIS
>
> - TIN consists of inflammatory disease primarily involving the renal tubules and interstitium.
> - *Acute pyelonephritis* is a bacterial infection caused either by ascending infection as a result of reflux, obstruction, or other abnormality of the urinary tract, or much less commonly by hematogenous spread of bacteria; it is characterized by abscess formation in the kidneys, sometimes with papillary necrosis.
> - *Chronic pyelonephritis* usually is associated with urinary obstruction or reflux; it results in scarring of the pelvicalyceal system and the interstium of the involved kidney and gradual progression of chronic kidney disease.
> - *Drug-induced interstitial nephritis* is an IgE- or T cell–mediated immune reaction to a drug; it is characterized by interstitial inflammation, often with abundant eosinophils, and edema.

Acute Tubular Injury/Necrosis

Acute tubular injury (ATI) is a clinicopathologic entity characterized by damage to tubular epithelial cells and an acute decline in renal function, often associated with shedding of granular casts and tubular cells into the urine. Clinicians use the term *acute tubular necrosis,* but frank necrosis is rarely observed in a kidney biopsy, so pathologists prefer the term *acute tubular injury.* The constellation of changes, broadly termed *acute kidney injury,* manifests clinically as decreased GFR with concurrent elevation of serum creatinine. ATI is the most common cause of acute kidney injury and may produce oliguria (defined as urine output of <400 mL/day).

There are two forms of ATI that differ in the underlying causes.

- *Ischemic ATI* is most often the result of a period of inadequate blood flow to all or some peripheral organs such as the kidney, sometimes in the setting of marked hypotension and shock. This can be caused by a variety of conditions, including severe trauma, blood loss, acute pancreatitis and septicemia. Ischemia to tubules may also result from reduced intrarenal blood flow, as in microscopic polyangiitis, malignant hypertension, and thrombotic microangiopathies. Mismatched blood transfusions and other hemolytic crises, as well as myoglobinuria, also produce a clinical picture resembling that of ischemic ATI.
- *Nephrotoxic ATI* is caused by a variety of poisons, including heavy metals (e.g., mercury); organic solvents (e.g., carbon tetrachloride); and a multitude of drugs such as gentamicin and other antibiotics, and radiographic contrast agents.

Pathogenesis

Proximal tubular epithelial cells are particularly sensitive to hypoxemia and also are vulnerable to toxins (Fig. 14.16). Several factors predispose these cells to toxic and ischemic injury, including elevated intracellular concentrations of various molecules that are resorbed or secreted across the proximal tubule, exposure to high concentrations of luminal solutes that are concentrated by the resorption of water from the glomerular filtrate, and a high rate of oxygen consumption, which is required to generate the ATP that is needed for transport and reabsorption functions.

Ischemia causes numerous structural alterations in epithelial cells. Loss of cell polarity is an early reversible event caused by ischemia. It leads to the redistribution of membrane proteins (e.g., Na⁺,K⁺-ATPase) from the basolateral to the luminal surface of tubular cells, resulting in decreased sodium reabsorption by proximal tubules and hence increased sodium delivery to distal tubules. The latter, through a tubuloglomerular feedback mechanism, contributes to afferent arteriolar vasoconstriction and a decrease in GFR, further worsening the perfusion (discussed below). Injury to the epithelial cells causes detachment of the damaged cells from the basement membranes, and their shedding into the urine. If sufficient tubular debris builds up, it can block the outflow of urine (obstruction by casts), increasing intratubular pressure and thereby exacerbating the decline in GFR. Additionally, fluid from the damaged tubules may leak back into the interstitium, resulting in decreased urine output, increased interstitial pressure, and collapse of the tubules. Ischemic tubular cells also express chemokines, cytokines, and adhesion molecules such as P-selectin that recruit leukocytes (interstitial inflammation) and can participate in tissue injury. Necrotic tubular cells also may elicit an inflammatory reaction that contributes to the tubular injury and functional derangements.

Tubular injury is exacerbated by severe hemodynamic alterations that cause reduced GFR. The major one is *intrarenal vasoconstriction,* which results in both reduced glomerular plasma flow and reduced oxygen delivery to the tubules in the outer medulla (thick ascending limb and straight segment of the proximal tubule) (see Fig. 14.16). Although a number of vasoconstrictor pathways have been implicated in this phenomenon (e.g., renin-angiotensin, thromboxane A₂, sympathetic nerve activity), the current opinion is that vasoconstriction is mediated by sublethal endothelial injury, leading to increased release of the endothelial vasoconstrictor endothelin and decreased production of vasodilatory nitric oxide and prostaglandins. Finally, some evidence points to a direct effect of ischemia or toxins on the glomerulus, causing a reduced effective glomerular filtration surface.

The patchiness of tubular necrosis and maintenance of the integrity of the basement membrane along many segments allow repair of the injured foci and recovery of function if the precipitating cause is removed. This repair is dependent on the capacity of reversibly injured epithelial cells to proliferate and differentiate.

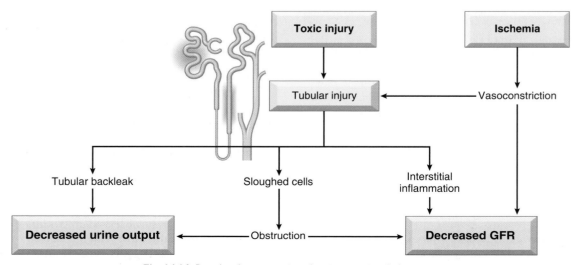

Fig. 14.16 Postulated sequence in ischemic or toxic tubular injury.

Ischemic ATI is characterized by lesions in the straight portions of the proximal tubule and the ascending thick limbs, but no segment of the proximal or distal tubules is spared. There is often a variety of **tubular injuries,** including attenuation of proximal tubular brush borders, blebbing and sloughing of brush borders, vacuolization of cells, and detachment of tubular cells from their underlying basement membranes with sloughing of cells into the urine (Fig. 14.17). A striking additional finding is the presence of proteinaceous casts in the distal tubules and collecting ducts, which consist of Tamm-Horsfall protein (normally secreted by tubular epithelium) along with hemoglobin and other plasma proteins. When crush injuries have produced ATI, the casts also contain myoglobin. The interstitium usually shows generalized edema along with a mild inflammatory infiltrate consisting of neutrophils, lymphocytes, and plasma cells. The histologic picture in **nephrotoxic ATI** is basically similar, with some differences. Overt necrosis is usually more prominent in the proximal tubule than in ischemic ATI, and the tubular basement membranes generally are spared.

If the patient survives, epithelial regeneration becomes apparent in the form of a low cuboidal epithelial covering and mitotic activity in the surviving tubular epithelial cells. In some cases, for reasons that are not entirely clear, acute kidney injury with underlying acute tubular injury as its cause may result in tubular atrophy and interstitial fibrosis rather than repair.

Clinical Features

The clinical course of ischemic ATI initially is dominated by the inciting medical, surgical or obstetric event. Affected patients often present with manifestations of acute kidney injury, including oliguria and decreased GFR. Not all patients have oliguria; both anuric and non-oligouric forms are seen. The clinical picture is often dominated by electrolyte abnormalities, acidosis, and the signs and symptoms of uremia and fluid overload. The prognosis varies depending upon the severity and nature of the underlying injury

and comorbid conditions. In the absence of supportive treatment or dialysis, patients may die. When the cause of acute kidney injury is ATI, repair and tubular regeneration lead to gradual clinical improvement. With supportive care, patients who survive have a good chance of recovering renal function, but a single severe episode of ATI also may result in chronic kidney disease. In those with preexisting chronic kidney disease, complete recovery is less frequent, and progression to end-stage renal disease is unfortunately common.

ACUTE TUBULAR INJURY

- ATI is the most common cause of acute kidney injury; its clinical manifestations are electrolyte abnormalities, acidosis, uremia, and signs of fluid overload, often with oliguria.
- ATI results from ischemic or toxic injury to renal tubules, and is associated with intrarenal vasoconstriction resulting in reduced GFR and diminished delivery of oxygen and nutrients to tubular epithelial cells.
- ATI is characterized morphologically by injury or necrosis of segments of the tubules (typically the proximal tubules), proteinaceous casts in distal tubules, and interstitial edema.

DISEASES INVOLVING BLOOD VESSELS

Nearly all diseases of the kidney affect the renal blood vessels secondarily. Systemic vascular diseases, such as various forms of vasculitis, also involve renal blood vessels, and often produce clinically important effects on renal function (Chapter 10). Conversely, the kidney is intimately involved in the pathogenesis of both essential and secondary hypertension. This section covers the renal lesions associated with hypertension.

Nephrosclerosis

Nephrosclerosis **refers to sclerosis of small renal arteries and arterioles that is strongly associated with hypertension.** The characteristic morphologic alterations of the small arterioles are called *hyaline arteriolosclerosis*, while the arteries show fibrous intimal and medial thickening often resulting in luminal narrowing. The vascular changes cause ischemia, which leads to various combinations of interstitial fibrosis, tubular atrophy, and focal global glomerulosclerosis. Some degree of nephrosclerosis, albeit mild, is present in many individuals older than 60 years of age. The frequency and severity of the lesions are increased at any age when hypertension or diabetes are present. Of note, many renal diseases cause hypertension, which in turn is associated with nephrosclerosis. Thus, this renal lesion often is superimposed on other primary kidney diseases.

Pathogenesis

The arterial lesions associated with hypertension are the result mainly of endothelial dysfunction and platelet

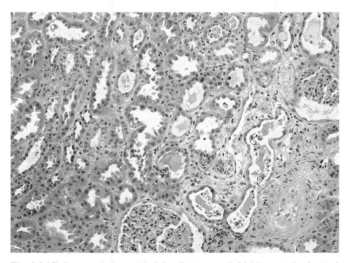

Fig. 14.17 Acute tubular epithelial cell injury with blebbing at the luminal pole, detachment of tubular cells from their underlying basement membranes, and granular casts.

activation (Chapter 10). Two processes participate in the arterial lesions of nephrosclerosis:

- Medial and intimal thickening, as a response to hemodynamic changes, aging, genetic defects, or some combination of these
- Hyalinization of arteriolar walls, caused by extravasation of plasma proteins through injured endothelium and by increased deposition of basement membrane matrix

MORPHOLOGY

Grossly, the kidneys are **symmetrically atrophic.** Typically the renal surface shows diffuse, fine granularity that resembles grain leather. Microscopically, the most prominent change is hyaline thickening of the walls of the arterioles, known as **hyaline arteriolosclerosis.** This appears as a homogeneous, pink hyaline thickening, at the expense of the vessel lumina, with loss of underlying cellular detail (Fig. 14.18). The narrowing of the lumen results in markedly decreased blood flow through the affected vessels, with consequent ischemia and renal atrophy. In advanced cases of arterionephrosclerosis, the glomerular tufts may become sclerosed. Diffuse tubular atrophy and interstitial fibrosis are present, but inflammatory infiltrates are absent or scant. The larger blood vessels (interlobar and arcuate arteries) show intimal thickening with replication of internal elastic lamina along with fibrous thickening of the media **(fibroelastic hyperplasia).**

Clinical Features

This renal lesion alone rarely causes damage severe enough to produce renal failure, except in individuals from some, possibly genetically susceptible, groups, such as African Americans, in whom it may lead to uremia and death. However, all patients usually show some functional impairment, such as loss of concentrating ability or a variably diminished GFR. A mild degree of proteinuria is a frequent finding.

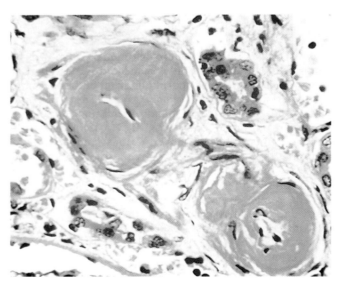

Fig. 14.18 Benign nephrosclerosis. High-power view of two arterioles with hyaline deposition, marked thickening of the walls, and a narrowed lumen. *(Courtesy of Dr. M.A. Venkatachalam, Department of Pathology, University of Texas Health Sciences Center, San Antonio, Texas.)*

Malignant Hypertension

Malignant hypertension, defined as blood pressure usually greater than 200/120 mm Hg, is far less common in the United States than essential hypertension and occurs in only about 5% of hypertensive individuals. It may arise de novo (i.e., without preexisting hypertension), or it may appear suddenly in an individual who had mild hypertension. The prevalence of malignant hypertension is higher in developing countries. It may present with severe acute kidney injury and renal failure. Renal changes are confined to the vasculature and may include thrombotic microangiopathy.

Pathogenesis

The renal changes are related to hypertension and the reactions to it.

- Injury resulting from long-standing hypertension causes increased permeability of the vessels to fibrinogen and other plasma proteins, endothelial injury, and platelet deposition. This leads to the appearance of *fibrinoid necrosis* of arterioles and small arteries and intravascular thrombosis
- Mitogenic factors from platelets (e.g., platelet-derived growth factor) and plasma cause intimal hyperplasia of vessels, resulting in *hyperplastic arteriosclerosis.* Because of the luminal narrowing, the kidneys become markedly ischemic, which leads to further elevation of blood pressure via the renin-angiotensin system.

MORPHOLOGY

The kidney may be normal in size or shrunken, depending on the duration and severity of the hypertensive disease. Small, **pinpoint petechial hemorrhages** may appear on the cortical surface from rupture of arterioles or glomerular capillaries, giving the kidney a peculiar, **flea-bitten appearance.**

The microscopic changes reflect the pathogenetic events discussed earlier. Damage to the small vessels is manifested as **fibrinoid necrosis** of the arterioles (Fig. 14.19A). The vessel walls show a homogeneous, granular eosinophilic appearance masking underlying detail. In the interlobular arteries and larger arterioles, proliferation of intimal cells after acute injury produces an *onion-skin* appearance (see Fig. 14.19B). This name is derived from the concentric arrangement of cells whose origin is believed to be intimal smooth muscle, although this issue has not been finally settled. This lesion, called **hyperplastic arteriolosclerosis,** causes marked narrowing of arterioles and small arteries, to the point of total obliteration. Necrosis also may involve glomeruli, with microthrombi within the glomeruli as well as necrotic arterioles. Similar lesions are seen in individuals with acute thrombotic microangiopathies (discussed later), and in patients with scleroderma in renal crisis.

Clinical Features

The full-blown syndrome of malignant hypertension is characterized by papilledema, encephalopathy, cardiovascular abnormalities, and renal failure. Most often, the early symptoms are related to *increased intracranial pressure* and include headache, nausea, vomiting, and visual impairment, particularly the development of scotomas, or "spots" before the

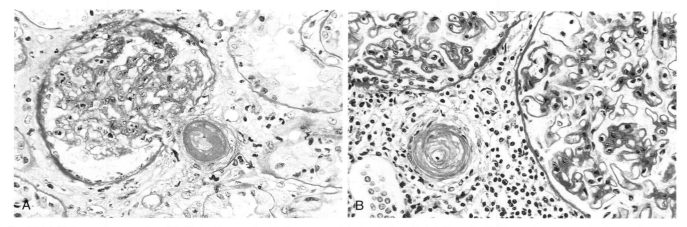

Fig. 14.19 Malignant hypertension. (A) Fibrinoid necrosis of afferent arteriole (periodic acid–Schiff stain). (B) Hyperplastic arteriolosclerosis (onion-skin lesion). *(Courtesy of Dr. H. Rennke, Department of Pathology, Brigham and Women's Hospital, Boston, Massachusetts.)*

eyes. At the onset of rapidly mounting blood pressure, there is marked proteinuria and microscopic, or sometimes macroscopic, hematuria but no significant alteration in renal function. Soon, however, *acute kidney injury* develops. The syndrome represents a true medical emergency that requires prompt and aggressive anti-hypertensive therapy before irreversible renal lesions develop. About 50% of patients survive at least 5 years; 90% of deaths are caused by uremia, and the other 10% are caused by cerebral hemorrhage or cardiac failure.

Thrombotic Microangiopathies

As discussed in Chapter 10, the term *thrombotic microangiopathy (TMA)* refers to lesions seen in various clinical syndromes characterized by microvascular thrombosis accompanied by *microangiopathic hemolytic anemia, thrombocytopenia*, and, in certain instances, *renal failure.* The primary forms of TMA include those with a known etiology, while the secondary forms develop in the background of other diseases or conditions without well-defined etiology. Common primary forms of TMA include *Shiga toxin–mediated hemolytic uremic syndrome (HUS); atypical HUS*, also called complement-mediated TMA because excessive complement activation is an important pathogenic mechanism; *thrombotic thrombocytopenic purpura (TTP);* and some of the *drug-mediated TMAs.* Malignant hypertension and scleroderma-associated TMA represent examples of the secondary forms.

Pathogenesis

The major pathogenetic factors in the thrombotic microangiopathies are endothelial cell injury and platelet activation and aggregation. They can be caused by diverse insults, including external toxins, drugs, autoantibodies, and inherited mutations, which can lead to excessive small vessel thrombosis in the capillaries and arterioles in various organs. Vascular compromise results in ischemic injury and organ dysfunction. The classic laboratory manifestations of thrombotic microangiopathy are thrombocytopenia caused by excessive platelet consumption, and microangiopathic hemolytic anemia due to mechanical injury (shearing) of red cells as they pass through vascular

channels narrowed by thrombi. In the primary forms of thrombotic microangiopathies, the etiology is well-defined (Table 14.4), while the secondary forms are associated with various underlying conditions and diseases, such as malignant hypertension, scleroderma, pregnancy, chemotherapy, anti-phospholipid antibodies, and transplant rejection, with less well-defined etiology and pathogenesis. Only the three major forms of primary thrombotic microangiopathies are sufficiently common to merit discusson.

- *Shiga toxin–mediated HUS.* As many as 75% of cases follow intestinal infection with Shiga toxin–producing *E. coli,* such as occurs following ingestion of contaminated ground meat (e.g., in hamburgers) and infections with *Shigella dysenteriae* type I. The pathogenesis is related to the effects of Shiga toxin. The basis for thrombus formation in small vessels, particularly in the kidney, is complex, but most studies suggest endothelial damage has a central role. Renal glomerular endothelial cells are vulnerable because they express the membrane receptor for Shiga toxin. At low doses, the toxin activates endothelial cells, leading to leukocyte adhesion,

Table 14.4 Etiologic Classification of the Major Forms of Primary Thrombotic Microangiopathy

	Forms	Etiology
Shiga toxin–mediated HUS	Acquired	Shiga toxin–producing *E. coli Shigella dysenteriae* serotype I
Atypical HUS (complement-mediated TMA)	Inherited	Complement dysregulation due to genetic abnormalities (relatively common)
	Acquired	Acquired complement dysregulation due to autoantibodies (rare)
TTP	Inherited	Genetic ADAMTS13 deficiency (rare)
	Acquired	ADAMTS13 deficiency due to autoantibodies (relatively common)

ADAMTS13, von Willebrand factor cleaving protease; *HUS*, hemolytic uremic syndrome; *TMA*, thrombotic microangiopathy; *TTP*, thrombotic thrombocytopenic purpura.

increased endothelin production and decreased nitric oxide production (both favoring vasoconstriction), as well as other changes that may promote platelet adhesion and activation. At high doses, the toxin causes endothelial cell death. All of these alterations may contribute to the formation of thrombi, which tend to be most prominent in glomerular capillaries, afferent arterioles, and interlobular arteries.

- *Atypical HUS* is caused by acquired or hereditary abnormalities of factors that dampen activation of complement by the alternative pathway. Their absence leads to excessive activation of complement, with ensuing microvascular injury and microvascular thrombosis. The C5-9 membrane attack complex appears to have a central role, as a therapeutic antibody that inhibits this complex turns off platelet consumption and improves renal function. Interestingly, abnormalities of the alternative pathway of complement activation also may lead to C3 glomerulonephritis and dense deposit disease, as discussed earlier.

- *TTP* is caused by acquired or inherited deficiencies in ADAMTS13 (a disintegrin and metalloprotease with thrombospondin-like motifs), a plasma protease that cleaves von Willebrand factor (vWF) multimers into smaller sizes. Acquired defects in ADAMTS13 are caused by inhibitory autoantibodies directed against ADAMTS13, while inherited deficiencies stem from mutations in the ADAMTS13 gene. Deficiencies of ADAMTS13 result in the formation of abnormally large vWF multimers that activate platelets spontaneously, leading to platelet aggregation and thrombosis in multiple organs, including the kidney.

MORPHOLOGY

The morphologic lesions are very similar in all forms of TMA regardless of the etiology. Thrombi are seen in glomerular capillaries and also the arterioles and sometimes the larger arteries in more severe cases. Additional glomerular changes resulting from endothelial injury include widening of the subendothelial space, duplication or splitting of GBMs, and lysis of mesangial cells. Cortical necrosis also may occur in severe cases. If TMA persists, scarring of glomeruli may develop. Except for varying amounts of fibrinogen in the glomeruli and arterioles, immunofluorescence studies are typically negative.

Clinical Features

The clinical course varies according to the etiology and the severity of the morphologic changes. More severe vascular changes are typically associated with a less favorable outcome.

Shiga toxin–associated HUS is characterized by the sudden onset, usually after a gastrointestinal or flulike prodromal episode, of bleeding manifestations (especially hematemesis and melena), severe oliguria, hematuria, microangiopathic hemolytic anemia, and (in some individuals) prominent neurologic changes. *This disease is one of the main causes of acute kidney injury in children.* If the acute kidney injury is managed properly with dialysis, most patients recover in a matter of weeks. The long-term prognosis (over 15–25 years), however, is not uniformly favorable, as about 25% of affected children eventually develop renal insufficiency.

The onset of atypical HUS is usually sudden, without prodromal diarrhea. The outcome is significantly poorer than in Shiga toxin–mediated HUS. The case-fatality ratio is approximately 20%, and only 60% to 70% of patients recover renal function. Plasma exchange can be used to temporarily restore missing factors (in those with inherited disease) or remove pathogenic antibodies. Since most complement factors are produced in the liver, liver transplantation can be curative. More recently, antibody inhibitors of the membrane attack complex have been shown to be effective in reducing thrombosis and improving renal function, and are now considered to be the first-line therapy in "complement-mediated" forms of HUS.

The typical onset of TTP is also sudden, with a dominant involvement of the central nervous system, and the kidneys are less commonly involved than in Shiga toxin and atypical HUS. Without therapy, TTP typically follows a rapidly fatal course, with survival rates of approximately 10%. With the advent of plasma exchange therapy that replaces ADAMTS 13, the prognosis has improved dramatically. In those patients who survive, residual renal abnormalities are rare.

SUMMARY

VASCULAR DISEASES OF THE KIDNEY

- *Arterionephrosclerosis:* Progressive, chronic renal damage associated with hypertension. Characteristic features are hyaline arteriolosclerosis and narrowing of vascular lumina with resultant cortical atrophy.
- *Malignant hypertension:* Acute kidney injury associated with severe elevation of blood pressure. Arteries and arterioles show fibrinoid necrosis and hyperplasia of smooth muscle cells; petechial hemorrhages appear on the cortical surface.
- *Thrombotic microangiopathies:* Disorders characterized by fibrin thrombi in glomeruli and small vessels resulting in acute kidney injury. Typical HUS is usually caused by endothelial injury by an *E. coli* toxin; TTP is often caused by abnormalities in von Willebrand factor leading to excessive thrombosis, with platelet consumption. The most common cause of atypical HUS is complement-mediated endothelial injury due to complement dysregulation.

CHRONIC KIDNEY DISEASE

Chronic kidney disease is a broad term that describes the final common pathway of progressive nephron loss resulting from any type of kidney disease. Alterations in the function of remaining intact nephrons are ultimately maladaptive and cause further scarring. This eventually results in an end-stage kidney with sclerosed glomeruli, tubules, interstitium and vessels, regardless of the anatomic site of the original injury. Unless the disorder is treated with dialysis or transplantation, death from uremia, electrolyte disturbances, or other complications of end-stage renal disease results.

Pathogenesis

As progressive renal damage destroys more and more nephrons, adaptive mechanisms are initiated that try to maintain renal function. Among such adaptive mechanisms, glomerular hyperfiltration tends to compensate for decreased glomerular filtration rate resulting from the loss of nephrons. An increase in the rate of excretion of solutes per nephron via increased plasma concentrations (for creatinine), decreased tubular reabsorption (for sodium, phosphate, and calcium), or increased tubular secretion (for potassium and hydrogen ions) helps to maintain homeostasis until the late stages of chronic kidney disease. The rate of functional decline varies based on the original disease; however, renal function often deteriorates progressively even when the original insult is controlled. Uncontrolled hypertension, regardless of the etiology, results in more rapid renal functional decline.

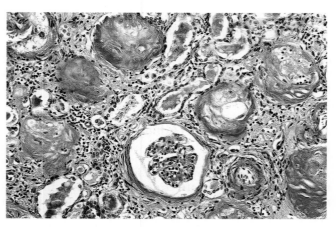

Fig. 14.20 Chronic glomerulonephritis. A Masson trichrome preparation shows complete replacement of virtually all glomeruli by blue-staining collagen. *(Courtesy of Dr. M.A. Venkatachalam, Department of Pathology, University of Texas Health Sciences Center, San Antonio, Texas.)*

MORPHOLOGY

Classically, the kidneys are **symmetrically contracted,** and their surfaces are red-brown and **diffusely granular** when the underlying disorder affects blood vessels or glomeruli. Kidneys damaged by chronic pyelonephritis are typically unevenly involved and have deep scars. Microscopically, the feature common to all cases is advanced scarring of the glomeruli, sometimes to the point of complete sclerosis (Fig. 14.20). This **obliteration of the glomeruli** is the end point of many diseases, and it is impossible to ascertain from such kidneys the nature of the initial lesion. There also is marked **interstitial fibrosis,** associated with atrophy and dropout of many of the tubules in the cortex, and diminution and loss of portions of the peritubular capillary network. The small- and medium-sized arteries frequently are thick-walled, with narrowed lumina, secondary to hypertension. Lymphocytic (and, rarely, plasma cell) infiltrates are present in the fibrotic interstitial tissue. As damage to all structures progresses, it may become difficult to ascertain whether the primary lesion was glomerular, vascular, tubular, or interstitial. Such markedly damaged kidneys have been designated **end-stage kidneys.**

Clinical Features

Chronic kidney disease may develop insidiously and be discovered late in its course, because it is often asymptomatic. Frequently, renal disease is first detected by the discovery of proteinuria, hypertension, or azotemia on routine medical examination. Disease-specific findings may precede development of chronic kidney disease. In patients with glomerular disease resulting in nephrotic syndrome, as the glomeruli undergo sclerotic changes and result in nephron loss, the avenue for protein loss is progressively lessened, and the nephrotic syndrome thus becomes less severe with advanced disease. Some degree of proteinuria, however, is present in almost all cases. Hypertension is very common. Although microscopic hematuria is usually present, grossly bloody urine is infrequent at this late stage.

Without treatment, the prognosis is poor; relentless progression to uremia and death is the rule. The rate of progression is extremely variable.

CYSTIC DISEASES OF THE KIDNEY

Cystic diseases of the kidney are a heterogeneous group comprising hereditary, developmental, and acquired disorders. They often present diagnostic problems for clinicians, radiologists, and pathologists and can occasionally be confused with malignant tumors. Some forms, such as adult polycystic disease, constitute major causes of chronic kidney disease.

An emerging theme in the pathophysiology of the hereditary cystic diseases is that the underlying defect is in the cilia-centrosome complex of tubular epithelial cells. Such defects may interfere with fluid absorption or cellular maturation, resulting in cyst formation. A brief overview of simple cysts, the most common form, is presented next, followed by a more detailed discussion of polycystic kidney disease. Renal dysplasia, the most common form of cystic renal disease in childhood, is discussed under congenital and developmental anomalies later in the chapter.

Simple Cysts

Simple cysts are generally innocuous lesions that occur as multiple or single cystic spaces of variable size. Commonly, they are 1 to 5 cm in diameter; translucent; lined by a gray, glistening, smooth membrane; and filled with clear fluid. On microscopic examination, these membranes are seen to be composed of a single layer of cuboidal or flattened cuboidal epithelium, which in many instances may be completely atrophic. The cysts usually are confined to the cortex. Rarely, massive cysts as large as 10 cm in diameter are encountered.

Simple cysts are a common postmortem finding that has no clinical significance. The main importance of cysts lies in their differentiation from kidney tumors, when they are discovered either incidentally or during evaluation of hemorrhage and pain. Radiographic studies show that in contrast with renal tumors, renal cysts have smooth contours, are almost always avascular, and produce fluid rather than solid tissue signals on ultrasonography.

Acquired cystic kidney disease occurs in patients with end-stage renal disease who have undergone dialysis for many years. Multiple cysts may be present in both the cortex and the medulla and may bleed, causing hematuria. The risk for renal neoplasms, particularly cystic ones, in this setting is over 100 times greater than in the general population.

Autosomal Dominant (Adult) Polycystic Kidney Disease

Adult polycystic kidney disease is characterized by multiple expanding cysts affecting both kidneys that ultimately destroy the intervening parenchyma. It is seen in approximately 1 in 500 to 1000 individuals and accounts for 10% of cases of chronic kidney disease. This disease is genetically heterogeneous. It can be caused by inheritance of one of at least two autosomal dominant genes of very high penetrance.

Pathogenesis

In 85% to 90% of families, *PKD1,* on the short arm of chromosome 16, is the defective gene. This gene encodes a large (460-kDa) and complex cell membrane–associated protein called *polycystin-1.* The polycystin-1 protein has a large extracelluar domain and multiple transmembrane regions. The extracellular domains have regions that can bind to extracellular matrix. Polycystin-1 localizes to the primary cilium of tubular cells (as do nephrocystins linked to medullary cystic disease, discussed later), giving rise to the concept of renal cystic diseases as a type of *ciliopathy.* Cilia are hairlike organelles that project into the lumina from the apical surface of tubular cells, where they serve as mechanosensors of fluid flow. Current evidence suggests that polycystin mutations produce defects in mechanosensing (Fig. 14.21). This, in turn, alters downstream signaling events involving calcium influx, leading to dysregulation of cell polarity, proliferation, and cell–cell and cell–matrix adhesion. The increase in intracellular calcium is thought to stimulate proliferation and secretion from the tubular epithelial cells, which together lead to the formation of cysts, which progressively enlarge over time. Mediators in cyst fluid derived from the epithelial cells can further enhance fluid secretion and induce inflammation. In addition, the calcium-induced signals alter the interaction of epithelial cells with extracellular matrix, and this too is thought to contribute to the cyst formation and interstitial fibrosis that are characteristic of progressive polycystic kidney disease. It is interesting to note that whereas germline mutations of the *PKD1* gene are present in all renal tubular cells of affected individuals, cysts develop in only some tubules. This is most likely due to loss of both alleles of *PKD1.* Thus, as with tumor suppressor genes, a second "somatic hit" is required for cyst development.

The *PKD2* gene, implicated in 10% to 15% of cases, resides on chromosome 4 and encodes *polycystin-2,* a smaller, 110-kDa protein. Polycystin-2 is thought to function as a calcium-permeable membrane channel, and is also localized to cilia. Although structurally distinct, polycystins 1 and 2 are believed to act together by forming heterodimers. Thus, mutation in either gene gives rise to essentially the same phenotype, although patients with

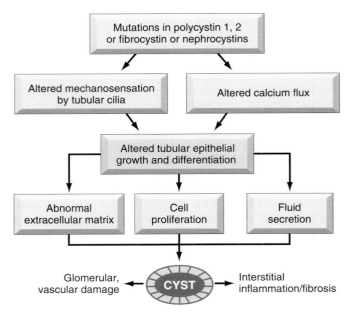

Fig. 14.21 Possible mechanisms of cyst formation in cystic kidney diseases (see text).

PKD2 mutations have a slower rate of disease progression compared to patients with *PKD1* mutations.

MORPHOLOGY

In autosomal dominant adult polycystic kidney disease, the kidney may reach enormous size; weights of up to 4 kg for each kidney have been recorded. These very large kidneys are readily palpable abdominally as masses extending into the pelvis. On gross examination, the kidney seems to be composed solely of cysts of up to 3 or 4 cm in diameter with no intervening parenchyma. The cysts are filled with fluid, which may be clear, turbid, or hemorrhagic (Fig. 14.22).

Cysts may arise at any level of the nephron, from tubules to collecting ducts, and therefore they have a variable, often atrophic, lining. Occasionally, Bowman's capsules are involved in the cyst formation, and in these cases glomerular tufts may be seen within the cystic space. The pressure of the expanding cysts leads to ischemic atrophy of the intervening renal substance. Some normal parenchyma may be dispersed among the cysts. Evidence of superimposed hypertension or infection is common. Asymptomatic liver cysts also occur in one-third of patients.

Clinical Features

Polycystic kidney disease in adults usually *does not produce symptoms until the fourth decade of life,* by which time the kidneys are quite large. The most common presenting complaint is *flank pain* or a heavy, dragging sensation. Acute distention of a cyst, either by intracystic hemorrhage or by obstruction, may cause excruciating pain. Sometimes attention is first drawn to the lesion on palpation of an abdominal mass. *Intermittent gross hematuria* commonly occurs. The most important complications, because of their deleterious effect on already marginal renal function, are *hypertension and urinary infection.* Hypertension of variable severity develops in about 75% of individuals with this

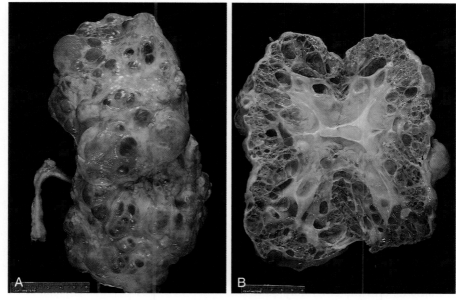

Fig. 14.22 Autosomal dominant adult polycystic kidney, viewed from the external surface (A) and bisected (B). The kidney is markedly enlarged (centimeter rule is shown for scale), with numerous dilated cysts.

disorder. Saccular aneurysms of the circle of Willis (Chapter 23) are present in 10% to 30% of patients and are associated with a high incidence of subarachnoid hemorrhage.

Although the disease is ultimately fatal, the outlook is generally more favorable than with most chronic kidney diseases. The condition progresses very slowly. End-stage renal disease occurs at about 50 years of age, but there is wide variation in the course, and nearly normal life spans are reported. Patients in whom the disease progresses to renal failure are treated by renal transplantation. Death usually results from uremia or hypertensive complications.

Autosomal Recessive (Childhood) Polycystic Kidney Disease

The childhood form of polycystic kidney disease is a rare autosomal recessive disorder that is genetically distinct from adult polycystic kidney disease. It occurs in approximately 1 in 20,000 live births. Perinatal, neonatal, infantile, and juvenile subcategories have been defined, depending on age at presentation and the presence of associated hepatic lesions. All types result from mutations in the *PKHD1* gene, coding for a putative membrane receptor protein called *fibrocystin*. Fibrocystin is found in cilia in tubular epithelial cells, but its function remains unknown.

MORPHOLOGY

In autosomal recessive polycystic kidney disease, **numerous small cysts** in the cortex and medulla give the kidney a sponge-like appearance. Dilated, elongated channels at right angles to the cortical surface completely replace the medulla and cortex. The cysts have a uniform lining of cuboidal cells, reflecting their origin from the collecting tubules. The disease is invariably bilateral. In almost all cases, findings include multiple epithelium-lined **liver cysts** and proliferation of portal bile ducts.

Clinical Features

Perinatal and neonatal forms are most common; serious manifestations usually are present at birth, and young infants may die quickly from hepatic or renal failure. Patients who survive infancy develop liver cirrhosis (congenital hepatic fibrosis).

Medullary Diseases With Cysts

There are two major types of cystic disease affecting the medulla: *medullary sponge kidney,* a relatively common and usually innocuous condition, occasionally associated with nephrolithiasis, which will not be discussed further, and *nephronophthisis-medullary cystic disease complex,* which is almost always associated with renal dysfunction.

Nephronophthisis–medullary cystic disease complex is an underappreciated cause of chronic kidney disease that usually begins in childhood. Four variants are recognized on the basis of the timing of onset: infantile, juvenile, and adolescent nephronophthisis, and medullary cystic disease developing later in adult life. The juvenile form is the most common. Approximately 15% to 20% of children with juvenile nephronophthisis have extrarenal manifestations, which most often appear as retinal abnormalities, including retinitis pigmentosa, and even early-onset blindness in the most severe form. Other abnormalities found in some individuals include oculomotor apraxia, mental retardation, cerebellar malformations, and liver fibrosis. In aggregate, the various forms of nephronophthisis are now thought to be the most common genetic cause of end-stage renal disease in children and young adults.

At least nine gene loci (NHP1 to NHP9) have been identified for the autosomal recessive forms of the nephronophthisis complex. The majority of these genes encode proteins that are components of epithelial cilia, as is the case with other types of polycystic disease. Two autosomal forms cause disease in adults; these are far less common.

MORPHOLOGY

Pathologic features of medullary cystic disease include **small contracted kidneys.** Numerous small cysts lined by flattened or cuboidal epithelium are present, typically at the corticomedullary junction. Other pathologic changes are nonspecific, but most notably include a chronic tubulointerstitial nephritis with tubular atrophy and thickened tubular basement membranes and progressive interstitial fibrosis.

Clinical Features

The initial manifestations are usually polyuria and polydipsia, a consequence of diminished tubular function. Progression to end-stage renal disease ensues over a 5- to 10-year period. The disease is difficult to diagnose because there are no serologic markers, and the cysts may be too small to be seen with radiologic imaging. Adding to this difficulty, cysts may not be apparent on renal biopsy if the corticomedullary junction is not well sampled. A positive family history and unexplained chronic renal failure in young patients should lead to suspicion of nephronophthisis.

SUMMARY

CYSTIC DISEASES

- *Adult polycystic kidney disease* is a disease of autosomal dominant inheritance caused by mutations in the genes encoding polycystin-1 or polycystin-2. It accounts for about 10% of cases of ESRD; the kidneys may be very large and contain many cysts.
- *Autosomal recessive (childhood) polycystic kidney disease* is caused by mutations in the gene encoding fibrocystin. It is less common than the adult form and strongly associated with liver abnormalities; the kidneys contain numerous small cysts.
- *Nephronophthisis–medullary cystic disease complex* is being increasingly recognized as a cause of chronic kidney disease in children and young adults. Of autosomal recessive inheritance, it is associated with mutations in several genes that encode epithelial cell proteins called *nephrocystins* that may be involved in ciliary function; the kidneys are contracted and contain multiple small cysts.

URINARY OUTFLOW OBSTRUCTION

Renal Stones (Urolithiasis)

Urolithiasis is calculus formation at any level in the urinary collecting system, but most often calculi arise in the kidney. Symptomatic urolithiasis is more common in men than in women. The stones occur frequently; it is estimated that by 70 years of age, 11% of men and 5.6% of women in the United States will have developed a symptomatic kidney stone. A familial tendency toward stone formation has long been recognized.

Table 14.5 Prevalence of Various Types of Renal Stones

Stone	Distribution (%)

Calcium oxalate and/or calcium phosphate
Idiopathic hypercalciuria (50%)
Hypercalcemia and hypercalciuria (10%)
Hyperoxaluria (5%)
   Enteric (4.5%)
   Primary (0.5%)
Hyperuricosuria (20%)
No known metabolic abnormality (15% to 20%)
	80

Struvite (Mg, NH$_3$, PO$_4$) Renal infection	10

Uric acid
   Associated with hyperuricemia
   Associated with hyperuricosuria
   Idiopathic (50% of uric acid stones)
	6–7

Cystine	1–2
Others or unknown	±1–2

Pathogenesis

There are three major types of renal stones:
- About 80% are composed of either calcium oxalate or calcium oxalate mixed with calcium phosphate.
- About 10% are composed of magnesium ammonium phosphate.
- Approximately 6% to 9% are either uric acid or cystine stones.

In all cases, an organic matrix of mucoprotein is present that makes up about 2.5% of the stone by weight.

The cause of stone formation is often obscure, particularly in the case of calcium-containing stones. Probably involved is a confluence of predisposing conditions, including the concentration of the solute, changes in urine pH, and bacterial infections. *The most important cause is increased urinary concentration of the stone's constituents,* so that it exceeds their solubility in urine (supersaturation). As shown in Table 14.5, 50% of patients who develop *calcium stones* have hypercalciuria that is not associated with hypercalcemia. Most patients in this group absorb calcium from the gut in excessive amounts (absorptive hypercalciuria) and promptly excrete it in the urine, and some have a primary renal defect of calcium reabsorption (renal hypercalciuria).

The causes of the other types of renal stones are better understood. *Magnesium ammonium phosphate (struvite) stones* almost always occur in individuals with a persistently alkaline urine resulting from UTIs. In particular, infections with urea-splitting bacteria, such as *Proteus vulgaris* and staphylococci, predispose individuals to urolithiasis. Moreover, bacteria may serve as particulate nidi for the formation of any kind of stone. In avitaminosis A, desquamated cells from the metaplastic epithelium of the collecting system act as nidi.

Gout and diseases involving rapid cell turnover, such as leukemias, lead to high uric acid levels in the urine and the possibility of *uric acid stones.* About one half of individuals with uric acid stones, however, have neither hyperuricemia nor increased urine urate but demonstrate an unexplained tendency to excrete a persistently acidic urine (with a pH < 5.5). This low pH favors uric acid stone formation, in contrast with the high pH that favors formation of stones containing calcium phosphate. *Cystine stones* are almost invariably associated with a genetically determined defect in the renal transport of certain amino acids, including cystine. Like uric acid stones, cystine stones are more likely to form when the urine is relatively acidic.

MORPHOLOGY

Stones are unilateral in about 80% of patients. Common sites of formation are the renal pelvis and calyces and the bladder. Often, many stones are found in one kidney. They tend to be small (average diameter, 2–3 mm) and may be smooth or jagged. Occasionally, progressive accretion of salts leads to the development of branching structures known as **staghorn calculi,** which create a cast of the renal pelvis and calyceal system. These massive stones usually are composed of magnesium ammonium phosphate.

Clinical Features

Stones may be present without producing symptoms or significant renal damage. This is particularly true with large stones lodged in the renal pelvis. Smaller stones may pass into the ureter, where they may lodge and produce intense pain, known as *renal or ureteral colic,* characterized by paroxysms of flank pain radiating toward the groin. Often at this time there is *gross hematuria.* The clinical significance of stones lies in their capacity to obstruct urine flow or to produce sufficient trauma to cause ulceration and bleeding. In either case, they *predispose the sufferer to bacterial infection.* In most cases, the diagnosis is readily made radiologically.

Hydronephrosis

Hydronephrosis refers to dilation of the renal pelvis and calyces, with accompanying atrophy of the parenchyma, caused by obstruction to the outflow of urine. The obstruction may be sudden or insidious, and it may occur at any level of the urinary tract, from the urethra to the renal pelvis. The most common causes are categorized as follows:

- *Congenital,* such as atresia of the urethra, valve formations in either the ureter or urethra, an aberrant renal artery compressing the ureter, renal ptosis with torsion, or kinking of the ureter
- *Acquired*
  - *Foreign bodies,* such as calculi or sloughed necrotic papillae
  - *Proliferative lesions,* such as benign prostatic hyperplasia, carcinoma of the prostate, bladder tumors (papilloma and carcinoma), contiguous malignant disease (retroperitoneal lymphoma, and carcinoma of the cervix or uterus)
  - *Inflammatory lesions,* such as prostatitis, ureteritis, urethritis, and retroperitoneal fibrosis
  - *Neurogenic,* such as paralysis of the bladder following spinal cord damage
  - *Normal pregnancy,* in which hydronephrosis is mild and reversible

Bilateral hydronephrosis occurs only when the obstruction is below the level of the ureters. If blockage is at the ureters or above, the lesion is unilateral. Sometimes obstruction is complete, allowing no urine to pass; usually it is only partial.

Pathogenesis

Even with complete obstruction, glomerular filtration persists for some time, and the filtrate subsequently diffuses back into the renal interstitium and perirenal spaces, from where it ultimately returns to the lymphatic and venous systems. Because of the continued filtration, the affected calyces and pelvis become dilated, often markedly so. The unusually high pressure thus generated in the renal pelvis, as well as that transmitted back through the collecting ducts, causes compression of the renal vasculature. Both arterial insufficiency and venous stasis result, although the latter probably is more important. The most severe effects are seen in the papillae, because they are subjected to the greatest increases in pressure. Accordingly, the initial functional disturbances are largely tubular, manifested primarily by impaired concentrating ability. Only later does glomerular filtration begin to diminish. Experimental studies indicate that serious irreversible damage occurs in about 3 weeks with complete obstruction, and in 3 months with incomplete obstruction. In addition to functional changes, the obstruction also triggers an interstitial inflammatory reaction, leading eventually to interstitial fibrosis.

MORPHOLOGY

Bilateral hydronephrosis (or unilateral hydronephrosis when the other kidney is already damaged or absent) leads to renal failure, and the onset of uremia tends to abort the natural course of the lesion. With subtotal or intermittent obstruction, the kidney may be massively enlarged (lengths in the range of 20 cm), and the organ may consist almost entirely of the greatly distended pelvicalyceal system. The renal parenchyma itself is compressed and atrophied, with obliteration of the papillae and flattening of the pyramids (Fig. 14.23). On the other hand, when obstruction is sudden and complete, glomerular filtration is compromised relatively early, and as a consequence, renal function may cease while dilation is still comparatively slight. Depending on the level of the obstruction, one or both ureters also may be dilated **(hydroureter).**

On microscopic examination, the early lesions show tubular dilation, followed by atrophy and fibrous replacement of the tubular epithelium with relative sparing of the glomeruli. Eventually, in severe cases the glomeruli also become atrophic and disappear, converting the entire kidney into a thin shell of fibrous tissue. With sudden and complete obstruction, there may be coagulative necrosis of the renal papillae, similar to the changes of papillary necrosis. In uncomplicated cases, the accompanying inflammatory reaction is minimal. Superimposed pyelonephritis, however, is common.

Clinical Features

Bilateral complete obstruction produces anuria. When the obstruction is distal to the bladder, the dominant symptoms are those of bladder distention. Paradoxically, incomplete bilateral obstruction causes polyuria rather

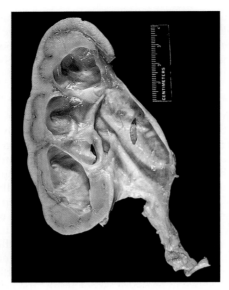

Fig. 14.23 Hydronephrosis of the kidney, with marked dilation of the pelvis and calyces and thinning of renal parenchyma.

than oliguria as a result of defects in tubular concentrating mechanisms, and this may obscure the true nature of the lesion. *Unilateral* hydronephrosis may remain completely silent for long periods unless the other kidney also is dysfunctional. Often the enlarged kidney is discovered on routine physical examination. Sometimes the underlying cause of the hydronephrosis, such as renal calculi or an obstructing tumor, produces symptoms that uncover the hydronephrosis. Removal of obstruction usually permits full return of function within a few weeks; however, with time the changes become irreversible.

CONGENITAL AND DEVELOPMENTAL ANOMALIES

Congenital and developmental abnormalities of the kidney and urinary tract represent the most common cause of end-stage renal disease in individuals younger than 21 years of age and account for 40% to 50% of pediatric renal failure worldwide. The abnormalities can affect the kidney (e.g., dysplasia, agenesis, and hypoplasia), collecting system (e.g., duplicated collecting system, hydronephrosis, and megaureter), bladder (e.g., ureterocele and vesicoureteral reflux), or urethra (e.g., posterior urethral valves). They may present as an isolated feature or as part of a syndrome in association with extrarenal manifestations. Most result from sporadic developmental defects of unknown cause. Others are caused by germline mutations in genes that impact the development of the kidney and especially the ureteric bud. The spectrum of clinical presentations is broad depending on the nature and severity of the underlying abnormalities. We restrict the discussion to a few forms affecting the kidney.

- *Multicystic dysplasia* is the most common form of renal cystic disease in childhood. The term *dysplasia* in this context refers to a developmental rather than a preneoplastic lesion. Because renal dysplasia is often

associated with obstruction in the lower urinary tract, increased hydrostatic pressure in the developing kidney is thought to play a role in its development. The kidneys are usually grossly distorted; the cysts range from microscopic to several centimeters in diameter. The histologic hallmarks are ducts and tubules lined by epithelial cells and surrounded by cuffs of cellular mesenchyme.

- *Renal agenesis:* Bilateral agenesis is incompatible with life and usually is encountered in stillborn infants. It is often associated with other congenital disorders (e.g., limb defects, hypoplastic lungs). Unilateral agenesis is uncommon and compatible with normal life if no other abnormalities exist.

- *Hypoplasia* may occur bilaterally, resulting in renal failure in early childhood, but is more commonly encountered as a unilateral defect. The hypoplastic kidney shows no scars and has a reduced number of renal lobes and pyramids, usually six or fewer.

NEOPLASMS

Many types of benign and malignant neoplasms occur in the urinary tract. In general, benign neoplasms such as small cortical papillary adenomas (<0.5 cm in diameter), which are found in up to 40% of adults in autopsies, have limited clinical significance. The most common malignant neoplasm of the kidney is renal cell carcinoma, followed in frequency by nephroblastoma (Wilms tumor) and by primary neoplasms of the calyces and pelvis. Other types of renal cancer are rare and are not discussed here. Neoplasms of the lower urinary tract are about twice as common as renal cell carcinomas. They are discussed in Chapter 18.

Neoplasms of the Kidney

Oncocytoma

Oncocytoma, a benign neoplasm that arises from the intercalated cells of collecting ducts, represents about 10% of renal neoplasms. These neoplasms are associated with genetic changes—loss of chromosomes 1 and Y—that distinguish them from other renal neoplasms. Oncocytomas are characterized by a plethora of mitochondria, providing the basis for their tan color and their finely granular eosinophilic cytoplasm, seen histologically. A central stellate scar, which is another feature of oncocytomas, provides a characteristic appearance on imaging studies.

Renal Cell Carcinoma

Renal cell carcinomas are derived from the renal tubular epithelium, and hence they are located predominantly in the cortex. These neoplasms represent 80% to 85% of all primary malignant neoplasms of the kidney and 2% to 3% of all cancers in adults. These data translate into about 65,000 cases per year in the United States; 40% of patients die of the disease. Carcinomas of the kidney are most common from the sixth to seventh decades, and men are affected about twice as commonly as women. The risk for developing these neoplasms is higher in smokers, hypertensive or obese patients, and those who have had occupational exposure to cadmium. The risk for developing renal cell cancer is increased 30-fold in individuals with acquired polycystic disease as a complication of chronic dialysis. The role of genetic factors in the causation of these cancers is discussed later.

Renal cell cancers are classified on the basis of morphology and growth patterns. However, recent advances in the understanding of the genetic basis of renal carcinomas have led to a new classification that takes into account the molecular origins of these tumors. The three most common forms, discussed next, are clear cell carcinoma, papillary renal cell carcinoma, and chromophobe renal carcinoma.

Clear Cell Carcinomas

Clear cell carcinomas are the most common type, accounting for 65% of renal cell cancers. Histologically, they are composed of cells with clear cytoplasm. Although most are sporadic, they also occur in familial forms or in association with von Hippel-Lindau (VHL) disease. It is the study of VHL disease that has provided molecular insights into the causation of clear cell carcinomas. VHL disease is inherited as an autosomal dominant trait and is characterized by predisposition to a variety of neoplasms, but particularly to hemangioblastomas of the cerebellum and retina. Hundreds of bilateral renal cysts and bilateral, often multiple, clear cell carcinomas develop in 40% to 60% of affected individuals. Those with VHL disease inherit a germline mutation of the VHL gene on chromosomal band 3p25 and lose the second allele by somatic mutation. The VHL gene also is involved in the majority of sporadic clear cell carcinomas. Cytogenetic abnormalities giving rise to loss of a segment on chromosome 3p that harbors the VHL gene are often seen in sporadic renal cell cancers. The second, nondeleted allele is inactivated by a somatic mutation or hypermethylation in 60% of sporadic cases. Thus, loss or inactivation of both copies of the VHL gene seems to be the common underlying molecular abnormality in both sporadic and familial forms of clear cell carcinomas. The VHL protein causes the degradation of hypoxia-induced factors (HIFs), and in the absence of VHL, HIFs are stabilized. HIFs are transcription factors that contribute to carcinogenesis by stimulating the expression of vascular endothelial growth factor (VEGF), an important angiogenic factor, as well as a number of other genes that drive tumor cell growth (Chapter 6). An uncommon familial form of clear cell carcinoma unrelated to VHL disease also is associated with cytogenetic abnormalities involving the short arm of chromosome 3 (3p). In addition, recent deep sequencing of clear cell carcinoma genomes has revealed frequent loss-of-function mutations in genes that encode proteins that regulate histone methylation, suggesting that changes in the "epigenome" have a central role in the genesis of this subtype of renal carcinoma.

Papillary Renal Cell Carcinomas

Papillary renal cell carcinomas account for 10% to 15% of all renal cancers and are defined in part by their papillary growth pattern. These neoplasms are frequently multifocal and bilateral and appear as early-stage tumors. Like clear cell carcinomas, they occur in familial and sporadic forms, but unlike these neoplasms, papillary renal cancers are not associated with abnormalities of chromosome 3. The culprit in most cases of hereditary papillary renal cell cancers is the MET proto-oncogene, located on chromosome 7q. The MET gene encodes a tyrosine kinase receptor for hepatocyte growth factor. The increased dosage of the MET gene due to duplications of chromosome 7 seems to spur abnormal growth in the proximal tubular epithelial cell precursors of papillary carcinomas. In familial cases, genetic analysis shows activating mutations of MET in the germ line, along with increased gene dosage in the cancers. Activating mutations of the MET gene also are found in a subset of patients with sporadic forms of papillary renal cell carcinoma.

Chromophobe Renal Carcinomas

Chromophobe renal carcinomas are the least common form, representing 5% of all renal cell carcinomas. They arise from intercalated cells of collecting ducts. Their name derives from the observation that the tumor cells stain more darkly (i.e., they are less clear) than cells in clear cell carcinomas. These neoplasms are unique in having multiple losses of entire chromosomes leading to extreme hypoploidy. Because of multiple losses, the "critical hit" has not been determined. In general, chromophobe renal cancers have a favorable prognosis.

MORPHOLOGY

Clear cell cancers (the most common form of renal carcinomas) usually are solitary and large when symptomatic (spherical masses 3 to 15 cm in diameter), but high-resolution radiographic techniques for investigation of unrelated problems sometimes detect smaller lesions incidentally. They may arise anywhere in the cortex. The cut surface of clear cell renal cell carcinomas is **yellow to orange to gray-white, with prominent areas of cystic softening or of hemorrhage,** either fresh or old (Fig. 14.24). The margins of the tumor are well defined. However, at times small processes project into the surrounding parenchyma and small satellite nodules are found, providing clear evidence of the aggressiveness of these lesions. As the tumor enlarges, it may fungate through the walls of the collecting system, extending through the calyces and pelvis as far as the ureter. Even more frequently, the **tumor invades the renal vein** and grows as a solid column within this vessel, sometimes extending in serpentine fashion as far as the inferior vena cava and even into the right side of the heart. Occasionally, direct invasion into the perinephric fat and adrenal gland may be seen.

Depending on the amounts of lipid and glycogen present, **the neoplastic cells of clear cell renal cell carcinoma may appear almost vacuolated or may be solid.** The classic vacuolated (lipid-laden) cells or clear cells are demarcated only by their cell membranes. The nuclei are usually small and round (Fig. 14.25). At the other extreme are granular cells, resembling the tubular epithelium, which have small, round, regular nuclei enclosed within granular pink cytoplasm. Some neoplasms are highly anaplastic, with numerous mitotic figures and markedly enlarged, hyperchromatic, pleomorphic nuclei. Between the extremes of clear cells and solid, granular cells, all intergradations may be found. The cellular arrangement, too, varies widely. The

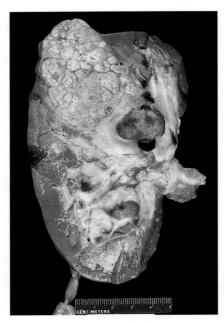

Fig. 14.24 Renal cell carcinoma: Representative cross-section showing yellowish, spherical neoplasm in one pole of the kidney. Note the tumor in the dilated, thrombosed renal vein.

cells may form abortive tubules or may cluster in cords or disorganized masses. The stroma is usually scant but highly vascularized.

Papillary renal cell carcinomas exhibit various degrees of papilla formation with fibrovascular cores. They tend to be bilateral and multiple. They also may show gross evidence of necrosis, hemorrhage, and cystic degeneration, but they are less vibrantly orange-yellow because of their lower lipid content. The cells may have a clear or, more commonly, pink cytoplasm. **Chromophobe-type renal cell carcinoma** tends to be grossly tan-brown. The cells usually have clear, flocculent cytoplasm with very prominent, distinct cell membranes. The nuclei are surrounded by halos of clear cytoplasm. Ultrastructurally, large numbers of characteristic macrovesicles are seen.

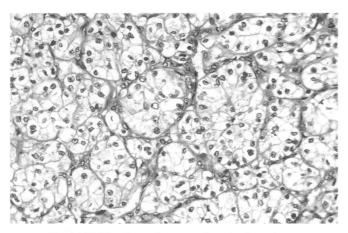

Fig. 14.25 The clear cell pattern of renal cell carcinoma.

Clinical Features

Renal cell carcinomas have several peculiar clinical characteristics that create especially difficult and challenging diagnostic problems. The signs and symptoms vary, but the *most frequent presenting manifestation is hematuria, occurring in more than 50% of cases.* Macroscopic hematuria tends to be intermittent and fleeting, superimposed on a steady microscopic hematuria. Less commonly, the tumor may declare itself simply by virtue of its size, when it has grown large enough to produce flank pain and a *palpable mass.* Because of the widespread use of imaging studies for unrelated conditions, even smaller tumors are detected. Extrarenal effects are *fever* and *polycythemia,* which, because they are nonspecific, may be misinterpreted for some time before their association with the renal tumor is appreciated. Polycythemia affects 5% to 10% of affected individuals and results from production of erythropoietin by the cancer cells. Uncommonly, these tumors produce other hormone-like substances, resulting in hypercalcemia, hypertension, Cushing syndrome, or feminization or masculinization. These, as noted in Chapter 6, are *paraneoplastic syndromes.* In some patients, the primary tumor remains silent and is discovered only after metastases produce symptoms. The common locations for metastases are the lungs and the bones. It must be apparent that renal cell carcinoma manifests in many ways, some quite devious, *but the triad of painless hematuria, a palpable abdominal mass, and dull flank pain is characteristic.*

SUMMARY

RENAL CELL CARCINOMA

Renal cell carcinomas account for 2% to 3% of all cancers in adults and are classified into three main types:
- *Clear cell carcinomas* are the most common and are associated with homozygous loss or inactivation of the VHL tumor suppressor protein; tumors frequently invade the renal vein.
- *Papillary renal cell carcinomas* frequently are associated with increased expression and activating mutations of the *MET* oncogene; they tend to be bilateral and multiple and show variable papilla formation.
- *Chromophobe renal cell carcinomas* are less common; neoplastic cells are not as clear as in the other renal cell carcinomas.

Wilms Tumor

Although Wilms tumor is rare in adults, it is the third most common solid (non-hematologic) cancer in children younger than 10 years of age. These neoplasms contain a variety of cell and tissue components, all derived from mesoderm. Wilms tumor, like retinoblastoma, may arise sporadically or be familial, with the susceptibility to tumorigenesis inherited as an autosomal dominant trait. This neoplasm is discussed in greater detail in Chapter 7 along with other tumors of childhood.

SUGGESTED READINGS

Bu F, Maga T, Meyer NC, et al: Comprehensive genetic analysis of complement and coagulation genes in atypical hemolytic uremic syndrome, *J Am Soc Nephrol* 25:55, 2014. [*An in-depth review of molecular abnormalities in hemolytic uremic syndrome.*]

Cornec-Le Gall E, Audrézet MP, Le Meur Y: Genetics and pathogenesis of autosomal dominant polycystic kidney disease: 20 years on, *Hum Mutat* 35:1393, 2014. *[A review of the discovery of the major genes leading to polycystic kidney disease, along with their phenotypic manifestations.]*

Cramer MT, Guay-Woodford LM: Cystic kidney disease: a primer, *Adv Chronic Kidney Dis* 22:297, 2015. *[An excellent review on the pathophysiology of renal cystic diseases, with emphasis on the role of ciliary dysfunction in tubular epithelial cells.]*

Crumley SM, Divatia M, Truong L, et al: Renal cell carcinoma: Evolving and emerging subtypes, *World J Clin Cases* 1:262, 2013. *[An up-to-date review of emerging subtypes of renal cell carcinoma.]*

D'Agati VD, Kaskel FJ, Falk RJ: Focal segmental glomerulosclerosis, *N Engl J Med* 365:2398, 2011. *[A comprehensive review of focal segmental glomerulosclerosis.]*

Dell KM: The role of cilia in the pathogenesis of cystic kidney disease, *Curr Opin Pediatr* 27:212, 2015. *[An up to date review of the normal functions of cilia and the pathogenesis of ciliopathies, with emphasis on cystic renal diseases.]*

Genovese G, Friedman DJ, Ross MD, et al: Association of trypanolytic ApoL1 variants with kidney disease in African Americans, *Science* 329:841, 2010. *[A landmark study of natural selection, linking a genetic variant of apolipoprotein L1 in African Americans to protection against sleeping sickness and risk for kidney disease.]*

George JN, Nester CM: Syndromes of thrombotic microangiopathy, *N Engl J Med* 371:1847, 2014. *[An excellent review of the classification of thrombotic microangiopathies.]*

Gubler MC: Inherited diseases of the glomerular basement membrane, *Nat Clin Pract Nephrol* 4:24, 2008. *[A superb review of the pathophysiology, clinical presentations, and diagnostic testing strategies for Alport syndrome, thin basement membrane disease, and other types of hereditary nephritis.]*

Jennette JC, Falk RJ: Pathogenesis of antineutrophil cytoplasmic autoantibody-mediated disease, *Nat Rev Rheumatol* 10:463, 2014. *[A good summary of the mechanisms of injury and clinical manifestations in antineutrophil cytoplasmic autoantibody–mediated disease.]*

Kambham N: Postinfectious glomerulonephritis, *Adv Anat Pathol* 19:338, 2012. *[An excellent review of the pathology and pathogenesis of postinfectious glomerulonephritis.]*

Kashtan CE, Segal Y: Genetic disorders of glomerular basement membranes, *Nephron Clin Pract* 118:c9, 2011. *[An excellent review of the genetic aspects of glomerular basement membrane diseases.]*

Knowles MA, Hurst CD: Molecular biology of bladder cancer: new insights into pathogenesis and clinical diversity, *Nat Rev Cancer* 15:25, 2015. *[A comprehensive review of the molecular changes in different types of bladder cancer.]*

Mathieson PW: Minimal change nephropathy and focal segmental glomerulosclerosis, *Semin Immunopathol* 29:415, 2007. *[An excellent overview of new insights into the pathogenesis and diagnosis of minimal change disease versus focal segmental glomerulosclerosis.]*

Miller O, Hemphill RR: Urinary tract infection and pyelonephritis, *Emerg Med Clin North Am* 19:655, 2001. *[An excellent review of acute urinary tract infections.]*

Murray PT, Devarajan P, Levey AS, et al: A framework and key research questions in AKI diagnosis and staging in different environments, *Clin J Am Soc Nephrol* 3:864, 2008. *[An excellent review outlining recent advances in early diagnosis and consequences of acute kidney injury.]*

Robert T, Berthelot L, Cambier A, et al: Molecular insights into the pathogenesis of IgA nephropathy. Review, *Trends Mol Med* 21:762, 2015. *[A concise summary of the pathogenesis of IgA glomerulonephritis.]*

Ronco P, Debiec H: Pathophysiological advances in membranous nephropathy: time for a shift in patient's care, *Lancet* 385:1983, 2015. *[An excellent summary of the novel developments in the field of membranous glomerulonephritis.]*

Schrier RW, Wang W, Poole B, et al: Acute renal failure: definitions, diagnosis, pathogenesis, and therapy, *J Clin Invest* 114:5, 2004. *[An insightful review covering all aspects of acute renal failure.]*

Sethi S, Haas M, Markowitz GS, et al: Mayo Clinic/Renal Pathology Society Consensus Report on Pathologic Classification, Diagnosis, and Reporting of GN, *J Am Soc Nephrol* 27:1278, 2016. *[An excellent summary of the consensus classification of glomerulonephritides.]*

Tryggvason K, Patrakka J, Wartiovaava J: Hereditary proteinuria syndromes and mechanisms of proteinuria, *N Engl J Med* 354:1387, 2006. *[An excellent review of the pathophysiology of defects in glomerular permeability.]*

Worcester EM, Coe FL: Calcium kidney stones, *N Engl J Med* 363:954, 2010. *[A comprehensive review of the pathophysiology and management of the most common types of kidney stones.]*

Oral Cavities and Gastrointestinal Tract

15

Oral Cavity 583
Diseases of Teeth and Supporting Structures 584
Oral Inflammatory Lesions 584
Aphthous Ulcers (Canker Sores) 584
Herpes Simplex Virus Infections 584
Oral Candidiasis (Thrush) 585
Proliferative and Neoplastic Lesions of the Oral Cavity 585
Fibrous Proliferative Lesions 585
Leukoplakia and Erythroplakia 585
Squamous Cell Carcinoma 586
Diseases of Salivary Glands 587
Xerostomia 587
Sialadenitis 588
Neoplasms 588
Odontogenic Cysts and Tumors 590
Esophagus 590
Obstructive and Vascular Diseases 590
Mechanical Obstruction 590
Functional Obstruction 591
Ectopia 591
Esophageal Varices 591
Esophagitis 591
Esophageal Lacerations, Mucosal Injury, and Infections 591

Reflux Esophagitis 593
Eosinophilic Esophagitis 594
Barrett Esophagus 595
Esophageal Tumors 596
Adenocarcinoma 596
Squamous Cell Carcinoma 596
Stomach 598
Gastropathy and Acute Gastritis 598
Stress-Related Mucosal Disease 599
Chronic Gastritis 599
Helicobacter pylori Gastritis 600
Autoimmune Gastritis 600
Complications of Chronic Gastritis 601
Peptic Ulcer Disease 601
Mucosal Atrophy and Intestinal Metaplasia 603
Dysplasia 603
Gastric Polyps and Tumors 603
Gastric Polyps 603
Gastric Adenocarcinoma 604
Lymphoma 605
Neuroendocrine (Carcinoid) Tumor 605
Gastrointestinal Stromal Tumor 606
Small and Large Intestines 607
Intestinal Obstruction 607
Intussusception 608
Hirschsprung Disease 608

Abdominal Hernia 609
Vascular Disorders of Bowel 609
Ischemic Bowel Disease 609
Hemorrhoids 610
Diarrheal Disease 611
Malabsorptive Diarrhea 611
Infectious Enterocolitis 614
Inflammatory Intestinal Disease 620
Sigmoid Diverticulitis 620
Inflammatory Bowel Disease 621
Colonic Polyps and Neoplastic Disease 626
Inflammatory Polyps 626
Hamartomatous Polyps 626
Hyperplastic Polyps 627
Adenomas 627
Familial Syndromes 629
Adenocarcinoma 630
Appendix 634
Acute Appendicitis 634
Tumors of the Appendix 635

The gastrointestinal tract is a hollow tube consisting of the esophagus, stomach, small intestine, colon, rectum, and anus. Each region has unique, complementary, and highly integrated functions that together serve to regulate the intake, processing, and absorption of ingested nutrients and the disposal of waste products. The intestines also are the principal site at which the immune system interfaces with a diverse array of antigens present in food and gut microbes. Thus, it is not surprising that the small intestine and colon frequently are involved by infectious and inflammatory processes. Finally, the colon is the most common site of gastrointestinal neoplasia in Western populations. In this chapter, we discuss the diseases that affect each section of the gastrointestinal tract. Disorders that typically involve more than one segment, such as Crohn disease, are considered with the most frequently involved region. We begin our discussion with diseases of the oral cavity, since that is where the journey of food begins.

Oral Cavity

Pathologic conditions of the oral cavity can be broadly divided into diseases affecting teeth their support structures, oral mucosa, salivary glands, and jaws. Discussed next are the more common conditions affecting these sites.

Odontogenic cysts and tumors (benign and malignant), which are derived from the epithelial and/or mesenchymal tissues associated with tooth development, are also discussed briefly.

DISEASES OF TEETH AND SUPPORTING STRUCTURES

Caries

Dental caries results from focal demineralization of tooth structure (enamel and dentin) caused by acids generated during the fermentation of sugars by bacteria. Worldwide, caries is the main cause of tooth loss before 35 years of age. The prevalence of caries used to be very high in developed countries where there is ready access to processed and refined foods containing large amounts of carbohydrates. However, the rate of caries has dropped markedly in countries such as the United States, where oral hygiene has improved and fluoridation of the drinking water is widespread. Fluoride is incorporated into the crystalline structure of enamel, forming fluoroapatite, which is resistant to degradation by bacterial acids. In contrast, with the globalization of the world's economy, processed foods are being increasingly consumed in developing nations; as a result, the rate of caries is increasing in these regions of the world.

Gingivitis

Inflammation involving the squamous mucosa, or gingiva, and associated soft tissues that surround teeth is defined as *gingivitis.* Poor oral hygiene, which facilitates buildup of dental plaque and calculus between and on the surfaces of teeth, is the most frequent cause of gingivitis. Dental plaque is a sticky biofilm composed of bacteria, salivary proteins, and desquamated epithelial cells. As it accumulates, plaque becomes mineralized to form calculus, or tartar. In chronic gingivitis, this is accompanied by gingival erythema, edema, and bleeding. Gingivitis may occur at any age but is most prevalent and severe in adolescence, where it is present in 40% to 60% of individuals, after which the incidence tapers off. Fortunately, gingivitis can be reversed, primarily by regular brushing and flossing of teeth which reduces accumulation of plaque and calculus.

Periodontitis

Periodontitis is an inflammatory process that affects the supporting structures of the teeth (periodontal ligaments), alveolar bone, and cementum. With progression, periodontitis may result in destruction of periodontal ligament and alveolar bone and eventual tooth loss. Periodontitis is associated with poor oral hygiene that affects the composition of gingival bacteria. Facultative Gram-positive organisms are found at healthy sites, while anaerobic and microaerophilic Gram-negative bacteria colonize plaque within areas of active periodontitis. Although about 300 bacterial species reside within the oral cavity, periodontitis is most closely associated with *Aggregatibacter (Actinobacillus) actinomycetemcomitans, Porphyromonas gingivalis,* and *Prevotella intermedia.*

⬤ SUMMARY

DISEASES OF TEETH AND SUPPORTING STRUCTURES

- Caries is the most common cause of tooth loss in individuals younger than 35 years of age. The primary cause is destruction of tooth structure by acid end products of sugar fermentation by bacteria.
- Gingivitis is a common and reversible inflammation of the mucosa surrounding the teeth. It is associated with buildup of dental plaque and calculus.
- Periodontitis is a chronic inflammatory condition that can lead to the destruction of the supporting structures of the teeth with eventual loss of dentition. It is associated with poor oral hygiene and altered oral microbiota.

ORAL INFLAMMATORY LESIONS

Aphthous Ulcers (Canker Sores)

These common superficial mucosal ulcerations affect up to 40% of the population. They are more frequent in the first 2 decades of life, extremely painful, and often recur. Although the cause of aphthous ulcers is unknown, they tend to be familal and may be associated with celiac disease, inflammatory bowel disease, and Behçet disease. Ulcers can be solitary or multiple; typically, they are shallow, with a hyperemic base covered by a thin exudate and rimmed by a narrow zone of erythema (Fig. 15.1). In most cases they resolve spontaneously in 7 to 10 days but can recur.

Herpes Simplex Virus Infections

Herpes simplex virus causes a self-limited primary infection that can be reactivated when there is a compromise in host resistance. Most orofacial herpetic infections are caused by herpes simplex virus type 1 (HSV-1), with the remainder being caused by HSV-2 (genital herpes). With changing sexual practices, oral HSV-2 is becoming increasingly common. Primary infections typically occur in children between 2 and 4 years of age and are often asymptomatic. However, in 10% to 20% of cases the primary infection manifests as acute herpetic gingivostomatitis, with abrupt onset of vesicles and ulcerations throughout the oral cavity. Most adults harbor latent HSV-1, and the virus can be reactivated, resulting in a

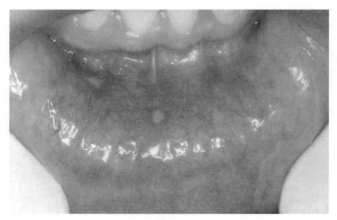

Fig. 15.1 Aphthous ulcer. Single ulceration with an erythematous halo surrounding a yellowish fibrinopurulent membrane.

so-called "cold sore" or recurrent herpetic stomatitis. Factors associated with HSV reactivation include trauma, allergies, exposure to ultraviolet light and extremes of temperature, upper-respiratory tract infections, pregnancy, menstruation, and immunosuppression. Recurrent lesions, which occur at the site of primary inoculation or in adjacent mucosa innervated by the same ganglion, typically appear as groups of small (1- to 3-mm) vesicles. The lips (herpes labialis), nasal orifices, buccal mucosa, gingiva, and hard palate are the most common locations. Although lesions typically resolve within 7 to 10 days, they can persist in immunocompromised patients, who may require systemic anti-viral therapy. Morphologically, the lesions resemble those seen in esophageal herpes (see Fig. 15.8 later in the chapter) and genital herpes (Chapter 19). The infected cells become ballooned and have large eosinophilic intranuclear inclusions. Adjacent cells commonly fuse to form large multinucleated polykaryons.

Oral Candidiasis (Thrush)

Candidiasis is the most common fungal infection of the oral cavity. *Candida albicans* is a normal component of the oral flora and only produces disease under unusual circumstances. Predisposing factors include the following:
- Immunosuppression
- The specific strain of *C. albicans*
- The composition of the oral microbial flora (microbiota)

Broad-spectrum antibiotics that alter the normal microbiota can promote oral candidiasis. The three major clinical forms of oral candidiasis are pseudomembranous, erythematous, and hyperplastic. The pseudomembranous form is most common and is known as *thrush*. This condition is characterized by a superficial, curdlike, gray to white inflammatory membrane composed of matted organisms enmeshed in a fibrinosuppurative exudate that can be readily scraped off to reveal an underlying erythematous base. In mildly immunosuppressed or debilitated individuals, such as diabetics, the infection usually remains superficial, but it may spread to deep sites in association with more severe immunosuppression, that may be seen in organ or hematopoietic stem cell transplant recipients, and in patients with neutropenia, chemotherapy-induced immunosuppression, or AIDS.

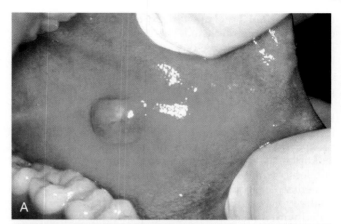

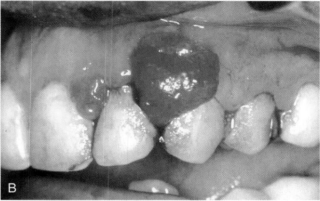

Fig. 15.2 Fibrous proliferations. (A) Fibroma. Smooth pink exophytic nodule on the buccal mucosa. (B) Pyogenic granuloma. Erythematous hemorrhagic exophytic mass arising from the gingival mucosa.

PROLIFERATIVE AND NEOPLASTIC LESIONS OF THE ORAL CAVITY

Fibrous Proliferative Lesions

Fibromas are submucosal nodular fibrous tissue masses that are formed when chronic irritation results in reactive connective tissue hyperplasia (Fig. 15.2A). They occur most often on the buccal mucosa along the bite line. Treatment is complete surgical excision and removal of the source of irritation.

Pyogenic granuloma (Fig. 15.2B) is an inflammatory lesion typically found on the gingiva of children, young adults, and pregnant women (pregnancy tumor). These lesions are richly vascular and typically ulcerated, which gives them a red to purple color. In some cases, growth can be rapid and raise fear of a malignant neoplasm. However, histologic examination demonstrates a proliferation of immature vessels similar to that seen in granulation tissue. Pyogenic granulomas may regress, mature into dense fibrous masses, or develop into a peripheral ossifying fibroma. Complete surgical excision is definitive treatment.

Leukoplakia and Erythroplakia

Leukoplakia is defined by the World Health Organization as "a white patch or plaque that cannot be scraped

● SUMMARY

ORAL INFLAMMATORY LESIONS

- Aphthous ulcers are painful superficial ulcers of unknown etiology that may in some cases be associated with systemic diseases.
- Herpes simplex virus causes a self-limited infection that presents with vesicles (cold sores, fever blisters) that rupture and heal, without scarring, and often leave latent virus in nerve ganglia. Reactivation can occur.
- Oral candidiasis may occur when the oral microbiota is altered (e.g., after antibiotic use). Invasive disease may occur in immunosuppressed individuals.

off and cannot be characterized clinically or pathologically as any other disease." This description is reserved for lesions that arise in the oral cavity in the absence of any known cause (Fig. 15.3A). Accordingly, white patches caused by obvious irritation or entities such as lichen planus and candidiasis are not considered leukoplakia. Approximately 3% of the world's population has leukoplakic lesions, of which 5% to 25% are dsyplastic and at risk for progression to squamous cell carcinoma. Thus, until proved otherwise by means of histologic evaluation, all leukoplakias must be considered precancerous. A related but less common entity, *erythroplakia,* is a red, velvety, sometimes eroded lesion that is flat or slightly depressed relative to the surrounding mucosa. Erythroplakia is associated with a much greater risk for malignant transformation than leukoplakia. While leukoplakia and erythroplakia may be seen in adults at any age, they typically affect individuals between 40 and 70 years of age, with a 2:1 male predominance. Although the etiology is multifactorial, tobacco use (cigarettes, pipes, cigars, and chewing tobacco) is the most common risk factor for leukoplakia and erythroplakia.

MORPHOLOGY

On histologic examination leukoplakia and erythroplakia show a spectrum of epithelial changes ranging from hyperkeratosis overlying a thickened, acanthotic but orderly mucosal epithelium to lesions with markedly dysplastic changes sometimes merging into carcinoma in situ (Fig. 15.3B). The most severe dysplastic changes are associated with erythroplakia, and more than 50% of these cases undergo malignant transformation. With increasing dysplasia and anaplasia, a subjacent inflammatory cell infiltrate of lymphocytes and macrophages is often present.

Squamous Cell Carcinoma

Approximately 95% of cancers of the oral cavity are squamous cell carcinomas, with the remainder largely consisting of adenocarcinomas of salivary glands. Squamous cell carcinoma, an aggressive epithelial malignancy, is the sixth most common neoplasm in the world today. Despite numerous advances in treatment, the overall long-term survival rate has remained less than 50% for the past 50 years. This dismal outlook is due to several factors, in large part because oral cancer often is diagnosed at an advanced stage.

Multiple primary tumors may be present at initial diagnosis but more often are detected later, at an estimated rate of 3% to 7% per year; patients who survive 5 years after diagnosis of the initial tumor have up to a 35% chance of developing at least one new primary tumor within that interval. The development of these secondary tumors can be particularly devastating for individuals whose initial lesions were small. Therefore, surveillance and early detection of new premalignant lesions are critical for the long-term survival of patients with oral squamous cell carcinoma.

The elevated risk for development of additional primary tumors in these patients has led to the concept of "field cancerization." This hypothesis suggests that multiple

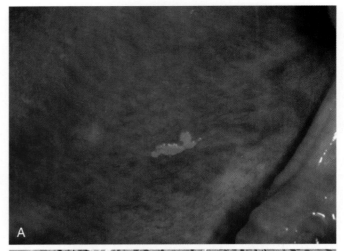

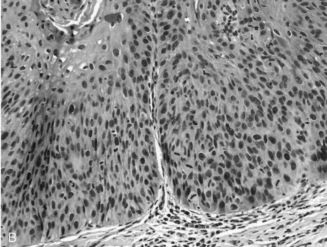

Fig. 15.3 Leukoplakia. (A) Gross appearance of leukoplakia is highly variable. In this example, the lesion is smooth with well-demarcated borders and minimal elevation. (B) Histologic appearance of leukoplakia showing dysplasia, characterized by nuclear and cellular pleomorphism and loss of normal maturation.

primary tumors develop independently as a result of years of chronic mucosal exposure to carcinogens such as alcohol or tobacco (described next).

Pathogenesis

Squamous cancers of the oropharynx arise through two distinct pathogenic pathways, one involving exposure to carcinogens, and the other related to infection with high risk variants of human papilloma virus (HPV). Carcinogen exposure mainly stems from chronic alcohol and tobacco (both smoked and chewed) use. In India and Southeast Asia, chewing of betel quid and paan are important predisposing factors. Betel quid is a "witch's brew" containing araca nut, slaked lime, and tobacco, all wrapped in betel nut leaf. It is likely that these tumors arise by a pathway similar to that characterized for tobacco use–associated tumors in the West. Deep sequencing of these cancers has revealed frequent mutations that bear a molecular signature consistent with exposure to carcinogens in tobacco. These mutations frequently involve *TP53* and genes that regulate cell proliferation, such as *RAS*. The HPV-related tumors tend to occur in the tonsillar crypts or the base of the tongue and harbor oncogenic "high-risk" subtypes, particularly HPV-16. These tumors carry far fewer mutations than those associated with tobacco exposure and often overexpress p16, a cyclin-dependent kinase inhibitor.

It is conservatively predicted that the incidence of HPV-associated oropharyngeal squamous cell carcinoma will surpass that of cervical cancer by 2020, in part because the anatomic sites of origin—tonsillar crypts, base of tongue, and oropharynx—are not readily accessible or amenable to cytologic screening (unlike the cervix). The prognosis for patients with HPV-positive tumors is better than for those with HPV-negative tumors. The HPV vaccine, which is protective against cervical cancer, offers hope to limit the increasing frequency of HPV-associated oropharyngeal squamous cell carcinoma.

The incidence of oral cavity squamous cell carcinoma (particularly in the tongue) has been on the rise in individuals younger than 40 years of age who have no known risk factors. The pathogenesis in this group of patients, who are nonsmokers and are not infected with HPV, is unknown

MORPHOLOGY

Squamous cell carcinoma may arise anywhere in the oral cavity. However, the most common locations are the ventral surface of the tongue, floor of the mouth, lower lip, soft palate, and gingiva (Fig. 15.4A). In early stages, these cancers may appear as raised, firm, pearly plaques or as irregular, roughened, or verrucous mucosal thickenings. Either pattern may be superimposed on a background of leukoplakia or erythroplakia. As these lesions enlarge, they typically form ulcerated and protruding masses that have irregular and indurated or rolled borders. Histopathologic analysis has shown that squamous cell carcinoma develops from dysplastic precursor lesions. Histologic patterns range from well-differentiated keratinizing neoplasms (Fig. 15.4B) to anaplastic, sometimes sarcomatoid tumors. However, the degree of histologic differentiation, as determined by the relative degree of keratinization, does not necessarily correlate with biologic behavior. Typically, oral squamous cell carcinoma infiltrates locally before it metastasizes. The cervical lymph nodes are the most common sites of regional metastasis; frequent sites of distant metastases include the mediastinal lymph nodes, lungs, and liver.

SUMMARY

LESIONS OF THE ORAL CAVITY

- Fibromas and pyogenic granulomas are common reactive lesions of the oral mucosa.
- Leukoplakia and eryhtroplakia are mucosal plaques that may undergo malignant transformation.
- The risk for malignant transformation is greater in erythroplakia (relative to leukoplakia).
- A majority of oral cavity cancers are squamous cell carcinomas.
- Oral squamous cell carcinomas are classically linked to tobacco and alcohol use, but the incidence of HPV-associated lesions is rising.

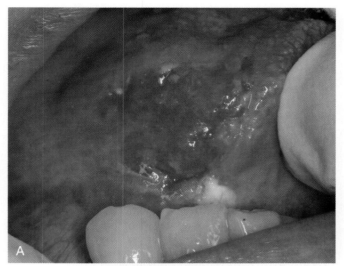

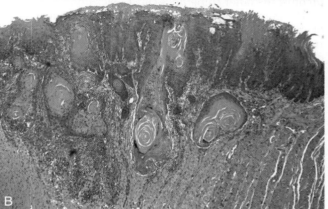

Fig. 15.4 Oral squamous cell carcinoma. (A) Gross appearance demonstrating ulceration and induration of the oral mucosa. (B) Histologic appearance demonstrating numerous nests and islands of malignant keratinocytes invading the underlying connective tissue stroma.

DISEASES OF SALIVARY GLANDS

There are three major salivary glands—parotid, submandibular, and sublingual—as well as innumerable minor salivary glands distributed throughout the oral mucosa. Inflammatory or neoplastic disease may develop within any of these.

Xerostomia

Xerostomia is defined as a dry mouth resulting from a decrease in the production of saliva. Its incidence varies among populations but has been reported in more than 20% of individuals older than 70 years of age. It is a major feature of the autoimmune disorder Sjögren syndrome, in which it usually is accompanied by dry eyes (Chapter 5). A lack of salivary secretions is also a major complication of radiation therapy. However, xerostomia is most frequently observed as a side effect of many common classes of medications including anti-cholinergic, anti-depressant/anti-psychotic, diuretic, anti-hypertensive, sedative, muscle relaxant, analgesic, and anti-histaminic agents. The oral cavity may reveal only dry mucosa and/or atrophy of the papillae of the tongue, with fissuring and ulcerations, or, in Sjögren syndrome, concomitant inflammatory enlargement of the salivary glands. Complications of xerostomia include increased rates of dental caries and candidiasis, as well as difficulty in swallowing and speaking.

Sialadenitis

Inflammation of the salivary glands, referred to as *sialadenitis*, may be induced by trauma, viral or bacterial infection, or autoimmune disease. The most common form of viral sialadenitis is *mumps,* which may produce enlargement of all salivary glands but predominantly involves the parotids. Mumps produces interstitial inflammation marked by a mononuclear inflammatory infiltrate. While mumps in children is most often a self-limited benign condition, in adults it can cause pancreatitis or orchitis; the latter sometimes causes sterility.

The *mucocele* is the most common inflammatory lesion of the salivay glands and results from either blockage or rupture of a salivary gland duct, with consequent leakage of saliva into the surrounding connective tissue stroma. Mucocele occurs most often in toddlers, young adults, and older adults, and typically manifests as a fluctuant swelling of the lower lip that may change in size, particularly in association with meals (Fig. 15.5A). Histologic examination demonstrates a cystlike space lined by granulation tissue or fibrous connective tissue that is filled with mucin and inflammatory cells, particularly macrophages (Fig. 15.5B). Complete excision of the cyst and the minor salivary gland constitutes definitive treatment.

Bacterial sialadenitis is a common infection that most often involves the major salivary glands, particularly the submandibular glands. The most frequent pathogens are *Staphylococcus aureus* and *Streptococcus viridans.* Duct obstruction by stones (sialolithiasis) is a common antecedent to infection; it may also be induced by impacted food debris or by edema consequent to injury. Dehydration and decreased secretory function can also predispose to bacterial invasion. Systemic dehydration, with decreased salivary secretions, may predispose to suppurative bacterial parotitis in older adult patients following major thoracic or abdominal surgery. Such obstruction and bacterial invasion lead to nonspecific inflammation of the affected glands that may be largely interstitial or, when induced by staphylococci or other pyogens, may be associated with suppurative necrosis and abscess formation.

Autoimmune sialadenitis, better known as Sjögren syndrome, is discussed in Chapter 5.

Neoplasms

Despite their relatively simple morphology, the salivary glands give rise to at least 30 histologically distinct tumors (Table 15.1). A small number of these neoplasms account for more than 90% of tumors. Overall, salivary gland tumors are relatively uncommon and represent less than 2% of all human tumors. Approximately 65% to 80% arise within the parotid, 10% in the submandibular gland, and the remainder in the minor salivary glands, including the sublingual glands. Approximately 15% to 30% of tumors

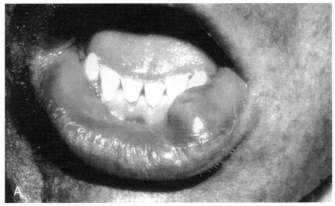

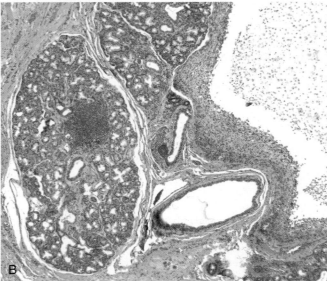

Fig. 15.5 Mucocele. (A) Fluctuant fluid-filled lesion on the lower lip subsequent to trauma. (B) Cystlike cavity *(right)* filled with mucinous material and lined by organizing granulation tissue. The normal gland acini are seen on the left.

in the parotid glands are malignant. By contrast, approximately 40% of submandibular, 50% of minor salivary gland, and 70% to 90% of sublingual tumors are cancerous. Thus, the likelihood that a salivary gland tumor is malignant is inversely proportional, roughly, to the size of the gland.

Salivary gland tumors usually occur in adults, with a slight female predominance, but about 5% occur in

Table 15.1 Histopathologic Classification and Prevalence of the Most Common Benign and Malignant Salivary Gland Tumors

Benign	Malignant
Pleomorphic adenoma (50%)	Mucoepidermoid carcinoma (15%)
Warthin tumor (5%)	Acinic cell carcinoma (6%)
Oncocytoma (2%)	Adenocarcinoma NOS (6%)
Cystadenoma (2%)	Adenoid cystic carcinoma (4%)
Basal cell adenoma (2%)	Malignant mixed tumor (3%)

NOS, Not otherwise specified.
Data from Ellis GL, Auclair PL, Gnepp DR: *Surgical pathology of the salivary glands, Vol 25: Major problems in pathology.* Philadelphia, 1991, Saunders.

children younger than 16 years of age. Whatever the histologic pattern, parotid gland neoplasms produce swelling in front of and below the ear. Benign tumors may be present for months to several years before coming to clinical attention, while cancers more often come to attention promptly, probably because of their more rapid growth. However, there are no reliable criteria to differentiate benign from malignant lesions on clinical grounds, and histopathologic evaluation is essential.

Pleomorphic Adenoma

Pleomorphic adenomas are benign tumors that consist of a mixture of ductal (epithelial) and myoepithelial cells, so they exhibit both epithelial and mesenchymal differentiation. Epithelial elements are dispersed throughout the matrix, which may contain variable mixtures of myxoid, hyaline, chondroid (cartilaginous), and even osseous tissue. In some pleomorphic adenomas, the epithelial elements predominate; in others, they are present only in widely dispersed foci. This histologic diversity has given rise to the alternative, albeit less preferred, name *mixed tumor*.

Pleomorphic adenomas represent about 60% of tumors in the parotid, are less common in the submandibular glands, and are relatively rare in the minor salivary glands. They present as slow-growing, painless, mobile discrete masses. They recur if incompletely excised. Recurrence rates approach 25% after simple enucleation of the tumor, but are only 4% after wider resection. In both settings, recurrence stems from a failure to recognize minute extensions of tumor into surrounding soft tissues.

Carcinoma arising in a pleomorphic adenoma is referred to variously as a *carcinoma ex pleomorphic adenoma* or *malignant mixed tumor*. The incidence of malignant transformation increases with time from 2% of tumors present for less than 5 years to almost 10% for those present for more than 15 years. The cancer usually takes the form of an adenocarcinoma or undifferentiated carcinoma. Unfortunately, these are among the most aggressive malignant neoplasms of salivary glands, with mortality rates of 30% to 50% at 5 years.

MORPHOLOGY

Pleomorphic adenomas typically manifest as rounded, well-demarcated masses rarely exceeding 6 cm in the greatest dimension. Although they are encapsulated, in some locations (particularly the palate), the capsule is not fully developed, and expansile growth produces protrusions into the surrounding tissues. The cut surface is gray-white and typically contains myxoid and blue translucent chondroid (cartilage-like) areas. The most striking histologic feature is their characteristic heterogeneity. Epithelial elements resembling ductal or myoepithelial cells are arranged in ducts, acini, irregular tubules, strands, or even sheets. These typically are dispersed within a mesenchyme-like background of loose myxoid tissue containing islands of chondroid and, rarely, foci of bone (Fig. 15.6). Sometimes the epithelial cells form well-developed ducts lined by cuboidal to columnar cells with an underlying layer of deeply chromatic, small myoepithelial cells. In other instances there may be strands or sheets of myoepithelial cells. Islands of well-differentiated squamous epithelium also may be present. In most cases, no epithelial

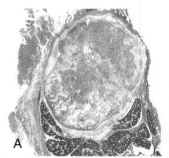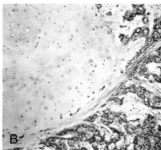

Fig. 15.6 Pleomorphic adenoma. (A) Low-power view showing a well-demarcated tumor with adjacent, deeply staining, normal salivary gland parenchyma. (B) High-power view showing epithelial cells as well as myoepithelial cells within chondroid matrix material.

dysplasia or mitotic activity is evident. No difference in biologic behavior has been observed between the tumors composed largely of epithelial elements and those composed largely of mesenchymal elements.

Mucoepidermoid Carcinoma

Mucoepidermoid carcinomas are composed of variable mixtures of squamous cells, mucus-secreting cells, and intermediate cells. These neoplasms represent about 15% of all salivary gland tumors, and while they occur mainly (60%–70%) in the parotids, they account for a large fraction of salivary gland neoplasms in the other glands, particularly the minor salivary glands. Overall, mucoepidermoid carcinoma is the most common form of primary malignant tumor of the salivary glands.

MORPHOLOGY

Mucoepidermoid carcinomas can grow as large as 8 cm in diameter and, although they are apparently circumscribed, they lack well-defined capsules and often are infiltrative. The cut surface is pale gray to white and frequently demonstrates small, mucinous cysts. On histologic examination, these tumors contain cords, sheets, or cysts lined by squamous, mucous, or intermediate cells. The latter is a hybrid cell type with both squamous features and mucus-filled vacuoles, which are most easily detected with mucin stains. Cytologically, tumor cells may be benign-appearing or highly anaplastic and unmistakably malignant.

Clinical course and prognosis depend on histologic grade. Low-grade tumors may invade locally and recur in about 15% of cases but metastasize only rarely and afford a 5-year survival rate of over 90%. By contrast, high-grade neoplasms and, to a lesser extent, intermediate-grade tumors are invasive and difficult to excise. As a result, they recur in 25% to 30% of cases, and about 30% metastasize to distant sites. The 5-year survival rate is only 50%.

SUMMARY

DISEASES OF SALIVARY GLANDS

- Sialadenitis (inflammation of the salivary glands) can be caused by trauma, infection (such as mumps), or an autoimmune reaction.

- Pleomorphic adenoma is a slow-growing neoplasm composed of a heterogeneous mixture of epithelial and mesenchymal cells. It is typically benign.
- Mucoepidermoid carcinoma is a malignant neoplasm of variable biologic aggressiveness that is composed of a mixture of squamous and mucous cells.

ODONTOGENIC CYSTS AND TUMORS

Odontogenic cysts usually are derived from remnants of odontogenic epithelium present within the jaws. In contrast to the rest of the skeleton, epithelium-lined cysts are quite common in the jaws. These cysts are subclassified as either inflammatory or developmental. Only the most common lesions are considered here, starting with developmental cysts.

The *dentigerous cyst* originates around the crown of an unerupted tooth and is thought to be the result of degeneration of the dental follicle (primordial tissue that makes the enamel surface of teeth). They are lined by a thin, stratified squamous epithelium that typically is associated with a dense chronic inflammatory infiltrate in the underlying connective tissue. Complete removal is curative.

Odontogenic keratocysts can occur at any age but are most frequent in individuals between 10 and 40 years of age, have a male predominance, and typically are located within the posterior mandible. Differentiation of the odontogenic keratocyst from other odontogenic cysts is important because it is locally aggressive and has a high recurrence rate. On histologic examination, the cyst lining consists of a thin layer of parakeratinized or orthokeratinized stratified squamous epithelium with a prominent basal cell layer and a corrugated luminal epithelial surface. Treatment requires aggressive and complete removal; recurrence rates of up to 60% are associated with inadequate resection.

In contrast with the developmental cysts just described, the *periapical cyst* has an inflammatory etiology. These extremely common lesions occur at the tooth apex as a result of long-standing pulpitis, which may be caused by advanced caries or trauma. Necrosis of the pulpal tissue, which can traverse the length of the root and exit the apex of the tooth into the surrounding alveolar bone, can lead to a periapical abscess. Over time, granulation tissue (with or without an epithelial lining) may develop. Periapical inflammatory lesions persist as a result of bacterial infection or necrotic tissue in the area. Successful treatment, therefore, necessitates the complete removal of the offending material followed by restoration or extraction of the tooth.

Odontogenic tumors are a complex group of lesions with diverse histologic appearances and clinical behaviors. Some are true neoplasms, either benign or malignant, while others are thought to be hamartomas. Odontogenic tumors are derived from odontogenic epithelium, ectomesenchyme, or both. The two most common and clinically significant tumors are ameloblastoma and odontoma.

Ameloblastomas arise from odontogenic epithelium. They are typically cystic, slow-growing and, despite being locally invasive, have an indolent course. The cysts are lined by palisading columnar epithelium that overlies a loose stroma with stellate cells. Odontoma, the most common type of odontogenic tumor, arises from epithelium but shows extensive deposition of enamel and dentin. Odontomas are cured by local excision.

SUMMARY

ODONTOGENIC CYSTS AND TUMORS

- The jaws are a common site of epithelium-lined cysts derived from odontogenic remnants.
- The odontogenic keratocyst is locally aggressive, with a high recurrence rate.
- The periapical cyst is a reactive, inflammatory lesion associated with caries or dental trauma.
- The most common odontogenic tumors are ameloblastoma and odontoma.

Esophagus

The esophagus develops from the cranial portion of the foregut. It is a hollow, highly distensible muscular tube that extends from the epiglottis to the gastroesophageal junction, located just above the diaphragm. Acquired diseases of the esophagus run the gamut from lethal cancers to the persistent "heartburn" of gastroesophageal reflux that may be chronic and incapacitating or merely an occasional annoyance.

OBSTRUCTIVE AND VASCULAR DISEASES

Mechanical Obstruction

Atresia, fistulas, and duplications may occur in any part of the gastrointestinal tract. When they involve the

esophagus, they are discovered shortly after birth, usually because of regurgitation during feeding. Prompt surgical repair is required. Absence, or agenesis, of the esophagus is extremely rare. Atresia, in which a thin, noncanalized cord replaces a segment of esophagus, is more common. It occurs most frequently at or near the tracheal bifurcation and usually is associated with a fistula connecting the upper or lower esophageal pouches to a bronchus or the trachea. This abnormal connection can result in aspiration, suffocation, pneumonia, or severe fluid and electrolyte imbalances.

Esophageal stenosis may be congenital or more commonly acquired. When acquired the narrowing generally is caused by fibrous thickening of the submucosa and atrophy of the muscularis propria. Stenosis due to inflammation and scarring may be caused by chronic gastroesophageal reflux, irradiation, ingestion of caustic agents, or other forms of severe injury. Stenosis-associated dysphagia usually is progressive; difficulty eating solids typically occurs long before problems with liquids.

Functional Obstruction

Efficient delivery of food and fluids to the stomach requires coordinated waves of peristaltic contractions. *Esophageal dysmotility* interferes with this process and can take several forms, all of which are characterized by discoordinated contraction or spasm of the muscularis. Because it increases esophageal wall stress, spasm also can cause small diverticula to form. Esophageal dysmotility can be separated into several forms depending on the character of the contractile abnormalities.

Achalasia is characterized by the triad of incomplete lower esophageal sphincter (LES) relaxation, increased LES tone, and esophageal aperistalsis. Primary achalasia is caused by failure of distal esophageal inhibitory neurons and is, by definition, idiopathic. Degenerative changes in neural innervation, either intrinsic to the esophagus or within the extraesophageal vagus nerve or the dorsal motor nucleus of the vagus, may lead to secondary achalasia. This occurs in Chagas disease, in which *Trypanosoma cruzi* infection causes destruction of the myenteric plexus, failure of LES relaxation, and esophageal dilatation. Duodenal, colonic, and ureteric myenteric plexuses also can be affected in Chagas disease. Achalasia-like disease may be caused by diabetic autonomic neuropathy, infiltrative disorders such as malignancy, amyloidosis, or sarcoidosis, and lesions of dorsal motor nuclei, which may be produced by polio or surgical ablation.

Ectopia

Ectopic tissues (developmental rests) are common in the gastrointestinal tract. The most frequent site of ectopic gastric mucosa is the upper third of the esophagus, where it is referred to as an *inlet patch*. Although the presence of such tissue generally is asymptomatic, acid released by gastric mucosa within the esophagus can result in dysphagia, esophagitis, Barrett esophagus, or, rarely, adenocarcinoma. *Gastric heterotopia*, small patches of ectopic gastric mucosa in the small bowel, particularly within a Meckel diverticulum, or colon, may present with occult blood loss due to local injury caused by acid secretion.

Esophageal Varices

Instead of returning directly to the heart, venous blood from the gastrointestinal tract is delivered to the liver via the portal vein before reaching the inferior vena cava. This circulatory pattern is responsible for the first-pass effect, in which drugs and other materials absorbed in the intestines are processed by the liver before entering the systemic circulation. **Diseases that impede portal blood flow cause portal hypertension, which can lead to the development of esophageal varices, an important cause of massive and frequently life-threatening bleeding.**

Pathogenesis

One of the few sites where the splanchnic and systemic venous circulations can communicate is the esophagus. Portal hypertension induces development of collateral channels that allow portal blood to shunt into the caval system. However, these collateral veins enlarge the subepithelial and submucosal venous plexi within the distal esophagus. These vessels, termed *varices*, develop in 50% of cirrhotic patients, most commonly in association with alcoholic liver disease. Worldwide, hepatic schistosomiasis is the second most common cause of varices. A more detailed consideration of portal hypertension is given in Chapter 16.

MORPHOLOGY

Varices can be detected by angiography, but are most commonly detected during endoscopy (Fig. 15.7A and B) and appear as tortuous dilated veins within the submucosa of the distal esophagus and proximal stomach (see Fig. 15.7C and D). The overlying mucosa can be intact or ulcerated and necrotic, particularly if rupture has occurred.

Clinical Features

Varices often are asymptomatic, but their rupture can lead to massive hematemesis and death. Variceal rupture therefore constitutes a medical emergency. Despite intervention, as many as half of the patients die from the first bleeding episode, either as a direct consequence of hemorrhage or due to hepatic coma triggered by the protein load that results from intraluminal bleeding as well as hypovolemic shock. Among those who survive, additional episodes of hemorrhage, each potentially fatal, occur in as many as 20% of cases.

ESOPHAGITIS

Esophageal Lacerations, Mucosal Injury, and Infections

The most common esophageal lacerations are *Mallory-Weiss tears*, which are often induced by severe retching or vomiting. Normally, a reflex relaxation of the gastroesophageal musculature precedes the anti-peristaltic contractile wave associated with vomiting. This relaxation may fail during prolonged vomiting, with the result that refluxing gastric contents cause the esophageal wall to stretch and tear. Patients usually present with hematemesis.

The roughly linear lacerations of Mallory-Weiss syndrome are longitudinally oriented and usually cross the gastroesophageal junction (Fig. 15.8A). These superficial tears generally heal quickly without surgical intervention. By contrast, severe, transmural esophageal tears *(Boerhaave syndrome)* result in mediastinitis, are catastrophic, and require prompt surgical intervention.

Chemical and Infectious Esophagitis

The stratified squamous mucosa of the esophagus may be damaged by a variety of irritants including alcohol, corrosive acids or alkalis, excessively hot fluids, and heavy

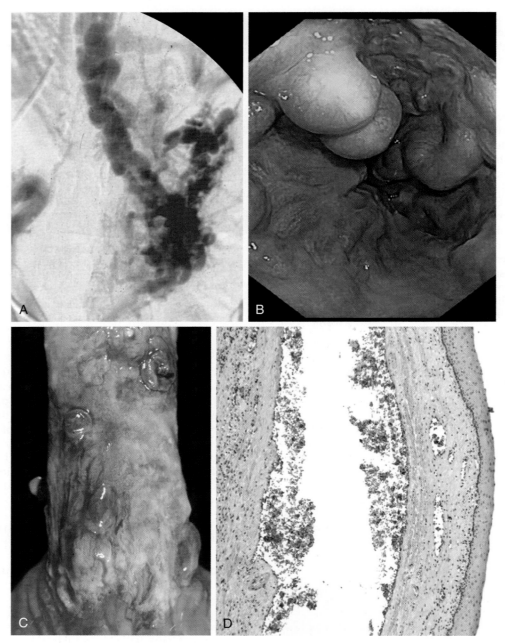

Fig. 15.7 Esophageal varices. (A) Angiogram showing several tortuous esophageal varices. (B) Although the angiogram is striking, endoscopy is more commonly used to identify varices. (C) Collapsed varices are present in this postmortem specimen corresponding to the angiogram in (A). The polypoid areas are sites of variceal hemorrhage that were ligated with bands. (D) Dilated varices beneath intact squamous mucosa.

smoking. Medicinal pills, most commonly doxycycline and bisphosphonates, may adhere to the esophageal lining and dissolve in the esophagus rather than passing immediately into the stomach, resulting in pill-induced esophagitis. Esophagitis due to chemical injury generally causes only self-limited pain, particularly odynophagia (pain with swallowing). Hemorrhage, stricture, or perforation may occur in severe cases. Iatrogenic esophageal injury may be caused by cytotoxic chemotherapy, radiation therapy, or graft-versus-host disease. The morphologic changes are nonspecific, consisting of ulceration and acute inflammation. Irradiation causes blood vessel damage adding an element of ischemic injury.

Infectious esophagitis may occur in otherwise healthy individuals but is most frequent in those who are debilitated or immunosuppressed. In these patients, esophageal infection by herpes simplex viruses, cytomegalovirus (CMV), or fungal organisms is common. Among fungi, Candida is the most common pathogen, although mucormycosis and aspergillosis may also occur. The esophagus may also be involved in desquamative skin diseases such as bullous pemphigoid and epidermolysis bullosa and, rarely, Crohn disease.

Infection by fungi or bacteria can be primary or complicate a preexisting ulcer. Nonpathogenic oral bacteria frequently are found in ulcer beds, while pathogenic organisms, which

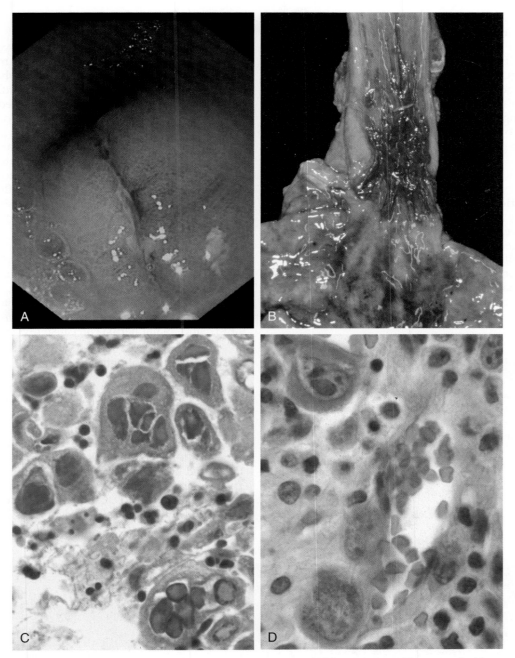

Fig. 15.8 Traumatic and viral esophagitis. (A) Endoscopic view of a longitudinally-oriented Mallory-Weiss tear. These superficial lacerations can range from millimeters to several centimeters in length. (B) Postmortem specimen with multiple herpetic ulcers in the distal esophagus. (C) Multinucleate squamous cells containing herpesvirus nuclear inclusions. (D) Cytomegalovirus-infected endothelial cells with nuclear and cytoplasmic inclusions. *(Endoscopic image courtesy of Dr. Ira Hanan, The University of Chicago, Chicago, Illinois.)*

account for about 10% of infectious esophagitis cases, may invade the lamina propria and cause necrosis of overlying mucosa. Candidiasis in its most advanced form is characterized by adherent, gray-white pseudomembranes composed of densely matted fungal hyphae and inflammatory cells covering the esophageal mucosa.

The endoscopic appearance often provides a clue to the identity of the infectious agent in viral esophagitis. Herpesviruses typically cause punched-out ulcers (Fig. 15.8B), and histopathologic analysis demonstrates nuclear viral inclusions within a rim of degenerating epithelial cells at the

ulcer edge (Fig. 15.8C). By contrast, CMV causes shallower ulcerations. Biopsy of these lesions show the characteristic nuclear and cytoplasmic inclusions within capillary endothelium and stromal cells (Fig. 15.8D). Immunohistochemical staining for viral antigens can be a useful ancillary diagnostic tool.

Reflux Esophagitis

Reflux of gastric contents into the lower esophagus is the most frequent cause of esophagitis and the most

common gastrointestinal ailment with which patients present in the out patient setting in the United States. The associated clinical condition is termed *gastroesophageal reflux disease (GERD)*. The stratified squamous epithelium of the esophagus is resistant to abrasion from foods but is sensitive to acid. The submucosal glands of the proximal and distal esophagus contribute to mucosal protection by secreting mucin and bicarbonate. More important, high lower esophageal sphincter tone protects against reflux of acidic gastric contents, which are under positive pressure.

Pathogenesis

Reflux of gastric juices is central to the development of mucosal injury in GERD. In severe cases, duodenal bile reflux may exacerbate the damage. Conditions that decrease lower esophageal sphincter tone or increase abdominal pressure contribute to GERD and include alcohol and tobacco use, obesity, central nervous system depressants, pregnancy, hiatal hernia (discussed later), delayed gastric emptying, and increased gastric volume. In many cases, no definitive cause is identified.

MORPHOLOGY

Simple hyperemia, evident to the endoscopist as redness, may be the only alteration. In mild GERD the mucosal histology is often unremarkable. With more significant disease, eosinophils are recruited into the squamous mucosa, followed by neutrophils, which usually are associated with more severe injury (Fig. 15.9A). Basal zone hyperplasia exceeding 20% of the total epithelial thickness and elongation of lamina propria papillae, such that they extend into the upper third of the epithelium, also may be present.

Clinical Features

GERD is most common in those over 40 years of age but also occurs in infants and children. The most frequently reported symptoms are heartburn, dysphagia, and, less often, noticeable regurgitation of sour-tasting gastric contents. Rarely, chronic GERD is punctuated by attacks of severe chest pain that may be mistaken for heart disease. Treatment with proton pump inhibitors reduces gastric acidity and typically provides symptomatic relief. While the severity of symptoms is not closely related to the degree of histologic damage, the latter tends to increase with disease duration. Complications of reflux esophagitis include esophageal ulceration, hematemesis, melena, stricture development, and Barrett esophagus, a precursor lesion to esophageal carcinoma.

Hiatal hernia is characterized by separation of the diaphragmatic crura and protrusion of the stomach into the thorax through the resulting gap. Congenital hiatal hernias are recognized in infants and children, but many are acquired in later life. Hiatal hernia is symptomatic in fewer than 10% of adults; symptoms when present resemble GERD since hiatal hernia can cause LES incompetence.

Eosinophilic Esophagitis

Eosinophilic esophagitis is a chronic immunologically mediated disorder that is being increasingly recognized. Symptoms include food impaction and dysphagia in adults and feeding intolerance or GERD-like symptoms in children. The cardinal histologic feature is epithelial infiltration by large numbers of eosinophils, particularly superficially (Fig. 15.9B) and at sites far from the gastroesophageal junction. Their abundance can help to differentiate eosinophilic esophagitis from GERD, Crohn disease, and other causes of esophagitis. Endoscopically evident rings in the upper and

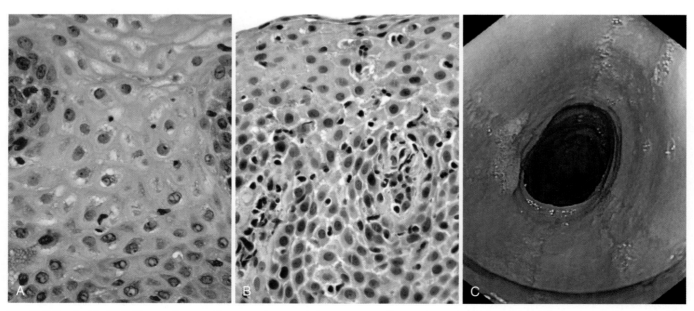

Fig. 15.9 Esophagitis. (A) Reflux esophagitis with scattered intraepithelial eosinophils. (B) Eosinophilic esophagitis with numerous intraepithelial eosinophils. (C) Endoscopy reveals circumferential rings in the proximal esophagus of this patient with eosinophilic esophagitis. *(Endoscopic image courtesy of Dr. Ira Hanan, The University of Chicago, Chicago, Illinois.)*

mid portions of the esophagus (Fig. 15.9C), may also help to distinguish eosinophilic esophagitis from GERD. Patients with eosinophilic esophagitis are typically refractory to high-dose proton pump inhibitor treatment. *Most patients are atopic, and many have atopic dermatitis, allergic rhinitis, asthma, or modest peripheral eosinophilia.* Treatments include dietary restrictions to prevent exposure to food allergens, such as cow milk and soy products, and topical or systemic corticosteroids.

Barrett Esophagus

Barrett esophagus is a complication of chronic GERD that is characterized by intestinal metaplasia within the esophageal squamous mucosa. The incidence of Barrett esophagus is rising; it is estimated to occur in as many as 10% of individuals with symptomatic GERD. White males are affected most often and typically present between 40 and 60 years of age. The greatest concern in Barrett esophagus is that *it confers an increased risk for development of esophageal adenocarcinoma.* Molecular studies suggest that Barrett epithelium may be more similar genetically to adenocarcinoma than to normal esophageal epithelium, consistent with the view that Barrett esophagus is a direct precursor of cancer. In keeping with this, epithelial *dysplasia*, considered to be a preinvasive lesion, develops in 0.2% to 1% of individuals with Barrett esophagus each year; its incidence increases with duration of symptoms and increasing patient age. Although the vast majority of esophageal adenocarcinomas are associated with Barrett esophagus, it should be noted that most individuals with Barrett esophagus do not develop esophageal cancer.

MORPHOLOGY

Barrett esophagus is recognized endoscopically as tongues or patches of red, velvety mucosa extending upward from the gastroesophageal junction (Fig. 15.10A). This metaplastic mucosa alternates with residual smooth, pale squamous (esophageal) mucosa proximally and interfaces with light-brown columnar (gastric) mucosa distally (Fig. 15.10B and C). High-resolution endoscopes have increased the sensitivity of Barrett esophagus detection.

Most experts require both endoscopic evidence of abnormal mucosa above the gastroesophageal junction and histologically documented gastric or intestinal metaplasia for diagnosis of Barrett esophagus. The defining feature of intestinal metaplasia, and a feature of Barrett esophagus, is the presence of goblet cells, which have distinct mucous vacuoles that stain pale blue by H&E and impart the shape of a wine goblet to the remaining cytoplasm (Fig. 15.10C). Dysplasia is classified as low-grade or high-grade on the basis of morphologic criteria. Intramucosal carcinoma is characterized by invasion of neoplastic epithelial cells into the lamina propria.

Clinical Features

Diagnosis of Barrett esophagus is usually prompted by GERD symptoms and requires endoscopy and biopsy. The best course of management is a matter of debate, but most clinicians recommend periodic surveillance endoscopy with biopsy to screen for dysplasia. Dysplasia is often treated and more advanced lesions, including high-grade dysplasia and intramucosal carcinoma, always require

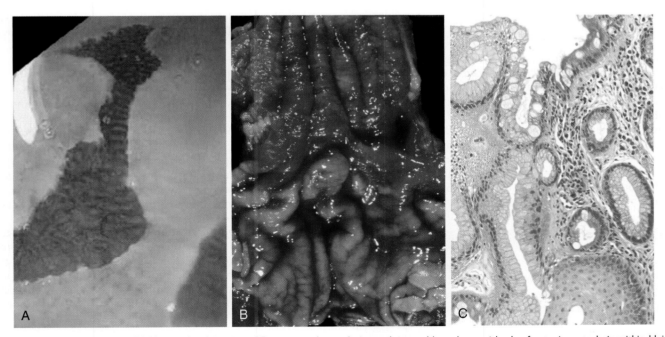

Fig. 15.10 Barrett esophagus. (A) Narrow band imaging of Barrett esophagus during endoscopy. Note the tan islands of ectopic metaplasia within bluish squamous mucosa. (B) Gross image of Barrett esophagus (compare to Fig. 15.7C). Only a few areas of pale squamous mucosa remain within the predominantly metaplastic, reddish mucosa of the distal esophagus. (C) Histologic appearance of the gastroesophageal junction in Barrett esophagus. Note the transition between esophageal squamous mucosa *(lower right)* and metaplastic mucosa containing goblet cells *(upper)*. *(Endoscopic image courtesy of Dr. Ira Hanan, The University of Chicago, Chicago, Illinois.)*

therapeutic intervention. Available modalities include surgical resection *(esophagectomy)*; newer approaches include photodynamic therapy, radiofrequency ablation, and endoscopic mucosectomy.

ESOPHAGEAL TUMORS

Two morphologic variants account for a majority of esophageal cancers: adenocarcinoma and squamous cell carcinoma. Worldwide, squamous cell carcinoma is more common, but adenocarcinoma is on the rise. Other rare tumors are not discussed here.

Adenocarcinoma

Esophageal adenocarcinoma typically arises in a background of Barrett esophagus and long-standing GERD. Risk for development of adenocarcinoma is greater in patients with documented dysplasia and in those who use tobacco, are obese, or who have had previous radiation therapy. In the United States, esophageal adenocarcinoma occurs most frequently in whites and shows a strong gender bias, being seven times more common in men than in women. However, the incidence varies by a factor of 60-fold worldwide, with rates being highest in Western countries, including the United States, the United Kingdom, Canada, Australia, and the Netherlands, and lowest in Korea, Thailand, Japan, and Ecuador. In countries where esophageal adenocarcinoma is more common, the incidence has increased markedly since 1970, more rapidly than for almost any other cancer. As a result, esophageal adenocarcinoma, which represented less than 5% of esophageal cancers before 1970, now accounts for half of all esophageal cancers in some Western countries, including the United States.

Pathogenesis

Molecular studies suggest that the progression of Barrett esophagus to adenocarcinoma occurs over an extended period through the stepwise acquisition of genetic and epigenetic changes. This model is supported by the observation that epithelial clones identified in nondysplastic Barrett metaplasia persist and accumulate mutations during progression to dysplasia and invasive carcinoma. Chromosomal abnormalities and *TP53* mutation are often present in the early stages of esophageal adenocarcinoma. Additional genetic changes and inflammation are thought to contribute to tumor progression.

MORPHOLOGY

Esophageal adenocarcinoma usually occurs in the distal third of the esophagus and may invade the adjacent gastric cardia (Fig. 15.11A). While early lesions may appear as flat or raised patches in otherwise intact mucosa, later tumors may form large exophytic masses, infiltrate diffusely, or ulcerate and invade deeply. On microscopic examination, Barrett esophagus frequently is present adjacent to the tumor. Tumors typically produce mucin and form glands (Fig. 15.11B).

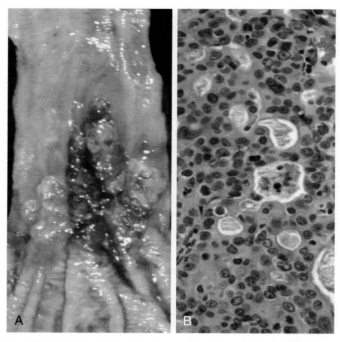

Fig. 15.11 Esophageal adenocarcinoma. (A) Adenocarcinoma usually occurs distally and, as in this case, often involves the gastric cardia. (B) Esophageal adenocarcinoma growing as back-to-back glands.

Clinical Features

Patients most commonly present with pain or difficulty in swallowing, progressive weight loss, chest pain, or vomiting. By the time signs and symptoms appear, the tumor usually has invaded submucosal lymphatic vessels. As a result of the advanced stage at diagnosis, the overall 5-year survival rate is less than 25%. By contrast, 5-year survival approximates 80% in the few patients with adenocarcinoma limited to the mucosa or submucosa.

Squamous Cell Carcinoma

In the United States, esophageal squamous cell carcinoma typically occurs in adults older than 45 years of age and affects males four times more frequently than females. Risk factors include alcohol and tobacco use, poverty, caustic esophageal injury, achalasia, Plummer-Vinson syndrome, frequent consumption of very hot beverages, and previous radiation therapy to the mediastinum. It is nearly six times more common in African Americans than in whites—a striking risk disparity that cannot be accounted for by differences in rates of alcohol and tobacco use. The incidence of esophageal squamous cell carcinoma can vary by more than 100-fold between and within countries, being more common in rural and underdeveloped areas. The countries with highest incidences are Iran, central China, Hong Kong, Argentina, Brazil, and South Africa.

Pathogenesis

A majority of esophageal squamous cell carcinomas in Europe and the United States are at least partially

related to the use of alcohol and tobacco, the effects of which synergize to increase risk. However, esophageal squamous cell carcinoma also is common in some regions where alcohol and tobacco use are uncommon due to religious or societal norms. In these areas, nutritional deficiencies, as well as exposure to polycyclic hydrocarbons, nitrosamines, and other mutagenic compounds, such as those found in fungus-contaminated foods, are suspected to be the risk factors. HPV infection also has been implicated in esophageal squamous cell carcinoma in high-risk but not in low-risk regions. The molecular pathogenesis of esophageal squamous cell carcinoma remains incompletely defined.

MORPHOLOGY

In contrast to the distal location of most adenocarcinomas, half of squamous cell carcinomas occur in the middle third of the esophagus (Fig. 15.12A). Squamous cell carcinoma begins as an in situ lesion in the form of **squamous dysplasia.** Early lesions appear as small, gray-white plaquelike thickenings. Over months to years, they grow into tumor masses that may be polypoid and protrude into and obstruct the lumen. Other tumors are either ulcerated or diffusely infiltrative lesions that spread within the esophageal wall, where they can cause thickening, rigidity, and luminal narrowing. These cancers may invade surrounding structures including the respiratory tree, causing pneumonia; the aorta, causing catastrophic exsanguination; or the mediastinum and pericardium.

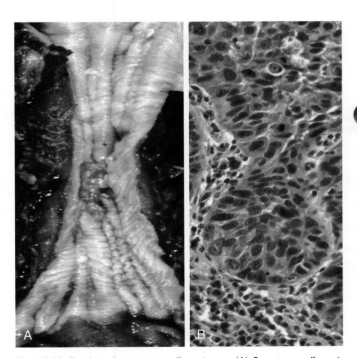

Fig. 15.12 Esophageal squamous cell carcinoma. (A) Squamous cell carcinoma most frequently is found in the mid-esophagus, where it commonly causes strictures. (B) Squamous cell carcinoma composed of nests of malignant cells that partially recapitulate the stratified organization of squamous epithelium.

Most squamous cell carcinomas are moderately to well-differentiated (Fig. 15.12B). Regardless of the histology symptomatic tumors have often invaded the esophageal wall at time of diagnosis. The rich submucosal lymphatic network promotes circumferential and longitudinal spread, and intramural tumor nodules may be present several centimeters away from the main mass. The sites of lymph node metastases vary with tumor location: Cancers in the upper third of the esophagus favor cervical lymph nodes; those in the middle third favor mediastinal, paratracheal, and tracheobronchial nodes; and those in the lower third spread to gastric and celiac nodes.

Clinical Features

Clinical manifestations of squamous cell carcinoma of the esophagus begin insidiously and include dysphagia, odynophagia (pain on swallowing), and obstruction. As with other forms of esophageal obstruction, patients may unwittingly adjust to the progressively increasing obstruction by altering their diet from solid to liquid foods. Extreme weight loss and debilitation may occur as consequences of both impaired nutrition and tumor-associated cachexia. As with adenocarcinoma, hemorrhage and sepsis may accompany tumor ulceration. Occasionally, squamous cell carcinomas of the upper and mid esophagus present with symptoms caused by aspiration of food via a tracheoesophageal fistula.

Increased use of endoscopic screening has led to earlier diagnosis of esophageal squamous cell carcinoma. Early detection is critical, because 5-year survival rates are 75% for patients with superficial esophageal carcinoma but much lower for patients with more advanced tumors. The overall 5-year survival rate remains a dismal 9%.

SUMMARY

DISEASES OF THE ESOPHAGUS

- *Esophageal obstruction* may occur as a result of mechanical or functional anomalies. Mechanical causes include developmental defects, fibrotic strictures, and tumors.
- *Achalasia,* characterized by incomplete LES relaxation, increased LES tone, and esophageal aperistalsis, is a common form of functional esophageal obstruction.
- *Esophagitis* can result from chemical or infectious mucosal injury. Infections are most frequent in immunocompromised individuals.
- The most common cause of esophagitis is *gastroesophageal reflux disease (GERD),* which must be differentiated from *eosinophilic esophagitis.*
- *Barrett esophagus,* which may develop in patients with chronic GERD, is associated with increased risk for development of esophageal adenocarcinoma.
- *Esophageal squamous cell carcinoma* is associated with alcohol and tobacco use, poverty, caustic esophageal injury, achalasia, tylosis, and Plummer-Vinson syndrome.

Stomach

Disorders of the stomach are a frequent cause of clinical disease, with inflammatory and neoplastic lesions being particularly common. In the United States, symptoms related to gastric acidity account for nearly one third of all health care spending on gastrointestinal disease. In addition, despite a decreasing incidence in certain locales, including the United States, gastric cancer remains a leading cause of death worldwide.

The stomach is divided into four major anatomic regions: the cardia, fundus, body, and antrum. The cardia is lined mainly by mucin-secreting *foveolar cells* that form shallow glands. The antral glands are similar but also contain endocrine cells, such as *G cells,* that release gastrin to stimulate luminal acid secretion by *parietal cells* within the gastric fundus and body. The well-developed glands of the body and fundus also contain *chief cells* that produce and secrete digestive enzymes such as pepsin.

GASTROPATHY AND ACUTE GASTRITIS

Gastritis results from mucosal injury. When neutrophils are present, the lesion is referred to as *acute gastritis.* When cell injury and regeneration are present but inflammatory cells are rare or absent, the term *gastropathy* is applied. Agents that cause gastropathy include nonsteroidal anti-inflammatory drugs, alcohol, bile, and stress-induced injury. Acute mucosal erosion or hemorrhage, such as Curling ulcers or lesions following disruption of gastric blood flow, for example, in portal hypertension, can also cause gastropathy that typically progresses to gastritis. The term *hypertrophic gastropathy* is applied to a specific group of diseases exemplified by Ménétrier disease and Zollinger-Ellison syndrome (discussed later).

Both gastropathy and acute gastritis may be asymptomatic or cause variable degrees of epigastric pain, nausea, and vomiting. In more severe cases, there may be mucosal erosion, ulceration, hemorrhage, hematemesis, melena, or, rarely, massive blood loss.

Pathogenesis

The gastric lumen is strongly acidic, with a pH close to 1 — more than 1 million times more acidic than the blood. This harsh environment contributes to digestion but also has the potential to damage the mucosa. Multiple mechanisms have evolved to protect the gastric mucosa (Fig. 15.13). Mucin secreted by surface foveolar cells forms a thin layer of mucus that prevents large food particles from directly touching the epithelium. The mucus layer also promotes formation of an "unstirred" layer of fluid over the epithelium that protects the mucosa; it has a neutral pH as a result of secretion of bicarbonate ions by surface epithelial cells. Finally, the rich blood supply of the gastric mucosa efficiently buffers and removes protons that back-diffuse into the lamina propria. Gastropathy, acute

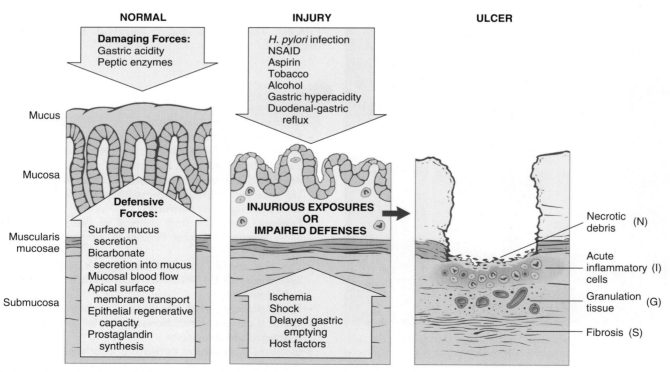

Fig. 15.13 Mechanisms of gastric injury and protection. This diagram illustrates the progression from mild forms of injury to ulceration that may occur with acute or chronic gastritis. Ulcers include layers of necrotic debris (N), inflammation (I), and granulation tissue (G); scarring (S), which develops over time, is present only in chronic lesions.

gastritis, and chronic gastritis can occur after disruption of any of these protective mechanisms. The main causes include:

- Nonsteroidal anti-inflammatory drugs (NSAIDs) inhibit cyclooxygenase (COX)-dependent synthesis of prostaglandins E2 and I2, which stimulate nearly all of the above defense mechanisms including mucus and bicarbonate secretion, mucosal blood flow, and epithelial restitution. Although COX-1 plays a larger role than COX-2, both isoenzymes contribute to mucosal protection. Thus, while the risk for development of NSAID-induced gastric injury is greatest with nonselective inhibitors, such as aspirin, ibuprofen, and naproxen, selective COX-2 inhibition, for example, by celecoxib, can also result in gastropathy or gastritis.
- The gastric injury that occurs in uremic patients and those infected with urease-secreting *H. pylori* may be due to inhibition of gastric bicarbonate transporters by ammonium ions.
- Reduced mucin and bicarbonate secretion have been suggested as factors that explain the increased susceptibility of older adults to gastritis.
- Hypoxemia and decreased oxygen delivery may account for an increased incidence of gastropathy and acute gastritis at high altitudes.
- Ingestion of harsh chemicals, particularly acids or bases, either accidentally or in a suicide attempt, leads to severe gastric mucosal damage as a result of direct injury to epithelial and stromal cells. Direct cellular damage also contributes to gastritis induced by excessive alcohol consumption, NSAID use, and radiation therapy. Agents that inhibit DNA synthesis or the mitotic apparatus, including those used in cancer chemotherapy, may cause generalized mucosal damage due to insufficient epithelial renewal.

MORPHOLOGY

Histologically, gastropathy and mild acute gastritis may be difficult to recognize, since the lamina propria shows only moderate edema and slight vascular congestion. The surface epithelium is intact, but hyperplasia of foveolar mucus cells is typically present. Neutrophils, lymphocytes, and plasma cells are not prominent.

The presence of neutrophils above the basement membrane in contact with epithelial cells is abnormal in all parts of the gastrointestinal tract and signifies active inflammation, or, at this site, gastritis (rather than gastropathy). The term *active inflammation* is preferred over acute inflammation throughout the luminal gastrointestinal tract, since active inflammation may be present in both acute and chronic disease states. With more severe mucosal damage, erosions and hemorrhage develop. Hemorrhage may manifest as dark punctae in an otherwise hyperemic mucosa. Concurrent presence of erosion and hemorrhage is termed **acute erosive hemorrhagic gastritis.**

Stress-Related Mucosal Disease

Stress-related gastric injury occurs in patients with severe trauma, extensive burns, intracranial disease, major surgery, serious medical disease, and other forms of severe physiologic stress. More than 75% of critically ill patients develop endoscopically visible gastric lesions during the first 3 days of their illness. In some cases, the associated ulcers are given specific names based on location and clinical associations. Examples are as follows:

- *Stress ulcers* affecting critically ill patients with shock, sepsis, or severe trauma.
- *Curling ulcers* occur in the proximal duodenum and are associated with severe burns or trauma.
- *Cushing ulcers* arise in the stomach, duodenum, or esophagus of those with intracranial disease and have a high incidence of perforation.

Pathogenesis

The pathogenesis of stress-related gastric mucosal injury is most often due to local ischemia. This may be caused by systemic hypotension or reduced blood flow resulting from stress-induced splanchnic vasoconstriction. Upregulation and increased release of the vasoconstrictor endothelin-1 also contributes to ischemic gastric mucosal injury, while increased COX-2 expression appears to be protective. Cushing ulcers are thought to be caused by direct stimulation of vagal nuclei resulting acid hypersecretion. Systemic acidosis may also contribute to mucosal injury by lowering the intracellular pH of mucosal cells.

MORPHOLOGY

Stress-related gastric mucosal injury ranges from shallow erosions caused by superficial epithelial damage to deeper lesions that penetrate the depth of the mucosa. Acute ulcers are rounded and typically less than 1 cm in diameter. The ulcer base frequently is stained brown to black by acid-digested extravasated red cells. Unlike peptic ulcers, which arise in the setting of chronic injury, acute stress ulcers are found anywhere in the stomach and are often multiple. They are sharply demarcated, with essentially normal adjacent mucosa, although there may be suffusion of blood into the mucosa and submucosa and some inflammatory reaction. The scarring and thickening of blood vessels that characterize chronic peptic ulcers are absent. Healing with complete reepithelialization occurs days or weeks after the injurious factors are removed.

Clinical Features

Most critically ill patients admitted to hospital intensive care units have histologic evidence of gastric mucosal damage. Ulcers are associated with nausea, vomiting, melena, and coffee-ground hematemesis. Bleeding from superficial gastric erosions or ulcers that may require transfusion develop in 1% to 4% of these patients. Other complications, including perforation, also may occur. Prophylaxis with proton pump inhibitors may blunt the impact of stress ulceration, but the most important determinant of outcome is the severity of the underlying condition.

CHRONIC GASTRITIS

The most common cause of chronic gastritis is infection with the bacillus *Helicobacter pylori*. *Autoimmune*

gastritis, typically associated with gastric atrophy, represents less than 10% of cases of chronic gastritis but is the most common cause in patients without *H. pylori* infection. Chronic NSAID use is a third important cause of gastritis in some populations, as discussed later. Less common causes include radiation injury and chronic bile reflux.

The signs and symptoms associated with chronic gastritis typically are less severe but more persistent than those of acute gastritis. Nausea and upper-abdominal discomfort may occur, sometimes with vomiting, but hematemesis is uncommon.

Helicobacter pylori Gastritis

The discovery of the association of *H. pylori* with peptic ulcer disease revolutionized the understanding of chronic gastritis. These spiral-shaped or curved bacilli are present in gastric biopsy specimens from almost all patients with duodenal ulcers and a majority of those with gastric ulcers or chronic gastritis. Acute *H. pylori* infection is subclinical in most cases; rather, it is the chronic gastritis that ultimately brings the afflicted person to medical attention. *H. pylori* infection most often presents as an *antral gastritis with increased acid production.* The increased acid production may give rise to peptic ulcer disease of the duodenum or stomach.

While in most cases *H. pylori* gastritis is limited to the antrum, in some individuals it progresses to involve the gastric body and fundus, resulting in reduced parietal cell mass and acid secretion. Reduced acid output results in hypergastrinemia, as in autoimmune atrophic gastritis. In addition, extension of the gastritis to the gastric body and fundus results in intestinal metaplasia and increased risk of gastric cancer.

Epidemiology

In the United States, *H. pylori* infection is associated with poverty, household crowding, limited education, residence in areas with poor sanitation, and birth outside of the United States. Infection is typically acquired in childhood and may then persist for life. Improved sanitation in many areas likely explains why *H. pylori* infection rates among younger individuals today are markedly lower than they were in similarly aged individuals 30 years ago. In the United States, the prevalence of *H. pylori* infection is also higher in African Americans and Mexican Americans. Worldwide, colonization rates vary from less than 10% to more than 80% as a function of age, geography, and social factors.

Pathogenesis

H. pylori organisms have adapted to the ecologic niche provided by gastric mucus. Although *H. pylori* may invade the gastric mucosa, the contribution of invasion to disease pathogenesis is not known. Four features are linked to *H. pylori* virulence:

- *Flagella,* which allow the bacteria to be motile in viscous mucus
- *Urease,* which generates ammonia from endogenous urea, thereby elevating local gastric pH around the organisms and protecting the bacteria from the acidic pH of the stomach

- *Adhesins,* which enhance bacterial adherence to surface foveolar cells
- *Toxins,* such as that encoded by cytotoxin-associated gene A *(CagA),* that may be involved in ulcer or cancer development

These factors allow *H. pylori* to create an imbalance between gastroduodenal mucosal defenses and damaging forces that overcome those defenses.

MORPHOLOGY

Gastric biopsy specimens generally demonstrate *H. pylori* in infected individuals (Fig. 15.14A). The organism is concentrated within mucus overlying epithelial cells in the surface and neck regions. The inflammatory reaction includes a variable number of neutrophils within the lamina propria, including some that cross the basement membrane to assume an intraepithelial location (Fig. 15.14B) and accumulate in the lumen of gastric pits to create pit abscesses. The superficial lamina propria includes large numbers of plasma cells, often in clusters or sheets, as well as increased numbers of lymphocytes and macrophages. When intense, inflammatory infiltrates may create thickened rugal folds, mimicking infiltrative lesions. Lymphoid aggregates, some with germinal centers, are frequently present (Fig. 15.14C) and represent an induced form of **mucosa-associated lymphoid tissue (MALT)** that has the potential to transform into lymphoma. **Intestinal metaplasia,** characterized by the presence of goblet cells and columnar absorptive cells (Fig. 15.14D), also may be present and is associated with increased risk of gastric adenocarcinoma. *H. pylori* shows tropism for gastric foveolar epithelium and generally is not found in areas of intestinal metaplasia, acid-producing mucosa of the gastric body, or duodenal epithelium. Antral biopsies are therefore preferred for evaluation of *H. pylori* gastritis.

Clinical Features

In addition to histologic identification of the organism, several diagnostic tests have been developed including a noninvasive serologic test for anti–*H. pylori* antibodies, a stool test for the organism, and the urea breath test, based on the generation of ammonia by bacterial urease. Gastric biopsy specimens also can be analyzed by the rapid urease test, bacterial culture, or polymerase chain reaction (PCR) assay for bacterial DNA. Effective treatments include combinations of antibiotics and proton pump inhibitors. Patients with *H. pylori* gastritis usually improve after treatment, although relapses can follow incomplete eradication or reinfection.

Autoimmune Gastritis

Autoimmune gastritis accounts for less than 10% of cases of chronic gastritis. In contrast *H. pylori*-associated gastritis, autoimmune gastritis typically spares the antrum and induces marked *hypergastrinemia* (Table 15.2). Autoimmune gastritis is characterized by the following:

- Antibodies to parietal cells and intrinsic factor that can be detected in serum and gastric secretions
- Reduced serum pepsinogen I levels
- Antral endocrine cell hyperplasia

stimulates gastrin release, resulting in hypergastrinemia and hyperplasia of antral gastrin-producing G cells. Lack of intrinsic factor disables ileal vitamin B_{12} absorption, leading to B_{12} deficiency and a particular form of megaloblastic anemia called pernicious anemia (Chapter 12). Reduced serum concentration of pepsinogen I reflects chief cell loss. Although *H. pylori* can cause hypochlorhydria, it is not associated with achlorhydria or pernicious anemia, because the parietal and chief cell damage is not as severe as in autoimmune gastritis.

MORPHOLOGY

Autoimmune gastritis is characterized by diffuse **damage of the oxyntic** (acid-producing) **mucosa** within the body and fundus. Damage to the antrum and cardia typically is absent or mild. With **diffuse atrophy,** the oxyntic mucosa of the body and fundus appears markedly thinned, and rugal folds are lost. Neutrophils may be present, but the inflammatory infiltrate more commonly is composed of lymphocytes, macrophages, and plasma cells; in contrast with ***H. pylori* gastritis,** the inflammatory reaction most often is deep and centered on the gastric glands. **Parietal and chief cell loss** can be extensive, and **intestinal metaplasia** may develop.

Clinical Features

Antibodies to parietal cells and intrinsic factor are present early in the disease, but B_{12} deficiency and pernicious anemia develop in only a minority of patients. The median age at diagnosis is 60 years, and there is a slight female predominance. Autoimmune gastritis often is associated with other autoimmune diseases but is not linked to specific human leukocyte antigen (HLA) alleles.

COMPLICATIONS OF CHRONIC GASTRITIS

There are three important complications of chronic gastritis: Peptic ulcer disease, mucosal atrophy and intestinal metaplasia, and dysplasia. Each of these is discussed shortly.

Peptic Ulcer Disease

Peptic ulcer disease (PUD) most often is associated with *H. pylori* infection or NSAID use. The imbalances of

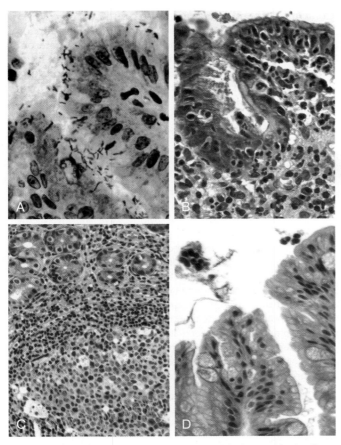

Fig. 15.14 Chronic gastritis. (A) Spiral-shaped *Helicobacter pylori* bacilli are highlighted in this Warthin-Starry silver stain. Organisms are abundant within surface mucus. (B) Intraepithelial and lamina propria neutrophils are prominent. (C) Lymphoid aggregates with germinal centers and abundant subepithelial plasma cells within the superficial lamina propria are characteristic of *H. pylori* gastritis. (D) Intestinal metaplasia, recognizable as the presence of goblet cells admixed with gastric foveolar epithelium, can develop and is a risk factor for development of gastric adenocarcinoma.

- Vitamin B_{12} deficiency leading to pernicious anemia and neurologic changes
- Impaired gastric acid secretion *(achlorhydria)*

Pathogenesis

Autoimmune gastritis is associated with immune-mediated loss of parietal cells and subsequent reductions in acid and intrinsic factor secretion. Deficient acid secretion

Table 15.2 Characteristics of *Helicobacter pylori*–Associated and Autoimmune Gastritis

Feature	*H. pylori*–Associated	Autoimmune
Location	Antrum	Body
Inflammatory infiltrate	Neutrophils, subepithelial plasma cells	Lymphocytes, macrophages
Acid production	Increased to slightly decreased	Decreased
Gastrin	Normal to markedly increased	Markedly increased
Other lesions	Hyperplastic/inflammatory polyps	Neuroendocrine hyperplasia
Serology	Antibodies to *H. pylori*	Antibodies to parietal cells (H^+,K^+-ATPase, intrinsic factor)
Sequelae	Peptic ulcer, adenocarcinoma, lymphoma	Atrophy, pernicious anemia, adenocarcinoma, carcinoid tumor
Associations	Low socioeconomic status, poverty, residence in rural areas	Autoimmune disease; thyroiditis, diabetes mellitus, Graves disease

mucosal defenses and damaging forces that cause chronic gastritis (see Fig. 15.13) are also responsible for PUD. In the United States, NSAID use is becoming the most common cause of gastric ulcers as *H. pylori* infection rates are falling and low-dose aspirin use in the aging population is increasing. PUD may occur in any portion of the gastrointestinal tract exposed to acidic gastric juices but is most common in the gastric antrum and first portion of the duodenum. Peptic (acid-induced) injury may occur in the esophagus as a result of acid reflux (GERD) or acid secretion by ectopic gastric mucosa. Peptic injury in the small intestine may also be associated with gastric heterotopia, including that within a Meckel diverticulum.

Epidemiology

PUD is common and is a frequent cause of physician visits worldwide. It leads to treatment of over 3 million individuals, 190,000 hospitalizations, and 5000 deaths in the United States each year. The lifetime risk for developing an ulcer is approximately 10% for males and 4% for females.

Pathogenesis

H. pylori infection and NSAID use are the primary underlying causes of PUD. More than 70% of PUD cases are associated with *H. pylori* infection and in these individuals PUD generally develops on a background of chronic gastritis. Because only 5% to 10% of *H. pylori*–infected individuals develop ulcers, it is probable that host factors as well as variation among *H. pylori* strains also contribute to the pathogenesis.

Gastric acid is fundamental to the pathogenesis of PUD. Hyperacidity may be caused by *H. pylori* infection, parietal cell hyperplasia, and excessive secretory responses. Insufficient inhibition of stimulatory mechanisms such as gastrin release may also contribute. For example, *Zollinger-Ellison syndrome*, characterized by multiple peptic ulcerations in the stomach, duodenum, and even jejunum, is caused by uncontrolled release of gastrin by a tumor and the resulting massive acid production.

Cofactors in peptic ulcerogenesis include chronic NSAID use, as noted; cigarette smoking, which impairs mucosal blood flow and healing; and high-dose corticosteroids, which suppress prostaglandin synthesis and impair healing. Peptic ulcers are more frequent in individuals with alcoholic cirrhosis, chronic obstructive pulmonary disease, chronic renal failure, and hyperparathyroidism. In the latter two conditions, hypercalcemia stimulates gastrin production and thereby increases acid secretion.

MORPHOLOGY

Peptic ulcers are four times more common in the proximal duodenum than in the stomach. Duodenal ulcers usually occur within a few centimeters of the pyloric valve and involve the anterior duodenal wall. Gastric peptic ulcers are predominantly located near the interface of the body and antrum.

Peptic ulcers are solitary in more than 80% of patients. Lesions less than 0.3 cm in diameter tend to be shallow, whereas those over 0.6 cm are likely to be deeper. The classic peptic ulcer is a round to oval, **sharply punched-out defect** (Fig. 15.15A and B). The base of peptic ulcers is smooth and clean as a result of peptic digestion of exudate and on histologic examination is composed of richly vascular granulation tissue (Fig. 15.15C). Ongoing bleeding within the ulcer base may cause life-threatening hemorrhage. **Perforation** is a complication that demands emergent surgical intervention.

Clinical Features

Peptic ulcers are chronic, recurring lesions that occur most often in middle-aged to older adults without obvious precipitating conditions, other than chronic gastritis. A majority of peptic ulcers come to clinical attention after patient complaints of *epigastric burning or aching pain*, although a significant fraction manifest with complications such as *iron deficiency anemia, frank hemorrhage*, or *perforation*. The pain tends to occur 1 to 3 hours after meals during the day, is worse at night, and is relieved by alkali or food. Nausea,

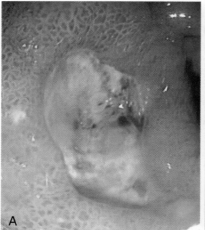
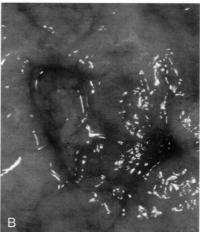
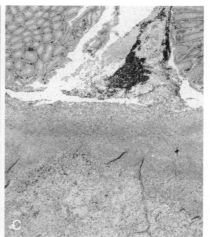

Fig. 15.15 Peptic ulcer disease. (A) Endoscopic view of typical antral ulcer associated with NSAID use. (B) Gross view of a similar ulcer that was resected due to gastric perforation, presenting as free air under the diaphragm. Note the clean edges. (C) The necrotic ulcer base is composed of granulation tissue overlaid by degraded blood. *(Endoscopic image courtesy of Dr. Ira Hanan, The University of Chicago, Chicago, Illinois.)*

vomiting, bloating, and belching may be present. Healing may occur with or without therapy, but the tendency to develop subsequent ulcers remains.

PUD causes much more morbidity than mortality. A variety of surgical approaches were formerly used to treat PUD, but current therapies are aimed at *H. pylori* eradication with antibiotics and neutralization of gastric acid, usually through use of proton pump inhibitors. These efforts have markedly reduced the need for surgical management, which is reserved primarily for treatment of ulcers with uncontrollable bleeding or perforation.

Mucosal Atrophy and Intestinal Metaplasia

Long-standing chronic gastritis may be associated with intestinal metaplasia, recognized by the presence of goblet cells. This is strongly associated with increased risk for development of gastric adenocarcinoma. In addition, the achlorhydria of gastric mucosal atrophy, which is commonly associated with intestinal metaplasia, permits overgrowth of bacteria that produce carcinogenic nitrosamines. Intestinal metaplasia caused by chronic *H. pylori* gastritis may regress after eradication of the organism.

Dysplasia

Chronic gastritis exposes the epithelium to inflammation-related free radical damage and proliferative stimuli. Over time, this can lead to the accumulation of genetic alterations that result in carcinoma. Preinvasive in situ lesions can be recognized histologically as dysplasia, which is marked by variations in epithelial size, shape, and orientation along with coarse chromatin texture, hyperchromasia, and nuclear enlargement. These overlap with and are sometimes difficult to distinguish from injury-associated regenerative changes.

SUMMARY

ACUTE AND CHRONIC GASTRITIS

- Gastritis is a mucosal inflammatory process. When inflammatory cells are absent or rare, the term *gastropathy* can be applied.
- The spectrum of acute gastritis ranges from asymptomatic disease to mild epigastric pain, nausea, and vomiting. Causative factors include any agent or disease that interferes with gastric mucosal protection. Acute gastritis can progress to gastric ulceration.
- The most common cause of chronic gastritis is *H. pylori* infection; most remaining cases are caused by NSAIDs, alcohol, or *autoimmune gastritis*.
- *H. pylori* gastritis typically affects the antrum and is associated with increased gastric acid production.
- *H. pylori* gastritis induces mucosa-associated lymphoid tissue (MALT) that can give rise to B-cell lymphomas (MALTomas).
- *Autoimmune gastritis* causes atrophy of the gastric body oxyntic glands, which results in decreased gastric acid production, antral G-cell hyperplasia, achlorhydria, and vitamin B_{12} deficiency. Anti–parietal cell and anti–intrinsic factor antibodies are typically present.

- *Intestinal metaplasia* develops in both forms of chronic gastritis and is a risk factor for development of gastric dysplasia and adenocarcinoma.
- Peptic ulcer disease can be caused by *H. pylori* chronic gastritis and the resultant hyperchlorhydria or NSAID use. Ulcers can develop in the stomach or duodenum and usually heal after suppression of gastric acid production, discontinuation of NSAID use, or, if present, *H. pylori* eradication.

GASTRIC POLYPS AND TUMORS

Gastric Polyps

Polyps are nodules or masses that project above the level of the surrounding mucosa. They are identified in up to 5% of upper gastrointestinal tract endoscopies. Polyps may develop as a result of epithelial or stromal cell hyperplasia, inflammation, ectopia, or neoplasia. Although many different types of polyps can occur in the stomach, only hyperplastic and inflammatory polyps, fundic gland polyps, and adenomas are considered here.

Inflammatory and Hyperplastic Polyps

Up to 75% of all gastric polyps are *inflammatory* or *hyperplastic polyps*. In the stomach, inflammatory and hyperplastic polyps represent opposite ends of the morphologic spectrum of a single entity; the distinction is based solely on the degree of inflammation. They most commonly affect individuals between 50 and 60 years of age, usually arising in a background of chronic gastritis that initiates the injury and reactive hyperplasia that cause polyp growth. If associated with *H. pylori* gastritis, polyps may regress after bacterial eradication.

The frequency with which dysplasia, a precancerous in situ lesion, develops in these polyps correlates with size; there is a significant increase in risk with polyps larger than 1.5 cm.

Fundic Gland Polyps

Fundic gland polyps occur sporadically and in individuals with familial adenomatous polyposis (FAP) Polyps associated with FAP (but not sporadic) may show dysplasia, but they almost never progress to become malignant. The incidence of sporadic lesions has increased markedly as a result of the widespread use of proton pump inhibitors. This likely results from increased gastrin secretion, in response to reduced acidity, and glandular hyperplasia driven by gastrin. Fundic gland polyps are nearly always asymptomatic, and are usually an incidental finding. These well-circumscribed polyps occur in the gastric body and fundus, often are multiple, and are composed of cystically dilated, irregular glands lined by flattened parietal and chief cells.

Gastric Adenoma

Gastric adenomas represent up to 10% of all gastric polyps. Their incidence increases with age and varies among different populations in parallel with that of gastric adenocarcinoma. Patients usually are between 50 and 60 years of age, and males are affected three times more often than females. Adenomas almost always occur on a background of chronic gastritis with atrophy and intestinal metaplasia. All gastrointestinal adenomas exhibit epithelial dysplasia, which can be classified as low- or high-grade. The risk for development of adenocarcinoma in gastric adenomas is related to the size of the lesion and is particularly elevated with lesions greater than 2 cm in diameter. Overall, the malignant potential of gastric adenomas is far greater than that of their colonic counterparts. Carcinoma may be present in up to 30% of gastric adenomas.

Gastric Adenocarcinoma

Adenocarcinoma is the most common malignancy of the stomach, comprising more than 90% of all gastric cancers. Early symptoms resemble those of chronic gastritis, including dyspepsia, dysphagia, and nausea. As a result, the cancer is often diagnosed at advanced stages when clinical manifestations such as weight loss, anorexia, altered bowel habits, anemia, and hemorrhage trigger diagnostic evaluation.

Epidemiology

Gastric cancer rates vary markedly with geography. The incidence is up to 20 times higher in Japan, Chile, Costa Rica, and Eastern Europe than in North America, northern Europe, Africa, and Southeast Asia. Mass endoscopic screening programs have been successful in regions of high incidence, such as Japan, where 35% of newly detected cases are *early gastric cancer* (i.e., tumors limited to the mucosa and submucosa). Unfortunately, mass screening programs are not cost-effective in regions in which the incidence is low, and less than 20% of cases are detected at an early stage in North America and northern Europe.

Gastric cancer is more common in lower socioeconomic groups and in individuals with *multifocal mucosal atrophy and intestinal metaplasia*. PUD does not impart an increased risk for development of gastric cancer, but patients who have had partial gastrectomies for PUD have a slightly higher risk for developing cancer in the residual gastric stump as a result of hypochlorhydria, bile reflux, and chronic gastritis.

In the United States, *gastric cancer rates have dropped by more than 85% during the 20th century.* Similar declines have been reported in many other Western countries, reflecting the importance of environmental and dietary factors. Despite this decrease in overall gastric adenocarcinoma incidence, *cancer of the gastric cardia is on the rise.* This trend probably is related to increased rates of Barrett esophagus and may reflect the growing prevalence of obesity and chronic GERD.

Pathogenesis

Gastric cancers are genetically heterogeneous, but certain molecular alterations are common. We will consider these first to be followed by the role of *H. pylori*–induced chronic inflammation and the association of a subset of gastric cancers with EBV infection.

- *Mutations.* While the majority of gastric cancers are not hereditary, mutations identified in familial gastric

cancer have provided important insights into the mechanisms of carcinogenesis in sporadic cases. Germ line mutations in *CDH1*, which encodes E-cadherin, a protein that contributes to epithelial intercellular adhesion, are associated with familial gastric cancers, usually of the diffuse type. By comparison, mutations in *CDH1* are present in about 50% of sporadic diffuse gastric tumors, while E-cadherin expression is drastically decreased in the rest, often by methylation of the *CDH1* promoter. *Thus, the loss of E-cadherin function seems to be a key step in the development of diffuse gastric cancer.*

In contrast to *CDH1*, patients with FAP who have germ line mutations in *adenomatous polyposis coli (APC) genes* have an increased risk for development of intestinal-type gastric cancer. Sporadic intestinal-type gastric cancer is associated with several genetic abnormalities including acquired mutations of β-catenin, a protein that binds to both E-cadherin and APC protein; microsatellite instability; and hypermethylation of genes including *TGFβRII, BAX, IGFRII,* and *p16/INK4a. TP53* mutations are present in a majority of sporadic gastric cancers of both histologic types.

- *H. pylori.* Chronic gastritis, most commonly due to *H. pylori* infection, promotes the development and progression of cancers that may be induced by diverse genetic alterations (Chapter 6). As is the case with many forms of chronic inflammation, *H. pylori*–induced chronic gastritis is associated with increased production of proinflammatory proteins, such as interleukin-1β (IL-1β) and tumor necrosis factor (TNF). It is therefore not surprising that polymorphisms of genes that encode such factors and enhance production of these cytokines confer increased risk for development of chronic gastritis-associated gastric cancer in those with coexisting *H. pylori* infection.

- *Epstein-Barr virus (EBV).* While *H. pylori* is most commonly associated with gastric cancer, approximately 10% of gastric adenocarcinomas are associated with Epstein-Barr virus (EBV) infection. Although the precise role of EBV in the development of gastric adenocarcinomas remains to be defined, it is notable that EBV episomes in these tumors frequently are clonal, suggesting that infection preceded neoplastic transformation. Further, *TP53* mutations are uncommon in EBV-positive gastric tumors, suggesting that the molecular pathogenesis of these cancers is distinct from that of other gastric adenocarcinomas. Morphologically, EBV-positive tumors tend to occur in the proximal stomach and most commonly have a diffuse morphology with a marked lymphocytic infiltrate.

MORPHOLOGY

Gastric adenocarcinomas are classified according to their location in the stomach as well as gross and histologic morphology. The **Lauren classification** that separates gastric cancers into **intestinal** and **diffuse** types correlates with distinct patterns of molecular alterations, as discussed earlier. Intestinal-type cancers tend to be bulky (Fig. 15.16A) and are composed of glandular structures similar to esophageal and colonic adenocarcinoma. Intestinal-type adenocarcinomas typically grow along broad cohesive fronts to form either an exophytic mass or an ulcerated tumor. The neoplastic cells often contain apical mucin vacuoles, and abundant mucin may be present in gland lumina.

Diffuse gastric cancers display an infiltrative growth pattern (Fig. 15.16B) and are composed of discohesive cells with large mucin vacuoles that expand the cytoplasm and push the nucleus to the periphery, creating a **signet ring cell** morphology (Fig. 15.16C). These cells permeate the mucosa and stomach wall individually or in small clusters. A mass may be difficult to appreciate in diffuse gastric cancer, but these infiltrative tumors often evoke a **desmoplastic** reaction that stiffens the gastric wall and may cause diffuse rugal flattening and a rigid, thickened wall that imparts a "leather bottle" appearance termed *linitis plastica.*

Clinical Features

Intestinal-type gastric cancer predominates in high-risk areas and develops from precursor lesions such as dysplasia and adenomas. The mean age at presentation is 55 years, and the male-to-female ratio is 2:1. By contrast, the incidence of diffuse gastric cancer is relatively uniform across countries, there are no identified precursor lesions, and the disease occurs at similar frequencies in males and females. Of note, *the decrease in gastric cancer incidence applies only to the intestinal type,* which is most closely associated with atrophic gastritis and intestinal metaplasia. As a result, the incidences of intestinal and diffuse types of gastric cancers are now similar in some regions.

The depth of invasion and the extent of nodal and distant metastasis at the time of diagnosis remain the most powerful prognostic indicators for gastric cancer. Local invasion into the duodenum, pancreas, and retroperitoneum is also characteristic. When possible, surgical resection remains the preferred treatment for gastric adenocarcinoma. After surgical resection, the 5-year survival rate for early gastric cancer can exceed 90%, even if lymph node metastases are present. By contrast, the 5-year survival rate for advanced gastric cancer remains below 20%, in large part because current chemotherapy regimens are have limited impact. This is changing slowly with individualized therapies. For example, patients whose tumors over-express the epidermal growth factor receptor HER2 benefit from agents that inhibit HER2 signaling. Nevertheless, most gastric cancers are discovered at advanced stage in the United States, and the overall 5-year survival rate is less than 30%.

Lymphoma

Although extranodal lymphomas can arise in virtually any tissue, they do so most commonly in the gastrointestinal tract, particularly the stomach. In allogeneic hematopoietic stem cell and organ transplant recipients, the bowel also is the most frequent site for Epstein-Barr virus–positive B cell lymphoproliferations. Nearly 5% of all gastric malignancies are primary lymphomas, the most common of which are indolent extranodal marginal zone B-cell lymphomas. In the gut, these tumors often are referred to as lymphomas of *MALT*, or *MALTomas*. This entity and the second most common primary lymphoma of the gut, diffuse large B cell lymphoma, are discussed in Chapter 12.

Neuroendocrine (Carcinoid) Tumor

Neuroendocrine tumors, also referred to as *carcinoid tumors,* arise from neuroendocrine organs (e.g., the endocrine pancreas) and neuroendocrine-differentiated gastrointestinal epithelia (e.g., G cells). A majority of these tumors are found in the gastrointestinal tract, and more than 40% occur in the small intestine. The tracheobronchial tree and lungs are the next most commonly involved sites. Gastric neuroendocrine tumors may be associated with endocrine cell hyperplasia, chronic atrophic gastritis, and Zollinger-Ellison syndrome. These tumors were called "carcinoid" because they are slower growing than carcinomas. The most current WHO classification describes these as low- or intermediate-grade neuroendocrine tumors. High-grade neuroendocrine tumors, termed *neuroendocrine carcinoma,* resemble small cell carcinoma of the lung (Chapter 13) and, in the gastrointestinal tract, are most common in the jejunum.

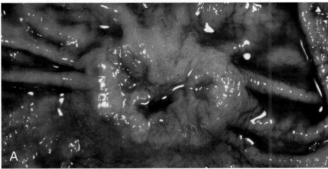
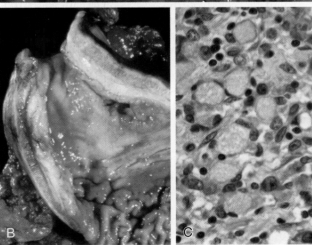

Fig. 15.16 Gastric adenocarcinoma. (A) Intestinal-type adenocarcinoma consisting of an elevated mass with heaped-up borders and central ulceration. Compare with the peptic ulcer in Fig. 15.15A. (B) Linitis plastica. The gastric wall is markedly thickened, and rugal folds are partially lost. (C) Signet ring cells with large cytoplasmic mucin vacuoles and peripherally displaced, crescent-shaped nuclei.

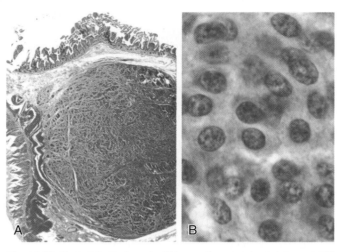

Fig. 15.17 Gastrointestinal carcinoid tumor (neuroendocrine tumor). (A) Carcinoid tumors often form a submucosal nodule composed of tumor cells embedded in dense fibrous tissue. (B) High magnification shows the bland cytology that typifies neuroendocrine tumors. The chromatin texture, with fine and coarse clumps, frequently assumes a "salt-and-pepper" pattern. Despite their innocuous appearance, tumors can be aggressive.

MORPHOLOGY

Neuroendocrine tumors are intramural or submucosal masses that create small polypoid lesions (Fig. 15.17A). The tumors are yellow or tan in appearance and elicit an intense desmoplastic reaction that may cause kinking of the bowel and obstruction. On histologic examination, neuroendocrine tumors are composed of islands, trabeculae, strands, glands, or sheets of uniform cells with scant, pink granular cytoplasm and a round-to-oval stippled nucleus (Fig. 15.17B).

Clinical Features

The peak incidence of neuroendocrine tumors is in the sixth decade, but they may appear at any age. Symptoms are determined by the hormones produced. For example, the *carcinoid syndrome* is caused by vasoactive substances secreted by the tumor that cause cutaneous flushing, sweating, bronchospasm, colicky abdominal pain, diarrhea, and right-sided cardiac valvular fibrosis. When tumors are confined to the intestine, the vasoactive substances released are metabolized to inactive forms by the liver—a "first-pass" effect similar to that seen with oral drugs. Thus, carcinoid syndrome occurs in less than 10% of patients and is *strongly associated with metastatic disease.*

The most important prognostic factor for gastrointestinal neuroendocrine tumors is location:

- *Foregut neuroendocrine (carcinoid) tumors* found within the stomach, duodenum proximal to the ligament of Treitz, and esophagus, rarely metastasize and are generally cured by resection. Rare duodenal gastrin-producing neuroendocrine tumors, also termed *gastrinomas,* may present with symptoms related to increased acid production, including pain and/or bleeding from gastroduodenal ulcers, refractory gastroesophageal reflux, and diarrhea due to inactivation of pancreatic enzymes by excessive gastric acid.

- *Midgut neuroendocrine (carcinoid) tumors* arise in the jejunum and ileum, are often multiple and tend to be aggressive. In these tumors, depth of local invasion, size, and the presence of necrosis and mitoses are associated with poor outcome.

- *Hindgut neuroendocrine (carcinoid)* tumors arising in the appendix and colorectum are typically discovered incidentally. Those in the appendix occur at any age and are almost uniformly pursue a benign course. Rectal tumors tend to produce polypeptide hormones and may manifest with abdominal pain and weight loss. Because they are usually discovered when small, metastasis of rectal neuroendocrine tumors is uncommon.

Gastrointestinal Stromal Tumor

Gastrointestinal stromal tumor (GIST) is the most common mesenchymal tumor of the abdomen, and more than half of these tumors occur in the stomach. A wide variety of other mesenchymal neoplasms may arise in the stomach. Many are named according to the cell type they most resemble; for example, smooth muscle tumors are called *leiomyomas* or *leiomyosarcomas,* nerve sheath tumors are termed *schwannomas,* and those resembling glomus bodies in the nail beds and at other sites are termed *glomus tumors.* These tumors are all rare and are not discussed here.

Pathogenesis

The most common genetic change underlying the pathogenesis of GISTs is gain-of-function mutations of the gene encoding the tyrosine kinase KIT, the receptor for stem cell factor. These are present in 75% to 85% of all GISTs. An additional 8% of GISTs have mutations that activate a related tyrosine kinase, platelet-derived growth factor receptor A (PDGFRA). The term *stromal* reflects historical confusion about the origin of this tumor, which is now recognized to arise from the interstitial cells of Cajal, or pacemaker cells, of the gastrointestinal muscularis propria. For unknown reasons, GISTs bearing *PDGFRA* mutations are overrepresented in the stomach. *KIT* and *PDGFRA* gene mutations are mutually exclusive, reflecting their activities within the same signal transduction pathway. Germ line mutations in these same genes are present in rare familial GISTs, in which patients develop multiple GISTs and may also have diffuse hyperplasia of Cajal cells.

Both sporadic and germ line mutations result in constitutively active KIT or PDGFRA receptor tyrosine kinases and produce intracellular signals that promote tumor cell proliferation and survival (Chapter 6). In GISTs without *KIT* or *PDGFRA* mutations, genes encoding components of the mitochondrial succinate dehydrogenase (SDH) complex are most commonly affected. These mutations result in loss of SDH function and confer increased risk for both GIST and paraganglioma. One mutant allele is often inherited, with the second copy of the gene being either mutated or otherwise lost in the tumor. The loss of SDH causes a number of metabolic changes, including increased production of reactive oxygen species, activation of hypoxia induced factor (HIF), and increased dependency on glycolysis for ATP production, but how these alterations lead to transformation is uncertain.

MORPHOLOGY

Primary gastric GISTs usually form a solitary, well-circumscribed, fleshy, submucosal mass. Metastases may form multiple small serosal nodules or fewer large nodules in the liver; spread outside of the abdomen is uncommon. GISTs can be composed of thin, elongated **spindle cells** or plumper **epithelioid cells.** The most useful diagnostic marker is KIT, which is immunohistochemically detectable in 95% of these tumors.

Clinical Features

The peak incidence of gastric GIST is around 60 years of age, with less than 10% occurring in individuals younger than 40 years of age. Overall, GISTs are slightly more common in males. Small GISTs may come to clinical attention incidentally during work-up of other GI symptoms, which are common. Larger GISTs may present with symptoms related to mass effects or mucosal ulceration, such as intestinal obstruction or gastrointestinal bleeding. Complete surgical resection is the primary treatment for localized gastric GIST. The prognosis correlates with tumor size, mitotic index, and location, *with gastric GISTs being somewhat less aggressive than those arising in the small intestine.* Recurrence or metastasis is rare for gastric GISTs less than 5 cm in diameter but common for mitotically active tumors larger than 10 cm. Tumors that are unresectable or metastatic often respond, sometimes for years, to tyrosine kinase inhibitors that are active against KIT and PDGFRA, such as imatinib. Unfortunately, as in chronic myeloid leukemia (Chapter 12), resistance to imatinib eventually arises due to outgrowth of subclones with additional mutations in KIT or PDGFRA. In some instances, these tumors respond to other tyrosine kinase inhibitors that retain activity against KIT and PDGFRA.

SUMMARY

GASTRIC POLYPS AND TUMORS

- *Inflammatory and hyperplastic gastric polyps* are reactive lesions associated with chronic gastritis. Risk for development of dysplasia increases with polyp size.
- *Gastric adenomas* develop in a background of chronic gastritis and are particularly associated with intestinal metaplasia and mucosal (glandular) atrophy. Adenocarcinoma frequently arises in gastric adenomas, which therefore require complete excision and surveillance to detect recurrence.
- *Gastric adenocarcinomas* are classified according to location and gross and histologic morphology. Those with an intestinal histologic pattern tend to form bulky tumors and may be ulcerated, whereas those composed of mucus-filled signet ring cells typically display a diffuse infiltrative growth pattern that may thicken the gastric wall (linitis plastica) without forming a discrete mass.
- *H. pylori* infection is the most common etiologic agent for gastric adenocarcinoma, but other associations, including chronic atrophic gastritis and EBV infection, suggest several possible pathways of neoplastic transformation.
- *Primary gastric lymphomas* most often are derived from the mucosa-associated lymphoid tissue whose development is induced by chronic gastritis.
- Low- or intermediate-grade *neuroendocrine (carcinoid) tumors* arise from the diffuse components of the endocrine system and are most common in the gastrointestinal tract, particularly the small intestine. Tumors of the small intestine tend to be most aggressive, while those of the appendix are almost always benign.
- *Gastrointestinal stromal tumor (GIST)*, the most common mesenchymal tumor of the abdomen, occurs most often in the stomach. GISTs arise from benign pacemaker cells, also known as the *interstitial cells of Cajal.* A majority of tumors have activating mutations in either the c-KIT or the PDGFRA tyrosine kinases and respond to kinase inhibitors.

Small and Large Intestines

The small intestine and colon are the sites of a wide variety of diseases, many of which affect nutrient and water transport. Perturbation of these processes may cause malabsorption and diarrhea. The intestines are also the principal site where the immune system interfaces with a diverse array of antigens present in food and gut microbes. Recent advances have defined the composition and diversity of the gut microbiome, which is largely unculturable, using molecular approaches. One common trend is the association of reduced microbial diversity in disease. The gut microbiome is also exquisitely sensitive to diet, which may partly explain the association between food allergy and other diet-induced diseases and altered composition of the microbiome. Thus, it is not surprising that the small intestine and colon frequently are involved by infectious and inflammatory processes. The colon is the most common site of gastrointestinal neoplasia in Western populations.

INTESTINAL OBSTRUCTION

Obstruction of the gastrointestinal tract may occur at any level, but the small intestine is most often involved because of its relatively narrow lumen. Collectively, *hernias, intestinal adhesions, intussusception,* and *volvulus* account for 80% of mechanical obstructions (Fig. 15.18), while tumors and infarction account for most of the remainder. The clinical manifestations of intestinal obstruction include abdominal pain and distention, vomiting, and constipation. Surgical intervention is usually required in cases involving

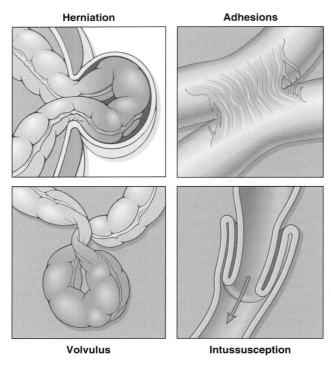

Fig. 15.18 Intestinal obstruction. The four major mechanical causes of intestinal obstruction are (1) herniation of a segment in the umbilical or inguinal regions, (2) adhesion between loops of intestine, (3) volvulus, and (4) intussusception.

mechanical obstruction or severe infarction. Volvulus and adhesions between bowel loops are well illustrated in Fig. 15.18. Brief comments are made next about the other causes of obstruction.

Intussusception

Intussusception occurs when a segment of the intestine, constricted by a wave of peristalsis, telescopes into the immediately distal segment. Once trapped, the invaginated segment is propelled by peristalsis and pulls the mesentery along. Untreated intussusception may progress to intestinal obstruction, compression of mesenteric vessels, and infarction. *Intussusception is the most common cause of intestinal obstruction in children younger than 2 years of age.* There usually is no underlying anatomic defect and the child is otherwise healthy. Other cases are associated with viral infection and rotavirus vaccines and may be related to reactive hyperplasia of Peyer patches, which can act as the leading edge of the intussusception. Contrast enemas are diagnostically useful and also are effective in correcting idiopathic intussusception in infants and young children. However, surgical intervention is necessary when an intraluminal mass or tumor serves as the initiating point of traction, as is typical in older children and in adults.

Hirschsprung Disease

Hirschsprung disease **occurs in approximately 1 of 5000 live births and stems from a congenital defect in colonic innervation.** It may be isolated or occur in combination with other developmental abnormalities. It is more common in males but tends to be more severe in females. Siblings are at increased risk for development of Hirschsprung disease.

Patients typically present as neonates with failure to pass meconium in the immediate postnatal period followed by obstructive constipation. The major threats to life are enterocolitis, fluid and electrolyte disturbances, perforation, and peritonitis. Surgical resection of the aganglionic segment with anastomosis of the normal colon to the rectum is effective, although it may take years for patients to attain normal bowel function and continence.

Pathogenesis

The enteric neuronal plexus develops from neural crest cells that migrate into the bowel wall during embryogenesis. Hirschsprung disease, also known as *congenital aganglionic megacolon,* results when the normal migration of neural crest cells from cecum to rectum is disrupted. This produces a distal intestinal segment that lacks both the Meissner submucosal plexus and the Auerbach myenteric plexus ("aganglionosis"), and thus fails to develop coordinated peristaltic contractions. **Mutations in the receptor tyrosine kinase RET account for a majority of familial cases** and approximately 15% of sporadic cases. Mutations in other genes, including disease-modifying genes, as well as environmental factors must also be involved.

MORPHOLOGY

Hirschsprung disease always affects the rectum, but the length of the additional involved segments varies. Most cases are limited to the rectum and sigmoid colon, but severe disease can involve the entire colon. The aganglionic region may have a grossly normal or contracted appearance, while the normally innervated proximal colon may undergo progressive dilation as a result of functional distal obstruction (Fig. 15.19). Diagnosis is made by demonstrating the absence of ganglion cells in the affected segment.

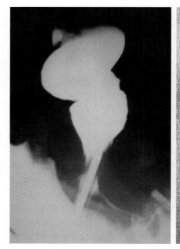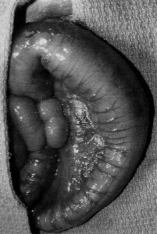

Fig. 15.19 Hirschsprung disease. (A) Preoperative barium enema study showing constricted rectum *(bottom)* and dilated sigmoid colon. Ganglion cells were absent in the rectum, but present in the sigmoid colon. (B) Corresponding intraoperative appearance of the dilated sigmoid colon. *(Courtesy of Dr. Aliya Husain, The University of Chicago, Chicago, Illinois.)*

Abdominal Hernia

Any weakness or defect in the wall of the peritoneal cavity may permit protrusion of a serosa-lined pouch of peritoneum called a *hernia sac.* Acquired hernias most commonly occur anteriorly, through the inguinal and femoral canals or umbilicus, or at sites of surgical scars. These are of concern because of visceral protrusion *(external herniation).* This is particularly true of inguinal hernias, which tend to have narrow orifices and large sacs. Small bowel loops herniate most often, but portions of omentum or large bowel also protrude, and any of these may become entrapped. Pressure at the neck of the pouch may impair venous drainage, leading to stasis and edema. These changes increase the bulk of the herniated loop, leading to permanent entrapment, or *incarceration,* and over time, arterial and venous compromise, or *strangulation,* can result in infarction.

SUMMARY

INTESTINAL OBSTRUCTION

- *Intussusception* is the most common cause of intestinal obstruction in children younger than 2 years of age and can usually be treated by barium enema or air enema.
- *Hirschsprung disease* is the result of defective neural crest cell migration from cecum to rectum. It gives rise to functional obstruction.
- *Abdominal herniation* may occur through any weakness or defect in the wall of the peritoneal cavity, including inguinal and femoral canals, umbilicus, and sites of surgical scarring.

VASCULAR DISORDERS OF BOWEL

The largest portion of the gastrointestinal tract is supplied by the celiac, superior mesenteric, and inferior mesenteric arteries. As they approach the intestinal wall, the superior and inferior mesenteric arteries fan out to form the mesenteric arcades. Interconnections between arcades, as well as collateral supplies from the proximal celiac and distal pudendal and iliac circulations make it possible for the small intestine and colon to tolerate slowly progressive loss of the blood supply from one artery. By contrast, acute compromise of any major vessel can lead to infarction of several meters of intestine.

Ischemic Bowel Disease

Ischemic damage to the bowel can range from mucosal infarction, extending no deeper than the muscularis mucosa; to mural infarction of mucosa and submucosa; to transmural infarction involving all three layers of the wall. While mucosal or mural infarctions often are secondary to acute or chronic hypoperfusion, transmural infarction is generally caused by acute vascular obstruction. Important causes of acute arterial obstruction include severe atherosclerosis (which is often prominent at the origin of mesenteric vessels), aortic aneurysm, hypercoagulable states, oral contraceptive use, and embolization of

cardiac vegetations or aortic atheromas. Intestinal hypoperfusion can also be associated with cardiac failure, shock, dehydration, or vasoconstrictive drugs. Systemic vasculitides also may damage intestinal arteries. While mesenteric venous thrombosis can lead to ischemic disease, it is uncommon. Other causes include invasive neoplasms, cirrhosis, portal hypertension, trauma, or abdominal masses that compress the portal drainage.

Pathogenesis

The severity of vascular compromise, time frame during which it develops, and vessels affected are the major variables that determine severity of ischemic bowel disease. Intestinal responses to ischemia occur in two phases. The initial hypoxic injury occurs at the onset of vascular compromise and, although some damage occurs, intestinal epithelial cells are relatively resistant to transient hypoxia. The second phase, reperfusion injury, is initiated by restoration of the blood supply and associated with the greatest damage. While the underlying mechanisms of reperfusion injury are incompletely understood, they involve free radical production, neutrophil infiltration, and inflammatory mediators such as complement and cytokines. Two aspects of intestinal vascular anatomy also contribute to the distribution of ischemic damage:

- *Watershed zones* refers to intestinal segments at the end of their respective arterial supplies that are particularly susceptible to ischemia. These zones include the splenic flexure, where the superior and inferior mesenteric arterial circulations terminate, and, to a lesser extent, the sigmoid colon and rectum where inferior mesenteric, pudendal, and iliac arterial circulations end. Generalized hypotension or hypoxemia can therefore cause localized injury at these sites, and ischemic disease should be considered in the differential diagnosis for focal colitis of the splenic flexure or rectosigmoid colon.
- *Patterns of intestinal microvessls.* Intestinal capillaries run alongside the glands, from crypt to surface, before making a hairpin turn at the surface to empty into the postcapillary venules. This configuration leaves the surface epithelium particularly vulnerable to ischemic injury. Thus, surface epithelial atrophy, or even necrosis and epithelial sloughing, with normal or hyperproliferative crypts constitutes a morphologic signature of ischemic intestinal disease.

MORPHOLOGY

Despite the increased susceptibility of watershed zones, **mucosal and mural infarction** may involve any level of the gut from stomach to anus. Involvement is frequently segmental and patchy, and the mucosa is hemorrhagic and often ulcerated. The bowel wall is thickened by edema that may involve the mucosa or extend into the submucosa and muscularis propria. With severe disease, pathologic changes include extensive mucosal and submucosal hemorrhage and necrosis, but serosal hemorrhage and serositis generally are absent. Damage is more pronounced in acute arterial thrombosis and **transmural infarction.** Blood-tinged mucus or blood accumulates within the lumen.

Coagulative necrosis of the muscularis propria occurs within 1 to 4 days and may be associated with purulent serositis and perforation.

Microscopic examination of ischemic intestine demonstrates **atrophy or sloughing of surface epithelium** (Fig. 15.20A). By contrast, crypts may be hyperproliferative. Inflammatory infiltrates are initially absent in acute ischemia, but neutrophils are recruited within hours of reperfusion. Chronic ischemia is accompanied by fibrous scarring of the lamina propria (Fig. 15.20B) and, uncommonly, stricture formation. In acute phases of ischemic damage, bacterial superinfection and enterotoxin release may induce pseudomembrane formation that can resemble *Clostridium difficile*–associated pseudomembranous colitis (discussed later).

Clinical Features

Ischemic bowel disease tends to occur in older adults with coexisting cardiac or vascular disease. Acute transmural infarction typically manifests with sudden, severe abdominal pain and tenderness, sometimes accompanied by nausea, vomiting, bloody diarrhea, or grossly melanotic stool. This presentation may progress to shock and vascular collapse within hours as a result of blood loss. Peristaltic sounds diminish or disappear, and muscular spasm creates boardlike rigidity of the abdominal wall. Because these physical signs overlap with those of other abdominal emergencies, including acute appendicitis, perforated ulcer, and acute cholecystitis, the diagnosis of intestinal infarction may be delayed or missed, with disastrous consequences. As the mucosal barrier breaks down, bacteria enter the circulation and sepsis can develop; the mortality rate in these cases may exceed 50%.

The overall progression of ischemic enteritis depends on the underlying cause and severity of injury:

- *Mucosal and mural infarctions* by themselves may not be fatal. However, these may progress to more extensive, transmural infarction if the vascular supply is not restored by correction of the insult or, in chronic disease, by development of adequate collateral supplies.
- *Chronic ischemia* may masquerade as inflammatory bowel disease, with episodes of bloody diarrhea interspersed with periods of healing.

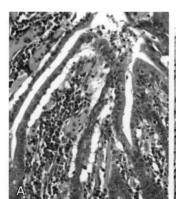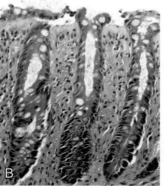

Fig. 15.20 Ischemia. (A) Characteristic attenuated and partially detached villous epithelium in acute jejunal ischemia. Note the hyperchromatic nuclei of proliferating crypt cells. (B) Chronic colonic ischemia with atrophic surface epithelium and fibrotic lamina propria.

- *Cytomegalovirus (CMV) infection* causes ischemic gastrointestinal disease as a consequence of the viral tropism for and infection of endothelial cells. CMV infection can be a complication of immunosuppressive therapy (Chapter 9).
- *Radiation enterocolitis* occurs when the gastrointestinal tract is irradiated. In addition to epithelial damage, radiation-induced vascular injury may be significant and produce changes that are similar to ischemic disease.
- *Necrotizing enterocolitis* is an idiopathic disorder of the small and large intestines that can result in transmural necrosis. It is the most common acquired gastrointestinal emergency of neonates, particularly those who are premature or of low birth weight. Its occurrence is often associated with initiation of oral feeding (Chapter 7). Although pathogenesis of necrotizing enterocolitis is not defined, ischemic injury is thought to contribute.
- *Angiodysplasia,* characterized by malformed submucosal and mucosal blood vessels, occurs most often in the cecum or right colon, and usually presents after the sixth decade of life. Although it affects less than 1% of the adult population, *angiodysplasia accounts for 20% of major episodes of lower intestinal bleeding.*

Hemorrhoids

Hemorrhoids are dilated anal and perianal collateral vessels that connect the portal and caval venous systems to relieve elevated venous pressure within the hemorrhoid plexus. Thus, although hemorrhoids are less serious than esophageal varices, the pathogenesis of these lesions is similar. They are common, affecting about 5% of the general population. Common predisposing factors include constipation and associated straining, which increase intraabdominal and venous pressures, venous stasis of pregnancy, and portal hypertension.

Collateral vessels within the inferior hemorrhoidal plexus are located below the anorectal line and are termed **external hemorrhoids,** while those that result from dilation of the superior hemorrhoidal plexus within the distal rectum are referred to as **internal hemorrhoids.** On histologic examination, hemorrhoids consist of thin-walled, dilated, submucosal vessels beneath anal or rectal mucosa. These vessels are subject to trauma, which leads to rectal bleeding. In addition, they can become thrombosed and inflamed.

Hemorrhoids often manifest with pain and rectal bleeding, particularly bright red blood seen on toilet tissue. Hemorrhoids also may develop as a result of portal hypertension, where the implications are more ominous. Hemorrhoidal bleeding generally is not a medical emergency; treatment options include sclerotherapy, rubber band ligation, and infrared coagulation. In severe cases, hemorrhoids may be removed surgically by *hemorrhoidectomy.*

SUMMARY

VASCULAR DISORDERS OF BOWEL

- Intestinal ischemia can occur as a result of either *arterial or venous obstruction.*
- Ischemic bowel disease resulting from hypoperfusion is most common at the splenic flexure, sigmoid colon, and rectum;

these are *watershed zones* where two arterial circulations terminate.

- Systemic vasculitides and infectious diseases (e.g., CMV infection) can cause vascular disease that is not confined to the gastrointestinal tract.
- Angiodysplasia is a common cause of lower gastrointestinal bleeding in older adults.
- Hemorrhoids are collateral vessels that form in response to venous hypertension.

DIARRHEAL DISEASE

Diarrhea is defined as an increase in stool mass, frequency, or fluidity, typically to amounts greater than 200 grams per day. In severe cases, stool volume can exceed 14 L per day and, without fluid resuscitation, result in death. Worldwide, diarrheal diseases account for greater than 700,000 deaths of children under 5 years of age, making them the second leading cause of death in this age group. Painful, bloody, small-volume diarrhea is known as *dysentery.* Diarrhea is a common symptom of many intestinal diseases, including those due to infection, inflammation, ischemia, malabsorption, and nutritional deficiency. It can be classified into four major categories:

- *Secretory diarrhea* is characterized by isotonic stool and persists during fasting.
- *Osmotic diarrhea,* such as that occurring with lactase deficiency, is due to osmotic forces exerted by unabsorbed luminal solutes. The diarrheal fluid is at least 50 mOsm more concentrated than plasma, and the condition abates with fasting.
- *Malabsorptive diarrhea* caused by inadequate nutrient absorption is associated with steatorrhea and is relieved by fasting.
- *Exudative diarrhea* is due to inflammatory disease and characterized by purulent, bloody stools that continue during fasting.

We begin our discussion with malabsorptive diarrhea. Other disorders associated with secretory and exudative types of diarrhea (e.g., cholera and inflammatory bowel disease, respectively) are addressed in separate sections.

Malabsorptive Diarrhea

Malabsorption manifests most commonly as *chronic diarrhea* and is characterized by defective absorption of fats, fat- and water-soluble vitamins, proteins, carbohydrates, electrolytes, minerals, and water. Chronic malabsorption causes weight loss, anorexia, abdominal distention, borborygmi, and muscle wasting. A hallmark of malabsorption is *steatorrhea,* characterized by excessive fecal fat and bulky, frothy, greasy, yellow, or clay-colored stools. *The chronic malabsorptive disorders most commonly encountered in Western countries are pancreatic insufficiency, celiac disease, and Crohn disease.* Environmental enteric dysfunction, or environmental enteropathy, which has a malabsorptive component, is pervasive in some communities within developing countries.

Malabsorption results from disturbance in at least one of the four phases of nutrient absorption:

- *Intraluminal digestion,* in which proteins, carbohydrates, and fats are broken down into absorbable forms
- *Terminal digestion,* which involves the hydrolysis of carbohydrates and peptides by disaccharidases and peptidases, respectively, in the brush border of the small-intestinal mucosa
- *Transepithelial transport,* in which nutrients, fluid, and electrolytes are transported across and processed within the small-intestinal epithelium
- *Lymphatic transport* of absorbed lipids

In many malabsorptive disorders, a defect in one of these processes predominates, but more than one usually contributes (Table 15.3). As a result, malabsorption syndromes resemble each other more than they differ. Signs and symptoms include diarrhea (from nutrient

Table 15.3 Defects in Malabsorptive and Diarrheal Disease

Disease	Intraluminal Digestion	Terminal Digestion	Transepithelial Transport	Lymphatic Transport
Celiac disease		+	+	
Tropical sprue		+	+	
Chronic pancreatitis	+			
Cystic fibrosis	+			
Primary bile acid malabsorption	+		+	
Carcinoid syndrome			+	
Autoimmune enteropathy		+	+	
Disaccharidase deficiency		+		
Mycobacterial infection, Whipple disease				+
Abetalipoproteinemia			+	
Viral gastroenteritis		+	+	
Bacterial gastroenteritis		+	+	
Parasitic gastroenteritis		+	+	
Inflammatory bowel disease	+	+	+	

+, Indicates that the process can be abnormal in the disease indicated. Other processes are not typically affected.

malabsorption and excessive intestinal secretion), flatus, abdominal pain, and weight loss. Inadequate absorption of vitamins and minerals can result in anemia and mucositis due to pyridoxine, folate, or vitamin B_{12} deficiency; bleeding due to vitamin K deficiency; osteopenia and tetany due to calcium, magnesium, or vitamin D deficiency; or neuropathy due to vitamin A or B_{12} deficiency. A variety of endocrine and skin disturbances may also occur. Mycobacterial infection, which can be lead to lymphatic transport defects, is discussed with infectious causes of diarrhea in the next section.

Cystic Fibrosis

Cystic fibrosis is discussed in greater detail elsewhere (Chapter 7). Only the malabsorption associated with cystic fibrosis is considered here. Owing to mutations of the epithelial cystic fibrosis transmembrane conductance regulator *(CFTR)*, individuals with cystic fibrosis have defects in intestinal and pancreatic ductal ion transport. This abnormality interferes with bicarbonate, sodium, and water secretion, ultimately resulting in inadequate luminal hydration. The viscous luminal contents may result in meconium ileus, which is present in up to 10% of newborns with cystic fibrosis. In the pancreas the ducts are plugged by thick mucus. This leads to obstruction, low-grade chronic autodigestion of the pancreas, and eventual *exocrine pancreatic insufficiency in more than 80% of patients.* The result is failure of the intraluminal phase of nutrient absorption, which can be effectively treated in most patients with oral enzyme supplementation.

Celiac Disease

Celiac disease, **also known as** *celiac sprue* **or** *gluten-sensitive enteropathy,* **is an immune-mediated enteropathy triggered by the ingestion of gluten-containing cereals, such as wheat, rye, or barley, in genetically predisposed individuals.** In countries whose populations consist predominantly of whites of European ancestry, celiac disease is a common disorder, with an estimated prevalence of 0.5% to 1%. The primary treatment for celiac disease is a *gluten-free diet*, which results in symptomatic improvement for most patients.

Pathogenesis

Celiac disease is an intestinal immune reaction to gluten, the major storage protein of wheat and similar grains. Gluten is digested by luminal and brush border enzymes into amino acids and peptides, including a 33–amino acid gliadin peptide that is resistant to degradation by gastric, pancreatic, and small-intestinal proteases (Fig. 15.21). Gliadin is deamidated by tissue transglutaminase and is then able to interact with HLA-DQ2 or HLA-DQ8 on antigen-presenting cells and be presented to CD4+ T cells. These T cells in lamina propria produce cytokines that likely contribute to the tissue damage and characteristic mucosal histopathology. An antibody response follows: This includes production of antibodies against tissue transglutaminase, deamidated gliadin, and, perhaps as a result of cross-reactive epitopes, anti-endomysial antibodies, which can be diagnostically useful. They may also be used to monitor disease, as titers typically fall after 3 to 6 months of gluten-free diet. However, whether these antibodies contribute to celiac disease pathogenesis or are merely markers of immune activation remains controversial. In addition to CD4+ cells, there is an accumulation of CD8+ cells that are not specific for gliadin but may play an ancillary role in causing tissue damage. It is thought that deamidated gliadin peptides induce epithelial cells to produce the cytokine IL-15, which in turn triggers activation and proliferation of CD8+ intraepithelial lymphocytes that become cytotoxic and kill

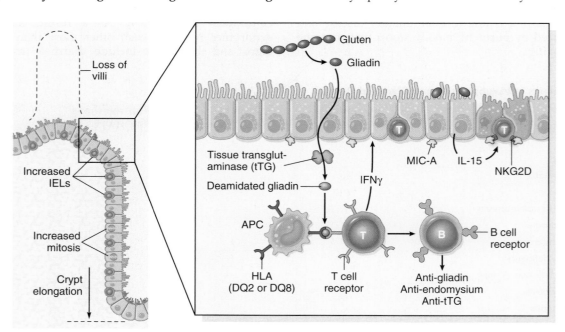

Fig. 15.21 The morphologic alterations that may be present in celiac disease, including varying degrees of villous atrophy, increased numbers of intraepithelial lymphocytes (IELs), and epithelial proliferation with crypt elongation *(left)*. A model for the pathogenesis of celiac disease *(right)*. Note that both innate and adaptive immune mechanisms are involved in the tissue responses to gliadin. CD4 T cells (producing IFNγ) are shown in lamina propria and CD8 T cells, expressing NKG2D receptor, in between epithelial cells.

enterocytes that have been induced by various stressors to express surface MIC-A. This molecule is recognized by the NKG2D receptor on activated CD8+ T cells. The damage caused by these immune mechanisms may increase the movement of gliadin peptides across the epithelium, which are then deamidated by tissue transglutaminase, thus perpetuating the cycle of disease.

While nearly all individuals eat grain and are exposed to gluten and gliadin, most do not develop celiac disease. Thus, host factors determine whether disease develops. Among these, HLA proteins seem to be critical, since almost all individuals with celiac disease carry the class II HLA-DQ2 or HLA-DQ8 alleles. There is also an association of celiac disease with other immune diseases including type 1 diabetes, thyroiditis, and Sjögren syndrome.

MORPHOLOGY

Biopsy specimens from the second portion of the duodenum or proximal jejunum, which are exposed to the highest concentrations of dietary gluten, are generally diagnostic in celiac disease. The histopathology is characterized by increased numbers of T lymphocytes, with **intraepithelial lymphocytosis, crypt hyperplasia**, and **villous atrophy** (Fig. 15.22). This loss of mucosal and brush-border surface area due to villous atrophy probably accounts for the malabsorption. In addition, increased rates of epithelial turnover, reflected in increased crypt mitotic activity, may limit the ability of absorptive enterocytes to fully differentiate and express proteins necessary for terminal digestion and transepithelial transport. Other histologic features of celiac disease can include increased numbers of plasma cells, mast cells, and eosinophils, especially within the upper part of the lamina propria. It should be noted that intraepithelial lymphocytosis and villous atrophy can be present in other disorders, including viral enteritis. The combination of histologic and serologic findings is, therefore, most specific for diagnosis of celiac disease.

Clinical Features

Pediatric celiac disease, which affects male and female children equally, may manifest with *classic symptoms,* typically between 6 and 24 months of age (after introduction of gluten to the diet) with irritability, abdominal distention, anorexia, diarrhea, failure to thrive, weight loss, or muscle wasting. Children with *nonclassic symptoms* tend to present at older ages with complaints of abdominal pain, nausea, vomiting, bloating, or constipation. A characteristic pruritic, blistering skin lesion, *dermatitis herpetiformis,* is also present in as many as 10% of patients, and the incidence of *lymphocytic gastritis* and *lymphocytic colitis* is increased as well.

In adults, celiac disease manifests most commonly between 30 and 60 years of age. However, many cases escape clinical attention for extended periods because of atypical presentations. Some patients have silent celiac disease, defined as positive serology and villous atrophy without symptoms, or latent celiac disease, in which positive serology is accompanied neither by villous atrophy nor symptoms. Symptomatic adult celiac disease is often associated with anemia (due to iron deficiency and, less commonly, B$_{12}$ and folate deficiency), diarrhea, bloating, and fatigue.

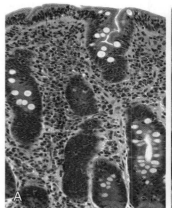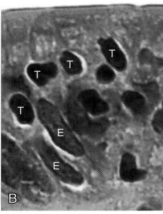

Fig. 15.22 Celiac disease. (A) Advanced cases of celiac disease show complete loss of villi, or total villous atrophy. Note the dense plasma cell infiltrates in the lamina propria. (B) Infiltration of the surface epithelium by T lymphocytes, which can be recognized by their densely stained nuclei (labeled *T*). Compare with elongated, pale-staining epithelial nuclei (labeled *E*).

Noninvasive serologic tests are generally performed before biopsy. The most sensitive tests are the presence of IgA antibodies to tissue transglutaminase or IgA or IgG antibodies to deamidated gliadin. Anti-endomysial antibodies are highly specific but less sensitive than other antibodies.

Patients with celiac disease exhibit a higher than normal rate of malignancy. The most common celiac disease–associated cancer is *enteropathy-associated T cell lymphoma,* an aggressive tumor of intraepithelial T lymphocytes. *Small-intestinal adenocarcinoma* also is more frequent in individuals with celiac disease. Thus, when symptoms such as abdominal pain, diarrhea, and weight loss develop despite a strict gluten-free diet, cancer or *refractory sprue,* in which the response to a gluten-free diet is lost, must be considered. It is, however, important to recognize that failure to adhere to a gluten-free diet is the most common cause of recurrent symptoms, and that most individuals with celiac disease do well with dietary restrictions and die of unrelated causes.

Environmental Enteric Dysfunction

The term *environmental enteric dysfunction, or environmental enteropathy,* **refers to a syndrome of stunted growth and impaired intestinal function that is common in developing countries,** including many parts of sub-Saharan Africa, such as Zambia; aboriginal populations within northern Australia; and some groups within South America and Asia, such as residents of impoverished communities within Brazil, Guatemala, India, and Pakistan. The impact of environmental enteric dysfunction, which was previously grouped under headings of *tropical enteropathy* or *tropical sprue,* cannot be overstated, as it is estimated to affect over 150 million children worldwide. Although malnutrition most likely contributes to the pathogenesis of this disorder, neither supplementary feeding nor vitamin and mineral supplementation are able to fully reverse the syndrome. Repeated bouts of diarrhea suffered within the first 2 or 3 years of life are most closely linked to environmental enteropathy, but no single infectious agent has been established as causal in these diarrheal episodes. Intestinal biopsy specimens have been examined in only a small number of cases, and the reported histopathology has some overlap with severe celiac disease as well as infectious enteritis.

Lactase (Disaccharidase) Deficiency

Lactase deficiency gives rise to osmotic diarrhea because, in its absence, osmotically active lactose remains in the lumen. The disaccharidases, including lactase, are located in the apical brush border membrane of villous absorptive epithelial cells. Because the defect is biochemical, biopsies are generally unremarkable. Lactase deficiency is of two types:

- *Congenital lactase deficiency* is an autosomal recessive disorder caused by mutations in the gene encoding lactase. The disease is rare and manifests as explosive diarrhea with watery, frothy stools and abdominal distention after milk ingestion. Symptoms abate when exposure to milk and milk products is terminated.
- *Acquired lactase deficiency* is caused by downregulation of lactase gene expression and is particularly common among Native Americans, African Americans, and Chinese populations. Downregulation of lactase occurs in the gut after childhood, perhaps reflecting the fact that, before farming of dairy animals, lactase was unnecessary after children stopped drinking mother's milk. Onset of acquired lactase deficiency is sometimes associated with enteric viral or bacterial infections.

Abetalipoproteinemia

Abetalipoproteinemia is an autosomal recessive disease characterized by an inability to secrete triglyceride-rich lipoproteins. Although rare, it is an example of a transepithelial transport defect leading to malabsorption. Mutation in the *microsomal triglyceride transfer protein* renders enterocytes unable to export lipoproteins and free fatty acids. As a result, monoglycerides and triglycerides accumulate within the epithelial cells. Abetalipoproteinemia manifests in infancy, and the clinical picture is dominated by failure to thrive, diarrhea, and steatorrhea. Failure to absorb essential fatty acids leads to deficiencies of fat-soluble vitamins, and lipid defects in plasma membranes often produce acanthocytic red blood cells (spur cells) in peripheral blood smears.

Microscopic Colitis

Microscopic colitis encompasses two entities, *collagenous colitis* and *lymphocytic colitis*. Both of these idiopathic diseases manifest with chronic, nonbloody, watery diarrhea without weight loss. Findings on radiologic and endoscopic studies typically are normal. Collagenous colitis, which occurs primarily in middle-aged and older women, is characterized by the presence of a dense subepithelial collagen layer, increased numbers of intraepithelial lymphocytes, and a mixed inflammatory infiltrate within the lamina propria. Lymphocytic colitis is histologically similar, but the subepithelial collagen layer is of normal thickness and the increase in intraepithelial, predominantly T lymphocytes, may be greater. Lymphocytic colitis is associated with celiac disease and autoimmune diseases, including thyroiditis, arthritis, and autoimmune or lymphocytic gastritis.

Graft-Versus-Host Disease

Graft-versus-host disease occurs after allogeneic hematopoietic stem cell transplantation. The small bowel and colon are involved in most cases. Although graft-versus-host disease is caused by donor T cell–mediated damage to the recipient's epithelial cells, the lymphocytic infiltrate in the lamina propria is typically sparse, suggesting that cytokines secreted by T cells may be the major mediators of tissue injury. Epithelial apoptosis, particularly of crypt cells, is the most common histologic finding. Intestinal graft-versus-host disease often manifests as watery diarrhea.

SUMMARY

MALABSORPTIVE DIARRHEA

- Diarrhea can be characterized as *secretory, osmotic, malabsorptive,* or *exudative.*
- The malabsorption associated with cystic fibrosis is the result of *pancreatic insufficiency* (i.e., inadequate pancreatic digestive enzymes) and *deficient luminal breakdown* of nutrients.
- *Celiac disease* is an immune-mediated enteropathy triggered by the ingestion of gluten-containing grains. The malabsorptive diarrhea in celiac disease is due to *loss of brush border surface area* and, possibly, deficient enterocyte maturation.
- *Lactase deficiency* causes an *osmotic diarrhea* owing to the inability to break down or absorb lactose.
- *Abetalipoproteinemia* is characterized by an inability to secrete triglyceride-rich lipoproteins due to an inherited transepithelial transport defect.
- The two forms of microscopic colitis, *collagenous colitis* and *lymphocytic colitis*, both cause chronic watery diarrhea. The intestines are grossly normal, and the diseases are identified by their histologic features.

Infectious Enterocolitis

This global problem is responsible for more than 1 million deaths annually and greater than 10% of all deaths in patients younger than 5 years of age worldwide. Enterocolitis presents with a broad range of signs and symptoms, including diarrhea, abdominal pain, urgency, perianal discomfort, incontinence, and hemorrhage. Bacterial infections, such as enterotoxigenic *Escherichia coli,* are frequently responsible, but the most common pathogens vary with age, nutrition, and host immune status, as well as environment (Table 15.4). For example, epidemics of cholera are common in areas with poor sanitation, as a result of inadequate public health measures, or as a consequence of natural disaster (e.g., the Haitian earthquake of 2010) or war. Pediatric infectious diarrhea, which may result in severe dehydration and metabolic acidosis, is commonly caused by enteric viruses. A summary of the epidemiology and clinical features of selected causes of bacterial enterocolitis is presented in Table 15.4. Representative bacterial, viral, and parasitic enterocolitides are discussed next.

Cholera

Vibrio cholerae organisms are comma-shaped, gram-negative bacteria that cause cholera, a disease that has

Table 15.4 Features of Bacterial Enterocolitides

Infection Type	Geography	Reservoir	Transmission	Epidemiology	Affected GI Sites	Symptoms	Complications
Cholera	India, Africa	Shellfish	Fecal-oral, water	Sporadic, endemic, epidemic	Small intestine	Severe watery diarrhea	Dehydration, electrolyte imbalances
Campylobacter spp.	Developed countries	Chickens, sheep, pigs, cattle	Poultry, milk, other foods	Sporadic; children, travelers	Colon	Watery or bloody diarrhea	Arthritis, Guillain-Barré syndrome
Shigellosis	Worldwide, endemic in developing countries	Humans	Fecal-oral, food, water	Children, migrant workers, travelers, nursing homes	Left colon, ileum	Bloody diarrhea	Reactive arthritis, urethritis, conjunctivitis, hemolytic-uremic syndrome
Salmonellosis	Worldwide	Poultry, farm animals, reptiles	Meat, poultry, eggs, milk	Children, older adults	Colon, small intestine	Watery or bloody diarrhea	Sepsis, abscess
Enteric (typhoid) fever	India, Mexico, Philippines	Humans	Fecal-oral, water	Children. adolescents, travelers	Small intestine	Bloody diarrhea, fever	Chronic infection, carrier state, encephalopathy, myocarditis, intestinal perforation
Yersinia spp.	Northern and central Europe	Pigs, cows, puppies, cats	Pork, milk, water	Clustered cases	Ileum, appendix, right colon	Abdominal pain, fever, diarrhea	Reactive arthritis, erythema nodosum
Escherichia coli							
Enterotoxigenic (ETEC)	Developing countries	Unknown	Food or fecal-oral	Infants, adolescents, travelers	Small intestine	Severe watery diarrhea	Dehydration, electrolyte imbalances
Enteropathogenic (EPEC)	Worldwide	Humans	Fecal-oral	Infants	Small intestine	Watery diarrhea	Dehydration, electrolyte imbalances
Enterohemorrhagic (EHEC)	Worldwide	Widespread, includes cattle	Beef, milk, produce	Sporadic and epidemic	Colon	Bloody diarrhea	Hemolytic-uremic syndrome
Enteroinvasive (EIEC)	Developing countries	Unknown	Cheese, other foods, water	Young children	Colon	Bloody diarrhea	Unknown
Enteroaggregative (EAEC)	Worldwide	Unknown	Unknown	Children, adults, travelers	Colon	Nonbloody diarrhea, afebrile	Poorly defined
Pseudomembranous colitis (*C. difficile*)	Worldwide	Humans, hospitals	Antibiotics allow emergence	Immunosuppressed, antibiotic-treated	Colon	Watery diarrhea, fever	Relapse, toxic megacolon
Whipple disease	Rural > urban	Unknown	Unknown	Rare	Small intestine	Malabsorption	Arthritis, CNS disease
Mycobacterial infection	Worldwide	Unknown	Unknown	Immunosuppressed, endemic	Small intestine	Malabsorption	Pneumonia, infection at other sites

CNS, Central nervous system; GI, gastrointestinal.

been endemic in the Ganges Valley of India and Bangladesh for all of recorded history. *V. cholerae* is transmitted primarily by contaminated drinking water. However, it can also be present in food and causes rare cases of seafood-associated disease. There is a marked seasonal variation in most locales due to rapid growth of *Vibrio* bacteria at warm temperatures. The only animal reservoirs are shellfish and plankton.

Pathogenesis

***Vibrio* organisms are noninvasive but cause disease by producing a toxin that interferes with the absorptive function of enterocytes.** Flagellar proteins, which are involved in motility and attachment, are necessary for efficient bacterial colonization, and a secreted metalloproteinase that also has hemagglutinin activity is important for bacterial detachment and shedding in the stool. However, it is the *preformed enterotoxin,* cholera toxin, which causes disease. The toxin, which is composed of five B subunits that direct endocytosis and a single active A subunit, is delivered to the endoplasmic reticulum by *retrograde transport.* A fragment of the A subunit is transported from the endoplasmic reticulum lumen into the cytosol, where it interacts with cytosolic ADP ribosylation factors to ribosylate and activate the G protein $G_{s\alpha}$. This stimulates adenylate cyclase, and the resulting increases in intracellular cyclic adenosine monophosphate (cAMP) open the cystic fibrosis transmembrane conductance regulator (CFTR), which releases chloride ions into the lumen. This creates an osmotic gradient that draws water into the lumen, leading to massive *secretory diarrhea.* Remarkably, mucosal biopsy specimens show only minimal morphologic alterations.

Clinical Features

Most exposed individuals are asymptomatic or suffer only mild diarrhea. Those with severe disease have an abrupt onset of watery diarrhea and vomiting after an incubation period of 1 to 5 days. The volume of diarrhea may reach 1 L per hour, leading to dehydration, hypotension, electrolyte imbalances, muscular cramping, anuria, shock, loss of consciousness, and death. Most deaths occur within the first 24 hours of presentation. Although the mortality rate for severe cholera is 50% to 70% without treatment, fluid replacement can save more than 99% of patients.

Campylobacter Enterocolitis

***Campylobacter jejuni* is the most common bacterial enteric pathogen in developed countries and is an important cause of traveler's diarrhea.** Most infections are associated with ingestion of improperly cooked chicken, but outbreaks also can be caused by unpasteurized milk or contaminated water.

Pathogenesis

The pathogenesis of *Campylobacter* infection remains poorly defined, but four major virulence properties contribute: motility, adherence, toxin production, and invasion. Flagella allow *Campylobacter* to be motile. This facilitates adherence and colonization, which are also necessary for mucosal invasion. Cytotoxins that cause epithelial damage and a cholera toxin–like enterotoxin are also released by

some *C. jejuni* isolates. *Dysentery* or bloody diarrhea, is generally associated with invasion and only occurs with a small minority of *Campylobacter* strains. *Enteric fever* occurs when bacteria proliferate within the lamina propria and mesenteric lymph nodes.

Campylobacter infection can result in reactive arthritis, primarily in patients with HLA-B27. Other extraintestinal complications, including erythema nodosum and Guillain-Barré syndrome (Chapter 22), a flaccid paralysis caused by autoimmune-induced inflammation of peripheral nerves, are not HLA-linked. Fortunately, Guillain-Barré syndrome develops in 0.1% or less of individuals infected with *Campylobacter*.

⬤ MORPHOLOGY

Campylobacter, Shigella, Salmonella, and many other bacterial infections, including ***Yersinia*** and ***E. coli,*** all induce a similar microscopic picture, termed ***acute self-limited colitis.*** Specific diagnosis is primarily by stool culture. The histology of acute self-limited colitis includes prominent lamina propria and intraepithelial neutrophil infiltrates (Fig. 15.23A); **cryptitis** (neutrophil infiltration of the crypts) and **crypt abscesses** (crypts with accumulations of luminal neutrophils) also may be present. The preservation of crypt architecture in most cases of acute self-limited colitis is helpful in distinguishing these infections from chronic inflammatory illnesses such as inflammatory bowel disease (Fig. 15.23B).

Clinical Features

Ingestion of as few as 500 *C. jejuni* organisms can cause disease after an incubation period of up to 8 days. Watery diarrhea, either acute or with onset after an influenza like prodrome, is the primary manifestation, and dysentery develops in 15% to 50% of patients. Patients may shed

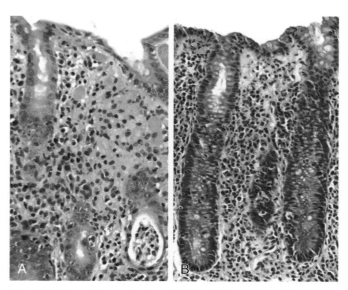

Fig. 15.23 Bacterial enterocolitis. (A) *Campylobacter jejuni* infection produces acute, self-limited colitis. Neutrophils can be seen within surface and crypt epithelium, and a crypt abscess is present *(lower right).* (B) Enteroinvasive *Escherichia coli* infection is similar to other acute, self-limited colitides. Note the maintenance of normal crypt architecture and spacing, despite abundant intraepithelial neutrophils.

bacteria for 1 month or more after clinical resolution. The disease is self-limited, and antibiotic therapy generally is not required.

Shigellosis

Shigella are gram-negative bacilli that are unencapsulated, nonmotile, facultative anaerobes responsible for one of the most common causes of bloody diarrhea. Shigellae are highly transmissible by the fecal-oral route or through ingestion of contaminated water and food; the *infective dose is fewer than 100 organisms,* and each gram of stool contains as many as 10^9 organisms during acute phases of the disease.

In the United States and Europe, children in day care centers, migrant workers, travelers to developing countries, and residents of nursing homes are most commonly affected. Most *Shigella*-associated infections and deaths occur in children younger than 5 years of age; in countries in which *Shigella* is endemic, it is responsible for approximately 10% of all cases of pediatric diarrheal disease and as many as 75% of diarrheal deaths.

Pathogenesis

Shigella organisms are resistant to the harsh acidic environment of the stomach, which partially explains the very low infective dose. Once in the intestine, organisms are taken up by M (microfold) epithelial cells, which are specialized for sampling and uptake of luminal antigens. After intracellular proliferation, the bacteria escape into the lamina propria. These bacteria then infect small-intestinal and colonic epithelial cells through the basolateral membranes, which express bacterial receptors. Alternatively, luminal shigellae can directly modulate epithelial tight junctions to expose basolateral bacterial receptors. The latter is partly mediated by virulence proteins, some of which are directly injected into the host cytoplasm by a type III secretion system. Some *Shigella dysenteriae* serotypes also release the Shiga toxin Stx, which inhibits eukaryotic protein synthesis and causes host cell death.

MORPHOLOGY

Shigella infections are most prominent in the left colon, but the ileum may also be involved, perhaps reflecting the abundance of M cells in the epithelium overlying Peyer patches. The histologic appearance in early cases is similar to that in other acute self-limited colitides. In more severe cases, the mucosa is hemorrhagic and ulcerated, and pseudomembranes may be present. Perhaps because of the tropism for M cells, aphthous-appearing ulcers similar to those seen in Crohn disease also may occur. The potential for confusion with chronic inflammatory bowel disease is substantial, particularly if there is distortion of crypt architecture.

Clinical Features

Shigella causes self-limited disease characterized by about 6 days of diarrhea, fever, and abdominal pain. After an incubation period of 1 to 7 days, the initial watery diarrhea progresses to a dysenteric phase in approximately 50% of patients, and constitutional symptoms can persist for as long as 1 month. A subacute presentation also can develop in a minority of adults. Antibiotic treatment shortens the clinical course and reduces the duration over which organisms are shed in the stool, but anti-diarrheal medications are contraindicated because they can prolong symptoms by delaying bacterial clearance.

Complications of *Shigella* infection are uncommon and include *reactive arthritis,* a triad of sterile arthritis, urethritis, and conjunctivitis that preferentially affects HLA-B27–positive men between 20 and 40 years of age. Hemolytic uremic syndrome, which typically is associated with *enterohemorrhagic Escherichia coli (EHEC),* also may occur after infection with shigellae that secrete Shiga toxin.

Escherichia coli

Escherichia coli are gram-negative bacilli that colonize the healthy gastrointestinal tract; most are nonpathogenic, but a subset cause human disease. The latter are classified according to morphology, mechanism of pathogenesis, and in vitro behavior (see Table 15.4). Here we summarize their pathogenic mechanisms:

- *Enterotoxigenic E. coli (ETEC) organisms* are the principal cause of traveler's diarrhea, and are spread by the fecal-oral route. They express a heat-labile toxin (LT) that is similar to cholera toxin and a heat-stable toxin (ST) that increases intracellular cGMP with effects similar to the cAMP elevations caused by LT.
- *Enteropathogenic E. coli (EPEC) organisms* are characterized by their ability to produce attaching and effacing (A/E) lesions in which bacteria attach tightly to the enterocyte apical membranes and cause local loss (i.e., effacement) of the microvilli. The proteins necessary for creating A/E lesions are all encoded by a large genomic pathogenicity island, the locus of enterocyte effacement (LEE). This locus also encodes a type III secretion system, similar to that in *Shigella,* that injects bacterial effector proteins into the epithelial cell cytoplasm. EPEC can cause endemic diarrhea as well as diarrheal outbreaks particularly in children younger than 2 years of age.
- *Enterohemorrhagic E. coli (EHEC) organisms* are categorized as O157:H7 and non-O157:H7 serotypes. Outbreaks of *E. coli* O157:H7 in developed countries have been associated with the consumption of inadequately cooked ground beef, milk, and vegetables. Both O157:H7 and non-O157:H7 serotypes produce Shiga-like toxins and can cause dysentery. They can also trigger hemolytic-uremic syndrome (Chapter 14).
- *Enteroinvasive E. coli (EIEC) organisms* resemble *Shigella* bacteriologically but do not produce toxins. They invade the gut epithelial cells and produce a bloody diarrhea.
- *Enteroaggregative E. coli (EAEC) organisms* attach to enterocytes by adherence fimbriae. Although they produce LT and Shiga-like toxins, histologic damage is minimal.

Salmonellosis

Salmonella species, which are members of the Enterobacteriaceae family of gram-negative bacilli, are divided into Salmonella typhi, the causative agent of typhoid fever and nontyphoid Salmonella strains that cause gastroenteritis. Nontyphoid *Salmonella* infection usually is due to *Salmonella enteritidis;* more than 1 million cases occur each year in the United States, which result in 2000 deaths; the prevalence is greater in many other countries. Infection is most common in young children and older adults, with a peak incidence in summer and fall. Transmission usually is through contaminated food, particularly raw or undercooked meat, poultry, eggs, and milk.

Pathogenesis

Very few viable *Salmonella* organisms are necessary to cause infection, and the absence of gastric acid, as in individuals with atrophic gastritis or those on acid-suppressive therapy, further reduces the required inoculum. Salmonellae possess *virulence genes that encode a type III secretion system* capable of transferring bacterial proteins into M cells and enterocytes. The transferred proteins activate host cell Rho GTPases, thereby triggering actin rearrangement and bacterial uptake into phagosomes where the bacteria can grow. Salmonellae also secrete a molecule that induces epithelial release of a chemoattractant eicosanoid that draws neutrophils into the lumen and potentiates mucosal damage. Stool cultures are essential for diagnosis.

Typhoid Fever

Typhoid fever, also referred to as *enteric fever,* is caused by *Salmonella typhi* and *Salmonella paratyphi.* It affects up to 30 million individuals worldwide each year. Infection by *S. typhi* is more common in endemic areas, where children and adolescents are most often affected. By contrast, *S. paratyphi* predominates in travelers and those living in developed countries. Humans are the sole reservoir for *S. typhi* and *S. paratyphi,* and transmission occurs from person to person or via contaminated food or water. Gallbladder colonization may be associated with gallstones and a chronic carrier state. Acute infection is associated with anorexia, abdominal pain, bloating, nausea, vomiting, and bloody diarrhea followed by a short asymptomatic phase that gives way to bacteremia and fever with flulike symptoms. It is during this phase that detection of organisms by blood culture may prompt antibiotic treatment and prevent further disease progression. Cultures are positive in 90% of cases during the febrile phase Without such treatment, the febrile phase is followed by up to 2 weeks of sustained high fevers with abdominal tenderness that may mimic appendicitis. *Rose spots,* small erythematous maculopapular lesions, are seen on the chest and abdomen. Systemic dissemination may cause *extraintestinal complications* including encephalopathy, meningitis, seizures, endocarditis, myocarditis, pneumonia, and cholecystitis. Patients with sickle cell disease are particularly susceptible to *Salmonella* osteomyelitis.

Like *S. enteritidis, S. typhi* and *S. paratyphi* are taken up by M cells and then engulfed by mononuclear cells in the underlying lymphoid tissue. Thus, infection causes Peyer patches in the terminal ileum to enlarge into plateau like elevations up to 8 cm in diameter. Mucosal shedding creates oval ulcers oriented along the long axis of the ileum. However, unlike *S. enteritidis, S. typhi* and *S. paratyphi* can disseminate via lymphatic and blood vessels. This causes reactive hyperplasia of draining lymph nodes, in which bacteria-containing phagocytes accumulate. In addition, the spleen is enlarged and soft with pale red pulp, obliterated follicular markings, and prominent phagocyte hyperplasia. Randomly scattered small foci of parenchymal necrosis with macrophage aggregates, termed *typhoid*

nodules, can be found in the liver, bone marrow, and lymph nodes. Definitive diagnosis depends on positive blood cultures. Serologic tests are of limited utility, especially in endemic areas unless rising titers of antibodies can be demonstrated.

Pseudomembranous Colitis

Pseudomembranous colitis, generally caused by *C. difficile,* also is referred to as *antibiotic-associated colitis* or *antibiotic-associated diarrhea.* While antibiotic-associated diarrhea also may be caused by other organisms such as *Salmonella, C. perfringens* type A, or *Staphylococcus aureus,* only *C. difficile* causes pseudomembranous colitis. It is likely that disruption of the normal colonic microbiota by antibiotics allows *C. difficile* overgrowth. Almost any antibiotic may be responsible; the most important determinants of the disease are frequency of use and the effect on colonic microbiota. Toxins released by *C. difficile* cause the ribosylation of small GTPases, such as Rho, and lead to disruption of the epithelial cytoskeleton, tight junction barrier loss, cytokine release, and apoptosis.

MORPHOLOGY

Fully developed *C. difficile*–associated colitis is accompanied by formation of **pseudomembranes** (Fig. 15.24A), made up of an adherent layer of inflammatory cells and debris at sites of colonic mucosal injury. The surface epithelium is denuded, and the superficial lamina propria contains a dense infiltrate of neutrophils and occasional fibrin thrombi within capillaries. Damaged crypts are distended by a mucopurulent exudate that "erupts" to the surface in a fashion reminiscent of a volcano (Fig. 15.24B).

Clinical Features

In addition to antibiotic exposure, risk factors for *C. difficile*–associated colitis include advanced age, hospitalization,

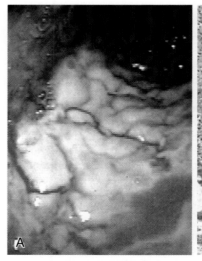
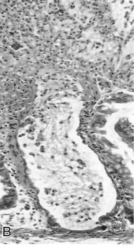

Fig. 15.24 *Clostridium difficile* colitis. (A) The colon is coated by tan pseudomembranes composed of neutrophils, dead epithelial cells, and inflammatory debris (endoscopic view). (B) Typical pattern of neutrophils emanating from a crypt is reminiscent of a volcanic eruption.

and immunosuppression. The organism is particularly prevalent in hospitals; as many as 20% of hospitalized adults are colonized with *C. difficile* (a rate 10 times higher than in the general population), but most colonized patients are free of disease. Individuals with *C. difficile*–associated colitis usually present with watery diarrhea and abdominal cramping; dehydration, fever, and leukocytosis may be seen in more severe cases. Fecal leukocytes and occult blood may be present, but grossly bloody diarrhea is rare. Diagnosis of *C. difficile*–associated colitis usually is accomplished by detection of *C. difficile* toxin, rather than culture, and is supported by the characteristic histopathologic findings. Regimens of metronidazole or vancomycin are generally effective treatments, but antibiotic-resistant and hypervirulent *C. difficile* strains are increasingly common, and the infection may recur in at-risk patients. Recent reports suggest that, particularly in patients with recurrent disease, fecal microbial transplantation may restore a normal microbiota and lead to lasting cure.

Mycobacterial Infection

Mycobacterial species, including *M. tuberculosis, M. bovis,* and *M. avium* species can involve the gastrointestinal tract primarily or be part of disseminated infection. Gastrointestinal tuberculosis is uncommon in Western countries, except in immunosuppressed individuals. In such cases, *M. avium* infection is most common. In endemic areas, including India and Pakistan, intestinal *M. tuberculosis* generally presents in the third and fourth decades of life and typically afflicts those of lower socioeconomic status. In such settings, primary intestinal infection is more common than disseminated disease. As the incidence of Crohn disease increases in these areas, differentiation between *M. tuberculosis* and Crohn disease has become more difficult.

M. avium tends to accumulate within the cytoplasm and distend lamina propria histiocytes. In some cases, this may result in a sheet-like expansion of histiocytes that fill the lamina propria and, in the small intestine, compress lympatic vessels leading to malabsorption. These cases can mimic Whipple disease clinically and morphologically. However, *M. avium* is positive by acid fast stain, while *Tropheryma whippelii* is not; both organisms are labelled by the periodic acid-Schiff (PAS) stain.

M. tuberculosis can present with granulomatous disease. In contrast to Crohn disease, these granulomas, which are generally multiple, often have caseous necrosis, but this can be difficult to determine on biopsies. Because the granulomas can be present in all layers of the bowel wall, transmural disease with fibrosis, perforation, and stenoses, or strictures, can be present. Patients may also have peritoneal dissemination with ascites.

Norovirus

Norovirus, **previously known as** *Norwalk-like virus,* **causes approximately half of all gastroenteritis outbreaks worldwide and is a common cause of sporadic gastroenteritis in developed countries.** Local outbreaks are usually related to contaminated food or water, but person-to-person transmission underlies most sporadic cases. Infections spread easily within schools, hospitals, nursing homes and, on other densely populated communities including cruise ships. After a short incubation period, affected individuals develop nausea, vomiting, watery diarrhea, and abdominal pain. Biopsy morphology is nonspecific. The disease is self-limited.

Rotavirus

The encapsulated *rotavirus* **infects 140 million individuals and causes 1 million deaths each year, making rotavirus the most common cause of severe childhood diarrhea and diarrhea-related deaths worldwide.** Children between 6 and 24 months of age are most vulnerable. Protection in the first 6 months of life is probably due to the presence of antibodies to rotavirus in breast milk, while protection beyond 2 years of age is due to immunity that develops after the first infection. Outbreaks in hospitals and day care centers are common, and infection spreads easily; the estimated minimal infective inoculum is only 10 viral particles. *Rotavirus selectively infects and destroys mature (absorptive) enterocytes in the small intestine, and the villus surface is repopulated by immature secretory cells.* This change in functional capacity results in loss of absorptive function and net secretion of water and electrolytes, compounded by an osmotic diarrhea from incompletely absorbed nutrients. Like norovirus, rotavirus infection becomes symptomatic after a short incubation period and manifests as several days of vomiting and watery diarrhea. Vaccines are now available, and their use is beginning to change the epidemiology of rotavirus infection. Unfortunately, oral rotavirus vaccines have been less effective in developing countries where they are most needed.

Parasitic Disease

Parasitic disease and protozoal infections affect over half of the world's population on a chronic or recurrent basis. The small intestine can harbor as many as 20 species of parasites, including nematodes, such as the roundworms *Ascaris* and *Strongyloides;* hookworms and pinworms; cestodes, including flatworms and tapeworms; trematodes (flukes); and protozoa.

- *Ascaris lumbricoides.* This nematode infects more than 1 billion individuals worldwide as a result of human fecal-oral contamination. Ingested eggs hatch in the intestine, and larvae penetrate the intestinal mucosa. From there, the larvae migrate via the splanchnic circulation to the liver, creating hepatic abscesses, and then through the systemic circulation to the lung, where they can cause *Ascaris* pneumonitis. In the latter case, larvae migrate up the trachea, are swallowed, and arrive again in the intestine to mature into adult worms. Diagnosis is made by detection of eggs in the stools.
- *Strongyloides.* The larvae of *Strongyloides* live in fecally contaminated ground soil and can penetrate unbroken skin. They migrate through the lungs to the trachea from where they are swallowed and then mature into adult worms in the intestines. Unlike other intestinal worms, which require an ovum or larval stage outside the human, the eggs of *Strongyloides* can hatch within the intestine and release larvae that penetrate the mucosa, creating a vicious cycle referred to as *autoinfection.* Hence, *Strongyloides* infection can persist for life,

and immunosuppressed individuals can develop over-whelming infections.

- *Necator americanus* and *Ancylostoma duodenale.* These hookworms infect 1 billion individuals worldwide and cause significant morbidity. Infection is initiated by larval penetration through the skin. After further development in the lungs, the larvae migrate up the trachea and are swallowed. Once in the duodenum, the larvae mature and the adult worms attach to the mucosa, suck blood, and reproduce. Hookworms are a leading cause of iron-deficiency anemia in the develop-ing world. Detection of eggs in the stools is used for diagnosis.

- *Giardia lamblia.* This flagellated protozoan, also referred to as *Giardia duodenalis* or *Giardia intestinalis,* is the *most common pathogenic parasite in humans* and is spread by fecally contaminated water or food. Infection may occur after ingestion of as few as 10 cysts and is characterized by acute or chronic malabsorptive diarrhea. Because cysts are resistant to chlorine, *Giardia* organisms are endemic in unfiltered public and rural water supplies. In the acidic environment of the stomach, excystation occurs and trophozoites are released. Secretory IgA and mucosal IL-6 responses are important for clearance of *Giardia* infections, and immunosuppressed, agamma-globulinemic, or malnourished individuals often are severely affected. *Giardia* evades immune clearance through continuous modification of the major surface antigen, variant surface protein, and can persist for months or years while causing intermittent symptoms. *Giardia* infection reduces expression of brush border enzymes, including lactase, and causes microvillous damage and apoptosis of small-intestinal epithelial cells. *Giardia* trophozoites are noninvasive and can be identified in duodenal biopsy specimens by their char-acteristic pear shape. The availability of a stool antigen assay for Giardia has simplified the diagnosis of Giardia infection.

- *Entamoeba histolytica.* This protozoan causes amebiasis and is spread by fecal-oral transmission. *E. histolytica* infects approximately 500 million people in countries such as India, Mexico, and Colombia, and causes 40 million cases of dysentery and liver abscess annually.

   While amebiasis affects the cecum and ascending colon most often, the sigmoid colon, rectum, and appen-dix can also be involved. Dysentery develops when the amebae attach to the colonic epithelium, induce apop-tosis, invade crypts, and burrow laterally into the lamina propria. This recruits neutrophils, causes tissue damage, and creates a flask-shaped ulcer with a narrow neck and broad base. Parasites may penetrate splanchnic vessels and embolize to the liver to produce abscesses in about 40% of patients with amebic dysentery. Amebic liver abscesses, which can exceed 10 cm in diameter, have a scant inflammatory reaction at their margins and a shaggy fibrin lining. The abscesses persist after the acute intestinal illness has passed and may rarely reach the lung and the heart by direct extension. Amebae may also spread to the kidneys and brain via the bloodstream.

   Individuals with amebiasis may present with abdom-inal pain, bloody diarrhea, or weight loss. Occasionally,

acute necrotizing colitis and megacolon occur, and both are associated with significant mortality.

⬤ SUMMARY

INFECTIOUS ENTEROCOLITIS

- *Vibrio cholerae* secretes a preformed toxin that causes massive chloride secretion. Water follows the resulting osmotic gradi-ent, leading to secretory diarrhea.
- *Campylobacter jejuni* is the most common bacterial enteric pathogen in developed countries and also causes traveler's diarrhea. Most isolates are noninvasive. *Salmonella* and *Shigella* spp. are invasive and associated with exudative bloody diar-rhea (dysentery). *Salmonella* infection is a common cause of food poisoning. *S. typhi* can cause systemic disease (typhoid fever).
- Pseudomembranous colitis is often triggered by antibiotic therapy that disrupts the normal microbiota and allows *C. dif-ficile* to colonize and grow. The organism produces toxins that disrupt epithelial function. Fecal microbial transplantation is becoming more common as a therapeutic approach in individu-als with recurrent disease.
- *Rotavirus* is the most common cause of severe childhood diar-rhea and diarrheal mortality worldwide. The diarrhea is sec-ondary to loss of mature enterocytes, resulting in malabsorption as well as secretion.
- *Parasitic* and *protozoal* infections affect over half of the world's population on a chronic or recurrent basis.

INFLAMMATORY INTESTINAL DISEASE

Sigmoid Diverticulitis

In general, diverticular disease refers to acquired pseudo-diverticular outpouchings of the colonic mucosa and sub-mucosa. Such *colonic diverticula* are rare in individuals younger than 30 years of age, but the prevalence approaches 50% in Western adult populations older than 60 years of age. Diverticula generally are multiple, and the condition is referred to as *diverticulosis.* This disease is much less common in developing countries, probably because of dietary differences.

Pathogenesis

Colonic diverticula tend to develop under conditions of elevated intraluminal pressure in the sigmoid colon. This is facilitated by the unique structure of the colonic muscu-laris propria, where nerves, arterial vasa recta, and their connective tissue sheaths penetrate the inner circular muscle coat to create discontinuities in the muscle wall. In other parts of the intestine, these gaps are reinforced by the external longitudinal layer of the muscularis propria, but in the colon, this muscle layer is discontinuous, being gath-ered into three bands termed *taeniae coli.* High luminal pressures may be generated by exaggerated peristaltic con-tractions, with spasmodic sequestration of bowel segments that may be exacerbated by diets low in fiber, which reduce stool bulk.

MORPHOLOGY

Anatomically, colonic diverticula are small, flasklike outpouchings, usually 0.5 to 1 cm in diameter, that occur in a regular distribution in between the taeniae coli (Fig. 15.25A and B). They are most common in the sigmoid colon, but other regions of the colon may be affected. Colonic diverticula have a thin wall composed of a flattened or atrophic mucosa, compressed submucosa, and attenuated muscularis propria—often, this last component is totally absent (Fig. 15.25C and D). Obstruction of diverticula with stasis of contents, leads to inflammatory changes, producing **diverticulitis** and peridiverticulitis. Because the wall of the diverticulum is supported only by the muscularis mucosa and a thin layer of subserosal adipose tissue, inflammation, increased pressure, and mucosal ulceration within an obstructed diverticulum can readily result in **perforation.** With or without perforation, recurrent diverticulitis may cause segmental colitis, fibrotic thickening in and around the colonic wall, or stricture formation.

Clinical Features

Most individuals with diverticular disease remain asymptomatic throughout their lives. About 20% of those affected

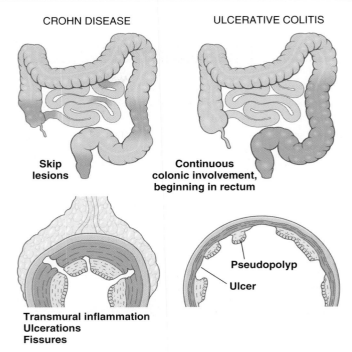

Fig. 15.26 Distribution of lesions in inflammatory bowel disease. The distinction between Crohn disease and ulcerative colitis is based primarily on morphology.

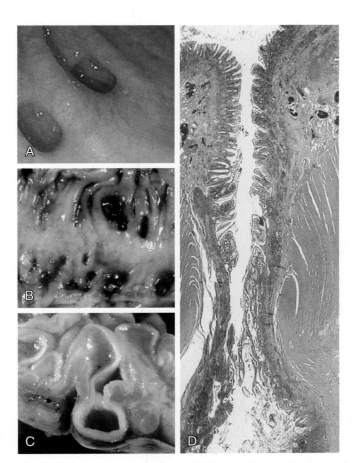

Fig. 15.25 Sigmoid diverticular disease. (A) Endoscopic view of two sigmoid diverticulae. Compare to B. (B) Gross examination of a resected sigmoid colon shows regularly spaced stool-filled diverticulae. (C) Cross-section showing the outpouching of mucosa beneath the muscularis propria. (D) Low-power photomicrograph of a sigmoid diverticulum showing protrusion of the mucosa and submucosa through the muscularis propria. *(Endoscopic image courtesy of Dr. Ira Hanan, The University of Chicago, Chicago, Illinois.)*

develop complaints including intermittent cramping, continuous lower abdominal discomfort, constipation, and diarrhea. Longitudinal studies have shown that while diverticula can regress early in their development they often become more numerous and larger over time. Whether a high-fiber diet prevents such progression or protects against diverticulitis is unclear. Even when diverticulitis occurs, it most often resolves spontaneously or after antibiotic treatment, and relatively few patients require surgical intervention.

Inflammatory Bowel Disease

Inflammatory bowel disease (IBD) is a chronic condition resulting from complex interactions between intestinal microbiota and host immunity in genetically predisposed individuals resulting an inappropriate mucosal immune activation. IBD encompasses two entities, *Crohn disease* and *ulcerative colitis*. The distinction between ulcerative colitis and Crohn disease is based, in large part, on the distribution of affected sites and the morphologic expression of disease at those sites (Fig. 15.26; Table 15.5). *Ulcerative colitis is limited to the colon and rectum and extends only into the mucosa and submucosa. By contrast, Crohn disease, also referred to as regional enteritis (because of frequent ileal involvement), may involve any area of the gastrointestinal tract and is frequently transmural.*

Epidemiology

Both Crohn disease and ulcerative colitis frequently present during adolescence or in young adults, although some studies suggest a second, smaller peak in the incidence of both diseases after the fifth decade. In Western

Table 15.5 Features of Crohn Disease and Ulcerative Colitis

Feature	Crohn Disease	Ulcerative Colitis
Macroscopic		
Bowel region affected	Ileum ± colon	Colon only
Rectal involvement	Sometimes	Always
Distribution	Skip lesions	Diffuse
Stricture	Yes	Rare
Bowel wall appearance	Thick	Thin
Inflammation	Transmural	Limited to mucosa and submucosa
Pseudopolyps	Moderate	Marked
Ulcers	Deep, knifelike	Superficial, broad-based
Lymphoid reaction	Marked	Moderate
Fibrosis	Marked	Mild to none
Serositis	Marked	No
Granulomas	Yes (~35%)	No
Fistulas/sinuses	Yes	No
Clinical		
Perianal fistula	Yes (in colonic disease)	No
Fat/vitamin malabsorption	Yes	No
Malignant potential	With colonic involvement	Yes
Recurrence after surgery	Common	No
Toxic megacolon	No	Yes

NOTE: Not all features may be present in a single case.

genetic, and clinical studies as well as data from laboratory models of IBD (Fig. 15.27).

- *Genetics.* Risk for disease is increased when there is an affected family member, and in Crohn disease, the concordance rate for monozygotic twins is approximately 50%. By contrast, concordance of monozygotic twins for ulcerative colitis is only 16%, suggesting that genetic factors are less dominant in this form of IBD.
  - Molecular linkage analyses of affected families have identified *NOD2* (nucleotide oligomerization binding domain 2) as a susceptibility gene in Crohn disease. *NOD2* encodes a protein that binds to intracellular bacterial peptidoglycans and subsequently activates NF-κB. Some studies suggest that the disease-associated form of NOD-2 is ineffective at defending against intestinal bacteria. The result is that bacteria are able to enter through the epithelium into the wall of the intestine, where they trigger inflammatory reactions. It should, however, be recognized that disease develops in less than 10% of individuals carrying specific *NOD2* polymorphisms, and these polymorphisms are uncommon in African and Asian patients with Crohn disease.
  - The search for IBD-associated genes using genome-wide association studies (GWAS) that assess single-nucleotide polymorphisms (SNPs) as well as high throughput sequencing and other approaches have yielded a rich harvest of over 200 genes associated with IBD. Among these, *NOD2*, discussed above, and two autophagy–related genes are of particular interest. They are *ATG16L1* (autophagy-related 16–like-1) and *IRGM* (immunity-related GTPase M)

industrialized nations, IBD is most common among whites and, in the United States, occurs three to five times more often among eastern European (Ashkenazi) Jews. This predilection is at least partly due to genetic factors, as discussed below. The geographic distribution of IBD is highly variable, but it is most prevalent in North America, northern Europe, and Australia. The incidence of IBD worldwide is on the rise and it is becoming more common in regions in which the prevalence was historically low. The *hygiene hypothesis*, first applied to asthma, says that childhood and even prenatal exposure to environmental microbes resets the immune system in a way that prevents excessive reactions. Extrapolated to IBD, it suggests that a reduced frequency of enteric infections due to improved hygiene has resulted in inadequate development of regulatory processes that limit mucosal immune responses early in life. While attractive and commonly stated, firm evidence is lacking and hence the increasing incidence of IBD remains mysterious.

Pathogenesis

Although precise causes are not yet defined, **most investigators believe that IBD results from the combined effects of alterations in host interactions with intestinal microbiota, intestinal epithelial dysfunction, aberrant mucosal immune responses, and altered composition of the gut microbiome.** This view is supported by epidemiologic,

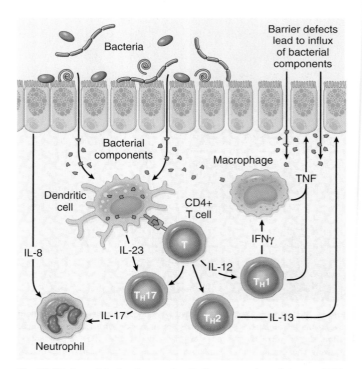

Fig. 15.27 A model of pathogenesis of inflammatory bowel disease (IBD). Aspects of both Crohn disease and ulcerative colitis are shown.

genes. Both are part of the autophagosome pathway and, like NOD-2, are involved in host cell responses to intracellular bacteria, supporting the hypothesis that inadequate defense against luminal bacteria may be important in the pathogenesis of IBD. None of these genes is associated with ulcerative colitis.

- *Mucosal immune responses.* Although the mechanisms by which mucosal immunity contributes to the pathogenesis of ulcerative colitis and Crohn disease are still being deciphered, immunosuppressive and immunomodulatory agents remain mainstays of IBD therapy. Polarization of helper T cells to the T_H1 type is well recognized in Crohn disease, and some data suggest that T_H17 T cells also contribute to disease pathogenesis. Consistent with this, certain polymorphisms of the IL-23 receptor confer protection from Crohn disease and ulcerative colitis (IL-23 is involved in the development and maintenance of T_H17 cells). However, agents that block IL-17 or its receptor have provided no benefit, whereas an antibody that inhibits both T_H1- and T_H17-inducing cytokines is effective, suggesting that the two T cell subsets may have a synergistic role in the disease. Some data suggest that mucosal production of the T_H2-derived cytokine IL-13 is increased in ulcerative colitis, and, to a lesser degree, Crohn disease.

  Defects in regulatory T cells, especially the IL-10-producing subset, are believed to underlie the inflammation especially in Crohn disease. Mutations in the IL-10 receptor are associated with severe, early-onset colitis. Thus, some combination of excessive immune activation by intestinal microbes and defective immune regulation likely is responsible for the chronic inflammation in both forms of IBD.

- *Epithelial defects.* A variety of epithelial defects have been described in Crohn disease, ulcerative colitis, or both. For example, defects in intestinal epithelial tight junction barrier function occur in patients with Crohn disease and a subset of their healthy first-degree relatives. This barrier dysfunction cosegregates with specific disease-associated *NOD2* polymorphisms, and experimental models demonstrate that barrier dysfunction can activate innate and adaptive mucosal immunity and sensitize subjects to disease. Interestingly, the Paneth cell granules, which contain anti-microbial peptides that can affect composition of the luminal microbiota, are abnormal in patients with Crohn disease carrying *ATG16L1* mutations, thus providing one potential mechanism in which a defective feedback loop between the epithelium and microbiota could contribute to disease pathogenesis.

- *Microbiota.* The quantity of microbial organisms in the gastrointestinal lumen is enormous, amounting to as many as 10^{12} organisms/mL of fecal material in the colon (50% of fecal mass). There is significant interindividual variation in the composition of this microbial population, which is modified by diet and disease. Microbial transfer studies are able to promote or reduce disease in animal models of IBD, and clinical trials suggest that probiotic (or beneficial) bacteria or even fecal microbial transplants from healthy individuals may benefit IBD patients.

One model that unifies the roles of intestinal microbiota, epithelial function, and mucosal immunity suggests a cycle by which transepithelial flux of luminal bacterial components activates innate and adaptive immune responses. In a genetically susceptible host, the subsequent release of TNF and other immune signals directs epithelia to increase tight junction permeability, which further increases the flux of luminal material. These events may establish a self-amplifying cycle in which a stimulus at any site may be sufficient to initiate IBD.

With this background of pathogenesis we will discuss next the morphologic and clinical features of each of the two forms of IBD.

Crohn Disease

MORPHOLOGY

Crohn disease, also known as *regional enteritis,* may occur in any area of the gastrointestinal tract but the most common sites involved at presentation are the **terminal ileum, ileocecal valve,** and **cecum.** Disease is limited to the small intestine alone in about 40% of cases; the small intestine and the colon both are involved in 30% of patients; and the remainder of cases are characterized by colonic involvement only. Infrequently, Crohn disease may involve the esophagus or stomach. The presence of multiple, separate, sharply delineated areas of disease, resulting in **skip lesions,** is characteristic of Crohn disease and may help in differentiation from ulcerative colitis. Strictures are common (Fig. 15.28A).

The earliest lesion, the **aphthous ulcer,** may progress, and multiple lesions often coalesce into elongated, serpentine ulcers oriented along the axis of the bowel. Edema and loss of normal mucosal folds are common. Sparing of interspersed mucosa results in a coarsely textured, **cobblestone** appearance in which diseased tissue is depressed below the level of normal mucosa (Fig. 15.28B). **Fissures** frequently develop between mucosal folds and may extend deeply to become sites of perforation or fistula tracts. The intestinal wall is thickened as a consequence of transmural edema, inflammation, submucosal fibrosis, and hypertrophy of the muscularis propria, all of which contribute to stricture formation. In cases with extensive transmural disease, mesenteric fat frequently extends around the serosal surface **(creeping fat)** (Fig. 15.28C).

The microscopic features of active Crohn disease include abundant neutrophils that infiltrate and damage crypt epithelium. Clusters of neutrophils within a crypt are referred to as a **crypt abscess** and often are associated with crypt destruction. Ulceration is common in Crohn disease, and there may be an abrupt transition between ulcerated and normal mucosa. Repeated cycles of crypt destruction and regeneration lead to **distortion of mucosal architecture;** the normally straight and parallel crypts take on bizarre branching shapes and unusual orientations to one another (Fig. 15.29A). Epithelial metaplasia, another consequence of chronic relapsing injury, often takes the form of gastric antral-appearing glands (pseudopyloric metaplasia). **Paneth cell metaplasia** may occur in the left colon, where Paneth cells are normally absent. These architectural and metaplastic changes may persist, even when active inflammation has resolved. Mucosal atrophy, with loss of crypts, may follow years of disease. **Noncaseating granulomas**

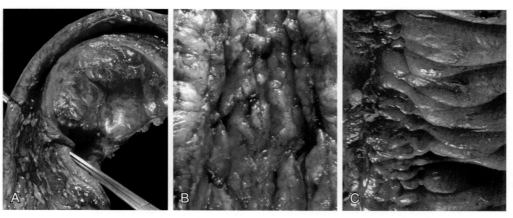

Fig. 15.28 Gross pathology of Crohn disease. (A) Small-intestinal stricture. (B) Linear mucosal ulcers and thickened intestinal wall. (C) Creeping fat.

(Fig. 15.29B), a hallmark of Crohn disease, are found in approximately 35% of cases and may arise in areas of active disease or uninvolved regions in any layer of the intestinal wall (Fig. 15.29C). Granulomas also may be found in mesenteric lymph nodes. Cutaneous granulomas form nodules that are referred to (misleadingly) as **metastatic Crohn disease. The absence of granulomas does not preclude a diagnosis of Crohn disease.**

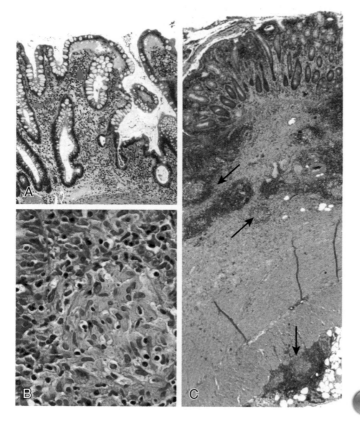

Fig. 15.29 Microscopic pathology of Crohn disease. (A) Haphazard crypt organization results from repeated injury and regeneration. (B) Noncaseating granuloma. (C) Transmural Crohn disease with submucosal and serosal granulomas *(arrows)*.

Clinical Features

The clinical manifestations of Crohn disease are extremely variable. In most patients, disease begins with intermittent attacks of relatively mild diarrhea, fever, and abdominal pain. Approximately 20% of patients present acutely with right lower-quadrant pain and fever, which may mimic acute appendicitis or bowel perforation. Patients with colonic involvement may present with bloody diarrhea and abdominal pain, creating a differential diagnosis with some colonic infections. Periods of disease activity typically are interrupted by asymptomatic intervals that last for weeks to many months. Disease reactivation can be associated with a variety of external triggers, including physical or emotional stress, specific dietary items, NSAID use, and cigarette smoking.

Iron-deficiency anemia may develop in individuals with colonic disease, while extensive small-bowel disease may result in serum protein loss and hypoalbuminemia, generalized nutrient malabsorption, or malabsorption of vitamin B₁₂ and bile salts. Fibrosing strictures, particularly of the terminal ileum, are common and require surgical resection. Disease often recurs at the site of anastomosis, and as many as 40% of patients require additional resections within 10 years. Fistulas develop between loops of bowel and may also involve the urinary bladder, vagina, and abdominal or perianal skin. Perforations and peritoneal abscesses can also occur.

Extraintestinal manifestations of Crohn disease include uveitis, migratory polyarthritis, sacroiliitis, ankylosing spondylitis, erythema nodosum, and clubbing of the fingertips, any of which may develop before intestinal disease is recognized. Pericholangitis and primary sclerosing cholangitis may occur in Crohn disease but are more common in ulcerative colitis. As discussed later, the risk for development of colonic adenocarcinoma is increased in patients with long-standing colonic Crohn disease.

Ulcerative Colitis

MORPHOLOGY

Ulcerative colitis always involves the rectum and extends proximally in a continuous fashion to involve part or the entire colon that can be diffusely ulcerated (Fig. 15.30A). Skip lesions are not seen (although focal appendiceal or cecal inflammation occasionally may be present in those with left-sided disease). Disease of the entire colon is termed *pancolitis* (Fig. 15.30B). Disease limited to the rectum or rectosigmoid may be referred to descriptively as **ulcerative proctitis** or **ulcerative proctosigmoiditis.** The small intestine is normal, although mild mucosal inflammation of the distal ileum, **backwash ileitis,** may be present in severe cases of pancolitis.

On gross evaluation, involved colonic mucosa may be slightly red and granular-appearing or exhibit extensive **broad-based ulcers.** The transition between diseased and uninvolved colon can be abrupt (see Fig. 15.30C). Ulcers are aligned along the long axis of the colon but typically do not replicate the serpentine ulcers of Crohn disease. Isolated islands of regenerating mucosa often bulge into the lumen to create small elevations, termed **pseudopolyps.** Chronic disease may lead to **mucosal atrophy** and a flat, smooth mucosal surface lacking normal folds. Unlike in Crohn disease, **mural thickening is absent, the serosal surface is normal, and strictures do not occur.** However, inflammation and inflammatory mediators can damage the muscularis propria and disturb neuromuscular function leading to colonic dilation and **toxic megacolon,** which carries a significant risk for perforation.

Histologic features of mucosal disease in ulcerative colitis are similar to those in colonic Crohn disease and include inflammatory infiltrates, crypt abscesses, crypt distortion, and epithelial metaplasia. However, **skip lesions are absent, and inflammation generally is limited to the mucosa and superficial submucosa** (Fig. 15.30D). This distinction may not be demonstrated by endoscopic biopsies, which typically sample the mucosa and little or no submucosa. In severe cases, mucosal damage may be accompanied by ulcers that extend more deeply into the submucosa, but the muscularis propria is rarely involved. Submucosal fibrosis, mucosal atrophy, and distorted mucosal architecture remain as residua of healed disease, but the histologic pattern also may revert to near normal after prolonged remission. **Granulomas are not present.**

Some extraintestinal manifestations of ulcerative colitis overlap with those of Crohn disease, including migratory polyarthritis, sacroiliitis, ankylosing spondylitis, uveitis, skin lesions, pericholangitis, and primary sclerosing cholangitis.

Clinical Features

Ulcerative colitis is a relapsing disorder characterized by attacks of bloody diarrhea with expulsion of stringy, mucoid material and lower abdominal pain and cramps that are temporarily relieved by defecation. These symptoms may persist for days, weeks, or months before they subside, and occasionally the initial attack may be severe enough to constitute a medical or surgical emergency. More than half of patients have mild disease, but almost all experience at least one relapse during a 10-year period. Colectomy cures intestinal disease, but extraintestinal manifestations may persist.

The factors that trigger ulcerative colitis are not known; infectious enteritis precedes disease onset in some cases. The onset of symptoms can occur shortly after smoking cessation in some patients, and smoking may partially relieve symptoms. Unfortunately, studies of nicotine as a therapeutic agent have been disappointing.

Colitis-Associated Neoplasia

One of the most feared long-term complications of ulcerative colitis and colonic Crohn disease is the development of neoplasia. This process begins as dysplasia, which, just as in Barrett esophagus and chronic gastritis, is a step along the road to full-blown carcinoma. The risk for development of dysplasia is related to several factors:

- *Duration of disease.* Risk increases beginning 8 to 10 years after disease initiation.
- *Extent of involvement.* Patients with pancolitis are at greater risk than those with only left-sided disease.

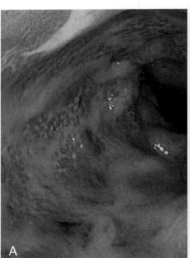
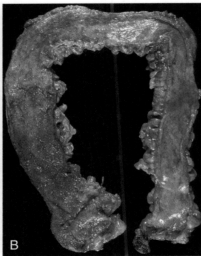
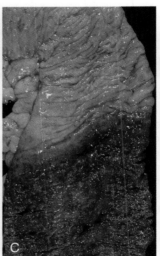
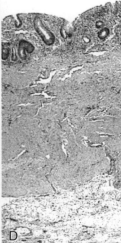

Fig. 15.30 Pathology of ulcerative colitis. (A) Endoscopic view of severe ulcerative colitis with ulceration and adherent mucopurulent material. (B) Total colectomy with pancolitis showing active disease, with red, granular mucosa in the cecum *(left)* and smooth, atrophic mucosa distally *(right)*. (C) Sharp demarcation between active ulcerative colitis *(bottom)* and normal *(top)*. (D) This full-thickness histologic section shows that disease is limited to the mucosa. Compare with Fig. 15.29C. *(Endoscopic image courtesy of Dr. Ira Hanan, The University of Chicago, Chicago, Illinois.)*

- *Inflammation.* Greater frequency and severity of active inflammation (characterized by the presence of neutrophils) may increase risk. This is another example of the enabling effect of inflammation on carcinogenesis (Chapter 6).

To facilitate early detection of neoplasia, patients typically are enrolled in surveillance programs approximately 8 years after diagnosis of IBD. An important exception to this approach is in patients with primary sclerosing cholangitis, who are at markedly greater risk for development of dysplasia and generally are enrolled for surveillance at the time of diagnosis. Surveillance requires regular and extensive mucosal biopsy, making it a costly practice. In many cases, dysplasia occurs in flat areas of mucosa that do not appear abnormal by eye. Thus, advanced endoscopic imaging techniques are being developed to try to enable the detection of early dysplastic changes.

SUMMARY

INFLAMMATORY BOWEL DISEASE

- Inflammatory bowel disease (IBD) is an umbrella term for Crohn disease and ulcerative colitis.
- Crohn disease most commonly affects the terminal ileum and cecum, but any site within the gastrointestinal tract can be involved; skip lesions and noncaseating granulomas are common.
- Ulcerative colitis is limited to the colon, is continuous from the rectum, and ranges in extent from only rectal disease to pancolitis; neither skip lesions nor granulomas are present.
- Both Crohn disease and ulcerative colitis can have extraintestinal manifestations.
- IBD is thought to arise from a combination of alterations in host interactions with intestinal microbiota, intestinal epithelial dysfunction, and aberrant mucosal immune responses.
- The risk for development of colonic epithelial dysplasia and adenocarcinoma is increased in patients who have had colonic IBD for more than 8 to 10 years.

COLONIC POLYPS AND NEOPLASTIC DISEASE

Polyps are most common in the colon but may occur in the esophagus, stomach, or small intestine. Those without stalks are referred to as *sessile*. As sessile polyps enlarge, proliferation of cells adjacent to the polyp and the effects of traction on the luminal protrusion may combine to create a stalk. Polyps with stalks are termed *pedunculated*. In general, intestinal polyps can be classified as *nonneoplastic* or *neoplastic*. The most common neoplastic polyp is the adenoma, which has the potential to progress to cancer. Nonneoplastic colonic polyps can be further classified as inflammatory, hamartomatous, or hyperplastic.

Inflammatory Polyps

The *solitary rectal ulcer syndrome* is associated with a purely inflammatory polyp. Patients present with the clinical triad of rectal bleeding, mucus discharge, and an inflammatory lesion of the anterior rectal wall. The underlying cause is impaired relaxation of the anorectal sphincter, creating a sharp angle at the anterior rectal shelf. This leads to recurrent abrasion and ulceration of the overlying rectal mucosa. Chronic cycles of injury and healing produce a polypoid mass composed of inflamed and reactive mucosal tissue.

Hamartomatous Polyps

Hamartomatous polyps occur sporadically and as components of various genetically determined or acquired syndromes (Table 15.6). As described previously, hamartomas are disorganized, tumorlike growths composed of mature cell types normally present at the site at which the polyp develops. Hamartomatous polyposis syndromes are rare, but they are important to recognize because of associated intestinal and extraintestinal manifestations and the need to screen family members.

Juvenile Polyps

Juvenile polyps are the most common type of hamartomatous polyp. They may be sporadic or syndromic. Sporadic juvenile polyps are usually solitary, but the number varies from 3 to as many as 100 in individuals with the autosomal dominant syndrome of juvenile polyposis. In adults, the sporadic form is sometimes also referred to as an *inflammatory polyp*, particularly when dense inflammatory infiltrates are present. The vast majority of juvenile polyps occur in children younger than 5 years of age. Juvenile polyps characteristically are located in the rectum and most manifest with rectal bleeding. In some cases, prolapse occurs and the polyp protrudes through the anal sphincter. Dysplasia occurs in a small proportion of (mostly syndrome-associated) juvenile polyps, and the juvenile polyposis syndrome is associated with an increased risk for development of adenocarcinoma within the colon and at other sites (Table 15.6). Colectomy may be required to limit the hemorrhage associated with polyp ulceration in juvenile polyposis.

MORPHOLOGY

Individual sporadic and syndromic juvenile polyps often are indistinguishable. They typically are pedunculated, smooth-surfaced, reddish lesions that are less than 3 cm in diameter and display characteristic cystic spaces on cut sections. Microscopic examination shows the spaces to be dilated glands filled with mucin and inflammatory debris (Fig. 15.31A). Some data suggest that mucosal hyperplasia is the initiating event in polyp development, and this mechanism is consistent with the discovery that mutations in pathways that regulate cellular growth, such as transforming growth factor-β (TGF-β) signaling, are associated with autosomal dominant juvenile polyposis.

Peutz-Jeghers Syndrome

Peutz-Jeghers syndrome is a rare autosomal dominant disorder defined by the presence of multiple gastrointestinal hamartomatous polyps and mucocutaneous hyperpigmentation that carries an increased risk for

Table 15.6 Gastrointestinal (GI) Polyposis Syndromes

Syndrome	Mean Age at Presentation (Years)	Mutated Gene(s)	GI Lesions	Selected Extragastrointestinal Manifestations
Peutz-Jeghers syndrome	10–15	LKB1/STK11	Arborizing polyps—small intestine > colon > stomach; colonic adenocarcinoma	Mucocutaneous pigmentation; increased risk for thyroid, breast, lung, pancreas, gonadal, and bladder cancers
Juvenile polyposis	<5	SMAD4, BMPR1A	Juvenile polyps; increased risk for gastric, small-intestinal, colonic, and pancreatic adenocarcinoma	Pulmonary arteriovenous malformations, digital clubbing
Cowden syndrome, Bannayan-Ruvalcaba-Riley syndrome	<15	PTEN	Hamartomatous polyps, lipomas, ganglioneuromas, inflammatory polyps; increased risk for colon cancer	Benign skin tumors, benign and malignant thyroid and breast lesions
Cronkhite-Canada syndrome	>50	Nonhereditary	Hamartomatous colon polyps, crypt dilatation and edema in nonpolypoid mucosa	Nail atrophy, hair loss, abnormal skin pigmentation, cachexia, anemia
Tuberous sclerosis	Infancy to adulthood	TSC1, TSC2	Hamartomatous polyps (rectal)	Facial angiofibroma, cortical tubers, renal angiomyolipoma
Familial adenomatous polyposis (FAP)				
Classic FAP	10–15	APC	Multiple adenomas	Congenital RPE hypertrophy
Attenuated FAP	40–50	APC	Multiple adenomas	
Gardner syndrome	10–15	APC	Multiple adenomas	Osteomas, desmoids, skin cysts
Turcot syndrome	10–15	APC	Multiple adenomas	CNS tumors, medulloblastoma

CNS, Central nervous system; *RPE*, retinal pigment epithelium.

development of several malignancies, including cancers of the colon, pancreas, breast, lung, ovaries, uterus, and testes, as well as other unusual neoplasms. Germ line loss-of-function mutations in the *LKB1/STK11* gene are present in approximately half of the patients with the familial form of Peutz-Jeghers syndrome, as well as a subset of patients with the sporadic form. *LKB1/STK11* encodes a tumor suppressive protein kinase that regulates cellular metabolism, yet another example of links between altered metabolism, abnormal cell growth, and cancer risk. Intestinal polyps are most common in the small intestine, although they may also occur in the stomach and colon and, rarely, in the bladder and lungs. On gross evaluation, the polyps are large and pedunculated with a lobulated contour. Histologic examination demonstrates a characteristic arborizing network of connective tissue, smooth muscle, lamina propria, and glands lined by normal-appearing intestinal epithelium (Fig. 15.31B).

Hyperplastic Polyps

Colonic hyperplastic polyps are common epithelial proliferations that typically are discovered in the sixth and seventh decades of life. The pathogenesis of hyperplastic polyps is incompletely understood, but formation of these lesions is thought to result from decreased epithelial cell turnover and delayed shedding of surface epithelial cells, leading to a "pileup" of goblet cells. Although these lesions have no malignant potential, they must be distinguished from sessile serrated adenomas, histologically similar lesions that have malignant potential, as described later.

MORPHOLOGY

Hyperplastic polyps are most commonly found in the left colon and typically are less than 5 mm in diameter. They are smooth, nodular protrusions of the mucosa, often on the crests of mucosal folds. They may occur singly but more frequently are multiple, particularly in the sigmoid colon and rectum. Histologically, hyperplastic polyps are composed of mature goblet and absorptive cells. The delayed shedding of these cells leads to crowding that creates the serrated surface architecture, the morphologic hallmark of these lesions (Fig. 15.32).

Adenomas

The most common and clinically important neoplastic polyps are colonic adenomas, benign polyps that give rise to a majority of colorectal adenocarcinomas. Most adenomas, however, do not progress to adenocarcinoma.

Colorectal adenomas are characterized by the presence of epithelial dysplasia. These growths range from small, often pedunculated polyps to large sessile lesions. There is no gender predilection, and they are present in nearly 50% of adults living in the Western world beginning at age 50. Because these polyps are precursors to colorectal cancer, current recommendations are that all adults in the United States undergo screening colonoscopy starting at 50 years of age. Because individuals with a family history are at risk for developing colon cancer earlier in life, they are typically screened at least 10 years before the youngest age at which a relative was diagnosed. While adenomas are less

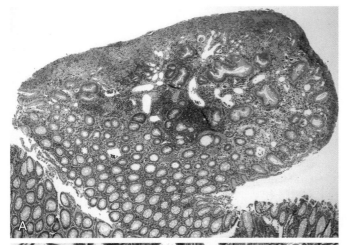

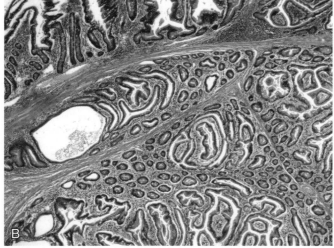

Fig. 15.31 Hamartomatous polyps. (A) Juvenile polyp. Note the surface erosion and cystically dilated crypts filled with mucus, neutrophils, and debris. (B) Peutz-Jeghers polyp. Complex glandular architecture and bundles of smooth muscle help to distinguish Peutz-Jeghers polyps from juvenile polyps.

common in Asia, their frequency has risen (in parallel with an increasing incidence of colorectal adenocarcinoma) as Western diets and lifestyles become more common.

MORPHOLOGY

Typical adenomas range from 0.3 to 10 cm in diameter and can be **pedunculated** (Fig. 15.33A) or **sessile,** with the surface of both types having a texture resembling velvet (Fig. 15.33B) or a raspberry, due to the abnormal epithelial growth pattern. Histologically, the cytologic hallmark of **epithelial dysplasia** (Fig. 15.34C) is nuclear hyperchromasia, elongation, and stratification. These changes are most easily appreciated at the surface of the adenoma, because the epithelium fails to mature as cells migrate out of the crypt. Pedunculated adenomas have slender fibromuscular stalks (see Fig. 15.33C) containing prominent blood vessels derived from the submucosa. The stalk usually is covered by nonneoplastic epithelium, but dysplastic epithelium is sometimes present.

Adenomas can be classified as **tubular, tubulovillous,** or **villous** on the basis of their architecture. These categories, however, have little clinical significance in isolation. Tubular

adenomas tend to be small, pedunculated polyps composed of small, rounded, or tubular glands (Fig. 15.34A). By contrast, villous adenomas, which often are larger and sessile, are covered by slender villi (Fig. 15.34B). Tubulovillous adenomas have a mixture of tubular and villous elements. Although foci of invasion are more frequent in villous adenomas than in tubular adenomas, villous architecture alone does not increase cancer risk when polyp size is considered.

The histologic features of **sessile serrated adenomas,** which are also referred to as sessile serrated polyps, overlap with those of hyperplastic polyps and lack typical cytologic features of dysplasia (Fig. 15.34D). Nevertheless, sessile serrated adenomas, which are most common in the right colon, have a malignant potential similar to that of conventional adenomas. The most useful histologic feature that distinguishes sessile serrated adenomas from hyperplastic polyps is the presence of serrated architecture throughout the full length of the glands, including the crypt base, associated with crypt dilation and lateral growth, in the former (Fig. 15.34D). By contrast, serrated architecture typically is confined to the surface of hyperplastic polyps.

Although most colorectal adenomas behave in a benign fashion, a small proportion harbor invasive cancer at the time of detection. **Size is the most important characteristic that correlates with risk for malignancy.** For example, while

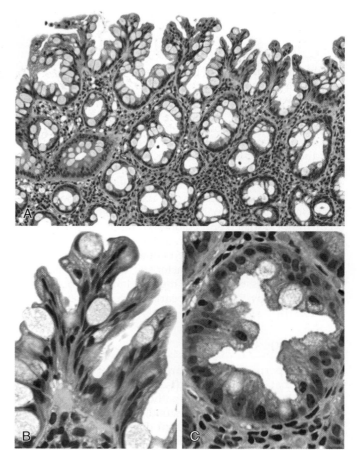

Fig. 15.32 Hyperplastic polyp. (A) Polyp surface with irregular tufting of epithelial cells. (B) Tufting results from epithelial overcrowding. (C) Epithelial crowding produces a serrated architecture when glands are cut in cross-section.

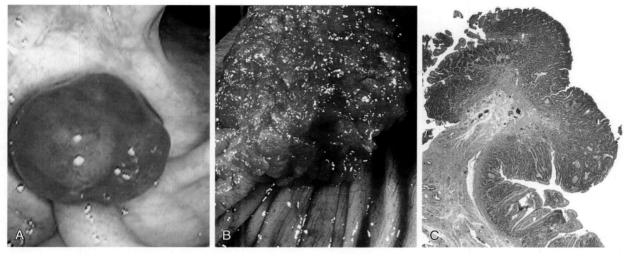

Fig. 15.33 Colonic adenomas. (A) Pedunculated adenoma (endoscopic view). (B) Adenoma with a velvety surface. (C) Low-magnification photomicrograph of a pedunculated tubular adenoma.

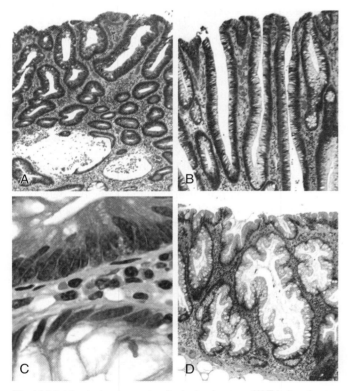

Fig. 15.34 Histologic appearance of colonic adenomas. (A) Tubular adenoma with a smooth surface and rounded glands. In this case, crypt dilation and rupture, with associated reactive inflammation, can be seen at the bottom of the field. (B) Villous adenoma with long, slender projections that are reminiscent of small-intestinal villi. (C) Dysplastic epithelial cells *(top)* with an increased nuclear-to-cytoplasmic ratio, hyperchromatic and elongated nuclei, and nuclear pseudostratification. Compare with the nondysplastic epithelium *(bottom)*. (D) Sessile serrated adenoma lined by goblet cells without typical cytologic features of dysplasia. This lesion is distinguished from a hyperplastic polyp by involvement of the crypts. Compare with the hyperplastic polyp in Fig. 15.32.

cancer is extremely rare in adenomas less than 1 cm in diameter, some studies suggest that nearly 40% of lesions larger than 4 cm in diameter contain foci of invasive cancer. In addition to size, high-grade dysplasia is a risk factor for cancer in an individual polyp (but not other polyps in the same patient).

Familial Syndromes

Several syndromes associated with colonic polyps and increased rates of colon cancer have been described. The genetic basis of these disorders has been established and has greatly enhanced the current understanding of sporadic colon cancer (Table 15.7).

Familial Adenomatous Polyps

Familial adenomatous polyposis (FAP) is an autosomal dominant disorder marked by the appearance of numerous colorectal adenomas by the teenage years. It is caused by mutations of the *adenomatous polyposis coli* gene *(APC)*. *A count of at least 100 polyps is necessary for a diagnosis of classic FAP,* and as many as several thousand may be present (Fig. 15.35). Except for their remarkable numbers, these growths are morphologically indistinguishable from sporadic adenomas. Colorectal adenocarcinoma develops in 100% of patients with untreated FAP, often before 30 years of age. As a result, prophylactic colectomy is standard therapy for individuals carrying *APC* mutations. However, patients remain at risk for *extraintestinal manifestations,* including neoplasia at other sites. Specific *APC* mutations are also associated with the development of other manifestations of FAP and explain variants such as *Gardner syndrome* and *Turcot syndrome*. In addition to intestinal polyps, clinical features of Gardner syndrome, a variant of FAP, may include osteomas of the mandible, skull, and long bones; epidermal cysts; desmoid and thyroid tumors; and dental abnormalities, including unerupted and supernumerary teeth. Turcot syndrome is rarer and is characterized by intestinal adenomas and tumors of the central nervous system. Two-thirds of

Table 15.7 Common Patterns of Sporadic and Familial Colorectal Neoplasia

Etiology	Molecular Defect	Target Gene(s)	Transmission	Predominant Site(s)	Histology
Familial adenomatous polyposis (70% of FAP)	APC/WNT pathway	APC	Autosomal dominant	None	Tubular, villous; typical adenocarcinoma
Hereditary nonpolyposis colorectal cancer	DNA mismatch repair	MSH2, MLH1	Autosomal dominant	Right side	Sessile serrated adenoma; mucinous adenocarcinoma
Sporadic colon cancer (80%)	APC/WNT pathway	APC	None	Left side	Tubular, villous; typical adenocarcinoma
Sporadic colon cancer (10%–15%)	DNA mismatch repair	MSH2, MLH1	None	Right side	Sessile serrated adenoma; mucinous adenocarcinoma

FAP, Familial adenomatous polyposis.

patients with Turcot syndrome have *APC* gene mutations and develop medulloblastomas. The remaining one-third have mutations in one of several genes involved in DNA repair and develop glioblastomas. Some patients with hundreds of adenomas lack APC mutations but instead have mutations of the base excision repair gene *MUTYH* (also called MUTYH polyposis). The role of these genes in tumor development is discussed later.

Hereditary Nonpolyposis Colorectal Cancer

Hereditary nonpolyposis colorectal cancer (HNPCC), also known as *Lynch syndrome*, originally was described as familial clustering of cancers at several sites including the colorectum, endometrium, stomach, ovary, ureters, brain,

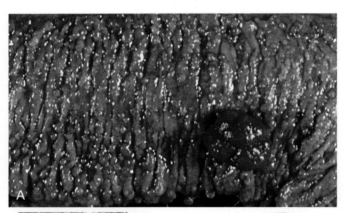

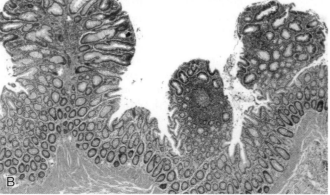

Fig. 15.35 Familial adenomatous polyposis. (A) Hundreds of small colonic polyps are present along with a dominant polyp *(right)*. (B) Three tubular adenomas are present in this single microscopic field.

small bowel, hepatobiliary tract, and skin. Colon cancers in patients with HNPCC tend to occur at younger ages than do sporadic colon cancers and often are located in the right colon (Table 15.7). Adenomas are present in HNPCC, but excessive numbers (i.e., polyposis) is not. In many cases, sessile serrated adenomas are associated with HNPCC, and mucin production may be a prominent in the subsequent adenocarcinomas.

Just as identification of *APC* mutations in FAP has provided molecular insights into the pathogenesis of a majority of sporadic colon cancers, dissection of the defects in HNPCC has shed light on the mechanisms responsible for most of the remaining sporadic cases. **HNPCC is caused by inherited germ line mutations in genes that encode proteins responsible for the detection, excision, and repair of errors that occur during DNA replication.** At least five such mismatch repair genes have been recognized, but a majority of HNPCC cases involve either *MSH2* or *MLH1*. Patients with HNPCC inherit one mutated DNA repair gene and one normal allele. When the second copy is lost through mutation or epigenetic silencing, defects in mismatch repair lead to the accumulation of mutations at rates up to 1000 times higher than normal, mostly in regions containing short repeating DNA sequences referred to as *microsatellite DNA*. The human genome contains approximately 50,000 to 100,000 microsatellites, which are prone to undergo expansion during DNA replication and represent the most frequent sites of mutations in HNPCC. The consequences of mismatch repair defects and the resulting *microsatellite instability* are discussed next in the context of colonic adenocarcinoma.

Adenocarcinoma

Adenocarcinoma of the colon is the most common malignancy of the gastrointestinal tract and is a major contributor to morbidity and mortality worldwide. By contrast, the small intestine, which accounts for 75% of the overall length of the gastrointestinal tract, is an uncommon site for benign and malignant tumors. Among malignant small-intestinal tumors, adenocarcinomas and carcinoid (neuroendocrine) tumors have roughly equal rates of occurrence, followed by lymphomas and sarcomas.

Epidemiology

Each year in the United States, there are more than 130,000 new cases and nearly 50,000 deaths from colorectal adenocarcinoma. This represents nearly 15% of all cancer-related deaths, second only to lung cancer. Colorectal cancer incidence peaks at 60 to 70 years of age; less than 20% of cases occur before 50 years of age. Males are affected slightly more often than females. Colorectal carcinoma is most prevalent in the United States, Canada, Australia, New Zealand, Denmark, Sweden, and other (so-called) developed countries that share lifestyles and diet. The incidence of this cancer is as much as 30-fold lower in India, South America, and Africa. In Japan, where incidence was previously very low, rates have now risen to intermediate levels (similar to those in the United Kingdom), presumably as a result of changes in lifestyle and diet.

The dietary factors most closely associated with increased colorectal cancer rates are low intake of unabsorbable vegetable fiber and high intake of refined carbohydrates and fat. In addition to dietary modification, pharmacologic chemoprevention has become an area of great interest. Several epidemiologic studies suggest that aspirin or other NSAIDs have a protective effect. This is consistent with studies showing that some NSAIDs cause polyp regression in patients with FAP in whom the rectum was left in place after colectomy. It is suspected that this effect is mediated by inhibition of the enzyme cyclooxygenase-2 (COX-2), which is highly expressed in 90% of colorectal carcinomas and 40% to 90% of adenomas and is known to promote epithelial proliferation, particularly in response to injury.

Pathogenesis

Studies of colorectal carcinogenesis have provided fundamental insights into the general mechanisms of cancer evolution. The combination of molecular events that lead to colonic adenocarcinoma is heterogeneous and includes genetic and epigenetic abnormalities. At least two distinct genetic pathways, the APC/β-catenin pathway and the microsatellite instability pathway, have been described. In simplest terms, mutations involving the APC/β-catenin pathway lead to increased WNT signaling, whereas those involving the microsatellite instability pathway are associated with defects in DNA mismatch repair (see Table 15.7). Both pathways involve the stepwise accumulation of multiple mutations, but the genes involved and the mechanisms by which the mutations accumulate differ. Epigenetic events, the most common of which is methylation-induced gene silencing, may enhance progression along both pathways.

- *The APC/β-catenin pathway.* The classic *adenoma-carcinoma sequence,* which accounts for as much as 80% of sporadic colon tumors, typically involves mutation of the *APC* tumor suppressor early in the neoplastic process (Fig. 15.36). For adenomas to develop, both copies of the *APC* gene must be functionally inactivated, either by mutation or epigenetic events. *APC is a key negative regulator of β-catenin, a component of the WNT signaling pathway* (Chapter 6). The APC protein normally binds to and promotes degradation of β-catenin. With loss of APC function, β-catenin accumulates and translocates to the nucleus, where it activates the transcription of genes, such as those encoding MYC and cyclin D1, that promote proliferation. This is followed by additional mutations, including activating mutations in *KRAS,* which also promote growth and prevent apoptosis. The conclusion that mutation of *KRAS* is a late event is supported by the observations that mutations are present in fewer than 10% of adenomas less than 1 cm in diameter, 50% of adenomas greater than 1 cm in diameter, and 50% of invasive adenocarcinomas. Neoplastic progression also is associated with mutations in other tumor suppressor genes such as *SMAD2* and *SMAD4,* which encode effectors of TGF-β signaling. Because TGF-β signaling normally inhibits the cell cycle, loss of these genes may allow unrestrained cell growth.

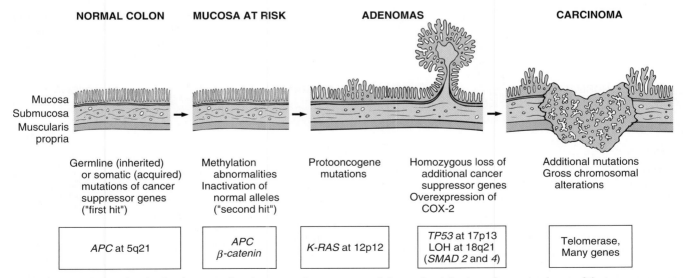

Fig. 15.36 Morphologic and molecular changes in the adenoma-carcinoma sequence. It is postulated that loss of one normal copy of the tumor suppressor gene *APC* occurs early. Individuals may be born with one mutant allele, making them extremely prone to the development of colon cancer, or inactivation of APC may occur later in life. This is the "first hit" according to Knudson's hypothesis. The loss of the intact copy of *APC* follows ("second hit"). Other mutations involving *KRAS, SMAD2, and SMAD4,* and the tumor suppressor gene *TP53,* lead to the emergence of carcinoma, in which additional mutations occur. Although there may be a preferred temporal sequence for these changes, it is the aggregate effect of the mutations, rather than their order of occurrence, that appears most critical.

The tumor suppressor gene *TP53* is mutated in 70% to 80% of colon cancers but is uncommonly affected in adenomas, suggesting that *TP53* mutations also occur at late stages of tumor progression. Loss of function of *TP53* and other tumor suppressor genes is often caused by chromosomal deletions, highlighting *chromosomal instability as a hallmark of the APC/β-catenin pathway*. Alternatively, tumor suppressor genes may be silenced by methylation of CpG islands, a 5′ region of some genes that frequently includes the promoter and transcriptional start site. Expression of telomerase also increases as lesions become more advanced.

- *The microsatellite instability pathway.* In patients with DNA mismatch repair deficiency (due to loss of mismatch repair genes, as discussed earlier), mutations accumulate in microsatellite repeats, a condition referred to as *microsatellite instability*. These mutations generally are silent, because microsatellites typically are located in noncoding regions, but other microsatellite sequences are located in the coding or promoter regions of genes involved in regulation of cell growth, such as those encoding the type II TGF-β receptor and the pro-apoptotic protein BAX (Fig. 15.37). Because TGF-β inhibits colonic epithelial cell proliferation, type II TGF-β receptor mutants can contribute to uncontrolled cell growth, while loss of *BAX* may enhance the survival of genetically abnormal clones.

- *CpG island hypermethylation phenotype (CIMP).* In a subset of colon cancers with microsatellite instability, there are no mutations in DNA mismatch repair enzymes. These tumors demonstrate the CpG island hypermethylation phenotype (CIMP). In these tumors, the MLH1 promoter region is typically hypermethylated, thereby reducing MLH1 expression and repair function. Activating mutations in the *BRAF* oncogene are common in these cancers. In contrast, KRAS and TP53 are not typically mutated. Thus, the combination of microsatellite instability, BRAF mutation, and methylation of specific targets, such as MLH1, is the signature of this pathway of carcinogenesis.

MORPHOLOGY

Overall, adenocarcinomas are distributed approximately equally over the entire length of the colon. **Tumors in the proximal colon often grow as polypoid, exophytic masses** that extend along one wall of the large-caliber cecum and ascending colon; these tumors rarely cause obstruction (Fig. 15.38A). By contrast, **carcinomas in the distal colon tend to be annular lesions that produce "napkin ring"** constrictions and luminal narrowing (Fig. 15.38B), sometimes to the point of obstruction. Both forms grow into the bowel wall over time and may be palpable as firm masses (Fig. 15.38C). The general microscopic characteristics of right- and left-sided colonic adenocarcinomas are similar. Most tumors are composed of tall columnar cells that resemble dysplastic epithelium found in adenomas (Fig. 15.39A). The invasive component of these tumors elicits a strong stromal desmoplastic response, which is responsible for their characteristic firm consistency. Some poorly differentiated tumors form few glands (Fig. 15.39B). Others may produce abundant mucin that accumulates within the intestinal wall, and these carry a poor prognosis. Tumors also may be composed of signet ring cells similar to those in gastric cancer (Fig. 15.39C).

Clinical Features

The availability of endoscopic screening combined with the recognition that most carcinomas arise within adenomas presents a unique opportunity for cancer prevention. Unfortunately, colorectal cancers develop insidiously and may therefore go undetected for long periods. Cecal and other *right-sided colon cancers* most often are called to clinical attention by the appearance of *fatigue and weakness due to iron-deficiency anemia*. **Thus, it is a clinical maxim that the underlying cause of iron-deficiency anemia in an older male or postmenopausal female is gastrointestinal cancer until proven otherwise.** *Left-sided colorectal adenocarcinomas* may produce *occult bleeding, changes in bowel habits, or cramping* left lower-quadrant discomfort.

Although poorly differentiated and mucinous histologic patterns are associated with poor prognosis, *the two most important prognostic factors are depth of invasion and the*

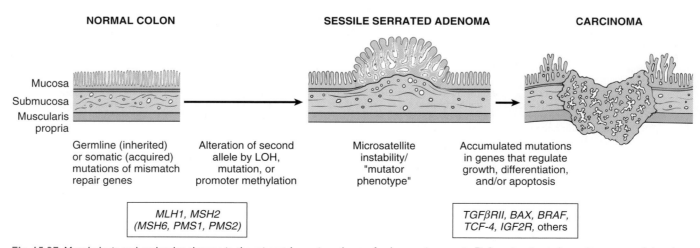

Fig. 15.37 Morphologic and molecular changes in the mismatch repair pathway of colon carcinogenesis. Defects in mismatch repair genes result in microsatellite instability and permit accumulation of mutations in numerous genes. If these mutations affect genes involved in cell survival and proliferation, cancer may develop. *LOH,* Loss of heterozygosity.

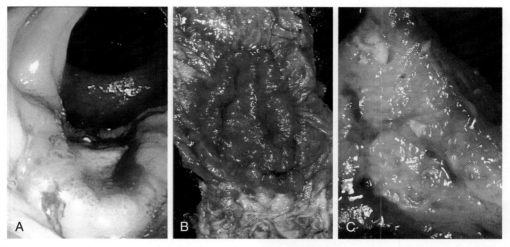

Fig. 15.38 Colorectal carcinoma. (A) Endoscopic view of ulcerated ascending colon adenocarcinoma. (B) Circumferential, ulcerated rectal cancer. Note the anal mucosa at the bottom of the image. (C) Cancer of the sigmoid colon that has invaded through the muscularis propria and is present within subserosal adipose tissue *(left)*. Areas of chalky necrosis are present within the colon wall *(arrow)*. *(Endoscopic image courtesy of Dr. Ira Hanan, The University of Chicago, Chicago, Illinois.)*

presence or absence of lymph node metastases. These factors were originally recognized by Dukes and Kirklin and form the core of the TNM (tumor-node-metastasis) classification and staging system from the American Joint Committee on Cancer. Staging systems have become more complex with time, reflecting more nuanced treatment approaches and personalized therapeutic strategies. The most important distinctions are:

- *Depth of invasion.* Tumors limited to the submucosa (i.e., those that do not cross the muscularis mucosae) have 5-year survival rates approaching 100%, while invasion into the submucosa or muscularis propria reduces 5-year survival to 95% and 70% to 90%, respectively (for tumors limited to the primary site). Invasion through the visceral serosal surface or into adjacent organs and tissues reduces survival further.
- *The presence of lymph node metastases* (Fig. 15.40A) further compromises survival. As a result, most cases with lymph node metastases receive radiation or

chemotherapy. In some cases, these treatments may be administered prior to primary tumor resection, a process termed neoadjuvant therapy. Molecular characterization of the tumor can be helpful in guiding the specific therapeutic approach.

- *Distant metastases* to lung (Fig. 15.40B), liver (Fig. 15.40C), or other sites also limits survival, and only 15% or fewer of patients with tumors at this stage are alive 5 years after diagnosis. Because of the portal drainage, the liver is the most common site of metastatic lesions. However, the rectum does not drain by way of the portal circulation, and metastases from carcinomas of the anorectum region often circumvent the liver.

Regardless of stage, however, some patients with small numbers of metastases do well for years after resection of distant tumor nodules. This is particularly true of metastases to liver or lung and emphasizes the clinical and molecular heterogeneity of colorectal carcinomas.

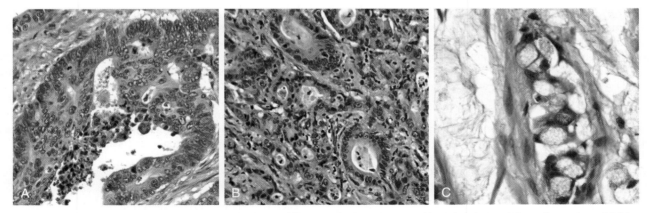

Fig. 15.39 Histologic appearance of colorectal carcinoma. (A) Well-differentiated adenocarcinoma. Note the elongated, hyperchromatic nuclei. Necrotic debris, present in the gland lumen, is typical. (B) Poorly differentiated adenocarcinoma forms a few glands but is largely composed of infiltrating nests of tumor cells. (C) Mucinous adenocarcinoma with signet ring cells and extracellular mucin pools.

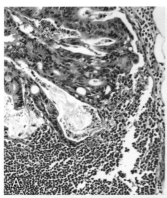
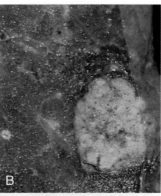
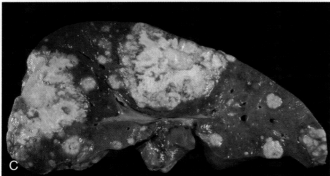

Fig. 15.40 Metastatic colorectal carcinoma. (A) Lymph node metastasis. Note the glandular structures within the subcapsular sinus. (B) Solitary subpleural nodule of colorectal carcinoma metastatic to the lung. (C) Liver containing two large and many smaller metastases. Note the central necrosis within metastases.

SUMMARY

COLONIC POLYPS, ADENOMAS, AND ADENOCARCINOMAS

- *Intestinal polyps* can be classified as *nonneoplastic* or *neoplastic*. The nonneoplastic polyps can be further defined as *inflammatory*, *hamartomatous*, or *hyperplastic*.
- *Inflammatory polyps* form as a result of chronic cycles of injury and healing.
- *Hamartomatous polyps* occur sporadically or as a part of genetic diseases. In the latter case, they often are associated with increased risk for malignancy.
- *Hyperplastic polyps* are benign epithelial proliferations most commonly found in the left colon and rectum. They are not reactive in origin, in contrast with gastric hyperplastic polyps; have no malignant potential; and must be distinguished from sessile serrated adenomas or polyps.
- *Benign epithelial neoplastic polyps* of the colon are termed *adenomas*. The hallmark feature of these lesions, which are the precursors of colonic adenocarcinomas, is cytologic dysplasia.
- In contrast with traditional adenomas, *sessile serrated adenomas*, or polyps, lack cytologic dysplasia and share some morphologic features with hyperplastic polyps.
- *Familial adenomatous polyposis (FAP)* and *hereditary nonpolyposis colorectal cancer (HNPCC)* are the most common forms of familial colon cancer. FAP is caused by *APC* mutations, and patients typically have over 100 adenomas and develop colon cancer before 30 years of age.
- HNPCC is caused by mutations in DNA mismatch repair genes. Patients with HNPCC have far fewer polyps and develop cancer at an older age than that typical for patients with FAP but at a younger age than in patients with sporadic colon cancer.
- The vast majority of colonic cancers are adenocarcinomas. They arise either by APC-β-catenin pathway or the microsatellite instability pathway. The two most important prognostic factors are depth of invasion and the presence or absence of metastases to lymph nodes or distant organs.

Appendix

The appendix is a normal true diverticulum of the cecum. Like any diverticulum, it is prone to acute and chronic inflammation, and acute appendicitis is a relatively common entity. Other lesions, including tumors, can also occur in the appendix but are far less common.

ACUTE APPENDICITIS

Acute appendicitis is most common in adolescents and young adults but may occur in any age group. The lifetime risk for appendicitis is 7%; males are affected slightly more often than females. Despite the prevalence of acute appendicitis, the diagnosis can be difficult to confirm preoperatively, and the condition may be confused with mesenteric lymphadenitis, acute salpingitis, ectopic pregnancy, mittelschmerz (pain associated with ovulation), and Meckel diverticulitis.

Pathogenesis

Acute appendicitis is thought to be initiated by progressive increase in intraluminal pressure that compromises venous outflow. In 50% to 80% of cases, acute appendicitis is associated with overt luminal obstruction, usually by a small, stone-like mass of stool, or *fecalith,* or, less commonly, a gallstone, tumor, or mass of worms. Ischemic injury and stasis of luminal contents, which favor bacterial proliferation, trigger inflammatory responses including tissue edema and neutrophilic infiltration of the lumen, muscular wall, and periappendiceal soft tissues.

MORPHOLOGY

In early acute appendicitis, subserosal vessels are congested, and a modest perivascular neutrophilic infiltrate is present within all layers of the wall. The inflammatory reaction transforms the normal glistening serosa into a dull, granular-appearing, erythematous surface. Although mucosal neutrophils and focal superficial ulceration often are present, these findings are not specific, and diagnosis of acute appendicitis requires neutrophilic infiltration of the muscularis propria. In more severe cases, focal abscesses may form within the wall **(acute suppurative appendicitis),** and these may even progress to large areas of hemorrhagic ulceration and gangrenous necrosis that extend to the serosa, creating **acute gangrenous appendicitis,** which often is followed by rupture and suppurative peritonitis.

Clinical Features

Typically, early acute appendicitis produces periumbilical pain that ultimately localizes to the right lower quadrant, followed by nausea, vomiting, low-grade fever, and a mildly elevated peripheral white blood cell count. A classic physical finding is *McBurney's sign,* deep tenderness noted at a location two-thirds of the distance from the umbilicus to the right anterior superior iliac spine (McBurney's point). These signs and symptoms however, are often absent, creating difficulty in clinical diagnosis.

TUMORS OF THE APPENDIX

The most common tumor of the appendix is the *carcinoid,* or well-differentiated neuroendocrine tumor. It usually is discovered incidentally at the time of surgery or on examination of a resected appendix. This neoplasm most frequently involves the distal tip of the appendix, where it produces a solid bulbous swelling up to 2 to 3 cm in diameter. Although intramural and transmural extension may be evident, nodal metastases are very infrequent, and distant spread is exceptionally rare. Conventional *adenomas* or *non–mucin-producing adenocarcinomas* also occur in the appendix and may cause obstruction and enlargement that mimics the changes of acute appendicitis. *Mucocele,* a dilated appendix filled with mucin, may simply stem from an obstructed appendix containing inspissated mucin or may be a consequence of *mucinous cystadenoma* or *mucinous cystadenocarcinoma.* In the latter instance invasion through the appendiceal wall can lead to intraperitoneal seeding and spread. In women, the resulting peritoneal implants may be mistaken for mucinous ovarian tumors. In the most advanced cases, the abdomen fills with tenacious, semisolid mucin, a condition called *pseudomyxoma peritonei.* This disseminated intraperitoneal disease may be held in check for years by repeated debulking, but ultimately is fatal in most instances.

SUMMARY

APPENDIX

- Acute appendicitis is most common in children and adolescents. It is thought to be initiated by increased intraluminal pressure consequent to obstruction of the appendiceal lumen, which compromises venous outflow.

- The most common tumor of the appendix, the *carcinoid,* or *well-differentiated neuroendocrine tumor,* is most often discovered incidentally and is almost always benign
- The clinical presentation of appendiceal adenocarcinoma can be indistinguishable from that of acute appendicitis, although the former tends to present in older patients.

SUGGESTED READINGS

Oral Cavity

Hennessey PT, Westra WH, Califano JA: Human papillomavirus and head and neck squamous cell carcinoma: recent evidence and clinical implications, *J Dent Res* 88:300, 2009. *[A discussion of head and neck cancers associated with HPV.]*

Leemans CR, Braakhuis BJ, Brakenhoff RH: The molecular biology of head and neck cancer, *Nat Rev Cancer* 11:9, 2011. *[A discussion of the molecular biology of head and neck cancer.]*

Leivo I: Insights into a complex group of neoplastic disease: advances in histopathologic classification and molecular pathology of salivary gland cancer, *Acta Oncol* 45:662, 2006. *[A good review of the histologic spectrum of salivary gland tumors.]*

Esophagus

Abonia JP, Rothenberg ME: Eosinophilic esophagitis: rapidly advancing insights, *Annu Rev Med* 63:421–434, 2012. *[A comprehensive review of eosinophilic esophagitis.]*

Boeckxstaens GE, Zaninotto G, Richter JE: Achalasia, *Lancet* 383:83–93, 2014. *[A clinically focused discussion of achalasia.]*

Clave P, Shaker R: Dysphagia: current reality and scope of the problem, *Nat Rev Gastroenterol Hepatol* 12:259–270, 2015. *[A brief review of dysphagia management.]*

McDonald SAC, Graham TA, Lavery DL, et al: The Barrett's gland in phenotype space, *Cell Mol Gastroenterol Hepatol* 1:41–54, 2015. *[A detailed diiscussion of Barrett esophagus and metaplasia.]*

Spechler SJ, Souza RF: Barrett's esophagus, *N Engl J Med* 371:836–845, 2014. *[A clinically oriented review of Barrett esophagus.]*

Stomach

Lin JT: Screening of gastric cancer: who, when, and how, *Clin Gastroenterol Hepatol* 12:135–138, 2014. *[A discussion of gastric cancer screening indications and efficacy.]*

Shaib YH, Rugge M, Graham DY, et al: Management of gastric polyps: an endoscopy-based approach, *Clin Gastroenterol Hepatol* 11:1374–1384, 2013. *[A discussion of gastric polyps and their management.]*

Wroblewski LE, Peek RM Jr: Helicobacter pylori in gastric carcinogenesis: mechanisms, *Gastroenterol Clin North Am* 42:285–298, 2013. *[A comprehensive review of gastritis-associated gastric cancer.]*

Intestinal Obstruction

Schappi MG, Staiano A, Milla PJ, et al: A practical guide for the diagnosis of primary enteric nervous system disorders, *J Pediatr Gastroenterol Nutr* 57:677–686, 2013. *[A clinically oriented review of dysmotility.]*

Diarrhea

Barzilay EJ, Schaad N, Magloire R, et al: Cholera surveillance during the Haiti epidemic—the first 2 years, *N Engl J Med* 368:599–609, 2013. *[A review of the Haitian cholera epidemic.]*

Camilleri M: Intestinal secretory mechanisms in irritable bowel syndrome—diarrhea, *Clin Gastroenterol Hepatol* 13:1051–1057, quiz e61–e62, 2015. *[A discussion of defects in secretion in patients with irritable bowel syndrome.]*

Ludvigsson JF, Green PH: The missing environmental factor in celiac disease, *N Engl J Med* 371:1341–1343, 2014. *[A review of celiac disease pathogenesis.]*

van Nood E, Vrieze A, Nieuwdorp M, et al: Duodenal infusion of donor feces for recurrent *Clostridium difficile*, *N Engl J Med* 368: 407–415, 2013. *[The first series showing efficacy of fecal microbial transplantation for recurrent C. difficile infection.]*

Sigmoid Diverticulitis
Mosadeghi S, Bhuket T, Stollman N: Diverticular disease: evolving concepts in classification, presentation, and management, *Curr Opin Gastroenterol* 31:50–55, 2015. *[A review of diverticulitis and approaches to its treatment.]*

Inflammatory Bowel Disease
Jostins L, Ripke S, Weersma RK, et al: Host-microbe interactions have shaped the genetic architecture of inflammatory bowel disease, *Nature* 491:119–124, 2012. *[A comprehensive review of polymorphisms linked to inflammatory bowel disease and their relationship to immune defense.]*

Rogler G: Chronic ulcerative colitis and colorectal cancer, *Cancer Lett* 345:235–241, 2014. *[A review of colitis-associated cancer.]*

Colonic Polyps and Neoplastic Disease
Brenner H, Kloor M, Pox CP: Colorectal cancer, *Lancet* 383:1490–1502, 2014. *[A clinically oriented review of colorectal cancer.]*

Corley DA, Levin TR: Doubeni CA: Adenoma detection rate and risk of colorectal cancer and death, *N Engl J Med* 370:2541, 2014. *[A study of adenoma detection and relationship to cancer risk.]*

Appendix
Cartwright SL, Knudson MP: Evaluation of acute abdominal pain in adults, *Am Fam Physician* 77:971, 2008. *[Clinically oriented approach to the acute abdomen.]*

Deschamps L, Couvelard A: Endocrine tumors of the appendix: a pathologic review, *Arch Pathol Lab Med* 134:871, 2010. *[Pathology-focused review of appendiceal carcinoid tumors.]*

Liver and Gallbladder 16

CHAPTER OUTLINE

The Liver and Bile Ducts 637
General Features of Liver Disease 638
Mechanisms of Injury and Repair 638
Liver Failure 639
Infectious Disorders 642
Viral Hepatitis 642
Bacterial, Parasitic, and Helminthic
  Infections 650
Autoimmune Hepatitis 651
Drug- and Toxin-Induced Liver
  Injury 651
Alcoholic and Nonalcoholic Fatty Liver
  Disease 652
Alcoholic Liver Disease 653
Nonalcoholic Fatty Liver Disease 655

Inherited Metabolic Liver Diseases 656
Hemochromatosis 656
Wilson Disease 657
α_1-Anti-Trypsin Deficiency 658
Cholestatic Syndromes 659
Bilirubin and Bile Formation 659
Pathophysiology of Jaundice 660
Defects in Hepatocellular Bilirubin
  Metabolism 661
Cholestasis 661
Neonatal Cholestasis 662
Biliary Atresia 663
Autoimmune Cholangiopathies 663
Circulatory Disorders 666
Impaired Blood Flow Into the Liver 666

Impaired Blood Flow Through the Liver 667
Hepatic Venous Outflow Obstruction 667
Passive Congestion and Centrilobular
  Necrosis 667
Nodules and Tumors 668
Focal Nodular Hyperplasia 668
Benign Neoplasms 669
Malignant Neoplasms 669
Gallbladder 672
Gallstone Disease 672
Cholecystitis 674
Acute Calculous Cholecystitis 674
Acute Acalculous Cholecystitis 674
Chronic Cholecystitis 674
Carcinoma of the Gallbladder 675

The Liver and Bile Ducts

The normal adult liver weighs 1400 to 1600 gm. It has a dual blood supply, with the portal vein providing 60% to 70% of hepatic blood flow and the hepatic artery supplying the remaining 30% to 40%. The portal vein and the hepatic artery enter the inferior aspect of the liver through the hilum, or *porta hepatis*. Within the liver, the branches of the portal veins, hepatic arteries, and bile ducts travel in parallel within *portal tracts*, ramifying variably through 10 to 12 orders of branches.

The most common terminology used to describe the hepatic microarchitecture is based on the lobular model (Fig. 16.1). This model divides the liver into lobules 1- to 2-mm in diameter that are centered on a terminal tributary of the hepatic vein and demarcated by portal tracts at their periphery. These lobules are often drawn as hexagonal structures, though in humans the shapes are far more variable; nonetheless, it is a useful simplification. A second model divides the liver into triangular acini (see Fig. 16.1) based on the position of hepatocytes relative to their blood supply. The hepatocytes in the vicinity of the terminal hepatic vein are called *centrilobular*; those near the portal tract are *periportal*. **Division of the lobular parenchyma into zones is an important concept because each zone differs with respect to its metabolic** **activities and susceptibility to certain forms of hepatic injury.**

Within the lobule, hepatocytes are organized into anastomosing sheets or "plates" extending from portal tracts to the terminal hepatic veins. Between the trabecular plates of hepatocytes are vascular *sinusoids*. Blood traverses the sinusoids and exits into the terminal hepatic veins through numerous orifices in the vein wall. Hepatocytes are thus bathed by well-mixed portal venous blood on one side and hepatic arterial blood on the other. The sinusoids are lined by a fenestrated endothelium that overlies a perisinusoidal space (the *space of Disse*) into which abundant hepatocyte microvilli protrude. Attached to the luminal face of the sinusoids are scattered *Kupffer cells*, specialized long-lived tissue macrophages that arise early in embryogenesis. Another specialized cell type, the *hepatic stellate cell*, is found in the space of Disse and has a role in the storage of vitamin A. Between abutting hepatocytes are *bile canaliculi*, channels 1 to 2 μm in diameter that are formed by grooves in the plasma membranes of adjacent hepatocytes and are separated from the vascular space by tight junctions. These channels drain successively into the intralobular *canals of Hering*, periportal *bile ductules*, and finally into the *terminal bile ducts* within the portal tracts.

Lobule

Acinus

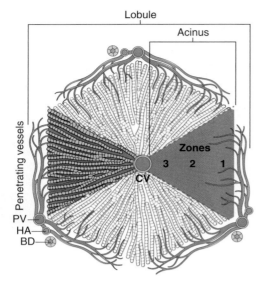

Fig. 16.1 Models of liver anatomy. In the lobular model, the terminal hepatic vein is at the center of a "lobule," while the portal tracts are at the periphery. Pathologists often refer to the regions of the parenchyma as "periportal and centrilobular." In the acinar model, on the basis of blood flow, three zones can be defined, zone 1 being the closest to the blood supply and zone 3 being the farthest. *BD,* Bile duct; *CV,* central hepatic vein; *HA,* hepatic artery; *PV,* portal tracts.

Table 16.1 Laboratory Evaluation of Liver Disease

Test Category	Blood Measurement*
Hepatocyte integrity	Cytosolic hepatocellular enzymes†
	Serum aspartate aminotransferase (AST)
	Serum alanine aminotransferase (ALT)
	Serum lactate dehydrogenase (LDH)
Biliary excretory function	Substances normally secreted in bile†
	Serum bilirubin
	Total: unconjugated plus conjugated
	Direct: conjugated only
	Urine bilirubin
	Serum bile acids
	Plasma membrane enzymes (from damage to bile canaliculus)†
	Serum alkaline phosphatase
	Serum γ-glutamyl transpeptidase (GGT)
Hepatocyte function	Proteins secreted into the blood
	Serum albumin‡
	Prothrombin time (PT)†
	Partial thromboplastin time (PTT)†
	Hepatocyte metabolism
	Serum ammonia†
	Aminopyrine breath test (hepatic demethylation)‡

*Most commonly used tests are in italics; †an elevation suggests liver disease; ‡a decrease suggests liver disease.

GENERAL FEATURES OF LIVER DISEASE

The major primary diseases of the liver are viral hepatitis, alcoholic liver disease, nonalcoholic fatty liver disease (NAFLD), and hepatocellular carcinoma (HCC). The liver also is frequently damaged secondarily in a variety of common disorders, such as cardiac disease, disseminated cancer, and extrahepatic infections. The functional reserve of the liver masks the clinical impact of mild liver damage, but severe diffuse liver disease often has life-threatening consequences.

With the rare exception of fulminant hepatic failure, liver disease is an insidious process in which the signs and symptoms of hepatic decompensation appear weeks, months, or even years after the onset of injury. The hepatic injury may be imperceptible to the patient and be manifest only by laboratory test abnormalities (Table 16.1), and liver injury and healing also may be subclinical. Hence, individuals with hepatic abnormalities who are referred to hepatologists most frequently have chronic liver disease.

Mechanisms of Injury and Repair

Injured hepatocytes may show several potentially reversible changes, such as accumulation of fat and bilirubin (cholestasis); when injury is not reversible, hepatocytes die by necrosis or apoptosis. Necrosis (Fig. 16.2) is commonly seen following hepatic injury caused by hypoxia and ischemia. Apoptotic cell death (Fig. 16.3) predominates in viral, autoimmune, and drug- and toxin-induced hepatitides.

Widespread death of hepatocytes may produce *confluent necrosis.* This may be seen in acute toxic or ischemic injuries or in severe chronic viral or autoimmune hepatitis. Confluent necrosis begins as a zone of hepatocyte dropout around the central vein. With increasing severity necrosis

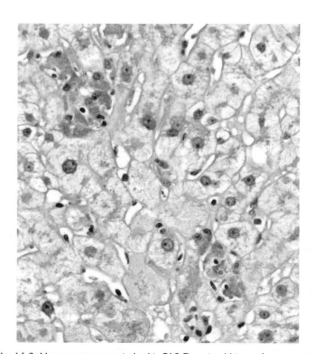

Fig. 16.2 Hepatocyte necrosis. In this PAS-D—stained biopsy from a patient with acute hepatitis B, clusters of pigmented hepatocytes with eosinophilic cytoplasm indicate foci of hepatocytes undergoing necrosis. *PAS-D,* Periodic acid-Schiff stain after diastase digestion.

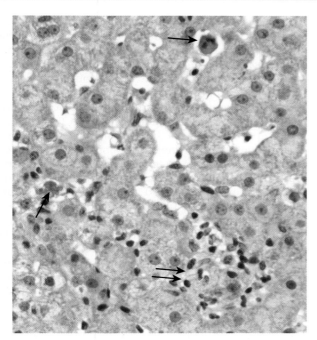

Fig. 16.3 Hepatocyte apoptosis. This biopsy from a patient with lobular hepatitis due to chronic hepatitis C shows scattered apoptotic hepatocytes ("acidophil bodies"; *single arrows*) and a patchy inflammatory infiltrate *(double arrows)*.

"bridges" central veins and portal tracts or adjacent portal tracts.

Regeneration of lost hepatocytes takes place primarily by mitotic replication of hepatocytes adjacent to those that have died. In more severe forms of acute liver injury hepatic stem cells located in a niche near the canal of Hering may also begin to divide, but the contribution of stem cells to the replenishment of hepatocytes in the setting of acute liver damage remains uncertain. In longstanding chronic liver diseases, however, there is clear evidence that stem cell proliferation and differentiation make significant contributions to parenchymal restoration, probably following the replicative senescence of preexisting hepatocytes. The differentiating progeny of these tissue stem cells produce duct-like structures, called *ductular reactions,* a morphologic marker of stem cell–mediated liver regeneration.

Scar formation may follow very severe acute injury, but occurs more often as a reaction to chronic injury. The principal cell type involved in scar deposition is the perisinusoidal hepatic stellate cell. Following liver injury, stellate cells may become activated and convert into highly fibrogenic myofibroblasts, which produce the fibrous scar. Stellate cell activation involves complex interactions between Kupffer cells, hepatocytes, and inflammatory cells. When there is severe injury that causes death of large number of hepatocytes and the drop out of liver cells, there may be collapse of the underlying reticulin, precluding orderly regeneration of hepatocytes. In such cases, there is activation of stellate cells, and the areas of liver cell loss are replaced by fibrous septae. Eventually, these fibrous septa encircle surviving, regenerating hepatocytes in late-stage chronic liver disease, many forms of which are described as *cirrhosis.*

Inflammation and immunologic reactions are involved in many forms of liver disease. Systemic inflammation alters the metabolic and biosynthetic activities of the liver, leading to increased secretion of acute-phase reactants such as C-reactive protein, serum amyloid A protein (a precursor of some forms of amyloid) and hepcidin, a key regulator of iron metabolism (Chapter 12). As we will discuss, adaptive immune cells play a critical role in viral hepatitis, with CD4+ and CD8+ T cells being particularly important in the eradication of virus-infected hepatocytes and, in chronic disease, liver injury.

Liver Failure

The most severe clinical consequence of liver disease is liver failure. It primarily occurs in three clinical scenarios: acute, chronic, and acute-on-chronic liver failure.

Acute Liver Failure

Acute liver failure is defined as a liver disease that produces hepatic encephalopathy within 6 months of the initial diagnosis. The condition is known as *fulminant liver failure* when the encephalopathy develops within 2 weeks of the onset of jaundice, and as *subfulminant liver failure* when the encephalopathy develops within 3 months. In the United States, accidental or deliberate ingestion of acetaminophen accounts for almost 50% of cases of acute liver failure, while autoimmune hepatitis, other drugs and toxins, and acute hepatitis A and B infections account for the remainder of cases. In Asia, acute hepatitis B and E predominate as causes of acute liver failure.

MORPHOLOGY

The clinical syndrome of acute liver failure is reflected anatomically and histologically as **massive hepatic necrosis.** The liver is small and shrunken due to loss of parenchyma (Fig. 16.4A). Microscopically, there are large zones of destruction surrounding occasional islands of regenerating hepatocytes (Fig. 16.4B). Scar is mostly absent given the acute nature of the process.

Clinical Features

Acute liver failure manifests with nausea, vomiting, jaundice, and fatigue, which are followed by the onset of life-threatening encephalopathy, coagulation defects, and portal hypertension associated with ascites. Typically, transaminase levels in the serum are elevated into the thousands. The liver is initially enlarged by swelling and edema related to inflammation, but then as parenchyma is destroyed the liver shrinks dramatically. Eventually, as hepatocytes are lost, serum transaminase values level off and then decline rapidly as their source disappears. Worsening jaundice, coagulopathy, and encephalopathy develop; with unabated progression, the end result is multiorgan failure and, without transplantation, death. Manifestations of acute liver failure include the following:

- *Jaundice* and *icterus* (yellow discoloration of the skin and sclera, respectively) due to retention of bilirubin, and *cholestasis* due to systemic retention of not only bilirubin but also other solutes eliminated in bile.

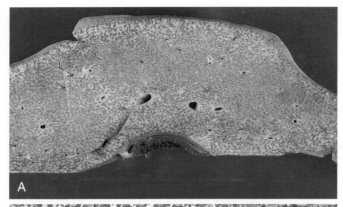

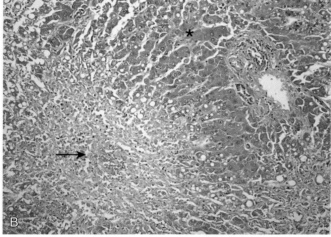

Fig. 16.4 Massive liver necrosis. (A) The liver is small (700 g), bile-stained, soft, and congested. (B) Hepatocellular necrosis caused by acetaminophen overdose. Confluent necrosis is seen in the perivenular region (zone 3, *arrow*). There is little inflammation. Residual normal tissue is indicated by the *asterisk*. *(Courtesy of Dr. Matthew Yeh, University of Washington, Seattle, Washington).*

- *Hepatic encephalopathy* encompasses a spectrum of disturbances in consciousness ranging from subtle behavioral abnormalities, to confusion and stupor, to coma and death. Encephalopathy may develop over days, weeks, or a few months after acute injury. Fluctuating neurologic signs, including rigidity, hyperreflexia, and *asterixis,* may develop. Asterixis refers to a nonrhythmic rapid extension-flexion movement of the head and extremities, best seen as "flapping" of the hands when the arms are held in extension with dorsiflexed wrists. Elevated ammonia levels in blood and the central nervous system correlate with impaired neuronal function and brain edema.
- *Coagulopathy.* The liver is the source of a number of coagulation factors that decline in the face of liver failure, leading to easy bruising and bleeding. Paradoxically, *disseminated intravascular coagulation* (Chapter 12) also may occur due to failure of the damaged liver to remove activated coagulation factors.
- *Portal hypertension* arises when there is diminished flow through the portal venous system, which may occur because of obstruction at the prehepatic, intrahepatic, or posthepatic level. While it can occur in acute live failure, portal hypertension is more commonly seen with

chronic liver failure and is discussed later. In acute liver failure, the obstruction is usually intrahepatic and the major clinical consequences are *ascites* and *hepatic encephalopathy.* In chronic liver disease, portal hypertension develops over months to years, and its effects are more complex and widespread (see later).

- *Hepatorenal syndrome* is a form of renal failure occurring in individuals with liver failure in whom there are no intrinsic morphologic or functional causes for kidney dysfunction. Sodium retention, impaired free-water excretion, and decreased renal perfusion and glomerular filtration rate are the main renal functional abnormalities. There is decreased renal perfusion pressure due to systemic vasodilation, activation of the renal sympathetic nervous system and vasoconstriction of the afferent renal arterioles, and increased activation of the renin-angiotensin axis, causing vasoconstriction that further decreases glomerular filtration. The syndrome's onset begins with a decrease in urine output and rising blood urea nitrogen and creatinine levels.

Chronic Liver Failure and Cirrhosis

Cirrhosis is the morphologic change most often associated with chronic liver disease; it refers to the diffuse transformation of the liver into regenerative parenchymal nodules surrounded by fibrous bands (Fig. 16.5). The leading causes of chronic liver failure worldwide include chronic hepatitis B, chronic hepatitis C, non-alcoholic fatty liver disease (NAFLD), and alcoholic liver disease. While cirrhosis is a common feature of a number of chronic liver diseases, it is not a specific entity, and it is important to recognize that not all chronic liver disease terminates in cirrhosis, and that not all cirrhosis leads to end-stage liver disease. For example, chronic biliary tract diseases often do not give rise to cirrhosis even at end stage, whereas patients with treated autoimmune hepatitis or cured hepatitis C may have adequate liver function in the face of cirrhosis. Even in diseases that are likely to give rise to cirrhosis, such as untreated viral hepatitis, alcoholic liver disease, NAFLD, and metabolic diseases, the morphology and pathophysiology of cirrhosis in each may be different.

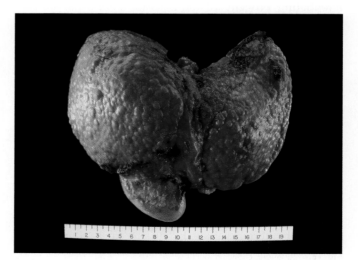

Fig. 16.5 Cirrhosis resulting from chronic viral hepatitis. Note the broad scars separating bulging regenerative nodules over the liver surface.

MORPHOLOGY

Liver failure in **chronic** liver disease is most often associated with cirrhosis, which is marked by the diffuse transformation of the entire liver into **regenerative parenchymal nodules surrounded by fibrous bands**. The nodular nature of the process is readily evident both grossly (Fig. 16.5) and microscopically (Fig. 16.6, A). The size of the nodules, the pattern of scarring (linking of portal tracts to each other vs. linking of portal tracts to central veins), the degree of parenchymal loss, and the frequency of vascular thrombosis (particularly of the portal vein) all vary between diseases and even, in some cases, between individuals with the same disease.

As mentioned earlier, stem cell activation and differentiation gives rise to duct-like structures, the so called ductular reactions. **In chronic liver disease, ductular reactions increase with disease progression and are usually most prominent in cirrhosis.** Ductular reactions may incite some of the scarring in chronic liver disease and thus may have a negative effect on progressive liver disease.

Regression of fibrosis and even of fully established cirrhosis may follow disease remission or cure. Scars become thinner, more densely compacted, and eventually start to fragment (see Fig. 16.6, B). As fibrous septa break apart, adjacent nodules of regenerating parenchyma coalesce into larger islands. All cirrhotic livers show elements of both progression and regression, with the balance being dictated by the severity and persistence of the underlying disease.

Clinical Features

About 40% of individuals with cirrhosis are asymptomatic until the most advanced stages of the disease. Even at late stages, they present with nonspecific clinical manifestations, such as anorexia, weight loss, weakness, and, eventually signs and symptoms of liver failure discussed earlier. Jaundice, encephalopathy, and coagulopathy may result from chronic liver disease, much the same as in acute liver failure. However, there are some significant additional features:

- Chronic severe jaundice can lead to *pruritus* (itching), the intensity of which may be so profound that patients scratch their skin raw and risk repeated bouts of potentially life-threatening infection. In some patients, severe pruritus is the primary indication for liver transplantation. Pruritus also is frequently seen in other disorders associated with cholestasis, suggesting that it is somehow related to the build up of bile salts in the body, but its precise pathogenesis is unknown.

- *Portal hypertension* is more frequent and manifests in more complex ways in chronic liver failure than in acute liver failure (Fig. 16.7). *Portosystemic shunts* develop when blood flow is reversed from the portal to systemic circulation. These shunts are principally produced by dilation of collateral vessels. Most notably, venous bypasses develop wherever the systemic and the portal circulations share common capillary beds, the most clinically important of which are *esophagogastric varices*, which appear in about 40% of individuals with advanced-stage liver disease. These often cause massive, frequently fatal hematemesis, particularly when there is compounding coagulopathy. Portal hypertension often occurs and may lead to congestive *splenomegaly,* which can lower the platelet count due to sequestration of these elements in the expanded red pulp.

- *Hyperestrogenemia* due to impaired estrogen metabolism in male patients with chronic liver failure can give rise to *palmar erythema* (a reflection of local vasodilatation) and *spider angiomas* of the skin. Such male hyperestrogenemia also leads to *hypogonadism* and *gynecomastia*. Hypogonadism also may occur in women from disruption of hypothalamic-pituitary axis functioning.

- Most chronic liver diseases predispose to development of *hepatocellular carcinoma* (HCC, discussed later).

The course and severity of chronic liver disease with cirrhosis vary widely from patient to patient. Even in instances in which cirrhosis regresses following disease remission or cure, portal hypertension may persist due to the presence of irreversible shunts. The causes of death are

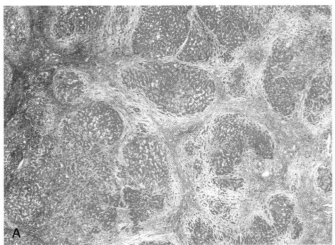
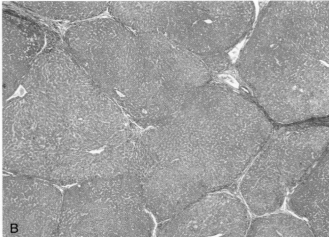

Fig. 16.6 Alcoholic cirrhosis in an active drinker (A) and following long-term abstinence (B). A, Thick bands of collagen separate rounded cirrhotic nodules. B, After 1 year of abstinence, most scars are gone (Masson trichrome stain). *(Courtesy of Drs. Hongfa Zhu and Isabel Fiel, Mount Sinai School of Medicine, New York, New York.)*

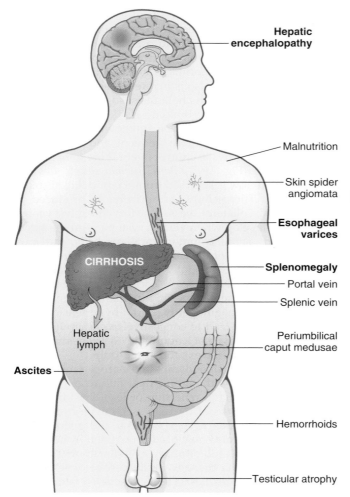

Fig. 16.7 Major clinical consequences of portal hypertension in the setting of cirrhosis, shown for the male. In females, oligomenorrhea, amenorrhea, and sterility are frequent as a result of hypogonadism.

liver failure (as in acute liver disease) and HCC. Clinical and laboratory findings are the main criteria used to gauge prognosis and disease progression. It some centers, portal venous wedge pressures are measured to assess the degree of vascular obstruction. Liver biopsy findings correlate with the presence and severity of portal hypertension. For example, specimens with thin fibrous septa and large islands of regenerated parenchyma are unlikely to be associated with portal hypertension, whereas broad bands of fibrosis and loss of parenchyma portend the development of portal hypertension and end-stage liver disease.

Acute-on-Chronic Liver Failure

Some individuals after years of stable, well-compensated, chronic disease suddenly develop signs of acute liver failure. In such patients, there is often established cirrhosis with extensive vascular shunting, or large volumes of functioning liver parenchyma with a borderline vascular supply, both of which leave the liver vulnerable to superimposed, potentially lethal insults. The short-term mortality of patients with this form of liver failure is around 50%.

Hepatic insults that cause sudden decompensation of patients with chronic liver disease include: hepatitis D superinfection in those with chronic hepatitis B; emergence of resistance to medical therapy in those with viral hepatitis; development of ascending bacterial cholangitis in patients with primary sclerosing cholangitis; or replacement of liver parenchyma by primary or metastatic carcinoma. In other instances the cause may be a systemic disorder, such as sepsis, acute cardiac failure or a superimposed toxic injury that tips a well-compensated cirrhotic patient into liver failure.

SUMMARY

LIVER FAILURE

- Liver failure may follow acute injury or chronic injury, or it may occur as an acute insult superimposed on otherwise well-compensated chronic liver disease.
- The mnemonic for causes of acute liver failure are as follows:
  - A: acetaminophen, hepatitis A, autoimmune hepatitis
  - B: hepatitis B
  - C: cryptogenic, hepatitis C
  - D: drugs/toxins, hepatitis D
  - E: hepatitis E, esoteric causes (Wilson disease, Budd-Chiari syndrome)
  - F: fatty change of the microvesicular type (fatty liver of pregnancy, valproate, tetracycline, Reye syndrome)
- Potentially fatal sequelae of liver failure include coagulopathy, encephalopathy, portal hypertension and ascites, hepatorenal syndrome, and portopulmonary hypertension.

INFECTIOUS DISORDERS

Viral Hepatitis

The terminology for acute and chronic viral hepatitis can be confusing, because the same word, *hepatitis,* can be used to describe several different entities; careful attention to context can clarify its meaning in any situation. Firstly, *hepatitis* is the name applied to viruses (hepatitis A, B, C, D, and E virus) that are *hepatotropic,* that is, have a specific affinity for the liver. Secondly, *hepatitis* is applied to patterns of acute and chronic hepatic injuries that are produced not only by hepatotropic viruses, but also by damage produced by other viruses such as EBV, CMV , and yellow fever as well as autoimmune reactions, drugs, and toxins. In this section, we will focus on the main features of hepatotropic viruses, which are summarized in Table 16.2, and we will then discuss the clinicopathologic characteristics of acute and chronic viral hepatitis.

Hepatitis A Virus (HAV)

HAV usually is a benign self-limited infection that does not cause chronic hepatitis and rarely (in about 0.1% of cases) produces fulminant hepatitis. HAV has an incubation period of 3-6 weeks. It is typically cleared by the host immune response, so it does not establish a carrier state. The infection occurs throughout the world and is endemic in countries with poor hygiene and sanitation.

Table 16.2 The Hepatitis Viruses

Virus	Hepatitis A (HAV)	Hepatitis B (HBV)	Hepatitis C (HCV)	Hepatitis D (HDV)	Hepatitis E (HEV)
Viral genome	ssRNA	partially dsDNA	ssRNA	Circular defective ssRNA	ssRNA
Viral family	Hepatovirus; related to picornavirus	Hepadnavirus	*Flaviviridae*	Subviral particle in *Deltaviridae* family	Calicivirus
Route of transmission	Fecal-oral (contaminated food or water)	Parenteral, sexual contact, perinatal	Parenteral; intranasal cocaine use is a risk factor	Parenteral	Fecal-oral
Incubation period	2–6 weeks	2–26 weeks (mean 8 weeks)	4–26 weeks (mean 9 weeks)	Same as HBV	4–5 weeks
Frequency of chronic liver disease	Never	5%–10%	>80%	10% (coinfection); 90%–100% for superinfection	In immunocompromised hosts only
Diagnosis	Detection of serum IgM antibodies	Detection of HBsAg or antibody to HBcAg; PCR for HBV DNA	ELISA for antibody detection; PCR for HCV RNA	Detection of IgM and IgG antibodies, HDV RNA in serum, or HDAg in liver biopsy	Detection of serum IgM and IgG antibodies; PCR for HEV RNA

ssRNA, Single-stranded RNA; *dsDNA*, double-stranded DNA; *HBcAg*, hepatitis B core antigen; *HBsAg*, hepatitis B surface antigen; *HDAg*, hepatitis D antigen; *ELISA*, enzyme-linked immunosorbent assay.
From Washington K: Inflammatory and infectious diseases of the liver. In Iacobuzio-Donahue CA, Montgomery EA, editors: *Gastrointestinal and liver pathology*, Philadelphia, 2005, Churchill Livingstone.

Acute HAV tends to cause a febrile illness associated with jaundice and nonspecific symptoms such as fatigue and loss of appetite. Overall, HAV accounts for about 25% of clinically evident acute hepatitis worldwide.

HAV is a small, nonenveloped, positive-strand RNA picornavirus that occupies its own genus, *Hepatovirus*. Ultrastructurally, HAV is an icosahedral capsid 27 nm in diameter. The receptor for HAV is HAVcr-1, a membrane glycoprotein that also may serve as a receptor for Ebola virus. *HAV is spread by ingestion of contaminated water and food and is shed in the stool for 2 to 3 weeks before and 1 week after the onset of jaundice.* Thus, close personal contact with an infected individual or fecal-oral contamination accounts for most cases and explains outbreaks in institutional settings such as schools and nurseries, as well as water-borne epidemics in places where people live in overcrowded, unsanitary conditions. HAV can also be detected in serum and saliva of infected individuals.

In developed countries, sporadic infections may be contracted by the consumption of raw or steamed shellfish that have concentrated the virus from seawater contaminated with human sewage. Infected workers in the food industry are another source of outbreaks. HAV itself does not seem to be cytopathic. The cellular immune response, particularly that involving cytotoxic CD8+ T cells, plays a key role in HAV-mediated hepatocellular injury.

Because HAV viremia is transient, blood-borne transmission is very rare; therefore, donated blood is not specifically screened for this virus. IgM antibody against HAV appears in blood at the onset of symptoms and is a reliable marker of acute infection (Fig. 16.8). Fecal shedding of the virus ends as the IgM titer rises. The IgM response usually declines in a few months followed by the appearance of IgG anti-HAV that persists for years, often conferring lifelong immunity. However, there are no routinely available tests for IgG anti-HAV; the presence of IgG anti-HAV is inferred from the difference between total and IgM

anti-HAV. The HAV vaccine, available since 1992, is effective in preventing infection.

Hepatitis B Virus (HBV)

The outcome of HBV infection varies widely, from (1) acute hepatitis with recovery and clearance of the virus; (2) nonprogressive chronic hepatitis; (3) progressive chronic disease ending in cirrhosis; (4) fulminant hepatitis with massive liver necrosis; and (5) an asymptomatic

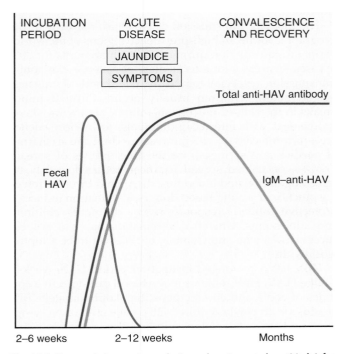

Fig. 16.8 Temporal changes in serologic markers in acute hepatitis A infection. *HAV*, Hepatitis A virus.

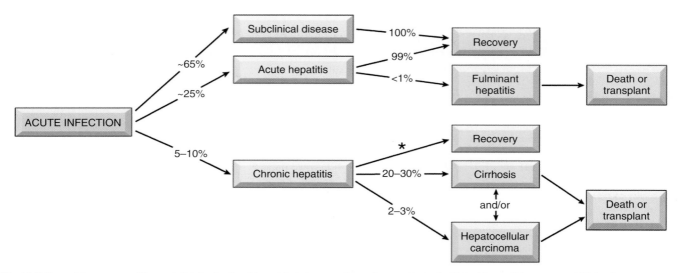

Fig. 16.9 Potential outcomes of hepatitis B infection in adults, with their approximate frequencies in the United States. *Spontaneous HBsAg clearance occurs during chronic HBV infection at an estimated annual incidence of 1% to 2% in Western countries. As mentioned in the text, fulminant hepatitis and acute hepatic failure are used interchangeably.

"healthy" carrier state. HBV-induced chronic liver disease is also an important precursor for the development of HCC. The approximate frequencies of various clinical outcomes of HBV infection are depicted in Fig. 16.9.

Liver disease due to HBV infection is an enormous global health problem. One-third of the world's population (2 billion individuals) has been infected with HBV, and 400 million individuals have chronic infections. Seventy-five percent of chronic carriers live in Asia and the Western Pacific rim. The global prevalence of chronic hepatitis B infection varies from greater than 8% in parts of Africa to less than 2% in Western Europe, North America, and Australia.

The mode of transmission of HBV also varies with the geographic locale. In high-prevalence regions of the world, perinatal transmission during childbirth accounts for 90% of cases. In areas with intermediate prevalence, horizontal transmission, especially in early childhood, dominates. Spread among children usually occurs through minor breaks in the skin or mucous membranes following physical contact with infected individuals. In low-prevalence areas, unprotected sex and intravenous drug abuse (sharing of needles and syringes) are the chief modes of spread. Transfusion-related spread has been reduced greatly by screening of donated blood for HBsAg and by cessation of the practice of paying blood donors. Vaccination induces a protective antibody response in 95% of infants, children, and adolescents. Universal vaccination has had notable success in Taiwan and Gambia, but has yet to be adopted worldwide.

HBV has a prolonged incubation period (2–26 weeks). Unlike HAV, HBV remains in the blood during active episodes of acute and chronic hepatitis. Approximately 70% of adults with newly acquired HBV have mild or no symptoms and do not develop jaundice. The remaining 30% have nonspecific constitutional symptoms such as anorexia, fever, jaundice, and right upper-quadrant pain. In most cases, the infection is self-limited and resolves without treatment, but chronic disease develops in 10% of infected individuals. Fulminant hepatitis is rare, occurring in approximately 0.1% to 0.5% of acutely infected individuals.

HBV is a member of *Hepadnaviridae*, a family of DNA viruses that cause hepatitis in multiple animal species. The HBV genome is a partially double-stranded, 3200-nucleotide, circular DNA with four open reading frames, which encode the following proteins:

- *Nucleocapsid "core" protein* (HBcAg, hepatitis B core antigen) and a longer polypeptide with a precore and core region, designated HBeAg (hepatitis B e antigen). The precore region directs the secretion of the HBeAg polypeptide into blood, whereas HBcAg remains in hepatocytes, where it participates in the assembly of virions.
- *Envelope glycoproteins* (HBsAg, hepatitis B surface antigen). Infected hepatocytes synthesize and secrete massive quantities of noninfective envelope glycoproteins (mainly small HBsAg).
- A *polymerase (Pol)* with both DNA polymerase activity and reverse transcriptase activity, which enables genomic replication to occur through a unique DNA → RNA → DNA cycle via an intermediate RNA template. This unusual polymerase is the target of drugs used to treat hepatitis B infection (described later).
- *HBx protein,* which is required for virus replication and which may act as a transcriptional transactivator for viral genes and a wide variety of host genes. It has been implicated in the pathogenesis of HBV-associated liver cancer.

The course of the disease can be followed clinically by monitoring certain serum markers (Fig. 16.10).
- HBsAg appears before the onset of symptoms, peaks during symptomatic disease, and then usually declines to undetectable levels in 12 weeks (though it may occasionally persist as long as 24 weeks).

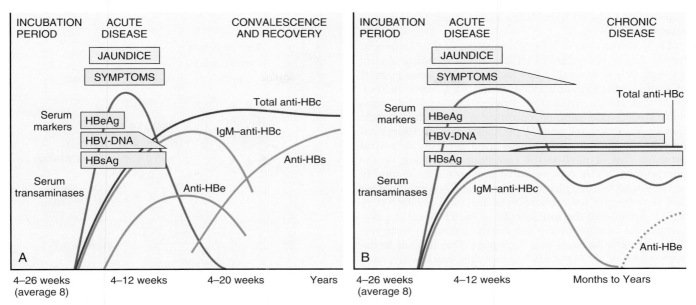

Fig. 16.10 Temporal changes in serologic markers for hepatitis B viral infection. (A) Acute infection with resolution. (B) progression to chronic infection. Note in some cases of chronic HBV infection, serum transaminases may become normal.

- Anti-HBs antibody appears after the acute disease is over and usually is not detected until a few weeks to several months after HBsAg disappears. Anti-HBs may persist for life and confers protection, which is the rationale for current vaccines containing HBsAg.
- HBeAg and HBV DNA appear in serum soon after HBsAg and signify ongoing viral replication. Persistence of HBeAg is an indicator of progression to chronic hepatitis. The appearance of anti-HBe antibodies implies that an acute infection has peaked and is on the wane.
- IgM anti-HBc becomes detectable in serum shortly before the onset of symptoms, concurrent with the onset of elevated serum aminotransferase levels (indicative of hepatocyte destruction). Over a period of months, the IgM anti-HBc antibody is replaced by IgG anti-HBc. As in the case of anti-HAV, there is no direct assay for IgG anti-HBc; its presence is inferred from decline of IgM anti-HBc in the face of rising total anti-HBc.

Occasionally, mutated strains of HBV emerge that do not produce HBeAg but are replication competent and express HBcAg. In such patients, the HBeAg may be low or undetectable despite the presence of serum HBV DNA. A second ominous development is the appearance of HBV mutants in vaccinated individuals that replicate in the presence of normally protective anti-HBs antibodies.

The host immune response is the main determinant of the outcome of the infection. Innate immune mechanisms protect the host during initial phases of the infection, and a strong response by virus-specific CD4+ and CD8+ interferon γ–producing cells is associated with the resolution of acute infection. HBV generally is not directly hepatotoxic, and most hepatocyte injury is caused by CD8+ cytotoxic T cells attacking infected cells.

Patient age at the time of infection is the best predictor of chronicity. In general, the younger the age at the time of HBV infection, the higher the chance of chronic infection. Treatment of chronic hepatitis B with viral polymerase inhibitors and interferon can slow disease progression, reduce liver damage, and prevent liver cirrhosis or liver cancer but does not eliminate the infection. As a result, treatment sometimes fails due to emergence of viruses bearing mutations that lead to drug resistance.

Hepatitis C Virus (HCV)

HCV is a major cause of liver disease, with approximately 170 million individuals affected worldwide. Approximately 4.1 million Americans (1.6% of the population) have chronic HCV infection. Notably, there has been a decrease in the annual incidence of infection from a mid-1980s peak of over 230,000 new infections per year to 30,000 new infections per year currently, due primarily to a reduction in transfusion-associated cases as a result of effective screening procedures. Until recently, the number of patients with chronic infection appeared likely to continue to increase, but new therapies (discussed later) are changing the outlook for the better.

According to data from the Centers for Disease Control and Prevention (CDC), the most common risk factors for HCV infection are as follows:

- Intravenous drug abuse
- Multiple sex partners
- Having had surgery within the last 6 months
- Needle stick injury
- Multiple contacts with an HCV-infected individual
- Employment in the medical or dental field

Currently, transmission of HCV by blood transfusion is close to zero in the United States; the risk for acquiring HCV by needle stick is about six times higher than that for HIV (1.8 vs. 0.3%). For children, the major route of infection is vertical perinatal transmission from the mother. Some patients have multiple risk factors, but one-third of individuals have no identifiable risk factors, an enduring mystery.

HCV, discovered in 1989, is a member of the *Flaviviridae* family. Just as in the case of HIV, an understanding of viral replication and assembly has facilitated the development of highly effective anti-HCV drugs (described below). HCV is a small, enveloped, single-stranded RNA virus with a 9600-base genome encoding a single polyprotein that is processed by several proteases into 10 functional proteins. Included among these viral proteins is a viral protease that is needed for complete processing of the polyprotein; NS5A, a protein that is essential for assembly of HCV into mature virions; and a viral RNA polymerase that is necessary for replication of the viral genome (Fig. 16.11). Because of the low fidelity of the HCV RNA polymerase, the viral genome is inherently unstable, giving rise to new genetic variants at a high pace. This has led to the appearance of six major HCV genotypes worldwide, each with one or more "subspecies." Infections in most individuals are due to a virus of a single genotype, but new genetic variants are generated in the host as long as viral replication persists. As a result, each patient usually comes to be infected with a population of divergent but closely related HCV variants known as *quasispecies.*

The incubation period for HCV hepatitis ranges from 4 to 26 weeks, with a mean of 9 weeks. In about 85% of individuals, the acute infection is asymptomatic and goes unrecognized. HCV RNA is detectable in blood for 1 to 3 weeks, coincident with elevations in serum transaminases (Fig. 16.12). In symptomatic acute HCV infection, anti-HCV antibodies are detected in only 50% to 70% of patients; in the remaining patients, the anti-HCV antibodies emerge after 3 to 6 weeks. The clinical course of acute HCV hepatitis is milder than that of HBV. It is not known why only a small minority of individuals is capable of clearing HCV infection.

Persistent infection and chronic hepatitis are the hallmarks of HCV infection, despite the generally asymptomatic nature of the acute illness. In contrast to HBV, chronic disease occurs in the majority of HCV-infected individuals (80%–90%), and cirrhosis eventually occurs in as many as one-third. The mechanisms leading to chronicity are not well understood, but it is clear that the virus uses multiple strategies to evade host anti-viral immunity. In addition to rapid generation of genetic variants, which may allow the virus to elude neutralizing antibodies, HCV encodes proteins that inhibit Toll-like receptor and interferon signaling in hepatocytes, activites that would otherwise allow hepatocytes to resist viral infection.

In chronic HCV infection, circulating HCV RNA persists in 90% of patients despite the presence of neutralizing antibodies (see Fig. 16.12). Hence, testing for HCV RNA must be done to confirm the diagnosis of chronic HCV infection. A characteristic clinical feature of chronic HCV infection is episodic elevations in serum aminotransferases separated by periods of normal or near-normal enzyme levels. However, even HCV-infected patients with normal transaminases are at high risk for developing permanent liver damage, and anyone with detectable serum HCV RNA needs treatment and long-term medical follow-up.

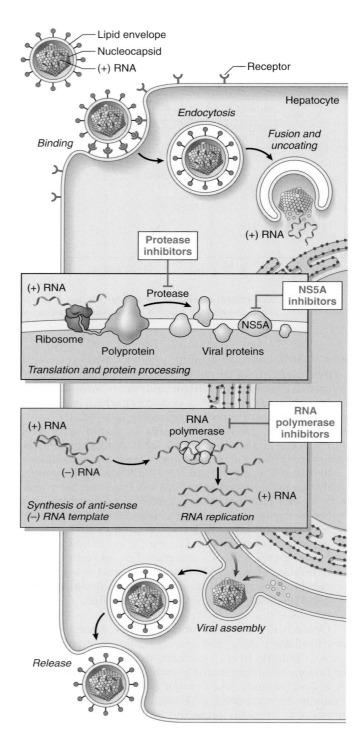

Fig. 16.11 Life cycle of hepatitis C. Viral entry, replication, assembly, and budding are shown, emphasizing steps that can be effectively targeted with anti-viral drugs.

Fortunately, **recent years have seen dramatic improvements in treatment of HCV infection that stem from development of drugs that specifically target the viral protease, RNA polymerase, and NS5A protein, all of**

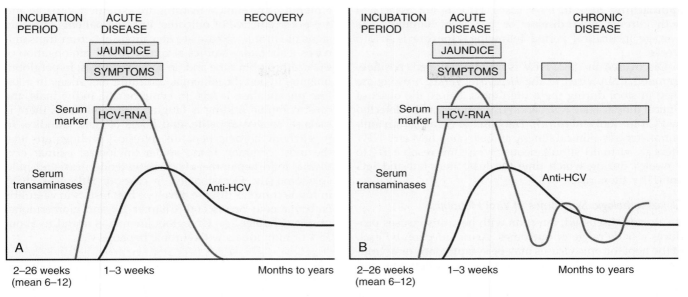

Fig. 16.12 Temporal changes in serologic markers in hepatitis C infection. (A) Acute infection with resolution; (B) progression to chronic infection.

which are required for production of virus (Fig. 16.11). Combination therapy with these drugs (a strategy akin to triple drug therapy for HIV) has proven to be remarkably effective. The goal of current treatment is to eradicate HCV RNA, which is defined by the absence of detectable HCV RNA in the blood 6 months after treatment is stopped and is associated with a high probability of cure. Currently, over 95% of HCV infections are curable, and this can be expected to improve further as new anti-viral drugs become available. The major downside of these advances is their very high cost; a curative course of drug therapy costs over $100,000, and it is estimated that treatment of HCV infections in the United States alone may generate expenses of over $50 billion over the next 5 years.

Hepatitis D Virus (HDV)

Also called the *delta agent*, HDV is a unique RNA virus that is dependent for its life cycle on HBV. Infection with HDV arises in the following settings:

- *Coinfection* by HDV and HBV. The HBV must become established first to provide the HBsAg, which is necessary for production of complete HDV virions. Coinfection with HBV and HDV is associated with higher rates of severe acute hepatitis and fulminant liver failure, particularly in intravenous drug abusers, and higher rates of progression to chronic infection, which is often complicated by emergence of liver cancer.
- *Superinfection* of a chronic HBV carrier by HDV. The superinfection presents 30 to 50 days later as severe acute hepatitis in a previously unrecognized HBV carrier or as an exacerbation of preexisting chronic hepatitis B. Chronic HDV infection occurs in 80% to 90% of such patients. The superinfection may have two phases: an acute phase with active HDV replication and suppression of HBV with high ALT levels, followed by a chronic phase in which HDV replication decreases, HBV replication increases, ALT levels fluctuate, and the

disease progresses to cirrhosis and hepatocellular cancer.

HDV infection occurs worldwide and affects an estimated 15 million individuals (about 5% of the 300 million individuals infected by HBV). Its prevalence varies, being highest in the Amazon basin, Africa, the Middle East, and Southern Italy, and lowest in Southeast Asia and China. In most western countries, it is largely restricted to intravenous drug abusers and those who have had multiple blood transfusions.

HDV RNA is detectable in the blood and liver at the time of onset of acute symptomatic disease. IgM anti-HDV is a reliable indicator of recent HDV exposure, but is frequently short-lived. Acute coinfection by HDV and HBV is associated with the presence of IgM against HDAg and HBcAg (denoting new infection with hepatitis B). With chronic delta hepatitis arising from HDV superinfection, HBsAg is present in serum, and anti-HDV antibodies (IgG and IgM) persist for months or longer. Because of its dependency on HBV, HDV infection is prevented by vaccination against HBV.

Hepatitis E Virus (HEV)

HEV is an enterically transmitted, water-borne infection that usually produces a self-limiting disease. The virus typically infects young to middle-aged adults. HEV is a zoonotic disease with animal reservoirs that include monkeys, cats, pigs, and dogs. Epidemics have been reported in Asia and the Indian subcontinent, sub-Saharan Africa, and Mexico, and sporadic cases are seen in Western nations, particularly where pig farming is common and in travelers returning from regions of high incidence. Of greater importance, HEV infection accounts for 30% to 60% of cases of sporadic acute hepatitis in India, exceeding the frequency of HAV. **A characteristic feature of HEV infection is the high mortality rate among pregnant women,**

approaching 20%. In most cases, HEV is not associated with chronic liver disease or persistent viremia. The average incubation period following exposure is 4 to 5 weeks.

Discovered in 1983, HEV is an unenveloped, positive-stranded RNA virus in the *Hepevirus* genus. Virions are shed in stool during the acute illness. Before the onset of clinical illness, HEV RNA and HEV virions can be detected by PCR in stool and serum. The onset of rising serum aminotransferases, clinical illness, and elevated IgM anti-HEV titers are virtually simultaneous. Symptoms resolve in 2 to 4 weeks, during which time the IgM titers fall and IgG anti-HEV titers rise.

Clinicopathologic Syndromes of Viral Hepatitis

As already discussed, infection with hepatitis viruses produces a wide range of outcomes. Acute infection by each of the hepatotropic viruses may be symptomatic or asymptomatic. HAV and HEV do not cause chronic hepatitis, and only a small number of HBV-infected adults develop chronic hepatitis. In contrast, HCV is notorious for producing chronic infections. Fulminant hepatitis is unusual and is seen primarily with HAV, HBV, or HDV infections. Although HBV and HCV are responsible for most cases of chronic hepatitis, there are many other causes of similar clinicopathologic presentations, including autoimmune hepatitis and drug- and toxin-induced hepatitis (discussed later). Therefore, serologic and molecular studies are essential for the diagnosis of viral hepatitis and for distinguishing between the various types.

Acute Asymptomatic Infection With Recovery. Patients in this group are identified incidentally on the basis of elevated serum transaminases or the presence of anti-viral antibodies. HAV and HBV infections, particularly in childhood, are frequently subclinical.

Acute Symptomatic Infection With Recovery. Whichever virus is involved, acute disease follows a similar course, consisting of: (1) an incubation period of variable length (see Table 16.2); (2) a symptomatic preicteric phase; (3) a symptomatic icteric phase; and (4) convalescence. Peak infectivity occurs during the last asymptomatic days of the incubation period and the early days of acute symptoms.

Fulminant Hepatic Failure. Viral hepatitis is responsible for about 12% of cases of fulminant hepatic failure; of these, two-thirds are caused by HBV infection and the rest by HAV. Survival for more than 1 week may permit recovery to occur via replication of residual hepatocytes. Activation of the stem/progenitor cells in the canals of Hering gives rise to very prominent ductular reactions but is usually insufficient to accomplish full restitution. Fulminant hepatic failure that follows acute viral hepatitis is treated supportively. Liver transplantation is the only option for patients whose disease does not resolve, as death from secondary infections and failure of other organs is otherwise inevitable.

Chronic Hepatitis. Chronic hepatitis is defined as persistent or relapsing hepatic disease for a period of more than 6 months. The clinical features are extremely variable and are not predictive of outcome. In some patients, the only signs of chronic disease are elevations of serum transaminases. Laboratory studies also may reveal prolongation of the prothrombin time and, in some instances, hyperglobulinemia, hyperbilirubinemia, and mild elevations in alkaline phosphatase levels. In symptomatic individuals, the most common finding is fatigue; less commonly, there is malaise, loss of appetite, and bouts of mild jaundice. In precirrhotic chronic hepatitis, physical findings are few, the most common being spider angiomas, palmar erythema, mild hepatomegaly, hepatic tenderness, and mild splenomegaly. Occasionally, in cases of HBV and HCV, immune complex disease develops that results in vasculitis (subcutaneous or visceral, Chapter 10) and glomerulonephritis (Chapter 14). Cryoglobulinemia is found in about 35% of individuals with chronic hepatitis C.

The Carrier State. A *carrier* is an individual who is chronically infected with a hepatropic virus and has no or subclinical evidence of liver disease. In both cases, particularly the latter, these individuals constitute reservoirs for infection. In the case of HBV, "healthy carriers" typically have serum studies that show an absence of HBeAg, the presence of anti-HBe, normal aminotransferases, and low or undetectable serum HBV DNA and liver biopsies showing a lack of significant inflammation or parenchymal injury. HBV infection acquired early in life in endemic areas (such as Southeast Asia, China, and sub-Saharan Africa) gives rise to a carrier state in more than 90% of cases, whereas in non-endemic regions the carrier state is rare. By contrast, it has been estimated that HCV infection in the United States produces a carrier state in 10% to 40% of cases.

HIV and Chronic Viral Hepatitis. Because of their similar transmission modes and overlapping risk factors, coinfection of HIV and hepatitis viruses is a common clinical problem. In the United States, 10% of HIV-infected individuals are coinfected with HBV and 25% with HCV, and, when untreated, chronic HBV and HCV infection are important causes of morbidity and mortality in HIV-infected individuals, even in those who receive effective anti-HIV therapy. Similarly, in individuals who progress to acquired immunodeficiency syndrome (AIDS), liver disease is the second most common cause of death. However, in adequately treated immunocompetent HIV patients, the severity and progression of HBV and HCV infection and response to anti–hepatitis virus therapy resembles that seen in non-HIV–infected individuals.

MORPHOLOGY

Clinical assessment of chronic hepatitis sometimes requires liver biopsy in addition to clinical and serologic data. Liver biopsy is helpful in confirming the clinical diagnosis, excluding common concomitant conditions (e.g., fatty liver disease, hemochromatosis), assessing histologic features associated with an increased risk for malignancy (discussed later), grading the extent of hepatocyte injury and inflammation, and staging the progression of scarring. Historically, histologic grading and staging of chronic hepatitis in liver biopsy specimens have been central to determinations of whether to attempt treatment of the underlying disease; however, with the new, highly effective targeted antiviral therapies for hepatitis C, fewer pretreatment biopsies are being performed.

The general morphologic features of acute and chronic viral hepatitis are depicted schematically in Fig. 16.13. **The morphologic changes in acute and chronic viral hepatitis are shared among the hepatotropic viruses and can be mimicked by drug reactions or autoimmune hepatitis.**

Acute viral hepatitis. Grossly, livers involved by mild acute hepatitis appear normal or slightly mottled. At the other end of the spectrum, massive hepatic necrosis may produce a greatly shrunken liver, as discussed earlier. Microscopically, there is considerable morphologic overlap in acute hepatitis caused by various hepatropic viruses. As is typical of many viral infections, mononuclear cells predominate in all phases of viral hepatitis. A subtle difference is that the mononuclear infiltrate in hepatitis A may be especially rich in plasma cells. Most parenchymal injury is scattered throughout the hepatic lobule as "spotty necrosis" or **lobular hepatitis.** Portal inflammation in acute hepatitis is minimal or absent. As discussed earlier, hepatocyte injury may result in necrosis or apoptosis. In the former, the cytoplasm appears empty, with only scattered wisps of cytoplasmic remnants, and eventual rupture of cell membranes leads to "dropout" of hepatocytes. In their place, collapsed sinusoidal collagen reticulin framework remains behind along with scavenger macrophages. With apoptosis, hepatocytes shrink, becoming intensely eosinophilic, and their nuclei become pyknotic and fragmented; effector T cells may be present in the immediate vicinity.

In severe acute hepatitis, confluent necrosis of hepatocytes is seen around central veins. In these areas, there may be cellular debris, collapsed reticulin fibers, congestion/hemorrhage, and variable inflammation. With increasing severity, there is central-portal bridging necrosis, followed by parenchymal collapse. In its most severe form, massive hepatic necrosis and fulminant liver failure ensue.

Chronic viral hepatitis. The defining histologic feature of chronic viral hepatitis is mononuclear portal infiltration. It may be mild to severe and variable from one portal tract to the other. There is often **interface hepatitis** as well, in addition to lobular hepatitis, distinguished by its location at the interface between hepatocellular parenchyma and portal tract stroma. The hallmark of progressive chronic liver damage is scarring. At first, only portal tracts exhibit fibrosis, but in some patients, with time, fibrous septa—bands of dense scar—will extend between portal tracts. In the most severe cases, continued scarring and nodule formation leads to the development of cirrhosis, as discussed earlier.

Certain histologic features point to specific viral etiologies in chronic hepatitis. In chronic hepatitis B, **"ground-glass" hepatocytes** (cells with endoplasmic reticulum swollen by HBsAg) are a diagnostic hallmark, and the presence of viral antigen in these cells can be confirmed by immunostaining (Fig. 16.14). Liver biopsies involved by chronic hepatitis C quite commonly show

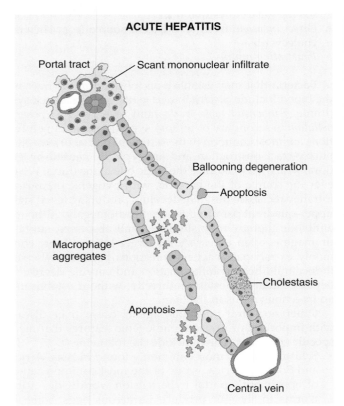

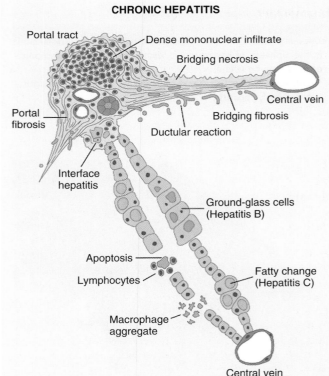

Fig. 16.13 Morphologic features of acute and chronic hepatitis. There is very little portal mononuclear infiltration in acute hepatitis (or sometimes none at all), while in chronic hepatitis portal infiltrates are dense and prominent—the defining feature of chronic hepatitis. Bridging necrosis and fibrosis are shown only for chronic hepatitis, but bridging necrosis may also occur in more severe acute hepatitis. Ductular reactions in chronic hepatitis are minimal in early stages of scarring, but become extensive in late-stage disease.

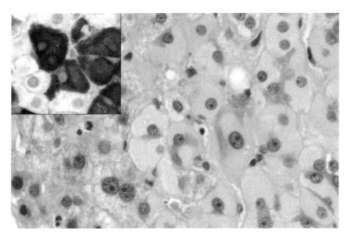

Fig. 16.14 Ground-glass hepatocytes in chronic hepatitis B, caused by accumulation of hepatitis B surface antigen. Hematoxylin-eosin staining shows the presence of abundant, finely granular pink cytoplasmic inclusions; immunostaining (inset) with a specific antibody confirms the presence of surface antigen (brown).

large lymphoid aggregates (Fig. 16.15). Often, hepatitis C, particularly genotype 3, is associated with fatty change in scattered hepatocytes. Bile duct injury is also prominent in some cases of hepatitis C and may mimic the histologic changes seen in primary biliary cholangitis (see later); clinical parameters distinguish these two diseases easily, however.

SUMMARY

VIRAL HEPATITIS

- In the alphabet of hepatotropic viruses, some easy mnemonic devices may be useful:
  - The vowels (hepatitis A and E) never cause chronic hepatitis, only AcutE hepatitis.
  - Only the consonants (hepatitis B, C, D) have the potential to cause chronic disease (C for consonant and for chronic).
  - Hepatitis B can be transmitted by blood, birthing, and "bonking" (as they say in the United Kingdom).
  - Hepatitis C is the single virus that is more often chronic than not (almost never detected acutely; 85% or more of patients develop chronic hepatitis, 20% of whom will develop cirrhosis).
  - Hepatitis D, the delta agent, is a defective virus, requiring hepatitis B coinfection for its own capacity to infect and replicate.
  - Hepatitis E is endemic in equatorial regions and frequently epidemic.
- The inflammatory cells in both acute and chronic viral hepatitis are mainly T cells; it is the pattern of injury that is different, not the nature of the infiltrate.
- Patients with long-standing HBV or HCV infections are at increased risk for development of HCC.

Bacterial, Parasitic, and Helminthic Infections

A multitude of organisms can infect the liver and biliary tree, including bacteria, fungi, helminths and other parasites, and protozoa. Infectious organisms can reach the liver through several pathways:

- *Ascending infection,* via the gut and biliary tract (ascending cholangitis)
- *Vascular seeding,* most often through the portal system via the gastrointestinal tract
- *Direct invasion,* from an adjacent source (e.g., bacterial cholecystitis)
- *Penetrating injury*

Bacteria that may establish an infection in the liver via the blood include *Staphylococcus aureus* in toxic shock syndrome, *Salmonella typhi* in typhoid fever, and *Treponema pallidum* in secondary or tertiary syphilis. Ascending infections are most common in the setting of partial or complete biliary tract obstruction and are typically caused by gut flora, which may colonize the static bile in the ducts. Whatever the source of the bacteria, with pyogenic organisms intrahepatic abscesses may develop, producing fever, right upper-quadrant pain, and tender hepatomegaly. Although antibiotic therapy may sterilize small abscesses, surgical drainage is often necessary for larger lesions. More commonly, extrahepatic bacterial infections, particularly sepsis, induce mild hepatic inflammation and varying degrees of hepatocellular cholestasis indirectly, without establishing an infectious nidus in the liver.

Other non-viral infectious agents cause liver disease with important or unusual pathogenic features that merit specific comment. These include the following:

- Schistosomiasis, most commonly found in Asia, Africa, and South America, is one of the most common causes of noncirrhotic portal hypertension worldwide. Adult worms in the gut produce numerous eggs, some of which find their way into the portal circulation, where they lodge and induce a granulomatous reaction associated with marked fibrosis.

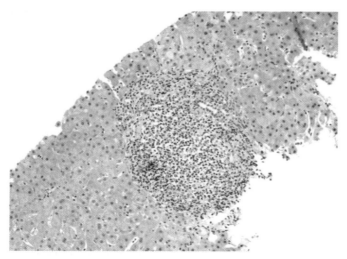

Fig. 16.15 Chronic viral hepatitis due to HCV, showing characteristic portal tract expansion by a dense lymphoid infiltrate.

- *Entamoeba histolytica*, an important cause of dysentery (Chapter 15), sometimes ascends to the liver through portal circulation and produces secondary foci of infection that can progress to large necrotic areas called amebic liver abscesses. Amebic abscesses are more common in the right lobe of the liver. The abscess cavity contains necrotic liver cells, but unlike pyogenic abscesses, neutrophils are absent.
- Liver fluke infection, most common in Southeast Asia, is associated with a high rate of cholangiocarcinoma. Responsible organisms include *Fasciola hepatica*, *Opisthorcis* species, and *Clonorchis sinensis*.
- Echinococcal infections may cause the formation of intrahepatic hydatid cysts that produce symptoms due to pressure on surrounding structures or following rupture.

AUTOIMMUNE HEPATITIS

Autoimmune hepatitis is a chronic, progressive hepatitis with all the features of autoimmune diseases in general: genetic predisposition, association with other autoimmune diseases, the presence of autoantibodies, and therapeutic response to immunosuppression. Risk for autoimmune hepatitis is associated with certain HLA alleles, such as the DRB1* allele in Caucasians, but as in other autoimmune disorders the mechanistic basis for this relationship is unclear. Triggers for the immune reaction may include viral infections or drug or toxin exposures.

Clinicopathologic Features

The annual incidence is highest among white northern Europeans at 1.9 in 100,000, but all ethnic groups are susceptible. There is a female predominance (78%). Autoimmune hepatitis is classified into two types, based on the patterns of circulating antibodies.

- *Type 1*, more common in middle-age and older individuals, is characterized by the presence of antinuclear (ANA), anti–smooth muscle actin (SMA), antimitochondrial (AMA), and anti–soluble liver antigen/liver-pancreas antigen (anti-SLA/LP) antibodies.
- *Type 2*, usually seen in children and teenagers, is characterized by the presence of anti–liver kidney microsome-1 antibodies and anti–liver cytosol-1 antibodies.

MORPHOLOGY

Although autoimmune hepatitis shares patterns of injury with acute or chronic viral hepatitis, the time course of histologic progression differs. In viral hepatitis, fibrosis typically follows many years of slowly accumulating parenchymal injury, whereas in autoimmune hepatitis, there is an early phase of severe parenchymal destruction followed rapidly by scarring. For unclear reasons, this early wave of hepatocyte damage is often subclinical. The following features are typical of autoimmune hepatitis:

- **Necrosis and inflammation**, indicated by extensive interface hepatitis or foci of confluent (perivenular or bridging) necrosis or parenchymal collapse

- **Plasma cell predominance** in the mononuclear inflammatory infiltrates
- **Hepatocyte "rosettes"** in areas of marked activity

An acute clinical illness is a common presentation (40%); sometimes the disease is fulminant, progressing to hepatic encephalopathy within 8 weeks of onset. Mortality for patients with severe untreated autoimmune hepatitis is approximately 40% within 6 months of diagnosis, and cirrhosis develops in at least 40% of survivors. Hence, diagnosis and intervention are imperative. Immunosuppressive therapy is usually effective, leading to remission in 80% of patients and enabling long-term survival. End-stage disease is an indication for liver transplantation. The 10-year survival rate after liver transplant is 75%, but recurrence in the transplanted organ occurs in 20% of cases.

SUMMARY

- There are two primary types of autoimmune hepatitis:
  - Type 1 autoimmune hepatitis is most often seen in middle-age women and is characteristically associated with antinuclear and anti–smooth muscle antibodies.
  - Type 2 autoimmune hepatitis is most often seen in children or teenagers and is associated with anti–liver kidney microsomal autoantibodies.
- Autoimmune hepatitis may either develop with a rapidly progressive acute disease or follow a more indolent path; if untreated, both are likely to lead to liver failure.
- Plasma cells are a prominent and characteristic component of the inflammatory infiltrate in biopsy specimens showing autoimmune hepatitis.

DRUG- AND TOXIN-INDUCED LIVER INJURY

As the major drug metabolizing and detoxifying organ in the body, the liver is subject to injury from an enormous array of therapeutic and environmental chemicals. Injury may result from direct toxicity, may occur through hepatic conversion of a xenobiotic compound to an active toxin, or may be produced by immune mechanisms, such as by the drug or a metabolite acting as a hapten to convert a cellular protein into an immunogen. A diagnosis of drug- or toxin-induced liver injury may be made on the basis of a temporal association of liver damage with drug or toxin exposure, recovery (usually) upon removal of the inciting agent, and exclusion of other potential causes. Exposure to a toxin or therapeutic agent should always be included in the differential diagnosis of any form of liver disease.

Principles of drug and toxic injury are discussed in Chapter 8. Here it suffices to note that drug reactions may be *predictable* (intrinsic) or *unpredictable* (idiosyncratic).

Table 16.3 Patterns of Injury in Drug- and Toxin-Induced Hepatic Injury

Pattern of Injury	Morphologic Findings	Examples of Associated Agents
Cholestatic	Bland hepatocellular cholestasis, without inflammation	Contraceptive and anabolic steroids, antibiotics, HAART
Cholestatic hepatitis	Cholestasis with lobular necrosis and inflammation; may show bile duct destruction	Antibiotics, phenothiazines, statins
Hepatocellular necrosis	Spotty hepatocyte necrosis	Methyldopa, phenytoin
	Massive necrosis	Acetaminophen, halothane
	Chronic hepatitis	Isoniazid
Fatty liver disease	Large and small droplet fat	Ethanol, corticosteroids, methotrexate, total parenteral nutrition
	"Microvesicular steatosis" (diffuse small droplet fat)	Valproate, tetracycline, aspirin (Reye syndrome), HAART
	Steatohepatitis with Mallory-Denk bodies	Ethanol, amiodarone
Fibrosis and cirrhosis	Periportal and pericellular fibrosis	Alcohol, methotrexate, enalapril, vitamin A and other retinoids
Granulomas	Noncaseating epithelioid granulomas	Sulfonamides, amiodarone, isoniazid
	Fibrin ring granulomas	Allopurinol
Vascular lesions	Sinusoidal obstruction syndrome (veno-occlusive disease): obliteration of central veins	High-dose chemotherapy, bush teas
	Budd-Chiari syndrome	Oral contraceptives
	Peliosis hepatis: blood-filled cavities, not lined by endothelial cells	Anabolic steroids, tamoxifen

HAART, Highly active anti-retroviral therapy
Adapted from Washington K: Metabolic and toxic conditions of the liver. In Iacobuzio-Donahue CA, Montgomery EA, editors: *Gastrointestinal and liver pathology*, Philadelphia, 2005, Churchill Livingstone.

Predictable drug or toxin reactions affect all individuals in a dose-dependent fashion. Unpredictable reactions depend on idiosyncrasies of the host, particularly the propensity to mount an immune response to the antigenic stimulus or the rate at which the agent can be metabolized. Both classes of injury may be immediate or take weeks to months to develop (Table 16.3).
- A classic, predictable hepatotoxin is *acetaminophen,* now the most common cause of acute liver failure necessitating transplantation in the United States. The toxic agent is not acetaminophen itself but rather toxic metabolites produced by the cytochrome P-450 system. The damage begins in centrilobular hepatocytes but extends to encompass entire lobules in the most severe cases.
- Examples of drugs that can cause *idiosyncratic reactions* include *chlorpromazine,* an agent that causes cholestasis in patients who are slow to metabolize it, and *halothane and its derivatives,* which can cause a fatal immune-mediated hepatitis after repeated exposure.

ALCOHOLIC AND NONALCOHOLIC FATTY LIVER DISEASE

Alcohol is a well-known cause of fatty liver disease in adults and can manifest histologically as steatosis, steatohepatitis, and cirrhosis. In recent years, it has become evident that another entity, so-called "nonalcoholic fatty liver disease (NAFLD)," can mimic the entire spectrum of hepatic changes associated with alcohol abuse. Since the morphologic changes of alcoholic and NAFLD are indistinguishable, they are discussed together, followed by the pathogenesis and distinctive clinical features of each entity.

MORPHOLOGY

Three types of liver alterations are observed in fatty liver disease: steatosis (fatty change), hepatitis (alcoholic or steatohepatitis), and fibrosis.

Hepatocellular steatosis. Hepatocellular fat accumulation typically begins in centrilobular hepatocytes. The lipid droplets range from small (microvesicular) to large (macrovesicular), the largest filling and expanding the cell and displacing the nucleus. As steatosis becomes more extensive, the lipid accumulation spreads outward from the central vein to hepatocytes in the midlobule and then the periportal regions (Fig. 16.16).

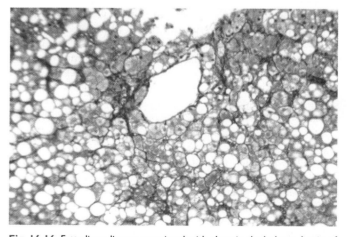

Fig. 16.16 Fatty liver disease associated with chronic alcohol use. A mix of small and large fat droplets (seen as clear vacuoles) is most prominent around the central vein and extends outward to the portal tracts. Some fibrosis *(stained blue)* is present in a characteristic perisinusoidal "chicken wire fence" pattern (Masson trichrome stain). *(Courtesy of Dr. Elizabeth Brunt, Washington University, St. Louis, Missouri.)*

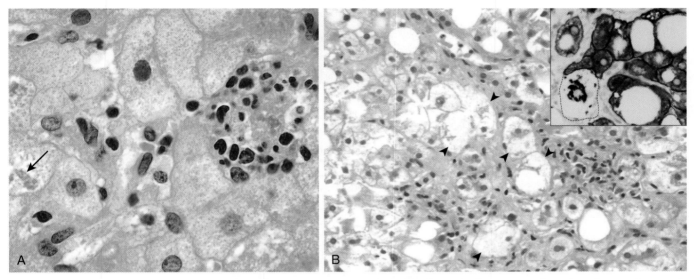

Fig. 16.17 Hepatocyte injury in fatty liver disease associated with chronic alcohol use. (A) Clustered inflammatory cells marking the site of a necrotic hepatocyte. A Mallory-Denk body is present in another hepatocyte *(arrow)*. (B) "Ballooned" hepatocytes *(arrowheads)* associated with clusters of inflammatory cells. The inset stained for keratins 8 and 18 *(brown)* shows a ballooned cell *(dotted line)* in which keratins have been ubiquitinylated and have collapsed into an immunoreactive Mallory-Denk body, leaving the cytoplasm "empty." *(Courtesy of Dr. Elizabeth Brunt, Washington University, St. Louis, Missouri.)*

Macroscopically, fatty livers with widespread steatosis are large (weighing 4–6 kg or more), soft, yellow, and greasy.

Steatohepatitis. These changes typically are more pronounced with alcohol use than in NAFLD, but can be seen in either:

- **Hepatocyte ballooning.** Single or scattered foci of cells undergo swelling and necrosis; as with steatosis, these features are most prominent in the centrilobular regions (Fig. 16.17A).
- **Mallory-Denk bodies.** These consist of tangled skeins of intermediate filaments (including ubiquitinylated keratins 8 and 18) and are visible as eosinophilic cytoplasmic inclusions in degenerating hepatocytes (see Fig. 16.17B).
- **Neutrophil infiltration.** Predominantly neutrophilic infiltration may permeate the lobule and accumulate around degenerating hepatocytes, particularly those containing Mallory-Denk bodies. Lymphocytes and macrophages also may be seen in portal tracts or parenchyma.

Steatofibrosis. Fatty liver disease of all kinds has a distinctive pattern of scarring. Like other changes, fibrosis appears first in the centrilobular region as **central vein sclerosis.** Perisinusoidal scarring appears next in the space of Disse of the centrilobular region and then spreads outward, encircling individual or small clusters of hepatocytes in a **chicken wire fence pattern** (see Fig. 16.16). Tendrils of fibrosis eventually link to portal tracts and then condense to create **central portal fibrous septa.** As these become more prominent, the liver takes on a nodular, cirrhotic appearance. Because in most cases the underlying cause persists, the continual subdivision of established nodules by new, perisinusoidal scarring leads to a classic **micronodular** or **Laennec cirrhosis.** Early in the course, the liver is yellow-tan, fatty, and enlarged, but with persistent damage over the course of years the liver is transformed into a brown, shrunken, nonfatty organ composed of cirrhotic nodules that are usually less than 0.3 cm in diameter—smaller than is typical for most chronic viral

hepatitis. The end-stage cirrhotic liver may enter into a "burned-out" phase devoid of fatty change and other typical features. A majority of cases of **cryptogenic cirrhosis,** without clear etiology, are now recognized as "burned-out" NAFLD.

Alcoholic Liver Disease

Excessive ethanol consumption causes more than 60% of chronic liver disease in Western countries and accounts for 40% to 50% of deaths due to cirrhosis. Among the most important adverse effects of chronic alcohol consumption are the overlapping forms of alcohol-related fatty liver disease already discussed: (1) hepatic steatosis, (2) alcoholic hepatitis, and (3) fibrosis and cirrhosis, collectively referred to as *alcoholic liver disease* (Fig. 16.18).

Between 90% and 100% of heavy drinkers develop fatty liver (i.e., hepatic steatosis), and of those, 10% to 35% develop alcoholic hepatitis, whereas only 8% to 20% of chronic alcoholics develop cirrhosis. Steatosis, alcoholic hepatitis, and fibrosis may develop sequentially or independently, so they do not necessarily represent a sequential continuum of changes. Hepatocellular carcinoma arises in 10% to 20% of patients with alcoholic cirrhosis.

Pathogenesis

Short-term ingestion of as much as 80 g of ethanol per day (5–6 beers or 8–9 ounces of 80-proof liquor) generally produces mild reversible hepatic changes, such as fatty liver. Chronic intake of 40 to 80 g/day is considered a borderline risk factor for severe injury. For reasons that may relate to decreased gastric metabolism of ethanol and differences in body composition, women are more susceptible than men to hepatic injury. It seems that how often and what one drinks may affect the risk for liver disease development. For example, binge drinking causes more

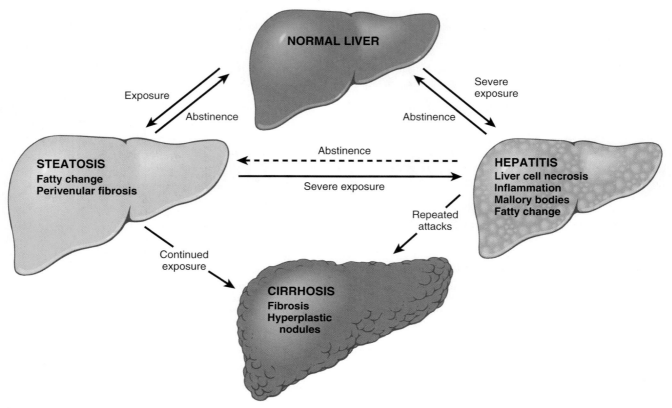

Fig. 16.18 Alcoholic liver disease. The interrelationships among hepatic steatosis, alcoholic hepatitis, and alcoholic cirrhosis are shown and key morphologic features are listed. As discussed in the text, steatosis, alcoholic hepatitis, and steatofibrosis may all develop independently and not along a continuum.

liver injury than that associated with steady, lower-level consumption. Since not everyone who drinks gets all the listed complications, individual, possibly genetic, risk factors must exist, but no reliable markers of susceptibility are known. In the absence of a clear understanding of the factors that influence liver damage, it is difficult to state what constitutes a safe level of alcohol consumption.

Hepatocellular steatosis is caused by alcohol through several mechanisms. First, metabolism of ethanol by alcohol dehydrogenase and acetaldehyde dehydrogenase generates large amounts of nicotinamide-adenine dinucleotide (NADH), which increases shunting of substrates away from catabolism and toward lipid biosynthesis. Second, ethanol impairs the assembly and secretion of lipoproteins. The net effect is to cause the accumulation of intracellular lipids.

The cause of *alcoholic hepatitis* is uncertain, but it may stem from one or more of the following toxic byproducts of ethanol and its metabolites:

- *Acetaldehyde* (a major metabolite of ethanol) induces lipid peroxidation and acetaldehyde-protein adduct formation, which may disrupt cytoskeleton and membrane function.
- *Alcohol* directly affects mitochondrial function and membrane fluidity.
- *Reactive oxygen species* generated during oxidation of ethanol by the microsomal ethanol oxidizing system react with and damage membranes and proteins. Reactive oxygen species also are produced by neutrophils, which infiltrate areas of hepatocyte necrosis.

Because generation of acetaldehyde and free radicals is maximal in the centrilobular region, this region is most susceptible to toxic injury. Pericellular and sinusoidal fibrosis develop first in this area of the lobule. Concurrent viral hepatitis, particularly hepatitis C, is a major accelerator of liver disease in alcoholics. The prevalence of hepatitis C among individuals with alcoholic liver disease is about 30% (and vice versa).

For unknown reasons, *cirrhosis* develops in only a small fraction of chronic alcoholics. With complete abstinence, at least partial regression of scarring occurs, and the micronodular liver transforms though parenchymal regeneration into a macronodular cirrhotic organ (see Figure 16.6); rarely, there is regression of cirrhosis altogether.

Clinical Features

Alcoholic steatosis may be innocuous or give rise to hepatomegaly with mild elevations of serum bilirubin and alkaline phosphatase. Severe hepatic compromise is unusual. Alcohol withdrawal and the provision of an adequate diet are sufficient treatment.

It is estimated that 15 to 20 years of excessive drinking are necessary to develop *alcoholic cirrhosis,* but *alcoholic hepatitis* can occur after just weeks or months of alcohol abuse. The onset is typically acute and often follows a bout of particularly heavy drinking. Symptoms and laboratory abnormalities range from minimal to severe. Most patients present with malaise, anorexia, weight loss, upper-abdominal discomfort, tender hepatomegaly, and fever. Typical findings include hyperbilirubinemia, elevated serum alkaline phosphatase levels, and neutrophilic leukocytosis. Serum alanine and aspartate aminotransferases are elevated but usually remain below 500 U/mL. The outlook is unpredictable; each bout of alcoholic hepatitis carries a 10% to 20% risk for death. With repeated bouts, cirrhosis appears in about one-third of patients within a few years.

The manifestations of alcoholic cirrhosis are similar to those of other forms of cirrhosis. In chronic alcoholics, ethanol may be the major source of calories in the diet, displacing other nutrients and leading to malnutrition and vitamin deficiencies (e.g., thiamine, vitamin B_{12}). Compounding these effects is impaired digestive function, primarily related to chronic gastric and intestinal mucosal damage and pancreatitis.

The long-term outlook for alcoholic patients with liver disease is variable. The most important aspect of treatment is abstinence from alcohol. The 5-year survival rate approaches 90% in abstainers who are free of jaundice, ascites, and hematemesis, but drops to 50% to 60% in individuals who continue to imbibe. Among those with end-stage alcoholic liver disease, the immediate causes of death are as follows:

- Hepatic failure
- Massive gastrointestinal hemorrhage
- Intercurrent infection (to which affected individuals are predisposed)
- Hepatorenal syndrome
- Hepatocellular carcinoma (3%–6% of cases)

SUMMARY

ALCOHOLIC LIVER DISEASE

- Alcoholic liver disease has three main manifestations, hepatic steatosis, alcoholic hepatitis, and cirrhosis, which may occur alone or in combination.
- Cirrhosis typically develops after more than 10 years of heavy drinking, but only occurs in a small proportion of chronic alcoholics; alcoholic cirrhosis has similar clinical signs and symptoms as cirrhosis caused by viral hepatitis.
- The multiple pathologic effects of alcohol include changes in lipid metabolism, decreased export of lipoproteins, and cell injury caused by reactive oxygen species and metabolites of alcohol.

Nonalcoholic Fatty Liver Disease

NAFLD is a common condition in which fatty liver disease develops in individuals who do not drink alcohol. The liver can show any of the three types of changes discussed earlier (steatosis, steatohepatitis, and cirrhosis), though on average inflammation is less prominent than in alcoholic liver disease. The term *nonalcoholic steatohepatitis (NASH)* is used to describe overt clinical features of liver injury, such as elevated transaminases, and the histologic features of hepatitis already discussed. NAFLD is consistently associated with insulin resistance and the metabolic syndrome (Chapter 8). Other commonly associated abnormalities are as follows:

- Type 2 diabetes (or family history of the condition)
- Obesity, primarily central obesity (body mass index >30 kg/m² in whites and >25 kg/m² in Asians)

- Dyslipidemia (hypertriglyceridemia, low high-density lipoprotein cholesterol, high low-density lipoprotein cholesterol)
- Hypertension

Pathogenesis

The key initiating events in NAFLD appear to be the development of obesity and insulin resistance, the latter within both adipose tissue and the liver. These factors combine to increase the mobilization of free fatty acids from adipose tissue, which are taken up by hepatocytes, and to stimulate the synthesis of fatty acids within hepatocytes. It is estimated that over half of the lipid found in hepatocytes in NAFLD is derived from adipose tissue, with most of the remainder coming from de novo synthesis in liver cells. Precisely how the accumulation of lipid in hepatocytes predisposes to the development of NASH is not known and may involve several interrelated mechanisms. Excessive intrahepatic lipids and their metabolic intermediates enhance insulin resistance in the liver and sensitize hepatocytes to the toxic effects of inflammatory cytokines, which are produced in increased amounts in the setting of the metabolic syndrome. In addition, hepatocytes in patients with NASH show evidence of inflammasome activation, possibly due to direct or indirect effects of particular lipids, leading to local release of the pro-inflammatory cytokine IL-1. Other products of lipid metabolism appear to be directly toxic to hepatocytes; proposed mechanisms include increased production of reactive oxygen species, induction of ER stress, and disruption of mitochondrial function. Liver injury resulting from these various insults causes stellate cell activation, collagen deposition, and hepatic fibrosis, which along with ongoing hepatocyte damage lead to full-blown NASH.

Clinical Features

NAFLD is the most common cause of incidental elevation of serum transaminases. Most individuals with steatosis are asymptomatic; patients with active steatohepatitis or fibrosis may also be asymptomatic, but some may have fatigue, malaise, right upper-quadrant discomfort, or more severe symptoms of chronic liver disease. Liver biopsy is required to identify NASH and distinguish it from uncomplicated NAFLD. Fortunately, the frequency of progression from steatosis to active steatohepatitis and then from active steatohepatitis to cirrhosis is low (Fig. 16.19). Nevertheless, NAFLD is considered to be a significant contributor to the pathogenesis of "cryptogenic" cirrhosis. Because they share common risk factors, the incidence of coronary artery disease also is increased in patients with NAFLD.

Current therapy is directed toward obesity reduction and reversal of insulin resistance. Lifestyle modifications that lead to weight loss (diet and exercise) appear to be the most effective form of treatment.

Pediatric NAFLD is becoming an increasing problem as obesity and metabolic syndrome approach epidemic proportions. In children, the appearance of the histologic lesions is somewhat different, as inflammation and scarring tend to be more prominent in the portal tracts and periportal regions, and mononuclear infiltrates rather than neutrophilic infiltrates predominate.

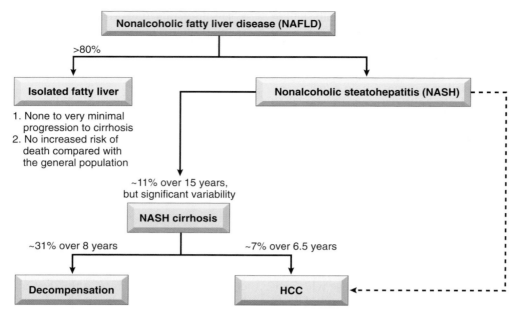

Fig. 16.19 Natural history of nonalcoholic fatty liver disease. Isolated fatty liver disease shows minimal risk for progression to cirrhosis or increased mortality, while nonalcoholic steatohepatitis shows increased overall mortality as well as increased risk for cirrhosis and hepatocellular carcinoma. *DM,* Diabetes mellitus.

SUMMARY

NONALCOHOLIC FATTY LIVER DISEASE

- Nonalcoholic fatty liver disease (NAFLD) is associated with the metabolic syndrome, obesity, type 2 diabetes, and dyslipidemia and/or hypertension.
- NAFLD may show all the changes associated with alcoholic liver disease: steatosis, nonalcoholic steatohepatitis (NASH), and cirrhosis, although the features of steatohepatitis (such as hepatocyte ballooning, Mallory-Denk bodies, and neutrophilic infiltration) often are less prominent than they are in alcohol-related injury.
- Pediatric NAFLD is increasingly being recognized as the obesity epidemic spreads to pediatric age groups, although its histologic pattern differs somewhat from that seen in adults.

INHERITED METABOLIC LIVER DISEASES

Although there are many inherited metabolic liver diseases, only some relatively common, pathogenically interesting entities are discussed here: hereditary hemochromatosis, Wilson disease, and alpha-1-anti-trypsin (α_1AT) deficiency.

Hemochromatosis

Hemochromatosis is caused by excessive absorption of iron, which is primarily deposited in parenchymal organs such as the liver and pancreas, as well as in the heart, joints, and endocrine organs. It results most commonly from an inherited disorder, *hereditary hemochromatosis.* When iron accumulation occurs as a consequence of

parenteral administration of iron, usually in the form of transfusions, it is called *acquired hemochromatosis.* Secondary iron overload also can complicate diseases that are associated with persistent ineffective erythropoiesis, particularly thalassemia and myelodysplastic syndromes (Chapter 12).

As discussed in Chapter 12, the total body iron pool ranges from 2 to 6 gm in normal adults; about 0.5 gm is stored in hepatocytes. In severe hemochromatosis, total iron may exceed 50 gm, one-third of which accumulates in the liver. Fully developed cases exhibit (1) micronodular cirrhosis; (2) diabetes mellitus (up to 80% of patients); and (3) abnormal skin pigmentation (up to 80% of patients).

Pathogenesis

Because there is no regulated iron excretion from the body, the total body content of iron is tightly regulated by intestinal absorption. As discussed in Chapter 12, hepcidin is a circulating peptide hormone that acts as a key negative regulator of intestinal iron uptake. **Diverse mutations in several genes have been described in hereditary hemochromatosis, all of which lower hepcidin levels or diminish hepcidin function.** Whatever the underlying defect, the net result is an increase in intestinal absorption of dietary iron, leading to an accumulation of 0.5 to 1 gm of iron per year.

The most frequently mutated gene in patients with hereditary hemochromatosis is *HFE,* which is located on chromosome 6 close to the *HLA* gene cluster. *HFE* encodes an HLA class I–like molecule that regulates the synthesis of hepcidin in hepatocytes. The most common HFE mutation is a cysteine-to-tyrosine substitution at amino acid 282 (C282Y). This mutation, which inactivates the HFE protein, is present in over 70% of patients diagnosed with hereditary hemochromatosis and is most common in European populations. Several other mutations can also give rise to hemochromatosis, including other mutations in HFE as well as mutations in transferrin receptor 2 and in hepcidin itself. The associated clinical condition is milder with some of these alternative mutations and more severe with others, sometimes manifesting in young adults or even during childhood.

Whatever the underlying cause, the onset of disease typically occurs after 20 gm of stored iron have accumulated. Excessive iron appears to be directly toxic to host tissues. Mechanisms of liver injury include the following:

- Lipid peroxidation via iron-catalyzed free radical reactions
- Stimulation of collagen formation by activation of hepatic stellate cells
- DNA damage by reactive oxygen species, leading to lethal cell injury or predisposition to HCC

The deleterious effects of iron on cells that are not fatally injured are reversible, and removal of excess iron with therapy promotes recovery of tissue function.

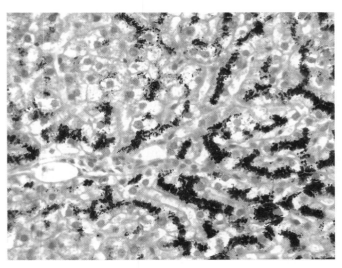

Fig. 16.20 Hereditary hemochromatosis. In this Prussian blue–stained section, hepatocellular iron appears blue. The parenchymal architecture is normal at this stage of disease, even with such abundant iron.

MORPHOLOGY

The morphologic changes in severe hemochromatosis are characterized principally by (1) **tissue deposition of hemosiderin** in the following organs (in decreasing order of severity): liver, pancreas, myocardium, pituitary gland, adrenal gland, thyroid and parathyroid glands, joints, and skin; (2) **cirrhosis**; and (3) **pancreatic fibrosis**. In the liver, iron becomes evident first as golden-yellow hemosiderin granules in the cytoplasm of periportal hepatocytes, which can be histochemically stained with Prussian blue (Fig. 16.20). With increasing iron load, there is progressive deposition in the rest of the lobule, the bile duct epithelium, and Kupffer cells. At this stage, the liver typically is slightly enlarged and chocolate brown. Fibrous septa develop slowly, linking portal tracts to each other and leading ultimately to **cirrhosis** in an intensely pigmented (very dark brown to black) liver.

The **pancreas** also becomes pigmented, acquires diffuse interstitial fibrosis, and may show parenchymal atrophy. Hemosiderin is found in the acinar and the islet cells and sometimes in the interstitial fibrous stroma. The **heart** often is enlarged, with hemosiderin granules within the myocardial fibers. The pigmentation may induce a striking brown coloration of the myocardium. A delicate interstitial fibrosis may appear. Although **skin pigmentation** is partially attributable to hemosiderin deposition in dermal macrophages and fibroblasts, most of the coloration results from increased epidermal melanin production. The combination of these pigments renders the skin slate-gray. With hemosiderin deposition in the joint synovial linings, an acute synovitis may develop. There is also excessive deposition of calcium pyrophosphate, which damages the articular cartilage and sometimes produces disabling polyarthritis, referred to as *pseudogout*. With the onset of cirrhosis, the testes may become atrophic.

Clinical Features

Symptoms usually appear earlier in men than in women since menstrual bleeding limits the accumulation of iron until menopause. This results in a male-to-female ratio of clinically significant iron overload of approximately 5:1 to 7:1. In the most common form caused by *HFE* mutations, symptoms usually appear in the fifth and sixth decades of life in men and later in women. With population screening, it has become clear that homozygosity for the most common *HFE* mutation (C282Y) shows variable penetrance; thus disease development is not inevitable, presumably because other genetic and environmental factors influence the rate of iron accumulation.

The principal manifestations include hepatomegaly, abdominal pain, skin pigmentation (particularly in sun-exposed areas), deranged glucose homeostasis or frank diabetes mellitus due to destruction of pancreatic islets, cardiac dysfunction (arrhythmias, cardiomyopathy), and atypical arthritis. In some patients, the presenting complaint is hypogonadism (e.g., amenorrhea in the female, impotence and loss of libido in the male). As noted, clinically apparent disease is more common in males and rarely becomes evident before 40 years of age. Death may result from cirrhosis or cardiac disease. In those with untreated disease, the risk for HCC is increased 200-fold, presumably because of ongoing liver damage and the genotoxic effects of oxidants generated by iron in the liver.

Fortunately, hemochromatosis can be diagnosed long before irreversible tissue damage has occurred. Screening of family members of probands is important. Heterozygotes also accumulate excessive iron, but not to a level that causes significant tissue damage. Currently most patients with hemochromatosis are diagnosed in the subclinical, precirrhotic stage due to routine serum iron measurements (as part of another diagnostic workup). Regular phlebotomy results in steady removal of excess tissue iron, and with this simple treatment life expectancy is normal.

Wilson Disease

Wilson disease is an autosomal recessive disorder caused by mutation of the *ATP7B* gene, which results in impaired copper excretion into bile and a failure to incorporate copper into ceruloplasmin. This disorder is marked by the accumulation of toxic levels of copper in many tissues and organs, principally the liver, brain, and eye. Normally, 40%

to 60% of ingested copper (2–5 mg/day) is absorbed in the duodenum and proximal small intestine, from where it is transported complexed with albumin and histidine to the liver. Here, free copper dissociates and is taken up by hepatocytes, where copper is incorporated into enzymes and α_2-globulin (apoceruloplasmin) to form *ceruloplasmin*, which is secreted into the blood. Ceruloplasmin carries 90% to 95% of plasma copper. Circulating ceruloplasmin is eventually desialylated, endocytosed by the liver, and degraded within lysosomes, after which the released copper is excreted into bile. This degradation/excretion pathway is the primary route for copper elimination.

The *ATP7B* gene, located on chromosome 13, encodes a transmembrane copper-transporting ATPase that is expressed on the hepatocyte canalicular membrane. The overwhelming majority of patients with Wilson disease are compound heterozygotes with different loss-of-function mutations affecting each *ATP7B* allele. The overall frequency of mutated alleles is 1:100, and the prevalence of the disease is approximately 1:30,000 to 1:50,000. Loss of ATP7B protein function impairs the transport of copper into the bile and the incorporation of copper into ceruloplasmin, which is not secreted in its apoceruloplasmin form. These abnormalities lead to copper accumulation in the liver and a decrease in plasma ceruloplasmin. Accumulating copper causes liver injury through the production of reactive oxygen species by the Fenton reaction (Chapter 3). Eventually, non-ceruloplasmin–bound copper is released from injured hepatocytes into the circulation, causing red cell hemolysis and allowing copper to deposit in other tissues, such as the brain, corneas, kidneys, bones, joints, and parathyroid glands. Concomitantly, urinary excretion of copper increases markedly from its normal minuscule levels.

MORPHOLOGY

The liver often bears the brunt of injury. The hepatic changes are variable, ranging from relatively minor to massive and mimic many other disease processes. There may be mild to moderate **fatty change (steatosis)** associated with focal hepatocyte necrosis. **Acute, fulminant hepatitis** can mimic acute viral hepatitis. **Chronic hepatitis** in Wilson disease exhibits moderate to severe inflammation and hepatocyte necrosis, areas of fatty change, and features of steatohepatitis (hepatocyte ballooning with prominent Mallory-Denk bodies). In advanced cases, **cirrhosis** may be seen. Copper deposition in hepatocytes can be demonstrated by special stains (rhodamine stain for copper, orcein stain for copper-associated protein).

Toxic injury to the brain primarily affects the basal ganglia. Nearly all patients with neurologic involvement develop eye lesions called **Kayser-Fleischer rings,** green to brown deposits of copper in Desçemet membrane in the limbus of the cornea.

Clinical Features

The age at onset and the clinical presentation of Wilson disease are extremely variable. Symptoms usually appear between 6 and 40 years of age. Acute or chronic liver disease are common presenting features. Neuropsychiatric manifestations are the initial features in most of the

remaining cases and stem from deposition of copper in the basal ganglia.

The diagnosis of Wilson disease is based on low levels of serum ceruloplasmin, an increase in hepatic copper content (the most sensitive test), and increased urinary excretion of copper (the most specific test). Hepatic copper content in excess of 250 μg per gram dry weight of liver is taken to be diagnostic, but is only about 80% sensitive. In those with lower liver copper levels, the diagnosis depends on other abnormalities, such as elevated urinary copper, low serum ceruloplasmin, and the presence of Kayser-Fleischer rings. Unlike hereditary hemochromatosis, where the limited number of genetic variants makes genetic testing fairly simple, the large number of different causative mutations in *ATP7B7* complicates the use of DNA sequencing as a diagnostic test. Serum copper levels also are of no diagnostic value, as they may be low, normal, or elevated, depending on the stage of the liver disease.

Early recognition and long-term copper chelation therapy (with D-penicillamine or Trientine) or zinc-based therapy (which inhibits copper uptake in the gut) has dramatically altered the usual progressive downhill course. Individuals with hepatitis or advanced cirrhosis require liver transplantation, which can be curative.

α_1-Anti-Trypsin Deficiency

α_1-Anti-trypsin deficiency is an autosomal recessive disorder marked by very low levels of circulating α_1-antitrypsin (α_1AT) that is caused by mutations that lead to misfolding of α_1AT. The major function of α_1AT is to inhibit proteases, particularly neutrophil elastase, cathepsin G, and proteinase 3, which are released from neutrophils at sites of inflammation. α_1AT deficiency leads to the development of pulmonary emphysema because the activity of destructive proteases is not inhibited (Chapter 13). It also causes liver disease as a consequence of hepatocellular accumulation of the misfolded α_1AT protein.

α_1AT is a small 394–amino acid plasma glycoprotein synthesized predominantly by hepatocytes. The gene, located on chromosome 14, is very polymorphic. At least 75 α_1AT variants have been identified, denoted alphabetically by their relative migration on an isoelectric gel. The general notation is "Pi" for "protease inhibitor" and an alphabetic letter for the position on the gel; two letters denote the genotype of the two alleles. The most common genotype is PiMM, occurring in 90% of individuals (the "wild-type").

The most common clinically significant mutation is PiZ; PiZZ homozygotes have circulating α_1AT levels that are only 10% of normal. These individuals are at high risk for developing clinical disease. Variant alleles are codominant, and, consequently, PiMZ heterozygotes have intermediate plasma levels of α_1AT. Among individuals of northern European descent, the PiZZ state affects 1 in 1800 live births. Because of the early presentation of the liver disease, α_1AT deficiency is the most commonly diagnosed genetic hepatic disorder in infants and children.

Pathogenesis

The PiZ polypeptide is prone to misfolding and aggregation due to a single amino acid glutamine-to-lysine

substitution at residue 342 (E342K). This in turn creates endoplasmic reticulum stress and triggers the unfolded protein response, which ultimately leads to apoptosis. It is worth emphasizing that the liver damage is caused by protein misfolding, whereas lung damage leading to emphysema stems from the loss of α_1AT function and excessive protease activity. Although all individuals with the PiZZ genotype accumulate α_1AT-Z in the endoplasmic reticulum of hepatocytes, only 10% to 15% develop overt clinical liver disease; thus, other genetic factors or environmental factors must also play a role in the development of liver disease.

MORPHOLOGY

α_1-Anti-trypsin deficiency is characterized by the presence of round-to-oval cytoplasmic **globular inclusions** in hepatocytes that are strongly periodic acid–Schiff (PAS) positive and diastase resistant (Fig. 16.21). Periportal hepatocytes are most affected in early and in mild forms of the disease, with central lobular hepatocytes being affected later or in more severe disease. Other pathologic features vary, ranging from hepatitis to fibrosis to full-blown cirrhosis.

Clinical Features

Neonatal hepatitis with cholestatic jaundice appears in 10% to 20% of newborns with α_1AT deficiency. In adolescence, presenting symptoms may be related to hepatitis or cirrhosis. Attacks of hepatitis may subside with apparent complete recovery, or they may become chronic and lead progressively to cirrhosis. Alternatively, the disease may remain silent until cirrhosis appears in middle to later adult life. HCC develops in 2% to 3% of PiZZ adults, usually in the setting of cirrhosis. The definitive treatment, for severe hepatic disease is liver transplantation. In patients with pulmonary disease, avoidance of cigarette smoking is crucial, because smoking results in accumulation of neutrophils and release of elastase in the

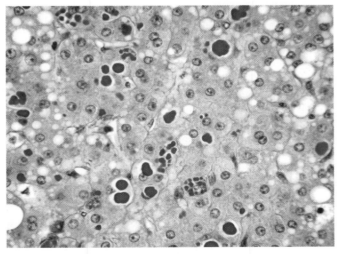

Fig. 16.21 α_1-Anti-trypsin deficiency. Periodic acid–Schiff (PAS) stain after diastase digestion of the liver, highlights the characteristic magenta cytoplasmic granules.

lung that is not inactivated because of lack of α_1AT. The unopposed action of neutrophil derived proteases destroys elastic fibers in alveolar walls, leading to emphysema (Chapter 13).

SUMMARY

INHERITED METABOLIC LIVER DISEASE

- Hemochromatosis is most commonly caused by mutations in the *HFE* gene and less commonly by mutations in other genes, all of which result in decreased hepcidin levels or function and increased intestinal iron uptake. It is characterized by accumulation of iron in the liver, pancreas, and other tissues.
- Wilson disease is caused by loss-of-function mutations in the metal ion transporter ATP7B, which results in accumulation of copper in the liver, brain (particularly basal ganglia), and eyes (Kayser-Fleischer rings).
- Wilson disease effects on the liver are protean, showing changes ranging from acute massive hepatic necrosis, to fatty liver disease, to chronic hepatitis and cirrhosis.
- α_1AT deficiency is a disease in which mutations in α_1AT lead to its misfolding, causing liver toxicity and a functional deficit of α_1AT in the plasma. This deficiency places affected individuals at high risk for emphysema, particularly smokers, due to the unopposed effects of proteases released from neutrophils.

CHOLESTATIC SYNDROMES

Hepatic bile serves two major functions: (1) the emulsification of dietary fat in the lumen of the gut through the detergent action of bile salts, and (2) the elimination of bilirubin, excess cholesterol, xenobiotics, and other waste products that are insufficiently water-soluble to be excreted into urine. Processes that interfere with excretion of bile lead to *jaundice* and *icterus* due to retention of bilirubin, and to *cholestasis* (discussed later).

Jaundice may occur in settings of increase bilirubin production (e.g., extravascular red cell hemolysis), hepatocyte dysfunction (e.g., hepatitis), or obstruction of the flow of bile (e.g., an impacted gallstone), any of which can disturb the equilibrium between bilirubin production and clearance (summarized in Table 16.4). The metabolism of bilirubin by the liver occurs in four steps: uptake from the circulation; intracellular storage; conjugation with glucuronic acid; and biliary excretion. These are discussed next.

Bilirubin and Bile Formation

Bilirubin is the end product of heme degradation (Fig. 16.22). Approximately 85% of daily production (0.2–0.3 gm) is derived from the breakdown of senescent red cells by macrophages in the spleen, liver, and bone marrow. The remainder is derived from the turnover of hepatic heme or hemoproteins (e.g., the P-450 cytochromes) and from destruction of red cell precursors in the bone marrow (Chapter 12). Whatever the source, intracellular heme oxygenase oxidizes heme to biliverdin (step 1 in Fig. 16.22),

Table 16.4 Major Causes of Jaundice

Predominantly Unconjugated Hyperbilirubinemia
Excess Production of Bilirubin
Hemolytic anemias
Resorption of blood from internal hemorrhage (e.g., alimentary tract bleeding, hematomas)
Ineffective erythropoiesis (e.g., pernicious anemia, thalassemia)
Reduced Hepatic Uptake
Drug interference with membrane carrier systems
Impaired Bilirubin Conjugation
Physiologic jaundice of the newborn
Diffuse hepatocellular disease (e.g., viral or drug-induced hepatitis, cirrhosis)
Predominantly Conjugated Hyperbilirubinemia
Decreased Hepatocellular Excretion
Drug-induced canalicular membrane dysfunction (e.g., oral contraceptives, cyclosporine)
Hepatocellular damage or toxicity (e.g., viral or drug-induced hepatitis, total parenteral nutrition, systemic infection)
Impaired Intrahepatic or Extrahepatic Bile Flow
Inflammatory destruction of intrahepatic bile ducts (e.g., primary biliary cirrhosis, primary sclerosing cholangitis, graft-versus-host disease, liver transplantation)
Gallstones
External compression (e.g., carcinoma of the pancreas)

which is immediately reduced to bilirubin by biliverdin reductase. Bilirubin thus formed is released and binds to serum albumin (step 2), which is critical since bilirubin is virtually insoluble in aqueous solutions at physiologic pH and also highly toxic to tissues. Albumin carries bilirubin to the liver, where bilirubin is taken up into hepatocytes (step 3) and conjugated with one or two molecules of glucuronic acid by bilirubin uridine diphosphate (UDP)–glucuronyltransferase (UGT1A1, step 4) in the endoplasmic reticulum. Water-soluble, nontoxic bilirubin glucuronides are then excreted into the bile. Most bilirubin glucuronides are deconjugated in the gut lumen by bacterial β-glucuronidases and degraded to colorless urobilinogens (step 5). The urobilinogens and the residue of intact pigment are largely excreted in feces. Approximately 20% of the urobilinogens formed are reabsorbed in the ileum and colon, returned to the liver, and reexcreted into bile. A small amount of reabsorbed urobilinogen is excreted in the urine.

Two-thirds of the organic materials in bile are bile salts, which are formed by the conjugation of bile acids with taurine or glycine. Bile acids, the major catabolic products of cholesterol, are a family of water-soluble sterols with carboxylated side chains. The primary human bile acids are cholic acid and chenodeoxycholic acid. Bile acids are highly effective detergents. Their primary physiologic role is to solubilize water-insoluble lipids secreted by hepatocytes into bile, and also to solubilize dietary lipids in the gut lumen. Ninety-five percent of secreted bile acids, conjugated or unconjugated, are reabsorbed from the gut lumen and recirculate to the liver (*enterohepatic circulation*), thus helping to maintain a large endogenous pool of bile acids for digestive and excretory purposes.

Pathophysiology of Jaundice

Both unconjugated bilirubin and conjugated bilirubin (bilirubin glucuronides) may accumulate systemically. As discussed earlier, unconjugated bilirubin is virtually insoluble and tightly bound to albumin. As a result, it cannot be excreted in the urine, even when blood levels are high. Normally, a very small amount of unconjugated bilirubin is present as a free anion in plasma. If unconjugated bilirubin levels rise, this unbound fraction may diffuse into tissues, particularly the brain in infants, and produce toxic injury. The unbound plasma fraction increases in severe hemolytic disease or when protein-binding drugs displace bilirubin from albumin. Hence, hemolytic disease of the newborn (erythroblastosis fetalis) may lead to accumulation of unconjugated bilirubin in the brain, which can cause severe neurologic damage, referred to as *kernicterus*

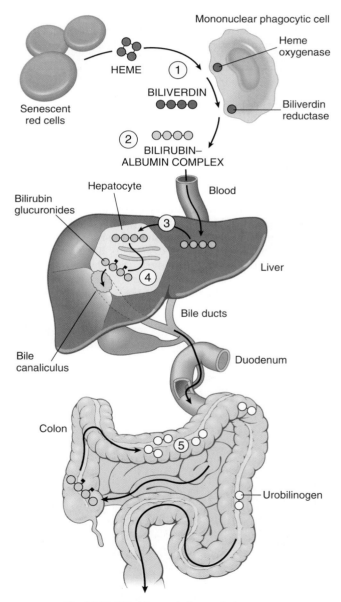

Fig. 16.22 Bilirubin metabolism and elimination.

(Chapter 7). In contrast, conjugated bilirubin is water-soluble, nontoxic, and only loosely bound to albumin. Because of its solubility and weak association with albumin, excess conjugated bilirubin in plasma can be excreted in urine.

Serum bilirubin levels in the normal adult vary between 0.3 and 1.2 mg/dL. Jaundice becomes evident when the serum bilirubin levels rise above 2 to 2.5 mg/dL; levels as high as 30 to 40 mg/dL can occur with severe disease. Causes of conjugated and unconjugated hyperbilirubinemia differ, and so measurement of both forms is of value in evaluating a patient with jaundice.

Defects in Hepatocellular Bilirubin Metabolism

Neonatal Jaundice

Because the hepatic machinery for conjugating and excreting bilirubin does not fully mature until about 2 weeks of age, almost every newborn develops transient and mild unconjugated hyperbilirubinemia, termed *neonatal jaundice* or *physiologic jaundice of the newborn*. This may be exacerbated by breastfeeding, due to the action of bilirubin-deconjugating enzymes in breast milk. Nevertheless, sustained jaundice in the newborn is abnormal and is discussed later in the "Neonatal Cholestasis" section.

Hereditary Hyperbilirubinemias

Jaundice also may result from inborn errors of metabolism, including the following:

- *Gilbert syndrome* is a common (7% of the population) inherited condition that manifests as fluctuating unconjugated hyperbilirubinemia of variable severity. The primary cause is mildly decreased hepatic levels of glucuronosyltransferase attributed to a mutation in the encoding gene, *UGT1A1*; polymorphisms in the gene may play a role in the variable expression of this disorder. Gilbert syndrome is not associated with any morbidity. By contrast, severe glucuronosyltransferase deficiency causes a rare disorder called *Crigler-Najjar Syndrome Type 1* that is fatal in infancy.

- *Dubin-Johnson syndrome* results from an autosomal recessive defect in the transport protein responsible for hepatocellular excretion of bilirubin glucuronides across the canalicular membrane. Affected individuals exhibit conjugated hyperbilirubinemia. Other than having a darkly pigmented liver (from polymerized epinephrine metabolites, not bilirubin) and hepatomegaly, patients are normal.

Cholestasis

Cholestasis is a condition caused by extrahepatic or intrahepatic obstruction of bile channels or by defects in hepatocyte bile secretion. Patients may have jaundice, pruritus, skin xanthomas (focal accumulation of cholesterol), or symptoms related to intestinal malabsorption, including nutritional deficiencies of the fat-soluble vitamins A, D, or K. A characteristic laboratory finding is elevated serum alkaline phosphatase and γ-glutamyl transpeptidase (GGT), enzymes that are present on the apical membranes of hepatocytes and cholangiocytes.

MORPHOLOGY

The morphologic features of cholestasis depend on its severity, duration, and underlying cause. Common to both obstructive and nonobstructive cholestasis is the accumulation of bile pigment within the hepatic parenchyma (Fig. 16.23). Elongated green-brown plugs of bile are visible in dilated bile canaliculi. Rupture of canaliculi leads to extravasation of bile, which is quickly phagocytosed by Kupffer cells. Droplets of bile pigment also accumulate within hepatocytes, which can take on a fine, foamy appearance referred to as *feathery degeneration*. Occasional apoptotic hepatocytes also may be seen.

Bile Duct Obstruction and Ascending Cholangitis

The most common cause of bile duct obstruction in adults is extrahepatic cholelithiasis (gallstones, discussed

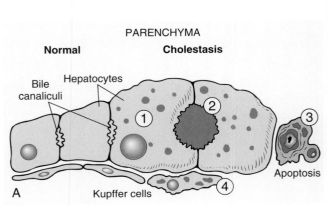
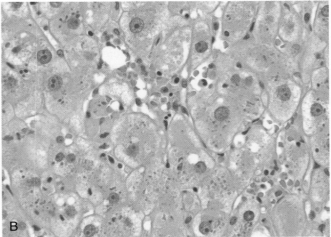

Fig. 16.23 Cholestasis. (A) Morphologic features of cholestasis *(right)* and comparison with normal liver *(left)*. Cholestatic hepatocytes (1) are enlarged and are associated with dilated canalicular spaces (2). Apoptotic cells (3) may be seen, and Kupffer cells (4) frequently contain regurgitated bile pigments. (B) Cholestasis, showing the characteristic accumulation of bile pigments in the cytoplasm.

later), followed by malignant obstructions, and post-surgical strictures. Obstructive conditions in children include biliary atresia, cystic fibrosis, choledochal cysts (a cystic anomaly of the extrahepatic biliary tree), and syndromes in which there are insufficient intrahepatic bile ducts (paucity of bile duct syndromes). The initial morphologic features of cholestasis have been discussed and are entirely reversible with correction of the obstruction. Prolonged obstruction can lead to biliary cirrhosis, discussed later.

Ascending cholangitis, secondary bacterial infection of the biliary tree, may complicate duct obstruction. Enteric organisms such as coliforms and enterococci are common culprits. Cholangitis usually presents with fever, chills, abdominal pain, and jaundice. The most severe form of cholangitis is *suppurative cholangitis,* in which purulent bile fills and distends bile ducts. Since sepsis rather than cholestasis tends to dominate this potentially grave process, prompt diagnostic evaluation and intervention are imperative.

Since extrahepatic biliary obstruction is frequently amenable to surgical treatment, correct and prompt diagnosis is imperative. In contrast, cholestasis due to diseases of the intrahepatic biliary tree or hepatocellular secretory failure (collectively termed *intrahepatic cholestasis*) is not benefited by surgery (short of transplantation), and the patient's condition may be worsened by an operative procedure. It is thus important to establish the underlying basis for jaundice and cholestasis.

MORPHOLOGY

Acute biliary obstruction, either intrahepatic or extrahepatic, causes distention of upstream bile ducts, which often become dilated. In addition, **ductular reactions** appear at the portal-parenchymal interface along with stromal edema and neutrophils. The hallmark of superimposed infection **(ascending cholangitis)** is the influx of periductular neutrophils into the bile duct epithelium and lumen (Fig. 16.24).

Left uncorrected, the inflammation and ductular reactions resulting **from chronic biliary obstruction** initiate periportal fibrosis, eventually generating **secondary or obstructive biliary cirrhosis** (Fig. 16.25). Cholestatic features in the parenchyma may be prominent. These take the form of extensive **feathery degeneration of periportal hepatocytes**, a type of cytoplasmic swelling often associated with **Mallory-Denk bodies** and **bile infarcts** caused by the detergent effects of extravasated bile.

Neonatal Cholestasis

Prolonged conjugated hyperbilirubinemia in the neonate, termed *neonatal cholestasis* (as opposed to the already discussed neonatal jaundice) affects approximately 1 in 2500 live births. The major conditions causing it are (1) cholangiopathies, primarily *biliary atresia* (discussed later), and (2) a variety of disorders causing conjugated hyperbilirubinemia in the neonate, collectively referred to as *neonatal hepatitis.*

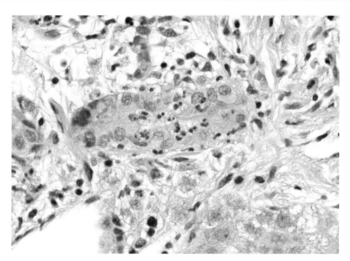

Fig. 16.24 Acute large-duct obstruction with ascending cholangitis. Superimposed on features of duct obstruction (edema, ductular reaction) is an infiltrate of neutrophils involving the bile duct, the hallmark of ascending cholangitis.

Neonatal hepatitis is not a specific entity, nor does it necessarily have an inflammatory basis. Rather it is an indication to conduct a diligent search for recognizable toxic, metabolic, and infectious liver diseases, as greater than 85% of cases have identifiable causes.

Differentiation of biliary atresia from nonobstructive neonatal cholestasis is very important, since definitive treatment of biliary atresia requires surgical intervention (Kasai procedure), whereas surgery may adversely affect a child with other disorders. Fortunately, discrimination can be made on the basis of clinical data in about 90% of cases. In 10% of cases, liver biopsy may be necessary to distinguish neonatal hepatitis from an identifiable cholangiopathy. Affected infants have jaundice, dark urine, light or acholic stools, and hepatomegaly. Variable degrees of hepatic synthetic dysfunction may be identified, such as hypoprothrombinemia.

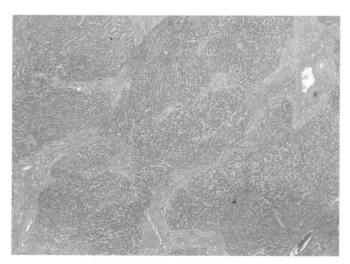

Fig. 16.25 Cirrhosis secondary to primary biliary cholangitis.

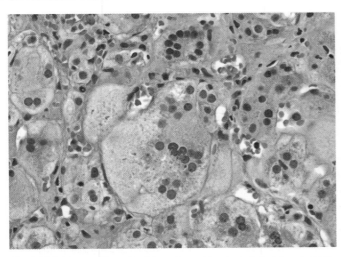

Fig. 16.26 Neonatal hepatitis. Note the multinucleated giant hepatocytes.

MORPHOLOGY

The morphologic features of neonatal hepatitis (Fig. 16.26) include striking giant-cell transformation of hepatocytes, associated with lobular disarray, focal liver cell apoptosis and prominent hepatocellular and canalicular cholestasis. In some cases, this parenchymal pattern of injury also is accompanied by ductular reaction and fibrosis of portal tracts.

Biliary Atresia

Biliary atresia is defined as a complete or partial obstruction of the extrahepatic biliary tree that occurs within the first 3 months of life. It underlies approximately one-third of cases of neonatal cholestasis and is the single most frequent cause of death from liver disease in early childhood. Approximately 50% to 60% of children referred for liver transplantation have biliary atresia.

Pathogenesis

Two major forms of biliary atresia are recognized; these are based on the presumed timing of luminal obliteration.

- The *fetal form* accounts for as many as 20% of cases and is commonly associated with other developmental anomalies involving the thoracic and abdominal organs, including malrotation of abdominal viscera, interrupted inferior vena cava, polysplenia, and congenital heart disease.
- Much more common is the *perinatal form* of biliary atresia, in which an apparently normally developed biliary tree is injured and obstructed following birth. The etiology of perinatal biliary atresia is unknown; viral infection and toxic exposures are considered prime suspects.

MORPHOLOGY

The salient features of biliary atresia include **inflammation and fibrosing stricture of the hepatic or common bile ducts;** in some individuals, periductular inflammation also extends into the intrahepatic bile ducts, leading to progressive destruction of the intrahepatic biliary tree as well. When biliary atresia is unrecognized or uncorrected, cirrhosis develops within 3 to 6 months of birth.

There is considerable variability in the pattern of biliary atresia. When the disease is limited to the common duct or right and/or left hepatic bile ducts with patent intrahepatic branches, the disease is surgically correctable (**Kasai procedure**). Unfortunately, in 90% of patients the obstruction also involves bile ducts at or above the porta hepatis. These cases are not correctable, since there are no patent bile ducts amenable to surgical anastomosis.

Clinical Features

Infants with biliary atresia present with neonatal cholestasis, but exhibit normal birth weight and postnatal weight gain. There is a slight female predominance. Initially stools are normal, but they become acholic as the disease progresses. Ascending cholangitis and/or intrahepatic progression of the disease may impede attempts at surgical resection of the obstruction and bypass of the biliary tree. Transplantation of a donor liver and its accompanying bile ducts is the primary hope for saving these young patients. Without surgical intervention, death usually occurs within 2 years of birth.

Autoimmune Cholangiopathies

Autoimmune cholangiopathies comprise two distinct immunologically-mediated disorders that involve intrahepatic bile ducts: primary biliary cholangitis and primary sclerosing cholangitis. The salient features of these are listed in Table 16.5.

Primary Biliary Cholangitis

Primary biliary cholangitis (PBC) is an autoimmune disease whose primary feature is nonsuppurative, inflammatory destruction of small- and medium-sized intrahepatic bile ducts. Large intrahepatic ducts and the extrahepatic biliary tree are not involved. Previously, this disease was known as primary biliary cirrhosis, but most patients do not progress to this stage, and the name primary biliary cholangitis is now preferred.

PBC is primarily a disease of middle-age women, with a female-to-male ratio of 6:1. Its peak incidence is between 40 and 50 years of age. The disease is most prevalent in Northern European countries (England and Scotland) and the Northern United States (Minnesota), where the prevalence is as high as 400 per 1 million cases. Recent increases in incidence and prevalence along with geographic clustering suggest that both environmental and genetic factors are important in its pathogenesis. Family members of PBC patients have an increased risk for developing the disease.

Pathogenesis

PBC is thought to be an autoimmune disorder, but as with other autoimmune diseases the triggers that initiate PBC are unknown. **Anti-mitochondrial antibodies are the most**

Table 16.5 Main Features of Primary Biliary Cholangitis and Primary Sclerosing Cholangitis

Parameter	Primary Biliary Cholangitis	Primary Sclerosing Cholangitis
Age	Median age 50 years	Median age 30 years
Gender	90% female	70% male
Clinical course	Progressive	Unpredictable, but progressive
Associated conditions	Sjögren syndrome (70%)	Inflammatory bowel disease (70%)
	Scleroderma (5%)	Pancreatitis (≤25%)
	Thyroid disease (20%)	Idiopathic fibrosing diseases (retroperitoneal fibrosis)
Serology	95% AMA-positive	0%–5% AMA-positive (low titer)
	20% ANA-positive	6% ANA-positive
	40% ANCA-positive	65% ANCA-positive
Radiology	Normal	Strictures and beading of large bile ducts; pruning of smaller ducts
Duct lesion	Florid duct lesions and loss of small ducts only	Inflammatory destruction of extrahepatic and large intrahepatic ducts; fibrotic obliteration of medium and small intrahepatic ducts

AMA, Anti-mitochondrial antibody; *ANA*, anti-nuclear anti-body; *ANCA*, anti-neutrophil cytoplasmic antibody.

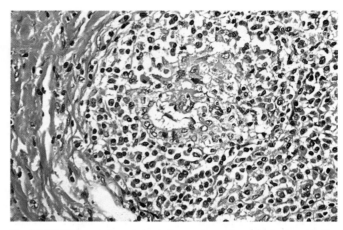

Fig. 16.27 Primary biliary cirrhosis. A portal tract is markedly expanded by an infiltrate of lymphocytes and plasma cells. Note the granulomatous reaction to the bile duct undergoing destruction (the "florid duct lesion").

characteristic finding in PBC. T cells specific for certain mitochondrial enzymes are another feature of the disease, supporting the notion of an immune-mediated process. Other findings suggestive of altered immunity include aberrant expression of MHC class II molecules on bile duct epithelial cells, accumulation of autoreactive T cells around bile ducts, and the frequent presence of other autoantibodies against nuclear pore proteins centromeric proteins, and other cellular components.

MORPHOLOGY

Interlobular bile ducts are actively destroyed by lymphoplasmacytic inflammation with or without granulomas (the *florid duct lesion*) (Fig. 16.27). Some biopsy specimens, however, do not have active lesions and only show the absence of bile ducts in portal tracts. The disease is quite patchy in distribution; it is common to see a single bile duct under immune attack in one level of a biopsy specimen, while other nearby ducts, are unaffected. **Ductular reactions** follow on this duct injury, and these in turn participate in the development of **portal-portal septal fibrosis.**

In the absence of treatment, the disease follows one of two paths to end-stage disease. In the first, most classic pathway, there is increasingly widespread duct loss, slowly leading to established cirrhosis and eventually to profound cholestasis. Alternatively, some patients eventually developed prominent portal hypertension rather than severe cholestasis. Fortunately, both of these outcomes are now rarely seen.

Clinical Features

Most patients are diagnosed while asymptomatic following a workup triggered by the identification of an elevated serum alkaline phosphatase level or severe itching. Hypercholesterolemia is common. Anti-mitochondrial antibodies are present in 90% to 95% of patients. They are highly characteristic of PBC, although other autoantibodies may be seen in a small number of cases. The disease is confirmed by liver biopsy, which is considered diagnostic if a florid duct lesion is present. When symptoms appear, their onset is insidious, with patients typically complaining of slowly increasing fatigue and pruritus.

In recent years, early treatment with oral ursodeoxycholic acid has dramatically improved outcomes by slowing disease progression. Its mechanism of action remains unclear, but is presumably related to the ability of ursodeoxycholate to enter the bile acid pool and alter the biochemical composition of bile.

With time, even with treatment, secondary features may emerge, including skin hyperpigmentation, xanthelasmas, steatorrhea, and vitamin D malabsorption–related osteomalacia and/or osteoporosis. Individuals with PBC may also have extrahepatic manifestations of autoimmunity, including the sicca complex of dry eyes and mouth (Sjögren syndrome), systemic sclerosis, thyroiditis, rheumatoid arthritis, Raynaud phenomenon, and celiac disease. Liver transplantation is the best treatment for individuals with advanced liver disease.

Primary Sclerosing Cholangitis

Primary sclerosing cholangitis (PSC) is characterized by inflammation and obliterative fibrosis of intrahepatic and extrahepatic bile ducts, leading to dilation of preserved segments. Irregular biliary strictures and dilations cause the characteristic "beading" of the intrahepatic and extrahepatic biliary tree seen by MRI. Inflammatory bowel disease (Chapter 15), most commonly ulcerative colitis, coexists in approximately 70% of individuals with PSC. Conversely, the prevalence of PSC in individuals with ulcerative colitis is about 4%. Like inflammatory bowel disease, PSC tends to occur in the third through fifth decades of life and has a 2:1 male predominance (see Table 16.5).

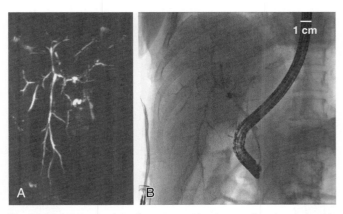

Fig. 16.28 Imaging studies of a patient with primary sclerosing cholangitis. (A) Magnetic resonance cholangiography of the bile ducts shows focal dilation in some ducts *(bright, broad areas)* and stricturing of others *(thinning or absence)*. (B) Endoscopic retrograde cholangiography of the same patient shows nearly identical features as in A. *(Courtesy of Dr. M. Edwyn Harrison, MD, Mayo Clinic, Scottsdale, Arizona.)*

Pathogenesis

Several features of PSC suggest immunologically mediated injury to bile ducts. T cells in the periductal stroma, the presence of autoantibodies, an association with HLA-B8 and other MHC alleles, and clinical linkage to ulcerative colitis all support an underlying, immunologic process. First-degree relatives of patients with PSC are at increased risk for developing the disease, suggesting that genetic factors also contribute.

In one model, it is proposed that T cells activated in the damaged mucosa of patients with ulcerative colitis migrate to the liver, where they recognize a cross-reacting bile duct antigen and initiate an autoimmune assault on bile ducts. Autoantibody profiles in PSC are not as characteristic as in PBC, but atypical perinuclear anti-neutrophil cytoplasmic antibodies (pANCA) that recognize a nuclear envelope protein are found in up to 80% of patients. The pathogenic relationship of pANCA to PSC is unknown.

MORPHOLOGY

Morphologic changes differ between large ducts (intrahepatic and extrahepatic) and smaller intrahepatic ducts. **Large duct inflammation** resembles that seen in ulcerative colitis, taking the form of neutrophils infiltrating into the epithelium superimposed on a chronic inflammatory background. Inflamed areas develop strictures as scarring narrows the lumen. The **smaller ducts,** however, often have little inflammation and show a striking **circumferential, "onion skin" fibrosis** around an atrophic duct lumen (Fig. 16.29), which eventually is obliterated, leaving a "tombstone" scar. Because the likelihood of sampling small-duct lesions on a random needle biopsy is small, diagnosis depends on radiologic imaging of the extrahepatic and large intrahepatic ducts. As the disease progresses, the liver becomes markedly cholestatic, culminating in cirrhosis. Biliary intraepithelial neoplasia often appear in the setting of chronic inflammation and cholangiocarcinoma develops in up to 7% of patients, usually with a fatal outcome.

Clinical Features

Patients may come to attention only because of persistent elevation of serum alkaline phosphatase, particularly in those with ulcerative colitis who are being routinely screened. Alternatively, progressive fatigue, pruritus, and jaundice may develop. Acute bouts of ascending cholangitis may also signal the presence or progression of PSC. Chronic pancreatitis and chronic cholecystitis due to involvement of the pancreatic ducts and gallbladder are also seen. In some patients, sclerosing cholangitis is associated with autoimmune pancreatitis. In such cases PSC may be one manifestation of IgG4 related chronic disease (Chapter 5).

PSC follows a protracted course of 5 to 17 years, and severely afflicted patients have symptoms typical of chronic cholestatic liver disease, including steatorrhea. Unlike with PBC, there is no satisfactory medical treatment. A variety of immunosuppressive agents have been tried, but none has been proven to alter the disease course. Endoscopic dilation with sphincterotomy or stenting is used to relieve obstruction. Liver transplantation is the only definitive treatment for individuals with end-stage liver disease.

SUMMARY

CHOLESTATIC DISEASES

- **Cholestasis** occurs with impaired excretion of bile, leading to jaundice and accumulation of bile pigment in the hepatic parenchyma. Causes include mechanical or inflammatory obstruction or destruction of the bile ducts or metabolic defects in hepatocyte bile secretion.
- **Large bile duct obstruction** is most commonly associated with gallstones and malignancies involving the head of the pancreas. Chronic obstruction can lead to cirrhosis.
- **Neonatal cholestasis** is not a specific entity; it is variously associated with cholangiopathies such as *biliary atresia* and a variety of disorders causing conjugated hyperbilirubinemia in the neonate, collectively referred to as *neonatal hepatitis*.
- **Primary biliary cholangitis** is an autoimmune disease with progressive, inflammatory, often granulomatous, destruction of

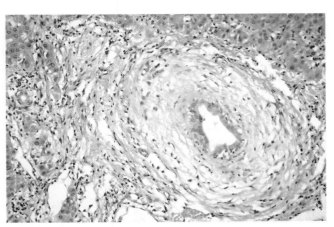

Fig. 16.29 Primary sclerosing cholangitis. A bile duct undergoing degeneration is entrapped in a dense, "onion-skin" concentric scar.

small to medium intrahepatic bile ducts. It most often occurs in middle-age women and is associated with anti-mitochondrial antibodies and often with other autoimmune diseases, such as Sjögren syndrome and Hashimoto thyroiditis.

- **Primary sclerosing cholangitis** is an autoimmune disease with progressive inflammatory and sclerosing destruction of intrahepatic and extrahepatic bile ducts of all sizes. Diagnosis is made by radiologic imaging of the biliary tree. It most often occurs in younger men and has a strong association with inflammatory bowel disease, particularly ulcerative colitis.

CIRCULATORY DISORDERS

Hepatic circulatory disorders can be grouped according to whether the disorder leads to abnormalities in the inflow, flow-through, or outflow of blood (Fig. 16.30).

Impaired Blood Flow Into the Liver

Hepatic Artery Compromise

Liver infarcts are rare, thanks to the double blood supply to the liver. Nonetheless, thrombosis or obstruction of an intrahepatic branch of the hepatic artery by embolism (Fig. 16.31), neoplasia, or an inflammatory process such as polyarteritis nodosa (Chapter 10) may produce an infarct, which may either be pale or hemorrhagic if suffused with blood from the portal circulation. Blockage of the main hepatic artery may not produce ischemic necrosis of the organ, particularly if the liver is otherwise normal, as retrograde arterial flow through accessory vessels and the portal venous supply is usually sufficient to sustain the liver parenchyma.

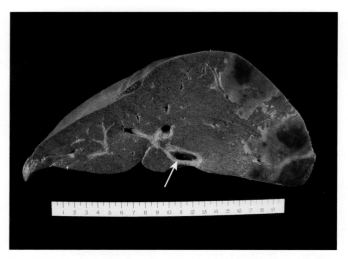

Fig. 16.31 Liver infarct. A thrombus is lodged in a peripheral branch of the hepatic artery (*arrow*) and compresses the adjacent portal vein; the distal hepatic tissue is pale, with a hemorrhagic margin.

Portal Vein Obstruction and Thrombosis

Blockage of the extrahepatic portal vein may cause only vague symptoms or may be a catastrophic and potentially lethal event; most cases fall somewhere in between. Occlusive disease of the portal vein or its major radicles typically produces abdominal pain and other manifestations of portal hypertension, principally esophageal varices that are prone to rupture. Ascites is not common (because the block is presinusoidal), but, when present, is often massive and intractable.

Extrahepatic portal vein obstruction may be idiopathic (approximately one-third of cases) or may arise from a number of conditions. Some of the most common settings for development of extrahepatic portal vein obstruction include the following:

- *Cirrhosis,* which is associated with portal vein thrombosis in 25% of patients, some of whom have other risk factors as well
- *Hypercoagulable states,* including myeloproliferative neoplasms such as polycythemia vera (Chapter 12), inherited thrombophilias such as factor V Leiden (Chapter 4), and miscellaneous hypercoagulable conditions such as paroxysmal nocturnal hemoglobinuria and antiphospholipid antibody syndrome
- *Inflammatory processes* involving the splenic vein or portal vein, such as pancreatitis and intraabdominal sepsis
- *Trauma,* surgical or otherwise

Obstruction of intrahepatic portal vein radicles may be caused by acute thrombosis. The thrombosis does not cause ischemic infarction but instead results in a sharply demarcated area of red-blue discoloration called *infarct of Zahn.* There is no necrosis, only severe hepatocellular atrophy and marked congestion of distended sinusoids. The most common cause of small portal vein branch obstruction is *schistosomiasis;* the eggs of the parasites lodge in and obstruct the smallest portal vein branches. The other

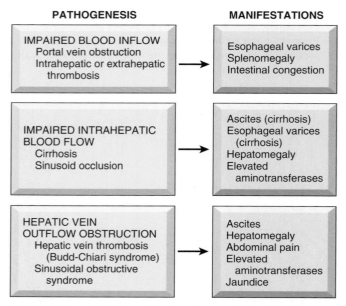

PATHOGENESIS	MANIFESTATIONS
IMPAIRED BLOOD INFLOW Portal vein obstruction Intrahepatic or extrahepatic thrombosis	Esophageal varices Splenomegaly Intestinal congestion
IMPAIRED INTRAHEPATIC BLOOD FLOW Cirrhosis Sinusoid occlusion	Ascites (cirrhosis) Esophageal varices (cirrhosis) Hepatomegaly Elevated aminotransferases
HEPATIC VEIN OUTFLOW OBSTRUCTION Hepatic vein thrombosis (Budd-Chiari syndrome) Sinusoidal obstructive syndrome	Ascites Hepatomegaly Abdominal pain Elevated aminotransferases Jaundice

Fig. 16.30 Hepatic circulatory disorders. Forms and clinical manifestations of compromised hepatic blood flow.

disorders producing this pattern of injury are now collectively referred to as *obliterative portal venopathy*, which often presents as noncirrhotic portal hypertension. Causes of obliterative portal venopathy are not well understood. It occurs in both untreated and treated HIV disease, and may in some instances be a complication of anti-retroviral therapy.

Impaired Blood Flow Through the Liver

The most common intrahepatic cause of blood flow obstruction is cirrhosis, as discussed earlier. In addition, physical occlusion of the sinusoids occurs in *sickle cell disease, disseminated intravascular coagulation, eclampsia*, and *intrasinusoidal metastasis* of solid tumors. If severe and unabated, all of these disorders may produce sufficient obstruction of blood flow to cause massive necrosis of hepatocytes and fulminant hepatic failure.

Hepatic Venous Outflow Obstruction

Hepatic Vein Thrombosis

Occlusive events can occur in any caliber of hepatic vein branches. If it occurs in the smallest intrahepatic branches, it produces *sinusoidal obstruction syndrome* (formally known as *veno-occlusive disease*). A rare, but well-known cause of this syndrome is consumption of pyrrolizidine alkaloid–containing Jamaican bush tea, but it now occurs primarily following allogeneic hematopoietic stem cell transplantation, usually within the first 3 weeks, or in cancer patients receiving chemotherapy, in whom it can have as high as 30% mortality.

The obstruction of two or more major hepatic veins produces liver enlargement, pain, and ascites, a condition known as *Budd-Chiari syndrome*. Obstruction of a single main hepatic vein by thrombosis is clinically silent. Hepatic damage is the consequence of increased intrahepatic blood pressure. Hepatic vein thrombosis is associated with the same hypercoagulable states as portal vein thrombosis as well as intraabdominal cancers, particularly HCC. As is often the case in those afflicted with various thrombotic disorders, Budd-Chiari syndrome often occurs in patients with several risk factors, such as pregnancy or oral contraceptive use combined with an underlying thrombophilic disorder.

MORPHOLOGY

In Budd-Chiari syndrome, the liver is swollen and red-purple and has a tense capsule (Fig. 16.32). There may be areas of hemorrhagic collapse alternating with areas of preserved or regenerating parenchyma, depending on which small and large hepatic veins are obstructed. Microscopically, the affected hepatic parenchyma reveals severe centrilobular congestion and necrosis. Centrilobular fibrosis develops in instances in which the thrombosis is more slowly developing. The major veins may contain fresh occlusive thrombi or, in chronic cases, organized adherent thrombi.

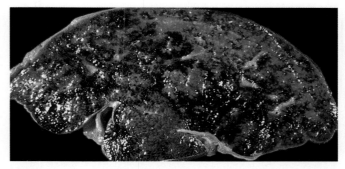

Fig. 16.32 Budd-Chiari syndrome. Thrombosis of the major hepatic veins has caused severe hepatic congestion.

The mortality of untreated acute hepatic vein thrombosis is high. The condition is rare, and treatments are largely empiric. They include anti-coagulation to prevent clot propagation; angioplasty to restore the patency of occluded veins; thrombolysis; and creation of portovenous shunts, using either invasive radiologic approaches or surgery, in order to decompress the liver. The chronic form is far less lethal, and more than two-thirds of patients are alive after 5 years.

Passive Congestion and Centrilobular Necrosis

These hepatic manifestations of systemic circulatory compromise—passive congestion and centrilobular necrosis—are considered together because they represent a morphologic continuum. Both changes are commonly seen at autopsy, as there is an element of preterminal circulatory failure in virtually every nontraumatic death.

MORPHOLOGY

Right-sided cardiac decompensation leads to passive congestion of the liver. The liver is slightly enlarged, tense, and cyanotic, with rounded edges. Microscopically there is congestion of **centrilobular sinusoids**. With time, centrilobular hepatocytes become atrophic, resulting in markedly attenuated liver cell plates. Left-sided cardiac failure or shock may lead to hepatic hypoperfusion and hypoxia, causing ischemic coagulative necrosis of hepatocytes in the central region of the lobule (**centrilobular necrosis**).

The combination of hypoperfusion and retrograde congestion acts synergistically to cause **centrilobular hemorrhagic necrosis**. The liver takes on a variegated mottled appearance, reflecting hemorrhage and necrosis in the centrilobular regions (Fig. 16.33A). This finding is known as **nutmeg liver** due to its resemblance to the cut surface of a nutmeg. There typically is a sharp demarcation between viable periportal and necrotic or atrophic pericentral regions that are suffused with blood (see Fig. 16.33B). Uncommonly, with sustained chronic severe congestive heart failure, centrilobular fibrosis (**cardiac sclerosis**) or even cirrhosis develops.

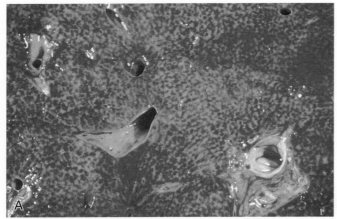

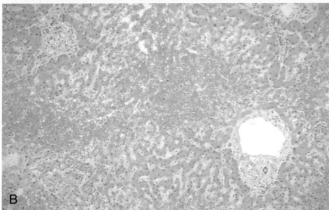

Fig. 16.33 Acute passive congestion ("nutmeg liver"). (A) The cut liver section, in which major blood vessels are visible, is notable for a variegated mottled red appearance, representing congestion and hemorrhage in the centrilobular regions of the parenchyma. (B) On microscopic examination, the centrilobular region is suffused with red blood cells, and atrophied hepatocytes are not easily seen. Portal tracts and the periportal parenchyma are intact.

SUMMARY

CIRCULATORY DISORDERS

- Circulatory disorders of the liver can be caused by impaired blood inflow, defects in intrahepatic blood flow, and obstruction of blood outflow.
- Portal vein obstruction by intrahepatic or extrahepatic thrombosis may cause portal hypertension, esophageal varices, and ascites.
- The most common cause of impaired intrahepatic blood flow is cirrhosis.
- Obstructions of blood outflow include hepatic vein thrombosis (Budd-Chiari syndrome) and sinusoidal obstruction syndrome, previously known as *veno-occlusive disease*.

NODULES AND TUMORS

Hepatic masses come to attention for a variety of reasons. They may generate epigastric fullness and discomfort or be detected by routine physical examination or radiographic studies for other indications. Hepatic masses include nodular hyperplasias and true neoplasms.

Focal Nodular Hyperplasia

Solitary or multiple hyperplastic hepatocellular nodules that may develop in the noncirrhotic liver are called *focal nodular hyperplasias*. These lesions arise from local alterations in hepatic parenchymal blood supply, such as arteriovenous malformations or inflammatory or posttraumatic obliteration of portal vein radicles and compensatory augmentation of arterial blood supply.

MORPHOLOGY

Focal nodular hyperplasia appears as a well-demarcated, poorly encapsulated nodule ranging up to many centimeters in diameter (Fig. 16.34A). It presents as a mass lesion in an otherwise normal liver, most frequently in young to middle-age adults. Typically, there is a central gray-white, depressed stellate

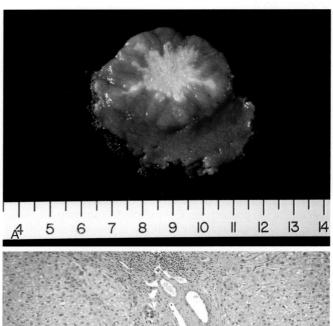

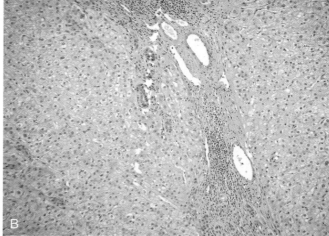

Fig. 16.34 Focal nodular hyperplasia. (A) Resected specimen showing lobulated contours and a central stellate scar. (B) Low-power photomicrograph showing a broad fibrous scar with mixed hepatic arterial and bile duct elements and chronic inflammation within hepatic parenchyma that lacks normal architecture due to hepatocyte regeneration.

scar from which fibrous septa radiate to the periphery (see Fig. 16.34B).

Microscopically, the central scar contains large abnormal vessels and ductular reactions along the spokes of scar. A vascular lesion is probably the initiating insult, as it is believed that hypoperfused parenchyma collapses to produce the septa, whereas hyperperfused regions undergo hyperplasia. The hyperplastic regions are composed of normal hepatocytes separated by thickened sinusoidal plates.

Benign Neoplasms

Cavernous hemangiomas are the most common benign liver tumors (Chapter 10). The chief clinical significance of cavernous hemangiomas is that they must be distinguished radiographically or intraoperatively from metastatic tumors.

Hepatocellular Adenomas

Benign neoplasms developing from hepatocytes are called hepatocellular adenomas (Fig. 16.35). They may be detected incidentally as a hepatic mass on abdominal imaging or when they cause symptoms. The most common symptom is pain, which may be caused by pressure placed on the liver capsule by the expanding mass or hemorrhagic necrosis of the tumor as it outstrips its blood supply. Hepatocellular adenomas occasionally rupture, an event that may lead to life-threatening intraabdominal bleeding.

Hepatic adenomas can be subclassified molecularly into tumors at low, intermediate, and high risk for malignant transformation. Sex hormone exposure (e.g., oral contraceptive pills, anabolic steroids) markedly increases the frequency of all types of hepatic adenoma, and cessation of exposure to sex hormones often—but not always—leads to tumor regression, clearly linking sex hormones to the growth and survival of tumor cells in some cases.

Malignant Neoplasms

Malignant tumors occurring in the liver can be primary or metastatic. The latter are far more common. Our discussion here is focused on primary hepatic tumors. Most primary liver cancers arise from hepatocytes and are termed *hepatocellular carcinoma (HCC)*. Much less common are cancers of bile duct origin, *cholangiocarcinomas*. Other types of primary liver cancers, such as *hepatoblastoma* (a childhood hepatocellular tumor) and *angiosarcoma*, are too rare to merit further discussion.

Hepatocellular Carcinoma (HCC)

Globally, HCC, also erroneously known as *hepatoma*, accounts for approximately 5.4% of all cancers, but its incidence varies widely in different parts of the world. More than 85% of cases occur in countries with high rates of chronic HBV infection. The incidence of HCC is highest in Asia (southeast China, Korea, Taiwan) and sub-Saharan Africa, areas in which HBV is transmitted vertically and, as already discussed, the carrier state starts in infancy. Moreover, many of these populations are exposed to aflatoxin, which when combined with HBV infection increases the risk for HCC dramatically. The peak incidence of HCC

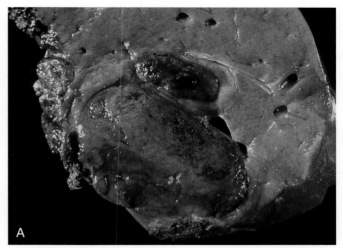

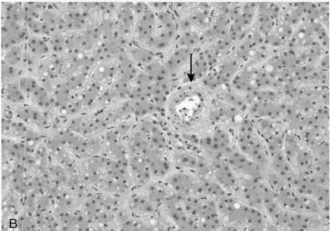

Fig. 16.35 Liver cell adenoma. (A) Resected specimen of the liver mass. (B) Microscopic view showing cords of hepatocytes, with an arterial vascular supply *(arrow)* and no portal tracts.

in these areas is between 20 and 40 years of age and, in almost 50% of cases, the tumor appears in the absence of cirrhosis.

In Western counties, the incidence of HCC is rapidly rising, largely owing to the increased prevalence of hepatitis C. The number of new HCC cases tripled in the United States in recent decades, but its incidence is still 8-fold to 30-fold lower than in some Asian countries. It is hoped that new, effective treatments for hepatitis C infection will stem the rising tide of HCC in the United States. In Western populations, HCC rarely manifests before 60 years of age, and in almost 90% of cases the malignancy emerges after cirrhosis becomes established. There is a pronounced male predominance throughout the world, about 3:1 in low-incidence areas and as high as 8:1 in high-incidence areas.

Pathogenesis

Chronic liver diseases are the most common setting for emergence of HCC. While usually identified in a background of cirrhosis, cirrhosis is not required for hepatocarcinogenesis. Rather, progression to cirrhosis and to hepatocellular cancer take place in parallel over many years to decades.

The most important underlying factors in hepatocarcinogenesis are viral infections (HBV, HCV) and toxic injuries (aflatoxin, alcohol). Thus, where HBV and HCV are endemic, there is a very high incidence of HCC. Coinfection further increases risk. *Aflatoxin* is a mycotoxin produced by *Aspergillus* species that contaminates staple food crops in Africa and Asia. Aflatoxin metabolites are present in the urine of individuals who consume these foods, as are aflatoxin-albumin adducts in serum. These biomarkers identify populations at risk and have helped to confirm the importance of aflatoxin in hepatocarcinogenesis. As discussed earlier, aflatoxin synergizes with HBV (and perhaps also with HCV) to increase risk further.

Other HCC risk factors all share the ability to cause chronic liver injury associated with varying degrees of inflammation. These factors include:

- *Alcohol consumption,* which synergistically increases risk with HBV, HCV, and possibly even cigarette smoking.
- *Inherited disorders,* particularly hereditary hemochromatosis and α_1AT deficiency, and to a lesser degree Wilson disease
- *Metabolic syndrome* and its attendant obesity, diabetes mellitus, and NAFLD, all of which increase the risk for HCC.

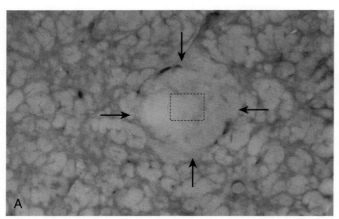

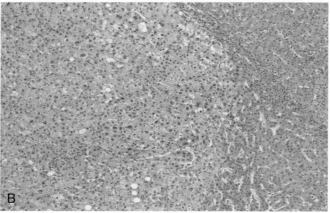

Fig. 16.36 (A) Hepatitis C–related cirrhosis with a distinctively large dysplastic nodule *(arrows)*. Nodule-in-nodule growth suggests an evolving cancer. (B) Histologically the region within the box in *A* shows a well-differentiated hepatocellular carcinoma *(right side)* and a subnodule of moderately differentiated hepatocellular carcinoma within it *(center, left)*. *(Courtesy of Dr. Masamichi Kojiro, Kurume University, Kurume, Japan.)*

As with all cancers, HCC is induced by acquired driver mutations in oncogenes and tumor suppressor genes. No single, universal sequence of molecular or genetic alterations leads to emergence of HCC. Gain of function mutations in beta-catenin and loss of function mutations in p53 are the two most common driver mutations. Beta-catenin mutations are identified in up to 40% of HCCs. These tumors are more likely to be unrelated to HBV and to demonstrate genomic instability. Inactivation of *TP53* is present in up to 60% of HCCs. These tumors are strongly associated with exposure to aflatoxin, which appears in many cases to be directly responsible for the causative *TP53* mutations.

HCC often appears to arise from premalignant precursors lesions. *Hepatic adenoma* has already been discussed, some of which carry beta-catenin–activating mutations. Chronic liver disease is associated with cellular dysplasias called *large-cell change* and *small-cell change*. These may be found at any stage of chronic liver disease, before or after development of cirrhosis, and serve to indicate which patients need more aggressive cancer surveillance. *Dysplastic nodules* are usually found in cirrhosis, either radiologically or in resected specimens (including explants). *Low-grade dysplastic nodules* may or may not undergo transformation to higher-grade lesions, but they indicate a higher risk for HCC. *High-grade dysplastic nodules* are probably the most important precursor of HCC in viral hepatitis and alcoholic liver disease. Overt HCC is often found in high-grade dysplastic nodules in biopsy or resection specimens.

MORPHOLOGY

HCC may appear grossly as (1) a unifocal (usually large) mass (Fig. 16.37); (2) multifocal, widely distributed nodules of variable size; or (3) a diffusely infiltrative cancer, permeating widely and sometimes involving the entire liver. Sometimes HCCs arise within dysplastic nodules (Fig. 16.37), eventually overgrowing these precursor lesions. Intrahepatic metastases by either vascular invasion or direct extension become more likely once tumors reach 3 cm in size. These metastases are usually small, satellite tumor nodules around a larger primary mass. Vascular invasion is also the most likely route for extrahepatic metastasis, especially by the hepatic venous system, usually only in advanced cases. Occasionally, long, snakelike masses of tumor invade the portal vein (causing portal hypertension) or inferior vena cava; in the latter instance, the tumor may extend all the way up into the right ventricle. Lymph node metastases are less common.

HCCs range from well differentiated to highly anaplastic lesions. Well-differentiated HCCs are composed of cells that look like normal hepatocytes and grow as thick trabeculae (recapitulating liver cell plates) or in pseudoglandular patterns that recapitulate poorly formed, ectatic bile canaliculi (see Fig. 16.37).

Clinical Features

The clinical manifestations of HCC are varied and in Western populations are often masked by symptoms related to underlying cirrhosis or chronic hepatitis. In areas of high incidence, such as tropical Africa where aflatoxin exposure is common, patients usually have no

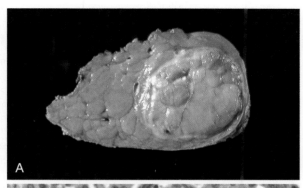

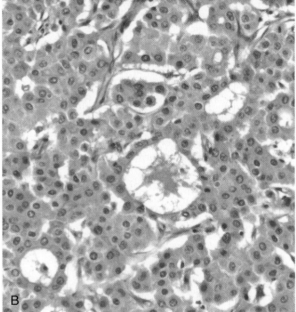

Fig. 16.37 Hepatocellular carcinoma. (A) Liver removed at autopsy showing a unifocal, massive neoplasm replacing most of the right hepatic lobe in a noncirrhotic liver. (B) Malignant hepatocytes growing in distorted versions of normal architecture: large pseudoacinar spaces, essentially malformed, dilated bile canaliculi, and thickened hepatocyte trabeculae.

clinical history of liver disease (although cirrhosis may be detected at autopsy). In both populations, most patients have ill-defined upper-abdominal pain, malaise, fatigue, weight loss, and sometimes awareness of an abdominal mass or abdominal fullness. Jaundice, fever, and gastrointestinal or esophageal variceal bleeding are inconstant findings.

Laboratory studies may provide clues but are rarely conclusive. Elevated serum levels of *α-fetoprotein* are found in 50% of individuals with advanced HCC, but this is neither a sensitive nor specific marker for premalignant or early well-differentiated cancers. Better tests for detection of small tumors are imaging studies, such as ultrasonography, computed tomography, and magnetic resonance imaging. Increasing arterialization during the development and progression of HCC can be identified by imaging and is so characteristic that its detection can be diagnostic, precluding the need for tissue biopsy.

The natural history of HCC involves the progressive enlargement of the primary mass until it disturbs hepatic function or metastasizes, most commonly to the lungs. Death usually occurs from (1) cachexia, (2) gastrointestinal or esophageal variceal bleeding, (3) liver failure with hepatic coma, or rarely (4) rupture of the tumor with fatal hemorrhage. The 5-year survival of large tumors is dismal, and the majority of patients die within 2 years of diagnosis.

With implementation of screening procedures and advances in imaging, the detection of HCCs less than 2 cm in diameter has increased in countries where such facilities are available. These small tumors can be removed surgically or ablated (e.g., through embolization, microwave radiation, or freezing) with good outcomes. If relatively small HCCs arise in the setting of advanced stage (cirrhotic) chronic liver disease, liver transplantation is a better option and may be curative. Radiofrequency ablation and chemoembolization are used for local control of unresectable tumors. The kinase inhibitor sorafenib can prolong the life of individuals with advanced-stage HCC.

Cholangiocarcinoma

Cholangiocarcinoma (CCA), the second most common primary malignant tumor of the liver after HCC, arises from intrahepatic and extrahepatic bile ducts. It accounts for 3% of gastrointestinal cancers in the United States, where there are approximately 2000 to 3000 new cases each year. However, in some regions of southeast Asia such as northeastern Thailand, Laos, and Cambodia where infestation with liver flukes is endemic, cholangiocarcinoma is much more common, occurring at rates 30 to 40 times higher than in areas of Asia without liver fluke infestation.

All risk factors for cholangiocarcinoma cause chronic inflammation and cholestasis, which presumably promote occurrence of somatic mutations or epigenetic alterations in cholangiocytes. The risk factors include infestation by liver flukes (particularly *Opisthorchis* and *Clonorchis* species), chronic inflammatory disease of the large bile ducts (such as primary sclerosing cholangitis), hepatolithiasis, and fibropolycystic liver disease. As with HCC, rates of cholangiocarcinoma also are elevated in patients with hepatitis B and C and NAFLD.

MORPHOLOGY

Extrahepatic cholangiocarcinomas are generally small lesions at the time of diagnosis, as they cause obstruction of the biliary tract early in their course. Most tumors appear as firm, gray nodules within the bile duct wall; some may be diffusely infiltrative, while others are papillary or polypoid. **Intrahepatic cholangiocarcinomas** occur in noncirrhotic livers (Fig. 16.38A) and may track along the intrahepatic portal tract system or produce a single massive tumor.

Cholangiocarcinomas are typical mucin-producing adenocarcinomas. Most are well to moderately differentiated, growing as glandular/tubular structures lined by malignant epithelial cells (see Fig. 16.38B). They typically incite marked desmoplasia. Lymphovascular invasion and perineural invasion are both common and often lead to extensive intrahepatic and extrahepatic metastases.

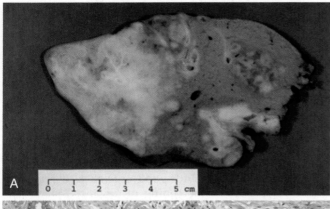

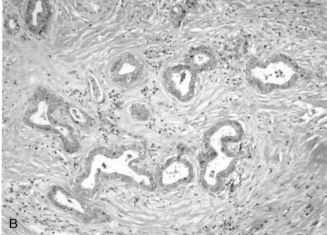

Fig. 16.38 Cholangiocarcinoma. (A) Multifocal cholangiocarcinoma in a liver from a patient with infestation by the liver fluke *Clonorchis sinensis* (flukes not visible) (B) Invasive malignant glands in a reactive, sclerotic stroma. *(A, Courtesy of Dr. Wilson M.S. Tsui, Caritas Medical Centre, Hong Kong.)*

SUMMARY

LIVER TUMORS

- The liver is the most common site of metastatic cancers from primary tumors of the colon, lung, and breast.
- **Hepatocellular adenomas** are benign tumors of hepatocytes. Most can be subclassified on the basis of molecular changes with varying degrees of malignant potential. They are associated with use of oral contraceptives and androgens.
- The two main types of malignant tumors are **hepatocellular carcinomas and cholangiocarcinomas**; HCCs are much more common.
  - HCC is a common tumor in regions of Asia and Africa, and its incidence is increasing in the United States.
  - The main etiologic agents for HCC are hepatitis B and C, alcoholic cirrhosis, hemochromatosis, and exposure to aflatoxins. In the Western population, about 90% of HCCs develop in cirrhotic livers; in Asia, almost 50% of cases develop in noncirrhotic livers.
  - The chronic inflammation and cellular regeneration associated with viral hepatitis are predisposing factors for the development of carcinomas.
  - HCC may be unifocal or multifocal, tends to invade blood vessels, and recapitulates normal liver architecture to varying degrees.
  - Cholangiocarcinoma is a tumor of intrahepatic or extrahepatic bile ducts that is relatively common in areas where liver flukes, such as *Opisthorchis* and *Clonorchis* species, are endemic.

Gallbladder

GALLSTONE DISEASE

Gallstones afflict 10% to 20% of adults residing in Western countries in the Northern Hemisphere, 20% to 40% in Latin American countries, and only 3% to 4% in Asian countries. In the United States, about 1 million new cases of gallstones are diagnosed annually, and two-thirds of individuals so affected undergo surgery, resulting in the removal of as much as 25 to 50 million tons of stones per year! There are two main types of gallstones: *cholesterol stones,* containing crystalline cholesterol monohydrate (80% of stones in Western countries), and *pigment stones,* made of bilirubin calcium salts.

Pathogenesis

Bile formation is the only significant pathway for elimination of excess cholesterol from the body, either as free cholesterol or as bile salts. Cholesterol is rendered water-soluble by aggregation with bile salts and lecithins. When cholesterol concentrations exceed the solubilizing capacity of bile (supersaturation), cholesterol can no longer remain dispersed and crystallizes out of solution. Cholesterol gallstone formation is enhanced by *hypomobility of the gallbladder* (stasis), which promotes nucleation, and by *mucus hypersecretion,* with consequent trapping of the crystals, thereby enhancing their aggregation into stones.

Pigment stones form when the bile contains a high concentration of unconjugated bilirubin in the biliary tree, as may occur in patients with chronic extravascular red cell hemolysis or with certain infections of the biliary tract, such as liver flukes. The precipitates are primarily insoluble calcium bilirubinate salts.

Prevalence and Risk Factors

The major risk factors for gallstones are listed in Table 16.6. In up to 80% of individuals with gallstones, the only identifiable risk factors are age and gender. Some elaboration on these risk factors follows:

- *Age and gender.* The prevalence of gallstones increases throughout life. In the United States, less than 5% to 6% of the population younger than 40 years of age has stones, in contrast with 25% to 30% of those older than

Table 16.6 Risk Factors for Gallstones

Cholesterol Stones
Demography: Northern Europeans, North and South Americans, Native Americans, Mexican Americans
Advancing age
Female sex hormones
Female gender
Oral contraceptives
Pregnancy
Obesity and insulin resistance
Rapid weight reduction
Gallbladder stasis
Inborn disorders of bile acid metabolism
Dyslipidemia syndromes

Pigment Stones
Demography: Asian more than Western, rural more than urban
Chronic hemolysis (e.g., sickle cell anemia, hereditary spherocytosis)
Biliary infection
Gastrointestinal disorders: ileal disease (e.g., Crohn disease), ileal resection or bypass, cystic fibrosis with pancreatic insufficiency

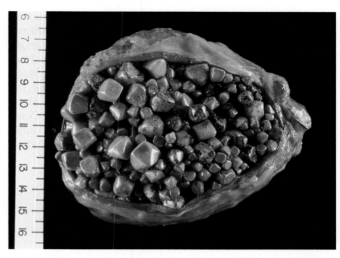

Fig. 16.39 Cholesterol gallstones. The wall of the gallbladder is thickened and fibrotic due to chronic cholecystitis.

80 years of age. The prevalence in women of all ages is about twice as high as in men.

- *Ethnic and geographic.* Cholesterol gallstone prevalence approaches 50% to 75% in certain Native American populations (Pima, Hopi, and Navajo), whereas pigment stones are rare. The high prevalence in these populations seems to be related to biliary cholesterol hypersecretion.
- *Heredity.* In addition to ethnicity, a positive family history imparts increased risk, as do a variety of inborn errors of metabolism, such as those associated with impaired bile salt synthesis and secretion.
- *Environment.* Estrogens increase hepatic cholesterol uptake and synthesis, leading to excess biliary secretion of cholesterol. These effects explain the increased risk for gallstone disease with oral contraceptive use and with pregnancy. Obesity, rapid weight loss, and treatment with the hypocholesterolemic agent clofibrate also are strongly associated with increased biliary cholesterol secretion and risk for gallstone disease.
- *Acquired disorders.* Any condition in which gallbladder motility is reduced predisposes to gallstones, such as pregnancy, rapid weight loss, and spinal cord injury. In most cases, however, gallbladder hypomotility is present without obvious cause.

MORPHOLOGY

Cholesterol stones arise exclusively in the gallbladder and consist of 50% to 100% cholesterol. Pure cholesterol stones are pale yellow; increasing proportions of calcium carbonate, phosphates, and bilirubin impart gray-white to black discoloration (Fig. 16.39). They are ovoid and firm; they can occur singly, but most often there are several, with faceted surfaces resulting from their apposition. Most cholesterol stones are radiolucent, although as many as 20% may contain sufficient calcium carbonate to be radiopaque.

    Pigment stones may arise anywhere in the biliary tree and are classified into black and brown stones. In general, black pigment stones are found in sterile gallbladder bile, while brown stones are found in infected intrahepatic or extrahepatic ducts.

The stones contain calcium salts of unconjugated bilirubin and lesser amounts of other calcium salts, mucin glycoproteins, and cholesterol. Black stones are usually small, numerous, and fragile to the touch (Fig. 16.40). Brown stones tend to be single or few in number and to have a soft, greasy, soaplike consistency owing to the presence of fatty acid salts released from biliary lecithins by bacterial phospholipases. Because of calcium carbonates and phosphates, 50% to 75% of black stones are radiopaque. Brown stones, which contain calcium soaps, are radiolucent.

Clinical Features

Gallstones may be present for decades without causing any symptoms, and 70% to 80% of individuals with gallstones remain asymptomatic throughout life. In an unfortunate minority, however, the symptoms are striking. There is usually right upper-quadrant or epigastric pain, often excruciating, which may be constant or, less

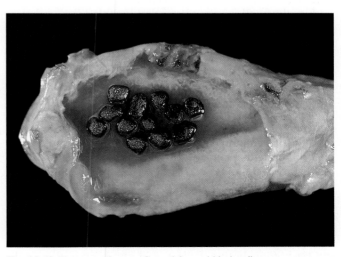

Fig. 16.40 Pigment gallstones. Several faceted black gallstones are present in this otherwise unremarkable gallbladder from a patient with a mechanical mitral valve prosthesis, leading to chronic intravascular hemolysis.

commonly, spasmodic. Such "biliary" pain is caused by gallbladder or biliary tree obstruction or by inflammation of the gallbladder itself. More severe complications include empyema, perforation, fistulas, inflammation of the biliary tree, obstructive cholestasis and pancreatitis. The larger the stone, the less likely it is to enter the cystic or common ducts to produce obstruction; thus, the very small stones, or "gravel," are dangerous. Occasionally a large stone may erode directly into an adjacent loop of small bowel, generating intestinal obstruction (*gallstone ileus*).

CHOLECYSTITIS

Inflammation of the gallbladder may be acute, chronic, or acute superimposed on chronic, and almost always occurs in association with gallstones. In the United States, cholecystitis is one of the most common indications for abdominal surgery. Its epidemiologic distribution closely parallels that of gallstones.

Acute Calculous Cholecystitis

Acute inflammation of a gallbladder that contains stones is termed *acute calculous cholecystitis* **and is precipitated in 90% of cases by obstruction of the gallbladder neck or cystic duct**. It is the most common major complication of gallstones and the most frequent indication for emergency cholecystectomy. Manifestations of obstruction may appear with remarkable suddenness and constitute a surgical emergency. In some cases, however, symptoms may be mild and resolve without intervention.

Acute calculous cholecystitis initially results from chemical irritation and inflammation of the gallbladder wall due to obstruction of bile outflow. Gallbladder injury in the setting of bile obstruction stems from several sources, including: phospholipases derived from the mucosa hydrolyze biliary lecithin to lysolecithin, which is toxic to the mucosa; the normally protective glycoprotein mucous layer is disrupted, exposing the mucosal epithelium to the detergent action of bile salts.; prostaglandins released within the wall of the distended gallbladder enhance mucosal and mural inflammation; and distention and increased intraluminal pressure may compromise blood flow to the mucosa. All of these effects occur in the absence of bacterial infection, which may be superimposed later.

Acute Acalculous Cholecystitis

Between 5% and 12% of gallbladders removed for acute cholecystitis contain no gallstones. Most cases occur in seriously ill patients. Some of the most common predisposing insults are as follows:

- Major surgery
- Severe trauma (e.g., from motor vehicle crashes)
- Severe burns
- Sepsis

Other contributing factors include dehydration, gallbladder stasis and sludging, vascular compromise, and bacterial contamination.

Chronic Cholecystitis

Chronic cholecystitis may be the sequel to repeated bouts of acute cholecystitis, but in most instances it develops without any antecedent history of acute attacks. Like acute cholecystitis, it is almost always associated with gallstones. However, gallstones do not seem to be an essential part of the initiation of inflammation or the development of pain, because chronic acalculous cholecystitis causes symptoms and morphologic alterations similar to those seen in the calculous form. Rather, supersaturation of bile appears to predispose to both chronic inflammation and, in most instances, stone formation. Microorganisms, usually *E. coli* and enterococci, can be cultured from the bile in only about one-third of cases. Unlike acute calculous cholecystitis, obstruction of gallbladder outflow by stones is not requisite in chronic cholecystitis. Most gallbladders removed at elective surgery for gallstones show features of chronic cholecystitis, making it likely that biliary symptoms emerge after long-term coexistence of gallstones and low-grade inflammation.

MORPHOLOGY

In **acute cholecystitis,** the gallbladder usually is enlarged and tense, and has a bright red or blotchy, violaceous color, the latter imparted by subserosal hemorrhages. The serosa frequently is covered by a fibrinous or, in severe cases, a fibrinopurulent exudate. In 90% of cases, stones are present, often obstructing the neck of the gallbladder or the cystic duct. The gallbladder lumen is filled with cloudy or turbid bile that may contain fibrin, blood, and pus. When the contained exudate is mostly pus, the condition is referred to as *empyema of the gallbladder.* In mild cases, the gallbladder wall is thickened, edematous, and hyperemic. In more severe cases, the gallbladder wall is green-black and necrotic—a condition termed *gangrenous cholecystitis.* On histologic examination, the inflammatory reactions are not distinctive and consist of some combination of the usual patterns of acute inflammation (i.e., edema, leukocytic infiltration, vascular congestion, abscess formation, gangrenous necrosis).

The morphologic changes in **chronic cholecystitis** are extremely variable and sometimes subtle. The mere presence of stones within the gallbladder, even in the absence of acute inflammation, often is taken as sufficient justification for a diagnosis. The gallbladder may be contracted, of normal size, or enlarged. Mucosal ulcerations are infrequent; the submucosa and subserosa often are thickened from fibrosis. In the absence of superimposed acute cholecystitis, collections of lymphocytes in the wall are the only sign of inflammation (Fig. 16.41A). Outpouchings of mucosal epithelium through the wall of the gallbladder (Rokitansky-Aschoff sinuses) may be quite prominent (see Fig. 16.41B).

Clinical Features

Acute calculous cholecystitis presents with biliary pain that lasts for more than 6 hours. The pain is severe, usually steady, upper abdominal in location, and often radiates to the right shoulder. Fever, nausea, leukocytosis, and prostration are classic; the presence of conjugated hyperbilirubinemia suggests obstruction of the common bile duct. The right subcostal region is markedly tender and rigid as a result of spasm of the abdominal muscles; occasionally a

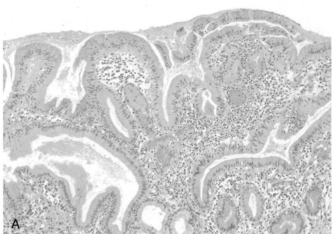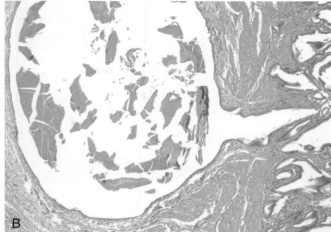

Fig. 16.41 Chronic cholecystitis. (A) The gallbladder mucosa is infiltrated by chronic inflammatory cells. (B) A Rokitansky-Aschoff sinus containing a fragmented bile pigment stone.

tender, distended gallbladder can be palpated. Mild attacks usually subside spontaneously over 1 to 10 days; however, recurrence is common. Approximately 25% of symptomatic patients are sufficiently ill to require surgical intervention.

The diagnosis of acute cholecystitis usually is based on the detection of gallstones by ultrasonography, typically accompanied by evidence of a thickened gallbladder wall. Attention to this disorder is important because of the potential for the following serious complications:

- Bacterial superinfection leading to cholangitis or sepsis
- Gallbladder perforation and local abscess formation
- Gallbladder rupture leading to diffuse peritonitis
- Biliary enteric (cholecystenteric) fistula, with drainage of bile into adjacent organs, entry of air and bacteria into the biliary tree, and potentially gallstone-induced intestinal obstruction (ileus)
- Aggravation of preexisting medical illness, with cardiac, pulmonary, renal, or liver decompensation

Symptoms arising from *acute acalculous cholecystitis* usually are obscured by another serious medical or surgical condition, which sets the stage for the development of cholecystitis. The diagnosis therefore rests on a high index of suspicion. *Chronic cholecystitis* lacks the striking manifestations of the acute forms and is usually characterized by recurrent attacks of steady epigastric or right upperquadrant pain. Nausea, vomiting, and intolerance for fatty foods are frequent accompaniments. Chronic cholecystitis is a pathologic diagnosis based on the examination of the resected gallbladder. Beyond signs and symptoms mentioned above, its principal importance may lie in the association of gallstones and chronic inflammation with carcinoma of the gallbladder (discussed next).

CARCINOMA OF THE GALLBLADDER

Carcinoma of the gallbladder is the most common malignancy of the extrahepatic biliary tract. It is slightly more common in women and occurs most frequently in the seventh decade of life. The incidence in the United States is 1 in 50,000. Only rarely is it discovered at a resectable stage, and the mean 5-year survival rate has remained unchanged at about 5% to 12% over the past many years. The most important risk factor associated with gallbladder carcinoma is gallstones (cholelithiasis), which are present in 95% of cases. Presumably, gallbladders containing stones or infectious agents develop cancer as a result of chronic inflammation, a known enabler of malignancy in several organs (Chapter 6). Carcinogenic derivatives of bile acids also are suspected to play a role. Primary sclerosing cholangitis is also a risk factor.

MORPHOLOGY

Carcinomas of the gallbladder show two patterns of growth: **infiltrating** and **exophytic.** The infiltrating pattern is more common and usually appears as a poorly defined area of diffuse wall thickening and induration. The exophytic pattern grows into the lumen as an irregular, cauliflower mass, but at the same time invades the underlying wall (Fig. 16.42). Most carcinomas of the gallbladder are adenocarcinomas. About 5% are squamous cell carcinomas or have adenosquamous differentiation.

Clinical Features

Preoperative diagnosis of carcinoma of the gallbladder is the exception rather than the rule, occurring in fewer than 20% of patients. Presenting symptoms are insidious and typically indistinguishable from those associated with cholelithiasis: abdominal pain, jaundice, anorexia, nausea and vomiting. There is no satisfactory treatment of gall bladder cancer due to the advanced stage at the time of diagnosis. Only 10% are diagnosed at a stage that is early enough to attempt curative surgery.

SUMMARY
GALLBLADDER DISEASES

- Gallbladder diseases include cholelithiasis and acute and chronic cholecystitis, and gall bladder cancer.

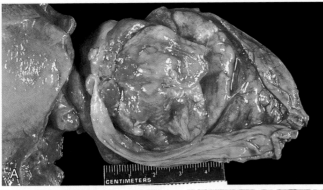

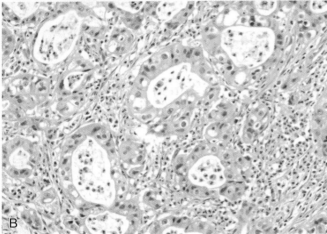

Fig. 16.42 Gallbladder adenocarcinoma. (A) The opened gallbladder contains a large, exophytic tumor that virtually fills the lumen. (B) Microscopically, the tumor has the same appearance as that of intrahepatic cholangiocarcinoma.

- Gallstone formation is a common condition in Western countries. The great majority of the gallstones are cholesterol stones. Pigmented stones containing bilirubin and calcium are most common in Asian countries, due to the higher incidence of chronic hemolytic disorders and liver fluke infestations in these locales.
- Risk factors for the development of cholesterol stones are advancing age, female gender, estrogen use, obesity, and heredity.
- Cholecystitis almost always occurs in association with cholelithiasis, although in about 10% of cases it occurs in the absence of gallstones.
- Acute calculous cholecystitis is the most common reason for emergency cholecystectomy.
- Gall bladder cancer is almost always associated with gall stones. Because of the advanced stage at diagnosis, it has a very poor prognosis.

SUGGESTED READINGS

Mechanisms of Liver Injury and Repair
Gouw ASW, Clouston AD, Theise ND: Ductular reactions in human livers: diversity at the interface, *Hepatology* 54:2011, 1853. [*A review of ductular reactions, the stem cell response of human livers in all liver diseases, that are related to mechanisms of regeneration, fibrogenesis, and neoplasia.*]

Kocabayoglu P, Friedman SL: Cellular basis of hepatic fibrosis and its role in inflammation and cancer, *Front Biosci (Schol Ed)* 5:217, 2013. [*Interweaves what is known about hepatic stellate cells and other myofibroblastic cells of the liver with inflammatory, fibrosing, and neoplastic disease processes.*]

Acute, Chronic, and Acute-on-Chronic Liver Failure
Bernal W, Wendon J: Acute liver failure, *New Engl J Med* 369:2525, 2013. [*An excellent clinical review.*]

Berzigotti A, Seijo S, Reverter E, et al: Assessing portal hypertension in liver diseases, *Expert Rev Gastroenterol Hepatol* 7:141, 2013. [*Evolving definitions and methodologies for evaluating portal hypertension.*]

Khungar V, Poordad F: Hepatic encephalopathy, *Clin Liver Dis* 16:301, 2012. [*A good overview of the one of the most ominous sequelae of all forms of liver failure.*]

Quaglia A, Alves VA, Balabaud C, et al: Role of aetiology in the progression, regression, and parenchymal remodelling of liver disease: implications for liver biopsy interpretation, *Histopathology* 68:953, 2016. [*A general review comparing and contrasting clinical and pathologic variants of advanced stages different acute and chronic liver diseases.*].

Yoon E, Babar A, Choudhary M, et al: Acetaminophen-induced hepatotoxicity: a comprehensive update, *J Clin Transl Hepatol* 4:131, 2016.

Viral Hepatitis
Chung RT, Baumert TF: Curing chronic hepatitis C — the arc of medical triumph, *New Engl J Med* 370:1576, 2014. [*An excellent perspective on why and how hepatitis C can be cured.*]

Trepo C, Chan HLY, Lok A: Hepatitis B infection, *Lancet* 384:2053, 2014. [*A thorough look at the continually evolving nature of hepatitis B and our attempts to prevent and treat it.*]

Ward JW, Lok AS, Thomas DL: Report on a single-topic conference on "Chronic viral hepatitis — strategies to improve effectiveness of screening and treatment," *Hepatology* 55:307, 2012. [*An overview of all aspects of chronic viral hepatitis and the relationship of pathology to disease course and management.*]

Autoimmune Liver Diseases
Carey EJ, Ali AH, Lindor KD: Primary biliary cirrhosis, *Lancet* 386:1565, 2015. [*A classic liver disease whose origins remain obscure — the latest in what is understood or hypothesized.*]

Lazaridis KN, LaRusso NF: Primary sclerosing cholangitis, *N Eng J Med* 375:1161, 2016. [*A comprehensive review of all aspects of this disease.*]

Manns MP, Lohse AW, Vergani D: Autoimmune hepatitis — update 2015, *J Hepatol* 62:S100, 2015. [*A review of pathogenesis, diagnosis, and treatment approaches.*]

Drug- and Toxin-Induced Liver Injury
Crawford JM: Histologic findings in alcoholic liver disease, *Clin Liver Dis* 16:699, 2012. [*A thorough look at the morphologic changes in alcoholic liver disease and the underlying mechanisms that produce them.*]

Kleiner DE: The pathology of drug-induced liver injury, *Semin Liver Dis* 29:364, 2009.

Louvet A, Mathurin P: Alcoholic liver disease: mechanisms of injury and targeted treatment, *Nat Rev Gastroenterol Hepatol* 12:231, 2015. [*A discussion of pathways of disease progression and possible interventions.*]

Metabolic Liver Diseases
Hardy T, Oakley F, Anstee QM, et al: Nonalcoholic fatty liver disease: Pathogenesis and disease spectrum, *Annu Rev Pathol* 11:451, 2016. [*A comprehensive discussion of NAFLD pathogenesis.*]

Pietrangelo A: Hereditary hemochromatosis: pathogenesis, diagnosis, and treatment, *Gastroenterology* 139:393, 2010. [*A comprehensive review.*]

Rosencrantz R, Schilsky M: Wilson disease: pathogenesis and clinical considerations in diagnosis and treatment, *Semin Liver Dis* 31:245, 2011. [*A still current review of basic and translational features of the disease.*]

Cholestatic Syndromes

Beuers U, Gershwin ME, Gish RG, et al: Changing nomenclature for PBC: From "cirrhosis" to "cholangitis", *Hepatology* 62:1620, 2015. [*A change in nomenclature by liver disease experts made in response to the needs of patients and their advocates.*]

Hirschfield GM, Heathcote EJ, Gershwin ME: Pathogenesis of cholestatic liver disease and therapeutic approaches, *Gastroenterology* 139:1481, 2010. [*A thorough overview of the most common features of liver disease.*]

Paumgartner G: Biliary physiology and disease: reflections of a physician-scientist, *Hepatology* 51:1095, 2010. [*How bench top work comes to exert an impact on clinical medicine, sometimes, slowly, over decades.*]

Benign and Malignant Liver Tumors

Bioulac-Sage P, Cubel G, Balabaud C: Revisiting the pathology of resected benign hepatocellular nodules using new immunohisto-chemical markers, *Semin Liver Dis* 31:91, 2011. [*From the team largely responsible for the new molecular subclassifications of hepatocellular adenomas.*]

Bosman F, Carneiro F, Hruban R, editors: *WHO Classification of Tumours of the Digestive System*, ed 4, Geneva, Switzerland, 2010, WHO Press. [*The current bible for tumors of the liver and biliary tree and the rest of the digestive tract.*]

Forner A, Llovet JM, Bruix J: Hepatocellular carcinoma, *Lancet* 379:1245, 2012. [*Clinical, radiologic, pathologic, and oncologic perspectives all woven together.*]

Razumilava N, Gores GJ: Cholangiocarcinoma, *Lancet* 383:2168, 2014. [*Update on pathogenesis and clinical features.*]

Shibata T, Aburatani H: Exploration of liver cancer genomes, *Nat Rev Gastroenterol Hepatol* 11:340, 2014. [*A review hepatocellular carcinoma pathogenesis seen through the prism of analysis of cancer genomes.*]

Pancreas 17

CHAPTER OUTLINE

Congenital Anomalies 680
Agenesis 680
Pancreas Divisum 680
Annular Pancreas 680

Ectopic Pancreas 680
Congenital Cysts 680
Pancreatitis 680
Acute Pancreatitis 680

Chronic Pancreatitis 683
Pancreatic Neoplasms 685
Cystic Neoplasms 685
Pancreatic Carcinoma 686

The pancreas is a transversely oriented retroperitoneal organ extending from the so-called "C loop" of the duodenum to the hilum of the spleen. Although the pancreas does not have well-defined anatomic subdivisions, adjacent vessels and ligaments serve to demarcate the organ into a head, body, and tail.

The pancreas is really two organs packaged into one. The islets of Langerhans scattered in the pancreas serve critical endocrine functions, and the exocrine portion that makes up the bulk of this organ is a major source of enzymes that are essential for digestion. Diseases affecting the pancreas can be the source of significant morbidity and mortality. Unfortunately, the retroperitoneal location of the pancreas and the generally vague nature of signs and symptoms associated with its injury or with dysfunction of the exocrine portion allow many pancreatic diseases to progress undiagnosed for extended periods of time; thus, recognition of pancreatic disorders requires a high degree of suspicion.

The pancreas gets its name from the Greek *pankreas,* meaning "all flesh," and is a complex lobulated organ. The endocrine portion constitutes only 1% to 2% of the pancreas and is composed of about 1 million cell clusters, the islets of Langerhans; these cells secrete insulin, glucagon, and somatostatin. The most significant disorders of the *endocrine pancreas* are diabetes mellitus and neoplasms; these are discussed in detail in Chapter 20 and are not discussed further here.

The *exocrine pancreas* is composed of *acinar cells* and the ductules and ducts that convey their secretions to the duodenum. The acinar cells are responsible for the synthesis of digestive enzymes, which are mostly made as inactive pro-enzymes that are stored in *zymogen granules.* When acinar cells are stimulated to secrete, the granules fuse with the apical plasma membrane and release their contents into the central acinar lumen. These secretions are transported to the duodenum through a series of anastomosing ducts.

The epithelial cells lining the ducts also are active participants in pancreatic secretion: The cuboidal cells that line the smaller ductules secrete bicarbonate-rich fluid, while the columnar cells lining the larger ducts produce mucin. The epithelial cells of the ducts also express the *cystic fibrosis transmembrane conductance regulator (CFTR);* aberrant function of this membrane protein affects the biochemical content and viscosity of pancreatic secretions. CFTR has a fundamental role in the pathophysiology of pancreatic disease in individuals with cystic fibrosis (Chapter 7).

As discussed later, autodigestion of the pancreas (e.g., in pancreatitis) can be a catastrophic event. A number of "fail-safe" mechanisms have evolved to minimize the risk for occurrence of this phenomenon:

- A majority of pancreatic enzymes are synthesized as inactive pro-enzymes and sequestered in membrane-bound zymogen granules, as mentioned earlier.
- Activation of pro-enzymes requires conversion of trypsinogen to trypsin by duodenal enteropeptidase (also called *enterokinase*).
- Trypsin inhibitors (e.g., SPINK1, also known as *pancreatic secretory trypsin inhibitor*) also are secreted by acinar and ductal cells.
- Trypsin cleaves and inactivates itself, a negative feedback mechanism that normally puts a limit on local levels of activated trypsin.
- Acinar cells are remarkably resistant to the action of activated enzymes such as trypsin, chymotrypsin, and phospholipase A_2.

Diseases of the exocrine pancreas include cystic fibrosis, congenital anomalies, acute and chronic pancreatitis, and

The contributions of those who authored this chapter in previous editions of this book are gratefully acknowledged.

neoplasms. Cystic fibrosis is discussed in detail in Chapter 7; the other pathologic processes are discussed in this chapter.

CONGENITAL ANOMALIES

Pancreatic development is a complex process involving fusion of dorsal and ventral primordia; subtle deviations in this process frequently give rise to congenital variations in pancreatic anatomy. While most of these do not cause clinical disease, variants (especially in ductal anatomy) can present challenges to the endoscopist and the surgeon. For example, failure to recognize idiosyncratic anatomy could result in inadvertent severing of a pancreatic duct during surgery, resulting in pancreatitis.

Agenesis

Very rarely, the pancreas may be totally absent, a condition usually (but not invariably) associated with additional severe malformations that are incompatible with life. *Pancreatic duodenal homeobox 1 (PDX1)* is a homeodomain transcription factor critical for normal pancreatic development, and germline mutations of this gene have been associated with pancreatic agenesis.

Pancreas Divisum

Pancreas divisum is the most common congenital anomaly of the pancreas, with an incidence of 3% to 10%. In most individuals, the main pancreatic duct (the duct of Wirsung) joins the common bile duct just proximal to the papilla of Vater, and the accessory pancreatic duct (the duct of Santorini) drains into the duodenum through a separate minor papilla. Pancreas divisum is caused by a failure of fusion of the fetal duct systems of the dorsal and ventral pancreatic primordia. As a result, the bulk of the pancreas (formed by the dorsal pancreatic primordium) drains into the duodenum through the small-caliber minor papilla. The duct of Wirsung in individuals with divisum drains only a small portion of the head of the gland through the papilla of Vater. More than 95% of individuals are asymptomatic. The remaining 5% develop acute or chronic pancreatitis, possibly related to inadequate drainage of pancreatic secretions through the minor papilla.

Annular Pancreas

Annular pancreas is a relatively uncommon variant of pancreatic fusion in which a ring of pancreatic tissue completely encircles the duodenum. It can manifest with signs and symptoms of duodenal obstruction such as gastric distention and vomiting.

Ectopic Pancreas

Aberrantly situated, or *ectopic,* pancreatic tissue occurs in about 2% of the population; favored sites are the stomach and duodenum, followed by the jejunum, Meckel diverticulum, and ileum. These embryologic rests typically are small (ranging from millimeters to centimeters in diameter) and are located in the submucosa; they are composed of normal pancreatic acini with occasional islets. Though usually incidental and asymptomatic, ectopic pancreas may become inflamed, leading to pain, or—rarely—can cause mucosal bleeding. Approximately 2% of pancreatic neuroendocrine tumors (Chapter 20) arise in ectopic pancreatic tissue.

Congenital Cysts

Congenital cysts result from anomalous development of the pancreatic ducts. In *polycystic disease,* the kidneys, liver, and pancreas may all contain cysts (Chapter 14). Congenital cysts generally are unilocular and range from microscopic to 5 cm in diameter. They are lined by either uniform cuboidal or flattened epithelium and are enclosed in a thin, fibrous capsule. These benign cysts contain clear *serous fluid*—an important point of distinction from pancreatic cystic neoplasms, which often are *mucinous* (discussed later).

PANCREATITIS

Inflammatory disorders of the pancreas are divided into acute and chronic forms. In *acute pancreatitis,* function can return to normal if the underlying cause of inflammation is removed. By contrast, *chronic pancreatitis* causes irreversible destruction of exocrine pancreas.

Acute Pancreatitis

Acute pancreatitis is a reversible inflammatory disorder that varies in severity, from focal edema and fat necrosis to widespread hemorrhagic necrosis. This is a relatively common condition, with an annual incidence of 10 to 20 per 100,000 people in the Western world.

Etiology
The most common cause of acute pancreatitis in the United States is the impaction of gallstones within the common bile duct, impeding the flow of pancreatic enzymes through the ampulla of Vater ("gallstone pancreatitis"); this is closely followed by pancreatitis secondary to excessive alcohol intake. *Overall, gallstones and alcoholism account for greater than 80% of acute pancreatitis cases,* with the remaining caused by a multitude of factors (Table 17.1). These include the following:

- *Non–gallstone-related obstruction* of the pancreatic ducts (e.g., due to pancreatic cancer or other periampullary neoplasms, pancreas divisum, biliary "sludge," or parasites, particularly *Ascaris lumbricoides* and *Clonorchis sinensis*)
- *Medications* including anti-convulsants, cancer chemotherapeutic agents, thiazide diuretics, estrogens, and more than 85 others in clinical use
- *Infections* with mumps virus or coxsackievirus, which can directly infect pancreatic exocrine cells
- *Metabolic disorders,* including hypertriglyceridemia, hyperparathyroidism, and other hypercalcemic states

Table 17.1 Etiologic Factors in Acute Pancreatitis

Metabolic
Alcoholism*
Hyperlipoproteinemia
Hypercalcemia
Drugs (e.g., azathioprine)

Genetic
Mutations in the cationic trypsinogen (PRSS1) and trypsin inhibitor (SPINK1) genes

Mechanical
Gallstones*
Trauma
Iatrogenic injury
Perioperative injury
Endoscopic procedures with dye injection

Vascular
Shock
Atheroembolism
Polyarteritis nodosa

Infectious
Mumps
Coxsackievirus

*Most common causes in the United States.

- *Ischemia* due to vascular thrombosis, embolism, vasculitis, or shock
- *Trauma,* both blunt force and iatrogenic during surgery or endoscopy
- *Germline mutations* involving genes encoding pancreatic enzymes or their inhibitors. For example, *hereditary pancreatitis* is a rare autosomal dominant disease with 80% penetrance that is characterized by recurrent attacks of severe pancreatitis, usually beginning in childhood. It is caused by mutations in the *PRSS1* gene, which encodes trypsinogen, the proenzyme of pancreatic trypsin. The pathogenic mutations alter the site through which trypsin cleaves and inactivates itself, abrogating an important negative feedback mechanism. This defect leads not only to the hyperactivation of trypsin, but also to the hyperactivation of many other digestive enzymes that require trypsin cleavage for their activation. As a result of this unbridled protease activity, the pancreas is prone to autodigestion and injury. Loss-of-function mutations in genes that encode protease inhibitors such as *SPINK1* are less commonly associated with hereditary pancreatitis.

Of note, 10% to 20% of cases of acute pancreatitis have no identifiable cause *(idiopathic pancreatitis),* although a growing body of evidence suggests that many may have an underlying genetic basis. For example, a subset of these so-called *idiopathic pancreatitis* patients has underlying germ line mutations of the *CFTR* gene with symptoms predominantly restricted to the pancreas (Chapter 7).

Pathogenesis

Acute pancreatitis appears to be caused by autodigestion of the pancreas by inappropriately activated pancreatic enzymes. As discussed earlier, once activated trypsin is capable of converting other zymogen forms of pancreatic enzymes to their active forms. Premature activation of trypsin within the substance of the pancreas can unleash these proenzymes (e.g., phospholipases and elastases), leading to tissue injury and inflammation. Trypsin also converts prekallikrein to its activated form, thus sparking the kinin system, and, by activation of factor XII (Hageman factor), also sets in motion the clotting and complement systems (Chapter 4). Three pathways can incite the initial enzyme activation that may lead to acute pancreatitis (Fig. 17.1):

- *Pancreatic duct obstruction.* Impaction of a gallstone or biliary sludge, or extrinsic compression of the ductal system by a mass blocks ductal flow, increases intraductal pressure, and allows accumulation of an enzyme-rich interstitial fluid. Since lipase is secreted in an active form, local fat necrosis may result. Injured tissues, periacinar myofibroblasts, and leukocytes then release proinflammatory cytokines that promote local inflammation and interstitial edema through a leaky microvasculature. Edema further compromises local blood flow, causing vascular insufficiency and ischemic injury to acinar cells.
- *Primary acinar cell injury.* This pathogenic mechanism comes into play in acute pancreatitis caused by ischemia, viral infections (e.g., mumps), drugs, and direct trauma to the pancreas.
- *Defective intracellular transport of proenzymes within acinar cells.* In normal acinar cells, digestive enzymes intended for zymogen granules (and eventually extracellular release) and hydrolytic enzymes destined for lysosomes are transported in discrete pathways after synthesis in the endoplasmic reticulum. However, at least in some animal models of metabolic injury, pancreatic proenzymes and lysosomal hydrolases become packaged together. This results in proenzyme activation, lysosomal rupture (action of phospholipases), and local release of activated enzymes. The role of this mechanism in human acute pancreatitis is not clear.

Alcohol consumption may cause pancreatitis by several mechanisms. Alcohol transiently increases pancreatic exocrine secretion and contraction of the sphincter of Oddi (the muscle regulating the flow of pancreatic juice through papilla of Vater). Alcohol also has direct toxic effects on acinar cells, including induction of oxidative stress in acinar cells, which leads to membrane damage (discussed later). Finally, chronic alcohol ingestion results in the secretion of protein-rich pancreatic fluid, which leads to the deposition of inspissated protein plugs and obstruction of small pancreatic ducts.

MORPHOLOGY

The basic alterations in acute pancreatitis are **(1) microvascular leakage causing edema, (2) necrosis of fat by lipases, (3) an acute inflammatory reaction, (4) proteolytic destruction of pancreatic parenchyma, and (5) destruction of blood vessels leading to interstitial hemorrhage.**

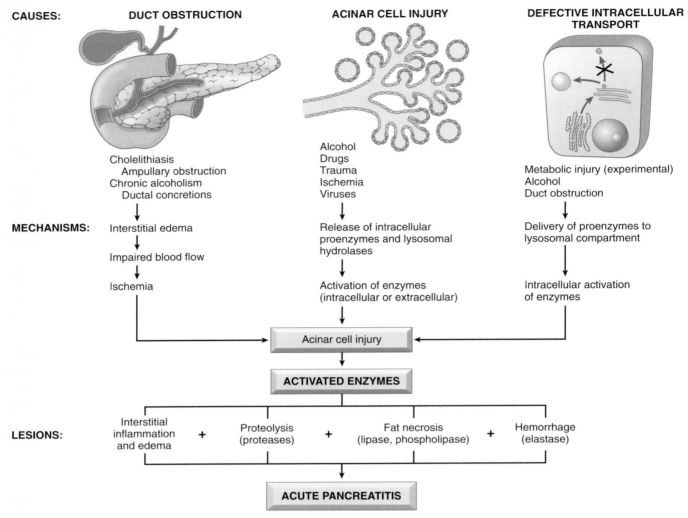

Fig. 17.1 Proposed pathogenesis of acute pancreatitis.

In mild forms, there is interstitial edema and focal areas of fat necrosis in the pancreas and peripancreatic fat (Fig. 17.2A). Fat necrosis results from enzymatic destruction of fat cells; the released fatty acids combine with calcium to form insoluble salts that precipitate in situ.

In more severe forms, such as **acute necrotizing pancreatitis,** the damage also involves acinar and ductal cells, the islets of Langerhans, and blood vessels. Macroscopically, the pancreas exhibits red-black hemorrhagic areas interspersed with foci of yellow-white, chalky **fat necrosis** (Fig. 17.2B). Fat necrosis also can occur in extrapancreatic fat, including the omentum and bowel mesentery, and even outside the abdominal cavity (e.g., in subcutaneous fat). In most cases, the peritoneum contains a serous, slightly turbid, brown-tinged fluid with globules of fat (derived from enzymatically digested adipose tissue). In the most severe form, **hemorrhagic pancreatitis,** extensive parenchymal necrosis is accompanied by diffuse hemorrhage within the substance of the gland.

Clinical Features

Abdominal pain is the cardinal manifestation of acute pancreatitis. Its severity varies from mild and uncomfortable to severe and incapacitating. Acute pancreatitis is diagnosed primarily by the presence of elevated plasma levels of amylase and lipase and the exclusion of other causes of abdominal pain. In 80% of cases, acute pancreatitis is mild and self-limiting; the remaining 20% develop severe disease.

Full-blown acute pancreatitis is a medical emergency of the first order. Affected individuals usually experience the sudden calamitous onset of an "acute abdomen" with pain, guarding, and the ominous absence of bowel sounds. Characteristically, the pain is constant, intense and referred to the upper back; it must be differentiated from pain of other causes such as perforated peptic ulcer, biliary colic, acute cholecystitis with rupture, and occlusion of mesenteric vessels with infarction of the bowel.

The manifestations of severe acute pancreatitis are attributable to systemic release of digestive enzymes and

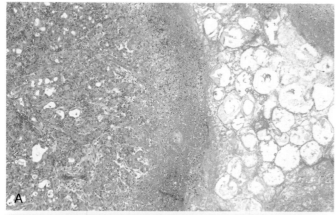

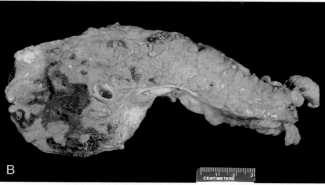

Fig. 17.2 Acute pancreatitis. (A) The microscopic field shows a region of fat necrosis *(right)* and focal pancreatic parenchymal necrosis *(center).* (B) The pancreas has been sectioned longitudinally to reveal dark areas of hemorrhage in the pancreatic substance and a focal area of pale fat necrosis in the peripancreatic fat *(upper left).*

explosive activation of the inflammatory response. The initial clinical evaluation may reveal leukocytosis, disseminated intravascular coagulation (Chapter 12), acute respiratory distress syndrome (due to diffuse alveolar damage) (Chapter 13), and diffuse fat necrosis. Peripheral vascular collapse (shock) can rapidly ensue as a result of increased microvascular permeability and resultant hypovolemia, compounded by endotoxemia (from breakdown of the barriers between gastrointestinal flora and the bloodstream), and renal failure due to acute tubular necrosis (Chapter 14).

Laboratory findings include markedly elevated serum amylase during the first 24 hours, followed (within 72–96 hours) by rising serum lipase levels. Hypocalcemia can result from precipitation of calcium in areas of fat necrosis; if persistent, it is a poor prognostic sign. The enlarged inflamed pancreas can be visualized by computed tomography (CT) or magnetic resonance imaging (MRI).

The crux of the management of acute pancreatitis is supportive therapy (e.g., maintaining blood pressure and alleviating pain) and "resting" the pancreas by total restriction of oral food and fluids. In 40% to 60% of cases of acute necrotizing pancreatitis, the necrotic debris becomes infected, usually by gram-negative organisms from the alimentary tract, further complicating the clinical course. Although most individuals with acute pancreatitis eventually recover, some 5% die from shock during the first week of illness; acute respiratory distress syndrome and acute

renal failure are ominous complications. In surviving patients, sequelae include sterile or infected *pancreatic "abscesses"* or *pancreatic pseudocysts.*

Pancreatic Pseudocysts

A common sequela of acute pancreatitis (and in particular, alcoholic pancreatitis) is a *pancreatic pseudocyst.* Liquefied areas of necrotic pancreatic tissue become walled off by fibrous tissue to form a cystic space, lacking an epithelial lining (hence the designation *pseudo*). The cyst contents are rich in pancreatic enzymes, and a laboratory assessment of the cyst aspirate can be diagnostic. Pseudocysts account for approximately 75% of all pancreatic cysts. While many pseudocysts spontaneously resolve, they can become secondarily infected, and larger pseudocysts can compress or even perforate into adjacent structures.

MORPHOLOGY

Pseudocysts usually are solitary; they commonly are attached to the surface of the gland and involve peripancreatic tissues such as the lesser omental sac or the retroperitoneum between the stomach and transverse colon or liver (Fig. 17.3A). They can range in diameter from 2 cm to 30 cm. Since pseudocysts form by walling off areas of hemorrhagic fat necrosis, they typically are composed of necrotic debris encased by walls of granulation tissue and fibroblasts lacking an epithelial lining (see Fig. 17.3B). If they get infected, a pancreatic abscess is formed.

Chronic Pancreatitis

Chronic pancreatitis is characterized by long-standing inflammation that leads to irreversible destruction of the exocrine pancreas, followed eventually by loss of the islets of Langerhans. Of note, recurrent bouts of acute pancreatitis regardless of etiology can evolve over time into chronic pancreatitis. The prevalence of chronic pancreatitis is difficult to determine but probably ranges between 0.04% and 5% of the U.S. population.

Etiology

By far **the most common cause of chronic pancreatitis is long-term alcohol abuse.** Middle-aged men constitute the bulk of patients in this etiologic group. Less common causes of chronic pancreatitis include the following:
- *Duct Obstruction.* Long-standing obstruction of pancreatic duct e.g., by pseudocysts, calculi, neoplasms, or pancreas divisum.
- *Tropical pancreatitis,* a poorly characterized heterogeneous disorder seen in Africa and Asia, with a subset of cases having a hereditary basis.
- *Hereditary pancreatitis* due to mutations in the pancreatic trypsinogen gene *(PRRS1)*, or the *SPINK1* gene encoding a trypsin inhibitor (see Table 17.1).
- *Chronic pancreatitis associated with CFTR mutations.* The pathophysiology of chronic pancreatitis in cystic fibrosis is discussed in detail in Chapter 7.
- *Autoimmune pancreatitis* is a pathogenically distinct form of chronic pancreatitis that is associated with the

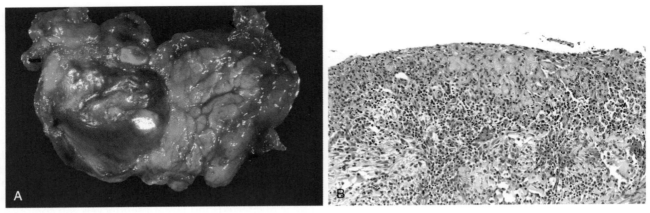

Fig. 17.3 Pancreatic pseudocyst. (A) Cross-section revealing a poorly defined cyst with a necrotic brownish wall. (B) Histologically, the cyst lacks an epithelial lining and instead is lined by fibrin and granulation tissue, with typical changes of chronic inflammation.

presence of IgG4-secreting plasma cells in the pancreas. Autoimmune pancreatitis is one manifestation of IgG-related disease (Chapter 5), which may involve multiple tissues. It is important to recognize because it responds to steroid therapy.

As many as 40% of individuals with chronic pancreatitis have no recognizable predisposing factors. As with acute pancreatitis, however, a growing number of these "idiopathic" cases are associated with inherited mutations in genes, such as *CFTR*, that are important for normal pancreatic exocrine function. Recent studies have also identified polymorphisms in genes encoding exocrine pancreatic enzymes, including carboxypeptidase A1 *(CPA1)* and lipase *(CEL)*, that may confer increased susceptibility to chronic pancreatitis.

Pathogenesis

Although the pathogenesis of chronic pancreatitis is not well defined, several hypotheses are proposed:

- *Ductal obstruction by concretions.* Many of the inciting agents in chronic pancreatitis (e.g., alcohol) increase the protein concentration of pancreatic secretions, and these proteins can form ductal plugs.
- *Toxic-metabolic.* Toxins, including alcohol and its metabolites, can exert a direct toxic effect on acinar cells, leading to lipid accumulation, acinar cell loss, and eventually parenchymal fibrosis.
- *Oxidative stress.* Alcohol-induced oxidative stress may generate free radicals in acinar cells, leading to membrane damage (Chapter 2), and subsequent expression of chemokines like interleukin-8 (IL-8), which recruits inflammatory cells. Oxidative stress also promotes the fusion of lysosomes and zymogen granules with resulting acinar cell necrosis, inflammation, and fibrosis.
- *Inappropriate activation of pancreatic enzymes* due to mutations affecting genes mentioned earlier.

In contrast to acute pancreatitis, a variety of profibrogenic cytokines, such as transforming growth factor-β (TGF-β), connective tissue growth factor, and platelet-derived growth factor, are secreted in chronic pancreatitis by infiltrating immune cells such as macrophages. These cytokines induce the activation and proliferation of peri-acinar myofibroblasts ("pancreatic stellate cells"), which deposit collagen and give rise to fibrosis.

MORPHOLOGY

Chronic pancreatitis is characterized by **parenchymal fibrosis, reduced number and size of acini, and variable dilation of the pancreatic ducts;** there is a relative sparing of the islets of Langerhans initially (Fig. 17.4A). **Acinar loss** is a constant feature, usually with a chronic inflammatory infiltrate around remaining lobules and ducts. The ductal epithelium may be atrophied or hyperplastic or exhibit squamous metaplasia, and ductal concretions may be noted (Fig. 17.4B). The remaining islets of Langerhans become embedded in the sclerotic tissue and may fuse and appear enlarged; eventually they also disappear. On gross evaluation, the gland is hard, sometimes with extremely dilated ducts and visible calcified concretions.

Autoimmune pancreatitis (AIP) is a distinct form of chronic pancreatitis that is characterized by striking infiltration of the pancreas by lymphocytes and plasma cells, many of which are positive for IgG4, accompanied by a "swirling" fibrosis and venulitis **(lymphoplasmacytic sclerosing pancreatitis).**

Clinical Features

Chronic pancreatitis manifests as repeated bouts of jaundice, vague indigestion, or persistent or recurrent abdominal and back pain, or it may be entirely silent until pancreatic insufficiency and diabetes mellitus develop (the latter as a consequence of islet destruction). Attacks can be precipitated by alcohol abuse, overeating (which increases demand on pancreatic secretions), or opiates or other drugs that increase the muscle tone of the sphincter of Oddi.

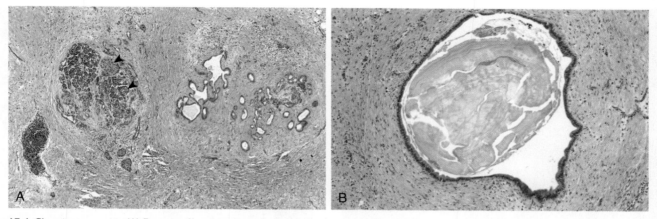

Fig. 17.4 Chronic pancreatitis. (A) Extensive fibrosis and atrophy have left only residual islets *(left)* and ducts *(right)*, with a sprinkling of chronic inflammatory cells and acinar tissue. (B) A higher-power view demonstrating dilated ducts with inspissated eosinophilic concretions in a patient with alcoholic chronic pancreatitis.

The diagnosis of chronic pancreatitis requires a high degree of clinical suspicion. During an attack of abdominal pain, there may be mild fever and modest elevations of serum amylase. In end-stage disease, however, acinar destruction may be so advanced that enzyme elevations are absent. Gallstone-induced obstruction may manifest as jaundice or elevated levels of serum alkaline phosphatase. A very helpful finding is visualization of calcifications within the pancreas by CT or ultrasonography. Weight loss and hypoalbuminemic edema from malabsorption caused by pancreatic exocrine insufficiency can also point to the disease.

Although chronic pancreatitis is usually not acutely life-threatening, the long-term outlook is poor, with a 50% mortality rate over 20 to 25 years. The most common long-term sequelae of chronic pancreatitis is insufficiency of pancreatic exocrine enzymes, with consequent malabsorption and deficiency of fat-soluble vitamins (Chapter 8). Exocrine insufficiency typically predates endocrine dysfunction, and patients with severe loss of islets can develop diabetes mellitus (Chapter 20). In other patients, *severe chronic pain* may dominate the clinical picture. *Pancreatic pseudocysts* (discussed earlier) develop in about 10% of patients. The most feared long-term complication of chronic pancreatitis is pancreatic cancer. The risk for malignant transformation in adult-onset disease is modest, with no more than 5% of patients developing cancer at 20 years. In contrast, chronic pancreatitis that begins in childhood, such as hereditary pancreatitis secondary to *PRSS1* mutations, confers a 40% to 55% lifetime risk for pancreatic cancer. It is not unusual for patients with *PRSS1* mutations to undergo prophylactic pancreatectomy.

necrosis to widespread parenchymal necrosis and hemorrhage; the clinical presentation varies widely, from mild abdominal pain to rapidly fatal vascular collapse.
- *Chronic pancreatitis* is characterized by irreversible parenchymal damage and scar formation; clinical presentations include chronic malabsorption (due to pancreatic exocrine insufficiency) and diabetes mellitus (due to islet cell loss).
- Both entities share similar pathogenic mechanisms, and indeed recurrent acute pancreatitis can result in chronic pancreatitis. *Ductal obstruction* and *long-term alcohol abuse* are the most common causes in both forms. Inappropriate activation of pancreatic digestive enzymes (due to mutations in genes encoding trypsinogen or trypsin inhibitors) and primary acinar injury (due to toxins, infections, ischemia, or trauma) also cause pancreatitis.

PANCREATIC NEOPLASMS

Pancreatic exocrine neoplasms can be cystic or solid. Some tumors are benign, while others are among the most lethal of all malignancies.

Cystic Neoplasms

Cystic neoplasms are diverse tumors that range from harmless benign cysts to invasive, potentially lethal, cancers. Approximately 5% to 15% of all pancreatic cysts are neoplastic; these constitute less than 5% of all pancreatic neoplasms. Some of these are almost always benign (e.g., serous cystadenoma); others, such as mucinous cystic neoplasms, can be benign or malignant.

Serous cystadenomas account for approximately 25% of all pancreatic cystic neoplasms; they are composed of glycogen-rich cuboidal cells surrounding small cysts containing clear, straw-colored fluid (Fig. 17.5). The tumors typically manifest in the seventh decade of life with nonspecific symptoms such as abdominal pain; the female-to-male ratio is 2:1. These tumors are almost uniformly benign, and surgical resection is curative in the vast majority of patients. Most serous

PANCREATITIS

- *Acute pancreatitis* is characterized by inflammation and reversible parenchymal damage that ranges from focal edema and fat

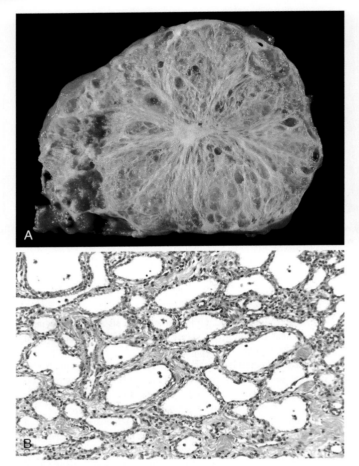

Fig. 17.5 Serous cystadenoma. (A) Cross-section through a serous cystadenoma. Only a thin rim of normal pancreatic parenchyma remains. The cysts are relatively small and contain clear, straw-colored fluid. (B) The cysts are lined by cuboidal epithelium without atypia.

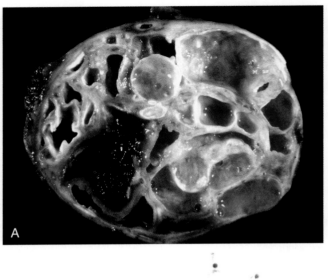

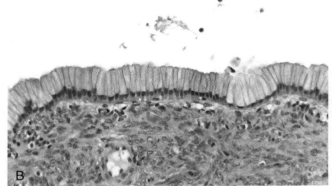

Fig. 17.6 Mucinous cystic neoplasm. (A) Cross-section through a mucinous multiloculated cyst in the tail of the pancreas. The cysts are large and filled with tenacious mucin. (B) The cysts are lined by columnar mucinous epithelium, with a densely cellular "ovarian" stroma.

cystadenomas carry somatic loss of function mutations of the von Hippel-Lindau *(VHL)* tumor suppressor gene, which you will recall is a negative regulator of hypoxia-inducible factor 1 alpha (HIF-1-alpha) (Chapter 6).

In contrast to serous cystic tumors, **close** *to 95% of mucinous cystic neoplasms arise in women, usually in the body or tail of the pancreas, and manifest as painless, slow-growing masses.* The cystic spaces are filled with thick, tenacious mucin, and the cysts are lined by a columnar mucinous epithelium with an associated densely cellular stroma resembling that of the ovary (Fig. 17.6). Based on the degree of cytologic and architectural atypia in the epithelial lining, noninvasive mucinous cystic neoplasms are classified as harboring *low-grade, moderate,* or *severe* dysplasia. Up to one-third of these cysts can be associated with an invasive adenocarcinoma, another important difference from the serous tumors. Distal pancreatectomy for noninvasive mucinous cysts typically is curative, even in the setting of severe dysplasia.

Intraductal Papillary Mucinous Neoplasms

In contrast with mucinous cystic neoplasms, intraductal papillary mucinous neoplasms (IPMNs) occur more frequently in men than in women and more frequently involve the head of the pancreas. IPMNs arise in the main pancreatic ducts, or one of its major branch ducts, and lack the cellular stroma seen in mucinous cystic neoplasms (Fig. 17.7). As with mucinous cystic neoplasms, the epithelia of noninvasive IPMNs harbor various grades of dysplasia, and a subset of lesions is associated with invasive adenocarcinoma. In particular, "colloid" carcinomas of the pancreas, which are adenocarcinomas associated with abundant extracellular mucin production, nearly always represent malignant transformation of an IPMN. Up to two-thirds of IPMNs harbor oncogenic mutations of *GNAS* on chromosome 20q13, which encodes the alpha subunit of a stimulatory G-protein, G_s (Chapter 20). Constitutive activation of this G-protein is predicted to result in an intracellular cascade that promotes cell proliferation.

Pancreatic Carcinoma

Infiltrating ductal adenocarcinoma of the pancreas (more commonly referred to as *pancreatic cancer*) is the third leading cause of cancer deaths in the United States, preceded only by lung and colon cancers. Although it is substantially less common than the other two malignancies, pancreatic carcinoma is near the top of the list of killers because it carries one of the highest mortality rates. Close to 49,000 Americans were diagnosed with pancreatic cancer in 2015, and virtually all will die in a short period after diagnosis; the 5-year survival rate is a dismal 8%.

Pathogenesis

Like all cancers, pancreatic cancer arises as a consequence of inherited and acquired mutations in cancer-associated

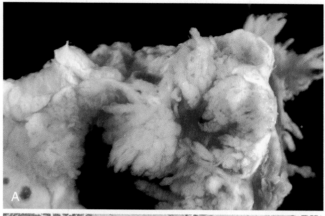

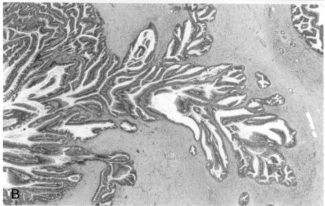

Fig. 17.7 Intraductal papillary mucinous neoplasm. (A) Cross-section through the head of the pancreas showing a prominent papillary neoplasm distending the main pancreatic duct. (B) The papillary mucinous neoplasm involves the main pancreatic duct *(left)* and is extending down into the smaller ducts and ductules *(right)*.

genes. In a pattern analogous to that seen in the multi-step progression of colon cancer (Chapter 6), there is a progressive accumulation of genetic changes in pancreatic epithelium as it proceeds from nonneoplastic, to noninvasive precursor lesions, to invasive carcinoma (Fig. 17.8). While both intraductal papillary mucinous neoplasms and mucinous cystic neoplasms can progress to invasive adenocarcinoma, **the most common antecedent lesions of pancreatic cancer arise in small ducts and ductules, and are called pancreatic intraepithelial neoplasias (PanINs).** Evidence in favor of the precursor relationship of PanINs to frank malignancy includes the observations that these microscopic lesions often are found adjacent to infiltrating carcinomas and the two share a number of genetic alterations. Moreover, the epithelial cells in PanINs show dramatic telomere shortening, potentially predisposing these lesions to pathogenic chromosomal abnormalities that may contribute to acquisition of the full spectrum of cancer hallmarks.

The recent sequencing of the pancreatic cancer genome has confirmed that **four genes are most commonly affected by somatic mutations in this neoplasm: *KRAS, CDKN2A/ p16, SMAD4,* and *TP53*:**

- *KRAS* is the most frequently altered oncogene in pancreatic cancer; it is activated by a point mutation in greater than 90% of cases. These mutations impair the intrinsic GTPase activity of the KRAS protein so that it is constitutively active. In turn, KRAS activates a number of intracellular signaling pathways that promote carcinogenesis (Chapter 6).
- The *p16 (CDKN2A)* gene is the most frequently inactivated tumor suppressor gene in pancreatic cancer, being turned off in 95% of cases. The p16 protein has a critical role in cell-cycle control; inactivation removes an important checkpoint.
- The *SMAD4* tumor suppressor gene is inactivated in 55% of pancreatic cancers and only rarely in other tumors; it codes for a protein that plays an important role in signal transduction downstream of the transforming growth factor-β receptor.
- Inactivation of the *TP53* tumor suppressor gene occurs in 50% to 70% of pancreatic cancers. Its gene

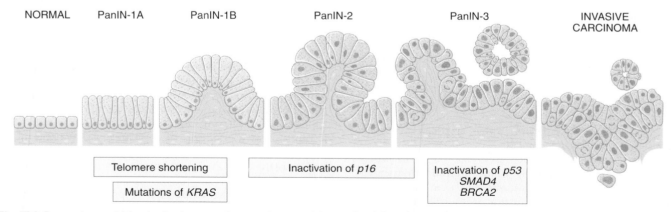

Fig. 17.8 Progression model for the development of pancreatic cancer. It is postulated that telomere shortening and mutations of the *KRAS* oncogene occur at early stages, inactivation of the p16 tumor suppressor gene occurs at intermediate stages, and inactivation of the *TP53, SMAD4,* and *BRCA2* tumor suppressor genes occurs at late stages. Note that while there is a general temporal sequence of changes, the accumulation of multiple mutations is more important than their occurrence in a specific order. PanIN, Pancreatic intraepithelial neoplasm. The numbers following the labels on the top refer to stages in the development of PanINs. *(Modified from Maitra A, Hruban RH: Pancreatic cancer,* Annu Rev Pathol Mech Dis *3:157, 2008.)*

product, p53, acts both to enforce cell-cycle check-points and as an inducer of apoptosis or senescence (Chapter 6). *BRCA2* is also mutated late in a subset of pancreatic cancers.

Pancreatic cancer is primarily a disease of older adults, with 80% of cases occurring between 60 and 80 years of age. The strongest environmental influence is smoking, which doubles the risk. Long-standing chronic pancreatitis and diabetes mellitus are also associated with a modestly increased risk for pancreatic cancer. These two entities have a bidirectional link with pancreatic cancer. Thus, for example, tumors arising in the head of the pancreas often cause chronic pancreatitis in the distal parenchyma, while diabetes caused by duct obstruction and subsequent pancreatitis may be the manifestation of an underlying neoplasm. In fact, approximately 1% of the older adult population with new-onset diabetes harbor an unsuspected pancreatic cancer. Familial clustering of pancreatic cancer has been reported, and a growing number of inherited genetic defects are now recognized that increase pancreatic cancer risk. For example, germ line mutations of the familial breast/ovarian cancer gene *BRCA2* are seen in approximately 10% of cases arising in individuals of Ashkenazi Jewish heritage.

MORPHOLOGY

Approximately 60% of pancreatic cancers arise in the head of the gland, 15% in the body, and 5% in the tail; in the remaining 20%, the neoplasm diffusely involves the entire organ. Carcinomas of the pancreas usually are hard, gray-white, stellate, poorly defined masses (Fig. 17.9A).

Two features are characteristic of pancreatic cancer: It is highly invasive (even "early" invasive pancreatic cancers invade peripancreatic tissues extensively), and it elicits an intense host reaction in the form of dense fibrosis **(desmoplastic response).**

Most carcinomas of the head of the pancreas obstruct the distal common bile duct as it courses through the head of the pancreas. In 50% of such cases, there is marked distention of the biliary tree, and patients typically exhibit jaundice. In contrast, carcinomas of the body and tail of the pancreas do not impinge on the biliary tract. Pancreatic cancers often extend through the retroperitoneal space, entrapping adjacent nerves (thus, accounting for the pain), and occasionally invade the spleen, adrenal glands, vertebral column, transverse colon, and stomach. Peripancreatic, gastric, mesenteric, omental, and portahepatic lymph nodes frequently are involved, and the liver often is enlarged with metastatic deposits. Distant metastases may occur, principally to the lungs and bones.

On microscopic examination, pancreatic carcinoma usually is a **moderately to poorly differentiated adenocarcinoma** forming abortive glands with mucin secretion or cell clusters and exhibiting an aggressive, deeply infiltrative growth pattern (see Fig. 17.9B). Dense stromal fibrosis accompanies tumor invasion, and there is a proclivity for perineural invasion within and beyond the organ. Lymphatic invasion also is commonly seen.

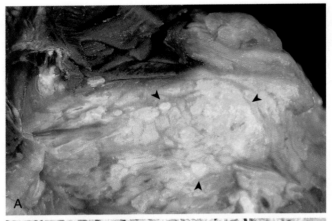

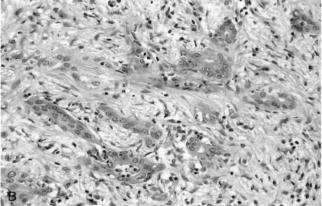

Fig. 17.9 Carcinoma of the pancreas. (A) Cross-section through the head of the pancreas and adjacent common bile duct showing both an ill-defined mass in the pancreatic substance *(arrowheads)* and the green discoloration of the duct resulting from total obstruction of bile flow. (B) Poorly formed glands are present in a densely fibrotic (desmoplastic) stroma within the pancreatic substance.

Less common variants of pancreatic cancer include **adeno-squamous carcinomas** with focal squamous differentiation in addition to glandular differentiation; and undifferentiated carcinomas with osteoclast-like giant cells of monocytic lineage intermixed within the neoplasm.

Clinical Features

Carcinomas of the pancreas typically remain silent until their extension impinges on some other structure. Pain usually is the first symptom, but by that point these cancers are often beyond cure. *Obstructive jaundice* can be associated with carcinoma in the head of the pancreas, but it rarely draws attention to the cancer soon enough for timely intervention. Weight loss, anorexia, and generalized malaise and weakness are manifestations of advanced disease. *Migratory thrombophlebitis (Trousseau syndrome)* occurs in about 10% of patients and is attributable to the elaboration of platelet-aggregating factors and pro-coagulants from the tumor or its necrotic products (Chapter 6). As previously stated, new-onset diabetes is the first manifestation of pancreatic cancer in some patients.

The clinical course of pancreatic carcinoma is rapidly progressive and often distressingly brief. Less than 20% of pancreatic cancers are resectable at the time of diagnosis. It has long been recognized that there is a profound need for biomarkers capable of detecting early, potentially curable, pancreatic cancers. Although serum levels of many enzymes and antigens (e.g., carcinoembryonic and CA19-9 antigens) are elevated, these markers are neither specific nor sensitive enough to be useful for screening. Several imaging techniques, such as endoscopic ultrasonography and high-resolution CT scans, are helpful for investigation in cases of suspected cancer but are not practical screening tests.

SUMMARY

PANCREATIC NEOPLASMS

- Pancreatic cancer probably arises from noninvasive precursor lesions (most commonly, PanINs), developing by progressive accumulation of mutations of oncogenes (e.g., *KRAS*) and tumor suppressor genes (e.g., *CDKN2A/p16*, *TP53*, and *SMAD4*).
- Typically, these neoplasms are ductal adenocarcinomas that produce an intense desmoplastic response.
- Most pancreatic cancers are diagnosed at an advanced stage, accounting for the high mortality rate.
- Obstructive jaundice is a feature of carcinoma of the head of the pancreas; many patients also experience debilitating pain.
- Carcinomas of the tail of the pancreas are often not detected until late in their course.

SUGGESTED READINGS

Andersen DK, Andren-Sandberg Å, Duell EJ, et al: Pancreatitis-diabetes-pancreatic cancer: summary of an NIDDK-NCI workshop, *Pancreas* 42:1227–1237, 2013. [*A white paper that summarizes the current state of evidence regarding the bidirectional and complex relationship between chronic pancreatitis or diabetes and pancreatic cancer. The recently described entity of pancreatogenic diabetes is also discussed.*]

Bailey P, Chang DK, Nones K, et al: Genomic analyses identify molecular subtypes of pancreatic cancer, *Nature* 531:47–52, 2016. [*A comprehensive genomic profiling of pancreatic cancer by the International Cancer Genome Consortium.*].

Dellinger EP, Forsmark CE, Layer P, et al: Determinant-based classification of acute pancreatitis severity: an international multidisciplinary consultation, *Ann Surg* 256:875–880, 2012. [*An international classification system for the clinical severity of acute pancreatitis, which represents the consensus of opinions from physicians spanning 49 countries.*]

Hart PA, Zen Y, Chari ST: Recent advances in autoimmune pancreatitis, *Gastroenterology* 149:39–51, 2015. [*An up-to-date review on the etiopathogenesis and clinical subtypes of autoimmune pancreatitis from one of the foremost expert groups on this subject.*]

Knudson ES, O'Reilly EM, Brody JR, et al: Genetic diversity of pancreatic ductal adenocarcinoma and opportunities for precision medicine, *Gastroenterology* 150:48–63, 2016. [*An up-to-date description of the molecular abnormalities in cancer of the pancreas revealed by next-generation sequencing and possible drug targets.*]

Ryan DP, Hong TS, Bardeesy N: Pancreatic adenocarcinoma, *N Engl J Med* 371:1039–1049, 2014. [*An outstanding clinically oriented update on pancreatic cancer, including newly emerging molecular targets for therapy.*]

Shelton CA, Whitcomb DC: Genetics and treatment options for recurrent acute and chronic pancreatitis, *Curr Treat Options Gastroenterol* 12:359–371, 2014. [*A comprehensive review on germ line mutations that result in recurrent pancreatitis, as well as recently identified polymorphisms that enhance the risk for pancreatitis.*]

Tanaka M, et al: International consensus guidelines 2012 for the management of IPMN and MCN of the pancreas, *Pancreatology* 12:183–197, 2012. [*An update to the 2006 consensus guidelines on how to identify the presence of malignancy within cystic precursor lesions of pancreatic cancer using imaging and other diagnostic criteria. Although not definitive, these guidelines are widely used for deciding which cyst patients require surgery versus observation.*]

Male Genital System and Lower Urinary Tract

CHAPTER OUTLINE

Penis 691
Malformations 691
Inflammatory Lesions 691
Neoplasms 691
Scrotum, Testis, and Epididymis 692
Cryptorchidism and Testicular Atrophy 692
Inflammatory Lesions 693
Vascular Disturbances 693
Testicular Neoplasms 693

Prostate 697
Prostatitis 697
Benign Prostatic Hyperplasia 698
Carcinoma of the Prostate 699
Ureter, Bladder, and Urethra 701
Ureter 702
Urinary Bladder 702
Sexually Transmitted Diseases 704
Syphilis 705

Gonorrhea 708
Nongonococcal Urethritis and Cervicitis 709
Lymphogranuloma Venereum 710
Chancroid (Soft Chancre) 710
Granuloma Inguinale 711
Trichomoniasis 711
Genital Herpes Simplex 711
Human Papillomavirus Infection 712

PENIS

Malformations

Among the most common malformations of the penis are those in which the distal urethral orifice is abnormally located. In *hypospadias,* the abnormal urethral opening is found on the ventral aspect of the penis anywhere along the shaft. This anomalous orifice is sometimes constricted, resulting in urinary tract obstruction and an increased risk for urinary tract infections. Hypospadias occurs in 1 in 300 live male births and may be associated with other congenital anomalies, such as inguinal hernia and undescended testis. In *epispadias,* which is less common, the abnormal urethral orifice is on the dorsal aspect of the penis.

Inflammatory Lesions

Balanitis and *balanoposthitis* refer to local inflammation of the glans penis and of the overlying prepuce, respectively. Among the more common agents are *Candida albicans,* anaerobic bacteria, *Gardnerella,* and pyogenic bacteria. Most cases occur as a consequence of poor hygiene in uncircumcised males, leading to the accumulation of desquamated epithelial cells, sweat, and debris, termed *smegma,* which acts as a local irritant. *Phimosis* is a condition in which the prepuce cannot be retracted easily over the glans penis. Phimosis may be a congenital anomaly, but most cases stem from scarring of the prepuce caused by balanoposthitis.

Neoplasms

More than 95% of penile neoplasms arise on squamous epithelium. In the United States, squamous cell carcinomas of the penis are relatively uncommon, accounting for about 0.4% of all cancers in males. In developing countries, however, penile carcinoma occurs at much higher rates. Most cases occur in uncircumcised patients older than 40 years of age. Several factors have been implicated in the pathogenesis of penile squamous cell carcinoma, including poor hygiene (with resultant exposure to potential carcinogens in smegma), smoking, and infection with human papillomavirus (HPV), particularly types 16 and 18.

Squamous cell carcinoma in situ of the penis (Bowen disease) occurs in older uncircumcised males and appears grossly as a solitary plaque on the shaft of the penis. Histologic examination reveals dysplastic cells throughout the epidermis with no invasion of the underlying stroma (Fig. 18.1). It gives rise to invasive squamous cell carcinoma in approximately 10% of patients.

Invasive squamous cell carcinoma of the penis appears as a gray, crusted, papular lesion, most commonly on the glans penis or prepuce. In many cases, infiltration of the underlying connective tissue produces an indurated, ulcerated lesion with irregular margins (Fig. 18.2). Histologically, the tumor is most often a typical keratinizing squamous cell carcinoma. The prognosis is related to the stage of the tumor. With localized lesions, the 5-year survival rate is 66%, whereas metastasis to inguinal lymph nodes carries a grim 27% 5-year survival rate. *Verrucous carcinoma* is a non-HPV–related variant of squamous cell

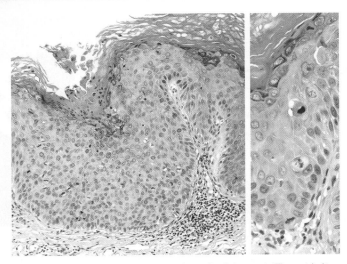

Fig. 18.1 Carcinoma in situ (Bowen disease) of the penis. The epithelium above the intact basement membrane shows delayed maturation and disorganization *(left)*. Higher magnification *(right)* shows several mitotic figures, some above the basal layer, and nuclear pleomorphism.

carcinoma characterized by papillary architecture, virtually no cytologic atypia, and rounded, pushing deep margins. Verrucous carcinomas are locally invasive but do not metastasize.

⬤ SUMMARY

LESIONS OF THE PENIS

- Squamous cell carcinoma and its precursor lesions are the most important penile lesions. Many are associated with HPV infection.
- Squamous cell carcinoma occurs on the glans or shaft of the penis as an ulcerated infiltrative lesion that may spread to inguinal nodes and infrequently to distant sites. Most cases occur in uncircumcised males.
- Other important penile disorders include congenital abnormalities involving the position of the urethra (epispadias, hypospadias) and inflammatory disorders (balanitis, phimosis).

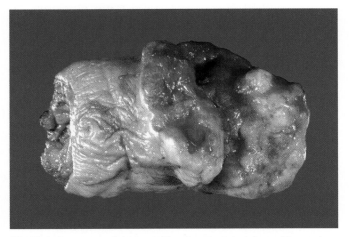

Fig. 18.2 Carcinoma of the penis. The glans penis is deformed by an ulcerated, infiltrative mass.

SCROTUM, TESTIS, AND EPIDIDYMIS

Several inflammatory processes may affect the skin of the scrotum, including local fungal infections and systemic dermatoses, such as psoriasis (Chapter 24). Neoplasms of the scrotal sac are unusual. *Squamous cell carcinoma,* the most common of these, is of historical interest in that it represents the first human malignancy associated with environmental exposures, dating from Sir Percival Pott's observation of a high incidence of the disease in chimney sweeps. The subsequent edict by the Chimney Sweeps Guild that its members must bathe daily remains one of the most successful public health measures for cancer prevention. Several disorders unrelated to the testes and epididymis may present as scrotal enlargement. *Hydrocele,* the most common cause of scrotal swelling, is caused by an accumulation of serous fluid within the tunica vaginalis. It may be idiopathic or arise in response to neighboring infections or tumors. The clear fluid of a hydrocele allows light to pass through (transluminescence), distinguishing it from collections of blood, pus, or lymph, all of which are cloudy or opaque. Accumulation of blood or lymphatic fluid within the tunica vaginalis, termed *hematocele* and *chylocele,* respectively, also may cause scrotal enlargement. In extreme cases of lymphatic obstruction, caused, for example, by filariasis, the scrotum and the lower extremities may enlarge to grotesque sizes—a condition termed *elephantiasis.*

Cryptorchidism and Testicular Atrophy

Cryptorchidism is a *failure of testicular descent* into the scrotum. Normally, the testes descend from the abdominal cavity into the pelvis by the third month of gestation and then through the inguinal canals into the scrotum during the last 2 months of intrauterine life. The diagnosis of cryptorchidism is only established with certainty after 1 year of age, particularly in premature infants, because testicular descent into the scrotum is not always complete at birth. Cryptorchidism affects 1% of the male population. In the vast majority of cases, the cause is unknown. The condition is bilateral in approximately 10% of affected patients, a small percentage of whom have chromosomal aberrations and other developmental abnormalities. Because undescended testes become atrophic, bilateral cryptorchidism results in sterility. For unclear reasons, even unilateral cryptorchidism may be associated with atrophy of the contralateral descended gonad.

In addition to infertility, failure of testicular descent is associated with a 3- to 5-fold increased risk for testicular cancer. Patients with unilateral cryptorchidism also are at increased risk for the development of cancer in the contralateral, normally descended testis, suggesting that some intrinsic abnormality, rather than simple failure of descent, underlies the increased cancer risk. Surgical placement of the undescended testis into the scrotum (orchiopexy) is recommended by 18 months of age to decrease the likelihood of testicular atrophy, infertility, and testicular cancer.

The cryptorchid testis may be of normal size early in life, but some degree of atrophy usually is evident by the onset of puberty. Microscopically, tubular atrophy begins to appear by 5 to 6 years of age, and is usually advanced by the time of puberty. *Germ cell neoplasia in-situ* (discussed later) may be present in cryptorchid testes and is a likely precursor of subsequent germ cell tumors. Atrophic changes similar to those in cryptorchid testes may be caused by other insults, including chronic ischemia, trauma, irradiation, and anti-neoplastic chemotherapy, as well as conditions associated with chronically elevated estrogen levels (e.g., cirrhosis).

SUMMARY

CRYPTORCHIDISM

- *Cryptorchidism* refers to incomplete descent of the testis from the abdomen to the scrotum and is present in about 1% of 1-year-old male infants.
- Bilateral or, in some cases, even unilateral cryptorchidism is associated with tubular atrophy and sterility.
- The cryptorchid testis carries a 3- to 5-fold higher risk for testicular cancer, which arises from foci of germ cell neoplasia in-situ within the atrophic tubules. Early orchiopexy reduces the risk for sterility and cancer.

Inflammatory Lesions

Inflammatory lesions of the testis are more common in the epididymis than in the testis proper. Sexually transmitted infectious disorders are discussed later in the chapter. Other causes of testicular inflammation include nonspecific epididymitis and orchitis, mumps, and tuberculosis. *Nonspecific epididymitis* and *orchitis* usually begin as a primary urinary tract infection that spreads to the testis through the vas deferens or the lymphatics of the spermatic cord. The involved testis is swollen and tender, and histologic examination reveals numerous neutrophils. *Mumps infection* involving the testes is rare in male children but occurs in roughly 20% of infected adults. Affected testes are edematous and congested, and contain a lymphoplasmacytic inflammatory infiltrate. Severe mumps orchitis may lead to extensive necrosis, loss of seminiferous epithelium, tubular atrophy, fibrosis, and sterility. Several conditions, including infections and autoimmune injury, may elicit granulomatous inflammation in the testis. Of these, *tuberculosis* is the most common. Testicular tuberculosis generally begins as an epididymitis, with secondary involvement of the testis. Histologically, there is granulomatous inflammation and caseous necrosis identical to that seen in active tuberculosis in other sites.

Vascular Disturbances

Torsion, or twisting of the spermatic cord, typically results in obstruction of testicular venous drainage while leaving the thick-walled and more resilient arteries patent. This leads to intense vascular engorgement and infarction unless the torsion is relieved. There are two types of testicular torsion. *Neonatal torsion* occurs either in utero or shortly after birth. There is no associated anatomic defect to account for its occurrence. *Adult torsion* typically is seen in adolescence and manifests with the sudden onset of testicular pain. In contrast with neonatal torsion, adult torsion results from a bilateral congenital anomaly whereby the testis is abnormally anchored in the scrotal sac giving rise to increased mobility (*bell clapper abnormality*). It often occurs without any inciting injury; sudden pain heralding the torsion may even awaken the patient from sleep.

Torsion constitutes one of the few urologic emergencies. If the testis is explored surgically and the cord is manually untwisted within approximately 6 hours, the testis will likely remain viable. To prevent the catastrophic occurrence of torsion in the contralateral testis, the unaffected testis typically is surgically fixed within the scrotum (orchiopexy).

Testicular Neoplasms

Testicular neoplasms occur in roughly 6 per 100,000 males. In the 15- to 34-year-old age group, when these neoplasms peak in incidence, they are the most common tumors in men. Neoplasms of the testis are heterogeneous and include germ cell tumors and sex cord–stromal tumors. **In postpubertal males, 95% of testicular tumors arise from germ cells, and almost all are malignant.** By contrast, sex cord-stromal tumors derived from Sertoli or Leydig cells are uncommon and usually benign. The focus of the remainder of this discussion is on testicular germ cell tumors.

The cause of testicular neoplasms is poorly understood. Testicular tumors are more common in whites than in blacks, and the incidence has increased in white populations over recent decades. As discussed earlier, cryptorchidism is associated with a 3- to 5-fold increase in the risk for cancer in the undescended testis, as well as an increased risk for cancer in the contralateral descended testis. A history of cryptorchidism is present in approximately 10% of cases of testicular cancer. Intersex syndromes, including androgen insensitivity syndrome and gonadal dysgenesis, also are associated with an increased frequency of testicular cancer. Family history is important, as brothers of males with germ cell tumors have an 8- to 10-fold increased risk, presumably owing to inherited factors. The development of cancer in one testis also is associated with a markedly increased risk for neoplasia in the contralateral testis. Extra copies of the short arm of chromosome 12, usually due to the presence of an isochromosome 12 [i(12p)], are found in virtually all germ cell tumors. Of note, point mutations that create oncogenes are relatively rare in germ cell tumors, occurring at the lowest frequency of any solid tumor in adults. Among these are oncogenic mutations in *KIT* which are found in up to 25% of tumors.

Most testicular tumors in postpubertal males arise from *germ cell neoplasia in situ*. This precursor lesion is present in conditions associated with a high risk for developing germ cell tumors (e.g., cryptorchidism, dysgenetic gonads) and exhibits the same abnormality of chromosome 12 that is characteristic of fully developed germ cell tumors. As might be expected, germ cell neoplasia in situ often is found in "normal" testis adjacent to full-blown germ cell tumors.

Testicular germ cell tumors are subclassified into seminomas and nonseminomatous germ cell tumors (Table 18.1). Seminomas are most common, accounting for about

Table 18.1 Summary of Testicular Tumors

Tumor	Peak Patient Age (years)	Morphology	Tumor Marker(s)
Seminoma	40–50	Sheets of uniform polygonal cells with cleared cytoplasm; lymphocytes in the stroma	10% of patients have elevated hCG
Embryonal carcinoma	20–30	Poorly differentiated, pleomorphic cells in cords, sheets, or papillary formation; most contain some yolk sac and choriocarcinoma cells	Negative (pure embryonal carcinoma)
Spermatocytic tumor	50-60	Small, medium, and large polygonal cells; no inflammatory infiltrate	Negative
Yolk sac tumor	3	Poorly differentiated endothelium-like, cuboidal, or columnar cells	90% of patients have elevated AFP
Choriocarcinoma	20–30	Cytotrophoblast and syncytiotrophoblast without villus formation	100% of patients have elevated hCG
Teratoma	All ages	Tissues from all three germ cell layers with varying degrees of differentiation	Negative (pure teratoma)
Mixed tumor	15–30	Variable, depending on mixture; commonly teratoma and embryonal carcinoma	90% of patients have elevated hCG and AFP

AFP, Alpha fetoprotein; *hCG*, human chorionic gonadotropin.

50% of testicular germ cell neoplasms. They are histologically identical to tumors called *dysgerminomas,* which occur in the ovary, and *germinomas,* which occur in the central nervous system and other extragonadal sites.

MORPHOLOGY

Germ cell tumors may be "pure" (i.e., composed of a single histologic type) or mixed (seen in 40% of cases). **Seminoma** presents as a soft, well-demarcated, gray-white tumor that bulges from the cut surface of the affected testis (Fig. 18.3). Large tumors may contain foci of coagulative necrosis, usually without hemorrhage. Seminomas are composed of **large, uniform cells with distinct cell borders, clear, glycogen-rich cytoplasm, round nuclei, and conspicuous nucleoli** (Fig. 18.4). The cells often are arrayed in small lobules with intervening fibrous septa. A lymphocytic infiltrate usually is present and may, on occasion, overshadow the neoplastic cells. Seminomas also may elicit a granulomatous reaction. In approximately 15% of cases, syncytiotrophoblasts are present; these cells are the source of the

minimally elevated serum human choriogonadotropin (hCG) that is encountered in approximately 10% of cases. Their presence has no bearing on prognosis.

Spermatocytic tumor (formerly called *spermatocytic seminoma*) is a distinct clinical and histologic entity. It is an uncommon tumor that occurs in older men than other testicular tumors; affected patients generally are beyond 50 years of age. In contrast with seminomas, spermatocytic tumors lack lymphocytic infiltrates, granulomas, and syncytiotrophoblasts; are not admixed with other germ cell tumor histologies; are not associated with germ cell neoplasia in-situ; and do not metastasize. The tumor usually comprises polygonal cells of variable size that are arranged in nodules or sheets.

Embryonal carcinoma presents as ill-defined, invasive masses containing foci of hemorrhage and necrosis (Fig. 18.5). The primary lesions may be small, even in patients with systemic metastases. **The tumor cells are large and have basophilic cytoplasm, indistinct cell borders, large nuclei, and prominent nucleoli.** The neoplastic cells may be arrayed in undifferentiated, solid sheets or may form primitive glandular

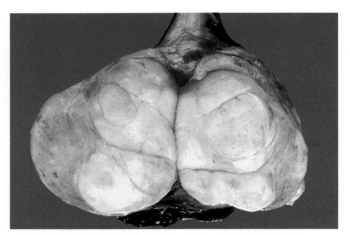

Fig. 18.3 Seminoma of the testis appearing as a well-circumscribed, pale, fleshy, homogeneous mass.

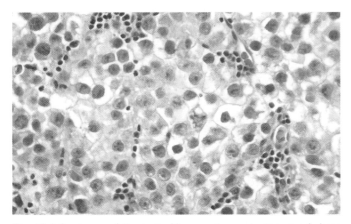

Fig. 18.4 Seminoma of the testis. Microscopic examination reveals large cells with distinct cell borders, pale nuclei, prominent nucleoli, and a sparse lymphocytic infiltrate.

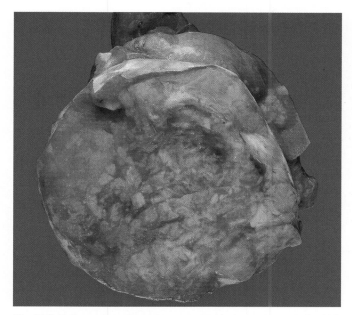

Fig. 18.5 Embryonal carcinoma. In contrast with the seminoma in Fig. 18.3, this tumor is hemorrhagic.

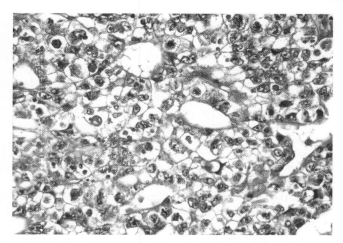

Fig. 18.6 Embryonal carcinoma. Note the sheets of undifferentiated cells and primitive glandlike structures. The nuclei are large and hyperchromatic.

structures and irregular papillae (Fig. 18.6). In most cases, cells characteristic of other germ cell tumors (e.g., yolk sac tumor, teratoma, choriocarcinoma) are admixed with the embryonal areas. Pure embryonal carcinomas account for only 2% to 3% of all testicular germ cell tumors.

Yolk sac tumor is the most common primary testicular neoplasm in children younger than 3 years of age; in this age group, it has a very good prognosis. In adults, yolk sac tumors most often are seen admixed with embryonal carcinoma. These tumors often are large and may be well demarcated. They are composed of low cuboidal to columnar epithelial cells that form microcysts, lacelike (reticular) patterns, sheets, glands, and papillae (Fig. 18.7). A distinctive feature is the presence of structures resembling primitive glomeruli, the so-called **Schiller-Duval bodies.** These tumors often have eosinophilic hyaline globules containing α_1-anti-trypsin and alpha fetoprotein (AFP), which can be demonstrated by immunohistochemical techniques.

Choriocarcinoma is a tumor in which the pluripotential neoplastic germ cells differentiate into cells resembling placental **trophoblasts.** The primary tumors often are small and nonpalpable, even in patients with extensive metastatic disease. The tumor is composed of sheets of small cuboidal **cytotrophoblast like cells** that are irregularly intermingled with or capped by large, eosinophilic **syncytiotrophoblast like cells** containing multiple dark, pleomorphic nuclei (Fig. 18.8). HCG can be identified in the syncytiotrophoblastic cells by immunohistochemical staining.

Teratoma is a tumor in which the neoplastic germ cells differentiate along multiple somatic cell lineages. These tumors form firm masses that often contain cysts and recognizable areas

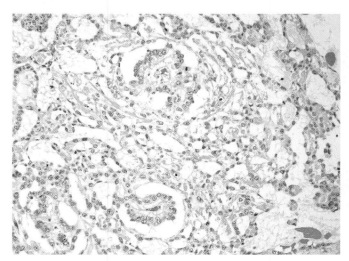

Fig. 18.7 Yolk sac tumor demonstrating areas of loosely textured, micro-cystic tissue and papillary structures resembling a developing glomerulus (Schiller-Duval bodies).

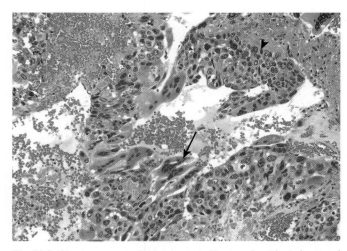

Fig. 18.8 Choriocarcinoma. Both cytotrophoblastic cells with single central nuclei (arrowhead, upper-right) and syncytiotrophoblastic cells with multiple dark nuclei embedded in eosinophilic cytoplasm (arrow, middle) are present. Hemorrhage and necrosis are prominent.

of cartilage. They may occur at any age from infancy to adult life. Pure forms of teratoma are fairly common in infants and children, being second in frequency only to yolk sac tumors. In adults, pure teratomas are rare, constituting 2% to 3% of germ cell tumors, and the remaining tumors are seen in combination with other histologic types. Teratomas are composed of a heterogeneous, helter-skelter collection of differentiated cells or organoid structures, such as neural tissue, muscle bundles, islands of cartilage, clusters of squamous epithelium, structures reminiscent of thyroid gland, bronchial epithelium, and bits of intestinal wall or brain substance, all embedded in a fibrous or myxoid stroma (Fig. 18.9). Elements may be mature (resembling various tissues within the adult) or immature (sharing histologic features with fetal or embryonal tissues). **In prepubertal males, teratomas are benign, whereas the majority of teratomas in postpubertal males are malignant, being capable of metastasis regardless of whether they are composed of mature or immature elements.**

Rarely, non–germ cell tumors may arise in teratoma—a phenomenon referred to as **teratoma with malignant transformation.** Examples of such neoplasms include squamous cell carcinoma, adenocarcinoma, and various sarcomas. These non–germ cell malignancies do not respond to therapies that are effective against metastatic germ cell tumors (discussed later); thus, the only hope for cure in such cases resides in surgical resection.

Clinical Features

Patients with testicular germ cell neoplasms present most frequently with a painless testicular mass that (unlike enlargements caused by hydroceles) is nontranslucent. Biopsy of a testicular neoplasm is associated with a risk for tumor spillage, which would necessitate excision of the scrotal skin in addition to orchiectomy. Consequently, the standard management of a solid testicular mass is radical orchiectomy, based on the presumption of malignancy. Some tumors, especially nonseminomatous germ cell neoplasms, may have metastasized widely by the time of diagnosis in the absence of a palpable testicular lesion.

Seminomas and nonseminomatous tumors differ in their behavior and clinical course.

- *Seminomas* often remain confined to the testis for long periods and may reach considerable size before diagnosis. Metastases most commonly are encountered in the iliac and paraaortic lymph nodes, particularly in the upper lumbar region. Hematogenous metastases occur late in the course of the disease.
- *Nonseminomatous germ cell neoplasms* tend to metastasize earlier, by lymphatic as well as hematogenous routes. Hematogenous metastases are most common in the liver and lungs. Metastatic lesions may be identical to the primary testicular tumor or may contain elements of other germ cell tumors.

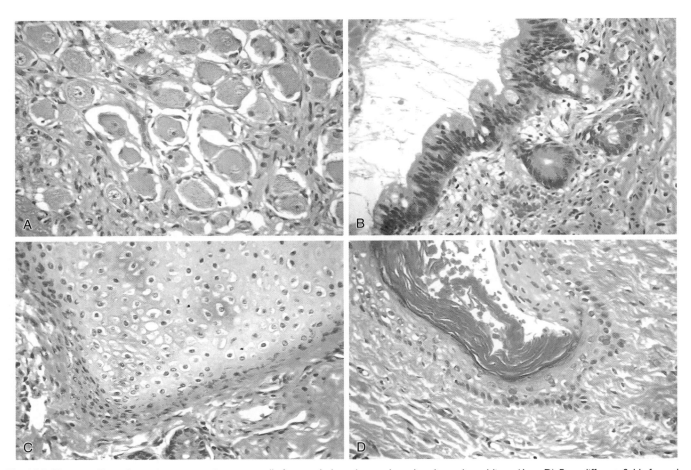

Fig. 18.9 Teratoma. Testicular teratomas contain mature cells from endodermal, mesodermal, and ectodermal lines. (A to D) Four different fields from the same tumor specimen contain neural (ectodermal) (A), glandular (endodermal) (B), cartilaginous (mesodermal) (C), and squamous epithelial (D) elements.

Assay of *tumor markers* secreted by germ cell tumors is important in two ways; these markers (summarized in Table 18.1, along with salient clinical and morphologic features) are helpful diagnostically and very valuable in following the response of tumors to therapy after the diagnosis is established. HCG is always elevated in patients with choriocarcinoma and, as noted, may be minimally elevated in individuals with other germ cell tumors containing syncytiotrophoblastic cells. Increased AFP in the setting of a testicular neoplasm indicates a yolk sac tumor component. The levels of lactate dehydrogenase (LDH) correlate with the tumor burden.

The treatment of testicular germ cell neoplasms is a remarkable clinical success story. Although roughly 8000 new cases of testicular cancer occur in the United States yearly, fewer than 400 men are expected to die of the disease. Seminoma, which is extremely radiosensitive and tends to remain localized for long periods, has the best prognosis. More than 95% of patients with early-stage disease can be cured. Among nonseminomatous germ cell tumors, the histologic subtype does not influence the therapy. Approximately 90% of patients achieve complete remission with aggressive chemotherapy, and most are cured. The exception is choriocarcinoma, which is associated with a poorer prognosis. With all testicular tumors, recurrences, typically in the form of distant metastases, usually occur within the first 2 years after treatment.

SUMMARY

TESTICULAR TUMORS

- Testicular neoplasms are the most common cause of painless testicular enlargement. They occur with increased frequency in association with undescended testes and with testicular dysgenesis.
- Germ cells are the source of 95% of testicular tumors, and the remainder arise from Sertoli or Leydig cells. Germ cell tumors may be composed of a single "pure" histologic pattern (60% of cases) or mixed patterns (40%).
- The most common histologic patterns of germ cell tumors are seminoma, embryonal carcinoma, yolk sac tumor, choriocarcinoma, and teratoma. Mixed tumors contain more than one element, most commonly embryonal carcinoma, teratoma, and yolk sac tumor.
- Clinically, testicular germ cell tumors are divided into two groups: seminomas and nonseminomatous tumors. Seminomas remain confined to the testis for a long time and spread mainly to paraaortic nodes; distant spread is rare. Nonseminomatous tumors tend to spread earlier, by both lymphatics and blood vessels.
- HCG is produced by syncytiotrophoblasts and is always elevated in patients with choriocarcinomas and those with seminomas containing syncytiotrophoblasts. AFP is elevated when there is a yolk sac tumor component.

PROSTATE

The prostate can be divided into biologically distinct regions, the most important of which are the peripheral and transition zones (Fig. 18.10). The types of proliferative

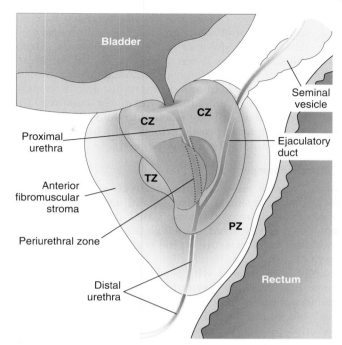

Fig. 18.10 Adult prostate. The normal prostate contains several distinct regions, including a central zone (CZ), a peripheral zone (PZ), a transitional zone (TZ), and a periurethral zone. Most carcinomas arise from the peripheral glands of the organ, whereas nodular hyperplasia arises from more centrally situated glands.

lesions are different in each region. For example, most hyperplastic lesions arise in the inner transition zone, while most carcinomas (70%–80%) arise in the peripheral zones. As a result, carcinomas are often detected by rectal examination, whereas hyperplasias are more likely to cause urinary obstruction. The normal prostate contains glands with two cell layers, a flat basal cell layer and an overlying columnar secretory cell layer. Surrounding prostatic stroma contains a mixture of smooth muscle and fibrous tissue. The prostate is involved by infectious, inflammatory, hyperplastic, and neoplastic disorders, of which prostate cancer is by far the most important clinically.

Prostatitis

Prostatitis is divided into three categories: (1) *acute bacterial prostatitis* (2%–5% of cases), caused by the same organisms associated with other acute urinary tract infections; (2) *chronic bacterial prostatitis* (2%–5% of cases), also caused by common uropathogens; and (3) *chronic pelvic pain syndrome* (90%–95% of cases). The latter can be subdivided into inflammatory cases, which are associated with leukocytes in prostatic secretions, and noninflammatory cases, in which leukocytes are absent.

The diagnosis of prostatitis is not typically based on biopsy, as the histologic findings are nonspecific and biopsy of an infected prostatitis can result in sepsis. The exception is *granulomatous prostatitis,* which may produce prostatic induration, leading to biopsy to rule out prostate cancer. In the United States, the most common cause of granulomatous prostatitis is instillation of Bacille Calmette-Guérin (BCG) within the bladder for treatment of superficial bladder cancer. BCG is an attenuated tuberculosis strain that produces a granulomatous immune reaction that is histologically indistinguishable from tuberculosis. Prostatic tuberculosis also occurs but is rare in the Western world. Fungal granulomatous prostatitis is typically seen only in immunocompromised hosts. *Nonspecific granulomatous prostatitis* is relatively common and stems from a foreign-body reaction to fluids that leak into tissue from ruptured prostatic ducts and acini. Postsurgical prostatic granulomas also may be seen.

Clinical Features

Acute bacterial prostatitis presents with sudden onset of fever, chills, dysuria, perineal pain, and bladder outlet obstruction; it may be complicated by sepsis. If acute prostatitis is suspected, digital rectal examination is contraindicated, as pressure on the boggy, exquisitely tender prostate can cause bacteremia. *Chronic bacterial prostatitis* usually is associated with recurrent urinary tract infections bracketed by asymptomatic periods. Presenting manifestations include low back pain, dysuria, and perineal and suprapubic discomfort. Both acute and chronic bacterial prostatitis is treated with antibiotics. *Chronic pelvic pain syndrome* is characterized by chronic pain localized to the perineum, suprapubic area, and penis. Pain during or after ejaculation is a prominent finding. The etiology is uncertain, and it is a diagnosis of exclusion; indeed, it is not even clear if the pain is related to an abnormality of the prostate. Therapy for chronic pelvic pain syndrome is empirical and depends on the nature of the symptoms.

SUMMARY

PROSTATITIS

- Bacterial prostatitis may be acute or chronic; the responsible organism usually is *E. coli* or another gram-negative rod.
- Chronic pelvic pain syndrome, despite shared symptomatology with chronic bacterial prostatitis, is of unknown etiology and difficult to treat.
- Granulomatous prostatitis may be either infectious (e.g., following treatment with BCG) or noninfectious.

Benign Prostatic Hyperplasia

Benign prostatic hyperplasia (BPH) is an extremely common cause of prostatic enlargement resulting from proliferation of of stromal and glandular elements. It is present in a significant number of men by 40 years of age, and its frequency rises progressively thereafter, reaching 90% by the eighth decade of life. The enlargement of the prostate in men with BPH is an important cause of urinary obstruction.

Although the cause of BPH is incompletely understood, excessive androgen-dependent growth of stromal and glandular elements has a central role. BPH does not occur in males who are castrated before the onset of puberty or in males with genetic diseases that block androgen activity. Dihydrotestosterone (DHT), the ultimate mediator of prostatic growth, is synthesized in the prostate from circulating testosterone by the action of the enzyme *5α-reductase,*

type 2. DHT binds to nuclear androgen receptors, which regulate the expression of genes that support the growth and survival of prostatic epithelium and stromal cells. Although testosterone can also bind to androgen receptors and stimulate growth, DHT is 10 times more potent.

MORPHOLOGY

BPH virtually always occurs in the inner transition zone of the prostate. The affected prostate is enlarged, typically weighing between 60 and 100 g, and contains many well-circumscribed nodules that bulge from the cut surface (Fig. 18.11). The nodules may appear solid or contain cystic spaces, the latter corresponding to dilated glands. The urethra is usually compressed, often to a narrow slit, by the hyperplastic nodules. In some cases, hyperplastic glandular and stromal elements lying just under the epithelium of the proximal prostatic urethra project into the bladder lumen as a pedunculated mass, producing a ball-valve type of urethral obstruction.

Microscopically, the hyperplastic nodules are composed of variable proportions of proliferating glandular elements and fibromuscular stroma. The hyperplastic glands are lined by tall, columnar epithelial cells and a peripheral layer of flattened basal cells (Fig. 18.12). The glandular lumina often contain laminated proteinaceous secretory material known as corpora amylacea.

Clinical Features

Because BPH preferentially involves the inner portions of the prostate, the most common manifestations are related to lower urinary tract obstruction, often in the form of difficulty in starting the stream of urine (hesitancy)

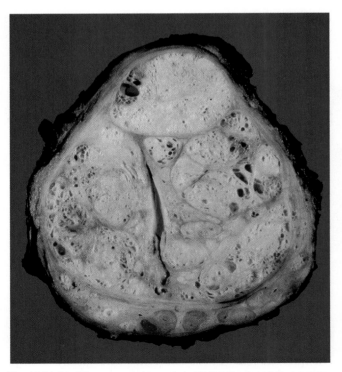

Fig. 18.11 Nodular prostatic hyperplasia. Well-defined nodules compress the urethra into a slitlike lumen.

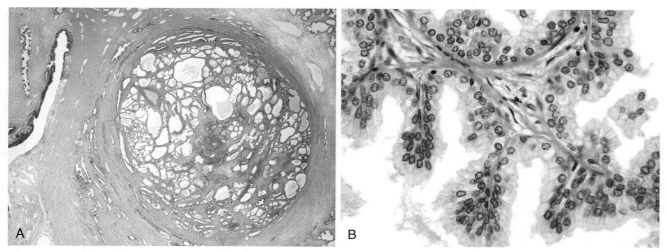

Fig. 18.12 Nodular hyperplasia of the prostate. (A) Low-power photomicrograph demonstrates a well-demarcated nodule at the right of the field, with a portion of urethra seen to the left. In other cases of nodular hyperplasia, the nodularity is caused predominantly by stromal, rather than glandular, proliferation. (B) Higher-power photomicrograph demonstrates the morphology of the hyperplastic glands, which are large and have papillary infoldings.

and intermittent interruption of the urinary stream while voiding. These symptoms frequently are accompanied by urinary urgency, frequency, and nocturia, all indicative of bladder irritation. Clinical manifestations of prostatic hyperplasia occur in only about 10% of men with pathologic evidence of BPH. The presence of residual urine in the bladder due to chronic obstruction increases the risk for urinary tract infections. In some affected men, BPH leads to complete urinary obstruction, with resultant painful distention of the bladder and, in the absence of appropriate treatment, hydronephrosis (Chapter 14). Initial treatment is pharmacologic, using targeted therapeutic agents that inhibit the formation of DHT from testosterone (such as 5-alpha reductase inhibitors) or that relax prostatic smooth muscle by blocking α_1-adrenergic receptors. Various surgical techniques are reserved for severely symptomatic cases that are recalcitrant to medical therapy.

SUMMARY

BENIGN PROSTATIC HYPERPLASIA

- BPH is characterized by proliferation of benign stromal and glandular elements. DHT, an androgen derived from testosterone, is the major hormonal stimulus for proliferation.
- BPH originates in the periurethral transition zone. The hyperplastic nodules exhibit variable proportions of stroma and glands. Hyperplastic glands are lined by two cell layers, an inner columnar layer and an outer layer composed of flattened basal cells.
- Clinical findings result from urinary tract obstruction and include hesitancy, urgency, nocturia, and poor urinary stream. Chronic obstruction predisposes to recurrent urinary tract infections.

Carcinoma of the Prostate

Adenocarcinoma of the prostate and is the most common form of cancer in men, accounting for 27% of cancer cases in the United States in 2014. Its is uncommon before the age of 50 years. Over the past several decades, mortality from prostate cancer has decreased significantly, and it currently causes only 10% of cancer deaths in the United States.

The relatively low rate of mortality in men with prostate cancer is related in part to increased detection of the disease through screening (discussed later), but how effective screening is at saving lives is controversial. This seeming paradox is related to the wide variation in the natural history of prostate cancer, from aggressive and rapidly fatal to indolent disease of no clinical significance. Indeed, prostate carcinoma commonly is found incidentally at autopsy in men dying of other causes, and many more men die with prostate cancer than of prostate cancer. It is not currently possible to identify the tumors that will be "bad actors" with certainty; thus, while some men are no doubt saved by early detection and treatment of their prostate cancers, it is equally certain that others are being "cured" of clinically inconsequential tumors.

Pathogenesis

Clinical and experimental observations suggest that androgens, heredity, environmental factors, and acquired somatic mutations have roles in the pathogenesis and progression of prostate cancer.

- *Androgens* are of central importance. Cancer of the prostate does not develop in males who are castrated before puberty, indicating that androgens somehow provide the "soil," the cellular context, within which prostate cancer develops. This dependence on androgens extends to established cancers, which often regress for a time in response to surgical or chemical castration. Notably, *tumors that are resistant to anti-androgen therapy often acquire androgen receptor gene amplifications or mutations that permit androgen receptors to activate the expression of their target genes despite therapy.* Thus, tumors that recur in the face of anti-androgen therapies still depend on gene products regulated by androgen receptors for their growth and survival. However, while prostate cancer, like normal prostate, is dependent on androgens for its survival, there is no evidence that androgens initiate carcinogenesis, nor are androgen levels associated with prostate cancer risk.

- *Heredity* also contributes, as there is an increased risk among first-degree relatives of patients with prostate cancer. Prostate cancer is uncommon in Asians and its incidence is highest among African-Americans and in Scandinavian countries. Aggressive, clinically significant disease is more common in African-Americans than in Caucasians. Genome-wide association studies have identified a number of genetic variants that are associated with increased risk for developing prostate cancer. Although each variant carries only a small increased risk, the effect is multiplicative, such that men with multiple risk alleles may have up to a 5-fold increase in risk compared to the general population.

- *Environment* also plays a role, as evidenced by the fact that in Japanese immigrants to the United States the incidence of the disease rises (although not to the level seen in native-born Americans). Also, as the diet in Asia becomes more westernized, the incidence of clinically significant prostate cancer in this region of the world is increasing. However, the relationship between specific dietary components and prostate cancer risk is unclear.

- *Acquired genetic aberrations,* as in other cancers, are the actual drivers of cellular transformation. Copy number variations in specific chromosomal regions and gene rearrangements are frequently seen in primary tumors. The most common gene rearrangements in prostate cancer create fusion genes consisting of the androgen-regulated promoter of the *TMPRSS2* gene and the coding sequence of *ETS* family transcription factors. **TMPRSS2-ETS fusion genes are found in approximately 40% to 60% of prostate cancers in Caucasian populations, and they occur relatively early in tumorigenesis.** Notably, the prevalence of these rearrangements is lower among African-Americans and other ethnic groups. Other mutations commonly lead to activation of the PI3K/AKT signaling pathway (Chapter 6); of these, the most common are loss-of-function mutations involving the tumor suppressor PTEN, which acts as a brake on PI3K activity.

MORPHOLOGY

Carcinomas detected clinically are usually not visible grossly. More advanced lesions appear as firm, gray-white lesions with ill-defined margins that infiltrate the adjacent gland (Fig. 18.13).

Most prostate cancers are **moderately differentiated adenocarcinomas** that produce well-defined glands. The glands typically are smaller than benign glands and are lined by a single uniform layer of cuboidal or low columnar epithelium, lacking the basal cell layer seen in benign glands. In further contrast with benign glands, malignant glands are crowded together and characteristically lack branching and papillary infolding. The cytoplasm of the tumor cells ranges from pale-clear (as in benign glands) to a distinctive amphophilic (dark purple) appearance. Nuclei are enlarged and often contain one or more prominent nucleoli (Fig. 18.14). Some variation in nuclear size and shape is usual, but in general, pleomorphism is not marked. Mitotic figures are uncommon. With increasing grade, irregular or ragged glandular

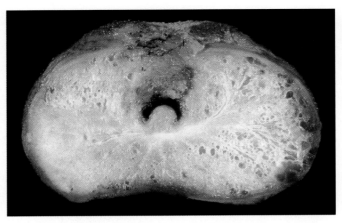

Fig. 18.13 Adenocarcinoma of the prostate. Carcinomatous tissue is seen on the posterior aspect *(lower left).* Note the solid whiter tissue of cancer, in contrast with the spongy appearance of the benign peripheral zone on the contralateral side.

structures, cribriform glands, sheets of cells, or infiltrating individual cells are present. In approximately 80% of cases, prostatic tissue removed for carcinoma also harbors presumptive precursor lesions, referred to as *high-grade prostatic intraepithelial neoplasia (HGPIN).* Many of the molecular changes seen in invasive cancers are also seen in HPIN.

Prostate cancer is graded by the **Gleason system,** created in 1967 and updated in 2014. According to this system, prostate cancers are stratified into five grades on the basis of glandular patterns of differentiation. Grade 1 represents the most well differentiated tumors, and grade 5 tumors show no glandular differentiation. Most tumors are patterns 3, 4, or 5. Since the majority of tumors contain more than one pattern, a primary grade is assigned to the dominant pattern and a secondary grade to the next most frequent pattern. The two numerical grades are then added to obtain a combined Gleason score. Tumors with only one pattern are treated as if their primary and secondary grades are the same, and, hence, the number is doubled. Thus, the most differentiated tumors have a Gleason score of 2 (1 + 1), and the least differentiated tumors merit a score of 10 (5 + 5). A new grading system also based on glandular pattern was recently accepted by the World Health Organization (WHO) to be used initially in conjunction with the Gleason system; it ranges from 1 (excellent prognosis) to 5 (poor prognosis).

Clinical Features

In the United States, most prostate cancers are small, nonpalpable, asymptomatic lesions discovered on needle biopsy performed to investigate an elevated serum prostate-specific antigen (PSA) level (discussed later). Some 70% to 80% of prostate cancers arise in the outer (peripheral) glands, and a subset of these may be palpable as irregular hard nodules on digital rectal examination. A minority of carcinomas is discovered unexpectedly during histologic examination of prostate tissue removed by transurethral resection for BPH. Because of the peripheral location, prostate cancer is less likely than BPH to cause urethral obstruction in its initial stages. Locally advanced cancers often infiltrate the seminal vesicles and periurethral zones

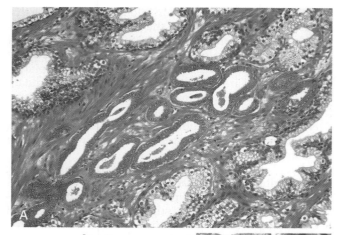

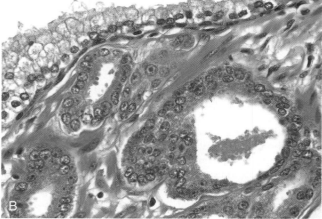

Fig. 18.14 (A) Adenocarcinoma of the prostate demonstrating small glands crowded in between larger benign glands. (B) Higher magnification shows several small malignant glands with enlarged nuclei, prominent nucleoli, and dark cytoplasm, as compared with the larger, benign gland *(top)*.

of the prostate and may invade the adjacent soft tissues, the wall of the urinary bladder, or (less commonly) the rectum. Bone metastases, particularly to the axial skeleton, are frequent late in the disease and typically cause osteoblastic (bone-producing) lesions that can be detected on *radionuclide bone scans*.

The PSA assay is the most widely used test in the diagnosis and management of prostate cancer, but it suffers from a number of limitations. PSA is a product of prostatic epithelium and is normally secreted in the semen. Although PSA screening can detect prostate cancers early in their course, studies of the natural history of the disease (so-called "watch-and-wait studies") have confirmed that many prostate cancers are clinically insignificant, requiring no treatment, sometimes for decades. Overtreatment of these indolent cancers can cause significant morbidity, particularly erectile dysfunction and incontinence. A second limitation of PSA as a biomarker is that it is not cancer-specific. BPH, prostatitis, prostatic infarcts, instrumentation of the prostate, and ejaculation all may increase serum PSA levels. Conversely, 20% to 40% of patients with organ-confined prostate cancer have PSA values below the cutoffs that are used to identify patients who are likely to have prostate cancer.

Because of these problems, PSA assays are being reappraised as screening tests. By contrast, once cancer is diagnosed, serial measurements of PSA are of great value in assessing the response to therapy. For example, a rising PSA level after radical prostatectomy or radiotherapy for localized disease is indicative of recurrent or disseminated disease.

The most common treatments for clinically localized prostate cancer are radical prostatectomy and radiotherapy. The prognosis after radical prostatectomy is based on the pathologic stage, whether the margins of the resected specimens are free of tumor, and Gleason grade. The Gleason grade, clinical stage, and serum PSA values are important predictors of outcome after radiotherapy. Because many prostate cancers follow an indolent course, active surveillance ("watchful waiting") is an appropriate approach for older men, patients with significant comorbidity, or even some younger men with low serum PSA values and small, low-grade cancers. Advanced metastatic carcinoma is treated by androgen deprivation, either by orchiectomy or by administration of synthetic agonists of luteinizing hormone–releasing hormone (LHRH). In addition, there are many new therapies that reduce androgen synthesis or signaling in metastatic prostate cancer. Although anti-androgen therapy induces remissions, androgen-independent clones almost invariably emerge, leading to rapid disease progression and death. As discussed earlier, these mutant clones commonly continue to express many genes that in normal prostate are androgen-dependent, suggesting that mechanisms arise to reactivate androgen signaling, even in the context of androgen deprivation therapy.

SUMMARY

CARCINOMA OF THE PROSTATE

- Carcinoma of the prostate is a common cancer of older men between 65 and 75 years of age.
- Prostate carcinomas range from indolent lesions that will never cause harm to aggressive fatal tumors, which are more common in African-Americans.
- The most common acquired mutations in prostatic carcinomas create *TPRSS2-ETS* fusion genes or act to enhance PI3K/AKT signaling, which promotes tumor cell growth and survival.
- Carcinomas of the prostate arise most commonly in the outer, peripheral zone of the gland and may be palpable by rectal examination.
- Grading of prostate cancer by the Gleason system correlates with pathologic stage and prognosis.
- Serum PSA measurement is a controversial cancer screening test, but has clear value in monitoring progressive or recurrent prostate cancer.

URETER, BLADDER, AND URETHRA

The renal pelves, ureters, bladder, and urethra are lined by specialized multi-layer transitional epithelium called urothelium. Beneath the mucosa are the lamina propria and, deeper yet, the muscularis propria (detrusor muscle), which makes up the bladder wall. Clinically significant disorders involving these organs include congenital aberrations, infectious and other inflammatory diseases, and neoplasms.

Ureter

Disorders of the ureter are uncommon and include congenital disorders, neoplasms, and reactive conditions. A few merit brief mention.

- *Ureteropelvic* junction (UPJ) obstruction, a congenital disorder, results in hydronephrosis. It usually manifests in infancy or childhood and is much more common in boys than in girls. It is the most frequent cause of hydronephrosis in infants and children.
- *Malignant* tumors of the ureter are pathologically similar to those arising in the renal pelvis, calyces, and bladder (discussed later). Most are urothelial carcinomas.
- *Retroperitoneal fibrosis* is an uncommon cause of ureteral narrowing or obstruction characterized by a fibrous proliferative inflammatory process encasing the retroperitoneal structures and causing hydronephrosis. The disorder occurs in middle to old age. At least a proportion of these cases occur in association with IgG4-related disease, characterized by fibroinflammatory lesions rich in IgG4-secreting plasma cells (Chapter 5). Other cases are associated with drug exposures (ergot derivatives, adrenergic blockers), radiation, infection, prior surgery, or malignant disease (lymphomas, urinary tract carcinomas). Most cases, however, have no obvious cause and are considered primary, or idiopathic (Ormond disease).

Urinary Bladder

Nonneoplastic Conditions

A bladder or vesical *diverticulum* consists of a pouchlike evagination of the bladder wall. Diverticula may be congenital but more commonly are acquired lesions that arise as a consequence of persistent urethral obstruction caused, for example, by benign prostatic hyperplasia. Although most diverticula are small and asymptomatic, they sometimes lead to urinary stasis predisposing to recurrent urinary tract infections and bladder stone formation.

Cystitis takes many forms.

- *Bacterial cystitis* is common, particularly in women. The most common etiologic agents are coliform bacteria.
- *Hemorrhagic cystitis* may occur in patients receiving cytotoxic anti-tumor drugs, such as cyclophosphamide, and sometimes complicates adenovirus infection.
- *Interstitial cystitis* causes a chronic pelvic pain syndrome, typically in women. It is characterized by suprapubic pain that increases with bladder filling and is relieved by bladder emptying, leading to very frequent urination during both day and night. Other symptoms include urgency, hematuria, and dysuria. Cystoscopic findings are nonspecific and include petechial hemorrhages. Up to 50% of patients have spontaneous remissions. Late in the course, transmural fibrosis may ensue, leading to a contracted bladder.

- *Malakoplakia* is an uncommon inflammatory disease that most commonly occurs in the bladder. It results from defects in the phagocytic or degradative function of macrophages. As a result of this defect, undigested bacterial products accumulate within distended phagosomes, which are seen in histologic sections as abundant granular material within the cytoplasm of macrophages. The abnormal macrophages also contain laminated mineralized concretions known as *Michaelis-Gutmann bodies,* which result from deposition of calcium salts in the enlarged lysosomes.
- *Polypoid cystitis* is an inflammatory condition resulting from irritation to the bladder mucosa in which the urothelium is thrown into broad bulbous polypoid projections as a result of marked submucosal edema. Polypoid cystitis may be confused with papillary urothelial carcinoma both clinically and histologically.

Transitional epithelium lining the bladder may undergo various forms of metaplasia. Nests of urothelium (*Brunn nests*) sometimes grow downward into the lamina propria. Here, their central epithelial cells may variously differentiate into a cuboidal or columnar epithelium lining (*cystitis glandularis*); cystic spaces filled with clear fluid lined by flattened urothelium (*cystitis cystica*); or goblet cells resembling intestinal mucosa (*intestinal metaplasia*). As a response to injury, the urothelium often undergoes *squamous metaplasia,* which must be differentiated from normal glycogenated squamous epithelium, commonly found at the trigone in women.

Neoplasms

Bladder cancer accounts for approximately 5% of cancers and 3% of cancer deaths in the United States. The vast majority of bladder cancers (95%–97% in the United States; 60%–90% in Africa) are urothelial carcinomas. Squamous cell carcinomas represent about 3% to 7% of bladder cancers in the United States but are much more common in countries such as Egypt, where urinary schistosomiasis is endemic. Adenocarcinomas of the bladder are rare. Carcinoma of the bladder is more common in men than in women, in industrialized than in developing nations, in urban than in rural dwellers, and in whites than in African-Americans. About 80% of patients are between 50 and 80 years of age.

Pathogenesis

Environmental factors are important in the pathogenesis of urothelial carcinoma and include *cigarette smoking, various occupational carcinogens, and prior cyclophosphamide or radiation therapy.* A family history of bladder cancer is a known risk factor. Squamous cell carcinoma is related to *Schistosoma haematobium* infections in areas where it is endemic. Cancers occurring in the setting of schistosoma infections arise in a background of chronic inflammation, which you will recall provides the "soil" for the development of a number of different cancers (Chapter 6).

Acquired genetic aberrations have been identified in urothelial carcinoma. Based on these observations, a model for bladder carcinogenesis has been proposed in which the tumor is initiated by deletions of tumor-suppressor genes on 9p and 9q, leading to the formation of superficial papillary tumors, which may then acquire *TP53* mutations and progress to invasive disease. A second pathway, possibly initiated by *TP53* mutations, leads first to carcinoma in situ and then, with loss of genes from chromosome 9, progresses to invasion. Additional genetic alterations in superficial tumors include mutations in telomerase, as well as mutations in fibroblast growth factor receptor 3 (FGFR3) and components of the RAS and PI3K/AKT pathways. Muscle invasive tumors often have mutations involving both *TP53* and *RB* (Chapter 6).

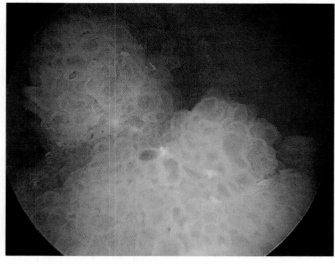

Fig. 18.16 Cystoscopic appearance of a papillary urothelial tumor, resembling coral, within the bladder.

MORPHOLOGY

Two distinct precursor lesions of invasive urothelial carcinoma are recognized (Fig. 18.15). The most common is a noninvasive papillary tumor (Fig. 18.16). The other precursor is carcinoma in situ (CIS), which is discussed later. In about one-half of patients with invasive bladder cancer, no precursor lesion is found; in such cases, it is presumed that the precursor lesion was overgrown by the high-grade invasive component.

The most important prognostic factor in noninvasive papillary urothelial neoplasms is their grade, which is based on both architectural and cytologic features. As shown in Table 18.2, the grading system subclassifies tumors as follows: (1) **papilloma;** (2) **papillary urothelial neoplasm of low malignant potential (PUNLMP);** (3) **low-grade papillary urothelial carcinoma;** and (4) **high-grade papillary urothelial carcinoma**

(Fig. 18.17). These exophytic papillary neoplasms are to be distinguished from **inverted urothelial papilloma,** which is entirely benign and not associated with an increased risk for subsequent carcinoma.

CIS is defined by the presence of overtly malignant-appearing cells within a flat urothelium (Fig. 18.18). Like high-grade papillary urothelial carcinoma, the tumor cells in CIS lack cohesiveness and are shed into the urine, where they can be detected by cytology. CIS commonly is multifocal and sometimes involves most of the bladder surface or extends into the ureters and urethra. Without treatment, 50% to 75% of CIS cases progress to invasive cancer.

Invasive urothelial cancer associated with papillary urothelial cancer (usually of high grade) or CIS may superficially invade the lamina propria or extend more deeply into underlying muscle. **The extent of invasion and spread (staging) at the time of initial diagnosis is the most important prognostic factor.** Almost all infiltrating urothelial carcinomas are high grade.

Squamous cell carcinomas of the bladder typically show extensive keratinization and are nearly always associated with chronic bladder irritation and infection. Adenocarcinomas of the bladder are histologically identical to adenocarcinomas seen in the gastrointestinal tract. Some arise from urachal remnants in the dome of the bladder or in association with extensive intestinal metaplasia.

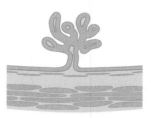
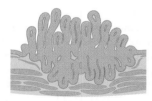
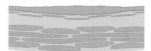

Papilloma

Invasive papillary carcinoma

Flat noninvasive carcinoma (CIS)

Flat invasive carcinoma

Fig. 18.15 Morphologic patterns of urothelial neoplasia.

Table 18.2 Noninvasive Papillary Urothelial Neoplasms

Neoplasm	Recurrences	Coexistent Invasion	Progression	Death
Papilloma	Rare	None	Rare*	None
PUNLMP	30%	None	2%	None
LGUC	45%	<10%	8%–10%	2%–3%
HGUC	45%	Up to 80%	30%	20%

HGUC, High-grade papillary urothelial carcinoma; *LGUC*, low-grade papillary urothelial carcinoma; *PUNLMP*, papillary urothelial neoplasia of uncertain malignant potential.
*Rare cases of progression have occurred in immunocompromised patients.

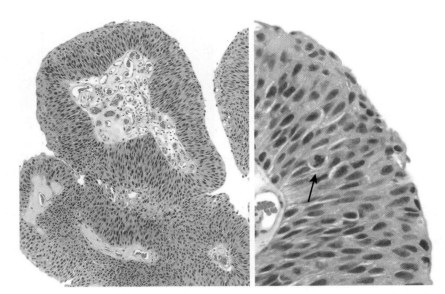

Fig. 18.17 Noninvasive low-grade papillary urothelial carcinoma. Higher magnification *(right)* shows slightly irregular nuclei with scattered mitotic figures *(arrow)*.

Clinical Features

Bladder tumors most commonly present with *painless hematuria.* Patients with urothelial tumors, whatever their grade, have a tendency to develop new tumors after excision, and recurrences may exhibit a higher grade. The risk for recurrence is related to several factors, including tumor size, stage, grade, multifocality, mitotic index, and associated dysplasia and/or CIS in the surrounding mucosa. Many recurrent tumors arise at sites different than that of the original lesion, yet share the same clonal abnormalities as those of the initial tumor; thus, these are true recurrences that stem from shedding and implantation of the original tumor cells at new sites. **Whereas high-grade papillary urothelial carcinomas frequently are associated with either concurrent or subsequent invasive urothelial carcinoma, lower-grade papillary urothelial neoplasms often recur but infrequently invade** (see Table 18.2).

Treatment of bladder cancer depends on tumor grade and stage and on whether the lesion is flat or papillary. For small, localized papillary tumors that are not high-grade, transurethral resection is both diagnostic and therapeutically sufficient. Patients with tumors that are at high risk for recurrence or progression typically receive topical immunotherapy consisting of intravesical instillation of an attenuated strain of the tuberculosis bacillus called *Bacillus Calmette-Guérin (BCG),* sometimes followed by intravesical chemotherapy. BCG elicits a granulomatous reaction that also triggers an effective local anti-tumor immune response. Patients are closely monitored for tumor recurrence with periodic cystoscopy and urine cytologic studies. Radical cystectomy is reserved for (1) tumor invading the muscularis propria; (2) CIS or high-grade papillary cancer refractory to BCG; and (3) CIS extending into the prostatic urethra and down the prostatic ducts, where BCG cannot come in contact the neoplastic cells. Advanced bladder cancer is treated using chemotherapy, which can palliate but is seldom curative.

SEXUALLY TRANSMITTED DISEASES

Sexually transmitted diseases (STDs) have complicated human existence for centuries. Globally, approximately 15 million new cases of STD occur every year; of these, 4 million affect 15- to 19-year-olds, and 6 million affect 20- to 24-year-olds. Women are far more likely to become infected by an STD and to be asymptomatic. Of the 10 leading infectious diseases that require notification of the Centers for Disease Control and Prevention (CDC) in the United States, five—chlamydial infection, gonorrhea, acquired immunodeficiency syndrome (AIDS), syphilis, and hepatitis B—are STDs (Table 18.3). In the United States, the two most common STDs are genital herpes and genital HPV infection, but these do not require CDC notification.

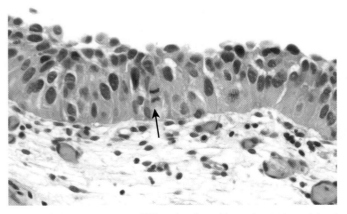

Fig. 18.18 Carcinoma in situ (CIS) with enlarged hyperchromatic nuclei and a mitotic figure *(arrow)*.

Table 18.3 Classification of Important Sexually Transmitted Diseases

| Pathogen | Associated Disease(s)—Distribution by Gender | | |
	Males	Both	Females
Viruses			
Herpes simplex virus		Primary and recurrent herpes, neonatal herpes	
Hepatitis B virus		Hepatitis	
Human papillomavirus	Cancer of penis (some cases)	Condyloma acuminatum, anal cancer, oropharyngeal carcinoma	Cervical dysplasia and cancer, vulvar cancer
Human immunodeficiency virus		Acquired immunodeficiency syndrome	
Chlamydiae			
Chlamydia trachomatis	Urethritis, epididymitis, proctitis	Lymphogranuloma venereum	Urethral syndrome, cervicitis, bartholinitis, salpingitis, and sequelae
Mycoplasmas			
Ureaplasma urealyticum	Urethritis		Cervicitis
Bacteria			
Neisseria gonorrhoeae	Epididymitis, prostatitis, urethral stricture	Urethritis, proctitis, pharyngitis, disseminated gonococcal infection	Cervicitis, endometritis, bartholinitis, salpingitis, and sequelae (infertility, ectopic pregnancy, recurrent salpingitis)
Treponema pallidum		Syphilis	
Haemophilus ducreyi		Chancroid	
Calymmatobacterium granulomatis		Granuloma inguinale (donovanosis)	
Protozoa			
Trichomonas vaginalis	Urethritis, balanitis		Vaginitis

Several of these entities, such as human immunodeficiency virus (HIV) infection, HPV infection, hepatitis B, and infection with *E. histolytica*, are discussed in other chapters.

Syphilis

Syphilis, or *lues*, is a chronic venereal infection caused by the spirochete *Treponema pallidum*. First recognized in epidemic form in 16th-century Europe as the Great Pox, syphilis is endemic in all parts of the world. In the United States, 20,000 cases of primary and secondary syphilis were reported to the CDC in 2014, representing almost a threefold increase since the year 2000. The increase for the most part can be attributed to the increased incidence in men who have sex with men. During 2013-2014, the incidence began to increase in women as well, raising the concern that there may be an impending increase in cases of congenital syphilis acquired from the mother. A strong racial disparity is evident; African Americans are affected six times more often than whites. Syphilis also is more common in HIV-infected patients, in whom syphilis is more likely to progress to organ involvement and neurosyphilis.

T. pallidum is a fastidious organism whose only natural host is man. The usual source of infection is contact with a cutaneous or mucosal lesion in a sexual partner in the early (primary or secondary) stages of syphilis. The organism is transmitted from such lesions during sexual activity through minute breaks in the skin or mucous membranes of the uninfected partner. In congenital cases, *T. pallidum* is transmitted across the placenta from mother to fetus, particularly during the early stages of maternal infection.

Once introduced into the body, the organisms rapidly disseminate to distant sites through lymphatics and the blood, even before the appearance of lesions at the primary inoculation site. This widespread dissemination accounts for the protean manifestations of the disease (Fig. 18.19), which in adults can be divided into primary, secondary, and tertiary stages.

- *Primary syphilis.* Several weeks after infection (mean, 21 days), a primary lesion, termed a *chancre,* appears at the point of spirochete entry. Systemic dissemination of organisms occurs during this period, while the host mounts an immune response. Two types of antibodies are formed: antibodies that cross-react with host constituents (nontreponemal antibodies) and antibodies to specific treponemal antigens. This humoral response, however, fails to eradicate the organisms.
- *Secondary syphilis.* The chancre of *primary syphilis* resolves spontaneously over a period of 4 to 6 weeks and is followed in approximately 25% of untreated patients by the development of secondary syphilis. The manifestations of secondary syphilis, discussed in greater detail later, include generalized lymphadenopathy and mucocutaneous lesions. *The mucocutaneous lesions of both primary and secondary syphilis are teeming with spirochetes and are highly infectious.* Like the chancre, the lesions of secondary syphilis resolve even without antimicrobial therapy, at which point patients are said to be in *early latent-phase syphilis.*
- *Tertiary syphilis.* Patients with untreated syphilis next enter an asymptomatic, *late latent* phase of the illness, defined as being more than 1 year after the initial infection. In about one third of cases, new symptoms develop over the next 5 to 20 years. This late symptomatic phase, or *tertiary syphilis,* is marked by the development of lesions in the cardiovascular system, central nervous system, or, less frequently, other organs. Spirochetes are much more difficult to demonstrate during the later

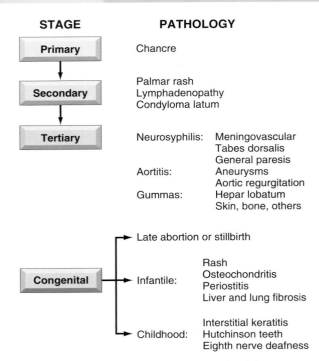

STAGE	PATHOLOGY	
Primary	Chancre	
↓		
Secondary	Palmar rash	
	Lymphadenopathy	
	Condyloma latum	
↓		
Tertiary	Neurosyphilis:	Meningovascular
		Tabes dorsalis
		General paresis
	Aortitis:	Aneurysms
		Aortic regurgitation
	Gummas:	Hepar lobatum
		Skin, bone, others

	Late abortion or stillbirth	
Congenital	Infantile:	Rash
		Osteochondritis
		Periostitis
		Liver and lung fibrosis
	Childhood:	Interstitial keratitis
		Hutchinson teeth
		Eighth nerve deafness

Fig. 18.19 Protean manifestations of syphilis.

stages of disease, and patients are accordingly much less likely to be infectious than are those in the primary or secondary stages of disease.

T. pallidum also may be transmitted across the placenta from an infected mother to the fetus at any time during pregnancy, leading to the development of *congenital syphilis*. The likelihood of transmission is greatest during the early (primary and secondary) stages of disease, when spirochetes are most numerous. Because the manifestations of maternal disease may be subtle, routine serologic testing for syphilis is mandatory in all pregnancies. The stigmata of congenital syphilis typically do not develop until after the fourth month of pregnancy. In the absence of treatment, as many as 40% of infected infants die in utero, typically after the fourth month. The incidence of congenital syphilis is expected to rise because infection rates in women have increased in recent years.

MORPHOLOGY

The pathognomonic microscopic lesion of syphilis is a proliferative endarteritis with an accompanying inflammatory infiltrate rich in plasma cells. Endarteritis has a central role in tissue injury at all sites involved by syphilis, but its pathogenesis is not understood; there is no evidence that the spirochetes cause any damage to host tissues directly. Instead, it is thought that the host immune response is responsible for the endothelial cell activation and proliferation that is the hallmark of the endarteritis, which eventually leads to perivascular fibrosis and luminal narrowing.

Both **primary and secondary syphilis** are associated with characteristic lesions. The **chancre** of primary syphilis is typically indurated and has been referred to as a hard chancre, to

distinguish it from the soft chancre of chancroid caused by *Haemophilus ducreyi* (discussed later). The primary chancre in males usually is on the glans, corona, or perianal region. In females, multiple chancres may be present, usually on the labia or vagina as well as the perianal region. The chancre begins as a small, painless, firm papule 2 to 4 weeks after sexual exposure, which gradually enlarges to produce a painless ulcer with well-defined, indurated margins and a "clean," moist base (Fig. 18.20). Regional lymph nodes often are slightly enlarged and firm. Microscopic examination of the ulcer reveals the typical lymphocytic and plasmacytic inflammatory infiltrate and endarteritis. Spirochetes are readily demonstrable in histologic sections of early lesions with the use of standard silver stains (e.g., Warthin-Starry stains) or immunohistochemical stains specific for spirochetes. Within approximately 2 months of resolution of the chancre, the lesions

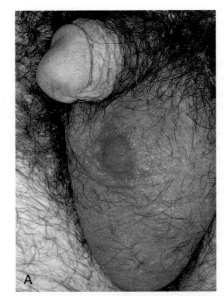

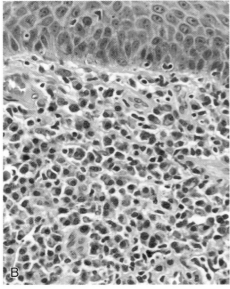

Fig. 18.20 (A) Syphilitic chancre of the scrotum. Such lesions typically are painless despite the presence of ulceration, and they heal spontaneously. (B) Histologic features of the chancre include a diffuse plasma cell infiltrate beneath squamous epithelium of skin.

of secondary syphilis appear. The manifestations of secondary syphilis are varied but typically include a combination of generalized lymph node enlargement and a variety of **mucocutaneous lesions**. Skin lesions usually are symmetrically distributed; may be maculopapular, scaly, or pustular; and characteristically involve the **palms of the hands and soles of the feet.** In moist skin areas, such as the anogenital region, inner thighs, and axillae, broad-based, elevated lesions termed **condylomata lata** may appear (not to be confused with condyloma acuminata caused by HPV) (Chapters 18 and 23). Superficial mucosal lesions resembling condylomata lata can occur anywhere but are particularly common in the oral cavity and pharynx and on the external genitalia. Histologic examination of mucocutaneous lesions during the secondary phase of the disease reveals the characteristic proliferative endarteritis and, with special stains or immunohistochemistry, spirochetes, which are often abundant. Lymphadenopathy is most common in the neck and inguinal areas. Histologic examination of enlarged nodes demonstrates hyperplasia of germinal centers accompanied by increased numbers of plasma cells or, less commonly, granulomas or neutrophils. Less common manifestations of secondary syphilis include hepatitis, renal disease, eye disease (iritis), and gastrointestinal abnormalities.

Lesions associated with **tertiary syphilis** develop in approximately one third of untreated patients, usually after a latent period of 5 years or more. These are divided into three major categories: cardiovascular syphilis, neurosyphilis, and so-called "benign" tertiary syphilis, which may occur singly or in combination. Cardiovascular syphilis takes the form of **syphilitic aortitis** and accounts for more than 80% of cases of tertiary disease; it is much more common in men than in women. Syphilitic aortitis is discussed further in Chapter 10. **Neurosyphilis** accounts for 10% of cases of tertiary syphilis overall but occurs at increased frequency in those with concomitant HIV infection; it is discussed in detail in Chapter 22. Large areas of parenchymal damage in tertiary syphilis result in the formation of a **gumma.** On microscopic examination, the gumma contains a central zone of coagulative necrosis surrounded by dense fibrous tissue containing a mixed inflammatory infiltrate composed of lymphocytes, plasma cells, activated macrophages (epithelioid cells), and occasional giant cells, features that suggest a delayed hypersensitivity reaction. Gummas occur most commonly in bone, skin, and the mucous membranes of the upper airway and mouth, but any organ may be affected. Spirochetes are only rarely demonstrable. Once common, gummas have become exceedingly rare thanks to effective antibiotics such as penicillin. They are reported now mostly in patients with AIDS.

Manifestations of **congenital syphilis** include stillbirth, infantile syphilis, and late (tardive) congenital syphilis.
- Among infants who are stillborn, the most common manifestations are hepatomegaly, bone abnormalities, pancreatic fibrosis, and pneumonitis. The liver often shows extramedullary hematopoiesis and portal tract inflammation. Changes in the bones include inflammation and disruption of the osteochondral junction in long bones and, on occasion, bone resorption and fibrosis of the flat bones of the skull. The lungs may be firm and pale as a result of the presence of inflammatory cells and fibrosis in the alveolar septa (pneumonia alba). With special stains, spirochetes are readily seen in tissue sections.
- **Infantile syphilis** refers to congenital syphilis in infants that manifests at birth or within the first few months of life. Affected infants present with chronic rhinitis (snuffles) and mucocutaneous lesions similar to those seen in secondary syphilis in adults. Visceral and skeletal changes resembling those seen in stillborn infants also may be present.
- **Late, or tardive, congenital syphilis** refers to cases of untreated congenital syphilis of more than 2 years' duration. Classic manifestations include the Hutchinson triad: notched central incisors, interstitial keratitis with blindness, and deafness from eighth cranial nerve injury. Other changes include a so-called "saber shin" deformity caused by chronic inflammation of the periosteum of the tibia, deformed molar teeth ("mulberry molars"), chronic meningitis, chorioretinitis, and gummas of the nasal bone and cartilage with a resultant "saddlenose" deformity.

Clinical Features

Syphilis remains highly sensitive to antibiotics such as penicillin, a short course of which is sufficient to treat all stages of the disease. Serology is the mainstay of diagnosis. Serologic tests for syphilis include nontreponemal antibody tests and antitreponemal antibody tests. Nontreponemal tests measure antibody to cardiolipin, an antigen that is present in both host tissues and the treponemal cell wall. These antibodies are detected by the rapid plasma reagin (RPR) and Venereal Disease Research Laboratory (VDRL) tests. Nontreponemal antibody tests are usually positive by 4 to 6 weeks of infection and are strongly positive in the secondary phase of infection. However, nontreponemal antibody test results may revert to negative during the tertiary phase or, conversely, may on occasion be persistently positive in some patients after successful treatment. Two additional points regarding nontreponemal antibody tests deserve emphasis:
- Nontreponemal antibody test results often are negative during the early stages of disease, even in the presence of a primary chancre. If there is a high degree of suspicion, these tests should be repeated in a few weeks.
- As many as 15% of positive VDRL test results are unrelated to syphilis. These false-positive results, which may be acute (transient) or chronic (persistent), increase in frequency with age and are associated with a variety of conditions, including the antiphospholipid antibody syndrome (Chapter 4).

Treponemal antibody tests also become positive within 4 to 6 weeks after an infection but (unlike those for nontreponemal antibody tests) they usually remain positive indefinitely, even after successful treatment. Historically, treponemal antibody tests have been used to confirm the diagnosis of syphilis in those with a positive nontreponemal antibody test. However, thanks to recent test improvements, some centers have reversed this algorithm and now use treponemal antibody tests for screening and nontreponemal antibody tests to confirm the diagnosis. As with all serologic tests for infection, certain pitfalls must be considered when interpreting these tests, including the timing of the test relative to the infection (e.g., too early for an antibody response to have been mounted) and the confounding influence of altered immunity, particularly in those who are HIV-infected.

SUMMARY

SYPHILIS

- Syphilis is caused by *T. pallidum* and has three stages.
  - Primary syphilis: A painless lesion called a *chancre* develops on the external genitalia along with regional lymph node enlargement.
  - Secondary syphilis: Generalized lymphadenopathy and mucocutaneous lesions that may be maculopapular or take the form of flat raised lesions called *condylomata lata*.
  - Tertiary syphilis: May cause proximal aortitis and aortic insufficiency; may involve the brain, meninges, and the spinal cord; or may cause focal granulomatous lesions called *gummas* in multiple organs.
- Congenital syphilis is caused by maternal transmission of the spirochetes during vaginal birth, mostly during the primary and secondary stages of disease in the mother. It may lead to stillbirth or cause widespread tissue injury in liver, spleen, lung, bones, and pancreas.
- Most syphilitic lesions demonstrate proliferative endarteritis and a plasma cell–rich inflammatory infiltrate. Gummas have a central area of necrosis surrounded by lymphoplasmacytic infiltrates, activated macrophages, and fibrosis.
- The diagnostic mainstay is serologic testing. Nontreponemal antibody tests (VDRL and RPR) are usually positive in early disease, but may be negative in advanced disease. Treponeme-specific antibody test results become positive later and remain positive indefinitely.

Gonorrhea

Gonorrhea is a sexually transmitted infection caused by *Neisseria gonorrhoeae*. It is second only to chlamydial infection (discussed later) among reportable communicable diseases in the United States. With an estimated 350,000 cases reported in 2014, it remains a major public health problem. Coinfection with other STDs is common, particularly *Chlamydia trachomatis,* which is found in 30% of males with gonorrhea. The gravity of gonococcal infections has increased with the emergence of strains of *N. gonorrhoeae* that are resistant to multiple antibiotics.

Humans are the only natural reservoir for *N. gonorrhoeae.* The organism is highly fastidious, and spread of infection requires direct contact with the mucosa of an infected individual, usually during sexual activity. The bacteria initially attach to mucosal epithelium, particularly of the columnar or transitional type, using a variety of membrane-associated adhesion molecules and structures termed *pili* (Chapter 9). Such attachment prevents the organism from being unceremoniously flushed away by body fluids such as urine or endocervical mucus. The organism then penetrates through the epithelial cells to invade the deeper tissues of the host.

MORPHOLOGY

N. gonorrhoeae provokes an intense, suppurative inflammatory reaction. In males, this manifests most often as a purulent urethral discharge, associated with an edematous, congested

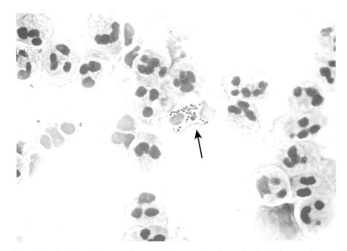

Fig. 18.21 *Neisseria gonorrhoeae.* Gram stain of urethral discharge demonstrates characteristic gram-negative, intracellular diplococci *(arrow). (Courtesy of Dr. Rita Gander, Department of Pathology, University of Texas Southwestern Medical School, Dallas, Texas.)*

urethral meatus. Gram-negative diplococci, many within the cytoplasm of neutrophils, are readily identified in Gram stains of the purulent exudate (Fig. 18.21). Ascending infection may result in the development of acute prostatitis, epididymitis (Fig. 18.22), or orchitis. Abscesses may complicate severe cases. Urethral and endocervical exudates tend to be less conspicuous in females, although acute inflammation of adjacent structures, such as the Bartholin glands, is fairly common. Ascending infection involving the uterus, fallopian tubes, and ovaries results in acute salpingitis, sometimes complicated by tuboovarian abscesses. The acute inflammatory process is followed by the development of granulation tissue and scarring, with resultant strictures and other permanent deformities of the involved structures, giving rise to *pelvic inflammatory disease* (Chapter 19).

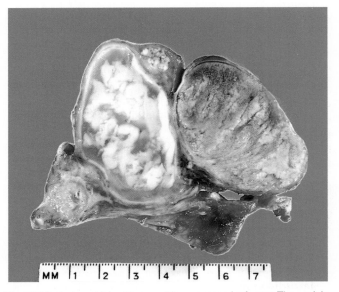

Fig. 18.22 Acute epididymitis caused by gonococcal infection. The epididymis is involved by an abscess. Normal testis is seen on the right.

Clinical Features

In most infected males, gonorrhea is manifested by the presence of *dysuria, urinary frequency, and a mucopurulent urethral exudate* within 2 to 14 days of the time of initial infection. However, urethral gonococcal infection can be detected in 40% of asymptomatic male contacts of women with symptomatic gonorrhea. Treatment with appropriate anti-microbial therapy results in eradication of the organism and prompt resolution of symptoms. Untreated infections may ascend to involve the prostate, seminal vesicles, epididymis, and testis. Neglected cases may be complicated by chronic urethral stricture and, in more advanced cases, by permanent sterility. Untreated men also may become chronic carriers of *N. gonorrhoeae*.

Among female patients, acute infections acquired by vaginal intercourse may be asymptomatic or may be associated with *dysuria, lower pelvic pain, and vaginal discharge*. Untreated cases may be complicated by ascending infection, leading to acute inflammation of the fallopian tubes (salpingitis) and ovaries. Scarring of the fallopian tubes may occur, with resultant infertility and an increased risk for ectopic pregnancy. Gonococcal infection of the upper genital tract may spread to the peritoneal cavity, where the exudate may extend up the right paracolic gutter to the dome of the liver, resulting in gonococcal perihepatitis. Depending on sexual practices, other sites of primary infection in both males and females include the oropharynx and the anorectal area, with resultant acute pharyngitis and proctitis, respectively.

Disseminated infection is much less common than local infection, occurring in 0.5% to 3% of cases of gonorrhea. It is more frequent in females than in males. Manifestations include, most commonly, tenosynovitis, arthritis, and pustular or hemorrhagic skin lesions. Endocarditis and meningitis are rare presentations. Strains that cause disseminated infection usually are resistant to the lytic action of complement, but rare patients with inherited complement deficiencies are susceptible to systemic spread regardless of the infecting strain.

Gonococcal infection may be transmitted to infants during passage through the birth canal. The affected neonate may develop purulent infection of the eyes (*ophthalmia neonatorum*), an important cause of blindness in the past. The routine application of antibiotic ointment to the eyes of newborns has markedly reduced this disorder.

Both culture and a variety of tests that detect organism-specific nucleic acids can be used to diagnose gonococcal infections. The advantage of culture is that it permits determination of antibiotic sensitivity. Nucleic acid–based tests are more rapid and somewhat more sensitive than culture, and are being used increasingly.

SUMMARY

GONORRHEA

- Gonorrhea is a common STD affecting the genitourinary tract. Control of dissemination requires an effective complement-mediated immune response.
- Gonorrhea presents with dysuria and a milky, purulent urethral discharge, although a high frequency of cases are asymptomatic.

- About 30% of men with gonococcal urethritis also are infected with *C. trachomatis*.
- Pregnant women can transmit gonorrhea to newborns during passage through the birth canal.
- Diagnosis can be made by culture of the exudates as well as by nucleic acid amplification techniques.

Nongonococcal Urethritis and Cervicitis

Nongonococcal urethritis (NGU) and cervicitis are the most common forms of STD. A variety of organisms are implicated in the pathogenesis of NGU and cervicitis, including *C. trachomatis, Mycoplasma genitalium, Trichomonas vaginalis,* and *Ureaplasma urealyticum*. **In the United States, most cases are apparently caused by *C. trachomatis*, and this organism is believed to be the most common bacterial cause of STD in the United States.** *Mycoplasma genitalium* is a close second as a cause of NGU. The frequency of causative agents varies geographically and in certain patient populations such a men having sex with men. In almost 50% of the cases world wide no pathogen can be identified. As discussed earlier, gonorrhea infection frequently is accompanied by chlamydial infection.

C. trachomatis is a small gram-negative bacterium that is an obligate intracellular pathogen. It exists in two forms. The infectious form, the *elementary body*, is capable of at least limited survival in the extracellular environment. The elementary body is taken up by host cells, primarily through a process of receptor-mediated endocytosis. Once inside the cell, the elementary body differentiates into a metabolically active form, termed the *reticulate body*. Using the energy sources of the host cell, the reticulate body replicates and ultimately forms new infectious elementary bodies, which have a tropism for columnar epithelial cells.

C. trachomatis infections are associated with a wide range of clinical features that are virtually indistinguishable from those caused by *N. gonorrhoeae*. Clinically, patients typically present 1 to 5 weeks after exposure with dysuria with or without urethral discharge. Patients may develop epididymitis, prostatitis, pelvic inflammatory disease, pharyngitis, conjunctivitis, perihepatic inflammation, and, among individuals who engage in anal sex, proctitis. It is the most common cause of epididymitis in young men. Similar to gonococcus, a large percentage of both men and women are asymptomatic. *C. trachomatis* also causes lymphogranuloma venereum (LGV), discussed in the next section. The infection may be transmitted to newborns during vaginal birth, where up to 15% of exposed newborns develop chlamydial pneumonia and 50% develop chlamydial conjunctivitis.

The morphologic and clinical features of chlamydial infection, with the exception of lymphogranuloma venereum, are virtually identical to those of gonorrhea. The primary infection is characterized by a watery to mucopurulent discharge that contains a predominance of neutrophils. Organisms are not visible in Gram-stained sections. In contrast with the gonococcus, *C. trachomatis* cannot be isolated with the use of conventional culture media. The diagnosis is best made by a nucleic acid amplification test on voided urine, which is now the gold standard. Another important manifestation of chlamydial infection is *reactive arthritis* (formerly known as *Reiter syndrome*), predominantly in patients who are HLA-B27 positive. This condition typically manifests as a combination of urethritis, conjunctivitis, arthritis, and generalized mucocutaneous lesions.

SUMMARY

NONGONOCOCCAL URETHRITIS AND CERVICITIS

- NGU and cervicitis are the most common forms of STD. Most cases are caused by *C. trachomatis*, and the rest by *T. vaginalis*, *M. genitalium* and *U. urealyticum*.
- *C. trachomatis* is a gram-negative intracellular bacterium that causes a disease that is clinically indistinguishable from gonorrhea in both men and women. Diagnosis can be made by sensitive nucleic acid amplification tests in urine samples or vaginal swabs.
- In patients who are HLA-B27 positive, *C. trachomatis* infection can cause reactive arthritis along with conjunctivitis and generalized mucocutaneous lesions.

Lymphogranuloma Venereum

LGV is a chronic, ulcerative disease caused by certain strains of *C. trachomatis* that are distinct from those causing the more common nongonococcal urethritis or cervicitis discussed earlier. It is endemic in parts of Asia, Africa, the Caribbean region, and South America. An increased incidence has been noted in the US in the past 15 years, due in large part of infections in men having sex with men, who are often co infected with HIV. As in the case of granuloma inguinale (discussed later), sporadic cases of LGV are seen most often among individuals with multiple sexual partners.

MORPHOLOGY

LGV may present as nonspecific urethritis or papular or ulcerative lesions involving the lower genitalia. Subsequently, tender enlarged matted inguinal and/or femoral lymphadenopathy ensues that typically is unilateral and is often associated with fistulous tracts. Proctocolitis also can be seen. The lesions contain a **mixed granulomatous and neutrophilic inflammatory response.** Variable numbers of chlamydial inclusions may be seen in the cytoplasm of epithelial cells or inflammatory cells with special staining methods. Regional lymphadenopathy is common, usually appearing within 30 days of the time of infection. Lymph node involvement is characterized by a granulomatous inflammatory reaction associated with irregularly shaped foci of necrosis and neutrophilic infiltration **(stellate abscesses).** With time, the inflammatory reaction gives rise to extensive fibrosis that can cause local lymphatic obstruction and strictures, producing **lymphedema.**

Clinical Features

Within 1 to 2 weeks of exposure, primary infection appears at the site of inoculation in the form of a genital ulcer or a mucosal inflammatory reaction. These primary lesions heal spontaneously, but the organisms at these sites seed draining lymph nodes, triggering a necrotizing lymphadenitis 2 to 6 weeks after the initial exposure. The lymphadenitis is usually unilateral and painful, and may lead to abscess formation. Abscesses sometimes rupture, spreading the inflammatory process into surrounding soft tissues. Rectal infections may progress to proctocolitis, associated with pain, constipation, fever, and bleeding, features that mimic inflammatory bowel disease. If untreated, rectal fissures and strictures may develop secondary to inflammation and fibrosis.

The diagnosis of LGV is difficult because laboratory tests are not standardized and serologic tests have low specificity. As with other chlamydial infections, nucleic acid amplification tests have the highest sensitivity and specific and are becoming more widely available. Culture and serologic tests are less sensitive but are still used, particularly in areas where nucleic acid amplification tests are not available.

Chancroid (Soft Chancre)

Chancroid, sometimes called the "third" venereal disease (after syphilis and gonorrhea), is an acute, ulcerative infection caused by *Haemophilus ducreyi*, a small, gram-negative coccobacillus. The disease is most common in tropical and subtropical areas and is more prevalent in lower socioeconomic groups, particularly among men who have regular contact with prostitutes. **Chancroid is one of the most common causes of genital ulcers in Africa and Southeast Asia, where it serves as an important cofactor in the transmission of HIV infection.** Chancroid probably is underdiagnosed in the United States because most STD clinics do not have facilities for isolating *H. ducreyi*, and PCR-based tests are not widely available.

MORPHOLOGY

The primary lesion of chanchroid appears first as a papule that rapidly breaks down to produce a ulcer. On microscopic examination, the ulcer of chancroid contains a superficial zone of neutrophilic debris and fibrin, with an underlying zone of granulation tissue containing areas of necrosis and thrombosed vessels. A dense, lymphoplasmacytic inflammatory infiltrate is present beneath the layer of granulation tissue. Secondarily involved draining lymph nodes also exhibit necrotizing inflammation that frequently progresses to abscess formation.

Clinical Features

The primary lesion of chanchroid appears within 4 to 7 days of inoculation. In male patients, the primary lesion is usually on the penis; in female patients, most lesions occur in the vagina or periurethral area. Over the course of several days, the surface of the primary lesion erodes to produce an irregular ulcer, which is more likely to be painful in males than in females. The regional lymph nodes, particularly in the inguinal region, become enlarged and tender in about 50% of cases within 1 to 2 weeks of the primary inoculation. In untreated cases, the inflamed and enlarged nodes (buboes) may erode the overlying skin to produce chronic, draining ulcers. A definitive diagnosis requires the identification of *H. ducreyi* on special culture media that are not widely available from commercial sources; even when such media are used, sensitivity is less than 80%. Therefore, the diagnosis often is based on clinical grounds alone.

Granuloma Inguinale

Granuloma inguinale is a chronic inflammatory disease caused by *Calymmatobacterium granulomatis,* a minute, encapsulated coccobacillus related to the *Klebsiella* genus. This disease is uncommon in the United States and Western Europe, but it is endemic in the rural parts of certain tropical and subtropical regions. When it occurs in urban settings, transmission of *C. granulomatis* typically is associated with a history of multiple sexual partners. Untreated cases are characterized by extensive scarring, often associated with lymphatic obstruction and lymphedema (elephantiasis) of the external genitalia. Culture of the organism is difficult, and PCR-based assays are not widely available.

MORPHOLOGY

Granuloma inguinale causes genital ulceration, accompanied by the development of abundant granulation tissue. Disfiguring scars may develop in untreated cases, sometimes associated with formation of urethral, vulvar, or anal strictures. In contrast with chancroid, regional lymph nodes typically are spared or show only nonspecific reactive changes.

Microscopic examination of active lesions reveals marked epithelial hyperplasia at the borders of the ulcer, sometimes mimicking carcinoma **(pseudoepitheliomatous hyperplasia).** A mixture of neutrophils and mononuclear inflammatory cells is present at the base of the ulcer and beneath the surrounding epithelium. The organisms are demonstrable in Giemsa-stained smears of the exudate as minute coccobacilli within vacuoles in macrophages **(Donovan bodies).** Silver stains (e.g., the Warthin-Starry stain) also may be used to demonstrate the organism.

SUMMARY

LYMPHOGRANULOMA VENEREUM, CHANCROID, AND GRANULOMA INGUINALE

- LGV is caused by *C. trachomatis* serotypes that are distinct from those that cause nongonococcal urethritis. LGV is associated with urethritis, ulcerative genital lesions, lymphadenopathy, and involvement of the rectum. The lesions show both acute and chronic inflammation; they progress to fibrosis, with consequent lymphedema and formation of rectal strictures. Diagnosis is made by nucleic acid amplification tests and serology.
- *H. ducreyi* infection causes an acute painful ulcerative genital infection called *chancroid*. Inguinal node involvement occurs in many cases and leads to their enlargement and ulceration. Ulcers show a superficial area of acute inflammation and necrosis, with an underlying zone of granulation tissue and mononuclear infiltrate. Diagnosis is possible by culture of the organism.
- *Granuloma inguinale* is a chronic fibrosing STD caused by *C. granulomatis*. The initial papular lesion on the genitalia expands and ulcerates, with formation of urethral, vulvar, or anal strictures in some cases. Microscopic examination reveals granulation tissue and intense epithelial hyperplasia that can mimic squamous cell carcinoma. Organisms are visible as small intracellular coccobacilli within vacuolated macrophages (Donovan bodies).

Trichomoniasis

T. vaginalis is a sexually transmitted protozoan that is a frequent cause of vaginitis. The trophozoite form adheres to the mucosa, where it causes superficial lesions. In females, *T. vaginalis* infection often is associated with loss of acid-producing lactobacilli. The incubation period is 4 to 28 days. It may be asymptomatic or be associated with pruritus and a profuse, frothy, yellow vaginal discharge. Urethral colonization may cause urinary frequency and dysuria. *T. vaginalis* infection typically is asymptomatic in males but in some cases may manifest as nongonococcal urethritis. The organism usually is demonstrable in smears of vaginal scrapings.

Genital Herpes Simplex

Genital herpes infection, or herpes genitalis, is a very common STD. According to CDC, approximately 800,000 people get new infections every year in the United States. One in six persons between the ages of 14 and 49 has HSV-2 infection in the US. With increasing rate of HSV-1 infections the overall prevalence of genital herpes is likely much higher. Although both herpes simplex virus 1 (HSV-1) and HSV-2 can cause anogenital or oral infections, most cases of anogenital herpes are caused by HSV-2. However, recent years have seen a rise in the number of genital infections caused by HSV-1, in part due to the increasing practice of oral sex. Genital HSV infection may occur in any sexually active population. As with other STDs, the risk for infection is directly related to the number of sexual contacts. Up to 95% of HIV-positive men who have sex with men are seropositive for HSV-1 and/or HSV-2. HSV is transmitted when the virus comes into contact with a mucosal surface or broken skin of a susceptible host. Such transmission requires direct contact with an infected individual, because the virus is readily inactivated at room temperature, particularly if dried.

MORPHOLOGY

The initial lesions of genital HSV infection are **painful, erythematous vesicles** on the mucosa or skin of the lower genitalia and adjacent extragenital sites. The anorectal area is a particularly common site of primary infection among men who have sex with men. Histologic changes include the presence of **intraepithelial vesicles** accompanied by necrotic cellular debris, neutrophils, and cells harboring characteristic intranuclear viral inclusions. The classic **Cowdry type A inclusion** appears as a light purple, homogeneous intranuclear structure surrounded by a clear halo. Infected cells commonly fuse to form multinucleate syncytia. The inclusions stain with antibodies to HSV, permitting a rapid, specific diagnosis of HSV infection in histologic sections or smears.

Clinical Features

As discussed earlier, both HSV-1 and HSV-2 can cause genital or oral infection, and both produce indistinguishable primary or recurrent mucocutaneous lesions. Primary infection with HSV-2 often may be asymptomatic or may produce a variety of signs and symptoms. Locally painful vesicular lesions may be accompanied by dysuria, urethral discharge, local lymph node enlargement and tenderness, and systemic manifestations, such as fever, muscle aches, and headache. HSV is actively shed during this period, and shedding continues until the mucosal lesions have completely healed. However, asymptomatic viral shedding can occur as long as 3 months after diagnosis. Signs and symptoms may last for several weeks during the primary phase of disease. Recurrences are milder and of shorter duration than in the primary episode. Diagnosis is most often made by viral culture or nucleic acid amplification testing of fluid collected after "unroofing" of a vesicular lesion.

In immunocompetent adults, herpes genitalis generally is not life-threatening. However, HSV poses a major threat to immunosuppressed patients, in whom fatal, disseminated disease may develop. Also life-threatening is *neonatal herpes infection,* which occurs in about one-half of infants delivered vaginally of mothers suffering from either primary or recurrent genital HSV infection. The viral infection is acquired during passage through the birth canal. Its incidence has risen in parallel with the rise in genital HSV infection. The manifestations of neonatal herpes vary from involvement of superficial sites (skin, eyes and mouth) to involvement of the CNS, with or without disseminated infection of other organs such as the liver and lungs. Approximately 60% of affected infants die of the disease, with significant morbidity occurring in about one-half of the survivors. PCR-based testing is far more sensitive and the preferred method for diagnosis of encephalitis.

Human Papillomavirus Infection

HPV causes a number of squamous proliferations in the genital tract, including condyloma acuminatum, as well as several precancerous lesions that commonly undergo transformation to carcinomas. The latter most commonly involve the cervix (Chapter 19), but also occur in the penis, vulva, oropharyngeal tonsil, and conjunctiva. *Condylomata acuminata,* also known as *venereal warts,* are caused by HPV types 6 and 11. These lesions occur on the penis as well as on the female genitalia. They should not be confused with the condylomata lata of secondary syphilis. Genital HPV infection may be transmitted to neonates during vaginal delivery. Recurrent and potentially life-threatening papillomas of the upper respiratory tract may develop subsequently in affected infants.

MORPHOLOGY

In males, condylomata acuminata usually occur on the coronal sulcus or inner surface of the prepuce, where they range in size from small, sessile lesions to large, papillary proliferations measuring several centimeters in diameter. In females, they commonly occur on the vulva. Examples of the microscopic appearance of these lesions are presented in Chapter 19.

SUMMARY

HERPES SIMPLEX VIRUS AND HUMAN PAPILLOMAVIRUS INFECTIONS

- HSV-2 and, less commonly, HSV-1 can cause genital infections. Initial (primary) infection may be asymptomatic or cause

painful, erythematous, intraepithelial vesicles on the mucosa and skin of external genitalia, along with painful regional lymph node enlargement. Recurrent lesions in general are less painful and less extensive than primary lesions.

- On histologic examination, the vesicles of HSV infection contain necrotic cells and fused multinucleate giant cells with intranuclear inclusions (Cowdry type A) that stain with antibodies to the virus.
- Neonatal herpes can be life-threatening and occurs in children born to mothers with genital herpes. Affected infants may have generalized herpes, often associated with encephalitis and consequent high mortality.
- HPV causes many proliferative lesions of the genital mucosa, including condyloma acuminatum, precancerous lesions, and invasive cancers.

SUGGESTED READINGS

Barbieri CE, Tomlins SA: The prostate cancer genome: perspectives and potential, *Urol Oncol* 32:53.e15, 2014. [*A review of molecular alterations in prostate cancer from recent sequencing data.*]

Boström PJ, Bjartell AS, Catto JW, et al: Genomic predictors of outcome in prostate cancer, *Eur Urol* 68:1033, 2015. [*A recent review of biomarkers that are useful for clinical decision making in prostate cancer.*]

Bushman W: Etiology, epidemiology, and natural history of benign prostatic hyperplasia, *Urol Clin North Am* 36:403, 2009.

Cuzick J, Thorat MA, Andriole G, et al: Prevention and early detection of prostate cancer, *Lancet Oncol* 15:e484, 2014. [*A review of the epidemiology and risk factors for prostate cancer as well as current screening methods and biomarkers.*]

Czerniak B, Dinney C, McConkey D: Origins of bladder cancer, *Annu Rev Pathol* 11:494, 2016. [*Reviews recent advances in molecular characterization of bladder cancer.*]

Donovan B: Sexually transmitted infections other than HIV, *Lancet* 363:545, 2004. [*A clinical review of STDs.*]

Epstein JI: An update of the Gleason grading system, *J Urol* 183:433, 2010.

Fanfair RN, Workowski KA: Clinical update in sexually transmitted diseases—2014, *Cleve Clin J Med* 81:91, 2014. [*A concise updated review with treatment recommendations.*]

Hanna NH, Einhorn LH: Testicular cancer—discoveries and updates, *N Engl J Med* 371:2005, 2014. [*A comprehensive review of current pathologic and clinical features of testicular germ cell tumors.*]

Le BV, Schaeffer AJ: Genitourinary pain syndromes, prostatitis and lower urinary tract symptoms, *Urol Clin North Am* 36:527, 2009. [*A recent review of the etiology, diagnosis, symptoms, and treatment of prostatitis and interstitial cystitis along with pelvic pain syndromes.*]

Lee PK, Wilkins KB: Condyloma and other infections including human immunodeficiency virus, *Surg Clin North Am* 90:99, 2010.

Patel AK, Chapple CR: Medical management of lower urinary tract symptoms in men: current treatment and future approaches, *Nat Clin Pract Urol* 5:211, 2008. [*This article clarifies the terminology used to evaluate men with lower urinary tract symptoms.*]

Rapley EA, Nathanson KL: Predisposition alleles for testicular germ cell tumour, *Curr Opin Genet Dev* 20:225, 2010. [*An update on inherited risk factors in germ cell tumors.*].

Spiess PE, Horenblas S, Pagliaro LC, et al: Current concepts in penile cancer, *J Natl Compr Canc Netw* 11:617, 2013. [*A systematic review of the epidemiology and current treatment of penile cancers.*]

Sulak PJ: Sexually transmitted diseases, *Semin Reprod Med* 21:399, 2003. [*An exhaustive review of STDs.*]

Female Genital System and Breast

19

CHAPTER OUTLINE

Vulva 713
  Vulvitis 713
  Nonneoplastic Epithelial Disorders 714
  Tumors 714
  Condylomas 714
  Carcinoma of the Vulva 715
  Extramammary Paget Disease 715
Vagina 716
  Vaginitis 716
  Malignant Neoplasms 716
  Squamous Cell Carcinoma 716
  Clear Cell Adenocarcinoma 716
  Sarcoma Botryoides 717
Cervix 717
  Cervicitis 717
  Neoplasia of the Cervix 717
  Squamous Intraepithelial Lesion (SIL, Cervical Intraepithelial Lesion) 718
  Invasive Carcinoma of the Cervix 720
  Endocervical Polyp 720
Uterus 721
  Endometritis 721
  Adenomyosis 721

Endometriosis 721
Abnormal Uterine Bleeding 722
Proliferative Lesions of the Endometrium and Myometrium 723
  Endometrial Hyperplasia 723
  Endometrial Carcinoma 724
  Endometrial Polyps 724
  Leiomyoma 725
  Leiomyosarcoma 726
Fallopian Tubes 726
Ovaries 727
  Follicle and Luteal Cysts 727
  Polycystic Ovarian Syndrome 727
  Tumors of the Ovary 727
  Surface Epithelial Tumors 727
  Serous Tumors 728
  Mucinous Tumors 729
  Endometrioid Tumors 729
  Brenner Tumor 729
  Other Ovarian Tumors 730
Diseases of Pregnancy 732
  Placental Inflammations and Infections 732

Ectopic Pregnancy 732
Gestational Trophoblastic Disease 733
  Hydatidiform Mole: Complete and Partial 733
  Invasive Mole 733
  Gestational Choriocarcinoma 734
  Placental Site Trophoblastic Tumor 735
  Preeclampsia/Eclampsia (Toxemia of Pregnancy) 735
Breast 736
  Clinical Presentations of Breast Disease 736
  Inflammatory Processes 737
  Stromal Neoplasms 738
  Benign Epithelial Lesions 738
  Carcinoma 739
  Epidemiology and Risk Factors 741

Vulva

The vulva is the external female genitalia and includes the hair-bearing skin (labia majora) and mucosa (labia minora). Disorders of the vulva most frequently are inflammatory, rendering them more uncomfortable than serious. Malignant tumors of the vulva, although life-threatening, are rare.

VULVITIS

One of the most common causes of vulvitis is reactive inflammation in response to an exogenous stimulus, which may be an irritant (contact irritant dermatitis) or an allergen (contact allergic dermatitis). Scratching-induced trauma secondary to associated intense "itching" (pruritus) often exacerbates the primary condition.

Contact irritant eczematous dermatitis manifests as well-defined erythematous weeping and crusting papules and plaques and may be a reaction to urine, soaps, detergents, antiseptics, deodorants, or alcohol. Allergic dermatitis has a similar clinical appearance and may result from allergy to perfumes; additives in creams, lotions, and soaps; chemical treatments on clothing; and other antigens.

Vulvitis also may be caused by infections, which often are sexually transmitted. The most important infectious agents in North America are human papillomavirus (HPV), the causative agent of condyloma acuminatum, vulvar intraepithelial neoplasia (VIN), and one type of vulvar squamous carcinoma (discussed later); herpes simplex virus (HSV-1 or HSV-2), the agent of genital herpes; *N. gonorrhoeae*, a cause of suppurative infection of the vulvovaginal glands; and *Treponema pallidum*, which causes primary chancre at vulvar sites of inoculation. Candida also is a cause of vulvitis, but is not sexually transmitted.

An important complication of vulvitis is obstruction of the excretory ducts of Bartholin glands. This blockage may result in painful dilation of the glands *(Bartholin cyst)* and abscess formation.

Nonneoplastic Epithelial Disorders

Lichen Sclerosus

Lichen sclerosus is characterized by thinning of the epidermis, disappearance of rete pegs, a zone of acellular, homogenized, dermal fibrosis, and a bandlike mononuclear inflammatory cell infiltrate (Fig. 19.1). It appears as smooth, white plaques (termed *leukoplakia*) or papules that in time may extend and coalesce. When the entire vulva is affected, the labia become atrophic and stiffened, and the vaginal orifice is constricted. Lichen sclerosus occurs in all age groups but most commonly affects postmenopausal women and prepubertal girls. The pathogenesis is uncertain, but the presence of activated T cells in the subepithelial inflammatory infiltrate and the increased frequency of autoimmune disorders in affected women suggest an autoimmune etiology. Lichen sclerosus is benign; however, 1% to 5% of women with symptomatic lichen sclerosus develop HPV negative squamous cell carcinoma of the vulva.

Lichen Simplex Chronicus

Lichen simplex chronicus is marked by epithelial thickening (particularly of the stratum granulosum) and hyperkeratosis. Increased mitotic activity is seen in the basal and suprabasal layers; however, there is no epithelial atypia (Fig. 19.1). Leukocytic infiltration of the dermis is sometimes pronounced. These nonspecific changes are a consequence of chronic irritation, often caused by pruritus related to an underlying inflammatory dermatosis. Lichen simplex chronicus appears as an area of leukoplakia. While no increased predisposition to cancer has been demonstrated when lesions are isolated, lichen simplex chronicus often is present at the margins of established vulvar cancer, suggesting some association with neoplastic disease.

Lichen sclerosus and lichen simplex chronicus may coexist in different areas of the body in the same person, and both lesions may take the form of leukoplakia. Similar white patches or plaques also are seen in a variety of other benign dermatoses, such as psoriasis and lichen planus (Chapter 24), as well as in malignant lesions of the vulva, such as squamous cell carcinoma in situ and invasive squamous cell carcinoma. Thus, biopsy and microscopic examination are often needed to differentiate these clinically similar-appearing lesions.

SUMMARY

NONNEOPLASTIC EPITHELIAL DISORDERS

- Lichen sclerosus is characterized by atrophic epithelium, subepithelial dermal fibrosis, and bandlike chronic inflammation.
- Lichen sclerosus carries a slightly increased risk for development of squamous cell carcinoma.
- Lichen simplex chronicus is characterized by thickened epithelium (hyperplasia), usually with a dermal inflammatory infiltrate.
- The lesions of lichen sclerosus and lichen simplex chronicus must be biopsied to distinguish them definitively from other causes of leukoplakia, such as squamous cell carcinoma of the vulva.

TUMORS

Condylomas

Condyloma **is the name given to any warty lesion of the vulva.** Most such lesions can be assigned to one of two distinctive forms. *Condylomata lata,* not commonly seen today, are flat, minimally elevated lesions that occur in secondary syphilis (Chapter 18). The more common *condylomata acuminata* may be papillary and distinctly elevated or somewhat flat and rugose. They may occur anywhere on the anogenital surface, sometimes as single but more often as multiple lesions. When located on the vulva, they range from a few millimeters to many centimeters in

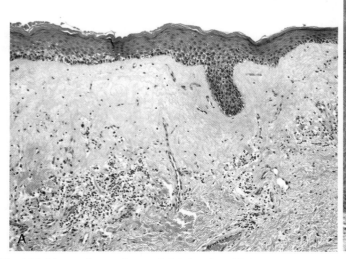
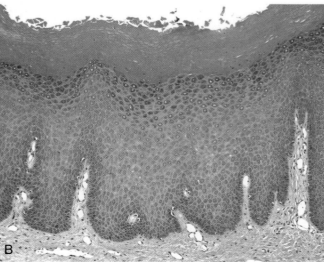

Fig. 19.1 Nonneoplastic vulvar epithelial disorders. (A) Lichen sclerosus. There is marked thinning of the epidermis, fibrosis of the superficial dermis, and chronic inflammatory cells in the deeper dermis. (B) Lichen simplex chronicus displaying thickened epidermis and hyperkeratosis.

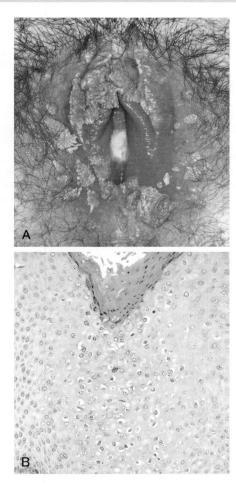

Fig. 19.2 (A) Numerous condylomas of the vulva. (B) Histopathologic features of condyloma acuminatum include acanthosis, hyperkeratosis, and cytoplasmic vacuolization (koilocytosis, *center*). *(A, Courtesy of Dr. Alex Ferenczy, McGill University, Montreal, Quebec, Canada.)*

diameter and are red-pink to pink-brown (Fig. 19.2). On histologic examination, the characteristic cellular feature is koilocytosis (a cytopathic change characterized by perinuclear cytoplasmic vacuolization and a wrinkled nuclear contour), a hallmark of HPV infection (Fig. 19.2). Indeed, more than 90% of condylomata acuminata are positive for HPV subtypes 6 and 11. HPV is sexually transmitted, and identical lesions occur in men on the penis and around the anus in men and women. HPV 6 and 11 are low-risk viral types, and hence, vulvar condylomas do not commonly progress to cancer. However, women with condyloma acuminata are at risk of having other HPV-related lesions in the vagina and cervix.

Carcinoma of the Vulva

Carcinoma of the vulva represents about 3% of all female genital tract cancers, occurring mostly in women older than age 60. Approximately 90% of carcinomas are squamous cell carcinomas; most of the other tumors are adenocarcinomas or basal cell carcinomas.

There appear to be two distinct forms of vulvar squamous cell carcinomas that differ in pathogenesis and course. The less common form is related to high-risk HPV strains (especially HPV type 16) and occurs in middle-aged women, particularly cigarette smokers. This form is often preceded by precancerous changes in the epithelium termed vulvar intraepithelial neoplasia (VIN). VIN progresses in many patients to greater degrees of atypia and eventually to carcinoma in situ; however, progression to invasive carcinoma is not inevitable and may occur only after many years. Environmental factors such as cigarette smoking and immunodeficiency appear to increase the risk of such progression.

A second form of squamous carcinoma occurs in older women, sometimes following a long history of reactive epithelial changes, principally lichen sclerosus. It is preceded by a subtle lesion, differentiated vulvar intraepithelial neoplasia (dVIN), characterized by cytologic atypia confined to the basal layer and abnormal keratinization. If left untreated it may give rise to HPV negative, well-differentiated, keratinizing squamous cell carcinoma.

MORPHOLOGY

VIN and early vulvar carcinomas commonly manifest as areas of **leukoplakia**. In about one-fourth of the cases, the lesions are pigmented owing to the presence of melanin. With time, these areas are transformed into overt exophytic or ulcerative endophytic tumors. HPV-positive tumors are often multifocal and warty and tend to be poorly differentiated **squamous cell carcinomas,** whereas HPV-negative tumors usually are unifocal and typically are well-differentiated keratinizing squamous cell carcinomas.

Both forms of vulvar carcinoma tend to remain confined to their site of origin for a few years but ultimately invade and spread, usually first to regional lymph nodes. The risk of metastasis correlates with the depth of invasion. As with most carcinomas, outcome is dependent on tumor stage. The overall 5-year survival is 70% to 93% for patients with negative lymph nodes but decreases to 25% to 41% for patients with lymph node metastases.

Extramammary Paget Disease

Paget disease is an intraepidermal proliferation of epithelial cells that can occur in the skin of the vulva or nipple of the breast (described later). However, unlike in the breast, where Paget disease is virtually always associated with an underlying carcinoma, only a minority of cases of vulvar (extramammary) Paget disease have an underlying tumor. Instead, vulvar Paget cells most commonly appear to arise from epidermal progenitor cells.

Paget disease manifests as a red, scaly, crusted plaque that may mimic the appearance of an inflammatory dermatitis. On histologic examination, large cells with abundant pale, finely granular cytoplasm and occasional cytoplasmic vacuoles infiltrate the epidermis, singly and in groups (Fig. 19.3). The presence of mucin, as detected by periodic acid–Schiff (PAS) staining, is useful in distinguishing Paget disease from vulvar melanoma, which lacks mucin.

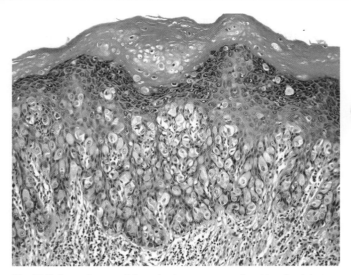

Fig. 19.3 Paget disease of the vulva. Large tumor cells with pale-pink cytoplasm are seen infiltrating the epidermis. Chronic inflammatory cells are present in the underlying dermis.

Intraepidermal Paget disease may persist for years or even decades without evidence of invasion. However, when there is an associated tumor involving skin appendages, the Paget cells may invade locally and ultimately metastasize. After metastasis occurs, the prognosis is poor.

SUMMARY

TUMORS OF THE VULVA

- HPV-related vulvar squamous cell carcinomas usually are poorly differentiated lesions and sometimes are multifocal. They often evolve from vulvar intraepithelial neoplasia.
- Non–HPV-related vulvar squamous cell carcinomas occur in older women and usually are well differentiated and unifocal. They are often preceded by "differentiated" vulvar intraepithelial neoplasia associated with lichen sclerosus.
- Vulvar Paget disease is characterized by a red, scaly plaque caused by proliferation of epithelial cells within the epidermis; usually, there is no underlying carcinoma, unlike Paget disease of the nipple.

Vagina

In adult females, the vagina is seldom a site of primary disease. More often, it is involved secondarily by cancer or infections arising in adjacent organs (e.g., cervix, vulva, bladder, rectum).

Congenital anomalies of the vagina fortunately are uncommon and include entities such as total absence of the vagina, a septate or double vagina (usually associated with a septate cervix and, sometimes, septate uterus), and congenital, lateral Gartner duct cysts arising from persistent wolffian duct rests.

VAGINITIS

Vaginitis is a common condition that is usually transient and of no clinical consequence. It is associated with the production of a vaginal discharge (leukorrhea). A large variety of organisms have been implicated, including bacteria, fungi, and parasites. Many are normal commensals that become pathogenic only in the setting of diabetes, systemic antibiotic therapy (which causes disruption of normal microbial flora), immunodeficiency, pregnancy, or recent abortion. In adults, primary gonorrheal infection of the vagina is uncommon. The other organisms worthy of mention, because they are frequent offenders, are *Candida albicans* and *Trichomonas vaginalis*. Candidal (monilial) vaginitis is characterized by a curdy white discharge. This organism is part of the normal vaginal flora in about 5% of women, so the appearance of symptomatic infection almost always involves one of the predisposing influences listed above or superinfection by a new, more aggressive strain. *T. vaginalis* is sexually transmitted; it produces a watery, copious gray-green discharge in which parasites can be identified by microscopy. Trichomonas also can be identified in about 10% of asymptomatic women; thus,

active infection usually stems from sexual transmission of a new strain.

MALIGNANT NEOPLASMS

Squamous Cell Carcinoma

Squamous cell carcinoma of the vagina is an extremely uncommon cancer that usually occurs in women older than 60 years in the setting of risk factors similar to those associated with carcinoma of the cervix (discussed later). Vaginal intraepithelial neoplasia (VAIN) is a precursor lesion that is nearly always associated with HPV infection. Invasive squamous cell carcinoma of the vagina is associated with the presence of HPV DNA in more than half of the cases, presumably derived from HPV-positive VAIN.

Clear Cell Adenocarcinoma

In 1970, clear cell adenocarcinoma, a very rare tumor, was identified in a cluster of young women whose mothers took diethylstilbestrol during pregnancy to prevent threatened abortion. Follow-up studies determined that the incidence of this tumor in persons exposed to diethylstilbestrol in utero is low (<1 per 1000, albeit about 40 times greater than in the unexposed population). In about one-third of exposed women, small glandular or microcystic inclusions develop in the vaginal mucosa. These lesions appear as red, granular foci lined by mucus-secreting or ciliated columnar cells. This condition is called vaginal adenosis and is benign but is important to recognize because it is from such precursor lesions that clear cell adenocarcinoma arises.

Sarcoma Botryoides

Sarcoma botryoides (embryonal rhabdomyosarcoma) is a rare form of primary vaginal cancer that manifests as soft polypoid masses. It usually is encountered in infants and children younger than 5 years of age, but may occur uncommonly in young women. It also may be found in other sites, such as the urinary bladder and bile ducts. It is discussed further with other soft tissue tumors in Chapter 21.

Cervix

Most cervical lesions are relatively banal inflammations (cervicitis), but the cervix also is the site of one of the most common cancers in women worldwide.

CERVICITIS

Inflammatory conditions of the cervix are extremely common and may be associated with a purulent vaginal discharge. Cervicitis can be subclassified as infectious or noninfectious, although differentiation is difficult owing to the presence of normal vaginal flora including incidental vaginal aerobes and anaerobes, streptococci, staphylococci, enterococci, and *Escherichia coli* and *Candida* spp.

Much more important are *Chlamydia trachomatis, Ureaplasma urealyticum, T. vaginalis, Neisseria gonorrhoeae,* HSV-2 (the agent of herpes genitalis), and certain types of HPV, all of which are often sexually transmitted. *C. trachomatis* is by far the most common of these pathogens, accounting for as many as 40% of cases of cervicitis encountered in sexually transmitted infection clinics. Although less common, herpetic infections are noteworthy because maternal–infant transmission during childbirth may result in serious, sometimes fatal systemic herpetic infection in the newborn.

Cervicitis commonly comes to attention on routine examination or because of leukorrhea. It often is treated empirically with antibiotics that are active against chlamydia and gonococcus. In some instances, nucleic acid amplification tests are used on vaginal fluid to identify the presence of these organisms as well as *Trichomonas vaginalis.*

NEOPLASIA OF THE CERVIX

Most tumors of the cervix are of epithelial origin and are caused by oncogenic strains of HPV. During development, the columnar mucus-secreting epithelium of the endocervix is joined to the squamous epithelial covering of the exocervix at the cervical os. With the onset of puberty, the squamocolumnar junction undergoes eversion, causing the columnar epithelium to become visible on the exocervix. The exposed columnar cells, however, eventually undergo squamous metaplasia, forming a region called the transformation zone, where tumors most commonly arise (Fig. 19.4).

Pathogenesis

HPV, the causative agent of cervical neoplasia, has a tropism for the immature squamous cells of the transformation zone. Most HPV infections are transient and are eliminated within months by the host immune response. A subset of infections persists, however, and some cause squamous intraepithelial lesions (SILs), which are precursors from which most invasive cervical carcinomas develop.

HPV is detectable by molecular methods in nearly all cases of cervical intraepithelial neoplasia (CIN) and cervical carcinoma. Important risk factors for the development of CIN and invasive carcinoma thus are directly related to HPV exposure and include:

- Early age at first intercourse
- Multiple sexual partners
- Male partner with multiple previous sexual partners
- Persistent infection by high-risk strains of papillomavirus

Like most other DNA viruses, HPV uses host cell DNA polymerases to replicate its genome and produce virions. Virions must be shed from the surface of the squamous mucosa, yet under normal circumstances squamous cell maturation is accompanied by a cessation of DNA replication, which would prevent virus production. HPV "solves" this problem through the action of two viral oncoproteins, E6 and E7. **The E6 and E7 proteins of "high risk" HPV variants inhibit p53 and RB, respectively** (Chapter 6), two potent tumor suppressors that act to suppress the division of squamous cells as they mature. E6 and E7 thus have a central role in the life cycle of HPV and largely explain the carcinogenic activity of HPV in the cervix and other sites that are prone to HPV infection (e.g., vulva, penis, oropharynx).

HPV variants are classified as high-risk or low-risk types based on their propensity to induce carcinogenesis.

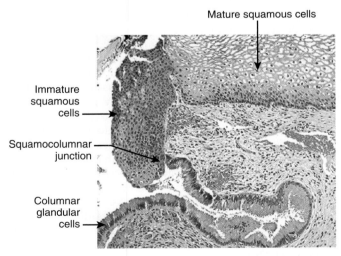

Fig. 19.4 Cervical transformation zone showing the transition from mature glycogenated squamous epithelium, to immature metaplastic squamous cells, to columnar endocervical glandular epithelium.

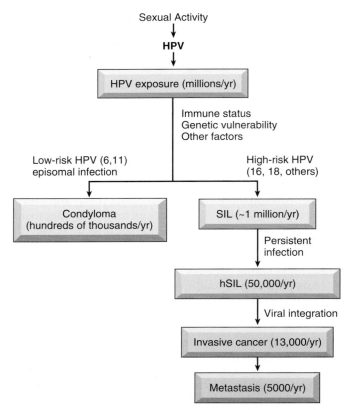

Fig. 19.5 Possible consequences of human papillomavirus (HPV) infection. Progression is associated with integration of virus and acquisition of additional mutations as discussed in the text. *SIL*, Squamous intraepithelial lesion; *hSIL*, High-grade cervical intraepithelial lesion.

High-risk HPV infection is the most important risk factor for the development of SIL that can progress to carcinoma. Two high-risk HPV viruses, types 16 and 18, account for approximately 70% of cases of SIL and cervical carcinoma. In general, infections with high-risk HPV types are more likely to persist, which is a risk factor for progression to carcinoma. These HPV types also show a propensity to integrate into the host cell genome, an event that is linked to progression. Low-risk HPV variants (e.g., types 6 and 11) associated with the development of condylomas of the lower genital tract (Fig. 19.5), by contrast, express E6 and E7 variants with different or weaker activities and do not integrate into the host genome, remaining instead as free episomal viral DNA. Despite the strong association of HPV infection with cancer of the cervix, HPV is not sufficient to drive the neoplastic process. As mentioned later, HPV-infected high-grade precursor lesions do not invariably progress to invasive cancer. Diverse other factors such as immune and hormonal status and coinfection with other sexually transmitted agents are suspected to play a role. Collectively these factors favor the acquisition of somatically acquired mutations that involve both oncogenes and tumor suppressor genes. Viral integration appear to contribute to transformation in two ways: 1) integration always disrupts an HPV gene that negatively regulates E6 and E7, which leads to their increased expression; and 2) sometimes HPV integrates near a host cell oncogene such as *MYC*, leading to its overexpression as well.

Squamous Intraepithelial Lesion (SIL, Cervical Intraepithelial Lesion)

HPV-related carcinogenesis begins with the precancerous epithelial change termed SIL, which usually precedes the development of an overt cancer by many years, sometimes decades. In support of this idea, SIL peaks in incidence at about 30 years of age, whereas invasive carcinoma peaks at about 45 years of age.

The classification of cervical precursor lesions has evolved with time. The current terminology is a two-tiered system that not only reflects the biology of the disease but also patient management, replacing a three-tiered system.

- SIL is divided into low-grade squamous intraepithelial lesion (LSIL), still often referred to as cervical intraepithelial neoplasia I (CIN I), and high-grade squamous intraepithelial lesion (HSIL), encompassing cervical intraepithelial neoplasia II and III (CIN II and III) of the previous three-tiered system.
- LSIL is associated with productive HPV infection and does not progress directly to invasive carcinoma. Actually, most LSILs regress and only a small percentage progress to HSIL.
- HSIL demonstrates increased proliferation, arrested epithelial maturation, and lower levels of viral replication. LSIL is not treated as a premalignant lesion, whereas HSIL is considered at high risk for progression to carcinoma.

Importantly, LSIL is 10 times more common than HSIL and while HSILs are precancerous, the majority of them fail to progress to cancer and may even regress. Patient management rests on the histopathologic diagnosis as discussed later. As shown in Table 19.1, the decision to treat HSIL and to observe LSIL is based on differences in the natural histories of these two groups of lesions.

Cervical precancerous lesions are associated with abnormalities in cytologic preparations that can be detected long before any abnormality is visible on gross inspection. Early detection of SIL is the rationale for the Papanicolaou (Pap) test, in which cells are scraped from the transformation zone and examined microscopically. **The Pap smear remains the most successful cancer-screening test ever developed.** In the United States, Pap screening has dramatically lowered the incidence of invasive cervical tumors to about 13,000 cases annually with a mortality of about 4000 per year; in fact, cervical cancer no longer ranks among the top 10 causes of cancer deaths in U.S. women. Paradoxically, the incidence of SIL has increased to its present level of more than 50,000 cases annually. Increased detection has certainly contributed to this. The U.S. Food and Drug Administration has approved testing for HPV DNA in cervical scrapings. This test is highly sensitive but has lower

Table 19.1 Natural History of Squamous Intraepithelial Lesions (SILs)

Lesion	Regress	Persist	Progress
LSIL (CIN I)	60%	30%	10% (to HSIL)
HSIL (CIN II, III)	30%	60%	10% (to carcinoma)[a]

[a]Progression within 10 years.
LSIL, Low-grade SIL; HSIL, high-grade SIL.

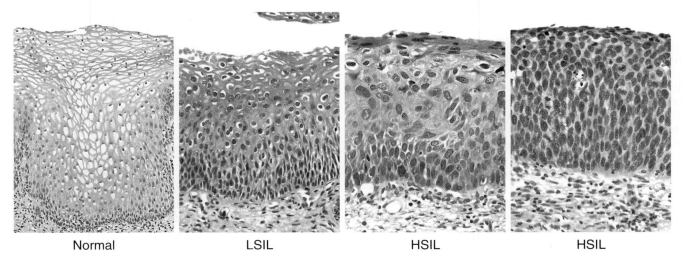

| Normal | LSIL | HSIL | HSIL |

Fig. 19.6 Spectrum of squamous intraepithelial lesions (SIL) with normal squamous epithelium for comparison: LSIL with koilocytotic atypia; HSIL with progressive atypia in all layers of the epithelium; and HSIL with diffuse atypia and loss of maturation (carcinoma in situ, *far right image*).

specificity than the Pap smear, and specific guidelines for its use have not been well established. One consideration is that while most women acquire HPV infections in their early 20s, these are usually cleared by the immune system and never progress to SIL, a process that occurs over many years. For this reason, HPV DNA screening is only recommended for women aged 30 or older, as a positive test at this age is more likely to identify an individual with a persistent infection that may lead to cervical neoplasia.

The quadrivalent HPV vaccine for types 6, 11, 16, and 18, and the more recently introduced 9-valent vaccine, are very effective in preventing HPV infections and are expected to greatly lower the frequency of genital warts and cervical cancers associated with these HPV genotypes. Despite its efficacy, vaccination does not supplant the need for routine cervical cancer screening—many at-risk women are already infected, and current vaccines protect against only some of the many oncogenic HPV genotypes.

MORPHOLOGY

Fig. 19.6 illustrates the three stages of SIL. LSIL is characterized by dysplastic changes in the lower third of the squamous epithelium and **koilocytotic change** in the superficial layers of the epithelium. In HSIL (CIN II), dysplasia extends to the middle third of the epithelium in the form of variation in cell and nuclear size, heterogeneity of nuclear chromatin, and the presence of mitoses, some atypical, above the basal layer extending into the middle third of the epithelium. The superficial layer of cells in CIN II still shows differentiation and occasional koilocytotic changes HSIL (CIN III) is marked by almost complete loss of differentiation, even greater variation in cell and nuclear size, chromatin heterogeneity, disorderly orientation of the cells, and abnormal mitoses, changes that affect virtually all layers of the epithelium. Koilocytotic change usually is absent. These histologic features correlate with the cytologic appearances shown in Fig. 19.7.

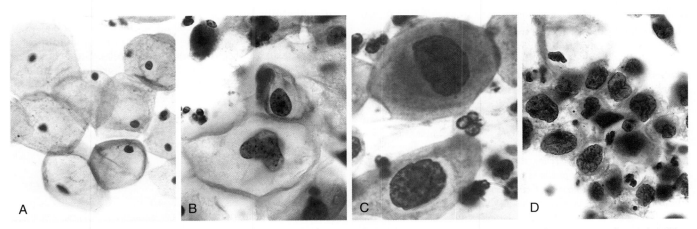

Fig. 19.7 Cytologic features of squamous intraepithelial lesion (SIL) in a Papanicolaou smear. Superficial squamous cells may stain either red or blue. (A) Normal exfoliated superficial squamous epithelial cells. (B) Low-grade squamous intraepithelial lesion (LSIL). (C and D) Both high-grade squamous intraepithelial lesions (HSILs). Note the reduction in cytoplasm and the increase in the nucleus-to-cytoplasm ratio as the grade of the lesion increases. This observation reflects the progressive loss of cellular differentiation on the surface of the cervical lesions from which these cells are exfoliated (see Fig. 19.6). *(Courtesy of Dr. Edmund S. Cibas, Brigham and Women's Hospital, Boston, Massachusetts.)*

SIL is asymptomatic and comes to clinical attention through an abnormal Pap smear result. These cases are followed up by colposcopy, in which acetic acid is used to highlight the lesions so they can be biopsied. Women with biopsy-documented LSIL are managed conservatively with careful observation, whereas HSILs and persistent LSIL are treated with surgical excision (cone biopsy). Follow-up smears and clinical examination are required in patients with HSIL, as these women remain at risk for HPV-associated cervical, vulvar, and vaginal cancers.

Invasive Carcinoma of the Cervix

The most common cervical carcinomas are squamous cell carcinomas (75%), followed by adenocarcinomas and mixed adenosquamous carcinomas (20%) and small cell neuroendocrine carcinomas (<5%). All of these types of carcinomas are associated with HPV. Of interest, the relative proportion of adenocarcinomas has been increasing in recent decades owing to the decreasing incidence of invasive squamous carcinoma and suboptimal detection of glandular lesions by Pap smear.

Squamous cell carcinoma has a peak incidence at the age of about 45 years, some 10 to 15 years after detection of precursor SIL. As already discussed, **progression of SIL to invasive carcinoma is variable and unpredictable and requires HPV infection as well as mutations in tumor suppressor genes and oncogenes.** Risk factors for progression include cigarette smoking and human immunodeficiency virus (HIV) infection, the latter finding suggesting that immune surveillance plays a role in preventing progression. Although risk factors may help identify patients who are likely to progress from SIL to carcinoma, the only reliable way to monitor the disease course is with frequent physical examinations coupled with Pap smears and biopsy of suspicious lesions.

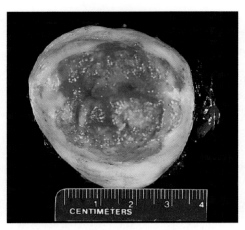

Fig. 19.8 Cervical os with surrounding, invasive, exophytic cervical carcinoma.

Clinical Features

Invasive cervical cancer most often is seen in women who have never had a Pap smear or who have not been screened for many years. In such cases, cervical cancer often is symptomatic, with patients coming to medical attention for unexpected vaginal bleeding, leukorrhea, painful coitus (dyspareunia), or dysuria. The primary treatment is hysterectomy and lymph node dissection; small microinvasive carcinomas may be treated with cone biopsy. Radiation and chemotherapy are also of benefit in instances where surgery alone is not curative. Mortality is most strongly predicted by tumor stage and, in the case of neuroendocrine carcinomas (which pursue an aggressive course) to cell type.

Endocervical Polyp

Endocervical polyps are benign polypoid masses seen protruding from the endocervical mucosa (sometimes through the exocervix). They can be as large as a few centimeters and have a smooth, glistening surface with underlying cystically dilated spaces filled with mucinous secretions. The surface epithelium and lining of the underlying cysts are composed of the same mucus-secreting columnar cells that line the endocervical canal. The stroma is edematous and may contain scattered mononuclear cells. Superimposed chronic inflammation may lead to squamous metaplasia of the overlying epithelium and ulcerations. These lesions may bleed, thereby arousing concern, but they have no malignant potential.

> ### MORPHOLOGY
>
> Invasive carcinomas of the cervix develop in the **transformation zone** and range from microscopic foci of stromal invasion to grossly conspicuous exophytic tumors (Fig. 19.8). Microscopically, the invasive tumors often consist of tongues and nests of squamous cells that produce a desmoplastic stromal response. Grading is based on the degree of squamous differentiation, which ranges from minimal to well-differentiated tumors that elaborate keratin pearls. Rare tumors with neuroendocrine differentiation resemble small cell carcinomas of the lung morphologically. Tumors encircling the cervix and penetrating into the underlying stroma produce a **barrel cervix,** which can be identified by direct palpation. Extension into the parametrial soft tissues can affix the uterus to the surrounding pelvic structures. The likelihood of spread to pelvic lymph nodes correlates with the depth of tumor invasion and the presence of tumor cells in vascular spaces. The risk of metastasis increases from less than 1% for tumors less than 3 mm in depth to more than 10% after invasion exceeds 3 mm.

> ### SUMMARY
> #### CERVICAL NEOPLASIA
>
> - Risk factors for cervical carcinoma are related to HPV exposure, such as early age at first intercourse, multiple sexual partners, and other factors including cigarette smoking and immunodeficiency.
> - Nearly all cervical carcinomas are caused by HPV infections, particularly high-risk HPV types 16, 18, 31, and 33;

- the HPV vaccine is effective in preventing infection resulting from the HPV types most commonly associated with carcinoma.
- HPV expresses E6 and E7 proteins that inactivate the p53 and RB tumor suppressors, respectively, resulting in increased cell proliferation and suppression of DNA damage–induced apoptosis.

- In cervical cancer, high-risk HPV is integrated in the host genome, an event that increases the expression of E6 and E7 and contributes to progression to cancer.
- The Pap smear is a highly effective screening tool for the detection of SIL and carcinoma and has significantly reduced the incidence of cervical carcinoma. HPV testing is currently being used in conjunction with the Pap smear.

Uterus

The body (corpus) of the uterus is composed of the endometrium, consisting of glands and stroma, and the myometrium, made up of smooth muscle. The more frequent and significant disorders of the uterus are considered here.

ENDOMETRITIS

Inflammation of the endometrium is classified as acute or chronic depending on whether a neutrophilic or a lymphoplasmacytic infiltrate predominates, respectively. The diagnosis of chronic endometritis generally requires the presence of plasma cells, as lymphocytes are present even in the normal endometrium.

Endometritis is a component of pelvic inflammatory disease and is frequently a result of *N. gonorrhoeae* or *C. trachomatis* infection. Histologic examination shows a neutrophilic infiltrate in the superficial endometrium coexisting with a stromal lymphoplasmacytic infiltrate. Prominent lymphoid follicles may be seen, particularly in chlamydial infection. Tuberculosis causes granulomatous endometritis, frequently with associated tuberculous salpingitis and peritonitis. Although seen in the United States mainly in immunocompromised persons, tuberculous endometritis is common in countries in which tuberculosis is endemic, and it should be included in the differential diagnosis for pelvic inflammatory disease in women who have recently emigrated from endemic areas.

Endometritis also may be a result of retained products of conception subsequent to miscarriage or delivery or the presence of a foreign body such as an intrauterine device. Retained tissue or foreign bodies act as a nidus for ascending infection by vaginal or intestinal tract flora. Removal of the offending tissue or foreign body typically results in resolution.

Clinically, all forms of endometritis manifest with fever, abdominal pain, and menstrual abnormalities. In addition, there is an increased risk of infertility and ectopic pregnancy due to damage and scarring of the fallopian tubes.

ADENOMYOSIS

Adenomyosis refers to the presence of endometrial tissue in the myometrium. Nests of endometrial stroma, glands, or both are found deep in the myometrium interposed between the muscle bundles. This endometrial tissue induces reactive hypertrophy of the myometrium, resulting in an enlarged, globular uterus, often with a thickened uterine wall. Extensive adenomyosis may produce menorrhagia, dysmenorrhea, and pelvic pain, particularly just prior to menstruation, and can coexist with endometriosis.

ENDOMETRIOSIS

Endometriosis is defined by the presence of endometrial glands and stroma in a location outside the uterus. It occurs in as many as 10% of women in their reproductive years and in nearly half of women with infertility. It frequently is multifocal and often involves pelvic structures (ovaries, pouch of Douglas, uterine ligaments, tubes, and rectovaginal septum). Less frequently, distant areas of the peritoneal cavity or periumbilical tissues are involved. Uncommonly, distant sites such as lymph nodes, lungs, and even heart, skeletal muscle, or bone are affected.

Four hypotheses have been put forth to explain the origin of dispersed endometriotic lesions, all of which are viable:

- The *regurgitation theory*, which is currently favored, proposes that menstrual backflow through the fallopian tubes leads to implantation.
- The *benign metastases theory* holds that endometrial tissue from the uterus can "spread" to distant sites via blood vessels and lymphatics.
- The *metaplastic theory*, on the other hand, posits endometrial differentiation of coelomic epithelium (mesothelium of pelvis and abdomen from which endometrium originates) as the source.
- The *extrauterine stem/progenitor cell theory*, proposes that circulating stem/progenitor cells from the bone marrow differentiate into endometrial tissue.

Studies suggest that endometriotic tissue is not just misplaced but is also abnormal (Fig. 19.9). As compared to normal endometrium, endometriotic tissue exhibits increased levels of inflammatory mediators, particularly prostaglandin E2. It is proposed that the inflammation results from the recruitment and activation of macrophages by factors made by endometrial stromal cells. Stromal cells also make aromatase, leading to local production of estrogen. These factors enhance the survival and persistence of the endometriotic tissue within a foreign location (a key feature in the pathogenesis of endometriosis) and help to explain the beneficial effects of COX-2 inhibitors and aromatase inhibitors in the treatment of endometriosis.

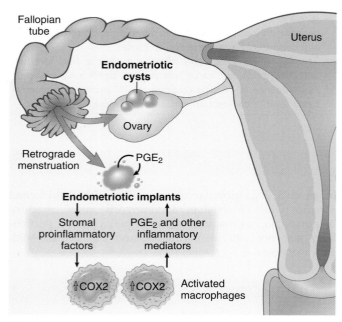

Fig. 19.9 Proposed origins of endometriosis.

MORPHOLOGY

Endometriosis typically consists of **functioning endometrium,** which undergoes cyclic bleeding. Because blood collects in these aberrant foci, they appear grossly as red-brown nodules or implants. They range in size from microscopic to 1 to 2 cm in diameter and lie on or just under the affected serosal surface. Often, individual lesions coalesce to form larger masses. When the ovaries are involved, the lesions may form large, blood-filled cysts that turn brown **(chocolate cysts)** as the blood ages (Fig. 19.10). With seepage and organization of the blood, widespread fibrosis occurs, leading to adhesions among pelvic structures, sealing of the tubal fimbriated ends, and distortion of the fallopian tubes and ovaries. The diagnosis depends on finding both endometrial glands and stroma at sites external to the endometrium.

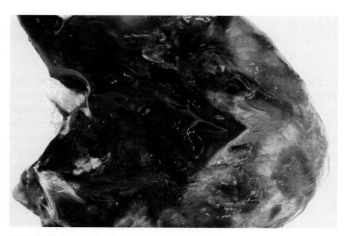

Fig. 19.10 Ovarian endometriosis. Sectioning of ovary shows a large endometriotic cyst with degenerated blood ("chocolate cyst").

Clinical Features

The clinical manifestations of endometriosis depend on the distribution of the lesions. Extensive scarring of the fallopian tubes and ovaries often produces discomfort in the lower abdomen and eventual sterility. Rectal wall involvement may produce pain on defecation, whereas involvement of the uterine or bladder serosa can cause dyspareunia (painful intercourse) and dysuria, respectively. Almost all cases feature severe dysmenorrhea and pelvic pain resulting from intrapelvic bleeding and intraabdominal adhesions.

ABNORMAL UTERINE BLEEDING

Women commonly seek medical attention for abnormal uterine bleeding, such as *menorrhagia* (profuse or prolonged bleeding at the time of the period), *metrorrhagia* (irregular bleeding between the periods), or postmenopausal bleeding. Common causes include dysfunctional uterine bleeding, endometrial polyps, leiomyomas, endometrial hyperplasia, and endometrial carcinoma.

The probable cause of uterine bleeding in any given case varies depending on the age of the patient (Table 19.2). Abnormal bleeding from the uterus in the absence of an organic uterine lesion is called *dysfunctional uterine bleeding.* The most common cause of dysfunctional uterine bleeding is anovulation (failure to ovulate). Anovulatory cycles result from hormonal imbalances and are most common at menarche and in the perimenopausal period because of fluctuations in the hypothalamus/pituitary/ovarian axis. Less common causes of anovulation are

- *Endocrine disorders,* such as thyroid disease, adrenal disease, or pituitary tumors.
- *Ovarian lesions,* such as a functioning ovarian tumor (granulosa cell tumors) or polycystic ovarian syndrome (see section on ovaries that follows).
- *Generalized metabolic disturbances,* such as obesity, malnutrition, or other chronic systemic disorders.

Dysfunctional uterine bleeding also may result from an inadequate luteal phase, which is thought to stem from

Table 19.2 Causes of Abnormal Uterine Bleeding by Age Group

Age Group	Cause(s)
Prepuberty	Precocious puberty (hypothalamic, pituitary, or ovarian origin)
Adolescence	Anovulatory cycle
Reproductive age	Complications of pregnancy (abortion, trophoblastic disease, ectopic pregnancy) Proliferations (leiomyoma, adenomyosis, polyps, endometrial hyperplasia, carcinoma) Anovulatory cycle Ovulatory dysfunctional bleeding (e.g., inadequate luteal phase)
Perimenopause	Anovulatory cycle Irregular shedding Proliferations (carcinoma, hyperplasia, polyps)
Postmenopause	Proliferations (carcinoma, hyperplasia, polyps) Endometrial atrophy

insufficient production of progesterone by the corpus luteum.

● SUMMARY

NONNEOPLASTIC DISORDERS OF ENDOMETRIUM

- Adenomyosis refers to growth of endometrium into the myometrium often with uterine enlargement.
- Endometriosis refers to endometrial glands and stroma located outside the uterus and most often involves the pelvic or abdominal peritoneum. Rarely, distant sites such as the lymph nodes and the lungs also are involved.
- The ectopic endometrium in endometriosis undergoes cyclic bleeding, and the condition is a common cause of dysmenorrhea and pelvic pain.

PROLIFERATIVE LESIONS OF THE ENDOMETRIUM AND MYOMETRIUM

The most common proliferative lesions of the uterine corpus are endometrial hyperplasia, endometrial carcinomas, endometrial polyps, and smooth muscle tumors. All tend to produce abnormal uterine bleeding as their earliest manifestation.

Endometrial Hyperplasia

An excess of estrogen relative to progestin, if sufficiently prolonged or marked, can induce exaggerated endometrial proliferation (hyperplasia), which is an important precursor of endometrial carcinoma. A common cause of estrogen excess is obesity, as adipose tissue converts steroid precursors into estrogens. Other potential causes of estrogen excess include failure of ovulation (such as in perimenopause), prolonged administration of estrogenic steroids without counterbalancing progestin, and estrogen-producing ovarian lesions (such as polycystic ovary syndrome and granulosa-theca cell tumors of the ovary).

Endometrial hyperplasia is placed in two categories based on the presence of cytologic atypia: hyperplasia without atypia and hyperplasia with atypia (Fig. 19.11). The importance of this classification is that the presence of cytologic atypia correlates with the development or concurrent finding of endometrial carcinoma. Hyperplasia without cellular atypia carries a low risk (between 1% and 3%) for progression to endometrial carcinoma, whereas hyperplasia with atypia, also called *endometrial intraepithelial neoplasia (EIN)*, is associated with a much higher risk (20%–50%). When hyperplasia with atypia is discovered, it must be carefully evaluated for the presence of cancer and usually warrants a hysterectomy in patients no longer desiring fertility. In younger patients, treatment with high-dose progestins may be used in an attempt to preserve the uterus.

Unopposed estrogen is also a risk factor for the most common type of endometrial carcinoma (see later), and inactivation of the *PTEN* tumor suppressor gene has been identified at a substantial frequency in hyperplasia with

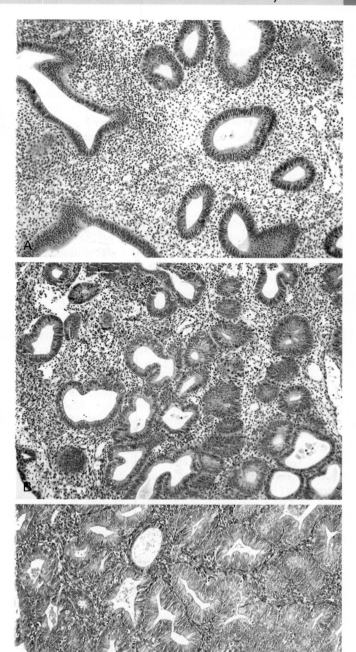

Fig. 19.11 Endometrial hyperplasia. (A) Anovulatory or "disordered" endometrium containing dilated glands. (B) Hyperplasia without atypia, characterized by nests of closely packed glands. (C) Hyperplasia with atypia, seen as glandular crowding and cellular atypia.

atypia (approximately 50%) and endometrioid carcinoma (>70%). Along with clinicopathologic and epidemiologic studies, these findings indicate that hyperplasia with atypia is a precursor lesion for endometrioid endometrial carcinoma.

Endometrial Carcinoma

In the United States and many other Western countries, endometrial carcinoma is the most frequent cancer occurring in the female genital tract. It generally appears between the ages of 55 and 65 years and is uncommon before age 40. Endometrial carcinoma can be broadly divided into two histologically and pathogenically distinct categories: endometrioid and serous carcinoma. There are other less common types of endometrial carcinoma, such as clear cell carcinoma and mixed Mullerian tumor (carcinosarcoma), but these will not be discussed further.

Pathogenesis

Endometrioid cancers arise in association with estrogen excess in the setting of endometrial hyperplasia in perimenopausal women, whereas serous cancers arise in the setting of endometrial atrophy in older postmenopausal women. The *endometrioid type* accounts for 80% of cases of endometrial carcinomas. These tumors are designated as endometrioid because of their histologic similarity to normal endometrial glands. Risk factors for this type of carcinoma include (1) obesity, (2) diabetes, (3) hypertension, (4) infertility, and (5) exposure to unopposed estrogen. Many of these risk factors result in increased estrogenic stimulation of the endometrium and are associated with endometrial hyperplasia. In fact, it is well recognized that prolonged estrogen replacement therapy and estrogen-secreting ovarian tumors increase the risk of the endometrioid type of endometrial carcinoma. **Mutations in mismatch repair genes and the tumor suppressor gene PTEN are early events in the stepwise development of endometrioid carcinoma.** Women with germline mutations in *PTEN* (Cowden Syndrome) and germline alterations in DNA mismatch repair genes (Lynch Syndrome) are at high risk for this cancer. *TP53* mutations occur but are relatively uncommon and are late events in the genesis of this tumor type.

The *serous type* of endometrial carcinoma is less common but also far more aggressive. It accounts, for roughly 15% of tumors and is not associated with unopposed estrogen or endometrial hyperplasia. Nearly all cases of serous carcinoma have mutations in the *TP53* tumor suppressor gene, whereas mutations in DNA mismatch repair genes and in *PTEN* are rare. Serous tumors are preceded by a lesion called serous endometrial intraepithelial carcinoma (SEIC) in which *TP53* mutations are often detected, suggesting an early role for such mutations in the development of this form of endometrial carcinoma.

MORPHOLOGY

Endometrioid carcinomas closely resemble normal endometrium and may be exophytic or infiltrative (Fig. 19.12A–B). They include a range of histologic types, including those showing mucinous, tubal (ciliated), and squamous differentiation. Endometrioid carcinomas often infiltrate the myometrium and can enter vascular spaces (lymphovascular invasion). They may also metastasize to regional lymph nodes. Endometrioid carcinomas are graded 1 to 3, based on the degree of differentiation.

Serous carcinomas typically grow in small tufts and papillae with marked cytologic atypia. They can also form glands that at times create confusion with endometrioid carcinoma, however serous carcinomas exhibit much greater cytologic atypia. Serous carcinomas behave aggressively and thus are by definition high grade. Immunohistochemistry often shows diffuse, strong staining for p53 in serous carcinoma (Fig. 19.12C–D), a finding that correlates with the presence of *TP53* mutations (mutant p53 accumulates and hence is more easily detected by staining).

Clinical Features

Endometrial carcinomas usually manifest with irregular or postmenopausal bleeding. With progression, the uterus enlarges and may become affixed to surrounding structures as the cancer infiltrates surrounding tissues. Endometrioid carcinoma usually is slow to metastasize, but if left untreated, eventually disseminates to regional nodes and more distant sites. With therapy, the 5-year survival rate for early-stage endometrioid carcinoma is 90%, but survival drops precipitously in higher-stage tumors. The prognosis with serous carcinomas is strongly dependent on operative staging but because of its aggressive behavior it often presents as high-stage disease with a poor prognosis.

SUMMARY

ENDOMETRIAL HYPERPLASIA AND ENDOMETRIAL CARCINOMA

- Endometrial hyperplasia results from unopposed endogenous or exogenous estrogen.
- Risk factors for developing endometrial hyperplasia include anovulatory cycles, polycystic ovary syndrome, estrogen-producing ovarian tumor, obesity, and estrogen therapy without counterbalancing progestin.
- Hyperplasia is classified based on cytologic atypia, which determines the risk of developing endometrioid carcinoma.
- On the basis of clinical and molecular data, two major types of endometrial carcinoma are recognized:
  - *Endometrioid carcinoma* is associated with estrogen excess and endometrial hyperplasia. Early molecular changes include inactivation of DNA mismatch repair genes and the *PTEN* gene.
  - *Serous carcinoma* of the endometrium arises in older women and usually is associated with endometrial atrophy and a distinct precursor lesion, serous intraepithelial carcinoma. Mutations in the *TP53* gene are an early event, usually being present in serous endometrial intraepithelial carcinoma as well as invasive serous carcinoma.
- Stage is the major determinant of survival in both types. Serous tumors tend to manifest more frequently with extrauterine extension and therefore have a worse prognosis than endometrioid carcinomas.

Endometrial Polyps

These polyps are usually sessile and range from 0.5 to 3 cm in diameter. Larger polyps may project from the

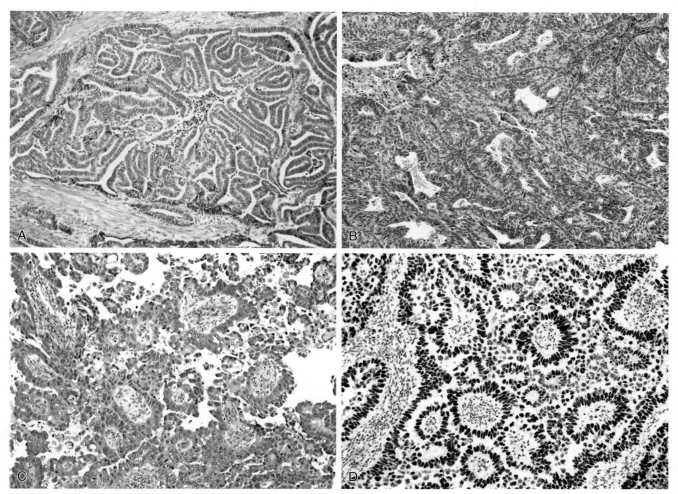

Fig. 19.12 Endometrial carcinoma. (A) Endometrioid type, grade 1, infiltrating myometrium and growing in a glandular pattern. (B) Endometrioid type, grade 3, has a predominantly solid growth pattern. (C) Serous carcinoma of the endometrium, with papilla formation and marked cytologic atypia. (D) Immunohistochemical staining shows accumulation of p53, a finding associated with *TP53* mutation.

endometrial mucosa into the uterine cavity. They are composed of endometrium resembling the basalis, frequently with small muscular arteries. Some glands are normal architecturally, but more often they are cystically dilated. The stromal cells are monoclonal, often with a rearrangement of chromosomal region 6p21, and thus constitute the neoplastic component of the polyp.

Although endometrial polyps may occur at any age, they are most common around the time of menopause. Their main clinical significance is that they may produce abnormal uterine bleeding.

Leiomyoma

Benign tumors that arise from the smooth muscle cells in the myometrium are properly termed *leiomyomas*, but because of their firmness often are referred to clinically as *fibroids*. Leiomyomas are the most common benign tumor in females, affecting 30% to 50% of women of reproductive age, and are considerably more frequent in black women. These tumors are associated with several different recurrent chromosomal abnormalities, including rearrangements of

chromosomes 6 and 12 that also are found in a variety of other benign neoplasms, such as endometrial polyps and lipomas. Mutations in the *MED12* gene, which encodes a component of the RNA polymerase transcription complex, have been identified in up to 70% of leiomyomas. The mechanism by which *MED12* mutations contribute to the development of leiomyomas is not presently understood. Estrogens and possibly oral contraceptives stimulate the growth of leiomyomas; conversely, these tumors shrink postmenopausally.

MORPHOLOGY

Leiomyomas are typically **sharply circumscribed,** firm gray-white masses with a characteristic **whorled cut surface.** They may occur singly, but more often occur as **multiple tumors** that are scattered within the uterus, ranging from small nodules to large tumors (Fig. 19.13) that may dwarf the uterus. Some are embedded within the myometrium (intramural), whereas others may lie immediately beneath the endometrium (submucosal)

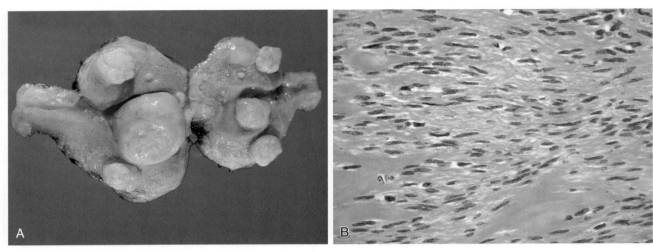

Fig. 19.13 Uterine leiomyomas. (A) The uterus is opened to show multiple submucosal, myometrial, and subserosal gray-white tumors, each with a characteristic whorled appearance on cut section. (B) Microscopic appearance of leiomyoma shows bundles of normal-looking smooth muscle cells.

or the serosa (subserosal). In the latter location, tumors may extend out on attenuated stalks and even become attached to surrounding organs, from which they may develop a blood supply (**parasitic** leiomyomas). On histologic examination, the tumors are characterized by **bundles of smooth muscle cells** mimicking the appearance of normal myometrium. Foci of fibrosis, calcification, and degenerative softening may be present.

Leiomyomas of the uterus often are asymptomatic, being discovered incidentally on routine pelvic examination. The most frequent presenting sign is menorrhagia, with or without metrorrhagia. Leiomyomas rarely, if ever, transform into sarcomas, and the presence of multiple lesions does not increase the risk of malignancy.

Leiomyosarcoma

Leiomyosarcomas of the uterus virtually always arise de novo from the mesenchymal cells of the myometrium. They are almost always solitary and most often occur in postmenopausal women, in contradistinction to leiomyomas, which frequently are multiple and usually arise premenopausally.

Recurrence after surgery is common with these cancers, and many metastasize, typically to the lungs, yielding a 5-year survival rate of about 40%. The outlook with anaplastic tumors is less favorable than with well-differentiated tumors.

MORPHOLOGY

Leiomyosarcomas typically take the form of **soft, hemorrhagic, necrotic masses.** The histologic appearance varies widely, from tumors that closely resemble leiomyoma to wildly anaplastic neoplasms. Well-differentiated tumors may lie at the morphologic interface between leiomyoma and leiomyosarcoma and are sometimes designated smooth muscle tumors of uncertain malignant potential. The diagnostic features of leiomyosarcoma include **tumor necrosis, cytologic atypia,** and **mitotic activity.** Because increased mitotic activity is sometimes seen in benign smooth muscle tumors, particularly in young women, an assessment of all three features is necessary to make a diagnosis of malignancy.

Fallopian Tubes

The most common disorder of the fallopian tubes is inflammation (salpingitis), almost invariably occurring as a component of pelvic inflammatory disease. Less common abnormalities are ectopic (tubal) pregnancy and endometriosis.

Inflammation of the fallopian tubes is almost always caused by infection. In addition to gonorrhea, nongonococcal organisms, such as *Chlamydia, Mycoplasma hominis,* coliforms, and (in the postpartum setting) streptococci and staphylococci are the major offenders. The morphologic changes produced by gonococci are similar to those in the male genital tract (Chapter 18). Infections with coliforms, streptococci, and staphylococci can penetrate the wall of the tubes, giving rise to blood-borne infections that seed to distant sites. Tuberculous salpingitis is far less common and is almost always encountered in combination with tuberculous endometritis. All forms of salpingitis may produce fever, lower abdominal or pelvic pain, and pelvic masses, which are the result of distention of the tubes with either exudate or inflammatory debris (Fig. 19.14). Adherence of the inflamed tube to the ovary and adjacent ligamentous tissues may produce a tuboovarian abscess. This may in turn result in adhesions between the ovary and the tubes when the inflammation subsides. Even more serious are adhesions of the tubal plicae, which are associated with increased risk of tubal ectopic pregnancy (discussed later).

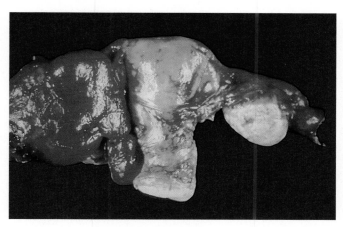

Fig. 19.14 Pelvic inflammatory disease, bilateral and asymmetric. The tube and ovary to the left of the uterus are totally obscured by a hemorrhagic inflammatory mass. The tube is adherent to the adjacent ovary on the other side.

Damage to or obstruction of the tubal lumina may produce permanent sterility.

Once thought to be uncommon, primary adenocarcinomas of the fallopian tube may be the site of origin for many of the high-grade serous carcinomas long thought to arise in the ovary. Studies have identified the presence of serous tubal intraepithelial carcinoma (STIC) in the fimbriated ends of fallopian tubes. Like the precursor of uterine serous carcinoma, STICs have mutations in *TP53* in more than 90% of cases. These lesions are found frequently in fallopian tubes removed prophylactically from women who carry mutations in *BRCA1* and *BRCA2* and less commonly in instances where tubes are removed from women without known genetic risk factors. This has led to the idea that sporadic "ovarian" serous carcinomas (discussed later) also originate in the fallopian tube. Because the fimbriated end of the fallopian tube is intimately associated with the ovary and has access to the peritoneal cavity, fallopian tube carcinomas frequently involve the ovary, omentum, and peritoneal cavity at presentation.

Ovaries

FOLLICLE AND LUTEAL CYSTS

Follicle and luteal cysts in the ovaries are so commonplace that they may be considered variants of normal physiology. These innocuous lesions originate from unruptured graafian follicles or from follicles that rupture and then immediately seal. Such cysts often are multiple and develop subjacent to the serosa of the ovary. They typically are small (1–1.5 cm in diameter) and are filled with clear serous fluid. Occasionally, they become sufficiently large (4–5 cm) to produce palpable masses and pelvic pain. When small, they are lined by granulosa lining cells or luteal cells, but as fluid accumulates, pressure may cause atrophy of these cells. Sometimes these cysts rupture, producing intraperitoneal bleeding and peritoneal symptoms (acute abdomen).

POLYCYSTIC OVARIAN SYNDROME

Polycystic ovarian syndrome (formerly called *Stein-Leventhal syndrome*) is a complex endocrine disorder characterized by hyperandrogenism, menstrual abnormalities, polycystic ovaries, chronic anovulation, and decreased fertility. It usually comes to attention after menarche in teenage girls or young adults who present with oligomenorrhea, hirsutism, infertility, and sometimes with obesity.

The ovaries are usually twice the normal size, graywhite with a smooth outer cortex, and studded with subcortical cysts 0.5 to 1.5 cm in diameter. Histologic examination shows a thickened, fibrotic ovarian capsule overlying innumerable cystic follicles lined by granulosa cells with a hyperplastic luteinized theca interna. There is a conspicuous absence of corpora lutea in the ovary.

TUMORS OF THE OVARY

In the United States it is estimated that there will be over 20,000 ovarian cancer cases diagnosed in 2016 leading to over 14,000 deaths, making ovarian cancer the fifth leading contributor to cancer mortality in women. Tumors of the ovary are remarkably varied as they may arise from any of the three cell types in the normal ovary: the multipotent surface (coelomic) epithelium, the totipotent germ cells, and the sex cord–stromal cells. Neoplasms of epithelial origin account for the great majority of ovarian tumors and, in their malignant forms, account for almost 90% of ovarian cancers (Table 19.3). Germ cell and sex cord–stromal cell tumors are much less frequent; although they constitute 20% to 30% of ovarian tumors, they are collectively responsible for less than 10% of malignant tumors of the ovary.

Surface Epithelial Tumors

The majority of ovarian tumors arise from the fallopian tube or epithelial cysts in the cortex of the ovary (Fig. 19.15). As mentioned, studies have shown that many of the tumors thought to arise from the coelomic epithelium that covers the surface of the ovary are now thought to arise from the fimbriated end of the fallopian tube (Fig. 19.15). The epithelium lining the cortical cysts may be derived from displaced ovarian surface epithelium or the lining of fallopian tube. These can become metaplastic or undergo neoplastic transformation to give rise to a number of different epithelial tumors. Benign lesions usually are cystic (cystadenoma) and may have an accompanying stromal component (cystadenofibroma). Malignant tumors also may be cystic (cystadenocarcinoma) or solid (carcinoma).

Table 19.3 Frequency of Major Ovarian Tumors

Type	Percentage of Malignant Ovarian Tumors	Percentage That Are Bilateral
Serous	47	
Benign (60%)		25
Borderline (15%)		30
Malignant (25%)		65
Mucinous	3	
Benign (80%)		5
Borderline (10%)		10
Malignant (10%)		<5
Endometrioid carcinoma	20	30
Undifferentiated carcinoma	10	—
Clear cell carcinoma	6	40
Granulosa cell tumor	5	5
Teratoma	1	
Benign (96%)		15
Malignant (4%)		Rare
Metastatic	5	>50
Others	3	—

Some ovarian epithelial tumors fall into an intermediate category currently referred to as borderline tumors. Although the majority of borderline tumors behave in a benign manner they can recur and some can progress to carcinoma.

Important risk factors for ovarian cancer include nulliparity, family history, and germline mutations in certain tumor suppressor genes. There is a higher incidence of carcinoma in unmarried women and married women with low parity. Of interest, prolonged use of oral contraceptives reduces the risk. Around 5% to 10% of ovarian cancers are familial, and most of these are associated with mutations in the *BRCA1* or *BRCA2* tumor suppressor genes. As will be discussed later, mutations in *BRCA1* and *BRCA2* also are associated with hereditary breast cancer. The average lifetime risk for ovarian cancer is approximately 30% in *BRCA1* carriers; the risk in *BRCA2* carriers is somewhat lower. In contrast with familial ovarian cancer, mutations in *BRCA1* and *BRCA2* are found in only 8% to 10% of sporadic ovarian cancers, which appear to arise through alternative molecular mechanisms.

Serous Tumors

Serous tumors are the most common of the ovarian epithelial tumors overall, and also make up the greatest fraction of malignant ovarian tumors. About 60% are benign, 15% are borderline, and 25% are malignant. Benign lesions are usually encountered in patients between 30 and 40 years of age, and malignant serous tumors are more commonly seen between 45 and 65 years of age.

There are two types of serous carcinomas, low-grade and high-grade. The former arise from benign or borderline lesions and progress slowly in a stepwise manner to become invasive carcinoma. These low-grade tumors are associated with mutations in genes encoding signaling proteins, such as *KRAS*, a member of the *RAS* gene family. The high-grade serous tumors develop rapidly. As already mentioned, many of these high-grade lesions arise in the fimbriated end of the fallopian tube via serous tubal intraepithelial carcinoma, rather than ovarian coelomic epithelium. *TP53* mutations are virtually ubiquitous in high-grade serous cancers, being present in over 95% of cases. Other frequently mutated genes include the tumor suppressors *NF1* and *RB*, as well as *BRCA1* and *BRCA2* in familial ovarian cancers.

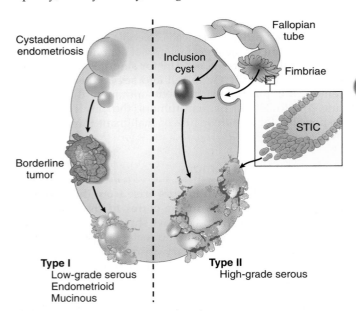

Fig. 19.15 Derivation, of various ovarian neoplasms. Type I tumors progress from benign tumors through borderline tumors that may give rise to a low-grade carcinoma. Type II tumors arise from inclusions cysts/fallopian tube epithelium via intraepithelial precursors that are often not identified. They demonstrate high-grade features and are most commonly of serous histology. STIC, serous tubal intraepithelial carcinoma.

● MORPHOLOGY

Most serous tumors are large, spherical to ovoid, cystic structures up to 30 to 40 cm in diameter. **About 25% of the benign tumors are bilateral.** In the benign tumors, the serosal covering is smooth and glistening. By contrast, the surface of adenocarcinomas often has nodular irregularities representing areas in which the tumor has invaded the serosa. On cut section, small cystic tumors may have a single cavity, but larger ones frequently are divided by multiple septa into multiloculated masses. The cystic spaces usually are filled with a clear serous fluid. Protruding into the cystic cavities are papillary projections, which are more prominent in malignant tumors (Fig. 19.16).

On histologic examination, benign tumors contain a single layer of **columnar epithelial cells** that line the cyst or cysts. The cells often are ciliated. **Psammoma bodies** (concentrically laminated calcified concretions) are common in the tips of papillae. In high-grade carcinoma the cells are markedly atypical, the papillary formations are usually complex and multilayered, and by definition nests or sheets of malignant cells invade the ovarian stroma. Between clearly benign and obviously malignant forms

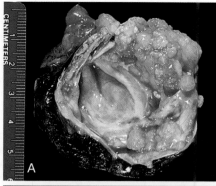

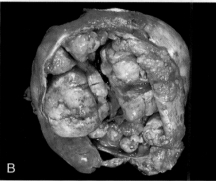

Fig. 19.16 Ovarian serous tumors. (A) Borderline serous cystadenoma opened to display a cyst cavity lined by delicate papillary tumor growths. (B) Cystadenocarcinoma. The cyst is opened to show a large, bulky tumor mass. (*Courtesy of Dr. Christopher Crum, Brigham and Women's Hospital, Boston, Massachusetts.*)

lie **borderline tumors,** which exhibit less cytologic atypia and typically no stromal invasion. Borderline tumors may seed the peritoneum, but fortunately the tumor implants usually are "noninvasive." In general, malignant serous tumors spread throughout the peritoneal cavity and to regional lymph nodes, including periaortic lymph nodes; distant lymphatic and hematogenous metastases are infrequent.

The prognosis for patients with high-grade serous carcinoma is poor, even after surgery and chemotherapy, and depends heavily on the stage of the disease at diagnosis. The 5-year survival for women with carcinoma confined to one ovary is about 90%, but falls precipitously with higher stage tumors to less than 40% depending on the exact stage. In contrast, borderline tumors are associated with nearly 100% survival. Of note, women with tumors containing BRCA1/2 mutations tend to have a better prognosis than women whose tumors lack these genetic abnormalities.

Mucinous Tumors

Mucinous tumors differ from serous tumors in two respects: the neoplastic epithelium consists of mucin-secreting cells; and mucinous tumors are considerably less likely to be malignant. Overall, only 10% of mucinous tumors are malignant; another 10% are borderline, and 80% are benign.

On gross examination, mucinous tumors produce cystic masses that may be indistinguishable from serous tumors except by the mucinous nature of the cyst contents. However, **they are more likely to be larger and** multicystic (Fig. 19.17A). **Serosal penetration and solid areas of growth are suggestive of malignancy.** Mucin-producing epithelial cells line the cysts (Fig. 19.17B). Malignant tumors are characterized by solid areas of growth, piling up (stratification) of lining cells, cytologic atypia, and stromal invasion.

Compared with serous tumors, mucinous tumors are much less likely to be bilateral. This feature is sometimes useful in differentiating mucinous tumors of the ovary from metastatic mucinous adenocarcinoma from a gastrointestinal tract primary (the so-called "**Krukenberg tumor**"), which more often produces bilateral ovarian masses.

Ruptured ovarian mucinous tumors may seed the peritoneum; however, these deposits typically regress spontaneously. Stable implantation of mucinous tumor cells in the peritoneum with production of copious amounts of mucin is called **pseudomyxoma peritonei;** in most cases, this disorder is caused by metastatic spread of tumors in the gastrointestinal tract, primarily the appendix (Chapter 15).

The prognosis of mucinous cystadenocarcinoma is somewhat better than that of its serous counterpart, although stage rather than histologic type (serous versus mucinous) is the major determinant of outcome. Mutations in *KRAS* are detected in approximately 50% of ovarian mucinous carcinomas, however this does not help distinguish them from metastatic GI tumors, which also have a high frequency of *KRAS* mutations.

Endometrioid Tumors

These tumors may be solid or cystic; they sometimes develop in association with endometriosis. On microscopic examination, they are distinguished by the formation of tubular glands, similar to those of the endometrium, within the lining of cystic spaces. Although benign and borderline forms exist, endometrioid tumors usually are malignant. They are bilateral in about 30% of cases, and 15% to 30% of women with these ovarian tumors have a concomitant endometrial carcinoma. Similar to endometrioid-type carcinoma of the endometrium, endometrioid carcinomas of the ovary frequently have mutations in the *PTEN* tumor suppressor gene as well as mutations in other genes that also act by upregulating PI3K-AKT signaling.

Brenner Tumor

The Brenner tumor is an uncommon, solid, usually unilateral ovarian tumor consisting of abundant stroma containing nests of transitional-type epithelium resembling that of the urinary tract. Occasionally, the nests are cystic and are lined by columnar mucus-secreting cells. Brenner tumors generally are smoothly encapsulated and gray-white on

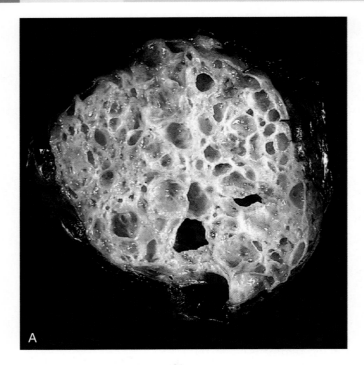

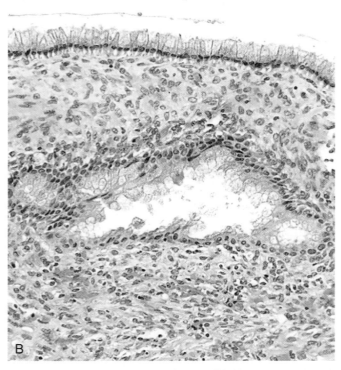

Fig. 19.17 Ovarian mucinous cystadenoma. (A) Mucinous cystadenoma with multicystic appearance and delicate septa. Note the presence of glistening mucin within the cysts. (B) Columnar cell lining of mucinous cystadenoma.

cut section, ranging from a few centimeters to 20 cm in diameter. These tumors may arise from the surface epithelium or from urogenital epithelium trapped within the germinal ridge. Although most are benign, both malignant and borderline tumors have been described.

Other Ovarian Tumors

Many other types of tumors of germ cell and sex cord–stromal origin also arise in the ovary, but only the teratomas of germ cell origin are sufficiently common to merit description. Table 19.4 presents some salient features of other neoplasms of germ cell and sex cord origin.

Teratomas

Teratomas constitute 15% to 20% of ovarian tumors. A distressing feature of these germ cell tumors is their predilection to arise in the first 2 decades of life; to make matters worse, the younger the person, the greater the likelihood of malignancy. More than 90% of these germ cell neoplasms, however, are benign mature cystic teratomas; the immature, malignant variant is rare.

Benign (Mature) Cystic Teratomas

Benign (mature) cystic teratomas are marked by the presence of mature tissues derived from all three germ cell layers: ectoderm, endoderm, and mesoderm. Usually these tumors contain cysts lined by epidermis replete with adnexal appendages—hence the common designation *dermoid cysts*. Most are discovered in young women as ovarian masses or are found incidentally on abdominal radiographs or scans because they contain foci of calcification produced by toothlike structures contained within the tumor. About 90% are unilateral, with the right side more commonly affected. Rarely do these cystic masses exceed 10 cm in diameter. On cut section, they often are filled with sebaceous secretion and matted hair that, when removed, reveal a hair-bearing epidermal lining (Fig. 19.18). Sometimes there is a nodular projection from which teeth protrude. Occasionally, foci of bone and cartilage, nests of bronchial or gastrointestinal epithelium, or other tissues are present.

For unknown reasons, these neoplasms sometimes produce infertility and are prone to undergo torsion (in 10%–15% of cases), which constitutes an acute surgical emergency. A rare, but fascinating, paraneoplastic complication is limbic encephalitis, which may develop in women with teratomas containing mature neural tissue and often remits with tumor resection. Malignant transformation, usually to a squamous cell carcinoma, is seen in about 1% of cases.

Immature Malignant Teratomas

Malignant (immature) teratomas are found early in life, the mean age at clinical detection being 18 years. They typically are bulky and appear solid on cut section, and they often contain areas of necrosis; uncommonly, cystic foci are present that contain sebaceous secretion, hair, and other features similar to those of mature teratomas. On microscopic examination, the distinguishing feature is the presence of immature elements or minimally differentiated cartilage, bone, muscle, nerve, or other tissues. As with other tumors, the prognosis depends on grade and stage.

Specialized Teratomas

A rare subtype of teratoma is composed entirely of specialized tissue. The most common example is struma ovarii,

Table 19.4 Salient Features of Ovarian Germ Cell and Sex Cord Neoplasms

Neoplasm	Peak Incidence	Usual Location	Morphologic Features	Behavior
Germ Cell Origin				
Dysgerminoma	Second to third decade of life Occur with gonadal dysgenesis	Unilateral in 80%–90%	Counterpart of testicular seminoma Sheets or cords of large clear cells Stroma may contain lymphocytes and occasional granulomas	All malignant but only one-third metastasize; all radiosensitive; 80% cure rate
Choriocarcinoma	First 3 decades of life	Unilateral	Identical to placental tumor Two types of epithelial cells: cytotrophoblast and syncytiotrophoblast	Metastasizes early and widely Primary focus may degenerate, leaving only metastases Resistant to chemotherapy
Sex Cord Tumors				
Granulosa-theca cell	Most postmenopausal, but may occur at any age	Unilateral	Composed of mixture of cuboidal granulosa cells and spindled or plump lipid-laden theca cells Granulosa elements may recapitulate ovarian follicle as Call-Exner bodies	May elaborate large amounts of estrogen Granulosa element may be malignant (5%–25%)
Thecoma-fibroma	Any age	Unilateral	Yellow (lipid-laden) plump thecal cells	Most hormonally inactive About 40% produce ascites and hydrothorax (Meigs syndrome) Rarely malignant
Sertoli-Leydig cell	All ages	Unilateral	Recapitulates development of testis with tubules or cords and plump pink Sertoli cells	Many masculinizing or defeminizing Rarely malignant
Metastases to Ovary				
	Older ages	Mostly bilateral	Anaplastic tumor cells, cords, glands, dispersed through fibrous background Cells may be "signet ring" mucin-secreting	Primaries are gastrointestinal tract (Krukenberg tumors), breast, and lung

which is composed entirely of mature thyroid tissue that may actually produce hyperthyroidism. These tumors appear as small, solid, unilateral brown ovarian masses. Other specialized teratomas include ovarian carcinoid, which in rare instances produces carcinoid syndrome.

Clinical Features

With all ovarian neoplasms, management poses a formidable clinical challenge, because symptoms or signs

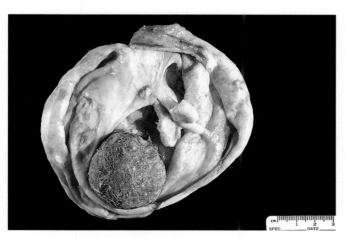

Fig. 19.18 Mature cystic teratoma (dermoid cyst) of the ovary. A ball of hair (bottom) and a mixture of tissues are evident. *(Courtesy of Dr. Christopher Crum, Brigham and Women's Hospital, Boston, Massachusetts.)*

usually appear only when tumors are well advanced. Ovarian tumors of surface epithelial origin usually are asymptomatic until they become large enough to cause local pressure symptoms (e.g., pain, gastrointestinal complaints, urinary frequency). Indeed, about 30% of all ovarian neoplasms are discovered incidentally on routine gynecologic examination. Larger masses, particularly the common epithelial tumors, may cause an increase in abdominal girth. Smaller masses, particularly dermoid cysts, sometimes twist on their pedicles (torsion), producing severe abdominal pain that mimics an acute abdomen. Metastatic seeding of malignant serous tumors often causes ascites, whereas functioning ovarian tumors often come to attention because of the endocrinopathies they produce.

Unfortunately, treatment of ovarian tumors remains unsatisfactory; only a modest increase in survival has been achieved since the mid-1970s. Screening methods that detect early tumors are badly needed, but those evaluated to date are of limited value. One such marker, the protein CA-125, is elevated in the sera of 75% to 90% of women with epithelial ovarian cancer. However, CA-125 is undetectable in up to 50% of women with cancer limited to the ovary; conversely, it often is elevated in a variety of benign conditions and nonovarian cancers. Hence, its usefulness as a screening test in asymptomatic postmenopausal women is limited. Currently, CA-125 measurements are of greatest value in monitoring response to therapy.

SUMMARY

OVARIAN TUMORS

- Tumors may arise from epithelium, sex cord–stromal cells, or germ cells.
- Epithelial tumors are the most common malignant ovarian tumor and are more common in women older than 40 years of age.
- The major types of epithelial tumors are serous, mucinous, and endometrioid. Each has a benign, malignant, and borderline counterpart.
- Serous carcinoma is the most common and many arise in the distal fallopian tube.
- Sex cord–stromal tumors may display differentiation toward granulosa, Sertoli, Leydig, or ovarian stromal cell type. Depending on differentiation, they may produce estrogens or androgens.
- Germ cell tumors (mostly cystic teratomas) are the most common ovarian tumor in young women; the vast majority are benign.
- Germ cell tumors may differentiate toward oogonia (dysgerminoma), primitive embryonal tissue (embryonal), yolk sac (endodermal sinus tumor), placental tissue (choriocarcinoma), or multiple tissue types (teratoma).

Diseases of Pregnancy

Diseases of pregnancy and pathologic conditions of the placenta are important contributors to morbidity and mortality for both mother and child. Discussed in this section are a limited number of disorders in which knowledge of the morphologic lesions contributes to an understanding of clinical disease.

PLACENTAL INFLAMMATIONS AND INFECTIONS

Infections may reach the placenta by either of two paths: (1) ascension through the birth canal or (2) hematogenous (transplacental) spread.

Ascending infections are by far the more common; in most instances they are bacterial and are associated with premature rupture of the fetal membranes. On microscopic examination, the chorioamnion shows neutrophilic infiltration associated with edema and congestion (acute chorioamnionitis). With extension beyond the membranes, the infection may involve the umbilical cord and placental villi, resulting in acute vasculitis of the cord (funisitis). Ascending infections are caused by *Mycoplasma, Candida,* and bacteria of the vaginal flora.

Uncommonly, placental infections may arise by *hematogenous spread* of bacteria and other organisms; on histologic examination, placental villi are the most frequently affected structures (villitis). Syphilis, tuberculosis, listeriosis, toxoplasmosis, and various viruses (rubella, cytomegalovirus, herpes simplex virus) all can cause placental villitis. Transplacental infections can affect the fetus and give rise to the so-called "TORCH" complex (toxoplasmosis, other infections, rubella, cytomegalovirus infection, herpes) (Chapter 7).

ECTOPIC PREGNANCY

Ectopic pregnancy is defined as implantation of a fertilized ovum in any site other than the uterus, which may occur in as many as 1% of pregnancies. In more than 90% of these cases, implantation occurs in the fallopian tube (tubal pregnancy); other sites include the ovaries and the abdominal cavity. Any factor that retards passage of the ovum through the fallopian tube predisposes to ectopic pregnancy. In about half of the cases, slowed passage results from chronic inflammation and scarring in the oviduct; intrauterine tumors and endometriosis may also hamper passage of the ovum. In the other 50% of tubal pregnancies, no anatomic cause is evident. Ovarian pregnancies probably result from rare instances in which the ovum is fertilized just as the follicle ruptures. Gestation within the abdominal cavity occurs when the fertilized egg drops out of the fimbriated end of the fallopian tube and implants on the peritoneum.

MORPHOLOGY

In all sites, early development of ectopic pregnancies proceeds normally, with formation of placental tissue, the amniotic sac, and decidual changes. With tubal pregnancies, the invading placenta eventually burrows through the wall of the fallopian tube, causing **intratubal hematoma (hematosalpinx), intraperitoneal hemorrhage,** or both. The tube is usually distended by freshly clotted blood containing bits of gray placental tissue and fetal parts. The histologic diagnosis depends on visualization of placental villi or, rarely, of the embryo.

Until rupture occurs, an ectopic pregnancy may be indistinguishable from a normal pregnancy, with cessation of menstruation and elevation of serum and urinary placental hormones. Under the influence of these hormones, the endometrium (in approximately 50% of cases) undergoes the characteristic hypersecretory and decidual changes of pregnancy. The absence of elevated gonadotropin levels does not exclude the diagnosis because poor attachment and necrosis of the ectopic placenta are common. Rupture of an ectopic pregnancy may be catastrophic, with the sudden onset of intense abdominal pain and signs of an acute abdomen, often followed by shock. Prompt surgical intervention is necessary.

SUMMARY

ECTOPIC PREGNANCY

- Ectopic pregnancy is defined as implantation of the fertilized ovum outside of the uterine corpus. Approximately 1% of pregnancies implant ectopically; the most common site is the fallopian tube.
- Chronic salpingitis with scarring is a major risk factor for tubal ectopic pregnancy.
- Rupture of an ectopic pregnancy is a medical emergency that, if left untreated, may result in exsanguination and death.

GESTATIONAL TROPHOBLASTIC DISEASE

Gestational trophoblastic disease refers to an abnormal proliferation of fetal trophoblast cells. The World Health Organization broadly divides these diseases into two categories: molar lesions and nonmolar lesions. The molar lesions are further divided into partial, complete, and invasive hydatidiform moles. The nonmolar category consists of choriocarcinoma and other more uncommon types of trophoblast-derived malignancies. All elaborate human chorionic gonadotropins (hCG), which is detected in the blood and urine at levels considerably higher than those found during normal pregnancy. In addition to aiding diagnosis, hCG levels in the blood or urine can be used to monitor treatment efficacy. Clinicians prefer the umbrella term gestational trophoblastic disease because the response to therapy, as judged by the hormone levels, is significantly more important than pathologic subtyping of lesions. However, the genetics, pathology, and natural history of these disorders are sufficiently distinct to merit discussion of each.

Hydatidiform Mole: Complete and Partial

The typical hydatidiform mole is a voluminous mass of swollen, sometimes cystically dilated, chorionic villi, appearing grossly as grapelike structures. Varying amounts of normal to highly atypical chorionic epithelium cover the swollen villi. There are two distinctive subtypes of hydatidiform moles: *complete* and *partial*. Complete hydatidiform moles are not compatible with embryogenesis and rarely contain fetal parts. All of the chorionic villi are abnormal, and the chorionic epithelial cells are diploid (46,XX or, uncommonly, 46,XY). The partial hydatidiform mole is compatible with early embryo formation and therefore may contain fetal parts, has some normal chorionic villi, and is almost always triploid (e.g., 69,XXY) (Table 19.5). Both types result from abnormal fertilization with an excess of paternal genetic material. In a complete mole the entire genetic content is supplied by two spermatozoa (or a diploid sperm), yielding diploid cells containing only paternal chromosomes, whereas in a partial mole a normal egg is fertilized by two spermatozoa (or a diploid sperm), resulting in a triploid karyotype with a preponderance of paternal genes.

Table 19.5 Features of Complete and Partial Hydatidiform Mole

Feature	Complete Mole	Partial Mole
Karyotype	46,XX (46,XY)	Triploid (69,XXY)
Villous edema	All villi	Some villi
Trophoblast proliferation	Diffuse; circumferential	Focal; slight
Serum hCG	Elevated	Less elevated
Tissue hCG	++++	+
Risk of subsequent choriocarcinoma	2%	Rare

hCG, Human chorionic gonadotropin.

The incidence of complete hydatidiform mole is about 1 to 1.5 per 2000 pregnancies in the United States and other Western countries. For unknown reasons, the incidence is much higher in Asian countries. Moles are most common before the age of 20 and after the age of 40 years, and a history of the condition increases the risk for molar disease in subsequent pregnancies. Although molar disease formerly was discovered at 12 to 14 weeks of pregnancy during investigation for a gestation that was "too large for dates," early monitoring of pregnancies by ultrasound has lowered the gestational age at detection. In both complete and partial moles, elevation of hCG in the maternal blood and absence of fetal heart sounds are typical.

MORPHOLOGY

In advanced cases the uterine cavity is expanded by a delicate, friable mass of thin-walled, translucent cystic structures (Fig. 19.19). Fetal parts are rarely seen in complete moles but are common in partial moles. On microscopic examination, the **complete mole** shows hydropic swelling of poorly vascularized chorionic villi with a loose, myxomatous, edematous stroma. The chorionic epithelium typically shows a proliferation of both cytotrophoblasts and syncytiotrophoblasts (Fig. 19.20). Histologic grading to predict the clinical outcome of moles has been supplanted by monitoring of hCG levels. In **partial moles**, villous edema involves only a subset of the villi, and the trophoblastic proliferation is focal and slight. In most cases of partial mole, some fetal cells are present, ranging from fetal red cells in placental villi to, in rare cases, a fully formed fetus.

Overall, 80% to 90% of moles do not recur after thorough curettage, but 10% of complete moles are invasive (described next). No more than 2% to 3% give rise to choriocarcinoma.

Invasive Mole

Invasive moles are complete moles that are locally invasive but lack the metastatic potential of choriocarcinoma. An invasive mole retains hydropic villi, which penetrate the uterine wall deeply, possibly causing rupture and sometimes life-threatening hemorrhage. On microscopic examination, the epithelium of the villi shows atypical changes, with proliferation of both trophoblastic and syncytiotrophoblast components.

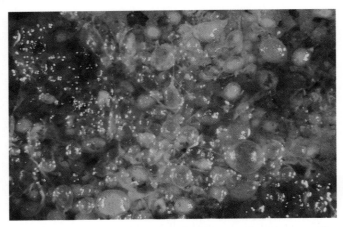

Fig. 19.19 Complete hydatidiform mole, consisting of numerous swollen (hydropic) villi.

Although the marked invasiveness of this lesion makes removal technically difficult, metastases do not occur. Hydropic villi may embolize to distant organs, such as lungs or brain, but these emboli do not behave like true metastases and may regress spontaneously. Because of deeper invasion into the myometrium, an invasive mole is difficult to remove completely by curettage, so if serum β-hCG remains elevated, further treatment is required. Fortunately, in most cases cure is possible with chemotherapy.

Gestational Choriocarcinoma

Choriocarcinoma, a very aggressive malignant tumor, arises from gestational chorionic epithelium or, less frequently, from totipotential cells within the gonads (as a germ cell tumor). These tumors are rare in the Western Hemisphere (they occur in about 1 per 30,000 pregnancies in the United States), but are much more common in Asian and African countries, reaching a frequency of 1 in 2000 pregnancies. Approximately 50% of choriocarcinomas arise from complete hydatidiform moles; about 25% arise after an abortion, while the remainder manifest following an apparently normal pregnancy. In most cases, choriocarcinoma presents as a bloody, brownish discharge accompanied by a rising titer of β-hCG in blood and urine, in the absence of marked uterine enlargement, such as would be seen with a mole. In general, the β-hCG titers are much higher than those associated with a mole.

MORPHOLOGY

Choriocarcinomas usually appear as hemorrhagic, necrotic uterine masses. Sometimes the necrosis is so extensive that little viable tumor remains. Indeed, the primary lesion may "self-destruct," and only the metastases tell the story. Very early, the tumor insinuates itself into the myometrium and into vessels. **In contrast with hydatidiform moles and invasive moles, chorionic villi are not formed; instead, the tumor is composed of anaplastic cuboidal cytotrophoblasts and syncytiotrophoblasts** (Fig. 19.21).

By the time a choriocarcinoma is discovered, widespread vascular spread usually has occurred to the lungs (50%), vagina (30%–40%), brain, liver, or kidneys. Lymphatic invasion is uncommon.

Clinical Features

Despite the extremely aggressive nature of placental choriocarcinoma, these tumors are remarkably sensitive to chemotherapy. Nearly 100% of affected patients are cured, even those with metastases at distant sites such as the lungs. By contrast, response to chemotherapy with choriocarcinomas that arise in the gonads (ovary or testis) is relatively poor. This striking difference in prognosis may be related to the presence of paternal antigens on placental choriocarcinomas that are lacking in gonadal lesions. Conceivably, a maternal immune response against the foreign (paternal) antigens helps clear the tumor by acting as an adjunct to chemotherapy.

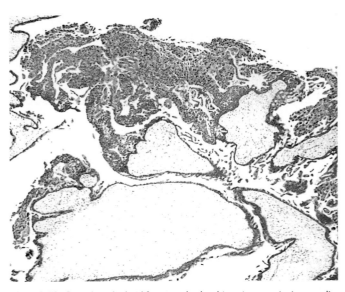

Fig. 19.20 Complete hydatidiform mole. In this microscopic image, distended hydropic villi *(below)* and proliferation of the chorionic epithelium *(above)* are evident. *(Courtesy of Dr. Kyle Molberg, Department of Pathology, University of Texas Southwestern Medical School, Dallas, Texas.)*

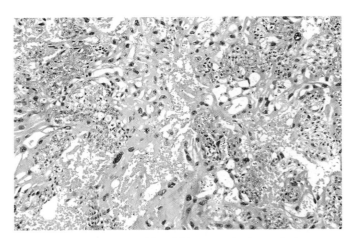

Fig. 19.21 Choriocarcinoma. This field contains both neoplastic cytotrophoblast and multinucleate syncytiotrophoblast. *(Courtesy of Dr. David R. Genest, Brigham and Women's Hospital, Boston, Massachusetts.)*

Placental Site Trophoblastic Tumor

Placental site trophoblastic tumors are derived from the placental site or intermediate trophoblast, a cell that has morphologic and functional features that overlap with those of trophoblasts and syncytiotrophoblasts. These uncommon diploid tumors, often XX in karyotype, typically arise a few months after pregnancy. Because intermediate trophoblasts do not produce hCG in large amounts, hCG concentrations are only slightly elevated. More typically, these tumors produce human placental lactogen. An indolent clinical course is typical, with a generally favorable outcome if the tumor is confined to the endomyometrium. Of note, however, placental site trophoblastic tumors are not as sensitive to chemotherapy as are other trophoblastic tumors, and the prognosis is poor when spread occurs beyond the uterus.

SUMMARY

GESTATIONAL TROPHOBLASTIC DISEASE

- Molar disease is a result of an abnormal contribution of paternal chromosomes to the conceptus.
- Partial moles are triploid and have two sets of paternal chromosomes. They typically are accompanied by fetal tissue. There is a low rate of persistent disease.
- Complete moles are diploid, and all chromosomes are paternal. Rarely are embryonic or fetal tissues associated with a complete mole.
- Among complete moles, 10% to 15% are associated with persistent disease that usually takes the form of an invasive mole. Only 2% of complete moles progress to choriocarcinoma.
- Gestational choriocarcinoma is a highly invasive and frequently metastatic tumor that, in contrast with ovarian choriocarcinoma, is responsive to chemotherapy and curable in most cases.
- Placental site trophoblastic tumor is an indolent tumor of intermediate trophoblast that produces human placental lactogen. It can be cured surgically but once it spreads it does not respond well to chemotherapy.

Preeclampsia/Eclampsia (Toxemia of Pregnancy)

The development of hypertension, accompanied by proteinuria and edema in the third trimester of pregnancy, is referred to as preeclampsia. This syndrome occurs in 5% to 10% of pregnancies, particularly with first pregnancies in women older than 35 years. In those severely affected, seizures may occur, and the symptom complex is then termed *eclampsia*. By long-existing precedent, preeclampsia and eclampsia sometimes are referred to as toxemia of pregnancy. No blood-borne toxin has been identified, and this historically sanctified term is a misnomer. Recognition and early treatment of preeclampsia have now made eclampsia, particularly fatal eclampsia, rare.

While exact triggering events initiating these syndromes are unknown, a common feature underlying all cases is insufficient maternal blood flow to the placenta secondary to inadequate remodeling of the spiral arteries of the uteroplacental vascular bed. In normal pregnancy, the musculoelastic walls of the spiral arteries are invaded by trophoblasts, permitting them to dilate into wide vascular sinusoids. In preeclampsia and eclampsia, this vascular remodeling is impaired, the musculoelastic walls are retained, and the channels remain narrow. Decreased uteroplacental blood flow appears to result in placental hypoxia, placental dysfunction, and the altered release of circulating factors that regulate angiogenesis. Specifically, increases in the anti-angiogenic factors soluble Flt1 (sFlt1) and soluble endoglin (sEng) and reductions in proangiogenic factors, such as VEGF, have been noted. These disturbances are hypothesized to result in endothelial cell dysfunction, vascular hyperreactivity, and end-organ microangiopathy. Although the exact basis of preeclampsia remains to be further defined, several serious consequences have been associated with this condition:

- *Placental infarction,* stemming from chronic hypoperfusion
- *Hypertension,* resulting from reduced endothelial production of the vasodilators prostacyclin and prostaglandin E_2 and from increased production of the vasoconstrictor thromboxane A2
- *Hypercoagulability,* due to endothelial dysfunction and release of tissue factor from the placenta
- *End-organ failure,* most notably of the kidney and the liver, which occurs in patients with full-blown eclampsia. Approximately 10% of the patients with severe preeclampsia develop the so-called "HELLP syndrome", characterized by elevated liver enzymes, microangiopathic hemolytic anemia, thrombocytopenia due to platelet consumption, and sometimes fullblown disseminated intravascular coagulation (DIC).

MORPHOLOGY

The morphologic changes of preeclampsia and eclampsia are variable and correlate to some degree with the severity of the disorder. **Placental abnormalities** include

- **Infarcts,** which can be a feature of normal pregnancy, but are much more numerous with severe preeclampsia or eclampsia
- **Retroplacental hemorrhages**
- **Premature maturation of placental villi** associated with villous edema, hypovascularity, and increased production of syncytial epithelial knots
- **Fibrinoid necrosis** and focal accumulation of lipid-containing macrophages (acute atherosis) of decidual vessels

Clinical Features

Preeclampsia presents insidiously during weeks 24 to 25 of gestation with edema, proteinuria, and rising blood pressure. Should the condition evolve into eclampsia, renal function is impaired, blood pressure rises further, and convulsions may occur. Prompt therapy early in the course aborts the associated organ changes, with all abnormalities resolving promptly after delivery or after cesarean section.

Breast

Three important features distinguish the breast from other organs. First, rather than being essential for survival, the major function is the nutritional support of another individual, the infant. Second, the structure of the organ undergoes marked changes throughout life: expansion of the lobular system after menarche, periodic remodeling during adulthood, especially during and after pregnancy, and ultimately involution and regression of lobules. Finally, breasts are visible and as a result have a social, cultural, and personal significance not shared by other organs. All of these features play a role when considering the origins, presentations, and treatment of breast disease.

The functional unit of the breast is the lobule, which is supported by a specialized intralobular stroma. The inner luminal epithelial cells produce milk during lactation. The basally located myoepithelial cells have contractile function to aid in milk ejection and also help support the basement membrane. The ducts are conduits for milk to reach the nipple. The size of the breast is determined primarily by interlobular stroma, which increases during puberty and involutes with age. Each normal constituent is a source of both benign and malignant lesions (Fig. 19.22).

CLINICAL PRESENTATIONS OF BREAST DISEASE

The predominant symptoms and signs of diseases of the breast are pain, inflammatory changes, nipple discharge, "lumpiness," or a palpable mass (Fig. 19.23A). However, few symptoms are so severe as to require treatment, and the primary reason for investigating their cause is to evaluate the possibility of malignancy. Most symptomatic breast lesions (>90%) are benign. Of women with cancer, about 45% have symptoms, whereas the remainder come to attention through screening tests (Fig. 19.23B).

- *Pain* (mastalgia or mastodynia) is a common symptom often related to menses, possibly due to cyclic edema and swelling. Pain localized in a specific area is usually caused by a ruptured cyst or trauma to adipose tissue (fat necrosis). Almost all painful masses are benign, but for unknown reasons a small fraction of cancers (about 10%) cause pain.
- *Inflammation* causes an edematous and erythematous breast. It is rare and is most often caused by infections, which only occur with any frequency during lactation and breastfeeding. An important mimic of

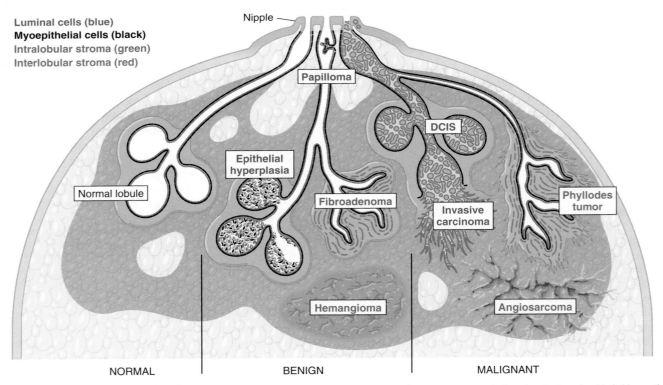

Luminal cells (blue)
Myoepithelial cells (black)
Intralobular stroma (green)
Interlobular stroma (red)

Nipple

Papilloma

DCIS

Epithelial hyperplasia

Normal lobule

Fibroadenoma

Invasive carcinoma

Phyllodes tumor

Hemangioma

Angiosarcoma

NORMAL   BENIGN   MALIGNANT

Fig. 19.22 Origins of breast disorders. Benign epithelial lesions include intraductal papillomas that grow in sinuses below the nipple and epithelial hyperplasia that arises in lobules. Malignant epithelial lesions are mainly breast carcinomas, which may remain in situ or invade into the breast and spread by metastasis. Specialized intralobular stroma *(green)* cells may give rise to fibroadenomas and phyllodes tumors, whereas interlobular stroma *(green)* may give rise to a variety of rare benign and malignant tumors.

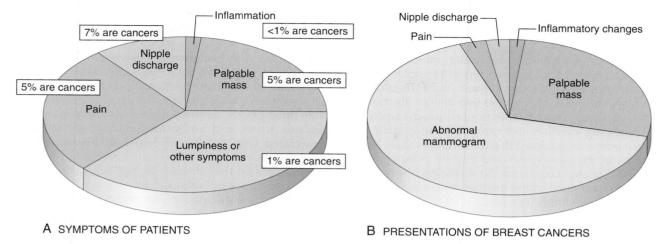

Fig. 19.23 Presenting symptoms of breast disease. (A) Common breast-related symptoms that bring patients to clinical attention. (B) Presentations of breast cancer.

inflammation is "inflammatory" breast carcinoma (discussed later).

- *Nipple discharge* may be normal when small in quantity and bilateral. The most common benign lesion producing a nipple discharge is a papilloma arising in the large ducts below the nipple (Fig. 19.22). Discharges that are spontaneous, unilateral, and bloody are of greatest concern for malignancy.
- *Lumpiness,* or a diffuse nodularity throughout the breast, is usually a result of normal glandular tissue. When pronounced, imaging studies may help to determine whether a discrete mass is present.
- *Palpable masses* can arise from proliferations of stromal cells or epithelial cells and are generally detected when they are 2 to 3 cm in size (Fig. 19.22). Most (~95%) are benign; these tend to be round to oval and to have circumscribed borders. In contrast, malignant tumors usually invade across tissue planes and have irregular borders. However, because some cancers grow deceptively as circumscribed masses, all palpable masses require evaluation.
- *Gynecomastia* is the only common breast symptom in males. There is an increase in both stroma and epithelial cells resulting from an imbalance between estrogens, which stimulate breast tissue, and androgens, which counteract these effects.

Regardless of presenting symptom, the likelihood of malignancy increases with age. For example, the risk of nipple discharge being due to cancer increases from 7% in women younger than 60 years of age to 30% in women older than 60. Similarly, only 10% of palpable masses in women younger than 40 years of age are carcinomas, as compared to 60% in women older than 50.

Mammographic screening was introduced in the 1980s as a means to detect early, nonpalpable asymptomatic breast carcinomas before metastatic spread has occurred. Mammography has met this promise, as the average size of invasive carcinomas detected by mammography is about 1 cm (significantly smaller than cancers identified by palpation), and only 15% will have metastasized to regional lymph nodes at the time of diagnosis. In the United States, most cancers in women more than 50 years of age are now detected by mammography (Fig. 19.23B). As with symptomatic breast lesions, the likelihood that an abnormal mammographic finding is caused by malignancy increases with age, from 10% at age 40 to more than 25% in women older than age 50.

<table>
<tr><td>🔴</td><td>SUMMARY</td></tr>
</table>

CLINICAL PRESENTATIONS OF BREAST DISEASE

- Symptoms affecting the breasts are evaluated primarily to determine if malignancy is present.
- Regardless of the symptom, the underlying cause is benign in the majority of cases.
- Breast cancer is most commonly detected by palpation of a mass in younger women and in unscreened populations and by mammographic screening in older women.

INFLAMMATORY PROCESSES

Inflammatory diseases of the breast are rare and may be caused by infections, autoimmune disease, or foreign body–type reactions. Symptoms include erythema and edema, often accompanied by pain and focal tenderness. Because inflammatory diseases are rare, the possibility that the symptoms are caused by inflammatory carcinoma should always be considered (discussed later).

The only infectious agent to cause breast disease with any frequency is *Staphylococcus aureus,* which typically gains entry via fissures in nipple skin during the first weeks of breastfeeding. The invading organisms may lead to the formation of "lactational abscesses," collections of neutrophils and associated bacteria in fibroadipose tissue. If untreated, tissue necrosis may lead to the appearance of fistula tracks opening onto the skin. Most cases are treated adequately with antibiotics and continued expression of milk. Rarely, surgical incision and drainage is required.

STROMAL NEOPLASMS

The two types of stroma in the breast, intralobular and interlobular, give rise to different types of neoplasms (Fig. 19.22). Historically, tumors derived from intralobular stroma have been cleanly divided into benign fibroadenomas and more cellular phyllodes tumors, which sometimes recur following excision and rarely pursue a malignant course. It is now appreciated that these tumors share driver mutations in the same genes and appear to be part of a spectrum of related neoplasms. Nevertheless, the old classification is engrained in the medical lexicon and we will follow it here for simplicity's sake.

MORPHOLOGY

Tumors derived from intralobular stroma are comprised of both stromal cells and epithelial cells (i.e., they are "biphasic"), as the neoplastic proliferation of specialized lobular fibroblasts also stimulates reactive proliferation of lobular epithelial cells. As the intralobular fibroblasts proliferate, they push and distort the epithelial cells so that they form elongated slitlike structures rather than round acini. In benign **fibroadenoma**, the tumor mass has circumscribed borders and low cellularity (Fig. 19.24A); mitoses are rare. By contrast, in **phyllodes tumors** the stromal cells tend to outgrow the epithelial cells, resulting in bulbous nodules of proliferating stromal cells that are covered by epithelium (Fig. 19.24B), the characteristic "phyllodes" (Greek for "leaflike") growth pattern. In high-grade phyllodes tumors epithelium may be scant or absent, producing a sarcomatous appearance. Overall, about 2% of phyllodes tumors metastasize to distant sites.

Lesions of interlobular stroma are monophasic (only comprised of mesenchymal cells) and include benign soft tissue tumors found elsewhere in the body, such as hemangiomas (Chapter 10) and lipomas (Chapter 21). The only malignancy derived from interlobular stromal cells of note is angiosarcoma (Chapter 21), which may arise in the breast after local radiotherapy. The morphologies of these lesions are described elsewhere.

BENIGN EPITHELIAL LESIONS

The majority of benign epithelial lesions are incidental findings detected by mammography. Their major clinical significance is their relationship to the subsequent risk of developing breast cancer. Benign changes are divided into three groups, *nonproliferative disease*, *proliferative disease without atypia*, and *proliferative disease with atypia*, each associated with a different degree of breast cancer risk (Table 19.6).

- Nonproliferative disease is not associated with an increased risk of breast cancer.
- Proliferative disease without atypia encompasses polyclonal hyperplasias that are associated with a slightly increased risk of breast cancer.
- Proliferative disease with atypia includes monoclonal "precancers" that are associated with a modest increase in the risk of breast cancer in both breasts; overall, 13% to 17% of women with these lesions develop breast cancer.

MORPHOLOGY

Nonproliferative disease consists of three major morphologic changes: cysts, fibrosis, and adenosis. It is termed "nonproliferative" because the lesions contain single layers of epithelial cells. The most common nonproliferative breast lesions are simple cysts lined by a layer of luminal cells that often undergo apocrine metaplasia (Fig. 19.25A). The apocrine secretions may calcify and be detected by mammography. When cysts rupture, chronic inflammation and fibrosis in response to the spilled debris may produce palpable nodularity of the breast (so-called "fibrocystic changes"). **Proliferative disease without atypia** includes epithelial hyperplasia, sclerosing adenosis, complex sclerosing lesion, and papilloma. Each is associated with varying degrees of epithelial cell proliferation. For example, in epithelial

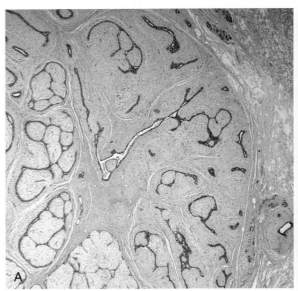
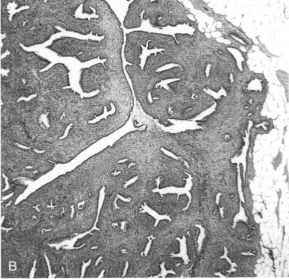

Fig. 19.24 Intralobular stromal neoplasms. (A) Fibroadenoma. This benign tumor has an expansile growth pattern with pushing circumscribed borders. (B) Phyllodes tumors. Proliferating stromal cells distort the glandular tissue, forming cleftlike spaces, and bulge into surrounding stroma.

Table 19.6 Factors Associated With Development of Invasive Carcinoma

Factor	Relative Risk[a]	Absolute Lifetime Risk[a]
Women with no risk factors	1.0	3%
First-degree relative(s) with breast cancer[b]	1.2–9.0	4%–30%
Germline tumor suppressor gene mutation (e.g., *BRCA1* mutation)	2.0–45.0	6% to >90%
Menstrual History		
Age at menarche <12 years	1.3	4%
Age at menopause >55 years	1.5–2.0	5%–6%
Pregnancy		
First live birth <20 years (protective)	0.5	1.6%
First live birth 20–35 years	1.5–2.0	5%–6%
First live birth >35 years	2.0–3.0	6%–10%
Never pregnant (nulliparous)	3.0	10%
Breast-feeding (slightly protective)	0.8	2.6%
Benign Breast Disease		
Proliferative disease without atypia	1.5–2.0	5%–6%
Proliferative disease with atypia (ALH and ADH)	4.0–5.0	13%–17%
Carcinoma in situ (ductal or lobular)	8.0–10.0	25%–30%
Ionizing radiation	1.1–1.4	3.6%–4.6%
Mammographic density	3.0–7.0	10%–23%
Postmenopausal obesity and weight gain	1.1–3.0	3.6%–10%
Postmenopausal hormone replacement	1.1–3.0	3.6%–10%
Alcohol consumption	1.1–1.4	3.6%–4.6%
Alcohol consumption	1.1–1.4	3.6%–4.6%

[a]Relative risk is the likelihood of developing cancer compared to a woman with no risk factors—whose relative risk is 1.0. Absolute lifetime risk is the fraction of women expected to develop invasive carcinoma without a risk reducing intervention. For women with no risk factors, there is about a 3% chance of developing invasive breast cancer.
[b]The most common family history is a mother who developed cancer after menopause. This history does not increase the risk of her daughters.

hyperplasia, increased numbers of both spindled myoepithelial cells and epithelioid luminal cells expand ductal and lobular spaces (Fig. 19.25B).

Proliferative disease with atypia includes atypical lobular hyperplasia (ALH) and atypical ductal hyperplasia (ADH). ALH closely resembles lobular carcinoma in situ (LCIS) and ADH closely resembles ductal carcinoma in situ (DCIS) (both described later), but are more limited in extent. The cells in ADH are uniform in appearance and form sharply marginated spaces or rigid bridges (Fig. 19.25C).

CARCINOMA

Breast carcinoma is the most common malignancy of women globally (excluding nonmelanoma skin cancer) and causes the majority of cancer deaths in women. Although the incidence in the United States decreased slightly in 2002 and then stabilized (changes attributed to a decrease in the use of postmenopausal hormone therapy and a plateau in the number of women undergoing mammographic screening), the worldwide incidence

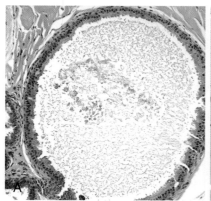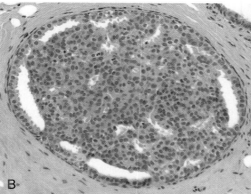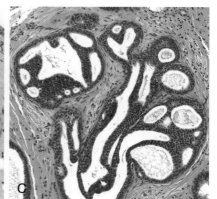

Fig. 19.25 Benign epithelial breast disease. (A) Nonproliferative disease. An apocrine cyst is shown that is a common feature of nonproliferative breast disease. (B) Proliferative breast disease is characterized by increased numbers of epithelial cells, as in this example of epithelial hyperplasia. (C) Proliferative breast disease with atypia. The proliferating epithelial cells are monomorphic in appearance and pile up to form abnormal architectural structures.

and mortality is increasing at an alarming rate. The major factors underlying this trend in developing countries are thought to be social changes that increase breast cancer risk—specifically, delayed childbearing, fewer pregnancies, and reduced breastfeeding—combined with a lack of access to optimal health care.

The lifetime risk of breast cancer is 1 in 8 for women living to age 90 in the United States. It is predicted that about 250,000 breast cancers will be diagnosed in 2016 and about 40,000 women will die of the disease—a toll among cancers second only to lung cancer. Since the mid-1980s the mortality rate has dropped from 30% to less than 20%. The decrease is attributed to both improved screening, which detects some cancers before they have metastasized, and more effective systemic treatment.

Almost all breast malignancies are adenocarcinomas (>95%). In the most clinically useful classification system, breast cancers are divided based on the expression of hormone receptors—estrogen receptor (ER) and progesterone receptor (PR)—and the expression of the human epidermal growth factor receptor 2 (HER2, also known as ERBB2), into three major groups:

- ER positive (HER2 negative; 50%–65% of cancers)
- HER2 positive (ER positive or negative; 10%–20% of cancers)
- Triple negative (ER, PR, and HER2 negative; 10%–20% of cancers)

These three groups show striking differences in patient characteristics, pathologic features, treatment response, metastatic patterns, time to relapse, and outcome (Table 19.7 and Fig. 19.26). Within each group are additional histologic subtypes (discussed later), some of which also have clinical importance.

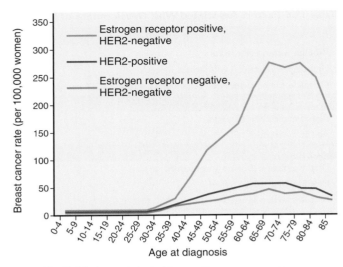

Fig. 19.26 Age and the incidence of breast cancer subtypes.

An alternative classification system with substantial overlap relies on gene expression profiling. This system, which is currently used mainly in the context of clinical research, divides breast cancers into four major types:

- *Luminal A.* The majority are lower-grade ER-positive cancers that are HER2 negative
- *Luminal B.* The majority are higher-grade ER-positive cancers that may be HER2 positive
- *HER2-enriched.* The majority overexpress HER2 and do not express ER
- *Basal-like.* The majority by gene expression profiling resemble basally located myoepithelial cells and are ER-negative, HER2-negative

Table 19.7 Summary of the Major Biologic Types of Breast Cancer

Feature	ER Positive/HER2 Negative	HER2 Positive (ER Positive or Negative)	Triple Negative (ER, PR, and HER2 Negative)
Overall frequency	50%–65%	20%	15%
Typical patient groups	Older women; men; cancers detected by screening; germline *BRCA2* mutation carriers	Young women; germline *TP53* mutation carriers	Young women; germline *BRCA1* mutation carriers
Ethnicity			
European/American	70%	18%	12%
African/American	52%	22%	26%
Hispanic	60%	24%	16%
Asian/Pacific Islander	63%	26%	11%
Grade	Mainly grade 1 and 2	Mainly grade 2 and 3	Mainly grade 3
Complete response to chemotherapy	Low grade (<10%), higher grade (10%)	ER positive (15%), ER negative (>30%)	30%
Timing of relapse	May be late (>10 years after diagnosis)	Usually short (<10 years after diagnosis)	Usually short (<8 years after diagnosis)
Metastatic sites	Bone (70%), viscera (25%), brain (<10%)	Bone (70%), viscera (45%), brain (30%)	Bone (40%), viscera (35%), brain (25%)
Similar group defined by mRNA profiling	Luminal A (low grade), luminal B (high grade)	Luminal B (ER positive), HER2-enriched (ER negative)	Basal-like
Common special histologic types	Lobular, tubular, mucinous, papillary	Apocrine, micropapillary	Carcinoma with medullary features
Common somatic mutations	*PIK3CA* (40%), *TP53* (26%)	*TP53* (75%), *PIK3CA* (40%)	*TP53* (85%)

PIK3CA encodes phosphoinositide 3-kinase (PI3K).

Epidemiology and Risk Factors

A large number of risk factors for breast cancer have been identified (Table 19.6). Some of the more important risk factors are summarized next.

Age and Gender. Breast cancer is rare in women younger than age 25, but increases in incidence rapidly after age 30 (Fig. 19.26); 75% of women with breast cancer are older than 50 years of age, and only 5% are younger than 40. The incidence in men is only 1% of that in women.

Family History of Breast Cancer. The greatest risk is for individuals with multiple affected first-degree relatives with early-onset breast cancer. In most families, it is thought that various combinations of low penetrance, "weak" cancer genes are responsible for increased risk. However, approximately 5% to 10% of breast cancers occur in persons who inherit highly penetrant germline mutations in tumor suppressor genes (discussed later). For these individuals, the lifetime risk of breast cancer may be greater than 90%.

Geographic Factors. Significant differences in the incidence and mortality rates of breast cancer have been reported in various countries. The risk is significantly higher in the Americas and Europe than in Asia and Africa. For example, the incidence and mortality rates are five times higher in the United States than in Japan. Some risk factors must be modifiable because migrants from low-incidence to high-incidence areas tend to acquire the rates of their new home countries. Diet, reproductive patterns, and breastfeeding practices are thought to be involved. In line with this, breast cancer rates appear to be rising in parts of the world that are adopting Western habits.

Race/Ethnicity. The highest rate of breast cancer is in women of European descent, largely because of a higher incidence of ER-positive cancers. Hispanic and African American women tend to develop cancer at a younger age and are more likely to develop aggressive tumors. Such disparities are thought to result from a combination of differences in genetics, social factors, and access to health care and are an area of intense study.

Reproductive History. Early age of menarche, nulliparity, absence of breastfeeding, and older age at first pregnancy are all associated with increased risk, probably because each increases the exposure of "at-risk" breast epithelial cells to estrogenic stimulation.

Ionizing Radiation. Radiation to the chest increases the risk of breast cancer if exposure occurs while the breast is still developing. For example, breast cancer develops in 25% to 30% of women who underwent irradiation for Hodgkin lymphoma in their teens and 20s, but the risk for women treated later in life is not elevated.

Other Risk Factors. Postmenopausal obesity, postmenopausal hormone replacement, mammographic density, and alcohol consumption also have been implicated as risk factors. The risk associated with obesity probably is due to exposure of the breast to estrogen produced by adipose tissue. In keeping with this, obesity is only associated with an increased risk of tumors that express ER.

Pathogenesis

The three major subtypes of breast cancer defined by differential expression of hormone receptors and HER2 arise through more-or-less distinct pathways that involve the stepwise acquisition of driver mutations in the epithelial cells of the duct/lobular system (Fig. 19.27). Factors that contribute directly to the development of breast cancer can be grouped into genetic, hormonal, and environmental categories.

Genetic. Driver mutations in cancer genes that contribute to breast carcinogenesis can be divided into those that are inherited and those that are acquired. **The major germline mutations conferring susceptibility to breast cancer affect genes that regulate genomic stability or that are involved in progrowth signaling pathways.** *BRCA1* and *BRCA2* are classic tumor suppressor genes, in that cancer arises only when both alleles are inactivated or defective (Chapter 6). *BRCA1* and *BRCA2* encode proteins that are required for repair of certain kinds of DNA damage. They are normally expressed in many different cells and tissues, and why germline mutations in these genes lead mainly to an increased risk of breast and serous ovarian cancer (discussed earlier) remains mysterious. The degree of penetrance, age of onset, and susceptibility to other types of cancers differ among the many *BRCA1* and *BRCA2* germline mutations, but most carriers develop breast cancer by the age of 70 years, as compared to about 12% of women with an average risk of breast cancer. For unclear reasons, *BRCA2* mutations are primarily associated with ER-positive tumors, whereas *BRCA1* mutations show a strong association with triple-negative cancers (Fig. 19.27). Other mutated genes associated with familial breast cancer include *TP53* (the so-called "guardian of the genome", Chapter 6) and *PTEN* (an important negative regulator of the pro-growth PI3K-AKT pathway), already mentioned earlier as a risk factor for endometrial carcinoma as part of *Cowden syndrome*.

As might be expected, **the pathways in which familial breast cancer genes function also are often disturbed in sporadic breast cancers.** Somatic mutations in *BRCA1* and *BRCA2* are rare in sporadic cancers, but *BRCA1* is inactivated by methylation in up to 50% of triple-negative cancers. Somatic mutations in *TP53* are common in breast cancer, particularly triple-negative and HER2-positive tumors (Table 19.7), whereas mutations that activate PI3K-AKT signaling are frequently found in sporadic ER-positive and HER2-positive breast cancers (Fig. 19.27).

A common clinically important driver mutation in breast cancer is amplification of the *HER2* gene. HER2 is a receptor tyrosine kinase that promotes cell proliferation and opposes apoptosis by stimulating the RAS- and PI3K-AKT signaling pathways. Cancers that overexpress HER2 are pathogenically distinct and highly proliferative. In the past they had a poor prognosis; however, the availability of therapeutic agents that specifically target HER2 has markedly improved the prognosis for patients with HER2-amplified tumors.

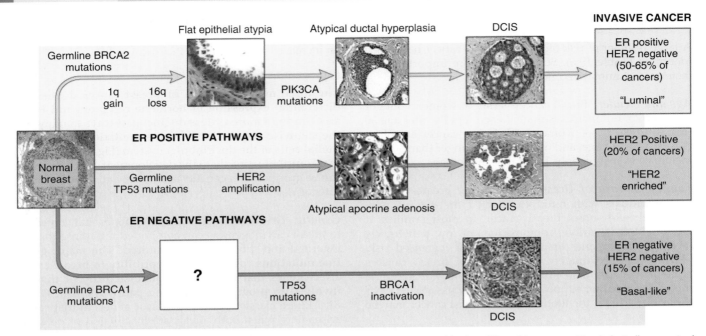

Fig. 19.27 Major pathways of breast cancer development. The most common pathway *(yellow arrow)* leads to ER-positive cancers. Morphologically recognized precursor lesions include flat epithelial atypia, ADH, and DCIS, all of which share certain genomic events with invasive ER-positive carcinomas, such gains of chromosome 1, losses of chromosome 16, and mutations of *PIK3CA* (the gene encoding PI3K). By gene expression profiling, these cancers are classified as "luminal." This is the type of cancer that arises most commonly in individuals with germline *BRCA2* mutations. Less common are cancers that overexpress HER2 because of gene amplification *(green arrow)*. These cancers may be positive or negative for ER and are usually associated with germline *TP53* mutations. A possible precursor lesion is atypical apocrine adenosis, which shares features with apocrine DCIS. The least common but molecularly most distinctive type of breast cancer is negative for ER and HER2 ("triple negative"; *blue arrow*). These cancers have loss of *BRCA1* and *TP53* function and are genomically unstable. The majority of triple-negative cancers are classified as "basal-like" by gene expression profiling.

Hormonal Influences. Estrogens stimulate the production of growth factors, such as transforming growth factor-α, platelet-derived growth factor, fibroblast growth factor, and others, which may promote tumor development through paracrine and autocrine mechanisms. In addition, ER regulates dozens of other genes in an estrogen-dependent fashion, some of which are important for tumor development or growth. Hormonal influences likely drive proliferation during the development of cancers from precursor lesions (which typically strongly express ER) to fully malignant and even metastatic carcinomas. The clearest measure of the importance of estrogen is found in the therapeutic benefits of estrogen antagonists, which reduce the development of ER-positive cancers in women at high risk and are mainstays in the treatment of established ER-positive tumors.

Environmental Factors. Environmental influences are suggested by the variable incidence of breast cancer in genetically homogeneous groups (e.g., Japanese women living in Japan and the United States) and the geographic differences in breast cancer incidence, as discussed earlier.

MORPHOLOGY

The most common location of tumors within the breast is in the upper outer quadrant (50%), followed by the central portion (20%). About 4% of women with breast cancer have bilateral primary tumors or sequential lesions in the same breast.

Breast cancers are classified morphologically according to whether they have penetrated the basement membrane. Those that remain within this boundary are termed *in situ carcinomas*, and those that have spread beyond it are designated *invasive carcinomas*. In this classification, the main forms of breast carcinoma are as follows:

A. Noninvasive
   1. Ductal carcinoma in situ
   2. Lobular carcinoma in situ
B. Invasive
   1. Invasive ductal carcinoma (includes all carcinomas that are not of a special type)—70% to 80%
   2. Invasive lobular carcinoma— ~10% to 15%
   3. Carcinoma with medullary features— ~5%
   4. Mucinous carcinoma (colloid carcinoma) — ~5%
   5. Tubular carcinoma— ~5%
   6. Other types

Noninvasive (in Situ) Carcinoma

There are two morphologic types of noninvasive breast carcinoma: ductal carcinoma in situ (DCIS) and lobular carcinoma in situ (LCIS). The terms *ductal* and *lobular* are misleading, as both types of CIS are thought to arise from cells in the terminal duct that give rise to lobules. LCIS usually expands involved lobules (Fig. 19.28A), whereas DCIS distorts lobules into ductlike spaces (Fig. 19.28B). By definition, both "respect" the basement membrane and do not invade into stroma or lymphovascular channels.

DCIS has a wide variety of histologic appearances, including solid, comedo, cribriform, papillary, micropapillary, and "clinging"

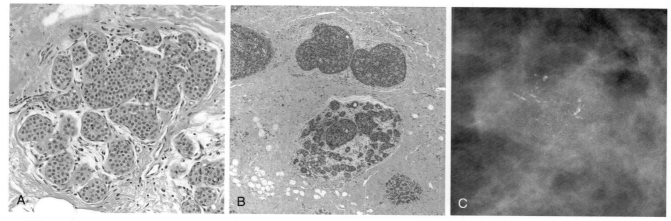

Fig. 19.28 Carcinoma in situ. (A) Lobular carcinoma in situ (LCIS). (B) Ductal carcinoma in situ (DCIS). DCIS partially involves the lobule in the lower half of this photo and has completely effaced the upper lobules, producing a ductlike appearance. (C) Mammographic detection of calcifications associated with DCIS.

types. Nuclear appearances range from bland and monotonous (low nuclear grade) to pleomorphic (high nuclear grade). The distinctive **comedo** subtype is characterized by extensive central necrosis, which produces toothpastelike necrotic tissue that extrudes from transected ducts on application of gentle pressure. **Calcifications frequently are associated with DCIS** (Fig. 19.28C), resulting from calcification of necrotic debris or secretory material. DCIS constitutes only 5% of breast cancers in unscreened populations but up to 30% in screened populations, largely because of the ability of mammography to detect calcifications. Current treatment strategies for DCIS use surgery and irradiation to eradicate the lesion. Treatment with anti-estrogenic agents such as tamoxifen also is used to decrease the risk of recurrence of ER-positive DCIS. The prognosis is excellent, with greater than 97% long-term survival. If untreated, DCIS progresses to invasive cancer in roughly one-third of cases, usually in the same breast and quadrant as the earlier DCIS.

Paget disease of the nipple is caused by the extension of DCIS up the lactiferous ducts and into the contiguous skin of the nipple, producing a unilateral crusting exudate over the nipple and areolar skin. Unlike Paget disease of the vulva (described earlier), Paget disease of the nipple stems from in situ extension of an underlying carcinoma. The prognosis of the carcinoma of origin is affected by the presence of Paget disease and is determined by other factors (discussed under Clinical Features).

LCIS has a uniform appearance. The cells are monomorphic, have bland, round nuclei, and are found in loosely cohesive clusters within the lobules (Fig. 19.28A). LCIS is virtually always an incidental finding because, unlike DCIS, it is only rarely associated with calcifications. Therefore, the incidence of LCIS has remained unchanged in mammographically screened populations. Approximately one-third of women with LCIS eventually develop invasive carcinoma. Unlike DCIS, invasive carcinomas following a diagnosis of LCIS may arise in either breast—⅔ in the same breast and ⅓ in the contralateral breast. Thus, **LCIS is both a marker of an increased risk of carcinoma in both breasts and a direct precursor of some cancers.** Current treatment options include close clinical and radiologic follow-up, chemoprevention with tamoxifen or, less commonly, bilateral prophylactic mastectomy.

Invasive (Infiltrating) Carcinoma

The distinctive histologic patterns of the subtypes of invasive carcinoma are described first, followed by grading, which is used for all.

Invasive ductal carcinoma is a term used for all carcinomas that cannot be subclassified into one of the specialized types described below. A majority (70%–80%) of cancers falls into this group. This type of cancer usually is associated with DCIS. The microscopic appearance varies, ranging from tumors with well-developed tubules and low-grade nuclei (Fig. 19.29A) to tumors consisting of sheets of anaplastic cells. Most invasive ductal carcinomas produce a desmoplastic response, which replaces normal breast fat (resulting in a mammographic density; Fig. 19.29B) and eventually leads to the appearance of a hard, palpable irregular mass. About 50% to 65% of ductal carcinomas are ER positive, 20% are HER2 positive, and 15% are negative for both ER and HER2 (Table 19.7).

Invasive lobular carcinoma consists of infiltrating cells that are morphologically similar to the tumor cells seen in LCIS; indeed, two-thirds of the cases are associated with LCIS. These tumors comprise 10% to 15% of all breast carcinomas. The cells invade stroma individually and often are aligned in "single-file" (Fig. 19.29C). Although most manifest as palpable masses or mammographic densities, a significant subgroup invade without producing a desmoplastic response; such tumors may be clinically occult and difficult to detect by imaging (Fig. 19.29D). The pattern of metastasis of lobular carcinoma is unique among breast cancers, as they frequently spread to cerebrospinal fluid, serosal surfaces, gastrointestinal tract, ovary, uterus, and bone marrow. Almost all lobular carcinomas express hormone receptors, whereas HER2 overexpression is rare.

Carcinomas with medullary features are a special type of triple-negative cancer comprising about 5% of all breast cancers. These carcinomas typically grow as rounded masses that can be difficult to distinguish from benign tumors on imaging (Fig. 19.29F). They consist of sheets of large anaplastic cells associated with pronounced lymphocytic infiltrates composed predominantly of T cells (Fig. 19.29E). The presence of lymphocytes is associated with a favorable prognosis, at least in part due to a better response to chemotherapy compared to poorly differentiated carcinomas without lymphoid infiltrates. This type

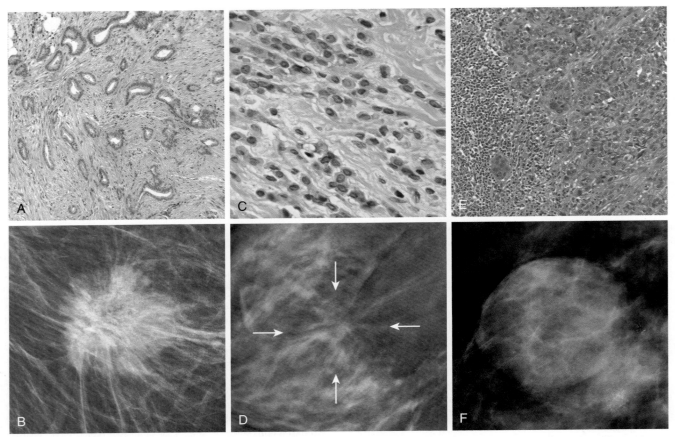

Fig. 19.29 Growth patterns of invasive breast carcinomas. (A) Most grow as tubules ("ductal" carcinoma) and stimulate a reactive desmoplastic stromal proliferation. In mammograms (B), these carcinomas appear as dense masses with spicular margins resulting from invasion of adjacent radiolucent breast tissue. (C) Lobular carcinomas are composed of noncohesive tumor cells that invade as linear cords of cells and induce little stromal response. Accordingly, in mammograms (D) lobular carcinomas often appear as relatively subtle, irregular masses *(arrows)*. (E) Uncommonly, carcinomas consist of tightly adhesive clusters of cells, as in this carcinoma with medullary features, or when there is abundant extracellular mucin production. (F) Such tumors may appear as well-circumscribed masses in mammograms, mimicking the appearance of a benign lesion.

of carcinoma is seen frequently in women with germline *BRCA1* mutations, but most women with these carcinomas are not carriers.

Mucinous (colloid) carcinoma is an ER-positive/HER2-negative tumor that produces abundant amounts of extracellular mucin. The tumors usually are soft and gelatinous because of the presence of mucin pools that create an expansile circumscribed mass.

Tubular carcinoma is another type of ER-positive/HER2-negative cancer and is almost always detected on mammography as a small irregular mass. The tumor cells are arranged in well-formed tubules and have low-grade nuclei. Lymph node metastases are rare, and the prognosis is excellent.

Inflammatory carcinoma is defined by its clinical presentation, rather than a specific morphology. Patients present with a swollen erythematous breast without a palpable mass. The underlying invasive carcinoma is generally poorly differentiated and diffusely infiltrates and obstructs dermal lymphatic spaces, causing the "inflamed" appearance; true inflammation is absent. Many of these tumors metastasize to distant sites; the overall 5-year survival is less than 50%, and understandably even lower in those with metastatic disease at diagnosis. About half express ER and 40% to 60% overexpress HER2.

All types of invasive breast carcinoma are assigned a grade from 1 (low-grade) to 3 (high-grade) based on nuclear pleomorphism, tubule formation, and proliferation. Low-grade nuclei are similar in appearance to the nuclei of normal cells. High-grade nuclei are enlarged and have irregular nuclear contours resulting from abnormal DNA content and structure. Most low-grade carcinomas form well-defined tubules and may be difficult to distinguish from benign lesions, whereas high-grade carcinomas lose this capacity and invade as solid sheets or single cells. Proliferation is evaluated by counting mitotic figures. The majority of HER2-positive and triple-negative carcinomas are highly proliferative, whereas ER-positive cancers show a wide range of proliferation.

Clinical Features

As previously discussed, in unscreened populations (including young women, for whom screening is not indicated) most breast cancers are detected as a palpable mass by the affected patient. Such carcinomas are almost all invasive and are typically at least 2 to 3 cm in size. At least half of these cancers will already have spread to regional lymph nodes. In older screened populations, approximately 60% of breast cancers are discovered before symptoms are present. About 20% are in situ carcinomas. Invasive carcinomas detected by screening in older women are 1 to 2 cm in size and only 15% will have metastasized to lymph nodes. Palpable cancers in the older age group are often "interval" cancers—cancers that appear suddenly between screening intervals. Understandably, interval cancers generally are highly proliferative and usually are high grade.

The clinical outcome for a woman with breast cancer can be predicted based on the molecular and morphologic features of the cancer and its stage at the time of diagnosis. Factors that influence outcome include the following:

- *Biologic type.* The biologic type of cancer is evaluated by a combination of histologic appearance, grade (including proliferative rate), expression of hormone receptors, and expression of HER2.

  Proliferation is evaluated by mitotic count and is closely tied to responsiveness to cytotoxic chemotherapy. This is because rapidly growing cancer cells are more sensitive to agents that damage DNA or otherwise interfere with cell division.

  Expression of estrogen or progesterone receptors predicts response to anti-estrogen therapy. The growth of hormone receptor–positive cancers can be inhibited for many years with therapy and it is possible for patients to survive for long periods with distant metastases. However, resistance often eventually develops—in some cancers because of mutations in the gene for ER. In contrast, there is no targeted therapy available for triple-negative cancers, which are treated with chemotherapy. Cancers that do not respond to initial therapy metastasize and usually cause the death of the patient.

  Overexpression of HER2 is seen in about 20% of breast cancers. HER2 remains one of the best-characterized examples of an effective therapy that is directed against a tumor-specific molecular lesion. Before targeted therapy, which may take the form of blocking antibodies or small

molecular inhibitors of HER2, outcomes were similar to patients with triple-negative carcinomas. However, complete response rates exceed 60% when targeted therapy is combined with chemotherapy, and the outlook for these patients has been markedly improved.

- *RNA expression profiling* is a newer method of subclassifying cancers. For breast cancers, many of the genes that predict prognosis are involved in proliferation. The greatest clinical value of these assays is their ability to identify patients with slow-growing, anti-estrogen-responsive cancers who can be spared the toxicity of chemotherapy.

- *Tumor stage.* "Stage" is a measure of the extent of tumor at the time of diagnosis and is important for all biologic types of carcinoma. It is based on features of the primary tumor (T), involvement of regional lymph nodes (N), and the presence of distant metastases (M) (Fig. 19.30). The AJCC/UICC staging system, used in the United States and Europe, classifies tumors as T1, T2, and T3 based on the tumor size, whereas T4 tumors have ulceration of the skin, involvement of the deep muscles of the chest wall, or are clinically diagnosed as inflammatory carcinoma. *The majority of cancers first metastasize to regional nodes*, and nodal involvement is a very strong prognostic factor. Lymphatic drainage goes to one or two sentinel lymph nodes in the axilla in most patients. If these nodes are not involved, the remaining axillary nodes are usually free of carcinoma. *Sentinel node biopsy* has become the standard for assessing nodal involvement, replacing more extensive lymph node dissections, which are associated with significant morbidity. *Distant metastases* (M) are only detected in 5% of newly diagnosed women. Stage 0 is CIS, which is associated with survival rates greater than 95%. Stage I includes women with smaller cancers and nodes either free of carcinoma or with only very small micrometastases. Survival is ~86% at 10 years. Carcinomas are classified as Stage II either because of larger tumor size or because of up to

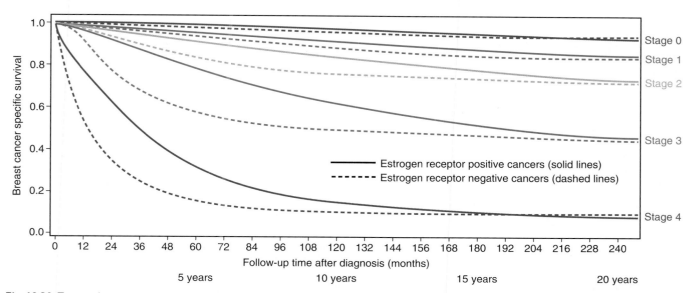

Fig. 19.30 Ten-year breast cancer specific survival according to AJCC stage for ER-positive and ER-negative cancers. Both stage and biologic type of cancer are important determinants of survival. ER-positive invasive cancers have improved survival over ER-negative cancers at all stages, but this advantage diminishes after 5 years because of late recurrences of ER-positive tumors. *(Graph courtesy of Dr. Stephanie Wong; data from SEER-18, 1992–2012. http://seer.cancer.gov.)*

three positive nodes. Survival declines to ~71% at Stage II. Stage III is the group of locally advanced cancers defined by large size, involvement of skin or chest wall, or by four or more positive nodes. Only ~54% of patients survive 10 years. Stage IV is reserved for patients with distant metastases, and survival is very poor (~11%). The most likely site of a distant recurrence varies with the biologic type of cancer. Triple-negative cancers and HER2 cancers are more likely to metastasize to the brain and viscera, in contrast to ER-positive cancers, which most often metastasize to bones (Table 19.7).

Combining stage and biologic factors may provide a more accurate assessment of outcome. For example, for each cancer stage, the survival of patients with ER-positive cancers is higher than patients with ER-negative cancers 5 years postdiagnosis, especially for Stages III and IV (Fig. 19.30). It must be noted, however, this advantage diminishes with time, with progressively smaller differences being seen at 10 years post-diagnosis and beyond (Fig. 19.30). This narrowing of survival differences is explained by two factors. First, most deaths from ER-negative cancers happen within 5 years of diagnosis (Fig. 19.31). Women who live beyond this point are those whose tumors have had excellent responses to treatment, and many of these women may be cured. Second, although the growth of ER-positive cancers is held in check for years by anti-estrogen therapy, this therapy is not curative and these cancers may eventually become resistant to treatment.

Historically, virtually all women with untreated breast cancer died within 3 to 4 years. However, great strides have been made in treatment and now 80% of women with breast cancer who receive optimal therapy will survive.

Endocrine therapy with tamoxifen and aromatase inhibitors is very effective for ER-positive cancers, which may remain dormant for many years.

Targeted therapy has the promise of being more effective and less toxic than conventional chemotherapy (Table

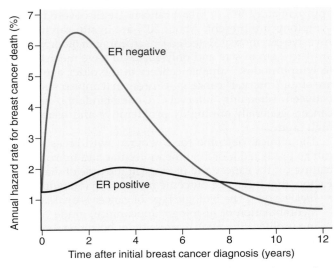

Fig. 19.31 Time to recurrence of breast cancers. The hazard ratio reflects the risk of recurrence of each molecular type of breast cancer at various points in time after diagnosis. ER-negative cancers usually recur within the first 8 years. Patients who survive beyond this interval are likely cured. In contrast, ER-positive cancers have a lower rate of recurrence, but remain at risk decades after the primary diagnosis.

19.8), as already proven by marked improvement in survival of women with HER2-positive carcinomas following the introduction of therapies that target HER2. Newer approaches to targeted therapy include inhibition of alternative DNA repair pathways in *BRCA*-mutated cancers and blockage of the PI3K-AKT-signaling pathway. Immune checkpoint blockade therapy (Chapter 6), is under evaluation in patients with breast cancer. It is hoped that such new approaches will improve outcomes in subtypes that currently have a generally poor prognosis, such as triple negative breast cancer.

Table 19.8 Targeted Treatment of Breast Cancer

Target	Treatment	Assay	Comments
ER	Estrogen deprivation (oophorectomy, aromatase inhibitors) Blockage of ER (tamoxifen)	IHC for nuclear ER	Effective cytostatic (but not cytotoxic) therapy for ER-positive cancer
HER2	Antibodies to HER2 Cytotoxic therapy linked to HER2 antibody Tyrosine kinase inhibitors	IHC for membrane HER2 ISH for HER2 gene amplification	Effective for HER2-positive cancers
Susceptibility to DNA damage resulting from BRCA 1 and BRCA2 mutations that cause defects in HRR	Chemotherapy with agents causing DNA damage that requires HRR (e.g., platinum agents) Inhibition of alternative DNA repair pathway (poly-ADP ribose polymerase or PARP inhibitors)	Sequencing of *BRCA1* and *BRCA2*	May be effective for carcinomas arising in patients with germline *BRCA1* or 2 mutations or cancers with somatic loss of BRCA function
PI3K/AKT pathway	Inhibition of proteins in the pathway	Activating mutations or pathway activation—not yet validated	>80% of breast cancers have alterations in this pathway Effectiveness of treatment not yet demonstrated
Immune checkpoint proteins	Blocking antibodies to PD-L1, PD-1, and other immune checkpoint proteins	IHC for immune checkpoint proteins—not yet validated	Under investigation in patients with triple-negative breast cancer

ER, Estrogen receptor; *HRR,* homologous recombination repair; *IHC,* immunohistochemistry; *ISH,* in situ hybridization.

SUMMARY

BREAST CARCINOMA

- The lifetime risk of developing breast cancer for an American woman is 1 in 8.
- A majority (75%) of breast cancers are diagnosed after the age of 50.
- The major risk factors for developing breast cancer are related to hormonal factors and inherited susceptibility.
- About 12% of all breast cancers are caused by identified germ-line mutations; *BRCA1* and *BRCA2* genes account for one-half of the cases associated with single-gene mutations.
- DCIS is a precursor to invasive ductal carcinoma and is most often found on mammographic screening as calcifications. When carcinoma develops in a woman with a previous diagnosis of untreated DCIS, it is usually is an invasive ductal carcinoma in the same breast.
- LCIS is both a marker of increased risk and a precursor lesion. When carcinoma develops in a woman with a previous diagnosis of LCIS, two-thirds are in the same breast and one-third is in the contralateral breast.
- Invasive carcinomas are classified according to histologic type and biologic type: ER-positive/HER2-negative, HER2-positive, and ER/PR/HER2-negative (triple-negative). The biologic types of cancer have important differences in patient characteristics, grade, mutation profile, metastatic pattern, response to therapy, time to recurrence, and prognosis.
- Prognosis is dependent on the biologic type of tumor, stage, and the availability of treatment modalities.

SUGGESTED READINGS

Bulun SE: Mechanism of disease: endometriosis, *N Engl J Med* 360:268, 2009. [*Excellent review of the molecular basis of endometriosis.*]

Cannistra S: Cancer of ovary, *N Engl J Med* 351:2519, 2004. [*A comprehensive review.*]

DiCristofano A, Ellenson LH: Endometrial carcinoma, *Annu Rev Pathol* 2:57, 2007. [*A comprehensive discussion of pathogenesis.*]

Ehrmann DA: Polycystic ovary syndrome, *N Engl J Med* 352:1223, 2004. [*A detailed review.*]

Fox H, Wells M: Recent advances in the pathology of the vulva, *Histopathology* 42:209, 2003. [*A short update on vulvar pathology.*]

Herrington CS: Recent advances in molecular gynaecological pathology, *Histopathology* 55:243, 2009. [*A review of molecular genetics of cervical, ovarian, and endometrial neoplasia.*]

Kathleen RC: Ovarian cancer, *Annu Rev Pathol Mech Dis* 4:287, 2009. [*A good review on the subject with discussion of molecular genetics.*]

Moody CA: Human papillomavirus oncoproteins: pathways to transformation, *Nat Rev Cancer* 10:550, 2010. [*A review of current opinion on cervical carcinogenesis.*]

Morice P, Leary A, Creutzberg C, et al: Endometrial cancer, *Lancet* 387:1094, 2016. [*A comprehensive review of the subject.*]

Rich TA, Woodson AH, Litton J, et al: Hereditary breast cancer syndromes and genetic testing, *J Surg Oncol* 111:6–80, 2015. [*Soon many individuals will know their entire DNA sequence. This review discusses the complexities of detecting low- and moderate-penetrance susceptibility genes.*]

Seckl MJ, Sebire NJ, Berkowitz RS: Gestational trophoblastic disease, *Lancet* 376:717, 2010. [*A review of gestation trophoblastic including discussion regarding management.*]

Sonnenblick A, Fumagalli D, Sotiriou C, et al: Is the differentiation into molecular subtypes of breast cancer important for staging, local and systemic therapy, and follow up? *Cancer Treat Rev* 40:1089–1095, 2014. [*The translation of the biologic types of cancer into clinical practice is discussed.*]

Endocrine System

20

CHAPTER OUTLINE

Pituitary 750
Anterior Pituitary Tumors 750
Pituitary Adenomas: General Features 750
Functioning Adenomas and
* Hyperpituatarism 753*
Other Anterior Pituitary Neoplasms 754
Hypopituitarism 754
Posterior Pituitary Syndromes 755
Thyroid 755
Hyperthyroidism 756
Hypothyroidism 757
Autoimmune Thyroid Disease 758
Chronic Lymphocytic (Hashimoto)
* Thyroiditis 758*
Subacute Granulomatous (de Quervain)
* Thyroiditis 759*
Subacute Lymphocytic Thyroiditis 760
Other Forms of Thyroiditis 760
Graves Disease 760
Diffuse and Multinodular Goiter 762
Thyroid Neoplasms 763

Adenomas 763
Carcinomas 764
Parathyroid Glands 769
Hyperparathyroidism 769
Primary Hyperparathyroidism 769
Secondary Hyperparathyroidism 771
Hypoparathyroidism 771
Endocrine Pancreas 772
Diabetes Mellitus 772
Normal Insulin Physiology and
* Glucose Homeostasis 773*
Pathogenesis of Type 1 Diabetes 774
Pathogenesis of Type 2 Diabetes 775
Monogenic Forms of Diabetes 776
Other Subtypes of Diabetes 776
Acute Metabolic Complications of
* Diabetes 777*
Chronic Complications of Diabetes 778
Pancreatic Neuroendocrine Tumors 784
Insulinomas 784
Gastrinomas 784

Adrenal Cortex 784
Adrenocortical Hyperfunction:
** Hyperadrenalism 785**
Hypercortisolism: Cushing Syndrome 785
Hyperaldosteronism 788
Adrenogenital Syndromes 789
Adrenal Insufficiency 790
Acute Adrenocortical Insufficiency 790
Chronic Adrenocortical Insufficiency: Addison
* Disease 790*
Secondary Adrenocortical Insufficiency 791
Adrenocortical Neoplasms 792
Adrenal Medulla 793
Tumors of the Adrenal Medulla 793
Pheochromocytoma 793
Neuroblastoma and Other Neuronal
* Neoplasms 794*
Multiple Endocrine Neoplasia
(MEN) Syndromes 795
Multiple Endocrine Neoplasia Type 1 795
Multiple Endocrine Neoplasia Type 2 795

The endocrine system is conprised of a widely distributed group of organs that work together to maintain the body's metabolic equilibrium, or homeostasis. The cells of the endocrine system achieve this by secreting molecules, which are frequently called *hormones,* that act on target cells distant from their site of synthesis. A hormone typically is carried by the blood from the endocrine gland to its target tissues. Most hormones are secreted in response to other, so-called trophic, hormones, which are produced in response to particular metabolic needs. Production of a hormone often downregulates the activity of the gland that secretes the stimulating trophic hormone, a process known as *feedback inhibition.*

Hormones can be classified into several broad categories, based on the nature of their receptors:

- *Hormones that act by binding to cell surface receptors:* This large class of compounds is composed of two groups: (1) peptide hormones, such as *growth hormone* and *insulin,* and (2) small molecules, such as *epinephrine.* Binding of these hormones to cell surface receptors leads to an increase in intracellular *second messengers,* such as cyclic adenosine monophosphate (cAMP), inositol 1,4,5-trisphosphate (IP3), and ionized calcium. Elevated levels of one or more of these compounds can activate intracellular signaling pathways that may stimulate cell growth or differentiation, or alter cell function.

- *Hormones that act by binding to intracellular receptors:* Many lipid-soluble hormones pass through the plasma membrane by diffusion to interact with receptors in the cytosol or the nucleus. The resulting hormone-receptor complexes bind specifically to regulatory elements in DNA, thereby affecting the expression of specific target genes. Hormones of this type include *steroids* (e.g., estrogen, progesterone, glucocorticoids), *retinoids* (vitamin A), and *thyroxine.*

Endocrine diseases generally are caused by: (1) *underproduction or overproduction* of hormones, with associated biochemical and clinical consequences; (2) *end-organ resistance* to the effects of a hormone; or (3) *neoplasms,* which may be nonfunctional or may be associated with overproduction or underproduction of hormones. In many settings, the study of endocrine diseases relies heavily on biochemical measurements of the levels of hormones, their regulators, and other metabolites.

Pituitary

The pituitary gland is a small, bean-shaped structure that lies at the base of the brain within the confines of the sella turcica. It is intimately related to the hypothalamus, with which it is connected by a stalk, composed of axons extending from the hypothalamus, and a rich venous plexus constituting a portal circulation. Along with the hypothalamus, the pituitary has a central role in the regulation of most of the other endocrine glands. The pituitary is composed of two morphologically and functionally distinct components: the anterior lobe (adenohypophysis) and the posterior lobe (neurohypophysis). Diseases of the pituitary, accordingly, can be divided into those that primarily affect the anterior lobe and those that primarily affect the posterior lobe.

The anterior pituitary, or adenohypophysis, produces trophic hormones that stimulate the production of hormones from the thyroid, adrenal, and other glands. The anterior pituitary is composed of epithelial cells derived embryologically from the developing oral cavity. In routine histologic sections, a colorful array of cells containing basophilic cytoplasm, eosinophilic cytoplasm, or poorly staining (chromophobic) cytoplasm is present (Fig. 20.1). Detailed studies using electron microscopy and immunohistochemical techniques have demonstrated that the staining properties of these cells are related to the presence of different polypeptide hormones within their cytoplasm that control the activity of other endocrine glands. The release of these pituitary hormones is under the control of factors produced in the hypothalamus; while most hypothalamic factors are stimulatory and promote pituitary hormone release, others (e.g., somatostatin and dopamine) are inhibitory (Fig. 20.2). Rarely, signs and symptoms of pituitary disease may be caused by overproduction or underproduction of hypothalamic factors, rather than a primary pituitary abnormality.

Symptoms and signs of pituitary disease fall into the following categories:

- *Hyperpituitarism* related effects: Hyperpituitarism arises from excessive secretion of trophic hormones. It most often results from an *anterior pituitary adenoma* but also may be caused by other pituitary and extrapituitary lesions, as discussed later. The symptoms and signs of hyperpituitarism are discussed in the context of individual tumors later in the chapter (see Table 20.1).
- *Hypopituitarism* related effects: Hypopituitarism is caused by deficiency of trophic hormones and results from a variety of destructive processes that may damage the pituitary, including ischemic injury, surgery, radiation, and inflammatory reactions. In addition, nonfunctional pituitary adenomas may encroach upon and destroy the normal anterior pituitary, causing hypopituitarism.
- *Local mass effects:* Among the earliest changes associated with pituitary neoplasms are radiographic abnormalities of the sella turcica, including sellar expansion, bony erosion, and disruption of the diaphragma sellae. Because of the close proximity of the optic nerves and chiasm to the sella, expanding pituitary lesions often compress decussating fibers in the optic chiasm. This can give rise to visual field abnormalities, classically in the form of defects in the lateral (temporal) visual fields—a so-called "bitemporal hemianopsia". As in the case of any expanding intracranial mass, pituitary tumors may produce signs and symptoms of elevated intracranial pressure, including headache, nausea, and vomiting. Pituitary neoplasms that extend beyond the sella turcica into the base of the brain produce seizures or obstructive hydrocephalus; involvement of cranial nerves can result in *cranial nerve palsy*. On occasion, acute hemorrhage into a pituitary neoplasm is associated with rapid enlargement of the lesion and loss of consciousness, a situation termed *pituitary apoplexy*. Acute pituitary apoplexy may be rapidly fatal and is therefore considered to be a neurosurgical emergency.

ANTERIOR PITUITARY TUMORS

The most common cause of anterior pituitary disorders are pituitary tumors, most of which are benign adenomas. Some of these produce hormones and result in endocrine abnormalities, and others are nonfunctional and produce mass effects. We discuss first the general features of pituitary adenomas, then specific tumors.

Pituitary Adenomas: General Features

The most common cause of hyperpituitarism is a hormone-producing adenoma arising in the anterior lobe. Other, less common, causes include hyperplasia and carcinomas of the anterior pituitary, secretion of hormones by some extrapituitary tumors, and certain hypothalamic disorders. Some salient features of pituitary adenomas are as follows:

- *Pituitary adenomas are classified on the basis of hormone(s) produced by the neoplastic cells*, which are detected by immunohistochemical stains performed on tissue sections (Table 20.1).

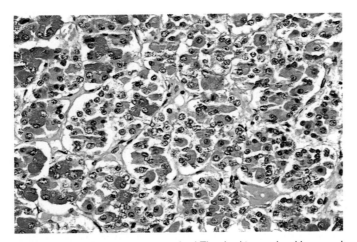

Fig. 20.1 Normal anterior pituitary gland. The gland is populated by several distinct cell types that express different peptide hormones. These hormones are basophilic (blue), eosinophilic (red), or nonstaining in routine sections stained with hematoxylin and eosin, which allows the various cell types to be identified. Note also the presence of a fine reticulin network between the cells.

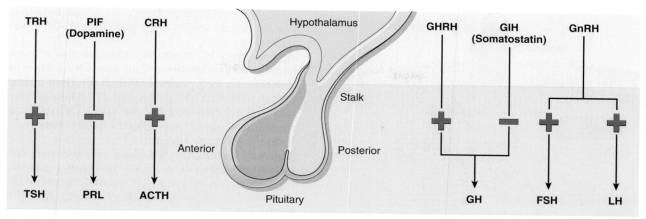

Fig. 20.2 The hypothalamic/pituitary axis. The hypothalamus regulates the secretion of hormones from the adenohypophysis (anterior pituitary gland) by releasing stimulatory (corticotropin-releasing hormone, CRH; growth hormone–releasing hormone, GHRH; gonadotropin-releasing hormone, GnRH; thyrotropin-releasing hormone (TRH) and inhibitory factors (growth hormone inhibitory hormone, GIH or somatostatin; prolactin inhibitory factor, PIF or dopamine). These in turn modulate the release of six hormones from the anterior pituitary: adrenocorticotropic hormone (ACTH or corticotropin); follicle-stimulating hormone (FSH); growth hormone (GH, or somatotropin); luteinizing hormone (LH); prolactin (PRL); and thyroid-stimulating hormone (TSH, or thyrotropin).

- Pituitary adenomas can be *functional* (hormone producing) or *nonfunctioning* (not producing hormone), or *silent* (i.e., demonstration of hormone production at the tissue level only, without clinical manifestations of hormone excess). Both functional and nonfunctioning pituitary adenomas usually are composed of a single cell type and produce at most a single predominant hormone, but there are exceptions. Some pituitary adenomas secrete two different hormones (growth hormone and prolactin being the most common combination); rarely, pituitary adenomas are plurihormonal.
- Pituitary adenomas are designated as *microadenomas* if they are less than 1 cm in diameter and *macroadenomas* if they exceed 1 cm in diameter.

- Nonfunctioning adenomas are likely to come to clinical attention at a later stage and are, therefore, more likely to be macroadenomas. Because of their larger size, nonfunctioning adenomas may encroach upon and destroy adjacent anterior pituitary parenchyma, leading to hypopituitarism.

Pathogenesis

Several genetic abnormalities associated with pituitary adenomas have been identified:

- **G-protein mutations are one of the most common genomic alterations in pituitary adenomas.** G-proteins play a critical role in signal transduction, transmitting signals from cell surface receptors e.g. growth

Table 20.1 Classification of Pituitary Adenomas

Pituitary Cell Type	Hormone	Adenoma Subtypes	Associated Syndrome*
Lactotroph	Prolactin	Lactotroph adenoma Silent lactotroph adenoma	Galactorrhea and amenorrhea (in females) Sexual dysfunction, infertility
Somatotroph	GH	Densely granulated somatotroph adenoma Sparsely granulated somatotroph adenoma Silent somatotroph adenoma	Gigantism (children) Acromegaly (adults)
Mammosomatotroph	Prolactin, GH	Mammosomatotroph adenomas	Combined features of GH and prolactin excess
Corticotroph	ACTH and other POMC-derived peptides	Densely granulated corticotroph adenoma Sparsely granulated corticotroph adenoma Silent corticotroph adenoma	Cushing syndrome Nelson syndrome
Thyrotroph	TSH	Thyrotroph adenomas Silent thyrotroph adenomas	Hyperthyroidism
Gonadotroph	FSH, LH	Gonadotroph adenomas Silent gonadotroph adenomas ("null cell," oncocytic adenomas)	Hypogonadism, mass effects, and hypopituitarism

ACTH, Adrenocorticotrophic hormone; FSH, follicle-stimulating hormone; GH, growth hormone; LH, luteinizing hormone; POMC, pro-opiomelanocortin; TSH, thyroid-stimulating hormone.

*Note that nonfunctional (silent) adenomas in each category express the corresponding hormone(s) within the neoplastic cells, as determined by special immunohistochemical staining on tissues. However, these adenomas do not produce the associated clinical syndrome, and typically present with *mass effects* accompanied by *hypopituitarism* due to destruction of normal pituitary parenchyma. These features are particularly common with gonadotroph adenomas. Partially adapted from Asa SL, Essat S: The pathogenesis of pituitary tumors. Annu Rev Pathol 4:97, 2009.

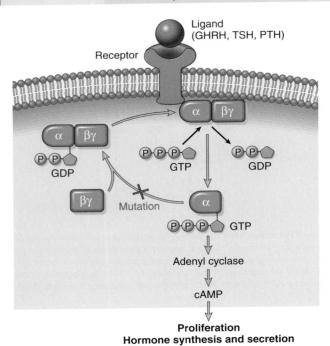

Fig. 20.3 G-protein signaling in endocrine neoplasia. Mutations that lead to G-protein hyperactivity are seen in a variety of endocrine neoplasms, including pituitary, thyroid, and parathyroid adenomas. G proteins play a critical role in signal transduction, transmitting signals from cell surface receptors (GHRH, TSH, or PTH receptor) to intracellular effectors (e.g., adenyl cyclase), which then generate second messengers (cAMP, cyclic adenosine monophosphate). *GDP,* Guanosine diphosphate; *GTP,* guanosine triphosphate; *P,* inorganic phosphate.

hormone–releasing hormone (GHRH) receptor, to intracellular effectors (e.g., adenyl cyclase), which then generate second messengers (e.g., cAMP). G-proteins are heterotrimeric proteins, composed of a specific α-subunit that binds guanine nucleotides and interacts with both cell surface receptors and intracellular effectors (Fig. 20.3); the β- and γ-subunits are noncovalently bound to the α-subunit. Gs is a stimulatory G protein that has a pivotal role in signal transduction in several endocrine organs, including the pituitary. The α-subunit of Gs (Gsα) is encoded by the *GNAS* gene. In the basal state, Gs exists in an inactive state, with guanosine diphosphate (GDP) bound to the guanine nucleotide-binding site of Gsα. On interaction with the ligand-bound cell surface receptor, GDP dissociates, and guanosine triphosphate (GTP) binds to Gsα, activating the G protein. The activation of Gsα results in the generation of cAMP, which is a potent mitogenic stimulus in several endocrine cells (e.g., pituitary somatotrophs and corticotrophs, thyroid follicular cells, parathyroid cells), promoting cellular proliferation and hormone synthesis and secretion. Normally, Gsα activation is transient because of an intrinsic GTPase activity in the α-subunit, which hydrolyzes GTP into GDP. *Approximately 40% of somatotroph cell adenomas bear GNAS mutations that abrogate the GTPase activity of Gsα, leading to constitutive activation of Gsα, persistent generation of cAMP, and unchecked cellular proliferation. GNAS* mutations also have been described in a minority of corticotroph adenomas; but are absent in thyrotroph, lactotroph, and gonadotroph

adenomas, which arise from cells whose hypothalamic release hormones do not signal via cAMP-dependent pathways.

- *Approximately 5% of pituitary adenomas arise as a result of an inherited predisposition.* Four genes have been identified thus far as a cause of familial pituitary adenomas: *MEN1, CDKN1B, PRKAR1A,* and *AIP.* These genes regulate transcription and the cell cycle. Of note, somatic mutations of these four genes are rarely encountered in sporadic pituitary adenomas.
- *Molecular abnormalities associated with aggressive behavior include aberrations in cell cycle checkpoint genes,* such as overexpression of cyclin D1, mutations of *TP53,* and epigenetic silencing of the retinoblastoma gene *(RB).* In addition, activating mutations of the *RAS* oncogene are observed in rare *pituitary carcinomas.* The functions of these genes were discussed in Chapter 6.

MORPHOLOGY

The usual pituitary adenoma is a well-circumscribed, soft lesion. Small tumors may be confined to the sella turcica, while larger lesions may compress the optic chiasm and adjacent structures (Fig. 20.4), erode the sella turcica and anterior clinoid processes, and extend locally into the cavernous and sphenoidal sinuses. In as many as 30% of cases, the adenomas are nonencapsulated and infiltrate adjacent bone, dura, and (uncommonly) brain. Foci of hemorrhage and/or necrosis are common in larger adenomas.

Pituitary adenomas are composed of relatively uniform, polygonal cells arrayed in sheets, cords, or papillae. Supporting connective tissue, or reticulin, is sparse. The nuclei of the neoplastic cells may be uniform or pleomorphic. **This cellular monomorphism and the absence of a significant reticulin network distinguish pituitary adenomas from**

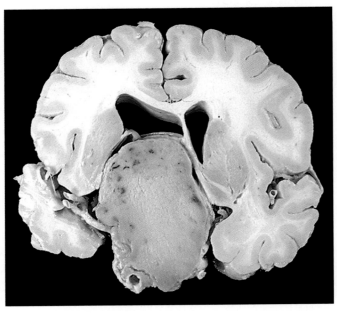

Fig. 20.4 Pituitary adenoma. This massive, nonfunctioning adenoma has grown far beyond the confines of the sella turcica and has distorted the overlying brain. Nonfunctioning adenomas tend to be larger at the time of diagnosis than those that secrete a hormone.

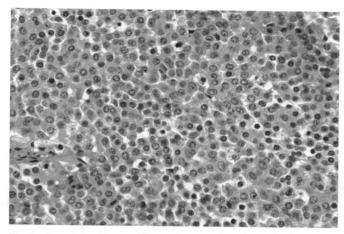

Fig. 20.5 Pituitary adenoma. The monomorphism of these cells contrasts with the admixture of cells seen in the normal anterior pituitary gland in Fig. 20.1. Note also the absence of the reticulin network.

non-neoplastic anterior pituitary parenchyma (Fig. 20.5). Mitotic activity usually is scanty. The cytoplasm of the constituent cells may be acidophilic, basophilic, or chromophobic, depending on the type and amount of secretory product within the cell, but it is fairly uniform throughout the neoplasm. The functional status of the adenoma cannot be predicted from its histologic appearance. Adenomas that harbor *TP53* mutations often demonstrate brisk mitotic activity and higher proliferation rates and are designated **atypical adenomas** because of their potential for aggressive behavior.

SUMMARY

PITUITARY ADENOMAS: GENERAL FEATURES

- The most common cause of hyperpituitarism is an anterior lobe pituitary adenoma.
- Pituitary adenomas can be macroadenomas (>1 cm in diameter) or microadenomas (<1 cm across), and on clinical evaluation, they can be functional or nonfunctioning.
- Macroadenomas may potentially lead to mass effects, including visual disturbances.
- Functioning adenomas are associated with distinct endocrine signs and symptoms.
- Mutation of the *GNAS* gene, which results in constitutive activation of a stimulatory G protein, is one of the more common genetic alterations.
- The two distinctive morphologic features of most adenomas are their cellular monomorphism and absence of a reticulin network.

Functioning Adenomas and Hyperpituatarism

Adenomas arising from different pituitary cells produce hormones characteristic of that cell type and cause clinical syndromes that reflect the activity of the hormones.

Lactotroph Adenomas

Prolactin-secreting lactotroph adenomas are the most frequent type of hyperfunctioning pituitary adenoma, accounting for about 30% of all clinically recognized cases. They range in size from microadenomas to large, expansile tumors associated with considerable mass effect. Prolactin is demonstrable within the cytoplasm of the neoplastic cells by immunohistochemical techniques. Prolactin secretion by lactotroph adenomas is highly efficient, such that even microadenomas can secrete sufficient hormone to induce systemic symptoms.

Hyperprolactinemia causes amenorrhea, galactorrhea, loss of libido, and infertility. Because manifestations of hyperprolactinemia (e.g., amenorrhea) are obvious in premenopausal women, prolactinomas are diagnosed at an earlier stage in women of reproductive age than in others with these tumors. By contrast, the effects of hyperprolactinemia are subtle in men and older women, in whom the tumor may reach a large size before coming to clinical attention. Hyperprolactinemia also is a feature of other conditions, including pregnancy, high-dose estrogen therapy, renal failure, hypothyroidism, hypothalamic lesions, and dopamine-inhibiting drugs (e.g., reserpine). In addition, any mass in the suprasellar compartment may disturb the normal inhibitory influence of hypothalamus on prolactin secretion, resulting in hyperprolactinemia—a mechanism known as the *stalk effect*. Thus, mild elevations of serum prolactin (<200 μg/L) in a patient with a pituitary adenoma do not necessarily indicate a prolactin-secreting neoplasm.

Somatotroph Adenomas

Growth hormone–secreting somatotroph adenomas are the second most common type of functioning pituitary adenoma, and cause gigantism in children or acromegaly in adults. Because the clinical manifestations of excess growth hormone may be subtle, somatotroph cell adenomas may be quite large by the time they come to clinical attention. On microscopic examination, growth hormone–producing adenomas are composed of densely or sparsely granulated cells, and immunohistochemical staining demonstrates growth hormone within the cytoplasm of the neoplastic cells. Small amounts of immunoreactive prolactin often are present as well.

Persistent growth hormone excess stimulates the hepatic secretion of insulin-like growth factor 1 (IGF1), which acts in conjunction with growth hormone to induce overgrowth of bones and muscle. If a growth hormone-secreting adenoma develops before the epiphyses close, as is the case in prepubertal children, excessive levels of growth hormone and IGF1 result in *gigantism*. This condition is characterized by a generalized increase in body size, with disproportionately long arms and legs. If elevated levels of growth hormone and IGF1 persist or develop after closure of the epiphyses, affected individuals develop *acromegaly,* in which growth is most conspicuous in soft tissues, skin, viscera, and the bones of the face, hands, and feet. Enlargement of the jaw results in its protrusion (*prognathism*), broadening of the lower face, and separation of the teeth. The hands and feet are enlarged, and the fingers are broad and sausage-like. In most instances gigantism is accompanied by evidence of acromegaly. These changes may develop slowly over decades before being recognized, hence the adenoma may be quite large before it is detected.

Persistent growth hormone excess also is associated with metabolic abnormalities, the most important of which is diabetes mellitus. This arises because of growth hormone–induced peripheral insulin resistance, which "blunts" the body's response to elevated glucose levels (see "Diabetes Mellitus", later). Failure to suppress growth hormone production in response to an oral load of glucose is one of the most sensitive tests for acromegaly. Other manifestations of growth hormone excess include gonadal dysfunction, generalized muscle weakness, hypertension, arthritis, congestive heart failure, and an increased risk for gastrointestinal cancers.

Corticotroph Adenomas

Excess production of ACTH by functioning corticotroph adenomas leads to adrenal hypersecretion of cortisol and the development of hypercortisolism (also known as *Cushing syndrome***).** Cushing syndrome (discussed later with diseases of the adrenal gland) may be caused by other conditions as well. When the hypercortisolism is caused by excessive production of ACTH by the pituitary, it is called *Cushing disease* after the neurosurgeon Harvey Cushing who first described the disorder.

Most corticotroph adenomas are small (microadenomas) at the time of diagnosis. These adenomas stain positively with periodic acid–Schiff (PAS) stains, as a result of the accumulation of glycosylated ACTH protein. ACTH also can be specifically detected by immunohistochemical methods. Large, clinically aggressive corticotroph cell adenomas may develop after surgical removal of the adrenal glands for treatment of Cushing syndrome. In most instances this condition, known as *Nelson syndrome*, results from loss of the inhibitory effect of adrenal corticosteroids on a preexisting corticotroph microadenoma. Because the adrenals are absent in individuals with Nelson syndrome, hypercortisolism does not develop. Instead, patients present with the mass effects of the pituitary tumor. Patients with Cushing syndrome often have hyperpigmented skin because of increased production of melanocyte stimulating hormone (MSH), which is derived from the same precursor as ACTH so its synthesis accompanies that of ACTH.

Other Anterior Pituitary Neoplasms

Other pituitary adenomas are associated with hormonal disorders not considered part of hyperpituitarism, or are nonfunctional and do not produce hormonal disturbances.

- *Gonadotroph adenomas* are so named because they produce hormones *(luteinizing hormone [LH] and follicle-stimulating hormone [FSH])* that act on reproductive organs (gonads). These adenomas can be difficult to recognize because they secrete hormones inefficiently and variably and the secretory products usually do not cause a recognizable clinical syndrome. They are typically detected when the tumors become large enough to cause signs and symptoms related to local mass effects, such as impaired vision, headaches, diplopia, or pituitary apoplexy. The neoplastic cells usually demonstrate immunoreactivity for the common gonadotropin α-subunit and the specific β-FSH and β-LH subunits; FSH usually is the predominant secreted hormone.
- *Thyrotroph (thyroid-stimulating hormone [TSH]–producing) adenomas* account for about 1% of all pituitary adenomas and constitute a rare cause of hyperthyroidism.

- *Nonfunctioning pituitary adenomas* are a heterogeneous group that constitutes 25% to 30% of all pituitary tumors. Not surprisingly, the typical presentation is characterized by mass effects. These lesions also may impinge on the residual anterior pituitary and produce hypopituitarism, which may appear slowly due to gradual enlargement of the adenoma or abruptly because of acute intratumoral hemorrhage (pituitary apoplexy).
- *Pituitary carcinomas are exceedingly rare.* In addition to local extension beyond the sella turcica, these tumors virtually always metastasize to distant sites.

SUMMARY

HYPERPITUITARISM-ASSOCIATED ADENOMAS

- *Prolactinomas:* amenorrhea, galactorrhea, loss of libido, and infertility
- *Growth hormone (somatotroph cell) adenomas:* gigantism (children), acromegaly (adults), and impaired glucose tolerance and diabetes mellitus
- *Corticotroph cell adenomas:* Cushing syndrome, hyperpigmentation
- All pituitary adenomas, particularly nonfunctioning adenomas, may be associated with mass effects and hypopituitarism.

HYPOPITUITARISM

Clinically significant hypopituitarism may occur with loss or absence of 75% or more of the anterior pituitary parenchyma. It may be ***congenital*** (exceedingly rare) or result from a wide range of ***acquired*** intrinsic abnormalities of the pituitary. Less frequently, disorders that interfere with the delivery of pituitary hormone–releasing factors from the hypothalamus, such as hypothalamic tumors, cause hypofunction of the anterior pituitary. ***Hypopituitarism accompanied by evidence of posterior pituitary dysfunction in the form of diabetes insipidus*** (discussed later) ***is almost always of hypothalamic origin.*** Most cases of anterior pituitary hypofunction are caused by the following:

- *Tumors and other mass lesions* (especially nonfunctioning pituitary adenomas)
- *Ischemic necrosis of the anterior pituitary,* called *Sheehan syndrome,* or postpartum necrosis of the anterior pituitary, is the most common form of clinically significant necrosis of the anterior pituitary. During pregnancy, the anterior pituitary enlarges, mainly because of an increase in the size and number of prolactin-secreting cells. This hyperplasia is not accompanied by an increase in blood supply from the low-pressure hypophyseal portal venous system. The enlarged gland is thus vulnerable to ischemic injury, especially in women who experience hypotension during the peripartal period. By contrast, the posterior pituitary receives its blood directly from arterial branches and is much less susceptible to ischemic injury. Pituitary necrosis also may occur in the setting of disseminated intravascular coagulation, sickle cell anemia, elevated intracranial pressure, traumatic injury, and shock of any origin.
- *Iatrogenic causes* include ablation of the pituitary by surgery or radiation

- Other, less common causes of anterior pituitary hypofunction include inflammatory lesions such as sarcoidosis or tuberculosis, trauma, and metastatic tumors involving the pituitary

The clinical manifestations of anterior pituitary hypofunction depend on the specific hormones that are lacking. In children, growth failure (*pituitary dwarfism*) may occur as a result of growth hormone deficiency. Gonadotropin or gonadotropin-releasing hormone (GnRH) deficiency leads to amenorrhea and infertility in women and to decreased libido, impotence, and loss of pubic and axillary hair in men. TSH and ACTH deficiencies result in hypothyroidism and hypoadrenalism, respectively (discussed later). Prolactin deficiency results in failure of postpartum lactation. The anterior pituitary also is a rich source of MSH, synthesized from the same precursor molecule that produces ACTH; therefore, one of the manifestations of hypopituitarism is pallor of skin from loss of stimulatory effects of MSH on melanocytes.

POSTERIOR PITUITARY SYNDROMES

The posterior pituitary, or neurohypophysis, is composed of modified glial cells (termed *pituicytes*) and axonal processes extending from nerve cell bodies in the supraoptic and paraventricular nuclei of the hypothalamus. The hypothalamic neurons produce two peptides: anti-diuretic hormone (ADH) and oxytocin. They are stored in axon terminals in the neurohypophysis and released into the circulation in response to appropriate stimuli. ADH is a nonapeptide hormone synthesized predominantly in the supraoptic nucleus. In response to several different stimuli, including increased plasma osmotic pressure, left atrial distention, exercise, and certain emotional states, ADH is released from axon terminals in the neurohypophysis into the general circulation. The hormone acts on the collecting tubules of the kidney to promote the resorption of free water. Oxytocin stimulates the contraction of smooth muscle in the pregnant uterus and of muscle surrounding the lactiferous ducts of the mammary glands. Impairment of oxytocin synthesis and release has not been associated with significant clinical abnormalities.

The clinically important posterior pituitary syndromes involve ADH under- or overproduction.

- **ADH deficiency causes *diabetes insipidus*, a condition characterized by excessive urination (polyuria) due to an inability of the kidney to resorb water properly from the urine.** Diabetes insipidus can result from several causes, including head trauma, neoplasms, and inflammatory disorders of the hypothalamus and pituitary, and from surgical procedures involving the hypothalamus or pituitary. The condition sometimes arises spontaneously (*idiopathic*). Diabetes insipidus from ADH deficiency is designated *central,* to differentiate it from *nephrogenic* diabetes insipidus, which is caused by renal tubular unresponsiveness to circulating ADH. The clinical manifestations of both diseases are similar and include the excretion of large volumes of dilute urine with an inappropriately low specific gravity. Serum sodium and osmolality are increased as a result of excessive renal loss of free water, resulting in thirst and polydipsia. Patients who can drink water generally compensate for urinary losses, but patients who are obtunded, bedridden, or otherwise limited in their ability to obtain water may develop life-threatening dehydration.
- **The syndrome of inappropriate ADH (SIADH) secretion is typically associated with ADH excess, which causes resorption of excessive amounts of free water, resulting in hyponatremia.** Causes of SIADH include the secretion of ectopic ADH by malignant neoplasms (particularly small-cell carcinomas of the lung), nonneoplastic diseases of the lung, and local injury to the hypothalamus or neurohypophysis. The clinical manifestations of SIADH are dominated by hyponatremia, cerebral edema, and resultant neurologic dysfunction. Although total body water is increased, blood volume remains normal, and peripheral edema does not develop.

Thyroid

The thyroid gland consists of two bulky lateral lobes connected by a relatively thin isthmus, usually located below and anterior to the larynx. The thyroid gland develops embryologically from an evagination of the developing pharyngeal epithelium that descends from the foramen cecum at the base of the tongue to its normal position in the anterior neck. This pattern of descent explains the occasional presence of ectopic thyroid tissue, most commonly located at the base of the tongue (lingual thyroid) or at other sites abnormally high in the neck.

The thyroid is divided into lobules, each composed of about 20 to 40 evenly dispersed follicles. The follicles are lined by cuboidal to low columnar epithelium, which is filled with thyroglobulin, the iodinated precursor protein of active thyroid hormone. In response to trophic factors from the hypothalamus, TSH (also called *thyrotropin*) is released by thyrotrophs in the anterior pituitary into the circulation. The binding of TSH to its receptor on thyroid follicular epithelial cells results in activation and conformational change in the receptor, allowing it to associate with a stimulatory G-protein (Fig. 20.6). As illustrated in Fig. 20.3, activation of stimulatory G-protein results in an increase in intracellular cAMP levels, which stimulates thyroid hormone synthesis and release. Thyroid follicular epithelial cells convert thyroglobulin into *thyroxine* (T_4) and lesser amounts of *triiodothyronine* (T_3). T_4 and T_3 are released into the systemic circulation, where most of these peptides are bound to circulating plasma proteins, such as T_4-binding globulin, for transport to peripheral tissues. The binding proteins maintain the serum unbound (free) T_3 and T_4 concentrations within narrow limits while ensuring that the hormones are readily available to the tissues.

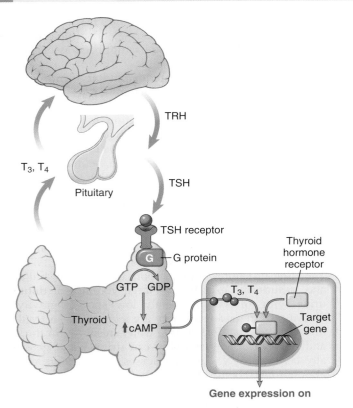

Fig. 20.6 Homeostasis in the hypothalamus-pituitary-thyroid axis and mechanism of action of thyroid hormones. Secretion of thyroid hormones (T_3 and T_4) is controlled by trophic factors secreted by both the hypothalamus and the anterior pituitary gland. Decreased levels of T_3 and T_4 stimulate the release of thyrotropin-releasing hormone (TRH) from the hypothalamus and thyroid-stimulating hormone (TSH) from the anterior pituitary, causing T_3 and T_4 levels to rise. Elevated T_3 and T_4 levels, in turn, suppress the secretion of both TRH and TSH. This relationship is termed a *negative-feedback loop.* TSH binds to the TSH receptor on the thyroid follicular epithelium, which causes activation of G proteins, release of cyclic AMP (cAMP), and cAMP-mediated synthesis and release of thyroid hormones (i.e., T_3 and T_4). In the periphery, T_3 and T_4 interact with the thyroid hormone receptor (TR) and form a complex that translocates to the nucleus and binds to so-called "thyroid response elements" (TREs) on target genes, thereby initiating transcription.

In the periphery, the majority of free T_4 is deiodinated to T_3; the latter binds to thyroid hormone nuclear receptors in target cells with 10-fold greater affinity than T_4 and has proportionately greater activity. Binding of thyroid hormone to its nuclear thyroid hormone receptor (TR) creates a hormone-receptor complex that regulates the transcription of a subset of cellular genes. This produces diverse cellular effects, including increased carbohydrate and lipid catabolism and protein synthesis in a wide range of cell types. The net result of these processes is an increase in the basal metabolic rate.

Clinical recognition of diseases of the thyroid is important, because most are amenable to medical or surgical management. Such diseases include conditions associated with excessive release of thyroid hormones (hyperthyroidism), thyroid hormone deficiency (hypothyroidism), and mass lesions of the thyroid. Considered next are the clinical consequences of disturbed thyroid function, followed by an overview of the disorders that generate these problems.

HYPERTHYROIDISM

Thyrotoxicosis is a hypermetabolic state caused by elevated circulating levels of free T_3 and T_4. Because it is caused most commonly by hyperfunction of the thyroid gland, thyrotoxicosis often is referred to as *hyperthyroidism.* In certain conditions, however, the oversupply either is related to excessive release of preformed thyroid hormone (e.g., in thyroiditis) or comes from an extrathyroidal source, rather than a hyperfunctioning gland (Table 20.2). *Thus, strictly speaking, hyperthyroidism is only one (albeit the most common) category of thyrotoxicosis.* Despite this clear distinction, the following discussion adheres to the common practice of using the terms *thyrotoxicosis* and *hyperthyroidism* interchangeably.

The three most common causes of thyrotoxicosis are associated with hyperfunction of the gland:
- Diffuse hyperplasia of the thyroid associated with Graves disease, a form of autoimmune thyroid disease (accounts for 85% of cases)
- Hyperfunctioning ("toxic") multinodular goiter
- Hyperfunctional ("toxic") adenoma of the thyroid

The clinical manifestations of thyrotoxicosis are protean and are mainly attributable to the *hypermetabolic state* induced by thyroid hormone and *overactivity of the sympathetic nervous system:*
- *Constitutional symptoms:* The skin of thyrotoxic individuals tends to be soft, warm, and flushed because of increased blood flow and peripheral vasodilation to increase heat loss; heat intolerance and excessive sweating are common. Increased sympathetic activity and hypermetabolism result in weight loss despite increased appetite.
- *Gastrointestinal:* Stimulation of the gut results in rapid transit time (hypermotility), which can cause fat malabsorption and steatorrhea.
- *Cardiac:* Palpitations and tachycardia are common due to both increased cardiac contractility and increased

Table 20.2 Causes of Thyrotoxicosis

Associated With Hyperthyroidism
Primary
Diffuse toxic hyperplasia (Graves disease)
Hyperfunctioning ("toxic") multinodular goiter
Hyperfunctioning ("toxic") adenoma
Iodine-induced hyperthyroidism
Secondary
TSH-secreting pituitary adenoma (rare)*
Not Associated With Hyperthyroidism
Granulomatous (de Quervain) thyroiditis *(painful)*
Subacute lymphocytic thyroiditis *(painless)*
Struma ovarii (ovarian teratoma with thyroid)
Factitious thyrotoxicosis (exogenous thyroxine intake)

TSH, Thyroid-stimulating hormone.
*Associated with increased TSH; all other causes of thyrotoxicosis associated with decreased TSH.

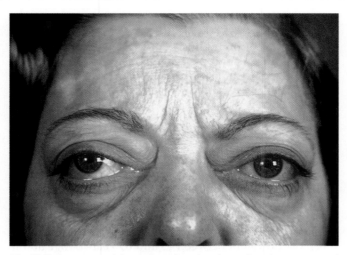

Fig. 20.7 A patient with hyperthyroidism. A wide-eyed, staring gaze, caused by overactivity of the sympathetic nervous system, is one of the classic features of this disorder. In Graves disease, one of the most important causes of hyperthyroidism, accumulation of loose connective tissue behind the orbits also adds to the protuberant appearance of the eyes.

peripheral oxygen requirements. Older adult patients with preexisting heart disease may develop congestive heart failure.
- *Neuromuscular:* Patients frequently experience nervousness, tremor, and irritability due to the sympathetic overactivity. Nearly 50% develop proximal muscle weakness *(thyroid myopathy).*
- *Ocular changes* often call attention to hyperthyroidism. A wide, staring gaze and lid lag are present because of sympathetic overstimulation of the superior tarsal muscle *(Müller's muscle),* which functions alongside the levator palpebrae superioris muscle to raise the upper eyelid (Fig. 20.7). However, fullblown *thyroid ophthalmopathy* associated with proptosis is a feature seen only in Graves disease (discussed later).
- *Thyroid storm* designates the abrupt onset of severe hyperthyroidism. It occurs most often in patients with Graves disease and probably results from an acute elevation in catecholamine levels, as might be encountered during infection, surgery, cessation of anti-thyroid medication, or any form of stress. Thyroid storm is a medical emergency, as a significant number of untreated patients die of cardiac arrhythmias.
- *Apathetic hyperthyroidism* refers to thyrotoxicosis occurring in older adults, in whom the typical features of thyroid hormone excess often are blunted. The underlying thyroid disease is usually detected during laboratory workup for unexplained weight loss or worsening cardiovascular disease.

The diagnosis of hyperthyroidism is based on clinical features and laboratory data. *The measurement of serum TSH is the most useful single screening test for hyperthyroidism,* because TSH levels are decreased even at the earliest stages, when the disease may still be subclinical. In rare cases of pituitary- or hypothalamus-associated (secondary) hyperthyroidism, TSH levels are either normal or raised. A low TSH value usually is associated with increased levels of free T_4. In the occasional patient, hyperthyroidism results

predominantly from increased circulating levels of T_3 (T_3 toxicosis). In such cases, free T_4 levels may be decreased, and direct measurement of serum T_3 may be useful. Once the diagnosis of thyrotoxicosis has been confirmed by a combination of TSH and free thyroid hormone assays, measurement of radioactive iodine uptake by the thyroid gland can be valuable in determining the etiology. For example, such scans may show diffusely increased uptake in Graves disease, increased uptake in a solitary nodule in toxic adenoma, or decreased uptake in thyroiditis.

HYPOTHYROIDISM

Hypothyroidism is caused by structural or functional derangements that interfere with thyroid hormone production. This disorder may be divided into primary and secondary categories, depending on whether it arises from an intrinsic abnormality in the thyroid or from hypothalamic or pituitary disease (Table 20.3). Primary hypothyroidism can be secondary to *congenital, autoimmune,* or *iatrogenic* causes.
- *Genetic defects* that perturb thyroid development (thyroid dysgenesis) or the synthesis of thyroid hormone (dyshormonogenetic goiter) are rare overall but the most common cause of congenital hypothyroidism in the U.S.
- *Endemic deficiency of dietary iodine* is typically manifested by hyothryoidism early in childhood and has been also called congenital, but is not caused by genetic defects. It is a common cause of hypothyroidism in infants and children worldwide.
- *Autoimmune thyroid disease* is a common cause of hypothyroidism in regions of the world where iodine is supplemented in dietary salt products. The vast majority of cases of autoimmune hypothyroidism are due to Hashimoto thyroiditis (discussed later).
- *Iatrogenic hypothyroidism* can be caused by either surgical or radiation-induced ablation of thyroid parenchyma, or as an unintended adverse effect of certain drugs.

The clinical manifestations of hypothyroidism include cretinism and myxedema.
- *Cretinism* refers to hypothyroidism developing in infancy or early childhood. This disorder formerly was

Table 20.3 Causes of Hypothyroidism

Primary
Postablative
Surgery, radioiodine therapy, or external irradiation
Autoimmune hypothyroidism
Hashimoto thyroiditis*
Iodine deficiency*
Drugs (lithium, iodides, p-aminosalicylic acid)*
Congenital biosynthetic defect (dyshormonogenetic goiter) (rare)*
Genetic defects in thyroid development (rare)
Thyroid hormone resistance syndrome (rare)

Secondary (Central)
Pituitary failure (rare)
Hypothalamic failure (rare)

*Associated with enlargement of thyroid ("goitrous hypothyroidism"). Hashimoto thyroiditis and postablative hypothyroidism account for the majority of cases of hypothyroidism in developed countries.

fairly common in areas of the world where dietary iodine deficiency is endemic, including mountainous areas such as the Himalayas and the Andes (*endemic cretinism*). It is now much less frequent because of the widespread supplementation of salt with iodine. By contrast, enzyme defects that interfere with thyroid hormone synthesis are a cause of *sporadic cretinism*. Clinical features of cretinism include impaired development of the skeletal system and central nervous system, severe mental retardation, short stature, coarse facial features, a protruding tongue, and umbilical hernia. The severity of the mental impairment in cretinism seems to be influenced by the time of onset of the deficient state in utero. Normally, maternal hormones that are critical to fetal brain development, including T_3 and T_4, cross the placenta. If maternal thyroid deficiency is present before the development of the fetal thyroid gland, mental retardation is severe. By contrast, reduction in maternal thyroid hormones later in pregnancy, after the fetal thyroid has developed, allows normal brain development.

- Hypothyroidism in older children and adults results in a condition known as *myxedema*. The initial symptoms include generalized fatigue, apathy, and mental sluggishness, which may mimic depression. Decreased sympathetic activity results in constipation and decreased sweating. The skin is cool and pale because of decreased blood flow. Reduced cardiac output contributes to shortness of breath and decreased exercise capacity, two frequent complaints. Thyroid hormones regulate the transcription of several sarcolemmal genes, such as calcium ATPases, whose encoded products are critical in maintaining efficient cardiac output. In addition, hypothyroidism promotes an atherogenic lipid profile—an increase in total cholesterol and low-density lipoprotein (LDL) levels—that may contribute to the adverse cardiovascular mortality rates in this disease. Histologically, there is an accumulation of matrix substances, such as glycosaminoglycans and hyaluronic acid, in skin, subcutaneous tissue, and viscera. This results in nonpitting edema, broadening and coarsening of facial features, enlargement of the tongue, and deepening of the voice.

The diagnosis of hypothyroidism is based on laboratory evaluation. As in the case of hyperthyroidism, *measurement of serum TSH is the most sensitive screening test*. The serum TSH concentration is increased in primary hypothyroidism because of a loss of feedback inhibition of thyrotropin-releasing hormone (TRH) and TSH production by the hypothalamus and pituitary, respectively. The TSH concentration is not increased in individuals with hypothyroidism caused by primary hypothalamic or pituitary disease. Serum T_4 is decreased in patients with hypothyroidism of any origin.

AUTOIMMUNE THYROID DISEASE

Autoimmunity is the underlying cause of a variety of thyroid diseases, which are collectively referred to as *autoimmune thyroid disease (AITD)*. These disorders include thyroiditis, and antibody-mediated disturbances in thyroid function that are not necessarily associated with inflammation (exemplified by Graves disease). We discuss first the various forms of thyroiditis.

Thyroiditis encompasses a diverse group of disorders characterized by some form of thyroid inflammation. This discussion focuses on the three most common and clinically significant subtypes: (1) Hashimoto thyroiditis, (2) granulomatous (de Quervain) thyroiditis, and (3) subacute lymphocytic thyroiditis.

Chronic Lymphocytic (Hashimoto) Thyroiditis

Hashimoto thyroiditis is the most common cause of hypothyroidism in areas of the world where iodine levels are sufficient. It is characterized by gradual thyroid failure secondary to autoimmune destruction of the thyroid gland. It is most prevalent between 45 and 65 years of age and is more common in women with a female to male ratio of 10:1 to 20:1. Although it is primarily a disease of older women, it can occur at any age, including childhood.

Pathogenesis

Hashimoto thyroiditis is an autoimmune disease caused by an immune response to thyroid autoantigens (Chapter 5). Circulating autoantibodies against thyroid antigens are present in the vast majority of patients. The immune response leads to progressive depletion of thyroid epithelial cells associated with lymphocytic infiltrates and fibrosis. The inciting events leading to the autoimmune response have not been fully elucidated, but multiple immunologic mechanisms that may contribute to thyroid cell damage have been identified (Fig. 20.8), including the following:
- CD8+ cytotoxic T-cell–mediated killing of thyroid epithelial cells.
- Cytokine-mediated cell death. T-cell activation leads to the production of inflammatory cytokines such as interferon-γ in the thyroid gland, with resultant recruitment and activation of macrophages and damage to follicles.
- Binding of anti-thyroid antibodies (anti-thyroglobulin, and anti-thyroid peroxidase antibodies), followed by antibody-dependent cell–mediated cytotoxicity (Chapter 5).

The disease appears to have a significant genetic component, based on a concordance rate of about 40% in monozygotic twins and the presence of anti-thyroid antibodies in approximately 50% of asymptomatic siblings of affected patients. Increased susceptibility to Hashimoto thyroiditis is associated with polymorphisms in immune regulation–associated genes, the most significant of which is the cytotoxic T lymphocyte–associated antigen-4 gene (*CTLA4*), which codes for a negative regulator of T-cell responses (Chapter 5).

MORPHOLOGY

The thyroid usually is diffusely and symmetrically enlarged. Microscopic examination reveals widespread infiltration of the parenchyma by a **mononuclear inflammatory infiltrate** containing small lymphocytes, plasma cells, and well-developed

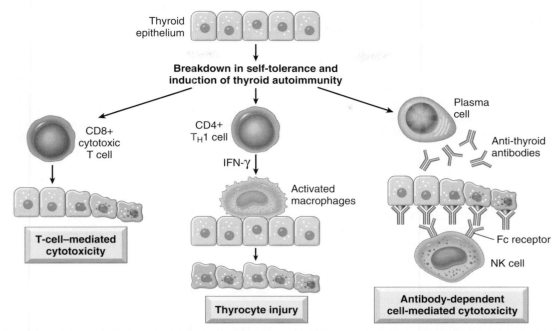

Fig. 20.8 Pathogenesis of Hashimoto thyroiditis. Breakdown of immune tolerance to thyroid autoantigens results in progressive autoimmune destruction of thyrocytes by infiltrating cytotoxic T cells, locally released cytokines, or antibody-dependent cytotoxicity.

germinal centers (Fig. 20.9). The thyroid follicles are atrophic and are lined in many areas by epithelial cells distinguished by the presence of abundant eosinophilic, granular cytoplasm, termed **Hürthle,** or **oxyphil, cells.** This is a metaplastic response of the normal low cuboidal follicular epithelium to ongoing injury; on ultrastructural examination, the Hürthle cells are characterized by numerous prominent mitochondria. Interstitial connective tissue is increased and may be abundant. Less commonly, the thyroid is small and atrophic as a result of more extensive fibrosis **(fibrosing variant).**

Clinical Features

Hashimoto thyroiditis comes to clinical attention as *painless enlargement of the thyroid, usually associated with some degree of hypothyroidism,* often in a middle-age woman.

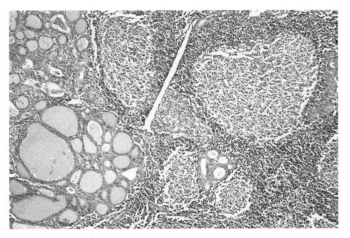

Fig. 20.9 Hashimoto thyroiditis. The thyroid parenchyma contains a dense lymphocytic infiltrate with germinal centers. Residual thyroid follicles lined by deeply eosinophilic Hürthle cells also are seen.

The enlargement of the gland usually is symmetric and diffuse, but in some cases it may be sufficiently localized to raise suspicion for neoplasm. In the usual clinical course, hypothyroidism develops gradually. In some cases, however, it may be preceded by transient thyrotoxicosis caused by disruption of thyroid follicles, with secondary release of thyroid hormones *(hashitoxicosis).* During this phase, free T_4 and T_3 concentrations are elevated, TSH is diminished, and radioactive iodine uptake is decreased. As hypothyroidism supervenes, T_4 and T_3 levels progressively fall, accompanied by a compensatory increase in TSH. Patients with Hashimoto thyroiditis often have *other autoimmune diseases* and are at *increased risk for the development of B-cell non-Hodgkin lymphomas* (Chapter 12), which typically arise within the thyroid gland. The relationship between Hashimoto disease and thyroid epithelial cancers remains controversial, with some morphologic and molecular studies suggesting a predisposition to papillary carcinomas.

Subacute Granulomatous (de Quervain) Thyroiditis

Subacute granulomatous thyroiditis, also known as *de Quervain thyroiditis,* is much less common than Hashimoto disease. De Quervain thyroiditis is most common between 30 and 50 years of age and, like other forms of thyroiditis, occurs more frequently in women than in men. Subacute thyroiditis is believed to be caused by a viral infection or an inflammatory process triggered by viral infections, and not by an autoimmune process. A majority of patients have a history of an upper-respiratory infection shortly before the onset of thyroiditis. Unlike in autoimmune thyroid disease, the immune response in subacute granulomatous thyroiditis is not self-perpetuating, so the process spontaneously remits.

MORPHOLOGY

The gland is firm, with an intact capsule, and may be unilaterally or bilaterally enlarged. Histologic examination reveals disruption of thyroid follicles, extravasation of colloid, and infiltrating neutrophils, which are replaced over time by lymphocytes, plasma cells, and macrophages. The extravasated colloid provokes an exuberant granulomatous reaction with giant cells, some containing fragments of colloid. Healing occurs by resolution of inflammation and fibrosis.

Clinical Features

The onset of this form of thyroiditis often is acute. It is characterized by *neck pain* (particularly with swallowing), fever, malaise, and variable enlargement of the thyroid. Transient hyperthyroidism may occur, as in other cases of thyroiditis, as a result of disruption of thyroid follicles and release of excessive thyroid hormone. The leukocyte count and erythrocyte sedimentation rates are increased. With progression of the gland destruction, a transient hypothyroid phase may ensue. The condition typically is self-limited, with most patients returning to a euthyroid state within 6 to 8 weeks.

Subacute Lymphocytic Thyroiditis

Subacute lymphocytic thyroiditis also is known as *silent* or *painless* thyroiditis; in a subset of patients, the onset follows pregnancy (*postpartum thyroiditis*). This disease is most likely autoimmune in etiology, as circulating antithyroid antibodies are found in a majority of patients. It mostly affects middle-aged women, who present with a painless neck mass or features of thyroid hormone excess. The initial phase of thyrotoxicosis (which is likely to be secondary to thyroid tissue damage) is followed by return to a euthyroid state within a few months. In a minority of affected individuals, the condition eventually progresses to hypothyroidism. Except for possible mild symmetric enlargement, the thyroid appears normal on gross inspection. The histologic features consist of lymphocytic infiltration and hyperplastic germinal centers within the thyroid parenchyma.

Other Forms of Thyroiditis

Riedel thyroiditis, a rare disorder that is a manifestation of IgG4-related disease (Chapter 5), is characterized by extensive fibrosis involving the thyroid and contiguous neck structures. Clinical evaluation demonstrates a hard and fixed thyroid mass, simulating a thyroid neoplasm. It may be associated with idiopathic fibrosis in other sites in the body, such as the retroperitoneum.

SUMMARY

THYROIDITIS

- Chronic lymphocytic (Hashimoto) thyroiditis is the most common cause of hypothyroidism in regions where dietary iodine levels are sufficient.

- Hashimoto thyroiditis is an autoimmune disease characterized by progressive destruction of thyroid parenchyma, Hürthle cell change, and mononuclear (lymphoplasmacytic) infiltrates, with or without extensive fibrosis.
- Multiple autoimmune mechanisms account for thyroid injury in Hashimoto disease, including cytotoxicity mediated by CD8+ T cells, cytokines (IFN-γ), and anti-thyroid antibodies.
- Subacute granulomatous (de Quervain) thyroiditis is a self-limited disease, probably secondary to a viral infection, and is characterized by pain and the presence of a granulomatous inflammation in the thyroid.
- Subacute lymphocytic thyroiditis is a self-limited disease that often occurs after a pregnancy (postpartum thyroiditis), typically is painless, and is characterized by lymphocytic inflammation in the thyroid.

Graves Disease

In 1835, Robert Graves reported on his observations of a disease characterized by "violent and long continued palpitations in females" associated with enlargement of the thyroid gland. **Graves disease is the most common cause of endogenous hyperthyroidism.** It is characterized by a triad of manifestations:

- *Thyrotoxicosis,* caused by a diffusely enlarged, hyperfunctional thyroid
- An infiltrative *ophthalmopathy* with resultant exophthalmos, noted in as many as 40% of patients
- A localized, infiltrative *dermopathy* (sometimes designated *pretibial myxedema*), seen in a minority of cases

Graves disease has a peak incidence between 20 and 40 years of age, with women being affected up to seven times more commonly than men. This is a common disorder, estimated to affect 1.5% to 2% of women in the United States. Genetic factors are important in Graves disease; the incidence is increased in relatives of affected patients, and the concordance rate in monozygotic twins is as high as 60%. As with other autoimmune disorders, a genetic susceptibility to Graves disease is associated with the presence of certain human leukocyte antigen (HLA) haplotypes, specifically HLA-DR3, and polymorphisms in genes whose products regulate T-cell responses, including the inhibitory T-cell receptor CTLA-4 and the tyrosine phosphatase PTPN22.

Pathogenesis

Many manifestations of Graves disease are caused by autoantibodies against the TSH receptor that bind to, and stimulate, thyroid follicular cells independent of endogenous trophic hormones. Multiple autoantibodies are produced in Graves disease, including the following:

- *Thyroid-stimulating immunoglobulin (TSI).* This IgG antibody binds to the TSH receptor and mimics the action of TSH, stimulating adenyl cyclase, with resultant increased release of thyroid hormones. Almost all individuals with Graves disease have detectable amounts of this autoantibody, which is relatively specific for Graves disease.

- *Thyroid growth-stimulating immunoglobulins.* Also directed against the TSH receptor, these antibodies have been implicated in the proliferation of thyroid follicular epithelium.
- *TSH-binding inhibitor immunoglobulins.* These anti-TSH receptor antibodies prevent TSH from binding to its receptor on thyroid epithelial cells and in so doing may inhibit thyroid cell function. The coexistence of stimulating and inhibiting immunoglobulins in the serum of the same patient is not unusual, and may explain why some patients develop episodes of hypothyroidism.

A T-cell–mediated autoimmune phenomenon also is involved in the development of the *infiltrative ophthalmopathy* characteristic of Graves disease. In Graves ophthalmopathy, the volume of the retroorbital connective tissues and extraocular muscles is increased due to (1) marked infiltration of the retroorbital space by mononuclear cells, predominantly T cells; (2) inflammatory edema and swelling of extraocular muscles; (3) accumulation of extracellular matrix components, specifically hydrophilic glycosaminoglycans such as hyaluronic acid and chondroitin sulfate; and (4) increased numbers of adipocytes (fatty infiltration). These changes displace the eyeball forward, potentially interfering with the function of the extraocular muscles.

Autoimmune thyroid diseases thus span a continuum in which Graves disease, characterized by hyperfunction of the thyroid, lies at one extreme and Hashimoto disease, manifesting as hypothyroidism, occupies the other end. Sometimes hyperthyroidism may supervene on preexisting Hashimoto thyroiditis, while at other times individuals with Graves disease may spontaneously develop thyroid hypofunction; occasionally, Hashimoto thyroiditis and Graves disease may coexist within an affected kindred. Not surprisingly, there is also an element of histologic overlap between the autoimmune thyroid disorders (most characteristically, prominent intrathyroidal lymphoid cell infiltrates with germinal center formation). In both disorders, the frequency of other autoimmune diseases, such as systemic lupus erythematosus, pernicious anemia, type 1 diabetes, and Addison disease, is increased.

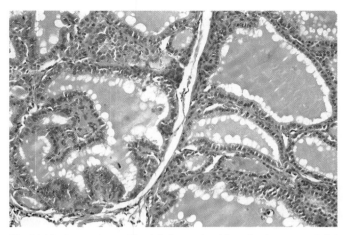

Fig. 20.10 Graves disease. The follicles are lined by tall columnar epithelial cells that are actively resorbing the colloid in the centers of the follicles, resulting in a "scalloped" appearance of the colloid.

hydrophilic glycosaminoglycans. In addition, there is infiltration by lymphocytes, mostly T cells. Orbital muscles initially are edematous but may undergo fibrosis late in the course of the disease. The dermopathy, if present, is characterized by thickening of the dermis, as a result of deposition of glycosaminoglycans and lymphocyte infiltration.

Clinical Features

The clinical manifestations of Graves disease include those common to all forms of thyrotoxicosis (discussed earlier), as well as those associated uniquely with Graves disease: *diffuse hyperplasia of the thyroid, ophthalmopathy,* and *dermopathy.* The degree of thyrotoxicosis varies from case to case, and the related changes may sometimes be less conspicuous than other manifestations of the disease. Increased flow of blood through the hyperactive gland often produces an audible bruit. Sympathetic overactivity produces a characteristic wide, staring gaze and lid lag. The ophthalmopathy of Graves disease results in abnormal protrusion of the eyeball *(exophthalmos).* The exophthalmos may persist or progress despite successful treatment of the thyrotoxicosis, sometimes resulting in corneal injury. The extraocular muscles often are weak. The infiltrative dermopathy most commonly involves the skin overlying the shins, where it manifests as scaly thickening and induration of the skin (pretibial myxedema). The skin lesions may be slightly pigmented papules or nodules and often have an orange peel texture. Laboratory findings in Graves disease include elevated serum free T_4 and T_3 and depressed serum TSH. Because of ongoing stimulation of the thyroid follicles by TSIs, radioactive iodine uptake is increased diffusely.

MORPHOLOGY

In the typical case of Graves disease, the thyroid gland is enlarged (usually symmetrically) due to **diffuse hypertrophy and hyperplasia** of thyroid follicular epithelial cells. The gland is usually smooth and soft, and its capsule is intact. On microscopic examination, the follicular epithelial cells in untreated cases are tall, columnar, and more crowded than usual. This crowding often results in the formation of small papillae, which project into the follicular lumen (Fig. 20.10). Such papillae lack fibrovascular cores, in contrast with those of papillary carcinoma. The colloid within the follicular lumen is pale, with scalloped margins. Lymphoid infiltrates, consisting predominantly of T cells, with fewer B cells and mature plasma cells, are present throughout the interstitium; germinal centers are common.

Changes in extrathyroidal tissues include generalized lymphoid hyperplasia. In individuals with ophthalmopathy, the tissues of the orbit are edematous because of the presence of

SUMMARY

GRAVES DISEASE

- Graves disease, the most common cause of endogenous hyperthyroidism, is characterized by the triad of thyrotoxicosis, ophthalmopathy, and dermopathy.

- Graves disease is an autoimmune disorder caused by autoantibodies to the TSH receptor that mimic TSH action and activate TSH receptors on thyroid epithelial cells.
- The thyroid in Graves disease is characterized by diffuse hypertrophy and hyperplasia of follicles and lymphoid infiltrates; glycosaminoglycan deposition and lymphoid infiltrates are responsible for the ophthalmopathy and dermopathy.
- Laboratory features include elevations in serum free T_3 and T_4 and decreased serum TSH.

DIFFUSE AND MULTINODULAR GOITER

Enlargement of the thyroid, or *goiter,* is the most common manifestation of thyroid disease. **Diffuse and multinodular goiters are the result of impaired synthesis of thyroid hormone,** most often caused by dietary iodine deficiency. Impairment of thyroid hormone synthesis leads to a compensatory rise in the serum TSH, which drives the hypertrophy and hyperplasia of thyroid follicular cells and, ultimately, enlargement of the thyroid gland. The degree of thyroid enlargement is proportional to the level and duration of thyroid hormone deficiency. These compensatory changes overcome the hormone deficiency and maintain a *euthyroid* metabolic state in the vast majority of affected individuals. However, if the underlying disorder is severe (e.g., a congenital biosynthetic defect), the compensatory responses may be inadequate, resulting in *goitrous hypothyroidism.*

Pathogenesis

Goiters can be endemic or sporadic.

- *Endemic goiter* occurs in geographic areas where the diet contains little iodine. The designation *endemic* is used when goiters are present in more than 10% of the population in a given region. Such conditions are particularly common in mountainous areas of the world, including the Himalayas and the Andes. With increased availability of dietary iodine supplementation, the frequency and severity of endemic goiter have declined significantly.
- *Sporadic goiter* occurs less frequently than endemic goiter. The condition is more common in females than in males, with a peak incidence in puberty or young adulthood, when there is an increased physiologic demand for T_4. Sporadic goiter may be caused by several conditions, including the excessive ingestion of substances that interfere with thyroid hormone synthesis, such as calcium and vegetables belonging to the *Brassicaceae* (also called *Cruciferae*) family (e.g., cabbage, cauliflower, Brussels sprouts, turnips). In other instances goiter may result from inherited enzymatic defects that interfere with thyroid hormone synthesis *(dyshormonogenetic goiter)*. In most cases, however, the cause of sporadic goiter is not apparent.

MORPHOLOGY

Early in its development, TSH-induced hypertrophy and hyperplasia of thyroid follicular cells usually result in diffuse, symmetric enlargement of the gland **(diffuse goiter).** The follicles are lined by crowded columnar cells, which may pile up and form projections similar to those seen in Graves disease. If dietary iodine subsequently increases, or if the demands for thyroid hormone decrease, the follicular epithelium involutes to form an enlarged, colloid-rich gland **(colloid goiter).** The cut surface of the thyroid in such cases usually is brown, glassy-appearing, and translucent. On microscopic examination, the follicular epithelium may be hyperplastic in the early stages of disease or flattened and cuboidal during periods of involution. Colloid is abundant during the latter periods.

With time, recurrent episodes of hyperplasia and involution combine to produce a more irregular enlargement of the thyroid, termed **multinodular goiter.** Virtually all long-standing diffuse goiters convert into multinodular goiters. Multinodular goiters are multilobulate, asymmetrically enlarged glands that may attain a massive size. On cut surface, irregular nodules containing variable amounts of brown, gelatinous colloid are

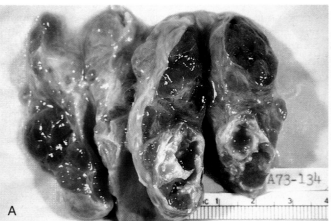
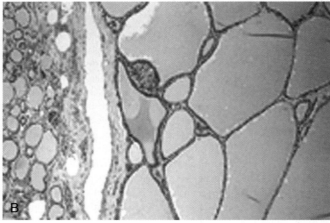

Fig. 20.11 Multinodular goiter. (A) Gross morphologic appearance. The coarsely nodular gland contains areas of fibrosis and cystic change. (B) Photomicrograph of a specimen from a hyperplastic nodule, with compressed residual thyroid parenchyma on the periphery. The hyperplastic follicles contain abundant pink "colloid" within their lumina. Note the absence of a prominent capsule, a feature distinguishing such lesions from neoplasms of the thyroid. (B, Courtesy of Dr. William Westra, Department of Pathology, Johns Hopkins University, Baltimore, Maryland.)

evident (Fig. 20.11A). Older lesions often show areas of fibrosis, hemorrhage, calcification, and cystic change. The microscopic appearance includes colloid-rich follicles lined by flattened, inactive epithelium and areas of follicular epithelial hypertrophy and hyperplasia, accompanied by the regressive changes just noted (see Fig. 20.11B).

Clinical Features

The dominant clinical features of goiter are those caused by the mass effects of the enlarged gland. In addition to the obvious cosmetic problem of a large neck mass, goiters also may cause airway obstruction, dysphagia, and compression of large vessels in the neck and upper thorax (so-called "superior vena cava syndrome").

Multinodular goiters typically are hormonally silent, but a minority (approximately 10% over 10 years) manifest with thyrotoxicosis secondary to the development of autonomous nodules that produce thyroid hormone independent of TSH stimulation. This condition, known as *toxic multinodular goiter* or *Plummer syndrome*, is not accompanied by the infiltrative ophthalmopathy and dermopathy of Graves disease–associated thyrotoxicosis. The incidence of malignancy in long-standing multinodular goiters is low (<5%) but not zero, and concern for malignancy arises with goiters that demonstrate sudden changes in size or associated symptoms (e.g., hoarseness).

THYROID NEOPLASMS

Thyroid tumors range from circumscribed, benign adenomas to highly aggressive, anaplastic carcinomas. From a clinical standpoint, the possibility of a tumor is of major concern in patients who present with thyroid nodules. Fortunately, the overwhelming majority of solitary nodules of the thyroid prove to be either benign adenomas or localized, non-neoplastic conditions (e.g., a dominant nodule in multinodular goiter, simple cysts, or foci of thyroiditis). Carcinomas of the thyroid, by contrast, are uncommon, accounting for less than 1% of solitary thyroid nodules. Several clinical criteria provide a clue to the nature of a given thyroid nodule:

- *Solitary nodules,* in general, are more likely to be neoplastic than are multiple nodules.
- *Nodules in very young (<20 years) or very old (>70 years) individuals* are more likely to be neoplastic.
- *Nodules in males* are more likely to be neoplastic than are those in females.
- A history of *radiation* exposure is associated with an increased incidence of thyroid malignancy.
- Nodules that take up radioactive iodine in imaging studies (*hot nodules*) are more likely to be benign.

Such associations, however, are of little significance in the evaluation of a given patient, in whom the timely recognition of a malignancy may be lifesaving. Ultimately, morphologic evaluation of a thyroid nodule by fine-needle aspiration, combined with the histologic study of surgically resected thyroid tissue, provide the most definitive information about the nature of the nodule.

Adenomas

Adenomas of the thyroid are benign neoplasms derived from follicular epithelium. Follicular adenomas usually are solitary. On clinical and morphologic grounds, they may be difficult to distinguish from a dominant nodule in multinodular goiter, for example, or from less common follicular carcinomas. Although the vast majority of adenomas are nonfunctional, a small proportion produce thyroid hormones *(toxic adenomas),* causing clinically apparent thyrotoxicosis. In general, follicular adenomas are not forerunners to carcinomas; nevertheless, shared genetic alterations support the possibility that at least a subset of follicular carcinomas arise in preexisting adenomas.

Pathogenesis

Driver mutations in the TSH receptor signaling pathway play an important role in the pathogenesis of toxic adenomas (see Fig. 20.6). Activating (gain-of-function) somatic mutations in one of two components of this signaling system—most often the gene encoding the TSH receptor itself *(TSHR)* and, less commonly, the α-subunit of Gs *(GNAS)*—allow follicular cells to secrete thyroid hormone independent of TSH stimulation (thyroid autonomy). The result of this overabundance is symptomatic hyperthyroidism, with a "hot" thyroid nodule seen on imaging studies. Overall, somatic mutations in the TSH receptor signaling pathway are present in slightly over half of toxic adenomas. Not surprisingly, such mutations also are observed in a subset of autonomous nodules that give rise to toxic multinodular goiters, discussed earlier. Thus, autonomy in both toxic goiter and toxic adenomas stems from the ability of follicular cells to release thyroid hormone independent of trophic factors (i.e., TSH). A minority of nonfunctioning follicular adenomas (<20%) exhibit mutations in *RAS* or other other genes, genetic alterations that are shared with follicular carcinomas (discussed later).

MORPHOLOGY

The typical thyroid adenoma is a **solitary,** spherical lesion that compresses the adjacent nonneoplastic thyroid. The neoplastic cells are demarcated from the adjacent parenchyma by a **well-defined, intact capsule** (Fig. 20.12A). On microscopic examination, the constituent cells are arranged in uniform follicles that contain colloid (see Fig. 20.12B). Occasionally, the neoplastic cells acquire brightly eosinophilic granular cytoplasm (oxyphil or Hürthle cell change) (Fig. 20.13). Similar to endocrine tumors at other anatomic sites, even benign follicular adenomas occasionally exhibit focal nuclear pleomorphism, atypia, and prominent nucleoli **(endocrine atypia);** by themselves, these features do not constitute evidence of malignancy. The hallmark of all follicular adenomas is the presence of an intact well-formed capsule encircling the tumor. **Careful evaluation of the integrity of the capsule is therefore critical in distinguishing follicular adenomas from follicular carcinomas,** which demonstrate capsular and/or vascular invasion (discussed later).

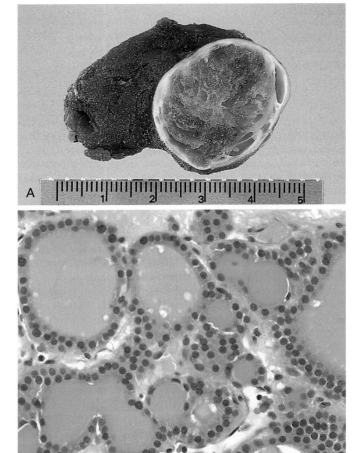

Fig. 20.12 Follicular adenoma of the thyroid gland. (A) A solitary, well-circumscribed nodule is visible in this gross specimen. (B) The photomicrograph shows well-differentiated follicles resembling those of normal thyroid parenchyma.

Clinical Features

Most adenomas of the thyroid manifest as painless nodules, often discovered during a routine physical examination. Larger masses may produce local symptoms such as difficulty in swallowing. Individuals with toxic adenomas may present with features of thyrotoxicosis. After injection of radioactive iodine, most adenomas take up iodine less avidly than normal thyroid parenchyma. On radionuclide scanning, therefore, adenomas appear as *cold* nodules relative to the adjacent normal thyroid gland. Toxic adenomas, however, appear as *warm* or *hot* nodules in the scan. As many as 10% of *cold* nodules eventually prove to be malignant. By contrast, malignancy is uncommon in *hot* nodules. Essential techniques used in the preoperative evaluation of suspected adenomas are ultrasonography and fine-needle aspiration biopsy. Because of the need for evaluating capsular integrity, *the definitive diagnosis of thyroid adenoma can be made only after careful microscopic examination of the resected specimen.* Suspected adenomas of the thyroid are therefore removed surgically to exclude malignancy. Thyroid adenomas carry an excellent prognosis and do not recur or metastasize.

Carcinomas

The detection of small , clinically asymptomatic cancerous nodules of the thyroid gland has increased dramatically in the United States over the last few years, largely due to the increasing use of thyroid ultrasound and other imaging studies. Nonetheless, deaths from thyroid cancer have remained relatively stable during this period, underscoring the favorable outcome for such incidentally detected thyroid carcinomas (and also raising questions about the value of detecting clinically insignificant cancers). A female predominance has been noted among patients who develop thyroid carcinoma in the early and middle adult years. By contrast, cases seen in childhood and late adult life are distributed equally between males and females. Most thyroid carcinomas (except medullary carcinomas) are derived from the thyroid follicular epithelium, and of these, the vast majority are well-differentiated lesions. The major subtypes of thyroid carcinoma and their relative frequencies are as follows:

- *Papillary carcinoma* (accounting for more than 85% of cases)
- *Follicular carcinoma* (5% to 15% of cases)
- *Anaplastic (undifferentiated) carcinoma* (<5% of cases)
- *Medullary carcinoma* (5% of cases)

Because of the unique clinical and biologic features associated with each type of thyroid carcinoma, these are described separately. Presented next is an overview of the molecular pathogenesis of all thyroid cancers.

Pathogenesis

Distinct molecular events are involved in the pathogenesis of the four major variants of thyroid cancer. Genetic alterations in the three follicular cell–derived malignancies are clustered along two oncogenic pathways that lie downstream of growth factor receptors and RAS—the mitogen-activated protein (MAP) kinase pathway and the phosphatidylinositol-3-kinase (PI-3K)/AKT pathway

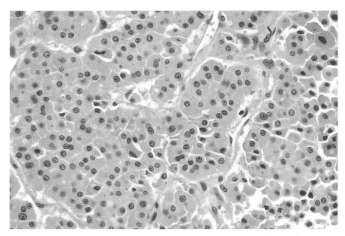

Fig. 20.13 Hürthle cell adenoma. On this high-power view, the tumor is composed of cells with abundant eosinophilic cytoplasm and small regular nuclei. *(Courtesy of Dr. Mary Sunday, Brigham and Women's Hospital, Boston, Massachusetts.)*

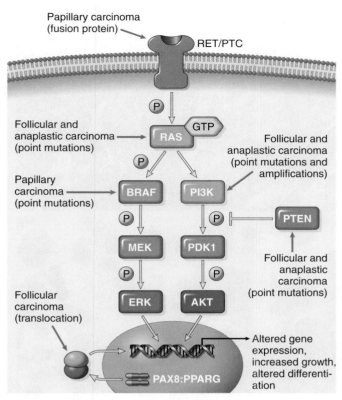

Fig. 20.14 Genetic alterations in follicular cell–derived malignancies of the thyroid gland.

(Fig. 20.14). In normal cells, these pathways are transiently activated by binding of growth factors to receptor tyrosine kinases, which results in signal transduction. In thyroid carcinomas, as with many solid cancers (Chapter 6), gain-of-function mutations in components of these pathways lead to constitutive activation, even in the absence of growth factors, thus promoting carcinogenesis.

- *Papillary thyroid carcinomas.* **Activation of the MAP kinase pathway is a feature of most papillary carcinomas.** The most common mechanisms of MAP kinase signaling are: (1) rearrangements in genes that encode the receptor tyrosine kinases RET and NTRK1 (neurotrophic tyrosine kinase receptor 1); and (2) activating point mutations in *BRAF*, whose product is a component of the MAP kinase pathway (see Fig. 20.14). One third to one half of papillary thyroid carcinomas harbor a gain-of-function mutation in *BRAF*, which is the most common driver mutation in this neoplasm. Since chromosomal rearrangements of the *RET* or *NTRK1* genes and mutations of *BRAF* have redundant effects, papillary thyroid carcinomas demonstrate either one or the other molecular abnormality, but not both.
- *Follicular thyroid carcinomas.* **Follicular thyroid carcinomas frequently harbor driver mutations in RAS or in components of the PI3K/AKT signaling pathway.** Both gain-of-function mutation in PI3K and loss-of-function mutations in PTEN, a negative regulator of PI3K, are seen. RAS and PI3K mutations also are found in benign follicular adenomas to and anaplastic carcinomas (see

next) suggesting a shared histogenesis. One third to one half of follicular carcinomas also have a unique (2;3) (q13;p25) translocation that disrupts *PAX8*, a paired homeobox gene that is important in thyroid development, and the peroxisome proliferator–activated receptor gene *(PPARG)*, whose gene product is a nuclear hormone receptor implicated in terminal differentiation of cells.

- *Anaplastic carcinomas.* **These highly aggressive tumors can arise de novo or, more commonly, by progression of a well-differentiated papillary or follicular carcinoma.** Molecular alterations present in anaplastic carcinomas include those also seen in well-differentiated carcinomas (e.g., *RAS* or *PIK3CA* mutations), as well as additional mutations that are specific to anaplastic carcinoma. The most common of these unique mutations are loss-of-function mutations in *TP53*, which are believed to have an important role in the development of anaplastic carcinomas.
- *Medullary thyroid carcinomas.* In contrast with the subtypes described earlier, these neoplasms arise from the parafollicular C cells, rather than the follicular epithelium. Familial medullary thyroid carcinomas occur in *multiple endocrine neoplasia type 2* (MEN-2) (see later) and are associated with germ line *RET* proto-oncogene mutations that lead to constitutive activation of the RET tyrosine kinase receptor. *RET* mutations are also seen in approximately one-half of nonfamilial (sporadic) medullary thyroid cancers.

***Environmental Factors.* The major risk factor predisposing to thyroid cancer is exposure to ionizing radiation, particularly during the first 2 decades of life.** In keeping with this finding, there was a marked increase in the incidence of papillary carcinomas among children exposed to ionizing radiation after the Chernobyl nuclear disaster in 1986. Deficiency of dietary iodine (and by extension, an association with goiter) is linked with a higher frequency of follicular carcinomas.

Papillary Carcinoma

As mentioned earlier, papillary carcinomas are the most common form of thyroid cancer. These tumors may occur at any age, and they account for the vast majority of thyroid carcinomas associated with previous exposure to ionizing radiation.

MORPHOLOGY

Papillary carcinomas are solitary or multifocal lesions. Some tumors may be well circumscribed and encapsulated; others infiltrate the adjacent parenchyma and have ill-defined margins. The cut surface sometimes reveals papillary foci that point to the diagnosis (Fig. 20.15A). The microscopic hallmarks of papillary neoplasms include the following:

- Branching **papillae** having a fibrovascular stalk covered by a single to multiple layers of cuboidal epithelial cells (see Fig. 20.15B). In most cases, the epithelium covering the papillae has well-differentiated, uniform, orderly cuboidal cells, but more pleomorphic or even anaplastic morphologies may be seen.

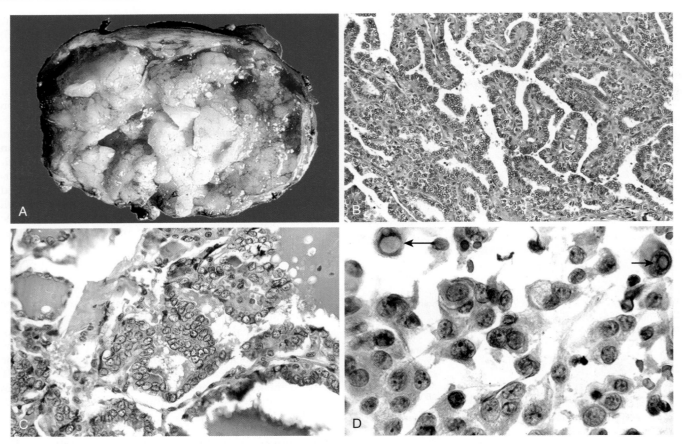

Fig. 20.15 Papillary carcinoma of the thyroid gland. (A to C) A papillary carcinoma with grossly discernible papillary structures. In this particular example, well-formed papillae (B) are lined by cells with characteristic empty-appearing nuclei, sometimes termed *Orphan Annie eye* nuclei (C). (D) Cells obtained by fine-needle aspiration of a papillary carcinoma. Characteristic intranuclear inclusions are visible in some of the aspirated cells *(arrows)*. *(Courtesy of Dr. S. Gokasalan, Department of Pathology, University of Texas Southwestern Medical School, Dallas, Texas.)*

- Nuclei with finely dispersed chromatin, which imparts an optically clear or empty appearance, giving rise to the designation **ground-glass** or **Orphan Annie eye nuclei** (see Fig. 20.15B). In addition, invaginations of the cytoplasm often give the appearance of intranuclear inclusions ("pseudo-inclusions") or intranuclear grooves (see Fig. 20.15D). **These nuclear features are sufficient for the diagnosis of papillary carcinoma,** even in the absence of papillary architecture.
- Concentrically calcified structures termed **psammoma bodies** are often present within the lesion, usually within the cores of papillae. These structures are almost never found in follicular and medullary carcinomas.
- Foci of lymphatic invasion by tumor are often present, but involvement of blood vessels is relatively uncommon, particularly in smaller lesions. Metastases to adjacent cervical lymph nodes occur in up to one-half of cases.
- There are over a dozen variants of papillary thyroid carcinoma, the most common of which is the so-called **encapsulated follicular variant,** comprised of follicles lined by cells harboring nuclear features of papillary cancers (discussed earlier).

Clinical Features

Papillary carcinomas are nonfunctional tumors, so they manifest most often as a painless mass in the neck, either within the thyroid or as a metastasis in a cervical lymph node. A preoperative diagnosis usually can be established by fine-needle aspiration based on the characteristic nuclear features described earlier. Papillary carcinomas are indolent lesions, with 10-year survival rates in excess of 95%. Of interest, the presence of isolated cervical node metastases does not have a significant influence on prognosis. In a minority of patients, hematogenous metastases are present at the time of diagnosis, most commonly to the lung. The long-term survival of patients with papillary thyroid cancer is dependent on several factors, including age (in general, the prognosis is less favorable among patients older than 40 years of age), presence of extrathyroidal extension, and presence of distant metastases (stage).

Recent studies have shown that follicular variants of papillary carcinoma that lack evidence of invasion have essentially no potential for malignant behavior. In recognition of this, forthcoming recommendations from the World Health Organization suggest the name carcinoma should be stripped from these tumors, which will henceforth be classified as benign neoplasms to prevent overtreatment.

Follicular Carcinoma

Follicular carcinomas account for 5% to 15% of primary thyroid cancers. They are more common in women (occurring in a ratio of 3:1) and manifest at an older age than papillary carcinomas, with a peak incidence between 40 and 60

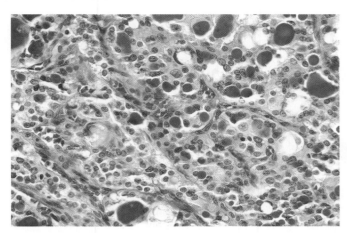

Fig. 20.16 Follicular carcinoma of the thyroid gland. A few of the glandular lumina contain recognizable colloid.

years of age. Follicular carcinoma is more frequent in areas with dietary iodine deficiency (accounting for 25%–40% of thyroid cancers), while its incidence has either decreased or remained stable in iodine-sufficient areas of the world.

MORPHOLOGY

On microscopic examination, most follicular carcinomas are composed of uniform cells forming small follicles, reminiscent of normal thyroid (Fig. 20.16); in other cases, follicular differentiation may be less apparent. As with follicular adenomas, Hürthle cell variants of follicular carcinomas may be seen. Follicular carcinomas may be widely invasive, infiltrating the thyroid parenchyma and extrathyroidal soft tissues, or minimally invasive. The latter type are sharply demarcated lesions that may be impossible to distinguish from follicular adenomas on gross examination. **The distinction between follicular adenoma and carcinoma requires extensive histologic sampling of the tumor capsule–thyroid interface, to exclude capsular and/or vascular invasion** (Fig. 20.17). As discussed earlier, invasive follicular lesions in which the nuclear features are typical of papillary carcinomas are regarded as follicular variants of papillary cancers.

Clinical Features

Follicular carcinomas manifest most frequently as *solitary cold thyroid nodules.* In rare cases, they may be hyperfunctional. These neoplasms tend to metastasize through the bloodstream *(hematogenous dissemination)* to the lungs, bone, and liver. In contrast with papillary carcinomas, regional nodal metastases are uncommon. As many as one-half of patients with widely invasive carcinomas succumb to their disease within 10 years, while less than 10% of patients with minimally invasive follicular carcinomas die within the same time span. Follicular carcinomas are treated with surgical excision. Well-differentiated metastases may take up radioactive iodine, which can be used to identify and also ablate such lesions.

Anaplastic Carcinoma

Anaplastic carcinomas are undifferentiated tumors of the thyroid follicular epithelium, accounting for less than 5%

of thyroid tumors. They are aggressive, with a mortality rate approaching 100%. Patients with anaplastic carcinoma are older than those with other types of thyroid cancer, with a mean age of 65 years. Approximately one-fourth of patients with anaplastic thyroid carcinomas have a history of a well-differentiated thyroid carcinoma, and another one-fourth harbor a concurrent well-differentiated tumor in the resected specimen.

MORPHOLOGY

Anaplastic carcinomas manifest as bulky masses that typically grow rapidly beyond the thyroid capsule into adjacent neck structures. On microscopic examination, these neoplasms are composed of highly anaplastic cells, which may be large and pleomorphic or spindle shaped and in some cases mixture of the two cell types.

Foci of papillary or follicular differentiation may be present in some tumors, suggesting origin from a better-differentiated carcinoma.

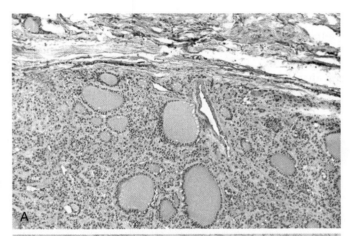

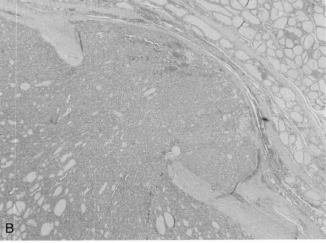

Fig. 20.17 Capsular invasion in follicular carcinoma. Evaluating the integrity of the capsule is critical in distinguishing follicular adenomas from follicular carcinomas. (A) In adenomas, a fibrous capsule, usually thin but occasionally more prominent, surrounds the neoplastic follicles and no capsular invasion is seen; compressed normal thyroid parenchyma usually is present external to the capsule *(top).* (B) By contrast, follicular carcinomas demonstrate capsular invasion that may be minimal, as in this case, or widespread, with extension into local structures of the neck.

Clinical Features

Anaplastic carcinomas grow with wild abandon despite therapy. Metastases to distant sites are common, but in most cases death occurs in less than 1 year as a result of aggressive local growth and compromise of vital structures in the neck.

Medullary Carcinoma

Medullary carcinomas of the thyroid are *neuroendocrine tumors* derived from the parafollicular cells, or C cells, of the thyroid. Like normal C cells, medullary carcinomas secrete calcitonin, measurement of which plays an important role in the diagnosis and postoperative follow-up of patients. In some cases, the tumor cells elaborate other polypeptide hormones such as somatostatin, serotonin, and vasoactive intestinal peptide. Medullary carcinomas arise *sporadically* in about 70% of cases. The remaining 30% are *familial*, occurring in the setting of multiple endocrine neoplasia (MEN) syndrome 2A or 2B, or familial medullary thyroid carcinoma without an associated MEN syndrome, as discussed later. Both familial and sporadic medullary forms are associated with gain-of-function driver mutations in the RET receptor tyrosine kinase. Sporadic medullary carcinomas, as well as familial cases without an associated MEN syndrome, occur in adults, with a peak incidence in the fifth and sixth decades. Cases associated with MEN-2A or MEN-2B, by contrast, tend to occur in younger patients, including children.

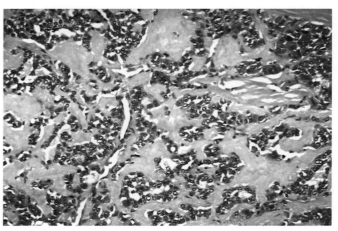

Fig. 20.18 Medullary carcinoma of the thyroid gland. These tumors typically contain amyloid, visible here as homogeneous extracellular material, derived from calcitonin molecules secreted by the neoplastic cells.

or *RET* mutations permits early detection of tumors in familial cases. As discussed later, all members of MEN-2 kindreds carrying *RET* mutations are offered prophylactic thyroidectomies to preempt the development of medullary carcinomas; often, the only histologic finding in the resected thyroid of these asymptomatic carriers is the presence of C cell hyperplasia or small (<1 cm) *micromedullary carcinomas*.

MORPHOLOGY

Medullary carcinomas may arise as a solitary nodule or may manifest as multiple lesions involving both lobes of the thyroid. **Multicentricity** is particularly common in familial cases. Larger lesions often contain areas of necrosis and hemorrhage and may extend through the capsule of the thyroid. On microscopic examination, medullary carcinomas are composed of polygonal to spindle-shaped cells, which may form nests, trabeculae, and even follicles. **Amyloid deposits**, derived from altered calcitonin molecules, are present in the adjacent stroma in many cases (Fig. 20.18) and are a distinctive feature. Calcitonin is readily demonstrable both within the cytoplasm of the tumor cells and in the stromal amyloid by immunohistochemical methods. One of the characteristic features of familial medullary carcinomas is the presence of **multicentric C cell hyperplasia** in the surrounding thyroid parenchyma, a feature usually absent in sporadic lesions. Foci of C cell hyperplasia are believed to represent the precursor lesions from which medullary carcinomas arise.

Clinical Features

In sporadic cases, medullary carcinoma manifests most often as a mass in the neck, sometimes associated with compression effects such as dysphagia or hoarseness. In some instances the initial manifestations are caused by the secretion of a peptide hormone (e.g., diarrhea caused by the secretion of vasoactive intestinal peptide). Screening of the patient's relatives for elevated calcitonin levels

SUMMARY

THYROID NEOPLASMS

- Most thyroid neoplasms manifest as *solitary thyroid nodules*, but only 1% of all thyroid nodules are neoplastic.
- *Follicular adenomas* are the most common benign neoplasms, while papillary carcinoma is the most common malignancy.
- Multiple genetic pathways are involved in *thyroid carcinogenesis*. Some of the driver mutations that are fairly unique to thyroid cancers include *PAX8/PPARG* fusion (in follicular carcinoma), chromosomal rearrangements involving the *RET* oncogene (in papillary cancers), and mutations of *RET* (in medullary carcinomas).
- *Follicular adenomas and carcinomas* both are composed of well-differentiated follicular epithelial cells; the latter are distinguished by presence of capsular and/or vascular invasion.
- *Papillary carcinomas* are recognized by nuclear features (ground-glass nuclei, pseudoinclusions), even in the absence of papillae. These neoplasms typically metastasize by way of the lymphatics, but the prognosis is excellent.
- *Anaplastic carcinomas* are thought to arise by progression of more differentiated neoplasms. They are highly aggressive, uniformly lethal cancers.
- *Medullary cancers* are nonepithelial neoplasms arising from the parafollicular C cells and can occur in either sporadic (70%) or familial (30%) settings. Multicentricity and C cell hyperplasia are features of familial cases. Amyloid deposits are a characteristic histologic finding.

Parathyroid Glands

The parathyroid glands are derived developmentally from pharyngeal pouches that also give rise to the thymus. They are most commonly located in close proximity to the upper and lower poles of each thyroid lobe but may be found anywhere along the pathway of descent of the pharyngeal pouches, including the carotid sheath, the thymus, and elsewhere in the anterior mediastinum. Most of the gland is composed of *chief cells* which have secretory granules containing *parathyroid hormone (PTH)*. *Oxyphil cells* are found throughout the normal parathyroid either singly or in small clusters. They are slightly larger than the chief cells, have acidophilic cytoplasm, and are tightly packed with mitochondria.

Parathyroid glands are key regulators of calcium homeostasis. The activity of the parathyroid glands is controlled by the level of free (ionized) calcium in the blood, rather than by trophic hormones secreted by the hypothalamus and pituitary. Normally, decreased levels of free calcium stimulate the synthesis and secretion of PTH, which has the following effects on its target tissues, the kidneys and the bones:

- Increased renal tubular reabsorption of calcium
- Increased urinary phosphate excretion, thereby lowering serum phosphate levels (since phosphate binds to ionized calcium)
- Increased conversion of vitamin D to its active dihydroxy form in the kidneys, which in turn augments gastrointestinal calcium absorption
- Enhanced osteoclastic activity (i.e., bone resorption, thus releasing ionized calcium), mediated indirectly by promoting the differentiation of osteoclast progenitor cells into mature osteoclasts

The net result of these activities is an increase in the level of free calcium in the blood, which inhibits PTH secretion from chief cells. Abnormalities of the parathyroids include both hyperfunction and hypofunction. *Tumors of the parathyroid glands, unlike thyroid tumors, usually come to attention because of excessive secretion of PTH, rather than mass effects.*

HYPERPARATHYROIDISM

Hyperparathyroidism occurs in two major forms, *primary* and *secondary,* and, less commonly, as *tertiary* hyperparathyroidism. The first condition represents an autonomous, spontaneous overproduction of PTH, while the latter two conditions typically occur as secondary phenomena in patients with chronic renal insufficiency.

Primary Hyperparathyroidism

Primary hyperparathyroidism is a common endocrine disorder and an important cause of hypercalcemia. There was a dramatic increase in the detection of cases in the latter half of the 20th century, mainly due to routine performance of serum calcium assays in hospitalized patients. The frequency of occurrence of the various parathyroid

lesions underlying primary hyperparathyroidism is as follows:

- Adenoma—85% to 95%
- Primary hyperplasia (diffuse or nodular)—5% to 10%
- Parathyroid carcinoma—1%

Pathogenesis

Abnormalities in two genes are commonly associated with parathyroid tumors:

- *Cyclin D1 gene rearrangements.* Cyclin D1 is a positive regulator of the cell cycle. An inversion on chromosome 11 repositions the *cyclin D1* gene (normally on 11q), so that it resides adjacent to genomic elements that regulate the *PTH* gene (on 11p). These elements drive abnormal expression of cyclin D1 in PTH-producing cells, leading to increased proliferation of these cells. Between 10% and 20% of adenomas have this acquired genetic defect. Cyclin D1 is overexpressed in approximately 40% of parathyroid adenomas, indicating the existence of additional mechanisms that lead to its dysregulation.
- *MEN1 mutations.* Approximately 20% to 30% of sporadic parathyroid tumors have mutations in both copies of the *MEN1* tumor suppressor gene (see later). The spectrum of *MEN1* mutations in the sporadic tumors is virtually identical to that in familial parathyroid adenomas.

MORPHOLOGY

The morphologic changes in primary hyperparathyroidism include those in the parathyroid glands and in other organs affected by hypercalcemia. In 75% to 80% of cases, one of the parathyroid glands harbors a solitary **adenoma.** The typical parathyroid adenoma is a well-circumscribed, soft, tan nodule, invested by a delicate capsule. **By definition, parathyroid adenomas are confined to a single gland** (Fig. 20.19). The other glands are normal in size or somewhat shrunken, as a result of feedback

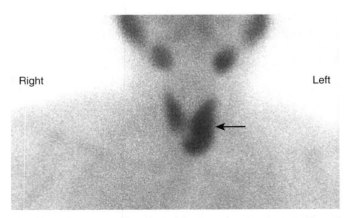

Right   Left

Fig. 20.19 Technetium-99 radionuclide scan demonstrates an area of increased uptake corresponding to the left inferior parathyroid gland *(arrow).* This proved to be a parathyroid adenoma. Preoperative scintigraphy is useful in localizing and distinguishing adenomas from parathyroid hyperplasia, in which more than one gland will demonstrate increased uptake.

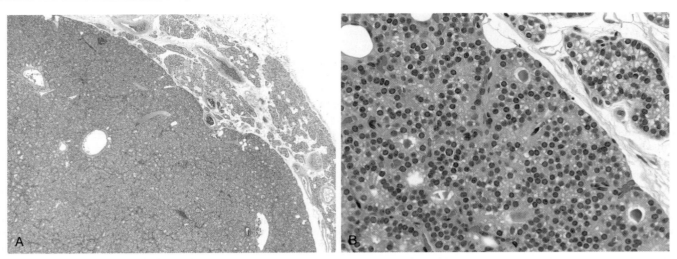

Fig. 20.20 Chief cell parathyroid adenoma. (A) In this low-power view, a solitary hypercellular adenoma is delineated from the residual normocellular gland on the upper right. (B) High-power detail shows minimal variation in nuclear size and occasional follicle formation. *(Courtesy of Dr. Nicole Cipriani, Department of Pathology, University of Chicago, Chicago, Illinois.)*

inhibition by elevated serum calcium. Most parathyroid adenomas weigh between 0.5 and 5 g. On microscopic examination, parathyroid adenomas are composed predominantly of chief cells (Fig. 20.20). A rim of compressed, non-neoplastic parathyroid tissue, generally separated by a fibrous capsule, often is visible at the edge of the adenoma. The chief cells of the adenoma are larger and show greater nuclear size variability than normal chief cells. Cells with bizarre and pleomorphic nuclei are often seen within adenomas (so-called "**endocrine atypia**") and must not be taken as a sign of malignancy. Mitotic figures are rare. In contrast with the normal parathyroid parenchyma, adipose tissue is inconspicuous within adenomas.

Parathyroid hyperplasia is typically a multiglandular process. In some cases, however, enlargement may be grossly apparent in only one or two glands, complicating the distinction between hyperplasia and adenoma. Microscopically, the most common pattern seen is that of chief cell hyperplasia, which may involve the glands in a diffuse or multinodular pattern. Less commonly, the constituent cells contain abundant clear cytoplasm as a consequence of the accumulation of glycogen—a condition designated water-clear cell hyperplasia. As in the case of adenomas, stromal fat is inconspicuous within foci of hyperplasia.

Parathyroid carcinomas may be circumscribed lesions that are difficult to distinguish from adenomas, or they may be clearly invasive neoplasms. These tumors enlarge one parathyroid gland and consist of gray-white, irregular masses that sometimes exceed 10 g in weight. The cells usually are uniform and resemble normal parathyroid cells. They are arrayed in nodular or trabecular patterns. The tumor mass is usually enclosed by a dense, fibrous capsule. There is general agreement that a **diagnosis of carcinoma based on cytologic detail is unreliable; invasion of surrounding tissues and metastasis are the only definitive criteria.** Local recurrence occurs in one-third of cases, and more distant dissemination occurs in another one-third.

Morphologic changes in other organs:
- **Skeletal changes** include increased osteoclastic activity, which results in erosion of bone matrix and mobilization of calcium salts, particularly in the metaphyses of long tubular bones. Bone

resorption is accompanied by increased osteoblastic activity and the formation of new bone trabeculae. In more severe cases, the cortex is grossly thinned and the bone marrow contains increased amounts of fibrous tissue accompanied by foci of hemorrhage and cysts **(osteitis fibrosa cystica)** (Chapter 21). Aggregates of osteoclasts, reactive giant cells, and hemorrhagic debris occasionally form masses that may be mistaken for neoplasms **(brown tumors** of hyperparathyroidism).
- **Renal changes.** PTH-induced hypercalcemia favors the formation of urinary tract stones **(nephrolithiasis)** as well as calcification of the renal interstitium and tubules **(nephrocalcinosis).**
- **Metastatic calcification** secondary to hypercalcemia also may be seen in other sites, including the stomach, lungs, myocardium, and blood vessels.

Clinical Features

Primary hyperparathyroidism usually is a disease of adults and is much more common in women than in men (gender ratio of nearly 4:1). *The most common manifestation of primary hyperparathyroidism is an increase in serum ionized calcium.* In fact, primary hyperparathyroidism is the most common cause of *clinically silent hypercalcemia.* Other conditions also may produce hypercalcemia (Table 20.4). The most common cause of clinically apparent hypercalcemia

Table 20.4 Causes of Hypercalcemia

Increased PTH	Decreased PTH
Hyperparathyroidism	Hypercalcemia of malignancy
Primary (adenoma >	Osteolytic metastases
hyperplasia)*	PTH-rP–mediated
Secondary†	Vitamin D toxicity
Tertiary†	Immobilization
Familial hypocalciuric	Drugs (thiazide diuretics)
hypercalcemia	Granulomatous diseases (sarcoidosis)

PTH, Parathyroid hormone; *PTH-rP,* PTH-related protein.
*Primary hyperparathyroidism is the most common cause of hypercalcemia overall.
†Secondary and tertiary hyperparathyroidism are most commonly associated with progressive renal failure.

in adults is cancer, which can cause hypercalcemia through a variety of mechanisms, including secretion of PTH-like polypeptides and osteolytic bone metastases (Chapter 6). The prognosis for patients with malignancy-associated hypercalcemia is poor, because it often occurs in those with advanced cancers. In individuals with hypercalcemia caused by parathyroid hyperfunction, serum PTH is inappropriately elevated, whereas serum PTH is low to undetectable in those with hypercalcemia caused by nonparathyroid diseases, including malignancy. Other laboratory alterations referable to PTH excess include hypophosphatemia and increased urinary excretion of both calcium and phosphate.

Primary hyperparathyroidism traditionally has been associated with a constellation of symptoms that include *painful bones, renal stones, abdominal groans, and psychic moans.* Pain, secondary to fractures of bones weakened by osteoporosis or osteitis fibrosa cystica and resulting from renal stones, with obstructive uropathy, was at one time a prominent manifestation of primary hyperparathyroidism. Because serum calcium is now routinely assessed in most patients who need blood tests for unrelated conditions, hyperparathyroidism is usually detected early in its course. Hence, many of the classic clinical manifestations, particularly those referable to bone and renal disease, are seen much less frequently. Additional signs and symptoms that may be encountered in some cases include the following:
- *Gastrointestinal disturbances,* including constipation, nausea, peptic ulcers, pancreatitis, and gallstones
- *Central nervous system alterations,* including depression, lethargy, and seizures
- *Neuromuscular abnormalities,* including weakness and hypotonia
- *Polyuria* and secondary polydipsia

Although some of these alterations (e.g., polyuria and muscle weakness) are clearly related to hypercalcemia, the pathophysiology of many of the other manifestations of the disorder remains poorly understood.

Secondary Hyperparathyroidism

Secondary hyperparathyroidism is caused by chronic depression of serum calcium levels, most often as a result of renal failure, leading to compensatory overactivity of the parathyroids. The mechanisms by which chronic renal failure induces secondary hyperparathyroidism are complex and not fully understood. Chronic renal insufficiency is associated with decreased phosphate excretion, which in turn results in hyperphosphatemia. The elevated serum phosphate levels directly depress serum calcium levels. In addition, loss of renal α_1-hydroxylase activity, which is required for the synthesis of the active form of vitamin D, reduces the intestinal absorption of calcium (Chapter 8). These alterations cause chronic hypocalcemia, which stimulates the activity of the parathyroid glands.

MORPHOLOGY

The parathyroid glands in secondary hyperparathyroidism are hyperplastic. As in primary hyperplasia, the degree of

glandular enlargement is not necessarily symmetric. On microscopic examination, the hyperplastic glands contain an increased number of chief cells, or cells with more abundant, clear cytoplasm **(water-clear cells),** in a diffuse or multinodular distribution. Fat cells are decreased in number. **Bone changes** similar to those seen in primary hyperparathyroidism also may be present. **Metastatic calcification** may be seen in many tissues.

Clinical Features

The clinical manifestations of secondary hyperparathyroidism usually are dominated by those related to chronic renal failure. Bone abnormalities *(renal osteodystrophy)* and other changes associated with PTH excess are, in general, less severe than those seen in primary hyperparathyroidism. Serum calcium remains near normal because the compensatory increase in PTH levels sustains serum calcium. The metastatic calcification of blood vessels (secondary to hyperphosphatemia) occasionally may result in significant ischemic damage to skin and other organs—a process referred to as *calciphylaxis.* In a minority of patients, parathyroid activity may become autonomous and excessive, with resultant hypercalcemia—a process sometimes termed *tertiary hyperparathyroidism.* Parathyroidectomy may be necessary to control the hyperparathyroidism in such patients.

SUMMARY
HYPERPARATHYROIDISM

- Primary hyperparathyroidism is the most common cause of asymptomatic hypercalcemia.
- In a majority of cases, primary hyperparathyroidism is caused by a sporadic parathyroid adenoma and, less commonly, by parathyroid hyperplasia.
- Parathyroid adenomas are solitary, while hyperplasia typically is a multiglandular process.
- Skeletal manifestations of hyperparathyroidism include bone resorption, *osteitis fibrosa cystica,* and *brown tumors.* Renal changes include nephrolithiasis (stones) and nephrocalcinosis.
- Most cases of hyperparathyroidism are clinically silent because of early detection of hypercalcemia during routine blood testing.
- Secondary hyperparathyroidism is caused by hypercalcemia most often secondary to renal failure, and the parathyroid glands are hyperplastic.
- Malignancies are the most important cause of symptomatic hypercalcemia, which results from osteolytic metastases or release of PTH-related protein from nonparathyroid tumors.

HYPOPARATHYROIDISM

Hypoparathyroidism is far less common than hyperparathyroidism. The major causes of hypoparathyroidism include the following:
- *Surgical ablation*: The most common cause is inadvertent removal of parathyroids during thyroidectomy or other surgical neck dissections.

- *Congenital absence:* This occurs in conjunction with thymic aplasia (Di George syndrome) and cardiac defects, secondary to deletions on chromosome 22q11.2 (Chapter 7).
- *Autoimmune hypoparathyroidism:* This is a hereditary polyglandular deficiency syndrome arising from autoantibodies to multiple endocrine organs (parathyroid, thyroid, adrenals, and pancreas). This condition is caused by mutations in the *autoimmune regulator (AIRE)* gene and is discussed more extensively later, in the context of autoimmune adrenalitis.

The major clinical manifestations of hypoparathyroidism are secondary to hypocalcemia. Acute cases (as may occur after surgical ablation) manifest as *increased neuromuscular irritability* (tingling, muscle spasms, facial grimacing, and sustained carpopedal spasm or tetany), *cardiac arrhythmias,* and, on occasion, *increased intracranial pressure* and *seizures.* Manifestations of chronic hypoparathyroidism include cataracts, calcification of the cerebral basal ganglia, and dental abnormalities.

Endocrine Pancreas

The endocrine pancreas consists of the islets of Langerhans, which contain four major cell types—beta, alpha, delta, and PP (pancreatic polypeptide) cells. *The beta cell produces insulin,* which regulates glucose utilization in tissues and reduces blood glucose levels, as will be detailed in the discussion of diabetes; *the alpha cell secretes glucagon,* which raises glucose levels through its glycogenolytic activity in the liver; *delta cells secrete somatostatin,* which suppresses both insulin and glucagon release; and *PP cells secrete pancreatic polypeptide,* which exerts several gastrointestinal effects, such as stimulation of secretion of gastric and intestinal enzymes and inhibition of intestinal motility. The most important disease of the endocrine pancreas is diabetes mellitus, caused by deficient production or action of insulin.

DIABETES MELLITUS

Diabetes mellitus is a group of metabolic disorders characterized by hyperglycemia. Hyperglycemia in diabetes (in common parlance, the suffix "mellitus" is often not used) results from defects in insulin secretion, insulin action, or, most commonly, both. The chronic hyperglycemia and attendant metabolic abnormalities of diabetes are often associated with secondary damage in multiple organ systems, especially the kidneys, eyes, nerves, and blood vessels. **In the United States, diabetes is the leading cause of end-stage renal disease, adult-onset blindness, and nontraumatic lower-extremity amputations resulting from atherosclerosis of arteries.**

According to the American Diabetes Association, diabetes affects over 29 million children and adults, or 9.3% of the population, in the United States, nearly one-third of whom are currently unaware that they have hyperglycemia. Approximately 1.4 million new cases of diabetes are diagnosed each year in the United States, and there is a wide variability in prevalence between different ethnic groups. For example, the prevalence of diabetes in American Indian/Alaskan Natives is almost twice that of Caucasians. Increasingly sedentary lifestyles and poor eating habits have contributed to the increases in diabetes and obesity, which some have termed the *diabesity epidemic.* A staggering 86 million adults in the United States have *prediabetes,* which is defined as *elevated blood sugar that does not reach the criterion accepted for an outright diagnosis of diabetes* (discussed next); individuals with prediabetes have an elevated risk for development of frank diabetes.

Diagnosis

Blood glucose is normally maintained in a very narrow range, usually 70 to 120 mg/dL. According to the American Diabetes Association (ADA) and the World Health Organization (WHO), **diagnostic criteria for diabetes include the following:**

1. A fasting plasma glucose greater than or equal to 126 mg/dL, and/or
2. A random plasma glucose greater than or equal to 200 mg/dL (in a patient with classic hyperglycemic signs, discussed later), and/or
3. A 2-hour plasma glucose greater than or equal to 200 mg/dL during an oral glucose tolerance test with a loading dose of 75 gm, and/or
4. A glycated hemoglobin (HbA1C) level greater than or equal to 6.5% (glycated hemoglobin is further discussed under chronic complications of diabetes)

All tests, except the random blood glucose test in a patient with classic hyperglycemic signs, need to be repeated and confirmed on a separate day. Of note, many acute conditions associated with stress, such as severe infections, burns, or trauma, can lead to transient hyperglycemia due to secretion of hormones such as catecholamines and cortisol that oppose the effects of insulin. The diagnosis of diabetes requires persistence of hyperglycemia following resolution of the acute illness.

Impaired glucose tolerance (prediabetes) is defined as:

1. A fasting plasma glucose between 100 and 125 mg/dL ("impaired fasting glucose"), and/or
2. A 2-hour plasma glucose between 140 and 199 mg/dL during an oral glucose tolerance test, and/or
3. HbA1C level between 5.7% and 6.4%

As many as one-fourth of individuals with impaired glucose tolerance will develop overt diabetes in the next 5 years, with additional risk factors such as obesity and family history compounding such risk. In addition, individuals with prediabetes have an elevated risk of cardiovascular disease.

Classification

Although all forms of diabetes share hyperglycemia as a common feature, the underlying causes of hyperglycemia vary widely. Previous classification schemes of diabetes were based on age at onset of the disease

Table 20.5 Simplified Classification of Diabetes

1. *Type 1 Diabetes*
   Beta cell destruction, usually leading to absolute insulin deficiency
2. *Type 2 Diabetes*
   Combination of insulin resistance and beta cell dysfunction
3. *Genetic Defects of Beta Cell Function*
   Maturity-onset diabetes of the young (MODY) (see text)
   Insulin gene mutations
4. *Genetic Defects in Insulin Action*
   Insulin receptor mutations
5. *Exocrine Pancreatic Defects*
   Chronic pancreatitis
   Pancreatectomy
   Cystic fibrosis
   Hemochromatosis
6. *Endocrinopathies*
   Growth hormone excess (acromegaly)
   Cushing syndrome
   Hyperthyroidism
   Pheochromocytoma
7. *Infections*
   Cytomegalovirus infection
   Coxsackievirus B infection
   Congenital rubella
8. *Drugs*
   Glucocorticoids
   Thyroid hormone
   β-Adrenergic agonists
9. *Gestational Diabetes*
   Diabetes associated with pregnancy

Modified from Diagnosis and classification of diabetes mellitus (American Diabetes Association). *Diabetes Care* 37:S81-S90; 2014.

or on the mode of therapy; in contrast, the current etiologic classification reflects a greater understanding of the pathogenesis of each variant (Table 20.5). *The vast majority of cases of diabetes fall into one of two broad classes:*

- *Type 1 diabetes is an autoimmune disease characterized by pancreatic β-cell destruction and an absolute deficiency of insulin.* It accounts for approximately 5% to 10% of all cases, and is the most common subtype diagnosed in patients younger than 20 years of age.
- *Type 2 diabetes is caused by a combination of peripheral resistance to insulin action and an inadequate secretory response by the pancreatic β cells ("relative insulin deficiency").* Approximately 90% to 95% of diabetic patients have type 2 diabetes, and many of them are overweight. Although classically considered "adult-onset," the prevalence of type 2 diabetes in children and adolescents is increasing at an alarming pace due to the increasing rates of obesity in these age groups.

A variety of monogenic and secondary causes are responsible for the remaining cases (discussed later). Of note, when combined, monogenic and secondary forms of diabetes account for >10% of diabetes (which together makes them more common than type 1 diabetes). An important point is that although the major types of diabetes arise by different pathogenic mechanisms, *the long-term complications in kidneys, eyes, nerves, and blood vessels are the same and are the principal causes of morbidity and death.*

Normal Insulin Physiology and Glucose Homeostasis

Before discussing the pathogenesis of the two major types of diabetes, we briefly review normal insulin physiology and glucose metabolism.

Normal glucose homeostasis is tightly regulated by three interrelated processes: (1) glucose production in the liver; (2) glucose uptake and utilization by peripheral tissues, chiefly skeletal muscle; and (3) the actions of insulin and counterregulatory hormones (especially glucagon).

The principal function of insulin is to increase the rate of glucose transport into certain cells in the body (Fig. 20.21). These are the striated muscle cells (including myocardial cells) and, to a lesser extent, adipocytes, representing collectively about two thirds of total body weight. Glucose uptake in other peripheral tissues, most notably the brain, is insulin-independent. In muscle cells, glucose is then either stored as glycogen or oxidized to generate adenosine triphosphate (ATP) and metabolic intermediates needed for cell growth. In adipose tissue, glucose is metabolized to lipids, which are stored as fat. Besides promoting lipid synthesis (lipogenesis), insulin also inhibits lipid degradation (lipolysis) in adipocytes. Similarly, insulin promotes amino acid uptake and protein synthesis while inhibiting protein degradation. Thus, the metabolic effects of insulin can be summarized as anabolic, with increased synthesis and reduced degradation of glycogen, lipid, and protein. In addition to these metabolic effects, insulin has several mitogenic functions, including initiation of DNA synthesis in certain cells and stimulation of their growth and differentiation.

Insulin reduces the production of glucose from the liver. Insulin and glucagon have opposing regulatory effects on glucose homeostasis. During *fasting* states, low

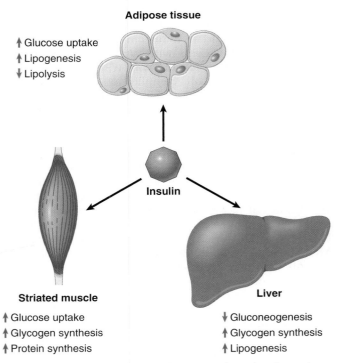

Fig. 20.21 Metabolic actions of insulin in striated muscle, adipose tissue, and liver.

insulin and high glucagon levels facilitate hepatic gluconeogenesis and glycogenolysis (glycogen breakdown) while decreasing glycogen synthesis, thereby preventing hypoglycemia. Thus, *fasting* plasma glucose levels are determined primarily by hepatic glucose output. After a meal, insulin levels rise and glucagon levels fall in response to the large glucose load.

The most important stimulus that triggers insulin release from pancreatic beta cells is glucose itself. Oral intake of food leads to secretion of multiple hormones, notably the incretins produced by cells in the intestines. These hormones stimulate insulin secretion from beta cells, and also reduce glucagon secretion and delay gastric emptying, which promotes satiety. The incretin effect is significantly blunted in patients with type 2 diabetes, and restoring incretin function can lead to improved glycemic control and loss of weight (through restoration of satiety). These observations have resulted in the development of new classes of drugs for patients with type 2 diabetes that mimic incretins or enhance the levels of endogenous incretins through delaying their degradation.

In peripheral tissues (skeletal muscle and adipose tissue), secreted insulin binds to the *insulin receptor*, triggering a number of intracellular responses that promote glucose uptake and postprandial glucose utilization, thereby maintaining glucose homeostasis. Abnormalities at various points along this complex signaling cascade, from synthesis and release of insulin by beta cells to insulin receptor interactions in peripheral tissues, can result in the diabetic phenotype.

Pathogenesis of Type 1 Diabetes

Type 1 diabetes is an autoimmune disease in which islet destruction is caused primarily by immune effector cells reacting against endogenous beta cell antigens. Although type 1 diabetes is the most common form of diabetes in childhood, it is important to remember that it can present at any age. Most patients with type 1 diabetes depend on exogenous insulin for survival; without insulin they develop serious metabolic complications such as ketoacidosis and coma. Although the clinical onset of type 1 diabetes is abrupt, it results from a chronic autoimmune attack on beta cells that usually starts years before the disease becomes evident (Fig. 20.22). The classic manifestations of the disease (such as ketoacidosis) occur late in its course, after more than 90% of the beta cells have been destroyed.

As with most autoimmune diseases, the pathogenesis of type 1 diabetes involves genetic susceptibility and environmental factors. Genome-wide association studies have identified over 20 susceptibility loci for type 1 diabetes. Of these, the strongest association is with class II MHC (HLA-DR) genes. Between 90% and 95% of white patients with type 1 diabetes have HLA-DR3, or DR4, or both, in contrast with about 40% of normal subjects, and 40% to 50% of patients are DR3/DR4 heterozygotes, in contrast with 5% of normal subjects. Of note, however, most individuals who inherit these HLA alleles do not develop diabetes, indicating that these genes contribute to the disease but do not, by themselves, cause it. Several non-HLA genes also increase susceptibility to type 1 diabetes, including polymorphisms within the gene encoding

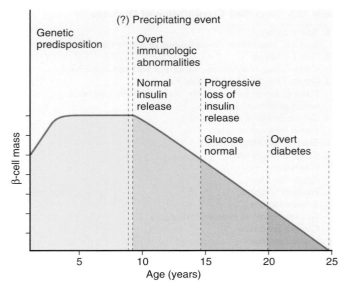

Fig. 20.22 Stages in the development of type 1 diabetes mellitus. The stages are listed from left to right, and hypothetical β cell mass is plotted against age. *(From Eisenbarth GE: Type 1 diabetes—a chronic autoimmune disease. N Engl J Med 314:1360, 1986.)*

insulin itself, as well as *CTLA4* and *PTPN22*. As discussed in Chapter 5, CTLA-4 is an inhibitory receptor of T cells, and PTPN-22 is a protein tyrosine phosphatase; both are thought to inhibit T-cell responses, so polymorphisms that interfere with their functional activity are expected to set the stage for excessive T-cell activation. Polymorphisms in the *insulin* gene may reduce its expression in the thymus, thus reducing the elimination of T cells reactive with this self protein (Chapter 5).

Additional evidence suggests that environmental factors, especially infections, are involved in type 1 diabetes. It has been proposed that certain viruses (mumps, rubella, and coxsackie B viruses, in particular) may be initiating triggers, perhaps because some viral antigens mimic beta cell antigens, leading to bystander damage to the islets, but this idea is not conclusively established. More recent advances in elucidating environmental contributions to the pathogenesis of type 1 diabetes have come from studies of the human microbiome. Studies in diabetic children have shown evidence for "intestinal dysbiosis" (change in composition of usual commensal flora), with reduction in diversity of the microbiome, and reduced abundance of certain bacterial species during progression of subclinical to clinical stages of the disease. Whether this is a cause or consequence of hyperglycemia remains unclear.

The fundamental immune abnormality in type 1 diabetes is a failure of self-tolerance in T cells specific for beta cell antigens. This failure of tolerance may result from some combination of defective clonal deletion of self-reactive T cells in the thymus and abnormalities of regulatory T cells (Tregs) that normally dampen effector T-cell responses (Chapter 5). One consequence of loss of self tolerance is the production of **autoantibodies** against a variety of beta cell antigens, including insulin and the beta cell enzyme glutamic acid decarboxylase, which are detected in the blood of 70% to 80% of patients. In the rare cases in which the pancreatic lesions have been examined

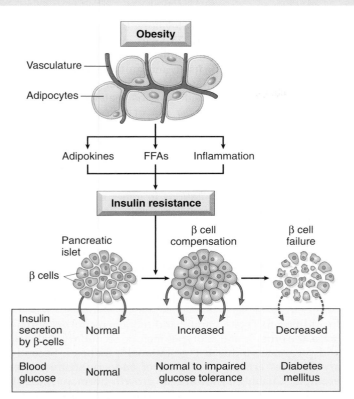

Fig. 20.23 Development of type 2 diabetes. Insulin resistance associated with obesity is induced by adipokines, free fatty acids, and chronic inflammation in adipose tissue. Pancreatic β cells compensate for insulin resistance by hypersecretion of insulin. However, at some point, β cell compensation is followed by β cell failure, and diabetes ensues. *(Reproduced with permission from Kasuga M: Insulin resistance and pancreatic β-cell failure. J Clin Invest 116:1756, 2006.)*

early in the disease process, the islets show necrosis of beta cells and lymphocytic infiltration (so-called "insulitis", described later).

Pathogenesis of Type 2 Diabetes

Type 2 diabetes is a heterogeneous and multifactorial complex disease that involves interactions of genetics, environmental risk factors, and inflammation. Unlike type 1 diabetes, however, there is no evidence of an autoimmune basis. **The two defects that characterize type 2 diabetes are: (1) a decreased ability of peripheral tissues to respond to insulin (insulin resistance) and (2) beta cell dysfunction that is manifested as inadequate insulin secretion in the face of insulin resistance and hyperglycemia** (Fig. 20.23). Insulin resistance predates the development of hyperglycemia and usually is accompanied by compensatory beta cell hyperfunction and hyperinsulinemia in the early stages of the evolution of diabetes.

Environmental factors, such as a sedentary lifestyle and dietary habits, unequivocally play a role, as described in the subsequent discussion of the association with obesity. Genetic factors also are involved, as evidenced by a concordance rate of 80% to 90% in monozygotic twins, which is even greater than that for type 1 diabetes (approximately 50% concordance rates in twins), suggesting perhaps an even larger genetic component in type 2 diabetes. Additional evidence for a genetic basis has emerged from recent large-scale genome-wide association studies, which have identified dozens of susceptibility loci called *diabetogenic genes.* Unlike type 1 diabetes, however, the disease is not linked to genes involved in immune tolerance and regulation (e.g., *HLA, CTLA4*).

Insulin Resistance

***Insulin resistance* is defined as the failure of target tissues to respond normally to insulin.** The liver, skeletal muscle, and adipose tissue are the major tissues where insulin resistance manifests as follows:

* Failure to inhibit endogenous glucose production (gluconeogenesis) in the liver, which contributes to high fasting blood glucose levels
* Abnormally low glucose uptake and glycogen synthesis in skeletal muscle following a meal, which contributes to a high postprandial blood glucose level
* Failure to inhibit hormone-sensitive lipase in adipose tissue, leading to excess circulating free fatty acids (FFAs), which, as will be discussed, exacerbates the state of insulin resistance

Obesity and Insulin Resistance

Few factors play as important a role in the development of insulin resistance as obesity. The association of obesity with type 2 diabetes has been recognized for decades, with visceral obesity being common in a majority of affected patients. Insulin resistance is present even with simple obesity unaccompanied by hyperglycemia, indicating a fundamental abnormality of insulin signaling in states of fat excess. The term *metabolic syndrome* has been applied to a constellation of findings dominated by visceral obesity, accompanied by insulin resistance, glucose intolerance, and cardiovascular risk factors such as hypertension and abnormal lipid profiles. Individuals with metabolic syndrome are at high risk for the development of type 2 diabetes.

It is not only the absolute amount but also the distribution of body fat that has an effect on insulin sensitivity: central obesity (abdominal fat) is more likely to be associated with insulin resistance than is peripheral (gluteal/subcutaneous) obesity. *Obesity can adversely impact insulin sensitivity in numerous ways* (see Fig. 20.23):

* *Excess FFAs.* Cross-sectional studies have demonstrated an inverse correlation between fasting plasma FFAs and insulin sensitivity. The level of intracellular triglycerides often is markedly increased in muscle and liver in obese individuals, presumably because excess circulating FFAs are taken up into these organs. Central adipose tissue is more "lipolytic" than peripheral adipose tissue, which might explain the particularly deleterious consequences of the central pattern of fat distribution. Intracellular triglycerides and products of fatty acid metabolism are potent inhibitors of insulin signaling and result in an acquired insulin resistance state.
* *Adipokines.* Adipose tissue is not merely a passive storage depot for fat; it also is an endocrine organ that releases hormones in response to changes in metabolic status. A variety of proteins secreted into the systemic circulation by adipose tissue have been identified that are known collectively as *adipokines* (or *adipose cytokines*). Some of these promote hyperglycemia, and others (such as leptin and adiponectin) decrease blood glucose, in

part by increasing the insulin sensitivity of peripheral tissues. Adiponectin levels are decreased in obesity, thus contributing to insulin resistance.

- *Inflammation.* Over the past several years, inflammation has emerged as an important contributor to the pathogenesis of type 2 diabetes. It is now known that a permissive inflammatory milieu (mediated by proinflammatory cytokines that are secreted in response to excess nutrients such as FFAs) results in both peripheral insulin resistance and beta cell dysfunction (discussed later). Excess FFAs within macrophages and beta cells can activate the *inflammasome,* a multiprotein cytoplasmic complex that leads to secretion of the cytokine interleukin (IL-1β; Chapter 5). IL-1β stimulates the secretion of additional proinflammatory cytokines from macrophages, islets, and other cells, and IL-1 as well as other cytokines promote insulin resistance in peripheral tissues. Thus, excess FFAs can impede insulin signaling directly, as well as indirectly through the release of cytokines.

Beta Cell Dysfunction

While insulin resistance by itself can lead to impaired glucose tolerance, **beta cell dysfunction is an essential component in the development of overt diabetes.** Beta cell function actually increases early in the disease process in most patients with type 2 diabetes, mainly as a compensatory measure to counter insulin resistance and maintain euglycemia. Eventually, however, beta cells are unable to adapt to the long-term demands of peripheral insulin resistance, and the hyperinsulinemic state gives way to a state of relative insulin deficiency.

Several mechanisms have been implicated in causing beta cell dysfunction in type 2 diabetes, including the following:

- Excess free fatty acids that compromise beta cell function and attenuate insulin release *(lipotoxicity)*
- Chronic hyperglycemia *(glucotoxicity)*
- Abnormal *incretin effect,* leading to reduced secretion of hormones that promote insulin release (discussed earlier)
- Amyloid replacement of islets, present in more than 90% of diabetic islets (see Morphology). It is unclear whether the amyloid is a cause or effect of beta cell "burnout."
- Polymorphisms associated with an increased lifetime risk for type 2 diabetes in genes that control insulin secretion.

Monogenic Forms of Diabetes

Type 1 and type 2 diabetes are genetically complex, and despite the associations with multiple susceptibility loci, no single-gene defect (mutation) can account for predisposition to these diseases. By contrast, monogenic forms of diabetes (see Table 20.5) are uncommon examples of the diabetes occurring as a result of loss-of-function mutations within a single gene. *Monogenic causes of diabetes* include primary defects in beta cell function and insulin receptor signaling. Monogenic diabetes can be classified based on age of onset into *congenital early onset diabetes* (manifesting in the neonatal period) and *maturity onset diabetes of*

the young (MODY), which develops beyond the neonatal period but usually before 25 years of age. Some of the underlying causes of congenital diabetes include mutations of the insulin gene itself, and mutations in mitochondrial DNA that lead to a syndrome of maternally inherited diabetes and bilateral deafness (the maternal pattern of inheritance being a *sine qua non* of mitochondrial DNA mutations). Rare instances of insulin receptor mutations that affect receptor synthesis, insulin binding, or downstream signal transduction can cause severe insulin resistance, accompanied by hyperinsulinemia (due to lack of feedback inhibition) and congenital diabetes. In contrast, MODY is caused by mutations in genes encoding factors driving beta cell function (see Table 20.5), and at least superficially, tends to resemble usual type 2 diabetes in many of its clinical features. Thus, it is not surprising that the diagnosis of MODY is often missed in individuals who harbor an underlying pathogenic mutation.

Other Subtypes of Diabetes

In addition to Types 1 and 2 and monogenic forms of diabetes, the other broad subtypes include secondary diabetes and pregnancy-induced ("gestational") diabetes. Secondary diabetes arising as a result of endocrinopathies (for example, Cushing syndrome or growth hormone excess) have been described in relevant portions of this chapter. Here, we will briefly discuss a form of secondary diabetes arising as a result of a variety of chronic exocrine pancreatic diseases ("pancreatogenic" diabetes), and the important subtype known as gestational diabetes.

- *Gestational diabetes.* Approximately 5% of pregnancies occurring in the United States are complicated by hyperglycemia. Pregnancy is a "diabetogenic" state in which the prevailing hormonal milieu favors a state of insulin resistance. In some euglycemic pregnant women this can give rise to gestational diabetes. Women with pregestational diabetes (where hyperglycemia is already present in the periconception period) have an increased risk for stillbirth and congenital malformations in the fetus (Chapter 7). Therefore, tight glycemic control is needed early in pregnancy to prevent congenital defects, and through the later trimesters of pregnancy to prevent fetal overgrowth (macrosomia). The latter occurs because maternal hyperglycemia can induce compensatory secretion of insulin-like growth factors in the fetus. Most pregnant women who develop gestational diabetes require insulin for glycemic control. Gestational diabetes typically resolves following delivery; however, there is an elevated risk for developing outright diabetes within the next ten years (highest in the first five years after pregnancy), after which the risk of diabetes reverts to that of women without antecedent gestational diabetes.
- *Pancreatogenic diabetes* is defined as hyperglycemia occurring as a result of a disorder of the exocrine pancreas (see Table 20.5). Pancreatogenic diabetes is heterogeneous, with underlying causes ranging from cystic fibrosis, to chronic pancreatitis, to pancreatic adenocarcinoma. In fact, evidence suggests that approximately 1% of new-onset diabetes in older adults is actually a manifestation of an occult pancreatic adenocarcinoma.

Acute Metabolic Complications of Diabetes

It is difficult to discuss with brevity the diverse clinical presentations of diabetes mellitus. We will discuss the most common initial presentation or mode of diagnosis for each of the two major subtypes, followed by a discussion of acute and chronic complications of diabetes.

Initial Presentation

In the initial 1 or 2 years after manifestation of overt type 1 diabetes (referred to as the *honeymoon period*), exogenous insulin requirements may be minimal because of residual insulin secretion, but eventually the beta cell reserve is exhausted and exogenous insulin becomes essential to control hyperglycemia. Although beta cell destruction is a gradual process, the transition from impaired glucose tolerance to overt diabetes may be abrupt, heralded by an event associated with increased insulin requirements such as infection. The onset of diabetes is marked by *polyuria, polydipsia, polyphagia* (known as the *classic triad of diabetes*), and in severe cases, *ketoacidosis*, all resulting from metabolic derangements (Fig. 20.24).

Since insulin is a major anabolic hormone, its deficiency has widespread effects. The assimilation of glucose into

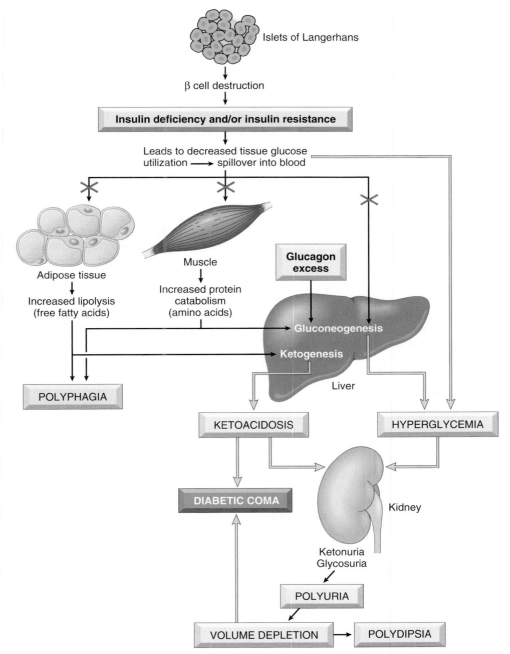

Fig. 20.24 Sequence of metabolic derangements leading to diabetic coma in type 1 diabetes mellitus. An absolute insulin deficiency leads to a catabolic state, eventuating in ketoacidosis and severe volume depletion. These derangements bring about sufficient central nervous system compromise to cause coma and, eventually, death if left untreated.

muscle and adipose tissue is sharply diminished or abolished. Storage of glycogen in liver and muscle ceases, and reserves are depleted by glycogenolysis. The resultant hyperglycemia exceeds the renal threshold for reabsorption, and glycosuria ensues. The glycosuria induces osmotic diuresis and polyuria, causing the loss of water and electrolytes. The renal water loss combined with hyperosmolarity due to increased levels of glucose in the blood depletes intracellular water, triggering osmoreceptors in the brain. This sequence of events generates intense thirst (polydipsia). The deficiency of insulin leads to the catabolism of proteins and fats. Gluconeogenic amino acids produced by proteolysis are taken up and by the liver and used as building blocks for glucose. The catabolism of proteins and fats induces a negative energy balance, which in turn leads to increasing appetite (polyphagia), thus completing the classic triad. Despite the increased appetite, catabolic effects dominate, resulting in weight loss and muscle weakness. *The combination of polyphagia and weight loss is paradoxical and should always point to the possibility of diabetes.*

Diabetic Ketoacidosis and Hyperosmolar Non-ketotic Coma

In patients with type 1 diabetes, significant deviations from normal dietary intake, unusual physical activity, infection, or any other forms of stress may worsen the metabolic imbalance, leading to *diabetic ketoacidosis. The plasma glucose usually is in the range of 500 to 700 mg/dL* as a result of absolute insulin deficiency and unopposed effects of counterregulatory hormones (epinephrine, glucagon). The marked hyperglycemia causes an osmotic diuresis and dehydration characteristic of the ketoacidotic state. The second major effect is activation of the ketogenic machinery. Insulin deficiency leads to activation of hormone-sensitive lipase, with resultant excessive breakdown of adipose stores, giving rise to increased FFAs, which are oxidized by the liver to produce ketones. Ketogenesis is an adaptive phenomenon in times of starvation, generating ketones as a source of energy for consumption by vital organs (e.g., the brain). The rate at which ketones are formed may exceed the rate at which they can be used by peripheral tissues, leading to ketonemia and ketonuria. If the urinary excretion of ketones is compromised by dehydration, the accumulating ketones decrease blood pH, resulting in metabolic acidosis.

Type 2 diabetes also may manifest with polyuria and polydipsia. In some cases, medical attention is sought because of unexplained weakness or weight loss. *Most frequently, however, the diagnosis is made after routine blood or urine testing in asymptomatic individuals.* In the decompensated state, patients with type 2 diabetes may develop *hyperosmolar nonketotic coma.* This syndrome is engendered by severe dehydration resulting from sustained osmotic diuresis and urinary fluid loss due to chronic hyperglycemia. Typically, the affected individual is an older adult diabetic who is disabled by a stroke or an infection and is unable to maintain adequate water intake. The absence of ketoacidosis and its symptoms (nausea, vomiting, respiratory difficulties) delays recognition of the seriousness of the situation until the onset of severe dehydration and coma.

Chronic Complications of Diabetes

The morbidity associated with long-standing diabetes of any type results from the chronic complications of hyperglycemia, and the resulting damage induced in both large- and medium-sized muscular arteries (diabetic macrovascular disease) and small-vessels (diabetic microvascular disease). Macrovascular disease causes accelerated atherosclerosis among diabetics, resulting in increased myocardial infarction, stroke, and lower-extremity ischemia. The effects of microvascular disease are most profound in the retina, kidneys, and peripheral nerves, resulting in diabetic retinopathy, nephropathy, and neuropathy, respectively (Fig. 20.25). The pathologic findings in these tissues and their clinical consequences are described next. There is extreme variability among patients in the time of onset of these complications, their severity, and the particular organ or organs involved. In individuals with tight control of their diabetes, the onset may be delayed (hence the need for tight control of hyperglycemia).

Pathogenesis of Chronic Complications of Diabetes

The pathogenesis of the long-term complications of diabetes is multifactorial, although persistent hyperglycemia (glucotoxicity) seems to be a key mediator. At least three distinct metabolic pathways seem to be involved in the pathogenesis of long-term complications; it is likely that all of them play a role in a tissue-specific manner.

1. *Formation of advanced glycation end products (AGEs).* AGEs are formed as a result of nonenzymatic reactions between intracellular glucose-derived precursors (glyoxal, methylglyoxal, and 3-deoxyglucosone) and the amino groups of proteins. The rate of AGE formation is greatly accelerated by hyperglycemia. AGEs bind to a specific receptor (RAGE), which is expressed on inflammatory cells (macrophages and T cells), endothelium and vascular smooth muscle. The detrimental effects of AGE-RAGE signaling within the vascular compartment include the following:
   - Release of cytokines and growth factors, including transforming growth factor β (TGFβ), which leads to deposition of excess basement membrane material, and vascular endothelial growth factor (VEGF), implicated in diabetic retinopathy (discussed later)
   - Generation of *reactive oxygen species (ROS)* in endothelial cells
   - Increased *procoagulant activity* on endothelial cells and macrophages
   - Enhanced *proliferation of vascular smooth muscle cells and synthesis of extracellular matrix*

   In addition to receptor-mediated effects, *AGEs can directly cross-link extracellular matrix proteins.* These cross-linked proteins can trap other plasma or interstitial proteins; for example, low-density lipoprotein (LDL) gets trapped within AGE-modified large-vessel walls, accelerating atherosclerosis (Chapter 10), while albumin can be trapped within capillary walls, accounting in part for the basement membrane thickening that is characteristic of diabetic microangiopathy (discussed later).

2. *Activation of protein kinase C.* Activation of intracellular protein kinase C (PKC) by calcium ions and the second messenger diacylglycerol (DAG) is an important

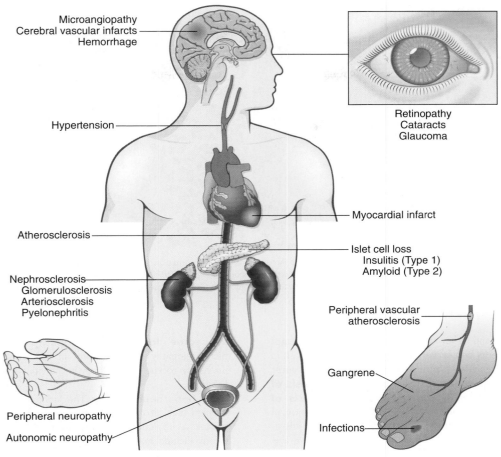

Fig. 20.25 Long-term complications of diabetes.

Microangiopathy
Cerebral vascular infarcts
Hemorrhage

Retinopathy
Cataracts
Glaucoma

Hypertension

Atherosclerosis

Myocardial infarct

Islet cell loss
Insulitis (Type 1)
Amyloid (Type 2)

Nephrosclerosis
Glomerulosclerosis
Arteriosclerosis
Pyelonephritis

Peripheral vascular
atherosclerosis

Gangrene

Peripheral neuropathy

Autonomic neuropathy

Infections

signal transduction pathway in many cellular systems. Intracellular hyperglycemia can stimulate the de novo synthesis of DAG from glycolytic intermediates and hence cause activation of PKC. The downstream effects of PKC activation are numerous and include production of *proangiogenic molecules* such as vascular endothelial growth factor (VEGF), implicated in the neovascularization seen in diabetic retinopathy, and profibrogenic molecules such as transforming growth factor β, leading to increased deposition of extracellular matrix and basement membrane material.

3. *Disturbances in polyol pathways.* In some tissues that do not require insulin for glucose transport (e.g., nerves, lens, kidneys, blood vessels), hyperglycemia leads to an increase in intracellular glucose that is then metabolized by the enzyme aldose reductase to sorbitol, a polyol, and eventually to fructose, in a reaction that uses NADPH (the reduced form of nicotinamide dinucleotide phosphate) as a cofactor. NADPH also is required by the enzyme glutathione reductase in a reaction that regenerates reduced glutathione (GSH). As described in Chapter 2, GSH is one of the important anti-oxidant mechanisms in the cell, and reductions in GSH increase cellular susceptibility to *oxidative stress.* In neurons, persistent hyperglycemia appears to be the major underlying cause of diabetic neuropathy (*glucose neurotoxicity*).

MORPHOLOGY

The most important morphologic changes are related to the many late systemic complications of diabetes. These changes are seen in both type 1 and type 2 diabetes (see Fig. 20.25).

Pancreas. Lesions in the pancreas are inconstant. One or more of the following alterations may be present:

- **Reduction in the number and size of islets.** This change most often is seen in type 1 diabetes, particularly with rapidly advancing disease. Most of the islets are small, inconspicuous, and not easily detected.
- **Leukocytic infiltrates in the islets** (insulitis) are principally composed of T lymphocytes (Fig. 20.26A). They are most often seen type 1 diabetes at the time of clinical presentation.
- **Amyloid deposition within islets in type 2 diabetes** begins in and around capillaries and between cells. At advanced stages, the islets may be virtually obliterated (see Fig. 20.26B); fibrosis also may be observed. Similar lesions may be found in older nondiabetics, apparently as part of normal aging.
- **An increase in the number and size of islets, especially characteristic of nondiabetic newborns of diabetic mothers.** Presumably, fetal islets undergo hyperplasia in response to the maternal hyperglycemia.

Diabetic macrovascular disease. The hallmark of diabetic macrovascular disease is **accelerated atherosclerosis**

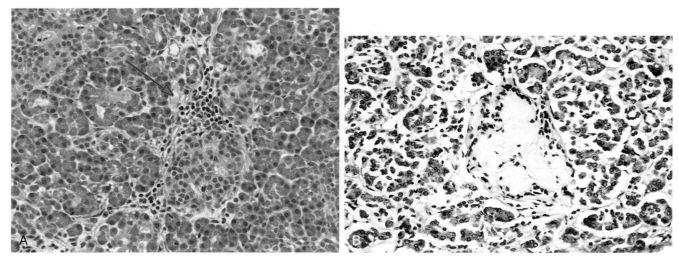

Fig. 20.26 (A) Autoimmune insulitis in a human pancreatic explant. Arrows point to inflammation surrounding islet of Langerhans, while the surrounding acinar structures are essentially normal. *(Photograph provided by Dr. Martha Campbell-Thompson, JDRF Network for Pancreatic Organ Donors, University of Florida., Gainesville, Florida.)* (B) Amyloidosis of a pancreatic islet in type 2 diabetes. Amyloidosis typically is observed late in the natural history of this form of diabetes, with islet inflammation noted at earlier observations.

affecting the aorta and large- and medium-sized arteries. Except for its greater severity and earlier age at onset, atherosclerosis in diabetics is indistinguishable from that in nondiabetics (Chapter 10). **Myocardial infarction, caused by atherosclerosis of the coronary arteries, is the most common cause of death in diabetics.** Significantly, it is almost as common in diabetic women as in diabetic men. By contrast, myocardial infarction is uncommon in nondiabetic women of reproductive age. **Gangrene of the lower extremities,** as a result of advanced vascular disease, is about 100 times more common in individuals with diabetes than in the general population. The larger renal arteries also are subject to severe atherosclerosis, but the most damaging effect of diabetes on the kidneys is exerted at the level of the glomeruli and the microcirculation, as discussed later.

Hyaline arteriolosclerosis, the vascular lesion associated with hypertension (Chapters 10 and 14), is both more prevalent and more severe in diabetics than in nondiabetics, but it is not specific for diabetes and may be seen in older adults who do not suffer from either diabetes or hypertension. It takes the form of an amorphous, hyaline thickening of the wall of the arterioles, which causes narrowing of the lumen (Fig. 20.27). Not surprisingly, in diabetic patients, its severity is related not only to the duration of the disease but also to the presence or absence of hypertension.

Diabetic microangiopathy. One of the most consistent morphologic features of diabetes is **diffuse thickening of basement membranes.** The thickening is most evident in the capillaries of the skin, skeletal muscle, retina, renal glomeruli, and renal medulla. However, it also may be seen in nonvascular structures such as renal tubules, the Bowman capsule, peripheral nerves, and placenta. By both light and electron microscopy, the basal lamina separating parenchymal or endothelial cells from the surrounding tissue is markedly thickened by concentric layers of hyaline material composed predominantly of type IV collagen (Fig. 20.28). Of note, despite the increase in the thickness of basement membranes, diabetic capillaries are leaky, leading to extravasation of plasma proteins. **The microangiopathy underlies the development of diabetic nephropathy, retinopathy,**

and some forms of neuropathy. An indistinguishable microangiopathy can be found in aged nondiabetic patients, but rarely to the extent seen in individuals with long-standing diabetes.

Diabetic nephropathy. The kidneys are prime targets of diabetes (see also Chapter 14). Renal failure is second only to myocardial infarction as a cause of death from this disease. The lesions include mainly: (1) glomerular lesions; (2) renal vascular lesions, principally arteriolosclerosis; and (3) pyelonephritis, including necrotizing papillitis.

The most important **glomerular lesions** are capillary basement membrane thickening, diffuse mesangial sclerosis, and nodular glomerulosclerosis. The glomerular capillary basement membranes are thickened along their entire length. This change can be detected by electron microscopy within a few years of

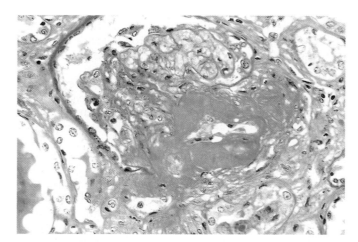

Fig. 20.27 Severe renal hyaline arteriolosclerosis in a periodic acid–Schiff stained specimen. Note the markedly thickened, tortuous afferent arteriole. The amorphous nature of the thickened vascular wall is evident. *(Courtesy of Dr. M.A. Venkatachalam, Department of Pathology, University of Texas Health Science Center, San Antonio, Texas.)*

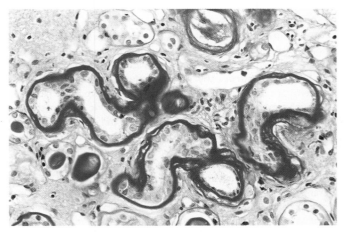

Fig. 20.28 Renal cortex showing thickening of tubular basement membranes in a specimen from a diabetic patient. (Periodic acid–Schiff stain.)

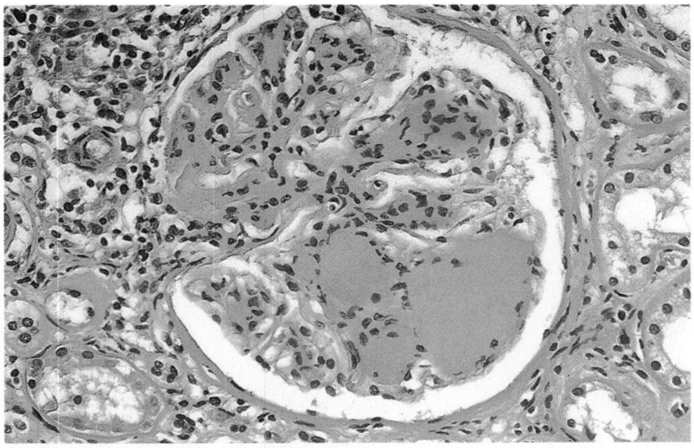

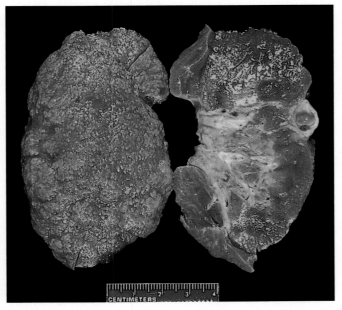

Fig. 20.30 Nodular glomerulosclerosis in a renal specimen from a patient with long-standing diabetes. (Courtesy of Dr. Lisa Yerian, Department of Pathology, University of Chicago, Chicago, Illinois.)

the onset of diabetes, sometimes without any associated change in renal function (Fig. 20.29).

Diffuse mesangial sclerosis refers to an increase in mesangial matrix associated with mesangial cell proliferation and basement membrane thickening. It is found in most individuals with disease of more than 10 years' duration. When glomerulosclerosis is severe, patients develop the nephrotic syndrome, characterized by proteinuria, hypoalbuminemia, and edema (Chapter 14).

Nodular glomerulosclerosis (Kimmelstiel-Wilson lesion) is a distinctive glomerular lesion characterized by ball-like deposits of a laminated matrix in the periphery of the glomerulus (Fig. 20.30). These nodules are PAS-positive and usually contain trapped mesangial cells. Nodular glomerulosclerosis is encountered in approximately 15% to 30% of individuals with long-term diabetes and is a major contributor to renal dysfunction. Diffuse

mesangial sclerosis also may be seen in association with old age and hypertension; by contrast, the nodular form of glomerulosclerosis is virtually pathognomonic of diabetes. Both the diffuse and the nodular forms of glomerulosclerosis induce sufficient ischemia to cause scarring of the kidneys, manifested by a finely granular–appearing cortical surface (Fig. 20.31).

Renal atherosclerosis and arteriolosclerosis constitute part of the macrovascular disease seen in diabetics. The kidney is one of the most frequently and severely affected organs; the changes in the arteries and arterioles are similar to those found throughout the body. Hyaline arteriolosclerosis affects not only the afferent but also the efferent arterioles. Such efferent arteriolosclerosis is rarely if ever encountered in individuals who do not have diabetes.

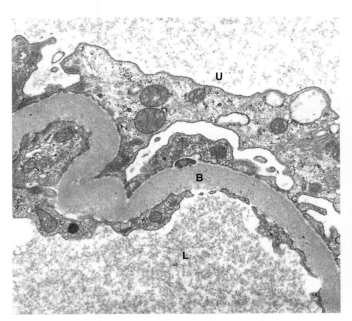

Fig. 20.29 Renal glomerulus showing markedly thickened glomerular basement membrane (B) in a diabetic. L, Glomerular capillary lumen; U, urinary space. (Courtesy of Dr. Michael Kashgarian, Department of Pathology, Yale University School of Medicine, New Haven, Connecticut.)

Fig. 20.31 Nephrosclerosis in a patient with long-standing diabetes. The bisected kidney demonstrates diffuse granular transformation of the surface (left) and marked thinning of the cortex (right). Additional features include some irregular depressions, the result of pyelonephritis, and an incidental cortical cyst (far right).

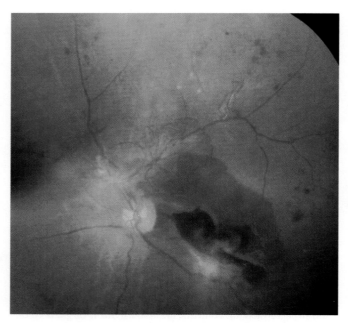

Fig. 20.32 Characteristic morphologic changes of diabetic retinopathy. Features include advanced proliferative retinopathy with retinal hemorrhages, exudates, neovascularization, and tractional retinal detachment *(lower-right corner). (Courtesy of Dr. Rajendra Apte, Washington University School of Medicine, St. Louis, Missouri.)*

Pyelonephritis is an acute or chronic inflammation of the kidneys that usually begins in the interstitial tissue and then spreads to involve the tubules. Both the acute and chronic forms of this disease occur in nondiabetics as well as in diabetics are more common in individuals with diabetes, and once affected, diabetics also tend to have more severe involvement. One special pattern of acute pyelonephritis, **necrotizing papillitis** (or papillary necrosis), is much more prevalent in diabetics than in nondiabetics.

Ocular complications of diabetes. Visual impairment, sometimes even total blindness, is one of the more feared consequences of long-standing diabetes. **The ocular involvement may take the form of retinopathy, cataract formation, or glaucoma.** Retinopathy, the most common pattern, consists of a constellation of changes that together are considered by many ophthalmologists to be virtually diagnostic of the disease. The lesion in the retina takes two forms: nonproliferative retinopathy and proliferative retinopathy.

Nonproliferative retinopathy includes intraretinal or preretinal hemorrhages, retinal exudates, microaneurysms, venous dilations, edema, and, most importantly, thickening of the retinal capillaries (microangiopathy). The retinal exudates can be "soft" (microinfarcts) or "hard" (deposits of plasma proteins and lipids) (Fig. 20.32). The microaneurysms are discrete saccular dilations of retinal choroidal capillaries that appear through the ophthalmoscope as small red dots. Dilations tend to occur at focal points of weakening, resulting from loss of pericytes. Retinal edema presumably results from excessive capillary permeability. Underlying all of these changes is the microangiopathy, which is thought to lead to loss of capillary pericytes and hence to focal weakening of capillary structure.

The so-called **proliferative retinopathy** is a process of neovascularization and fibrosis. This lesion leads to serious consequences, including blindness, especially if it involves the macula. Vitreous hemorrhages may result from the rupture of newly formed capillaries; the subsequent organization of the hemorrhage can pull the retina off its substratum (retinal detachment).

Diabetic neuropathy. The central and peripheral nervous systems are not spared by diabetes. The most frequent pattern of involvement is that of a peripheral, symmetric neuropathy of the lower extremities affecting both motor and sensory function, particularly the latter. Other forms include autonomic neuropathy, which produces disturbances in bowel and bladder function and sometimes sexual impotence, and diabetic mononeuropathy, which may manifest as sudden footdrop or wristdrop or isolated cranial nerve palsies. The neurologic changes may be the result of microangiopathy and increased permeability of the capillaries that supply the nerves, as well as direct axonal damage.

Clinical Features of Chronic Diabetes

As the previous discussion has emphasized, type 1 and type 2 diabetes are distinct pathophysiologic entities with the common manifestation of hyperglycemia. Table 20.6 summarizes some of the clinical, genetic and histopathologic features that distinguish the two diseases. Nonetheless, as previously stated, the long-term sequela of both types 1 and 2 diabetes, arising as a result of uncontrolled

Table 20.6 Type 1 Versus Type 2 Diabetes Mellitus

Type 1 Diabetes Mellitus	Type 2 Diabetes Mellitus
Clinical	
Onset usually in childhood and adolescence	Onset usually in adulthood; increasing incidence in childhood and adolescence
Normal weight or weight loss preceding diagnosis	Vast majority of patients are obese (80%)
Progressive decrease in insulin levels	Increased blood insulin (early); normal or moderate decrease in insulin (late)
Circulating islet autoantibodies	No islet autoantibodies
Diabetic ketoacidosis in absence of insulin therapy	Nonketotic hyperosmolar coma
Genetics	
Major linkage to MHC class I and II genes; also linked to polymorphisms in *CTLA4* and *PTPN22*	No HLA linkage; linkage to candidate diabetogenic and obesity-related genes
Pathogenesis	
Breakdown in self-tolerance to islet autoantigens	Insulin resistance in peripheral tissues, failure of compensation by beta cells Multiple obesity-associated factors (circulating nonesterified fatty acids, inflammatory mediators, adipocytokines) linked to pathogenesis of insulin resistance
Pathology	
Autoimmune "insulitis"	Amyloid deposition in islets (late)
Beta cell depletion, islet atrophy	Mild beta cell depletion

HLA, Human leukocyte antigen; *MHC,* major histocompatibility complex.

or poorly controlled hyperglycemia, are similar, and are responsible for much of the morbidity and mortality in diabetics. In most instances these complications appear approximately 15 to 20 years after the onset of hyperglycemia. The major chronic complications of the disease are described next.

- *Macrovascular complications, such as myocardial infarction, renal vascular insufficiency, and cerebrovascular accidents, are the most common causes of mortality in long-standing diabetes.* Diabetics have a two to four times greater incidence of coronary artery disease, and a fourfold higher risk of death from cardiovascular complications, than nondiabetics. Diabetes is often accompanied by underlying conditions that favor the development of adverse cardiovascular events, including hypertension and dyslipidemia (see earlier discussion on metabolic syndrome). The hallmark of cardiovascular disease is accelerated atherosclerosis of the large- and medium-sized arteries (i.e., macrovascular disease). The importance of obesity in the pathogenesis of insulin resistance has already been discussed, but it also is an independent risk factor for development of atherosclerosis.
- *Diabetic nephropathy is a leading cause of end-stage renal disease in the United States.* The earliest manifestation of diabetic nephropathy is the appearance of small amounts of albumin in the urine (>30 but <300 mg/day). Without specific interventions, approximately 80% of patients with type 1 diabetes and 20% to 40% of those with type 2 diabetes will develop overt nephropathy with macroalbuminuria (excretion of >300 mg/day) over the ensuing 10 to 15 years, usually accompanied by the appearance of hypertension. The progression from overt nephropathy to end-stage renal disease is highly variable and is evidenced by a progressive drop in glomerular filtration rate. By 20 years after diagnosis, more than 75% of individuals with type 1 diabetes and about 20% of those with type 2 diabetes with overt nephropathy will develop end-stage renal disease, necessitating dialysis or renal transplantation.
- *Visual impairment, sometimes even total blindness, is one of the more feared consequences of long-standing diabetes.* Diabetes is the fourth leading cause of acquired blindness in the United States. Approximately 60% to 80% of patients develop some form of diabetic retinopathy approximately 15 to 20 years after diagnosis. The fundamental lesion of retinopathy—neovascularization—is attributable to hypoxia-induced overexpression of VEGF in the retina. Current treatment for this condition includes intravitreous injection of anti-angiogenic agents. In addition to retinopathy, diabetic patients also have an increased propensity for glaucoma and cataract formation, both of which contribute to visual impairment in diabetes.
- *Diabetic neuropathy* can produce a variety of clinical syndromes, afflicting the central nervous system, peripheral sensorimotor nerves, and autonomic nervous system. The most frequent pattern of nerve involvement is a distal symmetric polyneuropathy of the lower extremities that affects both motor and sensory function, particularly the latter (Chapter 22). Over time, the upper extremities may be involved as well, thus approximating a "glove and stocking" pattern of polyneuropathy. Other forms include autonomic neuropathy, which produces disturbances in bowel and bladder function and sometimes sexual impotence, and diabetic mononeuropathy, which may manifest as sudden footdrop, wristdrop, or isolated cranial nerve palsies.
- Diabetic patients are plagued by an *increased susceptibility to infections of the skin, tuberculosis, pneumonia, and pyelonephritis.* Infections cause about 5% of diabetes-related deaths. In an individual with diabetic neuropathy, a trivial infection in a toe may be the first event in a long succession of complications (gangrene, bacteremia, pneumonia) that may ultimately lead to death.

Several large-scale prospective studies have convincingly demonstrated that the microvascular complications, and the associated morbidity and mortality, from diabetes are attenuated by strict glycemic control. For patients with type 1 diabetes, insulin replacement therapy is the mainstay of treatment, while nonpharmacologic approaches such as dietary restrictions and exercise (which improves insulin sensitivity) are often the "first line of defense" for type 2 diabetes. Most patients with type 2 diabetes eventually require therapeutic intervention to reduce hyperglycemia. Glycemic control is assessed clinically by measuring the percentage of glycosylated hemoglobin, also known as *HbA1C*, which is formed by nonenzymatic addition of glucose moieties to hemoglobin in red cells. Unlike blood glucose levels, HbA1C is a measure of glycemic control over long periods of time (2–3 months) and is relatively unaffected by day-to-day variations. The ADA recommends maintenance of HbA1C levels at less than 7% to reduce the risk for long-term complications. In addition, diabetics need to maintain LDL and HDL cholesterol and triglycerides at optimal levels to reduce the risk for macrovascular complications. The adoption of a healthy and active lifestyle remains one of the best defenses against this modern day scourge.

SUMMARY

DIABETES MELLITUS: PATHOGENESIS AND LONG-TERM COMPLICATIONS

- Type 1 diabetes is an autoimmune disease characterized by progressive destruction of islet beta cells, leading to absolute insulin deficiency. Both autoreactive T cells and autoantibodies are involved.
- Type 2 diabetes is caused by insulin resistance and beta cell dysfunction, resulting in relative insulin deficiency. Autoimmunity is not involved.
- Obesity has an important relationship with insulin resistance (and hence type 2 diabetes), mediated by various factors, including excess free fatty acids, aberrant levels of adipokines, and an altered inflammatory milieu within adipose tissue.
- Monogenic forms of diabetes are uncommon and are caused by single-gene defects that result in primary beta cell dysfunction or lead to abnormalities of insulin–insulin receptor signaling.
- The long-term complications of diabetes are similar in all types and affect mainly blood vessels, and the kidneys, nerves, and eyes. The development of these complications is attributed to three underlying mechanisms: formation of AGEs, activation of PKC, and disturbances in polyol pathways leading to oxidative stress.

PANCREATIC NEUROENDOCRINE TUMORS

Pancreatic neuroendocrine tumors (PanNETs), also known as *islet cell tumors,* are rare in comparison with tumors of the exocrine pancreas, accounting for only 2% of all pancreatic neoplasms. PanNETs are most common in adults and may be single or multifocal; when they are malignant, the liver is the most common site of metastases. These tumors have a propensity to elaborate pancreatic hormones, but some are nonfunctional. The latter typically are larger at the time of diagnosis, since they come to clinical attention later in their natural history than functional PanNETs, which often present with symptoms related to excessive hormone production. All PanNETs, with the exception of insulinomas (see later), are regarded as having malignant potential, and in fact, 60% to 90% of PanNETs manifest with overtly malignant features of biologic aggressiveness, such as invasion into local tissues or distant metastases. The tumors frequently have mutations in tumor suppressor genes *MEN1* and *PTEN,* or inactivating mutations in genes (e.g. *ATRX*) whose products maintain telomere length.

Insulinomas

Beta cell tumors (insulinomas) are the most common type of PanNET and elaborate sufficient insulin to induce attacks of hypoglycemia when blood glucose levels fall below 50 mg/dL. These attacks manifest as confusion, stupor, and loss of consciousness. They are precipitated by fasting or exercise and are promptly relieved by feeding or parenteral administration of glucose. Most insulinomas are cured by surgical resection.

MORPHOLOGY

The majority of insulinomas are identified while they are small (<2 cm in diameter) and localized to the pancreas. Most are solitary lesions, although multifocal tumors or tumors ectopic to the pancreas may be encountered. Malignancy in insulinomas occurs in less than 10% of cases, and is diagnosed on the basis of local invasion or metastases. On histologic examination, the benign tumors look remarkably like giant islets, with preservation of the regular cords of monotonous cells and their orientation to the vasculature. Malignant lesions also tend to be well-differentiated and may be deceptively encapsulated. **Deposition of amyloid** is a characteristic feature of many insulinomas (Fig. 20.33). Under the electron microscope, neoplastic beta cells, like their normal counterparts, display distinctive round granules.

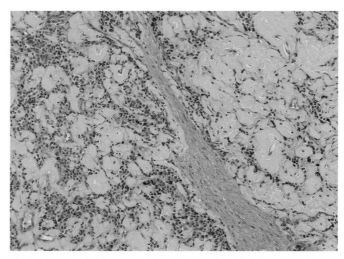

Fig. 20.33 Pancreatic neuroendocrine tumor (PanNET), also called *islet cell tumor.* The neoplastic cells are monotonous in appearance and demonstrate minimal pleomorphism or mitotic activity. There is abundant amyloid deposition, characteristic of an insulinoma.

Gastrinomas

Marked hypersecretion of gastrin usually has its origin in gastrin-producing tumors *(gastrinomas),* which are just as likely to arise in the duodenum and peripancreatic soft tissues as in the pancreas (the so-called "gastrinoma triangle"). *The Zollinger-Ellison syndrome refers to the association of pancreatic islet cell lesions with hypersecretion of gastric acid and severe peptic ulceration,* present in 90% to 95% of patients with gastrinomas. Hypergastrinemia from a pancreatic or duodenal tumor stimulates extreme gastric acid secretion, which, in turn, causes *peptic ulceration.* The duodenal and gastric ulcers often are multiple; although they are identical to those found in the general population, they often are unresponsive to usual therapy. In addition, ulcers may occur in unusual locations such as the jejunum; when intractable jejunal ulcers are found, Zollinger-Ellison syndrome should be considered. More than one-half of affected patients have diarrhea; in 30%, it is the presenting manifestation.

MORPHOLOGY

Gastrinomas may arise in the pancreas, the peripancreatic region, or the wall of the duodenum. **Over one-half of gastrin-producing tumors are locally invasive or have already metastasized at the time of diagnosis.** In approximately 25% of patients, gastrinomas arise in conjunction with other endocrine tumors, thus conforming to the MEN-1 syndrome (discussed later); MEN-1–associated gastrinomas frequently are multifocal, while sporadic gastrinomas usually are single. As with insulin-secreting tumors of the pancreas, gastrin-producing tumors are histologically bland and rarely exhibit marked anaplasia.

Adrenal Cortex

The adrenal glands are paired endocrine organs consisting of two regions, the cortex and medulla, which differ in their development, structure, and function. The *cortex* consists of three layers of distinct cell types. Beneath the capsule of the adrenal gland is the narrow layer of zona glomerulosa. An equally narrow zona reticularis abuts the medulla. Intervening is the broad zona fasciculata, which makes up about 75% of the total cortex.

The adrenal cortex synthesizes three different types of steroids:

- *Glucocorticoids* (principally cortisol), synthesized primarily in the zona fasciculata, with a small contribution from the zona reticularis
- *Mineralocorticoids,* the most important being aldosterone, generated in the zona glomerulosa
- *Sex steroids* (estrogens and androgens), produced largely in the zona reticularis

The *adrenal medulla* is composed of chromaffin cells, which synthesize and secrete *catecholamines,* mainly epinephrine. This section deals first with disorders of the adrenal cortex and then of the medulla. Diseases of the adrenal cortex can be conveniently divided into those associated with cortical hyperfunction or hypofunction.

ADRENOCORTICAL HYPERFUNCTION: HYPERADRENALISM

There are three distinctive hyperadrenal clinical syndromes, each caused by abnormal production of one or more of the hormones produced by the three layers of the cortex:

- *Cushing syndrome,* characterized by an excess of cortisol
- *Hyperaldosteronism,* caused by an excess of mineralocorticoid
- *Adrenogenital* or *virilizing syndromes,* caused by an excess of androgens

The clinical features of some of these syndromes show some similarities because of the shared functions of adrenal steroids.

Hypercortisolism: Cushing Syndrome

Hypercortisolism (Cushing syndrome) is caused by elevated glucocorticoid levels. In clinical practice, the vast majority of cases of Cushing syndrome are the result of administration of exogenous glucocorticoids (iatrogenic). The remaining cases are endogenous, and the three most common disorders are as follows (Fig. 20.34):

- Primary hypothalamic-pituitary diseases associated with hypersecretion of ACTH
- Secretion of ectopic ACTH by nonpituitary neoplasms
- Primary adrenocortical neoplasms (adenoma or carcinoma) and, rarely, primary cortical hyperplasia

Primary hypothalamic-pituitary disease associated with hypersecretion of ACTH, also known as *Cushing disease,*

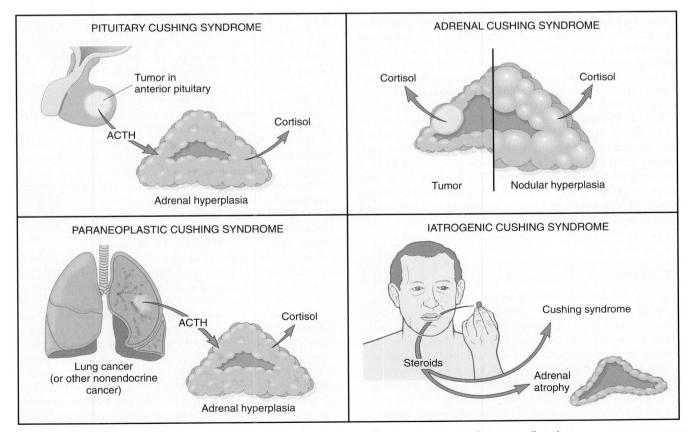

Fig. 20.34 Schematic representation of the various forms of Cushing syndrome: The three endogenous forms, as well as the more common exogenous (iatrogenic) form. *ACTH,* Adrenocorticotropic hormone.

accounts for approximately 70% of cases of spontaneous, endogenous Cushing syndrome. The prevalence of this disorder is about four times higher among women than among men, and it occurs most frequently during young adulthood (the twenties and thirties). In the vast majority of cases, the *pituitary gland contains an ACTH-producing micro-adenoma* that does not produce mass effects in the brain. In some cases there is a microadenoma and rarely, the anterior pituitary contains areas of *corticotroph cell hyperplasia* without a discrete adenoma. Corticotroph cell hyperplasia may be primary or, much less commonly, secondary to excessive ACTH release by a hypothalamic corticotropin-releasing hormone (CRH)–producing tumor. The adrenal glands in patients with Cushing disease show variable degrees of bilateral nodular cortical hyperplasia (discussed later), secondary to the elevated levels of ACTH ("ACTH-dependent" Cushing syndrome). The cortical hyperplasia is, in turn, responsible for the hypercortisolism.

Secretion of ectopic ACTH by nonpituitary tumors accounts for about 10% of cases of Cushing syndrome. In many instances the responsible tumor is a *small-cell carcinoma of the lung,* although other neoplasms, including carcinoids, medullary carcinomas of the thyroid, and PanNETs, have been associated with the syndrome. In addition to tumors that elaborate ectopic ACTH, occasional neuroendocrine neoplasms produce ectopic CRH, which, in turn, causes ACTH secretion and hypercortisolism. As in the pituitary variant, the adrenal glands undergo bilateral cortical hyperplasia secondary to elevated ACTH, but the rapid downhill course of patients with these cancers often cuts short the adrenal enlargement.

Primary adrenal neoplasms, such as adrenal adenoma and carcinoma, and rarely, *primary cortical hyperplasia,* are responsible for about 15% to 20% of cases of endogenous Cushing syndrome, also designated *ACTH-independent Cushing syndrome,* because the adrenals function autonomously. The biochemical hallmark of adrenal Cushing syndrome is elevated levels of cortisol and low serum levels of ACTH. In most cases, adrenal Cushing syndrome is caused by a unilateral adrenocortical neoplasm, which may be benign (adenoma) or malignant (carcinoma). Primary cortical hyperplasia of the adrenal cortices is a rare cause of Cushing syndrome. There are two variants of this entity; the first presents as macronodules of varying sizes (typically less than 3 cm in diameter) and the second as micronodules (1–3 mm).

MORPHOLOGY

The main lesions of Cushing syndrome are found in the pituitary and adrenal glands. The **pituitary** in Cushing syndrome shows changes that vary with different causes. The most common alteration, resulting from high levels of endogenous or exogenous glucocorticoids, is termed Crooke hyaline change. In this condition, the normal granular, basophilic cytoplasm of the ACTH-producing cells in the anterior pituitary is replaced by homogeneous, lightly basophilic material. This alteration is the result of the accumulation of intermediate keratin filaments in the cytoplasm. In pituitary Cushing syndrome, there is an adenoma (described under diseases of the pituitary).

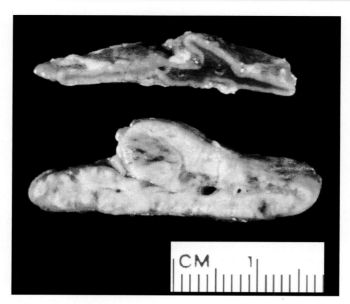

Fig. 20.35 Diffuse hyperplasia of the adrenal gland *(bottom)* contrasted with a normal adrenal gland *(top).* In a cross-section, the adrenal cortex is yellow and thickened, and a subtle nodularity is evident. The abnormal gland was from a patient with ACTH-dependent Cushing syndrome, in whom both adrenal glands were diffusely hyperplastic. *ACTH,* Adrenocorticotropic hormone.

Morphologic changes in the adrenal glands also depend on the cause of the hypercortisolism and include: (1) cortical atrophy, (2) diffuse hyperplasia, (3) macronodular or micronodular hyperplasia, or (4) an adenoma or carcinoma.

In patients in whom the syndrome results from exogenous glucocorticoids, suppression of endogenous ACTH results in bilateral **cortical atrophy,** due to a lack of stimulation of the zona fasciculata and zona reticularis by ACTH. The zona glomerulosa is of normal thickness in such cases, because this portion of the cortex functions independently of ACTH. In cases of endogenous hypercortisolism, by contrast, the adrenals either are hyperplastic or contain a cortical neoplasm.

Diffuse hyperplasia is found in patients with ACTH-dependent Cushing syndrome (Fig. 20.35). Both glands are enlarged, either subtly or markedly, each weighing up to 30 g. The adrenal cortex is diffusely thickened and variably nodular, although the latter is not as pronounced as in cases of ACTH-independent nodular hyperplasia. The yellow color of diffusely hyperplastic glands derives from the presence of **lipid-rich** cells, which appear vacuolated under the microscope.

In **primary cortical hyperplasia,** the cortex is replaced almost entirely by **macronodules** or 1- to 3-mm darkly pigmented **micronodules** (Fig. 20.36). The pigment is believed to be lipofuscin, a wear-and-tear pigment (Chapter 2).

Functional adenomas or carcinomas of the adrenal cortex are not morphologically distinct from nonfunctioning adrenal neoplasms (discussed later). Both the benign and malignant lesions are more common in women in their thirties to fifties. Adrenocortical **adenomas** are yellow tumors surrounded by thin or well-developed capsules, and most weigh less than 30 g (Fig. 20.37A). On microscopic examination, they are composed of cells similar to those encountered in the normal zona fasciculata (see Fig. 20.37B). The **carcinomas** associated with Cushing syndrome, by contrast, tend to be larger than the adenomas.

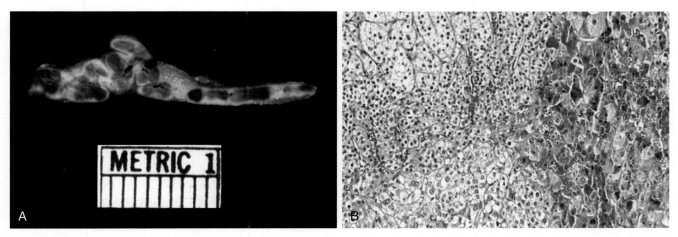

Fig. 20.36 (A) Primary pigmented nodular adrenocortical hyperplasia showing prominent pigmented nodules in the adrenal gland. (B) On histologic examination, the nodules are composed of cells containing lipofuscin pigment, seen in the right part of the field. *(Photographs courtesy of Dr. Aidan Carney, Department of Medicine, Mayo Clinic, Rochester, Minnesota.)*

These tumors are nonencapsulated masses frequently exceeding 200 to 300 g in weight, having all of the anaplastic characteristics of cancer, as detailed later. With functioning tumors, both benign and malignant, the adjacent adrenal cortex and that of the contralateral adrenal gland are atrophic, as a result of suppression of endogenous ACTH by high cortisol levels.

Clinical Features

The signs and symptoms of Cushing syndrome represent an exaggeration of the known actions of glucocorticoids. Cushing syndrome usually develops gradually and, like many other endocrine abnormalities, may be quite subtle in its early stages. A major exception to this insidious onset is Cushing syndrome associated with small-cell carcinomas of the lung, when the rapid course of the underlying disease precludes development of many of the characteristic features. Early manifestations of Cushing syndrome include *hypertension* and *weight gain*. With time, the more characteristic centripetal redistribution of adipose tissue becomes apparent, with resultant truncal obesity, "moon facies," and accumulation of fat in the posterior neck and back ("buffalo hump"). Hypercortisolism causes selective atrophy of fast-twitch (type II) myofibers, with resultant decreased muscle mass and proximal limb weakness. Glucocorticoids induce gluconeogenesis and inhibit the uptake of glucose by cells, resulting in secondary diabetes with its attendant *hyperglycemia*, *glucosuria*, and *polydipsia*. The catabolic effects of insulin resistance on proteins cause loss of collagen. Thus, the skin is thin, fragile, and easily bruised; *cutaneous striae* are particularly common in the abdominal area (Fig. 20.38). Cortisol also has diverse effects on calcium metabolism that lead to resorption of bone, which results in the development of *osteoporosis*, with consequent increased susceptibility to fractures. Because

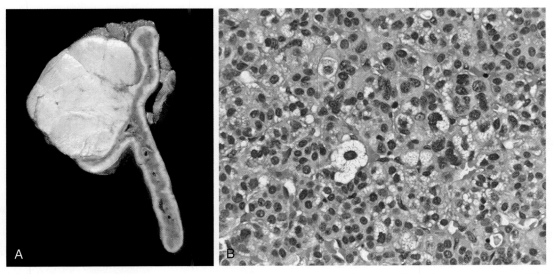

Fig. 20.37 Adrenocortical adenoma. (A) The adenoma is distinguished from nodular hyperplasia by its solitary, circumscribed nature. The functional status of an adrenocortical adenoma cannot be predicted from its gross or microscopic appearance. (B) Histologic features of an adrenal cortical adenoma. The neoplastic cells are vacuolated because of the presence of intracytoplasmic lipid. There is mild nuclear pleomorphism. Mitotic activity and necrosis are not seen.

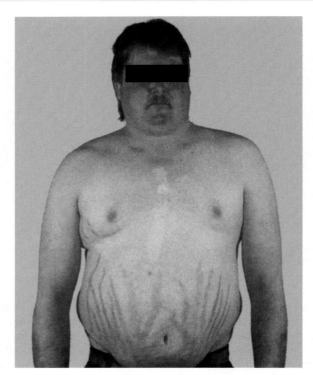

Fig. 20.38 A patient with Cushing syndrome. Characteristic features include central obesity, "moon facies," and abdominal striae. *(Reproduced with permission from Lloyd RV, et al: Atlas of nontumor pathology: endocrine diseases. Washington, DC, American Registry of Pathology, 2002.)*

glucocorticoids suppress the immune response, patients with Cushing syndrome also are at increased risk for a variety of infections. Additional manifestations include *hirsutism* and *menstrual abnormalities*, as well as a number of *psychiatric symptoms* including mood swings, depression, and frank psychosis. Extraadrenal Cushing syndrome caused by pituitary or ectopic ACTH secretion usually is associated with increased skin pigmentation secondary to melanocyte-stimulating activity in the ACTH precursor molecule.

In pituitary and ectopic Cushing syndrome, ACTH levels are elevated and the urine is characterized by high levels of excreted corticosteroids. In contrast, ACTH levels are low in Cushing syndrome secondary to adrenal tumors.

SUMMARY

HYPERCORTISOLISM (CUSHING SYNDROME)

- The most common cause of hypercortisolism is exogenous administration of steroids.
- Endogenous hypercortisolism most often is secondary to an ACTH-producing pituitary microadenoma *(Cushing disease)*, followed by primary adrenal neoplasms *(ACTH-independent hypercortisolism)* and paraneoplastic ACTH production by tumors (e.g., small-cell lung cancer).
- The morphologic features in the adrenal include bilateral cortical atrophy (in exogenous steroid-induced disease), bilateral diffuse or nodular hyperplasia (most common finding in endogenous Cushing syndrome), or an adrenocortical neoplasm.

Hyperaldosteronism

Hyperaldosteronism is the generic term for a group of closely related conditions characterized by chronic excess aldosterone secretion. Hyperaldosteronism may be primary, or it may be secondary to an extraadrenal cause.

Primary hyperaldosteronism refers to autonomous overproduction of aldosterone with resultant suppression of the renin-angiotensin system and decreased plasma renin activity. The causes of primary hyperaldosteronism are as follows (Fig. 20.39):

- *Bilateral idiopathic hyperaldosteronism*, characterized by bilateral nodular hyperplasia of the adrenal glands. This is the most common underlying cause of primary hyperaldosteronism, accounting for about 60% of cases. The pathogenesis of idiopathic hyperaldosteronism is unclear, although a subset harbors germ line mutations in the *KCNJ5* gene, which encodes a potassium channel protein that is expressed in the adrenal gland.
- *Adrenocortical neoplasm*, either an aldosterone-producing adenoma (the most common cause) or, rarely, an adrenocortical carcinoma. In approximately 35% of cases, primary hyperaldosteronism is caused by a solitary aldosterone-secreting adenoma, a condition referred to as *Conn syndrome*. Somatic mutations of *KCNJ5* (see earlier) are also present in a subset of aldosterone-secreting adenomas.
- Rarely, familial hyperaldosteronism may result from a genetic defect that leads to overactivity of the *aldosterone synthase gene, CYP11B2*.

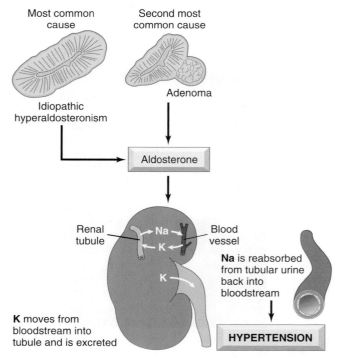

Fig. 20.39 The major causes of primary hyperaldosteronism and its principal effects on the kidney.

In *secondary hyperaldosteronism,* aldosterone release occurs in response to activation of the renin-angiotensin system. This condition is characterized by *increased levels of plasma renin* and is encountered in association with the following:

- Decreased renal perfusion (arteriolar nephrosclerosis, renal artery stenosis)
- Arterial hypovolemia and edema (congestive heart failure, cirrhosis, nephrotic syndrome)
- Pregnancy (caused by estrogen-induced increases in plasma renin substrate)

MORPHOLOGY

Aldosterone-producing adenomas are almost always solitary, small (<2 cm in diameter), well-circumscribed lesions. They are bright yellow on cut section and, surprisingly, are composed of lipid-laden cortical cells more closely resembling fasciculata cells than glomerulosa cells (the normal source of aldosterone). In general, the cells tend to be uniform in size and shape; occasionally there is some nuclear and cellular pleomorphism. A characteristic feature of aldosterone-producing adenomas is the presence of eosinophilic, laminated cytoplasmic inclusions, known as **spironolactone bodies.** These typically are found after treatment with the anti-hypertensive agent spironolactone, which is the drug of choice in primary hyperaldosteronism. In contrast with cortical adenomas associated with Cushing syndrome, those associated with hyperaldosteronism do not usually suppress ACTH secretion. Therefore, the adjacent adrenal cortex and that of the contralateral gland are not atrophic. **Bilateral idiopathic hyperplasia** is marked by diffuse or focal hyperplasia of cells resembling those of the normal zona glomerulosa.

Clinical Features

The most important clinical consequence of hyperaldosteronism is hypertension. With an estimated prevalence rate of 5% to 10% among unselected hypertensive patients, primary hyperaldosteronism may be the most common cause of secondary hypertension (i.e., hypertension secondary to an identifiable cause). The long-term effects of hyperaldosteronism-induced hypertension are cardiovascular compromise (e.g., left ventricular hypertrophy and reduced diastolic volumes) and an increase in the prevalence of adverse events such as stroke and myocardial infarction. *Hypokalemia* results from renal potassium wasting and, when present, can cause a variety of neuromuscular manifestations, including weakness, paresthesias, visual disturbances, and occasionally frank tetany. Hypokalemia was considered a mandatory feature of primary hyperaldosteronism, but almost 50% of normokalemic patients are now being diagnosed largely due to early detection.

In primary hyperaldosteronism, the therapy varies according to cause. Adenomas are amenable to surgical excision. By contrast, surgical intervention is not very beneficial in patients with primary hyperaldosteronism due to bilateral hyperplasia, which often occurs in children and young adults. These patients are best managed medically with an *aldosterone antagonist* such as spironolactone. The treatment of secondary hyperaldosteronism rests on correcting the underlying cause of the renin-angiotensin system hyperstimulation.

Adrenogenital Syndromes

Adrenogenital syndromes refer to a group of disorders caused by androgen excess, which may stem from a number of etiologies, including primary gonadal disorders and several primary adrenal disorders. The adrenal cortex secretes two compounds—dehydroepiandrosterone and androstenedione—which require conversion to testosterone in peripheral tissues for their androgenic effects. Unlike gonadal androgens, adrenal androgen formation is regulated by ACTH; thus, excessive secretion can present as an isolated syndrome or in combination with features of Cushing disease. The adrenal causes of androgen excess include *adrenocortical neoplasms* and an uncommon group of disorders collectively designated *congenital adrenal hyperplasia (CAH).* Adrenocortical neoplasms associated with symptoms of androgen excess *(virilization)* are more likely to be carcinomas than adenomas. They are morphologically identical to other functional or nonfunctional cortical neoplasms.

CAH represents a group of autosomal recessive disorders, each characterized by a hereditary defect in an enzyme involved in adrenal steroid biosynthesis, particularly cortisol. In these conditions, decreased cortisol production results in a compensatory increase in ACTH secretion due to absence of feedback inhibition. The resultant adrenal hyperplasia causes increased production of cortisol precursor steroids, which are then channeled into synthesis of androgens with virilizing activity. Certain enzyme defects also may impair aldosterone secretion, adding salt loss to the virilizing syndrome. *The most common enzymatic defect in CAH is 21-hydroxylase deficiency,* which accounts for more than 90% of cases. 21-hydroxylase deficiency may range in degree from a total lack to a mild loss, depending on the nature of the underlying mutation. In the adrenal glands cortisol, aldosterone and sex steroids are synthesized from cholesterol through various intermediates. 21-hydroxylase is required for synthesis of cortisol and aldosterone but not sex steroids. Thus, a deficiency of this enzyme reduces cortisol and aldosterone synthesis and shunts the common precursors into the sex steroid pathway.

MORPHOLOGY

In all cases of CAH, the adrenals are **hyperplastic bilaterally,** sometimes expanding to 10 to 15 times their normal weights. The adrenal cortex is thickened and nodular, and on cut section, the widened cortex appears brown as a result of depletion of lipid. The proliferating cells mostly are compact, eosinophilic cells intermixed with lipid-laden clear cells. Hyperplasia of corticotroph (ACTH-producing) cells is present in the anterior pituitary in most patients.

Clinical Features

The clinical manifestations of CAH are determined by the specific enzyme deficiency and include abnormalities related to androgen excess, with or without aldosterone and glucocorticoid deficiency. Depending on the nature and severity of the enzymatic defect, the onset of clinical symptoms may occur in the perinatal period, later childhood, or (less commonly) adulthood.

In 21-hydroxylase deficiency, excessive androgenic activity causes signs of masculinization in females, ranging from clitoral hypertrophy and pseudohermaphroditism in infants to oligomenorrhea, hirsutism, and acne in postpubertal girls. In males, androgen excess is associated with enlargement of the external genitalia and other evidence of precocious puberty in young patients. Most men with CAH are fertile but some have failure of Leydig cell development and oligospermia. In approximately one-third of individuals with 21-hydroxylase deficiency, the enzymatic defect is severe enough to produce aldosterone deficiency, with resultant salt (sodium) wasting. Concomitant cortisol deficiency places individuals with CAH at risk for acute adrenal insufficiency (discussed later).

CAH should be suspected in any neonate with ambiguous genitalia. Severe enzyme deficiency in infancy can be a life-threatening condition, with vomiting, dehydration, and salt wasting. In the milder variants, women may present with delayed menarche, oligomenorrhea, or hirsutism. In all cases, an androgen-producing ovarian neoplasm must be excluded. Treatment of CAH is with exogenous glucocorticoids, which, in addition to providing adequate levels of glucocorticoids, also suppress ACTH levels, thereby decreasing the excessive synthesis of the steroid hormones responsible for many of the clinical abnormalities. Mineralocorticoid supplementation is required in the salt-wasting variants of CAH.

SUMMARY

ADRENOGENITAL SYNDROMES

- The adrenal cortex can secrete excess androgens in either of two settings: adrenocortical neoplasms (usually *virilizing* carcinomas) or congenital adrenal hyperplasia (CAH).
- CAH consists of a group of autosomal recessive disorders characterized by defects in steroid biosynthesis, usually cortisol; the most common subtype is caused by deficiency of the enzyme 21-hydroxylase.
- Reduction in cortisol production causes a compensatory increase in ACTH secretion, which in turn stimulates androgen production. Androgens have virilizing effects, including masculinization in females (ambiguous genitalia, oligomenorrhea, hirsutism), precocious puberty in males, and, in some instances, salt (sodium) wasting and hypotension.
- Bilateral hyperplasia of the adrenal cortex is characteristic.

ADRENAL INSUFFICIENCY

Adrenocortical insufficiency, or hypofunction, may be caused by either primary adrenal disease (primary hypoadrenalism) or decreased stimulation of the adrenals resulting from ACTH deficiency (secondary hypoadrenalism). Primary adrenocortical insufficiency may be *acute* (called *adrenal crisis*), or *chronic (Addison disease)*.

Table 20.7 Causes of Adrenal Insufficiency

Acute
Waterhouse-Friderichsen syndrome
Sudden withdrawal of long-term corticosteroid therapy
Stress in patients with underlying chronic adrenal insufficiency

Chronic
Autoimmune adrenalitis (60%–70% of cases in developed countries)—includes APS1 (*AIRE* mutations) and APS2 (polygenic)

Infections
    Tuberculosis
    Acquired immunodeficiency syndrome
    Fungal infections

Hemochromatosis
Sarcoidosis
Systemic amyloidosis
Metastatic disease

APS1, APS2, Autoimmune polyendocrine syndrome types 1 and 2; *AIRE,* autoimmune regulator gene.

Acute Adrenocortical Insufficiency

Acute adrenocortical insufficiency occurs most commonly in the clinical settings listed in Table 20.7. Individuals with chronic adrenocortical insufficiency may develop an acute crisis after any stress that taxes their limited physiologic reserves. In patients maintained on exogenous corticosteroids, rapid withdrawal of steroids or failure to increase steroid doses in response to an acute stress may precipitate a similar adrenal crisis, because of the inability of the atrophic adrenals to produce glucocorticoid hormones. *Massive adrenal hemorrhage* may destroy enough of the adrenal cortex to cause acute adrenocortical insufficiency. This condition may occur in patients maintained on anti-coagulant therapy, in postoperative patients who develop disseminated intravascular coagulation, during pregnancy, and in patients suffering from overwhelming sepsis; in the latter setting, it is known as the *Waterhouse-Friderichsen syndrome* (Fig. 20.40). This catastrophic syndrome is classically associated with *Neisseria meningitidis* septicemia but can also be caused by other organisms. Waterhouse-Friderichsen syndrome can occur at any age but is somewhat more common in children. The basis for the adrenal hemorrhage is uncertain but may be attributable to direct bacterial seeding of small vessels in the adrenal, the development of disseminated intravascular coagulation (Chapter 4), endotoxin-induced vasculitis, or some form of hypersensitivity vasculitis.

Chronic Adrenocortical Insufficiency: Addison Disease

Addison disease, or chronic adrenocortical insufficiency, is an uncommon disorder resulting from progressive destruction of the adrenal cortex. More than 90% of all cases are attributable to one of four disorders: *autoimmune adrenalitis, tuberculosis,* the *acquired immune deficiency syndrome* (AIDS), or *metastatic cancer* (see Table 20.7).

- *Autoimmune adrenalitis* accounts for 60% to 70% of cases and is by far the most common cause of primary adrenal insufficiency in countries where infectious causes are

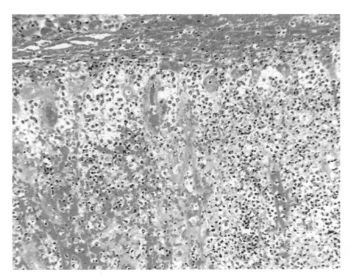

Fig. 20.40 Waterhouse-Friderichsen syndrome. Bilateral adrenal hemorrhage in an infant with overwhelming sepsis, resulting in acute adrenal insufficiency. At autopsy, the adrenal glands were grossly hemorrhagic and shrunken; in this photomicrograph, little residual cortical architecture is discernible.

uncommon. As the name implies, there is autoimmune destruction of steroid-producing cells, and autoantibodies to several key steroidogenic enzymes have been detected in affected patients. Autoimmune adrenalitis may occur in association with several distinct *auto-immune polyendocrine syndromes (APS)*. The best characterized of these is APS1, which is caused by mutations in the *autoimmune regulator (AIRE)* gene on chromosome 21. It is characterized by mucocutaneous candidiasis and abnormalities of skin, dental enamel, and nails (ectodermal dystrophy) occurring in association with a combination of organ-specific autoimmune disorders that result in destruction of target organs. The AIRE protein is involved in the expression of tissue antigens in the thymus and the elimination of T cells specific for these antigens (Chapter 5). Individuals with APS1 develop autoantibodies against IL-17 and IL-22, which are the principal effector cytokines secreted by T_H17 T cells (Chapter 5). Because these two T_H17-derived cytokines are crucial for defense against fungal infections, affected patients develop chronic mucocutaneous candidiasis.

- *Infections,* particularly tuberculosis and those produced by fungi, also may cause primary chronic adrenocortical insufficiency. Tuberculous adrenalitis, which once accounted for as many as 90% of cases of Addison disease, has become less common with improved anti-tuberculosis therapy. With the resurgence of tuberculosis mainly because of HIV infection and immunodeficiency, this cause of adrenal deficiency must be borne in mind. When present, tuberculous adrenalitis usually is associated with active infection in other sites, particularly the lungs and genitourinary tract. Among fungi, disseminated infections caused by *Histoplasma capsulatum* and *Coccidioides immitis* also may result in chronic adrenocortical insufficiency. Patients with AIDS are at risk for the development of adrenal insufficiency

from several other infectious (cytomegalovirus, *Mycobacterium avium-intracellulare*) and noninfectious (Kaposi sarcoma) complications of their disease.
- *Metastatic neoplasms* involving the adrenals are another potential cause of adrenal insufficiency. The adrenals are a fairly common site for metastases in patients with disseminated carcinomas, which sometimes destroy sufficient adrenal cortex to produce a degree of adrenal insufficiency. Carcinomas of the lung and breast are the source of a majority of metastases in the adrenals.

Secondary Adrenocortical Insufficiency

Any disorder of the hypothalamus and pituitary that reduces the output of ACTH, such as metastatic cancer, infection, infarction, or irradiation, leads to a syndrome of hypoadrenalism having many similarities to Addison disease. ACTH deficiency may occur alone, but in some instances, it is only one part of panhypopituitarism, associated with multiple pituitary hormone deficiencies. In patients with primary disease, the destruction of the adrenal cortex prevents a response to exogenously administered ACTH in the form of increased plasma levels of cortisol. By contrast, secondary adrenocortical insufficiency is characterized by low serum ACTH and a prompt rise in plasma cortisol levels in response to ACTH administration.

MORPHOLOGY

The appearance of the adrenal glands varies with the cause of the adrenocortical insufficiency. In **secondary hypoadrenalism,** the adrenals are reduced to small, flattened structures that usually retain their yellow color because of a small amount of residual lipid. A uniform, thin rim of atrophic yellow cortex surrounds a central, intact medulla. Histologic evaluation reveals atrophy of cortical cells with loss of cytoplasmic lipid, particularly in the zona fasciculata and zona reticularis. **Primary autoimmune adrenalitis** is characterized by irregularly shrunken glands, which may be exceedingly difficult to identify within the suprarenal adipose tissue. On histologic examination, the cortex contains only scattered residual cortical cells in a collapsed network of connective tissue. A variable lymphoid infiltrate is present in the cortex and may extend into the subjacent medulla (Fig. 20.41). The medulla is otherwise preserved. In **tuberculosis or fungal diseases,** the adrenal architecture may be effaced by a granulomatous inflammatory reaction identical to that encountered in other sites of infection. When hypoadrenalism is caused by **metastatic carcinoma,** the adrenals are enlarged, and their normal architecture is obscured by the infiltrating neoplasm.

Clinical Features

In general, clinical manifestations of adrenocortical insufficiency do not appear until at least 90% of the adrenal cortex has been compromised. The initial manifestations often include progressive weakness and easy fatigability, which may be dismissed as nonspecific complaints. *Gastrointestinal disturbances* are common and include anorexia, nausea, vomiting, weight loss, and diarrhea. In patients

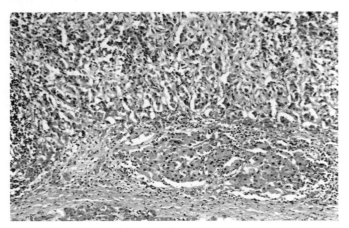

Fig. 20.41 Autoimmune adrenalitis. In addition to loss of all but a subcapsular rim of cortical cells, there is an extensive mononuclear cell infiltrate.

with primary adrenal disease, increased levels of ACTH precursor hormone stimulate melanocytes, with resultant *hyperpigmentation* of the skin and mucosal surfaces. The face, axillae, nipples, areolae, and perineum are particularly common sites of hyperpigmentation. By contrast, hyperpigmentation is not seen in patients with secondary adrenocortical insufficiency because melanotropic hormone levels are not increased. Decreased mineralocorticoid (aldosterone) activity in patients with primary adrenal insufficiency results in potassium retention and sodium loss, with consequent *hyperkalemia, hyponatremia, volume depletion,* and *hypotension,* whereas secondary hypoadrenalism is characterized by deficient cortisol and androgen output but normal or near-normal aldosterone synthesis. Hypoglycemia occasionally may occur as a result of glucocorticoid deficiency and impaired gluconeogenesis. It is more common in infants and children than adults. Stresses such as infections, trauma, or surgical procedures in affected patients may precipitate an acute adrenal crisis, manifested by intractable vomiting, abdominal pain, hypotension, coma, and vascular collapse. Death follows rapidly unless corticosteroids are replaced immediately.

SUMMARY

ADRENOCORTICAL INSUFFICIENCY (HYPOADRENALISM)

- Primary adrenocortical insufficiency can be acute (Waterhouse-Friderichsen syndrome) or chronic (Addison disease).
- Chronic adrenal insufficiency in the Western world most often is secondary to autoimmune adrenalitis, which occurs in the context of autoimmune polyendocrine syndromes.
- Tuberculosis and infections due to opportunistic pathogens associated with the human immunodeficiency virus and tumors metastatic to the adrenals are the other important causes of chronic hypoadrenalism.
- Patients typically present with fatigue, weakness, and gastrointestinal disturbances. Primary adrenocortical insufficiency also is characterized by high ACTH levels with associated skin pigmentation.

ADRENOCORTICAL NEOPLASMS

It should be evident from the discussion of adrenocortical hyperfunction that functional adrenal neoplasms may be responsible for any of the various forms of hyperadrenalism. **While functional adenomas are most commonly associated with hyperaldosteronism and with Cushing syndrome, a virilizing neoplasm is more likely to be a carcinoma**. Not all adrenocortical neoplasms, however, elaborate steroid hormones. Determination of whether a cortical neoplasm is functional or not is based on clinical evaluation and measurement of the hormone or its metabolites in the laboratory.

MORPHOLOGY

Adrenocortical adenomas were described earlier in the discussions of Cushing syndrome and hyperaldosteronism. Most cortical adenomas do not cause hyperfunction and usually are encountered as incidental findings at the time of autopsy or during abdominal imaging for an unrelated cause. In fact, the half-facetious appellation of **"adrenal incidentaloma"** has crept into the medical lexicon to describe these incidentally discovered tumors. On cut surface, adenomas usually are yellow to yellow-brown, owing to the presence of lipid within the neoplastic cells (see Fig. 20.37). As a general rule they are small, averaging 1 to 2 cm in diameter. On microscopic examination, adenomas are composed of cells similar to those populating the normal adrenal cortex. As with other endocrine tumors, pleomorphism may be encountered in benign tumors and is not a reliable marker of malignancy.

Adrenocortical carcinomas are rare neoplasms that may occur at any age, including in childhood. Two rare inherited causes of adrenal cortical carcinomas are Li-Fraumeni syndrome (Chapter 6) and Beckwith-Wiedemann syndrome (Chapter 7). In most cases, adrenocortical carcinomas are large, invasive lesions that efface the native adrenal gland. On cut surface, adrenocortical carcinomas typically are variegated, poorly demarcated lesions containing areas of necrosis, hemorrhage, and cystic change (Fig. 20.42). Microscopic examination typically shows these tumors

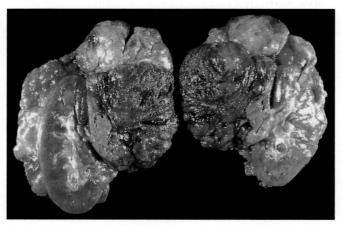

Fig. 20.42 Adrenal carcinoma. The tumor dwarfs the kidney and compresses the upper pole. It is largely hemorrhagic and necrotic.

to be composed of well-differentiated cells resembling those seen in cortical adenomas or bizarre, pleomorphic cells, which may be difficult to distinguish from those of an undifferentiated carcinoma metastatic to the adrenal gland (Fig. 20.43). Adrenal cancers have a strong tendency to invade the adrenal vein, vena cava, and lymphatics. Metastases to regional and periaortic nodes are common, as is distant hematogenous spread to the lungs and other viscera. Bone metastases are unusual. The median patient survival is about 2 years. Of note, **carcinomas metastatic to the adrenal cortex are significantly more frequent than a primary adrenocortical carcinoma.**

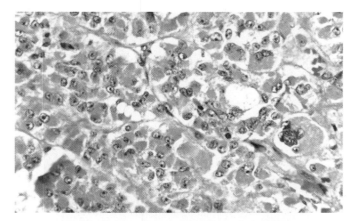

Fig. 20.43 Adrenal carcinoma with marked anaplasia.

Adrenal Medulla

The adrenal medulla is embryologically, functionally, and structurally distinct from the adrenal cortex. It is populated by cells derived from the neural crest (chromaffin cells) and their supporting (sustentacular) cells. The *chromaffin cells* are so named because of their brown-black color after exposure to potassium dichromate. They synthesize and secrete catecholamines in response to signals from preganglionic nerve fibers in the sympathetic nervous system. Similar collections of cells are distributed throughout the body in the extraadrenal paraganglion system. The most important diseases of the adrenal medulla are neoplasms, which include both neuronal neoplasms (including neuroblastomas and more mature ganglion cell tumors) and neoplasms composed of chromaffin cells (pheochromocytomas).

TUMORS OF THE ADRENAL MEDULLA

Pheochromocytoma

Pheochromocytomas are neoplasms composed of chromaffin cells, which, like their nonneoplastic counterparts, synthesize and release catecholamines and, in some cases, other peptide hormones. These tumors are of special importance because, although uncommon, they (like aldosterone-secreting adenomas) give rise to a surgically correctable form of hypertension.

Pheochromocytomas usually subscribe to a convenient "rule of 10s":

- *10% of pheochromocytomas are extraadrenal,* occurring in sites such as the organ of Zuckerkandl and the carotid body, where they usually are called *paragangliomas,* rather than pheochromocytomas.
- *10% of adrenal pheochromocytomas are bilateral;* this proportion may rise to 50% in cases that are associated with familial syndromes.
- *10% of adrenal pheochromocytomas are malignant,* although the associated hypertension represents a serious and potentially lethal complication of even benign tumors.

Frank malignancy is somewhat more common in tumors arising in extraadrenal sites.

- *10% of adrenal pheochromocytomas are not associated with hypertension.* Of the 90% that present with hypertension, approximately two-thirds have "paroxysmal" episodes associated with sudden rise in blood pressure and palpitations, which can, on occasion, be fatal.

One "traditional" 10% rule that has since been modified pertains to familial cases. It is now recognized that *as many as 25% of individuals with pheochromocytomas and paragangliomas harbor a germ line mutation* in one of at least six known genes, including *RET*, which causes type 2 MEN syndromes (described later); NF1, which causes type 1 neurofibromatosis (Chapter 22); VHL, which causes von Hippel-Lindau disease (Chapters 14 and 23); and three genes encoding subunits within the succinate dehydrogenase complex (*SDHB, SDHC,* and *SDHD*), which is involved in mitochondrial electron transport and oxygen sensing. It is postulated that loss of function in one or more of these subunits leads to stabilization of the transcription factor hypoxia-inducible factor 1α (HIF-1α), promoting tumorigenesis.

MORPHOLOGY

Pheochromocytomas range in size from small, circumscribed lesions confined to the adrenal to large, hemorrhagic masses weighing several kilograms. On cut surface, smaller pheochromocytomas are yellow-tan, well-defined lesions that compress the adjacent adrenal gland (Fig. 20.44). Larger lesions tend to be hemorrhagic, necrotic, and cystic and typically efface the adrenal gland. Incubation of the fresh tissue with potassium dichromate solutions turns the tumor dark brown, as noted earlier.

On microscopic examination, pheochromocytomas are composed of polygonal to spindle-shaped chromaffin cells and their supporting cells, compartmentalized into small nests, by a rich vascular network (Fig. 20.45). The cytoplasm of the neoplastic cells often has a finely granular appearance, highlighted by a

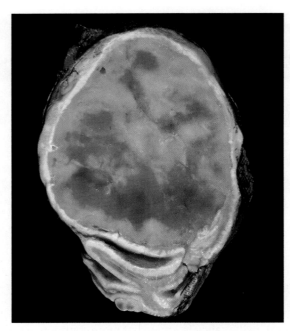

Fig. 20.44 Pheochromocytoma. The tumor is enclosed within an attenuated cortex and demonstrates areas of hemorrhage. The comma-shaped residual adrenal gland is seen *(lower portion)*.

variety of silver stains, because of the presence of granules containing catecholamines. Electron microscopy reveals variable numbers of membrane-bound, electron-dense granules, representing catecholamines and sometimes other peptides. The nuclei of the neoplastic cells are often quite pleomorphic. Both capsular and vascular invasion, as well as cellular pleomorphism, may be encountered in some benign lesions. **Therefore, the definitive diagnosis of malignancy in pheochromocytomas is based on the presence of metastases.** These may involve regional lymph nodes as well as more distant sites, including liver, lung, and bone.

Clinical Features

The dominant clinical manifestation of pheochromocytoma is hypertension, observed in 90% of patients. Approximately two-thirds of patients with hypertension demonstrate paroxysmal episodes, which are described as an abrupt, precipitous elevation in blood pressure, associated with tachycardia, palpitations, headache, sweating, tremor, and a sense of apprehension. These episodes may also be associated with pain in the abdomen or chest, nausea, and vomiting. Isolated paroxysmal episodes of hypertension occur in fewer than half of patients; more commonly, patients demonstrate a chronic, sustained elevation in blood pressure punctuated by the aforementioned paroxysms. The elevations of blood pressure are induced by the sudden release of catecholamines that may acutely precipitate congestive heart failure, pulmonary edema, myocardial infarction, ventricular fibrillation, and cerebrovascular accidents. The cardiac complications have been attributed to what has been called *catecholamine cardiomyopathy*, or *catecholamine-induced myocardial instability and ventricular arrhythmias*. In some cases, pheochromocytomas secrete other hormones such as ACTH and somatostatin and may therefore be associated with clinical features related to the effects of these and other peptide hormones. The laboratory diagnosis is based on demonstration of increased urinary excretion of free catecholamines and their metabolites, such as vanillylmandelic acid and metanephrines. Isolated benign pheochromocytomas are treated with surgical excision. With multifocal lesions, long-term medical treatment for hypertension may be required.

Neuroblastoma and Other Neuronal Neoplasms

Neuroblastoma is the most common extracranial solid tumor of childhood. These neoplasms occur most commonly during the first 5 years of life and may arise during infancy. Neuroblastomas may occur anywhere in the sympathetic nervous system and occasionally within the brain, but they are most common in the abdomen; a majority of these tumors arise in either the adrenal medulla or the retroperitoneal sympathetic ganglia. Most neuroblastomas are sporadic, although familial cases also have been described. These tumors are discussed in Chapter 7, along with other pediatric neoplasms.

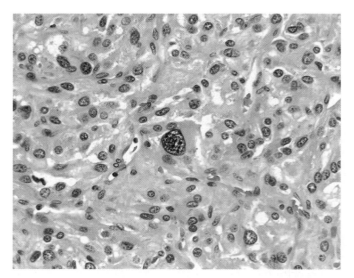

Fig. 20.45 Photomicrograph of pheochromocytoma, demonstrating characteristic nests of cells with abundant cytoplasm. Granules containing catecholamine are not visible in this preparation. It is not uncommon to find bizarre cells (such as the one in the center of this image), even in pheochromocytomas that are benign.

Multiple Endocrine Neoplasia (MEN) Syndromes

The MEN syndromes are a group of inherited diseases caused by proliferative lesions (hyperplasias, adenomas, and carcinomas) of multiple endocrine organs. Like other inherited cancer disorders (Chapter 6), endocrine tumors arising in the context of MEN syndromes have certain distinctive features that are not shared with their sporadic counterparts:

- These tumors occur at a younger age than that typical for sporadic cancers.
- They arise in multiple endocrine organs, either synchronously (at the same time) or metachronously (at different times).
- Even in one organ, the tumors often are multifocal.
- The tumors usually are preceded by an asymptomatic stage of endocrine hyperplasia involving the cell of origin of the tumor (e.g., patients with MEN-2 almost universally demonstrate C cell hyperplasia in the thyroid parenchyma adjacent to medullary thyroid carcinomas).
- These tumors are usually more aggressive and recur in a higher proportion of cases than similar endocrine tumors that occur sporadically.

MULTIPLE ENDOCRINE NEOPLASIA TYPE 1

MEN-1 syndrome is caused by germ line mutations in the *MEN1* tumor suppressor gene, which encodes a protein called Menin. Menin is a component of several different transcription factor complexes, and loss of Menin function leads to deregulation of the corresponding binding partners, promoting endocrine neoplasia. Organs most commonly involved are the parathyroid, the pancreas, and the pituitary—the "3 Ps."

- *Parathyroid. Primary hyperparathyroidism* is the most common manifestation of MEN-1 (80%–95% of patients) and is the initial manifestation of the disorder in most patients, appearing in almost all by 40 to 50 years of age. Parathyroid abnormalities include hyperplasia and adenomas.
- *Pancreas.* Endocrine tumors of the pancreas are the leading cause of death in MEN-1. These tumors usually are aggressive and present with metastatic disease. Pancreatic endocrine tumors often are functional (i.e., secrete hormones). Zollinger-Ellison syndrome, associated with gastrinomas, and hypoglycemia, associated with insulinomas, are common endocrine manifestations.
- *Pituitary.* The most frequent pituitary tumor in patients with MEN-1 syndrome is a prolactin-secreting macroadenoma. In some cases, acromegaly develops in association with somatotropin-secreting tumors.

MULTIPLE ENDOCRINE NEOPLASIA TYPE 2

MEN-2 syndrome actually comprises two distinct groups of disorders that are unified by the occurrence of activating (i.e., gain-of-function) mutations of the *RET* proto-oncogene at chromosomal locus 10q11.2. A strong genotype-phenotype correlation has been recognized for the MEN-2 syndromes, and differences in mutation patterns account for the variable features in the two subtypes. MEN-2 is inherited in an autosomal dominant pattern.

Multiple Endocrine Neoplasia Type 2A

Organs commonly involved in MEN-2A include the following:

- *Thyroid:* Medullary carcinoma of the thyroid develops in virtually all untreated cases, and the tumors usually occur in the first 2 decades of life. The tumors commonly are multifocal, and foci of C cell hyperplasia can be found in the adjacent thyroid. *Familial medullary thyroid cancer* is seen in a variant of MEN-2A, without the other characteristic manifestations listed here. In comparison with MEN-2, familial medullary carcinoma typically occurs at an older age and follows a more indolent course.
- *Adrenal medulla:* Adrenal pheochromocytomas develop in 50% of the patients; fortunately, no more than 10% of these tumors are malignant.
- *Parathyroid:* Approximately 10% to 20% of patients develop parathyroid gland hyperplasia with manifestations of primary hyperparathyroidism.

Multiple Endocrine Neoplasia Type 2B

A single amino acid change in RET, distinct from the mutations that are seen in MEN-2A, seems to be responsible for virtually all cases of MEN-2B. Patients develop medullary thyroid carcinomas, which are usually multifocal and more aggressive than in MEN-2A, and pheochromocytomas. MEN-2B has the following distinctive features:

- *Primary hyperparathyroidism does not develop* in patients with MEN-2B.
- *Extraendocrine manifestations* are characteristic in patients with MEN-2B. These include ganglioneuromas of mucosal sites (gastrointestinal tract, lips, tongue) and a *marfanoid habitus,* in which overly long bones of the axial skeleton give an appearance resembling that in Marfan syndrome (Chapter 7).

Before the advent of genetic testing, relatives of patients with the MEN-2 syndrome were screened with annual biochemical tests, which often lacked sensitivity. Now, routine genetic testing identifies *RET* mutation carriers earlier and more reliably in MEN-2 kindreds. All individuals carrying germ line RET mutations are advised to have prophylactic thyroidectomy to prevent the inevitable development of medullary carcinomas.

SUGGESTED READINGS

Andersen DK, Andren-Sandberg A, Duell EJ, et al: Pancreatitis-diabetes-pancreatic cancer: summary of a NCI-NIDDK workshop, *Pancreas* 42:1227–1237, 2013. [*This workshop summary discusses the complex relationship between diabetes and pancreatic cancer, as well as the recent emergence of the entity known as type 3c or pancreatogenic diabetes. One of the causes of type 3c diabetes is pancreatic cancer.]*

Asa SL, Ezzat S: Genomic approaches to problems in pituitary neoplasia, *Endocr Pathol* 25:209–213, 2014. *[A review on genomics of pituitary neoplasia from two of the best recognized authorities on these tumors.]*

Bancos I, Hahner S, Tomlinson J, et al: Diagnosis and management of adrenal insufficiency, *Lancet Diabetes Endocrinol* 3:216–226, 2015. *[A clinically oriented review on the etiology of acute and chronic adrenal insufficiency.]*

Bilezikian JP, Cusano NE, Khan AA, et al: Primary hyperparathyroidism, *Nat Rev Dis Primers* 2:16033, 2016. *[This review follows the format of other reviews in this journal that is heavy on summary figures and overviews written for a broad audience. The reader is encouraged to periodically browse the journal for discussions of other pertinent diseases.]*

Burman KD, Wartofsky L: Clinical practice. Thyroid nodules, *N Engl J Med* 373:2347–2356, 2015. *[An authoritative review on etiology and management of thyroid nodules. Useful supplement to the chapter discussion.]*

DeFronzo RA, Ferrannini E, Groop L, et al: Type 2 diabetes mellitus, *Nat Rev Dis Primers* 1:15019, 2015. *[An excellent overview of type 2 diabetes, again with overview figures on pathophysiology and complications. The level of discussion is beyond the scope of the chapter, so readers can use this review to supplement their knowledge.]*

De Leo S, Lee SY, Braverman LE: Hyperthyroidism, *Lancet* 388:906–918, 2016. *[An excellent and clinically oriented recent review on etiology of hyperthyroidism, including common and uncommon causes.]*

Dralle H, Machens A, Basa J, et al: Follicular cell-derived thyroid cancer, *Nat Rev Dis Primers* 1:15077, 2015. *[A timely review of thyroid cancers, including follicular and papillary neoplasms. As with reviews in this journal, the text spans genetics, symptoms, diagnosis, and management and can be a very useful supplement to the text for the curious reader.]*

Faillot S, Assie G: Endocrine tumors: the genomics of adrenocortical tumors, *Eur J Endocrinol* 174:R249–R265, 2016. *[In contrast to the TCGA paper below that is focused on adrenocortical cancers, this review also encompasses genetics of other adrenal pathologies, including adenomas and primary hyperplasia.]*

Higham CE, Johannsson G, Shalet SM: Hypopituitarism, *Lancet* 388:2403–2415, 2016. *[A current review on hypopituitarism including etiology and management.]*

Lacroix A, Feelders RA, Stratakis CA, et al: Cushing's syndrome, *Lancet* 386:913–927, 2015. *[A definitive review on Cushing syndrome, including genetics, pathophysiology, laboratory diagnosis, symptoms, and management. The text is exhaustive and can be used by the discerning for supplementing the text.]*

Nikiforov YE, Seethala RR, Tallini G, et al: Nomenclature revision for encapsulated follicular variant of papillary thyroid carcinoma: a paradigm shift to reduce overtreatment of indolent tumors, *JAMA Oncol* 2:1023–1029, 2016. *[The defining paper that led to changing the nomenclature for the erstwhile entity known as encapsulated follicular variant of papillary thyroid carcinoma. This paper is also important to understand the concept of "overdiagnosis," which is increasingly becoming a factor due to increasing use of imaging modalities in patients.]*

Pociot F, Lernmark A: Genetic risk factors for type 1 diabetes, *Lancet* 387:2331–2339, 2016. *[A recent review on the complex genetics of type 1 diabetes, especially the HLA alleles, and how these might interface with the environment.]*

Tuomi T, Santoro N, Caprio S, et al: The many faces of diabetes: a disease with increasing heterogeneity, *Lancet* 383:1084–1094, 2014. *[An excellent review underscoring the etiologic heterogeneity of the entity that we know as "diabetes" — and how so many diverse genetic and environmental factors contribute to the phenotype of hyperglycemia.]*

Zheng S, Cherniack AD, Dewal N, et al: Comprehensive pan-genomic characterization of adrenocortical carcinoma, *Cancer Cell* 29:723–736, 2016. *[The definitive study from The Cancer Genome Atlas (TCGA) on genomics of adrenocortical cancers.]*

Bones, Joints, and Soft Tissue Tumors

21

CHAPTER OUTLINE

Bone 797
**Basic Structure and Function of
    Bone 797**
Matrix 797
Cells 797
Development 798
Homeostasis and Remodeling 799
**Congenital Disorders of Bone and
    Cartilage 799**
Achondroplasia 800
Thanatophoric Dysplasia 800
*Type I Collagen Diseases (Osteogenesis
    Imperfecta) 800*
Osteopetrosis 800
Metabolic Disorders of Bone 801
Osteopenia and Osteoporosis 801
Rickets and Osteomalacia 802
Hyperparathyroidism 802
**Paget Disease of Bone (Osteitis
    Deformans) 803**

Fractures 805
Healing of Fractures 805
Osteonecrosis (Avascular Necrosis) 806
Osteomyelitis 806
Pyogenic Osteomyelitis 806
Mycobacterial Osteomyelitis 807
Bone Tumors and Tumorlike Lesions 808
Bone-Forming Tumors 808
Cartilage-Forming Tumors 810
Tumors of Unknown Origin 812
Lesions Simulating Primary Neoplasms 814
Metastatic Tumors 816
Joints 817
Arthritis 817
Osteoarthritis 817
Rheumatoid Arthritis 818
Juvenile Idiopathic Arthritis 821
Seronegative Spondyloarthropathies 822
Infectious Arthritis 822
Lyme Arthritis 822

Crystal-Induced Arthritis 823
**Joint Tumors and Tumorlike
    Conditions 826**
Ganglion and Synovial Cysts 826
Tenosynovial Giant Cell Tumor 826
Soft Tissue Tumors 827
Tumors of Adipose Tissue 828
Lipoma 828
Liposarcoma 828
Fibrous Tumors 828
Nodular Fasciitis 828
Fibromatoses 828
Skeletal Muscle Tumors 830
Rhabdomyosarcoma 830
Smooth Muscle Tumors 830
Leiomyoma 830
Leiomyosarcoma 831
Tumors of Uncertain Origin 831
Synovial Sarcoma 831
Undifferentiated Pleomorphic Sarcoma 831

Bone

BASIC STRUCTURE AND FUNCTION OF BONE

The functions of bone include mechanical support, transmission of forces generated by muscles, protection of viscera, mineral homeostasis, and providing a niche for the production of blood cells. The constituents of bone include an extracellular matrix and specialized cells responsible for production and maintenance of the matrix.

Matrix

Bone matrix is composed of an organic component known as osteoid (35%) and a mineral component (65%). Embedded within the bone matrix are a variety of bone cells including osteocytes that lay down bone and osteoclasts that reabsorb bone. These two cells types maintain bone homeostasis. Osteoid is made up predominantly of type I collagen with smaller amounts of glycosaminoglycans and other proteins. The unique feature of bone matrix, its hardness, is imparted by the inorganic moiety hydroxyapatite ($Ca_{10}[PO_4]_6[OH]_2$). The bone matrix is synthesized in one of two histologic forms, woven or lamellar (Fig. 21.1). Woven bone is produced rapidly, such as during fetal development or fracture repair, but the haphazard arrangement of collagen fibers imparts less structural integrity than the parallel collagen fibers in slowly produced lamellar bone. In an adult, the presence of woven bone is always abnormal, but it is not specific for any particular bone disease. A cross section of a typical long bone shows a dense outer cortex and a central medulla composed of bony trabeculae separated by marrow.

Cells

Bone contains three major cell types:
* *Osteoblasts,* located on the surface of the matrix, synthesize, transport and assemble bone matrix and regulate

797

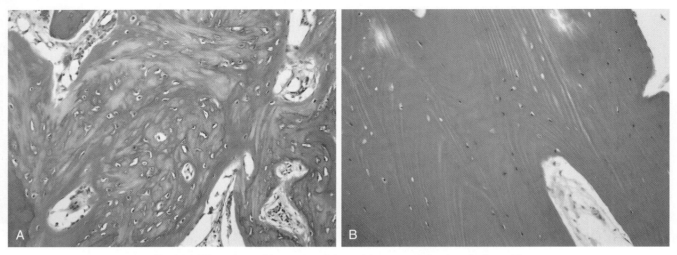

Fig. 21.1 Woven bone (A) is more cellular and disorganized than lamellar bone (B).

its mineralization (Fig. 21.2A). They are derived from mesenchymal stem cells that are located under the periosteum in the developing bone and additionally in the medullary space later in life.

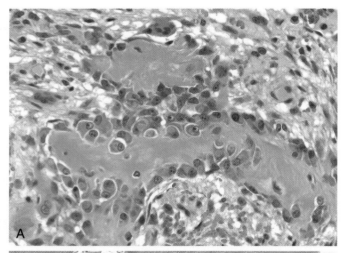

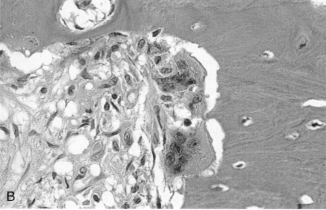

Fig. 21.2 (A) Active osteoblasts synthesizing bone matrix. The surrounding spindle cells represent osteoprogenitor cells. (B) Two osteoclasts resorbing bone.

- *Osteocytes*, located within the bone, are interconnected by an intricate network of cytoplasmic processes through tunnels known as canaliculi. Osteocytes help to control calcium and phosphate levels, detect mechanical forces, and translate them into biologic activity—a process called mechanotransduction.
- *Osteoclasts*, located on the surface of bone, are specialized multinucleated macrophages, derived from circulating monocytes, which are responsible for bone resorption (Fig. 21.2B). By means of cell surface integrins, osteoclasts attach to bone matrix and create a sealed extracellular trench (resorption pit). The cells secrete acid and neutral proteases (predominantly matrix metalloproteases [MMPs]) into the pit, and these enzymes resorb the bone.

Development

During embryogenesis, long bones develop from a cartilage mold by the process of endochondral ossification. A cartilage mold *(anlagen)* is synthesized by mesenchymal precursor cells. At approximately 8 weeks' gestation, the central portion of the anlagen is resorbed, creating the medullary canal. Simultaneously, at midshaft *(diaphysis)*, osteoblasts begin to deposit the cortex beneath the periosteum producing the *primary center of ossification* and growing the bone radially. At each longitudinal end *(epiphysis)*, endochondral ossification proceeds in a centrifugal fashion *(secondary center of ossification)*. Eventually, a plate of the cartilage becomes entrapped between the two expanding centers of ossification, forming the *physis* or *growth plate* (Fig. 21.3). The chondrocytes within the growth plate undergo sequential proliferation, hypertrophy, and apoptosis. In the region of apoptosis the matrix mineralizes and is invaded by capillaries, providing the nutrients for osteoblasts, which synthesize osteoid. This process produces longitudinal bone growth.

Intramembranous ossification, by contrast, is responsible for the development of flat bones. Bones of the cranium, for example, are formed by osteoblasts directly

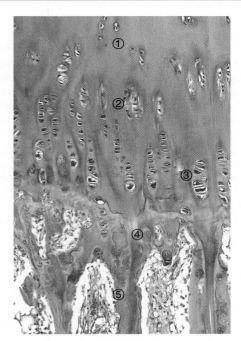

Fig. 21.3 Active growth plate with ongoing endochondral ossification. 1, Reserve zone. 2, Zone of proliferation. 3, Zone of hypertrophy. 4, Zone of mineralization. 5, Primary spongiosa.

from a fibrous layer of tissue, without cartilage anlagen. The enlargement of flat bones is achieved by deposition of new bone on a preexisting surface.

Homeostasis and Remodeling

The adult skeleton appears static but is actually constantly turning over in a tightly regulated process known as remodeling. Remodeling takes place at a microscopic locus known as the bone (or basic) multicellular unit (BMU), which consists of a unit of coupled osteoblast and osteoclast activity on the bone surface.

The events at the BMU are regulated by cell–cell interactions and cytokines (Fig. 21.4). An important signaling pathway that controls remodeling involves three factors: (1) the transmembrane receptor activator of NF-κB (RANK), which is expressed on osteoclast precursors; (2) RANK ligand (RANKL), which is expressed on osteoblasts and marrow stromal cells; and (3) osteoprotegerin (OPG), a secreted "decoy" receptor made by osteoblasts that can block RANK interaction with RANKL. RANK signaling activates the transcription factor NF-κB, which is essential for the generation and survival of osteoclasts. Other important pathways include monocyte-colony stimulating factor (M-CSF), produced by osteoblasts. WNT proteins produced by various cells bind to the LRP5 and LRP6 receptors on osteoblasts and trigger the production of OPG. The importance of these pathways is proven by rare but informative germline mutations in the *OPG, RANK, RANKL,* and *LRP5* genes, which cause severe disturbances of bone metabolism (described later).

Bone resorption or bone formation can be favored by tipping the RANK-to-OPG ratio. Systemic factors that affect this balance include hormones, vitamin D, inflammatory cytokines (e.g., IL-1), and growth factors (e.g., bone morphogenetic factors). The mechanisms are complex, but parathyroid hormone (PTH), IL-1, and glucocorticoids promote osteoclast differentiation and bone turnover. In contrast, BMPs and sex hormones (estrogen, testosterone) generally block osteoclast differentiation or activity by favoring OPG expression.

Peak bone mass is achieved in early adulthood after the cessation of skeletal growth. This set point is determined by many factors, including polymorphisms in the vitamin D and LRP5/6 receptors, nutrition, and physical activity. Beginning in the fourth decade, resorption exceeds formation, resulting in a decline in skeletal mass.

CONGENITAL DISORDERS OF BONE AND CARTILAGE

Congenital abnormalities of the skeleton frequently result from inherited mutations and first become manifest

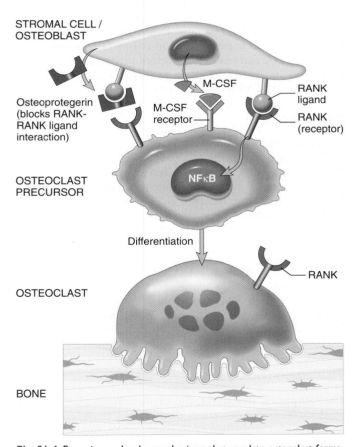

Fig. 21.4 Paracrine molecular mechanisms that regulate osteoclast formation and function. Osteoclasts are derived from the same mononuclear cells that differentiate into macrophages. Osteoblast/stromal cell membrane-associated RANKL binds to its receptor RANK located on the cell surface of osteoclast precursors. This interaction in the background of macrophage colony-stimulating factor (M-CSF) causes the precursor cells to produce functional osteoclasts. Stromal cells also secrete osteoprotegerin (OPG), which acts as a "decoy" receptor for RANKL, preventing it from binding the RANK receptor on osteoclast precursors. Consequently, OPG prevents bone resorption by inhibiting osteoclast differentiation.

during the early stages of bone formation. The spectrum of developmental disorders of bone is broad, and the classification system is not standardized. Here we will categorize the major diseases according to their perceived pathogenesis.

Congenital anomalies can result from localized abnormalities in the migration and condensation of mesenchyme (dysostosis) or global disorganization of bone and/or cartilage (dysplasia). Dysostoses result from defects in the formation of mesenchymal condensations and their differentiation into the cartilage anlage. The most common forms include the complete absence of a bone or a digit (*aplasia*), extra bones or digits (*supernumerary digit*), and abnormal fusion of bones (e.g., *syndactyly, craniosynostosis*). Genetic alterations that affect homeobox genes, cytokines, and cytokine receptors are especially common among the dysostoses. In contrast, dysplasias arise from mutations in genes that control development or remodeling of the entire skeleton. It is important to note that, as for developmental anomalies in other tissues, the term *dysplasia* implies abnormal growth rather than a premalignant lesion as used in the context of neoplasia (Chapter 6).

More than 350 skeletal dysostoses and dysplasias, most of them extremely rare, have been described. Examples of diseases with defined genetic abnormalities are discussed below. Note that various point mutations in a single gene (e.g., *COL2A1*) can result in different phenotypes, whereas mutations in diverse genes (e.g., *LRP5, RANKL*) can give rise to similar clinical phenotypes.

Achondroplasia

Achondroplasia, the most common skeletal dysplasia and a major cause of dwarfism, is an autosomal dominant disorder resulting from retarded cartilage growth. The disease is caused by gain-of-function mutations in fibroblast growth factor receptor 3 (FGFR3). Normally, FGF inhibits endochondral growth. FGFR3 mutation results in a constitutively active receptor, thereby exaggerating this effect and suppressing growth. Approximately 90% of cases stem from new mutations, almost all of which occur in the paternal allele. Affected individuals have shortened proximal extremities, a trunk of relatively normal length, and an enlarged head with bulging forehead and conspicuous depression of the root of the nose. The skeletal abnormalities are usually not associated with changes in longevity, intelligence, or reproductive status.

Thanatophoric Dysplasia

Thanatophoric dysplasia, the most common lethal form of dwarfism, results from diminished proliferation of chondrocytes and disorganization in the zone of proliferation. It also is caused by gain-of-function mutations in FGFR3, albeit ones that are distinct from those that cause achondroplasia. It occurs in about 1 of every 20,000 live births. Affected individuals have micromelic shortening of the limbs, frontal bossing, relative macrocephaly, a small chest cavity, and a bell-shaped abdomen. The underdeveloped thoracic cavity leads to respiratory insufficiency, and these individuals usually die at birth or soon thereafter.

Type I Collagen Diseases (Osteogenesis Imperfecta)

Osteogenesis imperfecta (OI), the most common inherited disorder of connective tissue, is a phenotypically diverse disorder caused by deficiencies in the synthesis of type I collagen. OI principally affects bone and other tissues rich in type I collagen (joints, eyes, ears, skin, and teeth). It usually results from autosomal dominant mutations in the genes that encode the α1 and α2 chains of type I collagen. These defects cause misfolding of the mutated collagen polypeptides, and they interfere with the proper assembly of wild-type collagen chains (a *dominant negative* loss of function).

The fundamental abnormality in OI is too little bone, resulting in extreme skeletal fragility. Other findings include blue sclerae caused by decreased collagen content, making the sclera translucent and allowing partial visualization of the underlying choroid; hearing loss related to a sensorineural deficit and impeded conduction due to abnormalities in the bones of the middle ear; and dental imperfections (small, misshapen, and blue-yellow teeth) secondary to a deficiency in dentin.

OI can be separated into multiple clinical subtypes that vary widely in severity. The type 2 variant is at one end of the spectrum and is uniformly fatal in utero or during the perinatal period. In contrast, individuals with the type 1 form have a normal life span despite a susceptibility to fractures, particularly during childhood.

Osteopetrosis

Osteopetrosis, also known as *marble bone disease*, refers to a group of rare genetic diseases that are characterized by reduced bone resorption and diffuse symmetric skeletal sclerosis resulting from impaired formation or function of osteoclasts. The term *osteopetrosis* reflects the stonelike quality of the bones. However, the bones are abnormally brittle and fracture easily, like a piece of chalk. Osteopetrosis is classified into variants based on both the mode of inheritance and the severity of clinical findings.

Most of the mutations underlying osteopetrosis interfere with the process of acidification of the osteoclast resorption pit, which is required for the dissolution of calcium hydroxyapatite within the matrix. These include autosomal recessive mutations in the enzyme carbonic anhydrase 2 (CA2), or mutations in the *TCIRG1* gene, which encodes a component of a vacuolar ATPase that helps to maintain acidic pH in osteoclasts, which is essential for breaking down bone. Bones involved by osteopetrosis lack a medullary canal, and the ends of long bones are bulbous (Erlenmeyer flask deformity) and misshapen. The neural foramina are small and compress exiting nerves. The primary spongiosa, which is normally removed during growth, persists and fills the medullary cavity, leaving no room for the hematopoietic marrow.

Severe infantile osteopetrosis is autosomal recessive and is often fatal because of leukopenia, despite extensive extramedullary hematopoiesis that can lead to prominent hepatosplenomegaly. The mild autosomal dominant form may not be detected until adolescence or adulthood, when it is discovered on radiographic studies for repeated fractures. These individuals also may have mild cranial nerve deficits and anemia.

SUMMARY

CONGENITAL DISORDERS OF BONE AND CARTILAGE

Abnormalities in a single bone or a localized group of bones are called **dysostoses** and arise from defects in the migration and condensation of mesenchyme. They manifest as absent, supernumerary, or abnormally fused bones. Global disorganizations of bone and/or cartilage are called **dysplasias**. Developmental abnormalities can be categorized by the associated genetic defect.

- FGFR3 mutations are responsible for achondroplasia and thanatophoric dysplasia, both of which manifest as dwarfism.
- Mutations in the genes for type I collagen underlie most types of osteogenesis imperfecta (brittle bone disease), characterized by defective bone formation and skeletal fragility.
- Mutations in CA2 and TCIRG1 result in osteopetrosis (in which bones are hard but brittle) and renal tubular acidosis.

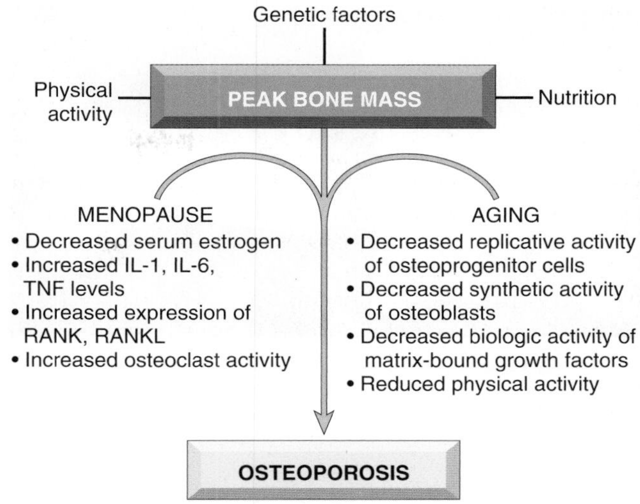

METABOLIC DISORDERS OF BONE

Osteopenia and Osteoporosis

The term *osteopenia* refers to decreased bone mass, while *osteoporosis* is defined as osteopenia that is severe enough to significantly increase the risk of fracture. Radiographically, osteoporosis is considered bone mass at least 2.5 standard deviations below mean peak bone mass, whereas osteopenia is 1 to 2.5 standard deviations below the mean. The disorder may be localized or generalized (involving the entire skeleton). Although osteoporosis can be secondary to endocrine disorders (e.g., hyperthyroidism), gastrointestinal disorders (e.g., malnutrition), or drugs (e.g., corticosteroids), most osteoporosis is primary.

The most common forms of osteoporosis are the senile and postmenopausal types. The following discussion relates largely to these forms of osteoporosis.

Pathogenesis

Peak bone mass is achieved during young adulthood. Its magnitude is influenced by hereditary factors, especially polymorphisms in the genes that influence bone metabolism (discussed later). Physical activity, muscle strength, diet, and hormonal state also make important contributions. After maximal skeletal mass is attained, bone turnover continues with a net deficit in bone formation resulting in an average loss of 0.7% of bone mass per year. Although much remains unknown, discoveries in the molecular biology of bone formation and resorption have provided new insights into the pathogenesis of osteoporosis (Fig. 21.5):

- *Age-related changes.* Osteoblasts from older individuals have reduced proliferative and biosynthetic potential and reduced response to growth factors compared to osteoblasts in younger individuals. The net result is a diminished capacity to make bone. This form of osteoporosis, known as *senile osteoporosis,* is categorized as a *low-turnover* osteoporosis.

Fig. 21.5 Pathophysiology of postmenopausal and senile osteoporosis (see text).

- *Reduced physical activity.* The decreased physical activity that is associated with normal aging contributes to senile osteoporosis. Mechanical forces stimulate normal bone remodeling as evidenced by bone loss in an immobilized or paralyzed extremity. The type of exercise is important, as load magnitude influences bone density more than the number of load cycles. Thus, resistance exercises such as weight training are more effective stimuli for increasing bone mass than repetitive endurance activities such as bicycling.
- *Genetic factors.* Single gene defects (e.g., *LRP5* mutations) account for only a small fraction of osteoporosis cases. Polymorphisms in other genes have been linked to osteoporosis by genome-wide association studies, in particular genes in the Wnt signaling pathway.
- *Calcium nutritional state.* Adolescents (particularly girls) tend to have low dietary calcium intake, a factor that restricts peak bone mass. Calcium deficiency, increased PTH concentrations, and reduced levels of vitamin D also may play a role in the development of senile osteoporosis.
- *Hormonal influences.* In the decade after menopause, yearly reductions in bone mass may be as much as 2% of cortical bone and 9% of medullary bone. *Estrogen deficiency* plays the major role in this phenomenon and close to 40% of postmenopausal women are affected by osteoporosis. Decreased estrogen levels after menopause increase both bone resorption and formation but the latter does not keep up with the former, leading to *high-turnover* osteoporosis. The decreased estrogen may increase secretion of inflammatory cytokines by monocytes. These cytokines stimulate osteoclast recruitment and activity by increasing the levels of RANKL, diminishing the expression of OPG, decreasing osteoclast proliferation, and preventing osteoclast apoptosis. Cytokines such as IL-6, TNF-α, and IL-1 also have been implicated in postmenopausal osteoporosis, either independently or as downstream mediators of estrogen signaling.

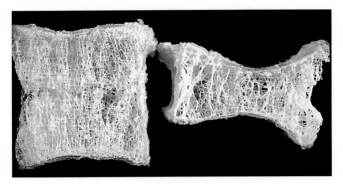

Fig. 21.6 Osteoporotic vertebral body *(right)* shortened by compression fractures compared with a normal vertebral body *(left)*. Note that the osteoporotic vertebra has a characteristic loss of horizontal trabeculae and thickened vertical trabeculae.

MORPHOLOGY

The hallmark of osteoporosis is histologically normal bone that is decreased in quantity. The entire skeleton is affected in postmenopausal and senile osteoporosis, but certain bones tend to be more severely impacted. In postmenopausal osteoporosis the increase in osteoclast activity affects mainly bones or portions of bones that have increased surface area, such as the cancellous compartment of vertebral bodies (Fig. 21.6). The trabecular plates become perforated, thinned, and lose their interconnections (Fig. 21.7), leading to progressive microfractures and eventual vertebral collapse.

Clinical Course

The clinical manifestations of osteoporosis depend on which bones are involved. Vertebral fractures that frequently occur in the thoracic and lumbar regions are painful, and, when multiple, can cause significant loss of height and various deformities, including lumbar *lordosis* and *kyphoscoliosis*. The immobility following fractures of the femoral neck, pelvis, or spine results in complications

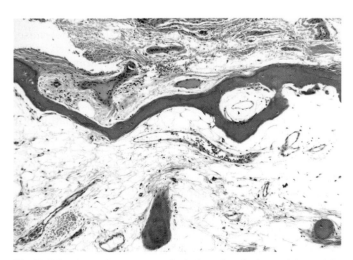

Fig. 21.7 In advanced osteoporosis, both the trabecular bone of the medulla *(bottom)* and the cortical bone *(top)* are markedly thinned.

such as pulmonary embolism and pneumonia, accounting for 40,000 to 50,000 deaths per year.

Osteoporosis cannot be reliably detected in plain radiographs until 30% to 40% of the bone mass is lost, and measurement of blood levels of calcium, phosphorus, and alkaline phosphatase are not diagnostic. Osteoporosis is thus a difficult condition to screen for in asymptomatic people. The best estimates of bone loss, aside from biopsy (which is rarely performed), are specialized radiographic imaging techniques, such as dual-energy x-ray absorptiometry and quantitative computed tomography, both of which measure bone density.

The prevention and treatment of senile and postmenopausal osteoporosis includes exercise, appropriate calcium and vitamin D intake, and pharmacologic agents that decrease resorption (bisphosphonates). Bisphosphonates reduce osteoclast activity and induce osteoclast apoptosis. Denosumab, an anti-RANKL antibody that blocks osteoclast activation, has shown promise in treating some forms of postmenopausal osteoporosis. The major challenge in pharmacotherapy of osteoporosis has been the inability to uncouple bone formation and resorption. Novel agents are currently undergoing clinical trials in an attempt to overcome this limitation. Although menopausal hormone therapy has been used to prevent fracture, complications, particularly deep venous thrombosis and stroke, have prompted the search for more selective estrogen receptor modulators.

Rickets and Osteomalacia

Both rickets and osteomalacia are manifestations of vitamin D deficiency or its abnormal metabolism (detailed in Chapter 8). *Rickets* refers to the disorder in children, in whom it interferes with the deposition of bone in the growth plates. *Osteomalacia* is the adult counterpart, in which bone formed during remodeling is undermineralized, resulting in a predisposition to fractures. The fundamental defect is an impairment of mineralization and a resultant accumulation of unmineralized matrix.

Hyperparathyroidism

Excess production and activity of PTH result in increased osteoclast activity, bone resorption, and osteopenia. Although the entire skeleton is affected, the osteopenia in some bones (e.g., phalanges) is more conspicuous radiographically. Isolated hyperparathyroidism peaks in middle adulthood and slightly earlier if presenting as a component of multiple endocrine neoplasia (MEN, types I and IIA).

Pathogenesis

As discussed in Chapter 20, PTH plays a central role in calcium homeostasis through the following effects:

- Osteoclast activation, increasing bone resorption, and calcium mobilization. PTH mediates the effect indirectly by increased RANKL expression on osteoblasts.
- Increased resorption of calcium by the renal tubules.
- Increased urinary excretion of phosphates.
- Increased synthesis of active vitamin D, $1,25(OH)_2$-D, by the kidneys, which in turn enhances calcium absorption

from the gut and mobilizes bone calcium by inducing RANKL on osteoblasts.

The net result of the actions of PTH is an elevation in serum calcium, which, under normal circumstances, inhibits further PTH production. However, excessive or inappropriate levels of PTH can result from autonomous parathyroid secretion *(primary hyperparathyroidism)* or can occur in the setting of underlying renal disease *(secondary hyperparathyroidism)* (see Chapter 20). PTH is directly responsible for the bone changes seen in primary hyperparathyroidism. Abnormalities stemming from chronic renal insufficiency that contribute to bone disease in secondary hyperparathyroidism include inadequate $1,25\text{-}(OH)_2\text{-D}$ synthesis, hyperphosphatemia, metabolic acidosis, and aluminum deposition in bone (in those undergoing renal dialsysis).

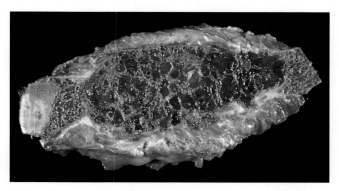

Fig. 21.9 Resected rib, harboring an expansile brown tumor adjacent to the costal cartilage.

Clinical Course

As bone mass decreases, affected patients are increasingly susceptible to fractures, bone deformation, and joint problems. Osteitis fibrosa cystica is now rarely encountered because hyperparathyroidism is usually diagnosed on routine blood tests and treated at an early stage. Restoration of PTH levels to normal can completely reverse the bone changes. Secondary hyperparathyroidism is usually not as severe or as prolonged as primary hyperparathyroidism, hence the skeletal abnormalities tend to be milder.

MORPHOLOGY

Symptomatic, untreated primary hyperparathyroidism manifests with three interrelated skeletal abnormalities: **osteoporosis, brown tumors,** and **osteitis fibrosa cystica.** Osteoporosis is generalized, but is most severe in the phalanges, vertebrae, and proximal femur. Osteoclasts may tunnel into and dissect centrally along the length of the trabeculae, creating the appearance of railroad tracks and producing what is known as *dissecting osteitis* (Fig. 21.8). The marrow spaces around the affected surfaces are replaced by fibrovascular tissue. The correlative radiographic finding is a decrease in bone density.

The bone loss predisposes to microfractures and secondary hemorrhages that elicit an influx of macrophages and an ingrowth of reparative fibrous tissue, creating a mass of reactive tissue, known as a **brown tumor** (Fig. 21.9). The brown color is the result of the vascularity, hemorrhage, and hemosiderin. These lesions often undergo cystic degeneration. The combination of increased bone cell activity, peritrabecular fibrosis, and cystic brown tumors is the hallmark of severe hyperparathyroidism and is known as **generalized osteitis fibrosa cystica.**

SUMMARY

METABOLIC DISORDERS OF BONE

- **Osteopenia** and **osteoporosis** represent histologically normal bone that is decreased in quantity. In osteoporosis the bone loss is sufficiently severe to significantly increase the risk of fracture. The disease is very common, with marked morbidity and mortality from fractures. Multiple factors including peak bone mass, age, activity, genetics, nutrition, and hormonal influences contribute to its pathogenesis.
- **Osteomalacia** is characterized by bone that is insufficiently mineralized. In the developing skeleton, the manifestations are characterized by a condition known as **rickets.**
- **Hyperparathyroidism** arises from either autonomous or compensatory hypersecretion of PTH and can lead to **osteoporosis, brown tumors,** and **osteitis fibrosa cystica.** However, in developed countries, where early diagnosis is the norm, these manifestations are rarely seen.

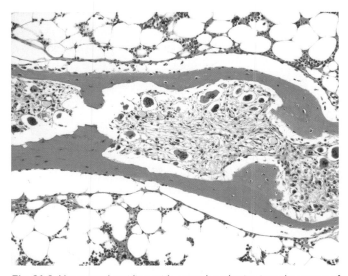

Fig. 21.8 Hyperparathyroidism with osteoclasts boring into the center of the trabecula resembling a train track (dissecting osteitis).

PAGET DISEASE OF BONE (OSTEITIS DEFORMANS)

Paget disease is a condition of increased, but disordered and structurally unsound, bone. This unique skeletal disease can be divided into three sequential phases: (1) an initial osteolytic stage, (2) a mixed osteoclastic–osteoblastic stage, which ends with a predominance of osteoblastic activity and evolves into (3) a final burned-out quiescent osteosclerotic stage (Fig. 21.10).

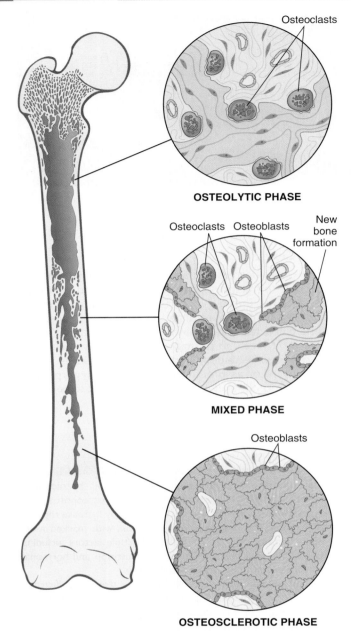

OSTEOLYTIC PHASE

Osteoclasts

MIXED PHASE

Osteoclasts Osteoblasts New bone formation

OSTEOSCLEROTIC PHASE

Osteoblasts

Fig. 21.10 Diagrammatic representation of Paget disease of bone demonstrating the three phases in the evolution of the disease.

Paget disease usually begins in late adulthood. An estimated 1% of the U.S. population older than age 40 is affected. An intriguing aspect is the striking geographic variation in the prevalence. Paget disease is relatively common in whites in England, France, Austria, regions of Germany, Australia, New Zealand, and the United States. In contrast, the disease is rare in the native populations of Scandinavia, China, Japan, and Africa.

Pathogenesis

Current evidence suggests both genetic and environmental causes of Paget disease. Approximately 50% of familial Paget disease and 10% of sporadic cases harbor mutations in the *SQSTM1* gene. The mutations increase the activity of

NF-κB, which, in turn increases osteoclast activity. Activating mutations in *RANK* and inactivating mutations in *OPG* account for some cases of juvenile Paget disease. The geographic distribution is suggestive of some environmental influence. Of note in this regard, cell culture studies have shown that infection of osteoclast precursors with viruses such as measles or other RNA viruses alters vitamin D sensitivity and IL-6 secretion, both of which can lead to increased bone resorption.

MORPHOLOGY

Paget disease shows remarkable histologic variation throughout time and from site to site. **The hallmark, seen in the sclerotic phase, is a mosaic pattern of lamellar bone** (Fig. 21.11). The jigsaw puzzle–like appearance is produced by unusually **prominent cement lines**, which join haphazardly oriented units of lamellar bone. In the sclerotic phase, the bone is thickened but lacks structural stability making it vulnerable to deformation and fracture. The findings during the other phases are less specific. The initial lytic phase is characterized by numerous large osteoclasts and resorption pits. The osteoclasts may have 100 or more nuclei. Osteoclasts persist in the mixed phase, but many of the bone surfaces are also lined by prominent osteoblasts.

Clinical Course

Paget disease is *monostotic* in about 15% of cases and *polyostotic* in the remainder. The axial skeleton or proximal femur is involved in up to 80% of cases. Most cases are asymptomatic and are discovered as an incidental radiographic finding. Pain localized to the affected bone is a common symptom. Pain is caused by microfractures or by bone overgrowth that compresses spinal and cranial nerve roots. Enlargement of the craniofacial skeleton may produce *leontiasis ossea* (lion face) and a cranium so heavy that is difficult for the person to hold the head erect. The weakened Pagetic bone may lead to invagination of the skull base (*platybasia*) and compression of the posterior fossa. Weight bearing causes anterior bowing of the femurs and tibiae

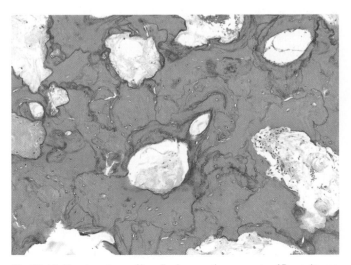

Fig. 21.11 Mosaic pattern of lamellar bone pathognomonic of Paget disease.

and distorts the femoral heads, resulting in the development of severe *secondary osteoarthritis*. *Chalk stick–type fractures* are another frequent complication and usually occur in the long bones of the lower extremities. Compression fractures of the spine result in spinal cord injury and the development of kyphosis. The diagnosis can frequently be made from the radiographic findings. Many affected individuals have elevated serum alkaline phosphatase levels but normal serum calcium and phosphorus.

A variety of tumor and tumorlike conditions develop in Pagetic bone. Secondary osteosarcoma occurs in less than 1% of all individuals with Paget disease, but appears in 5% to 10% of those with severe polyostotic disease. In the absence of malignant transformation, Paget disease is usually not a serious or life-threatening disease. Most affected individuals have mild symptoms that are readily suppressed by treatment with calcitonin and bisphosphonates.

FRACTURES

A fracture is defined as loss of bone integrity resulting from mechanical injury and/or diminished bone strength. Fractures are the most common pathologic conditions affecting bone. The following qualifiers describe fracture types and affect treatment:

- Simple: the overlying skin is intact
- Compound: the bone communicates with the skin surface
- Comminuted: the bone is fragmented
- Displaced: the ends of the bone at the fracture site are not aligned
- Stress: a slowly developing fracture that follows a period of increased physical activity in which the bone is subjected to repetitive loads
- Greenstick: extending only partially through the bone, common in infants when bones are soft
- Pathologic: involving bone weakened by an underlying disease process, such as a tumor

Healing of Fractures

Fracture repair involves regulated expression of a multitude of genes and can be separated into overlapping stages with particular molecular, biochemical, histologic, and biomechanical features.

Immediately after fracture, rupture of blood vessels results in a hematoma, which fills the fracture gap and surrounds the area of bone injury (Fig. 21.12). The clotted blood provides a fibrin mesh, sealing off the fracture site and creating a scaffold for the influx of inflammatory cells and the ingrowth of fibroblasts and new capillaries. Simultaneously, degranulated platelets and migrating inflammatory cells release PDGF, TGF-β, FGF, and other factors that activate osteoprogenitor cells in the periosteum, medullary cavity, and surrounding soft tissues and stimulate osteoclastic and osteoblastic activity. By the end of the first week, a mass of predominantly uncalcified tissue—called *soft callus* or *procallus*—provides anchorage between the ends of the fractured bones. After approximately 2 weeks, the soft callus is transformed into a *bony callus*. The

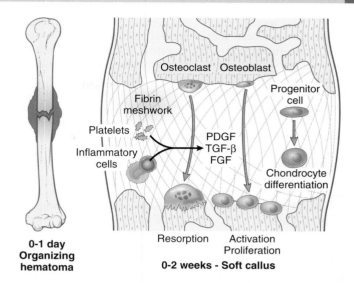

0-1 day
Organizing hematoma

0-2 weeks - Soft callus

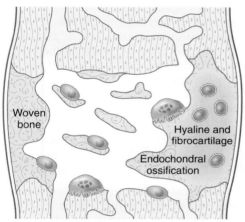

2-3 weeks - Bony callus

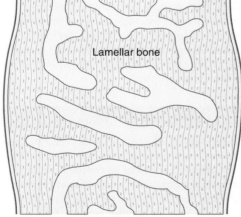

3 weeks-months - Bony callus

Fig. 21.12 The reaction to a fracture begins with an organizing hematoma. Within two weeks, the two ends of the bone are bridged by a fibrin meshwork in which osteoclasts, osteoblasts, and chondrocytes differentiate from precursors. These cells produce cartilage and bone matrix, which, with adequate immobilization, remodels into normal lamellar bone.

activated osteoprogenitor cells deposit *woven bone*. In some cases, the activated mesenchymal cells in the soft tissues and bone surrounding the fracture line also differentiate into chondrocytes that make fibrocartilage and hyaline cartilage. The newly formed cartilage along the fracture line undergoes endochondral ossification, forming a contiguous network of bone with newly deposited bone trabeculae in the medulla and beneath the periosteum. In this fashion, the fractured ends are bridged (Fig. 21.12).

As the callus matures and is subjected to weight-bearing forces, portions that are not physically stressed are resorbed. This remodeling reduces the size of the callus until the shape and outline of the fractured bone are reestablished as *lamellar bone*. The healing process is complete with restoration of the medullary cavity.

The sequence of events in the healing of a fracture can be easily impeded or blocked. Displaced and comminuted fractures frequently result in some deformity. Inadequate immobilization permits movement of the callus and prevents its normal maturation, resulting in *delayed union* or *nonunion*. If a nonunion persists, the malformed callus undergoes cystic degeneration, and the luminal surface may become lined by synovial-like cells, creating a false joint or *pseudoarthrosis*. Infection of the fracture site, especially common in open fractures, is a serious obstacle to healing. Malnutrition and skeletal dysplasia also hinder fracture healing.

OSTEONECROSIS (AVASCULAR NECROSIS)

Osteonecrosis refers to infarction (ischemic necrosis) of bone and marrow cells. A diverse set of conditions predisposes to bone ischemia, including vascular injury (e.g., trauma, vasculitis), drugs (e.g., corticosteroids), systemic disease (sickle cell crisis), and radiation. In about 25% of cases, the cause is unknown. The three suspected mechanisms causing osteonecrosis are mechanical disruption of vessels, thrombotic occlusion, and extravascular compression. Osteonecrosis has a wide age range but peaks in the 30s to 50s and accounts for about 10% of hip replacements in the United States.

MORPHOLOGY

Regardless of etiology, medullary infarcts are geographic and involve the trabecular bone and marrow. The cortex is usually not affected because of its collateral blood flow. In subchondral infarcts, a triangular or wedge-shaped segment of tissue that has the subchondral bone plate as its base undergoes necrosis. The overlying articular cartilage remains viable, as it can access nutrients that are present in synovial fluid. Microscopically, dead bone is recognized by empty lacunae surrounded by necrotic adipocytes that frequently rupture. In the healing response, osteoclasts resorb the necrotic trabeculae. Trabeculae that remain act as scaffolding for the deposition of new bone in a process known as creeping substitution. In subchondral infarcts, the pace of this substitution is too slow to be effective, so there is collapse of the necrotic bone and distortion, fracture, and even sloughing of the articular cartilage (Fig. 21.13).

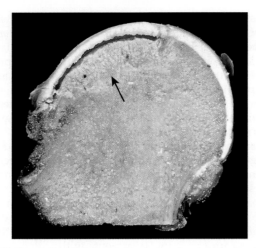

Fig. 21.13 Femoral head with a subchondral, wedge-shaped pale yellow area of osteonecrosis *(arrow)*. The space between the overlying articular cartilage and bone is caused by trabecular compression fractures without repair.

Clinical Course

The symptoms depend on the location and extent of infarct. Typically, subchondral infarcts cause pain that is initially associated only with activity but then becomes constant. Subchondral infarcts often collapse and may lead to severe, secondary osteoarthritis. Treatment ranges from conservative measures (limited weight bearing, immobilization) to surgery.

OSTEOMYELITIS

Osteomyelitis denotes inflammation of bone and marrow, virtually always secondary to infection. Osteomyelitis may be a complication of any systemic infection but frequently manifests as a primary solitary focus of disease. All types of organisms, including viruses, parasites, fungi, and bacteria, can produce osteomyelitis, but infections caused by certain pyogenic bacteria and mycobacteria are the most common.

Pyogenic Osteomyelitis

Pyogenic osteomyelitis is almost always caused by bacteria and rarely by fungi. Organisms may reach the bone by (1) hematogenous spread, (2) extension from a contiguous site, and (3) direct implantation after compound fractures or orthopedic procedures. In otherwise healthy children, most osteomyelitis is hematogenous in origin and develops in the long bones. In adults, however, osteomyelitis more often occurs as a complication of open fractures, surgical procedures, and infections of the feet in diabetics.

Staphylococcus aureus is responsible for 80% to 90% of the cases of culture-positive pyogenic osteomyelitis. These organisms express cell wall proteins that bind to bone matrix components such as collagen and facilitate adherence to bone. *Escherichia coli*, *Pseudomonas*, and *Klebsiella* are more frequently isolated from individuals with genitourinary tract infections or who are intravenous drug abusers. Mixed bacterial infections are seen in the setting of direct spread, inoculation of organisms during surgery, or into open fractures. In the neonatal period, *Haemophilus influenzae* and group B streptococci are frequent pathogens, and individuals with sickle cell disease are predisposed to *Salmonella* infection. In almost 50% of suspected cases, no organisms can be isolated.

The osseous vascular circulation, which varies with age, determines the location of infection in most long bones. In infants and adults, vascular communication allows the spread of infection between the metaphysis and the epiphysis. By contrast, the avascular growth plate in the child interrupts infection spread between the metaphysis and epiphysis.

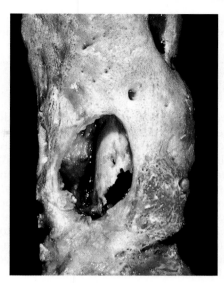

Fig. 21.14 Resected femur in a person with draining osteomyelitis. The drainage tract in the subperiosteal shell of viable new bone (involucrum) shows the inner native necrotic cortex (sequestrum).

MORPHOLOGY

Changes associated with osteomyelitis depend on the stage (acute, subacute, or chronic) and location of the infection. In the acute phase, bacteria proliferate and induce a neutrophilic inflammatory reaction. Necrosis of bone cells and marrow ensues within the first 48 hours. The bacteria and inflammation spread longitudinally and radially throughout the Haversian systems to reach the periosteum. In children, the periosteum is loosely attached to the cortex. Thus, sizable subperiosteal abscess may form that dissect for long distances along the bone surface. Lifting of the periosteum further impairs the blood supply to the affected region, contributing to the necrosis. The dead bone is known as a **sequestrum.** Rupture of the periosteum leads to a soft tissue abscess, which can channel to the skin, creating a draining sinus. Sometimes the sequestrum crumbles, releasing fragments that pass through the sinus tract.

In infants (and uncommonly in adults), epiphyseal infection may spread through the articular surface or along capsular and tendoligamentous insertions into a joint, producing septic or suppurative arthritis, which can cause destruction of the articular cartilage and permanent disability.

After the first week, chronic inflammatory cells release cytokines that stimulate osteoclastic bone resorption, ingrowth of fibrous tissue, and the deposition of reactive bone at the periphery. The newly deposited bone can form a shell of living tissue, known as an **involucrum,** around the segment of devitalized infected bone (Fig. 21.14). The histologic findings of chronic osteomyelitis are more protean but typically involve marrow fibrosis, sequestrum, and an inflammatory infiltrate of lymphocytes and plasma cells.

Clinical Course

Hematogenous osteomyelitis sometimes manifests as an acute systemic illness with malaise, fever, chills, leukocytosis, and marked throbbing pain over the affected region. In other instances the presentation is subtle, with only unexplained fever (most often in infants) or localized pain (most often in adults). The diagnosis is strongly suggested by the characteristic radiographic findings of a lytic focus of bone destruction surrounded by a zone of sclerosis. Biopsy and bone cultures are required to identify the pathogen in most instances. The combination of antibiotics and surgical drainage is usually curative.

In 5% to 25% of cases, acute osteomyelitis fails to resolve and persists as chronic infection. Chronic infections may

develop when there is delay in diagnosis, extensive bone necrosis, inadequate antibiotic therapy or surgical debridement, or weakened host defenses. The course of chronic infections may be punctuated by acute flare-ups; these are usually spontaneous and may occur after years of dormancy. Other complications of chronic osteomyelitis include pathologic fracture, secondary amyloidosis, endocarditis, sepsis, and the development of squamous cell carcinoma in the draining sinus tracts and sarcoma in the infected bone.

Mycobacterial Osteomyelitis

Mycobacterial osteomyelitis, historically a problem in developing countries, has increased in incidence in the developed world because of immigration patterns and immunocompromised patients. Overall, approximately 1% to 3% of individuals with pulmonary or extrapulmonary tuberculosis exhibit osseous infection.

The organisms are usually blood borne and originate from a focus of active visceral disease during the initial stages of primary infection. Direct extension (e.g., from a pulmonary focus into a rib or from tracheobronchial nodes into adjacent vertebrae) also may occur. The bone infection may persist for years before being recognized. Typically, affected individuals present with localized pain, low-grade fevers, chills, and weight loss. Infection is usually solitary except in immunocompromised individuals. The histologic findings, namely caseous necrosis and granulomas, are typical of tuberculosis. Mycobacterial osteomyelitis tends to be more destructive and resistant to control than pyogenic osteomyelitis.

Tuberculous spondylitis (Pott disease) is a destructive infection of vertebrae. The spine is involved in 40% of cases of mycobacterial osteomyelitis. The infection breaks through intervertebral discs to affect multiple vertebrae and extends into the soft tissues. Destruction of discs and vertebrae frequently results in permanent compression fractures that produce scoliosis or kyphosis and neurologic deficits secondary to spinal cord and nerve compression.

BONE TUMORS AND TUMORLIKE LESIONS

The rarity of primary bone tumors and the often-disfiguring surgery required to treat a bone malignancy make this group of disorders especially challenging. About 2400 primary bone sarcomas are diagnosed annually in the United States. Therapy aims to optimize survival while maintaining the function of affected body parts. The predilection of specific types of tumors for certain age groups and particular anatomic sites provides important diagnostic clues. For example, osteosarcoma peaks during adolescence and most frequently involves the knee, whereas chondrosarcoma affects older adults and involves the pelvis and proximal extremities.

Bone tumors may present in a number of ways. The more common benign lesions are often asymptomatic incidental findings. Many tumors, however, produce pain or a slow-growing mass. In some circumstances the first hint of a tumor's presence is a pathologic fracture. Radiographic imaging studies have an important role in diagnosing these lesions. In addition to providing the exact location and extent of the tumor, imaging studies can detect features that narrow the diagnostic possibilities. In almost all instances biopsy is necessary for definitive diagnosis.

When possible, bone tumors are classified according to the normal cell or matrix they produce. Lesions that do not have normal tissue counterparts are grouped according to their clinicopathologic features (Table 21.1). *Benign tumors greatly outnumber their malignant counterparts* and occur with greatest frequency within the first three decades of life. In older adults, a bone tumor is more likely to be malignant.

Bone-Forming Tumors

Tumors in this category all produce unmineralized osteoid or mineralized woven bone.

Osteoid Osteoma and Osteoblastoma
Osteoid osteoma and osteoblastoma are benign bone-producing tumors that have similar histologic features but differ clinically and radiographically. Osteoid osteomas are, by definition, less than 2 cm in diameter, and are most common in young men. About 50% of cases involve the femur or tibia, wherein they typically arise in the cortex. Usually, there is a thick rim of reactive cortical bone that may be the only clue radiographically. Despite their small size, they present with severe nocturnal pain that is relieved by aspirin and other nonsteroidal anti-inflammatory agents. The pain is probably caused by prostaglandin E_2 produced by osteoblasts. Osteoblastoma is larger than 2 cm and involves the posterior components of the vertebrae (laminae and pedicles) more frequently. The pain is unresponsive to aspirin, and the tumor usually does not induce a marked bony reaction. Osteoid osteoma is frequently treated by radiofrequency ablation, whereas osteoblastoma is usually curetted or excised. Malignant transformation is rare.

MORPHOLOGY

Osteoid osteoma and osteoblastoma are round-to-oval masses of hemorrhagic gritty tan tissue. They are well circumscribed and composed of randomly interconnecting delicate trabeculae

Table 21.1 Classification of Selected Primary Bone Tumors

Category	Behavior	Tumor Type	Common Locations	Age (yr)	Morphology
Cartilage forming	Benign	Osteochondroma	Metaphysis of long bones	10–30	Bony excrescence with cartilage cap
—	—	Chondroma	Small bones of hands and feet	30–50	Circumscribed hyaline cartilage nodule in medulla
—	Malignant	Chondrosarcoma (conventional)	Pelvis, shoulder	40–60	Extends from medulla through cortex into soft tissue, chondrocytes with increased cellularity and atypia
Bone forming	Benign	Osteoid osteoma	Metaphysis of long bones	10–20	Cortical, interlacing microtrabeculae of woven bone
—	—	Osteoblastoma	Vertebral column	10–20	Posterior elements of vertebra, histology similar to osteoid osteoma
—	Malignant	Osteosarcoma	Metaphysis of distal femur, proximal tibia	10–20	Extends from medulla to lift periosteum, malignant cells producing woven bone
Unknown origin	Benign	Giant cell tumor	Epiphysis of long bones	20–40	Destroys medulla and cortex, sheets of osteoclasts
—	—	Aneurysmal bone cyst	Proximal tibia, distal femur, vertebra	10–20	Vertebral body, hemorrhagic spaces separated by cellular, fibrous septae
—	Malignant	Ewing sarcoma	Diaphysis of long bones	10–20	Sheets of primitive small round cells

Adapted from Unni KK, Inwards CY: *Dahlin's Bone Tumors*, ed 6. Philadelphia, 2010, Lippincott-Williams & Wilkins; by permission of Mayo Foundation.

of woven bone that are prominently rimmed by a single layer of osteoblasts (Fig. 21.15). The stroma surrounding the neoplastic bone consists of loose connective tissue that contains many dilated and congested capillaries. The relatively small size, well-defined margins, and benign cytologic features of the neoplastic osteoblasts help distinguish these tumors from osteosarcoma. Osteoid osteomas elicit the formation of a large amount of reactive bone, which encircles the lesion.

Osteosarcoma

Osteosarcoma is a malignant tumor that produces osteoid matrix or mineralized bone. Excluding hematopoietic tumors (myeloma and lymphoma), osteosarcoma is the most common primary malignant tumor of bone. Osteosarcoma has a bimodal age distribution; 75% of osteosarcomas occur in persons younger than 20 years of age. The smaller second peak occurs in older adults, who frequently suffer from conditions known to predispose to osteosarcoma, such as Paget disease, bone infarcts, and previous radiation. These are referred to as secondary osteosarcomas. Overall, men are more commonly affected than women (1.6:1). The most common sites in adolescents are the metaphyseal regions of the distal femur and proximal tibia.

Osteosarcomas present as painful, progressively enlarging masses. Sometimes a pathologic fracture is the first indication. Radiographs usually show a large, destructive, mixed lytic and sclerotic mass with infiltrative margins (Fig. 21.16). The tumor frequently breaks through the cortex and lifts the periosteum, resulting in reactive subperiosteal bone formation. The triangular shadow between the cortex and raised ends of periosteum, known radiographically as *Codman triangle*, is indicative of an aggressive tumor, but is not pathognomonic of osteosarcoma.

Pathogenesis

Approximately 70% of osteosarcomas have acquired genetic abnormalities such as complex structural and numerical chromosomal aberrations. Molecular studies have shown that these tumors usually have mutations in well-known tumor suppressors and oncogenes:
- *RB* is a critical negative regulator of the cell cycle. Patients with germline mutations in *RB* have a 1000-fold

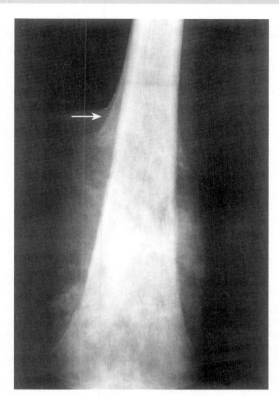

Fig. 21.16 Distal femoral osteosarcoma with prominent bone formation extending into the soft tissues. The periosteum, which has been lifted, has laid down a triangular shell of reactive bone known as a Codman triangle *(arrow)*.

increased risk of osteosarcoma, and somatic *RB* mutations are present in up to 70% of sporadic osteosarcomas.
- *TP53* is a gene whose product functions as the guardian of genomic integrity by promoting DNA repair and apoptosis of irreversibly damaged cells. Patients with Li-Fraumeni syndrome, who have germline *TP53* gene mutations, have a greatly elevated incidence of osteosarcoma, and abnormalities that interfere with p53 function are common in sporadic tumors.
- *CDKN2A* is inactivated in many osteosarcomas. This gene encodes two tumor suppressors, p16 (a negative regulator of cyclin-dependent kinases) and p14 (which augments p53 function).
- *MDM2* and *CDK4*, which are cell cycle regulators that inhibit p53 and RB function, respectively, are overexpressed in many low-grade osteosarcomas.

It also is noteworthy that osteosarcomas peak in incidence around the time of the adolescent growth spurt and occur most frequently in the region of the growth plate in bones with the fastest growth. The increased proliferation at these sites may predispose to osteosarcoma development.

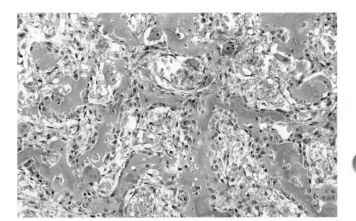

Fig. 21.15 Osteoid osteoma composed of haphazardly interconnecting trabeculae of woven bone that are rimmed by prominent osteoblasts. The intertrabecular spaces are filled by vascularized loose connective tissue.

MORPHOLOGY

Osteosarcomas are bulky tumors that are gritty, gray-white, and often contain areas of hemorrhage and cystic degeneration (Fig. 21.17). The tumors frequently destroy the surrounding cortices and produce soft tissue masses. They spread extensively in the medullary canal, infiltrating and replacing the marrow.

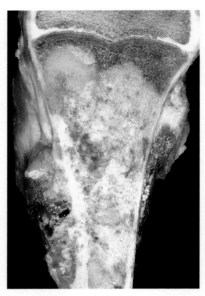

Fig. 21.17 Osteosarcoma of the proximal tibia. The tan-white tumor fills most of the medullary cavity of the metaphysis and proximal diaphysis. It has infiltrated through the cortex, lifted the periosteum, and formed soft tissue masses on both sides of the bone.

Infrequently they penetrate the epiphyseal plate or enter the joint.

The formation of osteoid matrix or mineralized bone by malignant tumor cells is diagnostic of osteosarcoma (Fig. 21.18). The neoplastic bone usually has a fine, lacelike configuration but also may be deposited in broad sheets or as primitive trabeculae. The tumor cells vary in size and shape (pleomorphic) and frequently have large hyperchromatic nuclei. Bizarre tumor giant cells, vascular invasion, and necrosis are common. Mitotic activity is high, including abnormal forms (e.g., tripolar mitoses).

Clinical Course

Osteosarcoma is treated with a multimodality approach that consists of (1) neoadjuvant chemotherapy, (2) surgery,

and (3) chemotherapy. The amount of chemotherapy-induced necrosis found at surgical resection is an important prognostic finding. These aggressive neoplasms spread hematogenously to the lungs. Although the prognosis has improved substantially since the advent of chemotherapy, with 5-year survival rates reaching 60% to 70% in patients without detectable metastases at initial diagnosis, the outcome for patients with metastases, recurrent disease, or secondary osteosarcoma is still poor.

Cartilage-Forming Tumors

These tumors are characterized by the formation of hyaline cartilage. Benign cartilaginous tumors are much more common than malignant ones.

Osteochondroma

Osteochondroma, known clinically as exostosis, is a benign cartilage-capped tumor that is attached to the underlying skeleton by a bony stalk. About 85% are solitary. The remainder are seen as part of the *multiple hereditary exostoses syndrome* (see later). Solitary osteochondromas are usually first diagnosed in late adolescence and early adulthood, but multiple osteochondromas become apparent during childhood. Men are affected three times more often than women. Osteochondromas develop in bones of endochondral origin and arise from the metaphysis near the growth plate of long tubular bones, especially near the knee (Fig. 21.19). They present as slow-growing masses, which can be painful if they impinge on a nerve or if the stalk is fractured. In many cases they are detected incidentally. In multiple hereditary exostoses, the underlying bones may be bowed and shortened, reflecting an associated disturbance in epiphyseal growth.

Pathogenesis

Hereditary exostoses are associated with germline loss-of-function mutations in either the *EXT1* or the *EXT2* gene and subsequent loss of the remaining wild-type allele in chondrocytes of the growth plate. Reduced expression of *EXT1* or *EXT2* also has been observed in sporadic osteochondromas. These genes encode enzymes that synthesize heparan sulfate glycosaminoglycans. The reduced or abnormal glycosaminoglycans may prevent normal diffusion of Hedgehog factors, which are local regulators of cartilage growth, thereby disrupting chondrocyte differentiation and skeletal development.

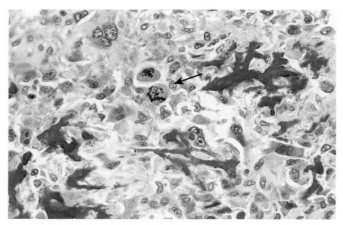

Fig. 21.18 Fine, lacelike pattern of neoplastic bone produced by anaplastic malignant tumor cells in an osteosarcoma. Note the abnormal mitotic figure *(arrow)*.

MORPHOLOGY

Osteochondromas are sessile or pedunculated, and they range in size from 1 to 20 cm. The cap is composed of benign hyaline cartilage (Fig. 21.20) and is covered peripherally by perichondrium. The cartilage has the appearance of a disorganized growth plate and undergoes endochondral ossification, with the newly made bone forming the inner portion of the head and stalk. The cortex of the stalk merges with the cortex of the host bone resulting in continuity between the medulla of the osteochondroma and the host bone.

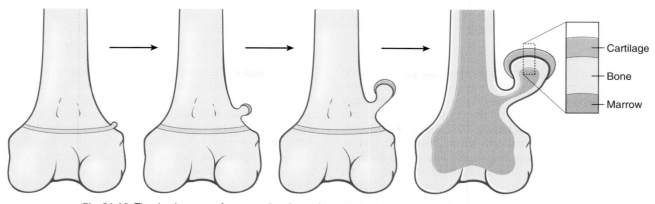

Fig. 21.19 The development of an osteochondroma, beginning with an outgrowth from the epiphyseal cartilage.

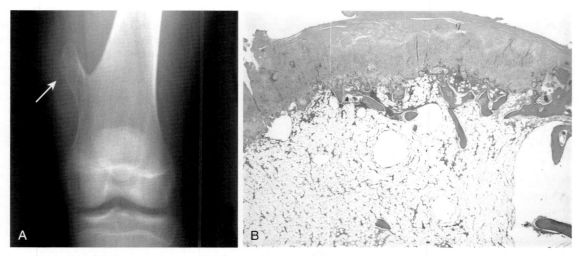

Fig. 21.20 Osteochondroma. (A) Radiograph of an osteochondroma arising from the distal femur *(arrow)*. (B) The cartilage cap has the histologic appearance of disorganized growth plate–like cartilage.

Clinical Course

Osteochondromas usually stop growing at the time of growth plate closure. Symptomatic tumors are cured by simple excision. Rarely in sporadic cases, but more commonly in those with multiple hereditary exostosis (5%–20%), osteochondromas progress to chondrosarcoma.

Chondroma

Chondromas are benign tumors of hyaline cartilage that usually occur in bones of endochondral origin. They arise within the medullary cavity *(enchondroma)* or on the cortical surface *(juxtacortical chondroma)*. Enchondromas are usually diagnosed in individuals 20 to 50 years of age. Typically, they appear as solitary metaphyseal lesions of the tubular bones of the hands and feet. The radiographic features consist of a circumscribed lucency with central irregular calcifications, a sclerotic rim, and an intact cortex (Fig. 21.21). *Ollier disease* and *Maffucci syndrome* are disorders characterized by multiple enchondromas (enchondromatosis). Maffucci syndrome also is associated with other rare tumors.

Most enchondromas of large bones are asymptomatic and are detected incidentally. Occasionally, they are painful and cause pathologic fracture. The tumors in

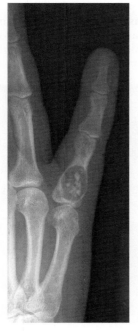

Fig. 21.21 Enchondroma of the proximal phalanx. The radiolucent nodule of cartilage with central calcification thins but does not penetrate the cortex.

enchondromatosis may be numerous and large, producing severe deformities, especially of the digits.

Pathogenesis

Heterozygous gain of function mutations in the *IDH1* and *IDH2* genes, coding for the enzymes isocitrate dehydrogenases, have been identified in the chondrocytes of syndromic and solitary enchondromas. Patients with enchondroma syndromes are mosaics, harboring *IDH* mutations in only a subset of otherwise normal cells throughout their bodies. The mutations confer a new enzymatic activity on the IDH proteins that leads to the synthesis of 2-hydroxyglutarate. As discussed in Chapter 6, this so-called "oncometabolite" interferes with regulation of DNA methylation and is also implicated in certain glial tumors and a subset of acute myeloid leukemias.

MORPHOLOGY

Enchondromas are usually smaller than 3 cm and are gray-blue and translucent. They are composed of well-circumscribed nodules of hyaline cartilage containing benign chondrocytes (Fig. 21.22). The peripheral portion of the nodules may undergo endochondral ossification, and the center can calcify and infarct. Syndromic enchondromas are sometimes more cellular with more atypia than sporadic enchondromas.

Clinical Course

The growth potential of chondromas is limited. Treatment depends on the clinical situation and usually includes observation or curettage. Solitary chondromas rarely undergo sarcomatous transformation, but those associated with enchondromatosis do so more frequently. Individuals with Maffucci syndrome also are at risk of developing other neoplasms, including brain gliomas.

Chondrosarcoma

Chondrosarcomas are malignant tumors that produce cartilage. They are subclassified into *conventional* (hyaline cartilage–producing), *dedifferentiated, clear cell,* and

mesenchymal types. Approximately 90% of chondrosarcomas are of the conventional type. Chondrosarcoma is about half as common as osteosarcoma. Individuals with conventional chondrosarcoma are usually in their 40s or older. These tumors affect men twice as frequently as women. The clear cell and especially the mesenchymal variants occur in children and young adults. Chondrosarcomas commonly arise in the axial skeleton, especially the pelvis, shoulder, and ribs. Unlike benign enchondroma, the distal extremities are rarely involved. On imaging, the calcified cartilage appears as foci of flocculent densities that may destroy the cortex and form a soft tissue mass. About 15% of conventional chondrosarcomas are secondary, arising from a preexisting enchondroma or osteochondroma.

Pathogenesis

Although chondrosarcomas are genetically heterogeneous, a few reproducible abnormalities have been identified. Chondrosarcomas arising in multiple osteochondroma syndrome exhibit mutations in the *EXT* genes, and both chondromatosis-related and sporadic chondrosarcomas may have *IDH1* and *IDH2* mutations. Mutation of the collagen *COL2A1* gene and silencing of the *CDKN2A* tumor

MORPHOLOGY

Conventional chondrosarcomas are large bulky tumors composed of nodules of glistening gray-white, translucent cartilage, along with gelatinous or myxoid areas (Fig. 21.23A). Spotty calcifications are typically present, and central necrosis may create cystic spaces. The tumor spreads through the cortex into surrounding muscle or fat. Histologically, the cartilage infiltrates the marrow space and entraps normal bony trabeculae (Fig. 21.23B). The tumors vary in cellularity, cytologic atypia, and mitotic activity and are assigned a grade from 1 to 3. Grade 1 tumors have relatively low cellularity, and the chondrocytes have plump vesicular nuclei with small nucleoli. By contrast, grade 3 chondrosarcomas are characterized by high cellularity, extreme pleomorphism with bizarre tumor giant cells, and mitoses.

suppressor gene by DNA methylation are also relatively common in sporadic tumors.

Clinical Course

Chondrosarcomas usually present as painful, progressively enlarging masses. Tumor grade predicts outcome, which ranges from 80% 5-year survival for Grade 1 tumors to 43% for Grade 3 tumors. Grade 1 chondrosarcomas rarely metastasize, whereas 70% of grade 3 tumors spread hematogenously, especially to the lungs. The treatment of conventional chondrosarcoma is wide surgical excision. The mesenchymal and dedifferentiated tumors are also excised and are additionally treated with chemotherapy because of their more aggressive clinical course.

Tumors of Unknown Origin

Ewing Sarcoma

Ewing sarcoma is a malignant tumor composed of primitive round cells with varying degrees of neuroectodermal

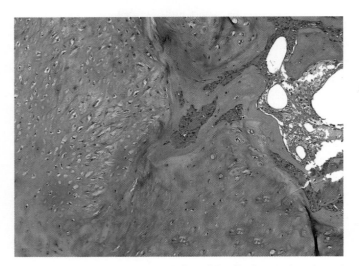

Fig. 21.22 Enchondroma composed of a nodule of hyaline cartilage encased by a thin layer of reactive bone.

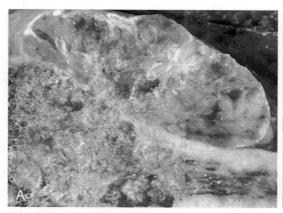

Fig. 21.23 Chondrosarcoma. (A) Nodules of hyaline and myxoid cartilage permeating throughout the medullary cavity, growing through the cortex, and forming a relatively well-circumscribed soft tissue mass. (B) Conventional chondrosarcoma entraps native lamellar bone as a confluent mass of cartilage.

differentiation and a characteristic molecular signature (see later). Entities previously classified as **primitive neuroectodermal tumor** (PNET) and Askin tumor have been unified into the single category of Ewing sarcoma.

Ewing sarcoma accounts for approximately 10% of primary malignant bone tumors and follows osteosarcoma as the second most common bone sarcoma in children. Of all bone sarcomas, Ewing sarcomas have the youngest average age at presentation (80% are younger than 20 years). Boys are affected slightly more frequently than girls, and there is a predilection for Caucasians. The tumors usually arise in the diaphysis of long tubular bones but 20% are extraskeletal. They present as painful enlarging masses, and the affected site is frequently tender, warm, and swollen. Plain radiographs show a destructive lytic tumor with permeative margins that extends into the surrounding soft tissues. The characteristic periosteal reaction produces layers of reactive bone deposited in an *onion-skin* fashion.

Pathogenesis

The vast majority (85%) of Ewing sarcomas contain a balanced (11;22) (q24;q12) translocation generating in-frame fusion of the *EWSR1* gene on chromosome 22 to the *FLI1* gene on chromosome 11. Variant translocations fuse *EWSR1* to other members of the ETS transcription factor family. How EWS fusion proteins contribute to transformation remains unsettled; effects on transcription, RNA splicing, and the cell cycle machinery have all been proposed. Similarly, the cell of origin still remains to be identified; the leading candidates are mesenchymal stem cells and primitive neuroectodermal cells.

⬤ MORPHOLOGY

Arising in the medullary cavity, Ewing sarcoma usually invades the cortex, periosteum, and soft tissue. The tumor is soft, tan-white, and frequently contains areas of hemorrhage and necrosis. It is one of the small, round blue cell tumors found in children (Chapter 7). Like other tumors in this group, Ewing sarcoma is composed of sheets of uniform small, round cells that are slightly larger and more cohesive than lymphocytes (Fig. 21.24). They have scant cytoplasm, which may appear clear because it is rich in glycogen. Homer-Wright rosettes (round groupings of cells with a central fibrillary core) may be present and indicate a greater degree of neuroectodermal differentiation. The tumor cells do not produce bone or cartilage.

Clinical Course

Ewing sarcomas are aggressive malignancies treated with neoadjuvant chemotherapy followed by surgical excision with or without radiation. With chemotherapy, 5-year survival of 75% and long-term cure in 50% of patients is possible.

Giant Cell Tumor

Giant cell tumor is so named because **multinucleated osteoclast-type giant cells dominate the histology.** It is a locally aggressive neoplasm that almost exclusively affects adults. Giant cell tumors arise in the epiphyses of long bones, most commonly the distal femur and proximal tibia. The typical location of these tumors near joints frequently

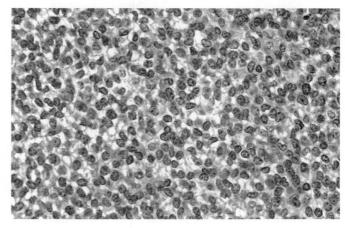

Fig. 21.24 Ewing sarcoma composed of sheets of small round cells with small amounts of clear cytoplasm.

causes arthritis-like symptoms. Occasionally, they present with pathologic fractures.

Pathogenesis

Experimental evidence suggests that the neoplastic cells of the giant cell tumor are osteoblast precursors, which represent only a minority of the cells in the tumor. The neoplastic cells express high levels of RANKL, which promotes the proliferation and differentiation of normal osteoclast precursors into osteoclasts. The osteoclasts in turn cause localized but highly destructive resorption of bone.

MORPHOLOGY

Giant cell tumors often destroy the overlying cortex, producing a bulging soft tissue mass delineated by a thin shell of reactive bone (Fig. 21.25). Grossly, they are red-brown masses that frequently undergo cystic degeneration. Microscopically, the tumor conspicuously lacks bone or cartilage, consisting of numerous osteoclast-type giant cells with 100 or more nuclei with uniform, oval mononuclear tumor cells in between (Fig. 21.26).

Clinical Course

Giant cell tumors are typically treated with curettage, but 40% to 60% recur locally. Up to 4% of tumors metastasize to the lungs, but these sometimes spontaneously regress and they are seldom fatal. The RANKL inhibitor, Denosumab, has shown promise in treating giant cell tumor.

Aneurysmal Bone Cyst

Aneurysmal bone cyst (ABC) is a benign tumor characterized by multiloculated blood-filled cystic spaces. ABC generally occurs during the first 2 decades of life and has

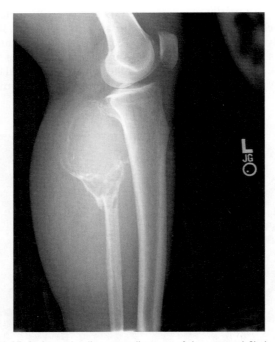

Fig. 21.25 Radiographically, giant cell tumor of the proximal fibula is predominantly lytic, expansile with destruction of the cortex. A pathologic fracture is also present.

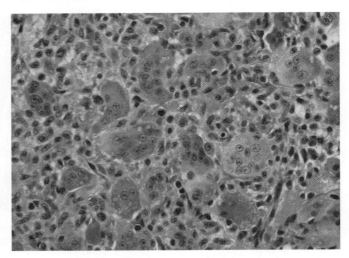

Fig. 21.26 Giant cell tumor illustrating an abundance of multinucleated giant cells with background mononuclear stromal cells.

no sex predilection. It most frequently develops in the metaphysis of long bones and the posterior elements of vertebral bodies. Pain and swelling are common.

Radiographically, ABC is usually an eccentric, expansile, lytic, metaphyseal lesion with well-defined margins (Fig. 21.27A). Computed tomography and magnetic resonance imaging may demonstrate internal septa and characteristic fluid-fluid levels (Fig. 21.27B).

Pathogenesis

The spindle-shaped cells of primary ABC frequently demonstrate rearrangements of chromosome 17p13 resulting in fusion of the coding region of *USP6* to the regulatory elements of genes that are highly expressed in osteoblasts, leading to USP6 overexpression. *USP6* encodes an enzyme that removes ubiquitin residues from proteins (a deubiquitinase). It is proposed that increased USP6 expression enhances the activity of the transcription factor NF-κB. Increased NF-κB activity may upregulate matrix metalloproteases, leading to cystic resorption of bone.

MORPHOLOGY

Aneurysmal bone cyst consists of multiple blood-filled cystic spaces separated by thin, tan-white septae (Fig. 21.28). The septae are composed of plump uniform fibroblasts, multinucleated osteoclast-like giant cells, and reactive woven bone, but they are not covered by endothelium.

Clinical Course

The treatment of ABC is surgical. Curettage is effective with low risk of recurrence.

Lesions Simulating Primary Neoplasms

Nonossifying Fibroma

Nonossifying fibroma (NOF) is a benign, likely reactive, mesenchymal proliferation that may be present in

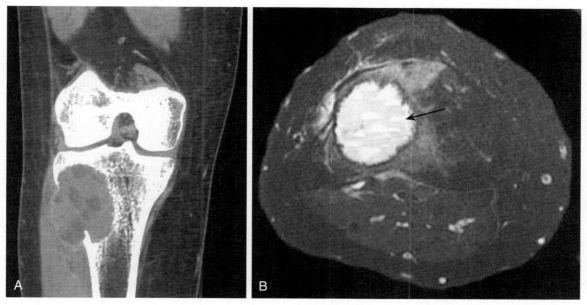

Fig. 21.27 (A) Coronal computed axial tomography scan showing eccentric aneurysmal bone cyst of tibia. The soft tissue component is delineated by a thin rim of reactive subperiosteal bone. (B) Axial magnetic resonance image demonstrating characteristic fluid-fluid levels *(arrow)*.

as many as 50% of children and young adults aged 2–25 years. It is synonymous with **fibrous cortical defect** or **metaphyseal fibrous defect** if localized to the cortex or medulla, respectively. The vast majority arises eccentrically in the metaphysis of the distal femur and proximal tibia. Plain radiographs show a sharply demarcated oval radiolucency with the long axis parallel to the cortex (Fig. 21.29). The findings are sufficiently specific on plain radiography that biopsy is rarely necessary. NOFs form gray to yellow-brown cellular lesions containing fibroblasts and macrophages. The cytologically bland fibroblasts are frequently arranged in a storiform (pinwheel) pattern, and the macrophages may take the form of clustered cells with foamy cytoplasm or multinucleated giant cells (Fig. 21.30). Hemosiderin is commonly present. Most small NOFs undergo spontaneous resolution within several years.

Fibrous Dysplasia

Fibrous dysplasia is a benign tumor that has been likened to a localized developmental arrest of bone constituents. The lesions arise during skeletal development, and they appear in several distinctive but sometimes overlapping clinical patterns:
- *Monostotic*: involvement of a single bone
- *Polyostotic*: involvement of multiple bones

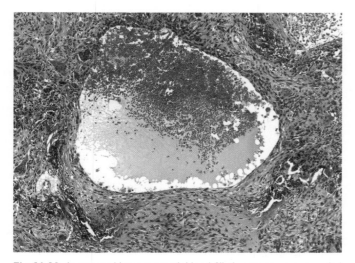

Fig. 21.28 Aneurysmal bone cyst with blood-filled cystic space surrounded by a fibrous wall containing proliferating fibroblasts, reactive woven bone, and osteoclast-type giant cells.

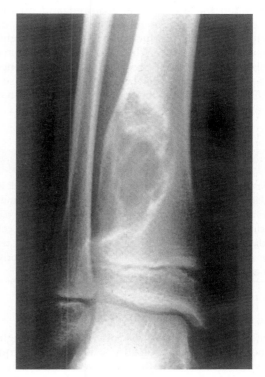

Fig. 21.29 Nonossifying fibroma of the distal tibia metaphysis producing an eccentric lobulated radiolucency surrounded by a sclerotic margin.

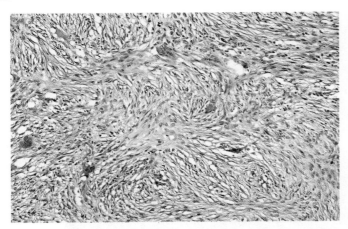

Fig. 21.30 Storiform pattern created by benign spindle cells with scattered osteoclast-type giant cells characteristic of a fibrous cortical defect.

- *Mazabraud syndrome*: fibrous dysplasia and soft tissue myxoma
- *McCune-Albright syndrome*: polyostotic fibrous dysplasia, café-au-lait skin pigmentations, and endocrine abnormalities, especially precocious puberty

Pathogenesis

All of the aforementioned variants result from a somatic gain-of-function mutation in *GNAS1*, the gene that is also mutated in pituitary adenomas (Chapter 20). The mutations produce a constitutively active G_s-protein that promotes cellular proliferation by increasing cellular levels of cAMP. The phenotype depends on the stage of embryogenesis when the mutation is acquired and on the fate of the cell harboring the mutation. A mutation during early embryogenesis produces the McCune-Albright syndrome, whereas a mutation during or after formation of the skeleton in an osteoblast precursor results in monostotic fibrous dysplasia. The skeletal manifestations arise from a cAMP–mediated interruption of normal osteoblast differentiation.

MORPHOLOGY

The lesions of fibrous dysplasia are well circumscribed, intramedullary, and vary greatly in size. Larger lesions expand and distort the bone. The lesional tissue is composed of curvilinear trabeculae of woven bone surrounded by a moderately cellular fibroblastic proliferation. The trabeculae lack prominent osteoblastic rimming (Fig. 21.31). Cystic degeneration, hemorrhage, and foamy macrophages are other common findings.

Clinical Course

Monostotic fibrous dysplasia often stops enlarging at the time of growth plate closure. The lesion is frequently asymptomatic and is usually discovered incidentally, but it may cause pain, fracture, and discrepancies in limb length. Symptomatic lesions are cured by curettage.

Polyostotic fibrous dysplasia may continue to cause problems into adulthood. If it involves the limb girdles, it can cause crippling deformities and fractures. The *McCune-Albright syndrome* usually presents with precocious sexual development, most often in girls. The skeletal manifestations are managed as for other polyostotic fibrous dysplasia, whereas the endocrinopathies are treated medically.

Metastatic Tumors

Metastatic tumors greatly outnumber primary bone cancers. The pathways of tumor spread to bone include (1) direct extension, (2) lymphatic or hematogenous dissemination, and (3) intraspinal seeding (via the Batson plexus of veins). Any cancer can spread to bone, but in adults more than 75% of skeletal metastases originate from cancers of the prostate, breast, kidney, and lung. In children, metastases to bone originate from neuroblastoma, Wilms tumor, and rhabdomyosarcoma.

Skeletal metastases are typically multifocal and involve the axial skeleton, especially the vertebral column. The radiographic appearance of metastases may be purely *lytic* (bone destroying), purely *blastic* (bone forming), or *mixed*. Bidirectional interactions between metastatic cancer cells and native bone cells account for the changes that manifest in the bone matrix. Tumor cells secrete substances such as prostaglandins, cytokines, and PTH-like peptide that upregulate RANKL on osteoblasts and stromal cells thereby stimulating osteoclast activity. At the same time, tumor cell growth is supported by the release of matrix-bound growth factors (e.g., TGF-β, IGF-1, and FGF) as bone is resorbed. Tumor cells secreting WNT proteins that stimulate osteoblastic bone formation may produce sclerotic metastases.

The presence of bone metastases carries a poor prognosis. Therapeutic options include systemic chemotherapy, radiation, and bisphosphonates. Surgery may be necessary to stabilize pathologic fractures.

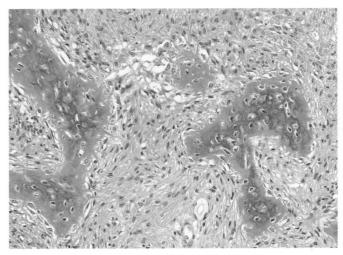

Fig. 21.31 Fibrous dysplasia composed of curvilinear trabeculae of woven bone that lack conspicuous osteoblastic rimming and arise in a background of fibrous tissue.

● SUMMARY

BONE TUMORS AND TUMORLIKE LESIONS

Primary bone tumors are classified according to the cell of origin or the matrix that they produce. The remainder is grouped according to clinicopathologic features. Most primary bone tumors are benign. Metastases, especially from lung, prostate, kidneys, and breast, are far more common than primary bone neoplasms.

Major categories of primary bone tumors include

- **Bone forming:** Osteoblastoma and osteoid osteoma consist of benign osteoblasts that synthesize osteoid. Osteosarcoma is an aggressive tumor of malignant osteoblasts, predominantly occurring in adolescents.
- **Cartilage forming:** Osteochondroma is an exostosis with a cartilage cap. Sporadic and syndromic forms arise from mutations in the *EXT* genes. Chondromas are benign tumors producing hyaline cartilage, usually arising in the digits. Chondrosarcomas are malignant tumors of chondroid cells that involve the axial skeleton in adults.
- **Ewing sarcomas** are aggressive, malignant, small round cell tumors most often associated with t(11;22).
- **Fibrous dysplasia** is an example of a disorder caused by gain-of-function mutations that occur during development.

Joints

Joints allow movement while providing mechanical stability. They are classified as *solid (nonsynovial)* and *cavitated (synovial)*. The solid joints, also known as *synarthroses*, provide structural integrity and allow only minimal movement. They lack a joint space and are grouped according to the type of connective tissue (fibrous tissue or cartilage) that bridges the ends of the bones. Fibrous synarthroses include the cranial sutures and the bonds between roots of teeth and the jawbones. Cartilaginous synarthroses (synchondroses) are represented by the symphyses between the sternum and the ribs and between bones of the pelvis. Synovial joints, in contrast, have a joint space that allows for a wide range of motion. Synovial membranes enclose these joints. The membranes are lined by type A synoviocytes that are specialized macrophages with phagocytic activity and type B synoviocytes that are similar to fibroblasts and synthesize hyaluronic acid and various proteins. The synovial lining lacks a basement membrane, which allows for efficient exchange of nutrients, wastes, and gases between blood and synovial fluid. Synovial fluid is a plasma filtrate containing hyaluronic acid produced by synovial cells that acts as a viscous lubricant and provides nutrition for the articular cartilage.

Hyaline cartilage is a unique connective tissue ideally suited to serve as an elastic shock absorber and wear-resistant surface. It lacks a blood supply, lymphatic drainage, and innervation. Hyaline cartilage is composed of water (70%), type II collagen (10%), proteoglycans (8%), and chondrocytes. The collagen resists tensile stresses and transmits vertical loads. The water and proteoglycans resist compression and limit friction. The chondrocytes synthesize the matrix as well as enzymatically digest it. Chondrocytes secrete degradative enzymes in inactive forms and enrich the matrix with enzyme inhibitors.

ARTHRITIS

Osteoarthritis

Osteoarthritis (OA), also called degenerative joint disease, is characterized by degeneration of cartilage that results in structural and functional failure of synovial joints. It is the most common disease of joints. Although the term *osteoarthritis* implies an inflammatory disease, it is considered an intrinsic disorder of cartilage in which chondrocytes respond to biochemical and mechanical stresses resulting in the breakdown of the matrix and failure of its repair. Nevertheless there is little doubt that inflammatory mediators (described later) whose release is triggered by joint injury perpetuate and worsen the damage.

In most instances OA appears insidiously, without apparent initiating cause, as an aging phenomenon (*idiopathic* or *primary osteoarthritis*). In these cases the disease is usually oligoarticular (affects few joints). In about 5% of cases, OA appears in younger individuals with some predisposing condition, such as joint deformity, a previous joint injury, or an underlying systemic disease that places joints at risk. In these settings the disease is called *secondary osteoarthritis*. The prevalence of OA increases exponentially beyond the age of 50, and about 40% of people older than 70 are affected.

Pathogenesis

The lesions of OA stem from degeneration of the articular cartilage and its disordered repair. Articular cartilage serves as a low-friction surface that transmits loads to the underlying bone. Cartilage resists compression through the viscoelastic properties of the extracellular matrix (principally type II collagen, proteoglycans, and water) secreted by chondrocytes. Repeated biomechanical stress contributes to development of OA, but genetic factors, including genes encoding components of the matrix and signaling molecules, also play a role. These factors are thought to predispose to chondrocyte injury, which in turn leads to alteration of the extracellular matrix (Fig. 21.32). Although chondrocytes proliferate and continuously synthesize and secrete proteoglycans, degradation ultimately exceeds synthesis, and the composition of proteoglycans changes as the disease progresses. Meanwhile, MMPs secreted by chondrocytes degrade the type II collagen network. Cytokines and diffusible factors from chondrocytes and synovial cells, particularly TGF-β (which induces MMPs), TNF, prostaglandins, and nitric oxide, have been implicated in OA (Fig. 21.32). Chronic, low-level inflammation contributes to the progression of the disease. Ultimately, chondrocyte loss and a severely degraded matrix mark the late stage of the disease.

Clinical Course

> ## MORPHOLOGY
>
> In the early stages of OA, chondrocytes proliferate, forming clusters. Concurrently, the water content of the matrix increases and the concentration of proteoglycans decreases. The normally horizontally arranged collagen type II fibers are cleaved, yielding fissures and clefts at the articular surface (Fig. 21.33). This
>
> manifests as a granular soft articular surface. Eventually, full-thickness portions of the cartilage are sloughed. The dislodged pieces of cartilage and subchondral bone tumble into the joint, forming loose bodies *(joint mice)*. The exposed subchondral bone plate becomes the new articular surface, and friction with the opposing surface burnishes the exposed bone, giving it the appearance of polished ivory *(bone eburnation)* (Fig. 21.33). Small fractures through the articulating bone are common, and the fracture gaps allow synovial fluid to be forced into the subchondral regions in a one-way, ball valve–like mechanism forming fibrous-walled cysts. Outgrowths *(osteophytes)* develop at the margins of the articular surface and are capped by fibrocartilage and hyaline cartilage that gradually ossify. The synovium is usually only mildly congested and fibrotic, and it may have scattered chronic inflammatory cells.

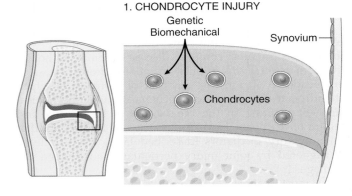

1. CHONDROCYTE INJURY

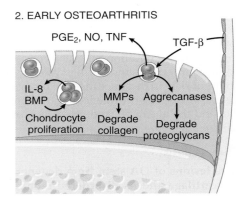

2. EARLY OSTEOARTHRITIS

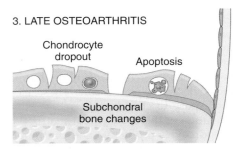

3. LATE OSTEOARTHRITIS

Fig. 21.32 Schematic view of osteoarthritis (OA). OA is thought to be initiated by chondrocyte injury (1) in a genetically predisposed patient leading to changes in the extracellular matrix. (2) Although chondrocytes may proliferate and attempt to repair damaged matrix, continued degradation exceeds repair in early OA. (3) Late OA is evidenced by loss of both matrix and chondrocytes with subchondral bone damage.

Primary OA usually presents in patients they are in their 50s. If a young person has significant manifestations of OA, a search for some underlying cause should be made. Characteristic symptoms include joint pain that worsens with use, morning stiffness, crepitus, and limitation of range of movement. Impingement on spinal foramina by osteophytes results in cervical and lumbar nerve root compression and radicular pain, muscle spasms, muscle atrophy, and neurologic deficits. The joints commonly involved include the hips (Fig. 21.34), knees, lower lumbar and cervical vertebrae, proximal and distal interphalangeal joints of the fingers, first carpometacarpal joints, and first tarsometatarsal joints. *Heberden nodes*, prominent osteophytes at the distal interphalangeal joints, are common in women (but not in men). With time, joint deformity can occur, but unlike rheumatoid arthritis (discussed next), joint fusion does not take place (Fig. 21.35). The level of disease severity detected radiographically, however, does not correlate well with pain and disability. There are still no satisfactory means of preventing primary OA, and there are no effective methods of halting its progression. Therapy includes management of pain, NSAIDs to reduce inflammation, intra-articular corticosteroids, activity modification, and, for severe cases, arthroplasty.

Rheumatoid Arthritis

Rheumatoid arthritis (RA) is a chronic inflammatory disorder of autoimmune origin that principally attacks the joints, producing a nonsuppurative proliferative and inflammatory synovitis. RA often progresses to the destruction of the articular cartilage and, in some cases ankylosis (adhesion) of the joints. Extraarticular lesions may occur in the skin, heart, blood vessels, and lungs. The prevalence in the United States is approximately 1%, and it is three times more common in women than in men. The peak incidence is in the third through fifth decades of life.

Pathogenesis

As in other autoimmune diseases, genetic predisposition and environmental factors contribute to the development, progression, and chronicity of the disease. The pathologic changes are mediated by antibodies against self-antigens

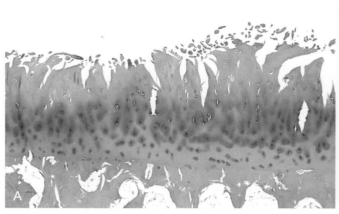
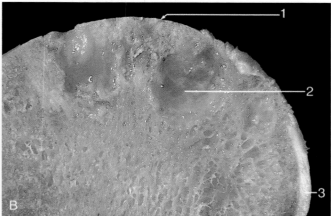

Fig. 21.33 Osteoarthritis. (A) Histologic demonstration of the characteristic fibrillation of the articular cartilage. (B) Eburnated articular surface exposing subchondral bone (1), subchondral cyst (2), and residual articular cartilage (3).

and inflammation caused by cytokines, predominantly secreted by CD4+ T cells (Fig. 21.36).

CD4+ T helper (T_H) cells may initiate the autoimmune response in RA by reacting with an arthritogen, perhaps microbial or a chemically modified self-antigen. The T cells produce cytokines that stimulate other inflammatory cells to effect tissue injury:

- IFN-γ from T$_H$1 cells activates macrophages and synovial cells.
- IL-17 from T$_H$17 cells recruits neutrophils and monocytes.

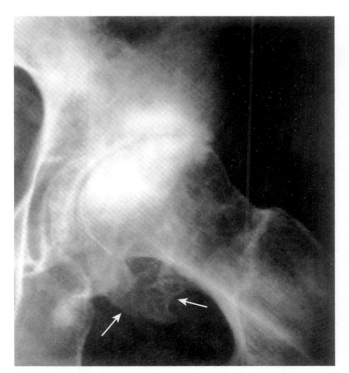

Fig. 21.34 Severe osteoarthritis of the hip. The joint space is narrowed, and there is subchondral sclerosis with scattered oval radiolucent cysts and peripheral osteophyte lipping (arrows).

- RANKL expressed on activated T cells stimulates osteoclasts and bone resorption.
- TNF and IL-1 from macrophages stimulate resident synovial cells to secrete proteases that destroy hyaline cartilage.

Of these, TNF has been most firmly implicated in the pathogenesis of RA, and TNF antagonists have proved to be effective therapies for the disease (see later).

The synovium of RA contains germinal centers with secondary follicles and abundant plasma cells that produce antibodies, some of which may be against self-antigens. Many of the serum autoantibodies detected in patients are specific for *citrullinated peptides* in which arginine residues are posttranslationally converted to citrulline. In RA, complexes of antibodies with citrullinated fibrinogen, type II collagen, α-enolase, and vimentin deposit in the joints. Evidence suggests that the anti-citrullinated protein antibodies (ACPA) in combination with a T cell response to the citrullinated proteins contribute to disease chronicity. Approximately 30% of RA patients do not have ACPA in the blood. About 80% of patients have serum IgM or IgA autoantibodies that bind to the Fc portions of their own IgG. These autoantibodies are called *rheumatoid factor* and may also deposit in joints as immune complexes, although they are not uniformly present in all patients with RA and can be found in patients without the disease.

It is estimated that 50% of the risk of developing RA is related to inherited genetic susceptibility. The *HLA* class II locus is associated with ACPA-positive RA. Evidence suggests that an epitope on a citrullinated protein, vinculin, mimics an epitope on many microbes and is the target of CD4+ T cells when presented by predisposing HLA-DQ alleles. A second gene linked to RA, *PTPN22*, encodes a protein tyrosine phosphatase that is postulated to inhibit T cell activation. Numerous other genetic associations have been reported.

Many candidate environmental factors whose antigens promote autoimmunity have been postulated. At least 70% of RA patients have ACPA in their blood, which may

OSTEOARTHRITIS   RHEUMATOID ARTHRITIS

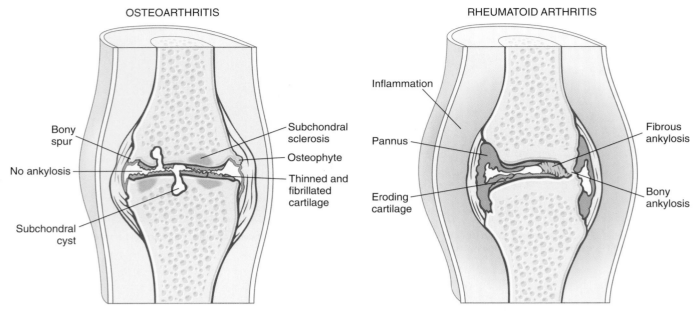

Fig. 21.35 Comparison of the morphologic features of rheumatoid arthritis and osteoarthritis.

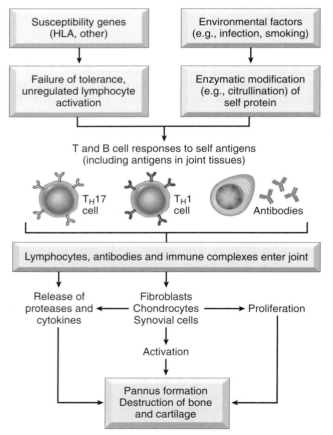

Fig. 21.36 Major processes involved in the pathogenesis of rheumatoid arthritis.

be produced during inflammation. Insults such as infection (including periodontitis) and smoking may promote citrullination of self-proteins, creating new epitopes that trigger autoimmune reactions.

The inflammation localizes to the joint, recruiting macrophages and triggering activation and/or proliferation of synovial cells, chondrocytes, and fibroblasts. The production of proteolytic enzymes and cytokines contributes to the destruction of cartilage and, through increased osteoclast activity, bone (Fig. 21.36).

MORPHOLOGY

RA typically manifests as symmetric arthritis principally affecting the small joints of the hands and feet. Grossly, the synovium becomes edematous, thickened, and hyperplastic, transforming its smooth contour to one covered by delicate and bulbous villi (Fig. 21.37A–B). The characteristic histologic features include (1) **synovial cell hyperplasia** and proliferation; (2) **dense inflammatory infiltrates** of CD4+ helper T cells, B cells, plasma cells, dendritic cells, and macrophages (Fig. 21.37C); (3) increased vascularity resulting from angiogenesis; (4) neutrophils and aggregates of organizing fibrin on the synovial and joint surfaces; (5) osteoclastic activity in underlying bone, allowing the synovium to penetrate into the bone, causing periarticular erosions and subchondral cysts. Together, the aforementioned changes produce a **pannus:** a mass of edematous synovium, inflammatory cells, granulation tissue, and fibroblasts that grows over the articular cartilage and causes its erosion. In advanced untreated cases the pannus can bridge the bones to form a **fibrous ankylosis,** which may later ossify as a **bony ankylosis** (Fig. 21.35).

Rheumatoid nodules are an infrequent manifestation of RA and typically occur in subcutaneous tissue including the forearm, elbows, occiput, and lumbosacral area. Microscopically, they resemble necrotizing granulomas (Fig. 21.38). Rarely, RA can involve the lungs (rheumatoid nodules, interstitial lung disease).

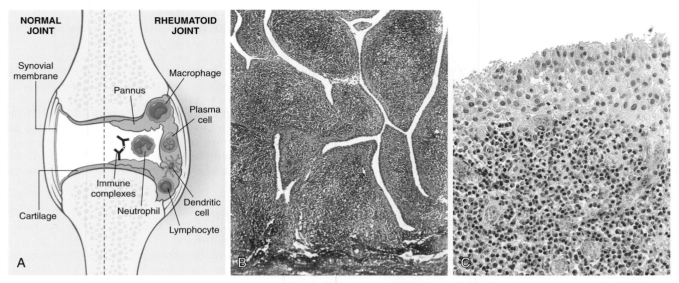

Fig. 21.37 Rheumatoid arthritis. (A) Schematic view of the joint lesion. (B) Low magnification shows marked synovial hypertrophy with formation of villi. (C) At higher magnification, subsynovial tissue containing a dense lymphoid aggregate. (A, *Modified from Feldmann M: Development of anti-TNF therapy for rheumatoid arthritis.* Nat Rev Immunol 2:364, 2002.)

Clinical Course

RA can be distinguished from other forms of polyarticular inflammatory arthritis by the presence of ACPA and by characteristic radiographic findings. In about half of patients, RA begins slowly and insidiously with malaise, fatigue, and generalized musculoskeletal pain. After several weeks to months, the joints become involved. The pattern of joint involvement is generally symmetrical and the hands and feet, wrists, ankles, elbows, and knees are most commonly affected. The metacarpophalangeal and proximal interphalangeal joints are frequently involved (in contrast to OA, see earlier).

Involved joints are swollen, warm, and painful. In contrast to OA, the joints are stiff when patient rises in the morning or following inactivity. The typical patient has progressive joint enlargement and decreased range of motion pursuing a chronic waxing and waning course. In a minority of patients, especially those lacking RF and ACPA, the disease may stabilize or even regress.

Inflammation in the tendons, ligaments, and occasionally the adjacent skeletal muscle frequently accompanies the arthritis and produces the characteristic ulnar deviation of the fingers and flexion-hyperextension of the fingers (swan-neck deformity, boutonnière deformity). Radiographic hallmarks are joint effusions and juxtaarticular osteopenia with erosions and narrowing of the joint space and loss of articular cartilage (Fig. 21.39).

The treatment for RA consists of corticosteroids, other immunosuppressants such as methotrexate, and, most notably, TNF antagonists. However, anti-TNF agents are not curative, and patients must be maintained on TNF antagonists to avoid disease flares. Long term treatment with TNF antagonists carries with it increased risk of infections with organisms such as *M. tuberculosis*.

Juvenile Idiopathic Arthritis

Juvenile idiopathic arthritis (JIA) is a heterogeneous group of disorders of unknown cause that present with arthritis before age 16 and persist for at least 6 weeks. In contrast to RA, in JIA: (1) oligoarthritis is more common, (2) systemic disease is more frequent, (3) large joints are affected more often than small joints, (4) rheumatoid nodules and rheumatoid factor are usually absent, and (5) anti-nuclear antibody (ANA) seropositivity is common. The pathogenesis is unknown but similar to adult RA; risk factors include *HLA* and *PTPN22* variants. Also, like adult RA, damage in JIA appears to be caused by T_H1 and T_H17 cells and cytokines produced by these and other inflammatory cells. Treatment is similar to adult RA with some success in using an IL-6 receptor antibody in the systemic form. Long-term prognosis of JIA is very variable. Although many affected individuals have

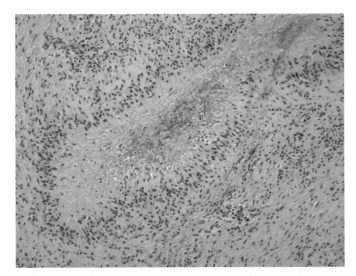

Fig. 21.38 Rheumatoid nodule composed of central necrosis rimmed by palisaded histiocytes.

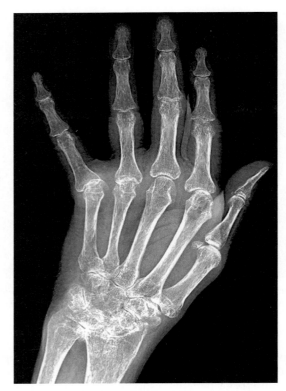

Fig. 21.39 Rheumatoid arthritis of the hand. Characteristic features include diffuse osteopenia, marked loss of the joint spaces of the carpal, metacarpal, phalangeal, and interphalangeal joints, periarticular bony erosions, and ulnar drift of the fingers.

chronic disease, only about 10% develop serious functional disability.

Seronegative Spondyloarthropathies

The spondyloarthropathies are a heterogeneous group of disorders that share the following features:

- Absence of rheumatoid factor
- Pathologic changes in the ligamentous attachments rather than synovium
- Involvement of sacroiliac joints, with or without other joints
- Association with HLA-B27
- Bony proliferation leading to ankylosis (fusion of joints)

The manifestations are immune mediated and are triggered by a T cell response presumably directed against an undefined antigen, possibly infectious, that may cross-react with antigens expressed on cells of the musculoskeletal system.

Ankylosing spondylitis, the prototypical spondyloarthritis, causes destruction of articular cartilage and bony ankylosis, especially of the sacroiliac joints. The disease becomes symptomatic in the second and third decades of life as lower back pain and spinal immobility. Involvement of peripheral joints, such as the hips, knees, and shoulders, occurs in at least one-third of affected individuals. Approximately 90% of patients are HLA-B27 positive, but how the B27 allele contributes to the disease is not known. An anti-IL-17 antibody has shown some efficacy in this disease.

Reactive arthritis is defined by a triad of arthritis, nongonococcal urethritis or cervicitis, and conjunctivitis. Most affected individuals are men in their 20s or 30s, and more than 80% are HLA-B27 positive. The disease is probably caused by an autoimmune reaction initiated by previous infection of the genitourinary system (*Chlamydia*) or the gastrointestinal tract (*Shigella, Salmonella, Yersinia, Campylobacter*). Within several weeks of urethritis or diarrhea, patients experience low back pain. The ankles, knees, and feet are affected most often, frequently in an asymmetric pattern. Patients with severe chronic disease have involvement of the spine that is indistinguishable from ankylosing spondylitis.

Infectious Arthritis

Joints can become infected from hematogenous dissemination, direct inoculation through the skin, or from contiguous spread from a soft tissue abscess or osteomyelitis. Infectious arthritis is potentially serious, because it can cause rapid, permanent joint destruction.

Suppurative Arthritis

Bacterial infections that cause acute suppurative arthritis usually enter the joints from distant sites by hematogenous spread. In neonates, however, contiguous spread from underlying epiphyseal osteomyelitis may occur. *H. influenza* arthritis predominates in children younger than 2 years of age, *S. aureus* is the main agent in older children and adults, and gonococcus is prevalent during late adolescence and young adulthood. Individuals with sickle cell disease are prone to infection with *Salmonella*. These joint infections affect the sexes equally except for gonococcal arthritis, which is seen mainly in sexually active women. Individuals with deficiencies of complement components (C5, C6, C7, or C9) are susceptible to disseminated gonococcal infections and hence arthritis.

The classic presentation is the sudden development of an acutely painful, warm, and swollen joint that has a restricted range of motion. Systemic findings of fever, leukocytosis, and elevated sedimentation rate are common. In 90% of nongonococcal cases, the infection involves only a single joint, most commonly the knee, followed in decreasing frequency by the hip, shoulder, elbow, wrist, and sternoclavicular joints. The axial joints are more often involved in drug users. Joint aspiration is diagnostic if it yields purulent fluid in which the causative agent can be identified. As mentioned earlier, cartilage has limited repair potential, so prompt recognition and effective anti-microbial therapy is vital to prevent permanent joint destruction.

Lyme Arthritis

Lyme arthritis is the leading arthropod-borne disease in the United States, predominantly affecting New England and mid-Atlantic states, but the geographic range and incidence are increasing. It is caused by infection with the spirochete *Borrelia burgdorferi*, which is transmitted by deer ticks of the *Ixodes ricinus* complex. In its classic form, Lyme disease progressively involves multiple organ systems through three clinical phases (Fig. 21.40). The initial infection of the skin, or *early localized stage*, is followed by *an*

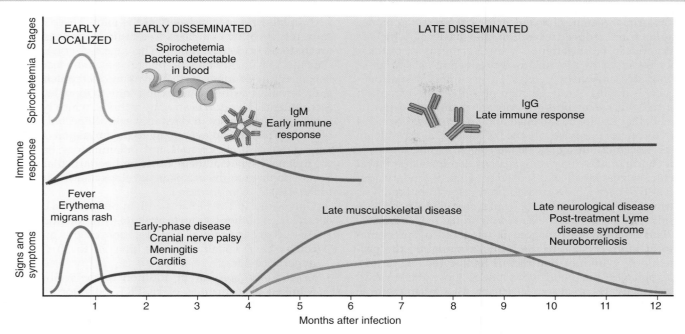

Fig. 21.40 Lyme disease progresses through three clinically recognizable phases: early localized, early disseminated, and late persistent. Although initial manifestations result directly from spirochete infection, later signs and symptoms are likely immune-mediated. *(Figure modified from Dr. Charles Chiu, University of California San Francisco, San Francisco, California. Used with permission.)*

early disseminated stage involving skin, cranial nerves, heart, and meninges. If left untreated, arthritis, especially of the knee, occurs weeks to months after infection.

Currently, arthritis occurs in less than 10% of cases because most patients are cured at an earlier stage. However, if left untreated approximately 60% to 80% of individuals develop a migratory arthritis *(Lyme arthritis)* lasting for weeks to months. Spirochetes can only be identified in about 25% of joints with arthritis, but the diagnosis can be confirmed by serologic testing for anti-*Borrelia* antibodies. Treatment of Lyme disease consists of antibiotics with activity against *Borrelia*. Cure rates of 90% have been achieved with standard regimens. A vaccine is under development. However, a chronic arthritis that is antibiotic refractory can develop in the *late disseminated stage*. In many of these patients, *Borrelia* cannot be detected in the joint fluid even by PCR. It has been proposed that cellular (especially T_H1) and humoral responses to *Borrelia* outer surface protein A may initiate this late, autoimmune, arthritis. The chronic manifestations, in addition to joint pain, can include nonspecific symptoms (fatigue, cognitive complaints), known collectively as *posttreatment Lyme disease syndrome* (PTLDS).

Infected synovium exhibits a chronic synovitis marked by synoviocyte hyperplasia, fibrin deposition, mononuclear cell infiltrates (especially CD4+ T cells), and onion-skin thickening of arterial walls. The morphology in severe cases can closely resemble that of RA.

Crystal-Induced Arthritis

Articular crystal deposits are associated with a variety of joint disorders. Endogenous crystals shown to be pathogenic include monosodium urate (MSU) *(gout)*, calcium pyrophosphate dehydrate *(pseudogout)*, and basic calcium phosphate. Exogenous crystals, such as silicone, polyethylene, and methyl methacrylate used in prosthetic joints, and the debris that accumulates with their erosion, may result in local arthritis. Crystals produce disease by triggering an inflammatory reaction that destroys cartilage.

Gout

Gout is marked by transient attacks of acute arthritis initiated by urate crystals deposited within and around joints. Whether gout is primary or secondary to some other underlying disease, the common feature is excessive uric acid in tissues and body fluids. In the primary form (90% of cases), gout is the major manifestation of the disease and the cause is usually unknown.

Pathogenesis

Hyperuricemia (plasma urate level above 6.8 mg/dL) is necessary, but not sufficient, for the development of gout. Uric acid metabolism can be summarized as follows:

- *Synthesis.* Uric acid is the end product of purine catabolism. Increased synthesis typically reflects some abnormality in purine production. The synthesis of purine nucleotides, in turn, involves two interlinked pathways. In the de novo pathway, purine nucleotides are synthesized from nonpurine precursors, and in salvage pathways they are synthesized from free purine bases obtained through the diet or the catabolism of purine nucleotides.
- *Excretion.* Uric acid is filtered from the circulation by the glomerulus and virtually completely resorbed by the proximal tubule of the kidney. A small fraction of the resorbed uric acid is secreted by the distal nephron and excreted in the urine.

In primary gout, elevated uric acid most commonly results from reduced excretion, the basis of which is unknown in most patients. A small minority of primary gout is caused by uric acid overproduction as a result of identifiable enzymatic defects. For example, partial deficiency of hypoxanthine guanine phosphoribosyl transferase (HGPRT) interrupts the salvage pathway, so purine metabolites cannot be salvaged and are, instead, degraded into uric acid. Complete absence of HGPRT also results in hyperuricemia, but significant neurologic manifestations of this condition (*Lesch-Nyhan syndrome*) dominate the clinical picture so it is classified as secondary gout. Secondary gout can also be caused by increased production (rapid cell lysis during chemotherapy for leukemia, so-called tumor lysis syndrome) or decreased excretion (chronic renal disease).

The inflammation in gout is triggered by precipitation of urate crystals in the joints, stimulating the production of cytokines that recruit leukocytes (Fig. 21.41). Macrophages and neutrophils phagocytose the crystals, which activates a cytosolic sensor, the inflammasome (Chapter 5). The inflammasome activates caspase-1, which is involved in the production of active IL-1β. IL-1 is proinflammatory, and promotes accumulation of more neutrophils and macrophages in the joint. These cells, in turn, release other cytokines, free radicals, proteases, and arachidonic acid metabolites. The ingested crystals also damage the membranes of phagolysosomes, leading to leakage of these mediators. Activation of complement by the alternative pathway may contribute to more leukocyte recruitment. The result is an acute arthritis, which typically remits spontaneously in days to weeks. Repeated attacks of acute arthritis lead eventually to the formation of tophi, aggregates of urate crystals and inflammatory tissue, in the inflamed synovial membranes and periarticular tissue. Severe damage to the cartilage develops and the function of the joints is compromised.

Only about 10% of patients with hyperuricemia develop clinical gout. Other factors contribute symptomatic gout:
- *Age* of the individual and duration of the hyperuricemia. Gout usually appears after 20 to 30 years of hyperuricemia.
- *Genetic predisposition*. In addition to the well-defined X-linked abnormalities of HGPRT, polymorphisms in genes involved with urate or ion transport and possibly inflammation are also associated with gout.
- *Alcohol* consumption.
- *Obesity*.
- *Drugs* (e.g., thiazides) that reduce excretion of urate.

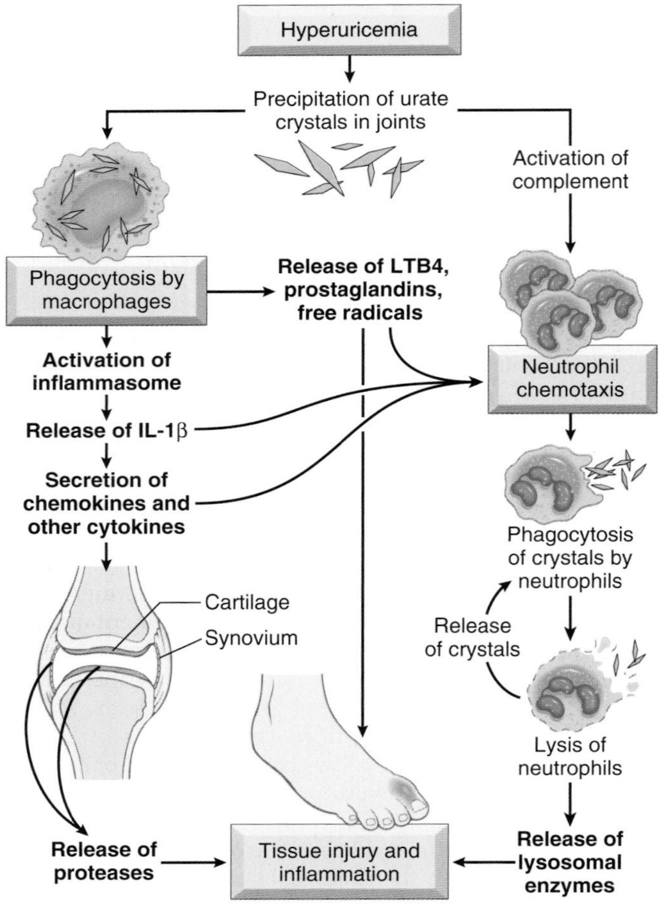

MORPHOLOGY

The distinctive morphologic changes in gout are (1) acute arthritis, (2) chronic tophaceous arthritis, (3) tophi in various sites, and (4) gouty nephropathy.

Acute arthritis is characterized by a dense inflammatory infiltrate that permeates the synovium and synovial fluid. Urate crystals are frequently found in the cytoplasm of the neutrophils and are arranged in small clusters in the synovium. They are long, slender, and needle-shaped, and are negatively birefringent. The synovium is edematous and congested, and it also contains scattered lymphocytes, plasma cells, and macrophages.

Chronic tophaceous arthritis evolves from the repetitive precipitation of urate crystals during acute attacks. The crystals encrust the articular surface and form visible chalky deposits in the synovium (Fig. 21.42A). The synovium becomes hyperplastic, fibrotic, and thickened by inflammatory cells and forms a pannus that destroys the underlying cartilage.

Tophi in the articular cartilage, ligaments, tendons, and bursae are pathognomonic of gout. They are formed by large aggregations of urate crystals surrounded by an intense foreign body giant cell reaction (Fig. 21.42B–C).

Gouty nephropathy refers to the renal complications caused by urate crystals or tophi in the renal medullary interstitium or tubules. Complications include uric acid nephrolithiasis and pyelonephritis.

Fig. 21.41 Pathogenesis of acute gouty arthritis. Urate crystals are phagocytosed by macrophages and stimulate the production of various inflammatory mediators that elicit the inflammation characteristic of gout. Note that IL-1, one of the major pro-inflammatory cytokines, in turn stimulates the production of chemokines and other cytokines from a variety of tissue cells. *LTB4*, Leukotriene B4; *IL-1β*, interleukin 1β.

Clinical Course

Gout is associated with male sex, obesity, metabolic syndrome, excess alchohol intake, renal failure, and age greater than 30 years. Four clinical stages are recognized:
- *Asymptomatic hyperuricemia* appears around puberty in men and after menopause in women.
- *Acute arthritis* presents after several years as sudden onset excruciating joint pain, localized hyperemia, and

warmth. Most first attacks are monoarticular; 50% occur in the first metatarsophalangeal joint. Untreated, acute gouty arthritis may last for hours to weeks, but gradually there is complete resolution.

- *Asymptomatic intercritical period*: Resolution of the acute arthritis leads to a symptom-free interval. In the absence of appropriate therapy, the attacks recur at decreasing intervals and frequently become polyarticular.

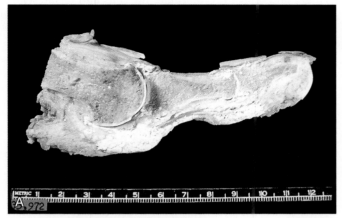

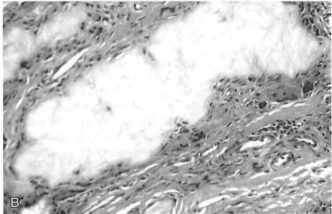

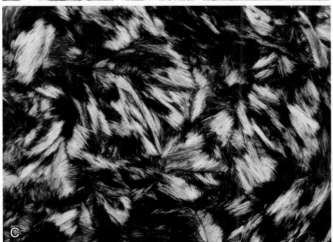

Fig. 21.42 Gout. (A) Amputated great toe with white tophi involving the joint and soft tissues. (B) Gouty tophus—an aggregate of dissolved urate crystals is surrounded by reactive fibroblasts, mononuclear inflammatory cells, and giant cells. (C) Urate crystals are needle shaped and negatively birefringent under polarized light.

- *Chronic tophaceous gout* develops on average about 12 years after the initial acute attack. At this stage, radiographs show characteristic juxtaarticular bone and loss of the joint space.

Treatment of gout aims at lifestyle modification and medication to reduce symptoms (e.g., NSAIDs) and lower urate levels (e.g., xanthine oxidase inhibitor).

Calcium Pyrophosphate Crystal Deposition Disease (Pseudogout)

Calcium pyrophosphate crystal deposition disease (CPPD), also known as *pseudogout,* usually occurs in individuals more than 50 years old and becomes more common with increasing age. The genders and races are equally affected. CPPD is divided into sporadic (idiopathic), hereditary, and secondary types. The autosomal dominant variant is caused by germline mutations in the pyrophosphate transport channel resulting in crystal deposition and arthritis relatively early in life. Various disorders, including previous joint damage, hyperparathyroidism, hemochromatosis, and diabetes, predispose to the secondary form. Studies suggest that articular cartilage proteoglycans, which normally inhibit mineralization, are degraded, allowing crystallization around chondrocytes. As in gout, inflammation is caused by activation of the inflammasome in macrophages.

MORPHOLOGY

The crystals first develop in the articular cartilage, menisci, and intervertebral discs, and as the deposits enlarge they may rupture and seed the joint. The crystals form chalky, white friable deposits, which are seen histologically in hematoxylin- and eosin-stained preparations as oval blue-purple aggregates (Fig. 21.43A). Individual crystals are rhomboid, 0.5 to 5 μm in greatest dimension (Fig. 21.43B), and are positively birefringent. Inflammation is usually milder than in gout.

Clinical Course

CPPD is frequently asymptomatic. However, it may produce acute, subacute, or chronic arthritis that can be confused clinically with OA or RA. The joint involvement may last from several days to weeks and may be monoarticular or polyarticular; the knees, followed by the wrists, elbows, shoulders, and ankles, are most commonly affected. Ultimately, approximately 50% of affected individuals experience significant joint damage. Therapy is supportive. There is no known treatment that prevents or slows crystal formation.

SUMMARY

ARTHRITIS

- **Osteoarthritis (OA, degenerative joint disease),** the most common disease of joints, is a degenerative process of articular cartilage in which matrix breakdown exceeds synthesis. Inflammation is minimal and typically secondary. Local production of inflammatory cytokines may contribute to the progression of joint degeneration.
- **Rheumatoid arthritis (RA)** is a chronic autoimmune inflammatory disease that affects mainly small joints, but can

be systemic. RA is caused by a cellular and humoral immune response against self-antigens, particularly citrullinated proteins. TNF plays a central role and antagonists against TNF are of clinical benefit.

- **Seronegative spondyloarthropathies** are a heterogeneous group of likely autoimmune arthritides that preferentially involve the sacroiliac and vertebral joints and are associated with HLA-B27.
- **Suppurative arthritis** describes direct infection of a joint space by bacterial organisms.
- **Lyme disease** is a systemic infection by *Borrelia burgdorferi*, which manifests, in part, as an infectious arthritis, possibly with an autoimmune component in chronic stages.
- **Gout and pseudogout** result from inflammatory responses triggered by precipitation of urate or calcium pyrophosphate, respectively.

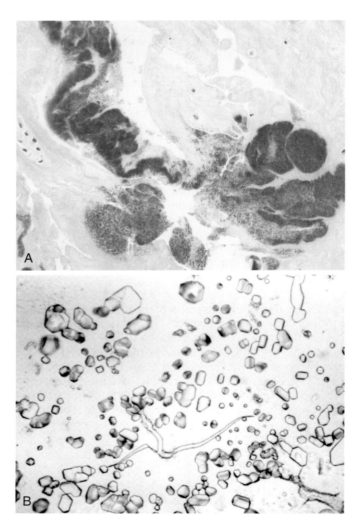

Fig. 21.43 Pseudogout. (A) Deposits are present in cartilage and consist of amorphous basophilic material. (B) Smear preparation of calcium pyrophosphate crystals.

JOINT TUMORS AND TUMORLIKE CONDITIONS

Reactive tumorlike lesions, such as ganglions, synovial cysts, and osteochondral loose bodies, commonly involve joints and tendon sheaths. They usually result from trauma or degenerative processes and are much more common than neoplasms. Primary neoplasms are rare, usually benign, and tend to recapitulate the cells and tissue types (synovial membrane, fat, blood vessels, fibrous tissue, and cartilage) native to joints and related structures. Synovial sarcoma, although once thought to be related to or derived from the tissues of the joint, is now recognized as a sarcoma of uncertain origin and is discussed later with soft tissue tumors.

Ganglion and Synovial Cysts

A *ganglion* is a small (1–1.5 cm) cyst that is almost always located near a joint capsule or tendon sheath. A common location is around the joints of the wrist, where it appears as a firm, fluctuant, pea-sized translucent nodule. It arises as a result of cystic or myxoid degeneration of connective tissue; hence the cyst wall lacks a cell lining. The lesion may be multilocular and enlarges through coalescence of adjacent areas of myxoid change. The fluid that fills the cyst is similar to synovial fluid; however, there is no communication with the joint space. Despite the name, the lesion is unrelated to ganglia of the nervous system.

Herniation of synovium through a joint capsule or massive enlargement of a bursa may produce a *synovial cyst*. A well-recognized example is the synovial cyst that forms in the popliteal space in the setting of RA or OA (*Baker cyst*). The synovial lining may be hyperplastic and contain inflammatory cells and fibrin.

Tenosynovial Giant Cell Tumor

Tenosynovial giant cell tumor is the term for a benign neoplasm that develops in the synovial lining of joints, tendon sheaths, and bursae. Clinical variants of tenosynovial giant cell tumor include the *diffuse type* (previously known as *pigmented villonodular synovitis*), and the *localized type*. Whereas the diffuse form tends to involve large joints, the localized type usually occurs as a discrete nodule attached to a tendon sheath, commonly in the hand.

Pathogenesis

Diffuse and localized types of this tumor both harbor a reciprocal somatic chromosomal translocation, t(1;2)(p13;q37), resulting in fusion of the type VI collagen α-3 promoter to the M-CSF gene. Consequently, the tumor cells overexpress M-CSF, which, through autocrine and paracrine effects, stimulates proliferation of macrophages in a manner similar to giant cell tumor of bone (described previously).

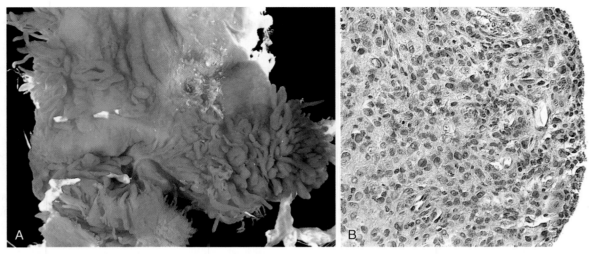

Fig. 21.44 Tenosynovial giant cell tumor, diffuse type. (A) Excised synovium with fronds and nodules typical of pigmented villonodular synovitis. (B) Sheets of proliferating cells in tenosynovial giant cell tumor bulging the synovial lining.

MORPHOLOGY

In diffuse tumors the normally smooth joint synovium is converted into a tangled mat by red-brown folds, fingerlike projections, and nodules (Fig. 21.44A). In contrast, localized (nodular) tumors are well circumscribed. The neoplastic cells, which account for only a minority of the cells in the mass, are polygonal, moderately sized, and resemble synoviocytes (Fig. 21.44B). Both diffuse and localized variants are heavily infiltrated by macrophages containing hemosiderin and foamy lipid, or are multinucleated.

Clinical Course

Diffuse tenosynovial giant cell tumor presents in the knee in 80% of cases. Affected individuals typically complain of pain, locking, and recurrent swelling similar to monoarticular arthritis. Sometimes, a palpable mass is appreciated. The localized variant manifests as a solitary, slow-growing, painless mass that frequently involves the hand. Both types are amenable to surgical excision, but recurrence is more common in the diffuse form. Clinical trials are investigating antagonists of the M-CSF signaling pathway for patients with unresectable disease.

Soft Tissue Tumors

By convention, soft tissue refers to non-epithelial tissue excluding the skeleton, joints, central nervous system, hematopoietic and lymphoid tissues Although nonneoplastic conditions can involve soft tissue, they are seldom confined to this compartment, so the area of soft tissue pathology is restricted to neoplasms.

With the exception of skeletal muscle neoplasms, benign soft tissue tumors outnumber their malignant counterparts, the sarcomas, by 100-fold. In the United States, the incidence of soft tissue sarcomas is approximately 12,000 per year, which is less than 1% of all cancers. Sarcomas, however, cause 2% of all cancer mortality, reflecting their aggressive behavior. Most soft tissue tumors arise in the extremities, especially the thigh. Approximately 15% arise in children but the incidence increases with age.

Pathogenesis

Most sarcomas are sporadic and have no known predisposing cause. A small minority of soft tissue neoplasms are associated with germline mutations in tumor suppressor genes (neurofibromatosis 1, Gardner syndrome, Li-Fraumeni syndrome, Osler-Weber Rendu syndrome). A few tumors can be linked to known environmental exposures such as radiation, burns, or toxins.

Unlike tumors such as colorectal carcinomas that usually arise from recognized precursor lesions, the origin of sarcomas is unknown. The best guess is that the tumors arise from pluripotent mesenchymal stem cells, which acquire somatic "driver" mutations. Despite heterogeneous mechanisms of tumorigenesis among sarcomas, some generalizations can be made based on their genomic complexity:

- *Simple karyotype* (15%–20% of sarcomas): Like many leukemias and lymphomas, sarcomas are often euploid tumors with a single or limited number of chromosomal changes that occur early in tumorigenesis and are specific enough to serve as diagnostic markers. Tumors with these features most commonly arise in younger patients and tend to have a monomorphic appearance microscopically. Examples include Ewing sarcoma, described earlier, and synovial sarcoma. In some cases, the oncogenic effect of these rearrangements is reasonably well understood. In others, the mechanisms are unknown. Oncogenic tumor-specific fusion proteins represent potential molecular targets for therapy.
- *Complex karyotype* (80%–85% of sarcomas): These tumors are usually aneuploid or polyploid and demonstrate multiple chromosomal gains and losses, a feature that suggests underlying genomic instability. Examples

include leiomyosarcoma and undifferentiated pleomorphic sarcoma. Such tumors are more common in adults and tend to be microscopically pleomorphic.

Classification of soft tissue tumors continues to evolve as new molecular genetic abnormalities are identified. Clinically, soft tissue tumors range from benign, self-limited lesions that require minimal treatment to intermediate grade, locally aggressive tumors with minimal metastatic risk to highly aggressive malignancies with significant metastatic risk and mortality. All highly aggressive malignancies are classified as *sarcomas* but this term is less consistently used among the locally aggressive, rarely metastasizing category. Pathologic classification integrates morphology (e.g., muscle differentiation), immunohistochemistry, and molecular diagnostics. In addition to accurate diagnosis, grade (degree of differentiation) and stage (size and depth) are important prognostic indicators.

With this as a primer, we will consider representative or especially illustrative soft tissue tumors.

TUMORS OF ADIPOSE TISSUE

Lipoma

Lipoma, a benign tumor of fat, is the most common soft tissue tumor in adults. The conventional lipoma is the most common subtype, from which rare variants are distinguished according to characteristic morphologic and/or genetic features. Conventional lipoma is a well-encapsulated mass of mature adipocytes. It usually arises in the subcutis of the proximal extremities and trunk, most frequently during middle adulthood. Infrequently, lipomas are large, intramuscular, and poorly circumscribed. Most lipomas are usually cured by simple excision.

Liposarcoma

Liposarcomas are malignant tumors of adipose tissue. Liposarcoma is one of the most common sarcomas of adulthood. It occurs mainly in people in their 50s to 60s in the deep soft tissues and retroperitoneum.

MORPHOLOGY

Liposarcomas are divided into three subtypes:
- Well-differentiated liposarcoma contains adipocytes with scattered atypical spindle cells (Fig. 21.45A). The tumors harbor amplification of chromosome region 12q13-q15, which includes the gene for *MDM2*. You will recall MDM2 encodes a potent inhibitor of p53.
- Myxoid liposarcoma contains abundant basophilic extracellular matrix, arborizing capillaries, and primitive cells at various stages of adipocyte differentiation reminiscent of fetal fat (Fig. 21.45B). The t(12;16) translocation characterizes myxoid liposarcoma. The resultant fusion gene arrests adipose differentiation.
- Pleomorphic liposarcoma consists of sheets of anaplastic cells, bizarre nuclei, and variable amounts of immature adipocytes (lipoblasts). These tumors have complex karyotypes.

Clinical Course

All types of liposarcoma recur locally and often repeatedly unless adequately excised. The well-differentiated variant is relatively indolent, the myxoid/round cell type is intermediate in its malignant behavior, whereas the pleomorphic variant usually is aggressive and frequently metastasizes.

FIBROUS TUMORS

Nodular Fasciitis

Nodular fasciitis is a self-limited fibroblastic and myofibroblastic proliferation that typically occurs the upper extremities of young adults. A history of trauma is present in approximately 25% to 50% of cases, and the tumors grow rapidly during a period of several weeks or months. Whereas nodular fasciitis was historically considered a purely reactive lesion, identification of a t(17;22) translocation producing a *MYH9-USP6* fusion gene indicates that it is a clonal, yet self-limited, proliferation. It is hypothesized that the proliferating cells lack some key hallmark of cancer, perhaps the ability to avoid senescence. Intriguingly, ABC (discussed earlier), another tumor that sits in a gray zone between reactive and neoplastic proliferations, also contains a *USP6* fusion gene. Nodular fasciitis can spontaneously regress and, if excised, rarely recurs. Malignant transformation is virtually nonexistent.

MORPHOLOGY

Nodular fasciitis arises in the deep dermis, subcutis, fascia, or muscle. Grossly the lesion is less than 5 cm, circumscribed, or slightly infiltrative. It is highly cellular containing plump, immature-appearing fibroblasts and myofibroblasts arranged in a pattern reminiscent of cultured fibroblasts (Fig. 21.46). A gradient of maturation *(zonation)* from cellular, loose, and myxoid to organized and fibrous is typical. The cells vary in size and shape (spindle to stellate) and have conspicuous nucleoli; mitotic figures are abundant. Lymphocytes and extravasated red blood cells are common but neutrophils are unusual.

Fibromatoses

Superficial Fibromatosis

Superficial fibromatosis is an infiltrative proliferation that can cause local deformity but has an innocuous clinical course. All forms of superficial fibromatosis affect males more frequently than females. They are characterized by nodular or poorly defined broad fascicles of fibroblasts in long, sweeping fascicles, surrounded by abundant dense collagen. Several clinical subtypes have been identified:
- *Palmar (Dupuytren contracture).* Irregular or nodular thickening of the palmar fascia either unilaterally or bilaterally.
- *Plantar.* Common in young patients, unilateral and without contractures.

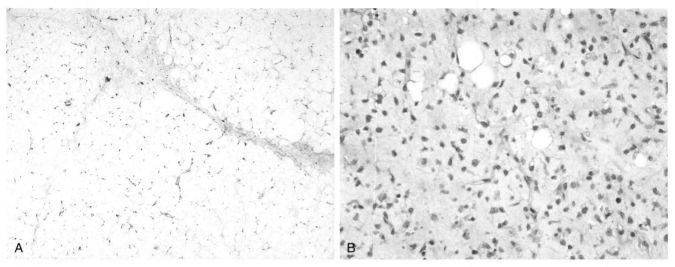

Fig. 21.45 Liposarcoma. (A) The well-differentiated subtype consists of mature adipocytes and scattered spindle cells with hyperchromatic nuclei. (B) Myxoid liposarcoma with abundant ground substance and a rich capillary network in which there are scattered immature adipocytes and more primitive round-to-stellate cells.

- *Penile (Peyronie disease).* Palpable induration or mass on the dorsolateral aspect of the penis.

In about 20% to 25% of cases, the palmar and plantar fibromatoses stabilize and do not progress, in some instances resolving spontaneously. Some recur after excision, particularly the plantar variant.

Deep Fibromatosis

Deep fibromatoses, also called desmoid tumors, are large, infiltrative masses that frequently recur but do not metastasize. They most frequently occur in the teenage years to 30s, predominantly in women. Abdominal fibromatosis generally arises in the musculoaponeurotic structures of the anterior abdominal wall but tumors can arise in the limb girdles or the mesentery. Deep fibromatoses contain mutations in the *CTNNB1* (β-catenin) or *APC* genes, leading to increased Wnt signaling. Most tumors are sporadic, but individuals with familial adenomatous polyposis (Gardner syndrome, Chapter 16) who have germline *APC* mutations are predisposed to deep fibromatosis.

MORPHOLOGY

Fibromatoses are gray-white, firm, poorly demarcated masses varying from 1 to 15 cm in greatest diameter. They are rubbery and tough, and have marked infiltration of surrounding muscle, nerve and fat. Cytologically bland fibroblasts arranged in broad sweeping fascicles amid dense collagen are the characteristic histologic pattern (Fig. 21.47). The histology resembles a scar.

Because of the extensively infiltrative nature, complete excision is often difficult. Recent efforts have concentrated on medical therapy and radiation as alternatives to surgery.

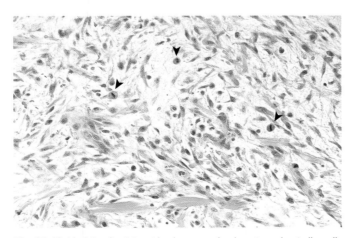

Fig. 21.46 Nodular fasciitis with plump, randomly oriented spindle cells surrounded by myxoid stroma. Note the mitotic activity *(arrowheads)*.

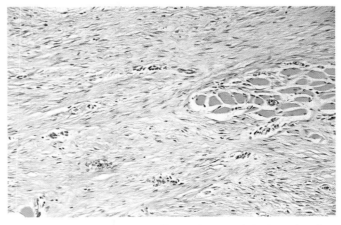

Fig. 21.47 Deep fibromatosis infiltrating between skeletal muscle cells.

SKELETAL MUSCLE TUMORS

Skeletal muscle neoplasms, in contrast to tumors of other lineages, are almost all malignant. The benign rhabdomyoma is more frequent in individuals with tuberous sclerosis.

Rhabdomyosarcoma

Rhabdomyosarcoma is a malignant mesenchymal tumor with skeletal muscle differentiation. Three main subtypes are recognized: *alveolar* (20%), *embryonal* (60%), and *pleomorphic* (20%). Rhabdomyosarcoma (alveolar and embryonal) is the most common soft tissue sarcoma of childhood and adolescence, usually appearing before age 20. Pleomorphic rhabdomyosarcoma is seen predominantly in adults. The pediatric forms often arise in the sinuses, head and neck, and genitourinary tract, locations that do not normally contain much skeletal muscle, underscoring the notion that sarcomas do not arise from mature, terminally differentiated mesenchymal cells. The embryonal and pleomorphic subtypes are genetically heterogeneous.

Alveolar rhabdomyosarcoma frequently contains fusions of the *FOXO1* gene to either the *PAX3* or the *PAX7* gene, rearrangements marked by the presence of (2;13) or (1;13) translocations, respectively. PAX3 is a transcription factor that initiates skeletal muscle differentiation, and it appears that the chimeric PAX3-FOXO1 fusion protein interferes with differentiation, a mechanism similar to many of the transcription factor fusion proteins that are found in acute leukemias.

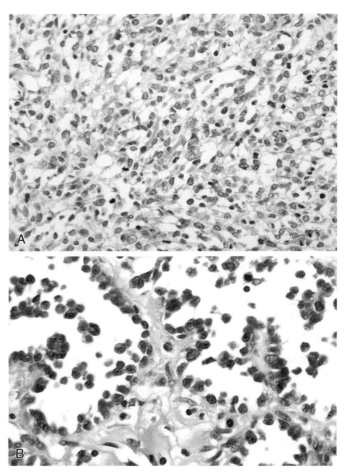

Fig. 21.48 Rhabdomyosarcoma. (A) Embryonal subtype composed of malignant cells ranging from primitive and round to densely eosinophilic with skeletal muscle differentiation. (B) Alveolar rhabdomyosarcoma with numerous spaces lined by discohesive, uniform round tumor cells.

MORPHOLOGY

Embryonal rhabdomyosarcoma presents as a soft gray infiltrative mass. The tumor cells mimic skeletal muscle at various stages of differentiation and consist of sheets of both primitive round and spindled cells (Fig. 21.48A). Rhabdomyoblasts with straplike cytoplasm and visible cross-striations may be present. **Sarcoma botryoides** is a variant of embryonal rhabdomyosarcoma that develops in the walls of hollow viscera such as the urinary bladder and vagina.

In **alveolar rhabdomyosarcoma,** a network of fibrous septae divide the cells into clusters or aggregates, creating a crude resemblance to pulmonary alveoli. The tumor cells are uniformly round with little cytoplasm and they are only minimally cohesive (Fig. 21.48B).

Pleomorphic rhabdomyosarcoma is characterized by numerous large, sometimes multinucleated, bizarre eosinophilic tumor cells that can resemble other pleomorphic sarcomas. Immunohistochemical identification of muscle specific proteins such as myogenin is usually necessary to confirm rhabdomyoblastic differentiation.

Rhabdomyosarcomas are aggressive neoplasms that are usually treated with surgery and chemotherapy, with or without radiation therapy. The botryoid variant of embryonal rhabdomyosarcoma has the best prognosis, whereas the pleomorphic subtype is often fatal.

SMOOTH MUSCLE TUMORS

Leiomyoma

Leiomyoma, a benign tumor of smooth muscle, is most common in the uterus but can arise in any soft tissue site. Uterine leiomyomas (Chapter 19) are common and may cause a variety of symptoms including infertility and menorrhagia. Leiomyomas also may arise from the erector pili muscles *(pilar leiomyomas)* in the skin and rarely in the deep somatic soft tissues or gastrointestinal tract. A germline loss-of-function mutation in the fumarate hydratase (FH) gene located on chromosome 1q42.3 leads to multiple cutaneous leiomyomas, uterine leiomyomas, and renal cell carcinoma. FH is an enzyme of the Krebs cycle, and this association constitutes another intriguing example of the link between metabolic abnormalities and neoplasia.

Soft tissue leiomyomas are usually 1 to 2 cm in size and are composed of fascicles of densely eosinophilic spindle cells that tend to intersect each other at right angles. The tumor cells have blunt-ended, elongated nuclei and show minimal atypia and few mitotic figures. Solitary lesions are cured with surgery.

Leiomyosarcoma

Soft tissue leiomyosarcoma accounts for 10% to 20% of soft tissue sarcomas. They occur in adults and affect women more frequently than men. Most develop in the deep soft tissues of the extremities and retroperitoneum or arise from the great vessels. Leiomyosarcomas have complex genotypes that stem from acquired defects that lead to profound genomic instability.

MORPHOLOGY

Leiomyosarcomas present as painless firm masses. Retroperitoneal tumors may be large and bulky and cause abdominal symptoms. They consist of eosinophilic spindle cells with blunt-ended, hyperchromatic nuclei arranged in interweaving fascicles. They express smooth muscle proteins (actin, desmin, caldesmon), which can be detected by immunohistochemistry. Unlike leiomyomas, mitotic activity and necrosis are common in leiomyosarcoma.

Clinical Course

Treatment depends on tumor size, location, and grade. Superficial leiomyosarcomas are usually small and have a good prognosis, whereas those of the retroperitoneum are difficult to control and cause death by both local extension and metastatic spread, especially to the lungs.

TUMORS OF UNCERTAIN ORIGIN

Although many soft tissue tumors can be assigned to recognizable histologic types, a large proportion of tumors do not recapitulate any known mesenchymal lineage. This group includes examples with simple or complex karyotypes; one of each type is described here.

Synovial Sarcoma

Synovial sarcoma was so-named because the first described cases arose in the soft tissues near the knee joint and a morphologic relationship to synovium was postulated. However, this name is a misnomer, as these tumors can present in locations that lack synovium and their morphologic features are inconsistent with an origin from synoviocytes. Synovial sarcomas account for approximately 10% of all soft tissue sarcomas. Most occur in people in their 20s to 40s. Patients usually present with a deep-seated mass that has been present for several years. Most synovial sarcomas show a characteristic chromosomal translocation t(x;18)(p11;q11) producing fusion genes composed of portions of the *SS18* gene and one of three *SSX* genes that encode chimeric transcription factors that derail cell cycle control.

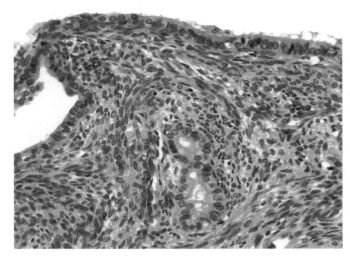

Fig. 21.49 Synovial sarcoma showing the classic biphasic spindle cell and glandlike histologic appearance.

MORPHOLOGY

Synovial sarcomas are microscopically monophasic or biphasic. Monophasic synovial sarcoma consists of uniform spindle cells with scant cytoplasm and dense chromatin growing in short, tightly packed fascicles. The biphasic type contains glandlike structures composed of cuboidal to columnar epithelioid cells in addition to the aforementioned spindle cell component (Fig. 21.49). Immunohistochemistry is helpful in identifying these tumors, since the tumor cells, especially in the biphasic type, are positive for epithelial antigens (e.g., keratins), differentiating them from many other sarcomas.

Synovial sarcomas are treated aggressively with limb-sparing surgery and frequently chemotherapy. The 5-year survival varies from 25% to 62%, related to stage and patient age. Common sites of metastases are the lung and, unusual for sarcomas, regional lymph nodes.

Undifferentiated Pleomorphic Sarcoma

Undifferentiated pleomorphic sarcoma (UPS) includes malignant mesenchymal tumors with high-grade, pleomorphic cells that cannot be classified into another category by a combination of histomorphology, immunophenotype, ultrastructure, and genetics. Most arise in the deep soft tissues of the extremity, especially the thigh of middle-aged or older adults. The diagnosis of *malignant fibrous histiocytoma* (MFH), sometimes used interchangeably with UPS, has fallen out of use because (1) the category included both undifferentiated tumors and others that could be reclassified with immunohistochemistry and genetics, and (2) no consensus exists for the morphologic definition of fibrohistiocytic lineage. Most tumors are aneuploid with multiple structural and numerical chromosomal changes.

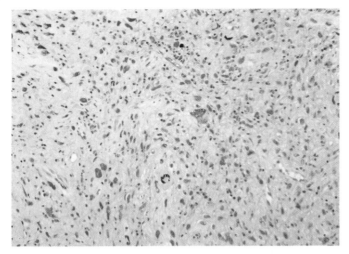

Fig. 21.50 Undifferentiated pleomorphic sarcoma showing anaplastic spindled to polygonal cells.

MORPHOLOGY

UPSs are usually large, grey-white fleshy masses that can grow quite large (10–20 cm) depending on the anatomic compartment. Necrosis and hemorrhage are common. Microscopically, they are some of the most pleomorphic malignancies encountered. UPSs consist of sheets of large, anaplastic, spindled to polygonal cells with hyperchromatic irregular, sometimes bizarre nuclei (Fig. 21.50). Mitotic figures, including atypical nonsymmetric forms, are abundant as is necrosis. By definition, tumor cells lack differentiation along recognized lineages or characteristic genetic defects.

UPSs are aggressive malignancies that are treated with surgery and adjuvant chemotherapy and/or radiation. The prognosis is generally poor, with metastases arising in 30% to 50% of cases.

SUMMARY

SOFT TISSUE TUMORS

- The category of soft tissue neoplasia describes tumors that arise from non-epithelial tissues, excluding the skeleton, joints, central nervous system, and hematopoietic and lymphoid tissues. A sarcoma is a malignant mesenchymal tumor.
- Although all soft tissue tumors probably arise from pluripotent mesenchymal stem cells, rather than mature cells, they can be classified as
  - Tumors that recapitulate a mature mesenchymal tissue (e.g., fat). These can be further subdivided into benign and malignant forms.
  - Tumors composed of cells for which there is no normal counterpart (e.g., synovial sarcoma, UPS).
- Sarcomas with simple karyotypes demonstrate reproducible, chromosomal, and molecular abnormalities that contribute to pathogenesis and are sufficiently specific to have diagnostic use.
- Most adult sarcomas have complex karyotypes, tend to be pleomorphic, and are genetically heterogeneous with a poor prognosis.

ACKNOWLEDGMENT

We thank Dr. Andrew Rosenberg for his outstanding contribution to previous editions of this chapter.

SUGGESTED READINGS

Basic Structure and Biology of Bone
Kogianni G, Noble BS: The biology of osteocytes, *Curr Osteoporos Rep* 5:81–86, 2007. *[Good review of the cellular basis of bone remodeling.]*
Olsen BR, Reginato AM, Wang W: Bone development, *Annu Rev Cell Dev Biol* 16:191–220, 2000. *[Update on the molecular and genetic basis of vertebrate skeletal development.]*
Zaidi M: Skeletal remodeling in health and disease, *Nat Med* 13:791–801, 2007. *[Excellent review of the genetics and pathophysiology of skeletal diseases.]*

Skeletal Dysplasias
Askmyr MK, Fasth A, Richter J: Towards a better understanding and new therapeutics of osteopetrosis, *Br J Haematol* 140:597–609, 2008. *[Nice summary of treatment options for osteoporosis including gene therapy.]*
Krakow D, Rimoin DL: The skeletal dysplasias, *Genet Med* 12:327–341, 2010. *[Comprehensive summary of the dysplasias with very useful summary table.]*
Van Dijk FS, Pals G, Van Rijn RR, et al: Classification of Osteogenesis Imperfecta revisited, *Eur J Med Genet* 53:1–5, 2010. *[An overview of the current classification of osteogenesis imperfecta based on clinical and molecular findings.]*

Osteoporosis
Mosekilde L: Mechanisms of age-related bone loss, *Novartis Found Symp* 235:150–166, discussion 66–71, 2001. *[Nice review of relationship between remodeling and osteoporosis.]*
Styrkarsdottir U, Halldorsson BV, Gretarsdottir S, et al: Multiple genetic loci for bone mineral density and fractures, *N Engl J Med* 358:2355–2365, 2008. *[Seminal paper elucidating the molecular pathways that underly osteoporosis.]*
Weitzmann MN, Pacifici R: Estrogen deficiency and bone loss: an inflammatory tale, *J Clin Invest* 116:1186–1194, 2006. *[Excellent review of current understanding of the relationship between estrogen and osteoporosis.]*

Hyperparathyroidism
Silva BC, Bilezikian JP: Parathyroid hormone: anabolic and catabolic actions on the skeleton, *Curr Opin Pharmacol* 22:41–50, 2015. *[Nice summary of effects of parathyroid hormone on calcium and bone metabolism.]*

Paget Disease
Roodman GD, Windle JJ: Paget disease of bone, *J Clin Invest* 115:200–208, 2005. *[Concise, nicely illustrated, summary of clinicopathologic manifestation of Paget disease.]*
Singer FR: The etiology of Paget's Disease of bone: viral and genetic interactions, *Cell Metab* 13:5–6, 2011. *[Very good review about the viral and genetic pathways in Paget disease.]*

Osteonecrosis
Seamon J, Keller T, et al: The pathogenesis of nontraumatic osteonecrosis, *Arthritis* 601763, 2012. *[Summarizes recent developments regarding pathophysiology of femoral head osteonecrosis.]*

Osteosarcoma
Klein MJ, Siegal GP: Osteosarcoma: anatomic and histologic variants, *Am J Clin Pathol* 125:555–581, 2006. *[Most recent update on classification of osteosarcoma.]*
Wagner ER, Luther G, Zhu G, et al: Defective osteogenic differentiation in the development of osteosarcoma, *Sarcoma* 2011:325238,

2011. [*Discusses molecular relationship between normal osteoblast development the pathogenesis of osteosarcoma.*]

Chondrogenic Tumors

Bovee JV, Hogendoorn PC, Wunder JS, et al: Cartilage tumours and bone development: molecular pathology and possible therapeutic targets, *Nat Rev Cancer* 10:481–488, 2010. [*A good review of the known genetic abnormalities in these tumors*]

Pansuriya TC, van Eijk R, d'Adamo P, et al: Somatic mosaic IDH1 and IDH2 mutations are associated with enchondroma and spindle cell hemangioma in Ollier disease and Maffucci syndrome, *Nat Genet* 43:1256–1261, 2011. [*Seminal article identifying IDH mutations in inherited cartilage tumors.*]

Wuyts W, Van Hul W: Molecular basis of multiple exostoses: mutations in the EXT1 and EXT2 genes, *Hum Mutat* 15:220–227, 2000. [*Discussion of genetic basis of multiple osteochondroma syndrome.*]

Ewing Sarcoma

Erkizan HV, Uversky VN, Toretsky JA: Oncogenic partnerships: EWS-FLI1 protein interactions initiate key pathways of Ewing's sarcoma, *Clin Cancer Res* 16:4077–4083, 2010. [*Excellent summary of molecular effects of the EWS-FLI1 fusion protein found in Ewing sarcoma.*]

Giant Cell Tumor of Bone

Robinson D, Einhorn TA: Giant cell tumor of bone: a unique paradigm of stromal-hematopoietic cellular interactions, *J Cell Biochem* 55:300–303, 1994. [*Nice discussion of molecular mechanisms underlying giant cell tumor and insight gained regarding normal bone remodeling.*]

Aneurysmal Bone Cyst

Oliveira AM, Chou MM: The TRE17/USP6 oncogene: a riddle wrapped in a mystery inside an enigma, *Front Biosci (Schol Ed)* 4:321–334, 2012. [*Excellent review of the USP6 clonal genetic rearrangement in various self-limited mesenchymal tumors.*]

Fibrous Dysplasia

Riminucci M, Robey PG, Saggio I, et al: Skeletal progenitors and the GNAS gene: fibrous dysplasia of bone read through stem cells, *J Mol Endocrinol* 45:355–364, 2010. [*Excellent discussion of how a mutation can affect skeletal progenitor cells and cause clinical expression of fibrous dysplasia.*]

Osteoarthritis

Goldring MB, Goldring SR: Articular cartilage and subchondral bone in the pathogenesis of osteoarthritis, *Ann N Y Acad Sci* 1192:230–237, 2010. [*A succint and thoughtful presentation of the role of articular structures in the development of osteoarthritis.*]

Valdes AM, Spector TD: Genetic epidemiology of hip and knee osteoarthritis, *Nat Rev Rheumatol* 7:23–32, 2011. [*Useful review of genome-wide association studies that have lead to candidate genes predisposing to osteoarthritis.*]

Rheumatoid Arthritis

Deane KD, El-Gabalawy H: Pathogenesis and prevention of rheumatic disease: focus on preclinical RA and SLE, *Nat Rev Rheumatol* 10:212–228, 2014. [*Recent, nicely illustrated, update on pathogenesis of RA and SLE.*]

Scott DL, Wolfe F, Huizinga TW: Rheumatoid arthritis, *Lancet* 376:1094–1108, 2011. [*Review of pathogenesis and treatment of the disease.*]

van Heemst J, Jansen DT, et al: Crossreactivity to vinculin and microbes provides a molecular basis for HLA-based protection against rheumatoid arthritis, *Nat Commun* 6:6681, 2015. [*Describes the relationship between autoimmunity, HLA alleles and microbes.*]

Lyme Disease

Iliopoulou BP, Huber BT: Infectious arthritis and immune dysregulation: lessons from Lyme disease, *Curr Opin Rheumatol* 22:451–455, 2010. [*Recent overview of immune mechanisms underlying Lyme arthritis*]

Marques A: Chronic Lyme disease: a review, *Infect Dis Clin North Am* 22:341–360, 2008. [*In-depth review of Lyme disease.*]

Gout and Pseudogout

Rosenthal AK: Update in calcium deposition diseases, *Curr Opin Rheumatol* 19:158–162, 2007. [*Recent, succint, review of crystal-induced arthritis.*]

VanItallie TB: Gout: epitome of painful arthritis, *Metabolism* 59(Suppl 1):S32–S36, 2010. [*Excellent summary of the recent developments in the molecular and cellular biology underlying gout.*]

Tenosynovial Giant Cell Tumor

Moller E, Mandahl N, Mertens F, et al: Molecular identification of COL6A3-CSF1 fusion transcripts in tenosynovial giant cell tumors, *Genes Chromosomes Cancer* 47:21–25, 2008. [*Seminal article identifying clonal chromosomal rearrangement in tenosynovial giant cell tumor.*]

Soft Tissue Sarcomas

Antonescu CR, Dal Cin P: Promiscuous genes involved in recurrent chromosomal translocations in soft tissue tumours, *Pathology* 46:105–112, 2014. [*Excellent review of specificity (or lack thereof) of genetic defects in soft tissue tumors.*]

Fletcher CD, Gustafson P, Rydholm A, et al: Clinicopathologic re-evaluation of 100 malignant fibrous histiocytomas: prognostic relevance of subclassification, *J Clin Oncol* 19:3045–3050, 2001. [*Seminal article reassessing the diagnosis of malignant fibrous histiocytoma (MFH) allowing more specific classification.*]

Peripheral Nerves and Muscles

22

Disorders of Peripheral Nerves 835
Patterns of Peripheral Nerve Injury 835
Disorders Associated With Peripheral Nerve
  Injury 837
Disorders of Neuromuscular
  Junction 839
Myasthenia Gravis 839
Lambert-Eaton Syndrome 839

Miscellaneous Neuromuscular Junction
  Disorders 839
Disorders of Skeletal Muscle 840
Patterns of Skeletal Muscle Injury and
  Atrophy 840
Inherited Disorders of Skeletal Muscle 841
Acquired Disorders of Skeletal Muscle 844
Peripheral Nerve Sheath Tumors 846

Schwannomas and Neurofibromatosis
  Type 2 846
Neurofibromas 846
Neurofibromatosis Type 1 846
Malignant Peripheral Nerve Sheath Tumors 846
Traumatic Neuroma 847

The peripheral nerves and skeletal muscles permit purposeful movement and provide the brain with sensory information about our surroundings. Both the anatomic distribution of lesions and their associated signs and symptoms are helpful in classifying neuromuscular diseases. The following discussion of neuromuscular disorders is organized along anatomic lines and traces the neuromuscular system from proximal to distal by discussing disorders of peripheral nerves, neuromuscular junctions, and skeletal muscle.

DISORDERS OF PERIPHERAL NERVES

The two major functional elements of peripheral nerves are axonal processes and their myelin sheaths, which are made by Schwann cells. Axonal diameter and myelin thickness are correlated with each other and with conduction velocity. These characteristics are used to distinguish different types of axons, which mediate distinct sensory inputs and motor function. Light touch, for example, is transmitted by thickly myelinated large-diameter axons with fast conduction velocities, whereas temperature sensation is transmitted by slow, unmyelinated thin axons. In the case of myelinated axons, one Schwann cell makes and maintains exactly one myelin segment, or internode, along a single axon (Fig. 22.1A). Adjacent internodes are separated by the nodes of Ranvier along which saltatory conduction occurs. Any given nerve contains axons of different sizes and axons serving different functions. These are arranged into fascicles ensheathed by a layer of perineurial cells. Perineurial cells form a barrier between endoneu-

rium on the inside of the fascicle and epineurium on the outside.

Patterns of Peripheral Nerve Injury

Peripheral neuropathies are often subclassified as axonal or demyelinating, even though many diseases exhibit mixed features. **Axonal neuropathies are caused by insults that directly injure the axon.** The entire distal portion of an affected axon degenerates. Axonal degeneration is associated with secondary myelin loss (Fig. 22.1B). The term *Wallerian degeneration* is borrowed from experimental studies involving the transection of nerves to describe analogous changes observed in axonal neuropathies. Regeneration takes place through axonal regrowth and subsequent remyelination of the distal axon (Fig. 22.1C). The morphologic hallmark of axonal neuropathies is a decrease in the density of axons, which in electrophysiologic studies correlates with a decrease in the signal strength or amplitude of nerve impulses.

Demyelinating neuropathies are characterized by damage to Schwann cells or myelin with relative axonal sparing, resulting in abnormally slow nerve conduction velocities but preserved amplitude. Demyelination typically occurs discontinuously, affecting individual internodes along the length of an axon in a random distribution. This process is termed *segmental demyelination* (Fig. 22.1B). Morphologically, demyelinating neuropathies show a relatively normal density of axons and features of segmental demyelination and repair. This is recognized by the presence of axons with abnormally thin myelin sheaths and short internodes (Fig. 22.1C). The discontinuous nature

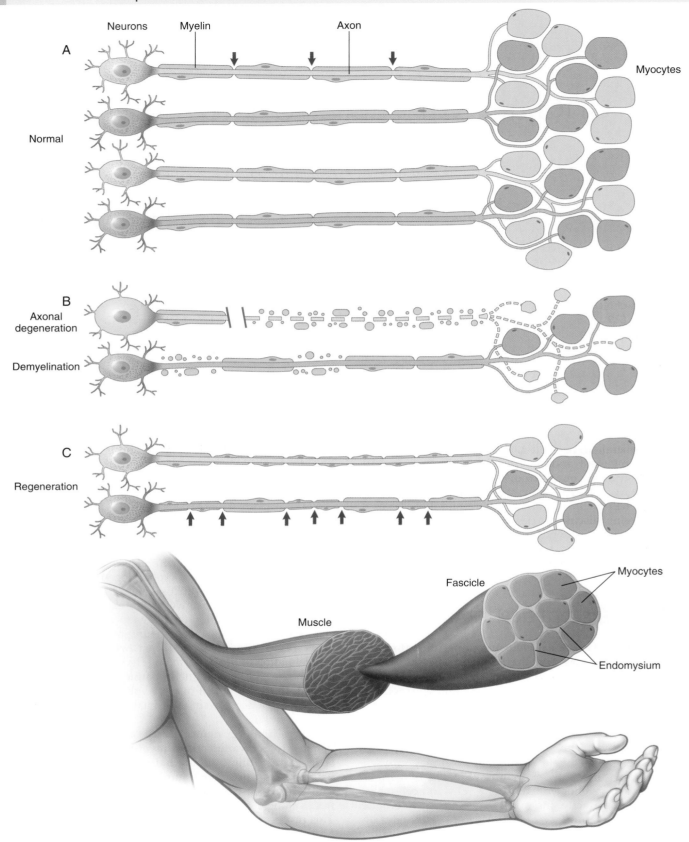

Fig. 22.1 Patterns of peripheral nerve damage. (A) In normal motor units, type I and type II myofibers (see Table 22.2 later) are arranged in a "checkerboard" distribution. The internodes, separated by nodes of Ranvier *(arrows)* along the motor axons are uniform in thickness and length. (B) Acute axonal injury *(upper axon)* results in degeneration of the distal axon and its associated myelin sheath, with atrophy of denervated myofibers. By contrast, acute demyelinating disease *(lower axon)* produces random segmental degeneration of individual myelin internodes, while sparing the axon. (C) Regeneration of axons after injury *(upper axon)* allows connections with myofibers to re-form. The regenerated axon is myelinated by proliferating Schwann cells, but the new internodes are shorter and the myelin sheaths are thinner than the original ones. (Nodes Ranvier are marked by *arrows*; compare with panel A.) Remission of demyelinating disease *(lower axon)* allows remyelination to take place, but the new internodes also are shorter and have thinner myelin sheaths than flanking normal undamaged internodes.

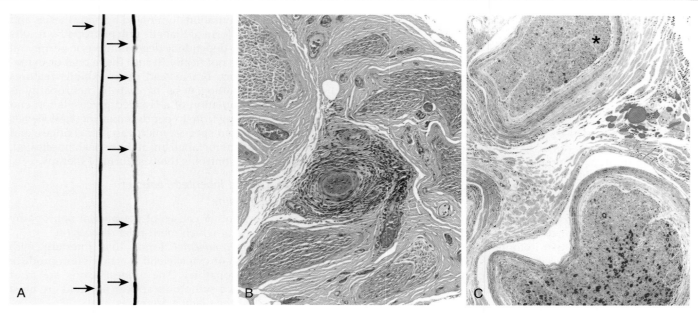

Fig. 22.2 Pathologic changes in peripheral neuropathies. (A) Regeneration after segmental demyelination. Teased fiber preparations allow for examination of individual axons of peripheral nerves. A normal axon *(left)* with a long thick dark myelin internode flanked by nodes of Ranvier *(arrows;* compare with Fig. 22.1A). All myelin internodes along his axon would be expected to be of similar length and width. The right axon, by contrast, shows a segment surrounded by a series of thinly myelinated internodes of uneven length flanked on both ends by normal thicker myelin internodes *(arrows* mark nodes of Ranvier; compare with Fig. 22.1C). (B–C) Vasculitic neuropathy. In (B), the perineurial connective tissue contains an inflammatory infiltrate around small blood vessels that has obliterated a vessel. In (C), a special stain that colors myelinated axons dark blue hue shows that the nerve fascicle in the upper portion of this field *(asterisk)* has lost almost all of its large myelinated axons, in contrast with the other fascicle shown. Such interfascicular variation in axonal density is often seen in neuropathies resulting from vascular injury.

of damage to random internodes is best visualized when examining a series of internodes along individual axons in teased fiber preparations (Fig. 22.2A).

Peripheral neuropathies exhibit several anatomic patterns.

- *Polyneuropathies* usually affect peripheral nerves in a symmetric, length-dependent fashion. Axonal loss is typically more pronounced in the distal segments of the longest nerves. Patients commonly present with loss of sensation and paresthesias that start in the toes and spread upward. By the time the sensory changes reach the level of the knees, the hands are also affected, resulting in a picture described as "stocking-and-glove" distribution. This pattern is often encountered with toxic and metabolic damage.
- *Mononeuritis multiplex,* in which the damage randomly affects individual nerves, resulting (for example) in a right radial nerve palsy and wrist drop and, at a separate point in time, a left foot drop. Mononeuritis multiplex is often caused by vasculitis.
- A simple *mononeuropathy* only involves a single nerve and is most commonly the result of traumatic injury, entrapment (e.g., carpal tunnel syndrome), or certain infections such as Lyme disease.

Disorders Associated With Peripheral Nerve Injury

Many different diseases may be associated with peripheral neuropathy (Table 22.1). We next discuss selected entities that are prototypical for a specific type of polyneuropathy or that are particularly common.

Table 22.1 Peripheral Neuropathies

Etiologic Category	Causative Disorders/Agents
Nutritional and metabolic	Diabetes mellitus Uremia Vitamin deficiencies—thiamine, vitamin B6, vitamin B12
Toxic	Drugs, including vinblastine, vincristine, paclitaxel, colchicine, and isoniazid Toxins—alcohol, lead, aluminum, arsenic, mercury, acrylamide
Vasculopathic	Vasculitis Amyloidosis
Inflammatory	Autoimmune diseases Guillain-Barré syndrome Chronic inflammatory demyelinating polyneuropathy (CIDP)
Infections	Herpes zoster Leprosy HIV infection Lyme disease
Inherited	Charcot-Marie-Tooth neuropathy, type I, type II, and X-linked Hereditary neuropathy with liability to pressure palsy
Others	Paraneoplastic, some leukodystrophies

Guillain-Barré Syndrome

Guillain-Barré syndrome is a rapidly progressive acute demyelinating disorder affecting motor axons, resulting in ascending weakness that can lead to death from failure of respiratory muscles within days of onset of symptoms. It is one of the most common life-threatening diseases of the peripheral nervous system. Guillain-Barré syndrome appears to be triggered by an infection or vaccination that breaks down self-tolerance, thereby leading to an autoimmune response. Associated infectious agents include Campylobacter jejuni, Epstein-Barr virus, cytomegalovirus, human immunodeficiency virus (HIV), and, most recently Zika virus. The injury is most extensive in the nerve roots and proximal nerve segments and is associated with mononuclear cell infiltrates rich in macrophages. Both humoral and cellular immune responses are believed to play a role in the disease process. Treatments include plasmapheresis (to remove offending antibodies), intravenous immunoglobulin infusions (which suppress immune responses through unclear mechanisms), and supportive care, such as ventilatory support. Patients who survive the initial acute phase of the disease usually recover with time.

Chronic Inflammatory Demyelinating Polyneuropathy (CIDP)

CIDP is the most common chronic acquired inflammatory peripheral neuropathy, characterized by symmetrical mixed sensorimotor polyneuropathy that persists for 2 months or more. Both motor and sensory abnormalities are common, such as weakness, difficulty in walking, numbness, and pain or tingling sensations. Like Guillain-Barré syndrome, CIDP is immune mediated. But in contrast to Guillain-Barré syndrome, CIDP follows a chronic, relapsing-remitting, or progressive course. It occurs with increased frequency in patients with other immune disorders, such as systemic lupus erythematosus and HIV infection. The peripheral nerves show segments of demyelination and remyelination (Fig. 22.2A). In long-standing cases, repeated activation and proliferation of Schwann cells with episodes of regeneration result in the concentric arrangement of multiple Schwann cells around individual axons to produce multilayered structures likened to onion bulbs. Treatment includes plasmapheresis and administration of immunosuppressive agents. Some patients recover completely, but more often recurrent bouts of symptomatic disease lead to permanent loss of nerve function.

Diabetic Peripheral Neuropathy

Diabetes is the most common cause of peripheral neuropathy, usually developing with long-standing disease. Diabetic neuropathies include several forms that can occur singly or together.

- *Autonomic neuropathy* is characterized by changes in bowel, bladder, cardiac, or sexual function.
- *Lumbosacral radiculopathy* usually manifests with asymmetric pain that can progress to lower extremity weakness and muscle atrophy.
- *Distal symmetric sensorimotor polyneuropathy* is the most common form of diabetic neuropathy. Sensory axons are more severely affected than motor axons, resulting

in a clinical presentation dominated by paresthesias and numbness. This form of diabetic polyneuropathy results from the length-dependent degeneration of peripheral nerves and does not neatly fit into the axonal or demyelinating category but instead often exhibits features of both. The pathogenesis of diabetic neuropathy is complex; accumulation of advanced glycosylation end products resulting from hyperglycemia, increased levels of reactive oxygen species, microvascular changes, and changes in axonal metabolism, all have been implicated. Strict glycemic control is the best form of therapy.

Toxic, Vasculitic, and Inherited Forms of Peripheral Neuropathy

There are diverse other causes of periperlal neuropathy (Table 22.1), some of which merit brief discussion.

- *Drugs* and *environmental toxins* that interfere with axonal transport or cytoskeletal function often produce peripheral neuropathies. The longest axons are most susceptible, hence symptoms appear first and are most pronounced in the distal extremities.
- Peripheral nerves are damaged in many different forms of *systemic vasculitis* (Fig. 22.2B) (Chapter 10), including polyarteritis nodosa, Churg-Strauss syndrome, and polyangiitis with granulomatosis. Overall, peripheral nerve damage is seen in about a third of all patients with vasculitis at the time of presentation. The most common clinical picture is that of *mononeuritis multiplex* with a painful asymmetric mixed sensory and motor peripheral neuropathy. Patchy involvement also is apparent at the microscopic level, as single nerves may show considerable interfascicular variation in the degree of axonal damage (Fig. 22.2C).
- *Inherited diseases of peripheral nerves* are a heterogeneous but relatively common group of disorders, with a prevalence of 1 to 4 in 10,000. They can be demyelinating or axonal. Many such disorders manifest in adulthood and follow a slowly progressive course that may mimic that of acquired polyneuropathies. The most common causes are mutations in the genes encoding myelin-associated proteins.

● SUMMARY

PERIPHERAL NEUROPATHIES

- Peripheral neuropathies may result in weakness and/or sensory deficits in patterns described as polyneuropathy, mononeuritis multiplex, and mononeuropathy.
- Axonal and demyelinating peripheral neuropathies can be distinguished on the basis of clinical and pathologic features. Some disorders are associated with a mixed pattern of injury.
- Diabetes is the most common cause of peripheral neuropathy.
- Guillain-Barré syndrome and chronic idiopathic demyelinating polyneuropathy are immune-mediated demyelinating diseases that follow acute and chronic courses, respectively.
- Metabolic diseases, drugs, toxins, connective tissue diseases, vasculitides, and infections all can result in peripheral neuropathy.
- A number of mutations cause peripheral neuropathy. Many of these are adult-onset diseases that may mimic acquired ones.

DISORDERS OF NEUROMUSCULAR JUNCTION

The neuromuscular junction is a complex specialized structure located at the interface of motor nerve axons and skeletal muscle that serves to control muscle contraction. Here the distal ends of peripheral motor nerves branch into small processes that terminate in bulbous synaptic boutons. Nerve impulses depolarize the presynaptic membrane, stimulating calcium influx and the release of acetylcholine into the synaptic cleft. Acetylcholine diffuses across the synaptic cleft to bind its receptor on the postsynaptic membrane, leading to depolarization of the myofiber and contraction through electromechanical coupling. Often disorders of the neuromuscular junction produce functional deficits in the absence of any significant alterations in morphology beyond ultrastructural changes. Considered in this section are some of the more common or pathogenically interesting disorders that disrupt the transmission of signals across the neuromuscular junction.

Myasthenia Gravis

Myasthenia gravis is an autoimmune disease with fluctuating muscle weakness that is caused by autoantibodies that target the neuromuscular junction. The most common antigenic target is the postsynaptic acetylcholine receptor (AChR). Other pathogenic antibodies recognize muscle-specific kinase (MuSK) and low-density lipoprotein receptor-related protein (LRP4). These antibodies lead to loss of receptors and damage to the structure of the junctions. The disease has an incidence of approximately 2 in 100,000 persons. Anti-AChR mediated cases have bimodal age distribution with somewhat distinctive clinical features. Early onset before age 50 years is more common in females and is frequently associated with enlargement of the thymus due to the presence of B cell follicles and germinal centers (follicular thymic hyperplasia). Late-onset cases show a more equal gender distribution and are associated with thymoma (Chapter 12), a neoplasm derived from thymic epithelium. Both of these thymic lesions are believed to perturb tolerance to self-antigens, setting the stage for the generation of autoreactive T and B cells.

Clinically, myasthenia gravis frequently manifests with *ptosis* (drooping eyelids) or *diplopia* (double vision) because of weakness in the extraocular muscles. This pattern of weakness is distinctly different from that of most primary myopathic diseases, in which there is relative sparing of facial and extraocular muscles. The severity of the weakness often fluctuates rapidly, sometimes over periods of a few minutes. Characteristically, repetitive firing of muscles makes the weakness more severe, whereas cholinesterase inhibitors improve strength markedly, features that are are diagnostically useful. Effective treatments include cholinesterase inhibitors, immunosuppression, plasmapheresis, and (in patients with thymic lesions) thymectomy. These interventions have improved the 5-year survival rate to greater than 95%.

Lambert-Eaton Syndrome

Lambert-Eaton syndrome is caused by autoantibodies that inhibit the function of presynaptic calcium channels, thereby reducing the release of acetylcholine into the synaptic cleft. Patients with Lambert-Eaton syndrome experience improvement in weakness with repetitive stimulation, in contrast to those suffering from myasthenia gravis. Repetitive stimulation serves to build up sufficient intracellular calcium to facilitate acetylcholine release. *Lambert-Eaton syndrome often arises as a paraneoplastic disorder,* particularly in patients with small cell lung carcinoma. Cholinesterase inhibitors are not effective, and therapy is therefore directed toward reducing the titer of causative antibodies, through either plasmapheresis or immunosuppression. The prognosis is worse than that of myasthenia gravis because of the frequent coexistence of an underlying malignancy.

Miscellaneous Neuromuscular Junction Disorders

Several other neuromuscular junction disorders merit brief mention.

- *Congenital myasthenic syndromes* comprise a heterogeneous group of diseases that result from mutations that disrupt the function of various neuromuscular junction proteins. Depending on the affected protein, the defects may occur at the level of acetylcholine release (presynaptic), the transport of acetylcholine across the synaptic cleft (synaptic), or the responsiveness of skeletal muscle (postsynaptic). Hence they may present with symptoms mimicking Lambert-Eaton syndrome or myasthenia gravis. Some forms respond to treatment with acetylcholinesterase inhibitors.
- *Infections with exotoxin-producing bacteria* may be associated with defects in neural transmission and muscle contraction. *Clostridium tetani* and *Clostridium botulinum* (Chapter 9) both release extremely potent neurotoxins that interfere with neuromuscular transmission. Tetanus toxin (known as tetanospasmin) blocks the action of inhibitory neurons, leading to the increased release of acetylcholine and sustained muscle contraction and spasm (tetanus). Botulinum toxin, by contrast, inhibits acetylcholine release, producing a flaccid paralysis. The purified toxin (Botox) is remarkably stable after injection, an attribute that has led to its widespread use as an antidote for wrinkles and a variety of other conditions associated with unwanted muscular activity (e.g., blepharospasm and strabismus).

SUMMARY

NEUROMUSCULAR JUNCTION DISORDERS

- Disorders of neuromuscular junctions manifest with weakness that often affects facial and extraocular muscles and may show rapid fluctuation in severity.
- Both myasthenia gravis and Lambert-Eaton syndrome, which are the most common forms, are immune mediated, being caused by antibodies that typically target postsynaptic acetylcholine receptors and presynaptic calcium channels, respectively.

- Myasthenia gravis often is associated with thymic hyperplasia or thymoma. Lambert-Eaton syndrome is a paraneoplastic disorder in the majority of the cases; the strongest association is with small cell lung cancer.
- Genetic defects in neuromuscular junction proteins and bacterial toxins also can cause symptomatic disturbances in neuromuscular transmission.

DISORDERS OF SKELETAL MUSCLE

Patterns of Skeletal Muscle Injury and Atrophy

The principal component of the motor system is the *motor unit*, which is composed of one lower motor neuron together with the associated axon, its neuromuscular junctions, and the skeletal muscle fibers it innervates. Skeletal muscle consists of different fiber types broadly classified as slow twitch type I and fast twitch type II fibers (Table 22.2). The fiber type is dependent on the innervation. All myofibers of a motor unit therefore share the same fiber type. Normally the fibers of different types are distributed in checkerboard patterns (Fig. 22.1A). A number of proteins and protein complexes are crucial for the unique structure and function of skeletal muscles. These include proteins that make up the sarcomeres and the dystrophin-glycoprotein complex (Fig. 22.3), as well as enzymes that allow muscle to meet it unusual metabolic requirements.

Primary muscle diseases or myopathies have to be distinguished from secondary neuropathic changes caused by disorders that disrupt muscle innervation. Both are associated with altered muscle function and morphology, but each has distinctive features (Fig. 22.4). Myopathic conditions are often associated with segmental necrosis and regeneration of individual muscle fibers (Fig. 22.4B). Some myopathies are also associated with other morphologic features, such as inflammatory infiltrates or intracellular inclusions. Disruption of muscle by endomysial fibrosis and fatty replacement is reflective of disease chronicity that can occur both in myopathic as well as neuropathic conditions.

Both neuropathic and myopathic processes cause *muscle fiber atrophy*. However, certain disorders are associated with particular patterns of atrophy, as follows:

- *Neuropathic changes.* Loss of innervation causes atrophy of myofibers. The two main morphologic hallmarks of neurogenic changes, *grouped atrophy* and *fiber type grouping* (Fig. 22.4C), are the result of multiple rounds of denervation and reinnervation. Loss of an axon or lower motor neuron results in atrophy of the myofibers that are part of this motor unit (Fig. 22.4C2). Atrophic myofibers can be reinnervated by axonal branches from adjacent motor units, increasing the size of these motor units and returning trophic input to the atrophic myofibers (Fig. 22.4C3). Multiple rounds of denervation and reinnervation result in a dwindling number of motor units of increasingly larger size. In this setting loss of innervation will therefore produce large clusters of atrophic myofibers, *grouped atrophy* (Fig. 22.4C5). Because

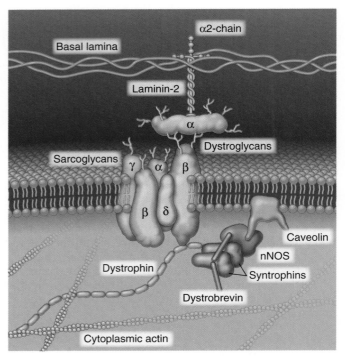

Fig. 22.3 The dystrophin-glycoprotein complex (DGC). This complex of glycoproteins serves to couple the cell membrane (the sarcolemma) to extracellular matrix proteins such as laminin-2 and the intracellular cytoskeleton. A key set of connections is made by dystrophin, a scaffolding protein that tethers the myofibrillar cytoskeleton to the transmembrane dystroglycans and sarcoglycans, and also binds signaling complexes containing dystrobrevin, syntrophin, neuronal nitric oxide synthetase (nNOS), and caveolin. Mutations in dystrophin are associated with X-linked Duchenne and Becker muscular dystrophies; mutations in caveolin and the sarcoglycan proteins with autosomal limb-girdle muscular dystrophies; and mutations in α2-laminin (merosin) with a form of congenital muscular dystrophy.

Table 22.2 Muscle Fiber Types

	Type I	Type II
Action	Sustained force	Fast movement
Activity type	Aerobic exercise	Anaerobic exercise
Power produced	Low	High
Resistance to fatigue	High	Low
Lipid content	High	Low
Glycogen content	Low	High
Energy metabolism	Low glycolytic capacity, high oxidative capacity	High glycolytic capacity, low oxidative capacity
Mitochondrial density	High	Low
Myosin heavy chain gene expressed	*MYH7*	*MYH2, MYH4, MYH1*
Color	Red (high myoglobin content)	Pale red / tan (low myoglobin content)

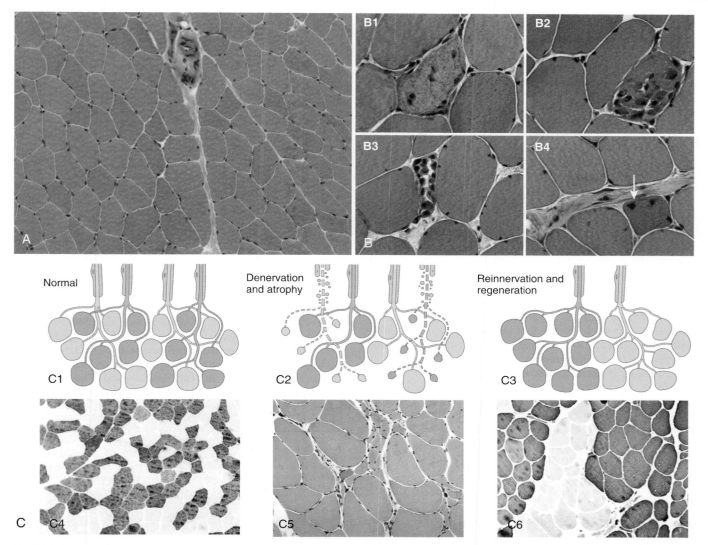

Fig. 22.4 Patterns of skeletal muscle injury. (A) Normal skeletal muscle has relatively uniform polygonal myofibers with peripherally placed nuclei that are tightly packed together into fascicles separated by scant connective tissue. A perimysial interfascicular septum containing a blood vessel is present *(top center)*. (B) Myopathic conditions often are associated with segmental necrosis and regeneration of individual myofibers. Necrotic cells (B1–B3) are infiltrated by variable numbers of inflammatory cells. Regenerative myofibers (B4, *arrow*) are characterized by cytoplasmic basophilia and enlarged nucleoli (not visible at this power). (C) Neurogenic changes. (C1) This diagrammatic representation of four normal motor units shows a checkerboard-type admixture of light and dark stained fibers of opposite type. (C2) Damage to innervating axons leads to a loss of trophic input and the atrophy of myofibers. (C3) Reinnervation of myofibers can result in a switch in fiber type and segregation of fibers of like type. As illustrated here, reinnervation is also often associated with an increase in motor unit size, with more myofibers innervated by an individual axon. (C4) Normal muscle has a checkerboard distribution of type I *(light)* and type II *(dark)* fibers on this ATPase reaction (pH9.4), corresponding to findings in (A). (C5) Clustered flattened "angulated" atrophic fibers *(grouped atrophy)* are a typical finding associated with disrupted innervation. (C6) With ongoing denervation and reinnervation, large clusters of fibers appear that all share the same fiber type *(fiber type grouping)*.

myofiber type depends on the innervating motor unit, reinnvervated fibers may change from type I to type II and vice versa. The presence of increasingly larger motor units alters the normal checkerboard type distribution of fibers by producing large clusters of the same type, *fiber type grouping* (Fig. 22.4C6).

• *Prolonged disuse of muscles* from any cause (e.g., prolonged bed rest in the sick, casting of a broken bone) may cause focal or generalized muscle atrophy, which tends to affect type II fibers more than type I fibers.

• *Glucocorticoid exposure,* whether exogenous or endogenous (e.g., in Cushing syndrome), also may cause muscle atrophy. Proximal muscles and type II myofibers are affected preferentially in this setting.

Inherited Disorders of Skeletal Muscle

Inherited mutations are responsible for a diverse collection of disorders marked by defects in skeletal muscle. In some of these disorders, skeletal muscle is the main site of disease, while in others multiple organs are involved. Of the other organs involved, the heart is of particular importance, because cardiac involvement is common and is often life-limiting. Included in this group of inherited muscular disorders are the following:

- *Muscular dystrophies* are associated with progressive muscle injury in patients who have normal muscle function at birth.
- *Congenital muscular dystrophies,* by contrast, are progressive, early-onset diseases. Some are also associated with malformations of the central nervous system.
- *Congenital myopathies* typically present in infancy with muscle defects that tend to be static or to even improve with time. They are often associated with distinct structural abnormalities of the muscle.

The discussion of muscular dystrophies may at first glance appear confusing because of different classification systems and terminologies. This is reflective of our evolving understanding of these diseases, from a description based on phenotype and inheritance pattern, to one based on underlying genetic mutations. An additional layer of complexity stems from the fact that there is not a simple one-to-one correspondence between genotypes and phenotypes. Instead mutations in several different genes can, for example, present as autosomal recessive limb-girdle muscular dystrophy; conversely different mutations in a single gene (such as dystrophin) can lead to very different clinical phenotypes, as illustrated by Duchenne and Becker types of muscular dystrophy.

Dystrophinopathies: Duchenne and Becker Muscular Dystrophy

The most common muscular dystrophies are X-linked and are caused by mutations that disrupt the function of a large structural protein called *dystrophin*. As a result, these diseases are referred to as *dystrophinopathies*. *Duchenne muscular dystrophy* (DMD) and *Becker muscular dystrophy* (BMD) are the two most important diseases in this group. DMD has an incidence of about 1 per 3500 live male births and follows an invariably fatal course. It becomes clinically evident in early childhood; most patients are wheelchair-bound by the time they are teenagers and are dead of their disease by early adulthood. The Becker type of muscular dystrophy is less common and less severe.

MORPHOLOGY

The histologic alterations in skeletal muscles affected by DMD and BMD are similar, except that the changes are milder in BMD (Fig. 22.5). The hallmarks of these as well as other muscular dystrophies are ongoing myofiber necrosis and regeneration. Progressive replacement of muscle tissue by fibrosis and fat is the result of degeneration outpacing repair. As a result of ongoing repair, muscles typically show marked variation in myofiber size and abnormal internally placed nuclei. Both DMD and BMD also affect cardiac muscles, which show variable degrees of myocyte hypertrophy and interstitial fibrosis.

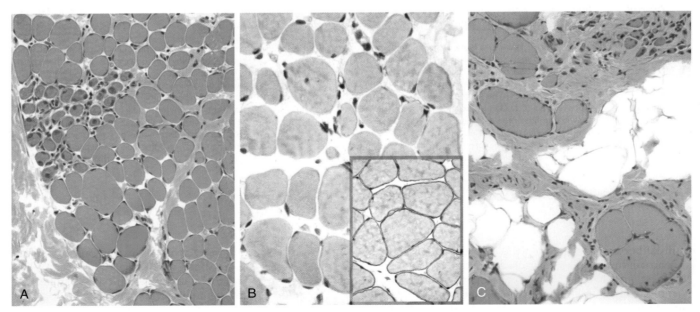

Fig. 22.5 Duchenne muscular dystrophy. Histologic images of muscle biopsy specimens from two brothers. (A–B) Specimens from a 3-year-old boy. (C) Specimen from his brother, 9 years of age. As seen in (A), at a younger age fascicular muscle architecture is maintained, but myofibers show variation in size. Additionally, there is a cluster of basophilic regenerating myofibers (left side) and slight endomysial fibrosis, seen as focal pink-staining connective tissue between myofibers. In (B), immunohistochemical staining shows a complete absence of membrane-associated dystrophin, seen as a brown stain in normal muscle (inset). In (C), the biopsy from the older brother illustrates disease progression, which is marked by extensive variation in myofiber size, fatty replacement, and endomysial fibrosis.

Pathogenesis

Both DMD and BMD are caused by mutations disrupting the function of the *dystrophin* gene located on the short arm of the X chromosome (Xp21). Dystrophin is a very large protein (427 kD in molecular weight) found in skeletal and cardiac muscle, brain, and peripheral nerves; it is part of the dystrophin-glycoprotein complex (Fig. 22.3). This complex stabilizes the muscle cell during contraction and may be involved in cell signaling through interactions with other proteins. Dystrophin-glycoprotein complex defects are thought to make muscle cells vulnerable to transient membrane tears during contraction that lead to calcium influx, and they may also disrupt intracellular signaling. The result is myofiber degeneration that with time outpaces the capacity for repair. The dystrophin-glycoprotein complex also is important for cardiac muscle function; this explains why cardiomyopathy eventually develops in many patients.

The dystrophin gene spans roughly 2.4 megabases (about 1% of the X chromosome), making it one of the largest human genes. Its enormous size may make it more prone to sporadic mutations, which all things being equal are more likely by chance to affect large genes. The most common mutations are deletions, followed by frameshift and point mutations. Patient with DMD usually have either of the first two and show complete absence of dystrohpin on a muscle biopsy. Patients with BMD often have point mutations and make residual but defective forms. The severity of disease therefore correlates with genotype and extent of dystrohpin deficiency.

Clinical Features

Often the first symptoms of DMD are clumsiness and an inability to keep up with peers because of muscle weakness. The weakness typically begins in the pelvic girdle and next involves the shoulder girdle. Enlargement of the calves, termed pseudohypertrophy, is an early physical finding. The increased muscle bulk initially stems from myofiber hypertrophy, but as myofibers progressively degenerate, an increasing part of the muscle is replaced by adipose tissue and endomysial fibrosis. Cardiac muscle damage and fibrosis may lead to heart failure and arrhythmias, which may prove fatal. Although no structural abnormalities in the central nervous system have been described, cognitive impairment also may occur and may be severe enough to be classified as mental retardation. Owing to ongoing muscle degeneration, high serum creatine kinase levels are present at birth and persist through the first decade of life but fall as muscle mass is lost as the disease progresses. Death results from respiratory insufficiency, pneumonia, and cardiac decompensation.

BMD becomes symptomatic later in childhood or adolescence and progresses at a slower and more variable rate. Many patients live well into adulthood and have a nearly normal life span. Cardiac involvement may be the dominant clinical feature and may result in death, even in the absence of significant skeletal muscle weakness.

Treatment of patients with dystrophinopathies is challenging. Current treatment consists primarily of supportive care. Definitive therapy requires restoration of dystrophin levels in skeletal and cardiac muscle fibers. Genetic approaches to accomplish this are being tested in clinical trials. One strategy involves the expression of anti-sense RNAs that alter RNA splicing so as to cause "skipping" of exons containing deleterious mutations, thus permitting the expression of a truncated, but partially functional, dystrophin protein. A second strategy involves the use of drugs that promote ribosomal "read-through" of stop codons, another ploy that may enable the synthesis of some functional dystrophin protein.

Other X-Linked and Autosomal Muscular Dystrophies

Other forms of muscular dystrophy share features with DMD and BMD but have distinct clinical, genetic, and pathologic features.

- *Myotonic dystrophy.* **Myotonia, the sustained involuntary contraction of a group of muscles, is the cardinal neuromuscular symptom in myotonic dystrophy.** Patients often complain of stiffness and difficulty in relaxing their grip, for example, after a handshake. Myotonic dystrophy is a nucleotide repeat expansion disease (Chapter 7) that is inherited as an autosomal dominant trait. More than 95% of patients with myotonic dystrophy have mutations in the gene that encodes the dystrophia myotonica protein kinase (DMPK). In normal subjects, this gene contains 5 to 37 CTG repeats, whereas affected patients usually carry 45 to several thousand. As with other nucleotide repeat expansion diseases, myotonic dystrophy exhibits *anticipation*, characterized by worsening of the disease manifestations with each passing generation because of further trinucleotide repeat expansion. The CTG repeat is located in the 3' untranslated region of the DMPK mRNA. Experimental studies suggest that the skeletal muscle phenotype stems from a "toxic" gain-of-function caused by the triplet repeat expansion. The mutant DMPK mRNA with the resulting CUG expansions sequesters muscleblind-like proteins involved in RNA splicing. This functional depletion of proteins involved in RNA splicing disrupts normal gene expression patterns and alters the function of diseased tissues like skeletal and cardiac muscle. Myotonic dystrophy often manifests in late childhood with gait abnormalities due to weakness of foot dorsiflexors, with subsequent progression to weakness of the intrinsic muscles of the hands and wrist extensors, atrophy of the facial muscles, and ptosis. Involvement of other organ systems results in potentially fatal cardiac arrhythmias, cataracts, early frontal balding, endocrinopathies, and testicular atrophy.
- *Limb-girdle muscular dystrophies.* **These muscular dystrophies preferentially affect the proximal musculature of the trunk and limbs.** Their genetic basis is heterogeneous. The growing list includes at least 7 dominant subtypes and 15 autosomal recessive subtypes. Some of the responsible mutations affect components of the dystrophin-glycoprotein complex other than dystrophin. Others affect proteins involved in vesicle transport and repair of cell membrane after injury (caveolin-3 and dysferlin), cytoskeletal proteins, or posttranslational modification of dystroglycan, a component of the dystrophin-glycoprotein complex.
- *Emery-Dreifuss muscular dystrophy* **(EMD) is a genetically heterogeneous disorder caused by mutations**

affecting structural proteins found in the nucleus. An X-linked form results from mutations in the gene encoding the protein emerin, whereas an autosomal dominant form is caused by mutations in the gene encoding lamin A/C. It is hypothesized that defects in these proteins compromise the structural integrity of the nucleus in cells that are subjected to repetitive mechanical stress (e.g., cardiac and skeletal muscle). These proteins may also regulate chromatin structure and thereby affect gene expression patterns. The clinical picture is characterized by progressive muscle weakness and wasting, contractures of the elbows and ankles, and cardiac disease. The cardiac involvement is severe, being associated with cardiomyopathy and arrhythmias that lead to sudden death in up to 40% of patients.

- *Facioscapulohumeral dystrophy* **is an autosomal dominant form of muscular dystrophy that is caused by complex genetic changes that allow expression of the transcription factor DUX4 that is normally repressed in mature tissues.** It is thought that the disease is caused by over expression of *DUX4* target genes, many of which are involved in the normal function of skeletal muscles. Most patients become symptomatic by the age of 20 years, usually owing to weakness in the facial muscles and the shoulder. Patients also exhibit weakness in the lower trunk and the dorsiflexors of the foot. Most affected persons have a normal life expectancy.

Channelopathies, Metabolic Myopathies, and Mitochondrial Myopathies

Other important inherited disorders of skeletal muscle are the result of defects in ion channels (channelopathies), metabolism, and mitochondrial function.

- *Ion channel myopathies* **are a group of familial disorders caused by inherited defects in ion channels that are characterized by myotonia, relapsing episodes of hypotonic paralysis associated with abnormal serum potassium levels, or both.** *Hyperkalemic periodic paralysis* results from mutations in the gene encoding the skeletal muscle sodium channel SCN4A, which regulates sodium entry during contraction. *Malignant hyperthermia* is a rare syndrome characterized by tachycardia, tachypnea, muscle spasms, and hyperpyrexia. It is triggered when patients carrying mutations in the ryanodine receptor RYR1, a calcium efflux channel, receive halogenated anesthetic agents or succinylcholine during surgery. On exposure to anesthetic, the mutated receptor leads to increased efflux of calcium from the sarcoplasmic reticulum, producing tetany and excessive heat production. There is some evidence that people carrying RYR1 mutations also are unusually susceptible to exertional hyperthermia (heat stroke).

- *Myopathies due to inborn errors of metabolism* **include disorders of glycogen synthesis and degradation** (Chapter 7) **and lipid handling.** The latter include disorders of the carnitine transport system and deficiencies of the mitochondrial dehydrogenase enzyme system, both of which can lead to accumulation of lipid in myocytes (lipid myopathies). These storage disorders may manifest as systemic disease or as a muscle-specific phenotype. Some are associated with muscle damage and weakness. Others manifest with recurring episodes of exercise- or fasting-induced muscle damage, which if severe may lead to necrosis of myoctyes (rhabdomyolysis), myoglobulinuria and acute renal failure.

- *Mitochondrial myopathies* **can stem from mutations in either the mitochondrial or nuclear genomes because both encode proteins and RNAs that are critical for mitochondrial function.** The variants caused by mitochondrial mutations show maternal inheritance (Chapter 7). Mitochondrial myopathies usually manifest in early adulthood with proximal muscle weakness and sometimes with severe involvement of the ocular musculature (external ophthalmoplegia). There may also be neurologic signs and symptoms, lactic acidosis, endocrinopathy, peripheral neuropathy, and cardiomyopathy. Some mitochondrial diseases are associated with normal muscle morphology, whereas others show aggregates of abnormal mitochondria; the latter impart a blotchy red appearance in special stains—hence the term *ragged red fibers*. On ultrastructural examination, these correspond to abnormal aggregates of mitochondria with abnormal shape and size, some containing crystalline inclusions.

Acquired Disorders of Skeletal Muscle

A diverse group of acquired disorders may manifest with muscle weakness, muscle cramping, or muscle pain. These include inflammatory myopathies, toxic muscle injuries, postinfectious rhabdomyolysis, and muscle infarction in the setting of diabetes. In most instances these are disorders of adults with acute or subacute onsets.

Inflammatory Myopathies

Polymyositis, dermatomyositis, and inclusion body myositis represent the traditional triad of inflammatory myopathies. This triad is a simplified view of complex diseases with variable phenotypes that are not always as well delineated as outlined here. Nevertheless, this approach still helps to outline key principles.

- *Polymyositis* is an autoimmune disorder associated with increased expression of MHC class I molecules on myofibers and predominantly endomysial inflammatory infiltrates containing CD8+ cytotoxic T cells. The autoimmune attack leads to myofiber necrosis and subsequent regeneration (Fig. 22.6A). Patients with polymyositis are often successfully treated with corticosteroids or other immunosuppressive agents.

- *Dermatomyositis* is the most common inflammatory myopathy in children, in whom it appears as an isolated entity. In adults, it often manifests as a paraneoplastic disorder. In both contexts, it is believed to have an autoimmune basis. The disease is typically associated with skin manifestations, as implied by the name, and may also have systemic manifestations such as interstitial lung disease. On microscopic examination and ultrastructural studies, it is associated with perivascular mononuclear cell infiltrates with plasma cells, "dropout" of capillaries, the presence of so-called "tubuloreticular inclusions" in endothelial cells, and myofiber damage in a paraseptal or perifascicular pattern (Fig. 22.6B).

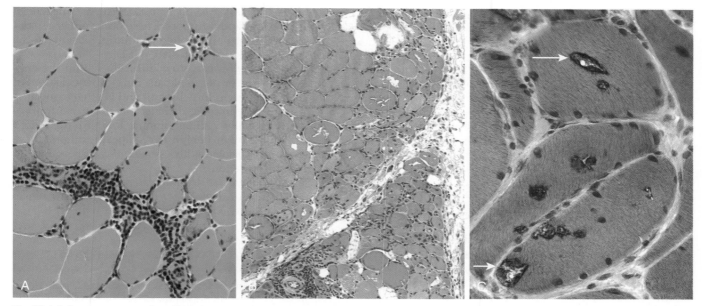

Fig. 22.6 Inflammatory myopathies. (A) Polymyositis is characterized by endomysial inflammatory infiltrates and myofiber necrosis *(arrow)*. (B) Dermatomyositis often shows prominent perifascicular and paraseptal atrophy. (C) Inclusion body myositis, showing myofibers containing rimmed vacuoles *(arrows)*. Modified Gomori trichrome stain.

As with some other autoimmune diseases such as SLE (Chapter 5), type 1 interferon-induced gene products are strongly upregulated in affected muscles. Some patients have autoantibodies that are relatively specific for dermatomyositis; these include antibodies against Mi-2 (a nuclear helicase) and p155 and p140, proteins with uncertain functions.

• *Inclusion body myositis* is the most common inflammatory myopathy in patients older than 60 years of age. It is grouped with other forms of myositis, but it has yet to be determined whether inflammation is a cause or an effect in this disorder. The morphologic hallmark of inclusion body myositis is the presence of rimmed vacuoles (Fig. 22.6C) that contain aggregates of the same proteins that accumulate in the brains of patients with neurodegenerative diseases—hyperphosphorylated tau, amyloid derived from β-amyloid precursor protein, and TDP-43 (Chapter 23)—leading some to speculate that this is a degenerative disorder of aging. Other features typical of chronic inflammatory myopathies, including myopathic changes, mononuclear cell infiltrates, endomysial fibrosis, and fatty replacement, also are evident. The disease follows a chronic, progressive course and generally does not respond well to immunosuppressive agents, another feature suggesting that inflammation is a secondary event.

Toxic Myopathies

A number of insults can cause toxic muscle injury, including intrinsic factors (e.g., thyroxine) and extrinsic factors (e.g., acute alcohol intoxication, various drugs).

• *Thyrotoxic myopathy* may take the form either of acute or chronic proximal muscle weakness, and it can be the first indication of thyrotoxicosis. Histologic findings include myofiber necrosis and regeneration.

• *Ethanol myopathy* occurs after an episode of binge drinking. The degree of rhabdomyolysis may be severe, sometimes leading to acute renal failure secondary to myoglobinuria. Patients usually complain of acute muscle pain, which may be generalized or confined to a single muscle group. Microscopically, there is myocyte swelling, necrosis, and regeneration.

• *Drug myopathy* can be produced by a variety of agents. For example, myopathy is the most common complication of statins (e.g., atorvastatin, simvastatin, pravastatin), occurring in approximately 1.5% of users. Two forms of statin associated myopathy are recognized: (1) toxicity of the drug and (2) statin-induced HMG-CoA reductase autoantibodies causing an immune mediated myopathy.

Tumors of Skeletal Muscles

These are discussed in Chapter 21 along with other tumors of soft tissues.

SUMMARY

DISORDERS OF SKELETAL MUSCLE

• Skeletal muscle function can be impaired by a primary (inherited or acquired) myopathy or secondarily because of problems with muscle innervation.
• The genetic forms of myopathy fall into several fairly distinct clinical phenotypes, including muscular dystrophy, congenital myopathy, and congenital muscular dystrophy.
• Dystrophinopathies are X-linked disorders caused by mutations in the dystrophin gene and disruption of the dystrophin-glycoprotein complex. Depending on the type of mutation, the disease may be severe, such as DMD, or mild (e.g., Becker dystrophy).
• Acquired myopathies have diverse causes, including inflammation and toxic exposures.

PERIPHERAL NERVE SHEATH TUMORS

A number of different tumors arise from peripheral nerves. Such tumors may manifest as soft tissue masses, with pain or loss of function related to impingement on nerves or other surrounding structures. In most peripheral nerve tumors, the neoplastic cells show evidence of Schwann cell differentiation. These tumors usually occur in adults and include both benign and malignant variants. An important feature is their frequent association with the familial tumor syndromes neurofibromatosis type 1 (NF1) and neurofibromatosis type 2 (NF2).

Schwannomas and Neurofibromatosis Type 2

Schwannomas are benign encapsulated tumors that may occur in soft tissues, internal organs, or spinal nerve roots. The most commonly affected cranial nerve is the vestibular portion of the eighth nerve. Tumors arising in a nerve root or the vestibular nerve may be associated with symptoms related to nerve root compression, which includes hearing loss in the case of vestibular schwannomas.

Most schwannomas are sporadic, but about 10% are associated with *familial neurofibromatosis type 2 (NF2)*. NF2 patients are at risk of developing multiple schwannomas, meningiomas, and ependymomas (the latter are described in Chapter 23). The presence of bilateral vestibular schwannomas is a hallmark of NF2; despite the name, neurofibromas (described later) are not found in NF2 patients. Affected patients carry a dominant loss of function mutation of the merlin gene on chromosome 22. Merlin is a cytoskeletal protein that functions as a tumor suppressor by facilitating E-cadherin–mediated contact inhibition (Chapter 6). With loss of merlin function, the tumor cells proliferate because contact inhibition is lost. Of note, merlin expression also is disrupted in sporadic schwannomas, possibly because of somatic mutations.

MORPHOLOGY

Most schwannomas appear as circumscribed masses abutting an adjacent nerve. On microscopic examination, these tumors often show an admixture of dense and loose areas referred to as Antoni A and B, respectively (Fig. 22.7A–B). They are comprised of a uniform proliferation of neoplastic Schwann cells. In the dense **Antoni A** areas, bland spindle cells with buckled nuclei are arranged into intersecting fascicles. These cells often align to produce nuclear palisading, resulting in alternating bands of nuclear and anuclear areas called Verocay bodies. Axons are largely excluded from the tumor. In the loose, hypocellular **Antoni B** areas, the spindle cells are spread apart by a prominent myxoid extracellular matrix. Thick-walled hyalinized vessels often are present. Hemorrhage or cystic changes also are sometimes seen.

Neurofibromas

Neurofibromas are benign peripheral nerve sheath tumors. Three important subtypes are recognized:

- *Localized cutaneous neurofibromas* arise as superficial nodular or polypoid tumors. These occur either as solitary sporadic lesions or often as multiple lesions in the context of neurofibromatosis 1 (NF1).
- *Plexiform neurofibromas* grow diffusely within the confines of a nerve or nerve plexus. Surgical enucleation of such lesions is therefore difficult and is often associated with lasting neurologic deficits. Plexiform neurofibromas are virtually pathognomonic for NF1 (discussed later). Unlike other benign nerve sheath tumors, these tumors are associated with a small but real risk of malignant transformation.
- *Diffuse neurofibromas* are infiltrative proliferations that can take the form of large, disfiguring subcutaneous masses. These also are often associated with NF1.

MORPHOLOGY

Unlike schwannomas, neurofibromas are not encapsulated. They may appear circumscribed, as in **localized cutaneous neurofibromas,** or may exhibit a diffusely infiltrative growth pattern. Also in contrast to schwannomas, the neoplastic Schwann cells in neurofibroma are admixed with other cell types, including mast cells, fibroblast like cells, and perineurial-like cells. The background stroma often contains loose wavy collagen bundles but also can be myxoid or can contain dense collagen (Fig. 22.7D). **Plexiform neurofibromas** involve multiple fascicles of individual affected nerves (Fig. 22.7C). **Diffuse neurofibromas** show an extensive infiltrative pattern of growth within the dermis and subcutis of the skin.

Neurofibromatosis Type 1

NF1 is an autosomal dominant disorder caused by mutations in the tumor suppressor neurofibromin, encoded on the long arm of chromosome 17 (17q). Neurofibromin is a negative regulator of the potent oncoprotein Ras (Chapter 6). Loss of neurofibromin function and the resulting Ras hyperactivity appear to be a cardinal feature of NF1-associated tumors. As would be anticipated for a tumor suppressor gene, the sole normal *NF1* allele is mutated or silenced in tumors arising in the setting of NF1. These include neurofibromas of all three main types, malignant peripheral nerve sheath tumors, "optic gliomas," and other glial tumors. In addition, patients with NF1 exhibit learning disabilities, seizures, skeletal abnormalities, vascular abnormalities with arterial stenoses, pigmented nodules of the iris (*Lisch nodules*), and pigmented skin lesions (axillary freckling and café-au-lait spots) in various degrees.

Malignant Peripheral Nerve Sheath Tumors

Malignant peripheral nerve sheath tumors are neoplasms seen in adults that typically show evidence of Schwann cell derivation and sometimes a clear origin from a peripheral nerve. They may arise from transformation of a neurofibroma, usually of the plexiform type. About one-half of such tumors arise in patients with NF1, and 3% to 10% of all patients with NF1 develop a malignant peripheral

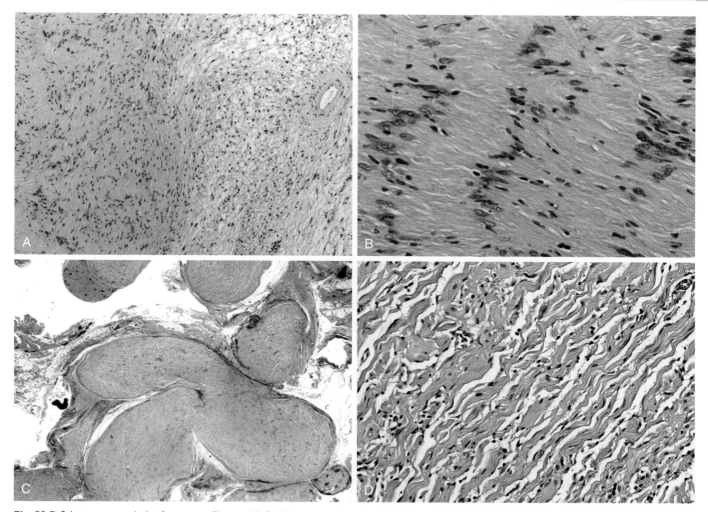

Fig. 22.7 Schwannoma and plexiform neurofibroma. (A–B) Schwannoma. As seen in (A), schwannomas often contain dense pink Antoni A areas *(left)* and loose, pale Antoni B areas *(right)*, as well as hyalinized blood vessels *(right)*. (B) Antoni A area with the nuclei of tumor cells aligned in palisading rows. (C–D) Plexiform neurofibroma. Multiple nerve fascicles are expanded by infiltrating tumor cells (C), which at higher power (D) are seen to consist of bland spindle cells admixed with wavy collagen bundles likened to carrot shavings.

nerve sheath tumor during their lifetimes. Histologically, these tumors are highly cellular and exhibit features of overt malignancy, including anaplasia, necrosis, infiltrative growth pattern, pleomorphism, and high proliferative activity.

Traumatic Neuroma

Traumatic neuroma is a nonneoplastic proliferation associated with a previous injury leading to transection of a peripheral nerve. Such injuries activate a regenerative program (see Fig. 22.1) characterized by sprouting and elongation of processes from the proximal axonal stump. With severe injuries that disrupt the perineurial sheath, these new processes may "miss" their target, the distal end of the transected nerve. The misguided elongating axonal processes can induce a reactive proliferation of Schwann cells, leading to the formation of a painful localized nodule that consists of a haphazard mixture of axons, Schwann cells, and connective tissue.

SUMMARY

PERIPHERAL NERVE SHEATH TUMORS

- In most peripheral nerve sheath tumors, the neoplastic cells show evidence of Schwann cell differentiation.
- Peripheral nerve sheath tumors are important features of the familial tumor syndromes NF1 and NF2.
- Schwannomas and neurofibromas are benign nerve sheath tumors.
- Schwannomas are circumscribed, usually encapsulated tumors that abut the nerve of origin and are a feature of NF2.
- Neurofibromas may manifest as a sporadic subcutaneous nodule, as a large, poorly defined soft tissue lesion, or as a growth within a nerve. Neurofibromas are associated with NF1.
- About 50% of malignant peripheral nerve sheath tumors occur de novo in otherwise normal persons, whereas the remainder arise from the malignant transformation of a preexisting NF1-associated neurofibroma.

SUGGESTED READINGS

Berrih-Aknin S, Le Panse R: Myasthenia gravis: a comprehensive review of immune dysregulation and etiological mechanisms, *J Autoimmun* 52:90–100, 2014. [*Review of subtypes and etiology of myasthenia gravis.*]

Briemberg HR: Peripheral nerve complications of medical disease, *Semin Neurol* 29:124, 2009. [*Review of the ways medical diseases including diabetes, connective tissue diseases, cancer, and infections affect peripheral nerves.*]

Dalakas MC: Inflammatory muscle diseases, *N Engl J Med* 372:18, 2015. [*Discussion of current concepts on the pathophysiology of idiopathic inflammatory myopathies.*]

Falzarano MS, Scotton C, Passarelli C, et al: Duchenne muscular dystrophy: from diagnosis to therapy, *Molecules* 20:18168, 2015. [*Molecular techniques for the diagnosis and treatment of this disease.*]

Habib AA, Brannagan TH III: Therapeutic strategies for diabetic neuropathy, *Curr Neurol Neurosci Rep* 10:92, 2010. [*Review focused especially on clinical features and therapy of diabetic neuropathy.*]

Kang PB, Griggs RC: Advances in muscular dystrophies, *JAMA* 72:741, 2015. [*An update on the molecular pathogenesis of muscular dystrophies and their treatment.*]

Mahadeva B, Phillips LH, Juel VC: Autoimmune disorders of neuromuscular transmission, *Semin Neurol* 28:212, 2008. [*Review of myasthenia gravis and Lambert-Eaton syndrome.*]

McClatchey AI: Neurofibromatosis, *Annu Rev Pathol* 2:191, 2007. [*Review of features that distinguish neurofibromatosis type 1, neurofibromatosis type 2, and schwannomatosis, with a focus on the genetics.*]

Obrosova IG: Diabetes and the peripheral nerve, *Biochim Biophys Acta* 1792:931, 2009. [*Detailed discussion of the pathophysiology of diabetic neuropathy.*]

Petrilli AM, Fernández-Valle C: Role of Merlin/NF2 inactivation on tumor biology, *Oncogene* 35:537–548, 2016. [*Mechanisms of action of the NF2 gene in the pathogenesis of neuronal tumors.*]

Ravenscroft G, Laing NG, Bönnemann CG: Pathophysiological concepts in the congenital myopathies: blurring the boundaries, sharpening the focus, *Brain* 138:246, 2015. [*A review of the overlapping and nonoverlapping genetic lesions in congenital myopathies.*]

Tawil R, van der Maarel SM, Tapscott SJ: Facioscapulohumeral dystrophy: the path to consensus on pathophysiology, *Skelet Muscle* 4:12, 2014. [*Review of FSHD including a discussion of the complex genetics.*]

van Adel BA, Tarnopolsky MA: Metabolic myopathies: update 2009, *J Clin Neuromuscul Dis* 10:97, 2009. [*Review of metabolic myopathies.*]

Vrablik M, Zlatohlavek L, Stulc T, et al: Statin-associated myopathy: from genetic predisposition to clinical management, *Physiol Res* 63(Suppl 3):S327, 2014. [*A discussion of the risk factors for statin-induced myopathy and its therapy.*]

Wang ET, Cody NA, Jog S, et al: Transcriptome-wide regulation of pre-mRNA splicing and mRNA localization by muscleblind proteins, *Cell* 150:710–724, 2012. [*Study of the transcriptional changes with myotonic dystrophy.*]

See Targeted Therapy available online at **studentconsult.com**

CHAPTER

Central Nervous System

23

CHAPTER OUTLINE

Edema, Herniation, and
  Hydrocephalus 850
Cerebral Edema 850
Hydrocephalus 851
Herniation 851
Cerebrovascular Diseases 852
Hypoxia, Ischemia, and Infarction 852
Intracranial Hemorrhage 854
Other Vascular Diseases 856
Central Nervous System Trauma 857
Traumatic Parenchymal Injuries 857
Traumatic Vascular Injury 858
Congenital Malformations and Perinatal
  Brain Injury 860
Malformations 860
Perinatal Brain Injury 861

Infections of the Nervous System 862
Epidural and Subdural Infections 862
Meningitis 862
Parenchymal Infections 864
Prion Diseases 869
Diseases of Myelin 870
Multiple Sclerosis (MS) 871
Other Acquired Demyelinating
  Diseases 871
Leukodystrophies 872
Genetic Metabolic Diseases 873
Acquired Metabolic and Toxic
  Disturbances 873
Nutritional Diseases 873
Metabolic Disorders 873
Toxic Disorders 874

Neurodegenerative Diseases 874
Alzheimer Disease 874
Frontotemporal Lobar Degeneration 877
Parkinson Disease 877
Huntington Disease 879
Spinocerebellar Ataxias 879
Amyotrophic Lateral Sclerosis 880
Tumors 881
Gliomas 881
Neuronal Tumors 883
Embryonal (Primitive) Neoplasms 884
Other Parenchymal Tumors 884
Meningiomas 885
Metastatic Tumors 885
Familial Tumor Syndromes 886

Degenerative, inflammatory, infectious, vascular, and neoplastic disorders of the central nervous system (CNS) are some of the most serious diseases of mankind. These diseases have many unique features that reflect the highly specialized structure and functions of the CNS. The principal functional unit of the CNS is the *neuron*. Neurons of different types and in different locations have distinct properties, including functional roles, distribution of their connections, neurotransmitters used, metabolic requirements, and levels of electrical activity at a given moment. A set of neurons, not necessarily clustered together in a region of the brain, may thus show *selective vulnerability* to various insults because it shares one or more of these properties. Since different regions of the brain participate in different functions, the pattern of clinical signs and symptoms that follow injury depend as much on the region of brain involved as on the pathologic process. Mature neurons are incapable of cell division, so destruction of even a small number of neurons essential for a specific function may leave the individual with a neurologic deficit. In addition to neurons the CNS contains other cells, such as *astrocytes* and *oligodendrocytes*, which make up the *glia*. The components of the CNS are affected by a number of unique neurologic disorders and also respond to common insults (e.g., ischemia, infection) in a manner that is distinct from other tissues.

Before delving into specific disorders, we will briefly review the characteristic morphologic changes that are often seen in the CNS in the setting of injury or infection.

MORPHOLOGY

Features of Neuronal Injury. In response to injury, a number of changes occur in neurons and their processes (axons and dendrites). Within 12 hours of an irreversible hypoxic-ischemic insult, **neuronal injury** becomes evident on routine hematoxylin and eosin (H&E) staining (Fig. 23.1A). There is shrinkage of the cell body, pyknosis of the nucleus, disappearance of the nucleolus, loss of Nissl substance, and intense eosinophilia of the cytoplasm ("red neurons"). Axonal injury also leads to cell body enlargement and rounding, peripheral displacement of the nucleus, enlargement of the nucleolus, and peripheral dispersion of Nissl substance **(central chromatolysis).** In addition, acute injuries typically result in breakdown of the blood-brain barrier and variable degrees of cerebral edema (discussed later).

Many neurodegenerative diseases are associated with specific **intracellular inclusions** (e.g., Lewy bodies in Parkinson disease and tangles in Alzheimer disease). Pathogenic viruses may form inclusions in infected neurons, just as in other cells, and such inclusions aid in the diagnosis. In some neurodegenerative diseases, neuronal processes become thickened and tortuous; these are termed **dystrophic neurites.**

849

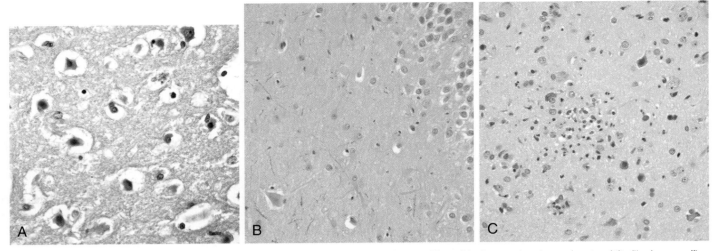

Fig. 23.1 Patterns of neuronal injury. (A) Acute hypoxic-ischemic injury in the cerebral cortex. The cell bodies are shrunken and eosinophilic ("red neurons"), and the nuclei are pyknotic. (B) Reactive astrocytes, with eosinophilic cytoplasm and multiple radiating processes. (C) Collection of microglial cells forming a poorly defined nodule, a common finding in viral infections.

Astrocyte Injury and Repair. Astrocytes are the principal cells responsible for repair and scar formation in the brain, a process termed **gliosis.** In response to injury, astrocytes undergo both hypertrophy and hyperplasia. The nucleus enlarges and becomes vesicular, and the nucleolus becomes prominent. The cytoplasm expands and takes on a bright pink hue, and the cell extends multiple stout, ramifying processes (called **gemistocytic astrocyte**; see Fig. 23.1B). Unlike elsewhere in the body, fibroblasts participate in healing after brain injury to a limited extent except in specific settings (penetrating brain trauma or around abscesses). In long-standing gliosis, the cytoplasm of reactive astrocytes shrinks in size, and the cellular processes become more tightly interwoven **(fibrillary astrocytes). Rosenthal fibers** are thick, elongated, brightly eosinophilic protein aggregates found in astrocytic processes in chronic gliosis and in some low-grade gliomas.

Oligodendrocytes, which produce myelin, exhibit a limited spectrum of specific morphologic changes in response to various injuries. In progressive multifocal leukoencephalopathy, viral inclusions can be seen in oligodendrocytes, with a smudgy, homogeneous-appearing enlarged nucleus.

Microglial cells are long-lived cells derived from the embryonic yolk sac that function as the resident phagocytes of the CNS. When activated by tissue injury, infection, or trauma, they proliferate and become more prominent histologically. Microglial cells take on the appearance of activated macrophages in areas of demyelination, organizing infarct, or hemorrhage; in other settings such as infections, they develop elongated nuclei **(rod cells).** Aggregates of elongated microglial cells at sites of tissue injury are termed **microglial nodules** (see Fig. 23.1C). Similar collections can be found congregating around and phagocytosing injured neurons **(neuronophagia).**

Ependymal cells line the ventricular system and the central canal of the spinal cord. Certain pathogens, particularly cytomegalovirus (CMV), can produce extensive ependymal injury, with typical viral inclusions. **Choroid plexus** is in continuity with the ependyma, and its specialized epithelial covering is responsible for the secretion of cerebrospinal fluid (CSF).

EDEMA, HERNIATION, AND HYDROCEPHALUS

The brain and spinal cord are encased within the skull and spinal canal, with nerves and blood vessels passing through specific foramina. The advantage of housing the delicate CNS within hard, rigid structures is obvious, but this arrangement provides little room for expansion of the brain in disease states. As a result, virtually any increase in the volume of the skull contents brings with it an increase in intracranial pressure. Substantial increases in the intracranial pressure compromise the ability of the cardiovascular system to deliver blood to the brain, resulting in decreased brain perfusion, with serious or fatal consequences. Disorders that may cause dangerous increases in the volume of intracranial contents include generalized cerebral edema, hydrocephalus, hemorrhages, ischemia, and mass lesions such as tumors.

Cerebral Edema

Cerebral edema is the accumulation of excess fluid within the brain parenchyma. There are two types, which often occur together, particularly after generalized injury.
- *Vasogenic edema* occurs when the integrity of the normal blood-brain barrier is disrupted, allowing fluid to shift from the vascular compartment into the extracellular spaces of the brain. Vasogenic edema can be localized (e.g., the result of increased vascular permeability due to inflammation or in tumors) or generalized.
- *Cytotoxic edema* is an increase in intracellular fluid secondary to neuronal and glial cell injury, as might follow generalized hypoxic or ischemic insult or exposure to certain toxins.

The edematous brain is softer than normal and often appears to "overfill" the cranial vault. In generalized

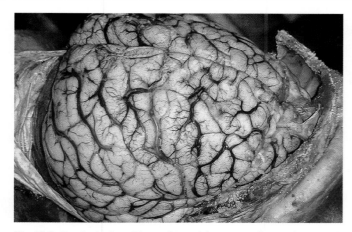

Fig. 23.2 Cerebral edema. The surfaces of the gyri are flattened as a result of compression of the expanding brain by the dura mater and inner surface of the skull. Such changes are associated with a dangerous increase in intra-cranial pressure.

edema, the gyri are flattened, the intervening sulci are narrowed, and the ventricular cavities are compressed (Fig. 23.2).

Hydrocephalus

After being produced by the choroid plexus within the ventricles, CSF circulates through the ventricular system and flows through the foramina of Luschka and Magendie into the subarachnoid space, where it is absorbed by arachnoid granulations. The balance between rates of generation and resorption regulates CSF volume.

Hydrocephalus refers to an increase in the volume of the CSF within the ventricular system. This disorder most often is a consequence of impaired flow or decreased resorption of CSF. If there is a localized obstacle to CSF flow within the ventricular system, then a portion of the ventricles enlarges while the remainder does not. This pattern is referred to as *noncommunicating hydrocephalus* and most commonly is caused by masses obstructing the foramen of Monro or compressing the cerebral aqueduct. In *communicating hydrocephalus,* the entire ventricular system is enlarged; it is usually caused by reduced CSF resorption.

If hydrocephalus develops in infancy before closure of the cranial sutures, the head enlarges. Once the sutures fuse, hydrocephalus causes ventricular expansion and increased intracranial pressure, but no change in head circumference (Fig. 23.3). In contrast to these disorders, in which increased CSF volume is the primary process, a compensatory increase in CSF volume *(hydrocephalus ex vacuo)* may occur secondary to a loss of brain volume from any underlying cause (e.g., infarction, neurode-generative disease). In such settings, the hydrocephalus merely reflects the primary disorder and is of no clinical significance.

Herniation

Herniation is the displacement of brain tissue from one compartment to another in response to increased intra-cranial pressure. The intra-cranial compartment is divided by rigid dural folds (falx and tentorium). If the pressure is sufficiently high, portions of the brain are displaced across these rigid structures. This herniation often leads to compromise of the blood supply to compressed tissue, producing infarction, additional swelling, and further herniation.

There are three main types of herniation (Fig. 23.4):

* *Subfalcine (cingulate) herniation* occurs when unilateral or asymmetric expansion of a cerebral hemisphere displaces the cingulate gyrus under the edge of the falx. This may compress the anterior cerebral artery.
* *Transtentorial (uncinate) herniation* occurs when the medial aspect of the temporal lobe is compressed against the free margin of the tentorium. As the temporal lobe is displaced, the third cranial nerve is compromised, resulting in pupillary dilation and impaired ocular movements on the side of the lesion ("blown pupil"). The posterior cerebral artery may also be compressed, resulting in ischemic injury to tissue supplied by that vessel, including the primary visual cortex. With further displacement of the temporal lobe, pressure on the mid-brain may compress the contralateral cerebral peduncle against the tentorium, resulting in hemiparesis ipsilateral to the side of the herniation. The compression of the peduncle creates a deformation known as *Kernohan's notch.* Compression of the midbrain and the ascending reticular activating system with transtentorial herniation leads to depressed consciousness. Progression of transtentorial herniation is often accompanied by linear or flame-shaped hemorrhages in the midbrain and pons, termed *Duret hemorrhages* (Fig. 23.5). These lesions usually occur in the midline and paramedian regions and are believed to be the result of tearing of penetrating veins and arteries supplying the upper brain stem.
* *Tonsillar herniation* refers to displacement of the cerebellar tonsils through the foramen magnum. This type of herniation causes brain stem compression and compromises vital respiratory and cardiac centers in the medulla, and is often fatal.

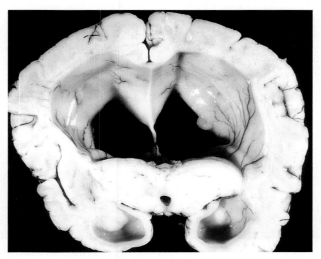

Fig. 23.3 Hydrocephalus. Dilated lateral ventricles seen in a coronal section through the mid-thalamus.

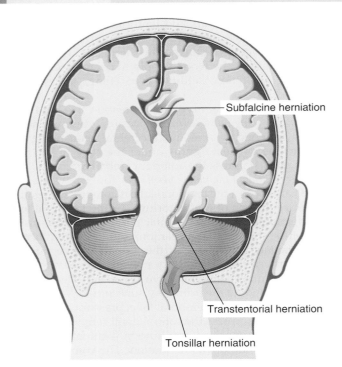

Fig. 23.4 Herniation syndromes. Displacement of brain parenchyma across fixed barriers can be subfalcine, transtentorial, or tonsillar (into the foramen magnum).

SUMMARY

EDEMA, HERNIATION, AND HYDROCEPHALUS

- Cerebral edema is the accumulation of excess fluid within the brain parenchyma. Hydrocephalus is defined as an increase in CSF volume within all or part of the ventricular system.
- Increases in brain volume (as a result of increased CSF volume, edema, hemorrhage, or tumor) raise the pressure inside the fixed capacity of the skull.
- Increases in pressure can damage the brain by decreasing perfusion or by displacing tissue across dural partitions inside the skull or through openings in the skull (herniations).

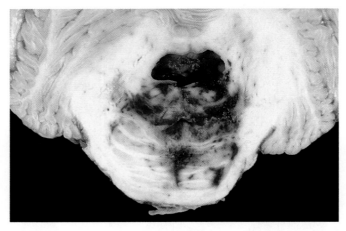

Fig. 23.5 Duret hemorrhage. As mass effect displaces the brain downward, there is disruption of the vessels that enter the pons along the midline, leading to hemorrhage.

CEREBROVASCULAR DISEASES

Cerebrovascular diseases are brain disorders caused by pathologic processes involving blood vessels. They are a major cause of death in the developed world and are the most prevalent cause of neurologic morbidity. The three main pathogenic mechanisms are (1) thrombotic occlusion, (2) embolic occlusion, and (3) vascular rupture. *Stroke* is the clinical designation applied to all of these conditions when symptoms begin acutely. Thrombosis and embolism have similar consequences for the brain: loss of oxygen and metabolic substrates, resulting in infarction or ischemic injury of regions supplied by the affected vessel. Similar injury occurs globally when there is complete loss of perfusion, severe hypoxemia (e.g., hypovolemic shock), or profound hypoglycemia. Hemorrhage accompanies rupture of vessels and leads to direct tissue damage as well as secondary ischemic injury. Traumatic vascular injury is discussed separately in the context of trauma.

Hypoxia, Ischemia, and Infarction

The brain is a highly oxygen-dependent tissue that requires a continual supply of glucose and oxygen from the blood. Although it constitutes no more than 2% of body weight, the brain receives 15% of the resting cardiac output and is responsible for 20% of total body oxygen consumption. Cerebral blood flow normally remains stable over a wide range of blood pressure and intracranial pressure because of autoregulation of vascular resistance. The brain may be deprived of oxygen by two general mechanisms:

- *Functional hypoxia,* caused by a low partial pressure of oxygen (e.g., high altitude), impaired oxygen-carrying capacity (e.g., severe anemia, carbon monoxide poisoning), or toxins that interfere with oxygen use (e.g., cyanide poisoning)
- *Ischemia,* either *transient* or *permanent,* due to tissue hypoperfusion, which can be caused by hypotension, vascular obstruction, or both

Global Cerebral Ischemia

Widespread ischemic-hypoxic injury can occur in the setting of severe systemic hypotension, usually when systolic pressures fall below 50 mm Hg, as in cardiac arrest and shock. The clinical outcome varies with the severity and duration of the insult. When the insult is mild, there may be only a transient postischemic confusional state, with eventual complete recovery. Neurons are more susceptible to hypoxic injury than are glial cells, and the most susceptible neurons are the pyramidal cells of the hippocampus and neocortex and Purkinje cells of the cerebellum. In some individuals, even mild or transient global ischemic insults may cause damage to these vulnerable areas. In severe global cerebral ischemia, widespread neuronal death occurs irrespective of regional vulnerability. Patients who survive often remain severely impaired neurologically and in a persistent vegetative state. Other patients meet the clinical criteria for so-called "brain death," in which all voluntary and reflex brain and brain stem function is absent, including respiratory drive. When patients with this form of irreversible injury are maintained on mechanical ventilation, the brain gradually undergoes autolysis, resulting in the so-called "respirator brain."

MORPHOLOGY

In the setting of global ischemia, the brain is swollen, with wide gyri and narrowed sulci. The cut surface shows poor demarcation between gray matter and white matter. The histopathologic changes that accompany irreversible ischemic injury (infarction) are grouped into three categories. **Early changes,** occurring 12 to 24 hours after the insult, include acute neuronal cell change (red neurons) (see Fig. 23.1A) characterized initially by microvacuolation, followed by cytoplasmic eosinophilia, and later nuclear pyknosis and karyorrhexis. Similar changes occur somewhat later in astrocytes and oligodendroglia. After this, the reaction to tissue damage begins with infiltration of neutrophils (Fig. 23.6A). **Subacute changes,** occurring at 24 hours to 2 weeks, include necrosis of tissue, influx of macrophages, vascular proliferation, and reactive gliosis (see Fig. 23.6B). **Repair,** seen after 2 weeks, is characterized by removal of necrotic tissue and gliosis (see Fig. 23.6C).

Border zone ("watershed") infarcts occur in regions of the brain and spinal cord that lie at the most distal portions of arterial territories. They are usually seen after hypotensive episodes. In the cerebral hemispheres, the border zone between the anterior and the middle cerebral artery distributions is at greatest risk. Damage to this region produces a wedge-shaped band of necrosis over the cerebral convexity a few centimeters lateral to the interhemispheric fissure.

Focal Cerebral Ischemia

Cerebral arterial occlusion leads first to focal ischemia and then to infarction in the distribution of the compromised vessel. The size, location, and shape of the infarct and the extent of tissue damage that results may be modified by collateral blood flow. Specifically, collateral flow through the circle of Willis or cortical-leptomeningeal anastomoses can limit damage in some regions. By contrast, there is little if any collateral blood flow to structures such as the thalamus, basal ganglia, and deep white matter, which are supplied by deep penetrating vessels.

Embolic infarctions are more common than infarctions due to thrombosis. Cardiac mural thrombi are a frequent source of emboli; myocardial dysfunction, valvular disease, and atrial fibrillation are important predisposing factors. Thromboemboli also arise in arteries, most often from atheromatous plaques in the carotid arteries or aortic arch. Emboli of venous origin may cross over to the arterial circulation through a patent foramen ovale and lodge in the brain (paradoxical embolism; see Chapter 4); these include thromboemboli from deep leg veins and fat emboli, usually following bone trauma. The territory of the middle cerebral artery, a direct extension of the internal carotid artery, is most frequently affected by embolic infarction. Emboli tend to lodge where vessels branch or in areas of stenosis, usually caused by atherosclerosis.

Thrombotic occlusions causing cerebral infarctions usually are superimposed on atherosclerotic plaques; common sites are the carotid bifurcation, the origin of the middle cerebral artery, and either end of the basilar artery. These occlusions may be accompanied by anterograde extension, as well as thrombus fragmentation and distal embolization. Thrombotic occlusions causing small infarcts of only a few millimeters in diameter, so-called "lacunar infarcts," occur when small penetrating arteries occlude due to chronic damage, usually from long-standing hypertension (discussed later).

Infarcts can be divided into two broad groups (Fig. 23.7). *Nonhemorrhagic infarcts* result from acute vascular occlusions and may evolve into *hemorrhagic infarcts* when there is reperfusion of ischemic tissue, either through collaterals or after dissolution of emboli.

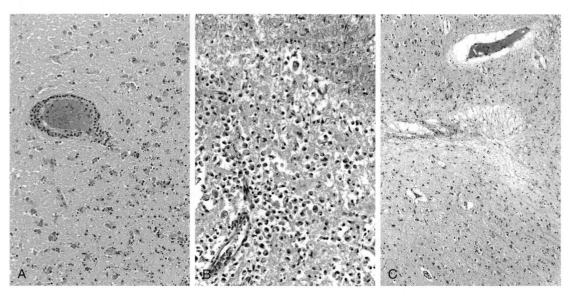

Fig. 23.6 Cerebral infarction. (A) Infiltration of a cerebral infarction by neutrophils begins at the edges of the lesion, where the vascular supply is intact. (B) By day 10, an area of infarction shows the presence of macrophages and surrounding reactive gliosis. (C) Old intracortical infarcts are seen as areas of tissue loss and residual gliosis.

MORPHOLOGY

Hemorrhagic infarcts usually manifest as multiple, sometimes confluent, petechial hemorrhages (Fig. 23.7A and B). The microscopic picture and evolution of hemorrhagic infarction parallel those of ischemic infarction, with the addition of blood extravasation and resorption. In individuals with coagulopathies, hemorrhagic infarcts may be associated with extensive intracerebral hematomas.

The macroscopic appearance of a **nonhemorrhagic infarct** evolves over time. During the first 6 hours, the tissue is unchanged in appearance, but by 48 hours, the tissue becomes pale, soft, and swollen. From days 2 to 10, the injured brain turns gelatinous and friable, and the boundary between normal and abnormal tissue becomes more distinct as edema resolves in the adjacent viable tissue. From day 10 to week 3, the tissue liquefies, eventually leaving a fluid-filled cavity, which gradually expands as dead tissue is resorbed (see Fig. 23.7C).

Microscopically, the tissue reaction follows a characteristic sequence. After the first 12 hours, ischemic neuronal change (red neurons) (see Fig. 23.1A) and cytotoxic and vasogenic edema appear. Endothelial and glial cells, mainly astrocytes, swell, and myelinated fibers begin to disintegrate. During the first several days neutrophils infiltrate the area of injury, but these are replaced over the next 2–3 weeks by macrophages. Macrophages containing myelin or red blood cell breakdown products may persist in the lesion for months to years. As the process of phagocytosis and liquefaction proceeds, astrocytes at the edges of the lesion progressively enlarge, divide, and develop a prominent network of cytoplasmic extensions. After several months, the striking astrocytic nuclear and cytoplasmic enlargement regresses. In the wall of the cavity, astrocyte processes form a dense feltwork of glial fibers admixed with new capillaries and a few perivascular connective tissue fibers.

Intracranial Hemorrhage

Hemorrhages within the brain are caused by (1) hypertension and other diseases leading to vascular wall injury, (2) structural lesions such as arteriovenous and cavernous malformations, and (3) tumors. Subarachnoid hemorrhages most commonly are the result of ruptured aneurysms but also occur with other vascular malformations. Subdural or epidural hemorrhages usually are associated with trauma.

Primary Brain Parenchymal Hemorrhage

Spontaneous (nontraumatic) intraparenchymal hemorrhages are most common in mid to late adult life, with a peak incidence at about 60 years of age. Most are due to the rupture of a small intraparenchymal vessel. Hypertension is the leading underlying cause, and brain hemorrhage accounts for roughly 15% of deaths among individuals with chronic hypertension. Intracerebral hemorrhage can be clinically devastating when it affects large portions of the brain or extends into the ventricular system; alternatively, it can affect small regions and be clinically silent. Hypertensive intraparenchymal hemorrhages typically occur in the basal ganglia, thalamus, pons, and

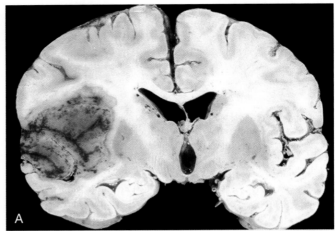

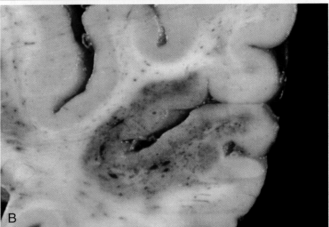

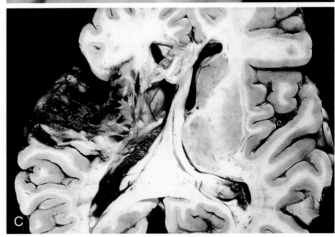

Fig. 23.7 Cerebral infarction. (A) Section of the brain showing a large, discolored, focally hemorrhagic region in the left middle cerebral artery distribution (hemorrhagic, or red, infarction). (B) An infarct with punctate hemorrhages, consistent with ischemia-reperfusion injury, is present in the temporal lobe. (C) Old cystic infarct shows destruction of cortex and surrounding gliosis.

cerebellum (Fig. 23.8), with the location and the size of the bleed determining its clinical manifestations. If the individual survives the acute event, gradual resolution of the hematoma ensues, sometimes with considerable clinical improvement.

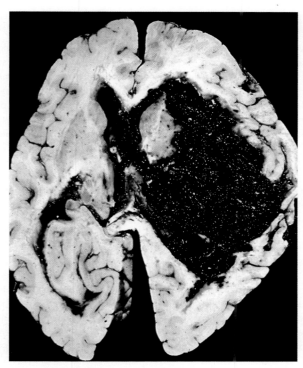

Fig. 23.8 Cerebral hemorrhage. Massive hypertensive hemorrhage rupturing into a lateral ventricle.

MORPHOLOGY

In acute intracerebral hemorrhage, the extravasated blood compresses the adjacent parenchyma. With time, hemorrhages are converted to a cavity with a brown, discolored rim. On microscopic examination, early lesions consist of clotted blood surrounded by edematous brain tissue containing neurons and glia displaying morphologic changes typical of anoxic injury. Eventually the edema resolves, pigment- and lipid-laden macrophages appear, and proliferation of reactive astrocytes becomes visible at the periphery of the lesion. The cellular events then follow the same time course observed after cerebral infarction.

Cerebral Amyloid Angiopathy

Cerebral amyloid angiopathy (CAA) is a disease in which the same amyloidogenic peptides as those found in Alzheimer disease (discussed later) deposit in the walls of medium- and small-caliber meningeal and cortical vessels. The amyloid confers a rigid, pipe-like appearance and stains with Congo red. Amyloid deposition weakens vessel walls and increases the risk for hemorrhages, which differ in distribution from those associated with hypertension. CAA-associated hemorrhages often occur in the lobes of the cerebral cortex (*lobar hemorrhages*). In addition to these symptomatic hemorrhages, CAA also results in small (<1 mm) cortical hemorrhages (*microhemorrhages*).

Subarachnoid Hemorrhage and Saccular Aneurysms

The most frequent cause of clinically significant nontraumatic subarachnoid hemorrhage is rupture of a saccular (berry) aneurysm. Hemorrhage into the subarachnoid space also may result from vascular malformation, trauma, rupture of an intracerebral hemorrhage into the ventricular system, coagulopathies, and tumors.

In about one-third of cases, rupture of a saccular aneurysm occurs at the time of an acute increase in intracranial pressure, such as occurs with straining at stool or sexual orgasm. Blood under arterial pressure is forced into the subarachnoid space, and the patient is stricken with sudden, excruciating headache (known as a *thunderclap headache,* often described as "the worst headache I've ever had") and rapidly loses consciousness. Between 25% and 50% of affected individuals die from the first bleed, and recurrent bleeds are common in survivors. Not surprisingly, the prognosis worsens with each bleeding episode.

About 90% of saccular aneurysms occur in the anterior circulation near major arterial branch points (Fig. 23.9); multiple aneurysms exist in 20% to 30% of cases. The aneurysms are not present at birth but develop over time because of underlying defects in the vessel media. There is an increased risk for aneurysms in patients with autosomal dominant polycystic kidney disease (Chapter 14) and genetic disorders of extracellular matrix proteins (e.g., Ehler-Danlos syndrome). Overall, roughly 1.3% of aneurysms bleed per year, with the probability of rupture increasing with size. For example, aneurysms larger than 1 cm in diameter have a roughly 50% risk for bleeding per year. In the early period after a subarachnoid hemorrhage, there is an additional risk for ischemic injury from vasospasm of other vessels. Healing and the attendant meningeal fibrosis and scarring sometimes obstruct CSF flow or disrupt CSF resorption, leading to hydrocephalus.

MORPHOLOGY

A saccular aneurysm is a thin-walled outpouching of an artery (Fig. 23.10). Beyond the neck of the aneurysm, the muscular wall and intimal elastic lamina are absent, such that the aneurysm sac is lined only by thickened hyalinized intima. The adventitia covering the sac is continuous with that of the parent artery. Rupture usually occurs at the apex of the sac, releasing blood into the subarachnoid space, the substance of the brain, or both..

In addition to saccular aneurysms, atherosclerotic, mycotic, traumatic, and dissecting aneurysms also occur intracranially. The last three types (like saccular aneurysms) most often are found in the anterior circulation, whereas atherosclerotic aneurysms frequently are fusiform and most commonly involve the basilar artery. Nonsaccular aneurysms usually manifest as cerebral infarction due to vascular occlusion instead of subarachnoid hemorrhage.

Vascular Malformations

Vascular malformations of the brain are classified into four principal types based on the nature of the abnormal vessels: arteriovenous malformations (AVMs), cavernous

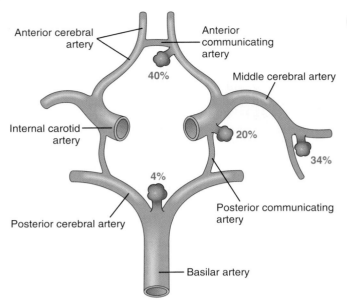

Fig. 23.9 Common sites of saccular aneurysms.

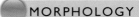

AVMs may involve subarachnoid vessels extending into brain parenchyma or occur exclusively within the brain. On gross inspection, they resemble a tangled network of wormlike vascular channels (Fig. 23.11). Microscopic examination shows enlarged blood vessels separated by gliotic tissue, often with evidence of previous hemorrhage. Some vessels can be recognized as arteries with duplicated and fragmented internal elastic lamina, while others show marked thickening or partial replacement of the media by hyalinized connective tissue.

Cavernous malformations consist of distended, loosely organized vascular channels with thin collagenized walls without intervening nervous tissue. They occur most often in the cerebellum, pons, and subcortical regions, and have a low blood flow without significant arteriovenous shunting. Foci of old hemorrhage, infarction, and calcification frequently surround the abnormal vessels.

Capillary telangiectasias are microscopic foci of dilated thin-walled vascular channels separated by relatively normal brain parenchyma that occur most frequently in the pons. **Venous angiomas** (varices) consist of aggregates of ectatic venous channels. These latter two types of vascular malformation are unlikely to bleed or to cause symptoms, and most are incidental findings.

malformations, capillary telangiectasias, and venous angiomas. AVMs, the most common of these, affect males twice as frequently as females and most commonly manifest between 10 and 30 years of age with seizures, an intracerebral hemorrhage, or a subarachnoid hemorrhage. In the newborn period, large AVMs may lead to high-output congestive heart failure because of blood shunting from arteries to veins. *The risk for bleeding makes AVM the most dangerous type of vascular malformation.* Multiple AVMs can be seen in the setting of hereditary hemorrhagic telangiectasia, an autosomal dominant condition often associated with mutations affecting the TGFβ pathway.

Other Vascular Diseases

Hypertensive Cerebrovascular Disease

Hypertension causes *hyaline arteriolar sclerosis* of the deep penetrating arteries and arterioles that supply the basal ganglia, the hemispheric white matter, and the brain stem. Affected arteriolar walls are weakened and are more vulnerable to rupture. In some instances, minute aneurysms *(Charcot-Bouchard microaneurysms)* form in vessels less than 300 μm in diameter. In addition to massive intracerebral

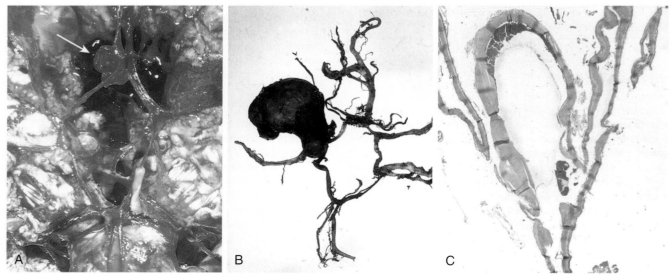

Fig. 23.10 Saccular aneurysms. (A) View of the base of the brain, dissected to show the circle of Willis with an aneurysm of the anterior cerebral artery *(arrow)*. (B) The circle of Willis is dissected to show a large aneurysm. (C) Section through a saccular aneurysm showing the hyalinized fibrous vessel wall. Hematoxylin-eosin stain.

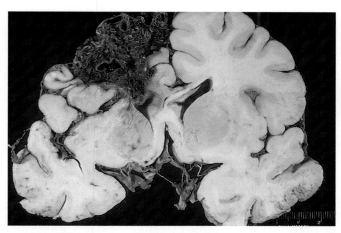

Fig. 23.11 Arteriovenous malformation.

hemorrhage (discussed earlier), several other pathologic outcomes are related to hypertension.

- *Lacunes* or *lacunar infarcts* are small cavitary infarcts, just a few millimeters in size, that are found most commonly in the deep gray matter (basal ganglia and thalamus), the internal capsule, the deep white matter, and the pons. They are caused by occlusion of a single penetrating branch of a large cerebral artery. Depending on their location, lacunes can be silent clinically or cause significant neurologic impairment.
- *Rupture of the small-caliber penetrating vessels* may occur, leading to the development of small hemorrhages. In time, these hemorrhages resorb, leaving behind a slit-like cavity *(slit hemorrhage)* surrounded by brownish discoloration.
- *Acute hypertensive encephalopathy* most often is associated with sudden sustained increases in diastolic blood pressure to greater than 130 mm Hg. It is characterized by increased intracranial pressure and global cerebral dysfunction, manifesting as headaches, confusion, vomiting, convulsions, and sometimes coma. Rapid therapeutic intervention to reduce the blood pressure is essential. Postmortem examination may show brain edema, with or without transtentorial or tonsillar herniation. Petechiae and fibrinoid necrosis of arterioles in the gray matter and white matter may be seen microscopically.

Vasculitis

Inflammatory processes involving blood vessels may compromise blood flow and cause cerebral dysfunction or infarction. Infectious arteritis of small and large vessels was previously seen mainly in association with syphilis and tuberculosis, but is now more often caused by opportunistic infections (such as aspergillosis, herpes zoster, or CMV) in the setting of immunosuppression. Some systemic forms of vasculitis, such as polyarteritis nodosa, may involve cerebral vessels and cause single or multiple infarcts. *Primary angiitis of the CNS* is a form of vasculitis that involves multiple small- to medium-sized parenchymal and subarachnoid vessels and is characterized by chronic inflammation, multinucleate giant cells (with or without granuloma formation), and destruction

of vessel walls. Affected individuals present with a diffuse encephalopathy, often with cognitive dysfunction. Treatment consists of immunosuppressive agents.

SUMMARY

CEREBROVASCULAR DISEASES

- *Stroke* is the clinical term for acute-onset neurologic deficits resulting from hemorrhagic or obstructive vascular lesions.
- Cerebral infarction follows loss of blood supply and can be widespread or focal, or affect regions with the least robust vascular supply ("watershed" infarcts).
- Focal cerebral infarcts are most commonly embolic; with subsequent dissolution of the embolus and reperfusion, a nonhemorrhagic infarct can become hemorrhagic.
- Primary intraparenchymal hemorrhages typically are due to either hypertension (most commonly in white matter, deep gray matter, or posterior fossa contents) or cerebral amyloid angiopathy (cerebral cortex).
- Spontaneous subarachnoid hemorrhage usually is caused by a structural vascular abnormality, such as an aneurysm or arteriovenous malformation.

CENTRAL NERVOUS SYSTEM TRAUMA

Trauma to the brain and spinal cord is a significant cause of death and disability. The severity and site of injury affect the outcome: injury of several cubic centimeters of brain parenchyma may be clinically silent (if in the frontal lobe), severely disabling (affecting the spinal cord), or fatal (involving the brain stem).

A blow to the head may be *penetrating* or *blunt*; it may cause an *open* or a *closed* injury. The magnitude and distribution of resulting traumatic brain lesions depend on the shape of the object causing the trauma, the force of impact, and whether the head is in motion at the time of injury. Severe brain damage can occur in the absence of external signs of head injury, and conversely, severe lacerations and even skull fractures do not necessarily indicate damage to the underlying brain. When the brain is damaged, the injuries may involve the parenchyma, the vasculature, or both.

Traumatic Parenchymal Injuries

When an object impacts the head, brain injury may occur at the site of impact—a *coup injury*—or opposite the site of impact on the other side of the brain—a *contrecoup injury*. Both coup and contrecoup lesions are contusions, with comparable gross and microscopic appearances. A *contusion* is caused by rapid tissue displacement, disruption of vascular channels, and subsequent hemorrhage, tissue injury, and edema. Since they are closest to the skull, the crests of the gyri are the parts of the brain that are most susceptible to traumatic injury. Contusions are common in regions of the brain overlying rough and irregular inner skull surfaces, such as the orbitofrontal regions and the temporal lobe tips. Penetration of the brain by a projectile such as a bullet or a skull fragment from a fracture causes a laceration, with tissue tearing, vascular disruption, and hemorrhage.

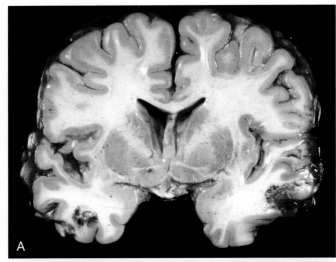

MORPHOLOGY

Contusions are wedge-shaped, with the widest aspect closest to the point of impact (Fig. 23.12A). Within a few hours of injury, blood extravasates throughout the involved tissue, across the width of the cerebral cortex, and into the white matter and subarachnoid spaces. Although functional effects are seen earlier, morphologic evidence of neruonal injury (nuclear pyknosis, cytoplasmic eosinophilia, cellular disintegration) takes about 24 hours to appear. The inflammatory response to the injured tissue follows its usual course, with neutrophils preceding the appearance of macrophages. In contrast with ischemic lesions, in which the superficial layer of cortex may be preserved, trauma affects the superficial layers most severely.

Old traumatic lesions characteristically appear as depressed, retracted, yellowish brown patches involving the crests of gyri (see Fig. 23.12B). These lesions show gliosis and residual hemosiderin-laden macrophages.

Although contusions are more easily seen, trauma may also cause more subtle but widespread injury to axons within the brain (called **diffuse axonal injury**), sometimes with devastating consequences. The movement of one region of brain relative to another is thought to disrupt axonal integrity and function. Angular acceleration, even in the absence of impact, may cause axonal injury as well as hemorrhage. As many as 50% of patients who develop coma shortly after trauma are believed to have white matter damage and diffuse axonal injury, usually in the form of axonal swellings that appear within hours of the injury.

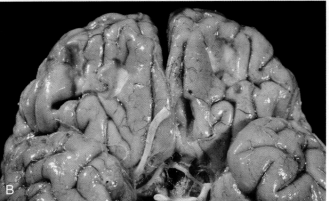

Fig. 23.12 Cerebral trauma. (A) Acute contusions are present in both temporal lobes, with areas of hemorrhage and tissue disruption. (B) Remote contusions, seen as discolored yellow areas, are present on the inferior frontal surface of this brain.

Concussion describes reversible altered brain function, with or without loss of consciousness, from head injury. The characteristic transient neurologic dysfunction includes loss of consciousness, temporary respiratory arrest, and loss of reflexes. Neurologic recovery is the norm, although amnesia for the event persists. The pathogenesis of the sudden disruption of nervous activity is unknown. Repeated episodes of concussion can result in persistent and profound neurologic deficits including cognitive impairment, parkinsonism, and others, and later development of neurodegenerative processes. Initially described in boxers *(dementia pugilistica)*, it is now recognized to occur in a wider range of settings, such as in athletes participating in contact sports. This syndrome is termed *chronic traumatic encephalopathy* and is characterized by accumulation of tangles in cerebral cortex and other brain regions (see the "Neurodegenerative Diseases" section later in the chapter).

Traumatic Vascular Injury

CNS trauma often directly disrupts vessel walls, leading to hemorrhage (Table 23.1). Depending on the affected vessel, the hemorrhage may be *epidural, subdural, subarachnoid,* or *intraparenchymal* (Fig. 23.13A), occurring alone or in combination. Subarachnoid and intraparenchymal hemorrhages most often occur at sites of contusions and lacerations.

Epidural Hematoma

Dural vessels—especially the middle meningeal artery—are vulnerable to traumatic injury. In infants, traumatic displacement of the easily deformable skull may tear a vessel, even in the absence of a skull fracture. In children and adults, by contrast, tears involving dural vessels almost always stem from skull fractures. Once a vessel tears, blood accumulates under arterial pressure and dissects the tightly applied dura away from the inner skull surface (see Fig. 23.13B), producing a hematoma that compresses the brain surface. Clinically, patients can be lucid for several hours after the traumatic event before neurologic signs appear. An epidural hematoma may expand rapidly and constitutes a neurosurgical emergency necessitating prompt drainage and repair to prevent death.

Subdural Hematoma

Rapid movement of the brain during trauma can tear the bridging veins that extend from the cerebral hemispheres

Table 23.1 Patterns of Vascular Injury in the Central Nervous System

Location	Etiology	Additional Features
Epidural space	Trauma	Usually associated with a skull fracture (in adults); rapidly evolving neurologic symptoms requiring intervention
Subdural space	Trauma	Level of trauma may be mild; slowly evolving neurologic symptoms, often with a delay from the time of injury
Subarachnoid space	Vascular abnormalities (arteriovenous malformation or aneurysm)	Sudden onset of severe headache, often with rapid neurologic deterioration; secondary injury may emerge due to vasospasm
	Trauma	Typically associated with underlying contusions
Intraparenchymal	Trauma (contusions)	Selective involvement of the crests of gyri where the brain contacts the skull (frontal and temporal tips, orbitofrontal surface)
	Hemorrhagic conversion of an ischemic infarction	Petechial hemorrhages in an area of previously ischemic brain, usually following the cortical ribbon
	Cerebral amyloid angiopathy	"Lobar" hemorrhage, involving cerebral cortex, often with extension into the subarachnoid space
	Hypertension	Centered in the deep white matter, thalamus, basal ganglia, or brain stem; may extend into the ventricular system
	Tumors (primary or metastatic)	Associated with high-grade gliomas or certain metastases (melanoma, choriocarcinoma, renal cell carcinoma)

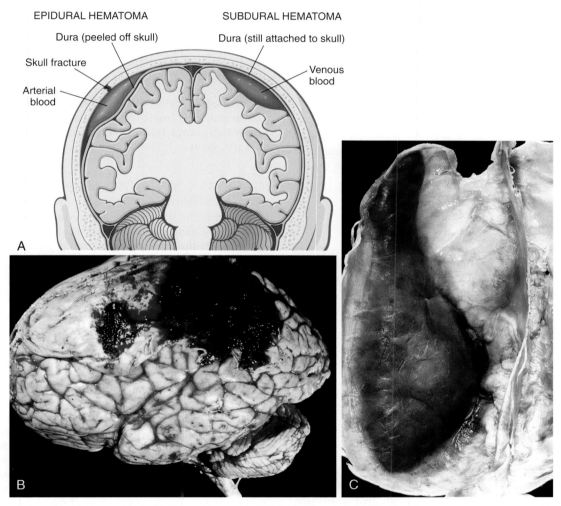

Fig. 23.13 Traumatic intracranial hemorrhages. (A) Epidural hematoma *(left)* in which rupture of a meningeal artery, usually associated with a skull fracture, has led to accumulation of arterial blood between the dura and the skull. In a subdural hematoma *(right)*, damage to bridging veins between the brain and the superior sagittal sinus has led to the accumulation of blood between the the two layers of dura. (B) Epidural hematoma covering a portion of the dura. (C) Large organizing subdural hematoma attached to the dura. *(B, Courtesy of the late Dr. Raymond D. Adams, Massachusetts General Hospital, Boston, Massachusetts.)*

through the subarachnoid and subdural space to the dural sinuses. Their disruption produces bleeding into the sub-dural space. Because the inner cell layer of the dura is quite thin and in very close proximity to the arachnoid layer, the blood appears to be between the dura and arach-noid, but in reality it is between the two layers of the dura. In patients with brain atrophy, the bridging veins are stretched out and the brain has additional space within which to move, accounting for the higher rate of subdural hematomas in older adults. Infants also are susceptible to subdural hematomas because their bridging veins are thin walled.

Subdural hematomas typically become manifest within the first 48 hours after injury. They are most common over the lateral aspects of the cerebral hemispheres and may be bilateral. Neurologic signs are attributable to the pressure exerted on the adjacent brain. Symptoms are most often nonlocalizing, taking the form of headache, confusion, and slowly progressive neurologic deterioration.

MORPHOLOGY

Acute subdural hematoma appears as a collection of freshly clotted blood apposed to the contour of the brain surface, without extension into the depths of sulci (see Fig. 23.13C). The underlying brain is flattened, and the subarachnoid space is often clear. Subdural hematomas organize by lysis of the clot (about 1 week), growth of granulation tissue from the dural surface into the hematoma (2 weeks), and fibrosis (1–3 months). Subdural hematomas commonly rebleed, presumably from the thin-walled vessels of the granulation tissue, leading to microscopic findings consistent with hemorrhages of varying ages. Symptomatic sub-dural hematomas are treated by surgical removal of the blood and associated reactive tissue.

SUMMARY

CENTRAL NERVOUS SYSTEM TRAUMA

- Physical injury to the brain can occur when the inside of the skull comes into forceful contact with the brain.
- In blunt trauma, there may be brain injury both at the original point of contact (coup injury) and on the opposite side of the brain (contrecoup injury) owing to impacts with the skull.
- Rapid displacement of the head and brain can tear axons (diffuse axonal injury), often causing severe, irreversible neu-rologic deficits.
- Traumatic tearing of blood vessels, depending on the location, leads to epidural, subdural, or intraparenchymal hematoma as well as subarachnoid hemorrhage.

CONGENITAL MALFORMATIONS AND PERINATAL BRAIN INJURY

The incidence of CNS malformations, giving rise to mental retardation, cerebral palsy, or neural tube defects, is estimated at 1% to 2%. Malformations of the brain are more common in the setting of multiple birth defects. Prenatal or perinatal insults may interfere with normal CNS develop-ment or cause tissue damage. During gestation, the timing of an injury determines the pattern of malformation, with earlier events typically leading to more severe phenotypes. Mutations affecting genes that regulate the differentiation, maturation, or intercellular communication of neurons or glial cells can cause CNS malformation or dysfunction. Additionally, various chemicals and infectious agents have teratogenic effects.

Some developmental disorders produce profound neu-ronal dysfunction in the absence of morphologic abnormal-ities. Genetic underpinnings for various forms of *autism* have emerged recently; many of the implicated genes con-tribute to the development or maintenance of synaptic con-nections. *Rett syndrome* is an X-linked dominant disorder associated with mutations in the gene encoding a regulator of epigenetic modifications of chromatin. Development in affected girls initially is normal, but neurologic deficits affecting cognition and movement appear by 1 to 2 years of age.

Malformations

Neural Tube Defects

One of the earliest steps in brain development is the for-mation of the neural tube, which gives rise to the ven-tricular system, brain, and spinal cord. **Partial failure or reversal of neural tube closure may lead to several malformations, each characterized by abnormalities involving neural tissue, meninges, and overlying bone or soft tissues**. Collectively, *neural tube defects* are the most frequent type of CNS malformation. Folate defi-ciency during the first trimester sharply increases risk through uncertain mechanisms and represents an impor-tant opportunity for prevention, as administration of folate to women of child-bearing age reduces the incidence of neural tube defects by up to 70%. The combination of imaging studies and maternal screening for elevated α-fetoprotein has increased the early detection of neural tube defects.

Neural tube defects include the following:
- The most common defects involve the posterior end of the neural tube, from which the spinal cord forms. These can range from asymptomatic bony defects (*spina bifida occulta*) to *spina bifida*, a severe malformation consisting of a flat, disorganized segment of spinal cord associated with an overlying meningeal outpouching.
- *Myelomeningocele* is an extension of CNS tissue through a defect in the vertebral column that occurs most com-monly in the lumbosacral region (Fig. 23.14). Patients have motor and sensory deficits in the lower extremi-ties and problems with bowel and bladder control. The clinical problems derive from the abnormal spinal cord segment and often are compounded by infections extending from the thin or ulcerated overlying skin.
- *Anencephaly* is a malformation of the anterior end of the neural tube that leads to the absence of the forebrain and the top of the skull. Varying amounts of posterior fossa structures may be present.

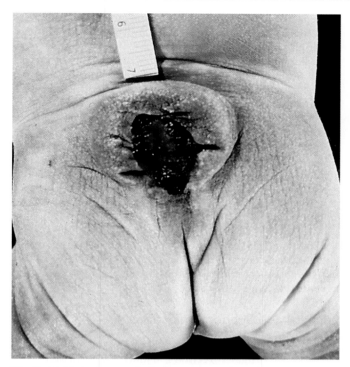

Fig. 23.14 Myelomeningocele. Both meninges and spinal cord parenchyma are included in the cystlike structure visible just above the buttocks.

- An *encephalocele* is a diverticulum of malformed CNS tissue extending through a defect in the cranium. It most often involves the occipital region or the posterior fossa. When it occurs anteriorly, brain tissue may extend into the sinuses.

Forebrain Malformations

Microencephaly describes the group of malformations in which the volume of brain is too small; usually it is associated with a small head as well (*microcephaly*). It has a wide range of associations, including chromosome abnormalities, fetal alcohol syndrome, and human immunodeficiency virus (HIV) and Zika virus infection acquired in utero. The unifying feature is decreased generation of neurons destined for the cerebral cortex. During the early stages of brain development, as progenitor cells proliferate in the subependymal ventricular zone, the balance between cells leaving the progenitor population to form the cortex and those remaining in the proliferating pool affects the overall number of neurons and glial cells generated. If too many cells leave the progenitor pool prematurely, there is inadequate generation of mature neurons, leading to a small brain. *Megalencephaly,* excessive brain volume that is always associated with a large head, is far less common and is mostly associated with rare genetic disorders.

Disruption of neuronal migration and differentiation during development can lead to abnormalities of gyration and neocortical architecture, often taking the form of neurons ending up in the wrong location. Mutations in various genes that control migration result in a variety of malformations. A representative example is *holoprosencephaly,* characterized by disruption of normal midline patterning. Mild forms show absence of the olfactory bulbs and related structures (*arrhinencephaly*). In severe forms, the brain is not divided into hemispheres or lobes, and there may be facial midline defects such as cyclopia. The best known genetic causes involve acquired or inherited loss of function mutations in components of the Hedgehog signaling pathway.

Other examples include loss of gyri, which may be complete (lissencephaly) or partial, and increased number of irregularly formed gyri (polymicrogyria).

Posterior Fossa Anomalies

The most common malformations in this region of the brain result in misplacement or absence of portions of the cerebellum.

- *Arnold-Chiari malformation* (Chiari type II malformation) combines a small posterior fossa with a misshapen midline cerebellum and downward extension of the vermis through the foramen magnum; hydrocephalus and a lumbar myelomeningocele typically are also present.
- The far milder *Chiari type I malformation* has low-lying cerebellar tonsils that extend through the foramen magnum. Excess tissue in the foramen magnum results in partial obstruction of CSF flow and compression of the medulla, with symptoms of headache or cranial nerve deficits often manifesting only in adult life. Surgical intervention can alleviate the symptoms.
- *Dandy-Walker malformation* is characterized by an enlarged posterior fossa, absence of the cerebellar vermis, and a large midline cyst.

Perinatal Brain Injury

Brain injury occurring in the perinatal period is an important cause of childhood neurologic disability. *Cerebral palsy* is a term for nonprogressive neurologic motor deficits characterized by spasticity, dystonia, ataxia or athetosis, and paresis attributable to injury occurring during the prenatal and perinatal periods. Signs and symptoms may not be apparent at birth and only declare themselves later, well after the causal event.

The two major types of injury that occur in the perinatal period are hemorrhages and infarcts. These differ from the otherwise similar lesions in adults in terms of their locations and the tissue reactions they engender. In premature infants, there is an increased risk for *intraparenchymal hemorrhage* within the germinal matrix, most often adjacent to the anterior horn of the lateral ventricle. Hemorrhages may extend into the ventricular system and from there to the subarachnoid space, sometimes causing hydrocephalus. Infarcts may occur in the supratentorial periventricular white matter (*periventricular leukomalacia*), especially in premature infants. The residua of these infarcts are chalky yellow plaques consisting of discrete regions of white matter necrosis and dystrophic calcification (Fig. 23.15). When severe enough to involve the gray matter and white matter, large cystic lesions can develop throughout the hemispheres, a condition termed *multicystic encephalopathy.*

Certain infections, which may be acquired transplacentally or during birth, have a propensity to cause destructive

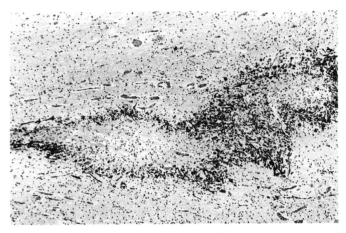

Fig. 23.15 Perinatal brain injury. This specimen from a patient with periventricular leukomalacia contains a central focus of white matter necrosis with a peripheral rim of mineralized axonal processes.

brain lesions. Agents in this group (commonly referred to as *TORCH*) include toxoplasmosis and CMV, which can both result in parenchymal calcifications along with the tissue injury; these are discussed in more detail later.

SUMMARY

CONGENITAL MALFORMATIONS AND PERINATAL BRAIN INJURY

- Malformations of the brain can occur because of genetic factors or external insults.
- The developmental timing and position of the injury determine its pattern and characteristics.
- Various malformations stem from failure of neural tube closure, improper formation of neural structures, and altered neuronal migration.
- Perinatal brain injury mostly takes one of two forms: (1) hemorrhage, often in the region of the germinal matrix with the risk for extension into the ventricular system; and (2) ischemic infarcts, leading to periventricular leukomalacia.
- Certain infections may affect the brain during development with subsequent tissue destruction and neurologic consequences.

INFECTIONS OF THE NERVOUS SYSTEM

The brain and its coverings can be sites of infection. Some infectious agents have a relative or absolute predilection for the nervous system (e.g., rabies), while others affect many other organs as well as the brain (e.g., *Staphylococcus aureus*). Damage to nervous tissue may be the consequence of direct injury of neurons or glial cells by the infectious agent or microbial toxins, or may be a consequence of the host immune response.

Infectious agents may reach the nervous system through several routes:

- *Hematogenous spread* by way of the arterial blood supply is the most common means of entry. There can also be retrograde venous spread through the anastomoses between the veins of the face and the venous sinuses of the skull.
- *Direct implantation* of microorganisms is almost invariably due to open or penetrating trauma; rare cases can be iatrogenic, as when microbes are introduced with a lumbar puncture needle or into a surgical field.
- *Local extension* can occur with infections of the skull or spine. Sources include air sinuses, most often the mastoid or frontal; infected teeth; cranial or spinal osteomyelitis; and congenital malformations, such as meningomyelocele.
- *Peripheral nerves* also may serve as paths of entry for a few pathogens—in particular, viruses such as rabies and herpes zoster.

Basic mechanisms of injury associated with infectious agents are discussed in Chapter 9; in the following sections we discuss infections that are specific to the central nervous system (Table 23.2).

Epidural and Subdural Infections

The epidural and subdural spaces can be involved by bacterial or fungal infections, usually as a consequence of direct local spread. *Epidural abscesses* arise from an adjacent focus of infection, such as sinusitis or osteomyelitis. When abscesses occur in the spinal epidural space, they may cause spinal cord compression and constitute a neurosurgical emergency. Infections of the skull or air sinuses may also spread to the subdural space, producing *subdural empyema*. The underlying arachnoid and subarachnoid spaces usually are unaffected, but a large subdural empyema may produce a mass effect. In addition, thrombophlebitis may develop in the bridging veins that cross the subdural space, resulting in venous occlusion and infarction of the brain. Most patients are febrile, with headache and neck stiffness, and if untreated may develop focal neurologic signs referable to the site of the infection, lethargy, and coma. With treatment, including surgical drainage, resolution of the empyema occurs from the dural side; if resolution is complete, a thickened dura may be the only residual finding. With prompt treatment, complete recovery is usual.

Meningitis

Meningitis **is an inflammatory process involving the leptomeninges within the subarachnoid space; if the infection spreads into the underlying brain, it is termed** *meningoencephalitis.* These terms are also used in non-infectious settings such as *chemical meningitis*, a response to a nonbacterial irritant such as debris from a ruptured epidermoid cyst, and *carcinomatous meningitis,* the spread of metastatic cancer cells to the subarachnoid space.

Infectious meningitis can be broadly divided into *acute pyogenic* **(usually bacterial),** *aseptic* **(usually viral), and** *chronic* **(usually tuberculous, spirochetal, or fungal) subtypes.** Examination of the CSF is often useful in distinguishing among the various causes of meningitis.

Table 23.2 Common Central Nervous System Infections

Type of Infection	Clinical Syndrome	Common Causative Organisms
Bacterial Infections		
Meningitis	Acute pyogenic meningitis	*Escherichia coli* or group B streptococci (infants) *Neisseria meningitidis* (young adults) *Streptococcus. pneumoniae* or *Listeria monocytogenes* (older adults)
	Chronic meningitis	*Mycobacterium tuberculosis*
Localized infections	Abscess	Streptococci and staphylococci
	Empyema	Polymicrobial (staphylococci, anaerobic gram-negative)
Viral Infections		
Meningitis	Acute aseptic meningitis	Enteroviruses Measles (subacute sclerosing panencephalitis) Influenza species Lymphocytic choriomeningitis virus
Encephalitis	Encephalitic syndromes	Herpes simplex (HSV-1, HSV-2) Cytomegalovirus Human immunodeficiency virus JC polyomavirus (progressive multifocal leukoencephalopathy)
	Arthropod-borne encephalitis	West Nile virus, other arboviruses
Brain stem and spinal cord syndromes	Rhombencephalitis Spinal poliomyelitis	Rabies Polio West Nile virus
Rickettsia, Spirochetes, and Fungi		
Meningitic syndromes	Rocky Mountain spotted fever	*Rickettsia rickettsii*
	Neurosyphilis	*Treponema pallidum*
	Lyme disease (neuroborreliosis)	*Borrelia burgdorferi*
	Fungal meningitis	*Cryptococcus neoformans* *Candida albicans*
Protozoa and Metazoa		
Meningitic syndromes	Cerebral malaria Amebic encephalitis	*Plasmodium falciparum* *Naegleria* species
Localized infections	Toxoplasmosis Cysticercosis	*Toxoplasma gondii* *Taenia solium*

Acute Pyogenic Meningitis (Bacterial Meningitis)

The most likely causes of bacterial meningitis vary with patient age. In neonates, common organisms are *Escherichia coli* and group B streptococci. In adolescents and young adults, *Neisseria meningitidis* is the most common pathogen; in older adults, *Streptococcus pneumoniae* and *Listeria monocytogenes* are more common. Across ages, patients typically show systemic signs of infection along with meningeal irritation and neurologic impairment, including headache, photophobia, irritability, clouding of consciousness, and neck stiffness. Lumbar puncture reveals an increased pressure; examination of the CSF shows abundant neutrophils, elevated protein, and reduced glucose. Untreated pyogenic meningitis is often fatal, but with prompt diagnosis and administration of antibiotics, most patients can be saved.

MORPHOLOGY

In acute meningitis, an exudate is evident within the leptomeninges on the surface of the brain (Fig. 23.16A). The meningeal vessels are engorged and prominent, and tracts of pus may extend along blood vessels. On microscopic examination, neutrophils may fill the entire subarachnoid space or, in less severe cases, may be confined to regions adjacent to leptomeningeal blood vessels. In untreated meningitis, Gram stain reveals varying numbers of the causative organism. Severe involvement of leptomeningeal veins (phlebitis) may lead to venous occlusion and hemorrhagic infarction of the underlying brain. When the meningitis is fulminant, the organisms and the associated inflammatory cells may spread into the substance of the brain (focal cerebritis), sometimes leading to the formation of abscesses, discussed later (see Fig. 23.16B). Extension to the ventricles (ventriculitis) also may occur. If treated early and effectively, resolved meningitis may leave little or no residuum.

Aseptic Meningitis (Viral Meningitis)

Aseptic meningitis is a clinical term for acute illness with meningeal signs and symptoms that is believed to be of viral origin. The clinical course is less fulminant than in pyogenic meningitis and is typically self-limiting. In contrast to pyogenic meningitis, examination of the CSF often shows lymphocytosis, moderate protein elevation, and a normal glucose level, but bacteria cannot be cultured. While an underlying viral agent is suspected, it is often difficult to identify the responsible virus by culture and serologic methods; application of nucleic acid sequencing has the potential to change our understanding of these cases. There are no distinctive macroscopic findings except for brain swelling, which may be seen in only some instances. On microscopic examination, there is either no recognizable abnormality or a mild to moderate leptomeningeal lymphocytic infiltrate.

Chronic Meningitis

Several pathogens, including mycobacteria, some spirochetes, and fungi, cause a chronic meningitis; infections with these organisms also may involve the brain parenchyma.

Tuberculous Meningitis

Tuberculous meningitis usually manifests with generalized signs and symptoms of headache, malaise, mental confusion, and vomiting. There is only a moderate increase in CSF cellularity, with mononuclear cells or a mixture of polymorphonuclear and mononuclear cells; the protein level is elevated, often strikingly so, and the glucose content typically is moderately reduced or normal. Infection with *Mycobacterium tuberculosis* also may result in a well-circumscribed intraparenchymal mass (*tuberculoma*), which may be associated with meningitis. Chronic tuberculous

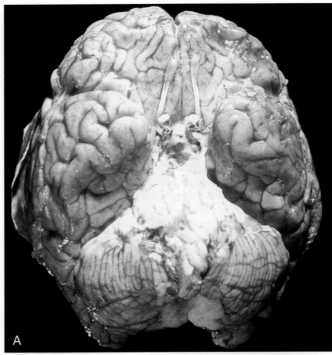

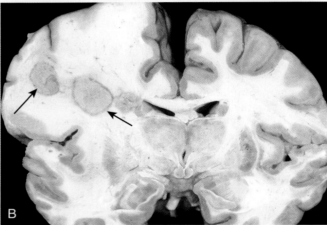

Fig. 23.16 Bacterial infections. (A) Pyogenic meningitis. A thick layer of suppurative exudate covers the brain stem and cerebellum and thickens the leptomeninges. (B) Cerebral abscesses in the frontal lobe white matter *(arrows).* (A, From Golden JA, Louis DN: Images in clinical medicine: acute bacterial meningitis. N Engl J Med 333:364, 1994. Copyright © 1994 Massachusetts Medical Society. All rights reserved.)

meningitis leads to arachnoid fibrosis and hydrocephalus from interference with resorption of CSF.

Spirochetal Infections

Neurosyphilis, a tertiary stage of syphilis, occurs in about 10% of individuals with untreated *Treponema pallidum* infection. Infection with HIV increases the risk for developing neurosyphilis, and the disease is often more aggressive in this setting. There are several patterns of CNS involvement by syphilis, which may be present alone or in combination.

- *Meningovascular neurosyphilis* is a chronic meningitis, usually involving the base of the brain, often with an obliterative endarteritis rich in plasma cells and lymphocytes.
- *Paretic neurosyphilis* stems from parenchymal involvement by spirochetes and is associated with neuronal loss and marked proliferation of microglial cells. Clinically, this form of the disease causes an insidious progressive loss of mental and physical functions, mood alterations (including delusions of grandeur), and eventually severe dementia.
- *Tabes dorsalis* results from damage to the sensory nerves in the dorsal roots. Consequences include impaired joint position sense and ataxia; loss of pain sensation, leading to skin and joint damage *(Charcot joints);* other sensory disturbances, particularly characteristic "lightning pains"; and the absence of deep tendon reflexes.

Neuroborreliosis refers to involvement of the nervous system by the spirochete *Borrelia burgdorferi,* the causative agent of Lyme disease. Neurologic signs and symptoms are highly variable and include aseptic meningitis, facial nerve palsies, mild encephalopathy, and polyneuropathies.

Fungal Meningitis

Fungal infection of the nervous system can give rise to chronic meningitis and, as with other pathogens, this can be associated at times with parenchymal infection. Immunosuppression increases the risk for these diseases, but it is not a requirement for infection to occur. Several fungal pathogens cause CNS disease:

- *Cryptococcus neoformans* can cause both meningitis and meningoencephalitis, often in the setting of immunosuppression. It may be fulminant and fatal in as little as 2 weeks or may be indolent, evolving over months or years. The CSF may have few cells but elevated protein, and the mucoid encapsulated yeasts can be visualized on India ink preparations. Extension into the brain follows vessels in the Virchow-Robin spaces. As organisms proliferate, these spaces expand, giving rise to a "soap bubble"–like appearance (Fig. 23.17).
- *Histoplasma capsulatum* commonly involves the nervous system in the setting of disseminated infection. There is an increased risk for disease in the setting of HIV infection. Histoplasmosis typically causes a basilar meningitis, with elevated CSF protein, mildly decreased glucose, and mild lymphocytic pleocytosis. Parenchymal lesions can occur, mostly from tracking of organisms along Virchow-Robin spaces.
- *Coccidioides immitis,* a fungus endemic to desert regions of the American Southwest, most commonly causes meningitis in the setting of disseminated infection. Diagnosis can be made by examining the CSF for specific antibody. Without treatment, coccidioidal meningitis has a high fatality.

Parenchymal Infections

The entire gamut of infectious pathogens (viruses to parasites) can infect the brain, often in characteristic patterns. In general, viral infections are diffuse, bacterial infections (when not associated with meningitis) are localized, while

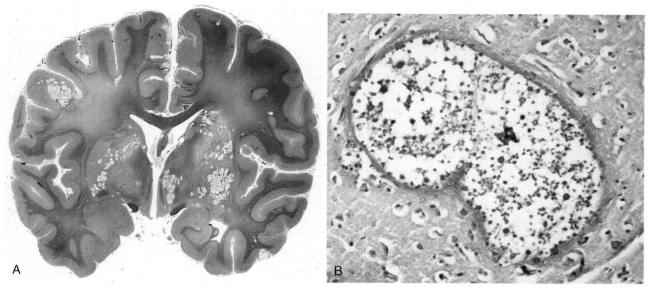

Fig. 23.17 Cryptococcal infection. (A) Whole-brain section showing the numerous areas of tissue destruction associated with the spread of organisms in the perivascular spaces. (B) At higher magnification, it is possible to see the cryptococci in the lesions.

other organisms produce mixed patterns. In immunosuppressed hosts, more widespread involvement with any agent is typical.

Brain Abscesses

Brain abscesses are most often caused by bacterial infections. These can arise by direct implantation of organisms, local extension from adjacent foci (mastoiditis, paranasal sinusitis), or hematogenous spread (usually from a primary site in the heart, lungs, or distal bones, or after tooth extraction). Predisposing conditions include *acute bacterial endocarditis*, from which septic emboli are released that may produce multiple abscesses; *cyanotic congenital heart disease*, associated with a right-to-left shunt and loss of pulmonary filtration of organisms; and *chronic pulmonary infections*, as in bronchiectasis, which provide a source of microbes that spread hematogenously.

Abscesses are discrete destructive lesions with central liquefactive necrosis surrounded by a rim of vascularized granulation and fibrous tissue (see Fig. 23.16B). Outside the fibrous capsule is a zone of reactive gliosis. Patients almost invariably present with progressive focal deficits as well as general signs related to increased intracranial pressure. While CSF white blood cell count and protein may be elevated, lumbar puncture has little role in the diagnosis of brain abscess since organisms are more reliably cultured by draining the abscess directly. In addition, if there is significant mass effect from the abscess, the decrease in lumbar CSF pressure following lumbar puncture can result in downward herniation of cerebral contents and neurologic deterioration. A systemic or local source of infection may or may not be apparent. The increased intracranial pressure may cause fatal brain herniation, and abscess rupture can lead to ventriculitis, meningitis, and venous sinus thrombosis. Surgery and antibiotics reduce the otherwise high mortality rate, with earlier intervention leading to better outcomes.

Viral Encephalitis

Viral encephalitis is a parenchymal infection of the brain that is almost invariably associated with meningeal inflammation (*meningoencephalitis*). While different viruses show varying patterns of injury, the most characteristic histologic features are perivascular and parenchymal mononuclear cell infiltrates, microglial nodules, and neuronophagia (Fig. 23.18A–B). Certain viruses also form characteristic inclusion bodies.

The nervous system is particularly susceptible to certain viruses such as rabies virus and poliovirus. Some viruses infect specific CNS cell types, while others preferentially involve particular brain regions (such as the medial temporal lobes, or the limbic system) that lie along the viral route of entry. Intrauterine viral infection following transplacental spread of rubella and CMV may cause destructive lesions, and Zika virus causes developmental abnormalities of the brain. In addition to direct infection of the nervous system, the CNS also can be injured by immune mechanisms after systemic viral infections.

Arboviruses

Arboviruses (arthropod-borne viruses) are an important cause of epidemic encephalitis, especially in tropical regions of the world, and are capable of causing serious morbidity and high mortality. Among the more commonly encountered types are Eastern and Western equine encephalitis and West Nile virus infection. Patients develop generalized neurologic symptoms, such as seizures, confusion, delirium, and stupor or coma, as well as focal signs, such as reflex asymmetry and ocular palsies. The CSF usually is colorless but with a slightly elevated pressure and an early neutrophilic pleocytosis that rapidly converts to a lymphocytosis; the protein concentration is elevated, but the glucose is normal. Thus, CSF examination helps to distinguish viral from bacterial infections of the CNS.

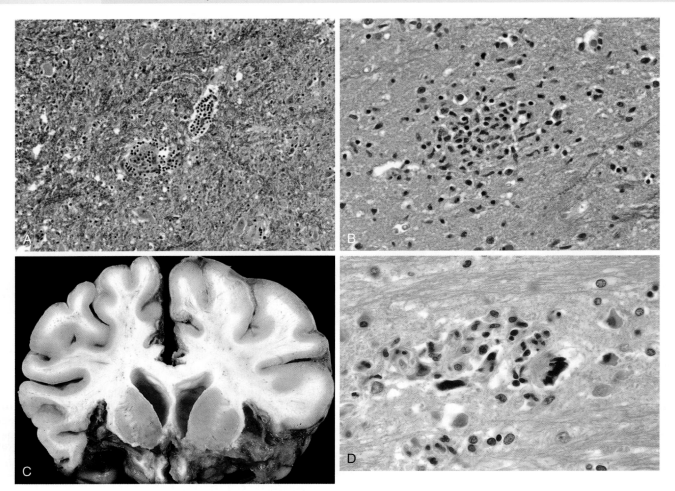

Fig. 23.18 Viral infections. (A and B) Characteristic findings in many forms of viral meningitis include perivascular cuffing of lymphocytes (A) and microglial nodules (B). (C) Herpes encephalitis showing extensive destruction of inferior frontal and anterior temporal lobes. (D) Human immunodeficiency virus (HIV) encephalitis. Note the accumulation of microglia forming a microglial nodule and multinucleate giant cell. *(C, Courtesy of Dr. T.W. Smith, University of Massachusetts Medical School, Worcester, Massachusetts.)*

MORPHOLOGY

Arbovirus encephalitides produce a similar histopathologic picture. Characteristically, there is a perivascular lymphocytic meningoencephalitis (sometimes with neutrophils) (see Fig. 23.18A). Multifocal gray matter and white matter necrosis is seen, often associated with neuronophagia, the phagocytosis of neuronal debris, as well as localized collections of microglia termed **microglial nodules** (see Fig. 23.18B). In severe cases, there may be a necrotizing vasculitis with associated focal hemorrhages.

Herpesviruses

HSV-1 encephalitis may occur in any age group but is most common in children and young adults. It typically manifests with alterations in mood, memory, and behavior, reflecting involvement of the frontal and temporal lobes. Recurrent HSV-1 encephalitis is sometimes associated with inherited mutations that interfere with Toll-like receptor signaling (specifically that of TLR-3), which has an important role in anti-viral defense.

MORPHOLOGY

Herpes encephalitis starts in and most severely involves the inferior and medial regions of the temporal lobes and the orbital gyri of the frontal lobes (see Fig. 23.18C). The infection is necrotizing and often hemorrhagic in severely affected regions. Perivascular inflammatory infiltrates usually are present, and large eosinophilic intranuclear viral inclusions (Cowdry type A bodies) can be found in both neurons and glial cells.

HSV-2 also affects the nervous system, usually in the form of meningitis in adults. Disseminated severe encephalitis occurs in many neonates born by vaginal delivery to women with active primary HSV genital infections.

Varicella-zoster virus (VZV) causes chickenpox during primary infection, usually without any evidence of neurologic involvement. The virus establishes latent infection in neurons of dorsal root ganglia. Reactivation in adults manifests as a painful, vesicular skin eruption in the distribution of one or a few dermatomes *(shingles)*. This usually is a self-limited process, but there may be a persistent pain syndrome in the affected region *(postherpetic neuralgia)*.

VZV also may cause a granulomatous arteritis that can lead to tissue infarcts. In immunosuppressed patients, acute herpes zoster encephalitis can occur. Inclusion bodies can be found in glial cells and neurons.

Cytomegalovirus

CMV infects the nervous system in fetuses and immuno-suppressed individuals. All cells within the CNS (neurons, glial cells, ependyma, and endothelium) are susceptible to infection. Intrauterine infection causes periventricular necrosis, followed later by microcephaly with periventricular calcification. When adults are infected, CMV produces a subacute encephalitis, which is also often most severe in the periventricular region. Lesions can be hemorrhagic and contain typical viral inclusion–bearing cells.

Poliovirus

Poliovirus is an enterovirus that most often causes a sub-clinical or mild gastroenteritis; in a small fraction of cases, it secondarily invades the nervous system and damages motor neurons in the spinal cord and brain stem *(paralytic poliomyelitis)*. The loss of motor neurons results in a flaccid paralysis with muscle wasting and hyporeflexia in the corresponding region of the body. In the acute disease, death can occur from paralysis of respiratory muscles. Long after the infection has resolved, typically 25 to 35 years after the initial illness, a poorly understood *post-polio syndrome* of progressive weakness associated with decreased muscle bulk and pain may appear. The re-emergent weakness has the same distribution as the prior polio infection.

Rabies Virus

Rabies is a fatal encephalitic infection transmitted to humans from rabid animals, usually by a bite. Various mammals are natural reservoirs. Exposure to some bat species, even without evidence of a bite, is also a risk factor. The virus enters the CNS by ascending along the peripheral nerves from the wound site, so the incubation period (usually a few months) depends on the distance between the wound and the brain. The disease manifests initially with non-specific symptoms of malaise, headache, and fever. As the infection advances, the patient shows extraordinary CNS excitability; the slightest touch is painful, with violent motor responses progressing to convulsions. Contracture of the pharyngeal musculature may create an aversion to swallowing even water *(hydrophobia)*. Periods of mania and stupor progress to coma and eventually death, typically from respiratory failure.

Human Immunodeficiency Virus

In the first 15 years or so after recognition of AIDS, neuropathologic changes were demonstrated at postmortem examination in as many as 80% to 90% of cases, owing to direct effects of the virus on the nervous system *(HIV encephalitis)*, along with opportunistic infections and primary CNS lymphoma. Introduction of highly active antiretroviral therapy (HAART) has decreased the frequency of these secondary effects of HIV infection. However, cognitive dysfunction ranging from mild to full-blown dementia that is lumped under the umbrella term *HIV-associated neurocognitive disorder (HAND)* continues to be a source of

morbidity. This syndrome is believed to stem from HIV infection of microglial cells in the brain and activation of innate immune responses. Neuronal injury likely stems from a combination of cytokine-induced inflammation and toxic effects of HIV-derived proteins.

Aseptic meningitis occurs within 1 to 2 weeks of onset of primary HIV infection in about 10% of patients; antibodies to HIV can be demonstrated, and the virus can be isolated from the CSF. The few neuropathologic studies of the early and acute phases of symptomatic or asymptomatic HIV invasion of the nervous system have shown mild lymphocytic meningitis, perivascular inflammation, and some myelin loss in the hemispheres.

When effective anti-HIV therapy is begun in the setting of established infection, there is a risk for neurologic involvement associated with the *immune reconstitution inflammatory syndrome (IRIS)*. Neurologic manifestations include rapidly developing cognitive impairment and cerebral edema. The pathogenesis of IRIS is unclear but it is thought to be due to the activation of a previously suppressed inflammatory response brought about by effective treatment of HIV infection. IRIS is often associated with the presence of a mycobacterial, fungal or viral opportunistic CNS infection, although it can also occur in the absence of any other inciting disease.

MORPHOLOGY

HIV encephalitis is a chronic inflammatory process with widely distributed **microglial nodules,** sometimes with associated foci of tissue necrosis and reactive gliosis (see Fig. 23.18D). The microglial nodules also are found in the vicinity of small blood vessels, which show abnormally prominent endothelial cells and perivascular foamy or pigment-laden macrophages. These changes are especially prominent in the subcortical white matter, diencephalon, and brain stem. An important component of the microglial nodule are macrophage-derived **multinucleate cells.** In some cases, there also is a disorder of white matter characterized by multifocal or diffuse areas of myelin pallor, axonal swellings, and gliosis. HIV is present in CD4+ mononuclear and multinucleate macrophages and microglia.

Unlike HIV encephalitis, the brain lesions of IRIS may be associated with a CD8+ T cell infiltrate, both around blood vessels and diffusely in the parenchyma, in the absence of significant HIV burden or multinucleated cells.

Polyomavirus and Progressive Multifocal Leukoencephalopathy

Progressive multifocal leukoencephalopathy (PML) is caused by JC virus, a polyomavirus, which preferentially infects oligodendrocytes, resulting in demyelination as these cells are injured and then die. Most people show serologic evidence of exposure to JC virus during childhood, and it is believed that PML results from virus reactivation, as the disease is restricted to immunosuppressed individuals. Patients develop focal and relentlessly progressive neurologic signs and symptoms, and imaging studies show extensive, often multifocal lesions in the hemispheric or cerebellar white matter.

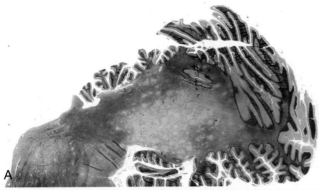

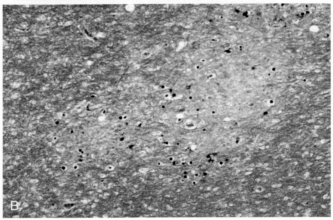

Fig. 23.19 Progressive multifocal leukoencephalopathy. (A) Section stained for myelin showing irregular, poorly defined areas of demyelination, which become confluent in places. (B) Enlarged oligodendrocyte nuclei stained for viral antigens surround an area of early myelin loss.

MORPHOLOGY

The lesions are patchy, irregular, ill-defined areas of white matter destruction that enlarge as the disease progresses (Fig. 23.19). Each lesion is an area of demyelination, in the center of which are scattered lipid-laden macrophages and a reduced number of axons. At the edges of the lesion are greatly enlarged oligodendrocyte nuclei whose chromatin is replaced by glassy-appearing amphophilic viral inclusions. The virus also infects astrocytes, leading to bizarre giant forms with irregular, hyperchromatic, sometimes multiple nuclei that can be mistaken for a tumor.

Fungal Encephalitis

Fungal infections usually produce parenchymal granulomas or abscesses, often associated with meningitis. The most common fungal infections have the following distinctive patterns:

- *Candida albicans* usually produces multiple microabscesses, with or without granuloma formation.
- *Mucormycosis,* caused by several fungi belonging to the order *Mucorales,* typically presents as an infection of the nasal cavity or sinuses in a diabetic patient with ketoacidosis. It may spread to the brain through vascular invasion or by direct extension through the cribriform plate. The proclivity of Mucor to invade the brain directly

sets it apart from other fungi, which reach the brain by hematogenous dissemination from distant sites.
- *Aspergillus fumigatus* tends to cause a distinctive pattern of widespread septic hemorrhagic infarctions because of its marked predilection for blood vessel wall invasion with subsequent thrombosis.

Other Meningoencephalitides

While a wide range of other organisms can infect the nervous system and its covering, only three relatively common entities are considered here.

Cerebral Toxoplasmosis

Cerebral infection with the protozoan *Toxoplasma gondii* can occur in immunosuppressed adults or in newborns who acquire the organism transplacentally from a mother with an active infection. The consequences include the triad of *chorioretinitis, hydrocephalus, and intracranial calcifications.* In adults, the clinical symptoms are subacute, evolving over weeks, and may be both focal and diffuse. Due to inflammation and breakdown of the blood-brain barrier at sites of infection, imaging studies often show edema associated with ring-enhancing lesions.

MORPHOLOGY

When the infection is acquired in immunosuppressed adults, the brain shows abscesses, frequently multiple, most often involving the cerebral cortex (near the gray-white junction) and deep gray nuclei. Acute lesions consist of central foci of necrosis surrounded by acute and chronic inflammation, macrophage infiltration, and vascular proliferation. Both free tachyzoites and encysted bradyzoites may be found at the periphery of the necrotic foci (Fig. 23.20).

Cysticercosis

Cysticercosis is the consequence of an end-stage infection by the tapeworm *Tenia solium.* If ingested larval organisms leave the lumen of the gastrointestinal tract, where they would otherwise develop into mature tapeworms, they encyst. Cysts can be found throughout the body and are common within the brain and subarachnoid space. Cysticercosis typically manifests as a mass lesion and can cause seizures. Symptoms can intensify when the encysted organism dies, as occurs after therapy.

The organism is found within a cyst with a smooth lining. The body wall and hooklets from mouth parts are most commonly recognized. Death of the encysted organism may produce an intense inflammatory reaction in the surrounding brain, often including eosinophils, and marked gliosis.

Amebiasis

Amebic meningoencephalitis manifests with different clinical syndromes, depending on the responsible pathogen. *Naegleria fowleri,* associated with swimming in stagnant warm fresh water ponds, causes a rapidly fatal necrotizing encephalitis. By contrast, various species of *Acanthamoeba* cause a chronic granulomatous meningoencephalitis.

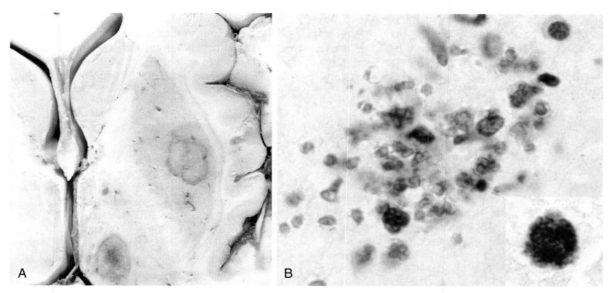

Fig. 23.20 Toxoplasma infection. (A) Abscesses are present in the putamen and thalamus. (B) Free tachyzoites are demonstrated by immunohistochemical staining. *Inset,* Bradyzoites are present as a pseudocyst, again highlighted by immunohistochemical staining.

Prion Diseases

Prion diseases are a group of infectious diseases in which the causative agent is an abnormal form of a cellular protein. These include sporadic, familial, iatrogenic, and variant forms of Creutzfeldt-Jakob disease (CJD), as well as animal diseases such as scrapie in sheep and bovine spongiform encephalopathy in cattle ("mad cow disease"). The causative protein, termed *prion protein (PrP),* may undergo a conformational change from its normal shape (PrP^c) to an abnormal conformation called *PrP^{sc}* (*sc* for *scrapie*). PrP normally is rich in α-helices, but PrP^{sc} has a high content of β-sheets, a characteristic that makes it resistant to proteolysis (hence an alternative term for the pathogenic form, *PrP^{res}*—i.e., protease-resistant). More important, when PrP^{sc} physically interacts with PrP molecules, it induces them to adopt the PrP^{sc} conformation (Fig. 23.21), a property that accounts for the "infectious" nature of PrP^{sc}. Over time, this self-amplifying process leads to the accumulation of a high burden of pathogenic PrP^{sc} molecules in the brain. Certain mutations in the gene encoding PrP^c *(PRNP)* accelerate the rate of spontaneous conformational change; these variants are associated with early-onset familial forms of prion disease (familial Creutzfeldt-Jakob disease [fCJD]). PrP^c also may change its conformation spontaneously (but at an extremely low rate), accounting for sporadic cases of prion disease (sporadic Creutzfeldt-Jakob disease [sCJD]). Accumulation of PrP^{sc} in neural tissue seems to be the cause of cell injury, but the mechanisms underlying the cytopathic changes and eventual neuronal death are still unknown.

Creutzfeldt-Jakob Disease (CJD)

CJD is a rapidly progressive dementing illness, with a typical duration from first onset of subtle changes in memory and behavior to death in only 7 months. It is sporadic in approximately 85% of cases and has a worldwide annual incidence of about 1 per million. While commonly

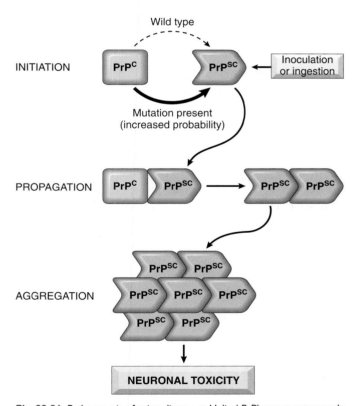

Fig. 23.21 Pathogenesis of prion disease. α-Helical PrP^c may spontaneously shift to the β-sheet PrP^{sc} conformation, an event that occurs at a much higher rate in familial disease associated with germ line PrP mutations. PrP^{sc} may also be from exogenous sources, such as contaminated food, medical instrumentation, or medicines. Once present, PrP^{sc} converts additional molecules of PrP^c into PrP^{sc} through physical interaction, eventually leading to the formation of pathogenic PrP^{sc} aggregates.

affecting individuals older than 70 years of age, familial forms caused by mutations in *PRNP* may present in younger individuals. In keeping with the infectious nature of PrP^{sc}, there are well-established cases of iatrogenic transmission by contaminated deep implantation electrodes and human growth hormone preparations.

MORPHOLOGY

The progression to death in CJD usually is so rapid that there is little, if any, macroscopic evidence of brain atrophy. On microscopic examination, the pathognomonic finding is a **spongiform transformation of the cerebral cortex and deep gray matter structures** (caudate, putamen); this multifocal process results in the uneven formation of small, apparently empty, microscopic vacuoles of varying sizes within the neuropil (the eosinophilic regions in grey matter that contain dendrites, axons, and synapses) and sometimes in the perikaryon of neurons (Fig. 23.22A). In advanced cases, there is severe neuronal loss, reactive gliosis, and sometimes expansion of the vacuolated areas into cystlike spaces ("status spongiosus"). No inflammatory infiltrate is present. Immunohistochemical staining demonstrates the presence of proteinase K–resistant PrP^{sc} in tissue, while western blotting of tissue extracts after partial protease digestion allows detection of diagnostic PrP^{sc}.

Variant Creutzfeldt-Jakob Disease

Starting in 1995, cases of a CJD-like illness appeared in the United Kingdom. The neuropathologic findings and molecular features of these new cases were similar to those of CJD, suggesting a close relationship between the two illnesses, yet this new disorder differed from typical CJD in several important respects: the disease affected young adults; behavioral disorders figured prominently in early disease stages; and the neurologic syndrome progressed somewhat more slowly than typical CJD. Multiple lines of evidence indicate that this new disease, termed *variant Creutzfeldt-Jakob disease (vCJD)* is a consequence of exposure to the prion disease of cattle, called *bovine spongiform encephalopathy*. Also, there is now documentation of

transmission by blood transfusion. This variant form has a similar pathologic appearance to that in other types of CJD, with spongiform change and absence of inflammation. In vCJD, however, there are abundant cortical amyloid plaques, surrounded by the spongiform change (see Fig. 23.22B).

SUMMARY

INFECTIONS OF THE NERVOUS SYSTEM

- Pathogens from viruses through parasites can infect the brain; in addition, prion disease is a protein-induced transmissible disease that is unique to the nervous system.
- Different pathogens use distinct routes to reach the brain, and they cause different patterns of disease.
- Bacterial infections may cause meningitis, cerebral abscesses, or a chronic meningoencephalitis.
- Viral infections can cause meningitis or meningoencephalitis.
- HIV can directly cause meningoencephalitis, or indirectly affect the brain by increasing the risk for opportunistic infections (toxoplasmosis, CMV) or CNS lymphoma.
- Prion diseases are transmitted by an altered form of a normal cellular protein. They can be sporadic, transmitted, or inherited.

DISEASES OF MYELIN

Within the CNS, axons are tightly ensheathed by myelin, an electrical insulator that allows rapid propagation of neural impulses. Myelin consists of multiple layers of highly specialized, closely apposed plasma membranes that are assembled by oligodendrocytes. Although myelinated axons are present in all areas of the brain, they are the dominant component in the white matter; therefore, most diseases of myelin are primarily white matter disorders. The myelin in peripheral nerves is similar to the myelin in the CNS, but with several important differences: (1) peripheral myelin is made by Schwann cells, not oligodendrocytes; (2) each Schwann cell in a peripheral nerve

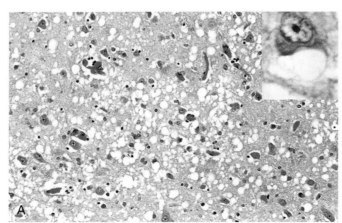
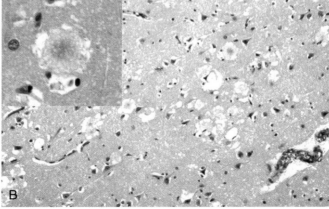

Fig. 23.22 Prion disease. (A) Histologic features of Creutzfeldt-Jakob disease (CJD) include spongiform change in the cerebral cortex. *Inset,* High magnification of a neuron with vacuoles. (B) Variant CJD (vCJD) is characterized by amyloid plaques *(inset)* that sit in the regions of greatest spongiform change.

provides myelin for only one internode, while in the CNS, many internodes are created by processes coming from a single oligodendrocyte; and (3) the specialized proteins and lipids are also different. Most diseases of CNS myelin do not involve the peripheral nerves to any significant extent, and vice versa.

In general, CNS diseases involving myelin are separated into two broad groups.

- Demyelinating diseases of the CNS are acquired conditions characterized by preferential damage to previously normal myelin. The most common diseases in this group result from immune-mediated injury, such as multiple sclerosis (MS) and related disorders. Other processes that can cause this type of disease include viral infection of oligodendrocytes, as in progressive multifocal leukoencephalopathy (see earlier), and injury caused by drugs and other toxic agents.
- By contrast, in other diseases, myelin is not formed properly or has abnormal turnover kinetics. As would be expected, most of these are caused by mutations that disrupt the function of proteins required for the formation of normal myelin sheaths. These diseases are grouped under leukodystrophy or dysmyelinating diseases.

Multiple Sclerosis (MS)

MS is an autoimmune demyelinating disorder characterized by episodes of disease activity, separated in time, that produce white matter lesions that are separated in space. It is the most common demyelinating disorder, having a prevalence of approximately 1 per 1000 individuals in the United States and Europe, and its incidence appears to be increasing. The disease may present at any age, but onset in childhood or after 50 years of age is rare. Women are affected twice as often as men.

Pathogenesis

The lesions of MS are caused by an autoimmune response directed against components of the myelin sheath. As in other autoimmune diseases (Chapter 5), the development of MS is related to genetic susceptibility and largely undefined environmental triggers. The incidence of MS is 15-fold higher when the disease is present in a first-degree relative and roughly 150-fold higher with an affected monozygotic twin. Only a portion of the genetic basis of the disease has been explained, and many of the identified loci are associated with other autoimmune diseases. There is a strong effect of the major histocompatibility complex; each copy of the *HLA-DRB1*1501* allele an individual inherits brings with it a roughly 3-fold increase in the risk for MS. Other genetic loci that are associated with MS include the IL-2 and IL-7 receptor genes and other genes encoding proteins involved in immune responses.

Immune mechanisms that underlie the destruction of myelin are the focus of much investigation. The available evidence indicates that the disease is initiated by T_H1 and T_H17 T cells that react against myelin antigens and secrete cytokines. Experimental autoimmune encephalomyelitis, an animal model of MS in which demyelination and inflammation occur after immunization of animals with myelin proteins, can be passively transferred to unimmunized animals with T_H1 and T_H17 cells that recognize myelin antigens. T_H1 cells secrete IFN-γ, which activates macrophages, and T_H17 cells promote the recruitment of leukocytes. The demyelination is caused by activated leukocytes and their injurious products. The infiltrate in plaques and surrounding regions of the brain consists of T cells (mainly CD4+, some CD8+) and macrophages. B lymphocytes and antibodies also play an important, but poorly defined, role in the disease, as indicated by the surprising success of B cell depleting therapies.

MORPHOLOGY

MS is primarily a multifocal white matter disease. Grossly, the characteristic lesions, termed **plaques**, are discrete, slightly depressed, glassy-appearing, and gray-tan in color (Fig. 23.23A). Plaques are common near the ventricles and also frequently occur in the optic nerves and chiasm, brain stem, ascending and descending fiber tracts, cerebellum, and spinal cord. The lesions have sharply defined borders at the microscopic level (see Fig. 23.23B). **Active plaques** contain abundant macrophages stuffed with myelin debris, evidence of ongoing myelin breakdown. Lymphocytes also are present, mostly as perivascular cuffs. Small active lesions often are centered on small veins. Axons are relatively preserved but may be reduced in number. When plaques become quiescent **(inactive plaques),** the inflammation mostly disappears, leaving behind little to no myelin, astrocytic proliferation, and gliosis.

Clinical Features

The course of MS is variable, but commonly there are multiple *relapses* followed by episodes of *remission;* typically, recovery during remissions is not complete. As a consequence, over time there is usually a gradual, often stepwise, accumulation of neurologic deficits. Imaging studies have demonstrated that there are often more lesions in the brains of patients with MS than might be expected from the clinical examination, and that lesions can come and go much more often than was previously suspected. Changes in cognitive function can be present, but are often much milder than the other deficits. In any individual patient, it is difficult to predict when the next relapse will occur; most current treatments, which are intended to control the immune response, aim at decreasing the rate and severity of relapses rather than recovering lost function.

The CSF in patients with MS shows a mildly elevated protein level with an increased proportion of immunoglobulin; in one-third of cases, there is moderate pleocytosis. When the immunoglobulin is examined further, *oligoclonal bands* usually are identified. These antibodies are directed against a variety of antigenic targets and can be used as markers of disease activity. The contribution of these antibodies to the disease process is unclear.

Other Acquired Demyelinating Diseases

Immune-mediated demyelination can occur after a number of systemic infectious illnesses, including

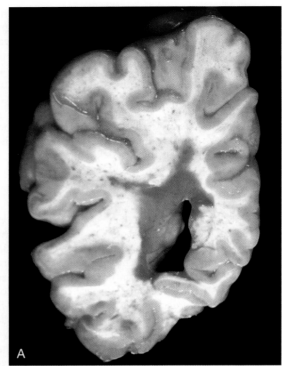

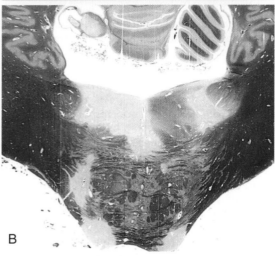

Fig. 23.23 Multiple sclerosis (MS). (A) Section of fresh brain showing a plaque around occipital horn of the lateral ventricle. (B) Unstained regions of demyelination (MS plaques) around the fourth ventricle. Luxol fast blue–periodic acid–Schiff stain for myelin.

relatively mild viral diseases. These are not thought to be related to direct spread of the infectious agents to the nervous system. Rather, it is believed that immune cells responding to pathogen-associated antigens cross-react against myelin antigens, resulting in myelin damage.

There are two general patterns of postinfectious autoimmune reactions to myelin; unlike MS, they both are associated with acute-onset monophasic illnesses. In *acute disseminated encephalomyelitis,* symptoms typically develop 1 or 2 weeks after an antecedent infection and are nonlocalizing (headache, lethargy, and coma), in contrast with the focal findings of MS. Symptoms progress rapidly, and the illness is fatal in as many as 20% of cases; in the remaining

patients, there is complete recovery. *Acute necrotizing hemorrhagic encephalomyelitis* is a more devastating related disorder, which typically affects young adults and children.

Other acquired diseases of myelin include *neuromyelitis optica (NMO),* an antibody-mediated demyelinating disease centered on the optic nerves and spinal cord, and *central pontine myelinolysis,* caused by nonimmune damage to oligodendrocytes typically after sudden correction of hyponatremia, that may result in a rapidly evolving quadriplegia.

As discussed earlier, *progressive multifocal leukoencephalopathy (PML)* is a demyelinating disease that occurs after reactivation of the JC virus in immunosuppressed patients.

Leukodystrophies

Leukodystrophies are inherited dysmyelinating diseases caused by abnormal myelin synthesis or turnover. They are caused by mutations of genes whose products are involved in the generation, turnover, or maintenance of myelin. Some of these mutations affect lysosomal enzymes, while others involve peroxisomal enzymes; a few are associated with mutations in myelin proteins. Most are of autosomal recessive inheritance, although X-linked diseases also occur. There is typically diffuse involvement of white matter leading to deterioration in motor skills, spasticity, hypotonia, or ataxia. Several clinical features separate leukodystrophies from demyelinating diseases. The leukodystrophies typically present with an insidious and progressive loss of function, often begin at younger ages, and are associated with diffuse and symmetric changes on imaging studies.

MORPHOLOGY

Much of the pathologic change of leukodystrophy is found in the white matter, which is diffusely abnormal in color (gray and translucent) and volume (decreased). Early in their course, some diseases may show patchy involvement, while others have a predilection for occipital lobe involvement. In the end, though, nearly all of the white matter usually is affected. With the loss of white matter, the brain becomes atrophic, the ventricles enlarge, and secondary changes can be found in the gray matter. Myelin loss is associated with infiltration of macrophages, which often become stuffed with lipid. Some of these diseases also show specific inclusions created by the accumulation of particular lipids.

SUMMARY

PRIMARY DISEASES OF MYELIN

- Because of the critical role of myelin in nerve conduction, diseases of myelin can lead to widespread and severe neurologic deficits.
- Multiple sclerosis, an autoimmune demyelinating disease, is the most common disorder of myelin, affecting young adults. It often pursues a relapsing-remitting course, with eventual progressive accumulation of neurologic deficits.
- Other, less common forms of immune-mediated demyelination often follow infections and are more acute illnesses.
- Leukodystrophies are genetic disorders in which myelin production or turnover is abnormal.

GENETIC METABOLIC DISEASES

Several genetic diseases disrupt metabolic processes in neurons and glia, resulting in progressive disorders that present early in life. These diseases can be grouped by the cells or compartment affected (neurons vs. white matter), the subcellular organelle affected (e.g., lysosome, peroxisome, or mitochondrion), or the metabolic pathway affected (e.g., sphingolipidoses, very long–chain fatty acid metabolism). The mutations underlying these diseases typically affect synthetic or degradation pathways that are specific to the nervous system.

- *Neuronal storage diseases* are characterized by the accumulation of storage material within neurons, typically leading to neuronal death. Cortical neuronal involvement leads to loss of cognitive function and may also cause seizures. Most commonly, they are autosomal recessive disorders caused by the deficiency of a specific enzyme involved in the catabolism of sphingolipids (including the gangliosides), mucopolysaccharides, or mucolipids; others appear to be caused by defects in protein or lipid trafficking within neurons. Several examples of these diseases, such as Tay-Sachs and Niemann-Pick diseases and mucopolysaccharidoses, are discussed in Chapter 7.
- *Mitochondrial encephalomyopathies* are disorders of oxidative phosphorylation, often affecting multiple tissues including skeletal muscle (Chapter 22). When they involve the brain, gray matter is more severely affected than white matter, as would be expected because of the greater metabolic requirements of neurons. These disorders may be caused by mutations in the mitochondrial or the nuclear genomes.

ACQUIRED METABOLIC AND TOXIC DISTURBANCES

Toxic and acquired metabolic diseases are relatively common causes of neurologic illnesses. **Because of its high metabolic demands, the brain is particularly vulnerable to nutritional diseases and alterations in metabolic state.** Some of these disorders have uneven pathologic lesions and distinct clinical presentations because of unique features or requirements of different anatomic regions of the brain. A few of the more common types of injury are discussed here.

Nutritional Diseases

Thiamine Deficiency

In addition to the systemic effects of thiamine deficiency *(beriberi)*, it also may be associated with the abrupt onset of confusion, abnormalities in eye movement and ataxia, syndrome termed *Wernicke encephalopathy.* Treatment with thiamine reverses these deficits, but if treatment is delayed the result is a largely irreversible profound memory disturbance called *Korsakoff syndrome.* Because the two syndromes are closely linked, the term *Wernicke-Korsakoff syndrome* is often used. The syndrome is particularly common in the setting of chronic alcoholism but also may be encountered in patients with thiamine deficiency resulting from gastric disorders, gastric bypass surgery, or persistent vomiting.

MORPHOLOGY

Wernicke encephalopathy is characterized by foci of hemorrhage and necrosis, particularly in the mammillary bodies but also adjacent to the ventricles, especially the third and fourth ventricles. Early lesions show dilated capillaries with prominent endothelial cells and progress to hemorrhage. As the lesions resolve, a cystic space appears along with hemosiderin-laden macrophages. Lesions in the medial dorsal nucleus of the thalamus seem to best correlate with the memory disturbance in Korsakoff syndrome.

Vitamin B$_{12}$ Deficiency

In addition to causing anemia, deficiency of vitamin B$_{12}$ may lead to neurologic deficits associated with changes in the spinal cord, resulting in a syndrome called *subacute combined degeneration of the spinal cord.* As the name implies, both ascending and descending tracts of the spinal cord are affected. Symptoms develop over weeks. Early clinical signs often include mild ataxia and lower-extremity numbness and tingling, which can progress to spastic weakness of the lower extremities; sometimes, complete paraplegia ensues. Prompt vitamin replacement therapy produces clinical improvement; however, if paraplegia has developed, recovery is poor.

Metabolic Disorders

Several systemic metabolic derangements may produce CNS dysfunction; only those associated with abnormal glucose levels and liver dysfunction are considered here.

Hypoglycemia

Since the brain requires glucose as a substrate for energy production, the cellular effects of diminished glucose generally resemble those of global hypoxia. Hippocampal neurons are particularly susceptible to hypoglycemic injury, while cerebellar Purkinje cells are relatively spared. As with anoxia, if the level and duration of hypoglycemia are sufficiently severe, there may be widespread injury to many areas of the brain.

Hyperglycemia

Hyperglycemia is most common in the setting of inadequately controlled diabetes mellitus and can be associated with either ketoacidosis or hyperosmolar coma. Patients develop confusion, stupor, and eventually coma associated with intracellular dehydration caused by the hyperosmolar state. The hyperglycemia must be corrected gradually, because rapid correction can produce severe cerebral edema.

Hepatic Encephalopathy

Decreased hepatic function may be associated with depressed levels of consciousness and sometimes coma. In the early stages, patients exhibit a characteristic "flapping" tremor *(asterixis)* when extending the arms with palms facing the observer. Elevated levels of ammonia, which the liver normally clears through the urea cycle, in combination with inflammation and hyponatremia, cause the changes in brain function. Because it is only one contributing factor, ammonia levels in symptomatic patients vary widely. Within the CNS, ammonia metabolism occurs only in astrocytes through the action of glutamine synthetase, and in the setting of hyperammonemia, astrocytes in the cortex and basal ganglia develop swollen, pale nuclei (referred to as Alzheimer type II cells).

Toxic Disorders

The list of toxins with effects on the brain is extremely long. Among the major categories of neurotoxic substances are *metals,* including lead, arsenic, and mercury; *industrial chemicals,* including organophosphates (in pesticides) and methanol (causing blindness from retinal damage); and *environmental pollutants* such as carbon monoxide (combining hypoxia with selective injury to the globus pallidus).

Ethanol has a variety of effects on the brain. While acute intoxication is reversible, excessive intake can result in profound metabolic disturbances, including brain swelling and death. Chronic alcohol exposure leads to cerebellar dysfunction in about 1% of cases, with truncal ataxia, unsteady gait, and nystagmus, associated with atrophy in the anterior vermis of the cerebellum.

Ionizing radiation, commonly used to treat intracranial tumors, can cause rapidly evolving signs and symptoms including headache, nausea, vomiting, and papilledema, even months to years after irradiation. Affected brain regions show large areas of coagulative necrosis, edema, and blood vessels with thickened walls containing intramural fibrin like material.

NEURODEGENERATIVE DISEASES

Neurodegenerative diseases are characterized by the progressive loss of neurons, typically affecting groups of neurons with functional interconnections. Different diseases tend to involve particular neural systems and therefore have relatively stereotypic presenting signs and symptoms (Table 23.3):

- Diseases that involve the hippocampus and associated cortices present with cognitive changes, often including disturbances of memory, behavior, and language. With time these progress to dementia, as occurs with Alzheimer disease.
- Diseases that affect the basal ganglia manifest as movement disorders; these may be hypokinetic, as with Parkinson disease, or hyperkinetic, as with Huntington disease.
- Diseases that affect the cerebellum or its input and output circuitry result in ataxia, as seen in the spinocerebellar ataxias.
- When the motor system bears the burden, weakness and difficulty with swallowing and respiration are often seen first, as with amyotrophic lateral sclerosis.

A pathologic process shared by most neurodegenerative diseases is the accumulation of protein aggregates,

Table 23.3 Features of the Major Neurodegenerative Diseases

Disease	Clinical Pattern	Protein Inclusions
Alzheimer disease (AD)	Dementia	Aβ (plaques) Tau (tangles)
Frontotemporal lobar degeneration (FTLD)	Behavioral changes, language disturbance	Tau TDP43 Others (rare)
Parkinson disease (PD)	Hypokinetic movement disorder	α-synuclein Tau
Huntington disease (HD)	Hyperkinetic movement disorder	Huntingtin (polyglutamine repeat expansions)
Spinocerebellar ataxias	Cerebellar ataxia	Various proteins (polyglutamine repeat expansions)
Amyotrophic lateral sclerosis (ALS)	Weakness with upper and lower motor neurons signs	SOD1 TDP43

which serve as histologic hallmarks of specific disorders (Table 23.3). Aggregates may arise because of mutations that alter the protein's conformation or that disrupt pathways involved in processing or clearance of the proteins. In other situations, there may be a subtle imbalance between protein synthesis and clearance (due to genetic, environmental, or stochastic factors) that allows gradual accumulation of proteins. The aggregates often are resistant to degradation by normal cellular proteases, accumulate within cells, elicit an inflammatory response, and may be directly toxic to neurons. As is evident from Table 23.3, the same proteins may be present as aggregates in multiple diseases. The clinical phenotype of the neurodegenerative disease is determined more by the distribution of the aggregates than by the nature of the aggregating protein.

Two other features are common to many neurodegenerative diseases:

- There is experimental evidence that many of the protein aggregates that accumulate in neurons affected in these diseases appear to be capable of spreading to healthy neurons. Thus, aggregates can seed the development of more aggregates, and the disease process can spread, like prions. However, there is no evidence for transmission from affected to healthy individuals.
- Activation of the innate immune system is a common feature of neurodegenerative diseases. The importance of this interaction between the brain and the immune system has been further strengthened by the identification of genes that confer risk for diseases (e.g., *TREM2* for Alzheimer disease) that encode components of immune regulatory pathways.

Alzheimer Disease

Alzheimer disease (AD) is the most common cause of dementia in older adults, with an increasing incidence as

a function of age. The incidence is about 3% in individuals 65 to 74 years of age, 19% in those 75 to 84 years of age, and 47% in those older than 84 years of age. Most cases of AD are sporadic, but at least 5% to 10% are familial. Sporadic cases rarely present before 50 years of age, but early onset is seen with some heritable forms.

The disease usually manifests with the insidious onset of impaired higher intellectual function, memory impairment, and altered mood and behavior. Over time, disorientation and aphasia, findings indicative of severe cortical dysfunction, often develop; those in the final phases of AD are profoundly disabled, often mute and immobile. Death usually occurs from intercurrent pneumonia or other infections.

Pathogenesis

The fundamental abnormality in AD is the accumulation of two proteins (Aβ and tau) in specific brain regions, in the forms of plaques and tangles, respectively; these changes result in secondary effects including neuronal dysfunction, neuronal death, and inflammatory reactions. Plaques are deposits of aggregated Aβ peptides in the neuropil, while tangles are aggregates of the microtubule binding protein tau, which develop intracellularly and then persist extracellularly after neuronal death. Both plaques and tangles appear to contribute to neural dysfunction. The details of the interplay between the processes that lead to the accumulation of these abnormal aggregates are a critical aspect of AD pathogenesis that has yet to be unraveled.

Clinical and experimental evidence strongly suggests that **Aβ generation is the critical initiating event for the development of AD.** Notably, mutations or alterations in copy number of the gene encoding the precursor protein for Aβ are associated with an elevated risk of AD, whereas mutations in the gene for tau do not give rise to AD but rather cause frontotemporal lobar degenerations. Overexpression of Aβ can replicate the disease in animal models.

The pathogenesis of AD involves Aβ and Tau deposits, as well as other risk factors and inflammatory reactions.

- *Role of Aβ.* Aβ is created when the transmembrane protein amyloid precursor protein (APP) is sequentially cleaved by the enzymes β-amyloid–converting enzyme (BACE) and γ-secretase (Fig. 23.24). APP also can be cleaved by α-secretase and γ-secretase, liberating a different peptide that is nonpathogenic. Mutations in APP or in components of γ-secretase (encoded by the presenilin-1 or presenilin-2 gene) lead to familial AD by increasing the rate at which Aβ, particularly its most aggregation-prone form, is generated. The *APP* gene is located on chromosome 21, and the risk for AD also is higher in those with an extra copy of the *APP* gene, such as patients with trisomy 21 (Down syndrome) and individuals with small interstitial duplications of *APP*, presumably because this too leads to greater Aβ generation. Once generated, Aβ is highly prone to aggregation; it first forms small oligomers, and these eventually propagate into large aggregates and fibrils. It is these aggregates that deposit in the brain and are visible as plaques. There is evidence that these oligomers decrease the number of synapses present and alter the function of those that remain so that the cellular processes felt to underlie learning and memory are disrupted.

- *Role of tau.* Because neurofibrillary tangles contain the tau protein, there has been much interest in the role of this protein in AD. Tau is a microtubule-associated protein present in axons in association with the microtubular network. With the development of tangles in AD, tau shifts to a somatic-dendritic distribution, becomes hyperphosphorylated, and loses the ability to bind to microtubules. The formation of tangles is an important component of AD, but the mechanism of tangle injury to neurons remains poorly understood. Two pathways have been suggested; 1) aggregates of tau protein elicit a stress response, which persists and eventually leads to cell death; and 2), the microtubule stabilizing function of tau protein is lost, leading to neuronal toxicity and death. It has been shown that tau aggregates can be passed across synapses from one neuron to the next; this may underlie some of the spread of lesions across the brain.

- *Other genetic risk factors.* The genetic locus on chromosome 19 that encodes apolipoprotein E (ApoE) has a strong influence on the risk for developing AD. Three alleles have been identified (ε2, ε3, and ε4) based on two amino acid polymorphisms. The dosage of the ε4 allele increases the risk for AD. This ApoE isoform promotes Aβ generation and deposition, although the mechanisms have not been established. Overall, this locus has been estimated to convey about one fourth of the risk for development of late-onset AD. Genome-wide association studies have identified multiple other loci that contribute to the risk for AD, but the roles of the encoded proteins in disease pathogenesis are not established.

- *Role of inflammation.* Both genetic and histologic studies have indicated that the innate immune system responds to Aβ and tau. Deposits of Aβ elicit an inflammatory response from microglia and astrocytes. This response probably assists in the clearance of the aggregated peptide, but also may stimulate the secretion of mediators that cause neuronal injury over time.

- *Basis for cognitive impairment.* Deposits of Aβ and tangles begin to appear in the brain well in advance of cognitive impairment. While there remains disagreement regarding the best correlate of dementia in individuals with AD, the presence of a large burden of plaques and tangles is strongly associated with severe cognitive dysfunction. The number of neurofibrillary tangles correlates better with the degree of dementia than does the number of neuritic plaques. Biochemical markers that have been correlated with the degree of dementia include amyloid burden.

MORPHOLOGY

Brains involved by AD show a variable degree of cortical atrophy, resulting in a widening of the cerebral sulci that is most pronounced in the frontal, temporal, and parietal lobes. The atrophy produces a compensatory ventricular enlargement (hydrocephalus ex vacuo). At the microscopic level, AD is diagnosed by the presence of **neuritic plaques** (an extracellular lesion) and **neurofibrillary tangles** (an intracellular lesion) (Fig. 23.25).

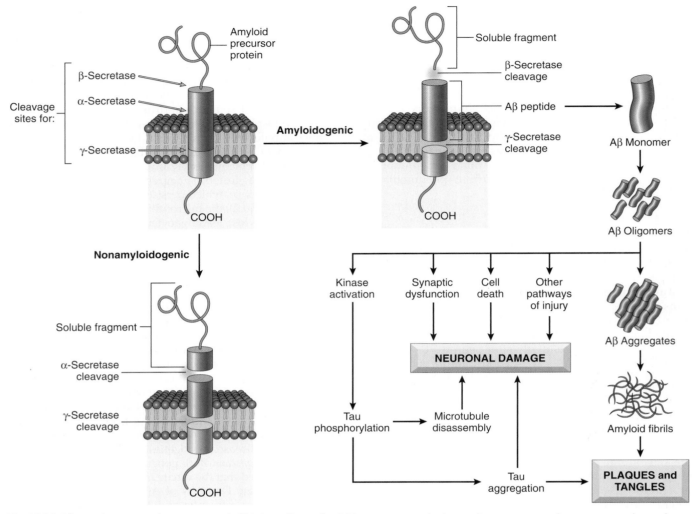

Fig. 23.24 Aβ peptide genesis and consequences in Alzheimer disease. Amyloid precursor protein cleavage by α-secretase and γ-secretase produces a harmless soluble peptide, whereas amyloid precursor protein cleavage by β-amyloid–converting enzyme (BACE) and γ-secretase releases Aβ peptides, which form pathogenic aggregates and contribute to the characteristic plaques and tangles of Alzheimer disease.

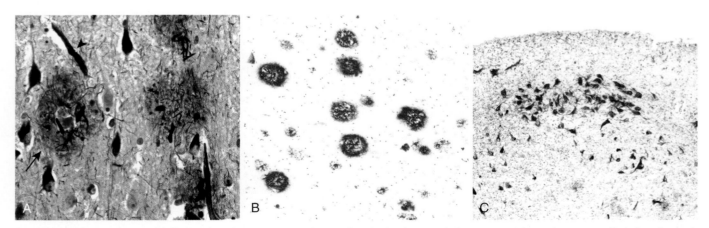

Fig. 23.25 Alzheimer disease. (A) Plaques *(arrow)* contain a central core of amyloid and a surrounding region of dystrophic neurites (Bielschowsky stain). (B) Immunohistochemical stain for Aβ. Peptide is present in the core of the plaques as well as in the surrounding region. (C) Neurons containing tangles stained with an antibody specific for tau.

Neuritic plaques are focal, spherical collections of dilated, tortuous, processes derived from dystrophic neurites, often around a central amyloid core (see Fig. 23.25A). Neuritic plaques range in size from 20 to 200 μm in diameter; microglial cells and reactive astrocytes are present at their periphery. Plaques can be found in the hippocampus and amygdala as well as in the neocortex, although there is relative sparing of primary motor and sensory cortices until late in the disease course. The amyloid core contains Aβ (see Fig. 23.25B). Aβ deposits also can be found that lack the surrounding neuritic reaction, termed **diffuse plaques;** these are found in the superficial cerebral cortex, the basal ganglia, and the cerebellar cortex and may represent an early stage of plaque development.

Neurofibrillary tangles are bundles of paired helical filaments visible as basophilic fibrillary structures in the cytoplasm of the neurons that displace or encircle the nucleus; tangles can persist after neurons die, becoming a form of extracellular pathology. They are commonly found in cortical neurons, especially in the entorhinal cortex, as well as in the pyramidal cells of the hippocampus, the amygdala, the basal forebrain, and the raphe nuclei. A major component of paired helical filaments is **hyperphosphorylated tau** (see Fig. 23.25C).

In individuals harboring autosomal dominant mutations that cause AD, deposition of Aβ and the formation of tangles precede the emergence of cognitive impairment by as much as 15 to 20 years. For this reason, the current diagnostic criteria consider the burden and distribution of amyloid deposits, tangles, and neuritic plaques—a constellation known as **Alzheimer disease neuropathologic changes.** The staging of each of these processes, which has a fairly consistent pattern across individuals, is then used to assess the likelihood that the observed lesions resulted in cognitive impairment.

Frontotemporal Lobar Degeneration

Frontotemporal lobar degeneration (FTLD) encompasses several disorders that preferentially affect the frontal and/or temporal lobes. As a result, these disorders have certain shared clinical features, such as progressive deterioration of language and changes in personality. The term *degeneration* is applied to describe the neuropathologic changes; clinically, these syndromes commonly are referred to as *frontotemporal dementias.* Depending on the disease distribution (frontal or temporal), behavioral changes or language problems may dominate. In general, behavioral and language problems precede memory disturbances, a distinction that assists in the clinical discrimination between FTLD and AD. The onset of symptoms occurs at younger ages for FTLD than for AD.

In addition to the clinical classification, two pathologic subgroups exist that are distinguished based on the composition of characteristic neuronal inclusions, which may contain tau or TDP43. One well-recognized subtype of FTLD-tau is *Pick disease,* which is associated with smooth, round inclusions known as *Pick bodies.* How tau aggregation may lead to neurodegeneration was discussed earlier, in the context of Alzheimer disease. The other major form of FTLD is characterized by aggregates containing the DNA/RNA-binding protein TDP43 (FTLD-TDP43). It is uncertain how this leads to neurodegeneration; both loss of TDP43 activity and a toxic gain-of-function related to the protein aggregates remain possibilities. TDP43 neuronal inclusions also are found in a large proportion of cases of amyotrophic lateral sclerosis (ALS). This overlap is manifest clinically, as many individuals with ALS also show evidence of FTLD.

MORPHOLOGY

The gross appearance is independent of the type of inclusions, with atrophy of frontal and temporal lobes of variable extent and severity, accompanied by neuronal loss and gliosis (Fig. 23.26A–B). In FTLD-tau, the characteristic additional lesion is the presence of tau-containing neurofibrillary tangles, similar to the tangles found in AD (see Fig. 23.26C). In FTLD-TDP, there is loss of nuclear staining for TDP43 associated with the appearance of TDP43-positive inclusions (see Fig. 23.26D).

Parkinson Disease

Parkinson disease (PD) is a neurodegenerative disease marked by a hypokinetic movement disorder that is caused by loss of dopaminergic neurons from the substantia nigra. *Parkinsonism* is a clinical syndrome characterized by tremor, rigidity, bradykinesia, and instability. These types of motor disturbances may be seen in a range of diseases that damage dopaminergic neurons, which project from the substantia nigra to the striatum and are involved in control of motor activity. Parkinsonism can be induced by drugs such as dopamine antagonists or toxins that selectively injure dopaminergic neurons. Among the neurodegenerative diseases, most cases of parkinsonism are caused by PD, which is associated with characteristic neuronal inclusions containing α-synuclein.

Pathogenesis

PD is associated with protein accumulation and aggregation, mitochondrial abnormalities, and neuronal loss in the substantia nigra and elsewhere in the brain. Based on the genetics of PD, it appears that abnormal protein and organelle clearance due to defects in autophagy and lysosomal degradation have a pathogenic role in the disease. One clue and diagnostic feature of the disease is the Lewy body, a characteristic inclusion containing *α-synuclein*, a protein involved in synaptic transmission. While PD in most cases is sporadic, point mutations and duplications of the gene encoding α-synuclein cause autosomal dominant PD. Synuclein aggregates are cleared by autophagy (Chapter 2), and several mutations associated with PD are in genes whose products (LRRK2, Parkin, others) all appear to have roles in endosomal trafficking pathways implicated in autophagy. It also has been demonstrated that heterozygosity for the Gaucher disease–causing mutation in glucocerebrosidase is a risk factor for PD. Glucocerebrosidase is a lysosomal enzyme, yet another clue suggesting that abnormal turnover of cellular constituents somehow sets the stage for the development of PD.

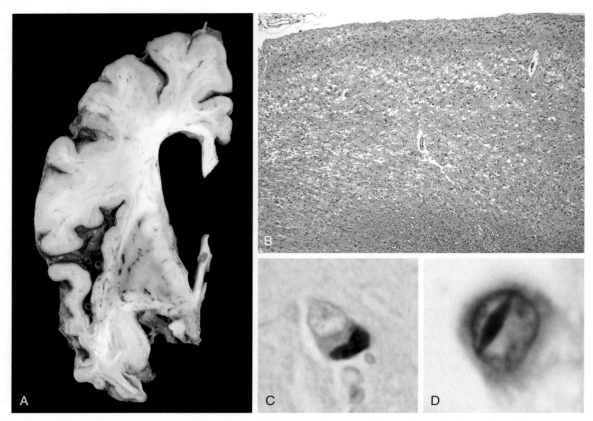

Fig. 23.26 Frontotemporal lobar degeneration (FTLD). (A) Atrophy of the temporal cortex can be seen in comparison to the relative preservation of frontal cortex. (B) Severe neuronal loss and gliosis in the region of atrophy. (C) FTLD-tau. Cytoplasmic inclusions containing TDP43 are seen in association with loss of normal nuclear immunoreactivity. (D) FTLD-TDP. Some forms of FTLD are associated with neuronal intranuclear inclusions containing TDP43.

MORPHOLOGY

A typical gross finding at autopsy is pallor of the substantia nigra (Fig. 23.27A–B) and locus ceruleus. Microscopic features include loss of the pigmented, catecholaminergic neurons in these regions associated with gliosis. **Lewy bodies** (see Fig. 23.27C) may be found in those neurons that remain. These are single or multiple, cytoplasmic, eosinophilic, round to elongated inclusions. On ultrastructural examination, Lewy bodies consist of fine filaments, composed of α-synuclein and other proteins, including neurofilaments and ubiquitin. The other major histologic finding is the presence of **Lewy neurites,** dystrophic neurites that also contain aggregated α-synuclein. Immunohistochemical staining for α-synuclein highlights more subtle Lewy bodies and Lewy neurites in many brain regions outside of the substantia nigra and in non-dopaminergic neurons, including regions of the medulla, the pons, the amygdala, and the cerebral cortex. Eventually they appear in the subcortical areas and the cerebral cortex. With involvement of the cerebral cortex, there is typically dementia present in addition to the movement disorder.

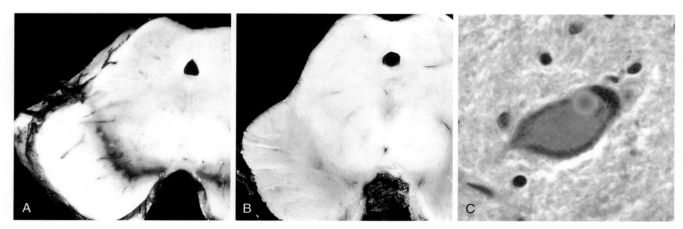

Fig. 23.27 Parkinson disease. (A) Normal substantia nigra. (B) Depigmented substantia nigra in idiopathic Parkinson disease. (C) Lewy body in a neuron from the substantia nigra stains pink.

Clinical Features

PD commonly manifests as a movement disorder in the absence of a toxic exposure or other known underlying etiology. The disease usually progresses over 10 to 15 years, eventually producing severe motor slowing to the point of near immobility. Death usually is the result of aspiration pneumonia or trauma from falls caused by postural instability.

Movement symptoms of PD initially respond to L-dihydroxyphenylalanine (L-DOPA), but this treatment does not slow disease progression. Over time, L-DOPA becomes less effective and begins to cause problematic fluctuations in motor function. Another treatment for the motor symptoms of PD is deep brain stimulation, in which electrodes are implanted in the globus pallidus or subthalamic nucleus to modulate basal ganglia circuitry, often allowing a significant reduction in L-DOPA dose.

While the movement disorder associated with loss of the nigrostriatal dopaminergic pathway is an important feature of PD, it is clear that the disease has more extensive clinical and pathologic manifestations. Lesions in the brain stem (in the dorsal motor nucleus of the vagus and in the reticular formation), in advance of nigral involvement, can give rise to behavioral sleep disorder often before the motor problems. Dementia, typically with a mildly fluctuating course and hallucinations, emerges in many individuals with PD and is attributable to involvement of the cerebral cortex. When dementia arises within 1 year of the onset of motor symptoms, it is referred to *Lewy body dementia (LBD)*.

Huntington Disease

Huntington disease (HD) is an autosomal dominant movement disorder associated with degeneration of the striatum (caudate and putamen). The disorder is characterized by involuntary jerky movements of all parts of the body; writhing movements of the extremities are typical. The disease is relentlessly progressive, resulting in death after an average course of about 15 years. Early cognitive symptoms include forgetfulness and thought and affective disorders, and there may be a progression to severe dementia. As a part of these early behavioral changes, HD carries an increased risk for suicide.

Pathogenesis

HD is caused by CAG trinucleotide repeat expansions in a gene located on 4p16.3 that encodes the protein huntingtin. Normal alleles contain 11 to 34 copies of the repeat; in disease-causing alleles, the number of repeats is increased, sometimes into the hundreds. There is a strong genotype-phenotype correlation, with larger numbers of repeats resulting in earlier-onset disease. Once the symptoms appear, however, the course of the illness is not affected by repeat length. Further expansions of the CAG (glutamine-encoding) repeats occur during spermatogenesis, so paternal transmission may be associated with earlier onset in the next generation, a phenomenon referred to as *anticipation* (Chapter 7).

HD appears to be caused by a toxic gain-of-function related to the expanded polyglutamine tract in huntingtin.

The mutant protein is subject to ubiquitination and proteolysis, yielding fragments that can form large intranuclear aggregates. As in other degenerative diseases, smaller aggregates of the abnormal protein fragments are suspected to be toxic. These aggregates have been shown to have a range of potentially injurious actions, including sequestration of transcription factors, disruption of protein degradation pathways, and perturbation of mitochondrial function. It is likely that some combination of these aberrations contributes to HD pathogenesis.

MORPHOLOGY

On gross examination, the brain is small and shows striking atrophy of the caudate nucleus and, sometimes less dramatically, the putamen (Fig. 23.28). The globus pallidus may be atrophied secondarily, and the lateral and third ventricles are dilated. Atrophy frequently also is seen in the frontal lobe, less often in the parietal lobe, and occasionally in the entire cortex.

Microscopic examination reveals severe loss of neurons from affected regions of the striatum along with gliosis. The medium-sized, spiny neurons that release the neurotransmitters γ-aminobutyric acid (GABA), enkephalin, dynorphin, and substance P are especially sensitive, disappearing early in the disease. There is a strong correlation between the degree of degeneration in the striatum and the severity of motor symptoms; there is also an association between cortical neuronal loss and dementia. In remaining striatal neurons and in the cortex, there are intranuclear inclusions that contain aggregates of ubiquitinated huntingtin protein (see Fig. 23.28, *inset*).

Spinocerebellar Ataxias

Spinocerebellar ataxias (SCAs) are a heterogeneous group of several dozen diseases with clinical findings that include a combination of cerebellar and sensory ataxia, spasticity, and sensorimotor peripheral neuropathy. They are distinguished from one another based on different

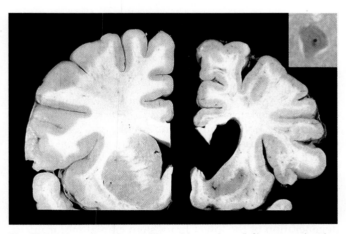

Fig. 23.28 Huntington disease. Normal hemisphere *(left)* compared with a hemisphere with Huntington disease *(right)* showing atrophy of the striatum and ventricular dilation. *Inset,* An intranuclear inclusion in a cortical neuron is strongly immunoreactive for ubiquitin. *(Gross photo courtesy of Dr. Vonsattel, Columbia University, New York, New York.)*

causative mutations, patterns of inheritance, age at onset, and signs and symptoms. This group of diseases affects, to a variable extent, the cerebellar cortex, spinal cord, other brain regions, and peripheral nerves. Degeneration of neurons, often without other distinctive histopathologic changes, occurs in the affected areas and is associated with mild gliosis. The additional clinical symptoms that accompany the ataxia can help distinguish between well-characterized subtypes. Although many distinct genetic types of SCA have been identified, there remain many cases that do not fall into one of the already characterized forms.

As with HD, several forms of SCA are caused by CAG repeat expansions encoding polyglutamine tracts in various genes. In these forms of SCA, as is true for HD, neuronal intranuclear inclusions are present containing the abnormal protein, and there is an inverse correlation between the degree of repeat expansion and age of onset. Other SCAs are caused by repeat expansions in untranslated regions or by other types of mutations.

Friedreich ataxia is an autosomal recessive disorder that generally manifests in the first decade of life with gait ataxia, followed by hand clumsiness and dysarthria. Most patients develop pes cavus and kyphoscoliosis, and there is a high incidence of cardiac disease and diabetes. The disease usually is caused by a GAA trinucleotide repeat expansion in the gene encoding frataxin, a protein that regulates cellular iron levels, particularly in the mitochondria. The repeat expansion results in decreased protein levels through transcriptional silencing; decreased frataxin leads to mitochondrial dysfunction as well as increased oxidative damage.

Amyotrophic Lateral Sclerosis

Amyotrophic lateral sclerosis (ALS) results from the death of lower motor neurons in the spinal cord and brain stem as well as upper motor neurons (Betz cells) in the motor cortex. The loss of lower motor neurons results in denervation of muscles, muscular atrophy (the "amyotrophy" of the condition), weakness, and fasciculations, while the loss of upper motor neurons results in paresis, hyperreflexia, and spasticity, along with a Babinski sign. An additional consequence of upper motor neuron loss is degeneration of the corticospinal tracts in the lateral portion of the spinal cord ("lateral sclerosis"). Sensation usually is unaffected, but cognitive impairment is not infrequent.

The disease affects men slightly more frequently than women and becomes clinically manifest in the fifth decade or later. It usually begins with subtle asymmetric distal extremity weakness. As the disease progresses, muscle strength and bulk diminish, and involuntary contractions of individual motor units, termed *fasciculations*, occur. The disease eventually involves the respiratory muscles, leading to recurrent bouts of pulmonary infection, which is the usual cause of death. The balance between upper and lower motor neuron involvement can vary, although most patients exhibit involvement of both. In some patients, degeneration of the lower brain stem cranial motor nuclei occurs early and progresses rapidly, a pattern of disease referred to as *bulbar amyotrophic lateral sclerosis*. With this disease pattern, abnormalities of swallowing and speaking dominate.

Pathogenesis

While most cases are sporadic, about 10% are familial, mostly with autosomal dominant inheritance. Familial disease begins earlier in life than sporadic disease, but once symptoms appear, the clinical course is similar in both forms. Mutations in the superoxide dismutase gene, *SOD1*, on chromosome 21 were the first identified genetic cause of ALS and account for about 20% of the familial forms. These mutations are thought to generate abnormal misfolded forms of the SOD1 protein, which may trigger the unfolded protein response and cause apoptotic death of neurons.

A number of other genetic loci have been identified as associated with ALS. The most common cause of familial ALS is hexanucleotide repeat expansion in a gene with the rather cumbersome name *C9orf72*, which is also frequently expanded in frontotemporal lobar degeneration. The protein encoded by *C9orf72* associates with RNA binding proteins; notably, two other genes that when mutated may cause ALS, TDP43 (also associated with FTLD) and FUS, encode RNA binding proteins. This convergence suggests that an abnormality of RNA processing directly or indirectly contributes to the pathogenesis of ALS, but it is uncertain how mutations in SOD1 fit into this picture, and much remains to be discovered. As expected from the genetic overlap, there is some clinical overlap between ALS and FTLD, such as cognitive impairment.

MORPHOLOGY

The most striking gross changes are found in anterior roots of the spinal cord, which are thin and gray. In especially severe cases, the precentral gyrus (motor cortex) is mildly atrophic due to the death of upper motor neurons. Microscopic examination demonstrates a **reduction in the number of anterior horn cell neurons** throughout the spinal cord associated with reactive gliosis and loss of anterior root myelinated fibers. Similar findings are found with involvement of motor cranial nerve nuclei except those supplying the extraocular muscles, which are spared in all but a few long term survivors. Cytoplasmic inclusions that contain TDP43 may be seen in a subset of cases. With the loss of innervation from the death of anterior horn cells, skeletal muscles show neurogenic atrophy.

SUMMARY

NEURODEGENERATIVE DISEASES

- Neurodegenerative diseases cause symptoms that depend on the pattern of brain involvement. Cortical disease usually manifests as cognitive change, alterations in personality, and memory disturbances; basal ganglia disorders usually manifest as movement disorders.
- Many of the neurodegenerative diseases are associated with various protein aggregates, which serve as pathologic hallmarks. Familial forms of these diseases are associated with mutations in the genes encoding these proteins or controlling their metabolism. Some of these protein aggregates can show prion like properties, facilitating spread from one cell to the next.

- Among dementias, Alzheimer disease (with plaques of Aβ and tangles of tau) is the most common; other predominantly dementing diseases include the various forms of FTLDs (both forms with tau-containing lesions and with other types of inclusions) and dementia with Lewy bodies (with α-synuclein containing lesions).
- Among the hypokinetic movement disorders, Parkinson disease is the most common, with α-synuclein containing inclusions.
- Amyotrophic lateral sclerosis (ALS) is the most common form of motor neuron disease, with diverse genetic causes as well as sporadic forms.

TUMORS

The annual incidence of CNS tumors ranges from 10 to 17 per 100,000 individuals for intracranial tumors and 1 to 2 per 100,000 individuals for intraspinal tumors; about one-half to three-fourths are primary tumors, and the rest are metastatic. Tumors of the CNS make up a larger proportion of childhood cancers, accounting for as many of 20% of all pediatric tumors. Childhood CNS tumors differ from those in adults in both histologic subtype and location. In childhood, tumors are likely to arise in the posterior fossa, whereas tumors in adults are mostly supratentorial.

Tumors of the nervous system have unique characteristics that set them apart from neoplastic processes elsewhere in the body.

- These tumors do not have morphologically evident premalignant or in situ stages comparable to those of carcinomas.
- Even low-grade lesions may infiltrate large regions of the brain, leading to serious clinical deficits, inability to be resected, and poor prognosis.
- The anatomic site of the neoplasm can influence outcome independent of histologic classification due to local effects (e.g., a benign meningioma may cause cardiorespiratory arrest from compression of the medulla).
- Even the most highly malignant gliomas rarely spread outside of the CNS.

Gliomas

Gliomas are tumors of the brain parenchyma that have long been classified as *astrocytomas, oligodendrogliomas,* **and** *ependymomas* **based on their morphologic resemblance to different types of glial cells.** With emerging genetic information, it has become clear that the gliomas are a molecularly distinct family of neoplastic lesions, independent of the histologic patterns. Nonetheless, histologic patterns continue to inform diagnosis and guide treatment, with refinement based on molecular characterization. The diffuse gliomas constitute the vast majority of gliomas that occur in adults, and include diffuse astrocytomas and oligodendrogliomas.

Diffuse Astrocytoma

Astrocytomas account for about 80% of adult gliomas. They are most frequent in the fourth through the sixth decades of life. They usually are found in the cerebral hemispheres. The most common presenting signs and symptoms are seizures, headaches, and focal neurologic deficits related to the anatomic site of involvement. **On the basis of histologic features, astrocytomas are stratified into three groups: diffuse astrocytoma (grade II), anaplastic astrocytoma (grade III), and glioblastoma (grade IV), with increasingly grim prognosis as the grade increases.** There is emerging evidence that genetic subtyping provides important additional prognostic information.

Diffuse astrocytomas can be static for several years, but at some point they progress; the mean survival is more than 5 years. Eventually, patients suffer rapid clinical deterioration that is correlated with the appearance of anaplastic features and more rapid tumor growth. Other patients present with glioblastoma from the outset. Once the histologic features of glioblastoma appear, the prognosis is very poor; with treatment (resection, radiotherapy, and chemotherapy), the median survival is only 15 months.

MORPHOLOGY

Grade II and III astrocytomas are poorly defined, gray, infiltrative tumors that expand and distort the invaded brain without forming a discrete mass (Fig. 23.29A). Infiltration beyond the grossly evident margins is always present. The cut surface of the tumor is either firm or soft and gelatinous; cystic degeneration may be seen. In glioblastoma, variation in the gross appearance of the tumor from region to region is characteristic (see Fig. 23.29B). Some areas are firm and white, others are soft and yellow (the result of tissue necrosis), and still others show regions of cystic degeneration and hemorrhage.

Microscopically, low-grade (WHO grade II) astrocytomas are characterized by a mild to moderate increase in the number of glial cell nuclei, somewhat variable nuclear pleomorphism, and an intervening feltwork of fine, glial fibrillary acidic protein (GFAP)-positive astrocytic cell processes that give the background a fibrillary appearance. The transition between neoplastic and normal tissue is indistinct, and tumor cells can be seen infiltrating normal tissue many centimeters from the main lesion. Anaplastic astrocytomas show regions that are more densely cellular and have greater nuclear pleomorphism; mitotic figures are present. Glioblastoma has a histologic appearance similar to that of anaplastic astrocytoma, as well as either necrosis (commonly present as serpiginous bands of necrosis with palisaded tumor cells along the border) or microvascular proliferation (see Fig. 23.29C).

Oligodendroglioma

Oligodendrogliomas account for 5% to 15% of gliomas and most commonly are detected in the fourth and fifth decades of life. Patients may have had several years of antecedent neurologic complaints, often including seizures. The lesions are found mostly in the cerebral hemispheres, mainly in the frontal or temporal lobes. The combination of surgery, chemotherapy, and radiotherapy yields an average survival of 10 to 20 years for well-differentiated (WHO grade II) oligodendrogliomas or 5 to 10 years for anaplastic (WHO grade III) oligodendrogliomas.

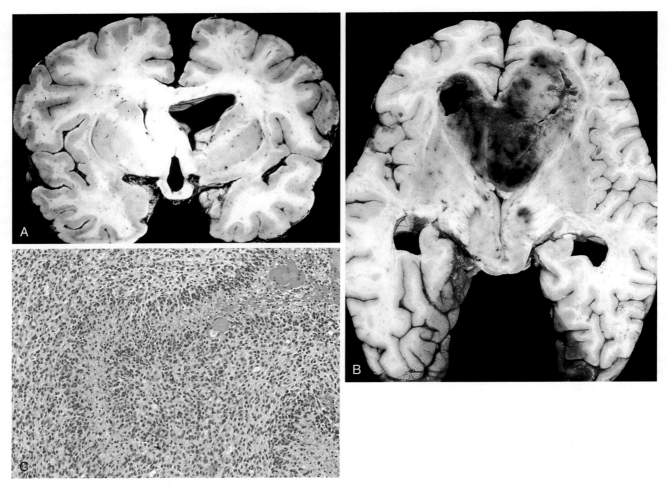

Fig. 23.29 Diffuse astrocytomas. (A) Grade II astrocytoma is seen as expanded white matter of the left cerebral hemisphere and thickened corpus callosum and fornices. (B) Glioblastoma appearing as a necrotic, hemorrhagic, infiltrating mass. (C) Glioblastoma is a densely cellular tumor with necrosis and pseudo-palisading of tumor cell nuclei along the edge of the necrotic zone.

MORPHOLOGY

Well-differentiated oligodendrogliomas (WHO grade II) are infiltrative tumors that form gelatinous, gray masses and may show cysts, focal hemorrhage, and calcification. On microscopic examination, the tumor is composed of sheets of regular cells with spherical nuclei containing finely granular chromatin (similar to that in normal oligodendrocytes) surrounded by a clear halo of cytoplasm (Fig. 23.30). The tumor typically contains a delicate network of anastomosing capillaries. Calcification, present in as many as 90% of these tumors, ranges in extent from microscopic foci to massive depositions. Mitotic activity usually is low. Anaplastic oligodendroglioma (WHO grade III) is a more aggressive subtype with higher cell density, nuclear anaplasia, increased mitotic activity, and often microvascular proliferation.

Genetics and Pathogenesis

Several classes of tumor-causing genetic alterations have been described in gliomas.

- Mutations in *isocitrate dehydrogenase (IDH)* genes are commonly observed in grade II astrocytomas and oligodendrogliomas. These mutations may occur in IDH1 or IDH2 and lead to increased production of 2-hydroxyglutarate, which interferes with the activity of several enzymes that regulate gene expression (Chapter 6).

- Mutations in the promoter for *telomerase*, which contribute to the immortalization of tumor cells (Chapter 6), are seen in glioblastomas and other astrocytic tumors. In tumors with IDH mutations, telomerase mutations are uncommon; instead, these tumors often have loss of function mutations in *ATRX*, which normally suppresses recombination events that can preserve telomere length, a mechanism called alternative lengthening of telomeres.

- Co-deletion of 1p and 19q chromosomal segments are present in oligodendrogliomas. The mechanism through which these chromosomal alterations shape tumor morphology and response to treatment is not known.

- Other genetic alterations, which are also common in tumors outside the CNS, include mutations that lead to overexpression of the EGF receptor and other receptor tyrosine kinases or disable p53 or RB (Chapter 6).

Midline Glioma

Midline gliomas arise most commonly in the brain stem (specifically in the pons) and also occur in the spinal cord

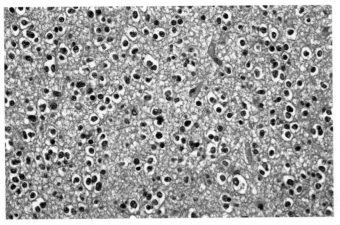

Fig. 23.30 In oligodendroglioma, tumor cells have round nuclei, often with a clear cytoplasmic halo. Blood vessels in the background are thin and can form an interlacing pattern.

and thalamus. They are infiltrative and result in significant neurologic impairment because of the disruption of critical nearby structures. Although they may not show typical high-grade features such as necrosis or vascular proliferation, they often behave aggressively. These lesions typically have acquired point mutations in histone H3, the consequence of which is loss of a lysine residue that is the target of post-translational modifications that regulate gene expression, another example of oncogenesis via alteration of the cancer cell "epigenome". Precisely how this mutation contributes to cellular transformation remains to be determined.

Pilocytic Astrocytoma

Pilocytic astrocytomas are relatively benign tumors that typically affect children and young adults. Most commonly located in the cerebellum, they also may involve the third ventricle, the optic pathways, the spinal cord, and occasionally the cerebral hemispheres. There is often a cyst associated with the tumor, and symptoms appearing after the incomplete resection of the lesions may be associated with cyst enlargement, rather than growth of the solid component. Tumors that involve the hypothalamus are especially problematic because they cannot be resected completely.

A high proportion of pilocytic astrocytomas have activating mutations or translocations involving the gene encoding the serine-threonine kinase BRAF, which result in activation of the MAPK signaling pathway. Pilocytic astrocytomas do not have mutations in *IDH1* and *IDH2*, supporting their distinction from the low-grade diffuse gliomas.

MORPHOLOGY

A pilocytic astrocytoma often is cystic, with a mural nodule in the wall of the cyst; if solid, it is usually well circumscribed. The tumor is composed of bipolar cells with long, thin "hairlike" processes that are GFAP-positive. Rosenthal fibers, eosinophilic granular bodies, and microcysts are often present, while necrosis and mitoses are rare.

Ependymoma

Ependymomas most often arise next to the ependyma-lined ventricular system, including the central canal of the spinal cord. In the first 2 decades of life, they typically occur near the fourth ventricle and constitute 5% to 10% of the primary brain tumors in this age group. In adults, the spinal cord is their most common location; tumors in this site are particularly frequent in the setting of neurofibromatosis type 2 (Chapter 22). The clinical outcome for completely resected supratentorial and spinal ependymomas is better than for those in the posterior fossa.

MORPHOLOGY

In the fourth ventricle, ependymomas typically are solid or papillary masses extending from the ventricular floor. The tumors are composed of cells with regular, round to oval nuclei and abundant granular chromatin. Between the nuclei is a variably dense fibrillary background. Tumor cells may form round or elongated structures (**rosettes, canals**) that resemble the embryologic ependymal canal, with long, delicate processes extending into a lumen (Fig. 23.31); more frequently present are **perivascular pseudorosettes** in which tumor cells are arranged around vessels with an intervening zone containing thin ependymal processes. Anaplastic ependymomas show increased cell density, high mitotic rates, necrosis, microvascular proliferation, and less evident ependymal differentiation.

Neuronal Tumors

Far less frequent than gliomas, tumors composed of cells with neuronal characteristics are typically lower-grade lesions that often present with seizures. While some neuronal differentiation can be observed in many tumors, lesions in this group are primarily composed of cells that express neuronal markers, such as synaptophysin and neurofilaments.

- *Central neurocytoma* is a low-grade neoplasm found within and adjacent to the ventricular system (most commonly the lateral or third ventricle); it is characterized by evenly spaced, round, uniform nuclei and often islands of neuropil.

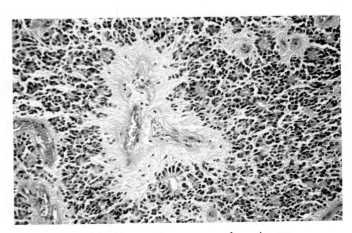

Fig. 23.31 Microscopic appearance of ependymoma.

- *Dysembryoplastic neuroepithelial tumor* is a distinctive, low-grade tumor of children and young adults that grows slowly, often manifests as a seizure disorder, and carries a favorable prognosis after resection. It typically is located in the superficial temporal lobe and consists of small, round neuronal cells arranged in columns and around central cores of processes.
- *Gangliogliomas* are tumors with a mixture of glial elements, usually a low-grade astrocytoma and mature-appearing neurons. Most of these tumors are slow growing, and often manifest with seizures. About 20% to 50% of gangliogliomas harbor point mutations in the *BRAF* gene.

Embryonal (Primitive) Neoplasms

Some tumors of neuroectodermal origin have a primitive "small round cell" appearance that is reminiscent of normal progenitor cells encountered in the developing CNS. Differentiation is often limited, but may progress along multiple lineages. The most common is the *medulloblastoma,* accounting for 20% of pediatric brain tumors.

Medulloblastoma

Medulloblastoma occurs predominantly in children and exclusively in the cerebellum. Neuronal and glial markers are nearly always expressed, at least to a limited extent. It is highly malignant, and the prognosis for untreated patients is dismal; however, medulloblastoma is exquisitely radiosensitive. With total excision, chemotherapy, and irradiation, the 5-year survival rate may be as high as 75%. There are a series of histologic patterns observed in medulloblastoma, which are informative about prognosis and correlate in part with the underlying genetics.

● MORPHOLOGY

In children, medulloblastomas are located in the midline of the cerebellum; lateral tumors occur more often in adults. The tumor often is well circumscribed, gray, and friable and may be seen extending to the surface of the cerebellar folia and involving the leptomeninges (Fig. 23.32A). Medulloblastomas are densely cellular, with sheets of anaplastic ("small blue") cells (see Fig. 23.32B). Individual tumor cells are small, with little cytoplasm and hyperchromatic nuclei; mitoses are abundant. Often, focal neuronal differentiation is seen in the form of rosettes, which closely resemble the rosettes encountered in neuroblastomas; they are characterized by primitive tumor cells surrounding central neuropil (delicate pink material formed by neuronal processes).

Pathogenesis

Genetic analysis of medulloblastoma has revealed several subtypes associated with different clinical outcomes. Current approaches separate medulloblastoma into distinct groups with different core pathogenic pathways or driver mutations. Examples of oncogenic pathways in these tumors are the following:

- *Wnt pathway activation,* most commonly associated with gain of function mutations in the gene for β-catenin; these have the most favorable prognosis of all of the genetic subtypes and are commonly classic-type tumors.
- *Hedgehog pathway activation,* most commonly associated with loss of function mutations in *PTCH1,* a negative regulator of the Hedgehog; these tumors have an intermediate prognosis, but the concomitant presence of *TP53* mutation confers a very poor prognosis.
- *MYC overexpression,* due to *MYC* amplification as well as other changes that result in increased expression; these tumors have the poorest prognosis.

Clinical trials are ongoing that seek to tailor therapy targeted to molecular alterations, with the goal of avoiding radiation therapy when possible.

Other Parenchymal Tumors

Primary Central Nervous System Lymphoma

Primary CNS lymphoma, occurring mostly as diffuse large B-cell lymphomas, accounts for 2% of extranodal lymphomas and 1% of intracranial tumors. It is the most common CNS neoplasm in immunosuppressed individuals, in

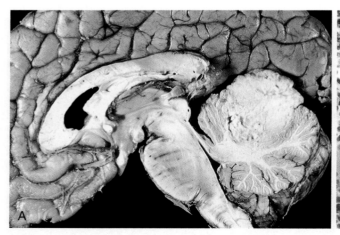
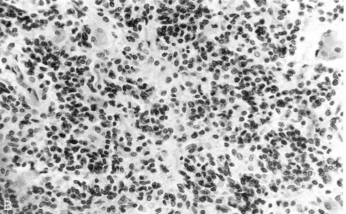

Fig. 23.32 Medulloblastoma. (A) Sagittal section of a brain showing medulloblastoma involving the superior vermis of the cerebellum. (B) Microscopic appearance of medulloblastoma, showing mostly small, blue, primitive-appearing tumor cells.

whom the tumors are nearly always positive for Epstein-Barr virus (EBV). In nonimmunosuppressed populations, the age spectrum is relatively wide, with the incidence increasing after 60 years of age. Regardless of the clinical context, primary brain lymphoma is an aggressive disease with a relatively poor response to chemotherapy as compared with peripheral lymphomas.

Patients with primary brain lymphoma often are found to have multiple tumor nodules within the brain parenchyma, yet involvement of sites outside of the CNS is uncommon. Conversely, lymphoma originating outside the CNS rarely spreads to the brain parenchyma; when this occurs, the tumor usually also involves the CSF or the meninges.

MORPHOLOGY

Lesions often involve deep gray structures, as well as the white matter and the cortex. Periventricular spread is common. The tumors are relatively well defined as compared with glial neoplasms, but they are not as discrete as metastases. EBV-associated tumors often show extensive areas of necrosis. The tumors are nearly always aggressive large B-cell lymphomas, although other histologic types may be encountered. Microscopically, malignant lymphoid cells accumulate around blood vessels and infiltrate the surrounding brain parenchyma. The diagnosis is confirmed by immunohistochemistry for B cell markers such as CD20, which also is a target of therapeutic antibodies.

Germ Cell Tumors

Primary brain *germ cell tumors* occur along the midline, most commonly in the pineal and the suprasellar regions. They account for 0.2% to 1% of brain tumors in individuals of European descent but in as many as 10% of brain tumors in individuals of Japanese ethnicity. They are a tumor of the young, with 90% occurring during the first 2 decades of life. Germ cell tumors in the pineal region show a strong male predominance. The most common primary CNS germ cell tumor is *germinoma,* a tumor that closely resembles testicular seminoma (Chapter 18). Secondary CNS involvement by metastatic gonadal germ cell tumors also occurs.

Meningiomas

Meningiomas are predominantly benign tumors that arise from arachnoid meningothelial cells. They usually occur in adults and are often attached to the dura. Meningiomas may be found along any of the external surfaces of the brain as well as within the ventricular system, where they arise from the stromal arachnoid cells of the choroid plexus. They often come to attention because of vague nonlocalizing symptoms, or with focal findings referable to compression of adjacent brain. Most meningiomas are easily separable from underlying brain, but some tumors are infiltrative, a feature associated with an increased risk for recurrence. The overall prognosis is determined by the lesion size and location, surgical accessibility, and histologic grade.

When an individual has multiple meningiomas, especially in association with eighth-nerve schwannomas or glial tumors, the diagnosis of neurofibromatosis type 2 (NF2) should be considered (Chapter 22). About half of meningiomas not associated with NF2 have somatic loss-of-function mutations in the *NF2* tumor suppressor gene on the long arm of chromosome 22 (22q). These mutations are found in all grades of meningioma, suggesting that they are involved in tumor initiation. Among sporadic tumors that lack mutations in *NF2,* several other driver mutations have been identified including in genes that regulate the Hedgehog pathway as well as in various signaling molecules and transcription factors.

MORPHOLOGY

Meningiomas (WHO grade I) grow as well-defined durabased masses that may compress the brain but do not typically invade it (Fig. 23.33A). Extension into the overlying bone may be present. The varied histologic patterns include: **meningothelial,** named for whorled, tight clusters of cells without visible cell membranes; **fibroblastic,** with elongated cells and abundant collagen deposition; **transitional,** with features of the meningothelial and fibroblastic types; **psammomatous,** with numerous psammoma bodies (see Fig. 23.33B); and **secretory,** with glandlike spaces containing PAS-positive eosinophilic material.

Atypical meningiomas (WHO grade II) are recognized by the presence of either an increased mitotic rate, or prominent nucleoli, increased cellularity, patternless growth, high nucleus-to-cytoplasm ratio, or necrosis. These tumors demonstrate more aggressive local growth and a higher rate of recurrence and may require therapy in addition to surgery. Some histologic patterns—clear cell and chordoid—also correlate with more aggressive behavior, as does the presence of brain invasion.

Anaplastic (malignant) meningiomas (WHO grade III) are highly aggressive tumors that may resemble a high-grade sarcoma or carcinoma morphologically. Mitotic rates are typically much higher than in atypical meningiomas.

Metastatic Tumors

Metastatic lesions, mostly carcinomas, account for approximately one-fourth to one-half of intracranial tumors. The most common primary sites are lung, breast, skin (melanoma), kidney, and gastrointestinal tract, which together account for about 80% of cases. Metastases form sharply demarcated masses, often at the grey-white matter junction, and elicit local edema (Fig. 23.34). The boundary between tumor and brain parenchyma is sharp at the microscopic level as well, with surrounding reactive gliosis.

In addition to the direct and localized effects produced by metastases, *paraneoplastic syndromes* may involve the peripheral and central nervous systems, sometimes even preceding the clinical recognition of the malignant neoplasm. Many patients with paraneoplastic syndromes have antibodies against tumor antigens. Some of the more common patterns include the following:

• *Subacute cerebellar degeneration* resulting in ataxia, with destruction of Purkinje cells, gliosis, and a mild inflammatory infiltrate

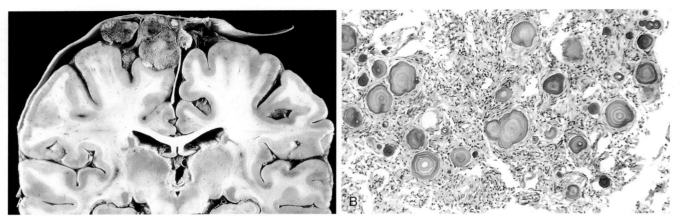

Fig. 23.33 Meningioma. (A) Parasagittal multilobular meningioma attached to the dura with compression of underlying brain. (B) Meningioma with a whorled pattern of cell growth and psammoma bodies.

- *Limbic encephalitis* causing a subacute dementia, with perivascular inflammatory cells, microglial nodules, neuronal loss, and gliosis, all centered in the medial temporal lobe
- *Subacute sensory neuropathy* leading to altered pain sensation, with loss of sensory neurons from dorsal root ganglia, in association with inflammation
- *Syndrome of rapid-onset psychosis, catatonia, epilepsy, and coma* associated with ovarian teratoma and antibodies against the *N*-methyl-D-aspartate (NMDA) receptor.

Familial Tumor Syndromes

Several inherited syndromes caused by mutations in various tumor suppressor genes are associated with an increased risk for particular types of cancers. Those with particular involvement of the CNS are discussed here; familial syndromes associated with tumors of the peripheral nervous system are covered in Chapter 22.

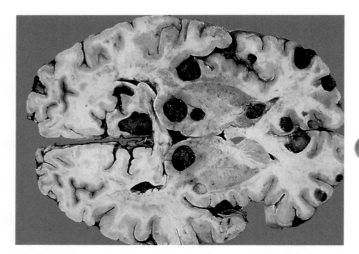

Fig. 23.34 Metastatic melanoma. Metastatic lesions are distinguished grossly from most primary central nervous system tumors by their multicentricity and well-demarcated margins. The dark color of the tumor nodules in this specimen is due to the presence of melanin.

Tuberous Sclerosis

Tuberous sclerosis is an autosomal dominant syndrome characterized by the development of hamartomas and benign neoplasms involving the brain and other tissues. CNS hamartomas variously consist of cortical tubers and subependymal hamartomas, including a larger tumefactive form known as *subependymal giant cell astrocytoma*. Because of their proximity to the foramen of Monro, they often present acutely with obstructive hydrocephalus, which requires surgical intervention and/or therapy with an mTOR inhibitor (see later). Seizures are associated with cortical tubers and can be difficult to control with anti-epileptic drugs. Extracerebral lesions include renal angiomyolipomas, retinal glial hamartomas, pulmonary lymphangiomyomatosis, and cardiac rhabdomyomas. Cysts may be found at various sites, including the liver, kidneys, and pancreas. Cutaneous lesions include angiofibromas, leathery thickenings in localized patches (shagreen patches), hypopigmented areas (ash leaf patches), and subungual fibromas.

Tuberous sclerosis results from disruption of either *TSC1*, which encodes hamartin, or *TSC2*, which encodes tuberin. The two TSC proteins form a dimeric complex that negatively regulates mTOR, a kinase that "senses" the cell's nutrient status and regulates cellular metabolism. Loss of either protein upregulates mTOR activity, which disrupts normal feedback mechanisms that restrict uptake of nutrients and leads to increased cell growth.

MORPHOLOGY

Cortical hamartomas are firmer than normal cortex and have been likened in appearance to potatoes—hence the appellation tubers. They are composed of haphazardly arranged large neurons that lack the normal cortical laminar architecture. These cells may exhibit a mixture of glial and neuronal features, having large vesicular nuclei with nucleoli (like neurons) and abundant eosinophilic cytoplasm. Similar abnormal cells are present in **subependymal nodules,** in which large astrocyte like cells cluster beneath the ventricular surface.

von Hippel–Lindau Disease

In this autosomal dominant disorder, affected individuals develop hemangioblastomas within the cerebellar hemispheres, retina, and, less commonly, the brain stem, spinal cord, and nerve roots. Patients also may have cysts involving the pancreas, liver, and kidneys and have an increased propensity to develop renal cell carcinoma. The disease frequency is 1 in 30,000 to 40,000. Therapy is directed at the symptomatic neoplasms, including surgical resection of cerebellar tumors and laser ablation of retinal tumors.

The affected gene, the tumor suppressor *VHL*, encodes a protein that is part of a ubiquitin-ligase complex that degrades the transcription factor hypoxia-inducible factor (HIF). Tumors arising in patients with von Hippel–Lindau disease generally have lost all VHL protein function. As a result, the tumors express high levels of HIF, which drives the expression of VEGF, various growth factors, and sometimes erythropoietin; the latter effect may produce a paraneoplastic form of polycythemia.

MORPHOLOGY

Hemangioblastoma, the principal neurologic manifestation of the disease, is a highly vascular neoplasm that occurs as a mural nodule associated with a large, fluid-filled cyst. These occur most commonly in the cerebellum, but can be found along the spinal cord and in the retina, and rarely at other sites in the brain. On microscopic examination, the lesion consists of numerous capillary-sized or somewhat larger thin-walled vessels separated by intervening stromal cells with a vacuolated, lightly PAS-positive, lipid-rich cytoplasm. These stromal cells express inhibin, a member of the TGF-β family, which serves as a useful diagnostic marker.

SUMMARY

TUMORS OF THE CENTRAL NERVOUS SYSTEM

- Tumors of the CNS may arise from the cells of the coverings (meningiomas), the brain (gliomas, neuronal tumors, choroid plexus tumors), or other CNS cell populations (primary CNS lymphoma, germ cell tumors), or they may originate elsewhere in the body (metastases).
- Even low-grade or benign tumors can have poor clinical outcomes, depending on where they occur in the brain.
- Distinct types of tumors affect specific brain regions (e.g., cerebellum for medulloblastoma, an intraventricular location for central neurocytoma) and specific age populations (medulloblastoma and pilocytic astrocytomas in pediatric age groups, and glioblastoma and lymphoma in older patients).
- Glial tumors are broadly classified into astrocytomas, oligodendrogliomas, and ependymomas. Increasing tumor malignancy is associated with more cytologic anaplasia, increased cell density, necrosis, and mitotic activity.
- Metastatic spread of brain tumors to other regions of the body is rare, but the brain is not comparably protected against the spread of distant tumors. Carcinomas are the dominant type of systemic tumors that metastasize to the nervous system.

SUGGESTED READINGS

Central Nervous System Trauma

McKee AC, Cairns NJ, Dickson DW, et al: The first NINDS/NIBIB consensus meeting to define neuropathological criteria for the diagnosis of chronic traumatic encephalopathy, *Acta Neuropathol* 131(1):75–86, 2016. [*The first effort to define objectively the neuropathologic changes which define CTI.*]

McKee AC, Stein TD, Kiernan PT, et al: The neuropathology of chronic traumatic encephalopathy, *Brain Pathol* 25(3):350–364, 2015. [*A summary of much of the descriptive work laying the basis for the emergence of CTE as a tauopathy associated with prior brain trauma.*]

Congenital Malformations and Perinatal Brain Injury

Guemez-Gamboa A, Coufal NG, Gleeson JG: Primary cilia in the developing and mature brain, *Neuron* 82(3):511–521, 2014. [*A discussion of the role of primary cilia in brain development, particularly the posterior fossa, as well as consideration of malformations that accompany disorders of this cilium.*]

Guerrini R, Dobyns WB: Malformations of cortical development: clinical features and genetic causes, *Lancet Neurol* 13(7):710–726, 2014. [*A clear review of many of the biological mechanisms that underlie cortical development as well as the genetic disorder that disrupt the process.*]

Infections of the Nervous System

Clifford DB: Neurological immune reconstitution inflammatory response: riding the tide of immune recovery, *Curr Opin Neurol* 28(3):295–301, 2015. [*Discusses the clinical and pathological aspects of the inflammatory syndrome which can accompany initiation of HAART as a result of recovery of aspects of the immune system.*]

Saylor D, Dickens AM, Sacktor N, et al: HIV-associated neurocognitive disorder—pathogenesis and prospects for treatment, *Nat Rev Neurol* 12(4):234–248, 2016. [*Summary of the underlying mechanisms for HIV-induced neurologic dysfunction and the impact of existing therapies on these complications of infection.*]

Demyelinating Diseases

Dendrou CA, Fugger L, Friese MA: Immunopathology of multiple sclerosis, *Nat Rev Immunol* 15(9):545–558, 2015. [*While the immune basis of MS has been accepted for many years, it has become clear that there are increasing complexities of this injury to myelin, axons, and oligodendrocytes than previously assumed.*]

Podestà MA, Faravelli I, Cucchiari D, et al: Neurological counterparts of hyponatremia: pathological mechanisms and clinical manifestations, *Curr Neurol Neurosci Rep* 15(4):18, 2015. [*The mechanistic relationship between alterations in serum osmolality and acute injury to myelin remains complex but is partially addressed in this discussion.*]

Yang X, Ransom BR, Ma JF: The role of AQP4 in neuromyelitis optica: More answers, more questions, *J Neuroimmunol* 298:63–70, 2016. [*While the presence of antibodies to aquaporin-4 helped clarify the syndrome of neuromyelitis optica, it remains a more complex disease than a simple autoimmune disorder.*]

Neurodegenerative Diseases

Barker RA, Williams-Gray CH: Review: the spectrum of clinical features seen with alpha synuclein pathology, *Neuropathol Appl Neurobiol* 42(1):6–19, 2016. [*Aggregation of α-synuclein marks several neurodegenerative diseases, and this review considers shared and distinct aspects of the pathologic findings.*]

Colonna M, Wang Y: TREM2 variants: new keys to decipher Alzheimer disease pathogenesis, *Nat Rev Neurosci* 17(4):201–207, 2016. [*One of the strongest links between Alzheimer disease and microglia is the risk associated with variants of TREM2 on the surfaces of microglia.*]

Ling SC, Polymenidou M, Cleveland DW: Converging mechanisms in ALS and FTD: disrupted RNA and protein homeostasis, *Neuron* 79(3):416–438, 2013. [*A clear summary of mechanisms associated with neurodegeneration that can be linked to the consequences of altered RNA dynamics within cells and the consequence of this for proteins.*]

Mackenzie IR, Neumann M: Molecular neuropathology of frontotemporal dementia: insights into disease mechanisms from postmortem studies, *J Neurochem* 138(Suppl 1):54–70, 2016. *[A consideration of the complex family of disorders that give rise to frontotemporal lobe degenerations, with different clinical pictures as well as different histologic findings and associated mechanisms.]*

Selkoe DJ, Hardy J: The amyloid hypothesis of Alzheimer's disease at 25 years, *EMBO Mol Med* 8(6):595–608, 2016. *[A current summary of the relationship of Aβ to the pathogenesis of Alzheimer disease.]*

Brain Tumors

Louis DN, Perry A, Reifenberger G, et al: The 2016 World Health Organization Classification of Tumors of the Central Nervous System: a summary, *Acta Neuropathol* 131(6):803–820, 2016. *[A concise summary of the most recent classification of brain tumors, including the concept of "layer" diagnoses that incorporate histologic findings as well as multiple types of molecular information in order to predict course and guide therapy.]*

CHAPTER

Skin 24

CHAPTER OUTLINE

Acute Inflammatory Dermatoses 889
Urticaria 889
Acute Eczematous Dermatitis 890
Erythema Multiforme 891
Chronic Inflammatory Dermatoses 892
Psoriasis 892
Lichen Planus 893

Lichen Simplex Chronicus 894
Infectious Dermatoses 894
Bacterial Infections 894
Fungal Infections 894
Verrucae (Warts) 895
Blistering (Bullous) Disorders 895
Pemphigus (Vulgaris and Foliaceus) 895

Bullous Pemphigoid 896
Dermatitis Herpetiformis 898
Tumors of the Skin 899
Benign and Premalignant Epithelial Lesions 899
Malignant Epidermal Tumors 900
Melanocytic Proliferations 903

Skin diseases are common and diverse, ranging from irritating acne to life-threatening melanoma. Many are intrinsic to the skin, but some are manifestations of diseases involving many tissues, such as systemic lupus erythematosus or genetic syndromes such as neurofibromatosis. In this sense, the skin is a uniquely accessible "window" through which numerous disorders can be recognized.

Skin is not a mere protective mantle but rather a complex organ, actually the largest in the body. It is constantly exposed to microbial and nonmicrobial antigens from the environment. Given this, it is not surprising that the skin is an active participant in immune responses. Environmentally derived antigens are processed by intraepithelial Langerhans cells, which bear their antigenic cargo to regional lymph nodes and initiate immune responses. Squamous cells (keratinocytes) help maintain skin homeostasis by providing a physical barrier to environmental insults and by secreting a plethora of cytokines that influence both the squamous and dermal microenvironments. The dermis contains resident populations of CD4+ helper and CD8+ cytotoxic T lymphocytes, some of which home to the skin by virtue of specialized receptors such as cutaneous lymphocyte antigen, as well as memory T cells, regulatory T cells (T_{regs}) and occasional B cells. The epidermis contains intraepithelial lymphocytes, including γ/δ T cells, while the dermis contains perivascular mast cells and scattered macrophages, all components of the innate immune system. Responses involving these immune cells and locally released cytokines account for the morphologic patterns and clinical expressions of inflammatory and infectious skin disorders.

This chapter focuses on common and pathogenically illustrative skin diseases. In considering these diseases, it is important to appreciate that the practice of

The contributions of Dr. George Murphy to this chapter in previous editions are gratefully acknowledged.

dermatopathology relies on close interactions with clinicians, particularly dermatologists, as the clinical history, gross appearance, and distribution of lesions are often as important as the microscopic findings in arriving at a specific diagnosis. Diseases of the skin can be confusing for the student, in part because dermatologists and dermatopathologists communicate using a large, "skin-specific" lexicon that students must become familiar with in order to understand skin diseases. The most important of these terms and definitions are listed in Table 24.1.

ACUTE INFLAMMATORY DERMATOSES

Thousands of inflammatory dermatoses exist, challenging the diagnostic acumen of even experienced clinicians. In general, acute lesions, defined as days to several weeks in duration, are characterized by inflammation, edema, and sometimes epidermal, vascular, or subcutaneous injury. Acute dermatoses are often marked by infiltrates consisting of mononuclear cells rather than neutrophils, unlike acute inflammatory disorders at most other sites. Some acute lesions may persist, transitioning to a chronic phase, while others are self-limited.

Urticaria

Urticaria ("hives") is a common disorder mediated by localized mast cell degranulation, which leads to dermal microvascular hyperpermeability. The resulting erythematous, edematous, and pruritic plaques are termed *wheals*.

Pathogenesis

In most cases, urticaria stems from an immediate (type 1) hypersensitivity reaction (Chapter 5), in which antigens trigger mast cell degranulation by binding to

Table 24.1 Nomenclature of Skin Lesions

Macroscopic Lesions	Definition
Excoriation	Traumatic lesion breaking the epidermis and causing a raw linear area (i.e., deep scratch); often self-inflicted
Lichenification	Thickened, rough skin (similar to a lichen on a rock); usually the result of repeated rubbing
Macule, patch	Circumscribed, flat lesion distinguished from surrounding skin by color. Macules are 5 mm in diameter or less, while patches are greater than 5 mm in size.
Papule, nodule	Elevated dome-shaped or flat-topped lesion. Papules are 5 mm in diameter or less, while nodules are greater than 5 mm in size.
Plaque	Elevated flat-topped lesion, usually greater than 5 mm in diameter (may be formed by coalescence of papules)
Pustule	Discrete, pus-filled, raised lesion
Scale	Dry, horny, platelike excrescence; usually the result of imperfect cornification
Vesicle, bulla, blister	Fluid-filled raised lesion 5 mm or less in diameter (vesicle) or greater than 5 mm in diameter (bulla). *Blister* is the common term for both lesions.
Wheal	Itchy, transient, elevated lesion with variable blanching and erythema formed as the result of dermal edema
Microscopic Lesions	**Definition**
Acanthosis	Diffuse epidermal hyperplasia
Dyskeratosis	Abnormal, premature keratinization within cells below the stratum granulosum
Hyperkeratosis	Thickening of the stratum corneum, often associated with a qualitative abnormality of the keratin
Papillomatosis	Surface elevation caused by hyperplasia and enlargement of contiguous dermal papillae
Parakeratosis	Retention of nuclei in the stratum corneum of a squamous epithelium. On mucous membranes, parakeratosis is normal.
Spongiosis	Intercellular edema of the epidermis

immunoglobulin E (IgE) antibodies attached to the mast cell surface through their Fc receptor. Responsible antigens include viruses, pollens, foods, drugs, and insect venom. IgE-independent urticaria also can result from exposure to substances that directly incite mast cell degranulation, such as opiates and certain antibiotics. In the vast majority of cases, no clinical cause is discovered even with extensive investigation.

MORPHOLOGY

The histologic features of urticaria often are subtle. There is usually a sparse superficial perivenular infiltrate of mononuclear cells, rare neutrophils, and sometimes eosinophils. Superficial dermal edema causes splaying of collagen bundles, making them appear to be more widely spaced than normal. Degranulation of mast cells, which reside around superficial dermal venules, is difficult to appreciate with routine hematoxylin-eosin (H&E) stains but can be highlighted using a Giemsa stain.

Clinical Features

Urticaria typically affects individuals between 20 and 40 years of age, but no age is immune. Individual lesions usually develop and fade within hours, but episodes can persist for days or even months. Lesions range in size and nature from small, pruritic papules to large, edematous, erythematous plaques. They may be localized to a particular part of the body or generalized. In a specific type of urticaria termed *pressure urticaria,* lesions are found only in areas exposed to pressure (such as the feet or buttocks). Although not life-threatening, severe pruritus and the social embarrassment of urticaria can compromise quality of life. Most cases respond to antihistamines, but more severe, refractory disease may require treatment with leukotriene antagonists, monoclonal antibodies that block the action of IgE, or immunosuppressive drugs.

Acute Eczematous Dermatitis

Eczema is a clinical term that embraces a number of conditions with varied underlying etiologies. New lesions take the form of erythematous papules, often with overlying vesicles, which ooze and become crusted. Pruritus is characteristic. With persistence, these lesions coalesce into raised, scaling plaques. The nature and degree of these changes vary among the clinical subtypes, which include the following:

- *Allergic contact dermatitis*—stems from topical exposure to an allergen and is caused by delayed hypersensitivy reactions.
- *Atopic dermatitis*—formerly attributed to allergen exposure, now thought to often stem from defects in keratinocyte barrier function, defined as skin with increased permeability to substances to which it is exposed, such as potential antigens
- *Drug-related eczematous dermatitis*—hypersensitivity reaction to a drug
- *Photoeczematous dermatitis*—appears as an abnormal reaction to UV or visible light
- *Primary irritant dermatitis*—results from exposure to substances that chemically, physically, or mechanically damage the skin

While atopic dermatitis reflects a genetic predisposition and can persist for years or decades, other forms of eczematous dermatitis resolve completely when the offending stimulus is removed or exposure is limited, stressing the importance of investigating the underlying cause. Only the most common form, *contact dermatitis,* is considered here.

Allergic contact dermatitis is triggered by exposure to an environmental contact-sensitizing agent, such as poison ivy, that chemically reacts with self-proteins, creating neoantigens that can be recognized by the T cell

arm of the adaptive immune system. The self-proteins modified by the agent are processed by epidermal Langerhans cells, which migrate to draining lymph nodes and present the antigen to naïve T cells. This sensitization event leads to acquisition of immunologic memory; on reexposure to the antigen, the activated memory CD4+ T lymphocytes migrate to the affected skin sites during the course of normal circulation. There they release cytokines that recruit additional inflammatory cells and also mediate epidermal damage, as in any delayed-type hypersensitivity reaction (Chapter 5).

MORPHOLOGY

As the name implies, skin involvement in contact dermatitis is limited to sites of direct contact with the triggering agent (Fig. 24.1A), whereas in other forms of eczema, lesions may be widely distributed. **Spongiosis,** or epidermal edema, characterizes all forms of acute eczematous dermatitis—hence the synonym **spongiotic dermatitis.** Edema fluid seeps into the epidermis, where it splays apart keratinocytes (Fig. 24.1B). Intercellular bridges are stretched and become more prominent and are easier to visualize. This change is accompanied by a superficial perivascular lymphocytic infiltrate, edema of dermal papillae, and mast cell degranulation. Eosinophils may be present and are especially prominent in spongiotic eruptions provoked by drugs, but in general the histologic features are similar regardless of cause, emphasizing the need for careful clinical correlation.

Clinical Features

Lesions of acute eczematous dermatitis are pruritic, edematous, oozing plaques, often containing vesicles and bullae. With persistent antigen exposure, lesions may become scaly (hyperkeratotic) as the epidermis thickens (acanthosis). Some changes are produced or exacerbated by scratching of the lesion (see "Lichen Simplex Chronicus", discussed later). The clinical causes of eczema are sometimes divided into "inside jobs"—reaction to an internal circulating antigen (such as an ingested food or drug)—and "outside jobs"—disease resulting from contact with an external antigen (such as poison ivy).

Susceptibility to atopic dermatitis is often inherited; the disorder is concordant in 80% of identical twins and 20% of fraternal twins. It usually appears in early childhood and remits spontaneously as patients mature into adults. Children with atopic dermatitis often have asthma and allergic rhinitis, termed the *atopic triad*. Recent genetic studies have identified polymorphisms associated with increased risk in genes that encode proteins involved in keratinocyte barrier function, innate immunity, and T cell function.

Erythema Multiforme

Erythema multiforme is characterized by epithelial injury mediated by skin-homing CD8+ cytotoxic T lymphocytes. It is an uncommon, usually self-limited disorder that appears to be a hypersensitivity response to certain infections and drugs. Antecedent infections include those

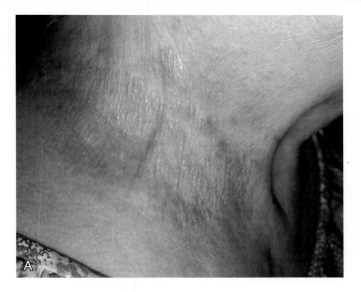

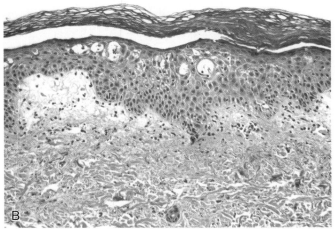

Fig. 24.1 Eczematous dermatitis. (A) Patterned erythema and scale stemming from a nickel-induced contact dermatitis produced by a necklace. (B) Microscopically, there is accumulation of fluid (spongiosis) between epidermal cells, which may progress to frank blister formation.

caused by herpes simplex, mycoplasma, and some fungi, while implicated drugs include sulfonamides, penicillin, salicylates, hydantoins, and anti-malarials. The cytotoxic T cell attack is focused on the basal cells of cutaneous and mucosal epithelia, presumably due to recognition of still unknown antigens. Certain human lymphocyte antigen (HLA) haplotypes are associated with the disease.

MORPHOLOGY

Affected individuals present with a wide array of lesions, which may include macules, papules, vesicles, and bullae (hence the term *multiforme*). Well-developed lesions have a characteristic "targetoid" appearance (Fig. 24.2A). Early lesions show a superficial perivascular lymphocytic infiltrate associated with dermal edema and margination of lymphocytes along the dermoepidermal junction in intimate association with apoptotic keratinocytes (see Fig. 24.2B). With time, discrete, confluent zones of basal

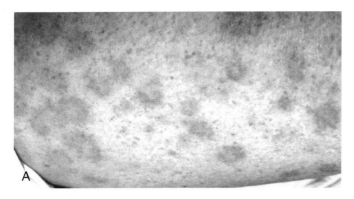

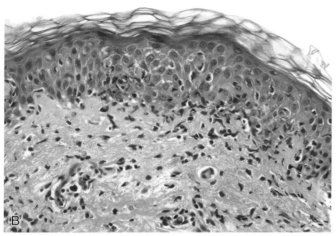

Fig. 24.2 Erythema multiforme. (A) Target like lesions consisting of a pale central blister or zone of epidermal necrosis surrounded by macular erythema. (B) Early lesions show lymphocytes along the dermoepidermal junction (interface dermatitis) associated with scattered apoptotic keratinocytes, marked by dark shrunken nuclei and eosinophilic cytoplasm.

epidermal necrosis appear, with concomitant blister formation. In a rarer and more severe form of this disease, **toxic epidermal necrolysis,** the necrosis extends through the full thickness of the epidermis.

Clinical Features

Erythema multiforme has a broad range of severity. The forms associated with infection (most often herpesvirus) are less severe. Erythema multiforme caused by medications may progress to more serious eruptions, such as Stevens-Johnson syndrome or toxic epidermal necrolysis. These forms can be life-threatening, as they may cause sloughing of large portions of the epidermis, resulting in fluid loss and infections complications similar to those seen in burn-injured patients.

CHRONIC INFLAMMATORY DERMATOSES

Chronic inflammatory dermatoses are persistent skin conditions that exhibit their most characteristic features over many months to years, although they may begin with an acute stage. The skin surface in some chronic inflammatory

dermatoses is roughened as a result of excessive or abnormal scale formation and shedding (desquamation).

Psoriasis

Psoriasis is a common chronic inflammatory dermatosis, affecting 1% to 2% of individuals residing in the United States. Recent epidemiologic studies have shown that psoriasis is associated with an increased risk for heart attack and stroke, a relationship that may be related to a chronic inflammatory state. Psoriasis also is associated in up to 10% of patients with arthritis, which in some cases may be severe.

Pathogenesis

Psoriasis is a T cell-mediated inflammatory disease, presumed to be autoimmune in origin, although the antigens are not well described. Both genetic (HLA types and other susceptibility loci) and environmental factors contribute to the risk. It is unclear whether the inciting antigens are self-antigens, environmental antigens, or some combination of the two. Sensitized populations of T cells home to the dermis, including CD4+ T_H17 and T_H1 cells and CD8+ T cells, and accumulate in the epidermis. These cells secrete cytokines and growth factors that induce keratinocyte hyperproliferation, resulting in the characteristic lesions. Psoriatic lesions can be induced in susceptible individuals by local trauma (Koebner phenomenon), which may induce a local inflammatory response that promotes lesion development. Genome-wide association studies (GWAS) have linked an increased risk for psoriasis to polymorphisms in HLA loci and genes affecting antigen presentation, TNF signaling, and skin barrier function. Several loci also are associated with the development of psoriatic arthritis, a more severe complication of this disease.

MORPHOLOGY

The typical lesion is a **well-demarcated, pink to salmon–colored plaque covered by loosely adherent silver-white scale** (Fig. 24.3A). There is marked epidermal thickening **(acanthosis),** with regular downward elongation of the rete ridges (see Fig. 24.3B). The pattern of this downward growth has been likened to "test tubes in a rack." Increased epidermal cell turnover and lack of maturation results in **loss of the stratum granulosum and extensive parakeratotic scale.** Also seen is thinning of the epidermal cell layer overlying the tips of dermal papillae (suprapapillary plates), and dilated and tortuous blood vessels within the papillae. These vessels bleed readily when the scale is removed, giving rise to multiple punctate bleeding points **(Auspitz sign).** Neutrophils form small aggregates within both the spongiotic superficial epidermis and the parakeratotic stratum corneum. Similar changes can be seen in superficial fungal infections, which need to be excluded with appropriate special stains.

Clinical Features

Psoriasis most frequently affects the skin of the elbows, knees, scalp, lumbosacral areas, intergluteal cleft, glans penis, and vulva. Nail changes on the fingers and toes occur in 30% of cases. In most cases psoriasis is limited in

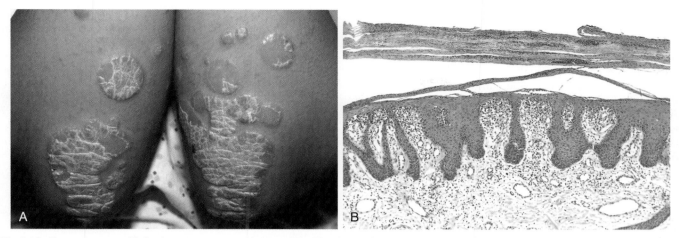

Fig. 24.3 Chronic psoriasis. (A) Erythematous psoriatic plaques covered by silvery-white scale. (B) Microscopic examination shows marked epidermal hyperplasia, downward extension of rete ridges (psoriasiform hyperplasia), and prominent parakeratotic scale with infiltrating neutrophils.

distribution, but it can be widespread and severe. The clinical subtypes are defined by pattern of involvement and severity. Treatment is aimed at preventing the release or actions of inflammatory mediators. Mild disease is treated topically with ointments containing corticosteroids or other immunomodulatory agents, whereas more severe disease is treated with phototherapy (which has immunosuppressive effects) or systemic therapy with immunosuppressive agents such as methotrexate or TNF antagonists.

Lichen Planus

"Pruritic, purple, polygonal, planar papules, and plaques" are the tongue-twisting *P*s that describe this disorder of skin and squamous mucosa. The lesions may result from a CD8+ T cell–mediated cytotoxic response against antigens in the basal cell layer and the dermoepidermal junction that are produced by unknown mechanisms, perhaps as a consequence of a viral infection or drug exposure.

MORPHOLOGY

Cutaneous lesions of lichen planus consist of **pruritic, violaceous, flat-topped papules** that may coalesce focally to form plaques (Fig. 24.4A). These papules are highlighted by white dots or lines termed **Wickham striae.** Hyperpigmentation may result from melanin loss into the dermis from damaged keratinocytes. Microscopically, lichen planus is a prototypical **interface dermatitis,** so called because the inflammation and damage are concentrated at the interface of the squamous epithelium and papillary dermis. There is a dense, continuous infiltrate of lymphocytes along the dermoepidermal junction (see Fig. 24.4B). The lymphocytes are intimately associated with basal keratinocytes, which often atrophy or become necrotic. Perhaps as a response to damage, the basal cells take on the appearance of the more mature cells of the stratum spinosum (squamatization). This pattern of inflammation causes the dermoepidermal interface to assume an angulated, zigzag contour **(sawtoothing).** Anucleate, necrotic basal cells are seen in the inflamed papillary dermis and are referred to as colloid bodies or **Civatte**

bodies. Although these changes bear some similarities to those in erythema multiforme (another type of interface dermatitis discussed earlier), lichen planus shows well-developed changes of chronicity, including epidermal hyperplasia, hypergranulosis, and hyperkeratosis.

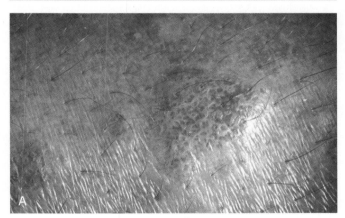

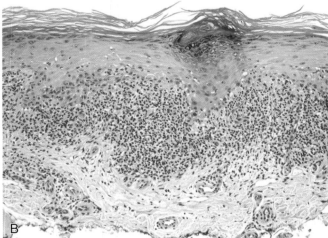

Fig. 24.4 Lichen planus. (A) Flat-topped pink-purple polygonal papule with white lacelike markings referred to as *Wickham striae.* (B) Microscopic examination shows a bandlike infiltrate of lymphocytes along the dermoepidermal junction, hyperkeratosis, hypergranulosis, and pointed rete ridges ("sawtoothing"), which results from chronic injury of the basal cell layer.

Clinical Features

Lichen planus is an uncommon disorder that usually presents in middle-aged adults. The cutaneous lesions are multiple and are usually symmetrically distributed, particularly on the extremities, and often occur around the wrists and elbows and on the vulva and glans penis. Approximately 70% of cases also involve the oral mucosa, where the lesions manifest as white papules with a reticulate or netlike appearance. The cutaneous lesions of lichen planus usually resolve spontaneously within 1 to 2 years, but the oral lesions may persist and be of sufficient severity to interfere with food intake.

Lichen Simplex Chronicus

Lichen simplex chronicus manifests as roughening of the skin, which takes on an appearance reminiscent of lichen on a tree. It is a response to local repetitive trauma, usually from rubbing or scratching. Nodular forms exist that are referred to as *prurigo nodularis*. The pathogenesis of lichen simplex chronicus is not understood, but the trauma probably induces epithelial hyperplasia and eventual dermal scarring.

MORPHOLOGY

Lichen simplex chronicus is characterized by **acanthosis, hyperkeratosis,** and **hypergranulosis.** Also seen are elongation of the rete ridges, fibrosis of the papillary dermis, and a dermal chronic inflammatory infiltrate (Fig. 24.5). Of interest, these lesions are similar in appearance to normal volar (palms and soles) skin, in which skin thickening serves as an adaptation to repetitive mechanical stress.

Clinical Features

The lesions often are raised, erythematous, and scaly and can be mistaken for keratinocytic neoplasms. Lichen simplex chronicus can be superimposed on and mask

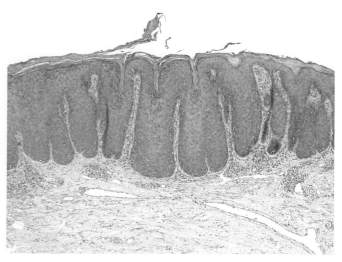

Fig. 24.5 Lichen simplex chronicus. Note the distinctive acanthosis, hyperkeratosis, and hypergranulosis. Superficial dermal fibrosis and vascular ectasia, both common features, also are present.

another (often pruritic) dermatosis. It is therefore important to rule out an underlying cause while recognizing that the lesion may be entirely trauma-related.

SUMMARY

INFLAMMATORY DERMATOSES

- Many specific inflammatory dermatoses exist and can be mediated by IgE antibodies (urticaria), antigen-specific T cells (eczema, erythema multiforme, and psoriasis), or trauma (lichen simplex chronicus).
- Underlying genetic susceptibility plays a role in atopic dermatitis and psoriasis.
- These disorders can be grouped based on patterns of inflammation (e.g., interface dermatitis in lichen planus and erythema multiforme).
- Clinical correlation is essential to diagnose specific skin diseases, since many have overlapping, nonspecific histologic features.

INFECTIOUS DERMATOSES

Bacterial Infections

Numerous bacterial infections occur in skin. These range from superficial infections known as *impetigo,* to deeper dermal abscesses associated with puncture wounds that are caused by bacteria such as *Pseudomonas aeruginosa.* The pathogenesis is similar to that for microbial infections elsewhere (Chapter 9). Only impetigo is discussed here.

MORPHOLOGY

Impetigo is characterized by an accumulation of neutrophils beneath the stratum corneum that often produces a subcorneal pustule. Nonspecific reactive epidermal alternation and superficial dermal inflammation accompany these findings. Bacterial cocci in the superficial epidermis can be demonstrated by Gram stain.

Clinical Features

Impetigo, one of the most common bacterial infections of the skin, is seen primarily in children. The causative organism is usually *Staphylococcus aureus* or, less commonly, *Streptococcus pyogenes,* and is typically acquired through direct contact with a source. Impetigo often begins as a single small macule, usually on the extremities or the face near the nose or the mouth, which rapidly evolves into a larger lesion (Fig. 24.6), often with a honey-colored crust of dried serum. Individuals who are colonized by *S. aureus* or *S. pyogenes* (usually nasal or anal) are more likely to be affected. A less common bullous form of childhood impetigo may mimic an autoimmune blistering disorder.

Fungal Infections

Fungal infections are varied, ranging from superficial infections with *Tinea* or *Candida* spp. to life-threatening

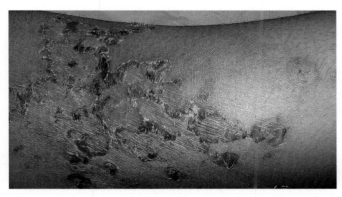

Fig. 24.6 Impetigo. A child's arm involved by a superficial bacterial infection showing the characteristic erythematous scablike lesions crusted with dried serum. *(Courtesy of Dr. Angela Wyatt, Bellaire, Texas.)*

Aspergillus spp. infections in immunosuppressed individuals. Fungal infections can be superficial (stratum corneum, hair, and nails), deep (dermis or subcutis), or systemic, the last type arising through hematogenous spread, often in an immunocompromised patient.

MORPHOLOGY

The histologic appearance varies depending on the organism, host response, and degree of superinfection. Superficial infections are often associated with a neutrophilic infiltrate in the epidermis. Deep fungal infections produce greater tissue damage and often elicit a granulomatous response. *Aspergillus* can be angioinvasive. Periodic acid–Schiff (PAS) and Gomori methenamine silver stains are helpful in identifying the fungal organisms.

Clinical Features

Superficial infections usually produce erythematous macules with superficial scale that can be pruritic, while deeper infections such as those seen with *Aspergillus* spp. are erythematous and often nodular and sometimes associated with local hemorrhage. Superficial fungal infections may have an annular appearance. However, they also may induce lesions that mimic other psoriasiform or eczematous dermatoses, so it is important to consider the possibility of fungal infection when these conditions are in the differential diagnosis.

Verrucae (Warts)

Verrucae are proliferative lesions of squamous epithelial cells that are caused by human papillomavirus (HPV). They are most common in children and adolescents, but may be encountered in any age group. HPV infection usually stems from direct contact with an infected individual or autoinoculation. Verrucae generally are self-limited, most often regressing spontaneously within 6 months to 2 years.

Pathogenesis

While some members of the HPV family are associated with preneoplastic and invasive cancers of the anogenital region (Chapters 6 and 18), cutaneous warts are mainly caused by low-risk HPV subtypes that lack transforming potential. Like high-risk HPV, low-risk viruses express viral E6 and E7 oncoproteins that lead to dysregulated epidermal cell growth and increased survival. Why low-risk viruses cause warts instead of cancer is likely due to structural variation in E6 and E7 proteins that affect their interactions with host proteins. Because the growth of warts is normally halted by the immune response, immunodeficiency is associated with more numerous and larger verrucae.

MORPHOLOGY

Different kinds of warts are identified on the basis of their gross appearance and location and generally are caused by distinct HPV subtypes. **Verruca vulgaris** (Fig. 24.7A), the most common type of wart, can occur anywhere but is found most frequently on the hands, particularly on the dorsal surfaces and periungual areas, where it appears as a gray-white to tan, flat to convex, 0.1- to 1-cm papule with a rough, pebble like surface. **Verruca plana**, or **flat wart**, is common on the face or dorsal surfaces of the hands. These warts are flat, smooth, tan macules. **Verruca plantaris** and **verruca palmaris** occur on the soles and palms, respectively. These rough, scaly lesions can reach 1 to 2 cm in diameter and may coalesce to form a surface that can be confused with ordinary calluses. **Condyloma acuminatum (venereal wart)** occurs on the penis, female genitalia, urethra, and perianal areas (Chapters 18 and 19). Histologic features common to verrucae include **epidermal hyperplasia,** which is often undulant in character (so-called **verrucous** or **papillomatous epidermal hyperplasia**) (Fig. 24.7B, *top panel*), and cytoplasmic vacuolization **(koilocytosis),** which preferentially involves the more superficial epidermal layers, producing halos of pallor surrounding infected nuclei. Infected cells also may demonstrate prominent keratohyalin granules and jagged eosinophilic intracytoplasmic protein aggregates as a result of impaired maturation (Fig. 24.7B, *bottom panel*).

BLISTERING (BULLOUS) DISORDERS

Although vesicles and bullae (blisters) occur as secondary phenomena in several unrelated conditions (e.g., herpesvirus infection, spongiotic dermatitis), there is a group of disorders in which blisters are the primary and most distinctive feature. Blistering in these diseases tends to occur at specific levels within the skin, a morphologic distinction that is critical for diagnosis (Fig. 24.8).

Pemphigus (Vulgaris and Foliaceus)

Pemphigus is an uncommon autoimmune blistering disorder resulting from loss of normal intercellular attachments within the epidermis and the squamous mucosal epithelium. There are three major variants:

- Pemphigus vulgaris (the most common type)
- Pemphigus foliaceus
- Paraneoplastic pemphigus

The last entity is associated with internal malignancy and is not discussed here.

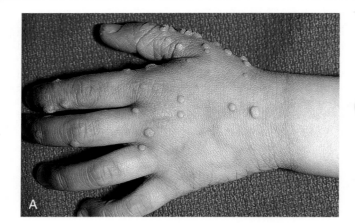

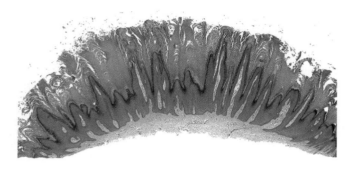

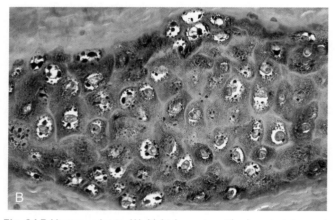

Fig. 24.7 Verruca vulgaris. (A) Multiple warts, with characteristic rough, pebble like surfaces. (B) Microscopically, common warts contain zones of papillary epidermal proliferation that often radiate symmetrically like the points of a crown *(top)*. Pallor or halos around nuclei, prominent keratohyalin granules, and related cytopathic changes are seen at higher magnification *(bottom)*.

Pathogenesis

Pemphigus vulgaris and pemphigus foliaceus are autoimmune diseases caused by antibody-mediated (type II) hypersensitivity reactions (Chapter 5). The pathogenic antibodies are IgG autoantibodies that bind to intercellular desmosomal proteins (desmoglein types 1 and 3) found in the skin and mucous membranes. The antibodies disrupt the intercellular adhesive function of desmosomes and may activate intercellular proteases as well. The distribution of desmoglein proteins within the epidermis determines the location of the lesions. By direct immunofluorescence study, lesional sites show a characteristic fishnet-like pattern of intercellular IgG deposits (Fig. 24.9). As with many other autoimmune diseases, pemphigus is associated with particular HLA alleles.

MORPHOLOGY

Pemphigus vulgaris involves both mucosa and skin, especially on the scalp, face, axillae, groin, trunk, and points of pressure. The lesions are superficial flaccid vesicles and bullae that rupture easily, leaving deep and often extensive erosions covered with a serum crust (Fig. 24.10A). **Pemphigus foliaceus,** a rare, milder form of pemphigus, results in bullae that are mainly confined to the skin, with only infrequent involvement of mucous membranes. The blisters in this disorder are superficial, such that more limited zones of erythema and crusting of ruptured blisters are seen (Fig. 24.11A).

The common histologic denominator in all forms of pemphigus is **acantholysis,** lysis of the intercellular adhesive junctions between neighboring squamous epithelial cells that results in the rounding up of detached cells. In pemphigus vulgaris, acantholysis selectively involves the layer of cells immediately above the basal cell layer, giving rise to a **suprabasal acantholytic blister** (Fig. 24.10B). In pemphigus foliaceus, acantholysis selectively involves the superficial epidermis at the level of the stratum granulosum (Fig. 24.11B). Variable superficial dermal infiltrates composed of lymphocytes, macrophages, and eosinophils accompany all forms of pemphigus.

Clinical Features

Pemphigus vulgaris is a rare disorder that occurs most commonly in older adults and more often in women than in men. Lesions are painful, particularly when ruptured, and frequently develop secondary infections. Most affected patients have oropharyngeal involvement at some point in their course. The mainstay of treatment is immunosuppressive therapy, sometimes for life. Medications can induce pemphigus, more often pemphigus foliaceus than pemphigus vulgaris. There is also an unusual endemic form of pemphigus foliaceus in South America *(fogo selvagem)* that is putatively associated with the bite of a black fly.

Bullous Pemphigoid

Bullous pemphigoid is another distinctive acquired blistering disorder with an autoimmune basis.

Pathogenesis

Blistering in bullous pemphigoid is triggered by the linear deposition of autoreactive IgG antibodies and complement in the epidermal basement membrane (Fig. 24.12A). Reactivity also occurs in the basement membrane attachment plaques (hemidesmosomes), where most bullous pemphigoid antigen (most commonly type XVII collagen) is located. The proteins that are recognized by the autoantibodies have structural roles in dermoepidermal adhesion. IgG autoantibodies to hemidesmosome components fix complement and cause tissue injury by recruiting neutrophils and eosinophils. Bullous pemphigoid and pemphigus vulgaris are thus caused by similar pathogenic

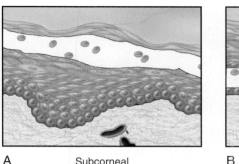
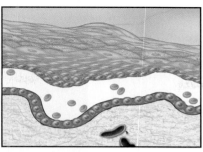
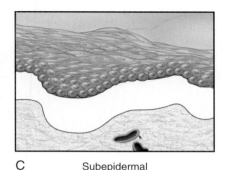

A Subcorneal   B Suprabasal   C Subepidermal

Fig. 24.8 Levels of blister formation. (A) Subcorneal (as in pemphigus foliaceus). (B) Suprabasal (as in pemphigus vulgaris). (C) Subepidermal (as in bullous pemphigoid or dermatitis herpetiformis).

mechanisms, but differ in their clinical presentation and course due to variation in the location of the target antigen (hemidesmosomes in bullous pemphigoid, desmosomes in pemphigus).

MORPHOLOGY

Bullous pemphigoid is associated with tense **subepidermal bullae** filled with clear fluid (Fig. 24.12B). The overlying epidermis characteristically lacks acantholysis. Early lesions show variable numbers of eosinophils at the dermal-epidermal junction, occasional neutrophils, superficial dermal edema, and associated basal cell layer vacuolization. The vacuolated basal cell layer eventually gives rise to a fluid-filled blister (Fig. 24.12C). The blister roof consists of full-thickness epidermis with intact intercellular junctions, a key distinction from the blisters seen in pemphigus.

Clinical Features

The lesions of bullous pemphigoid do not rupture as readily as in pemphigus and, if uncomplicated by infection, heal without scarring. The disease tends to follow a remitting and relapsing course and responds to topical or systemic immunosuppressive agents. Gestational pemphigoid (also known as *herpes gestationis,* a misnomer since there is no

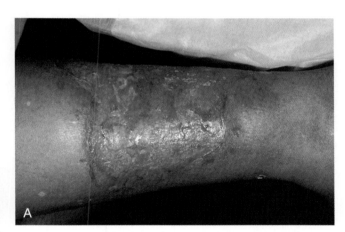

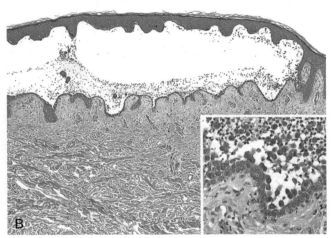

Fig. 24.10 Pemphigus vulgaris. (A) An erosion on the leg arising from coalescence of a group of "unroofed" blisters. (B) Suprabasal intraepidermal blister in which rounded, dissociated (acantholytic) keratinocytes are plentiful *(inset).*

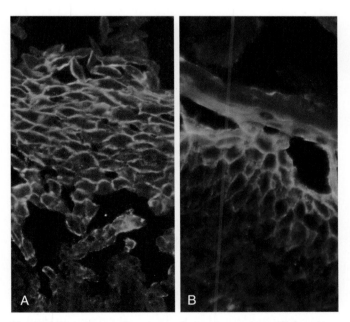

Fig. 24.9 Direct immunofluorescence findings in pemphigus. (A) Pemphigus vulgaris. Note the uniform deposition of immunoglobulin *(green)* along keratinocyte cell membranes in a characteristic "fishnet" pattern. (B) Pemphigus foliaceus. Immunoglobulin deposits are confined to superficial layers of the epidermis.

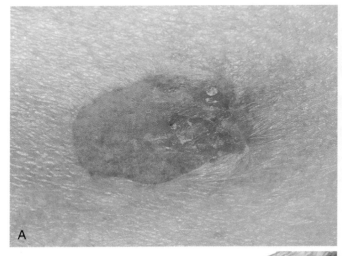

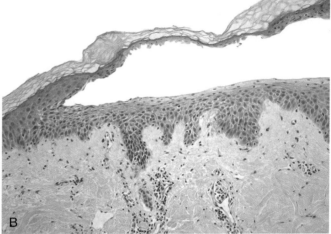

Fig. 24.11 Pemphigus foliaceus. (A) A typical blister, which is more superficial than those seen in pemphigus vulgaris. (B) Microscopic appearance of a characteristic subcorneal blister.

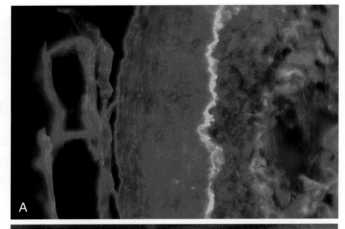

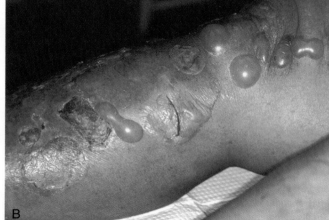

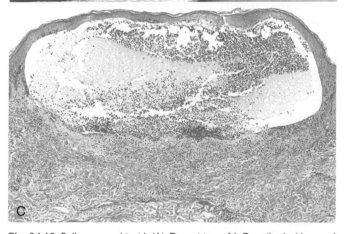

Fig. 24.12 Bullous pemphigoid. (A) Deposition of IgG antibody (detected by direct immunofluorescence) in the subepidermal basement membrane (epidermis is on the left side of the fluorescent band). (B) Gross appearance of characteristic tense, fluid-filled blisters. (C) Subepidermal vesicle with an eosinophil-rich inflammatory infiltrate. (*C, Courtesy of Dr. Victor G. Prieto, Houston, Texas.*)

viral etiology) is a clinically distinct subtype that appears suddenly during the second or third trimester of pregnancy. It also is caused by autoantibodies against bullous pemphigoid antigen. Gestational pemphigoid typically resolves after childbirth, but may recur with subsequent pregnancies.

Dermatitis Herpetiformis

Dermatitis herpetiformis is an autoimmune blistering disorder associated with gluten sensitivity that is characterized by extremely pruritic grouped vesicles and papules. The disease affects predominantly males, often in the third and fourth decades of life. Up to 80% of cases are associated with celiac disease; conversely, only a small fraction of patients with celiac disease develop dermatitis herpetiformis. Like celiac disease, dermatitis herpetiformis responds to a gluten-free diet.

Pathogenesis

The strong association of dermatitis herpetiformis with celiac disease provides a clue to its pathogenesis. Geneti-

cally predisposed individuals develop IgA antibodies to dietary gluten (derived from the wheat protein gliadin) as well as IgA autoantibodies that cross-react with endomysium and tissue transglutaminases, including epidermal transglutaminase expressed by keratinocytes. By direct immunofluorescence, the skin shows discontinuous, granular deposits of IgA selectively localized in the tips of dermal papillae (Fig. 24.13A). The resultant injury and inflammation produce a subepidermal blister.

MORPHOLOGY

The lesions of dermatitis herpetiformis are bilateral, symmetric, and grouped and preferentially involve the extensor surfaces, elbows, knees, upper back, and buttocks (Fig. 24.13B). Initially, neutrophils accumulate selectively at the **tips of dermal papillae,** forming small microabscesses (Fig. 24.13C). The basal cells overlying these microabscesses show vacuolization and focal dermoepidermal separation that ultimately coalesce to form a true **subepidermal blister.**

SUMMARY

BLISTERING DISORDERS

- Blistering disorders are classified based on the level of the epidermis that is affected.
- These disorders often are caused by autoantibodies specific for epithelial or basement membrane proteins that lead to unmooring of keratinocytes (acantholysis).
- Pemphigus is associated with IgG autoantibodies to various intercellular desmogleins (part of the desmosome), resulting in bullae that are either subcorneal (pemphigus foliaceus) or suprabasilar (pemphigus vulgaris).
- Bullous pemphigoid is associated with IgG autoantibodies to basement membrane proteins (part of the hemidesmosome) and produces a subepidermal blister.
- Dermatitis herpetiformis is associated with IgA autoantibodies to transglutaminase, and also is characterized by subepidermal blisters.

TUMORS OF THE SKIN

Benign and Premalignant Epithelial Lesions

Benign epithelial neoplasms are common and probably arise from stem cells residing in the epidermis and hair follicles. These tumors grow to a limited size and generally do not undergo malignant transformation.

Seborrheic Keratosis

These common pigmented epidermal tumors occur most frequently in middle-age or older individuals. They arise spontaneously and are particularly numerous on the trunk, although the extremities, head, and neck also may be sites of involvement.

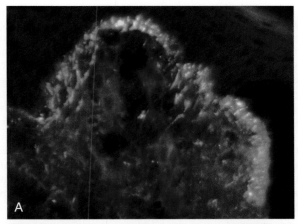

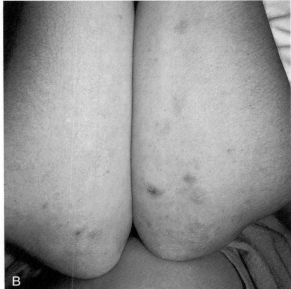

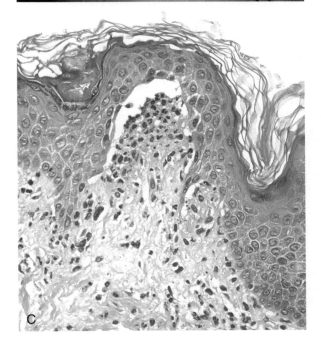

Fig. 24.13 Dermatitis herpetiformis. (A) Characteristic selective deposition of IgA autoantibody at the tips of the dermal papillae. (B) Lesions consist of intact and eroded (usually scratched) erythematous blisters, often grouped (seen here on elbows and arms). (C) Blisters associated with basal cell layer injury, initially caused by accumulation of neutrophils (microabscesses) at the tips of the dermal papillae. (A, Courtesy of Dr. Victor G. Prieto, Houston, Texas.)

Seborrheic keratoses are caused by acquired activating mutations in growth factor signaling pathways. A significant fraction of these tumors harbor activating mutations in fibroblast growth factor receptor 3 (FGFR3), which possesses a tyrosine kinase activity that stimulates RAS and the PI3K/AKT pathway, while others have activating mutations in downstream pathway components such as RAS and PI3K. Except for cosmetic concerns, seborrheic keratoses are usually of little clinical importance. However, in rare patients hundreds of lesions may appear suddenly as a paraneoplastic syndrome *(sign of Leser-Trelat)*. Patients with this presentation may harbor internal malignancies, most commonly gastrointestinal tract carcinomas, which produce growth factors that stimulate epidermal proliferation.

MORPHOLOGY

Seborrheic keratoses are **round, exophytic, coinlike plaques** that vary in diameter from millimeters to centimeters and have a **"stuck-on"** appearance (Fig. 24.14, *inset*). They are tan to dark brown and have a velvety- to granular-appearing surface. Occasionally, their dark color is suggestive of melanoma, leading to surgical removal.

Microscopically, seborrheic keratoses are composed of monotonous sheets of small cells that resemble the basal cells of the normal epidermis (see Fig. 24.14). Variable melanin pigmentation is present within these basaloid cells, accounting for the brown coloration seen grossly. Hyperkeratosis occurs at the surface, and the presence of small keratin-filled cysts (horn cysts) and downgrowth of keratin into the main tumor mass (pseudo–horn cysts) are characteristic features.

Actinic Keratosis

Actinic keratosis is a premalignant lesion caused by UV-induced DNA damage that is associated with mutations in *TP53* and other genes that also are frequently mutated in squamous cell carcinoma of the skin. Because such lesions usually are the result of chronic exposure to

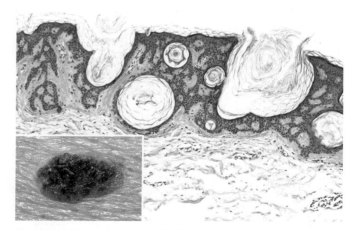

Fig. 24.14 Seborrheic keratosis. A characteristic roughened, brown, waxy lesion that appears to be "stuck on" the skin *(inset)*. Microscopic examination shows an orderly proliferation of uniform, basaloid keratinocytes that tend to form keratin microcysts (horn cysts).

sunlight and are associated with hyperkeratosis, they are called *actinic* (sun-related) *keratoses*. The rate of progression to squamous cell carcinoma is small, varying from 0.1% to 2.6% per year. Most regress or remain stable.

MORPHOLOGY

Actinic keratoses usually are less than 1 cm in diameter, tan-brown or red, and rough (sandpaper-like) to the touch (Fig. 24.15A). Microscopically, lower portions of the epidermis show **cytologic atypia,** often associated with hyperplasia of basal cells (see Fig. 24.15B) or with atrophy and diffuse thinning of the epidermal surface. The dermis contains thickened, blue-gray elastic fibers (solar elastosis), the result of chronic sun damage. The stratum corneum is thickened and shows abnormal retention of nuclei (parakeratosis). Uncommonly, full-thickness epidermal atypia is seen; such lesions are considered squamous cell carcinoma in situ (Fig. 24.15C).

Clinical Features

Actinic keratoses are very common in fair-skinned individuals and increase in incidence with age and sun exposure. As would be expected, there is a predilection for sun-exposed areas (face, arms, dorsum of the hands). Despite the low risk for malignant progression, actinic keratoses are often treated, either to prevent progression or for cosmetic reasons. Local eradication with cryotherapy (superficial freezing) or topical agents is effective and safe.

SUMMARY

BENIGN AND PREMALIGNANT EPITHELIAL LESIONS

- *Seborrheic keratosis:* Round, flat plaques made up of proliferating monotonous epidermal basal cells, which sometimes contain melanin. Hyperkeratosis and keratin-filled cysts are characteristic.
- *Actinic keratosis:* Present on sun-exposed skin, these lesions show cytologic atypia in lower parts of the epidermis and infrequently progress to carcinoma in situ.
- Although both of these lesions are associated with oncogenic mutations, malignant transformation is exceedingly rare in seborrheic keratoses and occurs in only a small subset of actinic keratoses.

Malignant Epidermal Tumors

Squamous Cell Carcinoma

Squamous cell carcinoma is a common tumor that typically arises on sun-exposed sites in older adults. These tumors have a higher incidence in men than in women.

Pathogenesis

Cutaneous squamous cell carcinoma is mainly caused by UV light exposure, which leads to widespread DNA damage and extremely high mutational loads (Chapter 6). As one might imagine, patients with the rare disorder *xeroderma pigmentosum*, which disrupts repair of UV-induced DNA damage, are at an exceptionally high risk. *TP53*

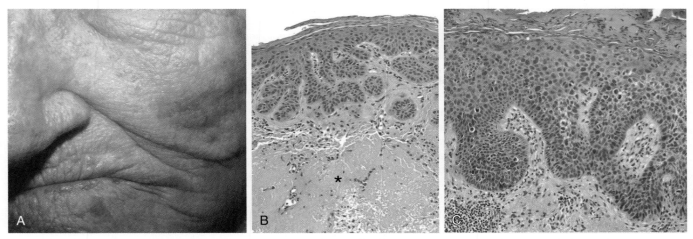

Fig. 24.15 Actinic keratosis. (A) Red, rough (sandpaper-like) lesions owing to excessive scale are present on the cheek and nose. (B) Basal cell layer atypia (dysplasia) with epithelial buds associated with marked hyperkeratosis, parakeratosis, and dermal solar elastosis *(asterisk)*. (C) Squamous cell carcinoma in situ lesion showing full-thickness epithelial atypia.

mutations are common, as are activating mutations in *RAS* and loss-of-function mutations in Notch receptors, which transmit signals that regulate the orderly differentiation of normal squamous epithelia.

Immunosuppression, particularly in organ transplant recipients, is associated with an increased incidence of cutaneous squamous cell carcinomas that are likely to be associated with HPV infection. Other predisposing factors include industrial carcinogens (tars and oils), chronic non-healing ulcers, old burn scars, ingestion of arsenicals, and ionizing radiation.

MORPHOLOGY

Squamous cell carcinomas in situ appear as sharply defined, red, scaling plaques; some appear to arise in association with prior actinic keratoses. Microscopically, squamous cell carcinoma in situ is characterized by highly atypical cells at all levels of the epidermis, with nuclear crowding and disorganization. More advanced, invasive squamous cell carcinomas are nodular, often scaly lesions that may undergo ulceration (Fig. 24.16A). Such tumors show variable degrees of differentiation, ranging from tumors with cells arranged in orderly lobules that exhibit extensive keratinization to neoplasms consisting of highly anaplastic cells with foci of necrosis and only abortive, single-cell keratinization (dyskeratosis) (Fig. 24.16B).

Clinical Features

Invasive squamous cell carcinomas of the skin often are discovered while small and resectable. Less than 1% will have metastasized to regional lymph nodes at diagnosis. The likelihood of metastasis is related to the thickness of the lesion and degree of invasion into the subcutis. Tumors arising from actinic keratoses may be locally aggressive but generally metastasize only after long periods of time, while those arising in burn scars, ulcers, and non–sun-exposed skin often behave more aggressively. Squamous cell carcinomas arising at internal sites (oropharynx, lung, esophagus, anus) are generally invasive and aggressive, possibly because (unlike in the skin) early lesions go unrecognized.

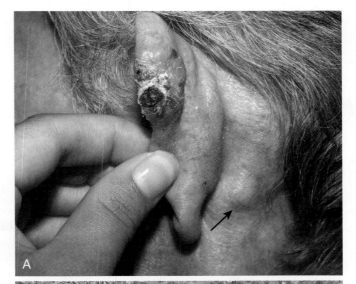

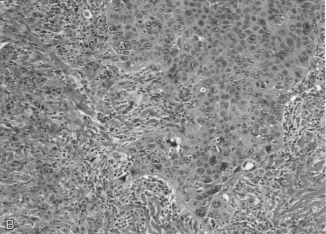

Fig. 24.16 Invasive squamous cell carcinoma. (A) A nodular, hyperkeratotic lesion occurring on the ear, associated with metastasis to a prominent postauricular lymph node *(arrow)*. (B) Tumor invades the dermal soft tissue as irregular projections of atypical squamous cells exhibiting acantholysis.

Basal Cell Carcinoma

Basal cell carcinoma is a common slow-growing cancer that rarely metastasizes. It tends to occur at sites subject to chronic sun exposure and in lightly pigmented individuals.

Pathogenesis

The molecular hallmark of basal cell carcinoma is loss-of-function mutations in _PTCH1_, a tumor suppressor gene that negatively regulates Hedgehog signaling; hence, tumors exhibit constitutive Hedgehog pathway activation. Excessive activation of Hedgehog in turn activates a host of downstream genes implicated in cell growth and survival and other phenotypes linked to malignant transformation. In sporadic basal cell carcinoma, _PTCH1_ mutations bear the telltale signs of UV light–induced DNA damage. The central role of increased Hedgehog signaling in basal cell carcinoma is further emphasized by _Gorlin syndrome_, an autosomal dominant disorder caused by inherited defects in _PTCH1_ that is associated with familial basal cell carcinoma. The Hedgehog pathway is an important regulator of embryonic development, and patients with Gorlin syndrome also often manifest subtle developmental anomalies. Mutations in _TP53_ caused by UV light–induced damage also are common in both familial and sporadic tumors.

MORPHOLOGY

Basal cell carcinomas manifest as **pearly papules**, often with prominent, dilated subepidermal blood vessels **(telangiectasia)** (Fig. 24.17A). Some tumors contain melanin pigment and can have an appearance similar to melanocytic nevi or melanomas. Microscopically, the tumor cells resemble the normal epidermal basal cell layer or follicular germinative elements. Because they arise from either the epidermis or the follicular epithelium, they are not encountered on mucosal surfaces. Two common patterns are seen: **multifocal superficial growths,** originating from the epidermis, and **nodular lesions** growing downward into the dermis as cords and islands of variably basophilic cells with hyperchromatic nuclei, embedded in a fibrotic or mucinous stromal matrix (Fig. 24.17B). Peripheral tumor cell nuclei align in the outermost layer (a pattern termed _palisading_), which often separates from the stroma, creating a characteristic cleft (Fig. 24.17C).

Clinical Features

It is estimated that more than 1 million basal cell carcinomas are treated in the United States annually. By far the most important risk factor is cumulative sun exposure; basal cell carcinoma is more common in warm southern regions of the United States, and its incidence is 40-fold higher in sunny climates near the equator, such as Australia, than it is in Northern European locales. Individual tumors usually are cured by local excision, but approximately 40% of patients develop another basal cell carcinoma within 5 years. Advanced lesions may ulcerate, and extensive local invasion of bone or facial sinuses may occur if the lesions are neglected. Metastasis is exceedingly rare. Hedgehog pathway inhibitors are used to treat locally advanced or metastatic tumors.

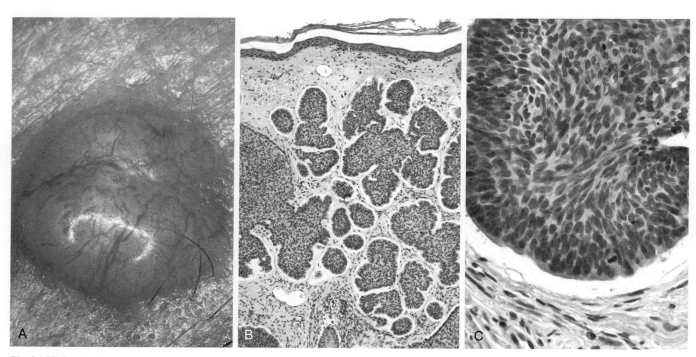

Fig. 24.17 Basal cell carcinoma. (A) A prototypical pearly, smooth-surfaced papule with telangiectatic vessels. (B) Tumor is composed of nests of basaloid cells infiltrating a fibrotic stroma. (C) Tumor cells with scant cytoplasm and small hyperchromatic nuclei that palisade on the outside of the nest. The cleft between the tumor cells and the stroma is a highly characteristic artifact of sectioning.

SUMMARY

MALIGNANT EPIDERMAL TUMORS

- The incidence of both basal cell and squamous cell carcinoma is strongly correlated with increasing lifetime sun exposure.
- Risk factors for cutaneous squamous cell carcinoma include fair skin, UV light exposure, exposure to carcinogenic chemicals, chronic skin inflammation and scarring, and HPV infection (in the setting of immunosuppression).
- Cutaneous squamous cell carcinoma has the potential for metastasis but usually is recognized and excised before it does so.
- Basal cell carcinoma, the most common malignancy worldwide, is a locally aggressive tumor associated with mutations in the Hedgehog pathway. Metastasis is very rare.

Melanocytic Proliferations

Melanocytic Nevi

Strictly speaking, the term *nevus* denotes any congenital lesion of the skin. *Melanocytic* nevus, however, refers to any benign congenital or acquired neoplasm of melanocytes.

Pathogenesis

Melanocytic nevi are benign neoplasms caused by somatic gain-of-function mutations in *BRAF* or *RAS*. Nevi are derived from melanocytes, pigment-producing cells with dendritic projections that are normally interspersed among basal keratinocytes. You will recall that *BRAF* encodes a serine/threonine kinase that lies downstream of RAS in the extracellular regulated kinase (ERK) pathway. Experimental evidence suggests that unbridled BRAF/RAS signaling initially induces melanocytic proliferation followed by senescence. How these opposing effects are coordinated is unclear, but it is believed that the "brake" on proliferation provided by induced senescence explains why very few nevi transform into malignant melanomas. Indeed, the growth and migration of nevus cells from the dermoepidermal junction into the underlying dermis is accompanied by morphologic changes that are taken as evidence of cellular senescence (Fig. 24.18). Superficial nevus cells are larger and tend to produce melanin pigment and grow in nests; deeper nevus cells are smaller, produce little or no pigment, and grow in cords or single cells. The deepest nevus cells have fusiform contours and grow in fascicles. This sequence of morphologic changes is of diagnostic importance, since they are absent from melanomas.

MORPHOLOGY

Common melanocytic nevi are tan-to-brown, uniformly pigmented, small papules (5 mm or less across) with well-defined, rounded borders (Fig. 24.19A). Early lesions are composed of round to oval cells that grow in "nests" along the dermoepidermal junction. Nuclei are uniform and round, and contain inconspicuous nucleoli with little or no mitotic activity. Such early-stage lesions are called **junctional nevi.** Eventually, most junctional nevi grow into the underlying dermis as nests or cords of cells **(compound nevi),** and in older lesions the epidermal nests may be lost entirely, creating **intradermal nevi** (Fig. 24.19B).

Clinical Features

There are numerous types of melanocytic nevi, with varied appearances. Although these lesions usually are of only cosmetic concern, they may cause irritation or mimic melanoma, requiring their surgical removal. Compound and intradermal nevi often are more elevated than junctional nevi.

Dysplastic Nevus

Dysplastic nevi may be sporadic or familial. The latter are important clinically because they identify individuals who

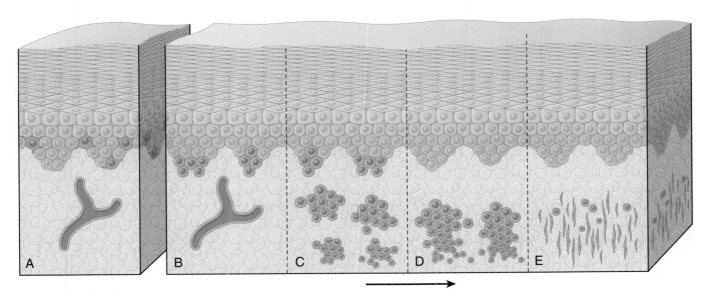

Fig. 24.18 Possible steps in the development of melanocytic nevi. (A) Normal skin shows only scattered melanocytes. (B) Junctional nevus. (C) Compound nevus. (D) Intradermal nevus. (E) Intradermal nevus with extensive cellular senescence.

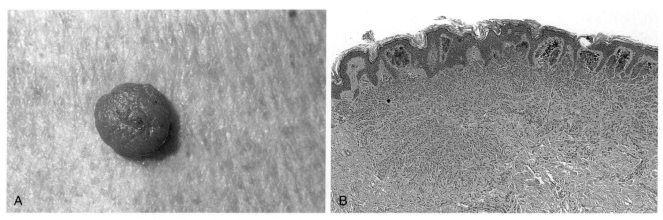

Fig. 24.19 Melanocytic nevus. (A) Melanocytic nevi are relatively small, symmetric, and uniformly pigmented. (B) A nevus composed of melanocytes that lose pigmentation and become smaller and more dispersed as they extend into the dermis—all signs that speak to the benign nature of the proliferation.

have an increased risk of developing melanoma. As with conventional melanocytic nevi, activating *RAS* or *BRAF* mutations are commonly found in dysplastic nevi and are believed to have a pathogenic role.

MORPHOLOGY

Dysplastic nevi are larger than most acquired nevi (often more than 5 mm across) and **may number in the hundreds** (Fig. 24.20A). They are flat macules to slightly raised plaques, with a "pebbly" surface. They usually have variable pigmentation (variegation) and irregular borders (Fig. 24.20A, *inset*).

Microscopically, dysplastic nevi are mostly compound nevi that exhibit both architectural and cytologic evidence of abnormal growth. Nevus cell nests within the epidermis may be enlarged and exhibit abnormal fusion or coalescence with adjacent nests (bridging). As part of this process, single nevus cells begin to replace the normal basal cell layer along the dermoepidermal junction, producing so-called "**lentiginous**

hyperplasia" (Fig. 24.20B). Cytologic atypia consisting of irregular, often angulated, nuclear contours and hyperchromasia is frequently observed (Fig. 24.20B-C). Associated alterations also occur in the superficial dermis. These consist of a sparse lymphocytic infiltrate, release of melanin pigment that is phagocytosed by dermal macrophages (melanin incontinence), and linear fibrosis surrounding epidermal nests of melanocytes. These dermal changes are elements of the host response to these lesions.

Clinical Features

Unlike ordinary nevi, dysplastic nevi have a tendency to occur on body surfaces not exposed to the sun as well as on sun-exposed sites. *Familial dysplastic nevus syndrome* is strongly associated with melanoma, as the lifetime risk for the development of melanoma in affected individuals is close to 100%. In sporadic cases, only individuals with 10 or more dysplastic nevi appear to be at an increased

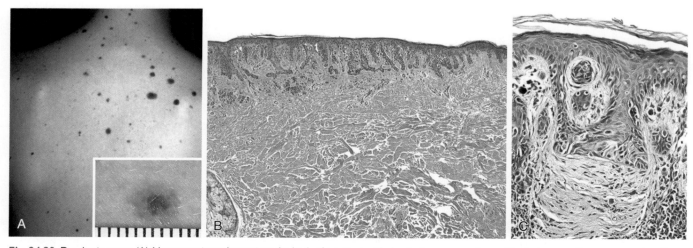

Fig. 24.20 Dysplastic nevus. (A) Numerous irregular nevi on the back of a patient with dysplastic nevus syndrome. The lesions usually are greater than 5 mm in diameter and have irregular borders and variable pigmentation *(inset)*. (B) Compound dysplastic nevus featuring a central dermal component and an asymmetric "shoulder" of exclusively junctional melanocytes (lentiginous hyperplasia). The former corresponds to the raised, more pigmented central zone seen in A *(inset)*, and the latter corresponds to the less pigmented flat peripheral rim. (C) Other important features are cytologic atypia (irregular, dark-staining nuclei) and characteristic parallel bands of fibrosis.

risk for melanoma. Transformation of dysplastic nevus to melanoma has been documented, both clinically and histologically. However, such cases are the exception, as most melanomas appear to arise *de novo* and not from a preexisting nevus. Thus, the likelihood that any particular nevus, dysplastic or otherwise, will develop into melanoma is low, and these lesions are best viewed as markers of melanoma risk.

Melanoma

Melanoma is less common but much more deadly than basal or squamous cell carcinoma. Today, as a result of increased public awareness of the earliest signs of skin melanomas, most melanomas are cured surgically. Nonetheless, the incidence of these lesions has increased dramatically over the past several decades, at least in part as a result of increasing sun exposure and/or higher detection rates resulting from vigorous surveillance.

Pathogenesis

As with other cutaneous malignancies, melanoma is mainly caused by UV light–induced DNA damage that leads to the stepwise acquisition of driver mutations. The incidence is highest in sun-exposed skin and in geographic locales such as Australia, where sun exposure is high and much of the population is fair-skinned. Intense intermittent exposure at an early age is particularly harmful. Hereditary predisposition also plays a role in an estimated 5% to 10% of cases, as already discussed under familial dysplastic nevus syndrome. For example, germ-line mutations in the *CDKN2A* locus (located on 9p21) are found in as many as 40% of the rare individuals who suffer from familial melanoma. This complex locus encodes two tumor suppressors: p16, a cyclin-dependent kinase inhibitor that regulates the G_1-S transition of the cell cycle by maintaining the retinoblastoma (RB) tumor suppressor protein in its active state; and p14, which augments the activity of the p53 tumor suppressor by preventing its degradation.

Key phases of melanoma development are marked by radial and vertical growth. The earliest recognizable phase of melanoma development is proposed to consist of lateral expansion of melanocytes along the dermoepidermal junction (lentiginous hyperplasia and lentiginous compound nevus; Fig. 24.21A-C). This then progresses to the phase of melanoma in situ, which is marked by *radial growth* within the epidermis, often for a prolonged period (Fig. 24.21D). During this stage, melanoma cells do not have the capacity to invade and metastasize. With time, a *vertical growth phase* supervenes, in which the tumor grows downward into the deeper dermal layers as an expansile mass lacking cellular maturation (Fig. 24.21E). This event often is heralded by the development of a nodule in a previously flat lesion and correlates with the emergence of metastatic potential.

DNA sequencing of familial and sporadic cases, including cases that appear to have arisen from benign nevi, has provided important insights into the molecular pathogenesis of melanoma (Fig. 24.22). The initiating event appears to be an activating mutation in *BRAF* or (less commonly) *RAS*. In the vast majority of cases, this produces only a benign nevus unless other mutations are superimposed. Sequencing of nevi with "atypical" morphologic features suggestive of melanoma as well as melanomas in the radial phase of growth (melanoma in situ) has shown that they commonly harbor mutations that activate the expression of telomerase, which is proposed to serve as an antidote to senescence (the usual fate of benign nevi). With additional mutations or epigenetic aberrations that lead to loss of

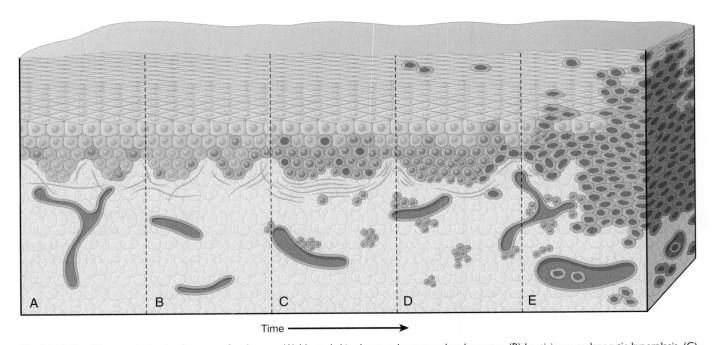

Fig. 24.21 Possible steps in the development of melanoma. (A) Normal skin shows only scattered melanocytes. (B) Lentiginous melanocytic hyperplasia. (C) Lentiginous compound nevus with abnormal architecture and cytologic features (dysplastic nevus). (D) Early or radial growth phase melanoma (large dark cells in epidermis) arising in a nevus. (E) Melanoma in vertical growth phase with metastatic potential. Note that no melanocytic nevus precursor is identified in most cases of melanoma. They are believed to arise de novo, perhaps all using the same pathway.

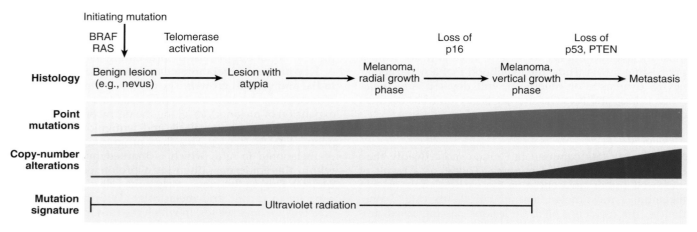

Fig. 24.22 Molecular evolution of cutaneous melanoma. The most important driver mutations and the overall mutational burden (point mutations and genomic copy-number variations) at various histologic phases of melanocytic lesion progression are indicated. Note that as the tumor metastasizes to internal sites, UV light–induced DNA damage leading to point substitutions ceases, and copy number changes related to aneuploidy increase.

CDNK2A and its encoded tumor suppressor p16, the tumor shifts to the invasive vertical phase of growth. Throughout this cutaneous phase of tumor evolution, exposure to UV light adds to the mutational burden and increases the chances of tumor progression. Finally, with additional mutations in genes such as tumor suppressors *TP53* and *PTEN,* the tumor acquires the capacity for metastasis. This phase is marked by the appearance of aneuploidy and genomic copy number alterations, which add to the genetic heterogeneity of the evolving tumor.

By contrast, the less common melanomas that arise in non–sun-exposed acral and mucosal sites follow different molecular courses. The most common initiating mutation in these tumors is a gain-of-function mutation in the KIT receptor tyrosine kinase. Similarly, melanomas arising the uvea of the eye also have a distinct set of driver gene mutations, most notably mutually exclusive mutations that activate the GTP-binding proteins GNAQ or GNA11.

In addition, it has long been speculated that melanomas express neoantigens that should be subject to recognition by the immune system. It follows that for melanoma to develop, tumor cells must acquire the ability to either suppress or evade the host immune response. **The importance of immune evasion has been proven by the response of many advanced melanomas to immune checkpoint inhibitors, agents that unleash muzzled melanoma-specific T cells, allowing them to attack the tumor** (described later).

MORPHOLOGY

Unlike benign nevi, melanomas often exhibit **striking variations in pigmentation,** including shades of black, brown, red, dark blue, and gray (Fig. 24.23A). The **borders are irregular** and often "notched." Microscopically, malignant cells grow as poorly formed nests or as individual cells at all levels of the epidermis (pagetoid spread) and in expansile dermal nodules; these constitute the radial and vertical growth phases, respectively (Fig. 24.23B-C). Of note, superficial spreading melanomas are often associated with a brisk lymphocytic infiltrate (Fig. 24.23B), a feature that may reflect a host response to tumor-specific antigens. **Increasing thickness strongly correlates with**

worse biologic behavior of melanomas (termed *Breslow thickness*). By recording and using these and other variables in aggregate, accurate prognostication is possible.

Individual melanoma cells usually are considerably larger than nevus cells. They have large nuclei with irregular contours, chromatin that is characteristically clumped at the periphery of the nuclear membrane, and prominent "cherry red" eosinophilic nucleoli (Fig. 24.23D). Immunohistochemical stains can be helpful in identifying metastatic deposits (Fig. 24.23D, *inset*).

Clinical Features

Although most of these lesions arise in the skin, they also may occur in the oral and anogenital mucosal surfaces, the esophagus, the meninges, and the eye. The following discussion applies to cutaneous melanomas.

Melanoma of the skin usually is asymptomatic, although pruritus may be an early manifestation. *The most important clinical sign is a change in the color or size of a pigmented lesion.* The main clinical warning signs are as follows:

1. Rapid enlargement of a preexisting nevus
2. Itching or pain in a lesion
3. Development of a new pigmented lesion during adult life
4. Irregularity of the borders of a pigmented lesion
5. Variegation of color within a pigmented lesion

These principles are expressed in the so-called "ABCs" of melanoma: *a*symmetry, *b*order, *c*olor, *d*iameter, and *e*volution (change of an existing nevus). It is vitally important to recognize melanomas and intervene as rapidly as possible. The vast majority of superficial lesions are curable surgically, while metastatic melanoma has a very poor prognosis.

The probability of metastasis is predicted by measuring the depth of invasion in millimeters of the vertical growth phase nodule from the top of the granular cell layer of the overlying epidermis (Breslow thickness). Metastasis risk also is increased in tumors with a high mitotic rate and in those that fail to induce a local immune response. When metastases occur, they involve not only regional lymph

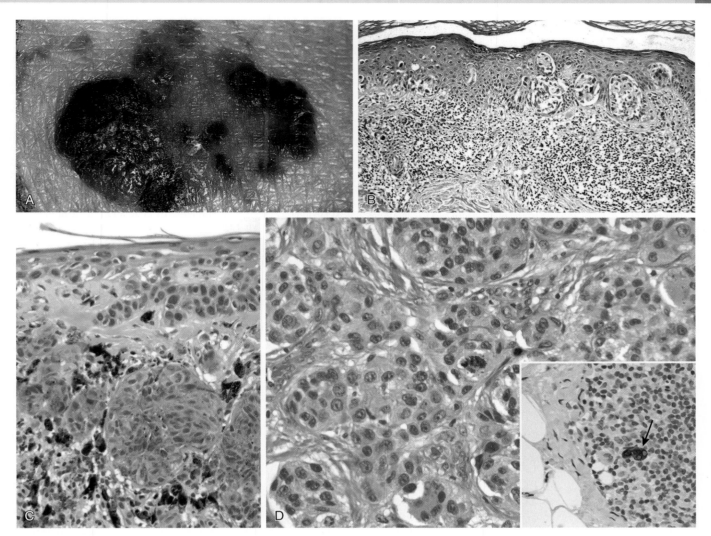

Fig. 24.23 Melanoma. (A) Lesions tend to be larger than nevi, with irregular contours and variable pigmentation. Macular areas indicate superficial (radial) growth, while elevated areas indicate dermal invasion (vertical growth). (B) Radial growth phase, with spread of nested and single melanoma cells within the epidermis. (C) Vertical growth phase, with nodular aggregates of infiltrating tumor cells within the dermis. (D) Melanoma cells with hyperchromatic irregular nuclei of varying size that have prominent nucleoli. An atypical mitotic figure is present in the center of the field). The *inset* shows a sentinel lymph node containing a tiny cluster of metastatic melanoma *(arrow)*, detected by staining for the melanocytic marker HMB-45.

nodes but also liver, lungs, brain, and virtually any other site that can be seeded hematogenously. Sentinel lymph node biopsy (of the first draining node[s] of a primary melanoma) at the time of surgery provides additional information on biologic aggressiveness.

Agents that selectively inhibit mutant BRAF and KIT have produced dramatic responses in patients with metastatic tumors with *BRAF* and *KIT* mutations, respectively, an encouraging development in a previously hopeless disease. More recently, immune checkpoint inhibitors have been shown to be effective at stabilizing metastatic disease and in some instances causing remarkable tumor regression and even clinical remissions. Immune checkpoint inhibitors are antibodies that interfere with the function of proteins found on the surface of T lymphocytes that abrogate cytotoxic T cell responsiveness. By blocking these pathways, checkpoint inhibitors reactivate the host T-cell response, which otherwise is held at bay. Current efforts are focused on building upon these successes by using combinations of different checkpoint inhibitors, as

well as checkpoint inhibitors together with other targeted therapies such as BRAF inhibitors.

SUMMARY

MELANOCYTIC LESIONS, BENIGN AND MALIGNANT

- Most *melanocytic nevi* have activating mutations in *BRAF* or less often *NRAS*, but the vast majority never undergoes malignant transformation.
- Most sporadic *dysplastic nevi* are best regarded as markers of melanoma risk rather than premalignant lesions. They are characterized by architectural disorder and cytologic atypia.
- *Melanoma* is a highly aggressive malignancy; tumors only a few millimeters in thickness can give rise to deadly metastases.
- In most cases, melanoma progresses from an intraepithelial (in situ) to an invasive (dermal) form. Characteristics of the dermal tumor such as depth of invasion and mitotic activity correlate with survival.

SUGGESTED READINGS

Bastian BC: The molecular pathology of melanoma: an integrated taxonomy of melanocytic neoplasia, *Ann Rev Pathol* 9:239, 2014. *[A modified classification of melanoma based on both clinical and genetic features. Such molecular classification schemes are critical for progress in targeted therapy.]*

Cancer Genome Atlas Network: Genomic classification of cutaneous melanoma, *Cell* 161:1681, 2015. *[A genomic study of cutaneous melanoma that highlights the different molecular subtypes and common pathogenic pathways.]*

Elder DE: Dysplastic nevi: an update, *Histopathology* 56:112, 2010. *[A balanced presentation of the histology and pathogenesis of dysplastic nevi and their relationship to melanoma.]*

Epstein EH: Basal cell carcinomas: attack of the hedgehog, *Nat Rev Cancer* 8:743, 2008. *[A succinct review of the epidemiology, clinical presentation, molecular pathogenesis, and novel treatment options for basal cell carcinoma.]*

Nestle FO, Kaplan DH, Barker J: Psoriasis, *N Engl J Med* 361:496, 2009. *[A discussion of the pathogenesis, clinical features, and targeted treatment options for psoriasis.]*

Ratushny V, Gober MD, Hick R, et al: From keratinocyte to cancer: the pathogenesis and modeling of cutaneous squamous cell carcinoma, *J Clin Invest* 122:464, 2012. *[Models of human epidermal carcinogenesis indicate that multiple mutations in specific pathways are required for malignant transformation.]*

Ujiie H, Shibaki A, Nishie W, et al: What's new in bullous pemphigoid, *J Dermatol* 37:194, 2010. *[A review of bullous pemphigoid pathogenesis.]*

Wargo JA, Cooper ZA, Flaherty KT: Universes collide: combining immunotherapy with targeted therapy for cancer, *Cancer Discov* 4:1377, 2014. *[A presentation of melanoma signaling pathways with therapeutic interventions and the role of the immune system.]*

Yokoyama T, Amagai M: Immune dysregulation of pemphigus in humans and mice, *J Dermatol* 37:205, 2010. *[A review of immune disturbances that may underlie pemphigus.]*

Index

A

AA protein, in amyloidosis, 184–185
Abdominal aortic aneurysm (AAA)
　clinical consequences of, 380
　inflammatory, 380
　mycotic, 380
　risk for rupture of, 380
Abetalipoproteinemia, 614
Aβ protein
　in Alzheimer disease, 875, 876f
　in diagnosis of AD, 875
ABL gene, 202
ABL proto-oncoprotein, 207, 208b
Abrasion, defined, 317–318
Abscesses
　in acute pyelonephritis, 565, 565f
　brain, 864f, 865, 866b
　in bronchopneumonia, 79f
　"cold", 70
　crypt, 623–624
　defined, 78–79
　epidural, 863
　lung, 525, 525b
　ring, 427, 428f
　stellate, 710
A-B toxins, in bacterial infection, 354
Acantholysis, in pemphigus, 896
Acanthosis, definition of, 890t
Acetaldehyde
　in alcohol metabolism, 310
　in ethanol metabolism, 311
Acetaminophen
　adverse reactions to, 314
　hepatotoxicity of, 651–652
　overdose of, 317b, 639, 640f
Achalasia, of esophagus, 591
Achondroplasia, 800
Acid aerosols, health effects of, 302t
Acinar cell injury, 681
Acinar cells, of pancreas, 679
Acinus, of lung, 498–500
Acquired immunodeficiency syndrome (AIDS), 172, 348
　central nervous system disease in, 181
　characteristics of, 173
　clinical features of, 177
　　effects of antiretroviral drug therapy, 181
　　opportunistic infections, 177
　　tumors, 177, 180–181
　epidemiology of, 172
　long-time prognosis for, 182
　morphology of, 182b
　Mycobacterium avium infection in, 359, 359f
　pathogenesis of, 173–174, 177b, 182b
　transmission of, 174
　tuberculosis in patients with, 532
Acromegaly, 753
Actinic keratosis, 900
　characteristics of, 900
　clinical features of, 900
　morphology of, 901b, 901f
Actin microfilaments, of cytoskeleton, 11
Activation-induced cytosine deaminase (AID), 227, 465
Acute chest syndrome, in sickle cell anemia, 447
Acute coronary syndrome, 409–410, 410f
Acute kidney injury, causes of, 567–568
Acute lymphoblastic leukemia (ALL), 478
　chromosomal aberrations in, 467
　flow cytometry results for, 467f
　morphology of, 465b–466b, 467f
　pathogenesis of, 466–467
　pediatric, 467
　prevalence of, 465
Acute lymphoblastic leukemia/lymphoma (ALLs), 466
　clinical features of, 467–468
　genetics of, 467
　immunophenotyping of, 467–468
Acute lymphoblastic lymphoma (ALL), 478
Acute myeloid leukemia (AML), 479–480, 480f, 484b
　bone marrow aspirate of, 480f
　classification of, 480–481, 480t
　clinical features of, 481
　epigenetic alterations in, 479–480
　flow cytometry results for, 480f
　immunophenotype for, 481

Acute myeloid leukemia (AML) *(Continued)*
　morphology of, 479b
　pathogenesis of, 480
Acute-phase response, in inflammation, 86
Acute postinfectious glomerulonephritis, 556t, 560–561
　clinical course of, 560–561
　morphology of, 560b, 561f
　pathogenesis of, 560
Acute respiratory distress syndrome (ARDS), 118, 496–497, 497b
　alveoli in, 497f
　from burns, 319
　clinical course of, 496
　clinical features of, 497
　DAD in, 498f
　inflammatory reaction in, 59t
　morphology of, 496b–497b, 498f
　pathogenesis of, 496
　radiation-induced, 322–323, 322f
Acute tubular injury (ATI), 567–569, 569b
　causes of, 568
　clinical course of, 569
　ischemic, 568–569
　morphology of, 569b, 569f
　pathogenesis of, 568, 568f
　toxic, 569
ADAMTS 13 deficiency, 488–489
Adaptations. *See also* Cellular responses
　cellular, 32
　pathologic, 48
　physiologic, 48
　to stress, 48–51, 51b
　　atrophy, 50
　　hyperplasia, 49–50
　　hypertrophy, 48–49, 48f–49f
　　metaplasia, 50–51
Adaptor proteins, in cell signaling, 18
Addison disease, 790–792
　causes of, 793
　hyperpigmentation of, 793
Adenocarcinoma in situ (AIS), of lung, 539, 540f
Adenocarcinomas
　of appendix, 635
　of bladder, 702
　of cervix, 720
　colon, 630–633, 634b
　　clinical features of, 632–633, 634f
　　epidemiology of, 630–631
　　morphology of, 632b, 633f
　　pathogenesis of, 631–632
　colorectal, 627, 629–630
　designation as, 190–191
　of fallopian tube, 727
　of female breast, 740
　gallbladder, 675b, 676f
　infiltrating ductal of pancreas of, 686–689
　poorly differentiated, 632, 633f
　of prostate, 699, 700f–701f
　of vagina, 716
　well-differentiated, 632, 633f
Adenocarcinomas, esophageal
　clinical features of, 596
　incidence of, 596
　morphology of, 596b, 596f
　pathogenesis of, 596
　risk for development of, 596
Adenocarcinomas, gastric, 604–605
　clinical features of, 605
　epidemiology of, 604
　morphology of, 604b–605b, 605f
　pathogenesis of, 604
Adenomas
　adrenocortical, 788f, 789, 795
　aldosterone-producing, 790
　of appendix, 635
　classification of, 628
　colonic, 627–628, 629f, 634b
　colorectal, 627–629
　corticotroph, 753–754
　hepatocellular, 669, 669f, 672
　histologic appearance of, 628, 629f
　lactotroph, 753–754
　morphology of, 628b–629b, 629f
　parathyroid, 770, 770f, 773f
　pituitary, 750
　　abnormalities associated with, 751–752, 756t
　　classification of, 750–751, 751t
　　clinical manifestations of, 754b
　　familial, 752

Adenomas *(Continued)*
　　functional or non functioning, 751
　　monomorphism of, 752–753, 753f
　　morphology of, 752b–753b, 752f
　　nonfunctioning, 751, 754
　somatotroph, 753
　of thyroid, 763–764
　thyrotroph or thyroid-stimulating hormone-producing, 754
Adenomas, pleomorphic, 191, 589
　defined, 589
　incidence of, 589
　morphology of, 589b, 589f
Adenomatous polyposis coli (APC), 213
Adenomatous polyposis coli *(APC)* gene, 213, 214f, 629–630
Adenomyosis, 721, 723
Adenosine deaminase (ADA), mutations in, 169
Adenosine diphosphate (ADP), 42–43
Adenosine triphosphate (ATP), source of, 7
Adipocytes, 336
Adiponectin
　and cancer, 337
　metabolic effects of, 336
Adipose tissue, 336
Adiposity, excess, 334–337
ADP. *See* Adenosine diphosphate
Adrenal aldosterone, in blood pressure regulation, 365
Adrenal cortex
　adrenal insufficiency, 789–790
　and adrenogenital syndromes, 789
　anatomy of, 786
　hyperaldosteronism of, 787–788
　hypercortisolism, 784–792
　hyperfunction of, 784
　steroids synthesized by, 786
Adrenal crisis, in adrenocortical insufficiency, 793–794
Adrenal glands, 786
Adrenal medulla, 786
　described, 795
　tumors of, 792
　　neuroblastoma, 794
　　pheochromocytoma, 793–794
Adrenocortical insufficiency, 789–790, 792b
　acute, 789–790, 792f
　causes of, 792
　chronic, 790–792
　clinical manifestations of, 793–794
　secondary, 790
　volume depletion in, 793–794
Adrenocortical neoplasms, 791–792
　adenomas, 795
　carcinomas, 795
Adrenogenital syndromes, 789, 790b
Adrenomedullary dysplasia, 790–791
Adult T Cell leukemia, 477
Adult T-cell leukemia/lymphoma (ATLL), 231–232, 232b
Adult T Cell lymphoma, 477
Adventitia, of blood vessels, 361–362, 362f
Adverse drug reactions (ADRs)
　to acetaminophen, 314
　to aspirin, 314–315
　common, 312–313, 313t
　defined, 312–313
　to exogenous estrogens, 313–314
　to OCs, 314
Affinity maturation, in humoral immunity, 132
Aflatoxin, 338, 670
Aflatoxin B₁, 229t, 230
African Americans
　esophageal tumor in, 596
　hypertension in, 366–367
Age
　and arteries, 362
　and atherosclerosis, 370–371
　and breast cancer incidence, 740f, 741
　and cancer, 199
Agenesis, use of term, 275
Aging
　amyloid of, 183–184
　cell injury caused by, 33
　and immune competence, 199
Aging, cellular, 54–56
　abnormalities contributing to, 55f, 56b
　causes of, 54–56
　mechanisms of, 55f
Agranulocytosis, 459–460
Agranulocytosis, in type II hypersensitivity, 139, 140f
AIRE gene, 145, 772, 795

Pages followed by *b, t,* or *f* refer to boxes, tables, or figures, respectively.

Air embolism, 113–114. *See also* Emboli
Air pollutants
  carbon monoxide, 303
  ozone, 302*t*, 303
  sulfur dioxide, 302*t*, 303
Air pollution, 302–303
  indoor, 303
  outdoor, 302–303, 302*t*
Airway, normal *vs.* asthmatic, 504*f*, 505*b*. *See also*
    Respiratory tract
Albumin, in plasma osmotic pressure, 99, 99*f*
Alcohol
  chronic consumption of, 654*f*
  effects of, 310–312, 312*b*
  malformations associated with, 275–276
  and oral cancer, 586–587
Alcohol abuse
  acute, 312*b*
  prevalence of, 310
Alcohol consumption
  and cancer risk, 198–199
  pancreatitis caused by, 681
  as risk factor for HCC, 670
  safe upper limit for, 653–654
Alcohol dehydrogenase, in alcohol metabolism, 310
Alcoholic liver disease, statistics for, 653–655
Alcoholics, chronic, 310
Alcoholism, chronic, 311–312, 312*b*, 324
Aldosterone
  in blood pressure regulation, 365
  metabolism of, 367
Alexander disease, 861
Alkylating agents, 229, 229*t*
ALL. *See* Acute lymphoblastic leukemia
Allergic alveolitis, 514
Allergic diseases, incidence of, 137
Allergic reactions. *See also* Hypersensitivity reactions
  to blood products, 492–493
  clinical manifestations of, 139*b*
Allergic rhinitis, 137, 138*t*
Allergies, development of, 136–139, 139*b*
Allografts
  defined, 162
  recognition and rejection of, 162
Allorecognition
  direct pathway of, 159–160, 162–163, 164*f*
  indirect pathway of, 162–163, 164*f*
All-trans-retinoic acid (ATRA), 276, 479, 481
Alpha₁ antitrypsin, 658
Alpha₁-antitrypsin deficiency
  clinical features of, 659
  defined, 658
  misfolded proteins in, 46*t*
  morphology of, 659, 659*f*
  pathogenesis of, 658–659
alphaα-thalassemia/mental-retardation-syndrome-X-linked
    gene (ATRX), in IDH mutations, 882
Alport syndrome, 556*t*, 562
Alveoli, 495
  in ARDS, 497*f*
  microscopic structure of, 496*f*
Alzheimer disease (AD), 46, 874–875
  clinical manifestations of, 875
  cognitive impairment in development of, 875
  inflammatory response in development of, 875
  misfolded proteins in, 46*t*
  morphology of, 875*b*, 877*b*
  neuropathologic changes in, 875
  pathogenesis of, 875
Amebiasis, 869
Ameloblastomas, 590
American Academy of Pediatrics, 280–281
American College of Rheumatology, 149–150
American Diabetes Association (ADA), 772
AML. *See* Acute myeloid leukemia
Amniocentesis, in fetal hydrops, 284
Amniotic fluid embolism, 113, 113*f*
Amyloid
  of aging, 183–184
  common forms of, 183
  endocrine, 183–185
  formation of, 183
  histology of, 185–186
  structure of, 183, 184*f*
  use of term, 182
Amyloidosis, 121, 134
  cardiac, 185, 187, 433
  characteristics of, 187*b*
  classification of, 181, 184*t*
  clinical features of, 184–185
  defined, 182
  diagnosis of, 187
  epidemiology of, 183
  gastrointestinal, 187
  of heart, 186
  hemodialysis-associated, 183–187
  heredofamilial, 183
  of kidney, 186
  in liver, 186
  localized, 183–187, 187*b*
  morphology of, 185*b*–186*b*
  pathogenesis of, 183, 186*f*
  pathogenesis of amyloid deposition in, 181, 184*f*
  primary, 181–182

Amyloidosis *(Continued)*
  primary or immunocyte-associated, 474
  prognosis for, 187
  reactive systemic, 182–187
  renal involvement in, 187
  secondary, 86–87
  of spleen, 186
  systemic, 187*b*
  vascular, 187
Amyotrophic lateral sclerosis (ALS), 880
  bulbar, 880
  causes of, 880
  characteristics of, 880
  morphology of, 880*b*
  pathogenesis of, 880
Anaphylatoxins, 76
Anaphylaxis, 137, 138*t*
Anaplasia
  defined, 192
  features of, 193, 193*f*
  of Wilms tumor, 290
Anaplastic lymphoma kinase (*ALK*) gene, and familial
    predisposition to neuroblastoma, 286
Anasarca, 98
Anchoring junctions (desmosomes), in cell-cell interactions,
    12
Ancylostoma duodenale, 620
Androgens, in prostate cancer, 699–700
Anemia, 441. *See also* Immunohemolytic anemia
  aregenerative, 442
  of blood loss, 443
  causes of, 443
  of chronic inflammation, 86–87, 455–456, 458
    clinical features of, 456
    pathogenesis of, 456
  classification of, 442, 442*t*
  clinical consequences of, 442–443
  clinical manifestations of, 443
  of diminished erythropoiesis, 453–458, 458*b*–459*b*
  fetal, 283
  hemolytic, 442–443
  iron deficiency, 453–455
  from lead exposure, 304–305
  megaloblastic, 458
  microangiopathic hemolytic, 452, 452*f*
  morphology of, 443
  myelophthisic, 458–459
  pathology of, 443*b*
  pernicious, 457
  radiation-caused, 322–323
  vitamin B₁₂ deficiency, 457–458
Anemia, aplastic, 458–459
  clinical course of, 458
  pathogenesis of, 458
  radiation-caused, 322–323
Anemia, hemolytic, 443–453, 453*b*
  classification of, 442*t*, 443–444
  glucose-6-phosphate dehydrogenase deficiency,
    450
  hallmarks of, 443
  hereditary spherocytosis, 444–445
  immunohemolytic anemia, 451
  malaria, 452–453, 452*f*
  from mechanical trauma to red cells, 451–452, 452*f*
  paroxysmal nocturnal hemoglobinuria, 450–451
  peripheral blood smear, 452*f*
  sickle cell anemia, 445–447
  thalassemia, 447–450
Anemia, megaloblastic, 456–458
  causes of, 456
  folate deficiency anemia, 456–457
  morphology of, 456*b*, 456*f*
  pathogenesis of, 456
  peripheral blood smear, 456*f*
Anencephaly, 860–861
Anergy, in immunologic tolerance, 145–146, 146*f*
Aneuploidy, 203, 262–263
Aneurysmal bone cyst (ABC), 814
  imaging of, 814, 815*f*
  morphology of, 814*b*, 815*f*
  pathogenesis of, 814
  treatment of, 814
Aneurysms. *See also* Saccular aneurysms
  abdominal aortic, 379–380
  berry, 364
  causes of, 382*b*
  classification of, 378, 378*f*
  defined, 378, 382*b*
  false, 378, 378*f*
  fusiform, 378, 378*f*
  intracranial, 855
  mycotic, 379, 389–390
  pathogenesis of, 378–379
  saccular, 378, 378*f*
  thoracic aortic, 380
  true, 378, 378*f*
Angelman syndrome, 273
  clinical characteristics of, 272
  genetics of, 272*f*
  molecular basis of, 272–273, 272*f*
  neurologic manifestations of, 272
  from uniparental disomy of parental chromosome 15,
    272
Angiitis, allergic, 389

Angina pectoris, 409, 419
  defined, 411
  variants of, 411
Angiodysplasia, lower intestinal bleeding in, 610
Angioedema, hereditary, 172
Angiogenesis
  defined, 90
  process of, 91
  role of VEGFs in, 20
  steps in, 90, 91*f*
  sustained, 219–220, 220*b*
  therapeutic agents blocking, 220
Angiomas, venous, 856
Angiomatosis, bacillary, 394, 394*f*
Angiosarcomas, 396
  etiology of, 396
  morphology of, 396*b*, 396*f*
Angiotensin-converting enzyme (ACE), in blood pressure
    regulation, 365
Anisocytosis, in thalassemia, 449–450
Anitschkow cells, in rheumatic fever, 425
Ankylosing spondylitis, 148*t*, 822
Anlagen, in bone development, 798
Anorexia nervosa, 334*b*
  clinical findings in, 326
  defined, 326
Anovulation, causes of, 722
Anthracosis
  asymptomatic, 509
  pulmonary, 509
  role in cell injury of, 52–53
Anthrax, extoxin action of, 354, 355*f*
Antibiotic resistance, 348
Antibiotic therapy, for infective endocarditis, 427–428
Antibodies, 134*b*, 135
  in humoral immunity, 132–133, 133*f*
  microbial overcoming of, 356
Antibody-mediated disorders (type II hypersensitivity), 135,
    135*f*. *See also* Hypersensitivity reactions
Anticitrullinated protein antibodies (ACPA), in RA, 819
Antidiuretic hormone (ADH), function of, 755
Antidiuretic hormone (ADH) deficiency, clinical
    manifestations of, 755
Antigenic drift, 524
Antigenic variation, of microbes, 355, 356*t*
Antigen-presenting cells (APCs), 127–129, 134*b*
  dendritic cells, 128
  macrophages, 128
Antiinflammatory drugs, 58
Anti-myeloperoxidase (MPO-ANCA), 384
Antineoplastic agents, 312–313, 317*b*
Anti-neutrophil cytoplasmic antibodies (ANCAs), 384
Anti-neutrophil cytoplasmic antibody (ANCA) vasculitis,
    384
Antinuclear antibodies (ANAs), 148–150, 151*t*, 152*f*
  in SLE, 149–150
  staining patterns of, 150, 152*f*
  in systemic sclerosis, 160
Antioxidant mechanisms, 68
Antiphospholipid antibody syndrome
  forms of, 109
  in SLE, 151, 153
Antiproteases, in acute inflammation, 68–69
Antiproteinase-3 (PR3-ANCA), 384
Aortic coarctation, 407–408
  classical forms of, 407, 407*f*
  clinical features of, 408
  morphology of, 408*b*, 408*f*
Aortic dissection, 380–382, 381*f*
  chronic dissection, 381
  classical clinical symptom of, 382
  classification of, 381–382, 382*f*
  clinical consequences of, 381–382
  pathogenesis of, 381
  survival rate for, 382
Aortic stenosis
  calcific, 423–424
  frequency of, 403*t*
APC-B-Catenin pathways, 213, 214*b*
APC/β-catenin pathway, in adenomacarcinoma sequence,
    631–632, 631*f*
Aphthous ulcers
  canker sores, 584, 584*f*
  in Crohn disease, 623
Aplasia, use of term, 275
Aplastic crises, in hereditary spherocytosis, 445
Apolipoprotein E (ApoE), in development of AD,
    875
Apoptosis, 12, 15*f*, 41, 41*b*
  causes of, 37–38, 38*t*
  defined, 37, 38*f*
  deletion by, 145
  features of, 34*t*
  genes regulating, 200
  and growth-promoting signals, 208
  in immunologic tolerance, 145
  in liver disease, 638, 639*f*
  massive, 218–219, 219*f*
  mechanisms of, 38–40, 38*t*, 39*f*
    clearance of apoptotic cells, 39–40
    death receptor (extrinsic) pathway in, 39
    mitochondrial (intrinsic) pathway in, 38–39
  p53-induced, 211
  process of, 34–35

Apoptosis (Continued)
in radiant energy damage, 322
role of mitochondria in, 15, 15f
two major pathways of, 41, 41b
Apoptotic cells
morphologic appearance of, 40, 40b, 40f
phagocytosis of, 39–40
Appendicitis, acute, 634–635, 635b
clinical features of, 635
morphology of, 634b–635b
pathogenesis of, 634
Appendix
lesions of, 634–635
tumors of, 635
APP gene, 875
Arboviruses, 865, 866b
Arnold-Chiari malformation, 862
Aromatic amines, 229t, 230
Array comparative genomic hybridization (aCGH), 293
Arrhythmias, 419–420, 420b
after MI, 417
causes of, 420
in MI, 412
sudden cardiac death, 420
Arrhythmogenic right ventricular cardiomyopathy (ARVC), 432, 433f
Arsenic
chronic exposure to, 306
exposure to, 305–306
toxicity of, 306
Arterial dissections, 378, 378f
Arteries
types of, 362
Arterioles, 362
Arteriolosclerosis, hyperplastic, 570, 571f
Arterionephrosclerosis, 572
Arteriosclerosis
in diabetics
hyaline, 781f, 783
renal, 783
hyaline, 367b–368b, 368f
hyperplastic, 367b–368b, 368f
types of, 369
Arteriovenous (AV) fistulas, 364
Arteriovenous malformations (AVMs), 855–856
morphology of, 857b, 857f
multiple, 855–856
Arthritis, 141t, 825b–826b
crystal-induced, 823–825
infectious, 822
classic presentation of, 822
suppurative arthritis, 822
inflammatory reaction in, 59t
of joints, 141
juvenile idiopathic arthritis, 821–822
Lyme, 822–823
osteoarthritis, 817–825
psoriatic, 892
reactive, 822
rheumatoid arthritis, 818–821
seronegative spondyloarthropathies, 822
Arthus reaction, 141, 141t
Artificial guide RNAs (gRNAs), 5–6, 6f
Asbestos
and lung carcinoma, 539
lung disease associated with, 509t
Asbestos bodies, 511
Asbestos fibers, 511
Asbestosis, 511–512
clinical features of, 511–512
morphology of, 511b, 511f
pathogenesis of, 511
pleural plaques in, 511, 512f
Asbestosis-related diseases, 511–512
Ascaris lumbricoides, 619
Aschoff bodies
microscopic appearance of, 426f
in rheumatic fever, 425
Ascites, 98
Ascorbic acid, antihistamine action of, 332
Askin tumor, 812–813
Aspergilloma ("fungus ball"), 537
Aspergillosis
allergic bronchopulmonary, 537
invasive, 536f, 537
Aspergillus, 229t, 230, 670
Aspirin, adverse reactions to, 314–315
Asteroid bodies, in sarcoidosis, 513
Asthma, 503–505, 505b
atopic, 503, 505
bronchial biopsy specimen in, 505, 505f
clinical features of, 505
and COPD, 499f
drug-induced, 503
hallmarks of, 503
inflammatory reaction in, 59t
morphologic changes in, 504f–505f, 505b
non-atopic, 503, 505
occupational, 503
pathogenesis of, 503
role of genetics in, 503
Astrocytes, 850, 850f

Astrocytomas
diffuse, 881
morphology of, 882f
pilocytic, 883, 883b
subependymal giant cell, 887
well-differentiated, 882
Ataxia telangiectasia, 171, 227, 227b–228b
defined, 495–496
forms of, 495–496
Atherogenesis, 378
contribution of diet to, 337–338
dyslipidemia in, 374
hypercholesterolemia in, 373–374
and hypertension, 367–368
Atheromas, 369, 374–376
calcification of, 375f
clinically silent, 410
Atheromatous plaque, basic structure of, 370, 370f
Atherosclerosis, 58, 110f, 111, 369–378, 370f
aortic aneurysms in, 379
and cigarette smoking, 309
clinical consequences of, 376–378, 377f
acute plaque change, 377–378, 377f
atherosclerotic stenosis, 376–377, 377f
in diabetics, 779, 783
endothelial injury in, 372–373, 373f
epidemiology of, 370–376, 370f, 371t
in familial hypercholesterolemia, 250b
fatty streaks in, 374, 375f
hemodynamic disturbances in, 373
inflammatory reaction in, 59t, 374
lipids in, 373–374, 373f
matrix synthesis in, 374–376
medial degeneration in, 379, 379f, 381
pathogenesis of, 372, 373f
renal, in diabetics, 783
risk factors for, 371–376
constitutional, 370–371, 371t
modifiable, 371
SMC proliferation in, 374–376
Atherosclerotic plaques, 374b–376b, 375f, 378
acute changes in, 377–378, 377f, 410, 410f
components of, 374–376
factors triggering erosion of, 410
inflammation of, 377–378
neovascularization of, 374–376, 375f
residual, 397, 397f
rupture of, 376f–377f, 377–378
stable, 378
thrombosis associated with, 409
ulcerated, 374, 375f
vasoconstriction in, 409
Atherosclerotic stenosis, 376–377, 377f
ATP. See Adenosine triphosphate
ATP7B gene, 658
Atresia, use of term, 275
Atrial fibrillation, 402, 420
Atrial septal defects (ASDs), 404, 404f
clinical features of, 405
in contrast to patent foramen ovale, 405
frequency of, 403t
morphology of, 405b
ostium primum, 405
ostium secundum, 405
pathogenesis of, 405
sinus venosus, 405
Atrioventricular septal defects, 403t
Atrophy, 51b
of brain, 50f
causes of, 50
in congenital heart disease, 404
defined, 50
ATRX (α-thalassemia/mental-retardation-syndrome-X-linked gene)
in development of AD, 875, 876f
in IDH mutations, 882
Atypical adenomatous hyperplasia (AAH), 539, 540f
Auer rods, 480, 480f
Auspitz sign, 892
Autism, 860
Autoantibodies
in autoimmune diseases, 151t
in SLE, 153
Autocrine signaling, 16
Autoimmune diseases and disorders, 58, 81, 134, 142–144
autoantibodies in, 151t
examples of, 145t
and immunologic tolerance, 143–144
incidence of, 145
non-HLA genes associated with, 147, 148t
organ-specific, 145, 145t
pulmonary hypertension associated with, 517
Autoimmune hemolytic anemia, 139, 139t, 140f
Autoimmune lymphoproliferative syndrome (ALPS), 145
Autoimmune myositis, autoantibodies in, 151t
Autoimmunity, 134, 145, 149b–150b
gender bias of, 148–149
HLA alleles in, 127
mechanisms of, 145–147
environmental insults, 148
generic factors, 146–147, 148t
role of infections in, 146–147
tissue injury, 149

Autoimmunity (Continued)
pathogenesis of, 145, 147f
in systemic sclerosis, 159
Autoinflammatory syndromes
excessive production of cytokine IL-1 in, 185
in inflammatory response, 60
Automatic cardioverter defibrillator, in chronic IHD, 420
Autophagy, 13, 14f, 40, 41f
defined, 216, 217b
extensive, 40
in lysosomal storage diseases, 255–256
Autosomal dominant inheritance disorders, 246–247, 247b
Autosomal recessive inheritance disorders, 246, 247b
Autosplenectomy, in sickle cell anemia, 446
Avian influenza, 524
Axonal neuropathies, 835, 836f
Axonal processes, 835
Azo dyes, 229t, 230
Azoospermia, in cystic fibrosis, 252–253
Azotemia, 549
in heart failure, 402
post-renal, 549
pre-renal, 549

B
BACE (β-amyloid-converting enzyme), in development of AD, 875, 876f
Bacillary angiomatosis, 394, 394f
Bacille Calmette-Guérin (BCG)
in bladder cancer, 704
in prostatitis, 697–698
"Back to Sleep" campaign, 280–281
Bacteria
and biofilms, 354
characteristics of, 342t
CRISPRs in, 6f
morphology of, 344f
quorum sensing of, 354
Bacterial infections
and adherence to host cells, 354
pathogens of, 342–343, 344t
of skin, 894
toxins, 354
virulence of, 353–354
Bacteriophages, and bacterial injury, 353–354
Balanitis, of penis, 691
Balanoposthitis, of penis, 691
Bannayan-Ruvalcaba-Riley syndrome, 627t
Barbiturates, protracted use of, 33–34
Barrett esophagus, 595–596, 595f
clinical features of, 595–596
and gastric cancer, 604
incidence of, 595
intestinal metaplasia of, 595, 595f
management of, 595–596
morphology of, 595b, 595f
Basal cell carcinoma of skin
clinical features of, 902
morphology of, 902b, 902f
pathogenesis of, 902
Basement membrane, formation of, 22
Basement membrane thickening
in diabetic microangiopathy, 781f, 783
in diabetic nephropathy, 781f, 783
diffuse mesangial sclerosis associated with, 783
Basic fibroblast growth factors (bFGF), in angiogenesis, 220, 220b
B (bone marrow-derived) lymphocytes, 124–125, 125f, 134b
B cell neoplasms
classification of, 465t
precursor, 466, 466t
B-cell receptor (BCR), 127–128, 128f, 132
B cells. See also B lymphocytes
APC properties of, 128
in HIV infection, 177
location of, 129–130, 129f
on skin, 889
B cell tumors, 464f, 465
BCL6 gene, 470
Bcl-2 proteins, 38–39, 39f
Bcl-xL proteins, 38–39, 39f
BCR gene, 202
Becker muscular dystrophy (BMD), 842–843
clinical features of, 843
morphology of, 842b
pathogenesis of, 843
Beckwith-Wiedemann syndrome (BWS), 289
Bell clapper abnormality, 693
Bence Jones proteins, 183, 473
the "bends", 113–114
Benign prostatic hyperplasia (BPH), 698, 699b
clinical features of, 698–699
morphology of, 698b, 698f–699f
treatment of, 698–699
Benzo[a]pyrene, 229–230, 229t
Berry aneurysms, 364
Beta-catenin mutations, in HCCs, 670
Betal quid, and oral cancer, 586–587
ß-carotene, 338
and vitamin A, 327
Bhopal, India, methyl isocyanate gas leak in, 299
Bicuspid aortic valve, abnormality of, 423, 423f
Bile, formation of, 660

Bile ducts
  anatomy of, 637
  obstruction of, 661–662
Biliary atresia
  clinical features of, 663
  defined, 663
  morphology of, 663b
  pathogenesis of, 663
Biliary cirrhosis, primary, 664t
Biliary obstruction
  acute, 662
  chronic, 662
  extrahepatic, 662
Bilirubin, production of, 659–660, 660f
Binding sites, for protein factors, 2
Bioaerosols, health effects of, 303
Bioterrorism, agents of, 348, 348t
Biotin
  deficiency syndrome for, 333t
  functions of, 333t
Bisphenol A (BPA), 307
  Schistosoma haematobium infection of, 358, 358f
  and tobacco smoke carcinogens, 309t
Bladder, male
  neo-neoplastic conditions of, 702
  neoplasms of, 702–704
    clinical features of, 704
    papillary urothelial tumor, 703, 703f–704f, 703t
    treatment for, 704
  urothelial carcinoma in
    morphology of, 703b
    pathogenesis of, 702–703
    precursor lesions of, 703, 703f–704f
Blastocysts, and role of stem cells, 27f
Blastomyces dermatitidis, 532
  epidemiology of, 532–533
  morphology of, 532, 533f
Blebs, in cell injury, 33f, 43
Bleeding, abnormal uterine, 722–723, 722t
Bleeding disorders, 441, 486–488, 491b. *See also* Hemorrhage
  coagulation disorders, 491
  disseminated intravascular coagulation, 486–487
  etiology of, 485
  thrombocytopenia, 489
Blister, definition of, 890t
Blistering (bullous) disorders, 895–899, 899b
  bullous pemphigoid, 896–898
  dermatitis herpetiformis, 898–899
  diagnosis of, 895, 897f
  pemphigus, 895–896
Blood
  exit of microbes via, 352
  in lead exposure, 304f, 305
  spread of microbes via, 351
Blood alcohol level, 310
Blood-brain barrier, role of ECs in, 363
Blood loss
  anemia of, 443
  chronic, 443
Blood pressure, in acute-phase response, 87. *See also* Hypertension
Blood products, 491
Blood vessels
  in acute inflammation, 60–62, 60b
  aneurysms and dissections, 378–382
  arteriosclerosis, 369
  atherosclerosis, 369–378, 370f
  blood pressure regulation in, 364–365, 365b, 365f
  concentric layers of, 361–362, 362f
  congenital anomalies in, 364
  disorders of blood vessel hyperreactivity, 390
    myocardial vessel vasospasm, 390
    Raynaud phenomenon, 390
  hypertensive vascular disease, 366–367, 367t, 368b, 368f
  intermediate-grade tumors of
    hemangioendotheliomas, 395–396
    Kaposi sarcoma, 394–395
  malignant tumors of, 396, 396f
  pathology of vascular intervention in, 397
    endovascular stenting, 397, 397f
    vascular replacement, 397
  structure and function of, 361–364, 364b
    endothelial cells, 363–364, 363f, 363t
    vascular organization, 362–363
    vascular smooth muscle cells, 364
  tumors of, 391–396, 392t
  vascular tumors of, 396b
  vascular wall response to injury of, 368–369, 369f
  vasculitis of, 382–390
  veins, 390–391
    phlebothrombosis, 391
    thrombophlebitis, 391
    varicose veins, 390
Blood volume, regulation of, 365, 366f
Bloom syndrome, 227, 227b–228b
"Blueberry muffin baby", 288–289
"Blue bloaters", 501
B lymphocytes, 124. *See also* B cells
  activation of, 132, 133f
  antigen receptors of, 130, 131f
  in chronic inflammation, 84
Body mass index (BMI), 334

Body weight
  edema in, 98
  and energy balance, 334, 335f
Bone
  bone-forming tumors of, 808–810, 808t, 817
    osteoblastoma, 808
    osteoid osteoma, 808
    osteosarcoma, 809–810
  cartilage-forming tumors of, 808t, 810–812, 817
    chondroma, 811–812, 811f
    chondrosarcoma, 812
    osteochondroma, 810–811
  congenital disorders of, 799–801, 801b
    achondroplasia, 800
    dysostoses, 800
    dysplasias, 800
    osteogenesis imperfecta, 800
    osteopetrosis, 800–801
    thanatophoric dysplasia, 800
  fractures of, 805–806
  homeostasis of, 799
  lesions simulating primary neoplasms of
    fibrous dysplasia, 815–816
    nonossifying fibroma, 814–815, 815f–816f
  metabolic disorders of, 801–803, 803b
    hyperparathyroidism, 802–803
    osteomalacia, 802
    osteopenia and osteoporosis, 801–802
    rickets, 802
  metastatic tumors of, 816
  osteomyelitis of, 806–808
  osteonecrosis of, 806
  Paget disease of, 803–805
  remodeling of, 799, 799f
  structure and function of, 797–799
    cells, 797–798
    development in, 798–799, 799f
    flat bones, 798–799
    matrix, 797, 798f
  tumors and tumorlike lesions of, 817b
  tumors of, 808–816
    classification of, 808, 808t
    clinical manifestations of, 808
    prevalence of, 808
  tumors of unknown origin of
    aneurysmal bone cyst, 814
    Ewing sarcoma, 812–813
    giant cell tumor, 813–814
  woven, 805–806
Bone destruction, in multiple myeloma, 475
Bone marrow
  in malnutrition, 326
  mesenchymal stem cells, 28
  in sarcoidosis, 513
Bone matrix
  lamellar, 798f
  woven, 798f
Bone multicellular unit (BMU), 799
Borrelia burgdorferi, in Lyme arthritis, 822–823
Bovine spongiform encephalopathy (BSE) (mad cow disease), 870
Bowel, vascular disorders of, 609–610, 610b–611b
  hemorrhoids, 610
  ischemic bowel disease, 609–610
"Boxcar nuclei", 421
BPH. *See* Benign prostatic hyperplasia
Bradycardia, 419–420. *See also* Arrhythmias
Bradykinin, 77
BRAF gene, 764, 765f
Brain. *See also* Central nervous system
  amyloid in, 186
  atrophy of, 50f
  blood flow for, 852
  diffuse axonal injury to, 858
  infarcts in, 115
  in lead exposure, 304f, 305
  in malnutrition, 326
  penetration of, 857–858
  respirator, 852–853
  trauma to, 857
Brain injury
  concussions, 858
  contusions, 857–858
Breast
  fibroadenoma of, 194–195, 194f
  invasive ductal carcinoma of, 195f
Breast, female
  benign epithelial lesions of, 738, 739f, 739t
  carcinoma of, 739–746, 747f
    classification of, 740, 740f, 740t
    clinical features in, 744–746
    incidence of, 739–740, 740f
    inflammatory, 744
    invasive, 739t
    invasive infiltrating, 743–744, 744f
    lifetime risk of, 740
    major types of, 740
    with medullary features, 743–744, 744f
    morphology of, 742b–744b, 743f–744f
    mucinous colloid, 744
    noninvasive (in situ) carcinoma, 742–743
    pathogenesis of, 741–742, 742f
    prognosis for, 745–746, 745f
    risk factors for, 739t, 741–746

Breast, female (Continued)
    staging for, 745–746
    survival rates for, 746, 746f
    targeted treatment for, 746, 746t
    tubular, 744
  functional unit of, 736, 736f
  function of, 736
  inflammatory processes of, 737
  origins of disorders of, 736f
  stromal tumors, 738, 738b, 738f
Breast cancer
  family history in, 741
  in Klinefelter syndrome, 267
  risk for, 200
  role of DNA repair genes in, 227, 227b–228b
Breast disease
  clinical presentations of, 736–737, 737b, 737f
  presenting symptoms of, 737f
Brenner tumor, 729–730
Breslow thickness, 906
Bridge-fusion-breakage cycles, 218–219, 219f
Bronchial asthma, 137, 138t
Bronchiectasis, 505–506
  clinical features of, 506
  conditions predisposed to, 505–506
  defined, 505–506
  histologic findings in, 506
  morphology of, 506b, 506f
  pathogenesis of, 506
  in patient with cystic fibrosis, 506, 506f
Bronchioalveolar stem cells (BASCs), in pulmonary adenocarinomas, 539
Bronchioles, 495
Bronchiolitis
  chronic, 502
  obliterans, 502
Bronchitis
  chronic, 502b
    clinical features of, 502
    and COPD, 499f
    defined, 498
    diagnosis of, 502
    lumen of bronchus in, 502b, 502f
    morphology of, 502b, 502f
    pathogenesis of, 502
  and smoking, 309
Bronchopneumonia, 522, 522f
Bronchopulmonary dysplasia (BPD), pathogenesis of, 279
Brown tumor, 803, 803f
Brunn nests, of male bladder, 702
Bruton disease, 168–173. *See also* X-linked agammaglobulinemia
Budd-Chiari syndrome, 483, 667, 667b, 667f
Buerger disease. *See* Thromboangiitis obliterans
"Buffalo hump," in Cushing syndrome, 789
Bulimia
  clinical manifestations of, 326
  defined, 326
Bulla, definition of, 890t
Bullous pemphigoid, 896–898
  clinical features of, 897–898
  compared with pemphigus vulgaris, 896–897
  morphology of, 897, 898f
  pathogenesis of, 896–897, 898f
Burkitt lymphoma, 202, 233–234, 233f, 234b, 466t, 471, 478–484
  chromosomal translocations and oncogenes in, 202, 202f
  clinical features of, 472–473
  immunophenotype for, 472
  morphology of, 471b, 471f
  pathogenesis of, 471–472
  possible evolution of EBV-induced, 233f
Burns
  appearance of, 318
  clinical severity of, 318
  defined, 318
  electrical, 320
  full-thickness, 318
  partial-thickness, 318

C
Cachexia, 326
  cancer and, 236, 237b
  defined, 238
  in thalassemia, 450
Cadherins, 213
Cadmium toxicity, 306
Calcification
  abnormal, 54b
  pathologic, 54b
    in cell injury, 53
    dystrophic calcification, 53, 53b–54b
    metastatic calcification, 53, 53b–54b
    morphology of, 53b–54b
Calciphylaxis, 771
Calcium pyrophosphate crystal deposition disease (CPPD), 825
  characteristics of, 825
  pseudogout, 825
Caliectasis, 566–567
Callus, in bone fracture, 805–806
Calyceal deformities, 566, 566f

Campylobacter infection
　clinical features of, 616–617
　morphology of, 616b, 616f
　pathogenesis of, 616
Campylobacter jejuni, 616
Campylobacter spp., 615t
CAMs. *See* Cellular adhesion molecules
Cancer, 16. *See also specific cancers*
　age and, 199
　characteristics of, 189–190
　in children, 199
　chronic inflammatory states associated with, 199, 199t
　and diet, 338
　epidemiology of, 189, 196–200, 200b
　　and acquired predisposing conditions, 199, 199t
　　and age, 199
　　environmental factors, 197–199, 198t
　　incidence, 197, 198f
　　and interactions between environmental and genetic
　　　factors, 200
　genetic alterations of, 189–190
　genetic lesions in, 201–204, 204b
　　aneuploidy, 203
　　deletions, 202–203, 204b
　　driver and passenger mutations, 201–204
　　epigenetic modifications, 203–204, 204b
　　gene amplifications, 203
　　gene rearrangements, 201–202, 204b
　　microRNAs and cancer, 203
　　point mutations, 201
　and host response to microbes, 355
　inherited predisposition to, 201t
　laboratory diagnosis of, 237–241
　　molecular diagnosis, 239, 240f
　　with molecular profiling in, 239–241, 241f
　　morphologic methods, 238, 238f
　　tumor markers, 238–239
　and obesity, 334, 337
　occupational, 198t
　secondary, 323
Cancer cells, self-sufficiency of, 206
Cancer genes, 200–201, 201t
　defined, 200
　functional classes of, 200
The Cancer Genome Atlas (TCGA), 240
Cancer hallmarks, 189–190, 204–228, 205f
　altered cellular metabolism
　　autophagy, 216, 217b
　　oncometabolism, 216–217, 216f, 217b
　　and Warburg effect, 214–217, 215f, 217b
　and enabling characteristics, 205
　evasion of cell death, 217f
　genomic instability as enabler of malignancy, 226,
　　227b–228b
　　cancers resulting from mutations induced by regulated
　　　genomic instability, 227, 227b–228b
　　diseases with defects in DNA repair by homologous
　　　recombination, 227, 227b–228b
　　hereditary nonpolyposis colon cancer syndrome, 227,
　　　227b–228b
　　xeroderma pigmentosum, 227, 227b–228b
　immune surveillance and escape, 226f
　insensitivity to growth inhibitory signals, 208–213
　　contact inhibition, 213, 214b
　　retinoblastoma gene, 208–211, 209f–210f, 211b
　　TP53, 211–212, 212b–213b, 212f
　　transforming growth factor-beta pathway, 213, 214b
　invasion and metastasis, 220–223
　　invasion of ECM, 220–222, 221f
　　metastasis, 223, 223b
　　vascular dissemination and homing of tumor cells in,
　　　222–223
　limitless replicative potential (immortality), 218–219, 219b,
　　219f
　self-sufficiency in growth signals, 205–208, 206f, 208b
　　ABL, 207, 208b
　　cyclins and cyclin-dependent kinases, 207–208, 208b
　　downstream signal-transducing proteins, 206–207
　　growth factor receptors, 206
　　growth factors, 206
　　nuclear transcription factors, 207, 208b
　　RAS, 206–207, 206f, 208b
　sustained angiogenesis, 219–220, 220b
　therapeutic targeting of, 229f
　tumor antigens, 225f
　tumor-promoting inflammation as enabler of malignancy,
　　228
Candida albicans, 535
Candidal vaginitis, 716
Candidiasis, 535–536
　and broad-spectrum antibiotics, 585
　chronic mucocutaneous, 535
　clinical features of, 535–536
　cutaneous, 535
　invasive, 535–536
　morphology of, 535b, 536f
　on muscosal surfaces of oral cavity, 535
　oral, 585
Canker sores, 584, 584f
Capillaries. *See also* Blood vessels
　fluid movement across, 98, 99f
　structure and function of, 362
Capillary hemangioblastoma, cerebellar, 887b
Capillary telangiectasias, 855–856

Capsid, 341–342
Carbon monoxide (CO), 303, 303b–304b
　acute poisoning by, 303
　chronic poisoning by, 303
Carbon tetrachloride (CCl₄), 33–34
Carcinogenesis, 204, 205f
　and ionizing radiation, 321, 321f
　mutations in, 604
Carcinogenic agents, 228–235, 229t, 231b
　chemical carcinogens, 228–230, 229t, 231b
　radiation carcinogenesis, 231, 231b
　viral and microbial oncogenesis, 231–235
Carcinogens. *See also* Chemical carcinogens; Pollutants;
　　Toxins
　endogenous synthesis of, 338
　exogenous, 338
Carcinoid, of appendix, 635
Carcinoid heart disease
　characteristics of, 438
　morphology of, 439b, 439f
　pathogenesis of, 439
Carcinoid tumors, 543–544, 605. *See also* Neuroendocrine
　　tumors
　atypical, 543–544
　classification of, 543
　morphology of, 543b–544b, 543f
　signs and symptoms of, 544
Carcinoma, 764–768
　adrenocortical, 793f–794f, 795
　of cervix, 720
　designation as, 190–191
　embryonal, 694–695, 694t, 695f
　endometrial, 724, 724b
　　categories of, 724
　　clinical features of, 724
　　exome sequencing of, 724
　　morphology of, 724b, 725f
　　pathogenesis of, 724
　endometrioid, 724, 725f
　of gallbladder, 675
　invasive ductal, 195f
　of larynx, 546–547, 547f
　　pathogenesis of, 547f
　of lung, 543b
　　adenocarcinomas, 540f
　　clinical features of, 540–543
　　etiology and pathogenesis for, 538–539
　　histologic types of, 538
　　incidence of, 537–538
　　large cell carcinomas, 539
　　morphology of, 539b–540b, 540f–542f
　　NSCLC *vs.* SCLC, 538, 542t
　　small cell carcinomas, 539–540, 542f
　　squamous cell carcinomas, 539, 541f
　　targeted therapy for, 538
　nasopharyngeal, 546
　of parathyroid, 770
　penile, 691
　renal cell, 578–580
　of thyroid, 762
　undifferentiated, 190–191
　urothelial, 702
　verrucous, 691–692
Carcinoma, mucoepidermoid
　clinical course and prognosis for, 589
　morphology of, 589b
　of salivary glands, 589
Carcinoma in situ (CIS), 194f
　defined, 193–194
　in male bladder, 703, 704f
Cardiac cirrhosis, 402
Cardiac diseases, economic impact of, 399. *See also* Heart
　　disease
Cardiac enlargement, cellular adaptation of, 48–49, 49f
Cardiac morphogenesis, 404
Cardiac output
　in blood pressure regulation, 364–365, 365f
　reduced, 99, 99f
Cardiac tamponade, 436–437
Cardiac transplantation, 439
　major complications of, 439
　survival rate for, 439
Cardiac tumors
　effects of noncardiac neoplasms on, 438–439, 438t, 439f
　primary neoplasms, 437–438
Cardiomyopathies, 429–435, 435b–436b
　arrhythmogenic right ventricular, 432, 433f
　characteristics of, 433
　classification of, 429, 430f, 430t
　dilated, 429–432, 430f
　hypertrophic, 432–433
　myocarditis, 434–435
　peripartum, 431
　restrictive, 430f, 433–434
　　forms of, 433–434
　　morphology of, 434b
Cardiorespiratory complications, in CF, 253–254
Cardiovascular disease, 399. *See also* Heart disease
　and climate change, 300
　and obesity, 334
Cardiovascular system, 247
　in chronic alcoholism, 312
　and cocaine use, 315
　in SLE, 156, 157f

Carditis, chronic rheumatic, 426–427
Carotenoids, 327
Cartilage, congenital disorders of, 799–801, 801b
Cas9 enzyme, 5–6, 6f
Cas (or CRISPR-associated genes), 5–6
Caspases, 353
CASR calcium-sensing receptor gene, in primary
　　hyperparathyroidism, 770
Catalase, in alcohol metabolism, 310
Catecholamine metabolites, in neuroblastoma, 288–289
Catenin, in cell-cell interactions, 12
Cat-scratch disease
　clinical features of, 462
　with granulomatous inflammation, 86b
　morphology of, 462b
Caveolae, in endocytosis, 9, 10f
Cavernous hemangiomas, of liver, 669
Cavernous malformations, 855–856
CCR5 gene, in HIV infection, 175
CD4+ helper T cells, 134b, 152
CD40L mutations, 170–171
CD4+ T cell-mediated hypersensitivity reactions,
　　142
CD4+ T cell-mediated inflammatory reactions, 142, 144f,
　　145b
CD4+ T cells
　in cell-mediated immunity, 131f
　and HIV infection, 124–125
　in HIV infection, 175, 178f
CD8+ cytotoxic T cells, 134b
　in emphysema, 500, 500f
　in erythema multiforme, 891
CD8+ T cell-mediated cytotoxicity, 142–145
CD8+ T lymphocytes (CTLs)
　activated, 131
　in cell-mediated immunity, 131f
CD21 cell, 127–128
CDH1 gene, mutations in, 604
CDKIs. *See* Cyclin-dependent kinase inhibitors
CD8+ T lymphocytes, in celiac disease, 613
Celiac disease, 612–613, 898
　clinical features of, 613
　and dermatitis herpetiformis, 898–899
　HLA alleles associated with, 148t
　morphologic alterations in, 612f
　morphology of, 613b, 613f
　pathogenesis of, 612–613
　pediatric, 613
Cell-cell interactions, 12
Cell communication
　cell signaling in, 16, 17f
　importance of, 16
Cell cycle, 24–25, 25f
　activators and inhibitors regulating, 25, 26f
　biosynthesis and growth in, 25
　checkpoints in, 25, 208
　landmarks of, 25f
Cell cycle control, loss of normal, 210–211, 211b
Cell death, 31–32, 34–35
　apoptosis, 37–40, 38f
　mechanisms of, 41–48, 42f
　　hypoxia and ischemia, 42–43, 43f
　　ischemia-reperfusion injury, 43
　　oxidative stress, 43–45, 44f, 44t
　necroptosis, 40
　necrosis, 35–37, 35b, 36f–37f
　patterns of, 41b
　process of programmed, 7
　pyroptosis, 40
　types of, 34, 34t
Cell growth and maintenance, 7–8
Cell injury, 31–40, 32f
　causes of, 32–33
　common events in, 47–48
　　defects in membrane permeability, 47–48, 48b
　　mitochondrial dysfunction, 47, 47f, 48b
　duration of, 35, 35f
　intracellular accumulations causing, 51–53,
　　52f–53f
　intracellular changes associated with, 33, 33f
　irreversible, 34
　mechanisms of, 41–48, 42f, 48b
　　caused by toxins, 45
　　DNA damage, 47
　　ER stress in, 45–46, 46f, 46t
　　hypoxia and ischemia, 42–43, 43f
　　inflammation, 47
　　ischemia-reperfusion injury, 43
　　oxidative stress, 43–45, 44f, 44t
　morphologic changes in irreversible, 34f
　patterns of, 41b
　persistent or excessive, 34
　reversible, 31–34, 32f, 33b, 34f
Cell junctions, types of, 12
Cell lysis, in complement system, 76, 76f
Cell-mediated immunity, in tuberculosis, 527
Cell polarity, 7
Cell proliferation
　normal, 205
　in scar formation, 90
Cells
　functions of, 6
　growth factor activity in, 19
　interaction with extracellular matrix of, 21–24, 21f

Cells *(Continued)*
    maintaining populations of, 24–28
        cell cycle in, 24–25, 25*f*
        cell proliferation, 24
        mechanisms regulating, 27*f*
        stem cells, 25–28, 27*f*–28*f*
    and mitochondrial function, 13–16
    waste disposal of, 13, 14*f*
Cell senescence, and growth-promoting signals, 208
Cell signaling, 16, 17*f*
    categories of receptors in, 16, 17*f*
    classification of, 16
    extracellular cell-cell, 16
    receptor proteins in, 16, 17*f*
    transduction pathways in, 16–18, 17*f*
        G-protein coupled receptors, 18
        modular signaling proteins, 18–19
        nonreceptor tyrosine kinase, 18
        Notch family receptors, 18
        nuclear receptors, 18
        receptors associated with kinase activity, 18
        receptor tyrosine kinases, 18
        transcription factors, 19
        Wnt protein ligands, 18
Cellular abnormalities, 1
Cellular adhesion molecules (CAMs), 23–24, 24*f*
Cellular dysfunction, in type II hypersensitivity, 139,
        140*f*
Cellular metabolism, altered, 214–217, 215*f*, 217*b*
Cellular proliferation, key elements of, 24
Cellular responses, 31–32, 32*f*. *See also* Adaptation
Center for Disease Control and Prevention (CDC)
    bioweapons ranked by, 348, 348*t*
    HIV classification of, 179, 179*t*
    on lead exposure, 304
    STD notification required by, 704–705
Central chromatolysis, 849
Central nervous system (CNS)
    acquired metabolic and toxic disturbances of, 873
    cerebral edema in, 850–851, 851*f*, 852*b*
    congenital malformations of, 860–861, 862*b*
        forebrain malformations, 861
        incidence of, 860
        neural tube deficits, 860–861
        neurologic deficits, 860
        posterior fossa anomalies, 861
        spinal cord abnormalities, 862–870
    demyelinating diseases of, 871–872
    diseases of, 849
    effects of cocaine on, 315, 316*f*
    genetic metabolic diseases of, 873
    herniation, 851, 852*b*, 852*f*
    in HIV infection, 177
    hydrocephalus, 851, 851*f*, 852*b*
    infections of, 863, 863*t*
        epidural and subdural infections, 862
        meningitis, 863, 863*t*
        parenchymal infections, 864–868
        spirochetal infections, 864–868
    metabolic disorders of, 873
    nutritional diseases affecting, 873
    perinatal brain injury, 861–862, 862*f*, 863*b*
    protective environment for, 850
    in SLE, 156
    toxic disorders of, 873–874
    trauma to, 857–862, 862*b*
        epidural hematoma, 858, 859*f*, 859*t*
        parenchymal injuries, 857–858, 858*f*
        subdural hematoma, 858–860, 859*f*, 859*t*, 860*b*
        traumatic vascular injury, 858–860, 859*f*, 859*t*
    tumors of, 881–887
        embryonal (primitive) neoplasms, 884
        familial tumor syndromes, 886–887
        germ cell tumors, 885
        gliomas, 881
        meningiomas, 885
        metastatic, 885–886, 886*f*
        neuronal tumors, 883–884
        primary central nervous system lymphoma, 884–885,
            885*b*
Central nervous system (CNS) disease, in AIDS, 181
Centrilobular necrosis, 402
Centromeres, 2, 2*f*
Cepacia syndrome, in cystic fibrosis, 252–253
Cerebral amyloid angiopathy (CAA), 855
Cerebral cavernous malformation (CCM) genes, 285
Cerebral edema, 850–851, 851*f*, 852*b*
Cerebral palsy, 862
Cerebrovascular accident (stroke), 97
Cerebrovascular diseases, 852–853, 858*b*
    and climate change, 300
    hypertensive cerebrovascular disease, 856–857
    hypoxia, 852
    intracranial hemorrhage, 854
        cerebral amyloid angiopathy, 855
        primary brain parenchymal hemorrhage, 854,
            855*f*
        secular aneurysms, 855
        subarachnoid hemorrhage, 855
        vascular malformations, 855–856
    ischemia, 852
    pathogenic mechanisms in, 852
    vasculitis, 857
Cervical cancer, decrease in, 197

Cervical intraepithelial neoplasia (CIN)
    of cervix, 717
    cytologic features of, 719*f*
    spectrum of, 719*f*
Cervical os, with surrounding invasive carcinoma, 720*f*
Cervicitis
    classification of, 717
    nongonococcal, 703*f*, 709–710
    pathogens in, 717
Cervix, diseases and disorders of
    cervicitis, 717
    neoplasia, 717–720, 717*f*, 720*b*–721*b*
        clinical features of, 720
        endocervical polyp, 720
        invasive carcinoma of, 720
        morphology of, 720*b*, 720*f*
        pathogenesis of, 717–718
        risk factors for, 720
        squamous intraepithelial lesion, 718–720
CFTR. *See* Cystic fibrosis transmembrane conductance
        regulator
CFTR gene, mutation in, 12
CFTR mutations, chronic pancreatitis associated with,
        683
Chagas disease, 434–435, 436*f*
Chamber dilation, after MI, 418
Chancre, of syphilis, 706*f*
Chancroid, 711*b*
    morphology of, 710*b*
    prevalence of, 710
Channelopathies, 844
Chaperone molecules, 12
Charcot joints, 868
Charcot-Leyden crystals, in asthma, 505
Chédiak-Higashi syndrome, 172, 172*t*
Chemical carcinogens, 228–230, 229*t*, 231*b*
    direct-acting agents, 229, 229*t*
    indirect-acting agents, 229–230, 229*t*
    mechanisms of action of, 230, 230*f*
Chemicals, 303*b*–304*b*
    metabolic activation of, 301–302
    potential health effects of, 301
    toxicology of, 301–302
Chemokines, 74–75
    activities of, 74–75
    in acute inflammation, 75
    classification of, 74
    functions of, 75
    in target tissues for metastasis, 222
Chemotaxis, of leukocytes, 65
Chernobyl nuclear accident, 299, 765
    and radiation carcinogenesis, 231
    survivors of, 323
Chiari type 1 malformation, 862
Chikungunya virus, 348
Childbirth, transmission of microbes during, 352
Children
    cancer deaths in, 467
    cancers in, 199
    type 2 diabetes in, 779
Childs-Pugh classification, 641–642
Chimney sweeps, scrotal cancers in, 306
Chlamydia, 343, 709–710
Chlamydia trachomatis, 705*t*, 709
    clinical features of, 709
    forms of, 709
    in NGU, 709
Chloride channel defect, in CF, 251–252, 251*f*,
        254
Chlorpromazine, hepatotoxicity of, 651–652
Chocolate cysts, 722
Cholangiocarcinoma (CCA), 671–672
    morphology of, 671*b*, 672*f*
    risk factors for, 671
Cholangiopathies, autoimmune, 663–665
    primary biliary cirrhosis, 663–664
    primary sclerosing cholangitis, 664–665
Cholangitis
    ascending, 662, 662*f*
Cholecystitis, 674–675
    acute acalculous, 674–675
    acute calculous, 674
    chronic, 674–675, 675*f*
    clinical features of, 674–675
    morphology of, 674
Cholelithiasis, and obesity, 337
Cholera, 614–616, 615*t*
    and climate change, 300
    clinical features of, 616
    pathogenesis of, 616
Cholestasis, 665–666, 665*b*–666*b*
    defined, 661
    intrahepatic, 662
    morphologic features of, 661*b*, 661*f*
    neonatal, 662, 665
Cholestatic syndromes, 659–665
    autoimmune cholangiopathies, 663–665
    biliary atresia, 663, 664*t*
    bilirubin and bile formation, 659–660, 660*f*
    cholestasis, 661–662
    defects in hepatocellular bilirubin metabolism,
        661
    neonatal cholestasis, 662
    pathophysiology of jaundice, 660–661

Cholesterol
    in atherosclerosis, 371
    in hypothyroidism, 757
    normal metabolism of, 248–249, 249*f*–250*f*
    in U.S. diet, 337–338
Cholesterol and cholesteryl esters, cell injury caused by, 51,
        52*f*
Cholesterol gallstones, in gallbladder, 673, 673*f*
Chondroma, 811–812, 811*f*
    clinical course for, 812
    morphology of, 812*b*, 812*f*
    pathogenesis of, 812
Chondrosarcoma, 812
    classification of, 812
    clinical course for, 812
    designation as, 190–191
    morphology of, 812*b*, 813*f*
    pathogenesis of, 812
Choriocarcinoma, 694*t*, 695, 695*f*
Choriocarcinoma, gestational, 734
    clinical features of, 734
    morphology of, 734*b*, 734*f*
Choristoma, 191, 285
Choroid plexus, 850
Christmas disease, 489
Chromatids, 2*f*
Chromatin
    erasers, 4
    structure, 3–4, 3*f*
Chromatin remodeling complexes, 4
Chromatin "writer", 4
Chromium, and lung carcinoma, 539
Chromosomal abnormalities, 262
Chromosomal disorders, general features of, 264
Chromosome count, human, 262–263
Chromosomes
    inversions of, 264, 264*f*
    in radiant energy damage, 322
    visualization of, 2*f*
Chronic granulomatous disease, 68, 171, 172*t*
Chronic inflammatory demyelinating polyneuropathy
        (CIDP), 837*t*, 838
Chronic interstitial lung diseases, 506–515, 508*b*
    categories for, 506–507, 507*t*
    fibrosing diseases, 507–512
    granulomatous diseases, 512–515
    pulmonary eosinophilia, 515
    smoking-related, 515
Chronic lymphocytic leukemia (CLL), 478
    clinical features of, 468
    course and prognosis of, 468
    immune dysregulation of, 468
    immunophenotype and genetics of, 468–469
    morphology of, 467*b*, 468*f*
    pathogenesis of, 468
    prevalence of, 467
Chronic myelogenous leukemia (CML), 481–483,
        482*f*
    clinical features of, 483–484
    morphology of, 482*b*
    pathogenesis of, 483
    peripheral blood smear, 482*f*
    targeted therapy for, 482
Chronic obstructive pulmonary disease (COPD), 498
    distinguished from asthma, 498, 521*t*
    pulmonary hypertension associated with, 517
    spectrum of, 499*t*
Chronic traumatic encephalopathy, 858
Churg-Strauss syndrome, 389
    characteristics of, 389
    etiology of, 389
Chyloceles, 692
Chylopericardium, 391
Chylothorax, 391, 544
Chylous ascites, 391
Cicatrization, in atelectasis, 496
Cigarette smoking. *See also* Tobacco
    and alcohol consumption, 309*f*
    in atherosclerosis, 371
    in chronic bronchitis, 502
    diseases caused by, 309–310
    interstitial lung diseases associated with, 515
    in pathogenesis of lung carcinoma, 538–539
Ciliopathy, renal cystic disease as, 574
C1 inhibitor (C1 INH), 77, 172
    alcoholic, 653–655
        following long-term abstinence, 641*f*
        manifestations of, 655
    biliary, 661–662
    causes of, 640
    in chronic alcoholics, 654
    from chronic viral hepatitis, 640*f*
    classification of, 641–642
    clinical features of, 641–642
    "cryptogenic", 653, 655
    in hemochromatosis, 657
    morphology of, 641*b*, 641*f*
    regression of fibrosis in, 641, 641*f*
Civatte bodies, 893
Class switching, 465
Clathrin, in endocytosis, 9, 10*f*
Clathrin-coated pit, 10–11
Clathrin-coated vesicle, 10–11
Claudin, in cell-cell interactions, 12

Clear cell cancers, 580
of kidney, 579
morphology of, 579–580
Cleft lip, 274f
Climate change
CO₂ levels in, 300, 300f
health effects of, 299–301
and human health, 300
recognition of catastrophic effects of, 300–301
temperature increases in, 300, 300f
CLL. See Chronic lymphocytic leukemia
Clostridium difficile, 346
Clostridium perfringens, gangrene caused by, 342–343
Clotting
fibrinolytic cascade in, 106f
inappropriate, 97
in laboratory vs. in vivo, 103, 104f
normal, 485
Clustered regularly interspaced short palindromic repeats
(CRISPRs), 5–6
Cluster of differentiation (CD) number, 465
CNS. See Central nervous system
Coagulation
final stage of, 106b
Coagulation, products of, as mediators of inflammation, 77
Coagulation cascade, in hemostasis, 103–105, 104f
Coagulation diseases, 243–244
Coagulation disorders, 491
deficiencies of factor VIII-von Willebrand factor complex,
491
hemophilia A–factor VIII deficiency, 491
hemophilia B–factor IX deficiency, 491
von Willebrand disease, 491
Coagulation factors, 106b
Coagulopathies
in liver failure, 640
tests for investigation of, 485
Coal dust, lung disease associated with, 509–510, 509t
Coal dust-induced disease, 512b
Coal worker's pneumoconiosis (CWP), 509
clinical features of, 509–510
spectrum of, 509–510
Coarctation of aorta, frequency of, 403t
Cobalamin deficiency, 457–458
Cocaine
characteristics of, 315–316
chronic use, 316
"crack", 315
toxicity, 315–316
in U.S., 315
Cocaine-and amphetamine-regulated transcript (CART)
neurons, 334
Coccidioides immitis, 532, 865
epidemiology of, 532–533
morphology of, 532, 533f
Cognitive impairment, in development of AD, 875
"Cold abscesses", 70
Colitis. See also Ulcerative colitis
antibiotic-associated, 618
C. difficile-associated, 618–619, 618f
microscopic, 614
Collagen bands, in Hodgkin lymphoma, 475f, 477
Collagens
composition of, 22–23
diseases of, 800
fibrillar, 22–23, 23f
non-fibrillar, 23
Collagen synthesis
in chronic inflammatory diseases, 95b
in wound healing, 91–92
Collagen vascular diseases
designation of, 145
Colon
metastatic disease in, 630–633, 634b
neoplastic disease of
adenomas, 627–628, 634b
familial colorectal neoplasia, 630t
familial syndromes, 629–630, 630t
hereditary nonpolyposis colorectal cancer, 630,
630t
Colon cancers
APC mutations in, 213
causation of, 338
right-sided, 632
TGF-beta pathway in, 213
Colony-stimulating factors, 27, 130
Colorectal adenocarcinomas, left-sided, 632
Colorectal cancers
Colorectal carcinomas
metastatic, 634f
precursor lesions associated with, 199
"Common cold", 545
Common variable immunodeficiency, 170
Communicating junctions (gap junctions), in cell-cell
interactions, 12
Comparative genome hybridization (CGH), 292
Complement activation
in antibody-mediated glomerular injury, 554
diseases caused by abnormal, 554
Complement system, 60, 172
activation of, 76, 76f
cleavage of C3 in, 75–76
defects in, 172t
defined, 75–77, 76f
and disease, 77

Complement system (Continued)
functions of, 76, 76f
microbial overcoming of, 356
regulatory proteins in, 76–77
Complex multigenic disorders, 261–262
GWASs in, 296
linkage analysis in, 295–296
molecular diagnosis of, 291–296
PCR analysis in, 294–295, 295f
Concussions, neurologic recovery from, 858
Condylomas, of vulva, 714–715, 715f
Condylomata acuminata (venereal wart), 712, 712b, 895
Congenital adrenal hyperplasia (CAH), 790
clinical manifestations of, 791
enzymatic defect in, 790
morphology of, 789b
in neonates, 791
treatment of, 791
Congenital anomalies
causes of, 277b
defined, 273
mortality associated with, 273, 273t
pathogenesis of, 276
terminology for, 273–275
Congenital cardiac malformations, frequency of, 403, 403t
Congenital diseases, 243–244
Congenital heart disease, 403–408, 408b
clinical features of, 404
cyanotic, 406
gene defects associated with, 404
obstructive lesions in, 407–408, 407f–408f
pathogenesis of, 403–404
prevalence of, 403
survivors of, 403
in trisomy 21 patients, 266
Congestion, 97
chronic, 97
mechanisms of, 97
morphology of, 97b–98b
Congestive heart failure (CHF), 366–367, 400
systemic edema in, 99
treatment for, 402
Connective tissue. See also Soft tissue tumors
Connective tissue deposition, in tissue repair, 88, 92
Connective tissue diseases, 145
Conn syndrome, 792
Contact dermatitis, 890–891, 891f
allergic, 890–891
example of, 142
Contact inhibition, 213, 214b
Contact sensitivity, 142–143, 143t
Contractile dysfunction, after MI, 417
Contracture, 94
Contusions, 317, 318f
to brain, 857–858, 858f
morphology of, 858f, 860b
Coombs test
in fetal hydrops, 284
in immunohemolytic anemia, 442
Copper
deficiency syndrome for, 333t
functions of, 333t
Copy number abnormalities
array-based genomic hybridization, 293–294, 294f
fluorescence in situ hybridization, 292–293, 293f
Copy number variations (CNVs), 2–3
Coronary arteries
collateral perfusion of, 409
critical stenosis of, 409
sequential progression of, 410, 410f
thrombosis within, 411
Coronary artery disease (CAD), 408
in familial hypercholesterolemia, 250b
in IHD, 420, 421f
and obesity, 336
risk factors for, 370, 370f
in SCD, 420
Coronary atherosclerosis, development of, 409
Coronary heart disease, and fish diet, 337–338
Cor pulmonale, 112, 420–421
acute and chronic, 422
disorders predisposing to, 422t
morphology of, 422b
pulmonary hypertensive heart disease, 422
Corticosteroids, as inflammatory agents, 73
Cough, in chronic bronchitis, 502
Cowden syndrome, 627t, 741
Cowdry type A inclusion, 711
CpG island hypermethylation phenotype (CIMP), 632
Cranial nerve palsy, 750
Craniotabes, 331
C-reactive protein (CRP), 86–87, 372f
Creatine kinase myocardial isoform (CK-MB), in myocardial
injury, 416–417, 417f
Crescentic glomerulonephritis, 553f, 554, 562–563, 563f
immune complex-mediated, 563
Pauci-immune type, 563
Cretinism, 757
Creutzfeldt-Jakob disease (CJD), 46t, 869–870
familial, 870
histologic features of, 870, 870f
morphology of, 870f, 871b
sporadic, 870
variant, 870

Crigler-Najjar syndrome type 1, 661
CRISPRs. See Clustered regularly interspaced short
palindromic repeats
Crohn disease, 623–624
clinical manifestations of, 624
compared with ulcerative colitis, 621, 621f, 622t
effect of smoking on, 623
epithelial defects in, 623
extraintestinal manifestations of, 624
genetics of, 622–623
with granulomatous inflammation, 86t
gross pathology of, 624f
microscopic pathology of, 624f
morphology of, 623b–624b, 624f
and mucosal immune responses, 623
noncaseating granulomas in, 623–624
Cronkhite-Canada syndrome, 627t
Crooke hyaline change, 789
Cross-matching, of blood types, 162
Croup, 546
Crypt abscess, in Crohn disease, 623–624
Cryptococcosis, 536–537
in AIDS, 180
clinical features of, 536–537
morphology of, 536b, 536f
Cryptococcus neoformans, 865, 865f
Cryptogenic fibrosing alveolitis, 507–508
Cryptorchidism, 692–693, 693b
Cryptosporidia, in GI tract, 350
Crystal-induced arthritis, 823–825
CSF. See Colony stimulating factors
C-type lectin receptors (CLRs), in innate immunity,
123
Culture, for diagnostic testing, 346
Curie (Ci), use of term, 320
Curschmann spirals, in asthma, 505
Cushing disease, 788
Cushing syndrome, 784–792, 788b
ACTH-dependent, 788
ACTH-independent, 788
carcinomas associated with, 789
clinical features of, 785–788, 788f
diffuse hyperplasia in, 787f, 789
ectopic, 789
etiology of, 788
morphology of, 786b–787b, 787f–788f
pituitary, 789
prevalence of, 788
primary adrenal neoplasms in, 788
primary cortical hyperplasia in, 787f, 789
secretion of ectopic ACTH in, 788
various forms of, 786f, 788
Cyclic adenosine monophosphate (cAMP), 749
Cyclin-dependent kinase inhibitors (CDKIs), 25, 207–208
Cyclin-dependent kinases (CDKs), 25, 26f, 207–208, 208b
Cyclin D1 gene inversions, in primary
hyperparathyroidism, 769
Cyclins, 25, 26f, 207–208, 208b
Cyclooxygenase-2 (COX-2), in colon cancer, 631
Cyclooxygenase inhibitors, as mediators of inflammation,
73
Cyclopamine, teratogenicity of, 276
Cyclopia, 276
CYP2E gene, in ethanol metabolism, 311
Cysticercosis, of brain, 868
Cystic fibrosis (CF), 12, 250–251
associated with malabsorptive diarrhea, 612
bronchiectasis in patient with, 506, 506f
clinical course of, 252f, 253–254
incidence of, 251
management of complications for, 253–254
misfolded proteins in, 46t
morphology of, 252b–253b, 252f
pathogenesis of, 251–252, 251f
pulmonary changes in, 252–253, 253f
Cystic fibrosis transmembrane conductance regulator
(CFTR), 612, 679
Cystic fibrosis transmembrane conductance regulator
(CFTR) gene, 251–252, 254
Cystic kidney disease, acquired, 574
Cystic medionecrosis, 247
Cystitis, of male bladder, 702
Cysts
congenital, of pancreas, 680
dentigerous, 590
of kidney, 573
odontogenic, 590
periapical, 590
synovial, 826
Cytochrome P-450 enzymes, in alcohol metabolism,
310
Cytochrome P-450 system, 200, 301–302
Cytogenetic disorders, 262–268
chromosomal disorders, 264
involving autosomes, 264–266, 265f, 267b
22q11.2 deletion syndrome, 266, 293f
trisomy 21, 264–266, 265f
involving sex chromosomes, 267–268
Klinefelter syndrome, 267
Turner syndrome, 267–268, 268f
numeric abnormalities, 262–263
structural abnormalities, 263–264, 264f
Cytokeratins, of cytoskeleton, 11
Cytokine-mediated inflammation, 144

Cytokines, 129–130
  in acute inflammation, 73–75, 74t, 75f
  in immediate hypersensitivity reactions, 136f, 137
  in immune responses, 130
  in inflammation, 74t
  in long-term diabetes, 783
  in rheumatoid arthritis, 819, 820f
  in SLE, 152
  therapeutic applications for, 130
Cytologic (Papanicolaou) smears, in diagnosis of cancer, 238, 238f
Cytomegalovirus (CMV) infection
  in CNS, 867
  disease manifestations of, 533
  in esophagitis, 593, 593f
  icshemic GI disease caused by, 610
  immunosuppression-related, 534
  in lung, 341–342, 342f
  morphology of, 534b, 534f
  transmission of, 533
Cytomegalovirus (CMV) mononucleosis, in immunocompromised host, 534
Cytopenias, 441
Cytoplasmic changes, in radiant energy damage, 322
Cytoskeleton, 11, 11f
Cytotoxic T lymphocytes (CTLs), 124–125, 125f
Cytotrophoblast-like cells, 695

D
Damage-associated molecular patterns (DAMPs), 60, 122
Danny-Walker malformation, 862
"Dark matter," genome, 1–2
Darwinian selection, in carcinogenesis, 204
Death rates, for various cancers, 197
Deaths, diarrhea-related, 619
Decay accelerating factor (DAF), 77
Deep venous thrombosis (DVT)
  clinical features of, 111
  etiology of, 391
  fragmented thrombi from, 112
  Leiden mutation in, 108–109
  lower-extremity, 108t, 111
  pulmonary embolism in, 391
Deformations, in congenital anomalies, 274
Degenerative joint disease (DJD)
  and obesity, 337
  osteoarthritis, 817–818
Delayed-type hypersensitivity (DTH), 142, 144f
Deletions, 202–203, 204b
  chromosome, 264, 264f
  in immunologic tolerance, 145
22q11.2 deletion syndrome, 293f
  clinical features of, 266
  FISH detection of, 293f
Delta agent. See Hepatitis D virus
Demyelinating diseases, 871–872
Demyelination, segmental, 835–837, 836f
Dendritic cells (DCs), 128, 130, 131f, 134b
  follicular, 128
  in HIV infection, 176–177
  plasmacytoid, 128
Dense deposit disease (DDD), 560
Dental caries, 584
Dentatorubropallidoluysian atrophy (DRPLA), 880
Denys-Drash syndrome (DDS), 289
Depositions, abnormal intracellular, 54b
De Quervain thyroiditis, 759
Dermatitis
  eczematous, 891
  interface, 893
  spongiotic, 891
Dermatitis herpetiformis, 898–899
  characteristics of, 898
  morphology of, 899b, 899f
  pathogenesis of, 898–899, 899f
Dermatomyositis, 844–845
Dermatopathology, 889
Dermatoses
  acute inflammatory, 889–892
    acute eczematous dermatitis, 890–891
    erythema multiforme, 891–892, 892f
    urticaria, 889–890
  chronic inflammatory, 892–894
    lichen planus, 893–894
    lichen simplex chronicus, 894
    psoriasis, 892–893
  infectious, 894–895
    bacterial infections, 894
    fungal infections, 894–895
    verrucae (warts), 895
  inflammatory, 894b
Desmin, of cytoskeleton, 11
Desmoids, 94
Desmoid tumor, 829
Desmosomes, in cell-cell interactions, 12
Desquamative interstitial pneumonia (DIP), 515, 515f
Destruction complex, 213
Developing countries, environmental diseases in, 299
Diabetes, 142–143, 143t, 772–773
  and arteries, 362
  in atherosclerosis, 371
  and celiac disease, 613
  chronic complications of, 778, 780f

Diabetes (Continued)
  classic triad of, 778, 779f
  classification of, 773–774, 782t
  clinical features of, 777–783, 790t
  defined, 772
  diagnosis of, 772–773
  gestational, 783
  HLA alleles associated with, 148t
  initial presentation of, 777–778
  long-term complications of, 788
  macrovascular disease of, 783
  malformations associated with, 275–276
  monogenic forms of, 776
  morphologic changes in, 779b–782b
  "pancreatogenic", 778
  pathogenesis of, 779, 783b
  prediabetes, 772
  secondary, 789
  stages in development of type 1, 775–776, 775f
  and tissue repair, 93
  type 1, 776, 782t, 785
    compared with type 2, 784, 790t
    environmental factors in, 776
    fundamental immune abnormality in, 776
    metabolic derangements in, 779, 779f
    pathogenesis of, 775–776
    susceptibility loci for, 776
    treatment for, 785
  type 2, 782t, 788
    association of obesity with, 776
    beta cell dysfunction in, 776
    compared with type 1, 776
    environmental factors in, 776
    increasing frequency of, 779
    and insulin resistance, 775–776
    lifetime risk for, 783
    and obesity, 334
    obesity and insulin resistance in, 776
    pathogenesis of, 775, 777f
    treatment for, 785
Diabetes, long-standing
  macrovascular complications in, 785
  susceptibility to infection in, 785
  visual impairment in, 785
Diabetes insipidus, clinical manifestations of, 755
Diabetic peripheral neuropathy, 837t, 838
Diabetogenic genes, 776
Diaphysis, in bone development, 798
Diarrhea
  antibiotic-associated, 618
  defined, 611
  malabsorptive, 614b
  secretory, 616
Diarrheal diseases, 341
  defects in, 611t
  infectious enterocolitis, 614–620, 615t
  malabsorptive diarrhea, 611–614
Diastolic dysfunction, 399–400
Dicer enzyme, 4, 5f
Dichlorodiphenyltrichloroethane (DDT), exposure to, 306–307
Diet
  in atherosclerosis, 371
  and cancer risk, 198–199, 338
  and colorectal adenocarcinoma, 627–628
  and colorectal cancer rates, 631
  healthy, 324
  and systemic diseases, 337–338
Differentiated vulvar intraepithelial neoplasia (dVIN), 715
Differentiation
  defined, 192
  and malignant potential, 192–193, 193f
Diffuse alveolar damage (DAD), 496, 498f
Diffuse alveolar hemorrhage syndrome, 519, 519f
Diffuse large B cell lymphomas, 470, 478
  clinical features of, 471
  immunophenotype for, 471
  morphology of, 470b, 470f
  pathogenesis of, 470
  special subtypes of, 471
DiGeorge syndrome, 173b, 266–267, 269b
  causes of, 170
  FISH detection of, 293f
  treatment of, 170
Dihydrotestosterone (DHT), in BPH, 698
1,25-dihydroxyvitamin D (1,25-(OH)2-D), 329–330
Dilated cardiomyopathies (DCMs)
  causes and consequences of, 431f
  causes of, 430t
  characteristics of, 429–432, 430f
  clinical features of, 431–432
  due to toxic exposure, 430–431
  end-stage, 430–431, 431f
  genetic causes of, 430, 431f
  histologic abnormalities in, 431
  infectious, 430
  from iron overload, 431
  morphology of, 431b, 432f
  pathogenesis of, 430–431
  secondary iron overload, 431
Dioxins, exposure to, 307
Dipeptidyl peptidases (DPPs), 775
Disaccharidase deficiency, 326

Diseases
  evolution of, 31, 32f
  pathologic basis of, 1
  study of, 1
  susceptibility to, 2
Disruptions, in congenital anomalies, 274, 274f
Disse, space of, 637
Dissections
  causes of, 382b
  defined, 382b
Disseminated bacterial infection, in AIDS, 180
Disseminated intravascular coagulation (DIC), 111–112, 486–487, 491–492
  acute, 487
  clinical features of, 488–489
  consequences of, 487, 487f
  etiology of, 486
  in liver failure, 640
  major disorders associated with, 486, 487t
  morphology of, 487b
  pathogenesis of, 487f, 488
Diverticular disease, 620–621. See also Sigmoid diverticulitis
Diverticulosis, and diet, 338
DNA (deoxyribonucleic acid)
  and ionizing radiation, 321, 321f
  at light microscopic level, 2f
  methylation, 3f, 4, 203–204
  noncoding, 1–3
  sequencing, 243
DNA (deoxyribonucleic acid) damage
  in cell injury, 48b
  cell injury induced by, 47
DNA (deoxyribonucleic acid) ploidy, in neuroblastoma, 288
Donovan bodies, 711
Down syndrome, 267
  clinical features of, 265f
  karyotype of, 265f
Dressler's syndrome, 436–437
Driver mutations, in carcinogenesis, 204, 205f
Drug abuse, 317, 317b
  adverse reactions to, 315–317
  with cocaine, 315–316
  commonly used drugs, 315t, 317b
  with heroin, 316–317
  with marijuana, 317
  with opioids, 316–317
Drug hypersensitivity vasculitis, 384
Drug reactions, mechanism responsible for, 142
Drugs
  adverse reactions to, 312–315
    acetaminophen, 314
    aspirin, 314–315
    exogenous estrogens, 313–314
    oral contraceptives, 314
  teratogenic, 275–276
  toxicology of, 301–302
Dubin-Johnson syndrome, 661
Duchenne muscular dystrophy (DMD), 842–843
  clinical features of, 843
  histologic images of, 842f
  morphology of, 842b
  pathogenesis of, 843
Ductal carcinoma in situ (DCIS), 742–743, 743f
Ductus arteriosus, pathogenesis of, 406
Duret hemorrhages, 851, 852f
Dutcher bodies, 474
Dwarfism, 800
Dysbiosis, 346
Dysembryoplastic neuroepithelial tumor, 884
Dysentery, 611
Dysgerminomas, 693–694
Dyskeratosis, definition of, 890t
Dyslipidemias
  in atherogenesis, 374
  and obesity, 334
Dysmorphogenesis, external, 274f
Dysostoses, 801
Dysplasia, 603, 801
  defined, 193–194
  presence of, 194
Dysplastic cortex, 862
Dysplastic nevi, 903–905
  clinical features of, 904–905
  morphology of, 904b, 904f
Dyspnea
  in emphysema, 501
  in heart failure, 402
Dystrophic neurites, 849
Dystrophin gene, 843
Dystrophin-glycoprotein complex (DGC), 840, 840f
Dystrophinopathies, 842–843

E
EBNA2 protein, and Burkitt lymphoma, 233
Ebola virus epidemic, in 2014, 348
Ecchymoses
  in bleeding disorders, 485
  in hemorrhage, 100–101
Eclampsia, 735
  causes of, 735
  clinical features of, 735
  morphologic changes of, 735b
ECM. See Extracellular matrix

"Ecstasy" (MDMA), 317
Ectasia, use of term, 392
Ectoparasites, 346
Ectopia lentis, 247
Eczema, 890–891
    clinical features of, 891
    clinical subtypes of, 890
    contact dermatitis, 890
    morphology of, 891b, 891f
Edema, 98–100
    causes of, 100b
        increased hydrostatic pressure, 99, 99f
        lymphatic obstruction, 99–100
        reduced plasma osmotic pressure, 99, 99f
        sodium and water retention, 100
    clinical features of, 100
    defined, 60, 97, 100b
    morphology of, 100b
    pathophysiologic causes of, 98t
    subcutaneous, 100
Edema, cerebral, 852
Edwards syndrome
    clinical features of, 265f
    karyotype of, 265f
Effector cells, 135
Effusions, 98
    defined, 78
    pericardial, 436
E2F transcription factor, release of, 210, 211b
Ehlers-Danlos syndrome (EDS), 22–23, 248, 248b, 378–379
    clinical features of, 248
    clinical heterogeneity of, 248
    common variants of, 248
Eicosanoids, 71, 72t
Eisenmenger syndrome, 404–405
Elastin
    function of, 23
    structure of, 23f
Electrical injury, 319–320
Elephantiasis, 99–100, 692
Emboli, 97, 112–114
    defined, 112
    paradoxical, 112, 405
    pulmonary, 112, 112f, 114b
    pulmonary thromboembolism, 112, 112f, 114b
    systemic thromboembolism, 112, 114b
        air embolism, 113–114
        amniotic fluid embolism, 113, 113f
        fat embolism, 112–113, 113f
    types of, 112
Embolization, systemic, 112
Embryonal neoplasms, 884
Embryonic stem cells, in regenerative medicine, 28
Embryopathy
    retinoic acid, 276
    valproic acid, 276
Emery-Dreifuss muscular dystrophy (EMD), 843–844
Emphysema, 498–501, 501b
    airway infection in, 500, 500f
    bullous, 501, 501f
    clinical features of, 501
    compensatory, 501
    conditions related to, 501
    and COPD, 499f
    defined, 498–500
    major patterns of, 499f
    mediastinal (interstitial), 501
    morphology of, 500f
    pathogenesis of, 500, 500f
    types of, 498–500, 499f
Empyema, 525
Encapsulated follicular variant of papillary thyroid
        carcinoma (EFVPTC), 766
Encephalitis
    fungal, 868
    herpes, 866f, 867, 868b
    HIV, 868
    viral, 865, 866f
Encephalocele, 860–861
Encephalomyelitis
    acute disseminated, 872
    acute necrotizing hemorrhagic, 872
Encephalomyopathies, mitochondrial, 873
Encephalopathy
    acute hypertensive, 857
    bovine spongiform, 870
    chronic traumatic, 858
    hepatic, 640, 873–874
    in liver failure, 639
    multicystic, 862
    Wernicke, 873, 873b
Enchondroma, 811, 812f. See also Chondroma
Endocarditis, vegetative, 427, 428f
Endocrine disruptors, exposure to, 306–307
Endocrine signaling, 16, 749
Endocrine system, 749
    adrenal cortex in, 784
    adrenal medulla in, 791–792
    diseases of, 749–750
    endocrine pancreas, 772–783
    hyperpituitarism, 750–754
    hypopituitarism, 754
    multiple endocrine neoplasia syndromes, 794
    pancreatic neuroendocrine tumors, 778–779

Endocrine system (Continued)
    parathyroid glands, 769–771
    pituitary gland, 750–755
    posterior pituitary syndromes, 754–755
    thyroid, 755
Endocytosis
    caveolae-mediated, 10–11, 10f
    fundamental mechanisms of, 9, 10f
    receptor-mediated, 10–11, 10f, 13
Endometrial carcinoma, precursor lesions associated with,
        199
Endometrial hyperplasia, 724b
    categories of, 723, 723f
    causes of, 723
Endometriosis
    clinical manifestations of, 722
    defined, 721
    morphology of, 722b, 722f
    pathogenesis of, 721
    proposed origins of, 721, 722f
Endometritis, 721
    causes of, 721
    clinical features of, 721
Endometrium, nonneoplastic disorders of, 723b
Endomyocardial fibrosis, 433–434
Endoplasmic reticulum (ER)
    composition of, 7f, 12
    editing function of, 12
    golgi apparatus in, 12–13
    hypertrophy of, 33–34
    intracellular catabolism in, 13, 14f
    membrane-bound ribosomes in, 12
    SER in, 13
    and unfolded protein response, 45–46, 46f, 46t
Endoscopy, to identify varices, 592f
Endosomal vesicles, regulation of, 7
Endosome, early, 10–11
Endothelial activation, 107–108
Endothelial cells (ECs)
    basal and activated states of, 363–364, 363f
    in blood vessels, 361, 362f
    of glomerular capillary wall, 551, 552f
    properties and function of, 363t
Endothelial dysfunction, 364
Endothelial injury
    and abnormal blood flow, 107f, 108
    in acute inflammation, 61–62
    initiated by DIC, 486
    and thrombosis, 107f, 108
Endothelium
    in hemostasis, 107f
Endotoxin
    bacterial, 354
    in ethanol metabolism, 311
End-stage renal disease (ESRD), 550, 575, 772
    and acute postinfectious glomerulonephritis, 561
    diabetic nephropathy in, 785
Energy balance
    and body weight, 334, 335f
    regulation of, 337
Engulfment, in phagocytosis, 67, 67f
Enhancers, 2, 2f
Entamoeba histolytica, 345, 350
Enteric (typhoid) fever, 615t
Enteritis, icshemic, 610
Enterocolitides, bacterial, 615t
Enterocolitis
    necrotizing, 610
    radiation, 610
Enterocolitis, infectious, 614–620, 615t, 620b
    Campylobacter, 616–617
    cholera, 614–616
    Escherichia coli, 617
    novovirus, 619
    parasitic disease, 619–620
    pseudomembranous colitis, 618–619, 618b, 618f
    rotavirus, 619
    salmonellosis, 617–618
    shigellosis, 617
    typhoid fever, 618
Enterohepatic circulation, 660
Enterotoxins, bacterial, 354
Environment
    and infectious disease, 348
    personal, 299
    in prostate cancer, 700
    use of term, 299
Environmental antigens, reactions against, 134
Environmental diseases, 299, 303b–304b
Environmental enteropathy, 613–614
Environmental exposure
    in breast cancer, 742
    and cancer development, 323
    in development of allergic diseases, 137
    susceptibility to, 2
Environmental hazards, 299
Environmental Protection Agency (EPA), 302
Enzymes. See also specific enzymes
    in angiogenesis, 91
    bacterial, 354
    granule, 68
Eosinophils
    in chronic inflammation, 84–85, 84f
    in late-phase hypersensitivity reactions, 137, 138f

Ependymal cells, 850
Ependymoma, 883, 883b, 883f
Epidermal growth factor (EGF), 20
Epidermal growth factor receptor (EGFR)
    in pathogenesis of lung carcinoma, 538
    in sequencing of signal transduction, 206
Epidermal hyperplasia, 895
Epididymis, 692–697
Epigenetic factors, 3–4
Epigenetic modifications, 203–204
Epigenetics, 3, 203–204
Epigenome, dysregulation of, 4
Epiphysis, in bone development, 798
Epispadias, 691
Epithelia, tissue regeneration in, 88–89
Epithelial cells, and vitamin A, 328–329
Epithelial sodium channel (ENaC), in blood pressure
        regulation, 365
Epithelial-to-mesenchymal transition (EMT), 223
Epithelioid cells, 85b
Epithelium, alveolar, 495
Epstein-Barr virus (EBV), 127–128, 181, 233–234, 233f, 234b,
        460
    in AIDS, 180
    gastric adenocarcinomas associated with, 604
    in human malignancies, 461
    in infectious mononucleosis, 461
    and tumor suppressors, 212
ER. See Endoplasmic reticulum
Erythema multiforme, 891–892, 892f
    clinical features of, 892
    morphology of, 891b–892b, 892f
Erythema nodosum, in sarcoidosis, 513
Erythroblastosis fetalis, 284, 284f
    and bilirubin in brain, 660–661
    in type II hypersensitivity, 139, 140f
Erythrocyte sedimentation rate (ESR), 86–87
Erythrocytosis, 459
Erythroplakia, 586b
    description of, 585–586
    morphology of, 586b
Erythropoietin, 442
Escherichia coli
    features of, 615t
    pathogenic mechanisms of, 617
Esophageal stenosis, 590–591
Esophageal varices
    clinical features of, 591
    development of, 591
    morphology of, 591b, 592f
    pathogenesis of, 591
Esophagitis
    Barrett esophagus, 595–596, 595f
    candida, 535
    eosinophilic, 594–595, 594f
    infectious, 592–593
    lacerations of, 591, 593f
    mucosal injury, 591–592
    reflux, 593–594
    in viral, 593, 593f
Esophagus, 309t
    diseases and disorders of, 590–597, 597b
        achalasia, 591
        esophagitis, 591–596, 593f–594f
        obstructive diseases of, 590–591
            functional obstruction, 591
            mechanical obstruction, 590–591
        tumors of, 596–597
            adenocarcinoma, 596, 596f
            squamous cell carcinoma, 596–597, 597f
        vascular diseases of
            ectopia, 591
            esophageal varices, 591, 592f
Estrogens
    adverse reactions to, 313–314
    unopposed, 723
Ethanol
    absorption of, 310
    CNS effects of, 874
    damage caused by, 310
    metabolism of, 310, 311f, 312b
    toxic effects from, 310–311
Ethanol abuse, adverse effects of, 311
Ethanol consumption, in atherosclerosis, 371
Ethnicity, and breast cancer, 741
Etiology, defined, 31
Euchromatin, 3–4, 3f
Ewing sarcoma, 812–813
    clinical course for, 813
    incidence of, 813
    morphology of, 813b, 813f
    pathogenesis of, 813
Excoriation, definition of, 890t
Exercise
    in atherosclerosis, 371
    and osteoporosis, 801
Exocytosis, process of, 9–10, 10f
Exostosis, 810
Exotoxins, bacterial, 354, 355f
Extracellular matrix (ECM)
    adhesive receptors of, 23–24, 24f
    basic forms of, 22f
    in blood vessels, 361, 362f
    and cell proliferation, 88

Extracellular matrix (ECM) (Continued)
  cellular interactions in, 24f
  cellular interaction with, 21–24, 21f
  components of, 22–24, 22f–24f
  excessive production of, 95b
  functions of, 21–22, 21f
  invasion of, 220–222, 221f
  local degradation of, 221–222
  in long-term diabetes, 783
  in tumor invasion, 222
  types of, 220–222, 221f
  valvular, 423
Extracellular matrix (ECM) proteins, in angiogenesis, 91
Extranodal marginal zone lymphoma, 466t, 470, 478
  clinical features of, 470
  immunophenotype for, 470
  morphology of, 470b
  pathogenesis of, 470
Extrinsic pathway, in apoptosis, 217f
Exudates
  defined, 60
  formation of, 61f
Exudation, defined, 60
Eye, in sarcoidosis, 513

F
Factor VIII deficiency, 491. See also Hemophila A
Factor IX deficiency, 491
Factor deficiencies, 105
Factor X, conversion to factor Xa of, 103, 104f
Factor XI deficiency, 105
Factor XII deficiency, 105
Fallopian tubes
  adenocarcinomas of, 727
  inflammation of, 726–727, 727f
Familial, use of term, 243–244
Familial adenomatous polyposis (FAP) syndrome, 603, 629–630, 630f
  common patterns of, 627t, 630t
  inheritance of, 214
Familial dysplastic nevus syndrome, 904–905
Familial hypercholesterolemia, 246, 248
  misfolded proteins in, 46t
  mutations causing, 249–250
  and normal cholesterol metabolism, 248–249, 249f–250f
  pathogenesis of, 249–250, 249f–250f
Familial mental retardation protein (FMRP), 269–271, 270f
Familial tumor syndromes, 886–887
Fanconi anemia, 227, 227b–228b
Fas (CD95) receptor, in apoptosis, 39, 39f
Fasciculations, of ALS, 880–881
Fascioscapulohumeral dystrophy, 844
Fat
  and colon cancer, 338
  mesenchymal stem cells in, 28
  in U.S. diet, 337–338
Fat embolism, 112–113, 113f
Fatty change (steatosis), cell injury caused by, 51, 52f
Fatty liver disease. See also Nonalcoholic fatty liver disease
  alcohol-related, 654f
  morphology of, 652
  nonalcoholic, 655
  and risk for malignant transformation, 669
Fatty streaks, in atherosclerosis, 374, 375f
FBN1 gene, 247, 247b
Feathery degeneration, of periportal hepatocytes, 661–662
Feedback inhibition, 749
Fenestrations (holes), in ECs, 363
Fetal abnormalities, in fetal growth restriction, 277. See also Congenital anomalies
Fetal alcohol syndrome (FAS)
  in chronic alcoholism, 312
  malformations associated with, 275–276
Fetal blood sampling, in fetal hydrops, 284
Fetal growth restriction, 277–278
Fetal hydrops, 285b
  causes of, 282–283, 282t, 285b
  clinical course for, 284
  clinical presentation of, 282f
  in fetal anemia, 283
  immune hydrops, 283
  morphology of, 282f, 284b
  nonimmune hydrops, 283–284, 283f
Fetus. See also Congenital anomalies
  effects of cocaine on, 315
  infections of, 277
Fever
  acute-phase response in, 86–87
  prostaglandins in, 73
FEV1 to FVC ratio, in emphysema, 501
Fibrillin-1, 247
Fibrinogen, 86–87
Fibrinolytic system, in coagulation cascade, 106f
Fibrinous inflammation, 78, 79f
Fibroadenoma, of breast, 191, 194–195, 194f
Fibroblast growth factor (FGF), 20
Fibroblast growth factor receptor 3 (FGFR3), 702–703
Fibroids, uterine, 725
Fibromatoses
  aggressive, 94
  deep, 829
  morphology of, 829b, 829f
  superficial, 828–829

Fibromuscular dysplasia, 364
Fibromuscular intimal hyperplasia, 369
Fibronectin, 23–24, 24f
Fibrosarcoma, designation as, 190–191
Fibrosing diseases
  idiopathic pulmonary fibrosis, 507–508
  nonspecific interstitial pneumonia, 508
  pneumoconioses, 508–509
Fibrosis
  mechanisms of, 95f
  morphology of, 92b, 92f
  in parenchymal organs, 94–95, 95f
  "pipe-stem", 358, 358f
  radiation induced, 321–322, 321f
  in systemic sclerosis, 159, 161f, 162b
Fibrous dysplasia, 815–816
  clinical course of, 816
  morphology of, 816b, 816f
  pathogenesis of, 816
Fibrous plaques, in atherosclerosis, 374–376
Fine-needle aspiration, in diagnosis of cancer, 238
Fish, in diet, 337–338
Flat wart, 895
Flexner-Wintersteiner rosettes, in pediatric retinoblastoma, 289, 290f
"Flint water crisis," in Michigan, 304
Floppy valve syndrome, 247
Flow cytometry, in classification of leukemias and lymphomas, 238
Flukes (trematodes), 345
Fluorescence in situ hybridization (FISH), for copy number abnormalities, 292–293, 293f
Fluoride
  deficiency syndrome for, 333t
  functions of, 333t
Foam cells, in atherosclerosis, 374–376
Focal adhesion complexes, in cell-cell interactions, 12
Focal nodular hyperplasia, 668, 668b–669b, 668f
Focal segmental glomerulosclerosis (FSGS), 556–557, 556t
  clinical course of, 557
  conditions associated with, 556
  morphology of, 557b, 558f
  pathogenesis of, 556–557
Folate (folic acid), functions of, 333t
Folate (folic acid) deficiency, 333t, 456–457
  causes of, 457
  clinical features of, 457
  pathogenesis of, 457
Follicle cysts, of ovaries, 727
Follicular helper T (Tfh) cells, in humoral immunity, 132
Follicular hyperplasia, morphology of, 462
Follicular lymphoma, 202, 466t, 468–469, 478
  clinical features of, 469
  immunophenotype for, 469
  morphology of, 468b, 469f
  pathogenesis of, 469
Food allergies, 137, 138t
Foramen ovale, in congenital heart disease, 405
Forced expiratory volume 1 (FEV1), 501
Forced vital capacity (FVC), in diffuse obstructive disorders, 498
Foreign bodies
  inflammation caused by, 59
  and tissue repair, 93
Foveolar cells, 598–599
FOXP3 gene, mutations in, 145
Fractures
  defined, 805
  healing of, 805–806, 805f
  types of, 805
Fragile X syndrome, 244, 271b
  causative mutation for, 269
  characteristic physical phenotype for, 269
  pathogenesis of, 269–270, 270f
  patterns of transmission for, 269
  pedigree for, 269, 270f
  permutations in, 269
Fragile X tremor/ataxia, 271b
  characteristics of, 270–271
  permutations in, 270
Frameshift mutations, 244
Framingham Heart Study, 370, 421
Frank-Starling mechanism, in CHF, 400
Free fatty acids (FFAs), in type 2 diabetes, 778
Friedreich ataxia, 880
Frontal bossing, 331
Frontotemporal dementias, 877
Frontotemporal lobar degeneration (FTLD), 877
  clinical classification of, 877
  morphology of, 877b, 878f
  pathologic subgroups of, 877
Frozen section diagnosis, in diagnosis of cancer, 238
Fukushima nuclear meltdown, 299
Fungal infections
  of CNS, 868
  of gastrointestinal tract, 350
  opportunistic
    candidiasis, 535–536, 536f
    cryptococcosis, 536–537
    molds, 537
  of skin, 894–895
    clinical features of, 895
    morphology of, 895b
  superficial, 345

Fungi
  characteristics of, 342t
  defined, 343–345
  endemic, 345
  opportunistic, 345, 345f

G
Galactosemia, 255
  clinical features of, 255
  dietary restrictions for, 255
Galactose-1-phosphate uridyltransferase (GALT), 255
Gallbladder
  carcinoma of, 675
    clinical features of, 675
    morphology of, 675b, 676f
  cholecystitis, 674–675
  empyema of, 674
Gallbladder disease, 675b–676b
Gallstone disease, 672–674
  clinical features of, 673–674
  morphology of, 673b, 673f
  pathogenesis of, 672
  prevalence of, 672–673
  risk factors for, 672–673, 673t
Gallstones
  and obesity, 337
  pigment, 673, 673f
Gangliogliomas, 884
Ganglion, 826
Ganglioneuroblastomas, 287
Ganglioneuromas, 287, 287f
Gangliosidoses, 256–257, 257t, 258f
Gangrene, in diabetics, 783
Gap junctions, in cell-cell interactions, 12
Gardner syndrome, 629–630
Garlic, and diet, 338
Gastrectomy, and vitamin B12 deficiency, 457–458
Gastric cancer, decline in, 197
Gastric injury
  NSAID-induced, 599
  severe, 599
Gastrinomas, 784
  clinical features of, 785–786
  morphology of, 784b
Gastritis
  acute erosive hemorrhagic, 599
  in chronic dysplasia, 603b
  susceptibility of older adults to, 599
Gastritis, autoimmune, 600–601
  characteristics of, 601t
  clinical features of, 601
  morphology of, 601b
  pantogenesis of, 601
Gastritis, chronic, 603b
  autoimmune gastritis, 600–601
  complications of, 601–603
    dysplasia, 603
    mucosal atrophy and intestinal metaplasia, 603
  Helicobacter pylori-associated, 599–600, 601t
  peptic ulcer disease, 601–603
Gastroenteritis, and climate change, 300
Gastroesophageal reflux disease (GERD), 593–594
  clinical features of, 594
  and gastric cancer, 604
  morphology of, 594b, 594f
  pathogenesis of, 594
  PUD in, 601–602
Gastrointestinal (GI) polyposis syndromes, 627t
Gastrointestinal (GI) tract
  in chronic alcoholism, 311
  diseases of, 583
  fungal infections of, 350
  infection via, 350
  in lead exposure, 304f, 305
  microbial infection of, 349–350, 349t
  normal defenses within, 350
  parasitic infections of, 350
Gastrointestinal stromal tumor (GIST), 606
  clinical features of, 607
  morphology of, 607b
  pathogenesis of, 606–607
Gaucher disease, 257t, 258–260
  etiology of, 258–259
  pathognomonic cytoplasmic appearance of, 257, 259f
  therapies for, 259
  variants of, 259
Gender, and breast cancer incidence, 740f, 741
Gender differences
  in atherosclerosis, 370–371
  in SLE, 149–150
Gene amplifications, 203
Gene editing, 5–6, 6f
Generations, and cancer incidence, 197
Gene rearrangements, 204b
  identification of pathogenic, 202
  malignancies associated with, 201–202
Genes. See also specific genes
  cancer, 200–201, 201t
  modifier, 245–246
  protein-encoding, 1
  regulating interactions between tumor cells and host cells, 200
Gene silencing, 4, 5f

Gene symbols, 205
Genetic aberrations, in prostate cancer, 700
Genetic abnormalities
    cell injury caused by, 32
    in human disease, 244–245
        alterations in non-coding RNAs, 244–245
        alterations in protein-coding genes, 244–245
        mutations in protein-coding genes, 244
Genetic alternations, acquired, 292
Genetic analysis
    indications for, 292
    postnatal, 292
    prenatal, 292
Genetic diseases, 243–272
    cytogenetic disorders, 262–268
    single-gene disorders, 269–272
Genetic disorders. See also Mendelian disorders
    categories of, 244–245
    complex multigenic disorders, 261–262
Genetic evolution, in carcinogenesis, 204
Genetic heterogeneity, 245
Genetics
    of atherosclerosis, 370–371
    of breast cancer, 741, 742f
Genital herpes virus infection, 705t, 711–712
    clinical features of, 711–712
    laboratory diagnosis of, 712
    morphology of, 711b
    transmission of, 711
Genital system, female
    cervix, 717–720
    and diseases of pregnancy, 732–735
    fallopian tubes, 726–727
    ovaries, 727–731
    uterus, 721–726
    vagina, 716–717
    vulva, 713–716
Genital system, male
    epididymis, 692–697
    penis, 691–692
    prostate gland, 697–701, 697f
    scrotum, 692–697
    and sexually transmitted diseases, 704–712
    testis, 692–697
Genital tract, exit of microbes via, 352
Genome, human
    and gene editing, 5–6, 6f
    histone organization of, 3–4, 3f
    micro-RNAs, 4–5
    noncoding DNA in, 1–3
    non-protein-coding sequences found in, 2, 2f
    regulation of, 4
    sequencing of, 1
Genome sequencing. See also Sanger sequencing;
        Sequencing technologies
Genome-wide association studies (GWAS), 293–294
    psoriasis in, 892
    results with, 296
Genomic alterations, systematic sequencing of, 240
Genomic analyses, 239–241, 241f
Genomic hybridization, array-based, 293–294, 294f
Genomic imprinting, 271–272, 273b
Geographic factors, and breast cancer, 741
GERD. See Gastroesophageal reflux disease
Germ cell neoplasia in situ, in cryptorchid testes, 692–693
Germ cell tumors
    of brain, 885
    of ovaries, 730, 731t
    tumor markers secreted by, 694t, 697
    classification of, 693–694, 694t
    clinical features of, 696–697
    molecular pathogenesis of, 693
    morphology of, 694
    treatment of, 697
Germinomas, 693–694
Gestational pemphigoid, 897–898
Gestational trophoblastic disease, 735b
    categories for, 733
    gestational choriocarcinoma, 734
    hydatidiform mole, 733
    invasive mole, 733–734
    placental site trophoblastic tumor, 735
Ghon complex, in primary tuberculosis, 528, 528f
Ghrelin, 336
Giant cell arteritis, 384–385
    clinical features of, 385
    morphology of, 385b
    pathogenesis of, 384–385, 385f
Giant cells, 85b
Giant cell tumors, 813–814
    clinical course of, 814
    morphology of, 814b, 814f
    pathogenesis of, 814
    tenosynovial, 826–827
Giardia lamblia, 620
    in GI tract, 350
    transmission of, 345
Giemsa stain (G banding) technique, 262
Gigantism, 753
Gilbert syndrome, 661
Gingivitis, 584
GIST. See Gastrointestinal stromal tumor
Glagov phenomenon, 369
Gleason system, for grading prostate cancer, 700

Glial fibrillary acidic protein (GFAP), 11, 882
Glioblastoma
    histologic appearance of, 882, 882f
    oncogenic pathways for, 882
Gliomas, 881
    classification of, 881
    diffuse astrocytomas, 881
    genetic studies of, 882
    midline, 882–883
    oligodendroglioma, 881–882
    pathogenesis of, 882–883
    and telomere integrity, 882
Global warming, 299
    evidence for, 299–300, 300f
    and infectious disease, 348
Glomangiomas, 394
Glomerular basement membrane (GBM)
    alterations in, 550
    anatomy of, 551, 551f–552f
    diffuse thickening of, 558, 558f
Glomerular basement membrane (GBM) proteins, mutations
        in genes encoding, 562
Glomerular diseases, 552, 552t
    major primary, 555, 556t
    primary, 552, 552t
    secondary, 552, 552t
    in SLE, 154
Glomerular filtration rate (GFR), 549
    diseases and disorders of, 552–563, 552t
        acute postinfectious (poststreptococcal)
            glomerulonephritis, 556t, 560–561
        antibody-associated injury, 553f
        anti-glomerular basement membrane antibody-
            mediated glomerulonephritis, 553f, 554
        C3 glomerulopathy, 560
        focal segmental glomerulosclerosis, 556–557, 556t
        glomerular diseases caused by abnormal complement
            activation, 554
        glomerulonephritis caused by circulating immune
            complexes, 552–553, 554f
        glomerulonephritis caused by circulating immune
            complexes formed in situ, 553–554
        hereditary nephritis, 562
        IgA nephropathy, 556t, 561–562
        immune mechanisms in, 552
        mechanisms of glomerular injury, 554–555
        mediators of immune injury, 554
        membranoproliferative glomerulonephritis, 556t,
            559–560
        membranous nephropathy, 556t, 557–559
        minimal-change disease, 555–556, 556t–557t
        rapidly progressive glomerulonephritis, 556t, 562–563
    permeability of, 552
Glomerular injury
    clinical syndromes and, 555b
    mechanisms of, 554–555
    membranoproliferative pattern of, 559
    nephron loss, 555
    podocyte injury, 554–555
Glomeruli
    basic strictures of, 550–552, 551f–552f
    disorders affecting, 550–552
    obliteration of, 573, 573f
C3 glomerulopathy (C3GN), 560
Glomerulonephritis (GN), 141, 141t, 550. See also Acute
        postinfectious glomerulonephritis;
        membranoproliferative glomerulonephritis
    antibody-mediated, 555
    anti-GBM antibody-mediated, 553f, 554
    anti-GBM antibody-mediated crescentic, 562–563
    associated with nephritic syndrome, 564
    caused by circulating immune complexes, 552–553,
        554f
    caused by circulating immune complexes formed in situ,
        553–554
    chronic, 573, 573f
    crescentic, 388
    inflammatory reaction in, 59t
    necrotizing, 388
Glomerulopathy
    C3, 560
        clinical course of, 560
        morphology of, 560b
        pathogenesis of, 560
    collapsing, 557
Glomerulosclerosis
    maladaptive alterations in, 555
    nodular, in long-standing diabetes, 781f–782f, 783
Glomus tumors (glomangiomas), 394
Glucagon, effects on glucose of, 775–776
Glucagon-like peptide-1 (GLP-1), 775
Glucocorticoids
    in bone remodeling, 799
    and muscle atrophy, 841
    and tissue repair, 93
Glucose-dependent insulinotropic polypeptide (GIP), 775
Glucose homeostasis, 774–775
Glucose-6-phosphate dehydrogenase (G6PD) deficiency,
        450, 453
    clinical features of, 450
    pathogenesis of, 450, 450f
    peripheral blood smear, 450f, 451
Gluten-free diet, 898
Glutensensitive enteropathy, 612–613

Glycemic control, assessment of, 785
Glycogen
    abnormal depositions of, 54b
    role in cell injury of, 52
Glycogen storage diseases (GSDs), 261b
    etiology of, 260
    forms of, 260, 261t
Glycolipids, 8
Glycolysis, aerobic, 15
Glycoproteins
    adhesive, 23–24, 24f
    HIV, 175
Glycosis, aerobic, 214
GN. See Glomerulonephritis
GNAS gene, 751–752, 756t
Goiter, 762–763
    clinical features of, 763
    colloid, 762b–763b, 762f
    diffuse, 762b–763b, 762f
    diffuse and multimodular, 762
    endemic, 762
    morphology of, 762b–763b, 762f
    multimodular, 762
    pathogenesis of, 762
    sporadic, 762
Goitrous hypothyroidism, 762
Golgi apparatus
    protein glycosylation in, 12–13
    proteins in, 6, 7f
Gomori methenamine silver stains, 895
Gonorrhea, 705t, 708–709, 709b
    among female patients, 709
    clinical features of, 709
    diagnosis of, 709
    disseminated infection of, 709
    morphology of, 708b, 708f
    transmission of, 708–709
Goodpasture syndrome, 139t, 519, 554, 556t, 562–563
Gout, 823
    calcium pyrophosphate crystal deposition disease, 825
    characteristics of, 823
    clinical course of, 824–825
    morphology of, 824b, 825f
    pathogenesis of, 823–824, 824f
    primary, 824
    symptomatic, 824
    treatment of, 825
G-protein mutations, in pituitary adenomas, 751–752, 752f
Grading of cancer, 236–237, 237b
Graft
    methods of increasing survival of, 162–166
    recognition of alloantigens in, 162, 164f
Graft rejection
    acute antibody-mediated, 164, 164b
    acute cellular, 162, 164b, 166f
    classification of, 163–165
    hyperacute, 162, 164, 165f
    mechanisms of, 162–168, 165f–166f
Graft vs. host disease (GVHD)
    forms of, 167–168, 169f
    with HSC transplants, 163–165
    watery diarrhea in, 614
Gram-negative infections, 342–343, 343f, 344t
Gram-positive bacteria, 342–343, 343f–344f, 344t
Granulation, exuberant, 94
Granulation tissue
    morphology of, 92b, 92f
    in wound healing, 90, 90f
Granule enzymes, in acute inflammation, 68
Granuloma inguinale, 711b
    incidence of, 711
    morphology of, 711b
Granulomas, 142, 144f
    in Crohn disease, 623–624
    eosinophilic, 485
    formation of, 85
    immune, 85
    in immune-mediated inflammatory diseases, 85
    irregular stellate necrotizing, 462
    of oral cavity, 585, 585f
    in sarcoidosis, 513, 513f
    tuberculous, 85, 85f
    types of, 85
Granulomatosis, allergic, 389
Granulomatosis with polyangiitis (GPA), 388
    characteristics of, 388
    clinical features of, 388–389
    morphology of, 388b, 388f
    pulmonary manifestations of, 519
    treatment of, 388–389
Granulomatous diseases, 512–515
    hypersensitivity pneumonitis, 514–515
    sarcoidosis, 512–514
Granulomatous inflammation, 85, 142, 144f
    Crohn disease, 85
    diseases with, 85, 86t
    in host response to microbes, 355
    in tuberculosis, 357f, 527–528
Graves disease (hyperthyroidism), 139t, 756–757,
        761b–762b
    clinical manifestations of, 761
    incidence of, 760
    laboratory findings in, 761
    manifestations of, 760

Graves disease (hyperthyroidism) *(Continued)*
  morphology of, 761*b*, 761*f*
  pathogenesis of, 760–761
  in type II hypersensitivity, 139, 140*f*
Graves ophthalmopathy, 760
Gray (Gy), use of term, 320
Greenhouse gases, 300
Growth factor receptor signaling, in Warburg effect, 215–216, 215*f*
Growth factors
  in angiogenesis, 91
  and cell proliferation, 88
  epidermal growth factor, 20
  fibroblast growth factor, 20
  hepatocyte growth factor, 20
  in long-term diabetes, 783
  major role of, 19
  platelet-derived growth factor, 20
  at steady state, 19–21
  transforming growth factor-α, 20
  transforming growth factor-ß, 20–21
  vascular endothelial growth factors, 20
Growth hormone, persistent excess of, 753
Growth plate, in bone development, 798, 799*f*
G₁/S transition, RB in, 210, 210*f*
Guillain-Barré syndrome, 837*t*, 838
Gull disease, 757
Gut hormones, 336
Gut microbiome, in obesity, 336
Gynecomastia, in breast disease, 737

H
HACEK group (Haemophilus, Actinobacillus, Cardiobacterium, Eikenella, and Kingella), in IE, 427
Haemophilus influenzae, 521
Hairy ears, inheritance of, 246–247
Halogenation, in acute inflammation, 68
Hamartoma
  CNS, 887
  cortical, 887
  of infancy and childhood, 285
  use of term, 191
Hand-foot syndrome, in sickle cell anemia, 447
Hand-Schüller-Christian triad, 485
HapMap project, 295–296
Harrison groove, 331
Hashimoto thyroiditis, 758–761
  clinical features of, 758
  genetics of, 758
  morphology of, 758*b*–759*b*, 759*f*
  pathogenesis of, 758–759, 759*f*
Hassall's corpuscles, 169*b*
Head, trauma to, 857. *See also* Brain; Central nervous system
Heart
  amyloidosis of, 186
  characteristics of, 399
  in hemochromatosis, 657
  in systemic sclerosis, 160
Heart disease, 408–419. *See also* Congenital heart disease; Hypertensive heart disease; ischemic heart disease
  arrhythmias, 419–420
  and cardiac transplantation, 439
  cardiomyopathies, 429–435
  in familial hypercholesterolemia, 250*b*
  pathophysiologic pathways in, 399
  pericardial disease, 436–437
  pulmonary hypertension associated with, 517
  valvular, 422–429
Heart failure, 400–403, 403*b*
  after MI, 418
  causes of, 400
  compensation in, 400
    hypertrophy, 400, 401*f*
    pathologic, 400–401
  left-sided, 401–402, 403*b*, 425
    clinical features of, 402
    morphology of, 401*b*–402*b*
  myocardial structural changes in, 400, 401*f*
  right-sided, 402–403, 403*b*
    clinical features of, 403
    morphology of, 402
Heart rate, in acute-phase response, 87
Heart transplantation procedures, 439
Heat cramps, 319
Heat exhaustion, 319
Heavy-chain class (isotype) switching, in humoral immunity, 132
Heavy-chain disease, 474
Heavy metals, toxic effects of, 306*b*
Helicobacter pylori
  and carcinogenesis, 604
  classified as carcinogen, 235, 235*b*
Helicobacter pylori gastritis, 599–600
  clinical features of, 600
  epidemiology of, 600
  morphology of, 600*b*, 601*f*
  pathogenesis of, 600
  secretion and peptic ulcer disease of, 600
HELLP syndrome, 735
Helminths, 345
  characteristics of, 342*t*, 345
  in GI tract, 350
  groups of, 345

Helper T cells, 124–125, 125*f*
Hemangioendotheliomas, 395–396
Hemangiomas
  capillary, 392, 393*f*
  cavernous, 393, 393*f*
  cavernous, of liver, 669
  characteristics of, 392–393
  juvenile, 392
  pediatric, 285, 285*f*
Hemarthroses, 490
Hematoceles, 692
Hematolymphoid system, dispersed nature of, 441
Hematopoiesis
  in CML, 481–482
  extramedullary, 442, 481–482
Hematopoietic stem cell (HSC) transplants, 162–163, 168*b*
  and graft *vs.* host disease, 163–165
  and immune deficiencies, 165–166
Hematopoietic stem cells (HSCs), harvesting of, 166
Hematopoietic system
  diseases affecting, 441
  radiation injury to, 322–323, 322*f*, 322*t*
Hematosalpinx, 732
Hematoxylin, in SLE, 156–157
Hematoxylin and eosin (H&E) staining, 849, 850*f*
Hematuria, in polycystic kidney disease, 574–575
Heme synthesis, effect of lead on, 304–305
Hemianopsia, bitemporal, 750
Hemochromatosis, 656
  clinical features of, 657
  diagnosis of, 657
  morphology of, 657*b*, 657*f*
  pathogenesis of, 656–657
  secondary, 442–443
Hemoglobin electrophoresis, 442
Hemoglobinopathies, 445
Hemolysis, 442
  extravascular, 443–444
  intravascular, 444
  traumatic, 452
Hemolytic disease in newborn, antibody-induced, 283
Hemolytic reactions, to blood products, 493
Hemolytic uremic syndrome (HUS), 172, 491–492
  atypical, 572
  defined, 488
  onset of atypical, 572
  pathogenesis of, 489
  Shiga toxin-associated, 572
  Shiga toxin-mediated, 571–572, 571*t*
Hemopericardium, 436
Hemophagocytic lymphohistiocytosis (HLH), 465–477
  clinical features of, 463
  treatment for, 463
Hemophilia, 492
Hemophilia A, 489–491
  clinical features of, 490
  prevalence of, 490
  treatment of, 490
Hemophilia B, 489, 491
Hemorrhage, 97, 100–101, 443
  clinical significance of, 101
  defined, 100
  intracerebral, 100–101, 101*f*
  manifestations of, 100–101
  risk of, 100
Hemorrhage, intracranial
  brain parenchymal hemorrhage, 854, 855*f*
  cerebral amyloid angiopathy, 855
  morphology of, 855*b*
Hemorrhagic diatheses, 441
Hemorrhoidectomy, 610
Hemorrhoids, 610
  pathogenesis of, 610
Hemosiderin
  in chronic pulmonary congestion, 97*b*–98*b*
  in hemochromatosis, 657
  role in cell injury, 52–53, 53*f*
Hemosiderosis, in thalassemia, 449*f*, 450
Hemostasis, 101–112
  coagulation cascade in, 103–105, 104*f*
  defined, 97, 101
  endothelium in, 107*f*
  inadequate, 97
  normal, 101–106, 102*f*
  platelets in, 102*f*, 103*b*
Hemothorax, 544
Heparin-induced thrombocytopenic (HIT) syndrome, 109
Heparin preparations, low-molecular-weight, 488
Hepatectomy, partial, proliferation of hepatocytes following, 89
Hepatic bile, functions of, 659
Hepatic circulatory disorders, 666–667, 666*f*, 668*b*
  hepatic venous outflow obstruction, 667
  impaired blood flow into liver, 666–667
    hepatic artery compromise, 666
    portal vein obstruction and thrombosis, 666–667
  impaired blood flow through liver, 667
  passive congestion and centrilobular necrosis, 667, 668*f*
Hepatic congestion
  acute, 97*b*–98*b*
  chronic, 97*b*–98*b*, 98*f*
Hepatic failure, fulminant, 648

Hepatic stellate cell (HSC), 637
Hepatic vein thrombosis, 667, 667*f*
Hepatitis, 650*b*
  AcutE, 650*b*
  acute viral, 357*f*
  alcoholic, 654
  chronic, 648, 650*b*
  neonatal, 662
Hepatitis, autoimmune, 651
  clinical presentation of, 651
  clinicopathologic features of, 651
  defined, 651
  morphology of, 651*b*
  types of, 651
Hepatitis, neonatal
  morphologic features of, 663*b*, 663*f*
  in α₁-antitrypsin deficiency, 659
Hepatitis, viral, 642–648, 650*b*
  acute, 649, 649*f*
  chronic, 649, 649*f*–650*f*
  clinicopathologic syndromes of, 648
    acute asymptomatic infection with recovery, 648
    acute symptomatic infection with recovery, 648
    carrier state, 648
    chronic hepatitis, 648
    fulminant hepatic failure, 648
    HIV and chronic viral hepatitis, 648
  hepatitis A virus, 642–643
  hepatitis B virus, 643–645
  hepatitis C virus, 645–647
  hepatitis D virus, 647
  hepatitis E virus, 647–648
  liver biopsy in, 649–650, 650*f*
  morphology of, 648*b*–650*b*
Hepatitis A virus (HAV), 642–643, 643*t*
  characteristics of, 643
  detection of, 643
  IgM antibody against, 643, 643*f*
  incidence of, 642
Hepatitis B virus (HBV), 640, 642–645, 643*t*
  clinical manifestations of, 342, 343*t*
  and hepatocarcinogenesis, 670
  and hepatocellular cancer, 234–235, 235*b*
  incubation period for, 644
  transmission of, 644
  and tumor suppressors, 212
Hepatitis B virus (HBV) genome, proteins encoded by, 644
Hepatitis B virus (HBV) infection
  chronicity of, 645
  as global health problem, 644
  potential outcomes of, 643–644, 644*f*
  serum markers for, 645*f*
Hepatitis C virus (HCV), 640, 642, 643*t*, 645–647
  and hepatocarcinogenesis, 670
  and hepatocellular cancer, 234–235, 235*b*
  and incidence of HCC, 669
  life cycle of, 646*f*
  and liver disease in alcoholics, 654
  properties of, 646
  transmission of, 645–646
Hepatitis C virus (HCV) infection
  chronicity of, 646, 647*f*
  clinical course of, 646
  incubation period for, 646
  risk factors for, 645
  treatment of, 646–647
Hepatitis D virus (HDV), 642, 643*t*, 647
Hepatitis D virus (HDV) infection
  prevalence of, 647
  and vaccination for HBV, 647
Hepatitis E virus (HEV), 643*t*, 647–648
Hepatitis E virus (HEV) infection, in pregnant women, 647–648
Hepatitis viruses, 643*t*
Hepatocellular cancer, etiology of, 234
Hepatocellular carcinoma (HCC), 669–672
  clinical manifestations of, 670–671
  detection of, 671
  etiologic agents for, 672
  gross appearance of, 670, 671*f*
  and incidence of, 669
  laboratory studies in, 671
  morphology of, 670*b*
  natural history of, 671
  pathogenesis of, 669
  precursors of, 670
  well differentiated, 670
Hepatocellular steatosis, 652–654, 652*f*
Hepatocyte growth factor (HGF), 20
Hepatocytes, 637
  ballooning, 653, 653*f*
  in fatty liver disease, 653*f*
  feathery degeneration of periportal, 662
  "groundglass", 649–650, 650*f*
  necrosis of, 638, 638*f*
  regeneration of lost, 639
Hepatolithiasis
Hepatoma, 669
Hepatomegaly, congestive, 402
Hepatorenal syndrome, in liver failure, 640
Hepcidin
  in acute-phase response, 86–87
  in iron deficiency anemia, 455
Hereditary disorders, 243–244

Hereditary nephritis, 562
  clinical course of, 562
  morphology of, 562b
  pathogenesis of, 562
Hereditary nonpolyposis colorectal cancer (HNPCC)
    syndrome, 227, 227b–228b
  common patterns of, 630, 630t
  sites of mutations in, 630
Hereditary predisposition, in diagnosis of cancer,
    239
Hereditary spherocytosis, 444–445, 453
  clinical features of, 445
  morphology of, 444b–445b, 445f
  pathogenesis of, 444–445, 444f
  treatment of, 445
Heredity, in prostate cancer, 700
HER2 gene, in breast cancer, 741
Hering, canals of, 89, 637
Hernias
  abdominal, 609
  inguinal, 609
Herniation, cerebral, 852b
  types of, 851, 852f
Herniation syndromes, 851, 852f
Heroin use
  adverse effects of, 316
  prevalence of, 316
Herpes genitalis, 711–712
Herpes simplex virus (HSV), 712b
  genital, 705t, 711–712
    clinical features of, 711–712
    morphology of, 711b
  vulvitis caused by, 713
Herpes simplex virus (HSV) infections, of oral cavity,
    584–585, 593f
Herpes viral infection, genital
  laboratory diagnosis of, 712
  transmission of, 711
Herpesviruses
  of brain, 866–867, 866f, 866b
  in esophagitis, 593, 593f
Herpes zoster virus, clinical manifestations of, 342,
    343t
Heterochromatin, 3–4, 3f
Heterotopia, of infancy and childhood, 285
HFE gene, 656–657
H5 influenza viruses, 348
HGF. See Hepatocyte growth factor
Hiatal hernia, 594
High-density lipoprotein (HDL) cholesterol, in
    atherosclerosis, 371
Highly active antiretroviral therapy (HAART),
    868
High mobility group box 1 protein (HMGB1), in septic
    shock, 116–117
Hip, severe osteoarthritis of, 819f
Hiroshima bombing
  and radiation carcinogenesis, 231
  survivors of, 323
Hirschsprung disease, 608, 608f
  morphology of, 608b, 608f
  pathogenesis of, 608
Histamine, as mediator of inflammation, 70t, 71
Histiocytic neoplasms, 486–488
Histology, 346
Histone modifying factors, 4
Histone organization, 3–4, 3f
Histoplasma capsulatum, 532, 865
  epidemiology of, 532–533
  morphology of, 532, 533f
HIV-associated neurocognitive disorder (HAND),
    868
Hives. See Urticaria
Hodgkin lymphoma, 463, 476–477, 479–480
  classification of, 465t, 477
  clinical features of, 477
  clinical staging of, 476t, 477
  compared with non-Hodgkin lymphoma, 476t,
    477
  EBV in pathogenesis of, 234
  etiology of, 476
  in HIV-infected individuals, 181
  lymphocyte-predominant, 475f, 476
  mixed-cellularity, 475f, 476
  morphology of, 474b–476b, 474f
  nodular sclerosis type, 475, 475f
  pathogenesis of, 477
  RS cells of, 477
Holoprosencephaly, 861
Homan sign, 391
Homeobox (HOX) proteins, 276
Homeostasis
  and endocrine system, 749
  in hypothalamus-pituitary-thyroid axis, 756f
  process of, 31–32
Homer-Wright pseudorosettes, in pediatric neuroblastomas,
    287, 287f
Homocysteine, in thrombosis, 109
Homovanillic acid (HVA), in neuroblastoma, 288–289
Honeycomb fibrosis, 507–508
"Honeycomb lung", 506–507
Hookworms, 620
Hormonal influences, on breast cancer, 742
Hormone replacement therapy (HRT), 317b

Hormones. See also specific hormones
  in bone development, 799
  categories of, 749
  gut, 336
  lipid-soluble, 749
Horner syndrome, 540
Human chorionic gonadotropins (hCG), 733
Human genome project, 243
Human herpesvirus 8 (HHV8), 181, 394–395
Human immunodeficiency virus (HIV), 173, 867
  and chronic viral hepatitis, 648
  life cycle of, 174–177, 178f
    infection of cells by HIV, 174–175, 178f
    vital replication in, 175
  properties of, 173
    forms of, 174
    structure of, 173–182, 176f
Human immunodeficiency virus (HIV) infection
  acute HIV syndrome in, 178
  CDC classification of, 179, 179t
  clinical course of, 183f
  clinical latency period in, 178
  complications associated with, 182
  effects of antiretroviral drug therapy on, 181
  life cycle of, 177b
  lymphoid involution in, 182
  natural history of, 177, 179f, 183f
  non-AIDS-related complications in, 182
  pathogenesis of, 173–174, 179f, 182b
    central nervous system involvement in, 177
    non-T immune cells in, 175–177
    T-cell depletion in, 175–176
  progression to AIDS in, 177, 179–180
  pulmonary disease in, 537
  spread of, 174
Human leukocyte antigen (HLA) complex
  location of, 126, 127f
  polymorphism of, 127
Human leukocyte antigen (HLA) proteins, in celiac disease,
    613
Human papillomavirus (HPV), 210–211, 211b
  clinical manifestations of, 342, 343t
  and E6 protein, 232, 232f
  and E7 protein, 232–233, 232f
  high-risk, 233
  oncogenic potential of, 232–233, 232f
  types of, 232
  vulvitis caused by, 713
  warts caused by, 895
Human papillomavirus (HPV) DNA, testing for, 718–719
Human papillomavirus (HPV) infection, 705t, 712, 712b
  of cervix, 717
  high-risk, 717–718
  immunosuppression in, 181
  possible consequences of, 718f
  precancerous lesions of, 712
Human papillomavirus (HPV) vaccine, 197, 719
Human T-cell leukemia virus type 1 (HTLV-1), 231–232,
    232b
Humoral immunity
  in host response to microbes, 355
  in myeloma, 475
Huntington disease (HD), 46, 270–271, 879
  characteristics of, 879
  morphology of, 879f, 880b
  pathogenesis of, 879–880
Hurler syndrome, 260. See also Mucopolysaccharidoses
Hürthle cell adenoma, 763, 764f
Hürthle cells, 758
Hyaline arteriolosclerosis, 367b–368b, 368f, 570, 856–857
Hyaline cartilage, 817
Hyaline membrane disease, 277–278, 279f. See also
    Respiratory distress syndrome
Hyaline membranes, eosinophilic, 278
Hyaluronan, 23, 23f
Hydatid cysts, 650
Hydatidiform mole, 733
  features of, 733, 733t
  incidence of, 733
  morphology of, 733b, 734f
  subtypes of, 733
Hydrocele, 692
Hydrocephalus, 851, 851f, 852b
  defined, 851
  in infancy, 851, 851f
Hydromyelia, 862
Hydronephrosis, 577–578
  bilateral, 577
  causes of, 577
  clinical course of, 577–578
  of kidney, 578f
  morphology of, 577b, 578f
  pathogenesis of, 577
Hydropericardium, 98
Hydroperitoneum, 98
Hydrostatic pressure
  increases in, 99, 99f
  vascular, 98, 99f
Hydrothorax, 98, 544
Hydroureter, 577
21-hydroxylase deficiency, 791
Hydroxyurea, in sickle cell disease, 447
Hygiene hypothesis, in epidemiology, 621–622
Hyperacidity, gastric, 602

Hyperaldosteronism, 787–788
  causes of, 790, 791f
  clinical features of, 788–789
  morphology of, 789b
  primary, 790
  secondary, 99, 790
  treatment for, 790
Hyperbilirubinemia
  hereditary, 661
  secondary to immune hydrolysis, 284, 284f
Hypercalcemia
  causes of, 53, 770, 773t
  in multiple myeloma, 473
Hypercholesterolemia, in atherogenesis, 373–374
Hypercoagulability
  defined, 108
  paraneoplastic syndromes as, 236
  primary (inherited), 108–109, 108t
  secondary (acquired), 108t, 109
Hypercortisolism, 788b
Hyperemia, 97
  mechanisms of, 97
  morphology of, 97b–98b
Hyperestrogenemia, in cirrhosis, 641
Hypergastrinemia, 600–601
Hyperglycemia
  CNS effects of, 873
  of diabetes mellitus, 772
  in pregnancy, 783
Hyperhomocysteinemia, in atherosclerosis, 372
Hyper-IgM syndrome
  characteristics of, 170
  treatment for, 170–171
Hyperinsulinemia, and obesity, 336
Hyperkalemia, in adrenocortical insufficiency, 793–794
Hyperkeratosis, definition of, 890t
Hyperlipidemia
  in atherosclerosis, 371
  genesis of, 550
Hypermetabolic state, with burns, 319
Hypermutation, somatic, 465
Hyperparathyroidism, 769–771, 771b, 803
  clinical course of, 803
  described, 802
  morphology of, 803b, 803f
  pathogenesis of, 802–803
  primary and secondary, 803
Hyperparathyroidism, primary, 769–771
  causes of, 769
  clinical features of, 771
  morphologic changes in, 769b–770b, 770f, 773f
  pathogenesis of, 770–771
Hyperparathyroidism, secondary, 771
  causes of, 771
  clinical features of, 771–772
  morphology of, 771b
Hyperparathyroidism, tertiary, 771
Hyperphosphatemia, 771
Hyperpituitarism, 750–751, 753b
Hyperplasia, 51b
  in cellular response to stress, 49
  control of, 50
  germinal center B-cell, 181
  pathologic, 49–50
  physiologic, 49–50
Hyperprolactinemia, 753
Hypersensitivity pneumonitis, 514–515
  antigens causing, 514t
  clinical features of, 515
  histologic appearance, 514f
  as immunologically mediated disease, 514
  morphology of, 514b, 514f
Hypersensitivity reactions, 81, 121, 132–134
  antibody-mediated (type II), 137–139, 139t, 140f
  causes of, 134
  cell-mediated (type IV), 135, 135t, 141–142, 143t
    CD8+ T cell-mediated cytotoxicity, 142–145
    CD4+ T cell-mediated inflammation, 142, 144f
    mechanisms of, 142, 143f, 145b
  classification of, 134–145, 135t
  delayed type, 81, 142, 144f
  immediate (type I), 135, 135t, 139b
    clinical and pathologic manifestations of, 136–137, 138f,
      139b
    development of allergies in, 136–139, 139b
    disorders caused by, 137, 138t
    genetic predisposition to, 503
    phases of, 138f
    sequence of events in, 135–136, 136f, 139b
  immune complex-mediated (type III), 139–140, 141f, 141t
    local, 141
    in SLE, 153
    systemic, 139–142, 141f
  mechanisms of, 135, 135t
  pathogenesis of, 142b
Hypersensitivity vasculitis, 387–388
Hypertension, 364, 366–367, 367b–368b
  aortic aneurysms in, 379
  arteries in, 362
  in atherosclerosis, 371
  in chronic alcoholism, 312
  complications of, 420–421
  in Cushing syndrome, 789
  diagnosing, 366

Hypertension (Continued)
 and diet, 338
 epidemiology of, 366–367
 essential, 366–367
 malignant, 367
 mechanisms of, 367
 and obesity, 334
 pathogenesis of, 367, 367t
 in pregnancy, 735
 pulmonary, 367b–368b, 368f
 types of, 367t
Hypertensive heart disease (HHD), 420–422, 422b
 diagnosis of, 421
 pulmonary hypertensive heart disease, 422
 systemic (left-sided), 421–422
  clinical features of, 422
  morphology of, 421b, 421f
Hypertensive vascular disease, 366–367, 367t, 368b, 368f
Hyperthermia, 319
Hyperthermia, malignant, 319
Hyperthyroidism, 755–768. See also Graves disease;
  Thyrotoxicosis
 apathetic, 757
 diagnosis of, 757
 multinodular goiters in, 762
Hypertriglyceridemia, and obesity, 336
Hypertrophic cardiomyopathy (HCM)
 causes and consequences of, 431f
 characteristics of, 432
 clinical features of, 433
 morphology of, 433b, 434f
 pathogenesis of, 432
Hypertrophy, 51f
 in adaptation to stress, 48–49, 48f–49f
 cardiac, 48–49, 49f
 and degenerative changes, 49
Hyperuricemia, 823
Hyperviscosity syndromes, 108, 474
Hypoadrenalism, secondary, 793
Hypoalbuminemia, 550
 of kwashiorkor, 325, 325f
 in nephrotic syndrome, 550
Hypocalcemia
 and vitamin D, 329
 and vitamin D deficiency, 330
Hypochromia, in thalassemia, 449–450
Hypoglycemia, CNS effects of, 873
Hypokalemia, in primary hyperaldosteronism, 790
Hyponatremia, in adrenocortical insufficiency, 793–794
Hypoparathyroidism, 772–784
 causes of, 771
 clinical manifestations of, 772
Hypophosphatemia, 329
Hypopituitarism, 750, 754
 causes of, 754
 clinical manifestations of, 755
Hypoplasia
 in congenital heart disease, 404
 of kidneys, 578
 use of term, 275
Hypoproteinemia, in CF, 253
Hypospadias, 691
Hypotension
 in adrenocortical insufficiency, 793–794
 effects of, 364
Hypothermia, 319
Hypothyroidism, 756–757
 causes of, 757, 770t
 clinical manifestations of, 757
 laboratory evaluation of, 757–758
 primary, 757
Hypoventilation syndrome, and obesity, 337
Hypovolemic shock, with burns, 318–319
Hypoxia
 in angiogenesis, 220, 220b
 in cell injury, 48b
 cell injury caused by, 32, 42f–43f
 functional, 852
 functional and morphologic consequences of, 42–43, 43f
 in ionizing radiation, 321
Hypoxia-inducible factor-1 (HIF-1) family, 42
Hypoxic encephalopathy, in heart failure, 402

I
Icterus, in acute liver failure, 639
Idiopathic pulmonary fibrosis (IPF), 507–508
 clinical features of, 508
 morphology of, 507b–508b, 508f
 pathogenesis of, 507, 507f
 proposed pathogenic mechanisms in, 507f
Idiopathic retroperitoneal fibrosis, 162
IgA, in humoral immunity, 132–133, 133f
IgA nephropathy, 556t, 561–562, 564
 clinical course of, 562
 mesangial deposition of IgA in, 562f
 morphology of, 561b–562b, 562f
 pathogenesis of, 561
 secondary, 561
IgE, in humoral immunity, 132–133, 133f
IgE antibodies
 helminths targeted by, 137
 in immediate hypersensitivity, 136, 136f
IgE-triggered reaction, 137

IgG, in humoral immunity, 132–133, 133f
IgG4-related disease (IgG4-RD), 162, 163f
IgM, in humoral immunity, 132–133, 133f
Ileitis, backwash, 624–625
Illness, PEM associated with, 324
Immune competence, and EBV, 233–234
Immune complex disease, 139–142, 141f
 deposition of immune complexes in, 141–142
 formation of immune complexes in, 140–142, 141f
 inflammation and tissue injury in, 141–142, 142b
Immune complex-mediated disorders (type III
  hypersensitivity), 135, 135f
Immune dysregulation, polyendocrinopathy, enteropathy,
  X-linked (IPEX), 145
Immune-privileged sites, antigens located in, 145
Immune reactions
 inflammation caused by, 59
 injurious, 134
Immune reconstitution inflammatory syndrome (IRIS),
  868
Immune responses
 adaptive, 130
  capture and display of antigens in, 130, 131f
  cell-mediated immunity, 130–134, 131f–132f
  decline of, 132
 innate, 133
 normal, 121–124, 134b
 in trisomy 21 patients, 266
Immune surveillance
Immune system, 121–122
 components of, 123–124
 innate, 134b
 lymphocytes in, 124
 microbe evasion of, 355–357, 356f, 357b
Immune thrombocytopenic purpura (ITP), 488–491
Immunity, 121
 adaptive, 122, 122f, 134b
  components of, 124
  types of, 124
 B lymphocytes in, 132, 133f
 cell-mediated, 130, 131f, 134b
  activation of T lymphocytes in, 130–131, 131f–132f
  elimination of intracellular microbes in, 131
 humoral, 134b
 innate, 121–124, 122f
  components of, 122–124
  C-type lectin receptors in, 123
  host defense in, 123
  NOD-like receptors in, 123
  pattern recognition receptors in, 122f, 123
  toll-like receptors in, 122–123
Immunodeficiencies, 121, 134, 166–168
 acquired, 359
 clinical manifestations of, 168
 defects in innate immunity, 171, 172t, 173b
  defects affecting complement system, 172
  defects in leukocyte function, 171
 in HSC transplants, 165–166
 infections in individuals with, 358–359
 primary (inherited) immunodeficiencies, 166–168, 173b,
  175f
  associated with systemic diseases, 171
  common variable immunodeficiency, 170
  with defects in lymphocyte activation, 170–171
  DiGeorge syndrome (thymic hypoplasia), 168–171
  hyper-IgM syndrome, 168–170
  isolated IgA deficiency, 170
  severe combined immunodeficiency, 168
  X-linked agammaglobulinemia, 168–173
 secondary (acquired) deficiencies, 172
  acquired immunodeficiency syndromes, 172
  causes of, 173t
 and vitamin A, 329
Immunoglobulin G4 (IgG4)-related disease, 380
Immunohemolytic anemia, 451, 453
 cause of, 451
 classification of, 451, 451t
 cold antibody immunohemolytic anemia, 451, 451t
 diagnosis of, 451
 warm antibody immunohemolytic anemia, 451, 451t
Immunohistochemistry, in diagnosis of cancer, 238
Immunologic memory, decline of, 132
Immunologic reactions, cell injury caused by, 32
Immunologic tolerance, 143–144, 149f–150b
 central tolerance, 145, 146f
 mechanisms of, 146f
 peripheral tolerance, 145–162
Immunosuppression
 and cutaneous squamous cell carcinomas, 901
 and infectious agents, 347
Impetigo, 894
 clinical features of, 894
 lesions of, 894, 895f
 morphology of, 894b
Incretins, 775
Induced pluripotent (iPS) cells, 28, 28f
Infancy, hazards of, 273
Infants, small-for-gestational-age, 277–278. See also Neonates
Infarctions, 97, 114–115, 115b
 causes of, 112
 development of, 115
 in polycythemia vera, 482
 septic, 115
 in sickle cell anemia, 446

Infarctions, cerebral, 853, 853f
 embolic, 853
 thrombotic occlusions causing, 853
Infarcts
 causes of, 114
 classification of, 114b–115b, 114f
 defined, 114
 histologic finding in, 114b–115b, 115f
 kidney, 115f
Infarcts, cerebral
 border zone (watershed), 853
 hemorrhagic, 853, 854f
 nonhemorrhagic, 853, 854b, 854f
Infections
 inflammation caused by, 59
 inflammatory responses to, 357–359, 357b, 357f
  chronic inflammation and scarring, 358, 358f
  cytopathic-cytoproliferative reaction, 357
  individuals with immunodeficiencies, 358–359
  mononuclear and granulomatous inflammation, 357,
   357b, 357f
  tissue necrosis, 358
 in opioid abuse, 316
 and tissue repair, 93
 vasculitis secondary to, 384
Infectious agents. See also Microbes
 and cancer risk, 198–199
 categories of, 341–346, 342t
  bacteria, 342–343, 343t
  ectoparasites, 346
  fungi, 343–345, 345f
  helminths, 345
  prions, 341
  protozoa, 345
  viruses, 341–342, 342f
 cell injury caused by, 32
 newly emerging, 347
Infectious agents, identification of
 culture, 346–347
 histology, 346
 molecular diagnostics, 347
 proteomics, 347
 serology, 346–347
 techniques for, 347t
Infectious diseases
 and antibiotic resistance, 348
 and climate change, 300
 emergence of, 348
 as global concern, 341
 manifestations of, 351
 rapid identification of, 292
Infective endocarditis (IE), 427
 classification of, 427
 clinical features of, 427–428
 morphology of, 427b, 428f
 pathogenesis of, 427
 prognosis for, 427–428
Inferior vena cava syndrome, 391
Infertility
 with cryptorchidism, 692
 in cystic fibrosis, 252–254
Inflammasome
 in innate immunity, 123, 123f
 microbial escaping from, 356
Inflammation
 in atherosclerosis, 371–372, 374
 causes of, 58–59, 60b
 in cell injury, 48b
 cell injury caused by, 47
 chronic, 57–58, 58t
 defective, 58–59
 defined, 57
 diseases caused by, 58, 59t
 external manifestations of, 58
 features of, 60b
 of female breast, 736–737
 and innate immunity, 121–122
 and obesity, 337
 recognition of microbes and damaged cells in, 59–60
 scar formation in, 89–90
 systemic effects of, 86–87, 87b
 termination of, 59
 in type II hypersensitivity, 139, 140f
Inflammation, acute, 57–58, 58t
 blood vessel reactions in, 60–62, 61f, 62b
 chemokines in, 75
 chemotaxis of leukocytes in, 65
 components of, 58f, 58t, 60–70
 and functional responses of activated leukocytes,
  70
 increased vascular permeability in, 61–62, 61f
 intracellular destruction of microbes and debris in,
  68–69
 leukocyte activation in, 66–67, 66f
 leukocyte adhesion to endothelium in, 62–65, 64t
 leukocyte-mediated tissue injury, 69–70
 leukocyte migration through endothelium in, 65
 leukocytes infiltrates in, 65, 66f
 lymphatic vessels and lymph nodes in, 62
 morphological patterns of, 78–79
  fibrinous inflammation, 78, 79f
  purulent inflammation, 78–79, 79f
  serous inflammation, 78, 78f
  ulcers, 79, 80f

Inflammation, acute (Continued)
  neutrophil extracellular traps, 69, 69f
  outcomes of, 79–81, 80f
  phagocytosis in, 67, 67f
  termination of, 70
  vascular flow and caliber changes in, 60–61
Inflammation, chronic, 81–85
  causes of, 81
  cells and mediators of, 82–85
  in collagen synthesis in chronic inflammatory diseases, 95b
  eosinophils in, 84, 84f
  granulomatous inflammation, 85
  macrophage-lymphocyte interactions in, 84f
  mast cells in, 84–85
  morphologic features of, 81–82, 81f
  neutrophils in, 85
  role of lymphocytes in, 83–84, 84f
  role of macrophages in, 82–83, 82f–83f
Inflammation, mediators of, 70–78, 70t
  actions of, 78b
  arachidonic acid metabolites, 70t, 71–73, 72f, 72t
  chemokines, 74–75
  complement system, 75–77, 76f
  cytokines, 73–75, 74t, 75f
  defined, 70–71
  histamine, 70t, 71
  kinins, 77
  leukotrienes, 70t, 72f, 72t, 73
  lipoxins, 72f, 73
  neuropeptides, 77–78
  origins of, 71
  platelet-activating factor, 77–78, 77t
  products of coagulation, 77
  prostaglandins, 71–73, 72f
  serotonin, 71
  vasoactive amines, 70t, 71
Inflammatory bowel disease (IBD), 142–143, 143t, 621–626, 626b
  and colitis-associated neoplasia, 625–626
  Crohn disease, 623–624
  epidemiology of, 621–622
  gastroenteritic dysbiosis in, 346
  genetics of, 622–623
  microbiota in, 623
  pathogenesis of, 622–623, 622f
  ulcerative colitis, 624–625
Inflammatory cells, cancer-enabling effects of, 228
Inflammatory diseases
  in host response to microbes, 355
  immune-mediated, 135
Inflammatory reaction
  sequence of events in, 58f
  steps in, 57
Inflammatory response
  in development of AD, 875
  physiological function of, 65
Inflammatory states, and cancer, 199, 199t
Influenza, 341
Influenza epidemics, 524
Influenza infections, 524
Inhalation injury, 319
Injuries
  electrical, 319–320
  from ionizing radiation, 320–323
  thermal, 318–319
Innate immune inflammation, in host response to microbes, 355
Innate immunity, defects in, 172t
Innate lymphoid cells (ILCs), 128
Insulin
  effects on glucose of, 775–776
  metabolic function of, 774f, 775
  mitogenic functions, 775
  production of, 772
  in regulation of adiposity, 336
Insulin-like growth factor 1 (IGF1), 753
Insulinlike growth factor-2 (IGF2), in Wilms tumor, 289
Insulinomas, 782–783
  characteristic clinical picture for, 785
  morphology of, 784b, 785f
Insulin physiology, normal, 774–775
Insulin resistance
  and cancer, 337
  defined, 776
  functional defects in, 776
  and obesity, 336
  obesity and, 776
Insulin-resistant diabetes, 139t
Insulitis, 776, 780f, 785
Integrins, 23–24, 24f
  in acute inflammation, 63–65, 64f, 64t
  in cell-cell interactions, 12
Interferon pathways, microbial disruption of, 356–357
Interferons, in SLE, 152
Interleukin-1 (IL-1), 73–74, 74t, 75f, 799
Interleukin 8 (IL-8), in ARDS, 496
Interleukins, 129–130. See also Cytokines
Intermediate filaments, of cytoskeleton, 11
International Labor Organization, 299
Interstitial lung disease, pulmonary hypertension associated with, 517

Intestinal disease, inflammatory
  inflammatory bowel disease, 621–626
  sigmoid diverticulitis, 620–621
Intestinal dysbiosis, in diabetic children, 776
Intestinal metaplasia, mucosal atrophy and, 603
Intestines, small and large, 607–633
  diarrheal disease in, 611–620
  inflammatory intestinal disease, 620–626
  intestinal obstruction, 607–609, 608f
  vascular disorders of bowel, 609–610
Intima
  of blood vessels, 361–362, 362f
  in vascular injury, 368
Intracellular accumulations, 51–53, 52f–53f
Intracranial pressure (ICP), elevation of, 850
Intraductal papillary mucinous neoplasms (IPMNs), 686, 687f
Intrinsic pathway, in apoptosis, 217f
Intussusception, 608, 608f
Invasion, by microbes, 351
Invasive mole, 733–734
Invasiveness, of tumors, 195, 195f
Involucrum, formation of, 807, 807f
Iodine
  deficiency syndrome for, 333t
  functions of, 333t
iPS. See Induced pluripotent cells
Iraq, mercury contamination in, 305
Iron
  deficiency syndrome for, 333t
  functions of, 333t
  in hemochromatosis, 656
  in Western diet, 455
Iron deficiency anemia, 458
  assessment of, 455
  clinical features of, 455, 455f
  in Crohn disease, 624
  pathogenesis of, 455
  peripheral blood smear, 455f
  prevalence of, 454–455
  and regulation of iron absorption, 454f, 455
Irritable bowel syndrome (IBS). See also Inflammatory bowel disease
Ischemia
  causes of, 852
  in cell injury, 48b
  cell injury caused by, 32, 42f–43f
  cerebral, 854–856
  functional and morphologic consequences of, 42–43, 43f
  global cerebral, 852–853, 853b, 853f
  myocardial, 408
Ischemia-reperfusion injury, 43, 48b
Ischemic bowel disease, 609–610
  clinical features of, 610
  morphology of, 609b–610b, 610f
  pathogenesis of, 609
Ischemic heart disease (IHD), 366–367, 419b
  acute plaque change in, 410, 410f
  angina pectoris, 411
  chronic, 409, 419
    morphology of, 419b
  in coronary artery disease, 420, 421f
  epidemiology of, 409
  and left-sided cardiac failure, 401
  manifestations of, 409
  myocardial infarction, 411–419
  pathogenesis of, 409
Islet cell tumors, 778–779
Islets of Langerhans, 679, 683
Isochromosomes, 263
Isocitrate dehydrogenase (IDH)
  mutations in, 216–217, 881
  oncogenic pathway of, 216, 216f
Isolated IgA deficiency, 170
Isoniazid, hepatotoxicity of, 651–652
Itai-itai disease, 306

J
Janeway lesions, 427
Japan, radiation carcinogenesis in, 231
Jaundice
  in acute liver failure, 639
  causes of, 659, 660t
  in hemorrhage, 100–101
  in liver failure, 639
  neonatal, 661
  pathophysiology of, 660–661
JC virus, in AIDS, 180
Joints, 817–827
  arthritis of, 817–825
  functions of, 817
  hyaline cartilage of, 817
  in SLE, 156
  tumorlike conditions of, 826–827
    ganglion, 826
    synovial cyst, 826
  tumors of, 826–827
Joubert syndrome, 862
"Jumping genes", 2
Juvenile idiopathic arthritis (JIA), 821–822
  characteristics of, 821–822
Juvenile polyposis, 627t

K
Kallikrein enzyme, 77
Kaplan-Meier survival curve, for infants with metastatic neuroblastoma, 288f
Kaposi sarcoma (KS), 394–395
  AIDS-associated, 394–395
  as AIDS-defining malignancy, 180
  classic, 394
  clinical presentation of, 181, 395
  endemic African, 394
  lesions of, 180–181, 395b, 395f
  morphology of, 395b, 395f
  pathogenesis of, 395
  transplantation-associated, 394
Kaposi sarcoma (KS) herpesvirus (KSHV), 181, 394–395
Karyotype
  defined, 262, 263f
  from normal male, 263f
Kasai procedure, 663
Kawasaki disease, 384, 387
  clinical features of, 387
  etiology of, 387
  morphology of, 387b
Kayser-Fleischer rings, 658
KCNJ5 gene, 792
Keratinocytes, 889
Keratoconjunctivitis, in Sjögren syndrome, 158
Kernicterus, in fetal hydrops, 284
Kernohan's notch, 851
Ketamine, 317
Ketoacidosis, 775–776, 779, 779f
Kidney disease, 574–575, 576b. See also Renal disease
  autosomal recessive polycystic, 575, 576b
  congenital and developmental anomalies, 578
  cystic diseases, 576b
  medullary diseases with cysts, 575–576
  neoplasms, 578–580
  in opioid abuse, 316
Kidney disease, chronic, 549–550, 572–573
  clinical course of, 573
  morphology of, 573b, 573f
  pathogenesis of, 573
Kidneys
  acute injury to, 550
  amyloidosis of, 186
  in blood pressure regulation, 365
  cystic diseases of, 573–576
    autosomal dominant polycystic, 574–575, 576b
    simple cysts, 573–574
  functions of, 549
  in lead exposure, 304f, 305
  neoplasms of, 578–580
    oncocytoma, 578–580
    renal cell carcinoma, 578–580
    Wilms tumor, 580
  in SLE, 154
  in systemic sclerosis, 160
  vascular diseases of, 572b
Kimmelstiel-Wilson lesion, 783
Kininogens, 77
Kinins, as mediators of inflammation, 77
Klebsiella pneumoniae, 521
Klinefelter syndrome, 269
  clinical manifestations of, 267
  defined, 267
  fertility in, 267
Knockdown technology, 4–5
Korsakoff psychosis, 324
Korsakoff syndrome, 311–312, 333t, 873–874
KRAS gene, mutation of, 631–632
KRAS oncogene, in pancreatic cancer, 687, 687f
Krukenberg tumor, 729
Kupffer cell, 637
Kupffer cell activation, in liver disease, 639
Kwashiorkor, 324–325, 325f, 334b
  clinical presentation of, 325
  prevalence of, 325

L
Lacerations, 317
  defined, 317–318
  of scalp, 318f
Lacrimal glands
  in sarcoidosis, 513
  in Sjögren syndrome, 158
Lactose deficiency, 614
Lacunar cells, in Hodgkin lymphoma, 475f, 477
Lacunes, 857
Lambert-Eaton syndrome, 839
Lamellar bone, mosaic pattern of, 804, 804f
Laminin, 23–24, 24f
LAMP1 gene, 233
Langerhans cell histiocytoses, 486–488
  clinicopathologic entities for, 484
  pathogenesis of, 484–485
Langerhans cells, 128
Large bile duct obstruction, 665
Large-cell change, in chronic liver disease, 670
Laryngeal cancer, carcinogenic interaction in, 309f
Laryngeal tumors, 546–547
  carcinoma of larynx, 546–547, 547f
  nonmalignant lesions, 546
Laryngitis, acute, 545–546

Laryngotracheobronchitis, 546
L-dihydroxyphenylalanine (L-DOPA), in Parkinson disease, 879
LDL. *See* Low-density lipoprotein
Lead
    absorbed, 304
    exposure to, 304
    health effects of, 304
Lead lines, radiodense, 304, 305f
Lead poisoning
    clinical features of, 304, 304f
    from contaminated drinking water, 299
    pathologic features of, 304, 304f
Lead toxicity, anatomic targets of, 305
Leber hereditary optic neuropathy, 271
Left anterior descending (LAD) artery, acute occlusion of, 412–413
Left circumflex (LCX) artery, acute occlusion of, 412–413
Legionella pneumophila, 521–522
Legionnaire disease, 521–522
Legs, bowing of, 331, 331f
Leiden mutation, 108–109
Leiomyomas, 197f, 725–726, 830–831
    development of, 725
    morphology of, 725b–726b, 726f
    parasitic, 725–726
Leiomyosarcomas, 726, 831
    clinical course for, 831
    morphology of, 726b, 831b
    recurrence of, 726
LEP gene, 334
Leprosy, granulomatous inflammation with, 86t
Leptin, 325
    functions of, 335–336
    net effect of, 334
    role of energy balance of, 337
Leptin gene, mutations of, 336
Leukemia, 463
    chromosomal translocations and oncogenes in, 202, 202f
    designation as, 190–191
    hairy cell, 477
    HTLV-1-associated, 232
    in trisomy 21 patients, 266
Leukemoid reactions, 87
Leukocyte adhesion deficiencies (LADs), 171, 172t
Leukocytes
    activation of, 66–67, 66f, 70b
    in acute inflammation, 61
        adhesion to endothelium of, 62–65, 64t
        leukocyte recruitment to sites of, 62–65, 64f, 65b
        migration through endothelium of, 65
        recruitment to sites of, 62–65, 64f, 65b
    chemotaxis of, 65
    defects in function of, 172t
    and functional responses of activated, 70
    infiltrates in inflammatory reactions, 65, 66f
    margination of, 62–63
    migration through blood vessels of, 64f
    recruitment to sites of inflammation, 65b
    and susceptibility to infections, 58–59
    tissue injury caused by, 69–70
Leukocytoclastic vasculitis, 387–388
Leukocytosis
    basophilic, 460t
    causes of, 460, 460t
    eosinophilic, 460t
    in inflammation reactions, 87
    monocytosis, 460t
    neutrophilic, 460t
Leukodystrophies, 872
Leukoencephalopathy, progressive multifocal, 868, 868f, 870b
Leukoerythroblastosis, 458
Leukomalacia, periventricular, 862, 862f
Leukopenia, 87, 459
Leukoplakia, 585–586, 586b
    defined, 585–586
    morphology of, 586b, 586f
Leukotriene receptor antagonists, as inflammatory agents, 73
Leukotrienes, 70t, 72f, 72t, 73
    pharmacologic inhibitors of, 73
    synthesis of, 73
Lewy bodies, in PD, 878f, 879
Lewy neurites, in PD, 879
Libman-Sacks endocarditis, 110, 156, 157f, 428f, 429
Lichenification of, 890t
Lichen planus, 893–894
    clinical features of, 894
    description of, 893
    morphology of, 893, 893f
Lichen simplex chronicus, 894
    clinical features of, 894
    morphology of, 894b, 894f
Liddle syndrome, 367
Life span, and diet, 338
Lifestyles, and colorectal adenocarcinoma, 627–628
Li-Fraumeni syndrome, 211–212, 809
Ligands, in cell signaling, 16, 17f
Limb-girdle muscular dystrophies, 843
Lipid mediators, in immediate hypersensitivity reactions, 136f, 137
Lipid rafts, 8

Lipids
    abnormal depositions of, 54b
    glycosylation of, 12–13
Lipofuscin, role in cell injury of, 52, 53f
Lipoma, 828
Lipoprotein(a) levels, in atherosclerosis, 372
Liposarcoma
    clinical course of, 828
    defined, 828
    morphology of, 828b, 829f
Lipoxins, as mediators of inflammation, 72f, 73
Lipoxygenase inhibitors, in treatment of asthma, 73
Lissencephaly (agyria), 861
Liver
    amyloidosis in, 186
    anatomy of, 637
    benign neoplasms of, 669
        cavernous hemangiomas, 669
        hepatocellular adenomas, 669
    in chronic alcoholism, 311
    in cystic fibrosis, 252–253
    focal nodular hyperplasia of, 668, 668b–669b, 668f
    hepatic masses, 668
    in kwashiorkor, 326
    lobular model of, 637, 638f
    malignant neoplasms of
        cholangiocarcinoma, 671
        hepatocellular carcinoma, 669
    metabolism of bilirubin by, 659
    metastatic cancer of, 195, 195f
    regeneration of, 89
    resistance to infarction of, 115
    in sarcoidosis, 513
    tissue regeneration in, 88–89
    tumors of, 672b
Liver cancer, and HCV, 235
Liver disease, 638–642. *See also* Fatty liver disease
    immunologic reactions in, 639
    infectious disorders
        bacteria, 650
        fungal, 650
        helminthic, 650
        parasitic, 650
    laboratory evaluation of, 638, 638t
    and liver failure, 639–642
    and mechanisms of injury and repair, 638–639
Liver disease, alcoholic, 640, 655b
    clinical features in, 654–655
    morphology of, 654f
    pathogenesis of, 653–654
    statistics for, 653
    treatment for, 655
Liver disease, chronic, 638
    with cirrhosis, 641–642
    ductular reactions in, 641
Liver disease, inherited metabolic, 656–659, 659b
    hemochromatosis, 656–657
    Wilson disease, 657–658
    α_1-antitrypsin deficiency, 658–659
Liver disease, nonalcoholic fatty, 656b
Liver failure, 639–642, 642b
    acute-on-chronic, 642
    fulminant, 639
    in viral hepatitis, 642–648
Liver failure, acute
    clinical course for, 639–640
    defined, 639
    morphology of, 639b, 640f
Liver failure, chronic, 640
Liver fluke infection, 650
Liver flukes, 671
Liver infarct, 666, 666f
Liver injury
    in hemochromatosis, 657
    toxin-induced, 651–652, 652t
Liver injury, drug-induced, 651–652, 652t
    diagnosis of, 651
    morphology of, 652b–653b
Liver injury, toxin-induced
    diagnosis of, 651
    morphology of, 652b–653b
Lobar pneumonia, 522, 522f
Lobular carcinoma in situ (LCIS), 742–743, 743f
Lobule, of lung, 498–500
Local invasion, of tumor, 194–195, 194f
Locomotion, in invasion of ECM, 222
Loeffler endomyocarditis, 434
Loeffler syndrome, 515
Long noncoding RNAs (lncRNA), 4–5, 5f
Lordosis, 331, 331f
Losartan, in Marfan syndrome, 247
Low-density lipoprotein (LDL), 11
    in atherosclerosis, 371
    in hypothyroidism, 757
    metabolism of, 248–249, 249f
Lumpiness, in breast disease, 737
Lung
    acute inflammation of, 81f
    chronic inflammation in, 81, 81f
    infarction of, 115
    tuberculosis of, 36–37, 37f
Lung abscess, 525
    clinical features of, 525
    morphology of, 525b

Lung cancer
    risk of developing, 309, 309f
    and tobacco, 307–308
Lung carcinoma
    causation of, 309
    precursor lesions associated with, 199
Lung fibrosis, 58
Lungs
    defense mechanisms of, 520f
    diseases and disorders of
        acute respiratory distress syndrome, 496–497
        atelectasis, 495–496
        chronic interstitial diseases, 506–515
        obstructive airway diseases, 498–506, 499t
        obstructive *vs.* restrictive, 498
        pleural lesions, 544–545
        pulmonary infections, 519–537
        upper-respiratory tract of, 545–547
        vascular origins of, 515–519
    function of, 495
    in left-sided heart failure, 401–402
    primary disease of, 495
    in sarcoidosis, 513
    in SLE, 156
    in systemic sclerosis, 160
Lung transplantation, sarcoidosis following, 513
Lung tumors, 537–544
    carcinoid tumors, 543–544
    carcinomas, 537–543
Lupus anticoagulant, 151
Lupus erythematosus (LE). *See also* Systemic lupus erythematosus
    chronic discoid, 153
    drug induced, 153–154
    subacute cutaneous, 157
Lupus erythematosus (LE) bodies, in SLE, 153, 156–157
Lupus nephritis, in SLE, 154, 155f
Luteal cysts, of ovaries, 727
Lyme arthritis, 822–823
Lyme disease
    myocarditis in, 435
    phases of, 823f
    PTLDS, 823
Lymph, spread of microbes via, 351
Lymphadenitis, 62, 461–463
    acute nonspecific, 461
    cat-scratch disease, 463–477
    chronic nonspecific, 462
    morphology of, 461b–462b
    reactive, 62
Lymphadenopathy, in infectious mononucleosis, 461
Lymphangiomas, 285, 393
Lymphangitis, 62, 391
Lymphatic drainage, impaired, 99–100
Lymphatics
    structure and function of, 363
    tumors of, 391–392, 392t
        bacillary angiomatosis, 394, 394f
        glomus tumors, 394
        lymphangiomas, 393
Lymphatic vessels, primary disorders of, 391
    lymphangitis, 391
    lymphedema, 391
Lymphedema, 99–100, 391
Lymph nodes, 128
    histology of, 129f
    in HIV infection, 182
    morphology of, 129f
    in sarcoidosis, 513
    sentinel, 196
Lymphocytes, 134b
    activation of, 134b
    B lymphocytes, 124–125, 125f (*see also* B lymphocytes)
    in chronic inflammation, 83–84, 84f
    innate lymphoid cells, 128
    in late-phase hypersensitivity reactions, 137, 138f
    and MHC molecules, 124–128
    natural killer cells, 128
    phases of, 124
    principal classes of, 124, 125f
    recirculation of, 129
    T lymphocytes, 124–130 (*see also* T lymphocytes)
Lymphocytosis, 87, 460t
Lymphogranuloma venereum (LGV), 711b
    defined, 710
    morphology of, 710b
Lymphoid neoplasms, 227, 227b–228b, 465–467, 477b–478b
    acute lymphoblastic leukemia/lymphoma, 466
    adult T Cell leukemia, 477
    adult T Cell lymphoma, 477
    Burkitt lymphoma, 466t, 471
    cancer hallmarks of, 478f
    characteristics of common, 466t
    chronic lymphocytic leukemia, 468
    classification scheme for, 464
    derivation of, 465
    diffuse large B cell lymphoma, 470
    extranodal marginal zone lymphoma, 466t, 470
    follicular lymphoma, 466t, 468–469
    hairy cell leukemia, 477
    Hodgkin lymphoma, 476–477
    lymphoplasmacytic lymphoma, 474
    mantle cell lymphoma, 466t, 469
    multiple myeloma, 473

Lymphoid neoplasms (Continued)
  mycosis fungoides, 477
  origin of, 464, 464f
  peripheral T cell lymphoma, 477
  plasma cell neoplasms, 472–473
  Sézary syndrome, 477
  small lymphocytic lymphoma, 468
  WHO classification of, 465, 465t
Lymphoid organs, tertiary, 84
Lymphoid systems, 441
  cutaneous, 128
  mucosal, 128
  radiation injury to, 322–323, 322f, 322t
Lymphoid tissues, 128–129, 134b
  cytokines, 129–130
  peripheral lymphoid organs, 129, 129t
Lymphoid tumors, gene rearrangements associated with, 202
Lymphomas, 463
  AIDS-defining, 180–182
  designation as, 190–191
  EBV-positive B-cell, 234
  in gastrointestinal tract, 605
  peripheral T cell, 477
  primary central nervous system, 884–885, 885b
  of stomach, 605
  two groups of, 463
  use of term, 191
Lymphoplasmacytic lymphoma, 474
  clinical features of, 476–477
  immunophenotype for, 474
  morphology of, 473b–474b, 474f
  pathogenesis of, 474
Lyon hypothesis, 267, 269
Lyonization, unfavorable, 451
Lysergic acid diethylamide (LSD), 317
Lysis, by microbes, 351
Lysosomal storage diseases (LSDs), 255–256
  categories for, 256, 257t
  clinical features of, 256
  frequency of, 256
  Gaucher disease, 257t, 258–259, 259f
  mucopolysaccharidoses, 257t, 259–260
  Niemann-Pick diseases, 257–258, 257t
  pathogenesis of, 256, 256f
  Tay-Sachs disease, 256–257, 257t, 258f
Lysosomes
  in cellular waste disposal, 13, 14f
  function of, 6, 7f

M
Macroorchidism, 269
Macrophage mannose receptor, in phagocytosis, 67
Macrophages
  APC properties of, 128
  in cerebral infarct, 854
  in chronic inflammation, 82–83, 82f–83f
  derivation of, 82, 82f
  in HIV infection, 175–176
  major pathways of, 82–83, 83f
  products of activated, 83
  tissue destruction of, 83
  in tuberculosis, 527
Macule, definition of, 890t
Maffucci syndrome, 811
Magnesium ammonium phosphate stones, 576
Major histocompatibility complex (MHC), 124
  Class I, 126
  Class II, 126
  function of, 124–128
Major histocompatibility complex (MHC) restriction, 126
Malabsorptive diarrhea, 611–614
  abetalipoproteinemia, 614
  causes of, 611–612
  celiac disease, 612–613
  cystic fibrosis associated with, 612
  environmental enteropathy, 613–614
  in graft vs. host disease, 614
  lactose (disaccharidase) deficiency, 614
  microscopic colitis, 614
Malabsorptive disease
  in CF, 253
  defects in, 611t
Malakoplakia, of male bladder, 702
Malaria, 341, 453
  causes of, 453
  clinical features of, 453
  and EBV, 233–234
  morphology of, 453b
  pathogenesis of, 452, 452f
  prevalence of, 453
Malformations
  causes of, 275t
  in congenital anomalies, 273–274, 274f
Malformation syndrome, 275
Malignancy
  and celiac disease, 613
  genomic instability as enabler of, 226, 227b–228b
  size in risk for, 628–629
  tumor-promoting inflammation as enabler of, 228

Malignant hypertension, 570–572
  clinical course of, 570–571
  morphology of, 570b, 571f
  pathogenesis of, 570
  renal manifestations of, 570
Malignant mesothelioma, 544–545
  asbestos associated with, 544–545
  morphology of, 545b, 545f
  pathogenesis of, 545
Malignant transformation, risk for, 199
Malignant tumors, nomenclature for, 190–191
Mallory-Denk bodies
  in biliary obstruction, 662
  in fatty liver disease, 653, 653f
  in PBC, 664
Mallory-Weiss syndrome, 591, 593f
Malnutrition, 324
  alcoholism associated with, 312
  causes of, 324
  and climate change, 300
  disease related to, 299
  primary, 324
  protein-energy, 324–326
  secondary, 324
  secondary protein-energy, 326
MALT. See Mucosa-associated lymphoid tissue
MALT lymphomas, 235
Mammographic screening, 737
Mammography, benign epithelial lesions on, 738
Mannose-binding lectin, 60, 67
Mannose-6-phosphate (M6P) receptor, 12–13
Mantle cell lymphoma, 466t, 469, 478
  clinical features of, 470
  immunophenotype for, 469–470
  morphology of, 469b
  pathogenesis of, 469
Marasmus, 325, 325f, 334b
  clinical presentation of, 325, 325f
  compared with kwashiorkor, 324
Marble bone disease, 800
Marfan syndrome, 245, 247–248, 247b–248b, 378–381, 424
  abnormalities in, 247
  morphology of, 247b
  type 2 (MFS2), 247
Marijuana
  CNS consequences of, 317
  components of, 317
  effect on lungs of, 317
  in U.S., 317
Marrow aplasia, radiation-caused, 322–323
Masses, palpable, in breast disease, 737
Mass spectrometry, 347
Mast cells, 137
  in chronic inflammation, 84–85
  in immediate hypersensitivity, 136, 136f
Maternal factors, in fetal growth restriction, 278
Maternal milk, transmission of infection during, 352
Matrix metalloproteinases (MMPs), collagen degraded by, 377
Maturity-onset diabetes of young (MODY), 778
Mazabraud syndrome, 816
McArdle disease, 260–261, 261t
McCune-Albright syndrome, 816
M cells, 350
Mean cell hemoglobin concentration (MCHC), 442, 443t
Mean cell hemoglobin (MCH), 442, 443t
Mean cell volume (MCV), 442, 443t
Mechanotransduction, 798, 798f
Meconium ileus, in CF, 252–253, 252f
Media layer, of blood vessels, 361–362, 362f
Medullary sponge kidney, 575
Medulloblastoma, 884
  morphology of, 884f, 885b
  pathogenesis of, 884–885
  survival rate for, 884
Megalencephaly, 861
Melanin, role in cell injury of, 52
Melanocytic nevi
  clinical features of, 903
  morphology of, 903b
  pathogenesis of, 903
Melanoma, 905
  ABCs of, 906
  of brain, 886, 886f
  clinical features of, 906–907
  and host immune response, 906
  immune checkpoint inhibitors in, 907
  molecular evolution of, 905–906, 906f
  morphology of, 906b, 907f
  pathogenesis of, 905–906, 906f
  probability of metastasis for, 906–907
  use of term, 191
Membranoproliferative glomerulonephritis (MPGN), 552–553, 556t, 559–560
  clinical course of, 559–560
  morphology of, 559b, 559f
  pathogenesis of, 559
  types of, 559, 559f
Membranous nephropathy, 556t, 557–559
  clinical course of, 558–559
  morphology of, 558b, 558f
  pathogenesis of, 558
  primary and secondary, 557–558
Memory cells, long-lived, 133

Mendelian disorders, 245–261
  compared with multifactorial disorders, 262
  GWASs in, 296
  inheritance patterns for, 245t
  linkage analysis in, 295–296
  molecular diagnosis of, 291–296
    with array-based genomic hybridization, 293–294, 294f
    with FISH, 292–293, 293f
  mutations in genes encoding enzyme proteins
    galactosemia, 255, 255b
    glycogen storage diseases (glycogenoses), 260, 261b, 261t, 262f
    lysosomal storage diseases, 255–260, 256f, 257t, 260b
    phenylketonuria, 254–255, 255b, 255f
    regulating cell growth, 261
  mutations in genes encoding receptor proteins or channels
    cystic fibrosis, 250–254, 251f–253f, 252b–254b
    familial hypercholesterolemia, 248–250, 249f–250f, 250b
  mutations in genes encoding structural proteins
    Ehlers-Danlos syndromes, 248, 248b
    Marfan syndrome, 247–248, 247b–248b
  PCR analysis in, 294–295, 295f
  prevalence of, 245t
  transmission patterns of
    autosomal dominant inheritance disorders, 246–247, 247b
    autosomal recessive inheritance disorders, 246, 247b
    X-linked disorders, 246–247, 247b
Ménétrier disease, 598
Meningiomas, 885
  anaplastic (malignant), 885
  atypical, 885
  morphology of, 885b, 886f
  and neurofibromatosis type 2, 885
Meningitis
  aseptic viral, 863
  acute pyogenic, 863–864, 863t
  chronic, 863, 863t
  defined, 862
  fungal, 864, 865f
  infections, 863–864
  morphology of, 864f, 866b
  tuberculous, 863–864
Meningoencephalitis, 866
  amebiasis, 868
  granulomatous, 870
MEN1 mutations, in primary hyperparathyroidism, 770
Menopausal hormone therapy (MHT), adverse reaction to, 313–314
Menopause, and incidence of atherosclerosis-related diseases, 370–371
Menorrhagia, 722
MEN-1 syndrome, 786
Mental retardation
  in fragile X syndrome, 269–270, 270f
  in Prader-Willi syndrome, 272
  in untreated phenylketonuric children, 254
Mercury
  medical disorders associated with, 305
  poisoning with, 305
  sources of exposure to, 305
  toxicity of, 306
Merlin protein, 846
Mesangial cells, of glomerular capillary wall, 551–552, 552f
Mesenchymal to epithelial transformation (MET), during renal morphogenesis, 290
Mesothelioma, use of term, 191. See also Malignant mesothelioma
Metabolic syndrome, 336–337
  in atherosclerosis, 372
  defined, 655
Metabolism, in cancer research, 214–215
Metals. See also Arsenic; Cadmium; Lead; Mercury
  effects on CNS of, 874
  as environmental pollutants, 304–306
Metaplasia, 51b
  defined, 50–51
  epithelial, 51, 51f
  squamous, 51
Metastasis
  of blood cancers, 195
  defined, 195
  distribution of, 222
  and enlargement of nodes, 196
  hematogenous spread of, 196
  limited, 222
  of liver, 195, 195f
  lymphatic vs. hematogenous spread, 196
  pathways for, 195–196
  prediction of sites for, 223
  sentinel lymph node in, 196
  site of, 222
  skip, 196
  systemic distributions of, 196
  within veins, 196
Metastatic cascade, 220–222, 221f
Methyl isocyanate gas leak, in Bhopal, India, 299
Methyl mercury contamination, of Minamata Bay, 299
Metrorrhagia, 722
MHC. See Major histocompatibility complex
Microangiopathy, diabetic, 781f, 783
Microarrays, high-resolution, 291–292

Microbes
  host responses to, 359
  immune evasion by, 355–357, 356f, 357b
  injurious effects of host immune responses to, 355
  reactions against, 134
  routes of entry of, 349–351, 349t, 351f
    gastrointestinal tract, 349–350, 349t
    respiratory tract, 349t, 350
    skin, 349, 349t
    urogenital tract, 349t, 351
  spread and dissemination of, 351, 351f
  transmission of, 352, 352b
  vertical transmission of, 352
Microbiome, 346
  and bacterial identification, 346
  defined, 346
  dysbiosis in, 346
Microcytosis, in thalassemia, 449–450
Microencephaly, 861
Microglial cells, 850, 850f
Microglial nodules, 850
Microorganisms, disease caused by, 352–355, 355b
  bacterial injury, 353–354, 355f
  mechanisms for, 352–353
  viral injury, 353
MicroRNAs (miRNAs), 4–5, 244
  and cancer, 203
  generation of, 5f
Microsatellite instability pathway, in adenomacarcinoma
  sequence, 632, 632f
Microscopic colitis, 614
Microscopic infarcts, 414
Microscopic polyangiitis, 387–388
  clinical features of, 387–388
  in immune disorders, 387
  morphology of, 388b
Microtubule organizing center (MTOC or centrosome), 11
Microtubules, of cytoskeleton, 11
Middle East respiratory syndrome coronavirus (MERS
  CoV), 347
Migration, in invasion of ECM, 222
Mikulicz syndrome
  in IgG4-RD spectrum, 162
  in sarcoidosis, 513
Milroy disease, 391
Minamata Bay, methyl mercury contamination of, 299
Minamata disease, 305–306
Mineral dusts, 307
Minimal-change disease, 555–556, 556t–557t
  clinical course of, 555–556
  morphology of, 555b, 557f
  pathogenesis of, 555
Minimal residual disease, in diagnosis of cancer, 239
Minocycline, adverse reaction to, 312–313, 312f
Mitochondria
  and cell death, 15–16
  energy generation of, 15
  evolution of, 13
  functions of, 15
  and immediate metabolism, 15
  metabolism of, 13–14
  and oxidative metabolism, 15
  roles of, 15f
  as source of reactive oxygen species, 15
Mitochondrial DNA
  inheritance of, 271
  maternally inherited, 13–14
Mitochondrial genes, diseases caused by mutations in, 271
Mitotic catastrophe, 218–219, 219f
Mixed connective tissue disease, 159–162
Mobile genetic elements, 2
Molecular diagnostics
  copy number abnormalities
    array-based genomic hybridization, 293–294, 294f
    fluorescence in situ hybridization, 292–293, 293f
  expansion of, 291–292
  in identification of infectious agents, 347
  indications for genetic analysis, 292
  linkage analysis and genomewide association studies,
    295–296
  polymerase chain reaction analysis, 294–295, 295f–296f
Molecular profiling, in cancer diagnosis, 239–241, 241f
Molecular techniques, in diagnosis of cancer, 239, 240f
Mönckeberg medial sclerosis, 369
Monoclonal gammopathy of undetermined significance
  (MGUS), 474
Monocytes, 65, 82, 82f
Mononeuritis multiplex, 837
Mononeuropathy, 837
Mononucleosis, infectious
  atypical lymphocytes in, 461, 461f
  cause of, 460–461
  clinical features of, 461
  morphology of, 461b, 461f
  pathogenesis of, 460–461
Monosodium urate (MSU) crystals, in gout, 823–824
Monosomy, 262–263
Monospot test, 461
"Moon facies," in Cushing syndrome, 788f, 789
Moraxella catarrhalis pneumonia, 521
Morphogenesis, errors in, 273–275
Mosaicism, 262–263
Motor system, 840
Motor unit, myofibers of, 840

M protein, in myeloma, 472
MTOC. See Microtubule organizing center
MUC5AC gene, 502
Mucinous tumors, of ovaries, 729, 729b, 730f
Mucocele, of appendix, 635
Mucopolysaccharidoses (MPSs), 257t, 260
  clinical features of, 259–260
  etiology of, 259
  type I, 260
  type II, 260
Mucormycosis, 537
  clinical features of, 537
  morphology of, 536f, 537b
Mucosa-associated lymphoid tissue (MALT), 235, 350, 605
Mucosal disease, stress-related
  clinical features of, 599
  incidence of, 599
  morphology of, 599b
  pathogenesis of, 599
Mucous plugs, in asthma, 505
Multicystic dysplasia, 578
Multifactorial disorders, 261–262
Multiple different proteases, in tumor cell invasion, 221–222
Multiple endocrine neoplasia (MEN) syndromes, 794
  type 1, 794
  type 2, 795
  type 2A, 795
  type 2B, 795
Multiple myeloma, 472–473, 479–480
  clinical features of, 474
  diagnosis of, 473
  morphology of, 472b, 473f
  pathogenesis of, 473–474
  prognosis for, 473–474
Multiple sclerosis (MS), 142–143, 143t
  cerebralspinal fluid in patients with, 871
  clinical features of, 871
  defined, 871
  HLA alleles associated with, 148t
  incidence of, 871
  morphology of, 871b, 872f
  pathogenesis of, 871
Mural thrombus, after MI, 418, 418f
Muscle, regenerative capacity for, 88
Muscle fiber atrophy, 840–841, 841f
Muscular dystrophy, 11, 842
  congenital, 842
  Emery-Dreifuss, 843–844
  limb-girdle, 843
  X-linked linked and autosomal, 843–844
Musculoskeletal system, in systemic sclerosis, 160
"Mutational signatures", 230
Mutations
  affecting cancer genes, 200–201
  in angiogenesis, 220, 220b
  causing hereditary spherocytosis, 444
  DNA with random vs. specific, 6, 6f
  driver, 201, 204b
  driver and passenger, 201–204
  examples of, 244
  gain-of-function, 208
  loss-of-function, 208
  passenger, 201, 204b
  point, 201
  RB, 209, 209f
  single-gene, 245–246
  toxic gain-of-function, 271
  use of term, 244
Myasthenia gravis, 139t
  causes of, 839
  clinical manifestations of, 839
MYC gene, 471
MYCN oncogene, in neuroblastomas, 287–288, 288f
Mycobacterial disease, nontuberculous, 532
Mycobacterial infection, 615t
Mycobacterium aviumintracellulare, in AIDS, 180
Mycobacterium tuberculosis, 526, 864
MYC oncogene, 207
  and EBV, 233–234, 234b
  in Warburg effect, 216
Mycoplasma, 343
Mycoplasma pneumoniae, 522–523
Mycosis fungoides, 477
MYD88 gene, 474, 519–520
Myelin
  in CNS, 870
  immune mechanisms in destruction of, 870–871
  in peripheral nerves, 870
  primary diseases of, 872b
Myelin sheaths, 835
Myelodyspastic syndrome (MDS), 481, 484b
  clinical features of, 481–482
  morphology of, 481b
  pathogenesis of, 481–482
Myeloid neoplasms, 479, 484b
  acute myeloid leukemia, 479–480
  categories of, 479
  myelodyspastic syndromes, 481
  myeloproliferative neoplasms, 482
Myeloma, "smoldering", 473–474. See also Multiple
  myeloma
Myelomeningocele, 860–861, 861f
Myeloperoxidase (MPO), in acute inflammation, 68
Myeloperoxidase (MPO) deficiency, 172t

Myeloproliferative neoplasms, 482, 484b
  chronic myelogenous leukemia, 481–483, 482f
  polycythemia vera, 484
  primary myelofibrosis, 484–485
Mylinolysis, central pontine, 872
Myocardial disease, causes of
  cardiotoxic drugs, 435
  catecholamines, 435
Myocardial infarction (MI), 97, 409, 411–419
  atherosclerotic plaque in, 376–377
  and cigarette smoking, 309
  clinical features of, 416–417
  consequences and complications of, 417–419, 418f
  coronary artery occlusion in, 411
  in diabetics, 783
  electrocardiographic abnormalities on, 416
  following healing, 414–415
  identification of, 414, 415f
  infarct modification by reperfusion, 415–417, 416f
  laboratory evaluation of, 416–417, 417f
  long-term prognosis after, 419
  microscopic appearance of, 414, 415f
  morphology of, 414b–415b, 414t
  myocardial response to ischemia in, 411–412, 412f
  pathogenesis of, 410f, 411
  patterns of infarction in, 412–414, 413f
  "silent", 416
  subendocardial infarctions in, 413–414, 413f
  transmural infarctions in, 413, 413f
Myocardial ischemia, 419
Myocardial natriuretic peptides, in blood pressure
  regulation, 365
Myocardial necrosis, progression of, 412, 412f, 414
Myocardial rupture, after MI, 417, 418f
Myocardial vessel vasospasm, 390
Myocarditis, 434–435
  Chagas, 435, 436f
  clinical features of, 435
  giant cell, 435, 436f
  hypersensitivity, 435, 436f
  morphology of, 435b
  noninfectious causes of, 435
  nonviral infectious causes of, 434–435
  pathogenesis of, 434–435
Myocardium
  necrotic, 414–415
  reversibly injured, 48–49, 49f
Myofibroblasts, 91–92
Myometrium, tumor of, 197f
Myopathies
  altered muscle function and morphology of, 840, 841f
  congenital, 842
  drug, 845
  ethanol, 845
  inflammatory, 159–162, 844–845, 845f
  ion channel, 844
  metabolic, 844
  mitochondrial, 844
  thyrotoxic, 845
Myositis, inclusion body, 845, 845f
Myotonic dystrophies, 843
Myxedema, 757
Myxomas, of heart, 437, 438f
  atrial, 438f
  characteristics of, 437
  clinical features of, 438

N
Nagasaki
  and radiation carcinogenesis, 231
  survivors of, 323
Nasopharyngeal carcinoma, 546
  and EBV infection, 234, 234b
  histologic variants of, 546
National Institute of Drug Abuse, on oxycodone, 316–317
Natural killer (NK) cells, 134b
  origins of, 128
Necator americanus, 620
Necroptosis, 40–41, 41b
Necrosis, 15f, 34–37, 34t, 41, 41b
  biochemical mechanisms of, 35
  caseous, 36–37, 37f, 85f
  coagulative, 36–37, 36f
  fat, 37, 37f
  features of, 34t
  fibrinoid, 37, 37f
  gangrenous, 36
  inflammation caused by, 59
  intracellular changes associated with, 33, 33f, 35
  ischemic coagulative, 48–49, 49f
  liquefactive, 36, 36f
  morphologic patterns of, 36–37, 36b–37b, 36f–37f
  morphology of, 33f–34f, 35b
  process of, 35
Necrotic lesions, in inflammatory response, 358
Necrotizing arteriolitis, 367b–368b, 368f
Necrotizing enterocolitis (NEC), 277, 279–280, 280f
  clinical course of, 280
  incidence of, 279–280
  presentation of, 280, 280f
Negative selection, in immunologic tolerance, 145
Neisseria gonorrhoeae, 708, 708f
Neonatal herpes infection, 712

Neonates, infections of, 277. *See also* Infants
Neoplasia
    clinical aspects of, 235–241, 237b, 237t
    colitis-associated, 625–626
    effects on host of, 235–236
        cancer cachexia, 236, 237b
        paraneoplastic syndromes, 236, 237b, 237t
    grading and staging of, 236–237, 237b
    laboratory diagnosis of cancer, 237–241
        molecular diagnosis, 239, 240f
        with molecular profiling, 239–241, 241f
        morphologic methods, 238, 238f
        tumor markers, 238–239
    nomenclature of, 190–191
Neoplasms
    histiocytic, 465
    kidney disease, 578–580
    lymphoid, 464
    myeloid, 202, 465
    terminology for, 191, 192t
    vascular, 396b
Neoplasms, pediatric
    benign
        hemangiomas, 285, 285f
        lymphangiomas, 285
        teratomas, 285–286, 286f
    malignant, 286–291, 286t
        histologic appearance of, 286
        neuroblastoma, 286–289, 289b
        retinoblastoma, 289, 290f
Neovascularization, of atherotic plaque, 374–376, 375f
C3 nephritic factor (C3NeF), 560
Nephritic syndrome, 555
Nephritis. *See also* Glomerulonephritis
    drug-induced tubulointerstitial, 567
        clinical course of, 567
        morphology of, 567b, 567f
        pathogenesis of, 567
    hereditary, 562
    interstitial, 564
    in SLE, 154, 155f
    tubulointerstitial, 564–567
Nephroblastoma, 289–291. *See also* Wilms tumor
Nephrocalcinosis, 770
Nephrogenic rests, of Wilms tumor, 290–291
Nephron loss, 555
Nephronophthisis-medullary cystic disease, 575–576
    clinical course of, 576
    morphology of, 576b
    variants of, 575
Nephropathy
    clinical manifestation of, 785
    diabetic, 779, 780f–781f, 783–785
    reflux, 566
Nephrosclerosis, 569–570
    clinical course of, 570
    morphology of, 570b, 570f
    pathogenesis of, 569–570
Nephrotic syndrome, 99, 99f, 550, 555
    causes of, 557t
    diseases associated with, 563b–564b
    leading to glomerular lesions, 550
Nerves, amyloidosis of, 186
Nervous system, 177. *See also* Central nervous system
    in HIV infection, 177
    infections of, 862–864, 872b
    patterns of injury of, 850–851, 850f
    prion diseases of, 869
    tumors of, 881
Neuofibromatosis type 2, 213
Neural tube deficits, 861, 861f
Neuroblastoma
    pediatric, 286–289, 289b
        clinical course and prognosis of, 287–289, 288f, 288t
        histological appearance of, 287, 287f
        locations of, 287
    staging of, 287–288, 288t
Neuroborreliosis, 864–865
Neurocytoma, central, 884
Neurodegenerative diseases/disorders, 849, 874–880, 880b–881b
    Alzheimer disease, 874–875
    amyotrophic lateral sclerosis, 880
    classification of, 874, 874t
    defined, 874
    frontotemporal lobar degenerations, 877
    Huntington disease, 879
    Parkinson disease, 877–879
    pathologic process of, 875
    protein misfolding in, 46
    related to trinucleotide repeat expansions, 270–271, 271f
    spinocerebellar ataxias, 879–880
    symptoms of, 880
Neuroendocrine tumors
    clinical features of, 606
    in gastrointestinal tract, 605
    morphology of, 606b, 606f
    prognostic factors for, 606
Neurofibromas
    morphology of, 846b, 847f
    subtypes of, 846
Neurofibromatosis type 1 (NF1), 846
Neurofibromatosis type 2 (NF2), 846, 885
Neurofilaments, of cytoskeleton, 11

Neurohypophysis, 755
Neuroma, traumatic, 836f, 847
Neuromuscular diseases, 835
Neuromuscular junction disorders, 839, 839b–840b
    congenital myasthenic syndromes, 839
    infections with exotoxin-producing bacteria, 839
    Lambert-Eaton syndrome, 839
    myasthenia gravis, 839
Neuromuscular system, peripheral nerves in, 835
Neuromyelitis optica (NMO), 872
Neuronal injury, features of, 849b, 850f
Neuronal storage diseases, of CNS, 872
Neuronal tumors, 883–884
Neuronophagia, 850
Neuropathies
    demyelinating, 835–837
    peripheral, 835, 838b
        causes of, 837t
        chronic inflammatory demyelinating polyneuropathy, 837t, 838
        diabetic peripheral neuropathy, 837t, 838
        Guillain-Barré syndrome, 837t, 838
        inherited forms of, 837t, 838
        pathologic changes in, 835–837, 837f
        toxic forms of, 837t, 838
        vasculitic forms of, 837t, 837t, 838
Neuropathologic changes, in trisomy 21 patients, 266
Neuropathy
    analgesic, 314–315
    peripheral demyelinating, 304f, 305
Neuropeptides, as mediators of inflammation, 77–78
Neurosyphilis, 864
Neurotoxins, bacterial, 354
Neutral proteases, in acute inflammation, 68
Neutroophil infiltration, in fatty liver disease, 653
Neutropenia, 459–460
    clinical features of, 460
    morphology of, 459b–460b
    pathogenesis of, 459–460
    radiation-caused, 322–323
Neutrophil extracellular traps (NETs), 69, 69f
Neutrophilia, 87
Neutrophils
    in acute inflammation, 61
    in ARDS, 496
    in chronic inflammation, 84–85
    granules of, 68
    in late-phase hypersensitivity reactions, 137, 138f
    migration through blood vessels of, 64f
    shift to left of, 87
Nevus flammeus (birthmark), 392
"Next Gen" sequencing, 296f
NF1 suppressor gene, in Warburg effect, 216
NF2 suppressor gene, 213
NHEJ. *See* Nonhomologous end joining
Niacin
    deficiency syndrome for, 333t
    functions of, 333t
Nickel, and lung carcinoma, 539
Nicotinamide adenine dinucleotide (NAD+), in ethanol metabolism, 310
Nicotine exposure, malformations associated with, 275–276
Niemann-Pick diseases, 260, 872
    type A, 257–258, 258f
    type B, 257–258
    type C, 258
Night blindness, 328
Nipple, Paget disease of, 743
Nipple discharge, in breast disease, 737
Nitric oxide (NO), in acute inflammation, 68
Nitric oxide synthase (NOS), in acute inflammation, 68
Nitrogen dioxide (NO₂), health effects of, 302t
Nitrosamides, 338
Nitrosamines, 229t, 230, 309, 338
NMYC gene, in neuroblastoma, 203f
NOD-like receptors (NLRs), 122f, 123
Nodular fasciitis
    defined, 828
    morphology of, 828b, 829f
Nodule, definition of, 890t
Nomenclature. *See also* Terminology
    for benign tumors, 190
    for malignant tumors, 190–191
    of skin lesions, 889, 890t
    for tumors, 192t
Nonalcoholic fatty liver disease (NAFLD), 336–337, 640, 652, 655, 656b
    clinical features of, 655, 656f
    natural history of, 656f
    pathogenesis of, 655
    pediatric, 655
Nonbacterial thrombotic endocarditis (NBTE), 428, 428f–429f
Nongonococcal urethritis (NGU), 709
Non-Hodgkin lymphoma, 463
    B-cell, 758
    clinical features of, 477
    clinical staging of, 476t, 477
    compared with Hodgkin lymphoma, 476t, 477
Nonhomologous end joining (NHEJ), 6, 6f
Nonossifying fibroma (NOF), 814–815, 815f–816f
Nonsense mediated decay, 244
Non-small cell lung carcinoma (NSCLC), 538, 542–543
Nonspecific interstitial pneumonia (NSIP), 508

Non-ST-segment elevated MIs (NSTEMIs), 413–414
Nontuberculous mycobacterial infection, 532
NOTCH1 gene, 204
Notch signaling, in angiogenesis, 91
Novovirus, 619
Nuclear factor-κB (NF-κB) pathway, in hepatocytes, 234
Nuclear membrane lamins, of cytoskeleton, 11
Nucleic acid tests, 347
Nucleosomes, 3–4, 3f
Nucleotide oligomerization binding domain 2 (NOD2), 622–623
Nutmeg liver, 97b–98b, 98f, 402, 667
Nutritional diseases, 323–338, 334b
    anorexia nervosa, 326
    bulimia, 326
    malnutrition, 324
    obesity, 334–337
    vitamin deficiencies, 326–332
Nutritional imbalances, cell injury caused by, 32
Nutritional status, and tissue repair, 93

O
Obesity, 334–337
    adiponectin in, 336
    adipose tissue in, 336
    and cancer, 337
    central, 336–337
    childhood, 336
    clinical consequences of, 336–337
    defined, 334
    etiology of, 334
    and gastric cancer, 604
    gut hormones in, 336
    and insulin resistance, 776
    and insulin sensitivity, 776, 777f
    leptin in, 335–336
    massive, 336
    role of gut microbiome in, 336
    untoward effects of, 334
    in U.S., 334
    and varicose veins, 390
Obesity genes, 334
Obstruction, intestinal, 607–608, 609b
    abdominal hernia, 609
    Hirschsprung disease, 608, 608f
    intussusception, 608, 608f
Obstructive lesions, of heart, 407–408, 407f–408f
Obstructive lung diseases
    asthma, 503–505
    bronchiectasis, 505–506
    chronic bronchitis, 502
    emphysema, 498–501
Obstructive overinflation, 501
Occludin, in cell-cell interactions, 12
Occluding junctions (tight junctions), in cell-cell interactions, 12
Occupational exposure
    and cancer development, 323
    human diseases associated with, 306–307, 307t
Occupational injuries and illnesses, 306–307
Occupations, cancers related to, 198t
Ocular complications, of diabetes, 783
Odds ratio, 147, 148t
Odontogenic cysts, 590
Oligodendrocytes, 850
Oligodendroglioma, 881–882
    histological appearance of, 883b, 883f
    survival rate for, 882
Oligohydramnios sequence, 274–275, 275f
Oligosaccharides
    N-linked, 12–13
    O-linked, 12–13
Omega-3 fatty acids, in atherosclerosis, 371
Oncocytoma, 578–580
Oncogenes, 200, 205, 208b
Oncogenesis, 231–235
    Helicobactor pylori, 235, 235b
    viral
        DNA viruses, 232–235, 234b
        Epstein-Barr virus, 233–234, 233f, 234b
        hepatitis B and hepatitis C viruses, 234–235, 235b
        human papillomavirus, 232–233
        RNA viruses, 231–232, 232b
Oncology, defined, 190
Oncometabolism, 216–217, 216f, 217b
Oncometabolite, 216–217
Oncoproteins, 205, 208b
Ophthalmopathy, of Graves disease, 760
Opioids
    adverse effects of, 316
    prevalence of, 316
Opportunistic infections, with AIDS, 177
Opsonins, in phagocytosis, 67
Opsonization
    in complement system, 76
    in type II hypersensitivity, 139, 140f
Oral cavity
    cancers of, 309t
    diseases and disorders of, 583–590
        odontogenic cysts and tumors, 590, 590b
        oral inflammatory lesions, 584–585, 585b
        salivary glands, 587–589, 588f, 589b–590b
        teeth and supporting structures, 584, 584b

Oral cavity (Continued)
  lesions of, 585–587, 587b
    erythroplakia, 585–586, 586b, 586f
    fibrous proliferative lesions, 585, 585f
    leukoplakia, 585–586, 586b, 586f
    squamous cell carcinoma, 586–587, 587b, 587f
Oral contraceptives (OCs), 314, 317b
Oral hygiene, 584
Oral inflammatory lesions
  aphthous ulcers (canker sores), 584, 584f
  herpes simplex virus infections, 584–585, 593f
  oral candidiasis (thrush), 585
Oral secretions, exit of microbes via, 352
Organellar biogenesis, 7–8
Organelles
  cellular functions within, 6
  regulation of, 7
  relative volumes of, 7f
Organic solvents, exposure to, 306
Organochlorines, exposure to, 306–307
Organ system failure, from sepsis, 319
Orthopnea, in heart failure, 402
Osler-Weber-Rendu disease, 392
Osmotic demyelination syndrome, 872
Osmotic pressure, colloid, 98, 99f
Osteitis, dissecting, 803, 803f
Osteitis deformans, 803–805
Osteitis fibrosa cystica, 770, 803
Osteoarthritis (OA), 817–818
  characteristics of, 817
  clinical course of, 818, 819f
  clinical presentation of, 817
  morphology of, 818b, 819f
  and obesity, 337
  pathogenesis of, 817–818, 818f
  primary vs. secondary, 817
Osteoblastoma
  clinical manifestations of, 808
  morphology of, 808b–809b
Osteoblasts, 797–798, 798f
Osteochondroma, 810–811
  clinical course for, 811, 811f
  morphology of, 810b, 811f
  pathogenesis of, 810
Osteoclasts, 798, 798f
Osteocytes, 798
Osteogenesis imperfecta (OI), 22–23, 246, 800
Osteoid osteoma
  clinical manifestations of, 808
  morphology of, 808b–809b, 809f
Osteomalacia, 802–803
  basic derangement in, 330–331
  morphological changes in, 331
  morphologic changes in, 330–331, 331f
  in vitamin D deficiency, 330
Osteomyelitis
  acute, 807
  chronic, 807
  clinical course of, 807
  hematogenous, 806–807
  manifestations of, 806
  morphology of, 807b, 807f
  mycobacterial, 807–808
  pyogenic, 806–807
    cause of, 806
    Staphylococcus aureus in, 806–807
Osteonecrosis
  causes of, 806
  clinical course of, 806
  morphology of, 806b, 806f
Osteopenia, 801, 803
Osteopetrosis, 800–801
  mutations underlying, 800
  severe infantile, 800–801
Osteoporosis, 803
  advanced, 802, 802f
  clinical manifestations of, 802
  common forms of, 801
  detection of, 802
  morphology of, 802b, 802f
  pathogenesis of, 801, 801f
  pharmacotherapy of, 802
  postmenopausal, 801, 801f
  senile, 801f, 823–825
  treatment of, 802
  use of term, 801
Osteoprotegerin (OPG), in bone remodeling, 799, 799f
Osteosarcoma
  clinical course of, 810
  clinical manifestations of, 809, 809f
  incidence of, 809
  morphology of, 809b–810b, 810f
  pathogenesis of, 809
Ostium primum, 405
Ostium secundum, 405
Ostium secundum defects, 405
Ovarian cancer, risk factors for, 728
Ovaries
  follicle cysts of, 727
  luteal cysts of, 727
  mucinous tumors of, 729, 730f
  polycystic ovarian syndrome, 727

Ovaries (Continued)
  tumors of, 727–731, 728t, 732b
    Brenner tumor, 729–730
    endometrioid, 729
    frequency of, 728t
    germ cell of, 717f, 730
    serous tumors, 728–729, 729f
    sex cord origin, 717f, 730
    surface epithelial, 727–728, 728f
    teratomas, 730–731
    treatment of, 731
Oxidation, in acute inflammation, 68
Oxidative metabolism, of cellular functions, 15
Oxidative phosphorylation, 13
Oxidative stress, 43
  in cell injury, 48b
  cell injury caused by ROS, 45
  in emphysema, 500, 500f
  removal of reactive oxygen species, 43–45, 44f, 44t
Oxycodone, abuse of, 316–317
Oxyphil cells, 758, 769
Oxytocin, function of, 755
Ozone
  in air pollution, 303b–304b
  health effects of, 302t, 303

P

Pacemaker, in chronic IHD, 420
Pachygyria, 861
Paget disease
  of bone, 803–805, 804f
  clinical course of, 804–805
  defined, 803
  extramammary, 715–716, 716f
  morphology of, 804b, 804f
  of nipple, 743
  pathogenesis of, 804
  phases of, 804f
  prevalence of, 804
Pain
  of female breast, 736
  prostaglandins in, 73
Pancoast tumors, 540
Pancreas, 309t
  annular, 680
  autodigestion of, 679
  cancer of
    clinical features of, 688–689
    environmental influence on, 688
    head of pancreas, 688–689
    morphology of, 688b, 688f
    pathogenesis of, 687–688, 687f
  congenital anomalies of, 680
    agenesis, 680
    annular pancreas, 680
    congenital cysts, 680
    ectopic pancreas, 680
    pancreas divisum, 680
  diabetic, 782
  ectopic, 680
  endocrine, 772
    diabetes mellitus, 772
    disorders of, 679
    functions of, 679
  exocrine
    composition of, 679
    diseases of, 679–680
  in hemochromatosis, 657
  infiltrating ductal adenocarcinoma of, 686–689
  location of, 679
Pancreas divisum, 680
Pancreatic abnormalities, in CF, 252, 252f, 254
Pancreatic cancers, TGF-beta pathway in, 213
Pancreatic duct obstruction, 681, 683
Pancreatic fibrosis, in hemochromatosis, 657
Pancreatic insufficiency, in cystic fibrosis, 254
Pancreatic intraepithelial neoplasias (PanINs), 687
Pancreatic neoplasms, 685–689, 689b
  cystic neoplasms, 685–686, 686f
  intraductal papillary mucinous neoplasms, 686, 687f
Pancreatic neuroendocrine tumors (PanNETs), 778–779
  gastrinomas, 784
  genomic sequencing of, 785
  insulinomas, 782–783
Pancreatitis, 680–685, 685b
  acute, 37, 37f, 680–683
    clinical features of, 682–683
    etiology of, 680–683, 681t
    laboratory findings in, 683
    management of, 683
    morphology of, 681b–682b, 683f
    pancreatic pseudocysts following, 683, 683b, 684f
    pathogenesis of, 681
  autoimmune, 162, 683–684
  chronic, 683–685
    clinical features of, 684–685
    diagnosis of, 685
    etiology of, 683–685
    morphology of, 684b, 685f
    pathogenesis of, 684
    prognosis for, 685
    in chronic alcoholism, 312
  hereditary, 683

Pancreatitis (Continued)
  idiopathic, 681
  idiopathic chronic, 253
  tropical, 683
Pandemics, influenza, 524
Paneth cell metaplasia, 623–624
Pantothenic acid
  deficiency syndrome for, 333t
  functions of, 333t
Papanicolaou (PAP) smear test, 197, 238, 238f, 718–719
Papillary muscle dysfunction, after MI, 417
Papillary urothelial neoplasm of low malignant potential (PUNLMP), 703
Papillomas
  laryngeal, 546
Papillomatosis, definition of, 890t
Pap smears, 238, 238f
Papules
  definition of, 890t
  of lichen planus, 893, 893f
Paracortical hyperplasia, morphology of, 462–463
Paracrine signaling, 16
Paradoxical embolism (PE), clinical and pathologic features of, 112
Parakeratosis, definition of, 890t
Paraneoplastic syndromes, 236, 237b, 237t, 543, 580, 886
Parasites, intestinal, 350
Parasitic disease, 619–620
Parathyroid
  adenoma, 770, 770f, 773f
  carcinoma, 770
  hyperplasia of, 770
Parathyroidectomy, 771
Parathyroid glands, 769–771
  abnormalities of, 769
  function of, 769
  hyperparathyroidism, 769–771
  hypoparathyroidism, 772–784
Parathyroid hormone (PTH), 769
  in bone remodeling, 799
  and hypercalcemia, 770, 773t
Parenchyma, 190
Parenchymal organs
  fibrosis in, 94–95, 95f
  tissue regeneration in, 88–89
Parental teratogenic insult, timing of, 276
Parkinson disease (PD), 46, 877–879
  causes of, 879
  clinical features of, 879
  morphology of, 878f, 879b
  pathogenesis of, 879
Parkinsonism, 879
Parotid gland enlargement, in Sjögren syndrome, 158
Parovirus B19, 283f
Paroxysmal nocturnal dyspnea, in heart failure, 402
Paroxysmal nocturnal hemoglobinuria (PNH), 172
  complications of, 451
  genetics of, 451
Partial thromboplastin time (PTT) assay, 104, 487
Particulates, health effects of, 302t
Patau syndrome
  clinical features of, 265f
  karyotype of, 265f
Patch, definition of, 890t
Patent ductus arteriosus (PDA), 404, 404f, 406
  clinical features of, 406
  frequency of, 403t
  pathogenesis of, 406
Patent foramen ovale, 405
Pathogen-associated molecular patterns (PAMPs), 59–60, 122
Pathogenesis, defined, 31, 32f
Pathogens
  blood-borne spread of, 351
  pyogenic, 78–79
Pathologists
  role of, 31
  surgical, 195
Pathology, 31
  defined, 1
  introduction to, 31
Pauci-immune glomerulonephritis, 556t
P16 (CDKN2A) gene, in pancreatic cancer, 687, 687f
PCP (1-(1-phenylcyclohexyl) piperidine), 317
PDGF. See Platelet-derived growth factor
Peanuts, infant exposure to, 137
Peau d'orange appearance, 99–100, 391
Pediatric diseases, 273–296
  and causes of death by age, 273t
    congenital anomalies, 273–276
    fetal hydrops, 282–284, 282f–283f
    necrotizing enterocolitis, 279–280, 280f
    perinatal infections, 277
    prematurity, 277
    respiratory distress syndrome of newborn, 278–279
    sudden infant death syndrome, 280–281
    tumors and tumorlike lesions of infancy and childhood, 285–291
Pelvic inflammatory disease (PID), 726–727, 727f
Pemphigus, 895–896
  clinical features of, 896
  pathogenesis of, 896
  variants of, 895
Pemphigus foliaceus, morphology of, 896, 896b, 898f

Pemphigus vulgaris
  as antibody-mediated disease, 139t
  morphology of, 896, 897f
Penis
  inflammatory lesions of, 691
  lesions of, 692b
  malformations of, 691
  neoplasms of, 691–692
P-450 enzymes, 302
Peptic ulcer disease (PUD), 601–602
  clinical features of, 602–603
  epidemiology of, 602
  morphology of, 602b, 602f
  pathogenesis of, 598f, 602
Peptide hormones, 749
Peptide YY (PYY), 336
  and satiety, 336
  secretion of, 336
Perfusion, poor, and tissue repair, 93
Pericardial diseases and disorders, 436
  effusions, 436
  pericarditis, 436–437
Pericarditis, 436–437
  acute bacterial, 437, 437f
  after MI, 417–418, 418f
  chronic, 437
  clinical features of, 437
  constrictive, 437
  morphology of, 437b
  in SLE, 156
Periodic acid-Schiff (PAS) stain, 895
Periodontitis, 584
Peripheral nerve injury
  disorders associated with, 837–838, 837t
  patterns of, 835–837, 836f
Peripheral nerves
  disorders of, 835–838
  functional elements of, 835
Peripheral nerve sheath tumors, 846–847, 847b
  malignant, 846–847
  neurofibromas, 846
  schwannomas, 846
Peripheral vascular resistance, in blood pressure regulation, 364–365, 365f
Permeability, increased
  in acute inflammation, 60–62, 61f
  principal mechanisms of, 61f
Pernicious anemia, 139t, 457
Peroxisome proliferator-activated receptors (PPARs), 328
Peroxisomes, function of, 6–7, 7f
Pesticides,, exposure to, 306–307
Petechiae
  in bleeding disorders, 485
  in hemorrhage, 100–101, 101f
  in SIDS autopsy, 281b
Peutz-Jeghers syndrome, 626–627, 627t, 628f
Peyer's patches, 128
Phagocytes, maturation of mononuclear, 82, 82f
Phagocytic receptors, 67, 67f
Phagocytosis, 13, 14f
  in acute inflammation, 67, 67f
  in complement system, 76, 76f
  microbial resistance to, 356
  in type II hypersensitivity, 139, 140f
Phase I reactions, in metabolism, 301–302
Phase II reactions, in metabolism, 301–302
Phenotypes, diversity of, 3
Phenylalanine hydroxylase (PAH) enzyme, 254
Phenylketonuria (PKU), 254
  biochemical abnormality in, 254, 255f
  clinical features of, 254, 255b
  variant forms of, 254–255, 255f
Pheochromocytoma
  clinical manifestations of, 793–794
  described, 795
  diagnosis of malignancy in, 795
  morphology of, 793b–794b, 794f
  "rule of 10s" for, 795
Philadelphia (Ph) chromosome, 202
Philadelphia (Ph) chromosome–translocation t(9;22), 244
Phimosis, 691
Phlebothrombosis, 111, 391
Phosphatidylinositol, 8
Phosphatidylserine, 8
Phospholipids, organization of, 8
Phosphotidyl inositide-3 kinase (PI3K), 232
Physical agents, cell injury caused by, 32
Pick disease, 877
PIGA gene, 451
Pigeon breast deformity, 247, 331
Pigments
  abnormal depositions of, 54b
  role in cell injury of, 52–53
"Pink puffers", 501
Pinocytosis, 10–11, 13
Pituitary
  diseases of, 750
    hyperpituitarism, 753b
    symptoms and signs of, 750
  genetic alterations in tumors of, 756t
Pituitary, anterior, 750
  corticotroph adenomas of, 753–754
  hormones relaxed by, 750, 751f
  hypofunction of, 754

Pituitary, anterior (Continued)
  lactotroph adenomas of, 753–754
  neoplasms of, 754
  normal architecture of, 750f
  somatotroph adenomas of, 753
Pituitary, posterior, 755
Pituitary apoplexy, 750
PiZ mutation, in inherited metabolic liver disease, 658
PKD1 gene, mutations of, 574
Placenta, transmission of microbes via, 352
Placental abnormalities, in fetal growth restriction, 277–278.
    See also Pregnancy, diseases of
Placental site trophoblastic tumor, 735
Plaques
  in AD development, 875, 876f
  definition of, 890t
  erythematous psoriatic, 892, 893f
  in MS, 872, 872f
Plaques, neuritic
  in AD, 876f, 877
  in staging of AD, 877
Plasma cell neoplasms, 463, 471–473
Plasma cells
  B cells differentiation into, 128
  in chronic inflammation, 84
Plasma membranes
  carriers and channels for transport across, 9, 10f
  components of, 8–9
  organization and asymmetry of, 8f
  passive diffusion across, 9
  phospholipids of, 8
  protection and nutrient acquisition functions of, 8–11
  receptor-mediated and fluid-phase uptake of, 9–11, 10f
Plasma osmotic pressure, reduced, 99, 99f
Plasmids, and bacterial injury, 353–354
Plasmin, in coagulation cascade, 106f
Plasmodium falciparum,, life cycle of, 452f, 453
Platelet-activating factor (PAF)
  as mediators of inflammation, 77–78, 77t
  in NEC, 279–280
Platelet aggregation, integrins in, 23–24
Platelet count, 487
Platelet-derived growth factor (PDGF), 20, 75f
Platelet endothelial cell adhesion molecule-1 (PECAM-1), 65
Platelet function, tests of, 487
Platelets
  deficiencies of, 485
  in glomerular injury, 554
  in hemostasis, 103b
  role in hemostasis of, 102f
Pleiotropy, 245
Pleura, diseases of, 544
  chylothorax, 544
  hemothorax, 544
  malignant mesothelioma, 544–545
  pleural effusion and pleuritis, 544
  pneumothorax, 544
Pleural effusions, 544
Pleural exudate formation, 544
Plummer syndrome, 762b–763b, 762f
Pneumoconioses, 307, 508–509, 512b
  coal worker's, 509–510
  morphology of, 509b, 510f
  pathogenesis of, 509
  use of term, 508–509, 509t
Pneumocystis, in immunocompromised host, 534–535
Pneumocystis jiroveci (formerly P. carinii), 534
Pneumocystis pneumonia
  diagnosis of, 534–535
  morphology of, 534b, 535f
Pneumonias, 341
  acute, 523f, 524b
  aspiration, 525
  from burns, 319
  chronic, 525–526
  eosinophilic, 515
  hospital-acquired, 524–525
  in immunocompromised host, 533–535
    CMV infection, 533
    CMV infection in immunosuppressed individuals, 534
    CMV mononucleosis, 534
    pneumocystis, 534–535
Pneumonias, bacterial
  classification of, 520
  community-acquired, 520–523
    clinical features of, 523
    Haemophilus influenzae, 521
    Klebsiella pneumoniae, 521
    Legionella pneumophila, 521–522
    Moraxella catarrhalis, 521
    Mycoplasma pneumoniae, 522–523
    Pseudomonas aeruginosa, 521
    Staphylococcus aureus, 521
    Streptococcus pneumoniae, 520–521
  complications of, 523
  morphology of, 522b–523b
Pneumonias, viral, 524
  clinical features of, 524
  community-acquired, 523–524
  influenza infections, 524
  morphology of, 523b, 524f
Pneumonia syndromes, 521t
Pneumothorax, 525, 544
Podocyte injury, 554–555

Podocytes
  effacement of foot processes of, 555, 557f
  of glomerular capillary wall, 551
Poikilocytosis, in thalassemia, 449–450
Point mutations, 244
Poison, definition of, 301–302
Poliovirus, in CNS, 867
Pollutants, effects on CNS of, 874
Pollution, environmental, 303b–304b
  air pollution, 302–303
    indoor air pollution, 303
    outdoor air pollution, 302–303, 302t
  industrial and agricultural exposure, 306–307, 307t
  from metals, 304–306
    arsenic, 305–306
    cadmium, 306
    lead, 304–305
    mercury, 305
Polyarteritis nodosa (PAN), 141t, 161–162, 386–387
  clinical features of, 387
  morphology of, 386b, 387f
Polychlorinated biphenyls (PCBs), exposure to, 306–307
Polycyclic hydrocarbons, 229–230, 229t, 309
  as carcinogen, 229t
  exposure to, 306
Polycystic kidney disease
  adult, 574–575, 576b
    clinical course of, 574–575
    morphology of, 574b, 575f
    pathogenesis of, 574, 574f
  childhood form of, 575
    clinical course of, 575
    morphology of, 575b
Polycystic ovarian syndrome, 727
Polycythemia, 459
  pathophysiologic classification of, 459t
  primary, 459
Polycythemia vera, 484
  clinical features of, 484–485
  diagnosis of, 483
  morphology of, 483b
Polydactyly, 274f
Polydipsia, 778, 779f
Polyendocrine syndromes, autoimmune adrenalitis in, 795
Polygenic disorders, 261–262
Polykaryons, 358b
Polymerase chain reaction (PCR) analysis, 294–295, 295f–296f, 347
  allele-specific, 294–295, 295f
  reverse transcriptions in, 294–295
Polymerase chain reaction (PCR) kits, 291–292
Polymicrogyria, 861
Polymorphisms, associated with disease, 2
Polymyositis, 844, 845f
Polyneuropathies, 837
Polyomavirus, 867, 868b
Polyphagia, 778, 779f
Polyploidy, 262–263
Polypoid cystitis, of male bladder, 702
Polyps
  designation as, 191f
  endocervical, 720
  endometrial, 724–725
  tumors, 607b
Polyps, colonic, 626–633, 634b
  hamartomatous, 626–627, 627t, 628f
    juvenile colonic polyps, 626, 628f
    morphology of, 626b, 628f
    Peutz-Jeghers syndrome, 626–627, 628f
  hyperplastic, 627
    morphology of, 627b, 628f
    pathogenesis of, 627
  inflammatory, 626
  juvenile, 626, 628f
Polyps, gastric, 603
  fundic gland, 603
  gastric adenoma, 603–604
  inflammatory and hyperplastic, 603
Polyribosomes, 12
Polyuria, 778, 779f
Pompe disease, 260, 261t
Pontiac fever, 521–522
"Popcorn" cells, 475f
Portal hypertension, 402
  in cirrhosis, 641
    clinical consequences of, 642f
  in liver failure, 640
Portal vein obstruction, 666–667
Port wine stain, 392
Positron emission tomography (PET) scanning, 214
Posttreatment Lyme disease syndrome (PTLDS), 823
Pott disease, 807–808
Prader-Willi syndrome, 273
  clinical characteristics of, 272
  cytogenetically normal patients with, 272
  genetics of, 272t
  molecular basis of, 272–273, 272f
"Precision medicine", 243
Precursor lesions, 199
Predisposing conditions, in cancer epidemiology, 199, 199t
Preeclampsia, 735
  causes of, 735
  clinical features of, 735
  morphologic changes of, 735b

Pregnancy
  anterior pituitary during, 754
  in chronic alcoholism, 312
  hyperglycemia in, 783
  hypertrophy of uterus during, 48-49, 48f
Pregnancy, diseases of, 732-735
  eclampsia, 735
  ectopic pregnancy, 732
  gestational trophoblastic disease, 733-735
  infections and inflammations, 732
  placental infections, 732
  preeclampsia, 735
Pregnancy, ectopic, 733b
  defined, 732
  morphology of, 732b
  rupture of, 732
Premature infants, perinatal brain injury in, 862,
    862f
Premature rupture of membrane (PPROM), 277
Prematurity
  immaturity of organ systems in, 277
  risk factors for, 277
Pressure sores, 93, 94f
Primary accumulation, in lysosomal storage diseases,
    255-256
Primary biliary cirrhosis (PBC), 665-666
  clinical features of, 664
  defined, 663
  morphology of, 664b, 664f
  pathogenesis of, 663-664
Primary myelofibrosis, 484-485
  clinical features of, 485-490
  marrow fibrosis in, 483
  morphology of, 483b
  peripheral blood smear, 484f
Primary progressive aphasia (PPA), 877
Primary sclerosing cholangitis (PSC), 664, 665f, 666
  clinical features of, 665
  imaging studies of patient with, 665f
  morphology of, 665b, 665f
  pathogenesis of, 665
Primitive neuroectodemal tumor (PNET), 812-813
Prinzmetal angina, 390
Prion diseases, 869
  causative agent, 869
  Creutzfeldt-Jakob disease, 869-870
  pathogenesis of, 869, 869f
Prion protein (PrP), 869
Prions, 342t
Procallus, in bone fracture, 805-806
Procoagulant activity, in long-term diabetes, 783
Procoagulants, in atherosclerosis, 372
Proctitis, ulcerative, 624-625
Proctosigmoiditis, ulcerative, 624-625
Progenitor cells, liver regeneration from, 89
Progeria, 11
Prognathism, 753
Prognosis and behavior, in diagnosis of cancer,
    239
Prognostic factors, for colon cancers, 632-633, 634f
Progressive massive fibrosis (PMF), 509, 512b
Progressive multifocal leukoencephalopathy (PML), 868,
    868f, 870b, 872
Prokaryotes, 342-343
Proliferation, in tissue repair, 88
Promoters, 2, 2f, 230, 231b
Proopiomelanocortin (POMC) neurons, 334
Proprotein convertase subtilisin/kexin type 9 (PCSK9), in
    familial hypercholesterolemia, 250
Prostaglandins (PGs), 72t
  in acute inflammation, 75f
  classification of, 72-73
  pharmacologic inhibitors of, 73
  production of, 71-72, 72f
Prostate gland
  benign prostatic hyperplasia of, 698
  biologically distinct regions of, 697-701, 697f
  carcinoma of, 699-701, 701b
    clinical features of, 700-701
    morphology of, 700b, 700f-701f
    pathogenesis of, 699-700
    screening for, 699
    treatments for, 701
Prostate-specific antigen (PSA) assay, 700-701
Prostatitis, 698b
  categories of, 697
  clinical features of, 698
  diagnosis of, 697-698
  nonspecific granulomatous, 697-698
Protease-activated receptor (PAR), 105
Protease-antiprotease imbalance, in emphysema, 500,
    500f
Proteasomes
  in cellular waste disposal, 13, 14f
  function of, 6
Protein-energy malnutrition (PEM), 324-326
  anatomic changes in, 326
  kwashiorkor, 324-325, 325f
  marasmus, 324-325, 325f
  primary, 334b
  victims of, 324-325
Protein misfolding, in cell injury, 48b
Protein products, 205
Protein-protein complexes, in cell signaling, 19

Proteins, 213
  abnormal depositions of, 54b
  acute-phase, 86-87
  cell injury caused by, 51-52, 52f
  cellular function of, 1
  circulating, 60
  clathrin, 9, 10f
  cytosolic, 6
  extracellular face of, 9
  glycosylation of, 12-13
  plasma membrane, 8-9
    carrier proteins in, 9, 10f
    channel proteins in, 9, 10f
    functioning together, 9
  of skeletal muscles, 840, 840f
Proteoglycans, 23, 23f
Proteolysis-inducing factor, in cancer patients, 236
Proteomics, 347
Prothrombin time (PT), 104, 487
Proto-oncogenes, 201-202, 205, 208b
Protozoa
  categories of, 345
  characteristics of, 342t
Pruritus, in cirrhosis, 641
Pseudoarthrosis, creation of, 806
Pseudocysts, pancreatic, 683, 683b, 684f
Pseudoepitheliomatous hyperplasia, 711
Pseudogout, 823
  characteristics of, 825
  morphology of, 825b
  pathogenesis of, 826b
Pseudomembranous colitis, 615t, 618-619, 618b, 618f
Pseudomonas aeruginosa, 521, 894
Pseudopolyps, in ulcerative colitis, 625
Pseudotumors, inflammatory, 162
Psoriasis, 142-143, 143t, 892-893
  clinical features of, 892-893
  morphology of, 892b, 893f
  pathogenesis of, 892
PTEN tumor suppressor, in Warburg effect, 216
Pulmonary congestion, acute, 97b-98b
Pulmonary disease. See also Chronic obstructive pulmonary
    disease
  drug-induced, 512
  in human immunodeficiency virus infection, 537
  in opioid abuse, 316
  radiation-induced, 512
  of vascular origin
    diffuse alveolar hemorrhage syndromes, 519
    infarction, 516, 516f
    pulmonary embolism, 515-517
    pulmonary hypertension, 517-518
Pulmonary edema
  with burns, 318-319
  noncardiogenic, 496
  in SIDS autopsy, 281b
Pulmonary emboli (PEs), 97, 515-517, 517b
  clinical features of, 516-517
  in DVT, 391
  incidence of, 515
  morphology of, 516b, 516f
  nonthrombotic, 517
  pathophysiologic consequences of, 516
  prophylactic therapy for, 517
  risk factors for, 515-516
  saddle embolus, 516, 516f
Pulmonary eosinophilia, 515
Pulmonary fibrosis, inflammatory reaction in, 59t
Pulmonary hemorrhage syndromes, 519, 519b, 519f
Pulmonary hypertension (PH), 367b-368b, 368f
  classification of, 517
  clinical features of, 518
  in emphysema, 501
  genetic basis of, 518
  in heart failure, 402
  morphology of, 518b, 518f
  pathogenesis of, 517-518
Pulmonary infections, 519-537. See also Tuberculosis
  aspiration pneumonias, 525
  bacterial pneumonias, 520-523
  candidiasis, 535-536
  chronic pneumonias, 525-526
  defined, 519-537
  fungal, 532-533
    clinical features of, 532-533
    epidemiology of, 532-533
    morphology of, 532b, 533f
  hospital-acquired pneumonias, 524-525
  lung abscess, 525
  opportunistic fungal infections, 535-537
  pneumonia in immunocompromised host, 533-535
  preventing, 519-520
  viral pneumonias, 523-524
Puncture wound, 317-318
Purified protein derivative (PPD) skin test, 142
Purpura, in hemorrhage, 100-101
Purulent inflammation, 78-79, 79f
Pus, defined, 60
Pustule, definition of, 890t
Pyelonephritis, 783
  acute, 564-567
    clinical course of, 566
    morphology of, 565b-566b, 565f
    pathogenesis of, 564-565, 565f

Pyelonephritis (Continued)
  chronic, 566-567
    clinical course of, 566-567
    morphology of, 566b, 566f
    obstructive, 566
    reflux-associated, 566
    scars of, 566f
  with papillary necrosis, 565-566
Pyogenic cocci infections, 342-343, 344t
Pyogenic granulomas, 392-393, 393f
Pyrogens, 86-87
  endogenous, 86-87
  exogenous, 86-87
Pyroptosis, 40-41, 41b

Q
Quantitative assays, 347

R
Rabies virus, in CNS, 867
Race, and breast cancer, 741
Rachitic process, 331
"Rachitic rosary", 331
Radiation, ionizing
  biological effects of
    carcinogenesis, 321
    DNA damage, 321
    fibrosis, 321-322, 321f
    main determinants of, 320-321
    on organ systems, 322-323, 322f, 322t
  and cancer risk, 323
  CNS effects of, 874
  injury caused by, 320-323, 323b
  threshold doses for, 322t
  total-body irradiation, 323, 323t
  whole-body, 323, 323t
Radiation carcinogenesis, 231, 231b
Radiation syndromes, acute, 323
Radon
  cancer risk with, 323
  health effects of, 303
Ranke complex, in primary tuberculosis, 528
RANK-to-OPG ratio, 799
Rapidly progressive glomerulonephritis (RPGN), 550, 562
  clinical course of, 563
  diseases associated with, 564
  morphology of, 563b, 563f
  pathogenesis of, 562-563
RAS-MAP kinase signaling pathway, mutations in, 288
RAS oncogene, 206-207, 206f, 208b, 230
RAS signaling, in Warburg effect, 216
Raynaud phenomenon, 390
RB. See Retinoblastoma gene
Reactive oxygen species (ROS), 301-302
  in acute inflammation, 68
  in cell injury, 44t
  generation and role of, 44f
  in ionizing radiation, 321
  in ischemia-reperfusion injury, 43
  in long-term diabetes, 783
  removal of, 43-45, 44f, 44t
  in septic shock, 116-117
Receptor activator of NF-κB ligand (RANKL), in bone
    remodeling, 799, 799f
Receptor activator of NF-κB (RANK), in bone remodeling,
    799, 799f
Receptor tyrosine kinases (RTKs), 18
Red cell disorders, 441-459
Red cell distribution width (RDW), 442, 443t
Red cell indices, 442, 443t
Reed-Sternberg (RS) cells, 181, 474-475, 474f
  characteristics of, 475
  in Hodgkin lymphoma, 475f, 476-477
Regeneration, tissue, 87-88
  of liver, 89
  mechanism of, 88-89
Regenerative medicine, 28
Regurgitation, in rheumatic heart disease, 425
Reidel thyroiditis, 162, 760
Relative risk, 147, 148t
Renal agenesis, 578
Renal cell carcinomas, 578-580, 580b
  chromophobe, 579-580
  clear cell carcinomas, 579
  clinical course of, 580
  morphology of, 579b-580b, 580f
  papillary, 579-580
  representative cross-section of, 580f
Renal disease, 555. See also Kidney disease
  affecting tubules and interstitium, 564-569
  clinical manifestations of, 549-550
  glomerular diseases, 550-563
  involving blood vessels, 569-572
    malignant hypertension, 570-571
    nephrosclerosis, 569-570
    thrombotic microangiopathies, 571-572
  urinary outflow obstruction, 576-578
Renal dysfunction, in myeloma, 473, 477
Renal failure, from burns, 319
Renal failure, pathways of, 565f
Renal injury, ischemic, 568f
Renal lesions, in GPA, 388

Renal stones
    clinical course of, 577
    morphology of, 577b
    pathogenesis of, 576–577
    various types of, 576t
Renin, in blood pressure regulation, 365
Renin-angiotensin system, in blood pressure regulation, 365
Repair
    reactions in, 87–88
Reperfusion injury, 415–416
Replicative potential, limitless (immortality), 218–219, 219b, 219f
Reproductive history
    and breast cancer, 741
    and cancer risk, 198–199
RER. See Rough endoplasmic reticulum
Respiratory burst, 68
Respiratory diseases. See also Pulmonary disease
    and climate change, 300
    infectious, 341
Respiratory distress syndrome (RDS), 277
Respiratory distress syndrome (RDS), neonatal, 279b
    causes of, 278
    clinical features of, 278–279
    fundamental defect in, 278
    morphology of, 278
    pathogenesis of, 278
    pathophysiology of, 278, 279f
    pediatric disease, 278–279
Respiratory secretions, exit of microbes via, 352
Respiratory tract. See also Upper respiratory tract
    amyloid of, 186
    anatomy of, 495
    microbial infection of, 349t, 350
Response-to-injury hypothesis, of atherosclerosis, 372, 373f
Reticulocytes, 442
Retinitis pigmentosa, 46t, 245
Retinoblastoma, pediatric, 289, 290f
    clinical features of, 289
    morphology of, 289b
Retinoblastoma (RB) gene
    antiproliferative effects of, 211
    cell cycle, 210, 210f
    discovery of, 208–211, 209f–210f, 211b
    importance of, 210
    pathogenesis of, 209, 209f
    risk for developing, 209
Retinoic acid, 276
Retinoic acid receptors (RARs), 327–328
Retinoic acid receptor α (RARA) gene, 479
Retinoic X receptor (RXR), 327–328
Retinoids, 327, 749
    clinical use of, 328
    metabolic effects of, 328
Retinol, 327, 327f
Retinol-binding protein (RBP), 327, 327f
Retinopathy
    of diabetes, 779, 780f, 783
    nonproliferative, 783
    proliferative, 783, 784f
    in sickle cell anemia, 447
Retinopathy of prematurity, pathogenesis of, 279
Retrolental fibroplasia, pathogenesis of, 279
Retroperitoneal fibrosis, in ureteral narrowing, 702
Rett syndrome, 860
Rhabdomyomas
    characteristics of, 438
    of heart, 437
Rhabdomyosarcoma, 193f, 830
    alveolar, 830
    embryonal, 830
    morphology of, 830b, 830f
    pleomorphic, 830
    subtypes of, 830
    treatment of, 830
Rheumatic fever, 139t
    acute, 425
    diagnosis of, 426
Rheumatic heart disease (RHD)
    acute rheumatic fever phase of, 427, 428f
    chronic, 425, 426f
    infective endocarditis in, 427–428
Rheumatic valvular disease, 425–427
    acute and chronic, 426f
    clinical features of, 425–427
    long-term prognosis for, 426–427
    morphology of, 425b
    pathogenesis of, 425
    as public health problem, 425
Rheumatoid arthritis (RA), 58, 142–143, 143t, 157, 818–821
    amyloidosis associated with, 184–185
    autoantibodies in, 151t
    autoimmune response in, 819
    chronicity of, 819
    clinical course of, 821, 822f
    defined, 818
    HLA alleles associated with, 148t
    inflammation of, 820, 820f
    morphology of, 820b, 821f
    pathogenesis of, 818–820, 820f
    synovium of, 819
    treatment for, 821
Rheumatoid nodules, 820
Rheumatoid vasculitis, 389

Rh-hemolytic disease of newborn
    pathogenesis of, 283
    prevention of, 283
Rhythm disorders, 419–420
Ribonucleic acid (RNA)
    non-coding, 244–245
    noncoding regulatory, 2
Rickets, 802
    morphologic changes in, 330–331, 331f
    in vitamin D deficiency, 330
Rickettsia, 343
Right ventricular infarction, after MI, 417
Ring abscess, 427, 428f
Ring chromosome, 264, 264f
Ring sideroblasts, 481
Ristocetin platelet agglutination test, 490
RNA. See Ribonucleic acid
RNA-induced silencing complex (RISC), 4, 5f
Rocky Mountain spotted fever, 343
Rolling, of cells, 62–63, 64f
Rosenthal fibers, 850
Roth spots, 427
Rotavirus, 619
Rough endoplasmic reticulum (RER), 7f
    composition of, 12
    proteins in, 6, 7f
Roundworms (nematodes), 345, 346f
RTKs. See Receptor tyrosine kinases
Rubella, maternal, 275–276
Russell bodies, 474

S
Saccular aneurysms, 855–856
    common sites of, 855, 856f
    morphology of, 856b, 856f
    risk for, 855
St. Vitus dance, 426
Salicylism, 314
Salivary glands, 587
    diseases and disorders of
        sialadenitis, 588, 588f
        xerostomia, 587–588
    neoplasms of, 588–589, 588t
        incidence of, 588–589
        mucoepidermoid carcinoma, 589
        pleomorphic adenoma, 589
    in Sjögren syndrome, 158
Salmonellosis, 615t, 617–618
Salpingitis, 727f
Sanger sequencing, 294
Sarcoidosis, 512–514, 514b
    classification of, 512
    clinical manifestations of, 514
    epidemiology of, 512
    etiology and pathogenesis of, 512–513
    with granulomatous inflammation, 85, 86t
    immunologic abnormalities in, 513
    morphology of, 513b, 513f
    remissions in, 514
Sarcoma botryoides, of vagina, 717
Sarcomas. See also Ewing sarcoma; Synovial sarcoma
    designation as, 190–191
    gene rearrangements in, 202
    origin of, 827–828
    soft tissue, 827
    synovial, 831
    undifferentiated pleomorphic, 831–832
Scale, definition of, 890t
Scar
    hypertrophic, 93–94
    morphology of, 92b, 92f
    use of term, 89
Scarring
    excessive, 93–94, 95f
    as response to infection, 358
    steps in scar formation, 89–90, 90f
    tissue repair by, 88–92, 92b–93b
Scavenger receptors, in phagocytosis, 67
Schaumann bodies, in sarcoidosis, 513
Schiller-Duval bodies, in yolk sac tumor, 695
Schistosomiasis, 650
Schwann cells, in pediatric neuroblastoma, 287
Schwannomas
    defined, 846
    familial neurofibromatosis type 2 associated with, 846
    histological appearance of, 846, 847f
    morphology of, 846b
Scleroderma, 159
Sclerosing cholangitis, primary, 664t
Screening colonoscopy, 627–628
Scrotal skin cancer, 228–230
Scrotum
    disorders of, 692–697
    neoplasms of, 692
Scurvy, 332, 379
Sea levels, rising, and human health, 300–301
Seborrheic keratosis, 899–900
    causes of, 900
    morphology of, 900b, 900f
Secondary accumulation, in lysosomal storage diseases, 255–256
Secretion, cells specialized for, 12–13
Selectins, in acute inflammation, 63, 64f, 64t

Selenium, 338
    deficiency syndrome for, 333t
    functions of, 333t
Self-tolerance
    definition for, 145
    failure in SLE of, 152
Sella turcica, radiographic abnormalities of, 750
Seminoma, 693–694, 694f, 694t
    clinical features of, 696
    use of term, 191
Senescence
    cellular, 33
    p53-induced, 211
    replicative, 54–55, 55f
Senile systemic amyloidosis, 185
Sepsis
    organ system failure from, 319
Septic shock
    from burns, 319
    inflammatory reaction in, 59t
    severity and outcome of, 118
Sequence, in congenital anomalies, 274–275, 275f
Sequencing technologies, 291–292
    "Next Gen", 296f
    Sanger sequencing, 294
    whole-genome, 240
SER. See Smooth endoplasmic reticulum
Serology, 346–347
Serotonin (5-hydroxytryptamine), as mediator of inflammation, 71
Serous endometrial intraepithelial carcinoma (SEIC), 724
Serous inflammation, 78, 78f
Serous tubal intraepithelial carcinoma (STIC), 727
Serous tumors of ovaries, 728
    morphology of, 728b–729b, 729f
    prognosis for, 729
    types of, 728
Serum amyloid A (SAA) protein, 86–87
Serum sickness, 141t
    acute, 139–142, 141f
    acute vs. chronic, 141
Severe acute respiratory syndrome (SARS) virus, 347–348
Severe combined immunodeficiency (SCID), 168, 173b
    autosomal recessive, 169
    histologic findings in, 169b
    treatment of, 169–170
    X-linked, 169
Sex cord neoplasms, of ovaries, 730, 731t
Sex cord-stromal tumors, 693
Sex hormone exposure, and hepatic adenoma, 669
Sexually transmitted diseases (STDs), 704–712
    chancroid, 710
    classification of, 705t
    genital herpes simplex, 705t, 711–712
    gonorrhea, 705t, 708–709, 709b
    granuloma inguinale, 711
    human papillomavirus infection, 705t, 712
    lymphogranuloma venereum, 710
    syphilis, 705–707, 705t, 708b
    trichomoniasis, 705t, 711
Sézary syndrome, 477
SF3B1 gene, 468
Sheehan postpartum pituitary necrosis, 487
Shigellosis, 615t, 617
    clinical features of, 617
    morphology of, 617b
    pathogenesis of, 617
Shingles, 867
Shock, 16, 115–119, 119b
    causes of, 116
    clinical manifestations of, 119
    defined, 115–116, 119
    major types of, 116t
    morphology of, 119b
    prognosis for, 119
    septic, 116–118, 119b
        endothelial activation and injury in, 117
        immunosuppressive mechanisms in, 116–117
        incidence of, 116
        induction of procoagulant state in, 104f–105f, 117–118
        inflammatory responses in, 116–117
        metabolic abnormalities in, 118
        organ dysfunction system in, 118
        pathogenesis of, 116–118, 116t, 117f
        stages of, 118–119
Short stature homeobox (SHOX) gene, 268
Shunts, in congenital heart disease, 404
    left-to-right, 404–406, 404f, 408b
        in atrial septal defects, 404, 404f
        in patent ductus arteriosus, 404, 404f
        in ventricular septal defects, 404, 404f
    right-to-left, 406–407, 408b
        tetralogy of Fallot, 406–407, 406f
        transposition of great arteries, 406f, 407
Sialadenitis, 588, 588f
    autoimmune, 588
    bacterial, 588
    mucocele in, 588f
Sicca syndrome, in sarcoidosis, 513
Sickle cell anemia, 108, 445–447, 453
    clinical course of, 446–447
    morphology of, 446b, 446f
    pathogenesis of, 445–447, 446f–447f
    peripheral blood smear, 445, 446f

Sickled cells, irreversibly, 445
Sickle hemoglobin (HbS), 445–446
Sick sinus syndrome, 420
Sievert (Sv), 320
Sigmoid diverticulitis, 620–621
　clinical features of, 621
　morphology of, 621b, 621f
　pathogenesis of, 620
the "silent killer", 58
Silica, lung disease associated with, 509t
Silicosis, 510–511, 512b
　advanced, 510f
　clinical features of, 511
　incidence of, 510
　morphology of, 510b–511b, 510f
Single-gene disorders, with atypical patterns of inheritance, 269–272
　alternations of imprinted regions, 271–272
　mutations in mitochondrial genes, 271
　triplet repeat mutations, 269–271, 270f–271f
Single-nucleotide polymorphisms (SNPs), 2–3, 293–294
　high-density, 295–296
　newer types of, 293–294
Sinus histiocytosis, morphology of, 463–485
Sinusitis, granulomatous, 388
Sjögren syndrome, 157, 159b
　autoantibodies in, 151t
　causes of, 158
　and celiac disease, 613
　characteristics of, 158
　clinical features of, 158
　enlargement of salivary gland, 158, 159f
　morphology of, 158b, 159f
　pathogenesis of, 157
Skeletal deformities, in thalassemia, 450
Skeletal muscle
　acquired disorders of, 844–845
　　inflammatory myopathies, 844–845, 845f
　　toxic myopathies, 845
　disorders of, 845b
　　inherited, 841–844
　　skeletal muscle injury and atrophy, 840–841
　fiber types in, 840–841, 841f
　grouped atrophy, 840–841, 841f
Skeleton
　diseases of, 800
　metastases of, 816
Skin
　malignant epidermal tumors of
　　basal cell carcinoma, 902
　　squamous cell carcinoma, 900–901
　melanocytic proliferations in, 907b
　　dysplastic nevus, 903–905
　　melanocytic nevi, 903
　　melanoma, 905–907
　microbe exit via, 352
　microbial infection of, 349, 349t
　in SLE, 156, 156f
　in systemic sclerosis, 159, 161f
　tumors of, 899–907
　　actinic keratosis, 900
　　benign epithelial neoplasms, 899
　　seborrheic keratosis, 899–900
Skin diseases, 889
Skin lesions
　in opioid abuse, 316
　in sarcoidosis, 513
Skin pigmentation, in hemochromatosis, 657
Sleep apnea, pulmonary hypertension associated with, 517
SLUG transcriptional regulators, 213
SMAD molecules, 213
SMAD4 tumor suppressor gene, in pancreatic cancer, 687, 687f
Small bowel, in kwashiorkor, 326. See also Intestines
Small-cell change, in chronic liver disease, 670
Small cell lung carcinoma (SCLC), 538–540, 542f
　clinical features of, 543
　compared with NSCLC, 542t
Small interfering RNAs (siRNAs), 4–5
Small lymphocytic lymphoma (SLL), 478
　clinical features of, 468
　course and prognosis of, 468
　immune dysregulation of, 468
　immunophenotype and genetics of, 468–469
　morphology of, 467b, 468f
　pathogenesis of, 468
　prevalence of, 467
Small nucleolar RNAs (snoRNAs), 272
Smallpox virus, as agent of terrorism, 348
Smog, health effects of, 303, 303b–304b
Smoke, tobacco. See also Tobacco
　constituents of, 308t
　exposure to environmental, 310
　noxious chemicals in, 308–309
　organ-specific carcinogens in, 309t
Smokers
　numbers for, 307–308
　survival of, 308, 308f
Smoking
　adverse effects of, 308, 308f
　and cancer risk, 198–199
　maternal, 310
　passive, 538

Smooth endoplasmic reticulum (SER), 7f, 12
　compounds metabolized by, 13
　functions of, 6
Smooth muscle cells (SMCs)
　in blood vessels, 361, 362f
　in intimal thickening, 368–369, 369f
　migratory and proliferative activities of, 364
　structure and function of, 364
SNAIL transcription factors, 223
SNPs. See Single-nucleotide polymorphisms
Soft tissue tumors, 827–832, 832b
　of adipose tissue
　　lipoma, 828
　　liposarcoma, 828
　chromosomal abnormalities in, 827–828
　classification of, 828
　fibrous tumors, 828–829
　　deep fibromatosis, 829
　　desmoid tumor, 829
　　nodular fasciitis, 828
　　superficial fibromatosis, 828–829
　pathogenesis of, 827–828
　skeletal muscle tumors, 830
　smooth muscle tumors, 830–831
　of uncertain origin, 831–832
　　synovial sarcoma, 831
　　undifferentiated pleomorphic sarcoma, 831–832
Solitary rectal ulcer syndrome, 626
Solvents, toxicology of, 301–302
Sonic hedgehog (SHH) pathway, 883
Spermatocytic tumor, 694
Sphingomyelin, 8
Spina bifida occulta, 860–861
Spinal cord
　subacute combined degeneration of, 874
　trauma to, 857
SPINK1, 679. See also Pancreatic secretory trypsin inhibitor
Spinocerebellar ataxias (SCAs), 879–880
　characteristics of, 881
　forms of, 880
Spleen
　amyloidosis of, 186
　disorders of, 493
　in hereditary spherocytosis, 444
　in immune responses, 128–129
　in infectious mononucleosis, 461
　in ITP, 488
　in sarcoidosis, 513
　in SLE, 156
Splenic infarcts, in CML, 481–482
Splenomegaly, 441, 493
　chronic, 492
　classification of, 492
　congestive, 402
　in hereditary spherocytosis, 444b–445b, 445
　in malaria, 453
　in sickle cell anemia, 446
　in thalassemia, 450
Spondyloarthropathies
　clinical features of, 822
　manifestations of, 822
　seronegative, 822
Spongiosis, 890t, 891
Squamous cell carcinoma (SCC)
　of cervix, 720
　designation as, 190–191
　esophageal, 596
　　clinical features of, 597
　　morphology of, 597b, 597f
　　pathogenesis of, 596–597
　keratin produced by, 193, 193f
　of lung, 539, 541f
　of oral cavity, 586–587, 587f
　　incidence of, 587
　　morphology of, 587b, 587f
　　pathogenesis of, 586–587
　penile, 691–692, 692f
　precursor lesions associated with, 199, 539, 541f
　sequential changes leading to, 539
　of skin, 193f
　of vagina, 716
　of vulva, 715, 716b
Squamous cell carcinoma (SCC), cutaneous, 900
　clinical features of invasive, 901, 901f
　morphology of, 901b, 901f
　pathogenesis of, 900–901
Squamous cell carcinoma (SCC) in situ, of penis, 691, 692f
Squamous cells (keratinocytes), 889
Squamous intraepithelial lesion (SIL)
　of cervix, 717
　classification of, 718
　early detection of, 718–719
　follow-up for, 720
　incidence of, 718–719
　morphology of, 719b, 719f
　natural history of, 718, 718t
Squamous metaplasia, 329
Staging, of solid cancers, 236–237, 237b
Staphylococcus aureus, in female breast, 737
Staphylococcus aureus pneumonia, 521
Stasis, in acute inflammation, 60–61
Statins
　in atherosclerosis, 371
　to lower plasma cholesterol, 250

Status asthmaticus, 505
Steatofibrosis, 652f, 653
Steatohepatitis, 653
Steatosis
　in cystic fibrosis, 252–253
　hepatic, 252–253
Stein-Leventhal syndrome, 727
Stellate abscesses, 710
Stellate cell activation, and liver fibrosis, 639
Stem cells
　adult, 25–27, 27f–28f
　cardiac, 419
　embryonic, 26–27, 27f–28f
　hematopoietic, 27
　homeostatic equilibrium of, 26, 27f
　induced pluripotent, 28, 28f
　location of, 28f
　mesenchymal, 28
　properties of, 26
　for regeneration, 88
　in regenerative medicine, 28
　tissue, 26–27, 27f–28f
　varieties of, 26–27, 27f–28f
Stenosis, in valvular heart disease, 422–423
Steroids, 749
　and cancer, 337
　and tissue repair, 93
Stevens-Johnson syndrome, 892
Stomach
　anatomy of, 598
　diseases and disorders of, 598–607
　gastropathy and gastritis of, 598–599
　　chronic gastritis, 599–601
　　morphology of, 599b
　　pathogenesis of, 598–599, 598f
　　use of terms, 598
　neoplastic disease of, 607b
　　gastric adenocarcinoma, 604–605
　　gastric polyps, 603–604
　　gastrointestinal stromal tumor, 606–607
　　lymphoma, 605
　　neuroendocrine (carcinoid) tumor, 605–606, 606f
Stomach carcinoma, death rate for, 197
Stool, exit of microbes via, 352
Strawberry hemangiomas, 392
Streptococcus pneumoniae, 520–521
Stress, cellular adaptations to, 48–51, 51b
　atrophy, 50, 50f
　hyperplasia, 49–50
　hypertrophy, 48–49, 48f–49f
　metaplasia, 50–51
Stroke
　designation of, 852
　heat, 319
　in sickle cell anemia, 447
Stroma, 190
Stromal tumors, of female breasts, 738, 738b, 738f
Strongyloides, 619–620
ST-segment elevated MIs (STEMIs), 413, 417
Sudden cardiac death (SCD), 409, 419–420, 420b
　causes in younger victims of, 420
　defined, 420
　HCM caused by, 433
　ultimate mechanism of, 420
Sudden death, in opioid abuse, 316
Sudden infant death syndrome (SIDS), 280–281, 281b–282b
　defined, 280
　factors associated with, 281t
　morphology for, 281b
　pathogenesis of, 280–281
　risk factors for, 280–281
Sudden unexpected infant death (SUID), factors associated with, 280
Sulfur dioxide, health effects of, 302t, 303
Superantigens
　bacterial, 354
　high levels of cytokines released by, 118
Superior vena cava syndrome, 391
Superoxide dismutase (SOD), 43–44
Suppurative inflammation, 78–79, 79f
Surface proteins, microbial modification of, 355–356
Surfactant, in newborn, 278
Surfactant synthesis, hormonal regulation of, 278
Surveillance programs, in IBD, 626
Sydenham chorea, 426
Synaptic signaling, 16
Synarthroses, 817
Syncytiotrophoblast-like cells, 695, 695f
Syndrome of inappropriate antidiuretic hormone (SIADH) secretion, 755
Synovial cyst, 826
Synovial sarcoma, 831
　incidence of, 831
　morphology of, 831b, 831f
　treatment for, 831
Syphilis, 705–707, 705t, 708b
　aortic aneurysms in, 379
　with granulomatous inflammation, 86t
　protean manifestations of, 706f
　secondary, 357f
Syringomyelia, 862
Syrinx, 862
Systemic inflammatory response syndrome (SIRS), 62, 486

Systemic lupus erythematosus (SLE), 141t, 147–150, 158b
  antinuclear antibodies, 148–150, 151t, 152f
  antiphospholipid antibodies, 151
  autoantibodies in, 147–148, 151, 151t
  changes in interstitium in, 154–156
  clinical features of, 153
  clinical and pathologic manifestations of, 154b–157b, 154t
  compared with chronic discoid lupus erythematosus, 153
  criteria for classification of, 150t
  endocarditis in, 428f, 429
  HLA alleles associated with, 148t
  morphologic changes in, 154b–157b, 155f–156f
  neuropsychiatric manifestations of, 153
  pathogenesis of, 150–157
    environmental factors, 151
    genetic factors, 151
    immunologic factors, 152
    model for, 152, 153f
  presentation of, 149–150
  prevalence of, 149–150
  tissue injury in, 152–153
Systemic sclerosis (scleroderma), 158
  alimentary tract in, 159–160
  autoantibodies in, 151t
  classification of, 159
  clinical features of, 158, 162b
  morphology of, 160b, 161f
  pathogenesis of, 158, 160f
Systolic dysfunction, 399–400

T

Tabes dorsalis, 868
Tachycardia, 419–420. *See also* Arrhythmias
Takayasu arteritis, 385–386
  clinical features of, 386
  defined, 385
  morphology of, 386b, 386f
Tangles, neurofibrillary
  in AD, 877
  in development of AD, 875, 876f
  in diagnosis of AD, 877
  in FTLD, 878f
Tapeworms (cestodes), 345
Targeted therapies, 239–241, 241f
tau protein, in development of AD, 875, 876f, 877
Tax protein, 232, 232b
Tay-Sachs disease, 256–257, 257t, 258f, 260, 872
  acute infantile variant of, 257
  epidemiology of, 256–257
  ganglion cells in, 258f
  misfolded proteins in, 46t
  pathologic changes in, 257, 258f
TCA. *See* Tricarboxylic acid
T-cell-mediated inflammation, in host response to microbes, 355
T cell neoplasms
  classification of, 465t
  precursor, 466, 466t
T-cell receptors (TCRs), 126f, 134b
  peptide antigens recognized by, 124, 126f
  in SLE, 152
T-cell recognition, microbial decreased, 357
T cells. *See also* T lymphocytes
  location of, 129–130, 129f
  in psoriasis, 892
  regulatory (Tregs)
    in type 1 diabetes, 776
  in rheumatoid arthritis, 819, 820f
  on skin, 889
  suppression by regulatory, 145
T cell tumors, 464f, 465
Teeth and supporting structures, diseases of
  caries, 584
  gingivitis, 584
  periodontitis, 584
Telangiectasia
  hereditary hemorrhagic, 392
  spider, 392
  use of term, 392
Telomerase, 54–55, 55f
Telomeres, 2, 54–55, 55f
Telomere shortening, mitotic catastrophe caused by, 189, 218–219, 219f
Telomeropathies
  defective protein homeostasis, 55
  persistent inflammation, 56
  signaling pathways, 55–56
Temporal arteritis, 384–385
Tenosynovial giant cell tumor, 826–827
  clinical course of, 827
  clinical variants of, 826
  morphology of, 827b, 827f
  pathogenesis of, 827
Teratogens, 277
Teratomas, 694t
  with malignant transformation, 696
  origins of, 191
  of ovaries, 730
    benign (mature) cystic, 730, 731f
    clinical features of, 731
    immature malignant, 730
    specialized, 730–731

Teratomas *(Continued)*
  sacrococcygeal, 285–286, 286f
  testicular, 695–696, 696f
Terminology, medical, 191. *See also* Nomenclature
Testes, 692–697
  atrophy of, 692–693
  cryptorchidism of, 692–693
  inflammatory lesions of, 693
  neoplasms of, 693–697, 694t, 697b
  vascular disturbances of, 693
Tetracyclines, adverse reactions to, 312–313, 312f, 317b
Tetralogy of Fallot, 406–407, 406f
  cardinal features of, 406
  clinical features of, 407
  frequency of, 403t
  morphology of, 406b–407b
Thalassemia, 447–450, 453
  cause of, 447
  classification of, 447–448, 448t
  clinical course of, 449–450
  morphology of, 448b–449b
  pathogenesis of, 447–448, 448t
  α-thalassemia, 448–450, 448t
  β-thalassemia, 448–450, 448t, 449f
Thalidomide, malformations associated with, 275–276
Thanatophoric dysplasia, 800
Th2 cells, in immediate hypersensitivity, 136, 136f
Th17 cells, 70, 130–131
Therapeutic decision-making, in diagnosis of cancer, 239, 240f
Therapeutic targets, classification of cancer according to, 239–241, 241f
Thermal injury, 318–319
  hyperthermia, 319
  thermal burns, 318
Thermogenin (or UCP-1), 15
Thiamine deficiency
  in chronic alcoholism, 311
  effects on CNS of, 873
Thoracic duct, structure and function of, 363
Th2 response, 137
Thrombi
  antemortem *vs.* postmortem, 110
  arterial, 110
  on heart valves, 110
  morphology of, 110
  mural, 110–111, 110f
  venous, 110
Thrombin
  enzymatic activities of, 105
  in glomerular injury, 554
  in hemostasis, 105, 105f
Thromboangiitis obliterans (Buerger disease)
  characteristics of, 389
  clinical features of, 389
  morphology of, 389b, 389f
Thrombocytopenia, 485, 489
  drug-induced, 488
  heparin-induced, 489–490
  immune thrombocytopenic purpura, 489–490
  major causes of, 488, 488t
  radiation-caused, 322–323
  thrombotic microangiopathies, 490
  in type II hypersensitivity, 139, 140f
Thrombocytopenic purpura, 139t
Thromboemboli
  pulmonary, 112, 112f, 114b
  pulmonary hypertension associated with, 517
  systemic, 112, 114b
    air embolism, 113–114
    amniotic fluid embolism, 113, 113f
    fat embolism, 112–113, 113f
  use of term, 112
Thrombomodulin, 108
Thrombophlebitis, 391
Thrombosis, 97, 101–112
  abnormalities leading to, 106–111, 107f
  arterial and cardiac, 111
  clinical features of, 111
  defined, 101
  DIC, 111–112
  endothelial injury in, 107–108, 107f
    with abnormal blood flow, 107f, 108
    hypercoagulability, 108–109, 108t
  fate of thrombus in, 110–111
  HIT syndrome, 109
  homocysteine in, 109
  in polycythemia vera, 482
  risk of, 109
  in sickle cell anemia, 446
  thrombus development in, 111b
  venous, 111
Thrombotic microangiopathies (TMAs), 490, 571–572
  clinical course of, 572
  etiologic classification of, 571t
  morphology of, 572b
  pathogenesis of, 571–572
  primary forms of, 571
Thrombotic thrombocytopenic purpura (TTP), 491–492, 571–572, 571t
  defined, 488
  pathogenesis of, 488–489
  typical onset of, 572
Thrush, 585

Thymoma
  classification of, 493
  morphology of, 493b
Thyroid gland
  adenomas of, 763–764
    clinical features of, 764
    morphology of, 763b, 764f
    pathogenesis of, 756f, 763
  anaplastic carcinomas of, 768
    clinical features of, 768
    morphology of, 767b
  anatomy of, 755
  autoimmune disorders of, 761
  carcinomas of, 762, 764–768
    anaplastic, 765
    environmental factors in, 765–766
    follicular, 764
    genetics of, 765
    medullary, 765
    papillary, 764, 765f, 766
    pathogenesis of, 764–765
    subtypes of, 763
  diseases of, 755
  follicular carcinomas of, 768
    clinical features of, 767–768
    incidence of, 767
    morphology of, 767b, 767f
  goiter, 762–763
  Graves disease, 760
  hyperthyroidism, 755–768
  hypothyroidism, 756–757
  lingual, 755
  medullary carcinomas of, 768–769
    clinical features of, 769–772
    morphology of, 768b, 768f–769f
  neoplasms of, 763–768, 768b
  papillary carcinomas of, 768
    clinical features of, 766–767
    diagnosis of, 765
    encapsulated follicular variant of, 766
    morphology of, 765b–766b, 766f
Thyroid hormone, secretion of, 755, 756f
Thyroid hormone receptor (TR), 755
Thyroid hormone response elements (TREs), 755
Thyroiditis, 757–758, 760b
  and celiac disease, 613
  chronic lymphocytic Hashimoto, 758–761
  Riedel, 760
  silent, 760
  subacute granulomatous, 759
    clinical features of, 760
    morphology of, 760b
  subacute lymphocytic, 760
Thyroid nodules
  "hot", 763
  solitary, 762
Thyroid-stimulating hormone (TSH), 754
Thyroid storm, 757
Thyrotoxicosis
  causes of, 756, 757t
  clinical manifestations of, 756, 757f
  diagnosis of, 757
  transient, 758
  use of term, 755–756
Thyrotropin, 755
Thyroxine, 749
Tight junctions, in cell-cell interactions, 12
Tissue damage, clinical markers of, 37
Tissue inhibitors of metalloproteinases (TIMPs), 92, 377
Tissue repair
  angiogenesis in, 90–91
  cell and tissue degeneration in, 88–89
  complications in, 93
  deposition of connective tissue in, 91–92
  factors influencing, 93
  fibroblasts in, 91–92
  mechanisms of, 87–88, 87f
  overview of, 87–88
  by regeneration, 89b
  remodeling of connective tissue in, 92
  role of cell proliferation in, 88
  by scarring, 89–92, 90f, 92b–93b
T lymphocytes (T cells), 124–130
  in acute inflammation, 70
  antigen receptors of, 130, 131f
  in apoptosis, 39
  in cell-mediated immunity, 130–134, 131f–132f
  cytotoxic T lymphocytes, 124–125, 125f
  effector, 135
  in glomerular injury, 554
  helper T cells, 124–125, 125f
  NKT cells, 125, 125f
  regulatory T lymphocytes, 125, 125f
Tobacco. *See also* Smoking
  health effects of, 307–310, 310b
  mortality associated with, 307–308, 308f
  and oral cancer, 586–587
Tobacco smoke
  constituents of, 308–309, 308t
  health effects of, 303
Toll-like receptors (TLRs), 122f
  in inflammatory response, 59–60
  in innate immunity, 122–123
  in septic shock, 116–117

Tongue, amyloid of, 186
Tonsils, pharyngeal, 128
Tophi, in gouty arthritis, 824, 825f
TORCH syndrome (toxoplasmosis, rubella, CMV, herpes simplex), 277, 732, 862
Torsion, testicular, 693
Totipotential cells, in regenerative medicine, 28
Toxemia of pregnancy, 735
Toxic agents, injury by nontherapeutic, 315–317, 315t
Toxic epidermal necrolysis, 891–892
Toxicology, defined, 301
Toxic shock syndrome, 118
Toxins
    cell injury caused by, 32, 45
    direct-acting, 45
    latent, 45
Toxoplasmosis, cerebral, 868, 868b, 869f
TP53 cells, mutation in, 321
TP53 mutations, 724, 725f
TP53 (tumor suppressor) gene, 211–212, 212b–213b, 212f
    in controlling carcinogenesis, 211–212
    and DNA damage, 211
    neoplastic transformation supported by, 211
    in pancreatic cancer, 687–688
Trace elements
    deficiency syndromes for, 333t
    function of, 333t
Transcription factors, in cardiac morphogenesis, 404
Transcription-mediated amplification, 347
Transcytosis, 10, 10f
    in acute inflammation, 62
    vacuolar, 363
Transferrin, 11
Transforming growth factor-alpha (TFG-α), 20
Transforming growth factor-β (TGF-β)
    associated with juvenile polyposis, 626b, 628f
    in fibrosis, 94
    in tissue repair, 91
Transforming growth factor-β (TGF-β) pathway, 213, 214b
Transfusion reactions, in type II hypersensitivity, 139, 140f
Transfusion-related acute lung injury (TRALI), 493
Transfusion therapy
    complications of, 492–493
        allergic reactions to blood products, 492–493
        hemolytic reactions to blood products, 493
        infectious complications of, 493
        and TRALI, 493
Translocation, of chromosomes, 263, 264f
Transplacental infections, 277
Transplantation candidates, 458
Transplant rejection, 162, 168b. See also Graft rejection
    chronic, 164, 165b, 167f
    and mechanisms of graft rejection, 162–168, 165f–166f
    and methods of increasing graft survival, 162–166
    and recognition and rejection of allografts, 162
Transplants. See also Allografts
    immune responses to, 130
    recognition and rejection of, 168b
Transplant surgery, immunosuppression of recipient in, 165–166
Transposition of great arteries, 406f, 407
    clinical features of, 407
    frequency of, 403t
    VSDs in, 407
Transposition of great vessels, 406, 406f
Transposons, 2
Transudates (effusions)
    defined, 60
    formation of, 61f
    in right-sided heart failure, 403
Trauma, mechanical, 317. See also Brain injury
Tricarboxylic acid (TCA) cycle, 15
Trichinella spiralis larva, 346f
Trichomonas vaginalis, 716
Trichomoniasis, 705t, 711
Trinucleotide repeat mutations, 244
Trisomies, 262–263
Trisomy 13 (Patau syndrome)
    clinical features of, 265f
    karyotype of, 265f
Trisomy 18 (Edwards syndrome)
    clinical features of, 265f
    karyotype of, 265f
Trisomy 21 (Down syndrome)
    characteristics of, 264–266
    clinical features of, 265f
    diagnostic clinical features of, 265f, 266
    karyotype of, 265f
    longevity of persons with, 266
    prenatal diagnosis of, 266
Tropical sprue, 613–614
Tropism, 341–342
Trousseau syndrome, 391, 688
T (thymus-derived) lymphocytes, 134b. See also T cells; T lymphocytes
Tubercle, granulomatous inflammation in, 85
Tubercular infection, immunity to, 528
Tuberculin (Mantoux) test, 526
Tuberculin reaction, 142
Tuberculosis (TB), 341, 526–532, 531b–532b
    defined, 531–532
    diagnosis of, 531
    epidemiology of, 526–528
    etiology of, 526

Tuberculosis (TB) (Continued)
    granulomatous inflammation in, 85, 86t
    infection vs. disease in, 526
    of lung, 36–37, 37f
    morphology of, 528b, 528f–529f
    mortality associated with, 525–526
    pathogenesis of, 526–528, 527f
    patterns of, 530, 531f
    poverty associated with, 526
    primary, 528
    prostatic, 697–698
    reactivation, 528–531
    secondary, 528–531
        caseation in, 529–530, 530f–531f
        clinical features of, 530–531
        in HIV-positive patients, 529
        intestinal, 530
        isolated-organ, 530
        localization in, 529
        lymphadenitis, 530
        miliary, 530, 530f–531f
        morphology of, 529b–530b, 530f–531f
    silicosis associated with, 511
    testicular, 693
    vitamin D supplements in, 331–332
Tuberculous spondylitis, 807–808
Tuberous sclerosis (TSC), 627t, 886
Tubules, in SLE, 154–156
Tubulointerstitial nephritis (TIN), 564–567, 567b
    acute pyelonephritis, 564–566
    chronic pyelonephritis, 566–567
    drug-induced tubulointerstitial nephritis, 567
Tumor antigens
    classification of, 225f
Tumor dormancy, 222
Tumor necrosis factor (TNF), 73–74, 75f
    in ARDS, 496
    in inflammation, 74t
Tumor necrosis factor (TNF) receptors, in apoptosis, 39, 39f
Tumor progression, 204
Tumor promoters, 230, 231b
Tumors. See also Cardiac tumors; specific tumors
    benign, 190
    blood supply for, 220, 220b
    components of, 190
    differentiation of benign and malignant, 196, 196b, 197f
    distinguishing features of, 192–196
        differentiation and anaplasia, 192–194, 193f–194f
        local invasion, 194–195, 194f
        metastasis, 195–196
    global molecular analysis of, 239–241, 241f
    immune responses to, 130
    malignant, 190
    mixed, 191, 191f
    nomenclature of, 192t
    odontogenic, 590
Tumors and tumorlike lesions, of infancy and childhood, 285–286, 285f
    benign neoplasm, 285–286, 285f
    malignant neoplasms, 286–291, 286t
Tumor suppressor genes, 200. See also RB
    antigrowth signals of, 208
    BRCA1, 741, 742f
    BRCA2, 741, 742f
    discovery of, 208–209
    and hypermethylation of promoter sequences, 203–204
    products of, 208
Turcot syndrome, 629–630
Turner syndrome, 269, 283
    chromosomes in, 268
    clinical features of, 267–268, 268f
    karyotype of, 267–268, 268f
    molecular pathogenesis of, 268
Twin studies, on diabetes development, 776
TWIST transcriptional regulators, 213
TWIST transcription factors, 223
Two-hit hypothesis, 208–209
Typhoid fever, 618
Typhus, epidemic, 343

U
Ulcerative colitis, 624–625
    clinical features of, 625
    compared with Crohn disease, 621, 621f, 622t
    effect of smoking on, 623
    epithelial defects in, 623
    genetics of, 622–623
    morphology of, 624b–625b, 625f
    mucosal disease in, 625
    and mucosal immune responses, 623
    pathology of, 625f
Ulcers
    aphthous, 584, 584f, 623
    arterial, 93, 94f
    defined, 79
    diabetic, 93, 94f
    gastric
        cause of, 601–602
        and NSAID use, 602f
    location of, 79
    morphology of, 80f
    venous leg, 93, 94f
Ultraviolet (UV) light, exposure to, in SLE, 152

Undernutrition, 299
Undifferentiated pleomorphic sarcoma (UPS), 831
    morphology of, 832b, 832f
    treatment for, 832
Unfolded protein response (UPR), 12, 45–46, 46f, 46t
Upper respiratory tract
    acute infections of, 545–546
        acute laryngitis, 545–546
        bacterial epiglottitis, 545
        "common cold", 545
        croup, 546
        pharyngitis, 545
    lesions of
        laryngeal tumors, 546–547
        nasopharyngeal carcinoma, 546
        ulcerative, 388
UPR. See Unfolded protein response
Uranium, and lung carcinoma, 539
Uremia, 549–550
    gastric injury in, 599
    with pericarditis, 436–437
Ureter, male, 702
    primary malignant tumors of, 702
    retroperitoneal fibrosis of, 702
Ureteropelvic junction (UPJ) obstruction, 702
Urethritis, nongonococcal, 703f, 709–710
Uric acid stones, 576–577
Urinary outflow obstruction
    hydronephrosis, 577–578
    renal stones, 576–578
Urinary tract, male
    bladder, 701–702
    ureter, 701–702
    urethra, 701–702
Urinary tract infection (UTI), 566
    causes of, 564–565
    risk factors for, 565
    and urolithiasis, 576
Urine, exit of microbes via, 352
Urobilinogens, 659–660
Urogenital tract, microbial infection of, 349t, 351. See also Genital system, female; Genital system, male
Urolithiasis, 576–578
Urothelial carcinoma, 702
    acquired genetic aberrations in, 702–703
    genesis of, 702
Urticaria ("hives")
    characteristics of, 889
    clinical features of, 890
    histologic features of, 890
    pathogenesis of, 889–890
Urticarial allergic reactions, 491
Usual interstitial pneumonia (UIP), 507, 508f
Uterus
    cellular adaptation of, 48, 48f
    disorders of
        abnormal uterine bleeding, 722–723, 722t
        adenomyosis, 721
        endometrial carcinoma, 724
        endometrial hyperplasia, 723
        endometrial polyps, 724–725
        endometriosis, 721–722
        endometritis, 721
        leiomyoma, 725–726
        leiomyosarcoma, 726
        proliferative lesions of, 723–726

V
Vaccination, 133
Vaculitides, systemic, 609
Vagina
    congenital anomalies of, 716
    malignant neoplasms of
        clear cell adenocarcinoma, 716
        sarcoma botryoides, 717
        squamous cell carcinoma, 716
Vaginal discharge, 716
Vaginitis
    candida, 535
    characteristics of, 716
Valproic acid, 276
Valvular heart disease (VHD), 422–429, 429b
    calcific aortic stenosis, 423–424, 424b
    clinical features of, 424–425
    degenerative, 423–425
    etiology of acquired, 423, 423t
    insufficiency in, 422–423
    Libman-Sacks endocarditis, 428f, 429
    morphology of, 424b, 424f
    myxomatous mitral valve, 424–425, 424f
    nonbacterial thrombotic endocarditis, 428, 428f–429f
    noninfected vegetations, 428–429
    outcome of, 423
    pathogenesis of, 424
    rheumatic, 425–427
Valvular stenosis, in rheumatic heart disease, 425
Vanillylmandelic acid (VMA), in neuroblastoma, 288–289
Varicella-zoster virus (VZV), 867
Varicose veins, 390
    clinical features of, 390
    esophageal varices, 390–391
    hemorrhoids, 390–391
Vascular congestion, in sickle cell anemia, 446

Vascular damage, in systemic sclerosis, 159
Vascular disease, mechanisms of, 361
Vascular ectasias, 396b
Vascular endothelial growth factor (VEGF), 20
  in angiogenesis, 220, 220b
  in long-term diabetes, 783
  in peripartum cardiomyopathy, 431
Vascular injury
  and intimal thickening, 368–369, 369f
  vascular wall response to, 368–369, 369f
Vascular malformations, of brain, 855–856
Vascular tone, regulation of, 365, 366f
Vasculitides
  common, 383f
  polyarteritis nodosa, 161–162
Vasculitis, 139t, 141
  acute, 141
  clinical manifestations of, 382
  defined, 390b
  forms of, 383f, 383t
  infectious, 389–390
  noninfectious, 382–389
    anti-endothelial cell antibodies, 384
    anti-neutrophil cytoplasmic antibodies, 384
    Churg-Strauss syndrome, 389
    giant cell (temporal) arteritis, 384–385, 385f
    granulomatosis with polyangiitis, 388–389
    immune complex-associated vasculitis, 382–384
    Kawasaki disease, 387
    microscopic polyangiitis, 387–388
    polyarteritis nodosa, 386–387
    Takayasu arteritis, 385–386
    thromboangiitis obliterans (Buerger disease), 389
  in SLE, 154
Vas deferens, in cystic fibrosis, 252–253
Vasoactive animes, in immediate hypersensitivity reactions, 136–137, 136f
Vasoconstriction, 362
Vasodilation
  in acute inflammation, 60
  control of, 362
Vegetable oils, 337–338
Vegetations, 110
VEGF. See Vascular endothelial growth factor
Vehicular accidents, injuries from, 318
Veins
  benign tumors of
    hemangiomas, 392–393
    vascular ectasias, 392
  inferior vena cava syndrome, 391
  structure and function of, 362–363
  superior vena cava syndrome, 391
Velocardiofacial syndrome, 266–267, 269b
Venereal warts, 895
Ventricular aneurysm, after MI, 418, 418f
Ventricular fibrillation, 419–420
Ventricular septal defects (VSDs), 404–406, 404f–405f
  clinical features of, 406
  frequency of, 403t
  morphology of, 405b
Verrucae (warts), 895
  morphology of, 895b, 896f
  pathogenesis of, 895
Vertebral body, osteoporotic, 802, 802f
Vesicle, definition of, 890t
Vesicoureteral reflux (VUR), 565
Vibrio cholerae, 349–350
Vimentin, of cytoskeleton, 11
Vinyl chloride
  and angiosarcoma of liver, 307
  and lung carcinoma, 539
Viral diseases, pathogens of, 343t
Viral infections, 342, 343t
  damage caused by, 353, 353f
  manifestations of, 353
Virchow triad, 106–107, 107f
Viremia, in HIV disease progression, 179
Viruses, 341–342, 342f
  cell-to-cell transmission of, 351
  characteristics of, 342t
  cytopathic-cytoproliferative reactions produced by, 357
  inclusion bodies of, 341–342, 342f
  tumors induced by, 180
Visual field abnormalities, 750
Vitamin A, 327–329
  deficiency states of, 328–329
  deficiency syndrome for, 333t
  dietary sources of, 327

Vitamin A (Continued)
  functions of, 327–328, 333t
  metabolism of, 327, 327f
  recommended dietary allowance for, 327
  and resistance to infections, 328
  toxicity of, 329
Vitamin B₁ (thiamine)
  deficiency syndrome for, 333t
  functions of, 333t
Vitamin B₂ (riboflavin)
  deficiency syndrome for, 333t
  functions of, 333t
Vitamin B₁₂ (cobalamin) deficiency
  CNS effects of, 873
Vitamin B₆ (pyridoxine)
  deficiency syndrome for, 333t
  functions of, 333t
Vitamin B₁₂ (cobalamin), functions of, 333t
Vitamin B₁₂ (cobalamin) deficiency, 333t, 457–458
  causes of, 457
  clinical features of, 457–458
  diagnosis of, 458
  metabolic defects in, 458
  pathogenesis of, 457–458
Vitamin C (ascorbic acid), 332, 338
  antioxidant properties of, 332
  deficiency of, 332, 332f, 333t, 485
  functions of, 332, 333t
  toxicity of, 332
Vitamin D, 329–332
  active form of, 329–330
  in bone development, 799
  deficiency states of, 330–332
  deficiency syndrome for, 333t
  effects on bone of, 330
  functions of, 329–330, 333t
  metabolism of, 329, 330f
  nonskeletal effects of, 331–332
  source of, 329
  toxicity, 332
Vitamin deficiencies, 326–332
Vitamin E, 338
  deficiency syndrome for, 333t
  functions of, 333t
Vitamin K
  deficiency syndrome for, 333t
  functions of, 333t
Vitamins, 334b
  deficiency syndrome for, 333t
  functions of, 333t
Vocal cord nodules ("polyps"), 546
von Gierke disease, 261, 261t
von Hippel-Lindau (VHL) disease, 285, 393, 887
von Hippel-Lindau (VHL) tumor suppressor gene, 685–686
von Willebrand disease, 489–492
  clinical findings in, 490
  common varieties of, 490
  diagnosis of, 490
Vulva
  disorders of, 713
    lichen sclerosus, 714, 714f
    lichen simplex chronicus, 714
    vulvitis, 713–714
  nonneoplastic epithelial disorders of, 714, 714b
  squamous cell carcinoma of, 716b
  tumors of
    carcinoma of, 715
    condylomas, 714–715, 715f
    extramammary Paget disease, 715–716, 716f
    morphology of, 715b
Vulvar intraepithelial neoplasia (VIN), 713, 715
Vulvitis
  causes of, 713
  complications of, 713–714

W
WAGR syndrome, 289
Waldenström macroglobulinemia, 474
Wallerian degeneration, 835
Warburg effect, 15, 25, 42, 214
Warts, venereal, 712. See also Verrucae
Waterhouse-Friderichsen syndrome, 118, 487, 792, 792f
Wegener granulomatosis, 519. See also Granulomatosis with polyangiitis
Weibel-Palade bodies, 63, 490
Weight gain, in Cushing syndrome, 789
Wernicke-Korsakoff syndrome, 873
West Nile virus, 348

West Nile virus infection, 867
Wheal, definition of, 890t
Whipple disease, 615t
White cell disorders, 441, 459–485
  neoplastic proliferations, 465
    classification of, 463
    histiocytic neoplasms, 486–488
    lymphoid neoplasms, 465–467
    myeloid neoplasms, 479
  nonneoplastic, 459–463
    leukopenia, 459–460
    reactive leukocytosis, 460–461
    reactive lymphadenitis, 461–463
Whole-genome sequencing, 240
Wickham striae, 893
Wilms tumor, 291b, 580
  characteristics of, 289
  clinical course for, 291
  histology of, 290, 291f
  morphology of, 290, 291f
  mutation of TP53 in, 290
  nonsyndrome, 290
  pediatric, 289–291
  risk for development of, 289
Wilson disease
  clinical features of, 658
  defined, 657–658
  morphology of, 658b
Wiskott-Aldrich syndrome, 171
Wiskott-Aldrich syndrome protein (WASP), 171
WNT signaling pathway, 213, 214f, 882
Wood smoke, health effects of, 303
Workplace, exposure to toxins in, 307
World Health Organization (WHO), 334
  diagnostic criteria for diabetes of, 772
  grading system for prostate cancer of, 700
Worms. See Helminths
Wound healing
  abnormal, 93–95
  classification of, 90
  contraction in, 94
  cutaneous, 95b
  defects in
    chronic wounds, 93
    excessive scarring, 93–94, 95f
    fibrosis in parenchymal organs, 94–95, 95f
  granulation tissue in, 90, 90f
  scarring in, 89
Wounds, puncture, 317–318
Woven bone, 805–806

X
Xenobiotics, 303b–304b
  defined, 301–302
  metabolism of, 301–302, 301f–302f
Xeroderma pigmentosum, 227, 227b–228b
Xerostomia, 587–588
  complications of, 587–588
  defined, 587–588
  in Sjögren syndrome, 158
XIST, 4–5
X-linked agammaglobulinemia (XLA), 168–173, 173b
  causative organisms in, 170
  treatment of, 170
X-linked disorders, 246–247, 247b
X-linked hyper-IgM syndrome, 173b
X-linked lymphoproliferative (XLP) syndrome, 461

Y
Yersinia spp., 615t
Yolk sac tumor, 694t, 695, 695f
Zahn, lines of, 110
Zellballen pattern, 795
Zinc
  deficiency syndrome for, 333t
  functions of, 333t

Z
Zollinger-Ellison syndrome, 598, 602, 784
Zonulin, in cell-cell interactions, 12
Zoonotic infections, 352
Zygote, and role of stem cells, 27f
B-amyloid-converting enzyme (BACE), in development of AD, 875, 876f
B-amyloid-converting enzyme (BACE), in development of AD, 875, 876f